Oxford Textbook of
Heart Failure

OXFORD TEXTBOOKS IN CARDIOLOGY SERIES

Oxford Textbook of
Heart Failure

SECOND EDITION

EDITED BY

Andrew L. Clark

Consultant Cardiologist and Chair of Clinical Cardiology, Hull University Teaching Hospitals NHS Trust, Castle Hill Hospital Cottingham, UK

Roy S. Gardner

Consultant Cardiologist, Scottish Advanced Heart Failure Service, Golden Jubilee National Hospital, and Honorary Professor at University of Glasgow, UK

Theresa A. McDonagh

Consultant Cardiologist in the School of Cardiovascular Medicine & Sciences, King's College Hospital, UK

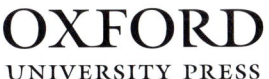

OXFORD
UNIVERSITY PRESS

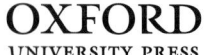

OXFORD
UNIVERSITY PRESS

Great Clarendon Street, Oxford, OX2 6DP,
United Kingdom

Oxford University Press is a department of the University of Oxford.
It furthers the University's objective of excellence in research, scholarship,
and education by publishing worldwide. Oxford is a registered trade mark of
Oxford University Press in the UK and in certain other countries

First Edition published in 2011

Second Edition Published in 2022

Impression: 1

Published in the United States of America by Oxford University Press
198 Madison Avenue, New York, NY 10016, United States of America

British Library Cataloguing in Publication Data
Data available

Library of Congress Control Number: 2021930546

ISBN 978–0–19–876622–3

DOI: 10.1093/med/9780198766223.001.0001

Printed in Great Britain by
Bell & Bain Ltd., Glasgow

Preface

The pace of scientific advance, the huge expansion in the number of scientific journals and scientific meetings, together with the range of different voices on social media mean that new information about heart failure is now rapidly disseminated. There's a darker side to the information boom, too, in the shape of predatory journals with few editorial controls and a weak peer review process, and widespread uninformed discussion in unmediated web fora.

It is inevitable that when any book is first published, it will be at the least several months out of date due to the time lags inherent in the process. An example is that during the preparation of this second edition of the Oxford Textbook of Heart Failure, the SGLT2 inhibitors have gone from being possible add on therapies in the management of type II diabetes to being one of the (current) pillars of heart failure management.

So what, then, is the role of the multi-author text book? New information and knowledge has to be assimilated and placed together with what is already known before it can be used to inform change, and that is particularly true of medical practice when ill-applied data can have catastrophic consequences. We are privileged to have colleagues joining us in this project who have an international reputation for their contribution to the scientific understanding of heart failure, but who are also superb communicators. They have the necessary ability to distil new developments and put them into context. They have a profound understanding of the subject and have the experience to distinguish the wheat from the chaff, what is important from the ephemeral.

We hope this expanded second edition, with its text thoroughly revised and rewritten and with more than 10 new chapters on the aetiology, investigation and management of heart failure, provides a definitive reference volume for all those interested in managing patients with heart failure. We would like to thank the contributors to the book: without their efforts the book would not have been possible; our mentors, whose unflagging support and example led us to become specialists in the most exciting medical specialty; and our patients, for whose benefit the book, we hope, is written.

ALC
RSG
TAM

Contents

Contributors

Stamatis Adamopoulos Director, Heart Failure-Transplant-Mechanical Circulatory Support Units, Onassis Cardiac Surgery Center, Athens, Greece

Cherry Alexander Institute of Cardiovascular and Medical Sciences, Glasgow Cardiovascular Research Centre, University of Glasgow, UK

Rafael Alonso-Gonzalez Director, Toronto ACHD Program Program Director, Adult Congenital Heart Disease Fellowship; Assistant Professor, Department of Medicine, University of Toronto, Toronto

Christopher Armstrong Consultant Emergency Physician, Department of Emergency, Royal Infirmary of Edinburgh, Edinburgh, UK

Nicholas R. Banner Consultant Cardiologist (Retired), Hairfield Hospital, UK

Jeroen J. Bax Professor in Cardiology, Cardiology Leiden University Medical Center, Leiden, The Netherlands

John Baxter Consultant in Care of the Elderly Medicine (Retired), Sunderland, UK

Simon A. S. Beggs Cardiology Registrar, Queen Elizabeth University Hospital, Glasgow, UK

Pushan Bharadwaj Department of Nuclear Medicine and Molecular Imaging, Singapore General Hospital, Singapore

Lynda Blue† Pioneer of the role of specialist heart failure nurses and made an outstanding contribution to lives of patients with heart failure

Margaret M. Burke Consultant Histopathologist (Retired), Harefield Hospital, Royal Brompton & Harefield NHS Trust, London, UK

Jane A. Cannon Consultant Cardiologist, Scottish National Advanced Heart Failure Service, Golden Jubilee National Hospital, Glasgow, UK

Andrew L. Clark Consultant Cardiologist and Chair of Clinical Cardiology, Hull University Teaching Hospitals NHS Trust, Castle Hill Hospital, Cottingham, UK

John G. F. Cleland Robertson Centre for Biostatistics, Institute of Health and Wellbeing, University of Glasgow, Glasgow, UK; Visiting Professor of Cardiology, Imperial College London, UK

Caroline Coats Consultant Cardiologist, Queen Elizabeth University Hospital, Glasgow, UK

Alison P. Coletta Castle Hill Hospital, Castle Road, Cottingham, UK

Derek T. Connelly Consultant Cardiologist, Golden Jubilee National Hospital and Glasgow Royal Infirmary, Honorary Clinical Professor, University of Glasgow, Scotland, UK

Peter J. Cowburn Consultant Cardiologist, Department of Cardiology, University Hospital Southampton, Southampton, Hampshire, UK

Martin R. Cowie Professor of Cardiology, Royal Brompton Hospital (Guy's & St Thomas' NHS Foundation Trust) & Faculty of Lifesciences & Medicine, King's College London, London, UK

Joseph J. Cuthbert Lecturer in Cardiology, Hull York Medical School, University of Hull, UK

Henry J. Dargie Professor of Cardiology and Honorary Senior Research Fellow (Institute of Cardiovascular & Medical Sciences), University of Glasgow, Glasgow, Scotland

Michiel A. de Graaf Cardiology Resident, Department of Cardiology, Leiden University Medical Centre, Leiden, The Netherlands

Victoria Delgado Associate Professor, Department of Cardiology, Leiden University Medical Centre, Leiden, The Netherlands

Kieran F. Docherty Institute of Cardiovascular and Medical Sciences, University of Glasgow, UK

Alison Duncan Consultant Cardiologist, Department of Cardiology, Royal Brompton Hospital, London, UK

Perry M. Elliott Professor in Inherited Cardiovascular Disease, University College London, London, UK

Carrie Ferguson Lecturer, School of Biomedical Sciences, University of Leeds, Leeds, UK

Gábor Földes Advanced Research Fellow, National Heart and Lung Institute, Imperial College London, London, UK; Associate Professor, Heart and Vascular Center, Semmelweis University, Budapest, Hungary, London, UK

Paul Forsyth Lead Pharmacist—Clinical Cardiology (Primary Care), Pharmacy, NHS Greater Glasgow & Clyde, Glasgow, UK

Michael P. Frenneaux Chief of AHS, Academic Health System, Hamad Medical Corporation, UK

Roy S. Gardner Consultant Cardiologist & Honorary Professor, Scottish National Advanced Heart Failure Service, Golden Jubilee National Hospital, Glasgow, UK

Aggeliki Gkouziouta Heart and Lung Transplantation Unit, Onassis Cardiac Surgery Center, Athens, Greece

Alasdair Gray Consultant and Honorary Professor in Emergency Medicine, Royal Infirmary of Edinburgh, Edinburgh, UK

Darren Green Professor of Nephrology, Department of Renal Medicine, Salford Royal Hospital, Northern Care Alliance NHS Foundation Trust and University of Manchester, Greater Manchester, UK

Michael Greenstone Castle Hill Hospital, Castle Road, Cottingham, UK

Kaushik Guha Consultant Cardiologist, Queen Alexandra Hospital, Portsmouth University Hospitals NHS Trust, UK

Brian P. Halliday Senior Clinical Lecturer in Cardiomyopathy and CMR, National Heart and Lung Institute, Imperial College and Honorary Consultant Cardiologist, Royal Brompton and Harefield Hospitals, Guys' and St Thomas' NHS Foundation Trust, UK

Sian E. Harding Professor, Department of NHLI, Imperial College, London, UK

Suzanna Hardman Consultant Cardiologist with an Interest in Community Cardiology, Whittington Health Honorary Senior Lecturer UCL Heart Failure Lead for Whittington Health, Whittington Hospital, London, UK

Andrew R. Harper Clinical Research Fellow, Radcliffe Department of Medicine, University of Oxford, Oxford, Oxfordshire, UK

Nathaniel M. Hawkins The University of British Columbia, Division of Cardiology, Vancouver, British Columbia, Canada

Paul M. Haydock Consultant Cardiologist, Department of Cardiology, University Hospital Southampton, UK

L. van Heerebeek Cardiologist, Department of Cardiology, OLVG Amsterdam, Amsterdam, Netherlands

Stephane Heymans Professor in Cardiomyopathies, Department of Cardiology, Maastricht University Medical Centre, Maastricht, Limburg, Netherlands

Richard J. Jabbour Department of Medicine, Faculty of Medicine, Imperial College London, London, UK

Alice Jackson Clinical Research Fellow, Institute of Cardiovascular and Medical Sciences, University of Glasgow, Glasgow, Scotland

Colette E. Jackson Consultant Cardiologist, Queen Elizabeth University Hospital Glasgow, UK

Andrew Jamieson Consultant Endocrinologist, Island Health Services, Hamilton, Bermuda; Honorary Senior Lecturer in Medicine, University of Glasgow, UK

Pardeep S. Jhund British Heart Foundation Cardiovascular Research Centre, University of Glasgow, Glasgow, UK

Miriam J. Johnson Professor of Palliative Medicine, Wolfson Palliative Care Research Centre, Hull York Medical School, University of Hull, Hull, UK

Paul R. Kalra Consultant Cardiologist and Honorary Professor of Cardiology, Portsmouth Hospitals University NHS Trust and University of Portsmouth, UK

Philip A. Kalra Professor of Nephrology, Department of Renal Medicine, Salford Royal Hospital, Northern Care Alliance NHS Foundation Trust and University of Manchester, Greater Manchester, UK

Georgios Karagiannis Consultant Cardiologist, Transplant Harefield Hospital, London, UK

Ahmad Khwanda Cardiology Consultant, Department of Cardiology, King's College Hospital NHS Foundation Trust, Orpington, Kent, UK

Matthew M. Y. Lee Institute of Cardiovascular and Medical Sciences, University of Glasgow, UK

Evangelos Leontiadis Attending Cardiologist, Heart Failure and Transplant Units, Onassis Cardiac Surgery Centre, Kallithea, Attica, Greece

Giuseppe Limongelli Ospedale Monaldi, A.O. Colli, Naples, Italy

Alexander R. Lyon Senior Lecturer in Cardiology, Royal Brompton Hospital, London, UK

Anna Maddison Liverpool Heart and Chest Hospital NHS Foundation Trust, Liverpool, UK

Hannah Z. R. McConkey Cardiology Registrar, Oxford Heart Centre, John Radcliffe Hospital, Oxford, UK

Theresa A. McDonagh Consultant Cardiologist and Professor of Heart Failure, Kings College, London, UK

Steve McGlynn Specialist Principal Pharmacist (Cardiology), Pharmacy Services, NHS Greater Glasgow and Clyde, Glasgow, UK

John McMurray Professor of Medical Cardiology, BHF Cardiovascular Research Centre, University of Glasgow, Scotland, UK

Rachel Myles Clinical Senior Lecturer in Cardiology, University of Glasgow and Honorary Consultant Cardiologist, Queen Elizabeth University Hospital Glasgow, UK

Ashley M. Nisbet British Heart Foundation Glasgow Cardiovascular Research Centre, University of Glasgow, Glasgow, UK; A consultant cardiologist, Bristol Heart Institute, Bristol Royal Infirmary, UK

Julian O.M. Ormerod Consultant Cardiologist, Oxford Heart Centre, John Radcliffe Hospital, Oxford, Oxfordshire, UK

Walter J. Paulus Emeritus Professor of Physiology, Amsterdam Cardiovascular Sciences, Amsterdam University Medical Centers, The Netherlands

John Pepper Consultant Surgeon, Cardiac Surgery, Royal Brompton Hospital, National Heart and Lung Institute, Imperial College, NIHR Imperial Biomedical Research Centre, London, UK

Mark Petrie Professor, Department of Cardiology, University of Glasgow, UK

Stephen Pettit Consultant Cardiologist, Heart Transplant Unit, Royal Papworth Hospital, Cambridge, UK

Susanna Price Professor, Royal Brompton Hospital, London, UK; National Heart & Lung Institute, Imperial College, London, UK

Massimo F. Piepoli Institute of Life Sciences, Sant'Anna School of Advanced Studies, Pisa, Italy

Susan Piper Consultant Cardiologist, Department of Cardiology, King's College Hospital, London, UK

Anne Pizard Researcher, IMRB (Institut Mondor de Recherche Biomédicale) PHYDES, France

Carla M. Plymen Consultant Cardiologist, Imperial College Healthcare NHS Trust, London, UK

Michael Pope Research Fellow, Cardiac Rhythm Management, John Radcliffe Hospital, Oxford University Hospitals NHS Foundation Trust, Winchester, Hampshire, UK

Sanjay K. Prasad Consultant Cardiologist, Royal Brompton Hospital, London, UK

Bernard Prendergast Professor, Consultant Cardiologist St Thomas' Hospital and Cleveland Clinic London, London, UK

J. Simon R. Gibbs Reader in Pulmonary Hypertension and Honorary Consultant Cardiologist, Imperial College Healthcare, London, UK

Anita K. Simonds Professor of Respiratory & Sleep Medicine, NHLI, Imperial College, London; Honorary Consultant in Respiratory & Sleep Medicine, Royal Brompton & Harefield Hospital, Guy's and St Thomas' NHS Foundation Trust, London, UK

S. Rekhraj Consultant Cardiologist, Department of Cardiology, Nottingham City Hospital, Nottingham, UK

S. Richard Underwood Emeritus Professor of Cardiac Imaging, National Heart & Lung Institute, Imperial College London, London, UK

Sam Rodgers Institute of Medical and Cardiovascular Sciences, University of Glasgow, Scotland, UK

Stuart D. Rosen Professor of Practice (Cardiology), National Heart and Lung Institute, Imperial College, London, Middlesex, UK

Sara Roversi Department of Respiratory Disease, University of Modena and Reggio Emilia, Modena, Italy

Diana Garcia Saez Resident Specialist, Department of Medicine, Mater Dei Hospital, Msida, Malta

John Sharp Consultant Psychologist, Golden Jubilee National Hospital, Glasgow, UK

André R. Simon Royal Brompton and Harefield NHS Foundation Trust Hill End Road, Harefield, Uxbridge, London, UK

Joanne Simpson Consultant Cardiologist, Institute of Cardiovascular and Medical Sciences, University of Glasgow, Scotland, UK

Arvind Singhal Royal Brompton Hospital London, UK

Godfrey Smith Professor of Cardiovascular Physiology (Institute of Cardiovascular & Medical Sciences), University of Glasgow, Glasgow, UK

Iain Squire Professor, Cardiovascular Sciences, Leicester NIHR Biomedical Research Institute, Leicester, UK

Allan D. Struthers Emeritus Professor of Cardiovascular Medicine, University of Dundee, Tayside, UK

Lorna Swan Consultant Cardiologist, Scottish Adult Congenital Cardiac Service, Golden Jubilee National Hospital, Glasgow, UK

Ben. R. Szwejkowski Consultant Cardiologist, Department of Cardiology, Ninewells Hospital and Medical School, Dundee, Tayside, UK

Laurens F. Tops Cardiologist, Department of Cardiology, Leiden University Medical Center, Leiden, The Netherlands

Shahana Uddin Consultant Intensive Care Medicine, King's College Hospital, London, UK

Ali Vazir Consultant Cardiologist, Royal Brompton Hospital, London, UK

Carol J. Whelan Consultant Cardiologist, National Amyloidosis Centre, London, UK

Niki L. Walker Consultant Cardiologist, Golden Jubilee National Hospital, Clydebank, Scotland, UK

Klaus K. Witte Professor of Cardiology, University Clinic of Aachen, Germany; and Senior Lecturer in Cardiology, Leeds Institute for Cardiovascular and Metabolic Medicine, University of Leeds, Leeds, UK

Lesley Young Consultant Geriatrician, Care of the Elderly, Sunderland Royal Hospital Sunderland, UK

Faiez Zannad Emeritus Professor of Therapeutics and Cardiology, Université de Lorraine, Inserm and CHRU de Nancy, France

List of abbreviations

ACCF	American College of Cardiology Foundation	ccTGA	congenitally corrected transposition of the great arteries
ACE	angiotensin converting enzyme	CDG	congenital disorders of glycosylation
ACEi	angiotensin converting enzyme inhibitor	CHD	congenital heart disease
ACHD	adults with congenital heart disease	CHF	chronic/congestive heart failure
ACS	acute coronary syndromes	CICR	$Ca2+$-induced $Ca2+$ release
ADBR	β-adrenergic receptor	6-CIT	Cognitive Impairment Test
AF	atrial fibrillation	CKD	chronic kidney disease
AFLP	acute fatty liver of pregnancy	CMR	cardiac magnetic resonance
AHA	American Heart Association	CNP	C-type natriuretic peptide
AHF	acute heart failure	COPD	chronic obstructive pulmonary disease
AHI	apnoea–hypopnoea index	COVID-19	coronavirus disease 2019
AKI	acute kidney injury	CPAP	continuous positive airways pressure
AL	light chain amyloidosis	CPCs	cardiac progenitor cells
AMI	acute myocardial infarction	CPET	cardiopulmonary exercise test
AMTS	Abbreviated Mental Test Score	CPFE	combined pulmonary fibrosis and emphysema
ANP	atrial natriuretic peptide	CRP	C-reactive protein
AP	action potential	CRT	cardiac resynchronization therapy
APA	American Psychiatric Association	CRU	$Ca2+$ release unit
APD	action potential duration	CSA	central sleep apnoea
APT	amiodarone pulmonary toxicity	CSD	cardiac support device
AR	adrenoceptor	CSR	Cheyne–Stokes respiration
ARB	angiotensin receptor blocker	CTA	computed tomography angiography
ARNI	angiotensin receptor–neprilysin inhibitor	CTEPH	chronic thromboembolic pulmonary hypertension
ART	antiretroviral therapy	CTGF	connective tissue growth factor
ARVC	arrhythmogenic right ventricular cardiomyopathy	CVC	central venous cannulation
ARVD	atherosclerotic renovascular disease	DAD	delayed afterdepolarization
AS	aortic stenosis	DCM	dilated cardiomyopathy
ASLVD	asymptomatic LV systolic dysfunction	DNP	D (dendroaspis)-type natriuretic peptide
ASV	adaptive servoventilation	DSM-5	Diagnostic and Statistical Manual of Mental Disorders, 5th edition
ATTR	transthyretin amyloidosis		
AV	atrioventricular	d-TGA	dextro-transposition of the great arteries
AVC	arrhythmogenic cardiomyopathy	EAD	early afterdepolarization
BMI	body mass index	E–C	excitation–contraction
BMNSCs	bone marrow mononuclear stem cells, skeletal myoblasts	ECG	electrocardiogram
		ECM	extracellular matrix
BNP	brain (B-type) natriuretic peptide	ECMO	extracorporeal membrane oxygenation
BP	blood pressure	ECPR	extracorporeal cardiopulmonary resuscitation
BPAP	biphasic positive airway pressure	ECT	electroconvulsive therapy
BUN	blood urea nitrogen	eGFR	glomerular filtration rate
$[Ca2+]i$	intracellular $Ca2+$ concentration	EHRA	European Heart Rhythm Association
CACT	carnitine/acylcarnitine translocase	ELISA	enzyme-linked immunosorbent assay
CAD	coronary artery disease	EMB	endomyocardial biopsy
CAM	cell adhesion molecules	EMF	endomyocardial fibrosis
CAV	cardiac allograft vasculopathy	EPAP	expiratory positive airway pressure
CBT	cognitive behaviour therapy		

ERT	enzyme replacement therapy	LABA	long-acting β2-agonists
ESC	European Society of Cardiology	LAMA	long-acting muscarinic antagonists
ESKD	end-stage kidney disease	LBBB	left bundle branch block
ESMO	European Society for Medical Oncology	LGE	late gadolinium enhancement
ESS	Epworth sleepiness score	LH	left ventricle
FAC	familial amyloid cardiomyopathy	LPA	Lasting Power of Attorney
FADD	Fas-associated death domain	LTCC	L-type Ca2+
FAOD	fatty acid oxidation disorders	LVEDP	left ventricular end-diastolic pressure
FAP	familial amyloid polyneuropathy	LVEF	left ventricular ejection fraction
FDA	US Food and Drug Administration	LVH	left ventricular hypertrophy
FDG-PET	18F-fluorodeoxyglucose positron emission tomography	LVMI	left ventricular mass index
		LVNC	left ventricular non-compaction
FGF	fibroblast growth factor	LVSD	left ventricular systolic dysfunction
FiO2	fraction of inspired oxygen	MAD	multiple acyl-CoA dehydrogenases
FLCs	free light chains	MAPK	mitogen-activated protein kinase
FOXO	forkhead box	MCP-1	monocyte chemoattractant protein-1
GAG	glycosaminoglycan	MELAS	mitochondrial encephalomyopathy with lactic acidosis and stroke-like episodes
GCM	giant cell myocarditis		
Gd-DPTA	gadolinium diethylenetriamine penta-acetic acid	MGUS	monoclonal gammopathy of undetermined significance
GFR	glomerular filtration rate		
GP	general practitioner	MIBG	meta-iodo-benzyl-guanidine (scan)
GSD	glycogen storage disorder	MMP	matrix metalloproteases
GWAS	genome-wide associated study	MMSE	Mini Mental State Examination
HAART	highly active antiretroviral therapy	MoCA	Montreal Cognitive Assessment
HbA1c	glycated haemoglobin	MPS	myocardial perfusion scintigraphy
HCM	hypertrophic cardiomyopathy	mPTP	mitochondrial permeability transition pore
HELLP	haemolysis, elevated liver enzymes, low platelets	MR	mitral regurgitation
HES	hypereosinophilic syndrome	MRA	mineralocorticoid receptor antagonist
HFA	heart failure anxiety	MRI	magnetic resonance imaging
HFA	Heart Failure Association	MSCs	mesenchymal stem cells
HFD	heart failure depression	MTP	mitochondrial trifunctional protein
HFmrEF	heart failure with mildly reduced ejection fraction	MUGA	multigated acquisition (nuclear) scanning
HFnEF	heart failure with normal ejection fraction	NAC	National Amyloidosis Centre
HFpEF	heart failure with preserved ejection fraction	NCX	sodium–calcium exchanger
HFrEF	heart failure with reduced ejection fraction	NF-κB	transcription nuclear factor NF-κB
HIV	human immunodeficiency virus	NGS	next-generation sequencing
HLA	human leukocyte antigen	NHS	National Health Service
HMG-CoA	3-hydroxy-3-methyl-glutaryl–Coenzyme A	NICE	National Institute for Health and Care Excellence
HRR	heart rate reserve	NIV	non-invasive ventilation
HRS	Heart Rhythm Society	NO	nitric oxide
ICD	implantable cardioverter–defibrillator	NP	natriuretic peptide
ICD-10	International Classification of Diseases, 10th edition	NPV	negative predictive value
		NSTEMI	non-ST-segment elevation myocardial infarction
ICI	immune checkpoint inhibitor	NT-proBNP	N-terminal pro B-type natriuretic peptide
ID	iron deficiency	NYHA	New York Heart Association
IFA	immunofluorescence antibody assay	OSA	obstructive sleep apnoea
IFN	interferon	PAC	pulmonary artery flotation catheter
IGF-1	insulin-like growth factor	PaCO$_2$	arterial partial pressure of carbon dioxide
IHD	ischaemic heart disease	PAH	pulmonary arterial hypertension
IL	interleukin	PCI	percutaneous coronary intervention
IMR	ischaemic mitral regurgitation	PCO$_2$	partial pressure of carbon dioxide
IPAP	positive airway pressure during inspiration	PCr	phosphocreatine
ISDN	isosorbide dinitrate	PCR	polymerase chain reaction
ISF	interstitial fluid	PCWP	pulmonary capillary wedge pressure
ISFC	International Society and Federation of Cardiology	PDE	phosphodiesterase
ISMN	isosorbide mononitrate	PDGF	platelet-derived growth factor
IVIG	intravenous immunoglobulin	PDH	pyruvate dehydrogenase
JVP	jugular venous pressure	PET	positron emission tomography

PKA	protein kinase A	SGLT-2	sodium–glucose-linked co-transporter 2 inhibitors
PKG	protein kinase G		
PLE	protein-losing enteropathy	SLE	systemic lupus erythematosus
PPAR	peroxisomal proliferator-activated receptor	SNP	single nucleotide polymorphism
PR	pulmonary regurgitation	SPECT	single-photon emission computed tomography
PSA	periodic acid–Schiff	SpO2	oxygen saturation
PVOD	pulmonary veno-occlusive disease	SR	sarcoplasmic reticulum
PVR	pulmonary vascular resistance	STEMI	ST-segment elevation myocardial infarction
QRS	Q, R, and S waves (combination of three of the graphical deflections)	SU	sulfonylurea drug
		SVR	systemic vascular resistance
RA	rheumatoid arthritis	T2w-STIR	T2-weighted short-τ inversion recovery
RAAS	renin–angiotensin–aldosterone system	TAT	transverse-axial tubular
RANTES	Regulated on Activation Normal T-cell Expressed and Secreted	TAVI	transcatheter aortic valve implantation
		TCM	takotsubo cardiomyopathy
RAS	renal artery stenosis	TGF	transforming growth factor
RAS	renin–angiotensin system	TLR	Toll-like receptor
RBBB	right bundle branch block	TMAO	trimethylamine-N-oxide
RCM	restrictive cardiomyopathy	TMS	tandem mass spectrometry
RCT	randomized controlled trial	TNFα	tumour necrosis factor-α
RNV	radionuclide ventriculography	ToF	tetralogy of Fallot
ROC	receiver operator characteristic	TSAT	transferrin saturation
ROS	reactive oxygen species	TTR	transthyretin
RRT	renal replacement therapy	TZD	thiazolidenedione drug
RV	right ventricle	UPR	unfolded protein response
RVEF	right ventricular ejection fraction	UPS	ubiquitin–proteasome system
RyR	ryanodine receptor	VAD	ventricular assist devices
SAA	acute-phase amyloid protein serum AA	VHD	valvular heart disease
SAP	serum amyloid P	VPB	ventricular premature beat
SARS-CoV-2	severe acute respiratory syndrome coronavirus 2	VSD	ventricular septal defect
SCD	sudden cardiac death	WES	whole exome sequencing
SCUBA	self-contained underwater breathing apparatus	WHO	World Health Organization
SDB	sleep-disordered breathing	WPW	Wolff–Parkinson–White syndrome
SERCA2a	sarcoendoplasmic reticulum Ca2+-ATPase channel	wt	wild type

SECTION 1
What is heart failure?

1

What is heart failure?

Andrew L. Clark

It is a commonplace in writings about heart failure that it has become an 'epidemic' in western societies in particular. In truth, the incidence is not rising, but the prevalence is. Heart failure is thus not a true epidemic which properly is a rise in the age-specific incidence of a condition followed by a decline. The major causes for its increasing prevalence are threefold: although the incidence of acute myocardial infarction may be falling, more patients survive acute coronary disease and go on to develop chronic heart failure; treatment of chronic heart failure has dramatically improved, and so many more patients survive for much longer; and the population generally is ageing—and heart failure is a disease of the elderly.

Although heart failure is a modern blight, it has been known for thousands of years. There is some suggestion from the Ebers papyrus (*c*.1550 BCE) that the ancient Egyptians recognized it ('When there is inundation of the heart, the saliva is in excess, and therefore the body is weak'), and Hippocrates (460–370 BCE) gave a much-quoted description of cardiac cachexia: 'The flesh is consumed and becomes water … the abdomen fills with water; the feet and legs swell; the shoulders, clavicles, chest, and thigh melt away.'[1]

It was not until after Harvey described the circulation of the blood that the heart failure syndrome truly began to be related to the heart, with Richard Lower perhaps giving the first textbook discussion of heart failure in 1669.[2] Treatment for heart failure with venesection, perhaps one of the few instances in which the procedure might be helpful, was formally described in 1696.[3] William Withering gave a medical description of the use of *Digitalis* extracts, giving birth to clinical pharmacology,[4] although cardiac glycosides had undoubtedly been used for hundreds, and perhaps thousands,[5] of years previously.

The modern era of heart failure treatment truly began with the discovery of mercurial,[6] and then thiazide and subsequently loop, diuretics in the late 1950s and early 1960s. Perhaps the most important single trial in heart failure therapy demonstrating the beneficial effects of angiotensin converting enzyme (ACE) inhibitors was published in 1987.[7]

Definition of heart failure

Neither the epidemiology of a condition nor its treatment can properly be understood unless properly defined. The term 'heart failure' is usually used freely between clinicians to describe what is wrong with individual patients, yet despite the fact that heart failure is so very common, it is very difficult to define it satisfactorily (**Box 1.1**).[8] Some difficulties arise because of the effects of modern treatment: whereas it might be reasonable to define *acute* heart failure in terms of some haemodynamic variable, the situation becomes very different in chronic *treated* heart failure.

Older general definitions of heart failure centred on haemodynamic changes, and were phrased in terms of inadequacy of cardiac output in response to normal filling pressure of the heart, with the inadequacy of the output thought of as being inadequate to meet the requirements of the metabolizing tissues.[9] These sorts of definition are of some value in thinking about the pathophysiology of patients being admitted acutely with salt and water retention or pulmonary oedema, but less so in thinking about patients with chronic heart failure.

Patients with chronic heart failure, particularly when adequately treated, may have normal resting cardiac output and normal left ventricular filling pressure. Their metabolizing tissues are well enough perfused that they are usually asymptomatic at rest: chronic treated heart failure is a condition of exercise limitation. Even so, for many patients, cardiac output and oxygen consumption go up as normal during modest exercise, only falling below normal towards peak exercise.

Ultimately, heart failure is a clinical syndrome characterized by a constellation of symptoms and signs, and not a discrete diagnosis. Much epidemiological work has defined heart failure in terms of those symptoms and signs, but taking such an approach may mistakenly include many patients without cardiac pathology.[10,11] The situation is even worse if simply considering *treatment* for heart failure as being adequate to define the presence of heart failure in epidemiological studies: such an approach may lead to gross overestimation of the prevalence of heart failure.[12]

The key is to recognize that the observed constellation of symptoms and signs should be coupled with objective evidence that there is an abnormality of the heart consistent with the diagnosis. This is the line now taken by the European Society of Cardiology,[13,14] with the added clause that in doubtful cases, a response to treatment directed at heart failure sustains the diagnosis.[13]

Such an approach is pragmatic, at least, and is rooted in clinical life. Some problems do arise in borderline cases. In an elderly patient, for example, breathlessness is a very common symptom, and peripheral oedema is a very common physical sign: if an echocardiogram shows left ventricular hypertrophy, can the patient truly be

---

Box 1.1 Some definitions of heart failure

A condition in which the heart fails to discharge its contents adequately
Thomas Lewis, 1933

A state in which the heart fails to maintain an adequate circulation for the needs of the body despite a satisfactory filling pressure
Paul Wood, 1950

A pathophysiological state in which an abnormality of cardiac function is responsible for the failure of the heart to pump blood at a rate commensurate with the requirements of the metabolizing tissues.
Eugene Braunwald, 1980

The state of any heart disease in which, despite adequate ventricular filling, the heart's output is decreased or in which the heart is unable to pump blood at a rate adequate for satisfying the requirements of the tissues with function parameters remaining within normal limits.
Denolin H, et al., 1983

A clinical syndrome caused by an abnormality of the heart and recognised by a characteristic pattern of haemodynamic, renal, neural and hormonal responses.
Philip Poole-Wilson, 1985

… syndrome … which arises when the heart is chronically unable to maintain an appropriate blood pressure without support.
Peter Harris, 1987

A syndrome in which cardiac dysfunction is associated with reduced exercise tolerance, a high incidence of ventricular arrhythmias and a shortened life expectancy.
Jay Cohn, 1988

… a complex clinical syndrome that can result from any structural or functional cardiac disorder that impairs the ability of the ventricle to fill with or eject blood.
ACC and AHA Task Force on Practice Guidelines. 2009 Focused Update Incorporated into the ACC/AHA 2005 Guidelines for the Diagnosis and Management of Heart Failure in Adults. Circulation 2009;**119**;e391–e479

A syndrome in which the patients should have the following features: symptoms of HF, typically shortness of breath at rest or during exertion, and/or fatigue; signs of fluid retention such as pulmonary congestion or ankle swelling, and objective evidence of an abnormality of the structure or function of the heart at rest.
Task Force for the Diagnosis and Treatment of Acute and Chronic Heart Failure 2008 of the European Society of Cardiology. Eur Heart J 2008;**29**:2388–442

HF is a clinical syndrome characterized by typical symptoms (e.g. breathlessness, ankle swelling and fatigue) that may be accompanied by signs (e.g. elevated jugular venous pressure, pulmonary crackles and peripheral oedema) caused by a structural and/or functional cardiac abnormality, resulting in a reduced cardiac output and/or elevated intracardiac pressures at rest or during stress.
Task Force for the Diagnosis and Treatment of Acute and Chronic Heart Failure of the European Society of Cardiology. Eur Heart J 2016;**37**:2129–200

HF, heart failure.

Source data from Poole-Wilson PA. History, definition and classification of heart failure. In Poole-Wilson, Colucci WS, Massie BM, Chatterjee K, Coast AJS (eds), *Heart Failure.* Churchill Livingstone, New York, 1997.

---

defined as having heart failure? The missing part of the equation is some objective test, independent of cardiac imaging, which allows the clinician to be sure that the cardiac abnormality is the cause of the patient's symptoms.

The natriuretic peptides offer at least a partial solution in this regard. These hormones and their derivatives, released from the heart in response to cardiac stretch, should be raised in patients with heart failure: if they are not, the diagnosis is likely to be wrong (or the heart failure to be extremely well treated). National and international guidelines all now acknowledge the importance of natriuretic peptide testing. However, their principle diagnostic role is as a 'rule out' test: below cut-off levels (which are different in different clinical scenarios), heart failure is excluded. Conversely, the higher the natriuretic peptide level, the more likely it is that heart failure is present.

Heart failure as an evolutionary disease

Why does heart failure present clinically as it does? This seems an odd question as clinicians are so familiar with the clinical syndrome, but it is not immediately obvious why a patient whose heart function declines should start to retain fluid and develop neurohormonal activation. Harris emphasized the importance of blood pressure in the evolution of terrestrial animals.[15] In order to perfuse a large body unsupported by water; in order to allow rapid movement of that body; and in order to excrete the high level of waste products incurred by having a large, rapidly moving body, high blood pressure is fundamental—certainly compared with the blood pressure needed to service a fish.

An array of very powerful defensive mechanisms has evolved to maintain that high blood pressure at more-or-less all costs. The responses of the body to a fall in blood pressure induced by, say, haemorrhage, are very similar to those induced by heart failure. Vasoconstriction, salt and water retention and neurohormonal activation are the responses to both conditions. The clinical pattern of heart failure can thus be viewed as a consequence of mammalian evolution and the vital importance of maintaining high blood pressure.

Descriptions of heart failure

Earlier textbooks of cardiology abound in paired descriptions of heart failure: forward versus backward; right versus left; high versus low output; systolic versus diastolic; acute versus chronic. Some of the terms are now largely redundant but are worth considering in brief.

Forward heart failure refers to the notion that there is primarily failure of forward pump function leading to inadequate perfusion of peripheral tissues, particularly skeletal muscle, causing fatigue and exercise intolerance. Conversely, backward failure is thought to arise from the need to maintain cardiac output via increased left ventricular filling pressure, which results in left atrial hypertension and thus lung congestion and breathlessness.

Right heart failure suggest that the heart failure is predominantly due to failure of the right ventricle with consequent systemic venous congestion and 'backward' failure, whereas left heart failure leads to pulmonary venous hypertension and pulmonary oedema together with the consequences of reduced pump function. Such a classification is not very helpful: the commonest cause of right heart failure is left heart failure and the two rarely occur as separate entities.

High-output cardiac failure is a rarity caused by excessive vasodilation together with salt and water retention; it should not be thought of as being primarily a cardiac condition. It is more correctly thought of as circulatory failure. Diastolic versus systolic heart failure remains a controversial distinction: some investigators report that up to half of patients with heart failure have impaired ventricular relaxation as their primary pathophysiological problem. In consequence, there is decreased stroke volume and the syndrome of heart failure. The implication is that had the heart been able to fill more completely, then there would be no heart failure.

The distinction between acute and chronic heart failure is clinically helpful, as long as the terms are understood correctly. The word 'acute' is often taken, wrongly, to mean 'severe', and should be used to mean 'presenting suddenly'. In very broad-brush terms, acute heart failure refers to patients presenting as emergencies to hospital, usually with either pulmonary oedema or with fluid retention. Such patients are often presenting for the first time, but may be patients having an exacerbation of their chronic, previously stable, heart failure. They have acutely abnormal haemodynamics.

By contrast, most patients with chronic heart failure have been treated medically and will usually have few if any symptoms or signs at rest. The term 'congestive' heart failure, often used to describe patients in this condition (particularly in North America), is inappropriate: patients with treated chronic heart failure should not be congested.[16]

Clinical course of heart failure

The prognosis of both acute and chronic heart failure was once bleak, with an average life expectancy from diagnosis of around three years (depending on the population studied),[17] and a prognosis worse than for many kinds of cancer.[18,19] Such statistics disguise the fact that modern medical therapy has greatly improved the prognosis for the individual patient, and that the course of heart failure can be highly variable. It is much less predictable than the course of other malignant diseases (Figure 1.1).

The initial presentation of heart failure is usually acute. The commonest cause of heart failure is coronary heart disease, and so an acute myocardial infarction is a common initial precipitant. With treatment, a number of outcomes are then possible: the patient might return to normal with impaired left ventricular function; the patient might reach a plateau of impaired function; or the patient might decline relentlessly toward death or transplantation.

Following an initial event and recovery or stabilization, a patient may continue unchanged for several years, or may have repeated episodes of decompensation of chronic heart failure. Each time, it is less likely that there will be complete recovery of the myocardium, and progressively left ventricular function worsens in a stuttering, stepwise course. As a general rule, such a trajectory often follows the pattern of a flat stone skimming across water: decompensation episodes become longer and the intervals between episodes shorten.[20]

For some patients, the decline in left ventricular function is more gradual than punctuated: in this scenario, a patient may enter a 'vicious cycle' of decline. An alarming feature of heart failure is that at any time in its clinical course, patients are at risk of sudden death.

A less common way for heart failure to present is with a less abrupt onset and gradually progressive symptoms of breathlessness, fatigue and peripheral oedema. The typical patient presenting this way may have had a remote myocardial infarct or have underlying valvular heart disease or dilated cardiomyopathy. Such a patient will usually present through primary care, and the diagnosis can be delayed in consequence—the range of causes of breathlessness is very broad.

Occasional patients appear completely to recover from an episode of heart failure. Such a recovery may happen in patients with a discrete episode of illness, such as acute myocarditis or postpartum cardiomyopathy. Some patients with dilated cardiomyopathy may apparently return to having normal left ventricular systolic function with medical therapy, or with cardiac resynchronization therapy,[21] and it can be difficult to judge in such circumstances whether medication should stop or continue indefinitely.[22]

Models of progression

Much of the thinking about the clinical course of heart failure has focused on potential vicious circles of decline (better thought of as spirals—the starting point is not regained!). With all of the potential spirals, an abnormality induced by heart failure results in further deterioration in heart function, thereby worsening the heart failure. These models are helpful in thinking about the pathophysiology of heart failure, and in suggesting avenues for therapeutic development.

The *haemodynamic model* of heart failure decline is the traditional way of looking at the pathophysiology of heart failure (Figure 1.2). Initial damage to the heart is detected by body systems (particularly via a fall in blood pressure and in renal perfusion) and the result is activation of a series of homeostatic mechanisms causing haemodynamic changes directed at maintaining tissue perfusion. Salt and water retention help to maintain output via the Frank–Starling relation by increasing preload; and vasoconstriction maintains blood pressure, but at a cost of increasing afterload. The increases in pre- and afterload, however, exacerbate the heart's problems, leading to further decline.

Treatments based on the haemodynamic understanding of heart failure have not proved very successful: positive inotropic drugs have almost uniformly proved harmful, and abrupt changes in haemodynamics (as with vasodilators or even heart transplantation) do not lead to immediate improvements in exercise function.

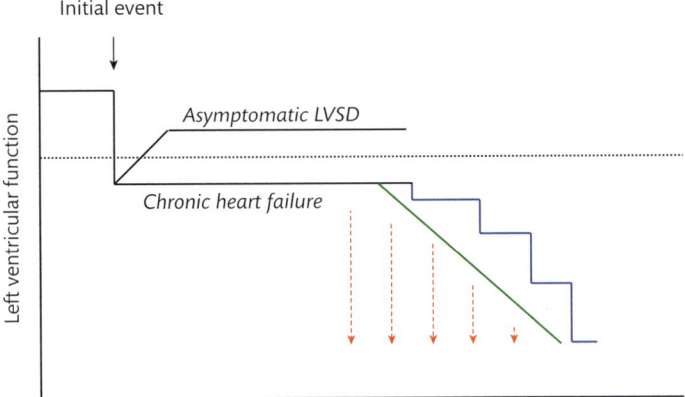

Figure 1.1 Possible trajectories of heart failure. Following an initial heart failure event, a patient might recover to a state of asymptomatic left ventricular dysfunction, or settle into a state of chronic heart failure. As time passes, left ventricular function tends to decline further, either gradually or in a stepwise manner. At any time, sudden death may occur.

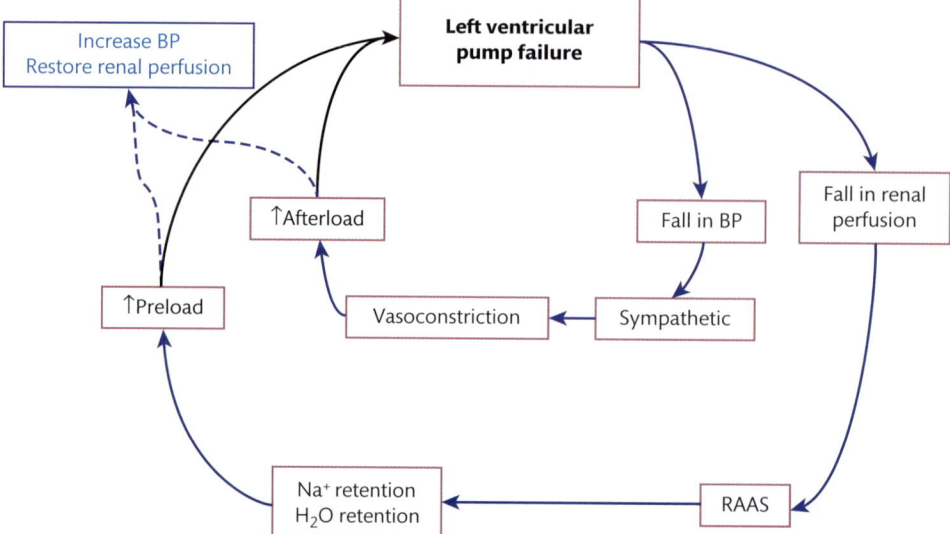

Figure 1.2 The traditional haemodynamic model of heart failure. Initial ventricular damage leads to haemodynamic responses that tend to preserve blood pressure and renal function (blue arrows), but at a cost of increasing preload and afterload and thereby feeding back to cause further damage to the heart (black arrows).

The *neurohormonal model*[23] has been particularly fruitful in guiding new treatments for heart failure. Note that the effectors in the neurohormonal model are the sympathetic nervous system and the renin–angiotensin system. These hormones have much more widespread effects than just their haemodynamic actions, causing direct harm to the heart, for example, by inducing programmed cell death and fibrosis. Thus neurohormonal activation leads to worsening heart failure.

As a guide to therapeutic advance, the neurohormonal model has been spectacularly successful, underlying the development of modern therapy with ACE inhibitors, β-blockers and mineralocorticoid receptor antagonists.

The *peripheral model*[24] (**Figure 1.3**) draws attention to the changes that happen in the periphery as a consequence of heart failure, particularly to skeletal muscle. Perhaps in part due to poor perfusion, perhaps due to lack of fitness, and perhaps due to neurohormonal and cytokine activation, a skeletal myopathy develops. The myopathy is a major cause of symptoms, particularly fatigue and breathlessness, but also causes sympathetic activation, leading to further damage to the heart.

The peripheral model suggests that intervention to preserve skeletal muscle function or to reverse the myopathy may be helpful in managing heart failure.

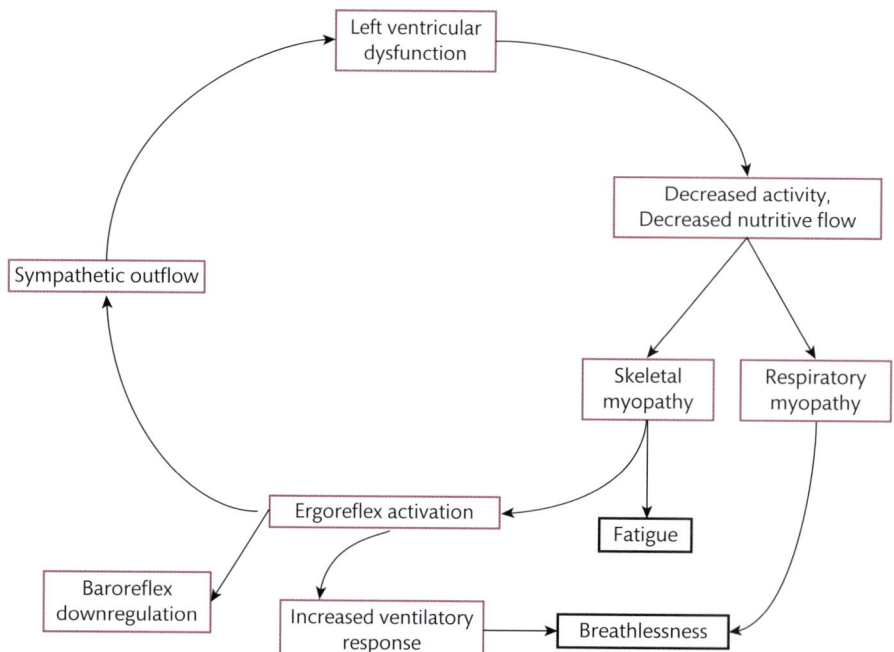

Figure 1.3 A peripheral model of heart failure. Heart failure leads to a skeletal myopathy which is responsible for the symptoms of heart failure. The resulting activation of the ergoreflex causes sympathetic nervous system activation which feeds back to cause further damage to the heart.

One problem in thinking about the pathophysiology of decline in terms of vicious cycles is the implication that there is a continuing rapid downhill spiral as heart failure inexorably declines. Untreated heart failure may behave in this way, but treated heart failure is typically much more stable—a punctuated equilibrium—presumably as a consequence of treatment.

REFERENCES

1. Katz AM, Kat PB. Diseases of heart in works of Hippocrates. *Br Heart J* 1962;**24**:257–64.
2. Lower R. *Tractatus de corde, item de motu, et colore sanguinis et chyli in eum transitu*, 1st edn. J Allestry, London, 1669.
3. Baglivi G. *De praxi medica*. Roma, 1696.
4. Withering W. An account of the foxglove and some of its medical uses—practical remarks on dropsy and other diseases, 1st edn. M. Swinney, Birmingham, 1785.
5. Somberg J, Greenfield D, Tepper D. Digitalis: 200 years in perspective. *Am Heart J* 1986;**111**:615–20.
6. Pugh LG, Wyndham CL. The circulatory effects of mercurial diuretics in congestive heart failure. *Clin Sci (Lond)* 1949;**8**:11–19.
7. CONSENSUS Trial Study Group. Effects of enalapril on mortality in severe congestive heart failure. Results of the Cooperative North Scandinavian Enalapril Survival Study (CONSENSUS). *N Engl J Med* 1987;**316**:1429–35.
8. Poole-Wilson PA. History, definition and classification of heart failure. In Poole-Wilson, Colucci WS, Massie BM, Chatterjee K, Coast AJS (eds), *Heart failure*. Churchill Livingstone, New York, 1997.
9. Denolin H, Kuhn H, Krayenbuehl HP, Loogen F, Reale A. The definition of heart failure. *Eur Heart J* 1983;**4**:445–8.
10. Remes J, Miettinen H, Reunanen A, Pyörälä K. Validity of clinical diagnosis of heart failure in primary health care. *Eur Heart J* 1991;**12**:315–21.
11. Marantz PR, Tobin JN, Wassertheil-Smoller S, et al. The relationship between left ventricular systolic function and congestive heart failure diagnosed by clinical criteria. *Circulation* 1988;**77**:607–12.
12. Clarke KW, Gray D, Hampton JR. Evidence of inadequate investigation and treatment of patients with heart failure. *Br Heart J* 1994;**71**:584–7.
13. Task Force for Diagnosis and Treatment of Acute and Chronic Heart Failure 2008 of European Society of Cardiology. ESC Guidelines for the diagnosis and treatment of acute and chronic heart failure 2008: the Task Force for the Diagnosis and Treatment of Acute and Chronic Heart Failure 2008 of the European Society of Cardiology. Developed in collaboration with the Heart Failure Association of the ESC (HFA) and endorsed by the European Society of Intensive Care Medicine (ESICM). *Eur Heart J* 2008;**29**:2388–442.
14. Ponikowski P, Voors AA, Anker SD, et al. 2016 ESC Guidelines for the diagnosis and treatment of acute and chronic heart failure: The Task Force for the diagnosis and treatment of acute and chronic heart failure of the European Society of Cardiology (ESC) developed with the special contribution of the Heart Failure Association (HFA) of the ESC. *Eur Heart J* 2016;**37**:2129–200.
15. Harris P. Evolution and the cardiac patient. *Cardiovasc Res* 1983;**17**:313–19 and 373–8 and 437–45.
16. Anand IS, Veall N, Kalra GS, et al. Treatment of heart failure with diuretics: body compartments, renal function and plasma hormones. *Eur Heart J* 1989;**10**:445–50.
17. Cowie MR, Wood DA, Coats AJ, et al. Survival of patients with a new diagnosis of heart failure: a population based study. *Heart* 2000;**83**:505–10.
18. Stewart S, MacIntyre K, Hole DJ, Capewell S, McMurray JJ. More 'malignant' than cancer? Five-year survival following a first admission for heart failure. *Eur J Heart Fail* 2001;**3**:315–22.
19. Mamas MA, Sperrin M, Watson MC, et al. Do patients have worse outcomes in heart failure than in cancer? A primary care-based cohort study with 10-year follow-up in Scotland. *Eur J Heart Fail* 2017;**19**:1095–104.
20. Braga JR, Tu JV, Austin PC, et al. Recurrent events analysis for examination of hospitalizations in heart failure: insights from the enhanced feedback for Effective Cardiac Treatment (EFFECT) Trial. *Eur Heart J Qual Care Clin Outcomes* 2018;**4**:18–26.
21. Hsu JC, Solomon SD, Bourgoun M, et al.; MADIT-CRT Executive Committee. Predictors of super-response to cardiac resynchronization therapy and associated improvement in clinical outcome: the MADIT-CRT (multicenter automatic defibrillator implantation trial with cardiac resynchronization therapy) study. *J Am Coll Cardiol* 2012;**59**:2366–73.
22. Anguita M, Arizón JM, Bueno G, Concha M, Vallés F. Spontaneous clinical and hemodynamic improvement in patients on waiting list for heart transplantation. *Chest* 1992;**102**:96–9.
23. Packer M. The neurohormonal hypothesis: a theory to explain the mechanism of disease progression in heart failure. *J Am Coll Cardiol* 1992;**20**:248–54.
24. Clark AL, Poole-Wilson PA, Coats AJS. Exercise limitation in chronic heart failure: the central role of the periphery. *J Am Coll Cardiol* 1996;**28**:1092–102.

2

Heart failure syndromes

Andrew L. Clark

Heart failure is a protean condition, presenting acutely to hospital in most cases, but often presenting with a more insidious course to primary care physicians.[1] Patients may only be diagnosed as having a primary cardiac problem after being seen by respiratory physicians or even, on occasion, after gastrointestinal work-up for hepatomegaly (with or without jaundice) or weight loss. Nevertheless, there are common presenting clinical syndromes in patients with heart failure (Box 2.1) which should prompt different initial treatment strategies.

Acute heart failure

As a pragmatic definition, acute heart failure is heart failure necessitating emergency admission to hospital. Attempts have been made to classify acute heart failure into different types,[2] but the classification schemes often read as arbitrary, and resemble Borges' classification system for animals.[3] For the majority of patients, the problem of acute heart failure is that of 'fluid in the wrong place'; if that fluid is in the lungs, the patient has pulmonary oedema, but if the fluid is predominantly in the tissues, the patient may present with anasarca (Greek ανα-, throughout; σαρχ, σαρκ-, flesh). Of course, patients will lie somewhere along a spectrum, often with fluid retention that has developed insidiously. Most patients admitted with heart failure are not breathless at rest,[4] but may have some degree of pulmonary congestion even if the dominant problem is one of fluid retention, and conversely, many patients with frank pulmonary oedema will have some evidence of ankle oedema.

Box 2.1 Heart failure syndromes

- Acute heart failure
  - Pulmonary oedema
  - Anasarca
  - Cardiogenic shock
- Chronic heart failure
- Cardiac cachexia
- Sudden death

Precipitants of acute heart failure

A large number of patients presenting with acute heart failure will have a background history of antecedent stable chronic heart failure. For patients presenting with pulmonary oedema, there will often be an obvious precipitant of the immediate crisis, and the trigger should be sought and treated (Box 2.2). Failure of compliance is the commonest identified trigger in several studies, with perhaps half of all admissions being potentially preventable if compliance had been better.[5,6]

Other common triggers include further ischaemic events in patients with ischaemic heart disease underlying their heart failure, and arrhythmia. Particularly in older patients, intercurrent illness, and especially chest infection, is a common precipitant (see Figure 2.1).[7] The immediate precipitant does affect prognosis. Where uncontrolled hypertension is the culprit, the prognosis is good: however, patients admitted because of pneumonia, worsening renal function, or ischaemia have a worse prognosis.[7]

The fact that poor compliance is such a common trigger in all populations studied emphasizes the importance of patient education and follow-up to try and prevent recurrences. Although it is difficult to demonstrate, increased numbers of admissions are certainly associated with a worse long-term prognosis,[8,9] and the pattern of admissions resembles that of a stone skimming

Box 2.2 Precipitants of acute heart failure

- Acute ischaemia
- Arrhythmia
  - Atrial fibrillation or flutter
  - Ventricular tachycardia
- Mechanical disaster
  - Papillary muscle rupture
- Intercurrent illness
  - Pneumonia
  - Influenza
- Non-compliance
- Pulmonary embolus
- Environment
  - Salt and or fluid load
  - Drugs

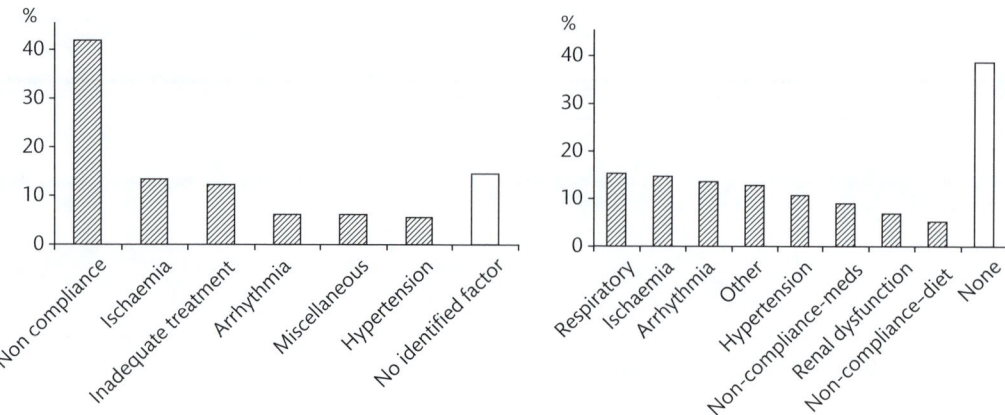

Figure 2.1 Precipitants of admission to hospital with acute heart failure in two patient cohorts. Note that the totals may exceed 100% as an individual patient may have more than one precipitant.

Source data from Michalsen A, Konig G, Thimme W. Preventable causative factors leading to hospital admission with decompensated heart failure. *Heart* 1998;**80**:437–41 (*left*) and Fonarow GC, *et al.* Factors identified as precipitating hospital admissions for heart failure and clinical outcomes: findings from OPTIMIZE-HF. *Arch Intern Med* 2008;**168**:847–54 (*right*).

across a pond, becoming more and more frequent as the disease progresses.[10]

Pulmonary oedema

Pathophysiology

If the left ventricle fails acutely, cardiac output is maintained by the Frank–Starling mechanism: an increase in the left ventricular end-diastolic pressure, representing the preload of the left ventricle, leads to an increase in stroke work. However, the increase in diastolic pressure inevitably causes an increase in left atrial, pulmonary venous, and then capillary, pressure.

The balance of forces keeping fluid within blood vessels is largely a balance between the hydrostatic pressure tending to force fluid out and the colloid osmotic pressure tending to keep fluid in. In a normal subject, there is a continuous flow of fluid from the pulmonary capillaries (at low rate) into the lung interstitium, which is then drained by the pulmonary lymphatics. If the left ventricle fails, the rise in pulmonary capillary pressure required to maintain left ventricular output will eventually exceed the combined resistance of the colloid osmotic pressure and the alveolar basement membrane and the capacity of the pulmonary lymphatics to drain tissue fluid.[11] At this point, fluid will start to accumulate in the pulmonary interstitium, then the alveoli, and ultimately the airways (see **Figure 2.2**).

This traditional explanation of the pathophysiology of acute pulmonary oedema does not explain one aspect: the rise in left ventricular end-diastolic pressure is often conceived to be a passive phenomenon, but for pressure rise, there must be an input of energy from somewhere. It thus cannot be that the left atrial pressure determines the pulmonary capillary pressure by a passive back-pressure effect. Following an initial insult, the stroke volume of the left ventricles falls—but that of the right is maintained. The imbalance between the two means that the right ventricle is inputting energy into the left system, raising the pulmonary capillary pressure (and hence left atrial pressure) until the left ventricular stroke volume is restored. The mismatch between right and left ventricular stroke volumes represents the fluid accumulating in the lung tissue.[12]

As fluid accumulates, so the lungs become stiffer and the work of breathing increases; bronchospasm (so-called 'cardiac asthma') can

be a prominent feature; and at the same time, gas exchange is hampered by fluid filling the alveoli. The sympathetic response worsens the situation by causing tachycardia and peripheral vasoconstriction, thereby increasing the afterload against which the failing left ventricle is trying to eject blood.

Clinical syndrome

Pulmonary oedema is an acute medical emergency and an exceptionally alarming experience for the patient. The typical clinical picture is well known. Symptoms tend to be of very abrupt onset, typically appearing over the course of less than an hour, but may be preceded by a day or so of worsening breathlessness and nocturnal dyspnoea. The patient rapidly becomes extremely breathless and distressed; speaking more than a few words at a time becomes impossible, and

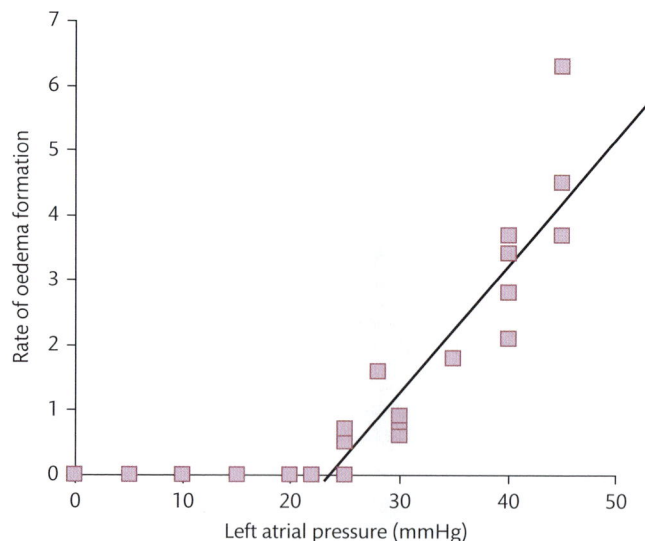

Figure 2.2 The rate of pulmonary oedema formation is dependent on exceeding a critical left ventricular end-diastolic pressure.

Source data from Guyton AC, Lindsey AW. Effect of elevated left atrial pressure and decreased plasma protein concentration on the development of pulmonary edema. *Circ Res* 1959;**7**:649–57.

the need to breathe becomes overwhelming. The fearful sensation of impending death, *angor animi*, is very common. The patient needs to sit upright, often forward, and might die if forced to lie flat. As the alveoli fill with fluid, the patient will cough, often violently, and will expectorate quantities of pink-tinged frothy fluid.

There is invariably a huge sympathetic nervous system response: the periphery becomes shut down due to vasoconstriction with associated pallor and coldness of the skin. Profuse sweating is commonly seen.

Common physical findings include sinus tachycardia, or arrhythmia, commonly atrial fibrillation or ventricular tachycardia. Hypertension is common, either as a precipitant or as a consequence of the sympathetic activity. The jugular venous pressure may be raised, but there are often no signs of peripheral oedema as the syndrome develops abruptly: there has been no time for the patient to become fluid-overloaded. The problem is not one of excess fluid, rather, fluid in the wrong body compartment. Some evidence suggests that there is a fall in intravascular volume during pulmonary oedema (as fluid accumulates in the lungs) which increases again as pulmonary oedema resolves.[13]

The cardiac findings depend upon the previous history, and may include a displaced and dyskinetic apex beat. A gallop rhythm is very common, with 3rd, 4th and summation sounds difficult to distinguish given the tachycardia. The chest may be silent *in extremis*, but is usually filled with a variety of fine and coarse crackles, and wheezes. In cases presenting early or with mild pulmonary oedema, the classical finding of fine late inspiratory crackles at the bases may be heard (see **Figure 2.3**).

Flash pulmonary oedema

Some patients have episodes of very abrupt onset pulmonary oedema, which may be recurrent, in the presence of apparently normal left ventricular systolic function. Renal artery stenosis is a common underlying cause.[14] Other causes include phaeochromocytoma, and swimming-induced pulmonary oedema. Although the latter is thought of as a rare event occurring in athletes, swimming-induced pulmonary oedema (and, more broadly, exercise-induced pulmonary oedema) may be more common: in a report of 30 Israeli soldiers performing a 2.4 km open water time trial, eight developed frothy sputum, dyspnoea, and haemoptysis consistent with pulmonary oedema.[15]

SCUBA divers (including recreational divers) are also at risk of immersion pulmonary oedema, which can be fatal.[16] The pathophysiological explanation is that cardiac output is greatly increased during exercise, and then immersion in cold water causes abrupt vasoconstriction and the increase in afterload precipitates pulmonary oedema.[17] In addition, immersion is associated with an increase in right relative to left ventricular stroke volume.[18]

Other rarer causes of pulmonary oedema include re-expansion pulmonary oedema following treatment for pneumothorax,[19] presumably as a large negative intrathoracic pressure abruptly increases the gradient between now negative alveolar and intravascular pressure.

Natural history

Modern treatment has changed the natural history of acute pulmonary oedema, and the outlook depends upon the severity of the syndrome as well as the underlying causes. Grading systems for recording severity are available, with the Killip class[20] and an assessment based on the combination of perfusion and congestion[21] commonly used (see **Table 2.1**). The gradings are primarily designed for use in people with heart failure following acute myocardial infarction, but are helpful in assessing prognosis whatever the underlying cause of the pulmonary oedema.

Patients with acute pulmonary oedema typically present outside office hours, and it is striking that they either improve rapidly or die, so that within a few hours, the immediate clinical outcome is obvious. In the EFICA study[22] of patients admitted to high-dependency units with acute severe HF (82% of whom had pulmonary oedema), mortality was 27.4% at four weeks and 46.5% at one year. When those who died *before* reaching hospital were included, mortality was 43.2% and 62.5% at the two time-points, respectively.

Table 2.1 Grading systems for severe heart failure

(a)

Killip class	Clinical state	Hospital mortality (%)
1	No signs of heart failure	6
2	Third heart sound, basal crackles	17
3	Acute pulmonary oedema	38
4	Cardiogenic shock	81

Source data from Killip T 3rd, Kimball JT. Treatment of myocardial infarction in a coronary care unit. A two year experience with 250 patients. *Am J Cardiol* 1967;**20**:457–64.

(b) Hazard ratio for the combined end-point of death or transplantation

		Congestion	
		No	Yes
Low perfusion	Yes	Warm and dry 1	Warm and wet 1.8
	No	Cool and dry	Cool and wet 2.5

Source data from Nohria A, Tsang SW, Fang JC, Lewis EF, Jarcho JA, Mudge GH, Stevenson LW. Clinical assessment identifies hemodynamic profiles that predict outcomes in patients admitted with heart failure. *J Am Coll Cardiol* 2003;**41**:1797–804.

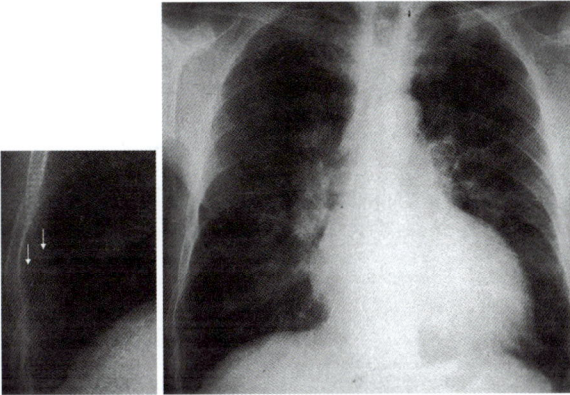

Figure 2.3 Plain chest X-ray of a patient presenting with early pulmonary oedema. The heart is enlarged and the hila prominent. The enlarged section highlights interstitial lines (arrowed) of developing interstitial fluid (known as Kerley B lines). On examination, the patient had fine late inspiratory crackles at the bases.

Anasarca

Pathophysiology

At the other end of the spectrum of acute heart failure from acute pulmonary oedema are patients presenting with fluid retention. This is a far more gradual process than that underlying acute pulmonary oedema. By the time patients present, they may have accumulated more than 20 L of excess fluid (and it requires approximately 5 L excess before ankle oedema appears).

The underlying pathophysiology is the neurohormonal response to poor renal perfusion and fall in arterial blood pressure. The kidneys 'try' to maintain normal perfusion by the release of renin, ultimately leading to aldosterone release and salt and water retention by the kidneys. In addition, antidiuretic hormone (ADH; arginine vasopressin) is released from the anterior pituitary gland. ADH is high relative to serum sodium, and causes water retention and the production of hypertonic urine, coupled with thirst, which results in increased fluid intake.[23]

The excess fluid increases the venous hydrostatic pressure which results in the Starling forces in the capillaries favouring fluid loss from the vessels and accumulation in the tissues.

Clinical syndrome

Where the excess fluid accumulates is a function of gravity. The ankles are usually first affected, commonly with swelling that increases during the day and may have gone by the next morning as a consequence of several hours' leg elevation. The oedema progressively rises up the legs, and then affects the abdominal wall. Pleural effusions and ascites are common at this stage, and pericardial effusions may become large.

The prominent physical finding is, of course, peripheral oedema, which is pitting. Sinus tachycardia or atrial fibrillation are usual findings together with low systemic blood pressure. The jugular venous pressure is invariably raised, and there may be evidence of tricuspid regurgitation in the jugular venous waveform. There is often a dilated heart with prominent third heart sound. The lung fields may be clear, or there may be some evidence of pulmonary oedema.

Natural history

There is some evidence that strict bed rest might result in a reduction in oedema,[24] but without therapy, anasarca or 'dropsy' becomes a chronic state. Surprisingly large volumes of excess fluid are sometimes tolerated for many months before a patient finally presents (see **Figure 2.4**). It does appear that congestion itself is harmful: data from the National Heart Failure Audit in England and Wales show that worsening oedema at presentation is associated with worse prognosis[25] (see **Figure 2.5**). Modern diuretic therapy means that most patients progress at this stage to having chronic heart failure, but even among patients with chronic heart failure, evidence of congestion is associated with a worse prognosis.[26,27] Although some earlier studies have suggested that clinical examination by an expert can reliably assess fluid status in chronic heart failure, perhaps half of pateints who are clinically euvolaemic have evidence of congestion based on ultrasound indices.[28] Although there is a well-known association between higher doses of diuretic and higher mortality,[29] the observation is confounded: patients with worse heart failure need higher doses of diuretic. The presence of subclinical congestion is associated with a worse outcome,[28] raising the possibility that

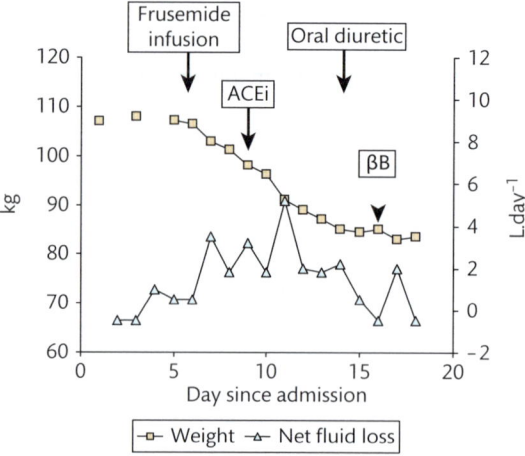

Figure 2.4 Clinical course of a patient presenting with anasarca. The patient lost 25 kg during his admission, representing 25 L of excess fluid. ACEi, ACE inhibitor; βB, β-blocker.

higher doses of diuretic might be beneficial for patients who can be shown to have congestion despite clinical euvolaemia.

Chronic heart failure

The vast majority of patients with heart failure receive active treatment so that following a presentation with an acute episode of heart failure, congestion is removed. The chronic heart failure syndrome is what affects patients with heart failure once they are taking appropriate combination therapy with diuretics (as needed), angiotensin converting enzyme inhibitors (or angiotensin receptor neprilysin inhibitors), β-blockers and sometimes mineralocorticoid receptor antagonists. For these patients, the term 'congestive' heart failure is inappropriate—they should not be congested at all with suitable use of diuretics.

The symptoms of chronic heart failure are most commonly breathlessness and fatigue on exertion, leading to exercise limitation and consequent decline in quality of life. Measuring the

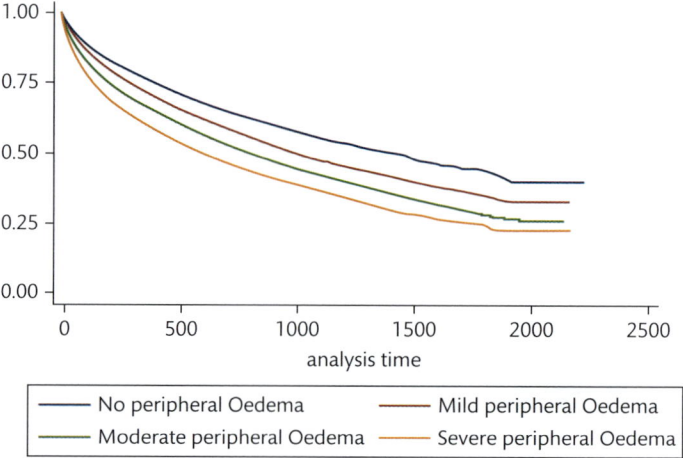

Figure 2.5 Relation between severity of congestion and outcome among 121 229 patients admitted to hospital with acute heart failure between 2007 and 2013.

Table 2.2 New York Heart Association classification of symptoms in chronic heart failure

Class	Symptoms
I	No symptoms during ordinary activity
II	Mild symptoms during activity with some limitation
III	Marked limitation in exercise capacity with symptoms on mild exertion
IV	Symptoms at rest

severity of symptoms is most commonly done with the New York Heart Association (NYHA) scale (see Table 2.2).[30] Unfortunately, the NYHA system is only weakly related to measures of exercise capacity, and bears no relation to left ventricular function at rest. It is often not clear from clinical studies as to whether the patients are recording their score (which should surely be the case as it is a subjective scoring system) or the physicians caring for the patients. When physicians score the patients, the NYHA system becomes a composite score of overall severity of heart failure rather than being a pure symptom score.[31]

Another limitation is that patients are forced into one of four categories, and in practice, most patients recruited to clinical trials are in either class II or class III (those in class I have no symptoms and might thus be thought not to have heart failure; those in class IV are bed-bound). Further, there is a temptation to describe populations of patients by their 'average' NYHA class. This is inappropriate—no individual patient can have anything other than an integer score, and the scale is non-linear.

Other scoring systems are better matched to the complexity of symptom assessment, and are better able to define subtle differences both between patients and in response to therapy. They are more cumbersome to administer in practice than the NYHA score. The Minnesota Living with Heart Failure self-assessment questionnaire is the most widely used, and is a series of 21 questions, each scored from 0 to 5.[32,33] The Kansas City questionnaire[34] has the advantage of asking patients about how symptoms have changed and gives a better idea of the trajectory of an individual's clinical course.

A functional assessment is very helpful in trying to get an objective measure of a patient's symptoms. Whereas incremental exercise tests with metabolic gas exchange measurements are often thought to be the best single assessment, the equipment required is not universally available. Many patients are unable to manage an incremental exercise test. The six-minute walk test[35,36] is easy to administer, can be attempted by the great majority of patients, and is reproducible.

Pathophysiology

Central haemodynamics

Why chronic heart failure causes shortness of breath and fatigue has traditionally been attributed to abnormal central haemodynamics. It might be supposed that 'forward' failure leads to inability adequately to perfuse exercising skeletal muscle, thereby resulting in fatigue; and 'backward' failure leads to a rise in pulmonary venous pressure, stiff (or even oedematous) lungs, thereby resulting in breathlessness. However, against this hypothesis is the fact that there is no relation between exercise capacity and central haemodynamics (at least at

rest); some patients with very severe left ventricular dysfunction have near-normal exercise capacity;[37] acute correction of central haemodynamics (with, for example, positive inotropic drug therapy or even heart transplantation[38]) does not result in acute correction of exercise limitation. During early stages of exercise, the cardiac output responses are often normal in heart failure.

Some light is thrown on the issue by the observation that different kinds of exercise can lead to different symptoms in the same individual: rapidly incremental tests are more likely to cause limiting breathlessness,[39] whereas slower tests, although eliciting the same exercise performance, are more likely to cause fatigue. Cycle exercise is more often stopped by fatigue than breathlessness compared with treadmill exercise, even when the same level of exercise is performed.[40,41]

Some work has suggested that right ventricular function and pulmonary haemodynamics might be key determinants of exercise capacity, but some patients with the Fontan circulation (who thus have no right ventricle in the circulation) have near-normal exercise capacity.[42]

Pulmonary physiology

The lungs are abnormal in many patients with chronic heart failure, both in terms of spirometric variables and diffusion capacity.[43] In some studies, exercise capacity correlates closely with some spirometric variables.[44] However, about one-third of patients being assessed for transplantation will have normal spirometry and diffusion.[45]

One possibility is that pulmonary dead space might be increased. Dead space is that component of air in the respiratory tract not available for gas exchange. Anatomical dead space is the fixed dead space formed from the airways. It could plausibly be increased by an altered ventilatory pattern: the same minute ventilation achieved with double the respiratory rate and half the tidal volume will double anatomical dead space. Physiological dead space, on the other hand, is made up of alveoli that are ventilated but not perfused—'wasted' or inefficient ventilation.

However, there is no dead space receptor that might sense the increase and drive an excessive ventilatory response. In contrast to what might be expected, patients with chronic heart failure have better than normal arterial blood gases during exercise,[46] suggesting that the primary abnormality driving an excessive ventilatory response to exercise must lie elsewhere.

Skeletal muscle

Abnormalities of skeletal muscle in chronic heart failure range from ultrastructural,[47] through histological[48] and metabolic,[49] to changes in gross function (weakness and early fatigue[50]), and reduction in bulk.[51] The key feature distinguishing patients with normal from abnormal exercise capacity is differences in skeletal muscle function: those with normal exercise capacity have normal (or near-normal) skeletal muscle.[37] That these changes might cause the sensation of fatigue is easy to picture.

A unifying picture to explain the origin of symptoms comes from the ergoreflex (Figure 1.3). The ergoreflex is neurally mediated and arises from exercising muscle in proportion to work done. The strength of the signal is also proportional to the amount of muscle doing the work—the stimulus is greater when arm muscle is used to perform a given workload compared with leg muscle.[52]

Stimulation of the ergoreflex both increases ventilation and causes sympathetic nervous system activation. In patients with chronic heart failure, the ergoreflex is enhanced in proportion to the degree of exercise limitation and ventilatory abnormality.[53]

The ergoreflex model explains the two common chronic heart failure symptoms, and helps to explain other features of the syndrome. The origin of the sympathetic activation is not immediately obvious as the baroreflexes are downregulated in heart failure.[54] Ergoreflex stimulation causes sympathetic activation. In addition, the chemoreflexes are enhanced in chronic heart failure, and they, too, are associated with baroreflex downregulation.[55] Indeed, the peripheral model gives a new understanding of autonomic nervous system changes in chronic heart failure;[56] in the normal state, the main inputs into autonomic nervous system control from the cardiovascular system are the baroreceptors and cardiopulmonary receptors, with parasympathetic modulation being the major output; in heart failure, chemoreceptors and ergoreceptors are the most important inputs, and sympathetic activation results.

Natural history

There is, of course, nothing 'natural' about the outcome of patients with chronic heart failure. The marked improvements in prognosis that have come with modern medical therapy[57] (**Figure 2.6**) are shown by the falling event rates among patients in clinical trials. For very many patients, chronic heart failure can be stable for many years, but for some, it can be a progressive illness resulting in early death or transplantation.

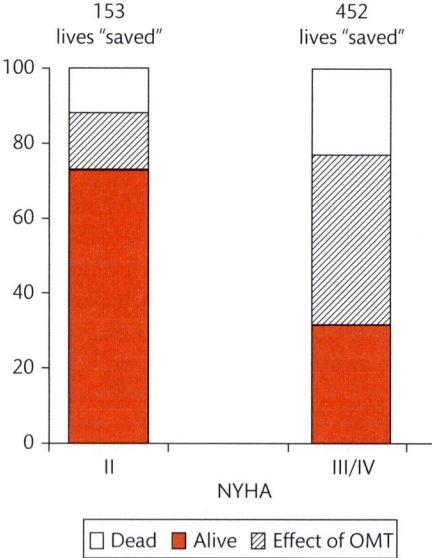

Figure 2.6 The effect of modern medical therapy in chronic heart failure. The bars represent the two-year outcome of 1000 patients with either mild (NYHA II/III) or severe (NYHA III/IV) heart failure. The red blocks represent the patients who would have survived and the white bars those who would have died without treatment. The shaded blocks represent the patients whose death would have been prevented by optimal medical therapy (OMT) with ACE inhibitor, β-blocker, and aldosterone antagonist.

Source data from Cleland JG, Clark AL. Delivering the cumulative benefits of triple therapy to improve outcomes in heart failure: too many cooks will spoil the broth. *J Am Coll Cardiol* 2003;**42**:1234–7.

Cardiac cachexia

That chronic heart disease can result in cachexia has been known for many hundreds of years. Quite how it comes about remains unknown, and anecdotally its frequency seems to be falling, perhaps as a consequence of widespread use of β-blockers. Part of the difficulty in discussing the syndrome is the lack of a universally recognized definition of cachexia. Clinicians know it when they see it, but defining it is a different matter. It is best thought of as a process of active weight loss rather than referring to a patient who is simply thin; but how much weight loss, and loss from which body compartment (fat, muscle or bone) is not satisfactorily determined.

Partly because of the lack of an agreed definition, the epidemiology of cardiac cachexia is unclear. Data from clinical trial databases suggest that weight loss is common,[58] with more than 40% of patients losing 5% or more of their body weight during three years of follow-up in the SOLVD trial (**Figure 2.7**).

The weight loss in cachexia is from all body compartments, not simply lean muscle. Muscle loss is common from early in the course of chronic heart failure,[59] but loss of non-lean tissue is also seen,[60] and patients are more prone to osteoporosis than normal subjects.[61] Patients with cachexia tend to have more advanced heart failure. The loss of bulk contributes to the general sense of fatigue and the activation of the ergoreflexes outlined above.

Origins of cachexia

Chronic heart failure seems to be an inherently catabolic state.[62,63] This is seen even at the level of increased hepatic fibrinogen synthesis.[64] Part of the explanation may be the continuous neurohormonal activation of heart failure. Sympathetic activation causes an increase in basal metabolic rate,[65,66] glycogenolysis, and lipolysis.[67]

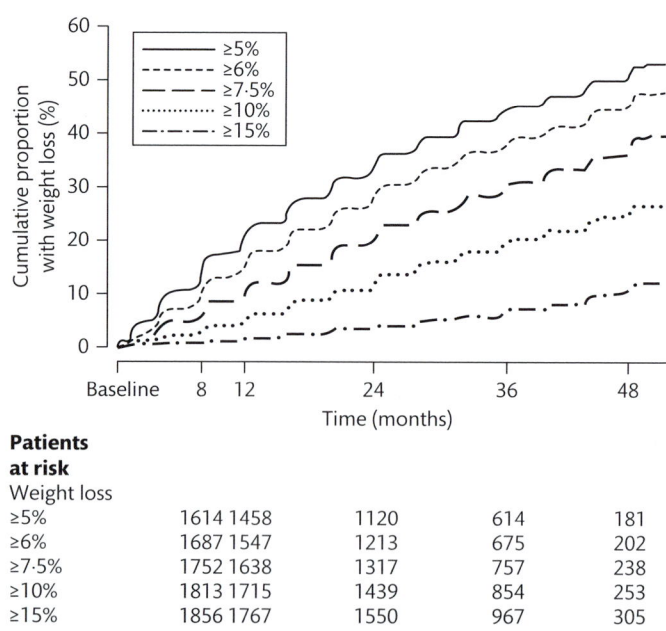

Patients at risk Weight loss					
≥5%	1614	1458	1120	614	181
≥6%	1687	1547	1213	675	202
≥7·5%	1752	1638	1317	757	238
≥10%	1813	1715	1439	854	253
≥15%	1856	1767	1550	967	305

Figure 2.7 Cumulative incidence of weight loss during follow-up in the SOLVD trial.

Reproduced from Anker SD, *et al*. Prognostic importance of weight loss in chronic heart failure and the effect of treatment with angiotensin-converting-enzyme inhibitors: an observational study. *Lancet* 2003;**361**:1077–83.

In animal models, high levels of angiotensin II are also associated with profound weight loss.[68,69] In normal subjects, infusions of catabolic hormones (hydrocortisone, glucagon, and adrenaline) induce hyperglycaemia, hyperinsulinaemia, insulin resistance, negative nitrogen balance—precisely the changes seen in the cachexia syndrome.[70,71]

Other neurohormonal changes are commonly seen in chronic heart failure which are much more prevalent in patients with cachexia. In general, there seems to be a shift in the normal balance between catabolic and anabolic hormonal factors, so that patients develop resistance to the effects of both insulin[72] and growth hormone[73] and a decrease in the ratio of anabolic to catabolic steroid.[74] Additional pro-catabolic changes include the production of tumour necrosis factor (TNF-α),[75] which is itself related to the changes in neurohormones.[76] These changes are strongly related to the alterations in body compartments,[77] suggesting that there is indeed an aetiological link between neurohormonal activation and weight loss.

One fascinating potential explanation which explains the otherwise slightly mysterious rise in TNF-α is the possibility that bowel wall oedema, possibly caused by recurrent episodes of decompensation, allows the translocation of bacterial endotoxin across the bowel wall.[78] Bacterial endotoxin is the most potent natural stimulus for TNF-α production. In support of this notion, circulating endotoxin is high during episodes of decompensation, and declines with treatment.[79] A further observation is that the endotoxin hypothesis may explain the apparent protective effects of cholesterol in patients with chronic heart failure:[80] endogenous lipoproteins act as a sump for endotoxin.[81]

Other potential contributors to cachexia are poor dietary intake, although there is only small-scale evidence for such a phenomenon.[82,83] There is some evidence that malabsorption (possibly as a consequence of gut oedema) may be a cause of impaired nutrition; fat malabsorption in particular.[84] Malaise, lethargy, nausea, lack of motivation and poor mobility may contribute, particularly in the elderly.[85] Frailty and signs of poor nutrition are common in patients admitted to hospital with acute heart failure.[86]

Treatment of cachexia

Hyperalimentation does not seem to offer any substantial benefit to stable patients with chronic heart failure,[80] but there is no large-scale intervention trial looking at its possible benefits in a cachectic population. There is some evidence that micronutrient supplementation may be helpful.[87] Other dietary approaches are being considered (reviewed[88] with many suggestions focusing on possible anti-inflammatory strategies), but none has so far proved to be effective.

Conventional heart failure therapy does affect cachexia. Angiotensin converting enzyme inhibitors, or, at least, enalapril, reduce the risk of weight loss (**Figure 2.8**).[89,90] Similar effects have been reported with the angiotensin receptor antagonist, candesartan.[91] Beta-adrenoceptor antagonism causes a fall in basal metabolic rate,[92] an effect that may underlie the increase in weight seen in some patients on long-term β-blocker therapy.[93,94] There is some evidence that β-blockers may reduce the risk of cardiac cachexia developing,[95] and may reverse it once it has occurred.[96]

Natural history

The major clinical impact of cachexia is on outcome. Defined as unintentional weight loss of at least 7.5%, cachexia was associated with

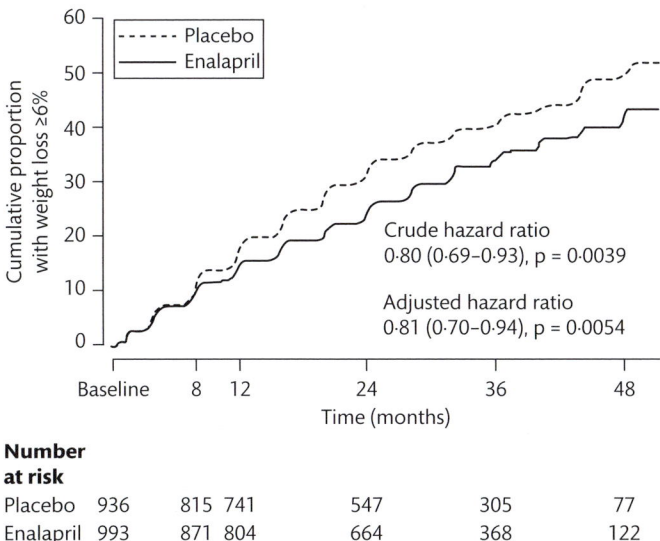

Figure 2.8 Effect of the ACE inhibitor, enalapril, on the risk of developing ≥6% weight loss in the SOLVD trial.

Reproduced from Anker SD, *et al. Prognostic importance of weight loss in chronic heart failure and the effect of treatment with angiotensin-converting-enzyme inhibitors: an observational study. Lancet* 2003;**361**:1077–83.

a mortality of 50% at 18 months.[97] In fact, decreasing body mass—not just an active process of cachexia—is inversely related to survival.[98,99] Increasing body mass is strongly associated with survival following left ventricular assist device implantation.[100] The situation following cardiac transplantation is more complex. Weight at transplantation does not have a major impact on outcome,[101] but because thinner patients have a worse prognosis, there is more to be gained from transplantation for underweight patients.

Sudden death

It may seem odd to consider 'sudden death' to be a clinical syndrome, but one of the peculiarities of chronic heart failure is that patients are at risk of dying suddenly at any point in their clinical course. Approximately half the patients dying from heart failure die from progressive disease, but the others die suddenly. The mode of death in heart failure depends upon the severity of the heart failure syndrome (see **Figure 2.9**). With worsening NYHA class of symptoms, so the likelihood of a death being sudden declines, with sudden death predominating as the mode of death in patients with milder symptoms. Note, however, that the likelihood of dying is much lower in the patients with mild symptoms, so the absolute number of sudden deaths increases with worsening symptoms.

Patients with chronic heart failure are prone to tachyarrhythmias, both atrial and ventricular. The cause of sudden death has traditionally been considered to be a ventricular arrhythmia—either ventricular tachycardia or fibrillation (see **Figure 2.10**). However, it is important to remember that conduction system disease is very common in heart failure, and so patients are at risk of bradycardia as well.[102,103]

A difficulty in understanding the pathophysiology of sudden death is the lack of an agreed definition of sudden death.[104] A further consideration is that most patients with chronic heart failure

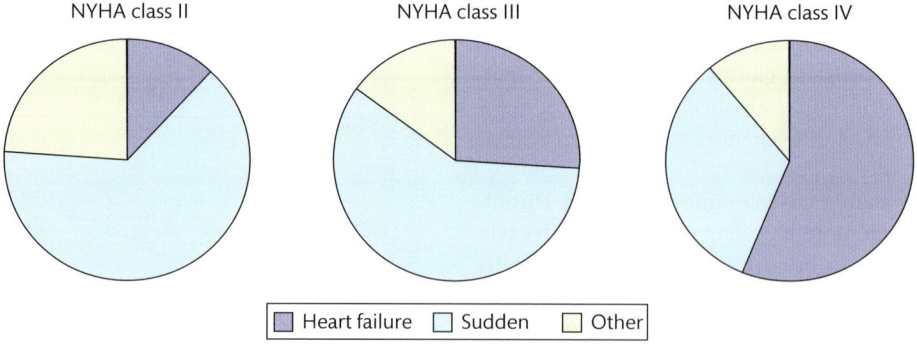

NYHA class II   NYHA class III   NYHA class IV

■ Heart failure □ Sudden □ Other

Figure 2.9 The proportion of patients dying suddenly by NYHA class. Note, however, that the proportion of patients dying falls with increasing NYHA class, and so the likelihood of dying suddenly actually increases.
Source data from *The Lancet*, **353**, 9161, MERIT-HF Study Group, Effect of metoprolol CR/XL in chronic heart failure: Metoprolol CR/XL Randomised Intervention Trial in Congestive Heart Failure (MERIT-HF), 2001–7, Copyright (1999).

have underlying coronary heart disease, and so are potentially at risk from further ischaemic events. Whilst sudden deaths are commonly presumed to be due to arrhythmia, postmortem studies of patients with heart failure dying suddenly show that very many are secondary to ischaemic events.[105,106] These ischaemic events are mostly not detected in life, leading to a false impression of how common arrhythmic death is. Among patients dying suddenly who have an implantable cardioverter–defibrillator implanted, arrhythmia is not the cause in a high proportion.[107–109]

The importance in understanding the causes of sudden death lies in appreciating that therapies targeted specifically at sudden death (with implantable cardioverter–defibrillators, for example) are not able to eradicate sudden death completely. Interestingly, the rate of sudden death (at least among patients recruited to clinical trials) has fallen by 44% between 1995 and 2014 independent of the use of the *International Classification of Diseases*,[110] presumably as a consequence of the cumulative effects of medical therapy.

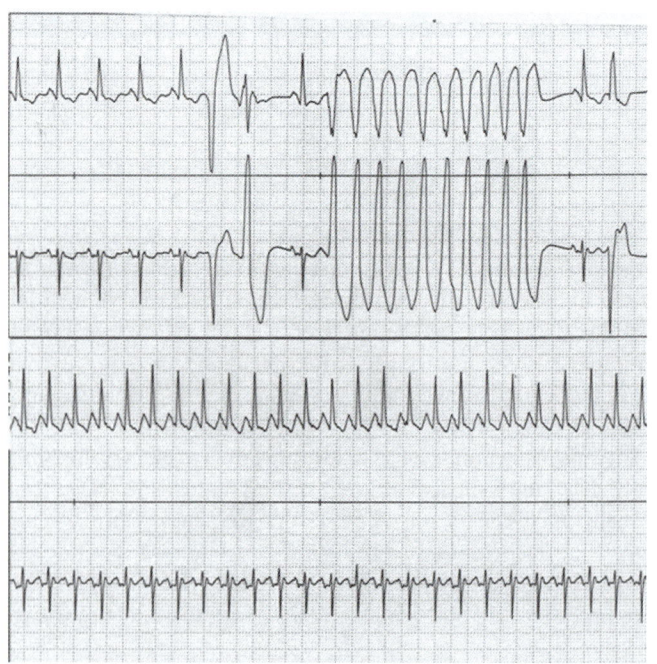

Figure 2.10 An extract from a 24 h Holter recording of a patient with chronic heart failure showing both non-sustained ventricular tachycardia (*top*) and atrial flutter (*bottom*).

Heart failure with normal ejection fraction

The vast majority of clinical trials in patients with chronic heart failure have been conducted in patients with left ventricular systolic dysfunction (LVSD). Although defining chronic heart failure can be difficult, its pragmatic definition requiring *symptoms* compatible with the syndrome in the *presence of cardiac dysfunction* makes LVSD relatively easy to identify. This is the appeal of the left ventricular ejection fraction as a measurement—a normal range can be established, and those people who are breathless on exertion and whose ejection fraction falls below the normal range are labelled as having heart failure.

This pragmatic approach to identifying patients who should be treated leaves a large group of people who have undoubted *symptoms* compatible with a diagnosis of chronic heart failure, but who have normal (or at most mildly impaired) left ventricular systolic function. There are many reports suggesting that perhaps half of all patients with heart failure fall into this category, and various labels are used.

- *Diastolic heart failure* implies that there is some objective abnormality of diastolic function to explain the symptoms: in turn, there is the implication that 'normal' diastolic function is well described, allowing *diastolic dysfunction* to be well defined.[111]
- *Heart failure with preserved systolic function* (sometimes 'HeFPEF' or variants thereof) implies that systolic function is as normal as it ever has been and that any abnormality must be restricted to diastole.
- *Heart failure with normal ejection fraction* (sometimes 'HeFNEF') is a more pragmatic description, but does imply that there is some way of being certain that the symptoms are due to the heart, even if the heart appears normal on imaging.

Despite the apparent commonness of HeFNEF in epidemiological studies,[112,113] many clinicians, even heart failure specialists, are sceptical about the diagnosis and its frequency.[114–116] Unlike the situation with clinical trials of patients with systolic left ventricular dysfunction, it has proved difficult to recruit patients to trials of HeFNEF, and the more stringent the requirements for objective evidence of diastolic dysfunction, the more difficult it has been to recruit. A further surprise, perhaps, is that no clinical trial has yet demonstrated robust survival evidence for any specific heart failure therapy in

patients with diastolic heart failure, suggesting that HeFNEF may be pathophysiologically distinct from heart failure with reduced ejection fraction.

Pathophysiology

Patients with systolic left ventricular dysfunction have impaired diastolic function, too, often due to increased fibrous tissue. In those with HeFNEF, there is predominant impairment of left ventricular filling because the ventricle is 'stiff' and has decreased compliance—that is, it requires a greater pressure than normal to increase the volume of the left ventricle prior to the next contraction. Ventricular filling (and subsequent stroke volume) is preserved, but at a cost of an increase in left ventricular diastolic pressure.

The increased left ventricular diastolic pressure is necessarily accompanied by an increase in left atrial pressure, and, in turn, pulmonary venous pressure. The pulmonary venous hypertension causes the lungs to stiffen, and can result in pulmonary oedema formation if it becomes very severe. Breathlessness is an obvious consequence.

Left ventricular hypertrophy is very common, and might be considered a defining feature of 'diastolic dysfunction'. Similarly, left atrial dilation is an almost inevitable consequence, and in its absence, an alternative for breathlessness should be sought.

End-diastolic pressure–volume relation

An increase in end-diastolic pressure would not constitute 'diastolic dysfunction', but could simply represent increased preload. In HeFNEF, there should be a shift in the end-diastolic pressure–volume relation of the left ventricle upward (see **Figure 2.11**).

However, where the end-diastolic pressure–volume relation has been specifically measured, there is little evidence of a consistent alteration in the relation: in fact, quite the reverse. In individual subjects with apparent heart failure and normal ejection fraction, the relation might be normal, increased or decreased.[114,117,118]

Transmitral flow

A major feature of diastolic dysfunction is an alteration in transmitral diastolic blood flow. In the normal (young) adult, most ventricular filling occurs early in diastole and is largely passive (although there is some evidence that there may be an active component from left ventricular suction). The contribution of left atrial contraction to left ventricular filling is small. The transmitral filling pattern seen on Doppler echocardiography is thus typically a large E or 'early' wave and a small A, or 'atrial', wave.

As diastolic heart failure develops and left ventricle compliance decreases, the E wave becomes relatively smaller and the A wave larger as atrial contraction becomes an important determinant of left ventricular filling. The A wave becomes larger than the E wave—so-called 'E:A reversal'. At the same time, the rate of decline of flow from the peak of the E wave, usually brisk, decreases, thus prolonging the E wave deceleration time and abbreviating the mid-diastolic diastasis.

Ultimately, a pattern of 'pseudonormalization' may develop in which the left ventricular diastolic pressure has risen sufficiently high that atrial contraction is no longer able to compensate for the decline in early filling. Left atrial pressure rises further and most left ventricular filling now reverts to being early and passive with a smaller contribution from atrial contraction: this time, however,

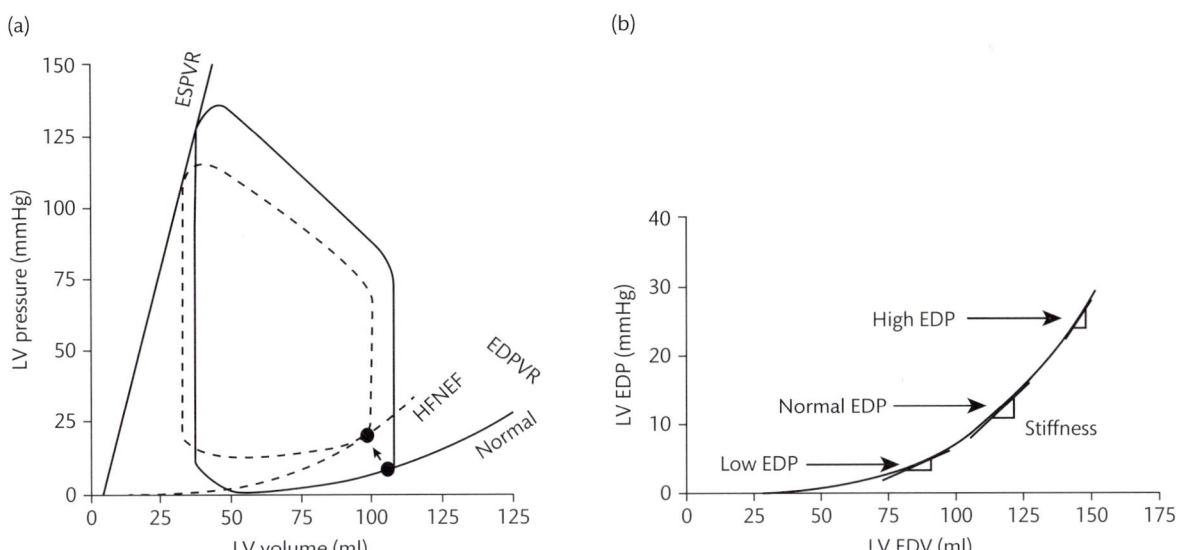

Figure 2.11 (a) Pressure–volume relations within the left ventricle (LV). For heart failure with normal ejection fraction (HFNEF) to be due to diastolic dysfunction, the end-diastolic pressure–volume relation (EDPVR) should be shifted upward and to the left so that to reach a given left ventricular volume, the pressure required is greater. (b) The EDPVR is non-linear: at higher volumes, the stiffness (measured as a tangent to the line) increases so that for a given increase in volume, the pressure change is greater than at smaller left ventricular volumes. Thus, simply demonstrating increased stiffness of the heart does not establish the presence of diastolic dysfunction. EDV, end-diastolic volume.

Reproduced from Burkhoff D, Maurer MS, Packer M. Heart failure with a normal ejection fraction: is it really a disorder of diastolic function? *Circulation* 2003;**107**:656–8 with permission from Wolters Kluwer.

at a cost of very high left atrial pressure and a very short E wave deceleration time.

Diagnosis of diastolic dysfunction

Measuring pressure–volume loops in the left ventricle during diastole is impractical for routine clinical practice, meaning that cardiac imaging, and in particular echocardiography with Doppler analysis of transmitral blood flow, has become the diagnostic method most widely used. However, transmitral blood flow is highly dependent on filling conditions,[119] and so the analysis of diastolic function must be broader. The key components of echocardiographic analysis are the assessment of transmitral flow; the assessment of motion of the mitral valve annulus; and assessment of pulmonary venous blood flow. In addition, evidence of cardiac structural changes (particularly left atrial dilation and left ventricular hypertrophy) is important.

Tissue Doppler interrogation of the mitral annulus targets long-axis function of the left ventricle. In health, there is a movement of the base towards the apex recorded as the S wave, and during diastole E and A motion corresponding to the transmitral E and A waves. The tissue movements are known as E' and A' (or E_m and A_m; or E_a and A_a: 'm' meaning mitral and 'a' annular).

There are two distinct pulses of blood flow into the left atrium from the pulmonary veins: one during systole (the larger in health) and one during diastole. There is some reversal of flow back into the pulmonary veins during atrial systole—the A wave.

Integrating these three movements is the major method for assessing diastolic function (see **Figure 2.3**). As left ventricular compliance falls and left atrial pressure rises, there is first a phase of abnormal relaxation during which there is reversal of the E:A ratio accompanied by reduction in E' and reversal of the E':A' ratio. The diastolic component of pulmonary venous flow increases. Then, as diastolic function worsens, 'pseudonormalization' of transmitral flow is accompanied by more and more marked reduction in mitral annular diastolic motion, greater increases in diastolic pulmonary venous flow, and more marked reversal of pulmonary venous flow during atrial contraction.

There is a linear relation between the ratio between transmitral E and mitral annular E' motion (E:E' ratio) and left ventricular filling pressure.[120] In health, the ratio is usually below 10, and a ratio above 20 strongly suggests that left atrial pressure is above 20 mmHg.

Epidemiology and clinical pattern

Perhaps as many as 60% of patients with chronic heart failure have HeFNEF[111,121] (see **Figure 2.12**). The cause of the heart failure is much more likely to be related to hypertension than in patients with systolic dysfunction.[122] Patients with HeFNEF compared with systolic heart failure are: older by about 10 years or so; have a lower haemoglobin; are more likely to be overweight; are more likely to have atrial fibrillation; more likely to have diabetes; and are far more likely to be female.[112,123,124] The proportion of patients with 'preserved systolic function' has increased with time.[108]

The strong association of HeFNEF with atrial fibrillation, especially incident atrial fibrillation,[117] and hypertension, lead to the suggestion that apparent HeFNEF might be an acute condition, more likely to present as acute pulmonary oedema and rapidly resolving with treatment.[125] In this scenario, an acute event

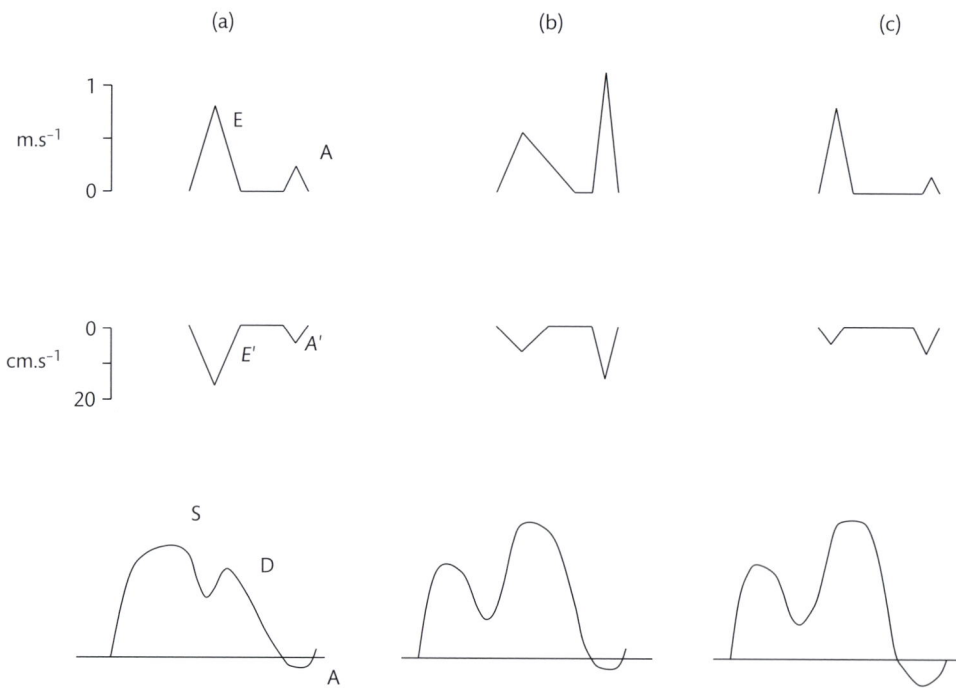

Figure 2.12 Schematic of echocardiographic changes in diastolic dysfunction. The top row is transmitral blood flow; the middle row is movement of the mitral valve annulus with tissue Doppler; and the bottom row is pulmonary venous blood flow. A is the normal state: The mitral E wave is much greater than the A wave; most pulmonary blood flow is in systole. With increasing diastolic dysfunction (B), the mitral A wave becomes larger than the E ('E:A reversal'); the mitral annular is similarly affected and most pulmonary vein flow is in diastole. Finally, with severe diastolic dysfunction, the E:A ratio reverses again ('pseudonormalization'), but with a very short E wave; mitral annular motion is much reduced, with the ratio of E to E' reduced. Pulmonary venous blood flow is further dominated by diastolic flow, with an increasing retrograde A wave.

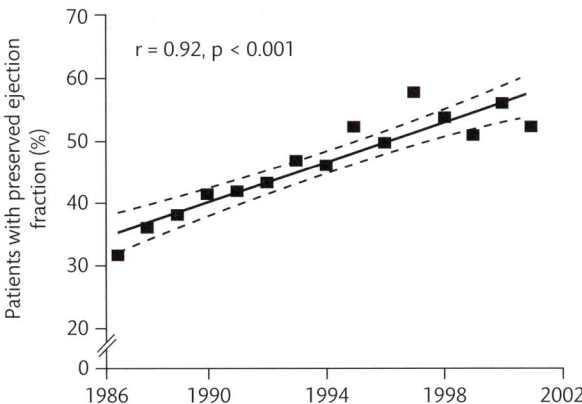

Figure 2.13 The proportion of patients with heart failure who have a normal ejection fraction has increased between 1986 and 2002.
Reproduced from Owan TE, Hodge DO, Herges RM, Jacobsen SJ, Roger VL, Redfield MM. Trends in prevalence and outcome of heart failure with preserved ejection fraction. *N Engl J Med* 2006;**355**:251–9.

precipitates an episode of heart failure and an admission to hospital, but the resolution of symptoms means that such patients are likely to be underrepresented in outpatient populations in chronic heart failure clinics.

The prognosis of patients with heart failure and normal ejection fraction remains controversial. Some studies suggest that the prognosis is just the same as for patients with impaired left ventricular systolic function,[113] slightly better,[112] or much better.[126] The general consensus is that the prognosis is similar regardless of ejection fraction (see **Figure 2.13**).

Diagnostic difficulties

Abnormal diastolic function estimated from echocardiography is extremely common in patients with left ventricular systolic dysfunction. Very grossly abnormal diastolic function in the absence of systolic dysfunction is much less common, and most patients diagnosed as having HeFNEF have much less marked abnormalities of diastolic function. A difficulty then arises as the changes of diastolic dysfunction are in many cases indistinguishable from the effects of ageing in which there is selective impairment of the longitudinal component of systolic contraction and consequent reduction in mitral annular velocities,[127] as compared with preservation of normal global indices of left ventricular systolic function.[128,129]

The final position might then seem to be that what distinguishes a patient with diastolic heart failure from an older person without heart failure is simply the presence of symptoms of breathlessness—in both, similar changes in the diastolic properties of the heart have happened.

An obvious problem with such an approach is that there is a long list of potential causes of breathlessness. This has led some to suggest that in many patients with supposed HeFNEF there may be another cause for breathlessness; for example, Caruana and colleagues suggest that more than 95% of such patients had an alternative explanation for symptoms of breathlessness.[130]

One cause of breathlessness in the elderly that is often overlooked is that of muscle wasting and lack of skeletal muscle fitness. Exercise capacity and breathlessness is strongly related to skeletal muscle bulk, and loss of bulk and muscle quality is extremely common with age (see review[131]). The relation between muscle bulk and quality,

and exercise capacity is a recurrent theme in studies of patients with chronic heart failure due to left ventricular systolic dysfunction,[132,133] but the issue is less well studied in patients with HeFNEF.

A further point to consider is that the definition of a 'normal' ejection fraction has largely arisen from the criteria used to define patients for inclusion into trials of *systolic* heart failure. The lower end of the normal range, conventionally taken as 45% or 50% when measured by echo, is almost certainly too low and does not consider change in ejection fraction: breathless patients whose ejection fraction has fallen from 75% to 50% may be labelled as having 'HeFNEF' when their systolic function is clearly markedly impaired compared with their normal (and is thus not 'preserved'). The solution might be to say that the lower end of the normal range should be 55%,[134] but such a definition immediately presents a new problem: perhaps as many as a quarter of apparently normal people might be labelled as having impaired left ventricular systolic function.[135]

It may be, too, that patients with 'diastolic heart failure' have more subtle abnormalities of systolic function than can simply be accounted for by measuring left ventricular ejection fraction. Many patients have abnormal long-axis systolic function with normal left ventricular ejection fraction,[136,137] and a key study of patients as they develop symptoms (that is, during exercise) demonstrates that most patients with HeFNEF have widespread abnormalities of both systolic and diastolic function that become much more obvious on exercise.[138]

Lessons from clinical trials

Clinical trials on the effectiveness of treatment for heart failure due to diastolic dysfunction have now been conducted. None has shown benefit for a specific treatment, but the data accumulated do shed some light on the problem. The trials have had different definitions of the heart failure syndrome, and invariably the more rigorous the definition of heart failure, the more difficult it was to recruit patients to the trial.

No clinical trial to date has convincingly shown benefit using any of the agents proven to be beneficial among patients with heart failure and reduced ejection fraction.[139–144]

Other points to note are that, where values are given, the N-terminal pro B-type natriuretic peptide (NT-proBNP) was not high, and, indeed, many of the patients had results in the normal range.[145] Where the data are given, the proportion of patients being treated with a loop diuretic is low for a population with chronic heart failure. Event rates were also low: in PEP-CHF,[146] for example, the sample size calculation was based on data suggesting that older patients with heart failure and a recent hospital admission had an annual mortality of 10–20%, a readmission rate for heart failure of 30%, and a risk of death or readmission of about 50%; but in the trial, only around 25% reached a primary end-point.

There is a strong relation between left ventricular ejection fraction and survival.[147,148] A similar finding was seen in a study of more than 200 000 patients having echocardiograms for a variety of clinical reasons, with the lowest risk of all-cause mortality seen at an ejection fraction of 60–65%.[149] The finding simply does not sit happily with the suggestion that the outcome for patients with chronic heart failure is the same regardless of left ventricular systolic function. A possible explanation is that there may be two groups of patients: those with 'systolic heart failure' in whom an increasing ejection fraction is beneficial; and a second, pathophysiologically

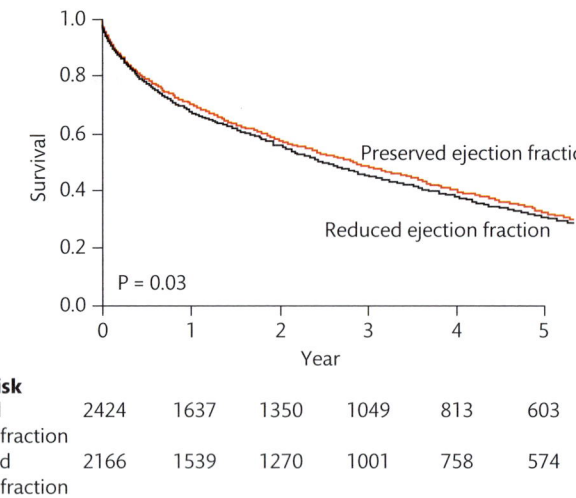

No. at risk

Reduced ejection fraction	2424	1637	1350	1049	813	603
Preserved ejection fraction	2166	1539	1270	1001	758	574

Figure 2.14 The prognosis of patients with heart failure appears to be similar regardless of whether left ventricular ejection fraction is reduced.
Reproduced from Owan TE, Hodge DO, Herges RM, Jacobsen SJ, Roger VL, Redfield MM. Trends in prevalence and outcome of heart failure with preserved ejection fraction. *N Engl J Med* 2006;**355**:251–9.

distinct, group with 'diastolic heart failure' in whom ejection fraction is irrelevant. Such a division does not seem very likely.

Unresolved issues

Do patients with 'diastolic heart failure' have heart disease at all?

Underlying many discussions of heart failure is the position that whereas many patients have symptoms of breathlessness and fatigue, there is no certainty that the symptoms come from the heart. The approach of comparing indices of diastolic function between elderly breathless women and young healthy men is not satisfactory: and where an appropriate comparator population is used, there is often no echocardiographic difference between patients and normal subjects.

Many of the patients included in clinical trials and epidemiological studies almost certainly did not have heart failure. That is not to say that they did not have symptoms of breathlessness, and nor is it to say that they did not have a poor prognosis: indeed, we may just be seeing that the presence of breathlessness is a poor prognostic feature in the elderly regardless of the underlying cause.

If they do have heart disease, is it 'heart failure'?

Even if an individual with symptoms of heart failure can definitely be labelled as having some cardiac pathology as the cause, the old mantra that heart failure is a syndrome, not a diagnosis, remains vitally important. It can be very easy to diagnose HeFNEF in someone presenting, say, with acute pulmonary oedema, and to assume that this represents a definitive statement. Such an approach will lead to patients with underlying acute ischaemia, mitral regurgitation, paroxysmal arrhythmia, or hypertension being mismanaged.

In practice, before a final diagnosis of HeNEF is reached, these alternatives must be treated as appropriate or excluded.

If they do have heart failure, is it 'diastolic'?

Some patients do have heart failure with a normal ejection fraction, but the distinction between 'diastolic' and 'systolic' heart failure

based on the single variable, left ventricular ejection, is to oversimplify the complex relations between all parts of the cardiac cycle. Detailed research into myocardial contraction has repeatedly demonstrated that most patients with diastolic heart failure have systolic abnormalities as well.

'HeFMREF'

In the latest iteration of its guidelines on heart failure, the European Society of Cardiology has introduced the concept of 'heart failure with mid-range ejection fraction' (HeFMREF).[150] The formulation does highlight the problem that there will be some patients with symptoms of heart failure who have neither clear-cut evidence of a reduced ejection fraction nor a clearly normal ejection fraction.

Around 15–20% of patients with heart failure have a mid-range ejection fraction. Perhaps not surprisingly, the clinical features of patients with HeFMREF are intermediate between those with HeFPEF and those with HeFREF:[151,152] patients with HeFMREF are older and more likely to be female (and to have a greater burden of co-morbidities) than patients with HeFREF, but they have a similar prevalence of ischaemic heart disease.[153,154] The causes of death (and potentially responses to medical therapy) among patients with HeFMREF are similar to those of patients with HeFREF.[153,154] The patients thus seem to be epidemiologically closer to HeFNEF, but behave as HeFREF.

It is not at all clear that HeFMREF is a useful descriptor. One problem is the high degree of variability in the measurement of ejection fraction by echocardiography, both inter- and intra-observer. A patient might have HeFMREF one day and HeFREF the next—or perhaps HeFPEF. Neither is it clear the extent to which ejection fraction is constant: medical therapy (and cardiac resynchronization therapy especially[154]) for HeFREF causes left ventricular ejection fraction to increase:[156] whether patients with HeFMREF are transitioning between HeFREF and HeFPEF (or vice versa) is another possibility.[157]

Conclusions

It is often said that heart failure is not a diagnosis in itself, but a syndrome.[158] Heart failure is, in fact, a suite of related syndromes and it is important to be certain what is being discussed in each circumstance. Our understanding of acute heart failure, in particular, is fogged by imprecision in the characterization of patients being recruited to clinical trials, because acute heart failure is imperfectly defined. Heart failure with normal ejection fraction continues to be an ill-defined entity, and, at least partly in consequence, is a syndrome for which there is no effective treatment. The beginning of wisdom is the definition of terms.[159]

REFERENCES

1. Cowie MR, Wood DA, Coats AJ, *et al*. Incidence and aetiology of heart failure; a population-based study. *Eur Heart J* 1999;**20**:421–8.
2. Nieminen MS, Böhm M, Cowie MR, *et al*.; ESC Committe for Practice Guideline (CPG). Executive summary of the guidelines on the diagnosis and treatment of acute heart failure: the

Task Force on Acute Heart Failure of the European Society of Cardiology. *Eur Heart J* 2005;**26**:384–416.

3. Borges JL. John Wilkins' analytical language. In Weinberger E, *et al.*, ed. and trans., *The total library: non-fiction 1922–86*. Penguin Books, London, 2001, pp. 229–232.

4. Shoaib A, Waleed M, Khan S, *et al.* Breathlessness at rest is not the dominant presentation of patients admitted with heart failure. *Eur J Heart Fail* 2014;**16**:1283–91.

5. Ghali JK, Kadakia S, Cooper R, Ferlinz J. Precipitating factors leading to decompensation of heart failure. Traits among urban blacks. *Arch Intern Med* 1988;**148**:2013–6.

6. Michalsen A, König G, Thimme W. Preventable causative factors leading to hospital admission with decompensated heart failure. *Heart* 1998;**80**:437–41.

7. Fonarow GC, Abraham WT, Albert NM, *et al.*; OPTIMIZE-HF Investigators and Hospitals. Factors identified as precipitating hospital admissions for heart failure and clinical outcomes: findings from OPTIMIZE-HF. *Arch Intern Med* 2008;**168**:847–54.

8. Setoguchi S, Stevenson LW, Schneeweiss S. Repeated hospitalizations predict mortality in the community population with heart failure. *Am Heart J* 2007;**154**:260–6.

9. Solomon SD, Dobson J, Pocock S, *et al.*; Candesartan in Heart failure: Assessment of Reduction in Mortality and morbidity (CHARM) Investigators. Influence of nonfatal hospitalization for heart failure on subsequent mortality in patients with chronic heart failure. *Circulation* 2007;**116**:1482–7.

10. Braga JR, Tu JV, Austin PC, *et al.* Recurrent events analysis for examination of hospitalizations in heart failure: insights from the enhanced feedback for effective cardiac treatment (EFFECT) Trial. *Eur Heart J Qual Care Clin Outcomes* 2018;**4**:18–26.

11. Guyton AC, Lindsey AW. Effect of elevated left atrial pressure and decreased plasma protein concentration on the development of pulmonary edema. *Circ Res* 1959;**7**:649–57.

12. MacIver DH, Clark AL. The vital role of the right ventricle in the pathogenesis of acute pulmonary edema. *Am J Cardiol* 2015;**115**:992–1000.

13. Figueras J, Weil MH. Blood volume prior to and following treatment of acute cardiogenic pulmonary edema. *Circulation* 1978;**57**:349–55.

14. Pickering TG, Herman L, Devereux RB, *et al.* Recurrent pulmonary oedema in hypertension due to bilateral renal artery stenosis: treatment by angioplasty or surgical revascularisation. *Lancet* 1988;**2**:551–2.

15. Weiler-Ravell D, Shupak A, Goldenberg I, *et al.* Pulmonary oedema and haemoptysis induced by strenuous swimming. *Br Med J* 1995;**311**:361–2.

16. Cochard G1, Arvieux J, Lacour JM, *et al.* Pulmonary edema in scuba divers: recurrence and fatal outcome. *Undersea Hyperb Med* 2005;**32**:39–44.

17. Casey H, Dastidar AG, MacIver D. Swimming-induced pulmonary oedema in two triathletes: a novel pathophysiological explanation. *J R Soc Med* 2014;**107**:450–2.

18. Castagna O, Gempp E, Poyet R, *et al.* Cardiovascular mechanisms of extravascular lung water accumulation in divers. *Am J Cardiol* 2017;**119**:929–32.

19. Yoon JS, Suh JH, Choi SY, *et al.* Risk factors for the development of reexpansion pulmonary edema in patients with spontaneous pneumothorax. *J Cardiothorac Surg* 2013;**8**:164.

20. Killip T 3rd, Kimball JT. Treatment of myocardial infarction in a coronary care unit. A two year experience with 250 patients. *Am J Cardiol* 1967;**20**:457–64.

21. Nohria A, Tsang SW, Fang JC, *et al.* Clinical assessment identifies hemodynamic profiles that predict outcomes in patients admitted with heart failure. *J Am Coll Cardiol* 2003;**41**:1797–804.

22. Zannad F, Mebazaa A, Juillière Y, *et al.*; EFICA Investigators. Clinical profile, contemporary management and one-year mortality in patients with severe acute heart failure syndromes: The EFICA study. *Eur J Heart Fail* 2006;**8**:697–705.

23. Anand IS, Ferrari R, Kalra GS, *et al.* Edema of cardiac origin. Studies of body water and sodium, renal function, hemodynamic indexes, and plasma hormones in untreated congestive cardiac failure. *Circulation* 1989;**80**:299–305.

24. McDonald CD, Burch GE, Walsh JJ. Prolonged bed rest in the treatment of idiopathic cardiomyopathy. *Am J Med* 1972;**52**:41–50.

25. Shoaib A, Mamas MA, Ahmad QS, *et al.* Characteristics and outcome of acute heart failure patients according to the severity of peripheral oedema. *Int J Cardiol* 2019;**285**:40–6.

26. Pellicori P, Kallvikbacka-Bennett A, Dierckx R, *et al.* Prognostic significance of ultrasound-assessed jugular vein distensibility in heart failure. *Heart* 2015;**101**:1149–58.

27. Pellicori P, Clark AL, Kallvikbacka-Bennett A, *et al.* Non-invasive measurement of right atrial pressure by near-infrared spectroscopy: preliminary experience. A report from the SICA-HF study. *Eur J Heart Fail* 2017;**19**:883–92.

28. Pellicori P, Shah P, Cuthbert J, *et al.* Prevalence, pattern and clinical relevance of ultrasound indices of congestion in outpatients with heart failure. *Eur J Heart Fail* 2019;**21**:904–16.

29. Pellicori P, Cleland JG, Zhang J, Kallvikbacka-Bennett A, Urbinati A, Shah P, Kazmi S, Clark AL. Cardiac dysfunction, congestion and loop diuretics: their relationship to prognosis in heart failure. *Cardiovasc Drugs Ther* 2016;**30**:599–609

30. Criteria Committee of the New York Heart Association. *Nomenclature and criteria for diagnosis*, 9th edn. Little, Brown, Boston, 1994.

31. Goode KM, Nabb S, Cleland JG, Clark AL. A comparison of patient and physician-rated New York Heart Association class in a community-based heart failure clinic. *J Card Fail* 2008;**14**:379–87

32. Rector TS, Francis GS, Cohn JN. Patients' self-assessment of their congestive heart failure. Part 1. Patient perceived dysfunction and its poor correlation with exercise tests. *Heart Fail* 1987;Oct/Nov:192–6.

33. Rector TS, Francis GS, Cohn JN. Patients' self-assessment of their congestive heart failure. Part 2: content, reliability and validity of a new measure, the Minnesota Living with Heart Failure questionnaire. *Heart Fail* 1987;Oct/Nov:196–209.

34. Green CP, Porter CB, Bresnahan DR, Spertus JA. Development and evaluation of the Kansas City Cardiomyopathy Questionnaire: a new health status measure for heart failure. *J Am Coll Cardiol* 2000;**35**:1245–55.

35. Olsson LG, Swedberg K, Clark AL, Witte KK, Cleland JG. Six minute corridor walk test as an outcome measure for the assessment of treatment in randomized, blinded intervention trials of chronic heart failure: a systematic review. *Eur Heart J* 2005;**26**:778–93.

36. Ingle L, Rigby AS, Carroll S, *et al.* Prognostic value of the 6 min walk test and self-perceived symptom severity in older patients with chronic heart failure. *Eur Heart J* 2007;**28**:560–8

37. Harrington D, Anker SD, Coats AJ. Preservation of exercise capacity and lack of peripheral changes in asymptomatic patients with severely impaired left ventricular function. *Eur Heart J* 2001;**22**:392–9.

38. Marzo KP, Wilson JR, Mancini DM. Effects of cardiac transplantation on ventilatory response to exercise. *Am J Cardiol* 1992;**69**:547–53.

39. Lipkin DP, Canepa-Anson R, Stephens MR, Poole-Wilson PA. Factors determining symptoms in heart failure: comparison of fast and slow exercise tests. *Br Heart J* 1986;**55**:439–45.

40. Fink LI, Wilson JR, Ferraro N. Exercise ventilation and pulmonary artery wedge pressure in chronic stable congestive heart failure. *Am J Cardiol* 1986;**57**:249–53.

41. Witte KKA, Clark AL. Cycle exercise causes a lower ventilatory response to exercise in chronic heart failure. *Heart* 2005;**91**:225–6.

42. Clark AL, Swan JW, Laney R, *et al*. The role of right and left ventricular function in the ventilatory response to exercise in chronic heart failure. *Circulation* 1994;**89**:2062–9.

43. Puri S, Baker BL, Dutka DP, *et al*. Reduced alveolar–capillary membrane diffusing capacity in chronic heart failure. *Circulation* 1995;**91**:2769–74.

44. Kraemer MD, Kubo SH, Rector TS, Brunsvold N, Bank AJ. Pulmonary and peripheral vascular factors are important determinants of peak exercise oxygen uptake in patients with heart failure. *J Am Coll Cardiol* 1993;**21**:641–8.

45. Wright RS, Levine MS, Bellamy PE, *et al*. Ventilatory and diffusion abnormalities in potential heart transplant recipients. *Chest* 1990;**98**:816–20.

46. Clark AL, Coats AJS. Usefulness of arterial blood gas estimations during exercise in patients with chronic heart failure. *Br Heart J* 1994;**71**:528–30.

47. Sullivan MJ, Green HJ, Cobb FR. Skeletal muscle biochemistry and histology in ambulatory patients with long-term heart failure. *Circulation* 1990;**81**:518–27.

48. Lipkin DP, Jones DA, Round JM, Poole-Wilson PA. Abnormalities of skeletal muscle in patients with chronic heart failure. *Int J Cardiol* 1988;**18**:187–95.

49. Massie BM, Conway M, Yonge R, *et al*. Skeletal muscle metabolism in patients with congestive heart failure: relation to clinical severity and blood flow. *Circulation* 1987;**76**:1009–19.

50. Buller NP, Jones D, Poole-Wilson PA. Direct measurements of skeletal muscle fatigue in patients with chronic heart failure. *Br Heart J* 1991;**65**:20–4.

51. Volterrani M, Clark AL, Ludman PF, *et al*. Determinants of exercise capacity in chronic heart failure. *Eur Heart J* 1994;**15**:801–9.

52. Clark AL, Piepoli M, Coats AJS. Skeletal muscle and the control of ventilation on exercise; evidence for metabolic receptors. *Eur J Clin Invest* 1995;**25**:299–305.

53. Piepoli M, Clark AL, Volterrani M, *et al*. Contribution of muscle afferents to the hemodynamic, autonomic, and ventilatory responses to exercise in patients with chronic heart failure: effects of physical training. *Circulation* 1996;**93**:940–52.

54. Ellenbogen KA, Mohanty PK, Szentpetery S, Thames MD. Arterial baroreflex abnormalities in heart failure: reversal after orthotopic cardiac transplantation. *Circulation* 1989;**79**:51–8.

55. Ponikowski P, Chua TP, Piepoli M, *et al*. Augmented peripheral chemosensitivity as a potential input to baroreflex impairment and autonomic imbalance in chronic heart failure. *Circulation* 1997;**96**:2586–94.

56. Clark AL, Cleland JGF. The control of adrenergic function in heart failure: therapeutic interventions. *Heart Fail Rev* 2000;**5**:101–14.

57. Cleland JG, Clark AL. Delivering the cumulative benefits of triple therapy to improve outcomes in heart failure: too many cooks will spoil the broth. *J Am Coll Cardiol* 2003;**42**:1234–7.

58. Anker SD, Negassa A, Coats AJ, *et al*. Prognostic importance of weight loss in chronic heart failure and the effect of treatment with angiotensin-converting-enzyme inhibitors: an observational study. *Lancet* 2003;**361**:1077–83.

59. Mancini DM, Walter G, Reichnek N, *et al*. Contribution of skeletal muscle atrophy to exercise intolerance and altered muscle metabolism in heart failure. *Circulation* 1992;**85**:1364–73.

60. Anker SD, Clark AL, Teixeira MM, Hellewell PG, Coats AJS. Loss of bone mineral in patients with cachexia due to chronic heart failure. *Am J Cardiol* 1999;**83**:612–15.

61. Shane E, Mancini D, Aaronson K, *et al*. Bone mass, vitamin D deficiency, and hypoparathyroidism in congestive heart failure. *Am J Med* 1997;**103**:197–207.

62. Riley M, Elborn JS, McKane WR, *et al*. Resting energy expenditure in chronic cardiac failure. *Clin Sci* 1991;**80**:633–9.

63. Poehlman ET, Scheffers J, Gottlieb SS, Fisher ML, Vaitekevicius P. Increased metabolic rate in patients with congestive heart failure. *Ann Intern Med* 1994;**121**:860–2.

64. Witte KK, Ford SJ, Preston T, Parker JD, Clark AL. Fibrinogen synthesis is increased in cachectic patients with chronic heart failure. *Int J Cardiol* 2008;**129**:363–7.

65. Staten MA, Matthews DE, Cryer PE, Bier DM. Physiological increments in epinephrine stimulate metabolic rate in humans. *Am J Physiol* 1987;**253**:E322–E330.

66. Simonsen L, Bulow J, Madsen J, Christensen, NJ. Thermogenic response to epinephrine in the forearm and abdominal subcutaneous adipose tissue. *Am J Physiol* 1992;**263**:E850–E855.

67. Lafontan M, Berlan M. Fat cell adrenergic receptors and the control of white and brown fat cell function. *J Lipid Res* 1993;**34**:1057–91.

68. Brink M, Wellen J, Delafontaine P. Angiotensin II causes weight loss and decreases circulating insulin- like growth factor I in rats through a pressor-independent mechanism. *J Clin Invest* 1996;**97**:2509–16.

69. Brink M, Price SR, Chrast J, *et al*. Angiotensin II induces skeletal muscle wasting through enhanced protein degradation and down-regulates autocrine insulin-like growth factor I. *Endocrinology* 2001;**142**:1489–96.

70. Bessey PQ, Watters JM, Aoki TT, Wilmore DW. Combined hormonal infusion simulates the metabolic response to injury. *Ann Surg* 1984;**200**:264–81.

71. Watters JM, Bessey PQ, Dinarello CA, Wolff SM, Wilmore DW. Both inflammatory and endocrine mediators stimulate host responses to sepsis. *Arch Surg* 1986;**121**:179–90.

72. Swan JW, Anker SD, Walton C, *et al*. Insulin resistance in chronic heart failure: relation to severity and aetiology of heart failure. *J Am Coll Cardiol* 1997:**30**:527–32.

73. Niebauer J, Pflaum C-D, Clark AL, *et al*. Deficient insulin-like growth factor-I in chronic heart failure predicts altered body composition, anabolic deficiency, cytokine and neurohormonal activation. *J Am Coll Cardiol* 1998;**32**:393–7.

74. Anker SD, Chua TP, Ponikowski P, *et al*. Hormonal changes and catabolic/anabolic imbalance in chronic heart failure and their importance for cardiac cachexia. *Circulation* 1997;**96**:526–34.

75. McMurray J, Abdullah I, Dargie HJ, Shapiro D. Increased concentrations of tumour necrosis factor in 'cachectic' patients with severe chronic heart failure. *Br Heart J* 1991;**66**:356–8.

76. Anker SD, Clark AL, Kemp M, *et al*. Tumour necrosis factor and steroid metabolism in chronic heart failure: possible relation to muscle wasting. *J Am Coll Cardiol* 1997;**30**:997–1001.

77. Anker SD, Ponikowski PP, Clark AL, *et al*. Cytokines and neurohormones relating to body composition alterations in

the wasting syndrome of chronic heart failure. *Eur Heart J* 1999;**20**:683–93.

78. Sandek A, Bauditz J, Swidsinski A, *et al*. Altered intestinal function in patients with chronic heart failure. *J Am Coll Cardiol* 2007;**50**:1561–9.

79. Niebauer J, Volk HD, Kemp M, *et al*. Endotoxin and immune activation in chronic heart failure: a prospective cohort study. *Lancet* 1999;**353**:1838–42.

80. Rauchhaus M, Clark AL, Doehner W, *et al*. The relationship between cholesterol and survival in patients with chronic heart failure. *J Am Coll Cardiol* 2003;**42**:1933–40.

81. Rauchhaus M, Coats AJ, Anker SD. The endotoxin–lipoprotein hypothesis. *Lancet* 2000;**356**:930–3.

82. Carr JG, Stevenson LW, Walden JA, Heber D. Prevalence and haemodynamic correlates of malnutrition in severe congestive heart failure secondary to ischaemic or idiopathic dilated cardiomyopathy. *Am J Cardiol* 1989;**63**:709–13.

83. Broqvist M, Arnqvist H, Dahlstrom U, *et al*. Nutritional assessment and muscle energy metabolism in severe chronic congestive heart failure-effects of long-term dietary supplementation. *Eur Heart J* 1994;**15**:1641–50.

84. King D, Smith ML, Chapman TJ, Stockdale HR, Lye M. Fat malabsorption in elderly patients with cardiac cachexia. *Age Ageing* 1996;**25**:144–9.

85. Bates CJ, Prentice A, Cole TJ, *et al*. Micronutrients: highlights and research challenges from the 1994–5 National Diet and Nutrition Survey of people aged 65 years and over. *Br J Nutr* 1999;**82**:7–15.

86. Sze S, Zhang J, Pellicori P, *et al*. Prognostic value of simple frailty and malnutrition screening tools in patients with acute heart failure due to left ventricular systolic dysfunction. *Clin Res Cardiol* 2017;**106**:533–41.

87. Witte KK, Nikitin NP, Parker AC, *et al*. The effect of micronutrient supplementation on quality-of-life and left ventricular function in elderly patients with chronic heart failure. *Eur Heart J* 2005;**26**:2238–44.

88. Kalantar-Zadeh K, Anker SD, Horwich TB, Fonarow GC. Nutritional and anti-inflammatory interventions in chronic heart failure. *Am J Cardiol* 2008;**101**(11A):89E–103E.

89. Adigun AQ, Ajayi AA. The effects of enalapril–digoxin–diuretic combination therapy on nutritional and anthropometric indices in chronic congestive heart failure: preliminary findings in cardiac cachexia. *Eur J Heart Fail* 2001;**3**:359–63.

90. Anker SD, Negassa A, Coats AJ, *et al*. Prognostic importance of weight loss in chronic heart failure and the effect of treatment with angiotensin-converting-enzyme inhibitors: an observational study. *Lancet* 2003;**361**:1077–83.

91. Kenchaiah S, Pocock SJ, Wang D, *et al*.; CHARM Investigators. Body mass index and prognosis in patients with chronic heart failure: insights from the Candesartan in Heart failure: Assessment of Reduction in Mortality and morbidity (CHARM) program. *Circulation* 2007;**116**:627–36.

92. Monroe MB, Seals DR, Shapiro LF, *et al*. Direct evidence for tonic sympathetic support for resting metabolic rate in healthy adult humans. *Am J Physiol* 2001;**280**:E740–E744.

93. Rossner S, Taylor CL, Byington RP, Furberg CD. Long term propranolol treatment and changes in body weight after myocardial infarction. *Br Med J* 1990;**300**:902–3.

94. Sharma AM, Pischon T, Hardt S, Kunz I, Luft FC. Hypothesis. Beta-adrenergic receptor blockers and weight gain: a systematic analysis. *Hypertension* 2001;**37**:250–4.

95. Clark AL, Coats AJ, Krum H, *et al*. Effect of beta-adrenergic blockade with carvedilol on cachexia in severe chronic heart failure: results from the COPERNICUS trial. *J Cachexia Sarcopenia Muscle* 2017;**8**:549–56.

96. Hryniewicz K, Androne AS, Hudaihed A, Katz SD. Partial reversal of cachexia by beta-adrenergic receptor blocker therapy in patients with chronic heart failure. *J Card Fail* 2003;**9**:464–8

97. Anker SD, Ponikowski P, Varney S, *et al*. Wasting as independent risk factor for mortality in chronic heart failure. *Lancet* 1997;**349**:1050–3.

98. Davos CH, Doehner W, Rauchhaus M, *et al*. Body mass and survival in patients with chronic heart failure without cachexia: the importance of obesity. *J Card Fail* 2003;**9**:29–35.

99. Horwich TB, Fonarow GC, Hamilton MA, *et al*. The relationship between obesity and mortality in patients with heart failure. *J Am Coll Cardiol* 2001;**38**:789–95.

100. Clark AL, Loebe M, Potapov EV, *et al*. Ventricular assist device in severe heart failure: effects on cytokines, complement and body weight. *Eur Heart J* 2001;**22**:2275–83.

101. Clark AL, Knosalla C, Birks E, *et al*. Heart transplantation in heart failure: the prognostic importance of body mass index at time of surgery and subsequent weight changes. *Eur J Heart Fail* 2007;**9**:839–44.

102. Luu M, Stevenson WG, Stevenson LW, Baron K, Walden J. Diverse mechanisms of unexpected cardiac arrest in advanced heart failure. *Circulation* 1989;**80**:1675–80.

103. Faggiano P, d'Aloia A, Gualeni A, Gardini A, Giordano A. Mechanisms and immediate outcome of in-hospital cardiac arrest in patients with advanced heart failure secondary to ischemic or idiopathic dilated cardiomyopathy. *Am J Cardiol* 2001;**87**:655–7.

104. Narang R, Cleland JG, Erhardt L, *et al*. Mode of death in chronic heart failure. A request and proposition for more accurate classification. *Eur Heart J* 1996;**17**:1390–403.

105. Uretsky BF, Thygesen K, Armstrong PW, *et al*. Acute coronary findings at autopsy in heart failure patients with sudden death: results from the assessment of treatment with lisinopril and survival (ATLAS) trial. *Circulation* 2000;**102**:611–16.

106. Orn S, Cleland JG, Romo M, Kjekshus J, Dickstein K. Recurrent infarction causes the most deaths following myocardial infarction with left ventricular dysfunction. *Am J Med* 2005;**118**:752–8.

107. Pires LA, Lehmann MH, Steinman RT, Baga JJ, Schuger CD. Sudden death in implantable cardioverter–defibrillator recipients: clinical context, arrhythmic events and device responses. *J Am Coll Cardiol* 1999;**33**:24–32.

108. Kinch Westerdahl A, Sjöblom J, Mattiasson AC, Rosenqvist M, Frykman V. Implantable cardioverter–defibrillator therapy before death: high risk for painful shocks at end of life. *Circulation* 2014;**129**:422–9.

109. Nikolaidou T, Johnson MJ, Ghosh JM, *et al*. Postmortem ICD interrogation in mode of death classification. *J Cardiovasc Electrophysiol* 2018;**29**:573–83.

110. Shen L, Jhund PS, Petrie MC, *et al*. Declining risk of sudden death in heart failure. *N Engl J Med* 2017;**377**:41–51.

111. Zile MR, Brutsaert DL. New concepts in diastolic dysfunction and diastolic heart failure: part I: diagnosis, prognosis, and measurements of diastolic function. *Circulation* 2002;**105**:1387–93.

112. Owan TE, Hodge DO, Herges RM, *et al*. Trends in prevalence and outcome of heart failure with preserved ejection fraction. *N Engl J Med* 2006;**355**:251–9.

113. Bhatia RS, Tu JV, Lee DS, *et al*. Outcome of heart failure with preserved ejection fraction in a population-based study. *N Engl J Med* 2006;**355**:260–9.

114. Burkhoff D, Maurer MS, Packer M. Heart failure with a normal ejection fraction: is it really a disorder of diastolic function? *Circulation* 2003;**107**:656–8.

115. Maurer MS, King DL, El-Khoury Rumbarger L, Packer M, Burkhoff D. Left heart failure with a normal ejection fraction: identification of different pathophysiologic mechanisms. *J Card Fail* 2005;**11**:177–87.

116. Brutsaert DL, De Keulenaer GW. Diastolic heart failure: a myth. *Curr Opin Cardiol* 2006;**21**:240–8.

117. Liu CP, Ting CT, Lawrence W, *et al*. Diminished contractile response to increased heart rate in intact human left ventricular hypertrophy: systolic versus diastolic determinants. *Circulation* 1993;**88**:1893–1906

118. Kawaguchi M, Hay I, Fetics B, Kass DA. Combined ventricular and arterial stiffening in patients with heart failure and preserved ejection fraction: implications for systolic and diastolic reserve limitations. *Circulation* 2003;**107**:714–20.

119. Stoddard MF, Pearson AC, Kern MJ, *et al*. Influence of alteration in preload on the pattern of left ventricular diastolic filling as assessed by Doppler echocardiography in humans. *Circulation* 1989;**79**:1226–36.

120. Nagueh SF, Mikati I, Kopelen HA, *et al*. Doppler estimation of left ventricular filling pressure in sinus tachycardia. A new application of tissue Doppler imaging. *Circulation* 1998;**98**:1644–50.

121. Hogg K, Swedberg K, McMurray J. Heart failure with preserved left ventricular systolic function: epidemiology, clinical characteristics, and prognosis. *J Am Coll Cardiol* 2004;**43**:317–27.

122. Yip GWK, Ho PPY, Woo KS, Sanderson JE. Comparison of frequencies of left ventricular systolic and diastolic heart failure in Chinese living in Hong Kong. *Am J Cardiol* 1999;**84**:563–7.

123. Hogg K, Swedberg K, McMurray J. Heart failure with preserved left ventricular systolic function; epidemiology, clinical characteristics, and prognosis. *J Am Coll Cardiol* 2004;**43**:317–27.

124. Owan T, Redfield M. Epidemiology of diastolic heart failure. *Prog Cardiovasc Dis* 2005;**47**:320–32.

125. Banerjee P, Clark AL, Nikitin N, Cleland JG. Diastolic heart failure. Paroxysmal or chronic? *Eur J Heart Fail* 2004;**6**:427–31.

126. Philbin EF, Rocco TA Jr, Lindenmuth NW, Ulrich K, Jenkins PL. Systolic versus diastolic heart failure in community practice: clinical features, outcomes, and the use of angiotensin-converting enzyme inhibitors. *Am J Med* 2000;**109**:605–13.

127. Nikitin NP, Witte KK, Ingle L, *et al*. Longitudinal myocardial dysfunction in healthy older subjects as a manifestation of cardiac ageing. *Age Ageing* 2005;**34**:343–9.

128. Klein AL, Leung DY, Murray RD, *et al*. Effects of age and physiologic variables on right ventricular filling dynamics in normal subjects. *Am J Cardiol* 1999;**84**:440–8.

129. Pfisterer ME, Battler A, Zaret BL. Range of normal values for left and right ventricular ejection fraction at rest and during exercise assessed by radionuclide angiocardiography. *Eur Heart J* 1985;**6**:647–55.

130. Caruana L, Petrie MC, Davie AP, McMurray JJ. Do patients with suspected heart failure and preserved left ventricular systolic function suffer from 'diastolic heart failure' or from misdiagnosis? A prospective descriptive study. *Br Med J* 2000;**321**:215–18.

131. Thompson LV. Age-related muscle dysfunction. *Exp Gerontol* 2009;**44**:106–11.

132. Anker SD, Swan JW, Volterrani M, *et al*. The influence of muscle mass, strength, fatigability and blood flow on exercise capacity in cachectic and non-cachectic patients with chronic heart failure. *Eur Heart J* 1997;**18**:259–69.

133. Harrington D, Clark AL, Chua TP, *et al*. Effect of reduced muscle bulk on the ventilatory response to exercise in chronic congestive heart failure secondary to idiopathic dilated and ischemic cardiomyopathy. *Am J Cardiol* 1997;**80**:90–3.

134. Lang RM, Bierig M, Devereux RB, *et al*.; Chamber Quantification Writing Group; American Society of Echocardiography's Guidelines and Standards Committee; European Association of Echocardiography. Recommendations for chamber quantification: a report from the American Society of Echocardiography's Guidelines and Standards Committee and the Chamber Quantification Writing Group, developed in conjunction with the European Association of Echocardiography, a branch of the European Society of Cardiology. *J Am Soc Echocardiogr* 2005;**18**:1440–63.

135. Mahadevan G, Davis RC, Frenneaux MP, *et al*. Left ventricular ejection fraction: are the revised cut-off points for defining systolic dysfunction sufficiently evidence based? *Heart* 2008;**94**:426–8.

136. Nikitin NP, Witte KK, Clark AL, Cleland JG. Color tissue Doppler-derived long-axis left ventricular function in heart failure with preserved global systolic function. *Am J Cardiol* 2002;**90**:1174–7.

137. Petrie MC, Caruana L, Berry C, McMurray JJ. 'Diastolic heart failure' or heart failure caused by subtle left ventricular systolic dysfunction? *Heart* 2002;**87**:29–31.

138. Tan YT, Wenzelburger F, Lee E, *et al*. The pathophysiology of heart failure with normal ejection fraction: exercise echocardiography reveals complex abnormalities of both systolic and diastolic ventricular function involving torsion, untwist, and longitudinal motion. *J Am Coll Cardiol* 2009;**54**:36–46.

139. Ahmed A, Rich MW, Fleg JL, *et al*. Effects of digoxin on morbidity and mortality in diastolic heart failure: the ancillary digitalis investigation group trial. *Circulation* 2006;**114**:397–403.

140. Yusuf S, Pfeffer MA, Swedberg K, *et al*.; CHARM Investigators and Committees. Effects of candesartan in patients with chronic heart failure and preserved left-ventricular ejection fraction: the CHARM-Preserved Trial. *Lancet* 2003;**362**:777–81.

141. Massie BM, Carson PE, McMurray JJ, *et al*.; I-PRESERVE Investigators. Irbesartan in patients with heart failure and preserved ejection fraction. *N Engl J Med* 2008;**359**:2456–67.

142. Cleland JG, Tendera M, Adamus J, *et al*.; PEP-CHF Investigators. The perindopril in elderly people with chronic heart failure (PEP-CHF) study. *Eur Heart J* 2006;**27**:2338–45.

143. Pitt B, Pfeffer MA, Assmann SF, *et al*.; TOPCAT Investigators. Spironolactone for heart failure with preserved ejection fraction. *N Engl J Med* 2014;**370**:1383–92.

144. Solomon SD, McMurray JJV, Anand IS, *et al*.; PARAGON-HF Investigators and Committees. Angiotensin–neprilysin inhibition in heart failure with preserved ejection fraction. *N Engl J Med* 2019;**381**:1609–20.

145. Raymond I, Groenning BA, Hildebrandt PR, *et al*. The influence of age, sex and other variables on the plasma level of N-terminal pro brain natriuretic peptide in a large sample of the general population. *Heart* 2003;**89**:745–51.

146. Cleland JG, Tendera M, Adamus J, *et al.* Perindopril for elderly people with chronic heart failure: the PEP-CHF study. The PEP investigators. *Eur J Heart Fail* 1999;**1**:211–17.

147. Curtis JP, Sokol SI, Wang Y, *et al.* The association of left ventricular ejection fraction, mortality, and cause of death in stable outpatients with heart failure. *J Am Coll Cardiol* 2003;**42**:736–42.

148. Pocock SJ, Wang D, Pfeffer MA, *et al.* Predictors of mortality and morbidity in patients with chronic heart failure. *Eur Heart J* 2006;**27**:65–75.

149. Wehner GJ, Jing L, Haggerty CM, *et al.* Routinely reported ejection fraction and mortality in clinical practice: where does the nadir of risk lie? *Eur Heart J* 2020;**41**:1249–57.

150. Ponikowski P, Voors AA, Anker SD, *et al.*; Authors/Task Force Members. 2016 ESC Guidelines for the diagnosis and treatment of acute and chronic heart failure: The Task Force for the diagnosis and treatment of acute and chronic heart failure of the European Society of Cardiology (ESC) developed with the special contribution of the Heart Failure Association (HFA) of the ESC. *Eur Heart J* 2016;**37**:2129–200.

151. Pascual-Figal DA, Ferrero-Gregori A, Gomez-Otero I, *et al.*; MUSIC and REDINSCOR I research groups. Mid-range left ventricular ejection fraction: clinical profile and cause of death in ambulatory patients with chronic heart failure. *Int J Cardiol* 2017;**240**:265–70.

152. Chioncel O, Lainscak M, Seferovic PM, *et al.* Epidemiology and one-year outcomes in patients with chronic heart failure and preserved, mid-range and reduced ejection fraction: an analysis of the ESC Heart Failure Long-Term Registry. *Eur J Heart Fail* 2017;**19**:1574–85.

153. Kapoor JR, Kapoor R, Ju C, *et al.* Precipitating clinical factors, heart failure characterization, and outcomes in patients hospitalized with heart failure with reduced, borderline, and preserved ejection fraction. *J Am Coll Cardiol* 2016;**4**:464–72.

154. Rickenbacher P, Kaufmann BA, Maeder MT, *et al.*; TIME-CHF Investigators. Heart failure with mid-range ejection fraction: a distinct clinical entity? Insights from the Trial of Intensified versus standard Medical therapy in Elderly patients with Congestive Heart Failure (TIME-CHF). *Eur J Heart Fail* 2017;**19**:1586–96.

155. Hsu JC, Solomon SD, Bourgoun M, *et al.*; MADIT-CRT Executive Committee. Predictors of super-response to cardiac resynchronization therapy and associated improvement in clinical outcome: the MADIT-CRT (multicenter automatic defibrillator implantation trial with cardiac resynchronization therapy) study. *J Am Coll Cardiol* 2012;**59**:2366–73.

156. Kalogeropoulos AP, Fonarow GC, Georgiopoulou V, *et al.* Characteristics and outcomes of adult outpatients with heart failure and improved or recovered ejection fraction. *JAMA Cardiol* 2016;**1**:510–18.

157. Ueda T, Kawakami R, Nishida T, *et al.* Left ventricular ejection fraction (EF) of 55% as cutoff for late transition from heart failure (HF) with preserved EF to HF with mildly reduced EF. *Circ J* 2015;**79**:2209–15.

158. Patel KC, Leyva F, Frenneaux MP. Heart failure is not a diagnosis. *Int J Clin Pract* 2008;**62**:526–8.

159. Socrates, b.470/469 BC, d.399 BC. Attributed.

SECTION 2
Epidemiology

3

The epidemiology of heart failure

Kaushik Guha and Theresa A. McDonagh

Introduction

When describing the epidemiology of heart failure, it is worth bearing in mind that estimates of incidence and prevalence will vary according to the definition of heart failure used and the type of cohort being studied. This is especially important when assessing work which has objectively measured left ventricular systolic function. Variables such as left ventricular ejection fraction are normally distributed, so the cut-point chosen is a critical determinant of the eventual results.

The first robust epidemiological data in the field came from the seminal publication on the natural history of heart failure from the Framingham Study in 1971 showing a prevalence of heart failure of 0.8% in those aged between 50 and 59 years, rising to 9.1% in those aged >80 years, with incidence rates of 0.2% at age 54 years and 0.4% at age 85 years (see **Figure 3.1**).[1] This was followed by a large European study—'The Men Born in 1913'—which found a similar prevalence of 2.1% in those aged 50 years and 13% at age 67 years; and incidence rates of 0.15% and 1%, respectively, at ages 50 and 67 years.[2] These landmark studies reported on a clinical diagnosis of heart failure, based on symptoms, signs, and scoring systems to identify cases. More modern epidemiological studies have used definitions of heart failure which include objective measures of cardiac function, in keeping with contemporary European and US guidelines for the diagnosis of heart failure. Initial studies focused on systolic dysfunction because they reported at much the same time as the heart failure treatment trials which enrolled patients with systolic heart failure. More recently, attention has turned also to describing the epidemiology of heart failure with preserved systolic function.

Prevalence studies

Community-based studies

Many studies have been conducted in primary care or across geographical health care communities to estimate the prevalence of heart failure in the community. One of the first was conducted in north west London which reviewed 30 204 case records, yielding a crude prevalence of 3.8 per 100 cases in the general population with a marked rise from those aged <65 to those >65 years, where the rate rose from 0.6 to 28.0 per 1000.[3]

More recent data are available from the Scottish Continuous Morbidity scheme, which covers 57 general practices in Scotland with access to GP Read Codes for heart failure in 307 741 patients.[4] The calculated prevalence within the general population in Scotland was 7.1 per 1000, increasing in those aged >85 years to 90.1 per 1000. The population identified by primary care were older and had more co-morbidities than other population-based studies or clinical trial populations. These findings have been corroborated in a European study based in Utrecht, Netherlands. It found that patients with heart failure who were under the supervision of a cardiologist were more likely to be male, younger (in their sixties) and to have an ischaemic aetiology, whereas those looked after in primary care were older and more likely to be female.[5] When considering such data it must be remembered that the signs and symptoms of heart failure are neither sensitive nor specific. Studies comparing referrals from primary care with expert cardiological assessment have revealed that only approximately 30% of patients diagnosed in primary care may actually have heart failure.[6,7]

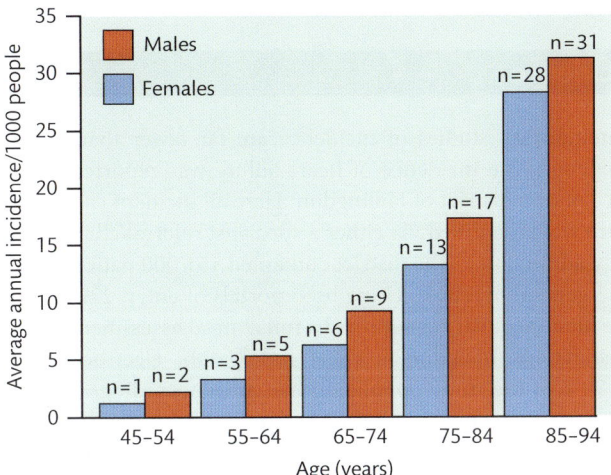

Figure 3.1 Incidence of heart failure within the Framingham cohort.
Source data from McKee PA, Castelli WP, McNamara PM, Kannel WB. The natural history of congestive heart failure. *N Engl J Med* 1971;**285**(26):1441–6.

A recent study in Sweden reiterated this salient point. Random primary health care centres were sampled from across the country. Medical records were interrogated and variables recorded. Only approximately 30% of the participants had an echocardiogram. The majority were labelled as having heart failure on the basis of signs and symptoms and basic investigations including chest radiographs and the electrocardiogram. There was also under-use of evidence-based therapies.[8]

Population-based studies using echocardiography

Systolic dysfunction

The North Glasgow MONICA study was the first to report on the prevalence of left ventricular systolic dysfunction in a random sample of the general population. Among 2000 men and women aged 25–74 years,[9] 2.9% had significant systolic dysfunction, of whom just over half had symptoms of breathlessness or were taking a loop diuretic. The estimated prevalence of heart failure was therefore 1.5% with 1.4% having the important precursor of heart failure, asymptomatic left ventricular systolic dysfunction (LVSD) (see Figure 3.2). The prevalence rose with age and was higher in men than women.

Many studies have reported since, both in Europe and the USA (see Table 3.1). Data from these cohorts are fairly consistent for the general population. Prevalence rates for LVSD were 1.8–3.5% in the ECHOES study from the English Midlands, with 50% of the LVSD being asymptomatic. In the US Olmsted County study, 2.2% of the population had heart failure validated using the Framingham criteria, of whom 56% had LVSD.[10]

When we look at population-based studies that have included much older subjects, the prevalence rates increase markedly. In the Helsinki Ageing Study of 501 subjects aged 75–86 years, clinical heart failure was found in 8.2% overall. However, only 28% of the cohort had LVSD and the majority of the population had heart failure secondary to a preserved ejection fraction. Notably

21% of the total population were noted to have heart failure secondary to significant valvular disease.[11] In the Rotterdam Study of 2267 men and women aged 55–95 years, 3.7% had fractional shortening ≤25% (5.5% of men and 2.2% of women) and 2.2% had asymptomatic LVSD (see Figure 3.3).[12] Similar findings were reported in a UK study of 817 randomly selected subjects aged 70–84 years from Poole which demonstrated that 7.5% had LVSD (12.2% men and 2.9% women) and 52% were previously undiagnosed.[13]

Heart failure with preserved systolic function

Many of the population-based cohorts reviewed above concentrated on finding systolic dysfunction as it is (to date) the only type of heart failure for which we have evidence-based treatment. Many of the studies have, however, by default or design been able to comment on the prevalence of heart failure with preserved systolic function. Hogg and colleagues reviewed the epidemiological data for preserved ejection fraction heart failure (HeFPEF). The prevalence ranged from 1.5% to 4.8% depending on the study. There was a definite increase in the proportion of heart failure due to HeFPEF in cohorts of older subjects.[14] In the ECHOES study (which sampled the general population), 1.1% had definite heart failure and an left ventricle ejection fraction (LVEF) >50%,[10] whereas in the Helsinki Ageing study, 72% of all the heart failure identified occurred among patients with a normal LVEF.[11] In the Rochester Epidemiology Project in the USA, in a random sample of 2042 subjects over 45 years, 216 patients had heart failure. Among the 137 with an assessment of ejection fraction, 44% had LVEF >50%.[15]

Even higher prevalence rates have been found in a recent large cross-sectional study from Portugal[16] which reported a prevalence of heart failure of 16.1% in those aged >80 years. The prevalence was roughly split equally between preserved and reduced ejection fraction.

The above studies all confirm the relationship between increasing prevalence of heart failure and increasing age. It is therefore unsurprising that the current burden of heart failure within the EU countries is estimated to be approximately 15 million; according to the American Heart Association, more than five million Americans have heart failure.[17,18]

Incidence

Contemporary studies of incidence are far fewer than those for prevalence. The incidence of heart failure was reported from the west London district of Hillingdon. Here all incident cases of heart failure were identified via either a specialist referral clinic or emergency admission.[19] The district contained 151 000 patients covered by 82 general practices. Using both portals of entry, 220 new cases were identified. Participants had a full clinical assessment, standard investigations including a chest radiograph, electrocardiogram, and 99% of the study population had an echocardiogram. The results were then shown to a panel of three cardiologists who made the reference standard diagnosis. The incidence rose from 0.02 per 1000 per year in the 25–34-year age group to 11.6 per 1000 in those aged >85 years (see Figure 3.4). There was a preponderance of impaired systolic function. The study confirmed that heart failure is

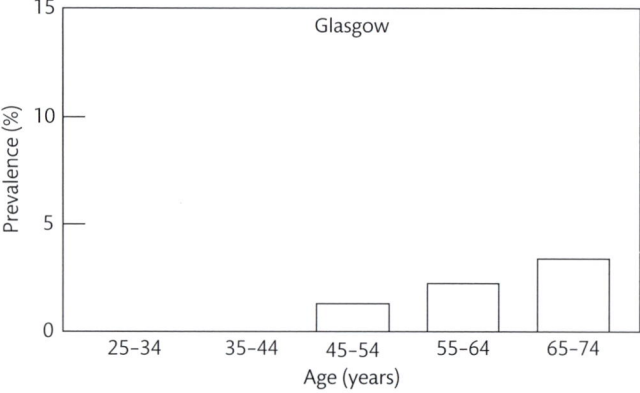

Figure 3.2 Prevalence of left ventricular systolic dysfunction in the North Glasgow MONICA cohort.

Source data from McDonagh TA, Morrison CE, Lawrence A, *et al.* Symptomatic and asymptomatic left ventricular systolic dysfunction in an urban population. *Lancet* 1997;**350**:829–33.

Table 3.1 Prevalence of symptomatic and asymptomatic LVSD in populations with a calculated prevalence of manifest heart failure where applicable

Authors	Name of study	No. of patients (no. of cases of heart failure)	Location	Age range (years)	Percentage symptomatic LVSD	Percentage ASLVD	Prevalence of HF aged >65 years	Prevalence of HF aged >65 years
Parameshwar et al., 1992	Prevalence of heart failure in 3 GP practices	30 204 (117)	North west London, UK	5–99	28% had echoes		0.6 per 1000	27.7 per 1000
Murphy et al., 2004	National survey of heart failure	307 741 (2186)	Scotland, UK	0 to >85	–		7.1 per 1000 (though not aged <65 years)	>85–90.1 per 1000
Rutten et al., 2003	A questionnaire-based survey of heart failure	(202)	Utrecht, Netherlands	40–95	53% had echoes 97% LVSD			
McDonagh et al., 1997	MONICA	1640 (43)	North Glasgow, UK	25–74	2.9% LVSD	1.4%	15 per 1000	
Davies et al., 2001	ECHOES	3960 (72)	West Midlands, UK		1.8% LVSD 3.5% preserved EF	0.9%	31 per 1000 (aged >45 years)	
Kupari et al., 1997	Helsinki Ageing Study	501 (41)	Helsinki, Finland	75–86	4.1% HEFPEF 3.9% LVSD	9%		(75–86) 82 per 1000
Mosterd et al., 1999	Rotterdam Heart Study	2267 (88)	Rotterdam, Netherlands	55–94	3.7% LSVD	1.4%	Men: 7 per 1000 (55–64). Women: 6 per 1000 (55–64)	Men: 37 per 1000 (65–74); 144 per 1000 (75–84); 59 per 1000 (85–94). Women: 16 per 1000 (65–74); 121 per 1000 (75–84); 140 per 1000 (85–94)
Morgan et al., 1999	Poole Heart Study	817 (61)	Poole, Dorset, UK	70–84	7.5% LVSD	3.9%		

ASLVD, asymptomatic left ventricular systolic dysfunction; HF, heart failure; LVSD, left ventricular systolic dysfunction.

predominantly a disease of the elderly with a median age of first presentation of 76 years.

Data for the USA are available from the Cardiovascular Health Study, showing an incidence of heart failure of 19.3 per 1000 person-years in 5.5 years of follow-up.[20] Data are also available for incidence from general practice records. Using the General Practice Research Database in the UK, which was officiated by the Office of National Statistics, 696 884 potential patients aged >45 years were identified.[21]

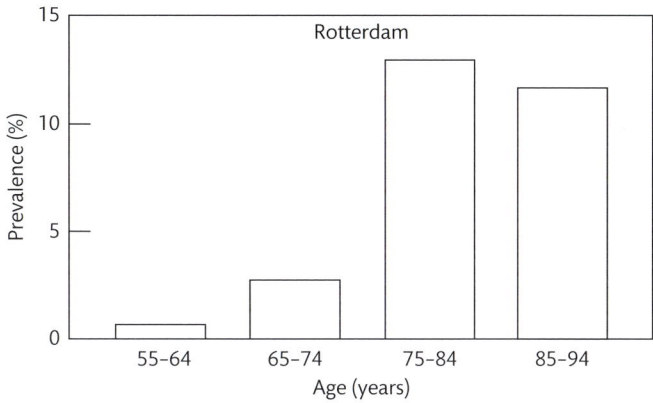

Figure 3.3 Prevalence of left ventricular systolic dysfunction within the Rotterdam study.
Source data from Mosterd A, Hoes AW, de Brunye DC, et al. Prevalence of heart failure and left ventricular dysfunction in the general population. *Eur Heart J* 1999;**20**:447–55.

Patients were categorized on the basis of interrogating records and medication prescription patterns: 6478 patients with definitive heart failure, 14 050 with possible heart failure, and 6076 with diuretics but a non-heart failure diagnosis were identified. The overall incidence of definitive heart failure was 9.3 per 1000 per year, but when the possible heart failure was included it increased to 20.2 per 1000 per year. The mean age of incident heart failure in the definite heart failure population was 77 years. More recent data from the Scottish continuous morbidity recording (CMR) data set showed an overall incidence of two per 1000 population per year—it was 25 per 1000 per year in men aged >85 years.[4]

The majority of epidemiological surveys have concentrated on Caucasian populations, with a bias towards relatively affluent areas of the west. However, further data have been accumulated on heart failure incidence within ethnic minority populations. Bibbins-Domingo and colleagues observed the rate of incident heart failure among 5115 individuals concentrated in six economically deprived sites in the USA. The cumulative incidence for Black men and women was 0.9% and 1.1%, respectively, significantly higher than among their White counterparts.[23] The work highlights the need for further characterization of the disease among both first and subsequent generation ethnic minorities in westernized populations. Recently efforts have been made to document the incidence of heart failure further on a global scale outside the intensively studied western health care environments. One such example is the INTER-CHF study which documents the incidence of heart failure within

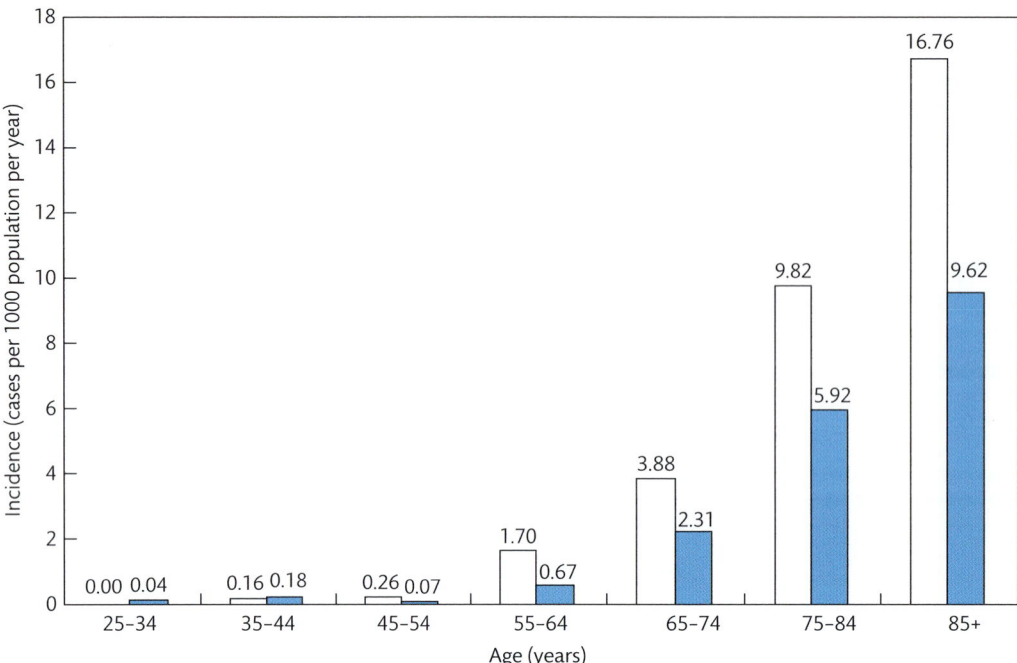

Figure 3.4 Incidence of heart failure by sex and age group in Hillingdon Heart Failure Study.
Source data from Cowie MR, Wood DA, Coats AJS, *et al.* Incidence and aetiology of heart failure: A population based study. *Eur Heart J* 1999;**20**:421–8.

Asia, Africa, the Middle East, and South America.[24] However, there is a paucity of such data, and more is needed.

Trends in incidence and prevalence

Data from the Framingham study have not shown any increase in heart failure incidence since the 1970s, dispelling the theory that we are experiencing an epidemic of heart failure. Similarly, data from Medicare records show a slight reduction in incidence from 57.5 per 1000 to 48.4 per 1000 person-years in the 80–84-year age group between 1994 and 2003. However, despite the slight reduction in incidence, the prevalence rose markedly from 90 per 1000 to 120 per 1000 as the *number* of older people increased.[25] Recent analysis from the Olmsted County project supports these findings. Using the historical Framingham diagnostic criteria, Redfield and colleagues highlighted a marked decrease in incident cases of heart failure during the period of 2000–2010. The overall rate of heart failure incidence declined from 315.8 per 100 000 in 2000 to 219.3 per 100 000 in 2010. There was a particularly marked reduction in patients with LVSD, with an increasing proportion of patients being diagnosed as having HeFPEF. The authors propose that the reduction in rates of LVSD might be due to better care of patients with acute myocardial infarction and greater access to primary percutaneous coronary intervention.[26]

A further, more detailed, contemporary analysis has been performed using the electronic health records of the Clinical Practice Research Datalink based within primary care in the UK. A total of four million health records were examined and cross-linkage performed to the Hospital Episodes Statistics. The study period ran for 12 years and documented the trend on both the incidence and prevalence of heart failure within the UK. There was an absolute small increase in numbers of incident heart failure from 170 727 in 2002 to 190 798 in 2014; however, the standardized age:gender ratio demonstrated a reduction in 7%. There was a large growth (23%) in the number of prevalent patients with an end result of 920 616 patients in 2014. The number of co-morbidities increased with age and patients were increasingly polymorbid. This survey is one of the first to chart the impact of the socio-economic gradient upon the rate of incident heart failure and it observed an increased incidence of heart failure within socio-economically deprived individuals who also possessed a larger number of baseline co-morbidities.[27]

Aetiology

Determining the exact aetiology of patients with heart failure in epidemiological studies can be difficult. The commonest cause in western societies currently is ischaemic heart disease (IHD), which is a change in aetiology over time: when the Framingham study first reported, the commonest aetiological factor was hypertension. Over time, coronary heart disease has increased as an aetiological factor by 40% in men and 20% in women.

In the North Glasgow MONICA study, >95% of patients with symptomatic LVSD had some evidence of prior IHD, although hypertension was also common, being present in 68%. In the ECHOES study, 53% of those with systolic dysfunction had evidence of IHD and 42% had hypertension; 54% had hypertension and 54% had IHD in the Helsinki Ageing Study. US data from the Cardiovascular Health Study report the population-attributable risk for heart failure for coronary heart disease to be 13.1% and for hypertension 12.8%. Both are clearly important aetiological factors.[20]

In the Hillingdon Study of incident heart failure, 41% of the heart failure cohort had underlying coronary artery disease and many

fewer (6%) had hypertension.[28] A subsequent study in Bromley, south London, identified 332 incident cases of heart failure and patients were referred to a specialist dedicated clinic or identified via tracking during hospitalization. A total of 99 out of the 136 patients aged <75 years also underwent coronary angiography. An ischaemic aetiology was eventually attributed to 52% of the 136 cases.[29]

Hypertension as a cause of heart failure does still seem to predominate in those with heart failure and preserved systolic function where IHD seems less prominent. Patients with HeFPEF tend to be older and a higher proportion are women than men for those with reduced ejection fraction. Both diseases are still common—a recent study by Zile showed a prevalence of hypertension of 82% and CHD of 45% among patients with preserved ejection fraction heart failure.[30]

The traditional risk factors associated with myocardial disease have been extensively studied in predominately white populations. Increasing awareness that the same diseases may manifest and act differently in different ethnic populations is the subject of recent studies. Hypertension is an important contributory factor in African-Americans aged <39 years who have a heart failure incidence rate 20 times that of age-matched Whites.[23] South Asians have a susceptibility to premature accelerated coronary artery disease.[31,32] A series of studies looking South Asians hospitalized with heart failure in Leicestershire, UK and Toronto, Canada has shown that admission rates for heart failure were higher, and diabetes and hypertension were more common, than among the White population in the same area. This may mean that the coronary artery disease leads to the development of heart failure at a younger age.[33–35]

The management of acute coronary syndromes and particularly those patients with ST elevation myocardial infarction has been revolutionized by primary revascularization. Primary percutaneous coronary intervention (PCI) programmes are now well established and have led to demonstrable reductions in cardiovascular mortality and morbidity.[36] However, the success of acute cardiovascular management means that there are more survivors of myocardial infarction who can go on to develop heart failure due to LVSD. Gho and colleagues recently presented the analysis of 24 745 patients from a primary care database from the UK who had an acute myocardial infarct between 1998 and 2010. In all, 6005 individuals (24.3%) were found to have developed heart failure following a median follow-up period of 3.7 years.[37] Although the study reported data collected over a long timespan during which services in the UK were reconfigured to deliver primary PCI, the statistics imply that a large number of patients will develop heart failure following acute myocardial infarction. More data are urgently needed to guide post-myocardial infarction care.

Heart failure in the developing world is often caused by either infective or nutritional disease. Rheumatic heart disease is still endemic in sub-Saharan Africa.[38] However, the epidemiological data from developing areas of the world is limited. Some previously 'developing' areas have undergone an epidemiological transition to a more affluent, sedentary urbanized population. The consequence is an epidemiological transition in cardiovascular disease from infective and nutritional heart disease to atherosclerosis and progressive coronary artery disease.

Co-morbidities

Heart failure is commonly associated with numerous co-morbidities, particularly because it affects older people. Co-morbidities include renal impairment, anaemia, diabetes mellitus, obstructive sleep apnoea, and chronic obstructive pulmonary disease. These all have an adverse impact on survival when associated with heart failure.[39]

Anaemia was present in 51% of patients with heart failure in the Rochester Epidemiology Project. Severely impaired renal function was present in 10%. These rates are increased in patients presenting with acute heart failure syndromes—renal dysfunction occurred in 20% of those admitted with decompensated heart failure in the Euroheart Failure Survey II.[40]

Prognosis

The mortality from heart failure is high, with a five-year prognosis worse than many common cancers.[41] The 32-year follow-up of the Framingham study highlighted the awful mortality rate associated with heart failure. The probability of dying from heart failure was 62% for men and 42% for women at five years of follow-up from initial diagnosis. However, data from the Framingham study have shown consistent improvements in survival over time for both men and women.[42] In Europe, the mortality of incident heart failure also seems to be falling. In the initial Hillingdon study (published 1999), 25% of patients had died at six months, but in the more recent cohort of the study from 2004 to 2005, the percentage had fallen to 14%.[43] The fall in mortality was independent of confounding variables and was linked to the increased usage of evidence-based pharmacotherapies.

Although mortality is higher in studies of incident heart failure, it is also poor in prevalent cases. In the ECHOES study, the five-year survival rate was 53% for those with heart failure due to systolic dysfunction (see **Figure 3.5**).[44] Survival for those with heart failure with preserved systolic function was a little better at 62%. This is in contrast to the Mayo Clinic data which showed that survival in

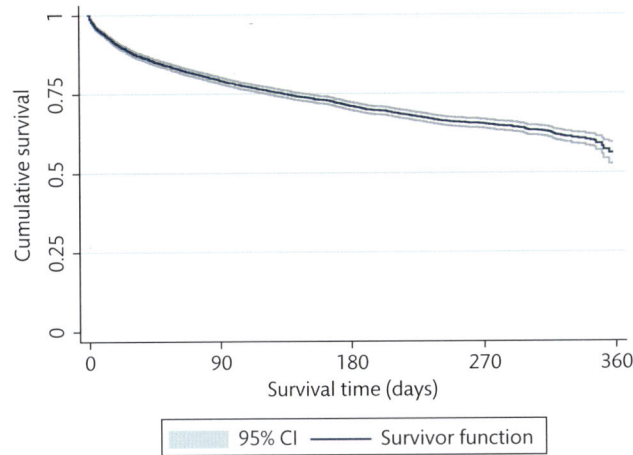

Figure 3.5 Overall annual mortality from the ECHOES study.

Source data from Hobbs FD, Roalfe AK, Davis RC, *et al. Prognosis of all-cause heart failure and borderline left ventricular systolic dysfunction: 5 year mortality follow-up of the Echocardiographic Heart of England Screening Study (ECHOES). Eur Heart J* 2007;**28**(9):1128–34.

the community with heart failure was similar for those with systolic and non-systolic heart failure.[15] However, the Mayo Clinic group reported on 4596 patients of whom 47% had preserved left ventricular function diagnosed between 1987 and 2001.[45] The survival rate was slightly better in the population with preserved systolic function. However, the mortality rate declined in the patients with systolic dysfunction during the study period, but did not change among the patients with normal ventricular function. The more recent meta-analysis group in heart failure (MAGGIC) has studied a cohort of more than 40 000 patients. Mortality was lower among the patients with preserved ejection fraction than among those with LVSD, but was high in both groups.[46]

'The mortality rate of subjects with asymptomatic left ventricular systolic dysfunction is also high. In the North Glasgow MONICA cohort, 21% of those with LVSD died by 4 years, with no difference in survival between those with and without symptoms.' This finding underscores the need for early detection and treatment of asymptomatic LVSD.

Data from patients hospitalized in Scotland also show a trend to improved survival. Between 1986 and 2003, median survival after a first admission with heart failure improved in men from 1.3 to 2.3 years and in women from 1.3 to 1.8 years (see **Figure 3.6**).[47]

The poorer survival of patients hospitalized with acute heart failure compared to patients with heart failure in the community is underscored by data from large European and US registries. In the Euro Heart Failure II survey, intrahospital mortality was 6.6%.[40] This varied with presentation but was nearly 40% in those presenting with cardiogenic shock. A historical audit of acute hospital admissions in the UK reported an in-hospital mortality of 15%.[48] Since the publication of the pilot audit data, the National Heart Failure Audit has been created, which covers England and Wales. The annual report from the audit represents an overview of patients hospitalized within the two countries with heart failure. In the most recent year of publication (2017–2018), more than 68,000 admissions were captured and data recorded. The in-hospital mortality rate was 10.1% with notable geographical and regional variation. The mortality rate for those aged <75 years was 5.7% and for those aged >75 years was 12%. The report also highlights the increased mortality rate of patients who are not managed by a specialist heart failure team or who are managed without access to cardiology input.[49] Patients cared for by specialists are, perhaps paradoxically, hospitalized for longer, presumably because they are more likely to be started on all three classes of disease-modifying drugs and the procedure takes time.

The in-hospital mortality in the USA is better, running at 4% in the OPTIMISE heart failure registry.[50] The differences in hospital mortality rates between the USA and Europe have to be viewed with caution, due to the method of case ascertainment, the clinical and racial background of the patients, and the composition of regional and national services. Hospital stay is much shorter in the USA (at around five days compared with 11 days in the UK), so in-hospital mortality is necessarily lower as there is less 'opportunity' for a patient to die.

Morbidity hospitalizations

Patients with heart failure have frequent admissions and readmissions to hospital. The rate of rehospitalization at six months is between 36% and 45%.[41,51] Data from the Netherlands, Scotland, and the USA in the 1990s all confirmed an increasing trend for heart

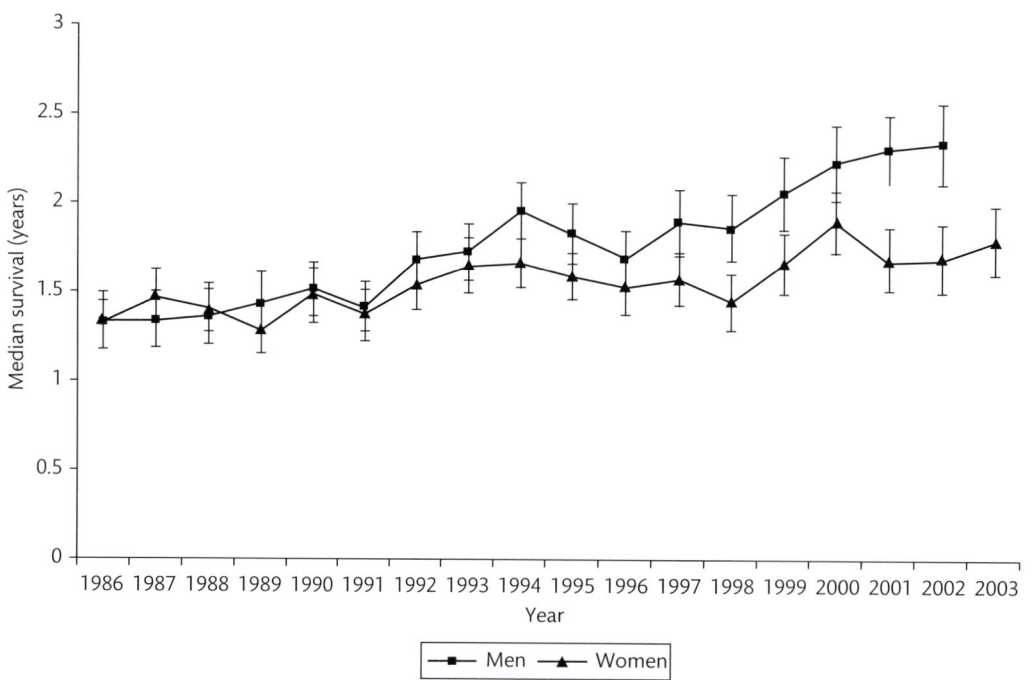

Figure 3.6 Trends in median survival in Scotland, 1986–2003.

Reproduced from Jhund PS, Macintyre K, Simpson CR, *et al.* Long term trends in first hospitalization for heart failure and subsequent survival between 1986–2003. A population study of 5.1 million people. *Circulation* 2009;**119**:515–23 with permission from Wolters Kluwer.

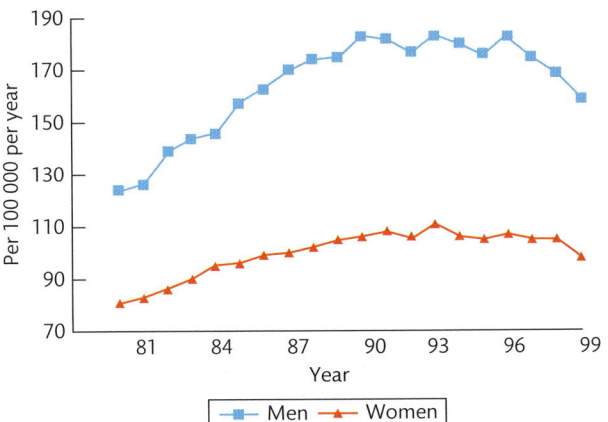

Figure 3.7 Heart failure hospitalization rate in the Netherlands, 1980–1999.

Source data from Mosterd A, Hoes AW. Clinical epidemiology of heart failure. *Heart* 2007;**93**:1137–46.

failure admissions.[52,53] The inexorable rise in admissions in the 1990s was associated with increasing expenditure.

However, data from more recent years suggests that heart failure admissions may have peaked in the 1990s. Data from Scotland on 116 556 patients identified from hospital discharge records between 1986 and 2003 showed that rates of heart failure admission peaked in the mid 1990s and fell by 2003.[46] This is also the case in the Netherlands (see **Figure 3.7**).[54]

The situation in the USA seems to lag behind the European data. The number of heart failure-related admissions tripled from 1 274 000 in 1979 to 3 860 000 in 2004 (see **Figure 3.8**).[55] However, the most recently available US data covering the period 2001–2009 demonstrate secular trends similar to the European studies. Using the National Inpatient Survey, the number of primary heart failure hospitalizations in the USA decreased from 1 137 944 in 2001 to 1 086 685 in 2009, while secondary heart failure hospitalisations increased from 2 753 793 to 3 158 179 over the same period. A secondary heart failure hospitalization was defined as the

acknowledgement of heart failure being present during the admission, but not entering the primary position on the discharge summary.[56] Agarwal and colleagues applied predictive modelling based on the Atherosclerosis Risk in Communities (ARIC) study to the National Inpatient Survey and found a rise in admissions for acute decompensated heart failure between 1998 and 2004, with a stabilization in the number of admissions between 2005 and 2011.[57]

Health economics

The increasing prevalence of patients with heart failure ensures that it continues to pose major challenges for health care economies. The frequent and lengthy hospitalizations are associated with enormous health care expenditure: perhaps 2% of western health care expenditure is on heart failure.

The US currently spends $31 billion on heart failure, with a predicted rise to potentially US$70 billion in 2030. The predictions also suggest that there will be eight million patients with heart failure in the US by 2030, with a prevalence of approximately of one in 33 of the total population.[58]

The statistics are similar in Europe. Heart failure consumes 1–2% of the National Health Service budget in the UK, which approximates at £1.2 billion (€1.3 billion, US$1.8 billion). It is the leading cause of hospitalisation in the elderly population within the UK. Approximately 60% of the total of heart failure costs are due to hospital admissions. In Europe more broadly, heart failure consumes approximately 1% of healthcare budgets. The length of stay also contributes to the expense, with median stay within the UK and Europe of 9–11 days. These are likely to be underestimates as true costs should include all primary care consultations, secondary care referrals, diagnostics, prescribing habits, further therapies including devices and care networks, and surgical intervention including transplantation.

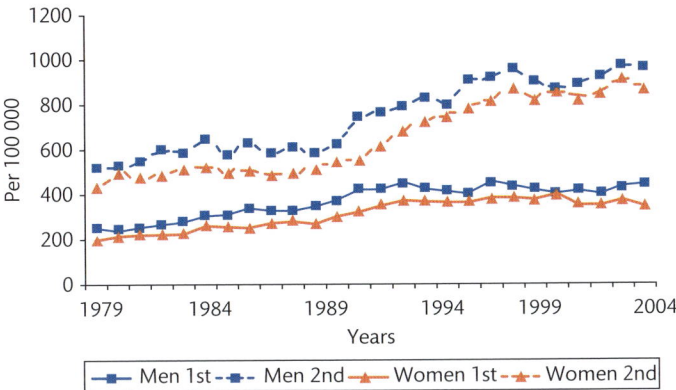

Figure 3.8 Age-adjusted hospitalization rates for heart failure, National Discharge Survey 1979–2004.

Reproduced from Fang J, Mensah GA, Croft JB, Keenan NL. Heart failure related hospitalization in the US, 1979–2004. *J Am Coll Cardiol* 2008;**52**:428–34 with permission from Elsevier.

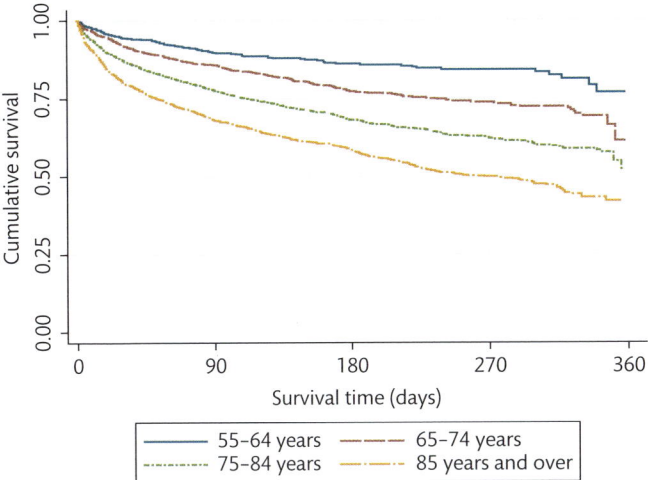

Figure 3.9 Overall annual mortality stratified by age, from the ECHOES study.

Source data from Hobbs FD, Roalfe AK, Davis RC, *et al.* Prognosis of all-cause heart failure and borderline left ventricular systolic dysfunction: 5 year mortality follow-up of the Echocardiographic Heart of England Screening Study (ECHOES). *Eur Heart J* 2007;**28**(9):1128–34.

Conclusions

Despite the advances made in its treatment over the course of the last 35 years, which have seen mortality rates for those in clinical trials of heart failure therapies fall to less than 10% per annum, epidemiological studies show that heart failure remains a common, lethal, disabling, and expensive condition. Its principal causes are IHD and hypertension, which often coexist. It also has a detectable asymptomatic precursor which is as common as manifest heart failure itself. As the burden of heart failure increases with the ageing of our populations, there needs to be an urgent focusing on the best heart failure disease management programmes that can cope with increasing numbers of elderly patients who have many co-morbidities and that can deliver equitable evidence-based health care. Even more challengingly, the delivery of health care needs to take place in an era of declining health care budgets but increasing absolute costs (see **Figure 3.9**).

REFERENCES

1. McKee PA, Castelli WP, McNamara PM, Kannel WB. The natural history of congestive heart failure: the Framingham study. *N Engl J Med* 1971;**285**(26):1441–6.
2. Eriksson H, Svardsudd K, Larsson B, et al. Risk factors for heart failure in the general population: the study of men born in 1913. *Eur Heart J* 1989;**10**(7):647–56.
3. Parameshwar J, Shackell MM, Richardson A, Poole-Wilson PA, Sutton GC. Prevalence of heart failure in three general practices in north west London. *Br J Gen Pract* 1992;**42**(360):287–9.
4. Murphy NF, Simpson CR, McAlister FA, et al. National survey of the prevalence, incidence, primary care burden, and treatment of heart failure in Scotland. *Heart* 2004;**90**(10):1129–36.
5. Rutten FH, Grobbee DE, Hoes AW. Diagnosis and management of heart failure: a questionnaire among general practitioners and cardiologists. *Eur J Heart Fail* 2003;**5**(3):345–8.
6. Cowie MR, Struthers AD, Wood DA, et al. Value of natriuretic peptides in assessment of patients with possible new heart failure in primary care. *Lancet* 1997;**350**(9088):1349–53.
7. Remes J, Miettinen H, Reunanen A, Pyorala K. Validity of clinical diagnosis of heart failure in primary health care. *Eur Heart J* 1991;**12**(3):315–21.
8. Dahlstrom U, Hakansson J, Swedberg K, Waldenstrom A. Adequacy of diagnosis and treatment of chronic heart failure in primary health care in Sweden. *Eur J Heart Fail* 2009;**11**(1):92–8.
9. McDonagh TA, Morrison CE, Lawrence A, et al. Symptomatic and asymptomatic left-ventricular systolic dysfunction in an urban population. *Lancet* 1997;**350**(9081):829–33.
10. Davies M, Hobbs F, Davis R, et al. Prevalence of left-ventricular systolic dysfunction and heart failure in the Echocardiographic Heart of England Screening study: a population based study. *Lancet* 2001;**358**(9280):439–44.
11. Kupari M, Lindroos M, Iivanainen AM, Heikkila J, Tilvis R. Congestive heart failure in old age: prevalence, mechanisms and 4-year prognosis in the Helsinki Ageing Study. *J Intern Med* 1997;**241**(5):387–94.
12. Mosterd A, Hoes AW, de Bruyne MC, et al. Prevalence of heart failure and left ventricular dysfunction in the general population; The Rotterdam Study. *Eur Heart J* 1999;**20**(6):447–55.

13. Morgan S, Smith H, Simpson I, et al. Prevalence and clinical characteristics of left ventricular dysfunction among elderly patients in general practice setting: cross sectional survey. *BMJ* 1999;**318**(7180):368–72.
14. Hogg K, Swedberg K, McMurray J. Heart failure with preserved left ventricular systolic function; epidemiology, clinical characteristics, and prognosis. *J Am Coll Cardiol* 2004;**43**(3):317–27.
15. Senni M, Tribouilloy CM, Rodeheffer RJ, et al. Congestive heart failure in the community: a study of all incident cases in Olmsted County, Minnesota, in 1991. *Circulation* 1998;**98**(21):2282–9.
16. Ceia F, Fonseca C, Mota T, et al. Prevalence of chronic heart failure in Southwestern Europe: the EPICA study. *Eur J Heart Fail* 2002;**4**(4):531–9.
17. Dickstein K, Cohen-Solal A, Filippatos G, et al. ESC guidelines for the diagnosis and treatment of acute and chronic heart failure 2008: the Task Force for the diagnosis and treatment of acute and chronic heart failure 2008 of the European Society of Cardiology. Developed in collaboration with the Heart Failure Association of the ESC (HFA) and endorsed by the European Society of Intensive Care Medicine (ESICM). *Eur J Heart Fail* 2008;**10**(10):933–89.
18. Hunt SA. ACC/AHA 2005 guideline update for the diagnosis and management of chronic heart failure in the adult: a report of the American College of Cardiology/American Heart Association Task Force on Practice Guidelines (Writing Committee to Update the 2001 Guidelines for the Evaluation and Management of Heart Failure). *J Am Coll Cardiol* 2005;**46**(6):e1–82.
19. Cowie MR, Wood DA, Coats AJ, et al. Incidence and aetiology of heart failure; a population-based study. *Eur Heart J* 1999;**20**(6):421–8.
20. Gottdiener JS, Arnold AM, Aurigemma GP, et al. Predictors of congestive heart failure in the elderly: the Cardiovascular Health Study. *J Am Coll Cardiol* 2000;**35**(6):1628–37.
21. De GF, Khaw KT, Cowie MR, et al. Incidence and outcome of persons with a clinical diagnosis of heart failure in a general practice population of 696,884 in the United Kingdom. *Eur J Heart Fail* 2005;**7**(3):295–302.
22. Kalogeropoulos A, Georgiopoulou V, Kritchevsky SB, et al. Epidemiology of incident heart failure in a contemporary elderly cohort: the health, aging, and body composition study. *Arch Intern Med* 2009;**169**(7):708–15.
23. Bibbins-Domingo K, Pletcher MJ, Lin F, et al. Racial differences in incident heart failure among young adults. *N Engl J Med* 2009;**360**(12):1179–90.
24. Dokainish H, Teo K, Zhu J, et al; INTER-CHF Investigators. Heart failure in Africa, Asia, Middle East and South America. INTER-CHF study. *Int J Cardiol* 2016;**204**:133–41.
25. Curtis LH, Whellan DJ, Hammill BG, et al. Incidence and prevalence of heart failure in elderly persons, 1994–2003. *Arch Intern Med* 2008;**168**(4):418–24.
26. Gerber Y, Weston SA, Redfield MM, et al. A contemporary appraisal of the heart failure epidemic in Olmsted County, Minnesota, 2000–2010. *JAMA Int Med* 2015;**176**(6):996–1004.
27. Conrad N, Judge A, Tran J, et al. Temporal trends and patterns in heart failure incidence: a population based study of 4 million individuals. *Lancet* 2018;**391**;572–80.
28. Parameshwar J, Poole-Wilson PA, Sutton GC. Heart failure in a district general hospital. *J R Coll Physns Lond* 1992;**26**(2):139–42.
29. Fox KF, Cowie MR, Wood DA, et al. Coronary artery disease as the cause of incident heart failure in the population. *Eur Heart J* 2001;**22**(3):228–36.

30. Zile MR, Simsic JM. Diastolic heart failure: diagnosis and treatment. *Clin Cornerstone* 2000;**3**(2):13–24.

31. Sheth T, Nair C, Nargundkar M, Anand S, Yusuf S. Cardiovascular and cancer mortality among Canadians of European, south Asian and Chinese origin from 1979 to 1993: an analysis of 1.2 million deaths. *CMAJ* 1999;**161**(2):132–8.

32. Wild S, McKeigue P. Cross sectional analysis of mortality by country of birth in England and Wales, 1970–92. *BMJ* 1997;**314**(7082):705–10.

33. Blackledge HM, Newton J, Squire IB. Prognosis for South Asian and white patients newly admitted to hospital with heart failure in the United Kingdom: historical cohort study. *BMJ* 2003;**327**(7414):526–31.

34. Blackledge HM, Tomlinson J, Squire IB. Prognosis for patients newly admitted to hospital with heart failure: survival trends in 12 220 index admissions in Leicestershire 1993–2001. *Heart* 2003;**89**(6):615–20.

35. Singh N, Gupta M. Clinical characteristics of South Asian patients hospitalized with heart failure. *Ethn Dis* 2005;**15**(4):615–19.

36. British Heart Foundation Heart and Circulatory Diseases. https://www.bhf.org.uk/what-we-do/our-research/heart-statistics/heart-statistics-publications/cardiovascular-disease-statistics-2020

37. Gho MH, Schmidt AF, Koudstaal S, et al. Heart failure following myocardial infarction: a cohort study of incidence and prognostic factors in 24 745 patients using linked electronic records. *Eur J Heart Fail Abstr* 2016;**18**(Suppl 1):442.

38. Brink AJ, Aalbers J. Strategies for heart disease in sub-Saharan Africa. *Heart* 2009;**95**(19):1559–60.

39. McMurray JJ, Pfeffer MA. Heart failure. *Lancet* 2005;**365**(9474):1877–89.

40. Nieminen MS, Brutsaert D, Dickstein K, et al. EuroHeart Failure Survey II (EHFS II): a survey on hospitalized acute heart failure patients: description of population. *Eur Heart J* 2006;**27**(22):2725–36.

41. Stewart S, MacIntyre K, Hole DJ, Capewell S, McMurray JJ. More 'malignant' than cancer? Five-year survival following a first admission for heart failure. *Eur J Heart Fail* 2001;**3**(3):315–22.

42. Ho KK, Anderson KM, Kannel WB, Grossman W, Levy D. Survival after the onset of congestive heart failure in Framingham Heart Study subjects. *Circulation* 1993;**88**(1):107–15.

43. Mehta PA, Dubrey SW, McIntyre HF, et al. Improving survival in the 6 months after diagnosis of heart failure in the past decade: population-based data from the UK. *Heart* 2009;**95**(22):1851–6.

44. Hobbs FD, Roalfe AK, Davis RC, Davies MK, Hare R. Prognosis of all-cause heart failure and borderline left ventricular systolic dysfunction: 5 year mortality follow-up of the Echocardiographic Heart of England Screening Study (ECHOES). *Eur Heart J* 2007;**28**(9):1128–34.

45. Owan TE, Hodge DO, Herges RM, et al. Trends in prevalence and outcome of heart failure with preserved ejection fraction. *N Engl J Med* 2006;**355**(3):251–9.

46. Meta-Analysis Global Group in Chronic Heart Failure (MAGGIC). The survival of patients with heart failure with preserved or reduced left ventricular ejection fraction:an individual patient data meta-analysis. *Eur Heart J* 2012;**33**:1750–7.

47. Jhund PS, MacIntyre K, Simpson CR, et al. Long-term trends in first hospitalization for heart failure and subsequent survival between 1986 and 2003: a population study of 5.1 million people. *Circulation* 2009;**119**(4):515–23.

48. Nicol ED, Fittall B, Roughton M, et al. NHS heart failure survey: a survey of acute heart failure admissions in England, Wales and Northern Ireland. *Heart* 2008;**94**(2):172–7.

49. National Heart Failure Audit 2017–2018. National Institutes of Cardiovascular Outcomes Research. https://www.nicor.org.uk/wp-content/uploads/2019/09/Heart-Failure-2019-Report-final.pdf

50. Fonarow GC, Abraham WT, Albert NM, et al. Day of admission and clinical outcomes for patients hospitalized for heart failure:findings from the Organized Program to Initiate Lifesaving Treatment in Hospitalized Patients With Heart Failure (OPTIMIZE-HF). *Circ Heart Fail* 2008;**1**(1):50–7.

51. Fonarow GC, Heywood JT, Heidenreich PA, Lopatin M, Yancy CW. Temporal trends in clinical characteristics, treatments, and outcomes for heart failure hospitalizations, 2002 to 2004: findings from Acute Decompensated Heart Failure National Registry (ADHERE). *Am Heart J* 2007;**153**(6):1021–8.

52. Stewart S, MacIntyre K, MacLeod MM, Bailey AE, Capewell S, McMurray JJ. Trends in hospitalization for heart failure in Scotland, 1990–1996. An epidemic that has reached its peak? *Eur Heart J* 2001;**22**(3):209–17.

53. Reitsma JB, Mosterd A, de Craen AJ, et al. Increase in hospital admission rates for heart failure in The Netherlands, 1980–1993. *Heart* 1996;**76**(5):388–92.

54. Mosterd A, Hoes AW. Clinical epidemiology of heart failure. *Heart* 2007;**93**(9):1137–46.

55. Fang J, Mensah GA, Croft JB, Keenan NL. Heart failure-related hospitalization in the U.S., 1979 to 2004. *J Am Coll Cardiol* 2008;**52**(6):428–34.

56. Blecker S, Paul M, Taksler G, Ogedegbe G, Katz S. Heart failure associated hospitalisations in the United States. *J Am Coll Cardiol* 2013;**61**(12):1259–67.

57. Agarwal SK, Wruck L, Quibrera M, et al. Temporal trends in hospitalization for acute decompensated heart failure in the United States, 1998–2011. *Am J Epidemiol* 2016;**183**(5):462–70.

58. Heidenreich PA, Albert NM, Allen LA, et al. Forecasting the impact of heart failure in the United States. A Policy Statement from the American Heart Association. *Circ Heart Fail* 2013;**6**:606–19.

SECTION 3
The aetiology of heart failure

4

The classical causes of heart failure

Colette E. Jackson and Roy S. Gardner

Introduction

Heart failure is the complex clinical syndrome that may result from a broad spectrum of structural or functional cardiac and non-cardiac diseases (see Table 4.1), often causing the classical triad of symptoms: breathlessness, fatigue, and fluid retention. It is not a single disease entity, but rather a process that may potentially complicate most forms of cardiac pathology, particularly in their final stages.

The aetiology of heart failure can be described in many ways. First, it can be categorized into a disorder of the myocardium, endocardium, pericardium, or great vessels. Myocardial disorders are the most common cause, and these are subdivided into those with reduced and those with normal, or preserved systolic function. Reduced systolic function heart failure can also be classed as ischaemic or non-ischaemic heart failure, the latter term only applied when an ischaemic cause has been excluded. Non-ischaemic causes of left ventricular systolic dysfunction (LVSD) include hypertension, genetic, valvular heart disease, arrhythmias, alcohol or drug-related, and peripartum cardiomyopathy.

The 'classical causes' of heart failure are the common cardiovascular conditions that result in heart failure. These exhibit geographical variation and depend on the population being studied. In western countries, coronary heart disease and hypertension are the commonest causes of heart failure.[1] However, valvular heart disease (particularly degenerative), arrhythmias, and alcohol are also frequently implicated. In Africans and African-Americans, hypertension is an important precursor of heart failure,[2] and heart failure secondary to Chagas disease is well recognized in South America.[3] In developing countries, heart failure more commonly develops because of rheumatic valvular heart disease and nutritional deficiencies.[4]

The prevalence of 'classical causes' of heart failure in the largest contemporary clinical trials and registries is shown in Table 4.2.[5–23] Whereas clinical trials often contain highly selective cohorts of patients, with reduced systolic function only, the large registries consistently demonstrate similar prevalence of the common aetiologies. Thus, the prevalence of the common causes of heart failure in real-life heart failure populations can be extrapolated from these studies, with coronary heart disease being the major cause in approximately two-thirds of patients. However, this has not always been the case. The original Framingham Heart Study, one of the earliest cardiovascular epidemiological studies, recorded hypertension as the most common cause of heart failure.[24] During the subsequent decades of follow-up, the proportion of cases of heart failure attributable to hypertension and valvular heart disease decreased, and those secondary to coronary artery disease rose (Figure 4.1). The changing aetiology of heart failure in recent decades is likely multifactorial. Improvements in survival post myocardial infarction[25] and wider availability of techniques for diagnosing coronary artery disease are plausible reasons for the increasing prevalence of heart failure secondary to coronary heart disease. The declining role of hypertension as the primary cause of heart failure may be explained by an appreciation of the need for population-level screening for hypertension, and advances in antihypertensive therapy preventing longer-term complications.[26]

At present, genetic and mitochondrial abnormalities are thought to be less frequent causes of heart failure, although increasingly it is apparent that many forms of 'idiopathic' dilated cardiomyopathy have a familial link. Heart failure may also result from less common aetiologies, such as metabolic conditions, infiltrative processes, infective conditions, and iatrogenic causes. These rarer causes will be addressed in subsequent chapters of this section. This rest of this chapter will focus on the 'classical' causes of heart failure in western countries.

The importance of establishing an aetiology

The appropriate management of the heart failure patient relies on establishing its aetiology, particularly with regards to the selection of investigations and most suitable treatment strategies. Many of the robust evidence-based therapies available for the treatment of heart failure are derived from cohorts of patients with specific causes of heart failure. Determining the cause of heart failure and identifying potential secondary contributing factors are also important for targeting ways to avoid future episodes of acute decompensation. Examples of this include addressing risk factors for myocardial infarction and enrolling patients with alcoholic cardiomyopathy in rehabilitation programmes to attempt to alleviate their addiction.

Table 4.1 Causes of heart failure and the common modes of presentation

Cause	Examples of presentations
Coronary heart disease	Myocardial infarction Chronic ischaemia Arrhythmias
Hypertension	Heart failure with preserved systolic function 'Burnt out' hypertensive cardiomyopathy Malignant hypertension/acute pulmonary oedema
Valve disease	Primary valvular disease, e.g. endocarditis Secondary valvular disease, e.g. functional regurgitation Congenital valvular disease
Arrhythmias	Incessant atrial arrhythmias Ventricular arrhythmias
Dilated cardiomyopathy	Idiopathic Inherited (familial) Toxins: alcohol, cocaine, iron, copper, amphetamines
Pregnancy	Peripartum cardiomyopathy Pre-eclampsia
Congenital heart disease	Corrected transposition of great arteries Repaired Tetralogy of Fallot Ebstein's anomaly
Infective	Viral myocarditis Chagas disease HIV Lyme disease
Iatrogenic	Anthracyclines Abstruzimab
Infiltrative	Amyloid Sarcoid Neoplastic
Storage disorders	Haemochromatosis Fabry disease Glycogen storage diseases
Endomyocardial disease	Radiotherapy Endomyocardial fibrosis Carcinoid
Pericardial disease	Calcification Infiltrative
Metabolic	Endocrine disease Nutritional disease (thiamine deficiency, selenium deficiency) Autoimmune disease
Neuromuscular disease	Friedreich's ataxia Muscular dystrophy
High-output	Anaemia Thyrotoxicosis Arteriovenous fistulae Paget's disease

Identifying the genetic abnormality in familial conditions is also important, as this may give prognostic information as well as having an impact on the lives of other members of an individual patient's family. Finally, establishing the cause of heart failure can be curative. An example of this is radiofrequency ablation for tachycardiomyopathy.

Challenge of attributing aetiology

Establishing the aetiology of heart failure is important, but it is often challenging for the clinician. Several causes of heart failure

frequently coexist and determining the primary aetiology can be difficult: one cause may obviously dominate, but commonly a patient may have multiple contributing aetiologies. An example of this is the hypertensive, diabetic patient with confirmed coronary artery disease on angiography who consumes excess alcohol. Secondary causes may contribute to the progression of heart failure and may be the primary reason for episodes of acute decompensation, although not the original primary cause of heart failure.

Coronary artery disease can be challenging to attribute as the primary cause of heart failure. Although coronary angiography may reveal the presence of atherosclerotic disease, this does not confirm an ischaemic cause for any cardiac dysfunction. Conversely, a myocardial infarction may result from plaque rupture or coronary vasospasm in the context of otherwise unobstructed coronary arteries. Cardiac magnetic resonance (CMR) imaging can help to clarify the underlying diagnosis by characterizing the myocardium, with late gadolinium-enhanced images useful in identifying areas of previous myocardial infarction. In the absence of a definite clinical myocardial infarction, or evidence of such from coronary angiography/CMR, coronary artery disease can only be suspected as a possible cause of heart failure.

A further challenge in accurately ascribing the primary aetiology of heart failure may be when the condition is no longer present. Patients with heart failure secondary to long-standing hypertension may have normal or low blood pressure at the time of their heart failure presentation. A subset of patients with hypertrophic cardiomyopathy develop progressive left ventricular dilatation with systolic dysfunction and thinning of the previously hypertrophied myocardium. This condition is often referred to as 'burnt out' hypertrophic cardiomyopathy and patients presenting at this stage of the disease may be incorrectly diagnosed as primary dilated cardiomyopathy.

Coronary heart disease

Coronary artery disease is the commonest cause of heart failure in western countries (Table 4.2). It may present in several different ways: acute myocardial infarction, chronic ischaemia, arrhythmia, and asymptomatic (occult) disease.

Acute physiological responses

An acute myocardial infarction initiates acute physiological mechanisms—the same processes that are used to enhance cardiac output in normal circumstances.[27] Activation of the sympathetic nervous system results in faster heart rates and enhanced cardiac output. Activation of systemic neurohumoral pathways leads to increases in circulating volume, enhancing venous return, and the effective maintenance of preload. Ultimately, these pathways act to preserve cardiac output via the Frank–Starling mechanism. Other physiological changes following myocardial infarction include systemic vasoconstriction, which maintains blood pressure at the expense of increasing the workload of the heart by increasing afterload. Often the outcome of these adaptive responses is the maintenance of normal cardiac output at rest but reduced reserve for any further demands in cardiac output. The consequence clinically is a reduction in exercise capacity and symptoms of heart failure on exertion for some patients. However, initially, many

Table 4.2 Aetiology of heart failure in contemporary randomized clinical trials and major registries

Study	RCT/REG	Size	Age (years)	Male (%)	Ischaemic (%)	Non-ischaemic (%)	HT (%)	IDCM (%)	Valve (%)	Other (%)	Unknown (%)
SOLVD[5]	RCT	2569	61	80	71	–	–	18	–	–	–
DIG[6]	RCT	6800	64	78	70	30	9	15	–	6	–
MERIT-HF[7]	RCT	3991	64	78	66	34	–	–	–	–	–
CIBIS-II[8]	RCT	2647	61	81	50	–	–	12	–	–	38
ATLAS[9]	RCT	3192	64	79	64	35	20	28	–	6	–
RALES[10]	RCT	1663	65	73	54	46	–	–	–	–	–
Val-HeFT[11]	RCT	5010	62	80	57	–	7	31	–	5	–
COPERNICUS[12]	RCT	2289	63	80	67	–	–	–	–	–	–
COMET[13]	RCT	3029	62	80	53	–	18	–	–	–	–
COMPANION[14]	RCT	1520	67	68	56	44	–	–	–	–	–
CARE-HF[15]	RCT	813	67	73	38	–	–	–	–	–	62
GISSI-HF[16]	RCT	4574	68	77	40	–	18	34	–	3	5
SHIFT[17]	RCT	6558	60	76	68	32	–	–	–	–	–
EMPHASIS[18]	RCT	2737	69	78	69	30.9	–	–	–	–	0.1
PARADIGM[19]	RCT	8442	64	78	60	–	–	–	–	–	40
SOLVD[20]	REG	6273	62	74	69	31	7	13	–	11	–
SPICE[21]	REG	9580	66	74	63	–	4	17	5%	–	6
ADHERE[22]	REG	105,388	72	48	57%	–	–	–	–	–	–
OPTIMIZE-HF[23]	REG	48,612	73	48	46%	–	23%	–	–	–	–

RCT, randomized clinical trial; REG, registry; age, mean age in years; HT, hypertension; IDCM, idiopathic dilated cardiomyopathy; valve, valvular heart failure.

patients remain asymptomatic in response to these compensatory adjustments.[27]

Chronic remodelling and progressive cardiac injury

After myocardial infarction, cardiac structure changes occur in parallel with, and are linked to, physiological changes in activated neurohormonal systems. Activation of the sympathetic nervous system and renin–angiotensin–aldosterone system (RAAS) lead to the release of cytokines and growth factors that stimulate structural alterations at the cellular and extracellular level. The alterations include cardiac myocyte hypertrophy and extracellular matrix changes which lead to regional alterations in ventricular wall and chamber sizes in order to preserve cardiac output.[28]

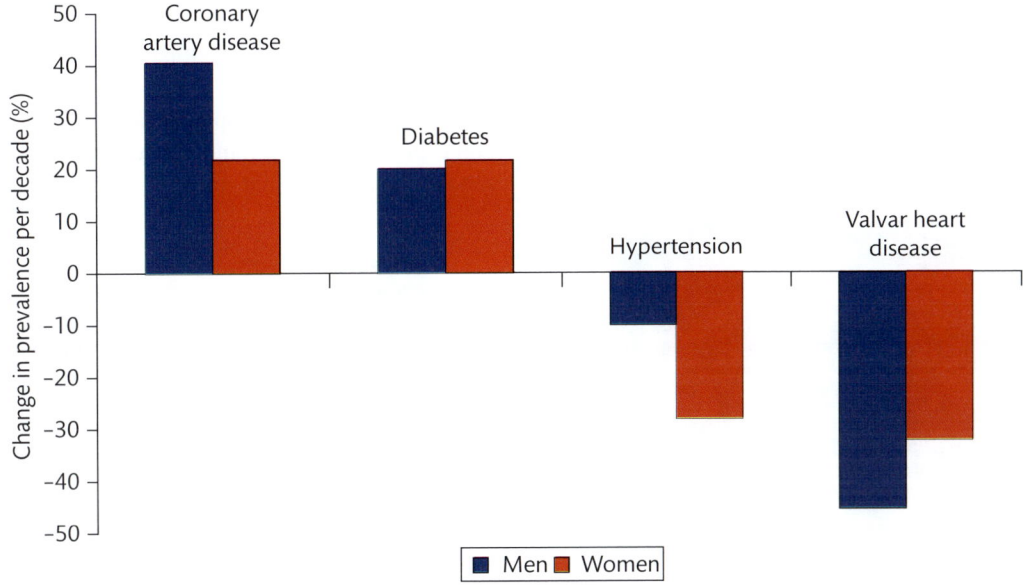

Figure 4.1 Changing pattern of aetiology of chronic heart failure in the Framingham study with time.

Republished with permission of BMJ Publishing Group Ltd, from McMurray JJ, Stewart S. Epidemiology, aetiology, and prognosis of heart failure. *Heart* 2000;**83**:596–602.

Although initially protective, compensatory mechanisms designed to maintain cardiac output may ultimately be deleterious. Chronic activation of compensatory neurohormonal processes can lead to the development of heart failure in the absence of any further ischaemic injury.[29]

Chronic catecholamine secretion promotes myocyte hypertrophy and interstitial fibrosis.[30] It also interferes with inter- and intracellular signalling pathways by inducing downregulation of adrenoreceptors and causing hyperphosphorylation of intracellular proteins. The consequence is hindrance of the ability of the adrenergic compensatory mechanisms to maintain cardiac output during future times of acute haemodynamic distress. Sympathetic nervous system activation also leads to further myocardial dysfunction by inducing the transcription of foetal genes and inducing cardiac myocyte death by promoting apoptosis and necrosis (see Chapter 12).

Chronic activation of the RAAS occurs in response to a variety of triggers including renal hypoperfusion, myocardial production of angiotensin and aldosterone in response to increased wall stress, and sympathetic nervous system activation stimulating renal renin release.[31] Although activation of the RAAS maintains blood pressure and enhances preload by stimulating vasoconstriction and renal sodium retention, harmful consequences arise from the effects of angiotensin and aldosterone on cardiac myocytes. These effects include enhancing myocardial fibrosis by promoting collagen deposition, cardiac myocyte hypertrophy, and cellular apoptosis and necrosis.

Ultimately, chronic activation of these systems damages cardiac structure and function.[27] Structural changes lead to ventricular dilatation and the heart remodels to a more globular shape (**Figure 4.2**), thereby altering atrioventricular valvular function, resulting in functional regurgitation and an increased ventricular preload. A vicious cycle ensues. Furthermore, increases in cardiac load which increase myocardial oxygen requirements may precipitate subendocardial ischaemia, exacerbating further reductions in cardiac contractility.

The transition from the index myocardial infarction to chronic heart failure is therefore complex, involving multiple regulatory mechanisms that, while initially protective and employed to maintain cardiac function, ultimately become maladaptive and destructive.

Acute complications post myocardial infarction

Acute myocardial infarction may cause acute heart failure. Particular complications include acute mitral valve incompetence secondary to papillary muscle rupture, hibernation and stunning of the left ventricle, ventricular septal defect, ventricular free wall rupture, right ventricular infarct syndrome, and cardiogenic shock.

Cardiogenic shock usually results from severe cardiac dysfunction, although the acute mechanical complications of myocardial infarction may contribute. It is defined as evidence of end-organ hypoperfusion and characterized by reduced blood pressure (systolic <90 mmHg) with raised ventricular filling pressure (pulmonary capillary wedge pressure >18 mmHg) and low cardiac output.[32]

Acute heart failure due to stunning or hibernation may completely return to normal when appropriately treated.[33] Stunning may occur following a prolonged ischaemic episode and can persist in the short term even after restoration of normal coronary blood flow. The amount and duration of stunning depends on the severity and duration of the preceding ischaemic event. Hibernation describes the state when cardiomyocytes fail to contract normally but remain structurally intact despite a significant reduction in coronary blood flow. Improving blood flow and oxygenation allows hibernating myocytes to return to normal function.

Hypertensive heart disease

Hypertension affects around a quarter of the population of the western world. It is an important cause of chronic heart failure in western societies,[1,4] and remains the most common cause in developing countries.[34] It is particularly prevalent in Africans and African-Americans.[2,35] Hypertension is proportionately more common in patients with heart failure and normal left ventricle ejection fraction (LVEF).[36]

Hypertension leads to an increase in afterload which consequently leads to concentric left ventricular hypertrophy (**Figure 4.3**). This compensatory mechanism preserves contractile function by recruiting additional sarcomere units of the muscle fibres to share the additional ventricular wall tension generated by the increased afterload, enabling higher forces and greater pressures to be generated.[37] The more hypertrophied the ventricular wall, the less tension experienced by each individual muscle fibre and consequently systolic function is not initially compromised. However, with

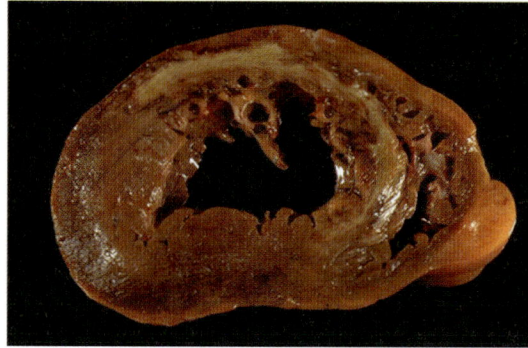

Figure 4.2 Gross pathological appearance of myocardial infarction at postmortem.

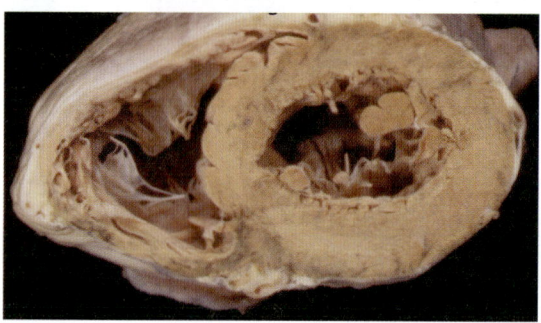

Figure 4.3 Gross pathological appearance of concentric left ventricular hypertrophy at postmortem.

progressive hypertrophy the compliance of the left ventricle reduces, producing a 'stiff' ventricle. This interferes with ventricular filling, leading to a reduction in end-diastolic volumes and an increase in left ventricular end-diastolic pressure (LVEDP). Rises in LVEDP lead to increased left atrial and pulmonary venous pressures. A consequence may be atrial arrhythmias and reduced exercise tolerance.

As left ventricular hypertrophy progresses, sarcomeres are added in parallel to established sarcomeres, leading to ventricular dilatation and systolic dysfunction. The progression from left ventricular hypertrophy to heart failure is complex, involving multiple pathophysiological processes including altered cellular signalling processes, myocyte apoptosis and increased collagen deposition.[38] As progressive pump failure develops, blood pressure may normalize, known as 'burnt out' hypertensive heart failure.

Malignant hypertension is an important cause of acute heart failure.[39] Malignant hypertension is the sudden development of severe high blood pressure with diastolic measurements often in excess of 130 mmHg. Characteristics of this condition include fundal changes (retinal haemorrhages, exudates, and papilloedema), central nervous system involvement (headache, confusion, seizures, and coma) and renal impairment (oliguria and uraemia). Malignant hypertension may present as 'flash pulmonary oedema' with very rapid onset of symptoms and signs. Flash pulmonary oedema is often seen in patients with normal LVEF. Malignant hypertension affects almost 1% of all people with essential hypertension[39] and is more common in younger adults (particularly those with secondary hypertension) and African-American men.[38,39] Although any cause of secondary hypertension may be a precursor to malignant hypertension, recurrent episodes of flash pulmonary oedema in the presence of significant hypertension is a classic presentation of renal artery stenosis. Other causes include phaeochromocytoma and Conn's syndrome.[39]

Valvular heart disease

Valvular dysfunction can be a cause (primary) or effect (secondary) of heart failure, with acquired valvular heart disease accounting for most cases. There is a geographical variation in valvular pathology; for example, rheumatic valvular heart disease is a common cause of heart failure in the developing world.[4] Valvular heart disease will be discussed in more detail in Chapter 36.

Primary valvular pathology causing heart failure

Aortic valve disease

Aortic stenosis and regurgitation are common valvular abnormalities. Both can have long, latent, asymptomatic stages but progression in severity will ultimately lead to heart failure if left untreated.

Aortic stenosis is the most common valvular heart disease in developed countries and a frequent cause of heart failure internationally.[41] The three main causes are congenital, rheumatic, and degenerative. Degenerative aortic stenosis is more common in western societies and tends to present in elderly populations (Figure 4.4), and as a result, the prevalence of this valvular pathology is increasing as the average life expectancy increases.[41] A chronic inflammatory process involving deposition of lipids in the valve leaflets is followed by calcification of the valve annulus and subsequently the valve leaflets, limiting the circulatory flow

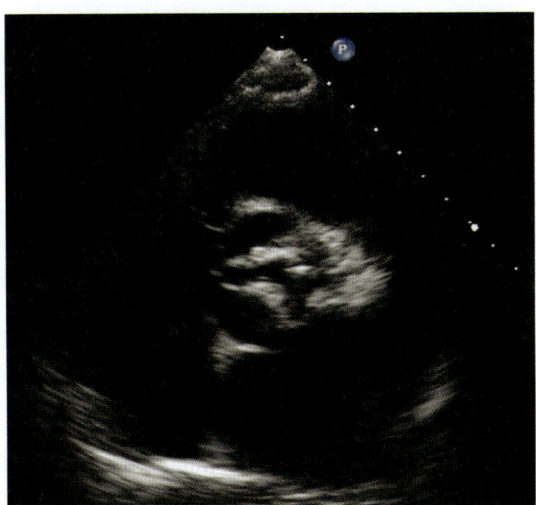

Figure 4.4 Short-axis parasternal view on transthoracic echocardiogram showing a calcified tricuspid aortic valve.

across the aortic valve.[42,43] Rheumatic aortic valve disease is more common in developing countries[41] and leads to stenosis by causing inflammatory-mediated fusion of the commissures and a reduction in the valve orifice area. Aortic stenosis causes heart failure by obstructing left ventricular outflow, resulting in an increased afterload, lower stroke volume, and reduced ejection fraction, with advanced disease suspected by the presence of symptoms. The severity of aortic stenosis is best assessed by calculating valve orifice area and using dobutamine stress echocardiograph.[44]

Aortic regurgitation may be acute or chronic. Acute severe aortic regurgitation (e.g. secondary to infective endocarditis, aortic dissection, or trauma) is potentially life-threatening by causing extremely elevated left ventricular filling pressures, severe pulmonary oedema, and inadequate cardiac output.[45] Chronic aortic regurgitation shares the same three main causes as aortic stenosis—congenital, rheumatic, and degenerative. Other less common causes include infective endocarditis, connective tissue or inflammatory diseases, antiphospholipid syndrome, anorectic drugs, and trauma.[46] Untreated, chronic aortic regurgitation slowly progresses from volume overload and left ventricular hypertrophy to left ventricular dilatation, then contractile dysfunction.[46] Patients are often asymptomatic in the early stages of disease and may remain so after the left ventricle has begun to dilate. LVSD is potentially reversible if valve repair/replacement is undertaken soon after the onset of contractile dysfunction.

Mitral valve disease

Mitral regurgitation may be caused by primary (e.g. rheumatic heart disease, infective endocarditis, mitral valve prolapse and connective tissue disease) or secondary valve disease.[47] Most patients with mitral regurgitation have a slow, insidious progression of their valve disease. Many are asymptomatic in the early stage, although the presentation may be more acute in cases of infective endocarditis. Progression to severe mitral regurgitation usually results in the development of symptoms of left-sided heart failure and pathophysiological consequences of left ventricular remodelling, left ventricular dysfunction, and pulmonary hypertension.[47] Sudden symptomatic deterioration is often seen with the subsequent development of atrial fibrillation secondary to left atrial dilatation.

Mitral stenosis is a primary valve disease, most commonly caused by rheumatic fever and persistent inflammatory valve disease in developing countries, and by degenerative disease with calcification of the annulus in developed countries.[48] As with mitral regurgitation, the early stages of this valve disease may be asymptomatic. As the severity of the stenosis progresses, a series of pathological changes ensues, ultimately leading to a rise in left atrial pressure with dilatation of the atrium and consequently development of pulmonary hypertension,[48] leading to symptoms of exertional breathlessness. The development of atrial fibrillation may be associated with pulmonary oedema. Left ventricular systolic function is usually preserved in severe mitral stenosis.

Tricuspid valve disease

Tricuspid stenosis is a more prevalent valvular pathology in developing countries, as the vast majority of cases are caused by rheumatic heart disease,[49] and it usually coexists with mitral stenosis. The main causes of solitary tricuspid stenosis are congenital heart disease, discussed below, and carcinoid syndrome.[49,50] Tricuspid stenosis may be detected by the auscultation of a diastolic murmur, loudest in inspiration. Clinical signs of heart failure are those of right heart failure.

Tricuspid regurgitation is most commonly functional. However, primary tricuspid regurgitation may be caused by infective endocarditis (particularly in intravenous drug users), or rheumatic valve disease, as well as carcinoid syndrome.[51] Symptoms and signs of tricuspid regurgitation are those of right-sided heart failure with a classic pan-systolic murmur accentuated by inspiration.

Pulmonary valve disease

Pulmonary stenosis is exclusively a form of congenital heart disease. Most cases of pulmonary regurgitation also occur in patients with congenital heart disease, the causes of which are outlined below. Acquired cases of pulmonary regurgitation are rare and include infective endocarditis or carcinoid syndrome.

Secondary valvular dysfunction causing heart failure

Valvular dysfunction may be the consequence of many other causes of heart failure. Any cause of left-ventricular dilatation can result in regurgitation of the aortic, mitral and tricuspid valves, known as functional regurgitation: the valve dysfunction is related to the abnormal ventricular shape and function. Functional mitral regurgitation is common in ischaemic cardiomyopathy, where dilatation of the valve annulus prevents coaptation of the valve leaflets (**Figure 4.5**).[52] Secondary mitral valve dysfunction can also result from failure of the valve apparatus following acute myocardial infarction if there is rupture or stretching of the chordae or papillary muscle,[52] often presenting with the sudden onset of pulmonary oedema. Functional tricuspid regurgitation may be caused by several pathologies including: right ventricular dysfunction, left-sided valvular disease causing pulmonary hypertension, left ventricular dysfunction, or chronic pulmonary disease.[51]

Adult congenital valvular heart disease

A detailed account of congenital heart disease as a cause of heart failure is given in Chapter 7. A brief summary of congenital valve disease follows.

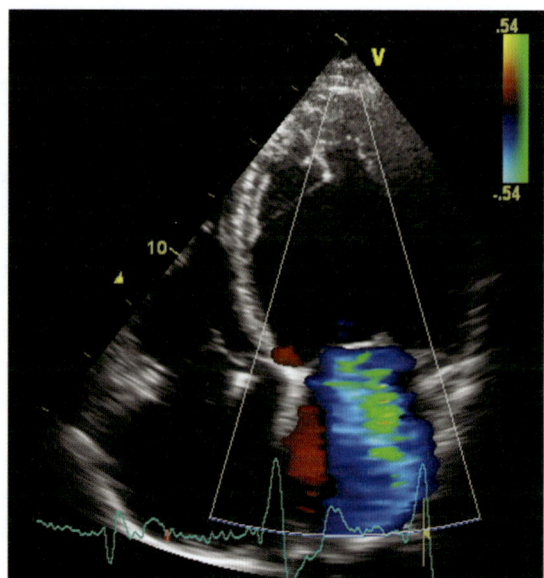

Figure 4.5 Four-chamber apical view on trans-thoracic echocardiogram showing a jet of severe mitral regurgitation.

Pulmonary valve disease is usually congenital and detected early in childhood. Pulmonary stenosis may occur as an isolated congenital abnormality or as a feature of Noonan's syndrome or Tetralogy of Fallot.[53] The symptomatic presentation is usually breathlessness with chronic progression to right heart failure.

Clinically significant pulmonary regurgitation occurs almost exclusively in patients with congenital heart disease. It may be a long-term complication of the repair of Tetralogy of Fallot[54] and occur secondary to transannular patching, commissurotomy of the pulmonary valve or failure of a pulmonary conduit. Progression in the severity of pulmonary regurgitation leads to right ventricular dilatation and subsequent right ventricular systolic dysfunction, reduced exercise tolerance, and ventricular arrhythmias.[54] Sudden death may be a sequela of this condition.

Congenital tricuspid valve disease most commonly occurs as part of Ebstein's anomaly,[55] a condition characterized by apical displacement of the septal and posterior valve leaflets, leading to atrialization of a portion of the right ventricle. The structural deformity of the valve leads to tricuspid regurgitation, and although often detected in childhood, Ebstein's anomaly may present in adulthood with symptoms of fatigue, exercise intolerance, palpitations, and dyspnoea. Signs include cyanosis, a tricuspid regurgitant murmur, and right-sided heart failure. Arrhythmias are common, with supraventricular tachycardias occurring in approximately one-third. Ventricular arrhythmias are due to the presence of accessory pathways and sudden death may occur.

Arrhythmias

Arrhythmias are common in patients with heart failure, and may be either be a cause or a consequence of it. Defining the cause-and-effect relationship can be difficult, particularly when tachycardia and cardiomyopathy present at the same time. Heart failure predisposes to arrhythmias due to structural and electrical remodelling (see Chapter 39).

Sustained tachycardias may lead to heart failure (a tachy-cardiomyopathy or tachycardia-related cardiomyopathy). The uncontrolled ventricular rate invariably results in systolic dysfunc-tion and is frequently accompanied by ventricular dilatation.[56] Thus, tachyarrhythmias may lead to a reduction in LVEF, an in-crease in end-diastolic and end-systolic volumes, and an increase in end-diastolic and pulmonary artery pressures. The degree of LVSD does not necessarily correlate with the duration or rate of the tachy-cardia.[57] Making the diagnosis is crucial, as treatment can be poten-tially curative (Figure 4.6).[58–60]

The most common causes of tachycardiomyopathy are inces-sant atrial arrhythmias. The cardiomyopathy and tachycardia often

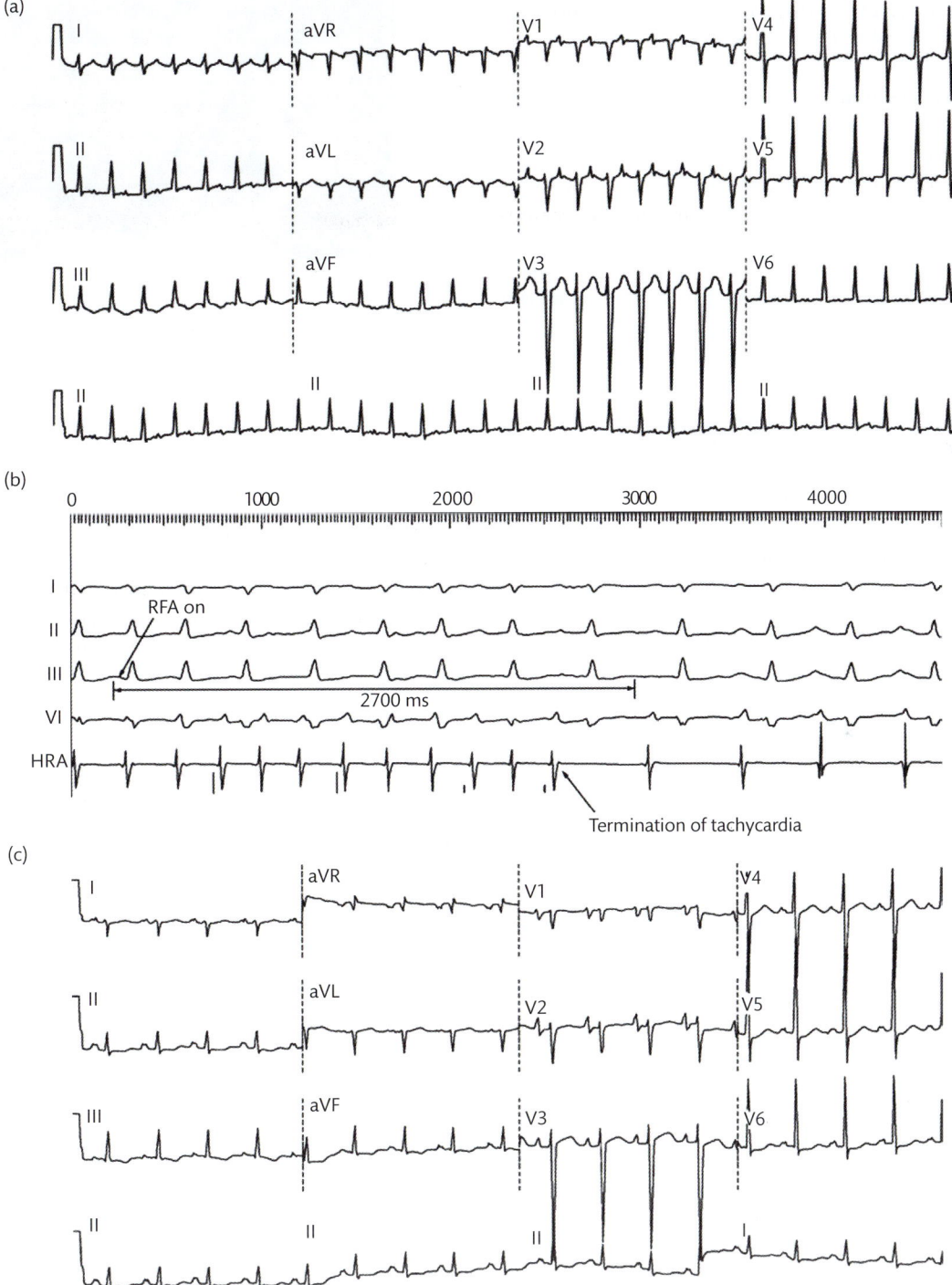

Figure 4.6 (a) Electrocardiogram (ECG) on admission for patient with tachycardiomyopathy. (b) Electrophysiological studies subsequently demonstrated an incessant right atrial tachycardia. Echocardiography showed a dilated, poorly contracting left ventricle. (c) Radiofrequency ablation (RFA) was curative for the atrial tachycardia and resulted in restoration of normal ventricular size and a significant improvement in ventricular function. ECG post RFA is displayed.

Reproduced from Walker NL, Cobbe SM, Birnie DH. Tachycardiomyopathy: a diagnosis not to be missed. *Heart* 2004;**90**:e7.

present simultaneously. Potential causes include atrial tachycardia, re-entrant tachycardia, and atrial fibrillation (AF).[61]

Atrial fibrillation is common in heart failure, with each condition predisposing to the other.[62] Some 10–50% of patients with LVSD have AF,[63] although AF is also common in patients with heart failure and preserved systolic function.[64] Haemodynamic disturbances associated with AF include the loss of atrial contraction (and subsequent contribution to ventricular filling), an irregular ventricular rhythm, tachycardia, and activation of the deleterious neurohumoral systems. These all contribute to a reduction in cardiac output.[65]

Ventricular tachyarrhythmias are also common in chronic heart failure (see Chapter 36). Although more commonly a consequence of heart failure, ventricular tachycardia can potentially cause a tachycardiomyopathy if there are frequent paroxysms or the tachycardia is incessant.[66] The likely focus of ventricular tachycardia that is stable enough to cause a tachycardiomyopathy is from the right ventricular outflow tract.[67] This form of ventricular tachycardia is identified by the pattern of left bundle branch block with an inferior axis. Recognition of this arrhythmia is extremely important as it can be potentially cured by radiofrequency ablation.[67]

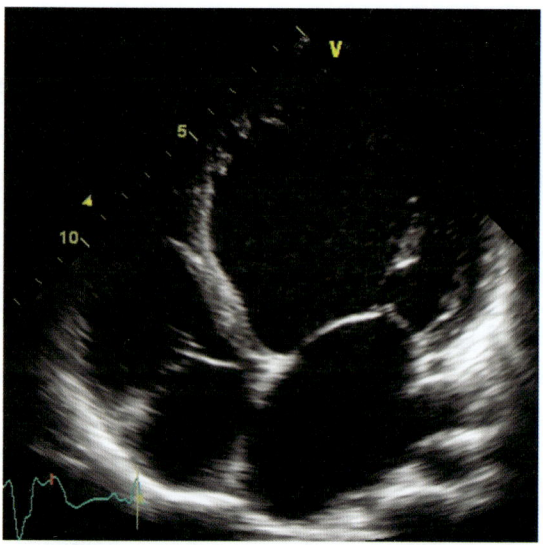

Figure 4.7 Four-chamber apical view on trans-thoracic echocardiogram showing a dilated cardiomyopathy of alcohol aetiology or pathology at postmortem of dilated ventricle of alcohol aetiology.

Alcohol

Alcohol excess is one of the commonest causes of a dilated cardiomyopathy and accounts for at least one-third of all cases.[68] There are no pathognomonic signs or specific tests for diagnosing alcoholic cardiomyopathy. It is impossible to differentiate it pathologically from other causes of dilated cardiomyopathy, and non-specific pathological findings include interstitial fibrosis, myocytolysis, small-vessel coronary artery disease, and myocyte hypertrophy.[68] The diagnosis depends on a history of excessive alcohol consumption and the absence of other causes of cardiomyopathy. Two distinct phases and modes of clinical presentation of alcoholic heart disease are recognized: asymptomatic and symptomatic. The latter may be further divided into acute and chronic stages. Consumption of more than 90 g of alcohol per day for at least five years increases the risk of asymptomatic alcoholic cardiomyopathy.[67,68] The asymptomatic phase is often associated with diastolic dysfunction, whereas continual consumption of excess alcohol increases the risk of developing symptomatic heart failure which is frequently associated with LVSD (Figure 4.7).[68] Importantly, in contrast with many other causes of cardiomyopathy, disease progression can be terminated or even reversed by complete abstinence from alcohol. However, the prognosis for patients with alcoholic cardiomyopathy who continue to consume excess alcohol is poor.[70]

Alcohol and its metabolites have direct toxic effects on cardiac myocytes, including disruption of: calcium transport and binding, mitochondrial respiration, lipid metabolism, myocardial protein synthesis, and cellular signal transduction[71] as well as apoptosis.[67] Alcohol excess may have other indirect toxic effects on the myocardium such as those derived from nutritional deficiencies (e.g. vitamin B_1 deficiency). Myocardial impairment due to cobalt sulphate (used as an additive) no longer occurs as this substance is no longer used in beer manufacturing.

Symptomatic alcoholic cardiomyopathy may present with any of the symptoms or signs of dilated cardiomyopathy of any aetiology, either as acute pulmonary oedema or more commonly with chronic heart failure. AF is a frequent finding in alcoholic cardiomyopathy (more so than other arrhythmias), and a paroxysm of AF is a common initial presenting sign. Stigmata of chronic liver disease may also be evident.

Approximately one-third of all alcoholics have evidence of LVSD. However, not all alcoholics develop a dilated cardiomyopathy and the reason for this is likely to be multifactorial. There is a genetic predisposition to alcohol cardiomyopathy. The DD genotype of the angiotensin converting enzyme gene polymorphism increases the risk of developing cardiomyopathy by 16 times in those who consume excess alcohol.[72]

Summary

Heart failure is the common endpoint of a diverse range of cardiovascular and non-cardiovascular conditions. The list of potential causes of this syndrome continues to expand as our knowledge of the pathophysiology of heart failure increases. In western societies, coronary heart disease and hypertension remain the commonest causes of heart failure. The prevalence of heart failure secondary to coronary heart disease has increased in recent years, due in part to improved survival following acute myocardial infarction. In addition to coronary disease and hypertension, valvular heart disease, arrhythmias, and alcohol are other common causes of heart failure in developed countries.

REFERENCES

1. McMurray JJ, Stewart S. Epidemiology, aetiology, and prognosis of heart failure. *Heart* 2000;**83**:596–602.
2. Kalinowski L, Dobrucki IT, Malinski T. Race-specific differences in endothelial function. Predisposition of African Americans to vascular diseases. *Circulation* 2004;**109**:2511–17.

3. Cubillos-Garzon LA, Casas JP, Morillo CA, Bautista LE. Congestive heart failure in Latin America: the next epidemic. *Am Heart J* 2004;**147**:412–17.

4. Cowie MR, Mosterd A, Wood DA, *et al*. The epidemiology of heart failure. *Eur Heart J* 1997;**18**:208–225.

5. SOLVD Investigators. Effect of enalapril in survival in patients with reduced left ventricular ejection fractions and congestive heart failure. *N Engl J Med* 1991;**325**:293–302.

6. Digitalis Investigation Group. The effect of digoxin on mortality and morbidity in patients with heart failure. *N Engl J Med* 1997;**336**:525–33.

7. MERIT Investigators. Effect of metoprolol CR/XL in chronic heart failure: metoprolol CR/XL randomised intervention trial in congestive heart failure (Merit-HF). *Lancet* 1999;**353**:2001–7.

8. CIBIS-II Investigators and Committees. The Cardiac Insufficiency Bisoprolol Study II (CIBIS-II): a randomised trial. *Lancet* 1999;**353**:9–13.

9. Packer M, Poole-Wilson PA, Armstrong PW, *et al*. Comparative effects of low and high doses of the angiotensin-converting enzyme inhibitor, lisinopril, on morbidity and mortality in chronic heart failure. ATLAS Study Group. *Circulation* 1999;**100**:2312–18.

10. Pitt B, Zannad F, Remme WJ, *et al*. The effect of spironolactone on morbidity and mortality in patients with heart failure. Randomized aldactone evaluation study investigators. *N Engl J Med* 1999;**341**:709–17.

11. Cohn J, Tognoni G; for the Valsartan Heart Failure Trial Investigators. A randomized trial of the angiotensin-receptor blocker valsartan in chronic heart failure. *N Engl J Med* 2001;**345**:1667–75.

12. Packer M, Coats AJ, Fowler MB, *et al*.; Carvedilol Prospective Randomized Cumulative Survival Study Group. Effect of carvedilol on survival in severe chronic heart failure. *N Engl J Med* 2001;**344**:1651–8.

13. Poole-Wilson PA, Swedberg K, Cleland JG, *et al*.; Carvedilol Or Metoprolol European Trial Investigators. Comparison of carvedilol and metoprolol on clinical outcomes in patients with chronic heart failure in the Carvedilol Or Metoprolol European Trial (COMET): randomized controlled trial. *Lancet* 2003;**362**:7–13.

14. Bristow MR, Saxon LA, Boehmer J, *et al*.; Comparison of Medical Therapy, Pacing, and Defibrillation in Heart Failure (COMPANION) Investigators. Cardiac-resynchronization therapy with or without an implantable defibrillator in advanced chronic heart failure. *N Engl J Med* 2004;**350**:2140–50.

15. Cleland JGF, Daubert JC, Erdmann E, *et al*.; for the Cardiac Resynchronization—Heart Failure (CARE-HF) Study Investigators. The effect of cardiac resynchronization on morbidity and mortality in heart failure. *N Engl J Med* 2005;**352**:1539–49.

16. GISSI-HF Investigators, Tavazzi L, Maggioni AP, Marchioli R, *et al*. Effect of rosuvastatin in patients with chronic heart failure (the GISSI-HF trial): a randomised, double-blind, placebo-controlled trial. *Lancet* 2008;**372**:1231–39.

17. Swedberg K, Komajda M, Böhm M, *et al*.; SHIFT Investigators. Ivabradine and outcomes in chronic heart failure (SHIFT): a randomised placebo-controlled study. *Lancet* 2010;**376**:875–85.

18. Zannad F, McMurray JJ, Krum H, *et al*.; EMPHASIS-HF Study Group. Eplerenone in patients with systolic heart failure and mild symptoms. *N Engl J Med* 2011;**364**:11–21.

19. McMurray JJ, Packer M, Desai AS, *et al*.; PARADIGM-HF Investigators and Committees. *N Engl J Med* 2014;**37**:993–1004.

20. SOLVD Investigators. Natural history and patterns of current practice in heart failure. *J Am Coll Cardiol* 1993;**4A**:14A–19A.

21. Bart BA, Ertl G, Held P, *et al*. Contemporary management of patients with left ventricular systolic dysfunction. Results from the study of patients intolerant of converting enzyme inhibitors (SPICE) registry. *Eur Heart J* 1999;**20**:1182–90.

22. Adams KF Jr, Fonarow GC, Emerman CL, *et al*.; ADHERE Scientific Advisory Committee and Investigators. Characteristics and outcomes of patients hospitalized for heart failure in the United States: rationale, design, and preliminary observations from the first 100,000 cases in the Acute Decompensated Heart Failure National Registry (ADHERE). *Am Heart J* 2005;**149**:209–16.

23. Fonarow GC, Abraham WT, Albert NM, *et al*.; OPTIMIZE-HF investigators and hospitals. Influence of a performance-improvement initiative on quality of care for patients hospitalized with heart failure. *Arch Intern Med* 2007;**167**:1493–1502.

24. Kannel WB, Ho KK, Thom T. Changing epidemiological features of cardiac failure. *Br Heart J* 1994;**72**(2 Suppl):S3–9.

25. Velagaleti RS, Pencina MJ, Murabito JM, *et al*. Long-term trends in the incidence of heart failure after myocardial infarction. *Circulation* 2008;**118**:2057–2062.

26. Furberg CD, Yusuf S. Effect of drug therapy on survival in chronic heart failure. *Adv Cardiol* 1986;**34**:124–30.

27. Mann DL, Bristow MR. Mechanisms and models in heart failure. The biomechanical model and beyond. *Circulation* 2005;**111**:2837–49.

28. Jessup M, Brozena S. Heart failure. *N Engl J Med* 2003;**348**:2007–18.

29. Pfeffer MA, Braunwald E. Ventricular remodelling after myocardial infarction: experimental observations and clinical implications. *Circulation* 1990;**81**:1161–72.

30. Bristow MR. β-Adrenergic receptor blockade in chronic heart failure. *Circulation* 2000;**101**:558–69.

31. Francis GS, Goldsmith SR, Levine TB, Olivari MT, Cohn JN. The neurohumoral axis in congestive heart failure. *Ann Intern Med* 1984;**101**:370–7.

32. Nieminen MS, Böhm M, Cowie MR, *et al*.; ESC Committe for Practice Guideline (CPG). Executive summary of the guidelines on the diagnosis and treatment of acute heart failure: the Task Force on Acute Heart Failure of the European Society of Cardiology. *Eur Heart J* 2005;**26**:384–416.

33. Dutka DP, Camici PG. Hibernation and congestive heart failure. *Heart Fail Rev* 2003;**8**:167–73.

34. Amoah AG, Kallen C. Aetiology of heart failure as seen from a National Cardiac Referral Centre in Africa. *Cardiology* 2000;**93**:11–18.

35. Kahn DF, Duffy SJ, Tomasian D, *et al*. Effects of black race on forearm resistance vessel function. *Hypertension* 2002;**40**:195–201.

36. Hogg K, Swedberg K, McMurray JJ. Heart failure with preserved left ventricular systolic function: epidemiology, clinical characteristics, and prognosis. *J Am Coll Cardiol* 2004;**43**:317–27.

37. James MA, Saadeh AM, Jones JV. Wall stress and hypertension. *J Cardiovasc Risk* 2000;**7**:187–90.

38. Lips DJ, deWindt LJ, van Kraaij DJW, Doevendans PA. Molecular determinants of myocardial hypertrophy and failure: alternative pathways for beneficial and maladaptive hypertrophy. *Eur Heart J* 2003;**24**:883–896.

39. Kitiyakara C, Guzman N. Malignant hypertension and hypertensive emergencies. *J Am Soc Nephrol* 1998;**9**:133–142.

40. Lip GY, Beevers M, Beevers G. The failure of malignant hypertension to decline: a survey of 24 years' experience in a multi-racial population in England. *J Hypertens* 1994;**12**:1297–305.

41. Carabello B, Paulus W. Aortic stenosis. *Lancet* 2009;**373**:956–66.

42. Otto CM, Kuusisto J, Reichenbach DD, Gown AM, O'Brien KD. Characterization of the early lesion of degenerative valvular aortic stenosis: histological and immunohistochemical studies. *Circulation* 1994;**90**:844–53.

43. Aronow WS, Ahn C, Kronzon I, Goldman ME. Association of coronary risk factors and use of statins with progression of mild valvular aortic stenosis in older persons. *Am J Cardiol* 2001;**88**:693–95.

44. deFilippi CR, Willett DL, Brickner ME, *et al.* Usefulness of dobutamine echocardiography in distinguishing severe from nonsevere valvular aortic stenosis in patients with depressed left ventricular function and low transvalvular gradients. *Am J Cardiol* 1995;**75**:191–4.

45. Cohn LH, Birjiniuk V. Therapy of acute aortic regurgitation. *Cardiol Clin* 1991;**9**:339–52.

46. Bekeredjian R, Grayburn PA. Valvular heart disease: aortic regurgitation. *Circulation* 2005;**112**:125–34.

47. Carabello B. The current therapy for mitral regurgitation. *J Am Coll Cardiol* 2008;**52**:319–26.

48. Chandrashekhar Y, Westaby S, Narula J. Mitral stenosis. *Lancet* 2009;**374**:1271–83.

49. Waller BF, Howard J, Fess S. Pathology of tricuspid valve stenosis and pure tricuspid regurgitation—Part 1. *Clin Cardiol* 1995;**18**:97–102.

50. Gustafsson BI, Hauso O, Drozdov I, Kidd M, Modlin IM. Carcinoid heart disease. *Int J Cardiol* 2008;**129**:318–324.

51. Shah P, Raney A. Tricuspid valve disease. *Curr Prob Cardiol* 2008;**33**:47–84.

52. Marwick TH, Lancellotti P, Pierard L. Ischaemic mitral regurgitation: mechanisms and diagnosis. *Heart* 2009;**95**:1711–18.

53. Bonow RO, Carabello BA, Chatterjee K, *et al.* ACC/AHA 2006 Guidelines for the Management of Patient With Valvular Heart Disease: A Report of the American College of Cardiology/American Heart Association Task Force on Practice Guidelines. *Circulation* 2006;**114**:e84–e231.

54. Apitz C, Webb GD, Redington AN. Tetralogy of Fallot. *Lancet* 2009;**374**:1462–71.

55. Paranon S, Acar P. Ebstein's anomaly of the tricuspid valve: from fetus to adult: congenital heart disease. *Heart* 2008;**94**:237–43.

56. Brugada P, Andries E. Tachycardiomopathy. The most frequently unrecognized cause of heart failure? *Acta Cardiol* 1993;**2**:165–169.

57. Packer DL, Bardy GH, Worley SJ, *et al.* Tachycardia-induced cardiomyopathy: a reversible form of LV dysfunction. *Am J Cardiol* 1986;**57**:563–570.

58. Rabbani LE, Wang PJ, Couper GL, Friedman PL. Time course of improvement in ventricular function after ablation of incessant automatic atrial tachycardia. *Am Heart J* 1991;**121**:816–19.

59. Tavernier R, De Pauw M, Trouerbach J. Incessant automatic atrial tachycardia: a reversible cause of tachycardiomyopathy. *Acta Cardiol* 1999;**54**:227–9.

60. Walker NL, Cobbe SM, Birnie DH. Tachycardiomyopathy: a diagnosis not to be missed. *Heart* 2004;**90**:e7.

61. Shinbane JS, Wood MA, Jensen DN, *et al.* Tachycardia-induced cardiomyopathy: a review of animal models and clinical studies. *J Am Coll Cardiol* 1997;**29**:709–15.

62. Wang TJ, Larson MG, Levy D, *et al.* Temporal relations of atrial fibrillation and congestive heart failure and their joint influence on mortality: the Framingham Heart Study. *Circulation* 2003;**107**:2920–5.

63. AF-CHF Trial Investigators. Rationale and design of a study assessing treatment strategies of atrial fibrillation in patients with heart failure: the Atrial Fibrillation and Congestive Heart Failure (AF-CHF) trial. *Am Heart J* 2002;**144**:597–607.

64. Olsson LG, Swedberg K, Ducharme A, *et al.*; CHARM Investigators. Atrial fibrillation and risk of clinical events in chronic heart failure with and without left ventricular systolic dysfunction: results from the Candesartan in Heart failure-Assessment of Reduction in Mortality and morbidity (CHARM) program. *J Am Coll Cardiol* 2006;**47**:1997–2004.

65. Efremidis M, Pappas L, Sideris A, Filippatos G. Management of atrial fibrillation in patients with heart failure. *J Cardiac Fail* 2008;**14**:232–7.

66. Umana E, Solares CA, Alpert MA. Tachycardia-induced cardiomyopathy. *Am J Med* 2003;**114**:51–5.

67. Jaggarao NS, Nanda AS, Daubert JP. Ventricular tachycardia induced cardiomyopathy: improvement with radiofrequency ablation. *Pacing Clin Electrophysiol* 1996;**19**:505–8.

68. Piano MR. Alcoholic cardiomyopathy: incidence, clinical characteristics, and pathophysiology. *Chest* 2002;**121**(5):1638–50.

69. Laonigro I, Correale M, Di Biase M, Altomare E. Alcohol abuse and heart failure. *Eur J Heart Fail* 2009;**11**:453–462.

70. Lazarevic AM, Nakatani S, Neskovic AN, *et al.* Early changes in left ventricular function in chronic asymptomatic alcoholics: relation to the duration of heavy drinking. *J Am Coll Cardiol* 2000;**35**:1599.

71. Duan J, McFadden GE, Borgerding AJ, *et al.* Overexpression of alcohol dehydrogenase exacerbates ethanol-induced contractile defect in cardiac myocytes. *Am J Physiol* 2002;**282**:H1216.

72. Fernandez-Sola J, Nicolas JM, Oriola J, *et al.* Angiotensin-converting enzyme gene polymorphism is associated with vulnerability to alcoholic cardiomyopathy. *Ann Intern Med* 2002;**137**:321.

5

The genetics of heart failure

Giuseppe Limongelli and Perry M. Elliott

Introduction

Heart failure, defined in its broadest sense as a syndrome characterized by symptoms and signs of ventricular dysfunction in the presence of structural and or functional abnormalities of heart function, affects millions of people worldwide; in addition, a substantial number of individuals have asymptomatic abnormalities of heart function that predispose them to symptomatic heart failure in later life. Coronary artery disease and hypertension are by far the most common causes of heart failure, but a substantial minority of cases is caused by a heterogeneous group of heart muscle diseases, the cardiomyopathies. These disorders differ in several important respects from other causes of heart failure in that they are often familial and present throughout life. With recent advances in the understanding of the molecular genetics of cardiomyopathies,[1–10] cardiologists are having to adapt diagnostic and treatment protocols in order to optimize management of individual patients and their families. This chapter reviews the clinical presentation and pathophysiology of the most common genetic forms of cardiomyopathy.

Cardiomyopathies

Definitions and nomenclature

In 1957 Wallace Brigden observed that when describing heart muscle disorders, 'adjectives such as isolated, idiopathic, non-specific, specific, interstitial, diffuse, and circumscribed abound in the literature; others, such as acute, subacute, chronic pernicious, and malignant, relate to the clinical picture; while still others, such as eosinophilic, allergic, idiosyncratic, and granulomatous hint at aetiology, as does familial cardiomegaly'.[11] His contribution to the resolution of this nosological confusion was to use the term cardiomyopathy to denote 'isolated non-coronary myocardial disease'. In 1961, John Goodwin promulgated this concept by defining cardiomyopathies as disorders of heart muscle 'of unknown or obscure aetiology, often with endocardial, and sometimes with pericardial involvement, but not atherosclerotic in origin'.[12] Subtypes of cardiomyopathy were defined using specific morphological and physiological features.[13] This scheme for classifying heart muscle disorders survived largely unchanged until a review by a joint World Health Organization (WHO)/International

Society and Federation of Cardiology (ISFC) panel in 1995,[14] in which the rigid distinction between primary and secondary disease was blurred and a new entity—arrhythmogenic right ventricular cardiomyopathy (ARVC)—was formally recognized.

In 2007, the Working Group on Myocardial and Pericardial Diseases of the European Society of Cardiology (ESC) proposed an update of the WHO/ISFC classification, defining cardiomyopathy as 'a myocardial disorder in which the heart muscle is structurally and functionally abnormal in the absence of coronary artery disease, hypertension, valvular disease and congenital heart disease sufficient to explain the observed myocardial abnormality'.[15] Cardiomyopathies were still grouped into specific morphological and functional phenotypes, but each phenotype was subclassified into familial/genetic and non-familial/non genetic forms; the distinction between primary and secondary forms was abandoned. This current scheme for grouping cardiomyopathies is still in use but continues to evolve. ARVC, in particular, is increasingly abbreviated to arrhythmogenic cardiomyopathy, in recognition of overlapping phenotypes that affect both ventricles. There is also a move towards more comprehensive disease nomenclatures that summarize aetiological, morphological, functional and clinical manifestations in a notation system similar to that used to describe cancers.[16]

Cardiomyopathy subtypes

Four major types of cardiomyopathy are recognized:

Dilated cardiomyopathy

Dilated cardiomyopathy (DCM) is defined by the presence of left ventricular dilation and systolic impairment in the absence of abnormal loading conditions (e.g. hypertension, valve disease) or coronary artery disease sufficient to cause systolic dysfunction.[9,10,15]

The term DCM encompasses a broad range of genetic and acquired disorders that manifest as a spectrum of electrical and functional abnormalities that change with time and often coexist with right ventricular dilatation and dysfunction. This applies particularly to genetic diseases that have delayed or incomplete cardiac expression, with mild or absent dilatation or systolic dysfunction in spite of the presence of clinically significant myocardial disease. Recently, the ESC Working Group on Myocardial and Pericardial

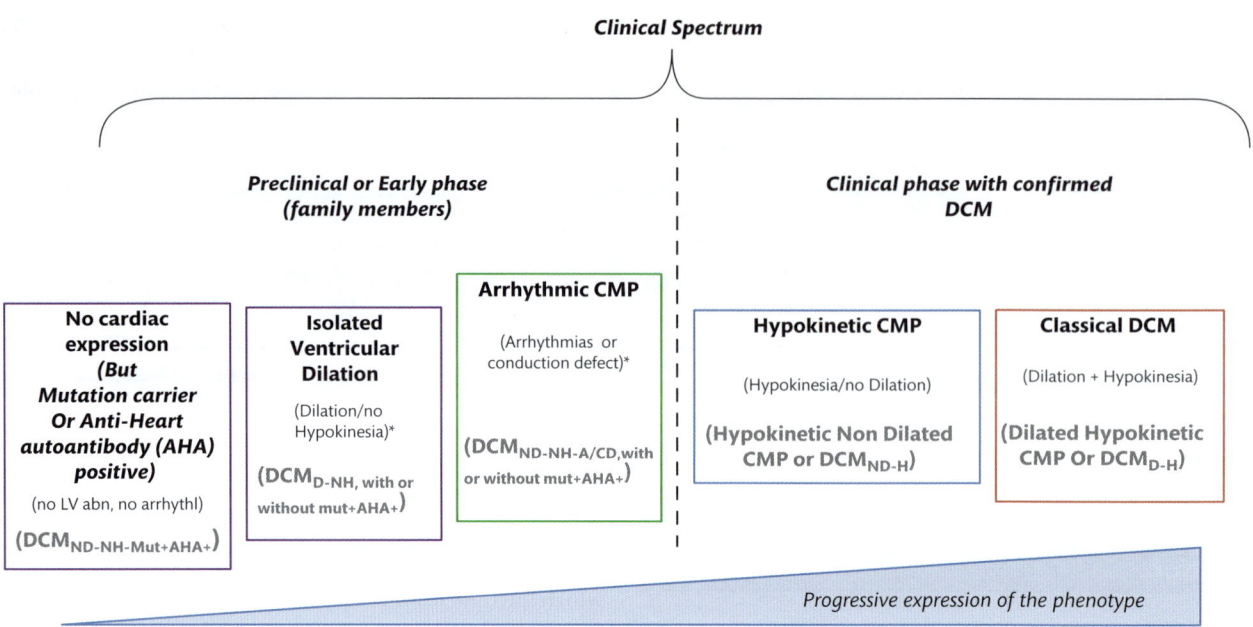

Figure 5.1 Dilated cardiomyopathy: new definition and clinical spectrum.

Diseases has proposed a new definition of DCM to take account of this heterogeneity.[17] The major innovation is the creation of a subcategory of hypokinetic non-DCM (i.e. left or biventricular systolic dysfunction without dilatation unexplained by abnormal loading conditions or coronary artery disease (**Figure 5.1**), which often represents the preclinical phase of disease in relatives.

The prevalence of DCM is estimated at one in 2500 adults, with an annual incidence of between five and eight per 100 000.[18] In children the incidence is much lower (0.5–0.8 per 100 000), but DCM is the commonest cardiomyopathy in the paediatric population.[19,20] Some 20–30% of adult patients with DCM have a familial predisposition.[21] The reported prevalence of familial DCM in paediatric studies is lower (up to 17%).[22,23] Most genetic forms are transmitted as an autosomal dominant trait, but other forms of inheritance, including autosomal recessive, X-linked, and matrilinear occur.[1,9,10] A variety of genes expressed within the cardiomyocyte is implicated in Mendelian forms of DCM, ranging from the cardiac sarcomere, the nuclear envelope, transcription factors, and the dystrophin-associated cytoskeletal complex.[1,9,10] DCM with a typical phenotype comprising bradycardia, conduction disorders, and atrial fibrillation has been associated with *SCN5A* mutations.[24]

Using a genome-wide association study (GWAS), a European consortium study on DCM[25] identified three DCM-associated single-nucleotide polymorphisms (SNPs). One identified locus involves rs2234962, a non-synonymous SNP (c.T757C, p. C151R) located within the coding sequence of BAG3 (BCL2-associated athanogene 3) on chromosome 10q26. The authors also identified rare variants in this gene, which segregated in families with familial DCM. This is one of the rare examples of the same genetic locus showing an association between rare variants with large effect and rare familial monogenetic disease on the one hand, and common variants with small effects with sporadic common diseases on the other. Next-generation sequencing (NGS) of candidate genes reveals definite

or probable causative mutations in 25–50% of patients with DCM depending on the presence of a family history.[9,10,26]

Hypertrophic cardiomyopathy

Hypertrophic cardiomyopathy (HCM)[27] is defined by the presence of increased left ventricular (LV) wall thickness that is not solely explained by abnormal loading conditions. Studies in North America, Europe, Japan, and China consistently report the prevalence of unexplained LV hypertrophy to be approximately one in 500 adults.[18,28–32] The prevalence of HCM in children is unknown, but two population studies report an annual incidence of 0.3–0.5 per 100 000.[19,20]

In most adolescents and adults, HCM is an autosomal dominant trait caused by mutations in cardiac sarcomere protein genes.[33–35] Mutations in genes encoding Z-disc proteins (myozenin (*MYOZ2*) and telethonin (*TCAP*)) are also reported.[36,37] Other genetic disorders that mimic the phenotypic expression of sarcomeric HCM include metabolic or storage disorders (mutations in the genes encoding the γ-2 regulatory subunit of adenosine monophosphate (AMP)-activated protein kinase (PRKAG2); lysosome-associated membrane protein 2 (LAMP2); or GLA-encoded α-galactosidase A), neuromuscular disorders (mutations in frataxin gene causing Friedreich ataxia), chromosome abnormalities (Down syndrome, trisomy 18) and genetic syndromes such as cardiofacial disorders (Noonan syndrome, LEOPARD syndrome, cardiofaciocutaneous syndrome, Costello syndrome) or phakomatoses (neurofibromatosis, tuberous sclerosis).[4,5,38–43]

Restrictive cardiomyopathy

Restrictive cardiomyopathy (RCM), the least common of all the cardiomyopathies, is characterized by increased stiffness of the myocardium that causes ventricular pressure to rise steeply with small increases in ventricular volume. This pathophysiology occurs in a number of different diseases, including HCM and DCM, but by

convention, the term RCM should only be used when systolic and diastolic volumes of one or both ventricles are normal or reduced and there is no increase in ventricular wall thickness.[15]

RCM may be idiopathic, familial, or result from various systemic disorders, notably amyloidosis, sarcoidosis, carcinoid heart disease, scleroderma, and anthracycline toxicity.[44] Familial disease is described in ~30% of patients with idiopathic restrictive cardiomyopathy.[45] Autosomal dominant RCM is commonly caused by sarcomeric gene defects (especially in cardiac troponin I).[46] Desmin gene defects cause RCM associated with atrioventricular block and skeletal myopathy.[47] Rarely, familial disease is associated with autosomal recessive inheritance (such as haemochromatosis caused by mutations in the HFE gene, or glycogen storage disease[44]).

Arrhythmogenic right ventricular cardiomyopathy

Arrhythmogenic right ventricular cardiomyopathy (ARVC) is a disorder characterized clinically by ventricular arrhythmia, heart failure, and sudden death, and histologically by cardiomyocyte loss and replacement with fibrous or fibro-fatty tissue.[48]

Clinically, features used to diagnose the condition are often non-specific. In 1994, an International Task Force proposed diagnostic criteria that integrated a number of different aspects of the disease.[49] With the improvement of cardiac imaging (notably cardiac magnetic resonance imaging) and molecular genetics analysis, the morphological characterization of the disease has been refined and the classification scheme revised to include isolated right ventricular form (ARVC), biventricular disease (so-called arrhythmogenic cardiomyopathy) (up to 50% of the cases) and an isolated left ventricular dominant form (ALVC; 5–10% of the cases).

The estimated prevalence of ARVC is one in 5000 of the population.[48] Systematic family studies have shown that ARVC is inherited in ~50% of cases.[48] The mode of transmission is usually autosomal dominant with variable penetrance, but rare autosomal recessive forms are recognized.[7,8,48,50] To date, most mutations occur in genes encoding proteins of the desmosome and adherens junction: specifically, plakoglobin (JUP); desmoplakin (DSP); plakophilin 2 (PKP2); desmoglein (DSG2); and desmocollin (DSC2).[7,8,48,50] Sarcomeric (titin), cytoskeletal (desmin), nuclear envelope (lamin A/C protein gene), calcium/sodium handling (phospholamban gene, PLN), and protein genes are associated with ARVC,[7,8,48,50] suggesting an overlap with other cardiomyopathy subtypes. Other associated genes include the α-T-catenin (CTNNA3), transforming growth factor β_3 (TGFβ_3), and the transmembrane protein 43 (TMEM43).[50,51]

Left ventricular non-compaction

Left ventricular non-compaction (LVNC) is a myocardial disorder defined by the presence of prominent trabeculations on the luminal surface of the ventricle associated with deep inter-trabecular recesses that extend into the ventricular wall.[15,52] LVNC often occurs in association with other congenital heart abnormalities, such as atrial and ventricular septal defects, congenital aortic stenosis and coarctation of the aorta. Isolated LVNC was thought to be extremely rare with a prevalence between 0.05 and 0.24%, but with improvements in diagnostic imaging, the frequency of the diagnosis has increased.[15,52] However, there is controversy with respect to the diagnostic criteria for LVNC and it is not clear whether it is a distinct cardiomyopathy or merely a congenital or acquired morphological trait shared by phenotypically distinct cardiomyopathies.[15,52,53]

Several genes have been implicated in LVNC.[7,52] These include TAZ/G4.5 located on the X chromosome which encodes for tafazzin, a protein involved in the maintenance of cardiolipin concentrations, expressed at high levels in cardiac and skeletal mucle cells.[15,52] Mutations in this gene cause Barth syndrome. Other genes implicated in isolated LVNC include: LDB3 encoding the LIM domain binding protein 3, a protein belonging to the Z-disc structure; α-dystrobrevin, a protein of the glycoprotein complex that interacts with other components of the complex conferring stability to the plasma membrane during the process of contraction and relaxation of the muscles; lamin A/C encoding a ubiquitously expressed protein found in the inner surface of the nuclear envelope; and sarcomeric genes encoding β-myosin heavy chain (MYH7), α-cardiac actin (ACTC) gene and cardiac troponin T (TNNT2).[52–54] An autosomal dominant LVNC phenotype is associated with germline mutations in human MIB1 (mindbomb homolog 1), which encodes an E3 ubiquitin ligase that promotes endocytosis of the NOTCH ligands DELTA and JAGGED, and implicating Notch signalling in LVNC.[55]

Pathophysiology

Most of the genes implicated in the cardiomyopathies are involved in force generation and propagation, energy production and regulation, calcium signalling, or transcription regulation (Table 5.1; Figures 5.2 and 5.3).[3–10,33–43,46–50]

Sarcomeric proteins

Genetic mutations in sarcomeric protein genes are implicated in a number of cardiomyopathy subtypes including HCM, RCM, DCM, and LVNC.[1–5,9,10,33–35,46,50,51] In HCM, more than 400 different sarcomeric mutations are known, the greatest number occurring in the genes encoding for β-myosin heavy chain (MYH7) and myosin-binding protein C (MYBPC3).[4,33–35] Most mutations are missense mutations, but nonsense, frameshift and in-frame insertion/deletion mutations are well described, particularly in MYBPC3.[4,33–35]

In general, sarcomeric protein gene mutations are characterized by incomplete penetrance and variable clinical expression, the explanation for which includes locus heterogeneity and the variable effect of mutations at different locations within the same gene on the structure and function of the encoded peptide (allelic heterogeneity).[4,5,33,35] It is thought that the majority of sarcomeric protein gene mutations have a dominant negative effect on sarcomere function, i.e. the mutant protein is incorporated into the sarcomere, but its interaction with the normal (wild-type) protein disrupts normal sarcomeric assembly and function; haploinsufficiency (i.e. when there is only a single functional copy of a gene, the other being inactivated by the mutation) may also be important.[4,5,33,35]

In HCM, hypertrophy may result from reduced contractile function, but studies of myocyte function in patients with mutations in sarcomere protein genes are inconsistent.[56–60] Murine models of sarcomeric mutations show increased calcium sensitivity and altered calcium cycling between the sarcomere and the sarcoplasmic reticulum. In-vitro studies using purified myosin filaments and skinned papillary muscle have demonstrated increased calcium sensitivity of force development, predicted to result in impaired ventricular relaxation in vivo.[56–59]

Sarcomere mutations that cause DCM occur in the same genes implicated in HCM, but the predominant mechanism leading to the phenotype seems to be the impairment of the transmission of

Table 5.1 Genes involved in cardiomyopathies

Gene	Symbol	Inheritance	Phenotype	Frequency
Sarcomeric proteins				
Cardiac β-myosin heavy chain	MYH7	AD	Variable: moderate to severe prognosis (apical HCM and LVNC), DCM and DCM in Laing distal myopathy	HCM 40–44%; DCM 3–4%
Cardiac troponin T	TNNT2	AD	HCM: possible higher risk of sudden deaths. DCM	HCM 5–15%; DCM 3%
Cardiac troponin I	TNNI3	AD	HCM with restrictive physiology; DCM; pure RCM	HCM 25%, DCM <1%
Cardiac troponin C	TNNC	AD	DCM	<1%
α-Tropomyosin	TPM1	AD	HCM, DCM	HCM; DCM 1–2%
Cardiac myosin binding protein C	MYBPC3	AD	Later onset of the disease and has generally a good prognosis; cases of children with a severe hypertrophy have also been reported, DCM	HCM 35–40%; DCM 2%
Titin	TTN	AD	DCM, HCM	DCM 15–20%; HCM rare
Cardiac actin	ACTC	AD (HCM/DCM)	DCM, LVNC, HCM	DCM <1%; HCM ~1%
Essential myosin light chain	MYL3	AD	HCM	~1%
Regulatory myosin light chain	MYL2	AD	HCM	1–2%
Z-disc proteins				
Metavinculin	VCL	AD	DCM, HCM	DCM: 1%; HCM <1%
LIM binding domain 3	LDB3	AD	DCM, HCM	DCM <1–1%; HCM 1–5%
Titin-cap or telethonin	TCAP	AD	DCM, HCM	DCM <1%–1%; HCM <1%
Myozenin 2	MYOZ2	AD	HCM	<1%
Muscle LIM protein	CSRP3	AD	DCM, HCM	DCM <1%; HCM <1%;
Nexilin	NEXN	AD	HCM	<1% NA
Cytoskeletal and nuclear envelope proteins				
Desmin	DES	AD	DCM	<1%
α- and β-dystroglycans	DAG1	NA	DCM	NA
α-, β-, γ- and δ-sarcoglycans	SGCA, SGCB, SGCG, SGCD	SGCD AD	DCM	SGCD <1%
Caveolin-3	CAV3	AD	DCM, HCM	HCM rare
Lamin A/C	LMNA	DCM AD; EMD2, AD; EMD3, AR; LGMD1B, AD	LVNC, DCM, DCM in Emery–Dreifuss muscular Dystrophy types 2 and 3 (EMD2 and EMD3), DCM in limb girdle muscular dystrophy (LGMD) 1B	DCM 4–8%
Syntrophin	SNT	NA	DCM	NA
Dystrobrevin	DTN	NA	DCM	NA
Dystrophin	DMD	XL	DCM in Duchenne muscular dystrophy (DMD), Becker muscular dystrophy (BMD)	NA
Filamin C	FLNC	AD	HCM DCM ARVC	HCM <1% DCM 1% ARVC <1%
Transmembrane protein 43	TMEM43	AD	ARVC	NA
Desmosomal proteins				
Plakoglobin	JUP	Naxos syndrome, AD	ARVC, ARVC in Naxos syndrome	Rare
Desmoplakin	DSP	Carvajal syndrome, AR	ARVC, DCM in Carvajal syndrome	ARVC/D 1–16%
Desmoglein 2	DSG2	AD	ARVC	3–20%

Table 5.1 *Continued*

Gene	Symbol	Inheritance	Phenotype	Frequency
Desmocollin 2	DSC2	AD	ARVC	1–13%
Plakophilin-2	PKP2	AD, AR	ARVC	AD 10–50%, AR rare
Sarcoplasmic reticulum				
Ryanodine receptor-2	RYR-2	AD	ARVC	Rare
Phospholamban	PLN	AD	DCM, HCM	DCM: NA HCM <1%
Sodium channel mutations				
α-subunit of the cardiac sodium channel	SCN5A	AD	DCM	2–3%
Metabolic proteins				
Protein kinase, AMP-activated, gamma 2 non-catalytic subunit	PRKAG2	AD	HCM in Wolf–Parkinson–White syndrome	
α-galactosidase A	GLA	XL	HCM in Fabry disease	
Lysosomal-associated membrane protein 2	LAMP2	XL	HCM in Danon disease	
Glucosidase A	GAA	AR	HCM in Pompe disease	Together with other HCM phenocopies account for 5–10% of HCM cases
Regulatory proteins				
RNA binding protein 20	RMB20	AD	DCM	2%
BCL2 associated athanogene 3	BAG3	AD	DCM	NA
Transforming growth factor-beta 3	TGFB3	AD	ARVC	NA
Others				
Hereditary haemochromatosis type 1	HFE	AR	DCM and RCM in hereditary haemochromatosis	NA
Hereditary haemochromatosis type 2	HAMP	AR		
Hereditary haemochromatosis type 3	TFR2	AR		
Hereditary haemochromatosis type 4	SLC40A1	AD		
Hereditary amyloidosis	TTR	AD	HCM and RCM in hereditary amyloidosis	NA
RAS–MAPK pathway genes	PTPN11/ RAF1/SOS1/KRAS/HRAS/ BRAF/MEK1–2 MAP2K1/MAP2K2/SHOC2/ RIT1	AD	HCM in Noonan (NS)/ Leopard (LS) syndromes/ Costello syndrome Cardio-facio-cutaneous syndrome	Together with other HCM phenocopies account for 5–10% of HCM cases
Frataxin	FRDA	AR	HCM in Friedreich ataxia	NA

HCM, hypertrophic cardiomyopathy; LVNC, left ventricular non-compression; DCM, dilated cardiomyopathy; RCM, restrictive cardiomyopathy; ARVC, arrhythmogenic right ventricular cardiomyopathy; AD, autosomic dominant; AR, autosomic recessive; XL, X-linked; NA, not available.

For each gene is reported the symbol, the inheritance pattern, the correspondent genotype/phenotypes and the frequency of the mutations. If multiple phenotype are present, eventually different inheritance and frequency are indicated.

Source data from Tester DJ, Ackerman MJ. Cardiomyopathic and channelopathic causes of sudden unexplained death in infants and children. *Annu Rev Med* 2009;**60**:69–84; Hershberger RE, Cowan J, Morales A, Siegfried JD. Progress with genetic cardiomyopathies: screening, counseling, and testing in dilated, hypertrophic, and arrhythmogenic right ventricular dysplasia/cardiomyopathy. *Circ Heart Fail* 2009;**2**(3):253–61; Akhtar M, Elliott P. The genetics of hypertrophic cardiomyopathy. *Glob Cardiol Sci Pract* 2018;2018(3):36; Aoki Y, Niihori T, Banjo T, Okamoto N, Mizuno S, Kurosawa K, Ogata T, Takada F, Yano M, Ando T, Hoshika T, Barnett C, Ohashi H, Kawame H, Hasegawa T, Okutani T, Nagashima T, Hasegawa S, Funayama R, Nagashima T, Nakayama K, Inoue S, Watanabe Y, Ogura T, Matsubara Y. Gain-of-function mutations in RIT1 cause Noonan syndrome, a RAS/MAPK pathway syndrome. *Am J Hum Genet* 2013;**93**(1):173–80; Elizabeth M. McNally and Luisa Mestroni. Dilated cardiomyopathy. Genetic determinants and mechanisms. *Circ Res* 2017;**121**:731–48.

contractile force.[35,60,61] The molecular basis of RCM phenotype arising from mutant sarcomeric proteins is unknown, but impaired ATP-mediated dissociation of myosin from actin (causing impaired myocardial relaxation and restrictive physiology), titin dysregulation by the mutant proteins, and phosphorylation of sarcomeric proteins have been suggested.[60,62] The recent discovery of sarcomeric mutations (*MYH7, ACTC, TNNT*) in patients with LVNC indicates that sarcomere proteins may also have a role in myocardial development.[54]

Z-disc proteins

Z-discs are the lateral boundaries of the sarcomere and their role is fundamental in mechanical stretch sensing.[63,64] Mutations in genes encoding Z-disc proteins have been implicated in DCM

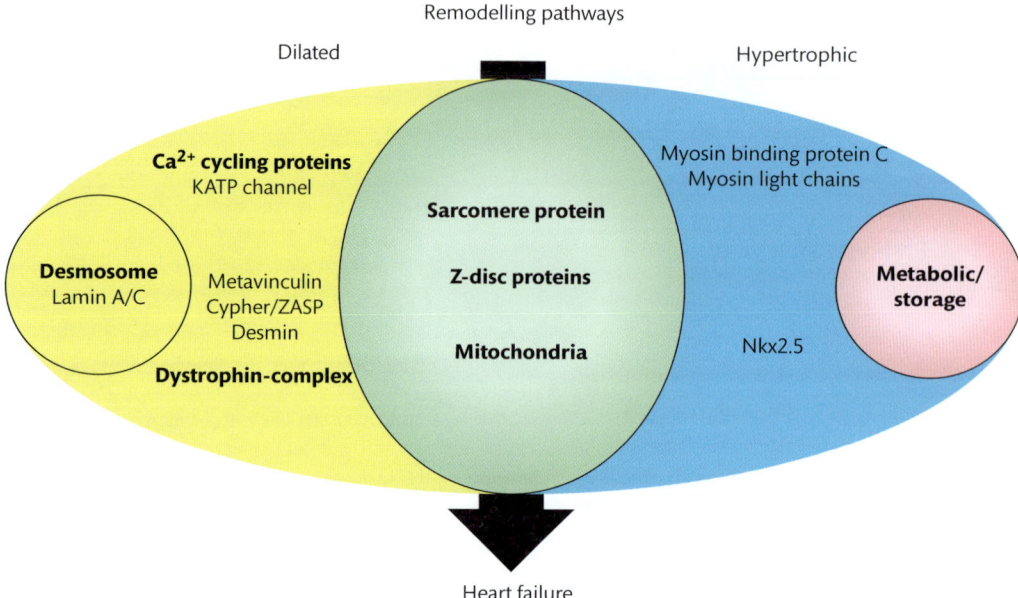

Figure 5.2 Human gene mutations and pathways causing inherited cardiomyopathies.

Source data from Morita H, Seidman J, Seidman CE. Genetic causes of human heart failure. *J Clin Invest* 2005;**115**(3):518–526. doi: 10.1172/JCI24351.

(e.g. metavinculin, which provides the direct connection to the plasma membrane and MLP which forms a complex with titin and telethonin) and in HCM (α-actinin which mediates the interaction between actin and titin, telethonin which interacts with muscle LIM protein, MLP and titin and has a structural function, and ZASP (LDB3) which interacts with α-actinin-2 and interferes with PKC-mediated signalling).[35–37,63,64] Mutations in LDB3 and actin have been found to cause LVNC.[65] Another protein involved in the development of cardiomyopathies is melusin (a muscle-specific integrin b1-interacting protein), which has a key role in mechanotransduction and development of hypertrophy.[64]

Cytoskeletal proteins

Cytoskeletal proteins act as an intracellular scaffold that passes on the contractile force from the sarcomere to the extracellular matrix and protects the cardiomyocyte from mechanical stress.[63,64] Mutations that compromise the cytoskeleton can increase ventricular stiffness and impair contractility of myocytes by reducing force transmission and resistance to stress.[63,64]

The dystrophin–glycoprotein complex is composed of dystrophin, sarcoglycans, dystroglycans, syntrophins, and sarcospan.[63,64] Mutations in genes that encode the various components of this complex are associated with DCM and neuromuscular disorders (dystrophinopathies).[63,64,66,67] Dystrophin itself is a large cytoskeletal protein expressed in skeletal, cardiac, and smooth muscle cells. Its interactions are with actin and dystrophin-associated glycoprotein complex (on the plasma membrane), while its function is force transduction, intracellular organization, and membrane stability.[63,64] The protein has an N-terminus that binds to the sarcomere via an actin-binding domain, a rod region composed of spectrin-like repeat sequences with interspersed hinge regions and a C-terminus that binds to the sarcolemma via a group of dystrophin-associated proteins, including the syntrophin and β-dystroglycan, as well as interacting with ion channels such as Nav 1.5, the cardiac sodium

channel encoded by the SCN5A gene.[64] When dystrophin is deficient (Becker muscular dystrophy) or absent (Duchenne muscular dystrophy), normal levels of mechanical stress result in increased cell membrane permeability, loss of membrane integrity, and progressive cell destruction.[64] Progressive myocyte destruction, whether in skeletal or cardiac muscle, results in a loss of muscle mass, fibrosis, and muscle weakness.[64] Dystrophin has also been associated with an X-linked DCM in which there is little or no clinical evidence of skeletal muscle weakness.[66,67] Interestingly, a similar pathology occurs when dystrophin is disrupted by acquired disease such as viral-induced myocarditis or coronary artery disease.[68] It has been suggested that dystrophin disruption may represent a 'final common pathway' of ventricular remodelling and failure.[68]

Genetic mutations in δ-sarcoglycan, one of the four proteins (α, β, γ, δ) that associate to form the sarcoglycan complex, cause sporadic and familial DCM.[66,67] The δ-component is expressed in striated and smooth muscles, with higher expression in the skeletal and cardiac muscles. The mutations described in human DCM are missense substitution (autosomal dominant transmission and sudden death at an early age) and two other mutations that delete the 238th codon corresponding to a lysine residue (no signs of heart failure before 20 years of age).[64,66,67] Absence of δ-sarcoglycan has been demonstrated to result in the loss of the entire complex.[64,66,67] δ-Sarcoglycan mutations are also associated with limb-girdle muscular dystrophy.[64,66,67]

Intermediate filaments connect the Z-disc to the sarcolemma.[63,64] Desmin is a muscle-specific intermediate filament that forms connections between Z-discs and myofibrils and between plasma membrane, nuclear envelope, and desmosomes.[42,64] Mutations in the gene encoding desmin cause skeletal muscle and cardiac disease by rendering the cells more susceptible to mechanical stress, impairing force transmission, and by leading to structural changes because of the formation of 'aggresomes' (aggregates of mutated proteins that associate with the sarcomere).[47,64] Intermediate filaments are linked

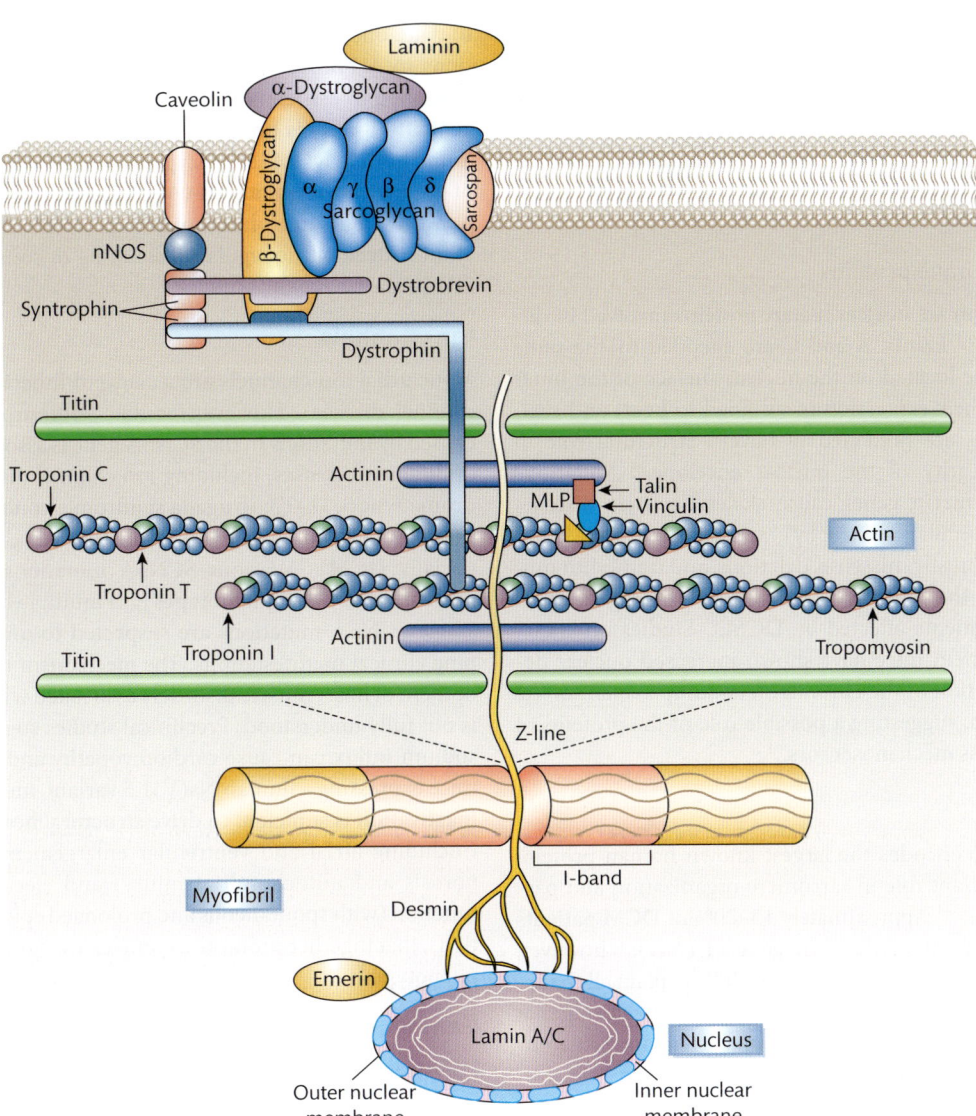

Figure 5.3 Proteins implicated in human inherited cardiomyopathies.
Reproduced from Towbin JA, Bowles NE. The failing heart. *Nature* 2002;**415**:227–233 with permission from Springer.

to dystrophin–glycoprotein complex (through α-dystrobrevin) and interruption of this interaction may be present in Duchenne dystrophy.[64,66,67] Filamin C is a large actin-cross-linking protein located at the myofibrillar intercalated Z-disk and has roles in sarcomere structural integrity, cell migration, cytoskeletal remodelling, and mechanosensitive signalling. Mutations in the *FLNC* gene may cause myofibrillar myopathy and several studies have reported cardiac involvement in the form of dilated, hypertrophic, and restrictive cardiomyopathies. Recent studies have shown that truncating variants in *FLNC* (FLNCtv) account for up to 4% of genetic DCM cases and are characterized by an arrhythmogenic phenotype with extensive left or biventricular myocardial fibrosis and dysfunction, malignant ventricular arrhythmia, and sudden cardiac death.[69]

Desmosomal proteins

The intercalated discs provide mechanical and electrical coupling between adjacent cardiomyocytes.[63,64] They are made up of three distinct structures: gap junctions, adherens junctions, and desmosomes.[64] The gap junction mediates the transfer of ions between cells, whereas the *adherens junction* (composed of cadherins, β-catenin, and γ-catenin (plakoglobin)) mediates the transmission of force between cells.[64] The *desmosome* provides mechanical attachment between cells by linking the desmosomal cadherins, desmocollin, and desmoglein with the intermediate filament cytoskeleton.[64] The intracellular components of the desmosomal cadherins interact with plakoglobin and plakophilin, which in turn bind to the N-terminal domain of a plakin protein, desmoplakin.[64] The C-terminal of desmoplakin anchors desmin intermediate filaments to the cell surface.

Mutations in desmosomal proteins cause ARVC and DCM.[1,2,7,8,70] More than 50 individual mutations have been identified to date, but the mechanism by which mutations result in disease is unclear.[2,7,8] It is suggested that mutations increase the susceptibility of the myocardium to the damaging effects of mechanical stress, thereby predisposing to cardiomyocyte detachment, death, and eventual replacement by fibro-fatty tissue.[8] In ARVC, the predilection for the

right ventricle has been explained by its thin wall and greater distensibility, but desmosomal proteins interact with many other proteins including components of the cellular cytoskeleton and intermediate filaments, and it is possible that dysfunction of either ventricle is the result of reduced cytoskeletal integrity and impaired force transduction.[7,43,63,64] Some desmosomal proteins (notably plakoglobin) are also important signalling molecules.[7]

Inner nuclear membrane proteins

Lamin A/C and emerin are nuclear matrix proteins involved in different myopathies.[6,63,64] Lamin A and C are encoded by the same gene (*LMNA*) and are located on the nuclear surface of the inner nuclear membrane; their expression is confined to heart and skeletal muscle.[64] Lamins are predicted to have a structural role in maintaining the integrity of the nuclear envelope.[64] Mutations in lamin A/C and emerin genes cause skeletal muscle diseases (Emery–Dreifuss muscular dystrophy) and isolated DCM.[6,63,64] About 19 mutations (mostly missense, deletions, and frameshift mutations), especially in the central rod domain in *LMNA* gene, have been described in patients affected by DCM.[64] Studies on transgenic lamin AC-deficient mice have shown increased nuclear deformation, fragmentation of the chromatin, and impairment of the mechanotransduction, suggesting a possible role of the proteins of the nuclear envelope as mechanosensors.[64]

Titin

The titin gene (TTN) encodes the largest known human protein, which plays an important role in sarcomere organization and passive myocyte stiffness.[63,64] Approximately 15–20% of DCM patients have a truncating variant in the titin gene (TTNtv);[71] however, haploinsufficiency caused by TTNtv does not fully explain all the associated molecular and physiological consequences, suggesting that other genetic and environmental mechanisms (pregnancy, chemotherapy, others) also contribute to disease pathogenesis.[72,73]

Calcium homeostasis

Calcium exchange between cytoplasm and extracellular matrix and between cytoplasm and storage organelles is fundamental to the regulation of the contraction–relaxation cycle in muscle cells.[64] Contraction of the sarcomere starts when calcium is released by sarcoplasmic reticulum; this step is regulated by a set of proteins localized within and on the membrane of the organelle, the most important of which are calsequestrin, which binds calcium into the sarcoplasmic reticulum, and the ryanodine-2 receptor that allows calcium exit into the cytoplasm (stimulated by the entry of calcium ions in the myocyte through L-type calcium channels).[64] Calcium ions diffused in the cytoplasm bind troponin C molecules in the sarcomere, triggering contraction; relaxation of the sarcomere is facilitated by the removal of calcium from the cytoplasm into the sarcoplamic endoreticulum by calcium ATPase (SERCA2a) and via the plasma membrane sodium/calcium exchanger.[64]

Dysregulation of calcium homeostasis has been described in HCM.[63,64,74] Calreticulin is a calcium-binding protein that acts as a chaperone in the sarcoplasmic reticulum. It is present in two forms, but its role in the cardiac tissue remains unknown.[64,74] Mutations in calreticulin gene have been found in two patients with DCM

to date: one had a unique mutation, the other also had two mutations in *MYBPC3*.[74] Mutations in calsequestrin (*CASQ2*) are also described in association with *MYBPC3* mutations but their pathogenicity (if any) is unclear.[74] Phospholamban mutations have been found both in DCM (homozygous) and HCM (heterozygous).[74] One of the identified mutations (Arg9Cys) causes abnormal interaction between PKA and phospholamban, so affecting the phosphorylation pattern of the regulator, resulting in constitutive inhibition of SERCA2a.

Ion channels

Myocardial ion channels are a cause of inherited arrhythmias (ion channel disease). However, cardiac sodium channel dysfunction caused by mutations in the SCN5A gene is associated with a number of different diseases, including ion channel diseases (long-QT syndrome type 3, LQT3; Brugada syndrome; conduction disease; sinus node dysfunction, and atrial standstill) and cardiomyopathies (especially DCM).[26] Various SCN5A mutations are now known to present with mixed phenotypes and multiple biophysical defects of single SCN5A mutations are suspected to underlie these overlapping clinical manifestations. The mechanism underlying the development of heart muscle disorders associated with SCN5A mutations is not fully understood. Preclinical studies suggest that an aberrant sodium influx can cause cardiomyopathy and atrial fibrillation. In mice expressing a human Na(V)1.5 variant, incomplete Na^+ channel inactivation is sufficient to drive structural heart muscle alterations (including atrial and ventricular enlargement, myofibril disarray, fibrosis and mitochondrial injury) and electrophysiological dysfunction (with spontaneous and prolonged episodes of atrial fibrillation), that together promote a complex cardiomyopathy/arrhythmic phenotype.[75]

Genetic, epigenetic, and environmental modifiers

Polymorphisms

Attempts have been made to investigate the effect of likely polymorphisms on disease expression in cardiomyopathies. Probably the best studied are genes involved in the renin–angiotensin–aldosterone system (RAAS). The deletion/insertion (D/I) polymorphism in the angiotensin converting enzyme (ACE) has been associated with several cardiovascular disorders including left ventricular hypertrophy in untreated hypertension and atherosclerosis.[76] Patients with HCM and the DD genotype have increased tissue levels of ACE, and small cohort studies have found that the D allele is over-represented in HCM patients.[76] Chronic β-adrenergic receptor (ADBR) activation is implicated in the pathogenesis of heart failure, and β-blockers improve survival in both ischaemic and non-ischaemic left ventricular systolic dysfunction.[77] Common functional polymorphisms in β-adrenergic receptor genes have been associated with diverse clinical features (e.g. functional status and exercise capacity) and outcome in heart failure patients, and with pharmacogenetic interaction with β-blockers.[77] A recent meta-analysis of the effect of ADRB1 Arg389Gly polymorphism on left ventricular remodelling with the use of β-blockers demonstrated a 5% improvement in left ventricular ejection fraction in Arg389 homozygotes.[77] There is accumulating evidence for a different functional response to β-blockers associated with this polymorphism.

Genome-wide association studies

Using genome-wide association studies (GWAS), some SNPs have been described in association with the risk of developing heart failure (including USP3 (ubiquitin-specific protease 3) in individuals of European ancestry and LRIG3 (leucine-rich, immunoglobulin like domain 3) in individuals of African ancestry); other SNPs (for example, CMTM7 (CKLF-like MARVEL transmembrane domain-containing-7) are associated with poorer prognosis in patients with heart failure.[78–80] Another study, using 50 000 SNPs in 2000 genes potentially associated with cardiovascular disorders, revealed an association between heart failure and the SNP rs1739843, located in an intronic region of the HSPB7 gene, which encodes a heat shock protein.[78,81] This finding was reproduced in a multicentre European study.[78,82] Given the absence of apparently functional SNPs upon re-sequencing of the HSPB7 gene and due to the fact that this gene is in high linkage disequilibrium with CLCNKA (renal ClC-Ka chloride channel), also located at 1p36, the latter gene was re-sequenced,[78,83] and the authors found a significant association with heart failure for a missense variant, Arg83Gly (OR 1.27). This means that the risk is increased by 54% in homozygotes. Importantly, one-quarter of Caucasians are homozygotes.

MicroRNA

MicroRNAs are a newly described class of RNA that have a basic role in regulating gene expression.[84] They are about 22 nucleotides long and are not translated into proteins. They inhibit the expression of target mRNA, binding in a sequence-specific manner. Some studies provide evidence for reactivation of a fetal microRNA program that can substantially contribute to alterations of gene expression in the failing human heart.[84] Microarray technology analysis has provided evidence that the pattern of expression of microRNAs is altered in stress/overload hypertrophy and heart failure.[84,85] These results argue for miRNAs having a fundamental role in the development of heart disease and as therefore being potential targets and/or agents of future novel therapies. To date, more than 1000 miRNA genes have been identified, and four miRNAs are highly expressed in the heart: miR-1, miR-133, miR-208, and miR-499.[86,87] Studies on mice and humans show promising results with miRNAs in relation to hypertrophy and heart failure:[84,87,88] in-vivo inhibition of miR-133 causes marked and sustained cardiac hypertrophy and may be a possible future therapeutic target.

Environmental

Physical activity may act as a modifier in inherited heart disease, favouring the development of hypertrophy, dilation, arrhythmias or worsening the outcome of a specific disease (HCM, DCM, ARVC). Long-term competitive sports have been suggested as predictors of adverse outcome in carriers with lamin A/C mutations[89] and some desmosomal mutations.[90] In addition, the effect of exercise in individuals with preclinical and/or manifest ARVC is thought to promote desmosome damage that eventually triggers fibro-fatty replacement. Indeed, endurance exercise and frequent exercise increase the risk of overt disease development and life-threatening ventricular arrhythmias in desmosomal mutation carriers. These findings support absolute and relative exercise restriction for ARVC patients and carriers, respectively. In addition, chemotherapy (TTNtv in DCM), pregnancy (TTNtv in DCM), and hypertension (MYL2 in HCM) have been reported as potential modifiers in cardiomyopathies.[72,73,91]

Clinical aspects of genetic cardiomyopathies

In routine clinical practice, the approach to the diagnosis of cardiomyopathies is relatively crude, with little emphasis given to the detection of specific disorders that cause heart muscle disease. However, a systematic approach to the assessment of family pedigree, symptoms and physical examination in combination with a detailed cardiac evaluation, and in some cases biochemical testing, can be helpful in identifying and managing some uncommon but clinically important forms of familial cardiomyopathy (Figure 5.4).[92,93]

Diagnosis

Age of onset

Age at diagnosis or presentation is an important clue to the differential diagnosis in all cardiomyopathies. In neonates and infants, the frequency of inborn errors of metabolism and congenital syndromes is much greater than in older children or adults. For example, in children presenting with HCM aged <18 years in a US paediatric registry, 8.7% had inborn errors of metabolism, 9% had inherited syndromes and 7.5% had neuromuscular disorders.[94] One exception is Anderson–Fabry disease, a lysosomal storage disorder that accounts for 1–4% of HCM in individuals aged >40 years but rarely if ever causes HCM in children and young adults.[38] Sarcomeric protein gene mutations represent the most common cause of HCM in individuals who present from adolescence onwards, although recent cohort studies have shown that sarcomeric gene mutations do occur in infants and children with otherwise unexplained left ventricular hypertrophy.[94,95] Children with HCM associated with inborn errors of metabolism and inherited syndromes have significantly worse survival.[96]

DCM is more likely to present in the first year of life than in older children or adolescents; most cases are idiopathic or caused by inborn errors of metabolism and malformation syndromes.[19,20,22,23] The most frequently reported causes of DCM in older children are myocarditis (46%) and neuromuscular disease (26%).[23] The 1- and 5-year rates of death or transplantation are 31% and 46%, respectively.[23] Most deaths or transplantation occurs within 2 years of DCM presentation, except with neuromuscular disease.[20,23] In adults, left ventricular systolic impairment is more likely to be caused by coronary artery disease (50–70%), hypertension (2–4%), and valve disease (1.5–4%).[94,97] Other important differentials include alcohol and drug abuse.[96] The relative contribution of myocarditis and genetic disease in adults with DCM remains controversial. Studies have shown that up to 64% of patients with DCM have inflammatory cardiomyopathy and 67% have inflammatory endothelial activation.[94] There is also at least circumstantial evidence that some of the inflammation relates to autoimmunity; in some patients, the inflammation is caused by viral persistence, but the prevalence of viral persistence in adults varies from zero to as many as 80% of patients with DCM in different series.[94] Against the viral hypothesis are the numerous studies that demonstrate a familial predisposition to DCM in 20–50% of cases.[94,97]

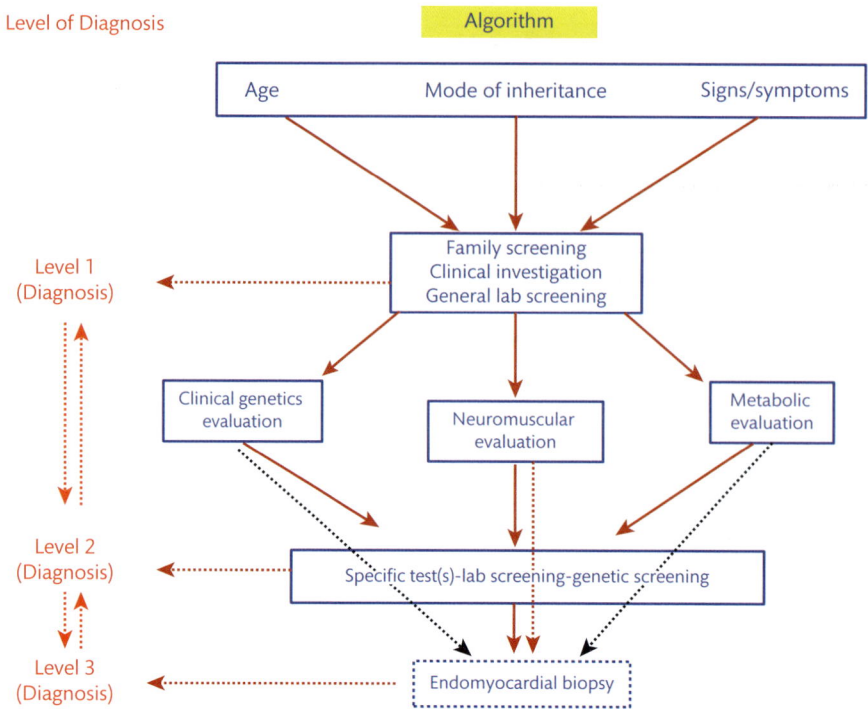

Figure 5.4 Clinical algorithm for the diagnosis of inherited cardiomyopathies.
Level 1. Age of onset (infants, children, adolescents, adults); inheritance (autosomal dominant, autosomal recessive, X-linked, matrilinear); cardiac signs or symptoms (dyspnoea, presyncope–syncope, palpitations, angina). Clinical investigations (history, ECG, echocardiography with new technologies, cardiopulmonary stress test, Holter, cardiac magnetic resonance imaging); general laboratory investigations (blood count, glycaemia, cardiac enzymes and isozymes, lipid profile, liver function, renal function, uric acid, Ca^{2+}, Mg^{2+}, K^+, Na^+, selenium, thyroid function, proteinuria, blood lactate and pyruvate, ammonaemia, ketonuria); family screening: screening of (at least) first degree relatives.
Level 2. Clinical genetics evaluation (dysmorphisms, including short stature or overgrowth; cutaneous anomalies such as lentigines, *café au lait* spots, cutis laxa, lipodystrophy, angiokeratomas; facial dysmorphia, coarse face, distinctive face, or face hypotonia; webbed neck, macroglossia, epicanthus, hypertelorism, ptosis, retinitis pigmentosa, cataract; cryptorchidism; encephalopathy, mental retardation; specific orthopaedic, endocrinological, radiological, metabolic, etc. examinations; karyotype and tailored genetic screening); neuromuscular evaluation (congenital hypotonia; muscle weakness beginning in infancy or after infancy; ataxia; myotonia; electroencephalogram, electromyography, muscle biospy with histology, immunohistochemistry, biochemical study, and genetics); metabolic evaluation (examples include: carnitine, acylcarnitine, fasting plasma fatty acids, amino acids, insulinaemia, hypoparathyroidism (parathyroid hormone), deficiency of coagulation factors, α-1,4-glucosidase (acid maltase), amylo-1,6-glucosidase deficiency, α-galactosidase A deficiency, 3-methylglutaconic aciduria, others).[101]
Level 3. Endomyocardial biopsy is indicated in specific conditions (e.g. suspect of giant cell myocarditis or infiltrative disorders or unexplained heart muscle disorders).[108]

Family history

A three- to four-generation family history should be obtained in all patients with a new diagnosis of cardiomyopathy.[1,92,93] This helps to determine the probability of familial disease and its mode of inheritance and may elicit clues to the possible aetiology. For example, the presence of male-to-male transmission effectively confirms autosomal dominant inheritance, whereas a pedigree in which there is female-to-male transmission with affected males and healthy affected mothers suggests X-linked recessive disease. Common pitfalls in pedigree interpretation include X-linked disorders (such as Anderson–Fabry disease and dystrophinopathies) in which female 'carriers' develop the same disease as affected males (albeit later in life) and autosomal dominant disorders with low clinical penetrance in some family members that give the appearance of sporadic disease. Disease caused by de-novo mutations may also be misattributed to environmental or acquired conditions.

A common finding is the presence of different cardiomyopathy phenotypes within the same family.[1,15,46,52,54,60,92,93,98] A dilated, failing heart may be the late evolution of different diseases such as familial DCM, arrhythmogenic cardiomyopathy with left ventricular involvement, and HCM.[1,9,15,48,92–95,97] Restrictive ventricular physiology may also occur in a number of different pathologies, including HCM and DCM.[1,44,45,46,59,95] Left ventricular hypertrabeculation/non-compaction has been associated with HCM and DCM, and it has been recently found to share a common genetic background (sarcomeric gene mutations) (**Figure 5.5**).[1,52,54,95]

Other examples of diagnostic clues that may be elicited from the family history include early onset supraventricular or ventricular arrhythmias, progressive atrioventricular block requiring pacemaker implantation, multiple sudden deaths suggesting laminopathy,[6,92,93,97] and a family history of sensorineural deafness and/or diabetes mellitus and/or retinitis pigmentosa consistent with mitochondrial disorders.[92,93,99]

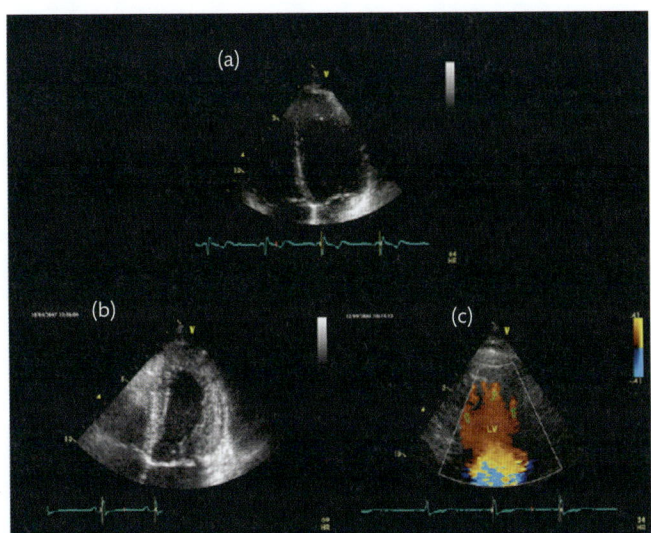

Figure 5.5 Genotype–phenotype correlation in inherited cardiomyopathies. Three apical four-chamber echocardiographic views from individuals within the same family are shown: (a) normal subject without mutation; (b) patient with *MYBPC3* mutation and classic hypertrophic cardiomyopathy; (c) patient with the same *MYBPC3* mutation and apical left ventricular noncompaction (intrafamilial heterogeneity).

Reproduced from Frisso G, Limongelli G, Pacileo G, et al. A child cohort study from southern Italy enlarges the genetic spectrum of hypertrophic cardiomyopathy. *Clin Genet* 2009;**76**(1):91–101. doi:10.1111/j.1399-0004.2009.01190.x with permission from Wiley.

Clinical examination

Many cardiomyopathies are associated with congenital dysmorphic syndromes.[1,18,19,20,42,43,92,93,99] One of the most common is Noonan syndrome, which is characterized by short stature, variable degrees of developmental delay, cutaneous abnormalities (café-au-lait spots) and other features (hypertelorism, ptosis, low-set posteriorly rotated ears, and a webbed neck).[99] Noonan syndrome shares many features with the less common LEOPARD syndrome (lentigines, deafness), Costello syndrome (coarse face, redundant skin of hands and feet, curly hair), and cardio-facio-cutaneous syndrome (distinctive craniofacial appearance, hyperkeratosis).[42,43,91,99] Recently, the term 'neurocardio-facial-cutaneous' syndrome has been introduced for all these conditions. Many are caused by germline mutations in some of the key components of the highly conserved RAS-MAPK cascade.[100] Missense PTPN11, KRAS, SOS1, RAF1, MEK1, BRAF, and RIT-1 gene mutations have been associated with HCM in the context of different neurocardio-facial-cutaneous syndromes.[100] Pulmonary stenosis and other valve dysplasias, septal and other congenital heart defects, HCM and rhythm disturbances are typically seen in patients with neurocardio-facial-cutaneous syndromes.[42,43,92,93,99,100] Somatic mutations in the RAS-MAPK gene pathway may also predispose patients to various neoplasia and lymphoproliferative disorders.[100–102]

Macroglossia, frequent respiratory infections or respiratory failure, hypotonia or proximal muscle weakness, hearing loss, hepatomegaly, splenomegaly, and cardiac failure (DCM or HCM with systolic dysfunction) are almost pathognomonic of Pompe disease (α-1,4-glucosidase deficiency).[92,93,99] Untreated, this disorder is fatal in infancy with rapid cardiac and respiratory failure.

Angiokeratomas, anhidrosis (less commonly, hyperhidrosis), Raynaud's-like symptoms with neuropathy (burning extremity pain), cutaneous angiokeratomata, ocular manifestations (cornea verticillata and retinal vascular dilation), tinnitus, diarrhoea, and proteinuria are typical features of Anderson–Fabry disease.[38,92,93]

Skeletal muscle weakness may indicate a primary neuromuscular disorder (cardioskeletal myopathy associated with creatine kinase elevation as in dystrophinopathy or with motor ataxia as in Friedreich ataxia), a mitochondrial disease (particularly if encephalopathy, ocular myopathy, or retinitis are present), a storage disorder (progressive exercise intolerance, cognitive impairment, and retinitis pigmentosa, as in Danon disease), or metabolic disorders (generally associated with hypoglycaemia, metabolic acidosis, hyperammonaemia or specific biochemical abnormalities).[92,93,99] In these patients, skeletal muscle weakness usually precedes cardiomyopathies and dominates the clinical picture. Occasionally, however, skeletal myopathy is subtle, and the first symptom of disease may be cardiac failure.

Cardiac features

ECG conduction abnormalities, including right bundle branch block, are reported in Noonan and LEOPARD syndrome, particularly when pulmonary stenosis or other congenital anomalies are present.[42,43,92,93,99] Supraventricular tachycardia, especially chaotic atrial rhythm/multifocal atrial tachycardia or ectopic atrial tachycardia are common in patients with Costello syndrome.

Ventricular pre-excitation on standard ECG is a common feature of storage diseases (Pompe disease, PRKAG2 mutations, Danon disease), and mitochondrial disorders (MELAS, MERFF).[38,39,40,92,93,99,103] Progressive atrioventricular conduction delay is a cardinal feature of nuclear envelope disorders (laminopathy and emerinopathy, in which the fibrosis often involves the myocardium around the atrioventricular node and the branches)[6] and in DCM and RCM is associated with desmin accumulation (desminopathy).[47,92,93]

There are few, if any, disease-specific changes on echocardiography but in context a number of features can point to a specific diagnosis. Concentric hypertrophy, often associated with a non-compaction with or without progressive systolic dysfunction, is common in metabolic/storage and mitochondrial disorders.[92,93,99] The coexistence of left ventricular non-compaction and localized inferobasal left ventricular akinesia is reported in dystrophinopathies (**Figure 5.6**).[104] Pericardial effusion associated with bi-atrial dilation, restrictive physiology, and an abnormal texture of the interventricular septum ('granular sparkling') is very suggestive of amyloid, although other infiltrative or storage diseases should be considered.[92,93,105] Finally, in HCM it has been suggested that septal morphology is preferentially sigmoidal in patients with Z-disc mutation, in contrast to myofilament HCM, which generally has a reverse-curve contour.[106]

Particular patterns of focal myocardial late gadolinium enhancement on cardiac magnetic resonance imaging have been reported in different cardiomyopathies (**Figure 5.7**).[107] Examples include: papillary muscles (sarcoid); the mid-myocardium in the postero-lateral left ventricle (Anderson–Fabry disease, glycogen storage disease, myocarditis, Becker muscular dystrophy); sub-endocardium (systemic sclerosis, Loeffler's endocarditis, amyloid, Churg–Strauss); and diffuse myocardial (cardiac amyloidosis)

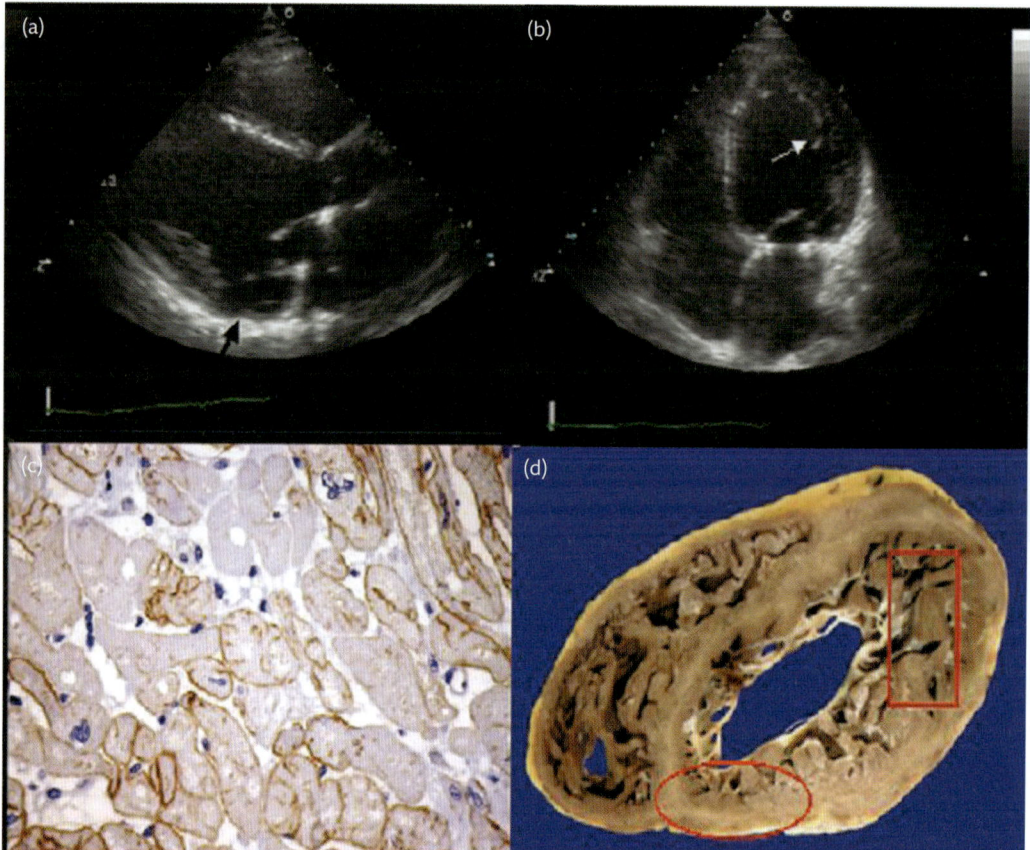

Figure 5.6 Clinical and pathological 'hallmarks' of dystrophin cardiomyopathy. (a) Localized inferobasal left ventricular akinesia and thinning. (b) Non-compaction appearance of the apicolateral left ventricular wall. (c) Immunostaining of myocardial tissue for detection of N-terminal domain of dystrophin (monoclonal antibody NCL-DYSB, clone 34C5, Novocastra) revealed discontinuous and partially disrupted positive myocytes (of varying intensity) interspersed with negative myocytes. (d) Macroscopic examination shows a localized inferobasal left ventricular thinning. From Rapezzi C, *et al. Heart* 2007;**93**;10.

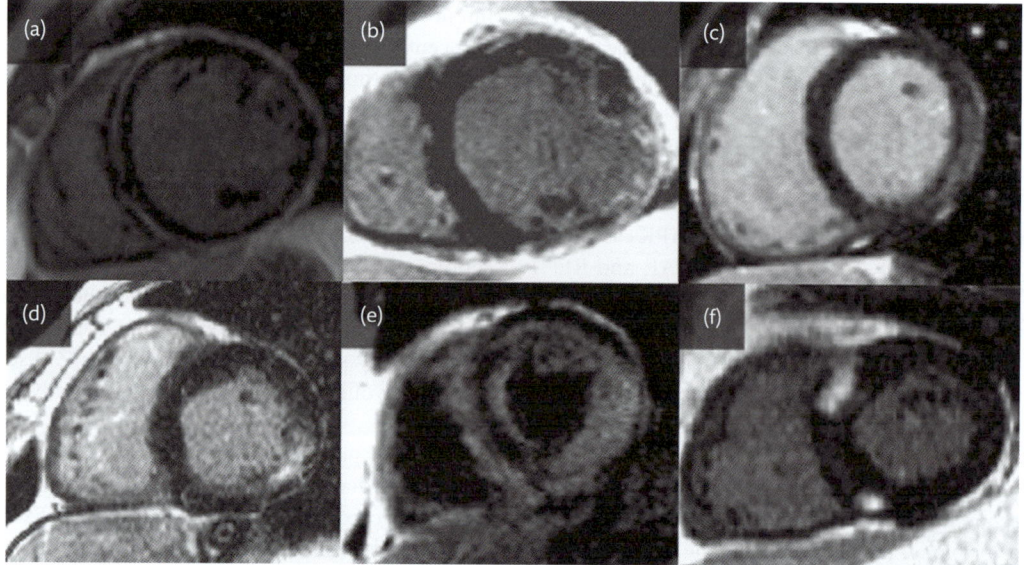

Figure 5.7 Cardiac magnetic resonance imaging with late gadolinium enhancement (LGE). Focal myocardial interstitial expansion may be visualized as LGE. The LGE extent and pattern may provide a clue to the underlying disease aetiology and stage. Characteristic cases here are from patients with (a) dilated cardiomyopathy; (b) dystrophinopathy; (c) left ventricular involvement in arrhythmogenic right ventricular cardiomyopathy; (d) Anderson–Fabry disease; (e) transthyretin amyloid, and (f) sarcomeric hypertrophic cardiomyopathy. Courtesy of Dr James Moon, University College London.

Endomyocardial biopsy/autopsy

Endomyocardial biopsy may be diagnostic for myocarditis and for some metabolic or mitochondrial disorders. Recent guidelines recommend that endomyocardial biopsy should be performed in the setting of new onset heart failure of less than 2 weeks duration with normal or enlarged left ventricular dimensions and haemodynamic compromise, or between 2 weeks and 3 months in the presence of left ventricular dilation and ventricular arrhythmias or higher degree heart block.[108] Occasionally, clinically unsuspected cardiomyopathy is diagnosed at necropsy or by molecular autopsy, and prompts investigation in family members at risk.[92,93,99]

Molecular genetics

Until recently, genetic analysis has been performed using Sanger sequencing in which the order of nucleotides is analysed in series, one after the other in each disease gene. Although the method is accurate and reproducible, it is also time-consuming and expensive. NGS uses a highly parallelized sequencing process, which makes it possible to investigate large numbers of genes simultaneously at greater speed and at lower cost, using 'targeted gene panels' (a set of known disease-causing genes). Other labs provide whole-exome sequencing (WES) which covers almost all protein-coding sequences, or whole-genome sequencing (WGS) which includes nearly all non-coding sequences as well, but to date these techniques are mostly used for research rather than for diagnostic purpose (i.e. not every part of the coding sequence is sufficiently covered, which may lead to false-negative results). In addition, issues related to management of the huge amount of data generated by WES and WGS remain to be solved before these approaches are suitable for routine clinical use.[109]

Genetic counselling

Genetic counselling is an essential component of the diagnostic process and management of inherited cardiomyopathies.[1,110] The process involves ascertainment of a three-generation family pedigree which includes information on individuals who have the same diagnosis as the index case, or other phenotypes that could represent expression of the same underlying genetic abnormality. This provides information on the heritability of the disease including mode of transmission and its clinical manifestations. It informs recommendations for clinical screening of at-risk relatives and discussion of the benefits, risks, limitations, and possible outcomes of genetic testing in the patient and their relatives.

The most important rationale for genetic testing in cardiomyopathy is to identify a disease-causing mutation in an index case in order to provide pre-symptomatic diagnosis in family members and thereby offer clinical surveillance, early medical intervention, and reproductive advice.[1,110] In selected cases, genetic testing can influence management (e.g. laminopathies, storage, and infiltrative diseases).[1,6,92,93,110] Whenever genetic testing is considered, individuals should be informed about the purpose of the test, the most probable mode of inheritance, its reliability, and the potential hazards and limitations including the psychological and social impact of the test result on the patient and their family. Rules on confidentiality of the result, especially in relation to insurance and employers, should be discussed.

Disease-specific management

Although over the last two decades major advances have been made both in our understanding of the molecular basis and in our ability to treat cardiomyopathies, the real impact of genetic testing in the clinical setting is only now emerging. Some examples of diseases in which disease-specific interventions should be considered are listed below.

Sarcomeric gene disease

New therapeutic options are under investigation in HCM due to sarcomeric gene disease. New insights from electrophysiological studies suggest that enhanced late sodium current, I(NaL), is a major contributor to the electrophysiological abnormalities of ventricular myocytes and trabeculae from patients with HCM, suggesting potential therapeutic implications of I(NaL) inhibition with specific blockers (e.g. ranolazine and its analogues).[111] Sarcomeric mutations increase myofilament Ca^{2+} sensitivity and force generation in patients with HCM, and decrease Ca^{2+} sensitivity and force generation in patients with DCM.[112]

Mavacamten is a first-in-class, selective allosteric inhibitor of cardiac myosin ATPase, which reduces actin–myosin cross-bridge formation, thereby reducing myocardial hypercontractility, a key pathophysiological abnormality in HCM, and improving myocardial energetics. In a phase 3, randomized, double-blind, placebo-controlled trial (EXPLORER-HCM), including 68 clinical cardiovascular centres in 13 countries, patients with HCM with an LVOT gradient of ≥50 mmHg and New York Heart Association (NYHA) class II/III symptoms were assigned (1:1) to receive mavacamten (starting at 5 mg) or placebo for 30 weeks.[113] Treatment with mavacamten improved exercise capacity, LVOT obstruction, NYHA functional class, and health status in patients with obstructive HCM.

Laminopathies

DCM associated with LMNA mutations seems to be a highly penetrant, age-dependent, malignant disease characterized by high rates of major cardiac events.[6] Many patients die suddenly even after pacing.[114] The current consensus recommendation is that when these patients require permanent pacing for bradycardia indications, an implantable defibrillator should be recommended.[114] Guidance on prophylactic ICD implantation in the absence of pacing indications is less certain, but should probably be considered in individuals with clear phenotypic expression, and particularly with non-sustained ventricular tachycardia, left ventricular ejection fraction <45% at the first clinical contact, male sex, and non-missense mutations (ins-del/truncating) or mutations affecting splicing.[88,114,115] Highly competitive sports should be discouraged in patients with laminopathies.[88,114,115]

Lysosomal storage diseases

Recombinant enzyme replacement in the infantile and childhood forms of Pompe disease appears to cause regression of left ventricular hypertrophy and is associated with improved survival.[116] Enzyme replacement therapy, however, has its limitations due to unsatisfactory access of recombinant α-glucosidase to the muscle cells and due to the formation of antibodies. Preclinical gene therapy experiments have shown that antibody formation limits long-term efficacy. Immunomodulatory gene therapy with a very low vector dose might enhance the efficacy of enzyme therapy in Pompe disease and other lysosomal storage disorders.[117] In Anderson–Fabry disease, treatment with recombinant α-galactosidase A improves renal and

neurological manifestations as well as quality of life, and probably retards the progression of cardiac manifestations.[118]

Amyloidosis

Light chain amyloidosis and transthyretin (TTR) amyloidosis (both mutant and wild type) are commonly associated with cardiac involvement, particularly HCM and RCM. Classical treatment for AL amyloidosis includes alkylating chemotherapy agents or high-dose melphalan followed by autologous stem cell transplantation.[119] However, novel therapeutic agents, including proteasome inhibitors, immunomodulators, and monoclonal antibodies, have shown promising activity for both initial treatment and after relapse.[119]

Transthyretin (TTR) amyloid cardiomyopathy, caused by the deposition of TTR amyloid fibrils in the myocardium, is a relatively common cause of heart failure with preserved ejection fraction (up to 13% cases).[120] Orthotopic liver transplantation has been the first-line treatment for familial TTR amyloidosis. However, progression of cardiac amyloidosis after transplantation is frequent due to deposition of wild-type TTR. Tafamidis, a novel drug that binds to the thyroxine-binding site of the TTR tetramer and inhibits its dissociation into monomers, block the rate-limiting step in the TTR amyloidogenesis cascade. In a multicentre, international, double-blind, placebo-controlled, phase 3 trial (ATTR-ACT ClinicalTrials. gov number, NCT01994889), tafamidis was associated with reductions in all-cause mortality and cardiovascular-related hospitalizations and reduced the decline in functional capacity and quality of life as compared with placebo.[121]

Respiratory chain disorders

Mitochondrial DNA

Mitochondria are the principal site of energy production in most eukaryotic cells.[98] Each cell contains more than one mitochondrion (the number is variable among cell types) and every mitochondrion contains between two and ten copies of a circular DNA molecule (mitochondrial DNA or mtDNA). Cardiomyocytes contain ~10 000 copies of mtDNA.

mtDNA is composed of ~16 500 base pairs and 37 genes encoding: 13 subunits of respiratory complexes I, III, IV, and V; 22 mitochondrial tRNAs (20 standard amino acids, plus an extra gene for leucine and serine); and two rRNAs.[99,122] With each cell division, mitochondria (and therefore mtDNA) are randomly distributed to daughter cells. Mitochondria can also replicate their DNA independently of the cell cycle in response to the energy needs of the cell. In humans, mitochondria are inherited exclusively from the mother.[98,122] After fertilization, sperm mitochondria are tagged with ubiquitin and actively destroyed.[98,122] This uniparental derivation means that recombination events are rare, a phenonemon that is exploited in the study of population genetics.

In healthy subjects, mtDNA copies are usually identical at birth (homoplasmy), but during life the mitochondrial genome is especially prone to somatic mutation because, unlike nuclear DNA, mtDNA is continuously replicated, even in non-dividing tissues such as myocardium. This may lead to the propagation of somatic mutations within single cells by a process called clonal expansion.[122,123] In addition, mtDNA lacks an extensive DNA repair mechanism and

histonic 'protection'. Deletions and duplications of mtDNA become pathogenic if they fall within genes involved in the respiratory chain or RNA genes.[98,122]

mtDNA and nDNA mutations

Many rearrangements (single deletions, duplications, large rearrangements) and point mutations of the mitochondrial genome have been described.[98,122] Patients with pathogenic mutations in mtDNA disease have cells that contain a mixture of mutated and wild-type (normal) mtDNA (heteroplasmy).[124] Unlike nuclear gene mutations (which are homozygous or heterozygous), the 'mtDNA mutation load' transmitted to offspring may vary from 1% to 100%. The development of disease in a specific tissue or organ is dependent on the so-called 'threshold' effect, determined by the proportion of mutated copies compared to wild-type copies of mtDNA.[124] The threshold varies with the energy requirements of different tissues and cells and on local factors influencing the effect of the genetic mutation. Tissues with high energy requirement such as heart, skeletal muscles, or central nervous system are particularly predisposed to develop disease.[124] The threshold at which pathogenic mutations become important may reduce over time with the accumulation of other functionally important somatic mutations in mtDNA with ageing, a sort of 'second hit' mechanism.[98,122–124]

A large number of nuclear genes are involved in the synthesis of respiratory chain subunits and essential co-factors required in normal respiratory chain function.[98,122] The transcription and translation of mtDNA is also dependent upon a number of nuclear genes.[98,122] Other critical nuclear genes relevant for mitochondrial cardiomyopathies include *TAZ*, which codes for the membrane protein tafazzin, and is disrupted in Barth syndrome;[125] and the various components of the coenzyme Q10 biosynthetic pathway.[126] Respiratory chain disease caused by nuclear gene mutations is transmitted as an autosomal dominant trait.[98,122]

Cardiac disease in respiratory chain defects

Mitochondrial disorders are clinically and genetically heterogeneous diseases. The same genetic defect may cause multisystem disorder with cardiac involvement, or an isolated cardiomyopathy with or without conduction disorders.[98,122] Conversely, a similar clinical syndrome may be caused by different genetic defects affecting nDNA or mtDNA.[98] An example of this extreme variability is the m.3243A→G mutation in the leucine (UUR) tRNA (MTTL1) gene, first described in a patient with mitochondrial encephalomyopathy with lactic acidosis and stroke-like episodes (MELAS).[127–130] Some families harbouring m.3243A→G have predominantly diabetes and deafness, whereas others have chronic progressive external ophthalmoplegia or HCM.[128–132] A summary of some of the more well-defined clinical syndromes is shown in Table 5.2.

Cardiovascular involvement is a common feature in adults and children with respiratory chain defects, with ECG abnormalities being the most common type.[130–132] Cardiac conduction defects are a defining feature of the Kearns–Sayre syndrome[130,131] and may occur in association with cardiomyopathy in patients with m.3243A→G.[130,131] Accessory pathways and the Wolff–Parkinson–White syndrome are also described in patients with Leber hereditary optic neuropathy and in patients with m.3243A→G.[130,131]

Echocardiographic evidence for cardiomyopathy is present in about one- to two-thirds of patients with mitochondrial disorders,

Table 5.2 Mitochondrial and nuclear defects leading to cardiomyopathies

Genome affected	Gene	Site of defect	Cardiac manifestation	Associated features
Mitochondrial	tRNA leucine	3260 A→G	HCM, WPW	MIMyCa, MELAS
		3303 C→T	Fatal infantile cardiomyopathy, HCM	Skeletal myopathy with ragged-red fibres.
		3243 A→G	HCM, WPW	The commonest mtDNA mutation: MELAS, diabetes, deafness, renal failure
	tRNA isoleucine	4269 A→G	Infantile DCM	Multisystem disorder (including: encephalomyopathy, epilepsy, short stature, deafness, focal glomerulosclerosis)
		4284 G→A	DCM	Multisystem disorder (including mental retard, deafness, and diabetes)
		4295 A→G	HCM	Isolated cardiomyopathy
		4300 A→G	HCM	Isolated cardiomyopathy
		4317 A→G	Fatal infantile cardiomyopathy	MELAS
		4320 A→G	HCM	Encephalopathy
	tRNA lysine	8348 A→G	HCM→DCM	Isolated, progressive cardiomyopathy
		8363 G→A	HCM→DCM	Cardiomyopathy and deafness
		8344 A→G	HCM	MERFF
		8361 G→A	HCM	MERFF
		8356 T→C	HCM	MERFF–MELAS overlap
	MTND1 (Complex I)	3460 G→A	HCM, WPW?	Leber optic atrophy
	MTND4 (Complex I)	11778G→A		
	MTND6 (Complex I)	14484 T→C		
Nuclear	SCO2	Different mutations	HCM	Fatal infantile cardioencephalomyopathy
	NDUFS2 (Complex I)	Different mutations	HCM	Leigh syndrome
	NDUFS4 (Complex I)			
	ACAD9 Acyl-CoA dehydrogenase 9	Different mutations	HCM	Skeletal myopathy
	TAZ	Different mutations	LVNC	Barth syndrome

HCM, hypertrophic myocardiopathy; WPW, Wolff–Parkinson–White syndrome; MIMyCa, Maternally Inherited disorder with adult-onset Myopathy and Cardiomyopathy; MELAS, mitochondrial encephalomyopathy with lactic acidosis and stroke-like episodes; MERFF, myoclonic epilepsy with ragged red fibres; LVNC, left ventricular non-compression. Numbers relate to base position in the mitochondrial genome.

Source data from Bindoff L. Mitochondria and the heart. *Eur Heart J* 2003;**24**(3):221–4; Aintablian HK, Narayanan V, Belnap N, Ramsey K, Grebe TA. An atypical presentation of ACAD9 deficiency: diagnosis by whole exome sequencing broadens the phenotypic spectrum and alters treatment approach. *Mol Genet Metab Rep* 2016;**10**:38–44.

the majority being hypertrophic.[130–132] ^{31}P-Magnetic resonance spectroscopy studies have shown that the myocardial bioenergetic defect precedes the hypertrophic phase.[133] Pure DCM is rarer, although progression to systolic impairment is frequently seen during follow-up.[130] The association between LVNC and RCD is relatively frequent, and LV hypertrabeculation/non-compaction in association with progressive systolic impairment has been suggested as an 'echocardiographic hallmark' of the disease.[53,130] Causative mutations associated with LVNC are the mtDNA mutations 3243A→G, 8381A→G and various ND1 and cytb mutations.[134,135]

Diagnosis

The presence of exclusively maternal inheritance or multisystem disease (visual problems, hearing loss, alopecia, muscle weakness, language disorders, seizures, endocrine abnormalities) in a family with a cardiomyopathy is always suspicious of respiratory chain disease.[130,134] The coexistance of left ventricular hypertrophy (or left ventricular dilation/non-compaction, with increased left ventricular mass on magnetic resonance imaging) and systolic dysfunction is typical.[130,134] Physical examination should look for clinical signs of multisystem involvement. The ECG may show signs of left ventricular hypertrophy and/or conduction disorders.[130,131] When respiratory chain disease is suspected, endocrine assessment (oral glucose tolerance test, thyroid function tests, alkaline phosphatase, fasting calcium, and parathyroid hormone levels) is mandatory.[130] The presence of an elevated serum creatine kinase and high levels of lactate in blood is also suggestive.[98,130,132] Additional metabolic investigations, including urinary organic and amino acids, are usually only necessary in neonates and young children.[98,130,132]

Peripheral neurophysiological investigations (electromyogram and nerve conduction studies) may identify myopathy or neuropathy which is usually axonal and mixed sensori-motor.[135] Electroencephalography may reveal diffuse slow-wave activity consistent with subacute encephalopathy, or it may reveal a predisposition to seizures.[135] Brain imaging may be normal, but may show atrophy, abnormal basal ganglia (including calcification), or leukoencephalopathy.[135]

Once a diagnosis is strongly suspected on clinical grounds, a skeletal muscle biopsy (or skin biopsy or fibroblast culture in children) is often performed to confirm and characterize the pattern of respiratory chain enzyme activity because some mtDNA defects (particularly mtDNA deletions) are not detectable in a DNA sample extracted from blood. The analysis of DNA extracted from muscle (or cardiac biopsy) is essential to establish the diagnosis.[92,93,98,135] Typical histological findings include the sub-sarcolemmal accumulation of mitochondria beneath the muscle cell membrane ('ragged-red' fibres) and cytochrome *c* oxidase (COX) deficiency.[135] Electron microscopy may identify paracrystalline inclusions in the intermembrane space (also seen in other non-mitochondrial disorders such as myotonic and other muscular dystrophies).[135] A mosaic histochemical defect generally points towards a primary mtDNA defect.[92,93,99,135] The presence of multiple respiratory chain defects usually points to a disorder of intra-mitochondrial protein synthesis, which could be of mtDNA or nuclear DNA origin. Specific isolated complex involvement suggests particular mtDNA genes, a nuclear structural subunit gene, or a nuclear-encoded respiratory chain assembly factor.[92,93,99,135]

The first step for molecular genetic analysis is Southern blot to look for mtDNA rearrangements or mtDNA depletion, followed by polymerase chain reaction and restriction fragment length polymorphism analysis for common point mutations, and then the entire sequencing of mtDNA.[92,99] Since mtDNA is highly polymorphic, a mutation can only be considered to be pathogenic if it has arisen independently several times in the population, it is not present in controls, and it has been associated with a specific disease mechanism.[92,99,135] Family, tissue segregation, and single-cell studies may show that higher levels of the mutation are associated with mitochondrial dysfunction and disease, which strongly suggests that the mutation is causing the disease.[92,99,135]

Some of the common nuclear genes are screened as part of standard procedures on blood samples, but a genetic diagnosis is not possible in many patients either because comprehensive screening is not possible, or because the underlying gene defects have not yet been identified.[92,99,135,136]

Management

There is currently no definitive treatment for patients with mitochondrial disease, except for patients with deficiency of coenzyme Q10.[137] According to recent guidelines of the Mitochondrial Medicine Society, nutritional supplement with ubidecarenone (coenzyme Q10), α-lipoic acid, and riboflavin should be used in all patients with a diagnosis of mitochondrial disease. Folinic acid should be considered in patients with central nervous system manifestations and L-carnitine should be administered only in patients with a documented deficiency. Patients with mitochondrial disease should avoid certain medications that interfere with mitochondrial function and which may precipitate acute or subacute multi-organ failure secondary to worsening mitochondrial respiratory chain

function (mitochondrial crisis): examples include metformin, valproic acid, statins, and propofol.[138]

Management is aimed at minimizing disability, preventing cardiac and systemic complications, and genetic counselling. Patients with mitochondrial disorders should undergo careful and repeated clinical assessment to diagnose and manage cardiovascular involvement.

The prognosis of cardiovascular disease differs between children and adults.[131–133] In paediatric patients with RCD, survival is poorer in patients with cardiomyopathy compared to patients with non-cardiac disease, particularly in those with cytochrome-*c* oxidase (complex IV) deficiency.[133] In contrast, the incidence of severe cardiovascular complications seems relatively low in adults[131,133] and most deaths are related to non-cardiac causes (mainly respiratory failure).[131] There may be a slighty higher mortality in adults with central nervous system manifestations[131,133,139,140] or with m.3243A→G patients in which life-threatening events may occur.[141]

Stringent glycaemic control in diabetes associated with m.3243A→G is imperative, as well as treatment of the cardiomyopathy with cardioprotective agents (such as angiotensin converting enzyme inhibitors) at an early stage.[131] Heart transplantation may be considered in mitochondrial cardiomyopathy in cases where the clinical expression of respiratory enzyme deficiency is limited to the myocardium.[141]

Summary

Inherited forms of heart muscle disease constitute a group of disorders characterized by substantial genetic and phenotypic heterogeneity. Evidence suggests that clinical phenotypes and outcome vary according to the disease gene and type of mutation. If this is correct, then there is the potential for condition-specific management strategies to delay disease progression and prevent complications such as sudden death. Even in the absence of specific therapies, cardiologists should be alert to symptoms and signs suggestive of genetic disease, and they need to become familiar with the general issues related to genetic counselling, screening, and genetic testing of families.

Acknowledgements

We are grateful to Dr Martina Caiazza for her help in the tables preparation and references check.

REFERENCES

1. Hershberger RE, Lindenfeld J, Mestroni L, *et al*. Genetic evaluation of cardiomyopathy: a Heart Failure Society of America Practice Guideline. *J Cardiac Fail* 2009;**15**:83–97.
2. Lambiase PD, Elliott PM. Genetic aspects and investigation of sudden death in young people. *Clin Med* 2008;**8**(6):607–10.
3. van Spaendonck-Zwarts KY, van den Berg MP, van Tintelen JP. DNA analysis in inherited cardiomyopathies: current status and clinical relevance. *Pacing Clin Electrophysiol* 2008;**31 Suppl 1**:S46–9.

4. Alcalai R, Seidman JG, Seidman CE. Genetic basis of hypertrophic cardiomyopathy: from bench to the clinics. *J Cardiovasc Electrophysiol* 2008;**19**(1):104–10.

5. Keren A, Syrris P, McKenna WJ. Hypertrophic cardiomyopathy: the genetic determinants of clinical disease expression. *Nat Clin Pract Card Med* 2008;**5**:158–68.

6. Mestroni L, Taylor M. Lamin A/C gene and the heart: how genetics may impact clinical care. *J Am Coll Cardiol* 2008;**52**:1261e2.

7. Awad MM, Calkins H, Judge DP. Mechanisms of disease: molecular genetics of arrhythmogenic right ventricular dysplasia/cardiomyopathy. *Nat Clin Pract Cardiovasc Med* 2008;**5**:258–67.

8. Sen-Chowdhry S, Syrris P, McKenna WJ. Role of genetic analysis in the management of patients with arrhythmogenic right ventricular dysplasia/cardiomyopathy. *J Am Coll Cardiol* 2007;**50**:1813–21.

9. Burkett EL, Hershberger RE. Clinical and genetic issues in familial dilated cardiomyopathy. *J Am Coll Cardiol* 2005;**45**:969–81.

10. Akinrinade O, Ollila L, Vattulainen S, *et al*. Genetics and genotype-phenotype correlations in Finnish patients with dilated cardiomyopathy. Eur Heart J 2015;**36**(34):2327–37.

11. Brigden W. Uncommon myocardial diseases: the non-coronary cardiomyopathies. *Lancet* 1957;**273**(7007):1179–84.

12. Goodwin JF, Gordon H, Hollman A, *et al*. Clinical aspects of cardiomyopathy. *Br Med J* 1961;**1**:69–79.

13. Report of the WHO/ISFC Task Force on the Definition and Classification of Cardiomyopathies. *Br Heart J* 1980;**44**:672–3

14. Richardson P, McKenna W, Bristow M, *et al*. Report of the 1995 World Health Organization/International Society and Federation of Cardiology Task Force on the Definition and Classification of cardiomyopathies. *Circulation* 1996;**93**(5):841–2.

15. Elliott P, Andersson B, Arbustini E, *et al*. Classification of the cardiomyopathies: a position statement from the European Society Of Cardiology Working Group on Myocardial and Pericardial Diseases. *Eur Heart J* 2008;**29**:270–6.

16. Arbustini E, Narula N, Tavazzi L, *et al*. The MOGE(S) classification of cardiomyopathy for clinicians. *J Am Coll Cardiol* 2014;**64**:304–18.

17. Pinto YM, Elliott PM, Arbustini E, *et al*. Proposal for a revised definition of dilated cardiomyopathy, hypokinetic non-dilated cardiomyopathy, and its implications for clinical practice: a position statement of the ESC working group on myocardial and pericardial diseases. *Eur Heart J* 2016;**37**:1850–8.

18. Codd MB, Sugrue DD, Gersh BJ, Melton LJ 3rd. Epidemiology of idiopathic dilated and hypertrophic cardiomyopathy. A population-based study in Olmsted County, Minnesota, 1975–1984. *Circulation* 1989;**80**:564–72.

19. Nugent AW, Daubeney PE, Chondros P, *et al*. The epidemiology of childhood cardiomyopathy in Australia. *N Engl J Med* 2003;**348**:1639–46.

20. Lipshultz SE, Sleeper LA, Towbin JA, *et al*. The incidence of pediatric cardiomyopathy in two regions of the United States. *N Engl J Med* 2003;**348**:1647–55.

21. Grunig E, Tasman JA, Kucherer H, *et al*. Frequency and phenotypes of familial dilated cardiomyopathy. *J Am Coll Cardiol* 1998;**31**:186–94.

22. Daubeney PE, Nugent AW, Chondros P, *et al*. Clinical features and outcomes of childhood dilated cardiomyopathy: results from a national population based study. *Circulation* 2006;**114**:2671–78.

23. Towbin JA, Lowe AM, Colan SD, *et al*. Incidence, causes, and outcomes of dilated cardiomyopathy in children. *JAMA* 2006;**296**:1867–76.

24. Remme CA, Wilde AA, Bezzina CR. Cardiac sodium channel overlap syndromes: different faces of SCN5A mutations. *Trends Cardiovasc Med* 2008;**18**:78–87.

25. Villard E, Perret C, Gary F, *et al*.; Cardiogenics Consortium. A genome-wide association study identifies two loci associated with heart failure due to dilated cardiomyopathy. *Eur Heart J* 2011;**32**:1065–76.

26. Haas J, Frese KS, Peil B, *et al*. Atlas of the clinical genetics of human dilated cardiomyopathy. *Eur Heart J* 2015;**36**:1123–35a.

27. Authors/Task Force members, Elliott PM, Anastasakis A, Borger MA, *et al*. ESC Guidelines on diagnosis and management of hypertrophic cardiomyopathy: the Task Force for the Diagnosis and Management of Hypertrophic Cardiomyopathy of the European Society of Cardiology (ESC). *Eur Heart J* 2014;**35**:2733–79.

28. Morita H, Larson MG, Barr SC, *et al*. Single-gene mutations and increased left ventricular wall thickness in the community: the Framingham Heart Study. *Circulation* 2006;**113**:2697–705.

29. Zou Y, Song L, Wang Z, *et al*. Prevalence of idiopathic hypertrophic cardiomyopathy in China: a population-based echocardiographic analysis of 8080 adults. *Am J Med* 2004;**116**:14–18.

30. Maron BJ, Gardin JM, Flack JM, *et al*. Prevalence of hypertrophic cardiomyopathy in a general population of young adults. Echocardiographic analysis of 4111 subjects in the CARDIA Study. Coronary Artery Risk Development in (Young) Adults. *Circulation* 1995;**92**:785–9.

31. Maron BJ, Peterson EE, Maron MS, Peterson JE. Prevalence of hypertrophic cardiomyopathy in an outpatient population referred for echocardiographic study. *Am J Cardiol* 1994;**73**:577–80.

32. Hada Y, Sakamoto T, Amano K, *et al*. Prevalence of hypertrophic cardiomyopathy in a population of adult Japanese workers as detected by echocardiographic screening. *Am J Cardiol* 1987;**59**:183–4.

33. Marian AJ, Roberts R. The molecular genetic basis for hypertrophic cardiomyopathy. *J Mol Cell Cardiol* 2001;**33**:655–70.

34. Richard P, Charron P, Carrier L, *et al*. Hypertrophic cardiomyopathy: distribution of disease genes, spectrum of mutations, and implications for a molecular diagnosis strategy. *Circulation* 2003;**107**:2227–32.

35. Seidman JG, Seidman C. The genetic basis for cardiomyopathy: from mutation identification to mechanistic paradigms. *Cell* 2001;**104**:557–67.

36. Bos JM, Poley RN, *et al*. Genotype–phenotype relationships involving hypertrophic cardiomyopathy-associated mutations in titin, muscle LIM protein, and telethonin. *Mol Genet Metab* 2006;**88**:78–85.

37. Osio A, Tan L, Chen SN, *et al*. Myozenin 2 is a novel gene for human hypertrophic cardiomyopathy. *Circ Res* 2007;**100**:766–8.

38. Sachdev B, Takenaka T, Teraguchi H, *et al*. Prevalence of Anderson-Fabry disease in male patients with late onset hypertrophic cardiomyopathy. *Circulation* 2002;**105**(12):1407–11.

39. Murphy RT, Mogensen J, McGarry K, *et al*. Adenosine monophosphate-activated protein kinase disease mimicks hypertrophic cardiomyopathy and Wolff–Parkinson–White syndrome: natural history. *J Am Coll Cardiol* 2005;**45**(6):922–30.

40. Maron BJ, Roberts WC, Arad M, *et al.* Clinical outcome and phenotypic expression in LAMP2 cardiomyopathy. *JAMA* 2009;**301**(12):1253–9.

41. Schulz JB, Boesch S, Bürk K, *et al.* Diagnosis and treatment of Friedreich ataxia: a European perspective. *Nat Rev Neurol* 2009;**5**(4):222–34.

42. Limongelli G, Sarkozy A, Pacileo G, *et al.* Genotype-phenotype analysis and natural history of left ventricular hypertrophy in LEOPARD syndrome. *Am J Med Genet A* 2008;**146A**(5):620–8.

43. Limongelli G, Pacileo G, Melis D, *et al.* Trisomy 18 and hypertrophy cardiomyopathy in an 18-year-old woman. *Am J Med Genet A* 2008;**146**(3):327–9.

44. Kushwaha SS, Fallon JT, Fuster V. Restrictive cardiomyopathy. N Engl J Med 1997;**336**:267–76.

45. Denfield, S.W. Restrictive cardiomyopathy and constrictive pericarditis. In Chang AC, Towbin JA (eds), *Heart failure in children and young adults: from molecular mechanisms to medical and surgical strategies*, pp. 264–27. Saunders Elsevier, Philadelphia, 2006.

46. Mogensen J, Kubo T, Duque M, *et al.* Idiopathic restrictive cardiomyopathy is part of the clinical expression of cardiac troponin I mutations. *J Clin Invest* 2003;**111**:209–16.

47. Dalakas MC, Park KY, Semino-Mora C, *et al.* Desmin myopathy, a skeletal myopathy with cardiomyopathy caused by mutations in the desmin gene. *N Engl J Med* 2000;**342**:770–80.

48. Basso C, Corrado D, Marcus FI, Nava A, Thiene G. Arrhythmogenic right ventricular cardiomyopathy. *Lancet* 2009;**373**(9671):1289–300.

49. Marcus FI, McKenna WJ, Sherrill D, *et al.* Diagnosis of arrhythmogenic right ventricular cardiomyopathy/dysplasia: proposed modification of the Task Force Criteria. *Eur Heart J* 2010;**31**:806–14.

50. Te Rijdt WP, Jongbloed JD, de Boer RA, *et al.* Clinical utility gene card for: arrhythmogenic right ventricular cardiomyopathy (ARVC). *Eur J Hum Genet* 2014;**22**(2).

51. Merner ND, Hodgkinson KA, Haywood AF, *et al.* Arrhythmogenic right ventricular cardiomyopathy type 5 is a fully penetrant, lethal arrhythmic disorder caused by a missense mutation in the TMEM43 gene. *Am J Hum Genet* 2008;**82**:809–21.

52. Sen-Chowdhry S, McKenna WJ. Left ventricular noncompaction and cardiomyopathy: cause, contributor, or epiphenomenon? *Curr Opin Cardiol* 2008;**23**:171–5.

53. Kohli SK, Pantazis AA, Shah JS, *et al.* Diagnosis of left-ventricular non-compaction in patients with left-ventricular systolic dysfunction: time for a reappraisal of diagnostic criteria? *Eur Heart J* 2008;**29**:89–95.

54. Klaassen S, Probst S, Oechslin E, *et al.* Mutations in sarcomere protein genes in left ventricular noncompaction. *Circulation* 2008;**117**;2893–901.

55. Luxán G, Casanova JC, Martínez-Poveda B, *et al.* Mutations in the NOTCH pathway regulator MIB1 cause left ventricular noncompaction cardiomyopathy. *Nat Med* 2013;**19**:193–201.

56. Redwood C, Lohmann K, Bing W, *et al.* Investigation of a truncated cardiac troponin T that causes familial hypertrophic cardiomyopathy: Ca(2+) regulatory properties of reconstituted thin filaments depend on the ratio of mutant to wild-type protein. *Circ Res* 2000;**86**:1146–52.

57. Blanchard E, Seidman C, Seidman JG, LeWinter M, Maughan D. Altered crossbridge kinetics in the alphaMHC403/+ mouse model of familial hypertrophic cardiomyopathy. *Circ Res* 1999;**84**:475–83.

58. Miller T, Szczesna D, Housmans PR, *et al.* Abnormal contractile function in transgenic mice expressing a familial hypertrophic cardiomyopathy-linked troponin T (I79N) mutation. *J Biol Chem* 2001;**276**:3743–55.

59. Prabhakar R, Petrashevskaya N, Schwartz A, *et al.* A mouse model of familial hypertrophic cardiomyopathy caused by a alpha-tropomyosin mutation. *Mol Cell Biochem* 2003;**251**:33–42.

60. Marian AJ. Phenotypic plasticity of sarcomeric protein mutations. *J Am Coll Cardiol* 2007;**49**:2427–9.

61. Senthil V, Chen SN, Sidhu JS, Roberts R, Marian AJ. Differences in protein-protein interactions as a basis for the contrasting phenotypes of hypertrophic and dilated cardiomyopathies resulting from different mutations in the same sarcomeric protein. *J Am Coll Cardiol* 2006;**47 Suppl A**:62A–3A.

62. Cazorla O, Freiburg A, Helmes M, *et al.* Differential expression of cardiac titin isoforms and modulation of cellular stiffness. *Circ Res* 2000;**86**:59–67.

63. Liew CC, Dzau VJ. Molecular genetics and genomics of heart failure. *Nat Rev Genet* 2004;**5**(11):811–25.

64. Fatkin D, Graham RM. Molecular mechanisms of inherited cardiomyopathies. *Physiol Rev* 2002;**82**(4):945–80.

65. Vatta M, Mohapatra B, Jimenez S, *et al.* Mutations in Cypher/ZASP in patients with dilated cardiomyopathy and left ventricular non-compaction. *J Am Coll Cardiol* 2003;**42**(11):2014–27.

66. Palmieri B, Sblendorio V. Duchenne muscular dystrophy: an update, Part I [Review]. *J Clin Neuromusc Dis* 2006;**8**:53–59.

67. Palmieri B, Sblendorio V. Duchenne muscular dystrophy: an update, Part II [Review]. *J Clin Neuromusc Dis* 2007;**8**:122–51.

68. Towbin JA, Vatta M. Myocardial infarction, viral infection, and the cytoskeleton final common pathways of a common disease? *J Am Coll Cardiol* 2007;**50**(23):2215–7.

69. Pecorari I, Mestroni L, Sbaizero O. Current understanding of the role of cytoskeletal cross-linkers in the onset and development of cardiomyopathies. *Int J Mol Sci* 2020;**21**(16):5865.

70. Posch MG, Posch MJ, Geier C, *et al.* A missense variant in desmoglein-2 predisposes to dilated cardiomyopathy. *Mol Genet Metab* 2008;**95**(1–2):74–80.

71. Herman DS, Lam L, Taylor MR, *et al.* Truncations of titin causing dilated cardiomyopathy. *N Engl J Med* 2012;**366**(7):619–28.

72. Linschoten M, Teske AJ, Baas AF, *et al.* Truncating titin (TTN) variants in chemotherapy-induced cardiomyopathy. *J Card Fail* 2017;**23**(6):476–9.

73. van Spaendonck-Zwarts KY, Posafalvi A, van den Berg MP, *et al.* Titin gene mutations are common in families with both peripartum cardiomyopathy and dilated cardiomyopathy. *Eur Heart J* 2014;**35**(32):2165–73.

74. Chiu C, Tebo M, Ingles J, *et al.* Genetic screening of calcium regulation genes in familial hypertrophic cardiomyopathy. *J Mol Cell Cardiol* 2007;**43**(3):337–43.

75. Wan E, Abrams J, Weinberg RL, *et al.* Aberrant sodium influx causes cardiomyopathy and atrial fibrillation in mice. *J Clin Invest* 2016;**126**(1):112–22.

76. Marian AJ, Yu QT, Workman R, Greve G, Roberts R. Angiotensin-converting enzyme polymorphism in hypertrophic cardiomyopathy and sudden cardiac death. *Lancet* 1993;**342**:1085–6.

77. Muthumala A, Drenos F, Elliott PM, Humphries SE. Role of beta adrenergic receptor polymorphisms in heart failure: systematic review and meta-analysis. *Eur J Heart Fail* 2008;**10**(1):3–13.

78. Lopes LR, Elliott PM. Genetics of heart failure. *Biochim Biophys Acta* 2013;**1832**(12):2451–61.

79. Smith NL, Felix JF, Morrison AC, *et al.*, Association of genome-wide variation with the risk of incident heart failure in adults of European and African ancestry: a prospective meta-analysis from the cohorts for heart and aging research in genomic epidemiology (CHARGE) consortium. *Circ Cardiovasc Genet* 2010;**3**:256–66.

80. Morrison AC, Felix JF, Cupples LA, *et al.* Genomic variation associated with mortality among adults of European and African ancestry with heart failure: the cohorts for heart and aging research in genomic epidemiology consortium. *Circ Cardiovasc Genet* 2010;**3**:248–55.

81. Cappola TP, Li M, He J, *et al.* Common variants in HSPB7 and FRMD4B associated with advanced heart failure. *Circ Cardiovasc Genet* 2010;**3**:147–54.

82. Stark K, Esslinger UB, Reinhard W, *et al.* Genetic association study identifies HSPB7 as a risk gene for idiopathic dilated cardiomyopathy. *PLoS Genet* 2010;**6**:e1001167.

83. Cappola TP, Matkovich SJ, Wang W, *et al.* Loss-of-function DNA sequence variant in the CLCNKA chloride channel implicates the cardio-renal axis in interindividual heart failure risk variation. *Proc Natl Acad Sci USA* 2010;**108**:2456–61.

84. Care A, Catalucci D, Felicetti F, *et al.* MicroRNA-133 controls cardiac hypertrophy. *Nat Med* 2007;**13**:613–18.

85. Marian AJ. Genetic determinants of cardiac hypertrophy. *Curr Opin Cardiol* 2008;**23**:199–205.

86. Meola N, Gennarino VA, Banfi S. Micrornas and genetic diseases. *Pathogenetics* 2009;**2**:7

87. Oliveira-Carvalho V, da Silva MM, Guimaraes GV, Bacal F, Bocchi EA. Micrornas: new players in heart failure. *Mol Biol Rep* 2013;**40**:2663–70.

88. van Rooij E, Olson EN. MicroRNAs: powerful new regulators of heart disease and provocative therapeutic targets. *J Clin Invest* 2007;**117**:2369–76.

89. Pasotti M, Klersy C, Pilotto A, *et al.* Long-term outcome and risk stratification in dilated cardiolaminopathies. *J Am Coll Cardiol* 2008;**52**(15):1250–60.

90. James CA, Bhonsale A, Tichnell C, *et al.* Exercise increases age-related penetrance and arrhythmic risk in arrhythmogenic right ventricular dysplasia/cardiomyopathy-associated desmosomal mutation carriers. *J Am Coll Cardiol* 2013;**62**:1290–7.

91. Claes GR, van Tienen FH, Lindsey P, *et al.* Hypertrophic remodelling in cardiac regulatory myosin light chain (MYL2) founder mutation carriers. *Eur Heart J* 2016;**37**(23):1815–22.

92. Rapezzi C, Arbustini E, Caforio AL, *et al.* Diagnostic work-up in cardiomyopathies: bridging the gap between clinical phenotypes and final diagnosis. A position statement from the ESC Working Group on Myocardial and Pericardial Diseases. *Eur Heart J* 2013;**34**(19):1448–58.

93. Limongelli G, Monda E, Tramonte S, *et al.* Prevalence and clinical significance of red flags in patients with hypertrophic cardiomyopathy. *Int J Cardiol* 2020;**299**:186–91.

94. Morita H, Rehm HL, Menesses A. *et al.* Shared genetic causes of cardiac hypertrophy in children and adults. *N Engl J Med* 2008;**358**:1899–908.

95. Frisso G, Limongelli G, Pacileo G, *et al.* A child cohort study from southern Italy enlarges the genetic spectrum of hypertrophic cardiomyopathy. *Clin Genet* 2009;**76**(1):91–101.

96. Colan SD, SE Lipshultz, AM Lowe, *et al.* Epidemiology and cause-specific outcome of hypertrophic cardiomyopathy in children: findings from the Pediatric Cardiomyopathy Registry. *Circulation* 2007;**115**:773–81.

97. Taylor MR, Carniel E, Mestroni L. Cardiomyopathy, familial dilated. *Orphanet J Rare Dis* 2006;**1**:27.

98. DiMauro S, Schon EA. Mitochondrial respiratory-chain diseases. *N Engl J Med* 2003;**348**(26):2656–68.

99. Schwartz ML, Cox GF, Lin AE, *et al.* Clinical approach to genetic cardiomyopathy in children. *Circulation* 1996;**94**:2021–38.

100. Aoki Y, Niihori T, Inoue S, Matsubara Y. Recent advances in RASopathies. *J Hum Genet* 2016;**61**(1):33–9.

101. Bentires-Alj M, Kontaridis MI, Neel BG. Stops along the RAS pathway in human genetic disease. *Nat Med* 2006;**12**:283–5.

102. Tidyman WE, Rauen KA. The RASopathies: developmental syndromes of Ras/MAPK pathway dysregulation. *Curr Opin Genet Dev* 2009;**19**(3):230–6.

103. Nikoskelainen EK, Savontaus ML, Huoponen K, Antila K, Hartiala J. Pre-excitation syndrome in Leber's hereditary optic neuropathy. *Lancet* 1994;**344**(8926):857–8.

104. Rapezzi C, Leone O, Biagini E, *et al.* Echocardiographic clues to diagnosis of dystrophin related dilated cardiomyopathy. *Heart* 2007;**93**:10.

105. Cueto-Garcia L, Reeder GS, Kyle RA, *et al.* Echocardiographic findings in systemic amyloidosis: spectrum of cardiac involvement and relation to survival. *J Am Coll Cardiol* 1985;**6**:737–43.

106. Binder J, Ommen SR, Gersh BJ, *et al.* Echocardiography-guided genetic testing in hypertrophic cardiomyopathy: septal morphological features predict the presence of myofilament mutations. *Mayo Clin Proc* 2006;**81**:459–67.

107. Silva C, Moon JC, Elkington AG, *et al.* Myocardial late gadolinium enhancement in specific cardiomyopathies by cardiovascular magnetic resonance: a preliminary experience. *J Cardiovasc Med* (Hagerstown) 2007;**8**:1076–9.

108. Cooper LT, Baughman KL, Feldman AM, *et al.* The role of endomyocardial biopsy in the management of cardiovascular disease: a scientific statement from the American Heart Association, the American College of Cardiology, and the European Society of Cardiology. *Circulation* 2007;**116**:2216–33.

109. Mogensen J, van Tintelen PJ, Fokstuen S, et al. The current role of next-generation DNA sequencing in routine care of patients with hereditary cardiovascular conditions: a viewpoint paper of the European Society of Cardiology working group on myocardial and pericardial diseases and members of the European Society of Human Genetics. *Eur Heart J* 2015;**36**(22):1367–70.

110. Hershberger RE, Cowan J, Morales A, Siegfried JD. Progress with genetic cardiomyopathies screening, counseling, and testing in dilated, hypertrophic, and arrhythmogenic right ventricular dysplasia/cardiomyopathy. *Circ Heart Fail* 2009;**2**:253–61.

111. Coppini R, Ferrantini C, Yao L, *et al.* Late sodium current inhibition reverses electromechanical dysfunction in human hypertrophic cardiomyopathy. Circulation 2013;**127**(5):575–84.

112. Watkins H, Ashrafian H, Redwood C. Inherited cardiomyopathies. *N Engl J Med* 2011;**364**(17):1643–56.

113. Olivotto I, Oreziak A, Barriales-Villa R, *et al.*; EXPLORER-HCM study investigators. Mavacamten for treatment of symptomatic obstructive hypertrophic cardiomyopathy (EXPLORER-HCM): a randomised, double-blind, placebo-controlled, phase 3 trial. *Lancet* 2020;**396**(10253):759–69.

114. Meune C, Van Berlo JH, Anselme F, *et al.* Primary prevention of sudden death in patients with lamin A/C Gene mutations. *N Engl J Med* 2006;**354**(2):209–10.

115. van Rijsingen IA, Arbustini E, Elliott PM, *et al.* Risk factors for malignant ventricular arrhythmias in lamin a/c mutation carriers a European cohort study. *J Am Coll Cardiol* 2012;**59**(5):493–500.

116. Beck M. Alglucosidase alfa: long term use in the treatment of patients with Pompe disease. *Ther Clin Risk Manag* 2009;**5**:767–72.

117. Koeberl DD, Kishnani PS. Immunomodulatory gene therapy in lysosomal storage disorders. *Curr Gene Ther* 2009;**9**(6):503–10.

118. Linhart A, Kampmann C, Zamorano JL, *et al.*; European FOS Investigators. Cardiac manifestations of Anderson–Fabry disease: results from the international Fabry outcome survey. *Eur Heart J* 2007;**28**(10):1228–35.

119. Chakraborty R, Muchtar E, Gertz MA. Newer therapies for amyloid cardiomyopathy. *Curr Heart Fail Rep* 2016;**13**(5):237–46.

120. González-López E, Gallego-Delgado M, Guzzo-Merello G, *et al.* Wild-type transthyretin amyloidosis as a cause of heart failure with preserved ejection fraction. *Eur Heart J* 2015;**36**(38):2585–94.

121. Maurer MS, Schwartz JH, Gundapaneni B, *et al.*; ATTR-ACT Study Investigators. Tafamidis treatment for patients with transthyretin amyloid cardiomyopathy. *N Engl J Med* 2018;**379**(11):1007–16.

122. Taylor RW, Turnbull DM. Mitochondrial DNA mutations in human disease. *Nat Rev Genet* 2005;**6**(5):389–402.

123. Brierley EJ, Johnson MA, Lightowlers RN, James OF, Turnbull DM. Role of mitochondrial DNA mutations in human aging: implications for the central nervous system and muscle. *Ann Neurol* 1998;**43**(2):217–23.

124. Chinnery PF, Thorburn DR, Samuels DC, *et al.* The inheritance of mitochondrial DNA heteroplasmy: random drift, selection or both? *Trends Genet* 2000;**16**(11):500–5.

125. Barth PG, Valianpour F, Bowen VM, *et al.* X-linked cardioskeletal myopathy and neutropenia (Barth syndrome): an update. *Am J Med Genet A* 2004;**126**(4):349–54.

126. Quinzii C, Naini A, Salviati L, *et al.* A mutation in para-hydroxybenzoate-polyprenyl transferase (COQ2) causes primary coenzyme Q10 deficiency. *Am J Hum Genet* 2006;**78**(2):345–9.

127. Goto Y, Nonaka I, Horai S. A mutation in the tRNA(Leu)(UUR) gene associated with the MELAS subgroup of mitochondrial encephalomyopathies. *Nature* 1990;**348**(6302):651–3.

128. Zeviani M, Gellera C, Antozzi C, *et al.* Maternally inherited myopathy and cardiomyopathy: association with mutation in mitochondrial DNA tRNALeu(UUR). *Lancet* 1991;**338**:143–7.

129. Reardon W, Ross RJ, Sweeney MG, *et al.* Diabetes mellitus associated with a pathogenic point mutation in mitochondrial DNA. *Lancet* 1992;**340**(8832):1376–9.

130. Limongelli G, Tome-Esteban M, Dejthevaporn C, *et al.* Prevalence and natural history of heart disease in adults with primary mitochondrial respiratory chain disease. *Eur J Heart Fail* 2010;**12**(2):114–21.

131. Anan R, Nakagawa M, Miyata M, *et al.* Cardiac involvement in mitochondrial diseases. A study on 17 patients with documented mitochondrial DNA defects. *Circulation* 1995;**91**(4):955–61.

132. Scaglia F, Towbin JA, Craigen WJ, *et al.* Clinical spectrum, morbidity, and mortality in 113 pediatric patients with mitochondrial disease. *Pediatrics* 2004;**114**(4):925–31.

133. Lodi R, Rajagopalan B, Blamire AM, *et al.* Abnormal cardiac energetics in patients carrying the A3243G mtDNA mutation measured in vivo using phosphorus MR spectroscopy. *Biochim Biophys Acta* 2004;**1657**(2–3):146–50.

134. Finsterer J. Cardiogenetics, neurogenetics, and pathogenetics of left ventricular hypertrabeculation/noncompaction. Cardiogenetics, neurogenetics, and pathogenetics of left ventricular hypertrabeculation/noncompaction. *Pediatr Cardiol* 2009;**30**(5):659–81.

135. Morris AA, Jackson MJ, Bindoff LA, Turnbull DM. The investigation of mitochondrial respiratory chain disease. *J R Soc Med* 1995;**88**(4):217P–22P.

136. Longley MJ, Clark S, Yu Wai Man C, *et al.* Mutant POLG2 disrupts DNA polymerase gamma subunits and causes progressive external ophthalmoplegia. *Am J Hum Genet* 2006;**78**(6):1026–34.

137. Chinnery P, Majamaa K, Turnbull D, Thorburn D. Treatment for mitochondrial disorders. *Cochrane Database Syst Rev* 2006(1):CD004426.

138. Parikh S, Goldstein A, Koenig MK, *et al.* Diagnosis and management of mitochondrial disease: a consensus statement from the Mitochondrial Medicine Society. *Genet Med* 2015;**17**:689–701.

139. Arpa J, Cruz-Martínez A, Campos Y, *et al.* Prevalence and progression of mitochondrial diseases: a study of 50 patients. *Muscle Nerve* 2003;**28**:690–5.

140. Wahbi K, Bougouin W, Béhin A, et al. Long-term cardiac prognosis and risk stratification in 260 adults presenting with mitochondrial diseases. *Eur Heart J* 2015;**36**:2886–93.

141. Robbins RC, Bernstein D, Berry GJ, *et al.* Cardiac transplantation for hypertrophic cardiomyopathy associated with Sengers syndrome. *Ann Thorac Surg* 1995;**60**(5):1425–7.

6

Metabolic disorders and heart failure

Carla M. Plymen

Inherited metabolic disorders are an important cause of heart failure, especially since many of them are amenable to treatment. It is therefore important that metabolic disorders are recognized and accurately diagnosed. The heart is dependent on normal metabolic function to provide a continuous source of energy at rest and even more so during exertion or stress. Many disorders of metabolism therefore affect cardiac function and may have devastating consequences (Table 6.1).

Heart failure in metabolic disorders is most commonly a consequence of cardiomyopathy. A phenotype of hypertrophic cardiomyopathy is typical of the glycogen and lysosomal storage diseases as well as the disorders of mitochondrial energy production. Dilated cardiomyopathy is a feature of some of the organic acidurias, disorders of carnitine metabolism, and some mitochondrial disorders. Often the distinction between hypertrophic and dilated phenotypes is unclear, with a transition from hypertrophic to dilated cardiomyopathy as the disease progresses.

Additional mechanisms leading to cardiac failure in metabolic disorders include valvular disease, arrhythmias and conduction disturbances, coronary artery disease, and pulmonary hypertension. It is not possible to discuss all metabolic disorders with associated cardiovascular manifestations however we will endeavour to discuss those most common below.

Biochemical basis

Fatty acid oxidation disorders: the carnitine shuttle and mitochondrial β-oxidation

The energy metabolism of the heart before birth relies more on glycolysis than on aerobic fatty acid metabolism. After birth, there is a transition to predominantly aerobic metabolism, with oxidation of long-chain free fatty acids as the preferred substrate.

Following their uptake from the blood, free fatty acids are activated by the acyl-CoA synthetase system. The entry of long-chain fatty acyl-CoA esters into the mitochondrion for subsequent β-oxidation is dependent upon the carnitine transport shuttle, using intracellular carnitine provided by the plasma membrane carnitine transporter (OCTN2). Fatty acids activated at the outer mitochondrial membrane are transesterified to their equivalent acylcarnitines by carnitine palmitoyl-transferase I (CPT1), translocated into the mitochondrial matrix by carnitine/acylcarnitine translocase (CACT), and reconverted to the original acyl-CoA ester by CPT2.

Within the mitochondrial matrix, chain-shortening by oxidative removal of two-carbon (acetyl) units occurs via repeated cycles of four sequential reactions catalysed by enzymes with varying and overlapping chain length specificities. The first reaction is an acyl-CoA dehydrogenation catalysed by very-long-chain, long-chain, medium-chain, or short-chain acyl-CoA dehydrogenases (VLCAD, LCAD, MCAD, and SCAD, respectively). These homologous enzymes use FAD (flavin adenine dinucleotide) as a cofactor which transfers electrons via the electron transfer flavoprotein (ETF) and its dehydrogenase (ETFDH) to the respiratory chain. Next, a hydration step catalysed by long-chain or short-chain 2-enoyl-CoA hydratase produces an L-3-hydroxyacyl-CoA which undergoes dehydrogenation by long-chain or short-chain L-3-hydroxyacyl-CoA. Finally, cleavage by long-chain (LKAT) or short-chain (SKAT) 3-ketoacyl-CoA thiolases generates an acyl-CoA ester shortened by two carbons and an acetyl-CoA which is available for ketogenesis (only in the liver) or oxidation in the Krebs cycle.

For long-chain oxidation, the last three reactions of the cycle are performed by a single multienzyme complex, the mitochondrial trifunctional protein (MTP), composed of four α-subunits performing the long-chain hydratase and hydroxyacyl-CoA dehydrogenase (LCHAD) activities, and four β-subunits performing the thiolase activity.

Defects in most of these enzymes have been identified. Cardiac disease (cardiomyopathy and/or arrhythmias) is a feature of carnitine transporter defects and of CPT2, CACT, VLCAD, and LCHAD/MTP deficiencies. Cardiomyopathy is not a feature of CPT1 and MCAD deficiencies. Defects in ETF or ETFDH produce a combined deficiency of multiple acyl-CoA dehydrogenases (MAD), with impaired oxidation of fatty acids of all chain lengths as well as organic acids (including glutaric and isovaleric). The pathogenesis of these disorders may be related to both deficiency of energy production and accumulation of toxic acyl-CoAs.

Disorders of amino and organic acid metabolism

The organic acidaemias are disorders of small-molecule intermediary metabolism, most of which result from defects in the

Table 6.1 Classification and summary of metabolic disorders with cardiovascular manifestations

Disease[a]	Abbreviation	OMIM[b]	Enzyme deficiency	Gene symbol	Major cardiovascular manifestations	Diagnostic approach	Treatment strategy
Disorders of the carnitine shuttle							
Carnitine deficiency, systemic primary (carnitine uptake defect)	CUD	#212140	OCTN2 (organic cation/carnitine transporter)	SLC22A5 (AR)	DCM/HCM, TA, SCD	Plasma carnitine ↓↓ Urine carnitine ↑↑; AC; transport assay; gene	Carnitine ++
Carnitine/ acylcarnitine translocase deficiency	CACT	#212138		SLC25A20 (AR)	DCM/HCM, TA	AC; enzyme; gene	Low-fat, high-CHO diet; MCT; carnitine?
Carnitine palmitoyl-transferase II deficiency	CPT2	*600650	Carnitine palmitoyltransferase 2	CPT2 (AR)	HCM/mixed, TA	AC; enzyme; gene	Low-fat, high-CHO diet; MCT; carnitine?
Mitochondrial and fatty acid β-oxidation disorders							
Very long-chain acyl-CoA dehydrogenase deficiency	VLCADD	#201475		ACADVL (AR)	HCM/other, TA	OA; AC; gene; enzyme	Low-fat, high-CHO diet; MCT; carnitine?
Long-chain 3-hydroxyacyl-CoA dehydrogenase deficiency	LCHAD	#609016		HADHA (AR)	HCM/other, TA	OA; AC; gene; enzyme	Low-fat, high-CHO diet; MCT; carnitine?
Mitochondrial trifunctional protein deficiency	MTP or TFP	#609015		HADHA (AR) HADHB (AR)	HCM/other/TA	OA; AC; gene; enzyme	Low-fat, high-CHO diet; MCT; carnitine?
Multiple acyl-CoA dehydrogenase deficiency (glutaric aciduria type II)	MADD (MAD deficiency)	#231680	Electron transfer flavoprotein (ETF), ETF dehydrogenase	ETFA (AR) ETFB (AR) ETFDH (AR)	HCM/DCM/fatty infiltration	OA; AC; gene; enzyme	Low-fat, high-CHO diet; carnitine? Riboflavin
Recurrent metabolic crises with rhabdomyolysis, cardiac arrhythmias, and neurodegeneration	MCECRCN	#61678		TANGO2 (AR)	TA, often fatal	Gene	High CHO diet, avoid fasting
Disorders of organic acid metabolism							
Propionic acidaemia	PA	#606054	Propionyl-CoA carboxylase	PCCA (AR) PCCB (AR)	HCM/DCM/ arrhythmias	OA; AC; gene; enzyme	ER; protein-modified diet; carnitine
Methylmalonic acidaemia	MMA	#251000	Methylmalonyl-CoA mutase	MUT, MMAA, MMAB, MCEE, MMADHC (all AR)	HCM/DCM arrhythmias	OA; AC; gene	ER; protein-modified diet; carnitine; OH-cobalamin; metronidazole
β-Ketothiolase deficiency	T2 deficiency	*607809	Acetoacetyl-CoA thiolase	ACAT1 (AR)	HCM/DCM	OA; AC; gene; enzyme	ER; carnitine;
Malonic aciduria	MA	#248360	Malonyl-CoA decarboxylase	MLYCD (AR)	HCM	OA; AC; gene	Low-fat, high-CHO diet; carnitine
D-2-Hydroxyglutaric aciduria	d2HGA	#600721	d-2-Hydroxyglutarate dehydrogenase	D2HGDH (AR)	DCM	OA; gene; enzyme	
Methylmalonic acidaemia and homocystinuria, cblC type	cblC	#277400	Homocysteine methyltetrahydrofolate methyltransferase	MMACHC (AR)	LVNC /DCM/ Other	Increased homocysteine; OA; AC; gene	OH-cobalamin, carnitine, diet
Barth syndrome (3-methyl-glutaconic aciduria type 2)	BTHS	#302060		TAZ (XLr)	DCM/LVNC/SCD	Increased urinary levels of 3-methylglutaconic acid, monolysocardiolipin/ cardiolipin; gene	
Hyperoxaluria, primary, type I		#259900	Alanine-glyoxylate aminotransferase	AGXT (AR)	DCM, heart block, vascular	Urine oxalic, glycolic acids; enzyme; gene	Pyridoxine, liver/ kidney transplant
Glycogen storage diseases							
Pompe disease	GSD II	#232300	Acid maltase	GAA (AR)	HCM, TA, short PR	Enzyme; gene	Enzyme RT

Table 6.1 *Continued*

Diseaseᵃ	Abbreviation	OMIMᵇ	Enzyme deficiency	Gene symbol	Major cardiovascular manifestations	Diagnostic approach	Treatment strategy
Glycogen debrancher enzyme deficiency (Cori disease)	GSD III	#232400	Amylo-1,6-glucosidase, 4-α-glucanotransferase	*AGL* (AR)	HCM	Enzyme; gene	High-CHO, high-protein diet; cornstarch
Glycogen branching enzyme deficency (Andersen disease)	GSD IV	#232500	Glucan (1,4-α-), Branching enzyme 1	*GBE1* (AR)	HCM/DCM	Enzyme; Gene	
Lethal congenital glycogen storage disease of the heart	CMH6	#261740	AMP-activated protein kinase, γ2 non-catalytic subunit	*PRKAG2* (AD)	HCM, WPW	Gene	
Danon disease (X-linked vacuolar CM and myopathy)		#300257		*LAMP2* (XLd)	HCM⇔DCM, WPW	Gene	
Lysosomal storage diseases							
Fabry disease		#310500	α-Galactosidase	*GLA* (XLd)	HCM, valves, coronary, hypertension, heart block	Enzyme (unreliable in carrier females); gene	Enzyme RT
Hurler syndrome Hurler–Scheie syndrome Scheie syndrome	MPS IH IH/S MPS IS	#607014 #607015 #607016	α-l-Iduronidase	*IDUA* (AR)	HCM, valves, coronary	GAGs: dermatan sulphate, heparan sulphate; enzyme; gene	Enzyme RT/HSCT
Hunter syndrome	MPS II	+309900	Iduronate 2-sulphatase	*IDS* (XLr)	Valves, HCM, coronary	GAGs: dermatan sulphate, heparan sulphate; enzyme; gene	Enzyme RT
Sanfilippo syndrome A Sanfilippo syndrome B Sanfilippo syndrome C Sanfilippo syndrome D	MPS IIIA MPS IIIB MPS IIIC MPS IIID	#252900 #252920 #252930 #252940	Heparan *N*-sulphatase *N*-Acetyl-α-glucosaminidase Heparin acetyl-CoA: α-Glucosaminide *N*-Acetyltransferase *N*-Acetylglucosamine-6-sulphatase	*SGSH* (AR) *NAGLU* (AR) *HGSNAT* (AR) *GNS* (AR)	Valves, HCM	GAGs: heparan sulphate; enzyme; gene	
Maroteaux–Lamy syndrome	MPS VI	#253200	Arylsulphatase B	*ARSB* (AR)	Valves, DCM	GAGs: dermatan sulphate; enzyme; gene	Enzyme RT
Pompe disease	GSD II	#232300	Acid maltase	*GAA* (AR)	HCM, TA, short PR	Enzyme; gene	Enzyme RT
Congenital disorders of glycosylationᶜ							
Congenital disorder of glycosylation, type Ia	CDG1a	#212065	Phosphomannomutase 2	*PMM2* (AR)	HCM/DCM, pericardial effusion; hyper-coagulability	Serum transferrin electrophoresis; enzyme; gene	

ᵃ Inheritance is autosomal recessive except where X-linked inheritance is indicated.
ᵇ Online Mendelian Inheritance in Man: http://www.ncbi.nlm.nih.gov/omim/.
ᶜ CDG type 1A only is presented, being the prototype and most common of this group of disorders.

AC, bloodspot or plasma acylcarnitines; CHO, carbohydrate; DCM, dilated cardiomyopathy; enzyme RT, enzyme replacement therapy; ER, emergency regimen; GAGs, urine glycosaminoglycans; HCM, hypertrophic cardiomyopathy; HSCT, haematopoietic stem cell transplantation; MCT, medium-chain triglycerides; OA, urine organic acids; TA, tachyarrhythmia; SCD, sudden cardiac death; AR, autosomal recessive; XLd, X-linked dominant; XLr, X-linked recessive.

degradation of amino acids. Of particular importance are the pathways of catabolism of the three branched-chain amino acids: leucine, isoleucine, and valine. Cardiomyopathy has been reported as a feature of the following organic acid disorders:

- propionic acidaemia
- methylmalonic acidaemia
- β-ketothiolase (T2) deficiency
- malonic aciduria
- D-2-hydroxyglutaric aciduria
- cblC (combined homocystinaemia and methylmalonic aciduria)

- Barth syndrome
- hyperoxaluria.

Disorders of glycogen and carbohydrate metabolism

Glycogen is the storage form of glucose used as a source of energy, particularly in skeletal and cardiac muscle and brain. Glycogen is composed of glucose residues joined in a straight chain by α-1,4 linkages, with branch points every 4–10 residues formed by α-1,6 linkages. The branching of the molecule gives it a compact spherical shape and confers solubility in water. Defects in the pathways of glycogen synthesis and degradation result in storage of abnormal

amounts and/or forms of glycogen. The glycogen storage disorders (GSD) with cardiac involvement are GSD II, GSD III, GSD IV, and Danon disease.

GSD II (Pompe disease)

Pompe disease is discussed in lysosomal storage disorders below.

GSD III (debranching enzyme deficiency; Forbes–Cori disease)

Debranching enzyme eliminates the branch points in glycogen during its degradation by performing two sequential activities, each with its own separate catalytic site on the enzyme. Following the shortening of the outer glycogen straight chain by the enzyme phosphorylase to within four glucosyl units of the α-1,6 branch point, the transferase activity of debranching enzyme transfers three outer units to the end of another chain into α-1,4 linkage, and the amylo-1,6-glucosidase activity then hydrolyses the remaining glucose residue at the branch point. Absence of debranching enzyme results in interruption of glycogen breakdown at branch points in the molecule and accumulation of abnormal glycogen (limit dextran) in affected tissues, most commonly skeletal and cardiac muscle, and less frequently in the liver. As a result of differential splicing, the *AGL* gene encodes four major isoenzymes which are variably expressed in liver and muscle—the resultant organ dysfunction can be quite varied. The majority of patients have the type IIIa variant affecting both liver and muscle; type IIIb disease is confined to the liver and has been associated specifically with mutations in exon 3 of the 35-exon *AGL* gene.[1]

GSD IV (branching enzyme deficiency; Andersen disease)

Branching enzyme, as its name suggests, generates the branch points in the glycogen molecule by transferring a segment of six or more glucosyl units from the outer end of a glycogen chain to an α-1,6-linkage branch point on the same or neighbouring chain. In its absence, glycogen contains fewer branch points and longer straight chains, resulting in storage of a poorly soluble molecule resembling amylopectin in cytoplasmic inclusion.

Danon disease

Danon was formerly believed to be a variant of Pompe disease, 'GSD IIB', but with normal acid maltase activity. It is now known to be caused by mutations in the *LAMP2* gene encoding the lysosome-associated membrane protein-2.

Mitochondrial respiratory chain disorders

Disorders of the mitochondrial respiratory chain, which is the final common pathway of aerobic fuel oxidation, are discussed in Chapter 5.

Lysosomal storage disorders

These disorders are characterized by the accumulation of complex macromolecules normally degraded in lysosomes.

GSD II (Pompe disease)

GSD II results from deficiency of the lysosomal enzyme α-glucosidase which degrades lysosomal glycogen to completion by cleavage of both α-1,4 and α-1,6 (branchpoint) glucosidic linkages. In contrast to other glycogen-metabolizing enzymes, it functions optimally at an acidic pH and hence is commonly known as acid maltase. Deficiency results in lysosomal storage of structurally normal glycogen in periodic acid–Schiff-positive vacuoles in all tissues. It is therefore classified as both a lysosomal and a glycogen storage disorder. In the most severe form with <1% residual enzyme activity, there is massive accumulation of glycogen in cardiac and skeletal muscle and liver, whereas in milder forms with higher residual activity, there is more moderate storage confined to skeletal muscle. The enzyme encoded by the *GAA* gene undergoes extensive post-translational modification in the endoplasmic reticulum by glycosylation at seven sites, followed by phosphorylation of mannose residues enabling its targeting to lysosomal mannose-6-phosphate receptors. The enzyme may be most reliably assayed in muscle or fibroblasts, showing good correlation of residual enzyme activity with age of onset and clinical severity. Blood lymphocytes or leucocytes may also be used, but the assay is complicated by the presence of α-glucosidases active at neutral pH.

Mucopolysaccharidoses

Defects in the pathway of lysosomal degradation of mucopolysaccharides (glycosaminoglycans, or GAGs) lead to the accumulation of dermatan sulphate, heparan sulphate, keratan sulphate, chondroitin sulphate, or hyaluronan, depending on the specific enzyme deficiency. Cardiac involvement, secondary to accumulation of GAGs in the myocardium, valves and coronary arteries, is most severe in:

- Hurler syndrome (mucopolysaccharidosis (MPS) I)
- Hunter syndrome (MPS II)
- Sanfilippo syndrome (MPS III)
- Maroteaux–Lamy syndrome (MPS VI).

Anderson–Fabry disease (α-galactosidase A deficiency)

This disorder is discussed in Chapter 5.

Congenital disorders of glycosylation

The congenital disorders of glycosylation (CDG) are a heterogeneous and expanding group of autosomal recessive inherited defects of protein glycosylation, the process by which oligosaccharides are linked to proteins, an essential step for ensuring their normal biological functioning. This is a complex process involving many steps in the synthesis of specific glycans, their linkage to the amide group of asparagine (*N*-glycosylation) or hydroxyl group of serine or threonine (*O*-glycosylation) residues in the protein backbone, and their subsequent remodelling. Cardiomyopathy has been reported in type I CDG disorders involving the early assembly pathway and type II defects in the later remodelling pathway of *N*-glycosylation. Readers are referred to Haeuptle and Hennet[2] for a detailed review of the *N*-glycosylation pathway and the clinical and molecular features of the different reported defects.

Clinical presentation

Cardiac involvement may be the dominant clinical feature of metabolic disorders or may be a relatively minor facet of a multisystem phenotype. A thorough history and complete physical examination may reveal important diagnostic clues (see **Table 6.2**).

Table 6.2 Diagnostic clues to metabolic cardiovascular disease

Clinical feature	Possible diagnoses
Psychomotor retardation	Lysosomal, mitochondrial, Danon, CDG, malonic, D-2-hydroxyglutaric
Coarse facies	Lysosomal
Corneal clouding	MPS
Pigment retinopathy	LCHAD/MTP
Macroglossia	Pompe, lysosomal
Angiokeratomata	Fabry
Tachyarrhythmia	Fatty acid oxidation, Barth, Pompe
Pre-excitation	Danon, PRKAG2
Sudden death	Fatty acid oxidation, MPS
Heart block	Hyperoxaluria, Fabry, MPS II, MPS VI
Valvular disease	MPS, Fabry
Pericardial effusion	CDG
Hepatosplenomegaly	Lysosomal, GSD IV
Hepatomegaly without splenomegaly	GSD II, III, CDG
Nephrolithiais	Hyperoxaluria
Impaired renal function	Methylmalonic, hyperoxaluria
Cystic renal disease	CPT2, MAD
Hypotonia, myopathy	Fatty acid oxidation, Pompe, GSD III, GSD IV, mitochondrial, Barth, Danon
Rhabdomyolysis	Fatty acid oxidation, mitochondrial
Skeletal dysplasia	MPS (stiff joints, dysostosis multiplex), CDG
X-linked inheritance	Danon, Fabry, Barth, MPS II (Hunter)
Reye-like episode	Fatty acid oxidation
Odour of sweaty feet	MAD deficiency
Thromboembolic	cblC, homocystinuria
Hypoglycaemia	Fatty acid oxidation, GSD III, CDG
Neutropenia	Barth syndrome, methylmalonic, propionic
Thrombocytopenia	cblC, methylmalonic, propionic
Metabolic acidosis	Methylmalonic, propionic, mitochondrial
Maternal pregnancy syndromes (HELLP, AFLP)	LCHAD/MTP, sometimes other fatty acid oxidation

See text and Table 6.3 for abbreviations.

Disorders of the carnitine shuttle and mitochondrial fatty acid β-oxidation

In general, the severity and clinical presentations of these disorders fall into three distinct phenotypes according to age of onset:

- in the newborn period, with prominent cardiomyopathy, multiorgan failure and high mortality;
- in later infancy or childhood, when fasting or a minor febrile or gastrointestinal illness in an apparently healthy child may precipitate a 'Reye-like' episode with acute encephalopathy, hepatic insufficiency, hypoketotic hypoglycaemia, hyperammonaemia, arrhythmias, and even sudden death;
- in later childhood or adulthood, with episodic rhabdmyolysis and myoglobinuria.

CPT2, VLCAD, and MAD deficiency

These presentations conform to the above phenotypes, with good correlation between severity of the mutation and clinical phenotype.[3,4] In their most severe forms, CPT2 and MAD deficiencies may be recognized on antenatal ultrasound examination due to multiple malformations, including multicystic kidneys and cerebral dysplasia.[5]

CACT deficiency

CACT deficiency usually presents in the newborn period with cardiomyopathy and multiorgan failure or as sudden death, presumably due to arrhythmia. Most of the reported *SCL25A20* gene mutations are private.[6]

Generalized MTP deficiency

This results from mutations in the genes encoding either the α-subunit or β-subunit, leading to deficiency of all three enzyme activities responsible for fatty acid oxidation. The clinical spectrum ranges from severe neonatal-onset disease with cardiomyopathy and early death, to mild, late-onset disease with peripheral neuropathy and/or intermittent rhabdomyolysis. There is good correlation between clinical severity and the biochemical phenotype in fibroblasts.[7] Prenatal diagnosis is possible in at-risk pregnancies.

Isolated LCHAD deficiency

This deficiency, with relative preservation of the hydratase and thiolase activities, is caused by mutations in the α-subunit at the LCHAD catalytic site, in particular the c.G1528C (p.Glu510Gln) mutation.[8] It causes moderate to severe disease, usually with cardiomyopathy.

Additional manifestations unique to LCHAD/MTP deficiency are pigmentary chorioretinopathy,[9] peripheral neuropathy,[10] neonatal cholestasis, and lactic acidosis.

Acute fatty liver of pregnancy (AFLP) and HELLP (haemolysis, elevated liver enzymes, low platelets) syndromes may develop in pregnant mothers with a foetus affected by LCHAD/MTP deficiency.[11]

TANGO2 deficiency

This rare and recently identified condition is characterized by episodic metabolic crises associated with encephalopathy and rhabdomyolysis. Crises are associated with QT prolongation and significant risk of malignant arrhythmia.[12]

The location and function of the protein TANGO2 has not yet been well defined however phenotpyes suggest a role both in Golgi apparatus to endoplasmic reticulum trafficking and mitochondrial pathways.[13]

Systemic primary carnitine deficiency

This may present early with a Reye-like hypoglycaemic episode, or later in the first year of life with progressive cardiomyopathy and myopathy leading to death by age 3 or 4 years unless diagnosed and appropriately treated. The cardiomyopathy may be hypertrophic or dilated, sometimes with features of endocardial fibroelastosis. Individuals with milder defects may remain asymptomatic despite significantly low plasma carnitine levels. Apparently asymptomatic adult females have been diagnosed after their infants were found on newborn screening to have low blood carnitine levels secondary to the primary carnitine deficiency in their mothers.[14,15]

Disorders of amino and organic acid metabolism

Cardiomyopathy may be an uncommon or relatively minor feature of these disorders but may occasionally assume primary importance.

Propionic acidaemia

This most commonly presents with life-threatening episodes of metabolic ketoacidosis. Dilated cardiomyopathy (DCM) develops in later childhood in approximately one in four patients who survive the first year of life, independent of the age of onset of the disorder, number of episodes of metabolic decompensation, or degree of metabolic control.[16] DCM is one of the most significant long-term complications of propionic acidaemia, sometimes with fatal outcome. It appears to be reversible following orthotopic liver transplantation, though peri- and postoperative complications are high.

Malonic aciduria

The major clinical manifestations of this very rare disorder are HCM and psychomotor retardation, in addition to seizures, hypotonia, and hypoglycaemia.[17,18]

d-2-Hydroxyglutaric aciduria

This neurometabolic disorder with extremely variable clinical presentation is characterized by epilepsy, psychomotor retardation, hypotonia, and characteristic neuroimaging findings. Cardiomyopathy, most commonly dilated, develops in about half of the patients with the more severe early-onset phenotype.[19] Prenatal diagnosis is possible.

Hyperoxaluria

Type I hyperoxaluria is characterized by urolithiasis and nephrocalcinosis leading to renal failure and deposition of oxalate crystals in extrarenal tissues, including the myocardium and conduction system, resulting in DCM and heart block. Age of symptom onset can vary from early childhood to age 40 or 50 years. Type II is milder and only rarely associated with cardiomyopathy.

Barth syndrome

This X-linked disorder is caused by mutations in the *TAZ* gene encoding taffazin,[20] a phospholipid transacylase located in the inner mitochondrial membrane which plays an important role in the remodelling of cardiolipin.

Children present with the following symptoms:

- cardiac disease is often the first presentation of Barth syndrome and it will often manifest before the age of 5 years. Dilated cardiomyopathy, often with non-compaction, is the most common cardiac feature, though patients are also at risk of tachyarrhythmias and sudden cardiac death;[21]
- skeletal myopathy leading to delayed motor milestones, positive Gower sign, and waddling gait;
- neutropenia with susceptibility to severe infections;
- poor growth and weight gain.

The biochemical phenotype includes:

- abnormal urine organic acids: increased 3-methylglutaconic/3-methylglutaric acids and 2-ethylhydracrylic acid. Why these metabolites of the leucine and isoleucine degradation pathways, respectively, are increased in Barth syndrome is not understood;

- hypocholesterolaemia;
- abnormal mitochondrial respiratory chain complex activities;
- decreased levels of the mitochondrial phospholipid cardiolipin, increased monolysocardiolipin, and a lower degree of unsaturation of the monolysocardiolipin acyl chains, reflecting the role of the inner mitochondrial membrane protein taffazin in cardiolipin remodelling.

Standard HF therapy, including advanced treatment options, as well as antibiotics and granulocyte colony-stimulating factor injections, help improve the outcome for those with this condition.[22]

The cblC cobalamin metabolism defect

This defect, resulting in combined methymalonic aciduria with homocystinaemia, is associated with risk of thrombus formation as well as structural heart defects.[23]

Glycogen storage disorders

GSD III

This presents in early childhood with marked hepatomegaly, without splenomegaly, and short stature. Fasting hypoglycaemia is variable, although when present is less severe than in GSD I and is not accompanied by lactic acidaemia. Patients with type IIIa disease have muscle involvement manifesting as skeletal muscle weakness and elevated plasma creatine kinase levels. Whereas the hepatomegaly, hypoglycaemia, and elevation of liver transaminases tend to improve with age, the myopathy may progressively worsen in later childhood and adulthood. About half of the patients develop a cardiomyopathy that resembles idiopathic HCM, although there is no correlation between the severity of the skeletal myopathy and the extent of cardiac involvement. The cardiomyopathy appears to progress with age but in most patients seems to be of little or no clinical significance,[24,25] although progression to heart failure or sudden death from arrhythmias has been reported. There is a suggestion that dietary management with cornstarch and a high protein intake may be effective.[26]

GSD IV

This disease is clinically variable. The hepatic form is most typical, presenting before age 2 years with hepatosplenomegaly and failure to thrive progressing to cirrhosis, portal hypertension, liver failure, and death by age 5 years. Fasting hypoglycaemia is rare. An uncommon variant presents in later childhood, predominantly as dilated cardiomyopathy with myopathy and hepatosplenomegaly.[27] Cardiac and muscle biopsies reveal massive accumulation of polyglucosan bodies. The most severe form is the congenital neuromuscular variant which can present during pregnancy with reduced foetal movements, polyhydramnios, and hydrops foetalis. At birth there is profound hypotonia with contractures and respiratory muscle failure leading to early death; cardiomyopathy is an inconsistent feature of this presentation. The adult-onset variant (adult polyglucosan body disease) may present with an isolated myopathy or combined central and peripheral nervous system involvement.

Lethal congenital glycogen storage disease of the heart: *PRKAG2*

Heterozygous mutations in this gene were identified in five unrelated patients with congenital onset and fatal outcome of massive non-lysosomal deposition of glycogen in the myocardium. As in previously reported infants with a similar phenotype, phosphorylase

kinase deficiency limited to the heart was identified in autopsy specimens. However, this appears to be a secondary or artefactual deficiency, as no mutations were identified in any of the eight genes encoding phosphorylase kinase subunits.[28] Milder mutations in the same gene are associated with dominantly inherited familial hypertrophic cardiomyopathy with Wolff–Parkinson–White (WPW) syndrome.[29] Glycogen-filled vacuoles are evident in myocytes.

Danon disease

This X-linked dominant inherited disorder is characterized by the early onset of HCM, skeletal myopathy, and mental retardation. HCM appears in affected males in childhood or teenage years with death before 30 years, whereas heterozygous females have milder cardiomyopathy, usually dilated, with later onset. Heart transplantation can prolong survival and implantable cardioverter defibrillators can help ameliorate the risk of SCD. Myopathy is usually mild in males with proximal limb and neck weakness and five- to tenfold elevation of creatine kinase level, and IQ varies from 60 to 90. About one-third of patients have pre-excitation which can be effectively treated with catheter ablation. Muscle histology reveals numerous intracytoplasmic autophagic vacuoles with glycogen particles and cytoplasmic debris.[30]

Lysosomal storage disorders

Pompe disease

Severe and progressive HCM together with generalized hypotonia, muscle weakness, and paucity of movement are the cardinal manifestations of infantile-onset Pompe disease. Hepatomegaly and macroglossia may be present. Massive cardiomegaly is evident on chest radiograph and the ECG characteristically reveals a short PR interval and very tall QRS complexes. Additional cardiac complications include left ventricular outflow obstruction and conduction system abnormalities. Cardiorespiratory failure or ventricular arrhythmias usually lead to death by the age of 1 year. Late-onset Pompe disease is predominantly a disorder of skeletal muscle weakness, without significant myocardial involvement. Prenatal diagnosis is available for Pompe disease.

Mucopolysaccharidoses

HCM is only one of many manifestations of the multisystem MPS disorders and may be masked by more obvious clinical features such as coarse facies, corneal clouding, hearing loss, developmental delay, short stature, hepatosplenomegaly, skeletal dysplasia (dysostosis multiplex), and stiff joints. Additional contributing factors to the cardiac dysfunction are coronary artery stenoses, and aortic and mitral valve thickening, leading to progressive regurgitation and/or stenosis. Pulmonary hypertension and *cor pulmonale* may develop secondary to obstructive upper airway disease. Typical storage cells are found in the myocardial interstitium, the intima of the coronary arteries and the thickened valves. Cardiomyopathy may occasionally be the presenting feature of MPS, but the majority of patients have normal systolic function. The conductive system may be histologically affected and arrhythmias are occasionally observed. Despite significant stenosis of the extramural coronary arteries, ischaemic events are rarely documented. Nevertheless, sudden and unexpected death occurs in a significant number of patients, suggesting an arrhythmia or acute ischaemic event.

MPS I

Hurler, Hurler–Scheie, and Scheie syndromes are the severe, intermediate, and mild variants of the phenotypic spectrum of MPS type I with onset of symptoms in infancy, early childhood and adolescence to adulthood, respectively. Cardiovascular involvement is largely limited to valvular disease.

MPS II (Hunter syndrome)

This differs from MPS I (Hurler syndrome) by virtue of X-linked inheritance, later onset and milder severity of disease, and the absence of corneal clouding.

MPS III (Sanfilippo syndrome)

This is a predominantly neurological disorder with relatively mild somatic features. Prenatal diagnosis is possible in at-risk pregnancies.

MPS VI (Maroteaux–Lamy syndrome)

Patients with this syndrome resemble those with Hurler syndrome, with the exception of having normal intelligence (as dermatan sulphate, unlike heparan sulphate, is not a component of the central nervous system).

Congenital disorders of glycosylation

Cardiac involvement in congenital disorders of glycosylation (CDG) may be in the form of DCM or HCM, in addition to pericardial effusion occasionally leading to cardiac tamponade, and sometimes structural heart defects. Presentation is usually in early life, or even prenatally with hydrops foetalis. These are multisystem disorders, with additional features including dysmorphism, hepatomegaly, psychomotor retardation, cerebellar hypoplasia, failure to thrive, skeletal dysplasia, inverted nipples, hypoglycaemia, coagulopathy, hepatic dysfunction, and protein-losing enteropathy. Because of the multiple subtypes of CDG type I and II and their phenotypic heterogeneity, a high index of clinical suspicion is required leading to screening for these disorders by transferrin electrophoresis.[2,31]

Diagnostic evaluation

Clinical suspicion

A high index of suspicion is essential if the possibility of a metabolic disorder is not to be missed. Acute presentations of metabolic disorders are often wrongly attributed to sepsis or asphyxia. Samples taken during crisis presentation are often the most informative. In cases of sudden or unexplained death, a metabolic diagnosis may be established retrospectively from samples collected postmortem, including skin and tissue biopsies.

Routine laboratory investigations

Readily available laboratory tests can provide important diagnostic information:

- hypoglycaemia with absent urine ketones in Reye-like presentation of fatty acid oxidation disorders (FAOD);
- metabolic acidosis and increased anion gap in organic acidaemias;
- lactic acidosis in mitochondrial disorders;
- hyperammonaemia in Reye-like presentation of FAOD;
- raised creatine kinase in GSD and in rhabdomyolysis due to FAOD;

- elevated liver transaminases and coagulopathy in Reye-like presentation of FAOD;
- elevated uric acid and triglycerides in GSD;
- neutropenia and hypocholesterolaemia in Barth syndrome;
- neutropenia and/or thrombocytopenia in acute presentations of organic acidurias.

Advanced investigations

Urine organic acids

Organic acids are extracted from a random urine sample, derivatized and analysed by gas chromatography–mass spectrometry. The following findings are of diagnostic significance (Table 6.3).

- Hypoketonuric dicarboxylic aciduria is characteristic of FAOD. The normal ketone body formation during fasting or hypoglycaemia is impaired in patients with deficient mitochondrial β-oxidation of fatty acids, whereas dicarboxylic acids can still be formed via the alternative pathway of fatty acid ω-oxidation in microsomes. This results in a significant dicarboxylic aciduria with relatively low ketones, although this may only be evident during stress or fasting. Hypoketonuric

dicarboxylic aciduria with a relative predominance of long-chain 3-hydroxydicarboxylic acids is suggestive of LCHAD/MTP deficiency.
- Specific organic acidurias have their own diagnostic pattern, including propionic, methylmalonic, malonic and D-2-hydroxyglutaric acidurias (see Table 6.3).
- 3-Methylglutaconic aciduria together with increased 2-ethylhydracrylate is characteristic of Barth syndrome;[20] 3-methylglutaconic aciduria is also a feature of the HCM associated with mitochondrial ATP synthase deficiency due to *TMEM70* mutations.[32]
- The combination of some or all of the following metabolites is suggestive of a mitochondrial respiratory chain defect: increased lactate, ketones, Krebs cycle intermediates, ethylmalonic acid, 3-methylglutaconic acid.

Carnitine, free and total

Although plasma carnitine levels are not necessarily an accurate reflection of tissue carnitine levels, their determination is important for assessment of primary or secondary carnitine deficiency. Total carnitine is made up of esterified carnitine (the sum of individual

Table 6.3 Abnormal findings on acylcarnitine and organic acid analysis[a]

Disease	Abbreviation	Urine organic acids	Blood/plasma acylcarnitine
Disorders of the carnitine shuttle			
Carnitine deficiency, systemic primary (carnitine uptake defect)	CUD		↓↓ C0; Plasma carnitine ↓↓ Urine carnitine ↑↑
Carnitine/acylcarnitine translocase deficiency	CACT		C16, C16:1, C18, C18:1, C14, C14:1
Carnitine palmitoyl transferase II deficiency	CPT2		C16, C16:1, C18, C18:1, C14, C14:1
Mitochondrial fatty acid β-oxidation disorders			
Very-long-chain acyl-CoA dehydrogenase deficiency	VLCAD	DC, ↓ ketones	C14:1
Long-chain 3-hydroxyacyl-CoA dehydrogenase deficiency	LCHAD	OH-DC, DC, ↓ ketones	C16OH, C18:1OH
Mitochondrial trifunctional protein deficiency	MTP or TFP	OH-DC, DC, ↓ ketones	C16OH, C18:1OH
Multiple acyl-CoA dehydrogenase deficiency (glutaric aciduria type II)	MAD	Glutaric, 2-OH-glutaric, ethylmalonic and dicarboxylic acids; isovaleryl-, isobutyryl- and hexanoyl-glycines	C4, C5, C5DC, C8, C12, C14
Disorders of organic acid metabolism			
Propionic acidaemia	PA	3-OH-propionic, methylcitric, tiglyl- and propionyl-glycines	C3, C3/C2
Methylmalonic acidaemia	MMA	Methylmalonic, 3-OH-propionic, methylcitric, tiglyl- and propionyl-glycines	C3
β-Ketothiolase deficiency	T2	Ketones, tiglylglycine, 2-methyl-3-OH-butyric, 2-methylacetoacetic	C5OH, C5:1
Malonic aciduria	MA	Malonic, methylmalonic	C3DC
D-2-Hydroxyglutaric aciduria	d2HGA	d-2-OH-glutaric	
Methylmalonic acidaemia and homocystinuria, cblC type	cblC	Methylmalonic total homocysteine	C3
Barth syndrome (3-methylglutaconic aciduria type 2)	BTHS	3-Methylglutaconic, 3-methylglutaric, 2-ethylhydracrylic	
Hyperoxaluria, primary, type I		Oxalic, glycolic	

[a]Metabolite levels are increased unless otherwise indicated.

Acylcarnitines: C0, free carnitine; C16, acylcarnitine with 16 carbon chain length (palmitoylcarnitine), C16:1, monounsaturated C16 carnitine; C16OH, hydroxy-C16 carnitine; C5DC, C5-dicarboxylic carnitine, etc.

Organic acids: DC, dicarboxylic acids; OH-DC, long-chain hydroxydicarboxylic acids.

acylcarnitine species) and free carnitine. In carnitine transporter defect, both free and total plasma carnitine levels are extremely low, whereas urine carnitine excretion is inappropriately high. This is best assessed by simultaneous determination of carnitine and creatinine levels in paired plasma and urine samples and calculation of the carnitine excretion index. In the organic acidurias and disorders of fatty acid β-oxidation, free carnitine is low while the ratio of esterified carnitine (the difference between total and free carnitine) to free carnitine is increased.

Acylcarnitines

By application of tandem mass spectrometry (TMS), individual acylcarnitine species can be quantified (not just total esterified carnitine as above), allowing recognition of specific diagnostic patterns (see Table 6.2). Long-chain (C16 and C18) acylcarnitines are elevated in CPT2 and translocase deficiencies (Figure 6.1d), long-chain hydroxyacylcarnitines in MTP/LCHAD deficiency (Figure 6.1f), C14:1 in VLCAD deficiency Figure 6.1e), and short-, medium-, and long-chain acylcarnitine species in MAD deficiency (Figure 6.1c). In the organic acidurias, C3 carnitine is elevated in propionic acidaemia (Figure 6.1b), C3-dicarboxylic in malonic acidaemia. Determination of acylcarnitines by TMS is highly sensitive, rapid, and relatively cheap, making it eminently suitable for universal screening of newborns by analysis of dried blood spots on filter paper (Guthrie) cards.[33] Analysis of plasma and urine samples is used for diagnostic testing. In-vitro acylcarnitine profiling of cultured fibroblasts fed with deuterated fatty acid substrates is a highly sensitive technique for identifying the defect in patients with borderline or equivocal results.[34]

Transferrin electrophoresis

Initial screening for CDG involving defects in *N*-glycosylation is by evaluation of transferrin glycosylation pattern in serum or dried blood spots. This is most commonly performed by isoelectric focusing, but capillary electrophoresis and TMS methods are also available.[33] Normal transferrin contains four sialic acid residues. Abnormal patterns reveal a reduced intensity of the normal tetrasiolatransferrin band, with the appearance of di- and asialotransferrin bands in type I CDG, and tri-, di-, mono- and asialotransferrin bands in type II CDG disorders. Transferrin isoelectrophoresis may give a false-negative result in the first months of life and should be repeated if there is clinical suspicion. CDG must be differentiated from abnormal patterns of transferrin glycosylation due to galactosaemia, hereditary fructose intolerance, and chronic alcoholism. Definitive diagnosis of the precise subtype is based on analysis of the specific enzyme and gene.[36]

Cardiolipin analysis

Abnormal cardiolipin remodelling in Barth syndrome patients is used as a diagnostic test based on demonstration of an increase in the ratio of monolysocardiolipin to cardiolipin, as determined by high-performance liquid chromatography–mass spectrometry. This assay can be performed on fibroblasts, muscle, lymphocytes,[37] or dried blood spots.[38]

Specific enzyme assay

In many disorders the diagnosis may already be established on the basis of a characteristic profile of metabolites as described above, in which case confirmation of the diagnosis by enzyme assay may be superfluous. There may still, however, be a role for enzyme assay when the degree of residual enzyme activity is known to be a predictor of clinical severity and outcome. In other disorders, especially the lysosomal storage disorders, enzyme assay remains the reference standard for diagnosis.

In contrast to metabolite and molecular testing, which are becoming increasingly available and cheaper as a result of technological advances and automation, enzyme assays for diagnosing metabolic disorders are for the most part manually performed, time-consuming, and expensive procedures. They must be individually developed and validated and require special reagents and a high degree of expertise. Their availability is therefore often limited to national or international reference laboratories, creating logistic difficulties in shipment of samples under appropriate conditions.

Selection of the appropriate tissue for assay is an important issue and is determined by the expression profile of the specific enzyme. Peripheral blood is the most practical and is appropriate when the enzyme can be assayed in serum or in isolated erythrocytes or leucocytes. Many enzymes are expressed in fibroblasts cultured from a skin biopsy. Although it can take several weeks until the fibroblast culture is established, fibroblasts provide an unlimited source of cells for testing, are easily shipped, and can be permanently cryopreserved. In some cases, however, diagnosis of an enzyme deficiency can only be established in the target organ for the disease, necessitating a liver, skeletal, or even myocardial biopsy.

Lysosomal enzymes have traditionally been assayed in peripheral blood leucocytes or fibroblasts, either individually or as a panel of enzymes. Recently, methodologies have been developed for assay of lysosomal enzymes in dried blood spots on standard cards used for newborn screening. This approach requires only small volumes of blood and the cards can be easily mailed to the laboratory under ambient conditions. The lysosomal enzyme activities remain stable during storage in this format. The use of TMS technology allows multiple enzymes to be assayed in a single analysis.[39] With the advent of enzyme replacement therapy for lysosomal disorders, this creates the very real prospect of including lysosomal storage disorders in newborn screening programmes, enabling early diagnosis and institution of treatment before irreparable damage has occurred.[40]

Mutation analysis

The causative genes for each disorder are listed in Table 6.1. Molecular testing is becoming increasingly available and is a powerful diagnostic tool for diagnosing metabolic disorders. However, there are numerous pitfalls in performing and interpreting molecular studies and it should not be used routinely simply because it exists. It is of particular value in the following circumstances:

- there is no available or reliable biochemical test, or when biochemical testing requires an invasive procedure;
- a single or limited number of pathogenic mutations are known to be responsible for the disease in a given family or community;
- there is a clear correlation between genotype and phenotype, allowing prediction of expected disease course and severity (e.g. VLCAD deficiency);
- prenatal diagnosis is requested, as molecular testing for a known mutation is often more rapid and reliable than biochemical testing;
- carrier testing of relatives is requested.

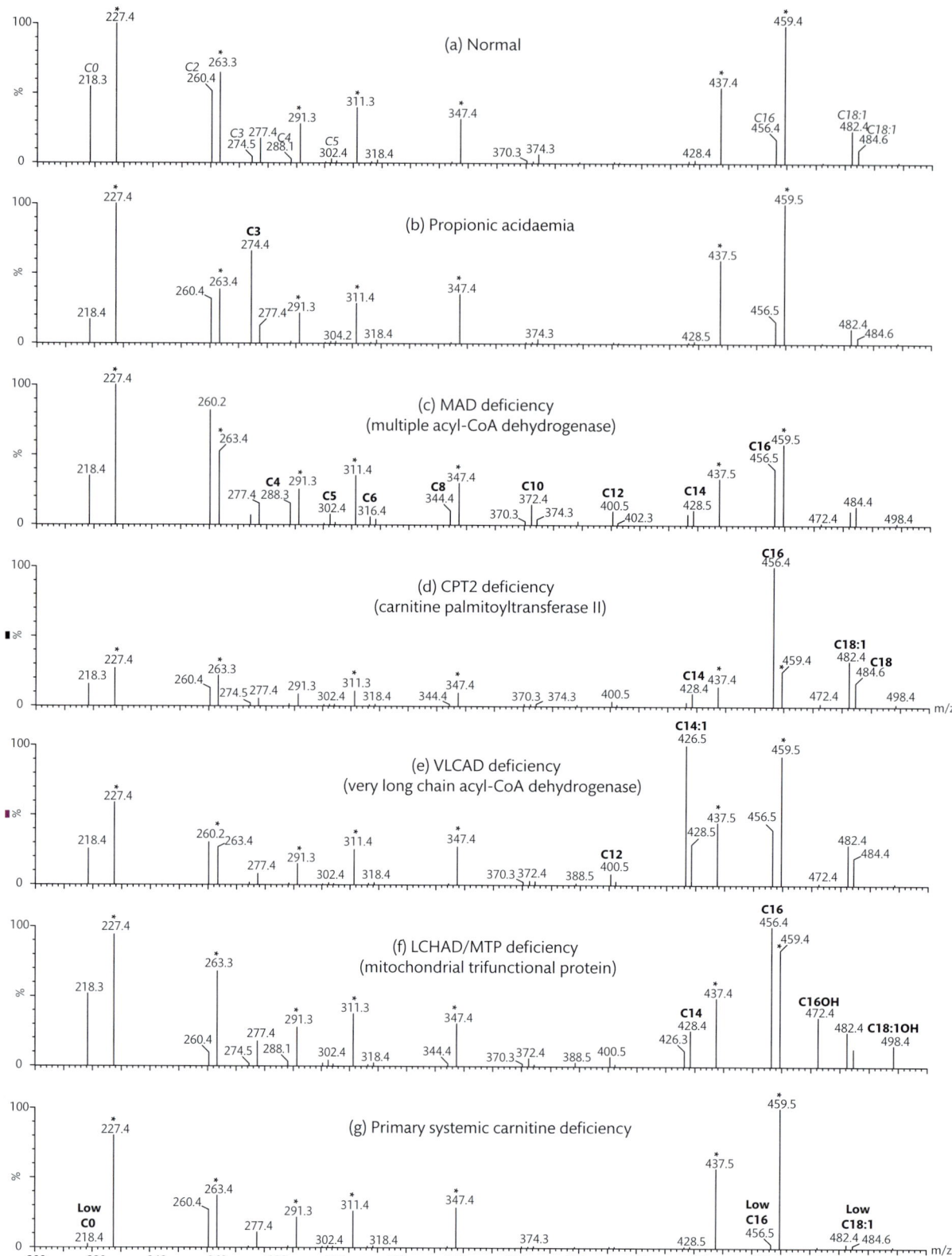

Figure 6.1 Dried blood spot acylcarnitine profiles by tandem mass spectrometry. (a) Normal profile. *Deuterated internal standard peaks; from left to right: free carnitine, C2, C3, C4, C5, C8, C14, C16 deuterated internal standards. The major acylcarnitine peaks are labelled in italics. C0, free carnitine. (g–f) From patients with organic acid and fatty acid oxidation disorders. Abnormally increased acylcarnitine peaks are labelled in bold.

Treatment

In contrast to many genetic disorders for which there are few or no therapeutic options, effective treatment is available for many of the inherited metabolic disorders. Development of an effective treatment depends on accurate diagnosis of the specific biochemical defect together with an understanding of its metabolic consequences and mechanism of disease pathogenesis. Some disorders have specific therapies, but general guidelines are applicable to many of these conditions.

Emergency management

Many metabolic disorders, especially those of fatty acid oxidation, organic and amino acid metabolism, and some of the GSDs, are characterized by acute episodes of decompensation on a background of relative well-being. These acute exacerbations can be life-threatening or lead to permanent sequelae. They are often precipitated by catabolic stress such as acute febrile illness, vomiting and/or diarrhoea, extended fasting, and surgery or other trauma. Management of these episodes therefore aims to:

- reduce the dietary sources and endogenous production of toxic metabolites;
- promote the elimination of toxic metabolites;
- reverse the catabolic process by provision of high energy intake.

The basic principles are to:

- give clear explanations to the family in advance, including a printed summary with a brief description of the illness and a list of instructions outlining the protocol for investigation and management of an acute crisis;
- stop oral intake of precursors of toxic metabolites, for example, protein in organic acidurias, long-chain fats in disorders of fatty acid oxidation;
- use intravenous glucose as the primary energy source, given as a 10% infusion (or higher concentration through a central line) to provide at least 8–10 mg/kg per min, with monitoring for hyperglycaemia, which is managed by addition of continuous insulin infusion (this has the added benefit of promoting the switch from a catabolic to anabolic state);
- use intravenous lipid infusion as an additional energy source, except in disorders of long-chain fatty acid oxidation, where MCT oil (medium-chain triglycerides) is an option;
- give carnitine (preferably intravenously) in organic acid disorders, but with extreme caution in long-chain FAOD;
- increase fluid intake above standard maintenance levels to facilitate clearance of toxic metabolites;
- treat aggressively any precipitating febrile illness with antipyretics, with or without antibiotics as appropriate;
- treat significant metabolic acidosis and hyperammonaemia.

'Emergency regimen' for initial home management

Early institution of home treatment at the very first signs of an acute intercurrent illness can often abort an acute decompensation crisis and avoid the need for hospital management as described above.[39] The emergency regimen is based on:

- clear instructions and training given to the parents in advance;
- cessation of regular feeds;
- use of an oral glucose polymer solution, thereby providing a large amount of rapidly absorbed calories in a relatively low osmolarity solution. Suitable products include Polycose (Abbott Nutrition), Caloreen (Nestlé), or Polyjoule (Nutricia). A 15–30% solution is used, depending on age;
- administration of small amounts at frequent intervals around the clock, thereby ensuring substantial absorption between episodes of vomiting;
- immediate referral to hospital if there is persistent vomiting or deterioration in conscious state;
- otherwise, reintroduction of regular feeds within 24 h.

High caloric intake and avoidance of fasting

A high caloric intake is essential to maintain patients in an anabolic rather than catabolic state. However, many factors make it difficult to achieve a high caloric intake, including recurrent vomiting, anorexia related to metabolic acidosis, unpalatable special diets, and feeding difficulties related to cardiac disease.

Fasting should be assiduously avoided. Even a normal overnight fast may be poorly tolerated in patients with metabolic disorders.

Management approaches to avoid fasting and achieve a high caloric intake may include the following.

Frequent diurnal and nocturnal feeds

Percutaneous endoscopic gastrostomy

This procedure can often resolve many of the feeding issues in severe patients, by allowing for:

- 'top-up' of oral feeds;
- continuous drip feedings which may be better tolerated than bolus feedings;
- nocturnal feeds, without the need to wake the child;
- emergency home administration of glucose during hypoglycaemia.

Uncooked cornstarch

This undergoes prolonged hydrolysis by amylase in the intestine, providing a more continuous source of glucose for absorption for 4–6 h. Cornstarch was originally introduced as treatment for GSD type I, where it replaced the requirement for overnight continuous intragastric glucose infusion. It has found wider application in patients with metabolic disorders as a source of 'slow release' glucose. One dose before bedtime and possibly a second during the night resolves the issue of overnight fasting.

Special diet

Manipulation of the content of the diet according to the specific metabolic defect can have a major therapeutic impact.

Substrate restriction

Restriction of the dietary source of substrate preceding the metabolic block reduces the production and accumulation of toxic metabolic intermediates.

- Natural protein intake is restricted in the organic acidurias to limit the intake of the amino acid(s) whose metabolism is blocked. The

diet may be supplemented with an otherwise nutritionally complete special formula devoid of the specific amino acids (e.g. methionine-, threonine-, valine- and isoleucine-free for propionic and methylmalonic acidaemia). Over-restriction of protein intake must be avoided, as this can exacerbate decompensation by inducing muscle protein catabolism to supply deficient essential amino acids.

- Long-chain fats are restricted in defects of the carnitine shuttle and long-chain fatty acid defects. Essential fatty acids must be supplemented when on a low-fat diet.

Use of alternative metabolic pathways

Functionally intact metabolic pathways can be exploited as an alternative metabolic route, such as a high-carbohydrate diet metabolized via glycolysis for patients with FAOD on a low-fat diet.

Bypassing the metabolic block

This can be achieved by providing an exogenous source of a distal metabolite.

- MCT oil contains medium-chain triglycerides which enter the mitochondrion directly for β-oxidation without requiring the carnitine shuttle. MCT is therefore used in patients with defects of the carnitine shuttle as well as long-chain fatty acid oxidation defects (VLCAD and LCHAD/MTP).[42]
- Triheptanoin has been proposed as an alternative to MCT in long-chain fatty acid disorders on the basis that medium-odd-chain rather than medium-even-chain fatty acids would supply both acetyl-CoA and anapleurotic propionyl-CoA and restore disturbed Krebs cycle dysfunction. Significant improvement of cardiomyopathy and rhabdomyolysis was reported in patients with VLCAD deficiency,[43] but confirmation of these initially promising results has not been forthcoming.
- 3-Hydroxybutyrate. In FAOD, ketone body production by the liver is impaired. Ketones exported from the liver normally serve as an important energy source for the myocardium and other tissues during fasting. Oral administration of the ketone sodium-D,L-3-hydroxybutyrate to two infants with MAD deficiency and critical cardiomyopathy unresponsive to other therapies resulted in progressive and sustained improvement.[44]

L-Carnitine

Carnitine is essential for the transport of long-chain fatty acids into the mitochondrion for subsequent β-oxidation.

Primary carnitine deficiency

In this disorder, administration of pharmacological doses of carnitine is life-saving.

Fatty acid β-oxidation disorders and organic acidurias

In these inherited disorders, carnitine has an essential function in the reverse direction, binding and enabling the removal from the mitochondrion of the accumulating toxic acyl-CoA compounds and the regeneration of essential free coenzyme A. The acylcarnitines thus formed are excreted into the urine, resulting in secondary carnitine depletion. Correction of carnitine deficiency is essential in the management of the organic acidurias, the usual starting dose being 100 mg/kg per day. However, in the long-chain fatty acid β-oxidation disorders such as LCHAD and VLCAD deficiency, use of carnitine supplementation is controversial. Although carnitine has been used to correct secondary carnitine depletion in these disorders, there is concern that its administration during acute metabolic crises may lead to sudden death due to the potentially toxic effects of long-chain acylcarnitines.

Supplementation of vitamins and cofactors

General supplementation of vitamins and minerals

This is important in patients with poor intake or restricted diets. When cornstarch is used as described above it may constitute a significant proportion of the caloric intake but is devoid of essential nutrients.

Specific vitamins in pharmacological doses

These may restore enzyme activity in vitamin-responsive defects or disorders of cofactor metabolism, e.g.:

- vitamin B_{12}-responsive methylmalonic acidemia;
- vitamin B_{12} in the cblC cobalamin metabolism defect;
- riboflavin (vitamin B_2)-responsive multiple acyl-CoA dehydrogenase deficiency.[45]

In hyperoxaluria type 1, a therapeutic trial of pyridoxine is recommended in all to try to reduce production of oxalate.[46]

Bezafibrate

Bezafibrate is a peroxisomal proliferator-activated receptor (PPAR) agonist widely used for its hypolipidaemic action; it increases gene expression, residual enzyme activity, and fatty acid oxidation capacity in fibroblast lines from patients with CPT2[47] and VLCAD deficiency.[48] A pilot trial in CPT2 deficiency patients produced encouraging results.[49] These effects were only apparent, however, in patients with significant residual enzyme activity in fibroblasts and a milder (predominantly muscular) clinical presentation. It is unlikely to benefit patients with cardiomyopathy, as they have severe enzyme deficiency.

Enzyme replacement therapy

Enzyme replacement therapy (ERT) has revolutionized the management of patients with lysosomal storage disorders, for whom previously there was little to offer beyond symptomatic and supportive treatment (see **Figure 6.2**). ERT was initially achieved for Gaucher disease. The two major breakthroughs allowing the development of ERT were the ability to produce large quantities of recombinant enzyme, and recognition of the critical importance of the mannose-6-phosphate (M6P) recognition marker for receptor-mediated uptake of lysosomal enzymes. The recombinant enzyme is modified by addition of mannose-6-phosphate (M6P) moieties for recognition by plasma membrane M6P receptors which sequester modified enzyme into lysosome-targeted transport vesicles, allowing delivery to and uptake by the lysosome.

ERT requires intravenous infusion of the recombinant enzyme every 1–2 weeks and involves a significant commitment by both the medical team and the patient. Common reactions include local irritation and infusion-related hypersensitivity responses. Treatment is usually initiated in a hospital outpatient setting, with the aim of eventual transfer to home infusion therapy. The high cost of this

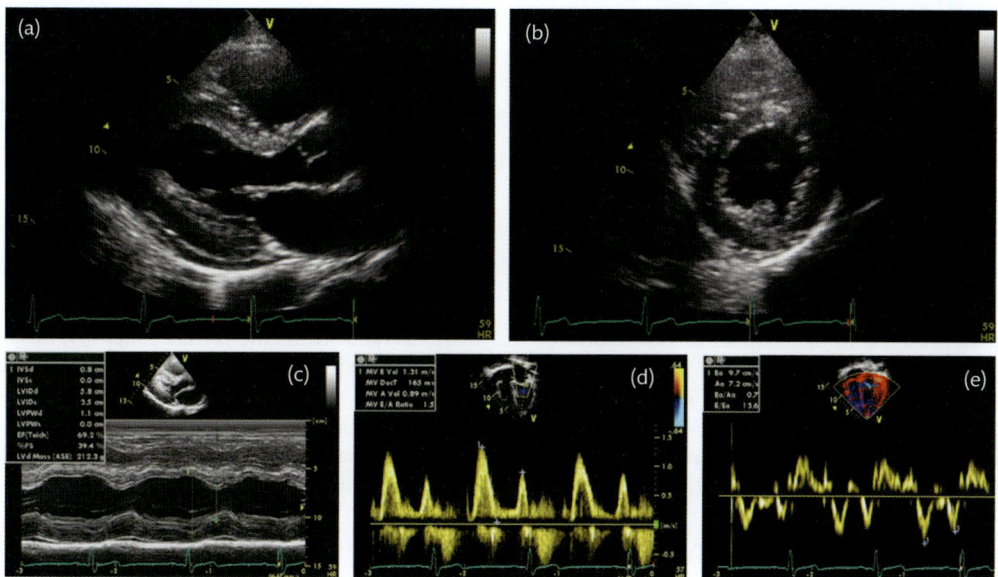

Figure 6.2 Typical echocardiographic findings in a 38-year-old patient with Anderson–Fabry disease who receives enzyme replacement therapy. Parasternal long-axis view (a), short-axis view (b), and M-mode recording (c) show concentric left ventricular hypertrophy (more pronounced in this case in the posterior wall) and small amount of posterior pericardial effusion. Pseudonormal E:A ratio on mitral Doppler (d) and low relaxation velocities on mitral annular tissue Doppler (e) are compatible with stage II diastolic dysfunction with elevated filling pressure.

lifelong treatment programme is a major issue in terms of insurance coverage, particularly where therapeutic benefit is only limited or where clinical manifestations are relatively minor. Enzyme infused intravenously does not cross the blood–brain barrier, limiting its use in treatment of lysosomal storage disorders with progressive neurological involvement.[50]

Pompe disease (GSD II)

Enzyme replacement therapy was initially performed using recombinant human enzyme derived from transgenic rabbit milk, and subsequently from genetically engineered Chinese hamster ovary cells. Myozyme (alglucoside-alfa; Genzyme Corp., Cambridge, MA, USA) has been approved for clinical use by the US Food and Drug Administration since 2006 for all patients with Pompe disease—children and adults. Targeting muscle is problematic, as most of the infused enzyme is taken up by liver and spleen, with only a small amount reaching heart and even less reaching skeletal muscle. High doses are therefore required to achieve a therapeutic effect. Current recommended dosage is 20 mg/kg body weight administered every 2 weeks, although up to 40 mg/kg has been used in individual patients. Clinical studies in patients with the severe infantile form show that the most dramatic effect is on the heart, with significant improvement in cardiac hypertrophy and function as well as prolonged survival beyond the expected age of 1 year in untreated infants. Serial muscle biopsies show clearing of glycogen, with good correlation between extent of glycogen clearance and clinical response. Many achieve motor milestones such as sitting, standing, and walking, which are not expected in the natural course of the disease. However, a significant proportion of treated infants in the initial studies died or remained ventilator dependent due to respiratory muscle failure. The most favourable results have been achieved in patients treated early, before irreversible muscle damage has occurred.[51–53]

The feasibility of newborn screening for Pompe disease created the possibility of initiating ERT before clinical deterioration has occurred. Indeed, a recently published study reported an encouraging outcome for ERT in six infants identified in a newborn screening programme in Taiwan. Five of the six, despite being still clinically asymptomatic in the first month of life, had the severe early-onset form of the disease as evidenced by significant cardiomyopathy, abnormal muscle histology, and severe enzyme deficiency in fibroblasts. Following early institution of ERT and follow-up for 14–32 months, all survived with normalization of cardiac size and muscle histology, normal growth, and normal age-appropriate motor development.[54]

MPS

Recombinant enzyme products are available for ERT of MPS I, II, and VI and can be of benefit in reducing the severity of the somatic manifestations including cardiac disease, but cannot affect the progression of central nervous system (CNS) disease. In contrast, haematopoietic stem cell transplantation with bone marrow or umbilical cord stem cells can arrest or even reverse CNS and somatic manifestations. The choice between these two therapeutic approaches depends on the age of the patient, extent of disease, and predicted rate of progression.[55]

Gene therapy

Gene therapy is being studied as a therapeutic option in many of the disorders of metabolism with the hope of preventing development and/or progression of disease. However, this is not currently a viable option.

Credits: This is a revision of the previous chapter written by Stanley H Korman and Andre Keren.

REFERENCES

1. Shen JJ, Chen YT. Molecular characterization of glycogen storage disease type III. *Curr Mol Med* 2002;**2**(2):167–75.
2. Haeuptle MA, Hennet T. Congenital disorders of glycosylation: an update on defects affecting the biosynthesis of dolichol-linked oligosaccharides. *Hum Mutat* 2009;**30**(12):1628–41.

3. Thuillier L, Rostane H, Droin V, *et al*. Correlation between genotype, metabolic data, and clinical presentation in carnitine palmitoyltransferase 2 (CPT2) deficiency. *Hum Mutat* 2003;**21**(5):493–501.

4. Andresen BS, Olpin S, Poorthuis BJ, *et al*. Clear correlation of genotype with disease phenotype in very-long-chain acyl-CoA dehydrogenase deficiency. *Am J Hum Genet* 1999;**64**(2):479–94.

5. Meir K, Fellig Y, Meiner V, *et al*. Severe infantile carnitine palmitoyltransferase II (cpt ii) deficiency in 19-week fetal sibs. *Pediatr Dev Pathol* 2009;**12**(6):481–6.

6. Korman SH, Pitt JJ, Boneh A, *et al*. A novel SLC25A20 splicing mutation in patients of different ethnic origin with neonatally lethal carnitine-acylcarnitine translocase (CACT) deficiency. *Mol Genet Metab* 2006;**89**(4):332–8.

7. Olpin SE, Clark S, Andresen BS, *et al*. Biochemical, clinical and molecular findings in LCHAD and general mitochondrial trifunctional protein deficiency. *J Inherit Metab Dis* 2005;**28**(4):533–44.

8. Tyni T, Pihko H. Long-chain 3-hydroxyacyl-CoA dehydrogenase deficiency. *Acta Paediatr* 1999;**88**(3):237–45.

9. Tyni T, Paetau A, Strauss AW, Middleton B, Kivela T. Mitochondrial fatty acid beta-oxidation in the human eye and brain: implications for the retinopathy of long-chain 3-hydroxyacyl-CoA dehydrogenase deficiency. *Pediatr Res* 2004;**56**(5):744–50.

10. Tein I, Vajsar J, MacMillan L, Sherwood WG. Long-chain L-3-hydroxyacyl-coenzyme A dehydrogenase deficiency neuropathy: response to cod liver oil. *Neurology* 1999;**52**(3):640–3.

11. Browning MF, Levy HL, Wilkins-Haug LE, Larson C, Shih VE. Fetal fatty acid oxidation defects and maternal liver disease in pregnancy. *Obstet Gynecol* 2006;**107**(1):115–20.

12. Laura S. Kremer, Felix Distelmaier, Bader Alhaddad, *et al*. Bi-allelic Truncating Mutations in TANGO2 Cause Infancy-Onset Recurrent Metabolic Crises with Encephalocardiomyopathy. *Am J Hum Genet* 2016;**98**(2):358–62.

13. Miroslav P. Milev, Djenann Saint-Dic, Khashayar Zardoui, et al. The phenotype associated with variants in TANGO2 may be explained by a dual role of the protein in ER-to-Golgi transport and at the mitochondria. *J Inherit Metab Dis* 2021;44:426–37.

14. Lee NC, Tang NL, Chien YH, *et al*. Diagnoses of newborns and mothers with carnitine uptake defects through newborn screening. *Mol Genet Metab* 2010;**100**(1):46–50.

15. El Hattab AW, Li FY, Shen J, *et al*. Maternal systemic primary carnitine deficiency uncovered by newborn screening: clinical, biochemical, and molecular aspects. *Genet Med* 2010;**12**(1):19–24.

16. Romano S, Valayannopoulos V, Touati G, *et al*. Cardiomyopathies in propionic aciduria are reversible after liver transplantation. *J Pediatr* 2010;**156**(1):128–34.

17. Ficicioglu C, Chrisant MR, Payan I, Chace DH. Cardiomyopathy and hypotonia in a 5-month-old infant with malonyl-CoA decarboxylase deficiency: potential for preclinical diagnosis with expanded newborn screening. *Pediatr Cardiol* 2005;**26**(6):881–3.

18. Salomons GS, Jakobs C, Pope LL, *et al*. Clinical, enzymatic and molecular characterization of nine new patients with malonyl-coenzyme A decarboxylase deficiency. *J Inherit Metab Dis* 2007;**30**(1):23–8.

19. van der Knaap MS, Jakobs C, Hoffmann GF, *et al*. D-2-hydroxyglutaric aciduria: further clinical delineation. *J Inherit Metab Dis* 1999;**22**(4):404–13.

20. Barth PG, Valianpour F, Bowen VM, *et al*. X-linked cardioskeletal myopathy and neutropenia (Barth syndrome): an update. *Am J Med Genet A* 2004;**126A**(4):349–54.

21. Spencer CT, Bryant RM, Day J, *et al*. Cardiac and clinical phenotype in Barth syndrome. *Pediatrics* 2006;**118**(2):e337–e346.

22. Jefferies JL. Barth syndrome. *Am J Med Genet* 2013;**163C**:198–205.

23. Profitlich LE, Kirmse B, Wasserstein MP, Diaz GA, Srivastava S. High prevalence of structural heart disease in children with cblC-type methylmalonic aciduria and homocystinuria. *Mol Genet Metab* 2009;**98**(4):344–8.

24. Carvalho JS, Matthews EE, Leonard JV, Deanfield J. Cardiomyopathy of glycogen storage disease type III. *Heart Vessels* 1993;**8**(3):155–9.

25. Lee PJ, Deanfield JE, Burch M, *et al*. Comparison of the functional significance of left ventricular hypertrophy in hypertrophic cardiomyopathy and glycogenosis type III. *Am J Cardiol* 1997;**79**(6):834–8.

26. Dagli AI, Zori RT, McCune H, *et al*. Reversal of glycogen storage disease type IIIa-related cardiomyopathy with modification of diet. *J Inherit Metab Dis* 2009;**32 Suppl 1**(01):S103–6.

27. Nase S, Kunze KP, Sigmund M, *et al*. A new variant of type IV glycogenosis with primary cardiac manifestation and complete branching enzyme deficiency. In vivo detection by heart muscle biopsy. *Eur Heart J* 1995;**16**(11):1698–704.

28. Burwinkel B, Scott JW, Buhrer C, *et al*. Fatal congenital heart glycogenosis caused by a recurrent activating R531Q mutation in the gamma 2-subunit of AMP-activated protein kinase (PRKAG2): not by phosphorylase kinase deficiency. *Am J Hum Genet* 2005;**76**(6):1034–49.

29. Arad M, Benson DW, Perez-Atayde AR, *et al*. Constitutively active AMP kinase mutations cause glycogen storage disease mimicking hypertrophic cardiomyopathy. *J Clin Invest* 2002;**109**(3):357–62.

30. Sugie K, Yamamoto A, Murayama K, *et al*. Clinicopathological features of genetically confirmed Danon disease. *Neurology* 2002;**58**(12):1773–8.

31. Footitt EJ, Karimova A, Burch M, *et al*. Cardiomyopathy in the congenital disorders of glycosylation (CDG): a case of late presentation and literature review. *J Inherit Metab Dis* 2009;**32 Suppl 1**:S313–19.

32. Cizkova A, Stranecky V, Mayr JA, *et al*. TMEM70 mutations cause isolated ATP synthase deficiency and neonatal mitochondrial encephalocardiomyopathy. *Nat Genet* 2008;**40**(11):1288–90.

33. Chace DH. Mass spectrometry in newborn and metabolic screening: historical perspective and future directions. *J Mass Spectrom* 2009;**44**(2):163–70.

34. Law LK, Tang NL, Hui J, *et al*. A novel functional assay for simultaneous determination of total fatty acid beta-oxidation flux and acylcarnitine profiling in human skin fibroblasts using (2)H(3)(1)-palmitate by isotope ratio mass spectrometry and electrospray tandem mass spectrometry. *Clin Chim Acta* 2007;**382**(1–2):25–30.

35. Babovic-Vuksanovic D, O'Brien JF. Laboratory diagnosis of congenital disorders of glycosylation type I by analysis of transferrin glycoforms. *Mol Diagn Ther* 2007;**11**(5):303–11.

36. Marklova E, Albahri Z. Screening and diagnosis of congenital disorders of glycosylation. *Clin Chim Acta* 2007;**385**(1–2):6–20.

37. Houtkooper RH, Rodenburg RJ, Thiels C, *et al.* Cardiolipin and monolysocardiolipin analysis in fibroblasts, lymphocytes, and tissues using high-performance liquid chromatography-mass spectrometry as a diagnostic test for Barth syndrome. *Anal Biochem* 2009;**387**(2):230–7.

38. Kulik W, van Lenthe H, Stet FS, *et al.* Bloodspot assay using HPLC–tandem mass spectrometry for detection of Barth syndrome. *Clin Chem* 2008;**54**(2):371–8.

39. Gelb MH, Turecek F, Scott CR, Chamoles NA. Direct multiplex assay of enzymes in dried blood spots by tandem mass spectrometry for the newborn screening of lysosomal storage disorders. *J Inherit Metab Dis* 2006;**29**(2–3):397–404.

40. Zhang XK, Elbin CS, Chuang WL, *et al.* Multiplex enzyme assay screening of dried blood spots for lysosomal storage disorders by using tandem mass spectrometry. *Clin Chem* 2008;**54**(10):1725–8.

41. Van Hove JL, Myers S, Kerckhove KV, Freehauf C, Bernstein L. Acute nutrition management in the prevention of metabolic illness: a practical approach with glucose polymers. *Mol Genet Metab* 2009;**97**(1):1–3.

42. Jones PM, Butt Y, Bennett MJ. Accumulation of 3-hydroxy-fatty acids in the culture medium of long-chain L-3-hydroxyacyl CoA dehydrogenase (LCHAD) and mitochondrial trifunctional protein-deficient skin fibroblasts: implications for medium chain triglyceride dietary treatment of LCHAD deficiency. *Pediatr Res* 2003;**53**(5):783–7.

43. Roe CR, Sweetman L, Roe DS, David F, Brunengraber H. Treatment of cardiomyopathy and rhabdomyolysis in long-chain fat oxidation disorders using an anaplerotic odd-chain triglyceride. *J Clin Invest* 2002;**110**(2):259–69.

44. Van Hove JL, Grunewald S, Jaeken J, *et al.* D,L-3-hydroxybutyrate treatment of multiple acyl-CoA dehydrogenase deficiency (MADD). *Lancet* 2003;**361**(9367):1433–5.

45. Olsen RK, Olpin SE, Andresen BS, *et al.* ETFDH mutations as a major cause of riboflavin-responsive multiple acyl-CoA dehydrogenation deficiency. *Brain* 2007;**130**(8):2045–54.

46. Clayton PT. B6-responsive disorders: a model of vitamin dependency. J Inherit Metab Dis 2006;**29**:317–26

47. Djouadi F, Bonnefont JP, Thuillier L, *et al.* Correction of fatty acid oxidation in carnitine palmitoyl transferase 2-deficient cultured skin fibroblasts by bezafibrate. *Pediatr Res* 2003;**54**(4):446–51.

48. Djouadi F, Aubey F, Schlemmer D, *et al.* Bezafibrate increases very-long-chain acyl-CoA dehydrogenase protein and mRNA expression in deficient fibroblasts and is a potential therapy for fatty acid oxidation disorders. *Hum Mol Genet* 2005;**14**(18):2695–703.

49. Bonnefont JP, Bastin J, Behin A, Djouadi F. Bezafibrate for an inborn mitochondrial beta-oxidation defect. *N Engl J Med* 2009;**360**(8):838–40.

50. Lim-Melia ER, Kronn DF. Current enzyme replacement therapy for the treatment of lysosomal storage diseases. *Pediatr Ann* 2009;**38**(8):448–55.

51. Schoser B, Hill V, Raben N. Therapeutic approaches in glycogen storage disease type II/Pompe disease. *Neurotherapeutics* 2008;**5**(4):569–78.

52. van der Ploeg AT, Reuser AJ. Pompe disease. *Lancet* 2008;**372**(9646):1342–53.

53. Chen LR, Chen CA, Chiu SN, *et al.* Reversal of cardiac dysfunction after enzyme replacement in patients with infantile-onset Pompe disease. *J Pediatr* 2009;**155**(2):271–5.

54. Chien YH, Lee NC, Thurberg BL, *et al.* Pompe disease in infants: improving the prognosis by newborn screening and early treatment. *Pediatrics* 2009;**124**(6):e1116–e1125.

55. Muenzer J, Wraith JE, Clarke LA. Mucopolysaccharidosis I: management and treatment guidelines. *Pediatrics* 2009;**123**(1):19–29.

7

Heart failure in congenital heart disease

Rafael Alonso-Gonzalez and Lorna Swan

Congenital heart disease (CHD) is the most common congenital abnormality, present in an estimated 8 cases per 1000 live births.[1,2] This prevalence varies significantly among continents, being higher in Asia with 9.3 per 1000 births (95% confidence interval (CI): 8.9–9.7) compared to Europe with 8.2 per 1000 births (95% CI: 8.1–8.3) or North America with 6.9 per 1000 births (95% CI: 6.7–7.1).[3] Whereas some defects are trivial, for example a septal defect that spontaneously closes during childhood, about 0.6 per 1000 adults will have a severe form of congenital heart disease.

Advances in cardiovascular diagnosis, surgical techniques, interventional cardiology, and postoperative care have increased survival in CHD patients. Recent data have shown that the number of adults living with CHD has already surpassed the number of children.[2] As a consequence there is now a large and growing population of adults with congenital heart disease (ACHD). However, many interventions are palliative rather than curative, and patients often are left with residual lesions which may lead to several cardiac complications, including heart failure. Heart failure management in the setting of CHD is challenged by the wide range of ages at which heart failure occurs, the heterogeneity of the underlying anatomy and surgical repairs, the wide spectrum of heart failure causes, the lack of validated biomarkers for disease progression, and the lack of reliable risk predictors or surrogate end-points. In addition there is little evidence demonstrating treatment efficacy.

Definition of heart failure in congenital heart disease

Defining heart failure in patients with CHD is challenging. By definition, patients with Fontan circulation will have low cardiac output immediately after the circuit is completed.[4,5] One even could consider that patients with CHD are born with heart failure since they already have structural heart disease at birth.[6] However, the reality is that the majority of patients will experience periods of exacerbation and remittance of different risks factors for heart failure that will eventually lead to symptoms of congestion or low cardiac output (Figure 7.1). In addition, patients with CHD may have signs of heart failure (e.g. low peak oxygen uptake (peak VO_2) or elevated brain natriuretic peptide (BNP)) in the absence of heart failure symptoms.

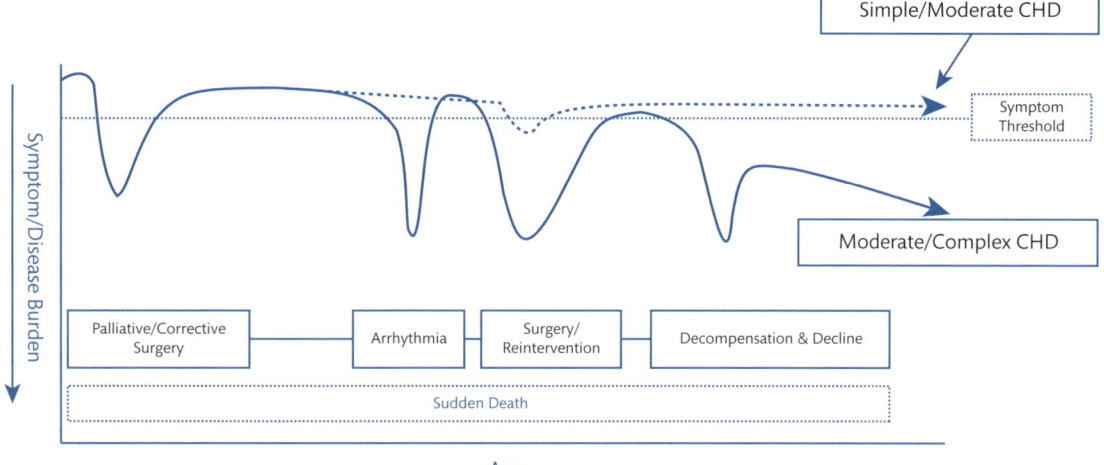

Figure 7.1 Schematic representation of pattern of heart failure presentation in simple and more complex forms of congenital heart. Possible causes of acute and chronic deterioration are listed in boxes below. Sudden death is a persistent, if low level, risk throughout the lifespan. CHD, congenital heart disease.

Reproduced with permission from Alshawabkeh LI, Opotowsky AR. Burden of heart failure in adults with congenital heart disease. *Curr Heart Fail Rep* 2016;**13**:247–254.

This makes it difficult to develop a universal definition of heart failure in these populations. The inconsistency of definitions of heart failure in ACHD patients in the published literature can be interpreted as an appropriate reflection of underlying complexity of the disease and its management.[7]

The American Heart Association has recently published a scientific statement in chronic heart failure in CHD.[8] The statement included a detailed definition of heart failure in CHD from the Heart Failure Society of America. This definition states that 'HF is a syndrome characterized by either one or both pulmonary and systemic venous congestion and/or inadequate peripheral oxygen delivery, at rest or during stress, caused by cardiac dysfunction.' While many symptomatic ACHD patients will be well classified using this definition, many asymptomatic ACHD patients with heart failure will not, e.g. Fontan patients with protein-losing enteropathy (PLE). Nonetheless, although this definition is not perfect, if we consider the complexity of this population, it is probably a good, clinically relevant solution.

Epidemiology

The absence of a national databases for CHD populations makes it difficult to know accurately the number of patients with ACHD in many countries including the UK. Data from the province of Quebec reports an increase in CHD prevalence of 11% in children and 57% in adults from 2000 to 2010. The overall prevalence of CHD in this study was 13.1 per 1000 (95% CI: 12.4–13.8) in children and 6.1 per 1000 (95% CI: 5.79–6.6) in adults. Assuming equivalent prevalences, there are currently at least 322 000 adults with CHD living in the UK, including 32 000 patients with complex CHD. Despite the success of their initial management, ACHD patients often have residual lesions or complications due to their palliative operations which may predispose to heart failure symptoms. Heart failure is therefore an important problem that is growing in this emerging population. One could say that we are paying the price of our own success.

Prevalence of heart failure in congenital heart disease

Although the majority of long-term survivors with CHD are patients with simple lesions such as atrial or ventricular septal defects, Marelli *et al.* reported an increase of 55% in patients with complex lesions between 2000 and 2010.[2] These patients will be at risk of developing heart failure and definitely need life-long care in specialized centres. Heart failure has been reported to develop during childhood in ~5% of all patients with CHD and up to 10–20% of patients after the Fontan procedure.[9–11] Recent data have suggested a prevalence of heart failure of nearly 50% in adult patients with Fontan procedure,[4,12,13] and between 25% and 35% in patients with systemic right ventricle (RV).[13]

According to the National Heart Failure Audit, there are currently at least 550 000 patients with heart failure in the UK. The in-hospital mortality is around 10% following an admission with heart failure per annum. Of those who survive, between one-quarter and one-third will die within one year of their admission. Patients with CHD contribute a minority of these patients, but the number of ACHD patients with heart failure-related hospitalization is increasing. From 1998 to 2005, the number of hospitalizations of ACHD patients in the USA increased 102% and heart failure-related hospitalizations

increased by 82%. The overall prevalence of heart failure among hospitalized patients with ACHD has been noted to be significantly greater than that reported for hospitalizations in the general adult population.[14] Hospitalization for heart failure identifies a population of ACHD patients at risk for subsequent hospitalizations and mortality over the next three years. A recent study from the Netherlands reported an incidence of first heart failure admission in ACHD patients of 1.2 per 1000 patient-years with an increase of fivefold risk of mortality in patients admitted with heart failure when compare with non-admitted ACHD patients.[15]

Heart failure and mortality in congenital heart disease

Heart failure is the most common cause of death in ACHD. From data for the Royal Brompton Hospital in 6969 ACHD patients, 524 (7.5%) patients died over a median follow-up time of 9.1 years. Heart failure was the leading cause of death (32%), followed by pneumonia (10%) and sudden cardiac death (SCD) (7%)[16] (**Figure 7.2**).

Data from the CONCOR registry reported 197 (2.8%) deaths in 6933 ACHD patients over a median follow-up of 24 865 patient-years. Heart failure was the most common underlying cause of death, in 26%, followed by non-cardiovascular causes in 23%, and sudden death in 19%.

The German National Registry for Congenital Heart Defects reported similar findings: 239 (9.2%) deaths in 2596 ACHD patients over a median follow-up of 14 114 patient-years. Heart failure was again the most common cause of death, accounting for 27.6% of the deaths followed by sudden cardiac death (23%) and non-CHD related causes (18%). Despite the differences in the overall mortality rate among the different publications, heart failure is clearly the leading cause of death in ACHD patients, accounting for 26–32% of deaths. Furthermore, the frequency of heart failure as a cause of death in these registries is likely to be underestimated because many patients who suffer sudden death have this in the context of ongoing underlying heart failure.[7]

Pathophysiology of heart failure in congenital heart disease

Heart failure in patients with CHD, both paediatric and adult, is complex and can originate from a monogenic aetiology. However, in the majority of patients, heart failure involves complex interactions between primary structural defects, the consequences of previous interventions (i.e. residual lesions), and the heart's response to enhanced myocardial mechanical stress which depends on many other genetic factors (i.e. gene modifiers).[17] Heart failure can be the result of valvular abnormalities, flow obstruction or myocardial dysfunction, as in patients with acquired heart diseases. However, some situations are specific to CHD patients, such as the presence of a systemic RV, chronic intracardiac shunts, or failure of the Fontan circulation.

Myocardial dysfunction in CHD can be the result of haemodynamic derangements such as abnormal pressure or volume loading, ventricular hypertrophy, myocardial ischaemia, or effects of prior cardiopulmonary bypass or ventriculotomy. Any of these may incite systolic or diastolic impairment, and clinical manifestations such as arrhythmia or exercise intolerance. In addition, pericardial

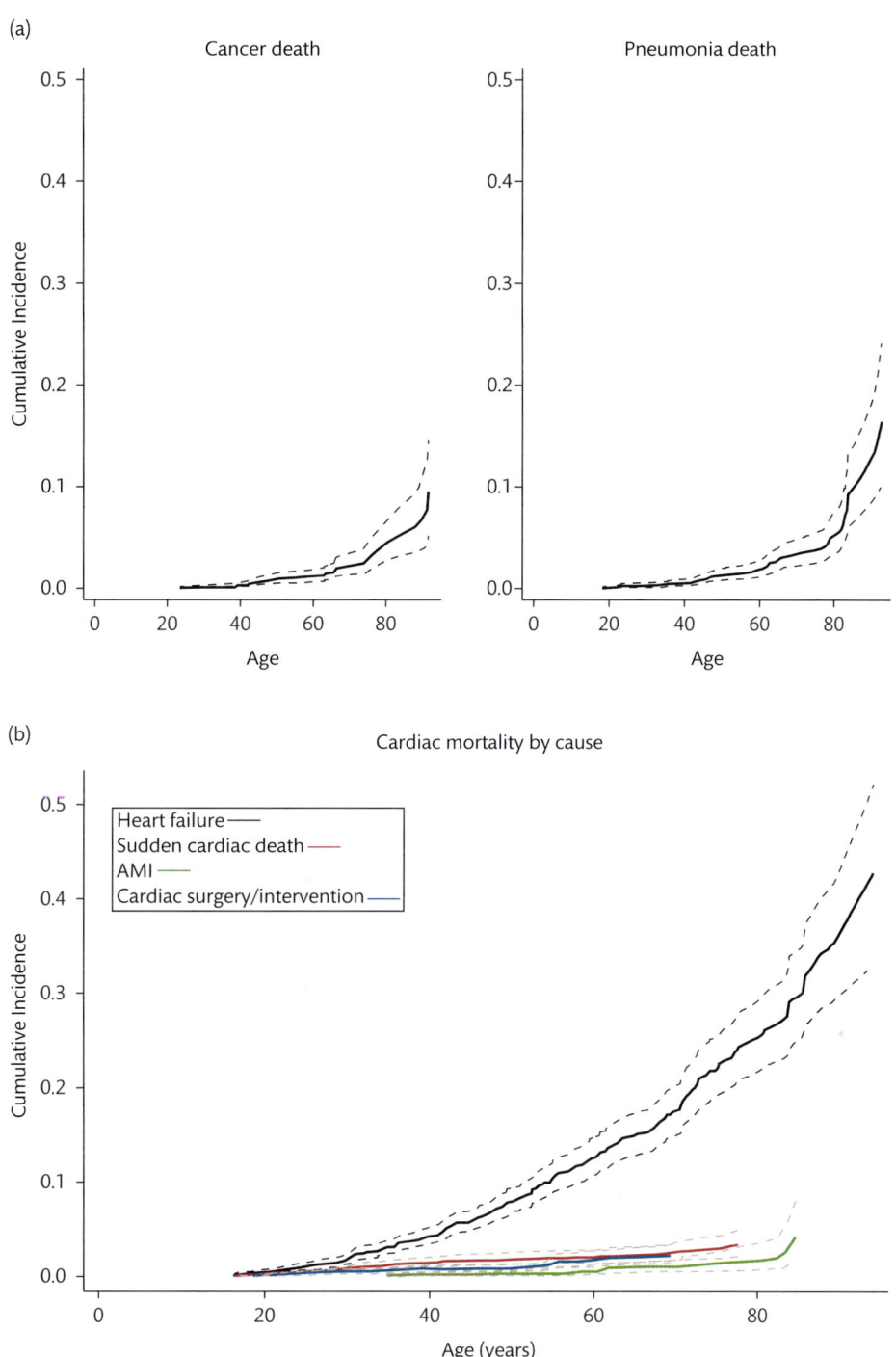

Figure 7.2 (a) Cumulative incidence of pneumonia and cancer death with 95% confidence intervals based on the results of competing risk model. (b) Cumulative incidence of various causes of cardiac mortality with 95% confidence intervals based on the results of competing risk model. AMI indicates acute myocardial infarction. AMI, acute myocardial infarction.

Reproduced with permission from Diller *et al*. Survival prospects and circumstances of death in contemporary adult congenital heart disease patients under follow-up at a large tertiary centre. *Circulation* 2015;**132**:2118–25. with permission from Wolters Kluwer.

constriction as a consequence of prior surgery may cause heart failure symptoms.[8]

Myocardial structure

The myocardial structure in CHD can exhibit disarray of ventricular myocardial fibres.[18] In an animal model of hypoplastic left heart syndrome, abnormal RV and left ventricle (LV) myocardial fibre orientation was noted prenatally, reflected in abnormal patterns of anisotropic RV and LV deformation.[19] Different myofibre and connective tissue architecture has also been observed in patients with tricuspid atresia.[8]

Many of the pathways involved in cardiac development *in utero* are also involved in myocardial structure and stability. Therefore, certain molecular perturbations can cause both a cardiac defect at

birth and a cardiomyopathy that can present later in life.[20] Noonan syndrome is the second most frequent syndromic form of CHD and can cause both CHD and cardiomyopathy. Mutations in the RAS–MAPK pathway have been identified in these patients, causing pulmonary stenosis and hypertrophic cardiomyopathy.[21] Another example of congenital cardiomyopathy is left ventricular non-compaction. In adults with CHD, left ventricular non-compaction occurs in up to 12% of cases, particularly in patients with left ventricular outflow tract obstruction, Ebstein anomaly, and Tetralogy of Fallot (ToF). This is caused by genes such as *MYH7* and the transcription factor *NKX2-5*, among others.[20,22,23]

Abnormal perfusion

Even in the absence of abnormal coronary arteries, patients with CHD might develop myocardial ischaemia. Coronary flow–demand mismatch is well-recognized in patients with systemic RV. Many studies demonstrated perfusion abnormalities in patients with a systemic RV in whom the typical coronary anatomy supplying the RV is insufficient for a hypertrophied, enlarged ventricle, although there are conflicting data on the frequency and clinical importance of these findings.[24-26] In addition, high wall stress from increased afterload in conjunction with decreased coronary flow reserve is associated with myocardial hypoperfusion and supply–demand mismatch, the effects of which may only become manifest over decades.[8] Chronic cyanosis is common in patients with CHD, which can result in significant myocardial ischaemia due to poor oxygen supply. Patients with cyanotic heart disease at birth might develop myocardial ischaemia until repair or palliation. The early period of ischaemia may not have a detectable impact on ventricular function in the short term but may jeopardize or preprogram the myocardium to more serious dysfunction later in life.[8]

Myocardial fibrosis

It is well recognized that one of the effects of neurohormonal and renin–angiotensin–aldosterone system (RAAS) activation is alteration in collagen turnover by myofibroblasts, leading to detectable myocardial fibrosis.[8] There are data to suggest that an abnormal accumulation of fibrous tissue from an early stage may be an inherent part of some CHD defects in hearts exposed to ischaemia and pressure and volume overload.[27,28] Cardiac magnetic resonance (CMR) with late gadolinium enhancement (LGE) has been used to assess fibrosis in CHD. Gadolinium increases signal intensity of extracellular material in myocardium late after injection, which correlates with fibrosis. The presence of fibrosis in several ACHD subgroups has been demonstrated: ToF (99%),[29] systemic RV (61%),[30] and patients with Eisenmenger syndrome (73%).[31] In patients with ToF, LGE is present mainly in the right ventricular outflow tract (99%) inferior wall of the RV (79%), trabeculated right ventricular myocardium (24%), and less common in the LV. Both in the ToF and systemic RV population, the extent of LGE correlates with systemic/subpulmonary right ventricular function, exercise intolerance, and the risk of developing clinical arrhythmias.[29,30] Patients with ToF with extensive LGE are more likely to have restrictive physiology.

While LGE detects macroscopic fibrosis, T1 mapping on CMR imaging demonstrates early diffuse fibrosis, and this technique is increasingly used in ACHD patients. Broberg *et al.* showed increased fibrosis beyond that demonstrated by LGE in a mixed cohort of 50 ACHD patients.[32] Such methods may help explain the time course and specific inciting causes of fibrosis across the CHD spectrum.

Interventricular interaction

Ventricular–ventricular interaction refers to the concept that size, shape and compliance of one ventricle will affect the function of the other. Animal experiments showed that the LV contributes approximately 20–40% of right ventricular systolic pressure, whereas the RV contributes little to the LV.[33] Increases in RV end-diastolic volume can lead to pericardial constraint affecting both LV and RV function. The systolic ventricular interdependence is mainly mediated by the interventricular septum, whereas the pericardium is more important in the diastolic interventricular interaction.

Interventricular interaction is an important mechanism of heart failure in ACHD patients. Abnormalities of left ventricular function, regardless of cause, all influence right ventricular function, depending on the degree to which they affect RV diastolic volume and function, RV systolic function, and RV afterload. In addition, in acute RV pressure, or volume-overload states, dilatation of the RV shifts the interventricular septum toward the left. This alters LV geometry and increases pericardial constraint. As a consequence, the LV preload can potentially decrease and lead to a low cardiac output state. This situation is common in patients with Ebstein anomaly and large atrialized portion of the RV or after ToF repair. Patients with ToF frequently have severe pulmonary regurgitation (PR) as a residual lesion. This will lead to RV dilatation and progressive RV dysfunction which, in the presence of pericardial constriction, will cause severe RV diastolic dysfunction and reduction in LV preload. Kempny *et al.* used CMR and speckle-tracking to describe a significant interrelation between the LV and RV in a small cohort of patients with ToF, half of them with severe PR.[34]

Neurohormonal activation

Neurohormonal activation is an integral part of the heart failure syndrome. In heart failure due to acquired heart disease, the degree of neurohormonal activation correlates to symptoms, severity of left ventricular dysfunction, and prognosis. It is also a major target for therapies.[35-37] There is emerging evidence on the usefulness of biomarkers in CHD. Bolger *et al.* described elevated plasma concentration of natriuretic peptides, endothelin-1, norepinephrine, renin, and aldosterone in adult patients with CHD.[6] Natriuretic peptides and endothelin concentration were related to New York Heart Association (NYHA) functional class, peak VO₂ and systemic ventricular function, as well as electrocardiographic and radiographic parameters.[38] Activation of the natriuretic peptides occurs in a wide spectrum of CHD patients and may remain elevated years after surgical repair of even relatively simple lesions.[39,40]

Even though a clear relation between neurohormonal activation and functional class has been demonstrated,[38] CHD patients who are asymptomatic often present with elevated levels of natriuretic peptides. Plasma atrial natriuretic peptide (ANP) concentration is high in patients with atrial septal defect even in the absence of heart failure symptoms and correlates with pulmonary blood flow/systemic blood flow ratio.[41] High sensitivity troponin T (hs-TnT) is also elevated in a significant proportion of stable ACHD patients and correlates with N-terminal pro B-type natriuretic peptide (NT-proBNP) and systemic and subpulmonary ventricular function.[42,43]

Recent studies suggested that biomarkers also predict outcome in patients with CHD.[44–47] Baggen *et al.* showed in a population of 595 stable ACHD patients, 90% in NYHA I, that NT-proBNP >33.3 pmol/L is strongly associated with cardiovascular events, risk of heart failure, or death.[44] In addition, NT-proBNP >14 pmol/L, hs-TnT >14 ng/L, and growth-differentiation factor 15 (GDF-15) >1109 ng/L identify ACHD patients at highest risk of developing cardiovascular events.[44]

Exercise intolerance in congenital heart disease

Exercise intolerance is a major problem in the ACHD population and it has a major impact on quality of life. ACHD patients, even those with simple lesions, have reduced exercise capacity when compared to the general population (Figure 7.3).[48]

Exercise intolerance is usually a result of a combination of cardiac and extracardiac contributors. The most important cardiac contributors include ventricular systolic or diastolic dysfunction (of either the systemic or the subpulmonary ventricle, or the function of a single ventricle), valvular stenosis or regurgitation, chronotropic incompetence, conduction abnormalities, significant arrhythmia burden, intracardiac shunt, and pericardial disease.[49] The most relevant extracardiac contributors include the presence of significant lung disease, pulmonary vascular disease, anaemia, iron deficiency, and deconditioning.[50]

Assessment of exercise capacity in patients with CHD is paramount. Although a simple exercise test without gas exchange may assist in identifying the cause of effort limitation in this population, the use of cardiopulmonary exercise test (CPET) is more informative. CPET is a powerful tool for the objective assessment of the cardiovascular, respiratory, and muscular systems and has become part of the routine clinical assessment of ACHD patients. Incremental protocols are used to assess functional and prognostic indices such as peak VO_2, VE/VCO_2 slope (the slope of the regression line between ventilation (VE) and rate of elimination of carbon dioxide (VCO_2)), anaerobic threshold, and heart rate and blood pressure response. Peak VO_2 may be reduced in several CHD conditions and worsens as the heart failure symptoms progress. Serial CPET are recommended as part of the assessment of patients with ToF and severe PR to help in the decision for elective pulmonary valve replacement. VE/VCO_2 slope may be influenced by multiple factors, but in CHD patients pulmonary flow distribution and consequent ventilation/perfusion (VQ) mismatch are probably the most important pathophysiologic processes in this population. Patients who have undergone repair of ToF may have residual branch pulmonary artery stenosis that causes maldistribution of the pulmonary blood flow, which in turn has been linked to VE/VCO_2 slope elevation and depressed peak VO_2. Patients with Eisenmenger syndrome and those with chronic cyanosis have the highest VE/VCO_2 slopes. Chronotropic incompetence, defined as the inability to achieve 80% of age-predicted maximal heart rate reserve (HRR) ([peak heart rate-resting heart rate]/[220-age-resting heart rate]) is common and associated with exercise limitation in patients with a systemic RV or univentricular circulation.[51]

CPET provides strong prognostic information in ACHD patients. However, prognostication should be approached differently depending on the presence of cyanosis, use of rate-lowering medications, and achieved level of exercise. Inuzuka *et al.* showed in a cohort of 1375 consecutive ACHD patients (aged 33 ± 13 years), who underwent CPET at a single centre over a period of 10 years, that peak VO_2, HRR, and oxygen saturation were independent predictors of mortality in ACHD patients. The risk of death increased with lower peak VO_2 and HRR. A higher VE/VCO_2 slope was also related to increased risk of death in non-cyanotic patients, but not in cyanotic patients. The combination of peak VO_2 and HRR provided the greatest predictive information after adjustment for clinical parameters such as negative chronotropic agents, age, and presence of cyanosis.[52]

The six-minute walk test is simpler to assess exercise capacity and can be used in selected ACHD patients. However, its utility and validity in patients with mild or moderate impairment are unclear.[49]

General considerations

Patients with ACHD are at risk of complications related to the original defect and/or subsequently repair. Due to the unique features of heart failure in this population, ACHD patients must be evaluated and managed by a physician with specialist knowledge in CHD. Thorough review of previous surgical interventions as well as thorough knowledge of individual patients' anatomy are paramount.

When examining CHD patients, basic principles used in acquired heart disease patients may not apply. For example, an elevated jugular venous pressure (JVP) will be a normal finding in a patient with a healthy Fontan circulation where the JVP is a marker of the pulmonary artery pressure and not a manifestation of an elevated right ventricular end-diastolic pressure. The presence of hypoalbuminaemia with or without peripheral oedema and/or diarrhoea in patients with Fontan circulation may suggest protein-losing enteropathy, a frequent condition in patients with chronically elevated right atrial pressures. Iron deficiency anaemia—a recognized cause of heart failure in CHD patients—must be ruled out in cyanotic patients with heart failure even in presence of normal haemoglobin.

Imaging assessment of ACHD patients is beyond the scope of this chapter. However, it is important to consider that accurate interpretation of imaging requires a high level of expertise even when assessing simple lesions. For example, the Doppler flow of a restrictive perimembranous ventricular septal defect may be misinterpreted as a tricuspid regurgitation jet, leading to an erroneous diagnosis of pulmonary hypertension. Involvement of imagers with CHD expertise is important and can help avoid erroneous treatments or unnecessary invasive procedures.[8]

Medical treatment

Despite the significant contribution of heart failure to premature morbidity and mortality in the ACHD population, no adequately powered clinical trials have been done to understand the role of medical therapies in heart failure. Although there are a handful of randomized control trials, most of the existing data in this population are derived from small observational studies with a heterogeneous population. In addition these studies often have short follow-up times and low event rates.

In a recent European Survey study, 39% of Fontan patients and 33% of systemic RV patients received angiotensin converting enzyme inhibitors (ACEi).[53] The corresponding rates for β-blockers

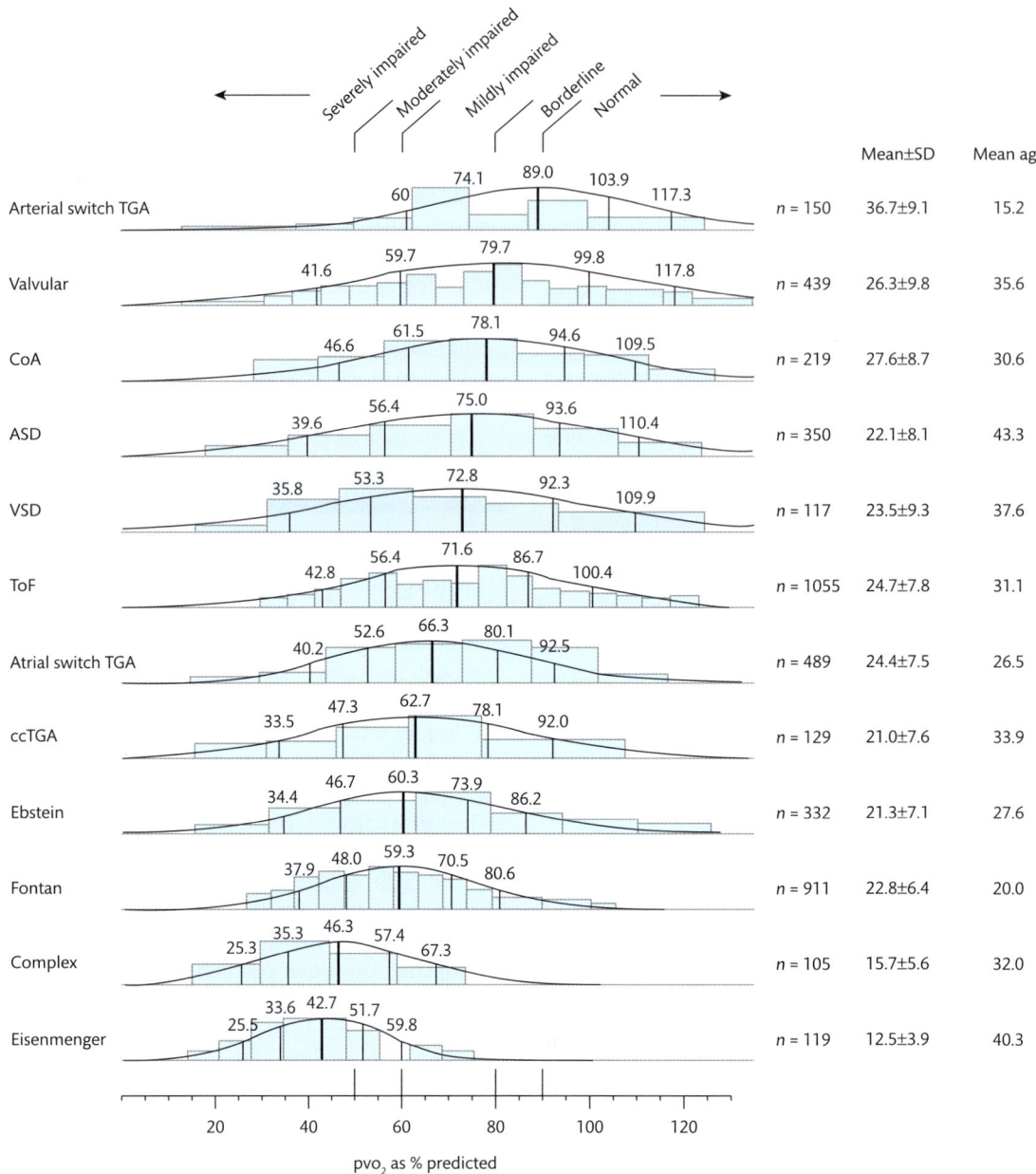

Figure 7.3 Peak oxygen uptake data expressed as percentage of predicted value. The density lines above histogram bars and the numbers to the right of the graph relate to all patients with a given diagnosis. The numbers above the density lines indicate percentage peak VO₂ values for the 10th, 25th, 50th, 75th and 90th centiles. ASD, atrial septal defect; ccTGA, congenitally corrected TGA; CoA, coarctation of aorta; Complex, complex congenital heart disease (including univentricular hearts); Ebstein, Ebstein anomaly; Eisenmenger, Eisenmenger syndrome; Fontan, patients after Fontan palliation; TGA, transposition of the great arteries; ToF, tetralogy of Fallot; Valvular, mixed collective of patients with congenital valvular heart disease; VSD, ventricular septal defect

Reproduced with permission from Khairy et al. (Khairy P, Van Hare GF, Balaji S, Berul CI, Cecchin F, Cohen MI, Daniels CJ, Deal BJ, Dearani JA, Groot N, Dubin AM, Harris L, Janousek J, Kanter RJ, Karpawich PP, Perry JC, Seslar SP, Shah MJ, Silka MJ, Triedman JK, Walsh EP and Warnes CA. PACES/HRS Expert Consensus Statement on the Recognition and Management of Arrhythmias in Adult Congenital Heart Disease: developed in partnership between the Pediatric and Congenital Electrophysiology Society (PACES) and the Heart Rhythm Society (HRS). Endorsed by the governing bodies of PACES, HRS, the American College of Cardiology (ACC), the American Heart Association (AHA), the European Heart Rhythm Association (EHRA), the Canadian Heart Rhythm Society (CHRS), and the International Society for Adult Congenital Heart Disease (ISACHD). *Heart Rhythm* 2014;**11**:e102–65.)

were 26% and 17%. When treating patients with CHD and heart failure, a good understanding of the anatomy and the physiology are paramount. Patients with dextro-transposition of the great arteries (d-TGA) corrected with an atrial switch (Mustard/Senning) normally develop heart failure secondary to systemic RV dysfunction with or without tricuspid regurgitation, but they also can develop

heart failure in the presence of a significant baffle obstruction. In this setting, afterload reduction medications might reduce ventricular filling instead of increasing stroke volume.

In ACHD patients with a biventricular circulation and left ventricular dysfunction (systemic ventricle) as the main mechanism of heart failure, it seems reasonable to apply the same treatment

strategies as in heart failure associated with acquired heart disease. However, these therapies may be detrimental in other subgroups of ACHD patients. For example, in patients with single ventricle physiology, mainly those palliated with Fontan circulation, the use of some of the standard heart failure drugs, such as ACEi or angiotensin receptor blockade inhibitors (ARB), may reduce preload and reduce cardiac output further. Stroke volume in patients with d-TGA corrected with an atrial switch depends significantly on heart rate; thus, β-blockers need to be used with caution in this population.

Resynchronization therapy in CHD

Cardiac resynchronization therapy (CRT) improves haemodynamic parameters and functional capacity, and reduces morbidity and mortality in patients with acquired heart failure. However, there is little evidence to support the use of CRT in ACHD patients. Janousek *et al.* demonstrated that CRT improves systemic RV function in patients with native or LV pacing-induced electromechanical delay.[54] However, CRT implantation in congenitally corrected transposition of the great arteries (ccTGA) or in d-TGA patients can be challenging due to the coronary sinus and coronary venous anatomy.[55] Adequate imaging of the coronary sinus anatomy is required before considering CRT implantation in these patients. Nonetheless, even when feasible, it is difficult to decide which patients will benefit from this therapy and clearly more data are needed in this area. Biventricular dyssynchrony may also be present in patients with right bundle branch block after ToF repair and commonly is associated with reduced global and regional LV function.[56] However, it is unclear how CRT can be successfully applied in this setting. Moreover, the presence of areas of RV late activation in the free wall, in portions of the interventricular septum, and in the outflow tract probably means that the exact target for RV resynchronization is different from patient to patient.[57,58]

Although there is not much evidence about the indication for CRT in ACHD patients, a PACES/HRS Expert Consensus Statement on the Recognition and Management of Arrhythmias in Adult Congenital Heart Disease was published in 2014. This statement, after reviewing the evidence, gave some recommendations regarding the indications for considering CRT in this population (Figure 7.3).[59]

Specific lesions

Right-sided heart failure

Right-sided heart failure is more common in CHD patients than in patients with acquired heart disease. Whereas in patients with acquired heart disease right sided-heart failure is generally secondary to left ventricular dysfunction, in CHD patients it is commonly related to a primary right-sided lesion. Right-sided lesions in this population can be primary or due to residual lesions after repair. Furthermore patients with CHD are more prone to develop right ventricular restriction which can lead to long-term complications and ultimately to heart failure.

Tetralogy of Fallot

ToF is the most common form of cyanotic CHD after the first year of life. Damage of the myocardial structure, sequelae from surgical repairs, conduction abnormalities, adverse ventricular–ventricular interaction, and coronary artery anomalies, may contribute to the development of heart failure in this population.[60]

The majority of patients with ToF undergo surgical repair early in life, which involves relief of the pulmonary stenosis and closure of the ventricular septal defect. Surgical repair of ToF often results in significant PR, the most common residual defect after ToF repair. Long-standing PR promotes a cascade of RV dilatation, ventricular dysfunction, and adverse clinical outcomes that include heart failure, tachyarrhythmias, and/or death. However, there is a long preclinical phase where symptoms and signs of overt heart failure are absent despite important underlying right heart dilation and dysfunction. This reflects the tremendous adaptive capacity of the RV as end-diastolic volume increases to maintain stroke volume and mass augments to maintain wall stress. If compensatory mechanisms of the RV fail, end-systolic volume will increase, ejection fraction will decrease, and mass-to-volume ratio will decrease, leading to clinical heart failure.[60] Long-standing PR causing severe RV dilatation will also reduce LV filling due the interventricular interaction. This leads to a reduction in cardiac output. In addition, a recent study of 511 adults with ToF revealed that LV systolic dysfunction is present in 21% of this population, which will also contribute to the development of heart failure.

The diagnosis of heart failure in patients with ToF may be challenging as 'usual' signs of right heart failure will be present only in few patients. Patients with severe PR will only become symptomatic when RV function becomes significantly impaired; thus, reliance only on symptoms for deciding timing of pulmonary valve replacement may be misleading. Objective assessment of exercise capacity may be more reliable and serial exercise testing may help identify changes in exercise capacity, which may not be perceived by the patient. Surgical intervention might also be considered when patients with severe PR and enlarged RVs develop moderate-to-severe tricuspid regurgitation (TR) or symptomatic atrial or ventricular arrhythmias. Indeed, no single parameter, but several variables, should be considered when deciding the correct timing of pulmonary valve replacement.[61]

Most patients with repaired ToF will not require heart failure medication; however, it may be necessary in the setting of RV or LV dysfunction. The use of ACEi and β-blockers may be reasonable in the few patients where LV dysfunction is significant, but the role of these therapies for RV failure is unknown. To date, there is only one double-blind, randomized, placebo-controlled trial of ACE inhibition in patients with repaired ToF. The APPROPRIATE trial enrolled 64 adults with repaired ToF and at least moderate PR and randomized them to 6 months of ramipril versus placebo. There was no difference in the primary outcome of right ventricular ejection fraction measured by CMR.[62] However, as more data become available, targeted surveillance and early referral to specialized centres has been shown to improve outcomes in these patients.[60]

Restrictive right ventricle

Right ventricle diastolic failure is not uncommon in CHD patients. In the setting of a restrictive RV the stiff right ventricle is acting as a conduit between the right atrium and the pulmonary artery at the end of diastole contributing to forward pulmonary flow, and thus cardiac output. Fibrosis likely contributes to restriction and impairment of diastolic filling.

RV restriction is more common in patients with ToF but also can be seen in those with long-standing right ventricular outflow tract obstruction. The effect of RV restriction after ToF repair remains somewhat controversial, especially in patients with residual PR. Increased RV end-diastolic pressure can limit pulmonary regurgitant volume and result in less RV dilation and better exercise tolerance. However, RV restriction is also likely to result in long-term complications including sequelae of increased central venous pressure, congestive heart failure and arrhythmias. Maintenance of sinus rhythm and effective right atrial contraction are particularly important in patients with a restrictive RV. Conditions that elevate PA pressure such as elevated left-sided pressures from LV restriction may impede antegrade flow into the PA during atrial systole and mask RV restriction.[63–65] As patients with restrictive RV and heart failure depend significantly on an adequate preload, diuretics should be managed carefully and patients should be offloaded slowly.

Ebstein anomaly

Ebstein anomaly is a rare and complex disorder accounting for <1% of all cases of CHD. Patients with Ebstein anomaly might have significant TR, which results in right atrial and right ventricular dilatation. The LV is typically small due to the septal displacement and is often intrinsically abnormal in its function.

The clinical presentation of Ebstein anomaly depends on the severity of TR, RV function, the size of the right atrium, right atrial pressure, and the presence of right to left shunting. Although most patients with Ebstein anomaly survive infancy, severe heart failure and cyanosis may occur early in life. Exercise intolerance with dyspnoea and/or fatigue, symptomatic arrhythmias and right-sided heart failure are the most common presenting symptoms and signs during adulthood. Generally, the younger the age at clinical presentation, the more severe the anatomic and haemodynamic derangement. When an atrial septal defect or patent foramen ovale is present, cyanosis may be noted at rest or during exercise and paradoxical embolism is possible. Tachyarrhythmias, related to right chamber enlargement or the presence of one or more accessory conduction pathways, are a more common mode of presentation of Ebstein anomaly in adults than heart failure, affecting 20–30% of patients. When examining patients with Ebstein anomaly, the JVP is rarely elevated, even in presence of severe TR, due to the severely enlarged right atrium, which does not allow propagation of regurgitant flow to the superior vena cava.

Patients with Ebstein anomaly will normally present with progressive decline of their exercise capacity but rarely with overt heart failure. In those patients with decompensated right heart failure, optimal fluid balance is paramount as both hypovolaemia and hypervolaemia can lead to low cardiac output. Loop-diuretics are first line therapy, and spironolactone should be added in order to achieve optimal diuresis. As occurs with other patients with primary RV failure, there is no evidence for the benefit of heart failure medications in this population. Appropriate timing for TV repair/replacement is important and should be decided by a centre with experience in managing CHD patients.

Systemic right ventricle

Systemic RV is an unique situation seen in patients with CHD where the RV is sub-aortic and therefore sustains the systemic circulation. Systemic RV is seen in patients with ccTGA, d-TGA after atrial switch repair (Mustard or Senning) and in some single ventricle conditions. Although almost half of the patients with Mustard/Senning repair will have moderate to severely impaired RV systolic function 25 years after the repair,[66] clinical heart failure will be only present in a quarter of them at this point in time.[13] In the atrial switch population, heart failure symptoms are associated with a 4.4-fold increase in the risk of sudden death.[67] Definitions of normal versus abnormal systemic RV function and methods to assess it are vague and inconsistent. This makes comparison of single-centre studies and interpretation of data challenging. Prognostic markers for the late development of heart failure or sudden death in the systemic RV population are also sparse.[8] However, when BNP is elevated in patients with systemic RV correlates with exercise capacity, systemic ventricular function and worsening TR.[68,69]

The usefulness of conventional heart failure treatment in the setting of a systemic RV is unknown and may be detrimental since vasodilatation can be counterproductive in patients with non-distensible atria or restrictive physiology. Altering venous capacitance may decrease ventricular filling rather than increasing cardiac output. Several small studies have assessed the effect of ACEi or ARBs in patients with systemic RV but the majority show neither benefit, nor harm. A small, prospective, crossover study of losartan in patients with TGA demonstrated improved EF and exercise duration in an adolescent/young adult population.[70] However, in the only two multicentre, randomized, placebo-controlled studies of ARBs in adults with TGA and a systemic RV, no significant benefit was demonstrated.[71,72] In the Van de Bom et al. study, however, there was an improvement of 4.5% in RV ejection fraction compared to the placebo group in a subgroup analysis of symptomatic patients. Furthermore, there was an improvement in RV volumes in asymptomatic patients.[72] Data on β-blockers in this population are even scarcer. Although small observational studies showed improvement in heart failure symptoms in patients with systemic RV after treatment with β-blockers, this also can be detrimental as patients with Mustard/Senning repair rely on heart rate to increase cardiac output. Thus, β-blockers can be used but care should be taken in this population. Some patients with systemic RV may also benefit from treatment with implantable cardioverter–defibrillator or CRT-D (**Figure 7.4**).

Currently, there is no evidence either in favour of, or against, using heart failure medications in patients with systemic RV. Therefore treatment needs to be individualized case by case. Although some randomized trials did not show benefit of heart failure treatment in these patients, it is important to consider that the majority of the studies included a mixed group of patients and most of them were asymptomatic. These factors have probably played a role in the outcome of the studies. Furthermore, the end-points used were not ideal and therefore new adequately powered randomized studies are needed before concluding that heart failure treatment is ineffective in this population.

A rather speculative therapeutic option for the treatment of heart failure in this setting is to band the pulmonary artery (effectively creating significant pulmonary stenosis) and render the left ventricle 'hypertensive'. This was initially done as a staging procedure towards a late arterial switch with the plan of training the LV prior to it becoming the systemic ventricle. However, in adults the results of late switch operations were disappointing. Incidentally, it was noted that a few patients with simple banding reported a symptomatic improvement. In these patients banding resulted in the septum moving towards the right ventricle and the right ventricular volumes and

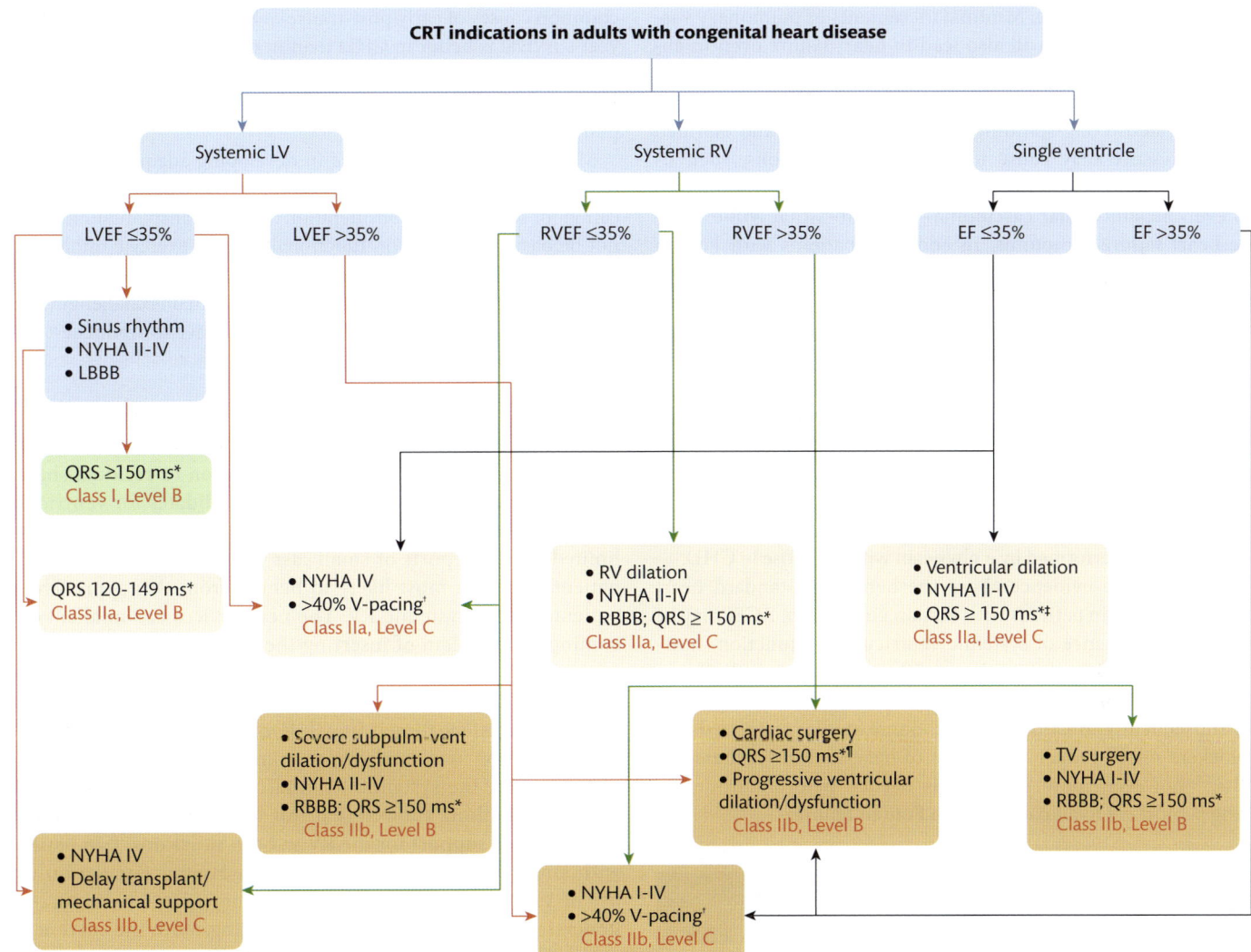

Figure 7.4 Overview of recommendations for cardiac resynchronization therapy (CRT) in adults with congenital heart disease.

EF, ejection fraction; LBBB, left bundle branch block; LV, left ventricle; NYHA, New York Association functional class; RBBB, right bundle branch block; supulm-vent: subpulmonary ventricle;TV, tricuspid valveV-pacing, ventricular pacing.

* Spontaneous or paced

† New or replacement device implantation with anticipated for >40% ventricular pacing, intrinsically narrow QRS complex; single site pacing from the systemic ventricular apex/mid-lateral wall may be considered as an alternative

‡ RBBB or LBBB

¶ Complete bundle branch block ipsilateral to the systemic ventricle

Reproduced with permission from Khairy *et al.* (Khairy P, Van Hare GF, Balaji S, Berul CI, Cecchin F, Cohen MI, Daniels CJ, Deal BJ, Dearani JA, Groot N, Dubin AM, Harris L, Janousek J, Kanter RJ, Karpawich PP, Perry JC, Seslar SP, Shah MJ, Silka MJ, Triedman JK, Walsh EP and Warnes CA. PACES/HRS Expert Consensus Statement on the Recognition and Management of Arrhythmias in Adult Congenital Heart Disease: developed in partnership between the Pediatric and Congenital Electrophysiology Society (PACES) and the Heart Rhythm Society (HRS). Endorsed by the governing bodies of PACES, HRS, the American College of Cardiology (ACC), the American Heart Association (AHA), the European Heart Rhythm Association (EHRA), the Canadian Heart Rhythm Society (CHRS), and the International Society for Adult Congenital Heart Disease (ISACHD). *Heart Rhythm* 2014;**11**:e102–65.)

geometry changing. The degree of tricuspid regurgitation was also reduced. These techniques have not been widely adopted and the long term role for such procedures is unknown.

Single ventricle physiology: Fontan circulation

One to the most severe forms of CHD occurs in those patients that fail to develop two ventricles and therefore, a functional single ventricle will supply both systemic and pulmonary circulations. The majority of these patients will undergo some form on initial palliation early in life followed by complete redirection of systemic venous return directly to the pulmonary arteries.

This type of repair is known as a Fontan circulation, named after the surgeon who initially described the operation. There are several modifications of the original operation but all of them share the same physiology. These patients do not have sub-pulmonary pumping chamber and therefore the flow to the pulmonary arteries is passive at expense of elevated systemic venous pressures. By definition the Fontan circulation is characterized by low cardiac output and several factors may favour the development of heart failure. Systolic or diastolic single ventricle dysfunction or atrioventricular valve regurgitation may lead to an increased left atrial pressure and subsequently reduction in single ventricle

preload and heart failure. Minimal increments in pulmonary vascular resistance (PVR) will also lead to heart failure even in absence of systolic or diastolic dysfunction as pulmonary blood flow will be compromised and systemic venous pressure will be significantly elevated. Long-standing low cardiac output and elevated venous pressure may cause long-term complications, such us chronic hepatic congestion, cirrhosis, ascites, renal dysfunction and even hepatocellular carcinoma—all factors that will exacerbate heart failure symptoms. In addition, patients with Fontan circulation may develop PLE, a condition that mimic heart failure symptoms including fatigue, peripheral oedema, effusions, and ascites. Arrhythmias are also common in these patients and one of the most common causes of decompensation.

The lack of a robust definition of Fontan failure has contributed to the limited understanding of the prevalence of heart failure in Fontan circulation.[8] Estimates of heart failure prevalence range from 10% to 20% early after Fontan surgery, rising to 50% in adults who underwent the Fontan operation many years previously.[12,13] Assessment and management of patients with Fontan circulation and heart failure has to be performed by a physician with expertise in CHD.

There is scarce evidence about the benefit of standard heart failure treatment in patients with Fontan circulation. ACEi may be beneficial in presence of systemic ventricular dysfunction, however may be detrimental in those with preserved systolic function, as increased veno-dilatation will lead to reduction in preload and subsequently in cardiac output. Some studies suggested that β-blockers might reduce symptoms of heart failure in these patients;[73] however, more evidence is needed before considering giving β-blockers to all patients with Fontan failure.

Transplant and devices in congenital heart disease

Heart or heart-lung transplant should always be considered in ACHD patients with refractory heart failure. Transplant numbers in ACHD patients have increased over the past two decades. Whereas, the proportion of transplants in patients with univentricular heart has not changed over the last 10 years, the number of patients with biventricular circulation and systemic right ventricle has doubled.[74] Standard risk factors used for listing patients with acquired heart disease for transplantation may not be applicable to ACHD patients. High sensitization, elevated PVR, distorted pulmonary artery anatomy, anatomical abnormalities including abnormal position of organs or vessels (e.g. situs inversus, malposition of the great arteries or venous anomalies) as well as previous cardiac operations that may add significant technical problems, are all factors that should be considered in the assessment of ACHD patients prior to transplantation. In addition, patients with Fontan circulation are prone to develop liver failure, thus a detailed assessment of the liver with a multidisciplinary team including cardiologists with expertise in ACHD and gastroenterologists with expertise in liver failure, is paramount.

Once listed, CHD patients are more likely to be listed at lower urgency (64% of CHD patients are listed as status 2 compared to 44% of non-CHD patients) despite a higher rate of complications once on the transplant list.[75] Early post-transplant mortality is increased in patients with CHD with bleeding and acute graft failure as the most

common causes of early post-transplant mortality. Nonetheless, 10-year survival is better in CHD than in non-CHD populations. Risk factors for adverse transplant outcomes in ACHD patients include prior Fontan operation, complex anatomy, re-do sternotomy and pulmonary hypertension.

More effort should be made in developing adequate criteria for referring ACHD patients to transplant. Perhaps, in ACHD, the indication for referring for consideration of heart transplantation should not be based primarily on functional class or exercise intolerance, but on evidence of organ failure, such as renal or liver dysfunction. The timely selection of optimal candidates remains challenging and large congenital centres need to work together to optimise transplant outcomes in ACHD.

Ventricular assist devices

heart failure patients with CHD are more likely to have right-sided heart failure, pulmonary hypertension or residual shunts, which may make them less attractive candidates for ventricular assist devices (VADs).[76,77] The use of VADs in ACHD patients is limited to case reports or small case series. The group of ACHD patients who are most likely to benefit from this approach are patients with a systemic RV. The new devices are smaller overcoming the problem of inserting them in a heavily trabeculated ventricle. Peng et al., recently reported a small series of seven patients with systemic RV failure who received the HeartWare (HeartWare International Inc., Framingham, MA, USA) VAD.[78] The indication was bridging to transplantation, with the aim of supporting the systemic RV and/or reduce pulmonary pressures. The authors showed that this third generation VAD provides durable support for the RV in both situations.[78] In patients with single ventricle physiology and a Fontan circulation, the use of VADs is more challenging and more data are required to understand the role of VADs in this setting. With the current advances in technology, smaller and more efficient VADs are on the market, which will hopefully increase exponentially the use of VADs in the ACHD population.

Conclusions

As the ACHD population ages the prevalence of heart failure is increasing dramatically. Specialist input is essential to fully assess and treat these patients. Although the evidence base for care lags behind that of acquired heart disease, there is increasing evidence to support using traditional tools of heart failure care to impact on the morbidity and mortality associated with heart failure in this patient group. However, the need for high quality multi-disciplinary care and ongoing research is of paramount importance.

REFERENCE

1. Hoffman JI, Kaplan S. The incidence of congenital heart disease. *J Am Coll Cardiol* 2002;**39**:1890–900.
2. Marelli AJ, Ionescu-Ittu R, Mackie AS, *et al.* Lifetime prevalence of congenital heart disease in the general population from 2000 to 2010. *Circulation* 2014;**130**:749–56.

3. van der Linde D, Konings EE, Slager MA, *et al*. Birth prevalence of congenital heart disease worldwide: a systematic review and meta-analysis. *J Am Coll Cardiol* 2011;**58**:2241–7.

4. Khairy P, Fernandes SM, Mayer JE, Jr, *et al*. Long-term survival, modes of death, and predictors of mortality in patients with Fontan surgery. *Circulation* 2008;**117**:85–92.

5. Law YM, Ettedgui J, Beerman L, Maisel A, Tofovic S. Comparison of plasma B-type natriuretic peptide levels in single ventricle patients with systemic ventricle heart failure versus isolated cavopulmonary failure. *Am J Cardiol* 2006;**98**:520–4.

6. Bolger AP, Coats AJ, Gatzoulis MA. Congenital heart disease: the original heart failure syndrome. *Eur Heart J* 2003;**24**:970–6.

7. Alshawabkeh LI, Opotowsky AR. Burden of heart failure in adults with congenital heart disease. *Curr Heart Fail Rep* 2016;**13**:247–254.

8. Stout KK, Broberg CS, Book WM, *et al*.; American Heart Association Council on Clinical Cardiology CoFG, Translational B, Council on Cardiovascular R and Imaging. Chronic heart failure in congenital heart disease: a scientific statement from the American Heart Association. *Circulation* 2016;**133**:770–801.

9. Mackie AS, Pilote L, Ionescu-Ittu R, Rahme E, Marelli AJ. Health care resource utilization in adults with congenital heart disease. *Am J Cardiol* 2007;**99**:839–43.

10. Opotowsky AR, Siddiqi OK, Webb GD. Trends in hospitalizations for adults with congenital heart disease in the U.S. *J Am Coll Cardiol* 2009;**54**:460–7.

11. Verheugt CL, Uiterwaal CS, van der Velde ET, *et al*. Mortality in adult congenital heart disease. *Eur Heart J* 2010;**31**:1220–9.

12. Norozi K, Wessel A, Alpers V, *et al*. Incidence and risk distribution of heart failure in adolescents and adults with congenital heart disease after cardiac surgery. *Am J Cardiol* 2006;**97**:1238–43.

13. Piran S, Veldtman G, Siu S, Webb GD, Liu PP. Heart failure and ventricular dysfunction in patients with single or systemic right ventricles. *Circulation* 2002;**105**:1189–94.

14. Rodriguez FH, 3rd, Moodie DS, Parekh DR, *et al*. Outcomes of heart failure-related hospitalization in adults with congenital heart disease in the United States. *Congenit Heart Dis* 2013;**8**:513–9.

15. Zomer AC, Vaartjes I, van der Velde ET, *et al*. Heart failure admissions in adults with congenital heart disease; risk factors and prognosis. *Int J Cardiol* 2013;**168**:2487–93.

16. Diller GP, Kempny A, Alonso-Gonzalez R, *et al*. Survival prospects and circumstances of death in contemporary adult congenital heart disease patients under follow-up at a large tertiary centre. *Circulation* 2015;**132**:2118–25.

17. Vanderlaan RD, Caldarone CA, Backx PH. Heart failure in congenital heart disease: the role of genes and hemodynamics. *Pflugers Arch* 2014;**466**:1025–35.

18. Sanchez-Quintana D, Climent V, Ho SY, Anderson RH. Myoarchitecture and connective tissue in hearts with tricuspid atresia. *Heart* 1999;**81**:182–91.

19. Tobita K, Keller BB. Right and left ventricular wall deformation patterns in normal and left heart hypoplasia chick embryos. *Am J Physiol Heart Circ Physiol* 2000;**279**:H959–69.

20. Fahed AC, Roberts AE, Mital S, Lakdawala NK. Heart failure in congenital heart disease: a confluence of acquired and congenital. *Heart Fail Clin* 2014;**10**:219–27.

21. Preuss C, Andelfinger G. Genetics of heart failure in congenital heart disease. *Can J Cardiol* 2013;**29**:803–10.

22. Ichida F, Tsubata S, Bowles KR, *et al*. Novel gene mutations in patients with left ventricular noncompaction or Barth syndrome. *Circulation* 2001;**103**:1256–63.

23. Stahli BE, Gebhard C, Biaggi P, *et al*. Left ventricular non-compaction: prevalence in congenital heart disease. *Int J Cardiol* 2013;**167**:2477–81.

24. Lubiszewska B, Gosiewska E, Hoffman P, *et al*. Myocardial perfusion and function of the systemic right ventricle in patients after atrial switch procedure for complete transposition: long-term follow-up. *J Am Coll Cardiol* 2000;**36**:1365–70.

25. Rutz T, de Marchi SF, Schwerzmann M, Vogel R, Seiler C. Right ventricular absolute myocardial blood flow in complex congenital heart disease. *Heart* 2010;**96**:1056–62.

26. Singh TP, Humes RA, Muzik O, *et al*. Myocardial flow reserve in patients with a systemic right ventricle after atrial switch repair. *J Am Coll Cardiol* 2001;**37**:2120–5.

27. Fuster V, Danielson MA, Robb RA, *et al*. Quantitation of left ventricular myocardial fiber hypertrophy and interstitial tissue in human hearts with chronically increased volume and pressure overload. *Circulation* 1977;**55**:504–8.

28. Hein S, Arnon E, Kostin S, *et al*. Progression from compensated hypertrophy to failure in the pressure-overloaded human heart: structural deterioration and compensatory mechanisms. *Circulation* 2003;**107**:984–91.

29. Babu-Narayan SV, Kilner PJ, Li W, *et al*. Ventricular fibrosis suggested by cardiovascular magnetic resonance in adults with repaired tetralogy of fallot and its relationship to adverse markers of clinical outcome. *Circulation* 2006;**113**:405–13.

30. Babu-Narayan SV, Goktekin O, Moon JC, *et al*. Late gadolinium enhancement cardiovascular magnetic resonance of the systemic right ventricle in adults with previous atrial redirection surgery for transposition of the great arteries. *Circulation* 2005;**111**:2091–8.

31. Broberg CS, Prasad SK, Carr C, *et al*. Myocardial fibrosis in Eisenmenger syndrome: a descriptive cohort study exploring associations of late gadolinium enhancement with clinical status and survival. *J Cardiovasc Magn Reson* 2014;**16**:32.

32. Broberg CS, Chugh SS, Conklin C, Sahn DJ, Jerosch-Herold M. Quantification of diffuse myocardial fibrosis and its association with myocardial dysfunction in congenital heart disease. *Circ Cardiovasc Imaging* 2010;**3**:727–34.

33. Santamore WP, Dell'Italia LJ. Ventricular interdependence: significant left ventricular contributions to right ventricular systolic function. *Prog Cardiovasc Dis* 1998;**40**:289–308.

34. Kempny A, Diller GP, Orwat S, *et al*. Right ventricular-left ventricular interaction in adults with Tetralogy of Fallot: a combined cardiac magnetic resonance and echocardiographic speckle tracking study. *Int J Cardiol* 2012;**154**:259–64.

35. Maisel AS, Krishnaswamy P, Nowak RM, *et al*. Rapid measurement of B-type natriuretic peptide in the emergency diagnosis of heart failure. *N Engl J Med* 2002;**347**:161–7.

36. Saremi A, Gopal D, Maisel AS. Brain natriuretic peptide-guided therapy in the inpatient management of decompensated heart failure. *Expert Rev Cardiovasc Ther* 2012;**10**:191–203.

37. Taub PR, Gabbai-Saldate P, Maisel A. Biomarkers of heart failure. *Congesti heart fail (Greenwich, Conn)* 2010;**16 Suppl 1**:S19–24.

38. Bolger AP, Sharma R, Li W, *et al*. Neurohormonal activation and the chronic heart failure syndrome in adults with congenital heart disease. *Circulation* 2002;**106**:92–9.

39. Iivainen TE, Groundstroem KW, Lahtela JT, *et al*. Serum N-terminal atrial natriuretic peptide in adult patients late after surgical repair of atrial septal defect. *Eur J Heart Fail* 2000;**2**:161–5.

40. Tulevski II, Groenink M, van Der Wall EE, *et al*. Increased brain and atrial natriuretic peptides in patients with chronic

right ventricular pressure overload: correlation between plasma neurohormones and right ventricular dysfunction. *Heart (Br Cardiac Soc)* 2001;**86**:27–30.

41. Kikuchi K, Nishioka K, Ueda T, *et al.* Relationship between plasma atrial natriuretic polypeptide concentration and hemodynamic measurements in children with congenital heart diseases. *J Pediatr* 1987;**111**:335–42.

42. Eindhoven JA, Roos-Hesselink JW, van den Bosch AE, *et al.* High-sensitive troponin-T in adult congenital heart disease. *Int J Cardiol* 2015;**184**:405–11.

43. Rybicka J, Dobrowolski P, Lipczynska M, *et al.* High sensitivity troponin T in adult congenital heart disease. *Int J Cardiol* 2015;**195**:7–14.

44. Baggen VJ, van den Bosch A, Eindhoven JA, *et al.* Prognostic value of N-terminal pro-B-type natriuretic peptide, troponin-T, and growth-differentiation factor 15 in adult congenital heart disease. *Circulation* 2016;**135**:264–79.

45. Diller GP, Alonso-Gonzalez R, Kempny A, *et al.* B-type natriuretic peptide concentrations in contemporary Eisenmenger syndrome patients: predictive value and response to disease targeting therapy. *Heart* 2012;**98**:736–42.

46. Giannakoulas G, Dimopoulos K, Bolger AP, *et al.* Usefulness of natriuretic peptide levels to predict mortality in adults with congenital heart disease. *Am J Cardiol* 2010;**105**:869–73.

47. Inai K, Nakanishi T, Nakazawa M. Clinical correlation and prognostic predictive value of neurohumoral factors in patients late after the Fontan operation. *Am Heart J* 2005;**150**:588–94.

48. Kempny A, Dimopoulos K, Uebing A, *et al.* Reference values for exercise limitations among adults with congenital heart disease. Relation to activities of daily life—single centre experience and review of published data. *Eur Heart J* 2012;**33**:1386–96.

49. Buber J, Rhodes J. Exercise physiology and testing in adult patients with congenital heart disease. *Heart Fail Clin* 2014;**10**:23–33.

50. Dimopoulos K, Alonso-Gonzalez R. Heart failure, exercise intolerance and physical training in congenital heart disease. In Gatzoulis M, Webb GD, Daubeney P (eds), *Diagnosis and management of congential heart disease*, 2nd edn, pp. 44–51. Elsevier/Saunders, Philadelphia, 2011.

51. Diller GP, Okonko DO, Uebing A, *et al.* Impaired heart rate response to exercise in adult patients with a systemic right ventricle or univentricular circulation: prevalence, relation to exercise, and potential therapeutic implications. *Int J Cardiol* 2009;**134**:59–66.

52. Inuzuka R, Diller GP, Borgia F, *et al.* Comprehensive use of cardiopulmonary exercise testing identifies adults with congenital heart disease at increased mortality risk in the medium term. *Circulation* 2012;**125**:250–9.

53. Engelfriet P, Boersma E, Oechslin E, *et al.* The spectrum of adult congenital heart disease in Europe: morbidity and mortality in a 5 year follow-up period. The Euro Heart Survey on adult congenital heart disease. *Eur Heart J* 2005;**26**:2325–33.

54. Janousek J, Tomek V, Chaloupecky VA, *et al.* Cardiac resynchronization therapy: a novel adjunct to the treatment and prevention of systemic right ventricular failure. *J Am Coll Cardiol* 2004;**44**:1927–31.

55. Diller GP, Okonko D, Uebing A, Ho SY, Gatzoulis MA. Cardiac resynchronization therapy for adult congenital heart disease patients with a systemic right ventricle: analysis of feasibility and review of early experience. *Europace* 2006;**8**:267–72.

56. Abd El Rahman MY, Hui W, Yigitbasi M, *et al.* Detection of left ventricular asynchrony in patients with right bundle branch

block after repair of tetralogy of Fallot using tissue-Doppler imaging-derived strain. *J Am Coll Cardiol* 2005;**45**:915–21.

57. Uebing A, Gibson DG, Babu-Narayan SV, *et al.* Right ventricular mechanics and QRS duration in patients with repaired tetralogy of Fallot: implications of infundibular disease. *Circulation* 2007;**116**:1532–9.

58. Vogel M, Sponring J, Cullen S, Deanfield JE, Redington AN. Regional wall motion and abnormalities of electrical depolarization and repolarization in patients after surgical repair of tetralogy of Fallot. *Circulation* 2001;**103**:1669–73.

59. Khairy P, Van Hare GF, Balaji S, *et al.* PACES/HRS Expert Consensus Statement on the Recognition and Management of Arrhythmias in Adult Congenital Heart Disease: developed in partnership between the Pediatric and Congenital Electrophysiology Society (PACES) and the Heart Rhythm Society (HRS). Endorsed by the governing bodies of PACES, HRS, the American College of Cardiology (ACC), the American Heart Association (AHA), the European Heart Rhythm Association (EHRA), the Canadian Heart Rhythm Society (CHRS), and the International Society for Adult Congenital Heart Disease (ISACHD). *Heart Rhythm* 2014;**11**:e102–65.

60. Wald RM, Valente AM, Marelli A. Heart failure in adult congenital heart disease: Emerging concepts with a focus on tetralogy of Fallot. *Trends Cardiovasc Med* 2015;**25**:422–32.

61. Alonso-Gonzalez R, Dimopoulos K, Ho S, Oliver JM, Gatzoulis MA. The right heart and pulmonary circulation (IX). The right heart in adults with congenital heart disease. *Rev Esp Cardiol* 2010;**63**:1070–86.

62. Babu-Narayan SV, Uebing A, Davlouros PA, *et al.* Randomised trial of ramipril in repaired tetralogy of Fallot and pulmonary regurgitation: the APPROPRIATE study (Ace inhibitors for Potential PRevention Of the deleterious effects of Pulmonary Regurgitation In Adults with repaired TEtralogy of Fallot). *Int J Cardiol* 2012;**154**:299–305.

63. Apitz C, Latus H, Binder W, *et al.* Impact of restrictive physiology on intrinsic diastolic right ventricular function and lusitropy in children and adolescents after repair of tetralogy of Fallot. *Heart* 2010;**96**:1837–41.

64. Chaturvedi RR, Shore DF, Lincoln C, *et al.* Acute right ventricular restrictive physiology after repair of tetralogy of Fallot: association with myocardial injury and oxidative stress. *Circulation* 1999;**100**:1540–7.

65. Helbing WA, Niezen RA, Le Cessie S, *et al.* Right ventricular diastolic function in children with pulmonary regurgitation after repair of tetralogy of Fallot: volumetric evaluation by magnetic resonance velocity mapping. *J Am Coll Cardiol* 1996;**28**:1827–35.

66. Roos-Hesselink JW, Meijboom FJ, Spitaels SE, *et al.* Decline in ventricular function and clinical condition after Mustard repair for transposition of the great arteries (a prospective study of 22–29 years). *Eur Heart J* 2004;**25**:1264–70.

67. Kammeraad JA, van Deurzen CH, Sreeram N, *et al.* Predictors of sudden cardiac death after Mustard or Senning repair for transposition of the great arteries. *J Am Coll Cardiol* 2004;**44**:1095–102.

68. Chow PC, Cheung EW, Chong CY, *et al.* Brain natriuretic peptide as a biomarker of systemic right ventricular function in patients with transposition of great arteries after atrial switch operation. *Int J Cardiol* 2008;**127**:192–7.

69. Koch AM, Zink S, Singer H. B-type natriuretic peptide in patients with systemic right ventricle. *Cardiology* 2008;**110**:1–7.

70. Lester SJ, McElhinney DB, Viloria E, *et al.* Effects of losartan in patients with a systemically functioning morphologic right

ventricle after atrial repair of transposition of the great arteries. *Am J Cardiol* 2001;**88**:1314–16.

71. Dore A, Houde C, Chan KL, *et al.* Angiotensin receptor blockade and exercise capacity in adults with systemic right ventricles: a multicenter, randomized, placebo-controlled clinical trial. *Circulation* 2005;**112**:2411–16.

72. van der Bom T, Winter MM, Bouma BJ, *et al.* Effect of valsartan on systemic right ventricular function: a double-blind, randomized, placebo-controlled pilot trial. *Circulation* 2013;**127**:322–30.

73. Ishibashi N, Park IS, Waragai T, *et al.* Effect of carvedilol on heart failure in patients with a functionally univentricular heart. *Circ J* 2011;**75**:1394–9.

74. Cohen S, Houyel L, Guillemain R, *et al.* Temporal trends and changing profile of adults with congenital heart disease undergoing heart transplantation. *Eur Heart J* 2016;**37**:783–9.

75. Davies RR, Russo MJ, Yang J, *et al.* Listing and transplanting adults with congenital heart disease. *Circulation* 2011;**123**:759–67.

76. Mulukutla V, Franklin WJ, Villa CR, Morales DL. Surgical device therapy for heart failure in the adult with congenital heart disease. *Heart Fail Clin* 2014;**10**:197–206.

77. Shah NR, Lam WW, Rodriguez FH, 3rd, *et al.* Clinical outcomes after ventricular assist device implantation in adults with complex congenital heart disease. *J Heart Lung Transplant* 2013;**32**:615–20.

78. Peng E, O'Sullivan JJ, Griselli M, *et al.* Durable ventricular assist device support for failing systemic morphologic right ventricle: early results. *Ann Thorac Surg* 2014;**98**:2122–9.

8

Infective and infiltrative causes of heart failure

Simon A. S. Beggs, Roy S. Gardner, and Andrew L. Clark

Heart failure can result from any form of cardiac injury. Infective and infiltrative causes are rare, but are important to identify since many are potentially reversible. An aetiological diagnosis is seldom chanced upon through 'routine' investigations, and will often require targeted testing. Therefore, a high index of suspicion is required.

Infective causes of heart failure

Myocarditis

Myocarditis is an inflammatory disease of the myocardium diagnosed by established histological, immunological, and immunohistological criteria. A vast array of causes has been reported (Tables 8.1 and 8.2). In developed countries, a viral aetiology—currently parvovirus B19—is most commonly implicated, but the principal offender changes with time.[1-3] Less commonly, myocarditis can be triggered by non-infective causes, including systemic disease, hypersensitivity drug reactions, and toxins. Both the clinical presentation and prognosis of myocarditis are variable, with the latter ranging from full recovery to sudden death, or the need for urgent cardiac transplantation or mechanical circulatory support. This variance appears to depend in part on the causative agent, as does the potential for treatment, meaning that aggressive pursuit of an aetiological diagnosis is sometimes warranted. The major long-term consequence of myocarditis is chronic heart failure (CHF) due to dilated cardiomyopathy.

Pathogenesis

The pathophysiology of myocarditis is incompletely understood. Murine models of (entero)viral myocarditis suggest that three distinct phases may occur:[4]

- Phase 1: viral invasion of the myocardium results in cell injury and myocyte necrosis, leading to exposure of intracellular antigens, immune activation and the influx of natural killer cells, macrophages and T lymphocytes. This acute phase takes place over days.
- Phase 2: a subacute immune-mediated process of viral elimination occurs, led by activated T lymphocytes. In some cases, molecular mimicry may result in antibodies targeting host cardiac proteins, potentiating further myocyte damage. In the

majority of hosts, immune response lessens over time and cardiac function recovers. This subacute phase takes place over weeks.
- Phase 3: in some hosts, autoimmune processes continue despite the absence of detectable viral genomes, leading to ongoing fibrosis, dilation and contractile dysfunction. This chronic phase occurs over weeks to months.

This pathological sequence illustrates why myocarditis is thought to underlie up to 30% of dilated cardiomyopathies.[5]

A set of distinct clinicopathological classifications by Lieberman *et al.*[6] gives prognostically useful information:[7,8]

- Fulminant: preceding flu-like illness, with a distinct onset of cardiac symptoms and rapid deterioration. Patients present with shock or symptoms and signs of severe left ventricular systolic

Table 8.1 Infective causes of myocarditis

Infecting agent	Examples
Viral	Adenovirus, arbovirus (dengue fever, yellow fever), arenavirus (Lassa fever), coronavirus (SARS-CoV-2), coxsackie virus, echovirus, Epstein–Barr virus, hepatitis B, herpesvirus (including cytomegalovirus, Epstein-Barr virus), HIV-1, influenza virus, mumps virus, poliomyelitis virus, rabies, respiratory syncytial virus, rubella virus, rubeola virus, vaccinia virus, varicella virus, variola virus covid-19
Bacterial	Brucella, campylobacter, clostridia, diphtheria, francisella (Tularensis), gonococcus, haemophilus, legionella, meningococcus, mycobacteria, mycoplasma, nocardia, pneumococcus, psittacosis, salmonella, staphylococcus, streptococcus, *Tropheryma whippelii* (Whipple's disease)
Fungal	Actinomycetes, aspergillus, blastomyces, candida, coccidioides, cryptococcus, histoplasma, sporothrix
Rickettsial	Rocky Mountain spotted fever, Q fever, scrub typhus, typhus
Spirochetal	Borrelia (Lyme disease), leptospira, syphilis
Helminthic	Cysticercus, echinococcus, schistosoma, toxocara (visceral larva migrans), trichinella
Protozoal	Entamoeba, leishmania, trypanosoma (Chagas disease), toxoplasmosis

Adapted from Pisani B, Taylor DO, Mason JW. Inflammatory myocardial diseases and cardiomyopathies. *Am J Med* 1997;**102**:459–469.

Table 8.2 Non-infective causes of myocarditis

Cause	Subgroup	Examples
Drug-induced	Toxic myocarditis	Amphetamines, anthracyclines*, arsenic, catecholamines, chloroquine, cocaine*, cyclophosphamide*, emetine, 5-fluorouracil, α-interferon, interleukin-2*, lithium, paracetamol, thyroid hormone
	Hypersensitivity myocarditis	Acetazolamide, allopurinol, amitriptyline, amphotericin B, ampicillin*, carbamazepine, cephalothin, chlorthalidone, clozapine, colchicine, diclofenac, diphenhydramine, furosemide, hydrochlorothiazide*, indomethacin, isoniazid, lidocaine, methyldopa*, methysergide, oxphenbutazone, para-aminosalicyclic acid, penicillins*, phenindione, phenylbutazone, phenytoin, procainamide, pyribenzamine, reserpine, spironolactone, streptomycin, sulfadiazine*, sulfamethoxizole*, sulfisoxazole*, sulfonylureas, tetracycline, trimethaprim
Toxins		Arsenic, carbon monoxide, copper, iron, lead, mercury, phosphorus, scorpion stings, snake venom, spider bites, wasp sting
Systemic diseases		Arteritis (giant cell, Takayasau), β-thalassaemia major, eosinophilic granulomatosis with polyangiitis (Churg–Strauss vasculitis), Crohn's disease, cryoglobulinaemia, dermatomyositis, diabetes mellitus, Hashimoto's thyroiditis, Kawasaki's disease*, mixed connective tissue disorder, myasthenia gravis, periarteritis nodosa, pernicious anaemia, phaeochromocytoma, polymyositis, rheumatoid arthritis, sarcoidosis*, scleroderma, Sjögren's syndrome, systemic lupus erythematosis*, thymoma, ulcerative colitis, granulomatosis with polyangiitis (Wegener granulomatosis)
Other		Cardiac rejection*, eosinophilic myocarditis, genetic, giant cell myocarditis*, granulomatous myocarditis, head trauma, hypothermia, hyperpyrexia, ionizing radiation, mononuclear myocarditis, peripartum myocarditis*

*Denotes more common causes.
Source data from Pisani B, Taylor DO, Mason JW. Inflammatory myocardial diseases and cardiomyopathies. *Am J Med* 1997;**102**:4594–69.

dysfunction (LVSD). The clinical course is variable and patients either recover over the space of a few weeks or deteriorate rapidly requiring consideration of cardiac transplantation. Endomyocardial biopsy shows active myocarditis. Immunosuppressive therapy is ineffective.

- Acute: unclear onset with gradual decline in cardiac function. Patients present with symptoms of progressive heart failure and ventricular dilation with LVSD. There is active or borderline myocarditis on biopsy, which resolves with time. Patients either respond to congestive heart failure (CHF) therapy or progress to dilated cardiomyopathy.
- Chronic active: onset indistinct with progressive deterioration, present with CHF with LVSD. Initial biopsy shows active or borderline myocarditis, and subsequent biopsy shows continued inflammation, fibrosis, giant cells, with eventual development of a dilated cardiomyopathy.
- Chronic persistent: no distinct onset of symptoms (primarily chest pain or palpitations) characterized by a persistent infiltrate on biopsy, often with foci of myocyte necrosis, but without ventricular dysfunction. Immunosuppressive therapy does not affect myocardial infiltrate or clinical outcome.

Clinical features

It is usually not possible to arrive at a diagnosis of myocarditis based on clinical presentation alone. In the European Study of the Epidemiology and Treatment of Inflammatory Heart Disease,[9] 72% had dyspnoea, 32% chest pain, and 18% arrhythmias. Chest pain is particularly common in myopericarditis, but myocarditis can also mimic myocardial ischaemia (from coronary artery spasm) and therefore should be considered in patients with an acute coronary syndrome and unobstructed coronary arteries.[10] Other presentations include palpitations, syncope, aborted sudden cardiac death, and unexplained cardiogenic shock (see Table 8.3).

The underlying cause of myocarditis may be even more difficult to divine from the presentation. Although viral myocarditis is classically associated with a prodromal viral illness with fever, myalgia,

fatigue, and respiratory, or gastrointestinal symptoms, reported symptoms are highly variable.[11]

Table 8.3 Diagnostic criteria for clinically suspected myocarditis

Myocarditis should be suspected in the presence of:
≥1 of the following clinical presentations and ≥1 of the following diagnostic criteria*
or
≥2 diagnostic criteria when the patient is asymptomatic*
Clinical presentations
Acute chest pain, pericarditic or pseudo-ischaemic
New-onset (up to 3 days) or worsening of dyspnoea or fatigue
Subacute/chronic (>3 months) or worsening of dyspnoea or fatigue
Palpitations and/or unexplained symptoms of possible arrhythmia and/or syncope and/or aborted sudden cardiac death
Unexplained cardiogenic shock
Diagnostic criteria
(i) ECG/Holter/stress test features — new abnormal features including atrioventricular block (any type), or bundle branch block, ST/T wave changes, sinus arrest, ventricular tachycardia or fibrillation and asystole, atrial fibrillation, reduced R wave height, intraventricular conduction delay (widened QRS complex), abnormal Q waves, low voltage, frequent premature beats, supraventricular tachycardia
(ii) Elevated cardiac troponin concentrations
(iii) New, otherwise unexplained LV and/or RV structural or functional abnormalities (including incidental finding in apparently asymptomatic subjects), including regional wall motion abnormalities, global systolic impairment, or diastolic dysfunction.
(iv) Characteristic myocarditic CMR findings

*These criteria require the absence of angiographically significant coronary artery disease (≥50% stenosis) or known pre-existing conditions that could explain the presentation.
Source data from Caforio ALP, Pankuweit S, Arbustini E, *et al*. Current state of knowledge on aetiology, diagnosis, management, and therapy of myocarditis: a position statement of the European Society of Cardiology Working Group on Myocardial and Pericardial Diseases. *Eur Heart J* 2013;**34**:2636–2648.

Investigation and diagnosis

Table 8.3 presents the diagnostic criteria recently proposed by the European Society of Cardiology for patients in whom myocarditis should be suspected. Biomarkers of cardiac injury, particularly the cardiac troponins (I or T), may be raised in acute myocarditis, but have limited diagnostic sensitivity.[12,13] This also applies to natriuretic peptides, circulating cytokines, and novel biomarkers. Markers of inflammation, such as white cell count and C-reactive protein, may also be raised. Antibodies to an assortment of cardiac and muscle-specific autoantigens may be detected in myocarditis but at present their use in clinical practice remains limited.

The ECG often shows sinus tachycardia and non-specific ST/T wave abnormalities. Occasionally, changes consistent with an acute ST elevation myocardial infarction are seen, and may reflect pericarditis or coronary artery spasm.[14]

The chest radiograph may be normal, or show evidence of cardiomegaly and/or pulmonary oedema. Echocardiography reveals global dysfunction or regional wall motion abnormalities, with variable degrees of cardiac dysfunction. Mitral and tricuspid regurgitation are common. Fulminant myocarditis may be differentiated from acute myocarditis by a smaller left ventricular cavity size and greater wall thickness.[15] Loss of right ventricular function is a powerful predictor of adverse outcome.[16]

Cardiac magnetic resonance (CMR) imaging is increasingly used in suspected myocarditis due to its capacity to detect myocardial inflammation, oedema, necrosis, and fibrosis. Non-invasive diagnostic criteria for myocarditis based on CMR findings (the 'Lake Louise Criteria') have been proposed and are presented in **Box 8.1**. The presence of any two of these three characteristic CMR findings confers a 63% sensitivity, 89% specificity, and 63% negative predictive value for biopsy-proven myocarditis. The presence of LV dysfunction or pericardial effusion provide ancillary evidence for diagnosing myocarditis. Newer techniques such as extracellular volume mapping promise to improve the diagnostic performance of CMR in the coming years. Identifying areas of active myocarditis with CMR may also be helpful in localizing sites for endomyocardial biopsy (**Figure 8.1**).

Endomyocardial biopsy (EMB) remains the reference standard for confirming the diagnosis of myocarditis, although its status in this respect is less than ideal given the possibility of false-negative results due to sampling error.[17] The Dallas histopathological

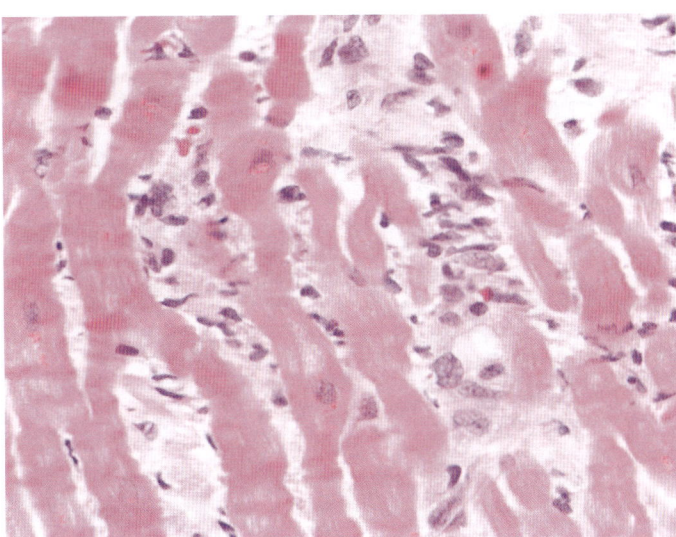

Figure 8.1 Viral myocarditis. The myocardium contains focal interstitial infiltration by mononuclear cells with associated cardiac myocyte degeneration. Haematoxylin and eosin ×400.
Courtesy of Dr Allan McPhaden, Queen Elizabeth University Hospital, Glasgow.

criteria, devised in 1986, were an initial attempt to standardize the diagnosis:[18]

- Active myocarditis: an inflammatory infiltrate of the myocardium with necrosis and/or degeneration of adjacent myocytes 'not typical of the ischaemic damage associated with coronary heart disease'. The infiltrates are usually mononuclear, but may be neutrophilic or, occasionally, eosinophilic.
- 'Borderline myocarditis' is the term used when the inflammatory infiltrate is less intense, or myocyte injury is not demonstrated, and a repeat biopsy may be indicated.

However, the Dallas criteria are limited by inter-observer variability, and because non-cellular infiltrative processes are not considered.[19] Contemporary tools including immunohistochemistry and viral genome analysis (which still require tissue via EMB) are now recommended.[5] According to the current consensus, an immunohistochemical diagnosis of active myocarditis is achieved in the presence of focal or diffuse mononuclear infiltrates (T lymphocytes and macrophages) with a cut-off of ≥14 leucocytes per mm^2 (including up to 4 monocytes per mm^2) with the presence of CD3$^+$ T-lymphocytes ≥7 cells per mm^2.[5]

EMB may also identify the underlying aetiology and type of inflammation (which CMR does not). Infiltrates are most commonly lymphocytic (including viral and autoimmune forms) (**Figure 8.1**), but may also be neutrophilic (bacterial, fungal, and early forms of viral myocarditis) or eosinophilic (hypersensitivity myocarditis or the hypereosinophilic syndrome), and invariably include macrophages. Other findings include giant cells (giant cell myocarditis) (**Figure 8.2**) and granulomas (cardiac sarcoidosis). Since these infiltrates favour specific underlying aetiologies, which may alter the management strategy, EMB carries a class IIa guideline recommendation in certain scenarios wherein a progressive myocarditis is suspected.[20]

Box 8.1 Diagnostic criteria for myocarditis based on cardiac magnetic resonance findings (Lake Louise Criteria)

In the setting of clinically suspected myocarditis, CMR findings are consistent with this diagnosis if ≥2 of the following criteria are present:
(i) Increased signal intensity in T2-weighted oedema images
(ii) Increased early gadolinium enhancement ratio between myocardial and skeletal muscle in T1-weighted images
(iii) Late gadolinium enhancement in ≥1 focal area of non-ischaemic distribution in inversion recovery gadolinium-enhanced T1-weighted images

Source data from Friedrich MG, Strohm O, Schulz-Menger J, *et al.* Contrast media-enhanced magnetic resonance imaging visualizes myocardial changes in the course of viral myocarditis. *Circulation* 1998;**97**:1802–9.

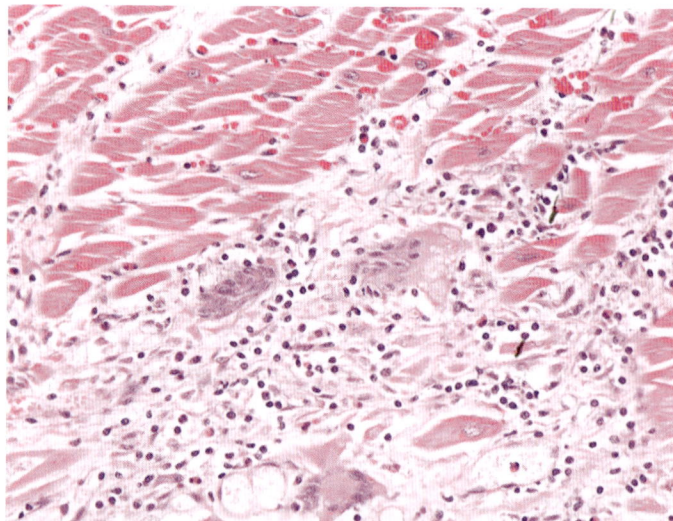

Figure 8.2 Giant cell myocarditis. The myocardium is being damaged by a marked chronic inflammatory infiltrate that includes prominent multinucleated giant cells in the lower half of the image. Haematoxylin and eosin ×200.

Courtesy of Dr Allan McPhaden, Queen Elizabeth University Hospital, Glasgow.

Treatment

Patients who present with acute heart failure and LVSD due to myocarditis should be treated with rest and—once stable—established on prognostic heart failure pharmacotherapy, as well as diuretics where appropriate. Although most patients will improve, some patients will require supportive therapy for cardiogenic shock with inotropes or mechanical circulatory support, and possible urgent listing for cardiac transpantation.[21,22] At this juncture, consideration of the underlying aetiology of myocarditis, and thus the recoverability of LV function, is important. Patients with sustained or symptomatic ventricular arrhythmias may need to be treated with anti-arrhythmic medication, or an implantable cardioverter–defibrillator (ICD),[23] although acute myocarditis could be considered a transient and reversible illness. There is currently little evidence of significant benefit from immunosuppressive therapy.[24,25]

Viral myocarditis

Polymerase chain reaction (PCR) and in-situ hybridization techniques permit the identification of viral genomic sequences in biopsied myocardium. The viruses most frequently implicated are parvovirus B19, coxsackie B, human herpes virus 6, and adenoviruses 2 and 5. They appear to enter cardiac myocytes or macrophages through specific receptors and co-receptors,[26] triggering an innate immune response through several mechanisms, as well as causing a proinflammatory cytokine release.[27]

The causal association between detectable viral DNA/RNA and myocardial dysfunction in any individual patient is uncertain—viruses can also be detected in the myocardium of patients in the absence of myocarditis. It is poorly understood why the vast majority of infections with these viruses do not lead to myocarditis or a dilated cardiomyopathy. However, in those patients who are clinically affected, a persistently detectable viral load at repeat EMB is associated with progressive LV dysfunction, whereas viral clearance is associated with recovery of myocardial function.[28]

Viral serology is usually of limited utility due to false-positive results but may be helpful in specific clinical scenarios, including suspected hepatitis C, rickettsial phase 1 and phase 2, Lyme disease in endemic areas, and human immunodeficiency virus (HIV) infection.[5] Survival in patients with biopsy-proven viral myocarditis has been reported as 80% and 44% at 1 and 4.3 years, respectively.[29] No pathogen-targeted antiviral therapy has yet been approved for use in viral myocarditis. Acyclovir, ganciclovir or valacyclovir may be considered in herpesvirus infection, and there is limited evidence that interferon-α and interferon-β encourage viral clearance and clinical improvement; however, evidence from large randomized trials is lacking. For similar reasons, treatments such as intravenous immunoglobulin and immunoadsorption are not currently recommended.

At the time of writing, there are widespread reports of acute myocardial injury and suspected acute myocarditis in association with the novel severe acute respiratory syndrome coronavirus 2 (SARS-CoV-2) virus.[30,31] To date, evaluation by CMR and EMB have demonstrated inflammation, oedema, and cellular infiltrates in patients with suspected SARS-CoV-2 myocarditis; however, viral genome has not yet been demonstrated within the myocardium of these subjects, and at present the pathogenesis of this phenomenon remains uncertain.

Giant cell myocarditis

Giant cell myocarditis (GCM) is a rare form of myocarditis that presents with rapidly deteriorating cardiac function and arrhythmias.[32] Approximately 20% of patients have coexisting autoimmune disease, and the great majority of affected individuals (~90%) are White. The histological diagnosis requires a diffuse or multifocal inflammatory infiltrate of lymphocytes and characteristic multinucleated giant cells, in the absence of granuloma formation (GCM and cardiac sarcoid were once considered the same entity) (Figure 8.2).[33] The sensitivity of EMB in patients who present early in the course of fulminant disease is ~85%.[31]

The prognosis of giant cell myocarditis is very poor (<6 months) and identifying such patients early will allow the immediate administration of multidrug immunosuppressive therapy—a combination of prednisolone, ciclosporin, azathioprine, or muromonab-CD3 (OKT3). If OKT3 is unavailable, there are observational reports of efficacy with alemtuzumab.[33] Due to the rapid deterioration of myocardial function, patients may require mechanical circulatory support (intra-aortic balloon pump therapy or ventricular assist device therapy) as a bridge to recovery, or as a bridge to transplantation. It should be noted that a recurrence of giant cells occurs in 25% of transplanted hearts, but this is usually an asymptomatic histological recurrence several years after surgery, and generally responds to a temporary augmentation of immunosuppression.

HIV cardiomyopathy

The survival of patients with HIV infection has improved markedly with the use of highly active antiretroviral therapy (HAART) and the incidence of AIDS-defining events has significantly fallen.[34]

Cardiac involvement occurs in around 50% of patients with HIV, although it is frequently asymptomatic. HIV itself can cause myocarditis, although most cases are clinically silent.[35] The pathogenesis of HIV cardiomyopathy is not fully established but thought to include infection of myocardial cells with HIV type 1 (HIV-1),[36] as HIV-1

Table 8.4 Cardiovascular problems in HIV infection

	Aetiology	Comment
Pericardium and effusions	Pericarditis	Pericardial effusion frequent, although tamponade is rare; tuberculous effusion (may be associated with myocarditis) frequent in developing countries; other causes: bacterial pericarditis, Kaposi's sarcoma, and lymphoma
	Kaposi sarcoma	Often disseminated; cardiac problems are infrequent
Myocardium	Cardiomyopathy	LVSD usually clinically silent; complex pathogenesis (direct virus effect, inflammatory response, autoantibodies)
	Myocarditis	Specific cause in <20% of patients; rare causes: toxoplasmosis, tuberculosis, cryptococcosis, histoplasmosis, aspergillosis, candidosis, cytomegalovirus, and herpes simplex; HIV itself can cause myocarditis
	Lymphoma	Non-Hodgkin's B-cell lymphoma; primary cardiac lymphoma is extremely rare
	Drug toxicity	Drug toxicity: amphotericin B, doxorubicin, foscarnet, interferon-α, zidovudine
Pulmonary hypertension	Inflammation and genetic factors	Possibly leading to right HF; histologically plexogenic arteriopathy is most commonly similar to the immunocompetent patient
Endocardium and valves	Infective endocarditis	Bacterial aetiology in intravenous drug abusers, is most often *Staph. aureus* and *Strep. viridans*; HIV infection itself is not associated with bacterial endocarditis
	Non-bacterial/marantic	Tricuspid valve often involved; embolization of thrombus (frequently clinically silent)
Atherosclerosis	HAART	HAART may cause metabolic syndrome and lipodystrophy; premature atherosclerosis of coronary, cerebral, and peripheral arteries
Arrhythmia	No specific association with HIV infection	Arrhythmia caused by cardiomyopathy or myocarditis, myocardial infiltration in cardiac lymphoma; HIV itself does not cause rhythm disturbances
	Drug toxicity	Ganciclovir (against cytomegalovirus) may induce ventricular tachycardia; interferon-α can cause AV block and sudden death; pentamidine and pyrimethamine (for toxoplasmosis) cause QT prolongation, torsade de pointes; trimethoprim-sulfomethoxazole (*Pneumocystis carinii* prophylaxis) causes QT prolongation, torsade de pointes
Aneurysmal vascular disease	Inflammation	Premature aortic and cerebrovascular aneurysms described in patients with HIV infection

Source data from Sudano I, Spieker LE, Noll G, Corti R, Weber R, Lüscher TF. Cardiovascular disease in HIV infection. *Am Heart J* 2006;**151**:11475–5.

genomic material has been demonstrated within cardiac myocytes in patients with cardiomyopathy at autopsy. Other possible causes for cardiovascular problems include subsequent opportunistic infection, neoplasia, and cardiotoxicity from pharmacologic agents, e.g. nucleoside analogues and pentamidine (Table 8.4). Heart failure can also result from endocarditis (principally right sided) in intravenous drug misusers. It should also be borne in mind that antiretroviral therapy can lead to premature coronary artery disease by inducing a syndrome akin to the metabolic syndrome.[37]

In a five-year echocardiographic follow-up study of 952 asymptomatic HIV patients, 8% developed a dilated cardiomyopathy (DCM).[38] The incidence was higher if the CD4 count was <400 cells/mm³. A histological diagnosis of active or borderline myocarditis was made in 83% of those who developed DCM, with inflammatory infiltrates predominantly composed of CD3 and CD8 lymphocytes. HIV nucleic acid sequences were detected in the myocardium of 76% of DCM patients, and 57% of the subgroup with myocarditis. In those with active myocarditis, patients were also infected with: Coxsackie B (17%), cytomegalovirus (6%), and Epstein–Barr virus (3%). Although this study was published in the *New England Journal of Medicine*, the work was later retracted by the journal's editors[39] and therefore the validity of the data is uncertain.

A rare but important differential diagnosis of HIV cardiomyopathy is infective myocarditis (e.g. myocardial toxoplasmosis, aspergillosis, tuberculosis, cryptococcosis, histoplasmosis, candidosis, herpes simplex, and cytomegalovirus).

Treatment

Conventional heart failure treatment may help improve cardiac function, even in asymptomatic HIV-positive patients. Physicians should also be aware of the possible interaction between protease inhibitors and β-adrenoreceptor antagonists, digoxin, or non-dihydropyridine calcium antagonists due to possible prolongation of atrioventricular (AV) conduction (although non-dihydropyridine calcium antagonists should not in any case be used in patients with LVSD). Protease inhibitors should be used with caution in patients with pre-existing conduction system disease.

Cardiovascular risk factors should be addressed,[40] but caution should be employed when initiating lipid-lowering therapy, because of interactions between HIV protease inhibitors (e.g. ritonavir, atazanavir, and saquinavir) and statins affecting cytochrome P450 function.[41] For this reason, simvastatin, atorvastatin, and lovastatin should be avoided, and pravastatin used with careful dose adjustment.

Although HIV is not a contraindication for cardiac transplantation, few patients ultimately receive a new heart. Immunosuppressive agents such as ciclosporin and tacrolimus appear to slow virus replication and interleukin-2-induced T-cell replication,[42] and the incidence of opportunistic infections is not increased by pharmacological immunosuppression in HIV patients. However, there are pharmacological interactions between HAART and both ciclosporin and tacrolimus, with the need for careful dose adjustment.

Chagas disease

Chagas disease is caused by the protozoan parasite *Trypanosoma cruzi*, most often transmitted by triatomine insects. Vector-borne transmission occurs only in the Americas, where the burden of disease in endemic areas is substantial. It is the most important parasitic disease in the Western Hemisphere.

Acute Chagas disease tends to be diagnosed most frequently in children, although individuals of all ages may be infected. It can cause a severe myocarditis, particularly in the young, resulting in heart failure and a high risk of death.[43] However, if chronic disease occurs, the manifestations are usually delayed and typically do not arise until 20 years later.

Transmission and epidemiology

The major route of transmission of *T. cruzi* is directly from the triatomine reduviid bug. However, the infection can also arise from other routes, including blood transfusion, organ transplantation, and vertical transmission. Public health measures in Latin American countries have substantially reduced the spread of the disease, with the estimated global prevalence falling from 18 million people in 1991 to 5.7 million in 2010.[44]

Pathophysiology and clinical features

In the vast majority of patients, the acute phase of infection—during which there is detectable parasitaemia—passes without detection. Rarely, acute infection may precipitate a life-threatening myocarditis (or meningoencephalitis). Once parasitaemia resolves, patients move into the chronic phase of *T. cruzi* infection, with an estimated 20–30% of people infected developing Chagas cardiomyopathy over a time-course ranging to decades.[44] The pathogenesis of this disease phase is poorly understood, but thought to involve an inflammatory host immune response, with eventual diffuse organ fibrosis due to antibody and cell-mediated immunity against *T. cruzi* antigens. The earliest clinical manifestations of the chronic disease phase are often ECG abnormalities, particularly progressive conduction system problems, with subsequent clinical features including myocardial dysfunction, ventricular arrhythmias, and sudden death. Thromboembolic disease may also be a feature, as are the usual symptoms and signs of heart failure. Patients may also develop gastrointestinal Chagas disease, resulting in mega-oesophagus and/or mega-colon.

Investigation

Echocardiography may reveal either global LVSD or regional wall motion abnormality. In advanced disease there may be posterior hypokinesis with relative sparing of the septal wall. A left ventricular apical aneurysm is also frequently a feature. A diagnosis of acute *T. cruzi* infection can be made by microscopic visualization or PCR. In the chronic phase, indirect immunofluorescence antibody assay or enzyme-linked immunosorbent assay (ELISA) may aid the diagnosis.

Treatment

Two antiparasitic medications—benznidazole and nifurtimox—are effective at clearing parasitaemia during acute infection, with the former considered the first-line agent. Their use in the chronic phase is an area of uncertainty, with the benefit of treating infected adults with antitrypanosomal therapy called into question by a recent, large, double-blinded, randomized, placebo-controlled trial.[45] Although not evidence-based, standard heart failure therapy, the control of ventricular arrhythmias with antiarrhythmic drugs (e.g. amiodarone), and anticoagulation to reduce the risk of thromboembolic disease should be considered. Of note, where cardiac transplantation is required to treat Chagas cardiomyopathy, serial post-transplantation PCR testing may be used to monitor for *T. cruzi* reactivation.

Lyme disease

Lyme disease is a multisystem disease caused by infection from a tick-borne spirochete (*Borrelia burgdorferi*). Early features include erythema migrans and constitutional upset, but the development of cardiac, neurological, and joint involvement may follow after weeks to months. In the USA, cardiac involvement occurs in up to 10% of untreated adults during the early disseminated phase of the disease—usually within the first two months after infection. Lyme carditis is less common in Europe, possibly relating to infection by different organisms. Interestingly, although Lyme disease itself has a slight female predominance, the cardiac manifestations are much more common in males (3:1).

Clinical features

Erythema migrans is found in approximately 90% of people with Lyme disease. The early disseminated features occur days to months later, with these including myocarditis, lymphocytic meningitis, cranial nerve palsies, and migratory polyarthritis.

Myocarditis most commonly manifests as conduction system disease—often progressing rapidly from first degree to higher degrees of block over a relatively short period of time, frequently requiring temporary transvenous pacing.[46] Myopericarditis and cardiomyopathy may also develop, but these are generally mild and self-limiting. Late features occur weeks to years later, and include chronic arthritis and neurological problems (e.g. dementia). Lyme myocarditis should be suspected in patients with a history of a tick bite, particularly if they have conduction system abnormalities.

Investigations and diagnosis

Serological studies with ELISA and western blot help to confirm the diagnosis.

Treatment

Lyme disease should generally be treated by those experienced in its management. Doxycycline is currently the antibacterial of choice for early disease, and intravenous ceftriaxone is recommended for Lyme disease associated with moderate-to-severe cardiac or neurological abnormalities, late Lyme disease, and Lyme arthritis. The duration of treatment is generally two to four weeks, although Lyme arthritis requires longer treatment with oral antibacterial drugs. With appropriate treatment, the prognosis of patients with Lyme carditis is favourable. Although temporary pacing is often required, the underlying conduction defect usually reverses, such that the requirement for a permanent pacemaker is rare. Very few deaths worldwide have been attributed to Lyme carditis.[47]

Infiltrative causes of heart failure

Infiltrative cardiomyopathies are characterized by the deposition of abnormal material into the ventricular myocardium, causing it to become increasingly stiff, with reduced ventricular compliance.[48] The restrictive physiology impedes ventricular filling, leading to impaired diastolic function. However, systolic function usually remains normal, at least early in the disease process.

Table 8.5 Infiltrative cardiac conditions that present with increased left ventricle mass and thick ventricular walls

Condition	Age at presentation	History and clinical presentation	Echocardiography	ECG profile	CMR LGE	Biopsy
Cardiac amyloid	>30 years	Heart failure symptoms, nephrotic syndrome, idiopathic peripheral neuropathy, unexplained hepatomegaly	Symmetrical increase in LV and RV wall thickness, dilated LA and RA, granular appearance of myocardium, pericardial effusion, decreased EF in advanced cases	Decreased or normal QRS complex voltage, pseudoinfarction in inferolateral leads (AL amyloidosis)	Global, diffuse, pronounced in subendocardium; RV and LV walls	Myocyte atrophy, amyloid replaces normal cardiac tissue
Fabry disease	Male: 11 ± 7 years; female: 23 ± 16 years	Neuropathic pain, impaired sweating, skin rashes	Symmetrical increase in LV and RV wall thickness, normal EF	Increased or normal QRS complex voltage, short or prolonged PR interval	Focal, midwall, inferolateral wall	Enlarged myocytes with clusters of concentric glycolipid (myelinoid bodies) within lysosomes
Danon disease	<20 years	Heart failure, skeletal myopathy, mental retardation	Very thick LV (20–60 mm), RV may or may not be thick, decreased EF	Increased or normal QRS complex voltage, short PR interval (delta wave)	Subendocardial, does not correspond to perfusion territory	Sarcoplasmic vacuolization, focal storage of PAS-positive material, myofibrillar disarray
Friedreich ataxia	25 years (range: 2–51 years)	Gait abnormality	Increase in LV septal and posterior wall thickness, normal EF	Normal QRS complex voltage, ventricular tachycardia		Non-specific
Cardiac oxalosis	>20 years	Juvenile urolithiasis and nephrocalcinosis	Symmetrical increase in LV and RV wall thickness; patchy, echodense speckled reflection; normal EF	Increased or normal QRS complex voltage, complete heart block	Increased myocardium attenuation on CT	Intra- and extracellular deposition of oxalate crystals without concomitant inflammation and necrosis
Mucopolysaccharidoses	1–24 years (median: 10)	Variable depending on subtype, coarse facial features, delayed mental development, skeletal deformities, corneal clouding, hepatosplenomegaly	Asymmetrical septal hypertrophy, mitral and/or aortic valve stenosis or insufficiency, normal EF	Increased or decreased QRS complex voltage, malignant arrhythmia		Swollen myocytes with clear cytoplasm due to accumulation of mucopolysaccharides within lysosomes
Differential diagnosis						
Hypertrophic cardiomyopathy	17–18 years	May be asymptomatic, dyspnoea, angina, syncope, sudden death	Asymmetrical hypertrophy small LV cavity, LVOT obstruction, normal EF	Increased QRS complex voltage pseudo-delta wave, giant T-wave inversion	Patchy, mid-wall, junctions of the ventricular septum and RV	Myocyte hypertrophy, myofibrillar disarray, and interstitial fibrosis
Hypertensive heart disease	Adults	History of hypertension	Symmetrical increase in LV wall thickness, mild LV dilation, normal EF	Increased QRS complex, non-specific ST-T-wave changes	No pattern, predominantly subendocardial	Enlarged myocytes with enlarged or replicated nuclei

EF, ejection fraction; LA, left atrium; LV, left ventricle; RA, right atrium; RV, right ventricle.
Source data from Seward JB, Casaclang-Verzosa G. Infiltrative cardiovascular diseases: cardiomyopathies that look alike. *J Am Coll Cardiol* 2010;**55**:17697–9.

Infiltrative cardiac diseases either increase ventricular wall thickness (Table 8.5), or cause chamber enlargement with secondary wall thinning (Table 8.6). However, infiltrative disorders can be mistaken for other cardiac conditions. A good example is cardiac amyloidosis, where the increased wall thickness, small ventricular volume, and occasional dynamic left ventricular outflow obstruction can mimic conditions with true myocyte hypertrophy such as hypertrophic cardiomyopathy and hypertensive heart disease.

Infiltrative cardiac conditions often result in a restrictive cardiomyopathy (Box 8.2), although this is uncommon in western countries. However, in certain geographical locations (particularly the tropics—Africa, India, South and Central America, and Asia),

restrictive cardiomyopathy is a more important cause of heart failure and death due to a higher incidence of endomyocardial fibrosis. Here we concentrate on the acquired causes of myocardial and endocardial infiltration.

Clinical features

Patients with restrictive cardiomyopathy often complain of exercise intolerance due to a fixed stroke volume limiting any increase in cardiac output. Elevated filling pressures and Kussmaul's sign (inspiratory increase in jugular venous pressure (JVP)) may be apparent. Other clinical features include an impalpable apex beat (unlike constrictive pericarditis), third or fourth heart sound, peripheral oedema, hepatomegaly, and ascites.

Table 8.6 Infiltrative cardiac conditions that present with dilated left ventricle and infarct pattern

Condition	Age at presentation	History	Echocardiography	ECG	CMR LGE	Cardiac biopsy
Sarcoidosis	Young adults	Heart failure, arrhythmia	Variable wall thickness, focal or global hypokinesia, LV aneurysm	Infrahisian block, atypical infarction pattern	Patchy, basal and lateral LV walls	Non-caseating, multinucleated giant cell granuloma surrounded by band of dense collagen fibres
Granulomatosis with polyangiitis	Young adults	Chronic upper and lower respiratory tract infections	Regional hypokinesis pericardial effusion, mild, MR, LV systolic dysfunction	Atrial fibrillation, atrioventricular block, atypical infarction pattern	Diffuse, midwall	Vasculitis with necrotizing granulomatous inflammation
Haemochromatosis	Hereditary haemochromatosis: >30 years in men, older in women; secondary haemochromatosis: any age	Hereditary haemochromatosis: liver function abnormalities, weakness and lethargy, skin hyperpigmentation, diabetes mellitus, arthralgia, impotence in men; secondary haemochromatosis: haemolytic anaemia, multiple blood transfusions	Dilated LV with global systolic dysfunction	Supraventricular arrhythmia, ventricular conduction abnormality is rare	T2* values substantially reduced	Iron deposits within the myocyte
Differential diagnoses						
Ischaemic cardiomyopathy	Adult	Coronary artery disease, heart failure	Dilated LV, regional hypokinesis corresponding to perfusion territory, decreased systolic function	Multiform premature ventricular complexes, non-sustained ventricular tachycardia	Subendocardial, different degrees of transmural extension, corresponds to perfusion territory	
Dilated cardiomyopathy	Adult	Heart failure, no known cardiovascular disease	Dilated LV with global systolic dysfunction	Atrial fibrillation	No LGE, or if present, mid-wall and patchy	

Source data from Seward JB, Casaclang-Verzosa G. Infiltrative cardiovascular diseases: cardiomyopathies that look alike. *J Am Coll Cardiol* 2010;**55**:17697–9.

Investigations

The ECG may show P mitrale/pulmonale, low precordial QRS amplitudes, and atrial arrhythmias. Echocardiography may initially appear unremarkable, with normal ventricular dimensions and systolic function. However, there is often marked bi-atrial enlargement secondary to elevated atrial pressures and a restrictive inflow pattern seen on mitral Doppler. Features that may help differentiate restrictive cardiomyopathy from constrictive pericarditis are shown in Table 8.7. On cardiac catheterization, left ventricular and right ventricular pressure tracings are in phase and right ventricular peak pressure is frequently in excess of 40 mmHg. CMR is very useful in the assessment of patients with infiltrative myocardial

and endomyocardial disease, and may help identify areas likely to have a high diagnostic yield on endomyocardial biopsy.

Treatment

The mainstay of medical therapy for restrictive cardiomyopathy is diuretics, although caution should be taken to avoid under-filling patients, as a fall in filling pressure will have a marked adverse impact on cardiac output. Avoidance of atrial fibrillation (AF) or optimal rate control of AF will help maintain ventricular filling time. It is also important to identify and treat the underlying cause.

Prognosis

The prognosis of restrictive cardiomyopathy is generally poor, and some patients will ultimately need cardiac transplantation if appropriate.

Cardiac sarcoidosis

Sarcoidosis is a multisystem, non-caseating, granulomatous disease of unknown aetiology. It is estimated to affect one in 10 000 people, with marked geographical and racial variation, being three to four times more common in Black people. It typically affects young adults, and most commonly affects the lung (90%), presenting with either evidence of bilateral hilar lymphadenopathy or pulmonary infiltrates. Pulmonary hypertension carries an ominous prognosis. Skin, joint, or eye involvement is also common. However, clinical cardiac involvement is uncommon, affecting only around 2–5% of

Box 8.2 Causes of restrictive cardiomyopathy

- Myocardial
  - Infiltrative (e.g. amyloid, sarcoid, Gaucher's disease)
  - Non-infiltrative (e.g. scleroderma)
  - Storage diseases (e.g. haemochromatosis, glycogen and lysosomal storage disease)
- Endomyocardial
  - Endomyocardial fibrosis
  - Hypereosinophilic syndrome (Löffler's endocarditis)
  - Carcinoid and metastatic disease
  - Radiation
  - Anthracycline therapy

Table 8.7 Features differentiating constrictive pericarditis from restrictive cardiomyopathy

Feature	Constrictive pericarditis	Restrictive cardiomyopathy
Past medical history	Previous pericarditis, cardiac surgery, trauma, radiotherapy, connective tissue disease	These items rare
Jugular venous waveform	X and Y dips brief and 'flicking', not conspicuous positive waves	X and Y dips less brief, may have conspicuous A wave or V wave
Extra sounds in diastole	Early S3, high pitched 'pericardial knock'. No S4	Later S3, low pitched, 'triple rhythm', S4 in some cases
Mitral or tricuspid regurgitation	Usually absent	Often present
ECG	P waves reflect intra-atrial conduction delay. Atrioventricular or intraventricular conduction defects rare	P waves reflect right or left atrial hypertrophy or overload. Atrioventricular or intraventricular conduction defects not unusual
Plain chest radiograph	Pericardial calcification in 20–30%	Pericardial calcification rare
Ventricular septal movement in diastole	Abrupt septal movement ('bounce') in early diastole in most cases	Abrupt septal movement in early diastole seen only occasionally
Ventricular septal movement with respiration	Notable movement towards left ventricle in inspiration usually seen	Relatively little movement towards left ventricle in most cases
Atrial enlargement	Slight or moderate in most cases	Pronounced in most cases
Respiratory variation in mitral and tricuspid flow velocity	>25% in most cases	<15% in most cases
Equilibration of diastolic pressures in all cardiac chambers	Within 5 mmHg in nearly all cases, often essentially the same	Within 5 mmHg in a small proportion of cases
Dip-plateau waveform in the right ventricular pressure waveform	End-diastolic pressure more than one-third of systolic pressure in many cases	End-diastolic pressure often less than one-third of systolic
Peak right ventricular systolic pressure	Nearly always <60 mmHg, often <40 mmHg	Frequently >40 mmHg and occasionally >60 mmHg
Discordant respiratory variation of ventricular peak systolic pressures	Right and left ventricular peak systolic pressure variations are out of phase	Right and left ventricular peak systolic pressure variations are in-phase
Paradoxical pulse	Often present to a moderate degree	Rarely present
MR/CT imaging	Shows thick pericardium in most cases	Shows thick pericardium only rarely
Endomyocardial biopsy	Normal, or non-specific abnormalities	Shows amyloid in some cases, rarely other specific infiltrative disease

Source data from Hancock EW. Differential diagnosis of restrictive cardiomyopathy and constrictive pericarditis. *Heart* 2001 Sep;**86**(3):343–9.

patients with sarcoidosis, although autopsy studies suggest that subclinical cardiac involvement is more common. Cardiac sarcoidosis generally affects the basal septum, conduction system, papillary muscles, and patchy regions on the ventricular free wall.

Pathophysiology

The aetiology of sarcoidosis is not clear, and several potential antigens have been suggested as triggers, including *Mycobacterium tuberculosis*, mycoplasma, aluminium, and pollen. T-Helper cell activation leads to the formation of granuloma lesions and interleukin-6 is thought to be involved in the maintenance of inflammation by inducing T-cell proliferation. A positive association between cardiac sarcoidosis and HLA-DQB1*0601 has been reported.

Clinical features

The clinical consequences of cardiac sarcoidosis range from asymptomatic conduction abnormalities to fatal ventricular arrhythmias, depending upon the location and extent of granulomatous inflammation. Complete heart block is frequently seen, and patients are at risk of both supraventricular and ventricular tachycardias (**Figure 8.3**). Heart failure symptoms may also develop due initially to restrictive physiology, although left ventricular dilation and systolic dysfunction can develop. Cardiac imaging in sarcoidosis

frequently demonstrates dyskinetic or akinetic segments interspersed with normal segments.[49] Pericardial effusions can occur, but rarely cause tamponade. There may also be valve dysfunction, including mitral valve prolapse. Patients with cardiac sarcoidosis have a poorer prognosis than those with no cardiac involvement, with depressed left ventricular ejection fraction (LVEF) being the major adverse risk factor. Patients in this group ultimately die from ventricular tachyarrhythmia, conduction disturbances, or progressive heart failure.

Investigations

The clinical findings of cardiac sarcoidosis are largely non-specific. The only absolute test for organ involvement in sarcoidosis is histological examination of tissue for non-caseating granulomatous inflammation, in the absence of an alternative explanation for this finding. Since EMB carries an inherent procedural risk and lacks sensitivity (non-caseating granulomas (**Figure 8.4**) are revealed in less than 25% of patients with cardiac sarcoidosis),[50] the diagnosis of cardiac sarcoidosis is challenging (**Box 8.3**). However, the diagnosis of systemic sarcoidosis has often already been made from another system involvement (commonly lung).

Precursor investigations that may suggest systemic sarcoidosis include serum angiotensin converting enzyme and a chest radiograph,

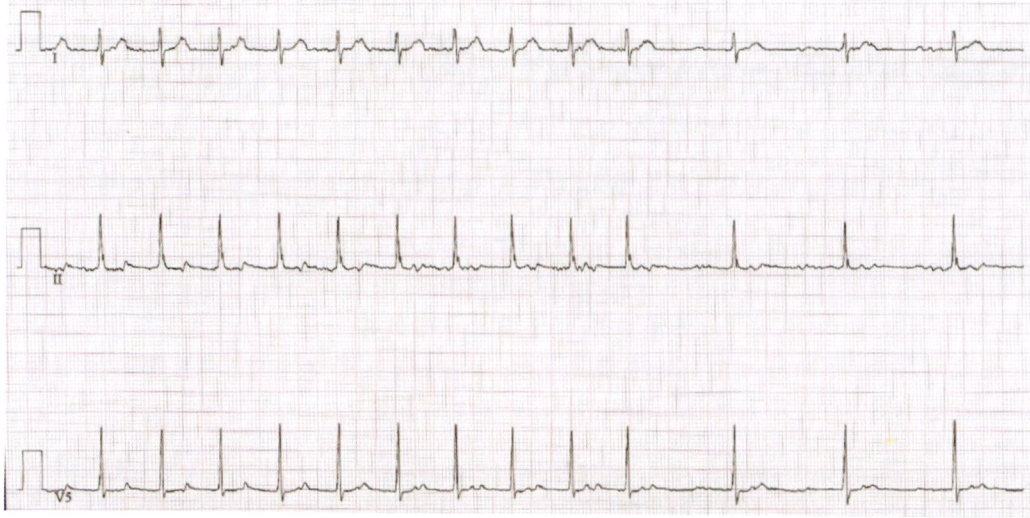

Figure 8.3 Electrocardiographic monitoring of a patient with cardiac sarcoidosis during exertion. Note the very long PR interval progressing to 2:1 heart block as the sinus node rate increases.
Courtesy of Prof. Andrew Clark, Castle Hill Hospital, Hull.

which commonly demonstrates hilar lymphadenopathy. A 12-lead ECG and 24 h Holter monitor will help to identify patients at risk of brady- or tachyarrhythmia. Echocardiography is not sensitive or specific enough to identify early or small areas of myocardial involvement, although it is more useful in advanced disease.[51] The ventricular septum often appears thinned and hyperechogenic, and there may be evidence of LVSD or left ventricular aneurysm. More rarely, wall thickening that mimics left ventricular hypertrophy or hypertrophic cardiomyopathy is seen. As mentioned above, dyskinetic or akinetic segments are commonly interspersed with normal segments, typically in a non-coronary distribution. Nuclear imaging (particularly thallium-201 scintigraphy) has largely been superseded by contrast-enhanced CMR and ^{18}F-fluorodeoxyglucose–positron

emission tomography (FDG-PET). Late gadolinium enhancement is patchy and typically involves the basal and lateral left ventricle walls, with sparing of the endocardial border.[52] This may help target subsequent endomyocardial biopsy, particularly as specimens are usually obtained from the apical septum. Fluorodeoxyglucose is a glucose analogue that helps identify inflammatory lesions via their higher metabolic rate and glucose utilization. No individual FDG-PET finding is pathognomonic for cardiac sarcoidosis, but focal uptake patterns are in keeping with active disease.[53] Simultaneous

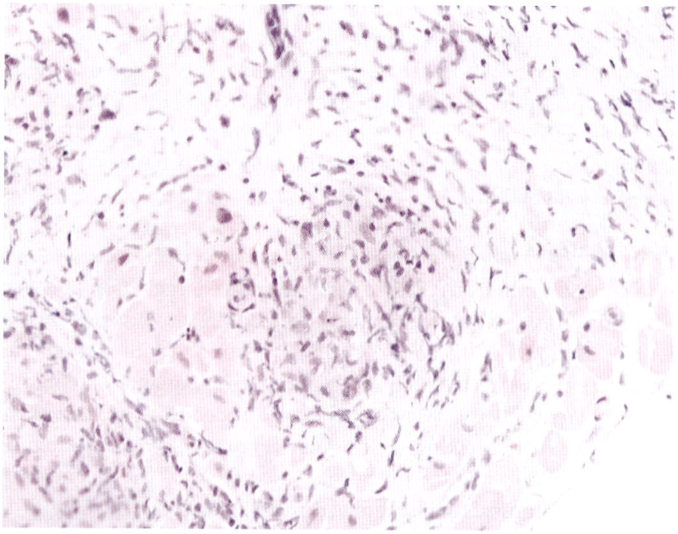

Box 8.3   Heart Rhythm Society recommendations for the diagnosis of cardiac sarcoidosis

1 Histologic diagnosis of cardiac sarcoidosis from myocardial tissue (Endomyocardial biopsy specimens with non-caseating granuloma and no alternative cause identified)

2 Clinical diagnosis of 'probable' cardiac sarcoidosis from invasive and non-invasive studies

   a Histological diagnosis of extra-cardiac sarcoidosis; and

   b One or more of the following:
- steroid ± immunosuppressant responsive cardiomyopathy or heart block
- unexplained reduced LVEF (<40%)
- unexplained sustained (spontaneous or induced) VT
- Mobitz type II 2nd degree heart block or 3rd degree heart block
- patchy uptake on dedicated cardiac PET (in a pattern consistent with cardiac sarcoidosis)
- LGE on CMR (in a pattern consistent with cardiac sarcoidosis)
- positive gallium uptake (in a pattern consistent with cardiac sarcoidosis); and

   c Other causes for cardiac manifestations have been reasonably excluded

In general, 'probable' involvement is considered sufficient evidence to establish a clinical diagnosis of cardiac sarcoidosis

Source data from Birnie DH, Sauer WH, Bogun F, *et al*. HRS expert consensus statement on the diagnosis and management of arrhythmias associated with cardiac sarcoidosis. *Heart Rhythm* 2014;**11**:1305–23.

Figure 8.4 Sarcoidosis. A central non-caseating granuloma is disrupting the myocardium with myocyte destruction and early replacement fibrosis. A second granuloma is present at the lower left. Haematoxylin and eosin ×400.
Courtesy of Dr Allan McPhaden, Queen Elizabeth University Hospital, Glasgow.

whole-body FDG-PET may also identify extracardiac lesions that are appropriate for biopsy and there is emerging interest in whether disease activity on FDG-PET could be used to guide treatment for cardiac sarcoidosis.

Treatment

Corticosteroids are thought capable of halting or slowing the progression of inflammation and fibrosis in sarcoidosis although there is no trial evidence to support their use. The initial starting dose is usually 30–40 mg of prednisolone daily, with response to treatment evaluated after 1–3 months and the dose adjusted as needed. Gradual tapering to a maintenance level of 5–15 mg per day is common, with treatment extended for another 9–12 months.[53] However, a possible association between corticosteroid treatment and formation of ventricular aneurysms has been described. In refractory cases—or if a steroid-sparing strategy is required—alternative agents include methotrexate, azathioprine, cyclophosphamide, and infliximab.

A permanent pacemaker is indicated in patients with complete heart block or other high-grade conduction system disease. An ICD is recommended in survivors of sudden death or patients with refractory ventricular tachyarrhythmias. Some also recommend an ICD for primary prevention due to the high rate of sudden death (presumed due to ventricular tachyarrhythmias) in cardiac sarcoidosis. In this scenario—given the likely need for future pacing for bradycardia in such patients—a dual-chamber ICD or cardiac resynchronization therapy–defibrillator should be considered. Catheter ablation may be considered for refractory ventricular arrhythmias.

Cardiac transplantation for cardiac sarcoidosis is rare, but it remains a possibility for younger patients with severe end-stage irreversible cardiac failure or resistant ventricular tachyarrhythmia, although disease can recur in the transplanted heart. Other types of surgery may be occasionally required such as correction of mitral valve disease or resection of ventricular aneurysms.

Haemochromatosis

Haemochromatosis is an autosomal recessive disorder in which mutations in the *HFE* gene (most commonly C282Y, on the short arm of chromosome 6) cause increased intestinal iron absorption. The clinical manifestations are related to excessive tissue iron deposition, particularly in the liver, pancreas, and pituitary, but also in the heart.

Clinical features

The clinical manifestations of iron accumulation include liver disease (ultimately leading to cirrhosis and an increased risk of hepatocellular carcinoma), skin pigmentation, diabetes mellitus, arthropathy, and hypogonadism. Cardiac effects can be the presenting manifestation in 15% of patients including heart failure, most commonly due to systolic rather than diastolic dysfunction, and conduction system disease.

Investigations

Investigation should begin with routine biochemistry including thyroid and liver function tests and iron studies (ferritin, transferrin saturation, serum iron, total iron binding concentration). However, although plasma transferrin saturation >55% and serum ferritin >200 ng/mL and 300 ng/mL (for women and men respectively) have

been proposed to identify patients with iron overload, reliance on these tests is risky (ferritin is falsely elevated in numerous other conditions, for instance, and transferrin saturations may not identify *HFE* gene homozygotes).[54] Genetic testing for C282Y homozygosity is important where iron overload is suspected. Although the ECG can appear normal initially, the QRS complexes can be low voltage with repolarization abnormalities.[55] CMR is the imaging modality of choice as echocardiography is poor at distinguishing haemochromatosis from dilated cardiomyopathy. T_2^* CMR can detect and quantify myocardial iron load and distribution.[56] Ultimately, a liver biopsy is the definitive test for iron overload, although with cardiac involvement a right ventricular endomyocardial biopsy will show evidence of stainable sarcoplasmic iron (**Figure 8.5**), where normally this should not be present.

Treatment

Venesection and chelation therapy are associated with an improvement in ventricular dysfunction.[57] However, irreversible myocardial dysfunction can occur with advanced disease. Some patients may require combined heart and liver transplantation, although this is currently a rare occurrence because of the lack of available organs.

Granulomatosis with polyangiitis (Wegener granulomatosis)

Granulomatosis with polyangiitis (formerly Wegener granulomatosis) is a vasculitis affecting small-to-medium-sized vessels characterized by necrotizing granulomatous inflammation that principally affects the lungs and the kidneys.[58] However, in a case series of 85 patients with confirmed granulomatosis with polyangitiis, 36% had cardiac abnormalities on echocardiography attributable to the disease.[59] Of these 26 patients, regional wall motion abnormalities were found in 65%, mild mitral regurgitation in 54%, LVSD in 50%, and pericardial effusion in 19%. Patients with cardiac abnormalities had a higher mortality rate than those without. On CMR, late gadolinium enhancement (LGE) in the mid-wall rather than the subendocardium is consistent with fibrosis

Figure 8.5 Haemochromatosis. Granular intracellular cardiac myocyte deposits of haemosiderin are stained blue. Perls stain ×400.
Courtesy of Dr Allan McPhaden, Queen Elizabeth University Hospital, Glasgow.

rather than infarction.[60] The diagnostic reference standard for granulomatosis with polyangiitis is histological examination, but positive antineutrophil cytoplasmic antibodies may suggest the disease.

Management requires a multidisciplinary approach. Patients with cardiac involvement have 'severe', life-threatening disease.[61] Cyclophosphamide or rituximab alongside steroids and plasma exchange are usually the treatments of choice to induce remission. Complete recovery of ventricular function following immunosuppression has been reported.[59]

Tropical endomyocardial fibrosis

Tropical endomyocardial fibrosis (EMF) is characterized by the deposition of fibrous tissue in the ventricular endocardium resulting in restrictive physiology, with involvement of either or both ventricles, and often with associated atrioventricular valvular regurgitation. EMF typically occurs in equatorial Africa, where it is a frequent cause of CHF. It is also recognized elsewhere, but generally within 15° of the equator. No consensus has been reached on the underlying pathophysiology but it appears to involve recurrent phases of inflammatory activation in susceptible individuals, progressively resulting in chronic fibrosis. EMF is the leading cause of restrictive cardiomyopathy worldwide.[62]

Clinical features and investigation

EMF most frequently causes biventricular involvement (50%), although single-chamber involvement does occur, either left ventricular (40%) or right ventricular (10%). Subsequently, atrial enlargement occurs, particularly where there is mitral or tricuspid regurgitation. The symptoms and signs are primarily those of left/right ventricular failure, and marked ascites out of proportion to peripheral oedema is often a striking feature of EMF. Peripheral blood eosinophilia may be present. The 12-lead ECG shows small QRS voltages with non-specific ST/T wave abnormalities. Echocardiography is the key investigation and may show apical obliteration of the involved ventricle, dilated atria, mitral or tricuspid regurgitation, and a pericardial effusion which may be large. Mural thrombi are common. Criteria for the diagnosis of EMF and assessment of disease severity of EMF have been developed, based on echocardiographic findings (see **Table 8.8**).

Treatment

The mainstay of treatment is diuretics. Anticoagulation should be considered in view of the risk of mural thrombi, and particularly so if AF is present. AF can be rate-controlled with digoxin, although its occurrence heralds a poor prognosis. Corticosteroids and immunosuppression agents may be used in the early phases of disease, but evidence supporting this approach is lacking. Surgical removal of fibrotic endocardium can lead to a significant improvement in symptoms, although recurrent fibrosis invariably occurs.

Löffler's endocarditis and the hypereosinophilic syndrome

The hypereosinophilic syndrome (HES) is a clinical diagnosis wherein there is a sustained eosinophil count >1500/mm³ for at least 6 months, with multi-organ dysfunction. Most patients with HES have biventricular cardiac involvement—this complication of HES

Table 8.8 Criteria for diagnosis and assessment of the severity of endomyocardial fibrosis*

Criteria	Score
Major criteria	
Endomyocardial plaques >2 mm in thickness	2
Thin (≤1 mm) endomyocardial patches affecting >1 ventricular wall	3
Obliteration of right ventricular or left ventricular apex	4
Thrombi or spontaneous contrast without severe ventricular dysfunction	4
Retraction of the right ventricular apex (right ventricular apical notch)	4
Atrioventricular valve dysfunction due to adhesion of valvular apparatus to ventricular wall	1–4†
Minor criteria	
Thin endomyocardial patches localized to one ventricular wall	1
Restrictive flow pattern across mitral or tricuspid valves	2
Pulmonary valve diastolic opening	2
Diffuse thickening of the anterior mitral valve leaflet	1
Enlarged atrium with normal ventricular dimensions	2
M-movement of interventricular septum and flat posterior wall	1
Enhance density of moderator band or other intraventricular bands	1

*Diagnosis of EMF is made in the presence of two major criteria or one major criterion associated with two minor criteria. Severity of EMF is graded in relation to total score as follows: <8: mild; 8–15: moderate; >15: severe.
†Score assigned according to severity of valvular regurgitation.
Source data from Mocumbi AO, Ferreira MB, Sidi D, *et al*. A population study of endomyocardial fibrosis in a rural area of Mozambique. *N Eng J Med* 2008;**359**(1):43–9.

being termed Löffler's endocarditis—with eosinophilic myocarditis, mural thrombosis, and fibrotic change, resulting in a restrictive cardiomyopathy. Associated involvement of the lungs, bone marrow, brain, and kidneys also occurs. Classically, HES is idiopathic, but other causes of hypereosinophilia such as drug allergy, parasitic infection, and bone marrow malignancy must be excluded.

Clinical features and investigations

The syndrome is frequently heralded by systemic upset, including fever, weight loss, rash, and cough. Symptoms and signs of heart failure then develop, and AF and thromboembolic disease are common. The 12-lead ECG shows non-specific T wave abnormalities, and the echocardiogram reveals localized thickening of the left ventricle basal posterior wall with restricted motion of the posterior mitral valve leaflet (**Figure 8.6**). Left ventricular systolic function is invariably preserved, and atrial dilatation and apical thrombus are common.

Treatment

The mainstay of treatment for Löffler's endocarditis is corticosteroid therapy, with a myelosuppressive agent such as hydroxyurea used in resistant cases. Interferon-α or the tyrosine kinase inhibitor imatinib are alternative options. Diuretics are important for symptomatic relief and conventional heart failure therapy is often used, with anticoagulation frequently mandated by either AF or mural thrombi. Attempts can also be made to remove fibrotic endocardium surgically.

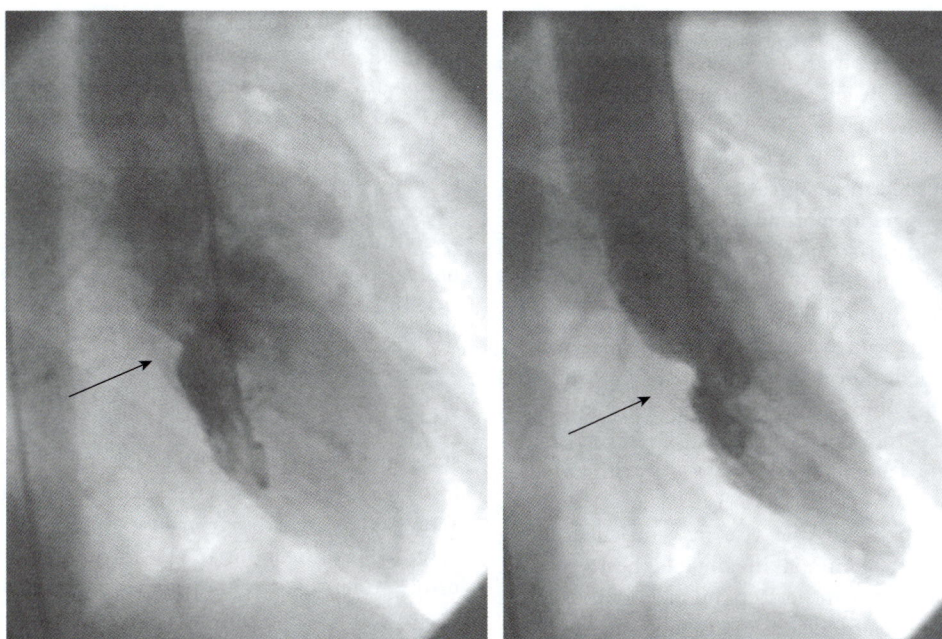

Figure 8.6 End-diastolic and end-systolic frames from the left ventricular angiogram of a woman with hypereosinophilic cardiac disease. The arrows point to the dense material involving and immobilizing the posterior mitral valve leaflet.

Amyloidosis

Amyloid proteins are normal proteins which can become insoluble polymers forming β-pleated sheets in tissues. What leads to an amyloid precursor protein causing amyloidosis (see Chapter 9) depends upon circumstances: most commonly, it may be an intrinsically abnormal protein, as in inherited abnormalities of the transthyretin gene; or it may be a protein being produced in large quantities, as happens with AL and AA amyloidosis (see below).

As an amyloid protein is deposited in tissue, it is partly stabilized by serum amyloid P (SAP),[63] a normal circulating factor, which binds to amyloid proteins and makes them resistant to normal proteolytic mechanisms.[64] The systemic illness, amyloidosis, may develop, with the symptoms depending on the site of amyloid deposition. Not all types of amyloid affect the heart.

Classification of amyloidosis

The classification of amyloidosis has changed several times, and can be confusing. The modern system uses an abbreviation starting with A (for amyloid) followed by the abbreviation for the protein involved (Table 8.9). The most important from the perspective of the heart are AL and ATTR amyloidosis. In AL amyloidosis, a white cell clone inappropriately produces large quantities of an aberrant immunoglobulin light chain. ATTR amyloidosis can be inherited as an autosomal dominant trait due to pathogenic mutations in the transthyretin gene TTR (ATTRm) or secondary to deposition of wild-type transthyretin protein (ATTRwt). The latter disease was formerly referred to as 'senile' systemic amyloidosis.

Presentation

AL amyloidosis presents very insidiously and patients frequently give a long history of general malaise and weight loss and have often undergone a wide range of investigations before the correct diagnosis is reached. Overt heart failure can be a late presenting feature.

Suggestive features include periorbital purpura (so-called 'panda eyes') and macroglossia. Neuropathies, autonomic and sensory, can occur, as well as carpal tunnel syndrome. The autonomic neuropathy contributes to orthostatic hypotension and frequent syncope. Renal involvement is more or less constant and causes proteinuria, which is frequently in the nephrotic range.

Table 8.9 Types of amyloidosis

Abbreviation	Amyloid protein	Source of protein	Clinical tissue deposition
AL	Immunoglobulin light chains	White cell dyscrasia	Heart, kidneys
AA	Serum amyloid protein A; acute phase reactants	Chronic inflammation	Kidneys, spleen, adrenal glands, liver, and gut (cardiac involvement rare)
ATTR (variant)	Transthyretin	Abnormal gene	Heart, neurological
ATTR (wild type)	Transthyretin	Age	Heart

There are other forms of amyloidosis, e.g. those associated with renal dialysis (β_2-microglobulin), prion disease, and Alzheimer's disease.

Cardiac involvement

The heart is almost always involved histologically in patients with AL amyloid, but clinical involvement is present in around 50%. In patients with cardiac involvement, death is commonly due to heart failure, or sudden, due to arrhythmia or pulseless electrical activity.

Amyloid can be deposited in small cardiac vessels, resulting in cardiac chest pain with apparently normal epicardial vessels.[65] More typically, patients have a restrictive cardiomyopathy in which the physical presence of the amyloid deposits prevents adequate diastolic relaxation of the ventricles. Interestingly, the light chains themselves may have a direct effect on the myocardium.[66,67] The clinical picture is dominated by right-sided clinical signs with raised JVP and fluid retention. A gallop rhythm or loud third sound is frequent. Patients often have a low cardiac output state with very limited exercise capacity and marked fatigue. Patients may also present with a dilated cardiomyopathy, presumably reflecting late disease.

The atria dilate in response to the rise in ventricular filling pressures, making AF very common in amyloid heart disease. Thromboembolic complications are very common, even in patients in sinus rhythm. Sudden death occurs, presumably due to more complex arrhythmia, at least in some patients.[68]

Investigations

The ECG is typically abnormal and frequently—but not always—shows low-voltage complexes (**Figure 8.7**), and commonly AF. The echocardiogram is extremely helpful. There is usually concentric left ventricular thickening (often labelled 'hypertrophy' but due to infiltration). The combination of left ventricular hypertrophy with small-voltage complexes on the ECG is characteristic, but not universal.[69] The atrial walls are often thickened, together with the interatrial septum (**Figure 8.8**). The texture of myocardium is abnormal and frequently 'speckled'. Diastolic flow across the mitral valve is grossly abnormal with a tall E wave and very short E wave deceleration time. The patient may be in sinus rhythm, but with no atrial mechanical activity.[70]

Cardiac catheterization shows a restrictive filling pattern in both ventricles with a dip-and-plateau pattern in diastole. In contrast to the pathophysiology of pericardial disease, the ventricular traces are often not identical (**Figure 8.9**).

Imaging for amyloidosis itself is now possible using radiolabelled SAP scanning and is helpful for assessing the burden of extracardiac deposits, but cannot be used to image the heart because of blood pool uptake.[71,72] The findings on CMR are characteristic in advanced disease, with subendocardial LGE together with abnormal gadolinium kinetics.[73] Less is known about CMR earlier in the progress of the disease, although this is a developing field.

Ultimately, the diagnosis often has to be made by tissue histology. Abdominal fat aspiration is said to be sensitive, and is certainly a safe first site for biopsy.[74] Other sites include rectal and gingival biopsies. Cardiac biopsy, usually from the right ventricle, may be necessary (see Figures 24.17 and 24.18) but it is worth remembering to stain any other available tissue for amyloid as it is widely deposited (see **Figure 8.10**). Amyloid takes up Congo Red dye very readily and shows apple-green birefringence under polarized light.

Other investigations in AL amyloid should include serum and urine protein electrophoresis for a paraprotein and/or free light chains (more commonly λ than κ). Bone marrow biopsy may be necessary (one in ten patients will have myeloma). Urine protein estimation is important to assess renal involvement. Early involvement of expert haematologists is vital.

ATTR amyloid may be restricted to the heart and historically myocardial biopsy was often necessary to make the diagnosis. The emergence of ^{99m}Tc-DPD (^{99m}-technetium-3,3-diphosphono-1,2-propanodicarboxylic acid) scintigraphy now permits the non-invasive diagnosis of cardiac ATTR amyloidosis with remarkable sensitivity, limiting the need for proof from myocardial histology.[75]

Treatment

The prognosis in AL amyloid is bleak, death within two years being usual.[76]

The presence of heart failure reduces median survival to months.[77] Cardiac involvement in amyloidosis is not treatable specifically. The heart failure syndrome itself is treated symptomatically with diuretics, but there is no evidence to suggest that other therapy helps. Patients are particularly prone to develop hypotension with

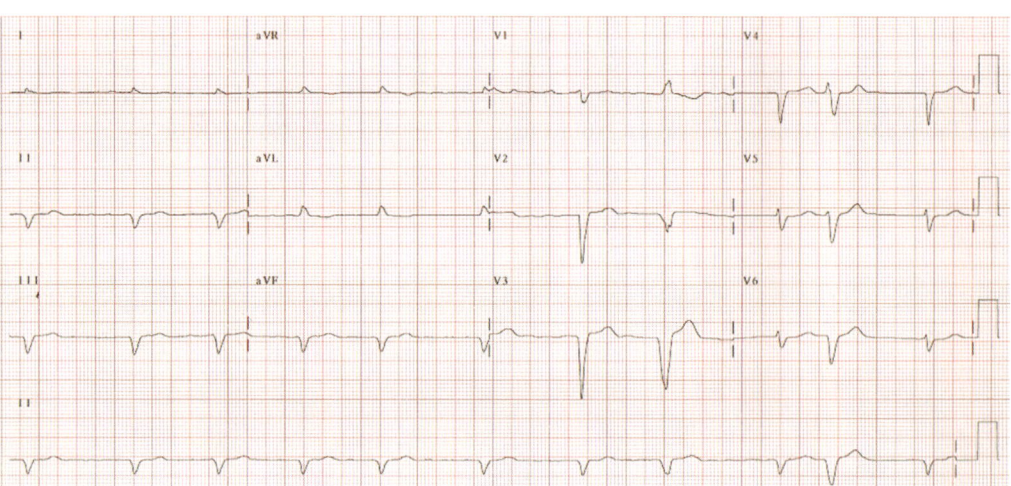

Figure 8.7 Twelve-lead ECG in patient with light-chain amyloidosis, showing atrial fibrillation, left axis deviation, and broad low-voltage complexes.

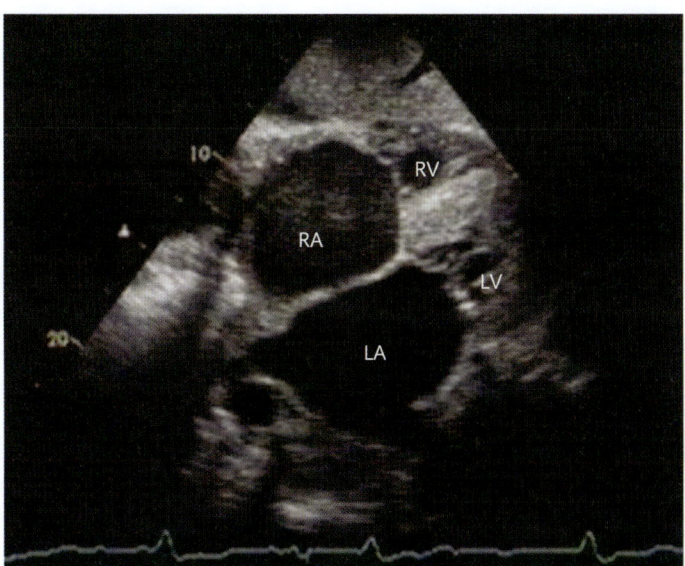

Figure 8.8 Subcostal echocardiographic view of the heart in the same patient as in Figure 8.6. Note the greatly dilated atria and relatively small, apparently hypertrophied ventricles. The interatrial septum is thickened.

standard treatment, perhaps in part due to autonomic and small-vessel involvement, and administration by default of the usual pharmacotherapeutic options for LVSD is not advised. It is suggested that digoxin should be used with caution as it binds avidly to amyloid protein. It may help control heart rate in some patients. Similarly, non-dihydropyridine calcium channel blockers bind avidly to amyloid fibrils and are contraindicated due to the risk of syncope and severe hypotension. Anticoagulation is recommended in all patients with atrial fibrillation and cardiac amyloidosis: the need to calculate the risk of thromboembolic events with the CHA_2DS_2-VASc score does not apply in these patients. The role for an ICD in patients with amyloidosis is controversial, driven by a paucity of evidence in parallel with a high incidence of sudden death.[78]

Any successful treatment is aimed at the underlying cause—a plasma cell dyscrasia—and high-dose chemotherapy with or without subsequent autologous bone marrow transplant can in some cases be successful.[79] These treatment strategies are toxic and only around half of patients may be suitable. Toxicity seems to be

worse in patients with cardiac involvement. Chemotherapeutic and immunomodulatory strategies include bortezomib-based regimens, thalidomide-like drugs, and monoclonal antibody therapies. Doxycycline—the tetracycline antibiotic—is also increasingly administered due to its effect in inhibiting the matrix metalloproteinases that dysregulate the cardiac extracellular matrix in amyloidosis. The addition of doxycycline to standard chemotherapy regimens was associated with greater survival and a threefold increase in cardiac response to therapy in one retrospective study of cardiac light chain amyloidosis.[80] Prospective efficacy data are being sought.

Treatment of the underlying clonal plasma cell disorder may not successfully restore organ function, and, for a very few patients, chemotherapy followed by bone marrow transplant and then heart transplant may be appropriate.

An intriguing possibility exploits the fact that SAP is always involved in amyloid formation. There is some evidence that clearing circulating SAP from the blood can in turn reduce SAP in tissue deposits, exposing the amyloid itself to proteolysis.[81]

Patients with transthyretin amyloidosis, although clinically very similar to patients with AL amyloidosis, have a much better prognosis.[82] ATTR is much more common than once thought. The treatment of cardiac amyloidosis secondary to ATTR has evolved rapidly over recent years, with most emerging therapies broadly classed into transthyretin tetramer stabilizers and synthesis inhibitors. The most important development has been the tetramer stabilizer tafamidis, which binds to the thyroxine site of TTR, slowing dissociation of TTR tetramers into pathogenic monomers and thus inhibiting amyloid fibril aggregation. In the Transthyretin Amyloidosis Cardiomyopathy Clinical Trial (ATTR-ACT), randomization to tafamidis was associated with a reduction in all-cause mortality and cardiovascular readmission, as well as markers of better quality of life, in patients with cardiomyopathy due to ATTRm or ATTRwt.[83] In May 2019, tafamidis was the first drug to receive US Food and Drug Administration approval for the treatment of both ATTRm and ATTRwt. Other transthyretin tetramer stabilizers include the non-steroidal anti-inflammatory drug diflunisal, the small-molecule transthyretin ligand AG-10, and the catechol-methyltransferase inhibitor tolcapone. None has high-level evidence of treatment efficacy to match tafamidis at the time of writing, although all are under active investigation. The most clinically relevant transthyretin synthesis inhibitor is patisiran, an interfering RNA which inhibits

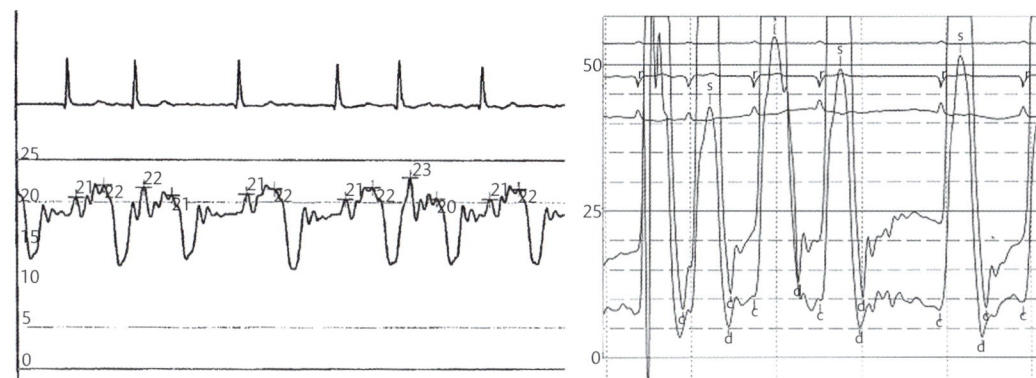

Figure 8.9 Pressure trace from the right atrium (*left*) showing raised mean atrial pressure and a striking y-descent. The patient is in atrial fibrillation. Simultaneous pressure traces from left and right ventricles (*right*). The diastolic pressures are widely separated, but show the features of restrictive filling. There is pulmonary hypertension.

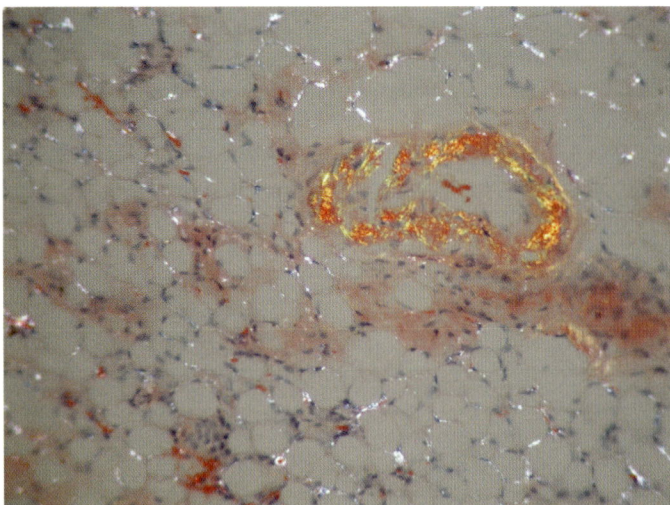

Figure 8.10 Amyloid detected as apple-green birefringence on a pleural biopsy specimen. The biopsy had been taken as part of a diagnostic work-up for pleural effusion about two years prior to presentation with a restrictive cardiomyopathy.

expression of both ATTRm and ATTRwt. Patisiran significantly improves neuropathy and quality of life in ATTR amyloidosis and ameliorates natriuretic peptide concentrations and echocardiographic markers of cardiac structure and function in patients with cardiac involvement.[84,85] Inotersen–another transthyretin synthesis inhibitor–improves the course of neurological disease and quality of life in patients with ATTR.[86]

ATTRwt amyloidosis tends to be a disease of elderly men, making transplantation inappropriate for most. In this form of the disease, conduction system disturbance is common, and permanent pacing may be needed. In some forms of familial disease, liver transplantation may be successful by removing the source of abnormal protein.

REFERENCES

1. Mahrholdt H, Wagner A, Deluigi CC, *et al*. Presentation, patterns of myocardial damage, and clinical course of viral myocarditis. *Circulation* 2006;**114**:1581–90.
2. Kühl U, Pauschinger M, Noutsias M, *et al*. High prevalence of viral genomes and multiple viral infections in the myocardium of adults with 'idiopathic' left ventricular dysfunction. *Circulation* 2005;**111**:887–93.
3. Kindermann I, Kindermann M, Kandolf R, *et al*. Predictors of outcome in patients with suspected myocarditis. *Circulation* 2008;**118**:639–48.
4. Kindermann I, Barth C, Mahfoud F, *et al*. Update on myocarditis. *J Am Coll Card* 2012;**59**(9):779–92.
5. Caforio ALP, Pankuweit S, Arbustini E, *et al*. Current state of knowledge on aetiology, diagnosis, management, and therapy of myocarditis: a position statement of the European Society of Cardiology Working Group on Myocardial and Pericardial Diseases. *Eur Heart J* 2013;**34**:2636–48.
6. Lieberman EB, Hutchins GM, Herskowitz A, Rose NR, Baughman KL. *J Am Coll Cardiol* 1991;**18**:1617–26.
7. Hare JM, Baughman KL. Fulminant and acute lymphocytic myocarditis: the prognostic value of clinicopathological classification. *Eur Heart J* 2001;**22**:269–70.
8. McCarthy RE III, Boehmer JP, Hruban RH, *et al*. Long-term outcome of fulminant myocarditis as compared with acute (nonfulminant) myocarditis. *N Engl J Med* 2000;**342**:690–5.
9. Hufnagel G, Pankuweit S, Richter A, Schönian U, Maisch B. The European Study of Epidemiology and Treatment of Cardiac Inflammatory Diseases (ESETCID): first epidemiological results. *Herz* 2000;**25**:279–85.
10. McCully RB, Cooper LT, Schreiter S. Coronary artery spasm in lymphocytic myocarditis: a rare cause of acute myocardial infarction. *Heart* 2005;**91**:202.
11. Magnani JW, Dec GW. Myocarditis: current trends in diagnosis and treatment. *Circulation* 2006;**113**:876–90.
12. Smith SC, Ladenson JH, Mason JW, Jaffe AS. Elevations of cardiac troponin I associated with myocarditis: experimental and clinical correlates. *Circulation* 1997;**95**:163–8.
13. Lauer B, Niederau C, Kühl U, *et al*. Cardiac troponin T in patients with clinically suspected myocarditis. *J Am Coll Cardiol* 1997;**30**:1354–9.
14. Morgera T, Di Lenarda A, Dreas L, *et al*. Electrocardiography of myocarditis revisited: clinical and prognostic significance of electrocardiographic changes. *Am Heart J* 1992;**124**:455–67.
15. Felker GM, Boehmer JP, Hruban RH, *et al*. Echocardiographic findings in fulminant and acute myocarditis. *J Am Coll Cardiol* 2000;**36**:227–32.
16. Mendes LA, Dec GW, Picard MH, *et al*. Right ventricular dysfunction: an independent predictor of adverse outcome in patients with myocarditis. *Am Heart J* 1994;**128**:301–7.
17. Cooper LT, Baughman KL, Feldman AM, *et al*. The role of endomyocardial biopsy in the management of cardiovascular disease: a scientific statement from the American Heart Association, the American College of Cardiology, and the European Society of Cardiology. *Circulation* 2007;**116**:2216–33.
18. Aretz HT, Billingham ME, Edwards WD, *et al*. Myocarditis: a histopathologic definition and classification. *Am J Cardiovasc Pathol* 1987;**1**:3–14.
19. Baughman KL. Diagnosis of myocarditis. Death of the Dallas Criteria. *Circulation* 2006;**113**:593–5.
20. Ponikowski P, Voors AA, Anker SD, *et al*. 2016 ESC Guidelines for the diagnosis and treatment of acute and chronic heart failure: the Task Force for the diagnosis and treatment of acute and chronic heart failure of the European Society of Cardiology (ESC). Developed with the special contribution of the Heart Failure Association (HFA) of the ESC. *Eur J Heart Fail* 2016;**18**(8):891–975.
21. Topkara VK, Dang NC, Barili F, *et al*. Ventricular assist device use for the treatment of acute viral myocarditis. *J Thorac Cardiovasc Surg* 2006;**131**:1190–1.
22. Moloney ED, Egan JJ, Kelly P, Wood AE, Cooper LT Jr. Transplantation for myocarditis: a controversy revisited. *J Heart Lung Transplant* 2005;**24**:1103–10.
23. Priori SG, Blomstrom-Lundqvist C, Mazzanti A, *et al*. 2015 ESC Guidelines for the management of patients with ventricular arrhythmias and the prevention of sudden cardiac death. The Task Force for the Management of Patients with Ventricular Arrhythmias and the Prevention of Sudden Cardiac Death of the European Society of Cardiology (ESC). *Eur Heart J* 2015;**36**(41):2757–9.
24. Wojnicz R, Nowalany-Kozielska E, Wojciechowska C, *et al*. Randomized, placebo-controlled study for immunosuppressive treatment of inflammatory dilated cardiomyopathy: two-year follow-up results. *Circulation* 2001;**104**:39–45.

25. Parrillo JE, Cunnion RE, Epstein SE, *et al*. A prospective, randomized, controlled trial of prednisone for dilated cardiomyopathy. *N Engl J Med* 1989;**321**:1061–8.

26. Coyne CB, Bergelson JM. Virus-induced Abl and Fyn kinase signals permit coxsackie virus entry through epithelial tight junctions. *Cell* 2006;**124**:119–31.

27. Fairweather D, Frisancho-Kiss S, Rose NR. Viruses as adjuvants for autoimmunity: evidence from Coxsackie virus-induced myocarditis. *Rev Med Virol* 2005;**15**:17–27.

28. Kühl, U, Pauschinger M, Seeberg B, *et al*. Viral persistence in the myocardium is associated with progressive cardiac dysfunction. *Circulation* 2005;**112**:1965–70.

29. Mason JW, O'Connell JB, Herkowitz A, *et al*. A clinical trial of immunosuppressive therapy for myocarditis. The Myocarditis Treatment Trial Investigators. *N Engl J Med* 1995;**333**:269–75.

30. Inciardi RM, Lupi L, Zaccone G, *et al*. Cardiac involvement in a patient with coronavirus disease 2019 (COVID-19). *JAMA Cardiol* 2020;**5**(7):819–24.

31. Sala S, Peretto G, Gramegna M, *et al*. Acute myocarditis presenting as a reverse Tako-Tsubo syndrome in a patient with SARS-CoV-2 respiratory infection. *Eur Heart J* 2020;**41**:1861–2.

32. Cooper LT Jr, Berry GJ, Shabetai R. Idiopathic giant-cell myocarditis—natural history and treatment. *N Engl J Med* 1997;**336**:1860–6.

33. Blauwet LA, Cooper LT. Idiopathic giant cell myocarditis and cardiac sarcoidosis. *Heart Fail Rev* 2013;**18**:733–46.

34. d'Arminio Monforte A, Sabin CA, Phillips A, *et al*. The changing incidence of AIDS events in patients receiving highly active antiretroviral therapy. *Arch Intern Med* 2005;**165**:416–23.

35. Pugliese A, Isnardi D, Saini A, *et al*. Impact of highly active antiretroviral therapy in HIV-positive patients with cardiac involvement. *J Infect* 2000;**40**:282–4.

36. Chen F, Shannon K, Ding S, *et al*. HIV type 1 glycoprotein 120 inhibits cardiac myocyte contraction. *AIDS Res Hum Retroviruses* 2002;**18**:777–84.

37. Sudano I, Spieker LE, Noll G, Corti R, Weber R, Luscher TF. Cardiovascular disease in HIV infection. *Am Heart J* 2006;**151**:1147–55.

38. Barbaro G, Di Lorenzo G, Grisorio B, Barbarini G. Incidence of dilated cardiomyopathy and detection of HIV in myocardial cells of HIV-positive patients. Gruppo Italiano per lo Studio Cardiologico dei Pazienti Affetti da AIDS. *N Engl J Med* 1998;**339**:1093–9.

39. Drazen JM, Curfman GD. Retraction: Barbaro, *et al*. Incidence of dilated cardiomyopathy and detection of HIV in myocardial cells of HIV-positive patients. *N Engl J Med* 1998;**339**:1093–9. *N Engl J Med* 2002;**347**:140.

40. Friis-Moller N, Weber R, Reiss P, *et al*. Cardiovascular disease risk factors in HIV patients—association with antiretroviral therapy. Results from the DAD study. *AIDS* 2003;**17**:1179–93.

41. Hulgan T, Sterling TR, Daugherty J, *et al*. Prescribing of contraindicated protease inhibitor and statin combinations among HIV infected persons. *J Acquir Immune Defic Syndr* 2005;**38**:277–82.

42. Sekigawa I, Koshino K, Hishikawa T, *et al*. Inhibitory effect of the immunosuppressant FK506 on apoptotic cell death induced by HIV-1 gp120. *J Clin Immunol* 1995;**15**:312–17.

43. Rassi A Jr, Rassi A, Little WC, *et al*. Development and validation of a risk score for predicting death in Chagas' heart disease. *N Engl J Med* 2006;**355**:799–808.

44. Bern C. Chagas' disease. *N Eng J Med* 2015;**373**(5):456–66.

45. Morillo CA, Marin-Neto JA, Avezum A, *et al*. for the BENEFIT Investigators. Randomized trial of benznidazole for chronic Chagas' cardiomyopathy. *N Engl J Med* 2015;**373**:1295–1306.

46. McAlister HF, Klementowicz PT, Andrews C, *et al*. Lyme carditis: an important cause of reversible heart block. *Ann Intern Med* 1989;**110**:339–45.

47. Scheffold N, Herkommer B, Kandolf R, *et al*. Lyme carditis—diagnosis, treatment and prognosis. *Dtsch Arztebl Int* 2015;**112**(12):202–8.

48. Seward JB, Casaclang-Verzosa G. Infiltrative cardiovascular diseases: cardiomyopathies that look alike. *J Am Coll Cardiol* 2010;**55**:1769–79.

49. Yazaki Y, Isobe M, Hiramitsu S, *et al*. Comparison of clinical features and prognosis of cardiac sarcoidosis and idiopathic dilated cardiomyopathy. *Am J Cardiol* 1998;**82**:537–40.

50. Birnie DH, Sauer WH, Bogun F, *et al*. HRS expert consensus statement on the diagnosis and management of arrhythmias associated with cardiac sarcoidosis. *Heart Rhythm* 2014;**11**:1305–23.

51. Doughan AR, Williams BR. Cardiac sarcoidosis. *Heart* 2006;**92**:282–8.

52. Smedema JP, Snoep G, van Kroonenburgh MP, *et al*. Evaluation of the accuracy of gadolinium-enhanced cardiovascular magnetic resonance in the diagnosis of cardiac sarcoidosis. *J Am Coll Cardiol* 2005;**45**:1683–90.

53. Birnie DH, Kandolin R, Nery PB, *et al*. Cardiac manifestations of sarcoidosis: diagnosis and management. *Eur Heart J* 2016; doi:10.1093/eurheartj/ehw328.

54. Gujja P, Rosing DR, Tripodi DJ et al. Iron overload cardiomyopathy, better understanding of an increasing disorder. *J Am Coll Cardiol* 2010;**56**(13):1001–12.

55. Hoffbrand AV. Diagnosing myocardial iron overload. *Eur Heart J* 2001;**22**:2140–1.

56. Masci PG, Dymarkowski S, Bogaert J. The role of cardiovascular magnetic resonance in the diagnosis and management of cardiomyopathies. *J Cardiovasc Med* 2008;**9**:435–49.

57. Alexander J, Kowdley KV. Hereditary hemochromatosis: genetics, pathogenesis, and clinical management. *Ann Hepatol* 2005;**4**:240–7.

58. Hoffman GS, Kerr GS, Leavitt RY, *et al*. Wegener granulomatosis: an analysis of 158 patients. *Ann Intern Med* 1992;**116**:488–98.

59. Oliveira GH, Seward JB, Tsang TS, Specks U. Echocardiographic findings in patients with Wegener granulomatosis. *Mayo Clin Proc* 2005;**80**:1435–40.

60. Edwards NC, Ferro CJ, Townend JN, Steeds RP. Myocardial disease in systemic vasculitis and autoimmune disease detected by cardiovascular magnetic resonance. *Rheumatology* 2007;**46**:1208–9.

61. Seo P, Min YI, Holbrook JT, *et al*. Damage caused by Wegener's granulomatosis and its treatment: prospective data from the Wegener's Granulomatosis Etanercept Trial (WGET). *Arthritis Rheum* 2005;**52**:2168–78.

62. Mocumbi AO, Ferreira MB, Sidi D, *et al*. A population study of endomyocardial fibrosis in a rural area of Mozambique. *N Engl J Med* 2008;**359**(1):43–9.

63. Cathcart ES, Shirahama T, Cohen AS. Isolation and identification of a plasma component of amyloid. *Biochim Biophys Acta* 1967;**147**:392–393.

64. Tennent GA, Lovat LB, Pepys MB. Serum amyloid P component prevents proteolysis of the amyloid fibrils of Alzheimer

disease and systemic amyloidosis. *Proc Natl Acad Sci USA* 1995;**92**:4299–4303.

65. Al Suwaidi J, Velianou JL, Gertz MA, *et al.* Systemic amyloidosis presenting with angina pectoris. *Ann Intern Med* 1999;**131**:838–41.

66. Liao R, Jain M, Teller P, *et al.* Infusion of light chains from patients with cardiac amyloidosis causes diastolic dysfunction in isolated mouse hearts. *Circulation* 2001;**104**:1594–7.

67. Brenner DA, Jain M, Pimentel DR, *et al.* Human amyloidogenic light chains directly impair cardiomyocyte function through an increase in cellular oxidant stress. *Circ Res* 2004;**94**:1008–10.

68. Reisinger J, Dubrey SW, Lavalley M, *et al.* Electrophysiologic abnormalities in AL (primary) amyloidosis with cardiac involvement. *J Am Coll Cardiol* 1997;**30**:1046–51.

69. Dubrey SW, Cha K, Skinner M, *et al.* Familial and primary (AL) cardiac amyloidosis: echocardiographically similar diseases with distinctly different clinical outcomes. *Heart* 1997;**78**:74–82.

70. Dubrey S, Pollak A, Skinner M, *et al.* Atrial thrombi occurring during sinus rhythm in cardiac amyloidosis: evidence for atrial electromechanical dissociation. *Br Heart J* 1995;**74**:541–4.

71. Hawkins PN, Pepys MB. Imaging amyloidosis with radiolabelled SAP. *Eur J Nucl Med* 1995;**22**:595–9.

72. Hazenberg BP, van Rijswijk MH, Piers DA, *et al.* Diagnostic performance of 123I-labeled serum amyloid P component scintigraphy in patients with amyloidosis. *Am J Med* 2006;**119**:355.e15–355.e24.

73. Maceira AM, Joshi J, Prasad SK, *et al.* Cardiovascular magnetic resonance in cardiac amyloidosis. *Circulation* 2005;**111**:195–202.

74. Arbustini E, Verga L, Concardi M, *et al.* Electron and immuno-electron microscopy of abdominal fat identifies and characterizes amyloid fibrils in suspected cardiac amyloidosis. *Amyloid* 2002;**9**:108–14.

75. Gillmore J, Maurer MS, Falk RH, *et al.* Nonbiopsy diagnosis of cardiac transthyretin amyloidosis. *Circulation* 2016;**133**:2404–12.

76. Kyle RA, Gertz MA, Greipp PR, *et al.* A trial of three regimens for primary amyloidosis: colchicine alone, melphalan and prednisone, and melphalan, prednisone, and colchicine. *N Engl J Med* 1997;**336**:1202–7.

77. Kyle RA, Gertz MA. Primary systemic amyloidosis: clinical and laboratory features in 474 cases. *Semin Hematol* 1995;**32**:45–59.

78. Kristen AV, Dengler TJ, Hegenbart U, *et al.* Prophylactic implantation of cardioverter-defibrillator in patients with severe cardiac amyloidosis and high risk for sudden cardiac death. *Heart Rhythm* 2008;**5**:235–40.

79. Dember LM, Sanchorawala V, Seldin DC, *et al.* Effect of dose-intensive intravenous melphalan and autologous blood stem-cell transplantation on AL amyloidosis-associated renal disease. *Ann Intern Med* 2001;**134**:746–53.

80. Wechalekar A, Whelan C. Encouraging impact of doxycycline on early mortality in cardiac light chain (AL) amyloidosis. *Blood Cancer J* **2017**;7(3):e546.

81. Pepys MB, Herbert J, Hutchinson WL, *et al.* Targeted pharmacological depletion of serum amyloid P component for treatment of human amyloidosis. *Nature* 2002;**417**:254–9.

82. Grogan M, Gertz MA, Kyle RA, Tajik AJ. Five or more years of survival in patients with primary systemic amyloidosis and biopsy-proven cardiac involvement. *Am J Cardiol* 2000;**85**:664–5.

83. Maurer MS, Schwartz JH, Gundapaneni B. Tafamidis treatment for patients with transthyretin amyloid cardiomyopathy. *N Engl J Med* 2018;**379**:1007–16.

84. Adams D, Gonzalez-Duarte A, O'Riordan WD, *et al.* Patisiran, an RNAi therapeutic, for hereditary transthyretin amyloidosis. *New Engl J Med* 2018;**379**(1):11–21.

85. Solomon SD, Adams D, Kristen A, *et al.* Effects of patisiran, an RNA interference therapeutic, on cardiac parameters in patients with hereditary transthyretin-mediated amyloidosis. *Circulation* 2019;**139**(4):431–43.

86. Benson MD, Waddington-Cruz M, Berk JL, *et al.* Treatment for patients with hereditary transthyretin amyloidosis. *N Engl J Med* 2018;**379**:22–31.

9

Amyloidosis

Carol J. Whelan

Introduction

Amyloidosis is a clinical disorder caused by extracellular deposition of insoluble abnormal fibrils, derived from aggregation of misfolded, normally soluble, protein. Systemic amyloidosis, with amyloid deposits in the viscera, blood vessel walls, and connective tissue, is usually fatal and is the cause of around one per 1000 deaths in developed countries.[1] Patients may present to almost any specialty, as a result of the variable involvement of organs and tissues, and diagnosis is frequently delayed.[2–4] Cardiac involvement is a leading cause of morbidity and mortality, especially in primary light chain (AL) amyloidosis and in both wild-type and hereditary transthyretin amyloidosis (ATTR). The heart is also occasionally involved in acquired AA amyloidosis and other rare hereditary types. The clinical phenotype varies greatly between different types of amyloidosis, and even the cardiac presentation has a great spectrum. Not all types of amyloid affect the heart. In this chapter, therefore, we concentrate on systemic AL and TTR amyloidosis where cardiac involvement is common. Outcomes have improved in recent years in AL amyloidosis with developments in diagnosis, investigations and treatment. Several novel therapies are on the horizon for various types of amyloidosis, including antibody-based therapy and silencing RNA treatment. However, in patients presenting with advanced organ involvement, management is a challenge with almost a third of all AL amyloidosis patients dying within a few months of diagnosis.[5] Early diagnosis of amyloidosis remains an elusive goal and requires education of both physicians and patients.

Classification

Amyloidosis is classified according to the amyloid fibril precursor protein. More than 30 different amyloid-forming precursor proteins have been identified. They share a pathognomonic structure although they are associated with clinically distinct conditions.[1]

The fibril protein is always designated protein A plus a suffix. The suffix is an abbreviation of the precursor protein. As examples, the fibril protein AL is derived from immunoglobulin light (L) chains and the fibril protein ATTR is derived from the precursor protein transthyretin (TTR). The fibril protein AA is derived from the acute-phase amyloid protein serum AA (SAA). This biochemical nomenclature also allows more detailed designations. For example, specific mutations can be mentioned in the name. ATTR V122I is the name of the mutant amyloid fibril protein of transthyretin origin where the normal valine residue at position 122 has been substituted with isoleucine.[6]

Pathophysiology

The process of amyloidogenesis involves substantial unfolding of the native protein structure and aberrant misfolding into an alternative highly ordered aggregated form with a predominant β-sheet fold. Under light microscopy, all types of amyloid appear in tissue sections as homogeneous amorphous eosinophilic material that stains with Congo Red dye to produce characteristic apple-green birefringence when viewed under cross-polarized filters. Under electron microscopy, amyloid appears as a meshwork of randomly dispersed non-branching fibrils of around 7–10 nm diameter and indeterminate length.[7]

All amyloid deposits contain several minor non-fibrillary components, including glycosaminoglycans (GAGs) and serum amyloid P component (SAP).[8] Their presence provides the basis for specific imaging (SAP scintigraphy) and novel therapeutic approaches targeting GAGs[9] or amyloid-associated SAP.[10]

Confirmation of the type of amyloid is crucial as this will guide therapy. Immunohistochemical staining (the most commonly used method) using a panel of antifibril protein antibodies enables, in most cases, determination of amyloid type.[11] Its diagnostic value is very high in AA amyloidosis and to a lesser extent in ATTR amyloidosis, but in AL amyloidosis the results are often not definitive. The proteomic method of mass spectrometric analysis of amyloidotic material has recently been described as the new reference standard for fibril typing. This involves laser microdissection using a laser capture microscope of Congo Red-stained deposits from a fixed tissue section. Computer algorithms then match the peptides to a protein reference database.[5]

Amyloid accumulates in the extracellular space, progressively disrupting the structure and function of the organ affected, ultimately leading to organ failure. Treatment that reduces production of

the respective amyloid precursor protein inhibits further amyloid formation and can facilitate clearance of existing deposits with potential to stabilize and even reverse organ dysfunction. If significant organ damage has already occurred, however, loss of function may be irreversible and progressive organ failure inevitable.

Epidemiology

The incidence of systemic AL amyloidosis has been estimated as three to five cases per million population based on a population study in Olmstead, Minnesota, USA, in 1992.[12] A more recent UK study indicated an incidence of about one per 100 000 population.[13] Of 5100 individuals referred to the National Amyloidosis Centre (NAC), London, over a 25-year period, 1987–2012, 68% had AL amyloidosis, 12% had AA amyloidosis, 6.6% had hereditary ATTR amyloidosis, and 3.2% had acquired (or wild-type) ATTR amyloidosis. (Others had rare hereditary types of amyloidosis such as Afib (fibrinogen A α-chain) amyloidosis.)

Of interest, patterns of referrals to the NAC over this time-period have changed substantially. Although the number of referrals with AL amyloidosis, as a proportion of the total, has remained the same, there has been a decrease in the number of patients referred with AA amyloidosis from 32% of cases during 1987–1995 to 6.8% between 2009 and 2012. This is likely to reflect an improvement in the treatment of inflammatory arthropathies with biological drugs. Referrals of patients with wild-type ATTR amyloidosis (ATTRwt) have risen from 0.2% cases in 1988–9 to 6.4% cases in 2009–12. This probably reflects increased awareness of amyloidosis and the increased use of cardiac magnetic resonance imaging to aid diagnosis. The incidence of ATTRwt remains unknown but cardiac amyloid deposits of transthyretin type have been detected at autopsy in 25% of people aged ≥80 years, suggesting that this type of amyloidosis is underdiagnosed.[14,15]

Little is known regarding the epidemiology of hereditary amyloidosis except familial amyloid polyneuropathy (ATTR-FAP)

which results from a mutation in TTR. More than 100 genetic TTR variants have been identified that enhance amyloidogenesis. Overall in Europe, ATTR-FAP occurs with a frequency of less than one in 100 000. However, the frequency of some TTR mutations is high in certain populations. The T60A variant is found in around 1% of the population of County Donegal in northwest Ireland.[16] The V30M variant has a prevalence of one in 538 in northern Portugal[17] and 4% in Sweden[18] but penetrance differs between the two countries: 80% in Portugal compared with 11% in Sweden[19] for reasons that are not clear. The V122I variant is carried by 3–4% of the African-American population and is associated with late onset familial amyloid cardiomyopathy (FAC)[20] but the disease penetrance seems to be low.[21]

Clinical features

Cardiac amyloidosis, irrespective of type, presents as a restrictive cardiomyopathy characterized by increased biventricular wall thickening with progressive diastolic and subsequently systolic biventricular dysfunction and bi-atrial dilation leading to heart failure and arrhythmias.[22]

It should be noted, however, that early cardiac amyloidosis may be difficult to detect clinically and classic 'right-sided' heart failure signs (raised jugular venous pressure, peripheral oedema, and congestive hepatomegaly) are features of advanced disease.

The two most common forms of cardiac amyloidosis are the AL and TTR types. AL amyloidosis can involve almost any organ in the body whereas hereditary TTR amyloidosis (ATTR-FAP) only involves the autonomic and peripheral nerves and the heart. ATTRwt has a predominant cardiac phenotype (although either a past medical history of, or coexistent, carpal tunnel syndrome is common) (Table 9.1).[23]

Pulmonary oedema is not common early in the disease process,[24] but pleural and pericardial effusions and atrial arrhythmias are often seen.[23,25] Presence of an atrial thrombus is common, particularly

Table 9.1 Characteristics of the commonest types of cardiac amyloidosis

Characteristic	AL	ATTRwt (SSA)	ATTR V122I	ATTR T60A	ATTR V30M
Precursor/amyloidogenic protein	Monoclonal immunoglobulin light chain	Wild-type transthyretin	Variant transthyretin	Variant transthyretin	Variant transthyretin
Average age at presentation (years)	60–70	70–80	≥60	≥60	30–40 or 50–60
Common ethnicity	Any	Caucasian	African-American	Caucasian (Irish)	Any (Portugese, Swedish, Japanese)
Frequency of cardiac involvement	40–50%	Almost all	Almost all	Detectable in up to 90%	Uncommon in early onset group
Other systemic involvement	Kidney, liver, soft tissue, nerves, spleen, gastrointestinal	Carpal tunnel, (bladder, spine)	Carpal tunnel	Nerves	Nerves
Treatment	ASCT or chemotherapy. Consider cardiac transplantation followed by ASCT in select cases	Supportive	Supportive. Cardiac transplantation in young patients	Supportive	Liver transplantation (+ cardiac transplantation) in select cases
Prognosis/median survival from diagnosis	Generally poor but variable	3–5 years	2–3 years	2.5–5.5 years	Good with liver transplantation but variable

AL, monoclonal immunoglobulin light chain amyloidosis; ATTR, transthyretin amyloidosis; ATTRwt, transthyretin associated with wild-type transthyretin formerly known as senile systemic amyloidosis (SSA); ASCT, autologous peripheral blood stem cell transplantation.

in AL amyloidosis, sometimes before atrial fibrillation occurs.[26] Thromboembolism causes transient ischaemic attacks or strokes and may be an early or even presenting feature.[27] Anticoagulation carries greater risk than usual risk due to amyloid-induced coagulopathy, gastrointestinal amyloidosis, erratic oral absorption, increased risk of falling, and intracranial vascular amyloid involvement.[28] Disproportionate ventricular septal amyloid accumulation mimicking hypertrophic cardiomyopathy with dynamic left ventricular outflow tract obstruction[29] is rare, but well documented. Syncope is common and a poor prognostic sign.[30] It is typically exertional or postprandial as part of either restrictive cardiomyopathy, sensitivity to intravascular fluid depletion from loop diuretics, combined with autonomic neuropathy, or conduction tissue involvement (atrioventricular (AV) or sinus nodes) or ventricular arrhythmia.[31] The latter may rarely cause recurrent syncope. Amyloid deposits can also obliterate the lumens of distal coronary arteries and give rise to balanced cardiac ischaemia[32] that is sufficient to cause angina or a positive stress test in up to 10% of patients. Rarely, acute coronary syndromes such as ST elevation myocardial infarction can occur.[24]

AL amyloidosis

AL amyloidosis is the most commonly diagnosed form of cardiac amyloidosis. It is associated with a B-cell dyscrasia and AL amyloid fibrils are composed of fragments of either κ or λ monoclonal immunoglobulin light chains. In 10% of patients, overt myeloma may coexist and carries a poorer prognosis.[33] These patients may have bone involvement and a history of recurrent infection.

Cardiac involvement occurs in around 50% of cases and is the leading cause of morbidity and mortality with a prognosis of six to 12 months from diagnosis. Despite advances in treatment and improvement in overall survival over time, the one-year mortality remains unchanged at approximately 45%. In a small proportion, the heart is the sole organ involved.[34] Patients may present with reduced exercise tolerance and progressive heart failure. However, since almost any organ can be involved, patients may present with a wide range of symptoms ranging from nephrotic syndrome to hepatosplenomegaly, autonomic neuropathy (postural hypotension, syncope, diarrhoea), soft tissue infiltrations (macroglossia, carpal tunnel syndrome), bleeding (e.g. cutaneous such as periorbital or gastrointestinal), and cachexia from malnutrition. This potential array of symptoms and signs can lead to delays in diagnosis as findings may be non-specific depending on the severity and nature of organ involvement. Hoarseness of the voice due to amyloid deposition on the vocal cords may be observed.

The combination of macroglossia and periorbital purpura ('panda eyes') is virtually pathognomonic of AL amyloidosis but occurs in less than a third of cases.[5] Isolated periorbital purpura can occasionally occur in other types of amyloidosis.

Patients with AL amyloidosis often have much more symptomatic heart failure than those with other types of amyloidosis such as ATTRwt despite a similar or even lesser degree of amyloid deposition in the heart. This supports in-vitro evidence of myocardial cell toxicity of the amyloidogenic light chains.[35]

Neuropathy is a recognized feature of AL amyloidosis. Amyloid peripheral neuropathy is mainly axonal and involves small and large fibres. It typically begins with loss of the small fibre-mediated sensations of heat or cold, and can be painful. It can be mistaken for the more common chronic inflammatory demyelinating polyneuropathy. Autonomic neuropathy causes impotence in men as an early symptom, syncope due to postural hypotension, and gastrointestinal disturbance, typically alternating constipation and diarrhoea.

ATTR amyloidosis

The precursor protein in TTR amyloidosis is transthyretin encoded by a gene on chromosome 18. It is a homo-tetrameric plasma protein and each monomer subunit comprises 127 amino acids. More than 100 amyloidogenic mutations have been described in the literature (www.amyloidosismutations.com). Genetic sequencing using DNA extracted from blood is performed in patients with suspected or proven ATTR amyloidosis. TTR is produced mainly in the liver but can also be found in the retina and choroid plexus. Its physiological function is to transport retinol-binding protein and thyroxine (although thyroxine-binding globulin is the main transporter for the latter).

Whereas wild-type ATTR amyloidosis is a sporadic disease among older people (typically men), hereditary ATTR amyloidosis presents from the third decade onwards and is inherited in an autosomal dominant fashion, with most patients being heterozygous for normal and variant transthyretin.[36] The genetic mutations, which mostly result in single amino acid substitutions, are thought to promote greatly the weak inherent amyloidogenic propensity of wild-type TTR through destabilizing the tetrameric protein and increasing the abundance of dissociated TTR monomers that are able to self-assemble in the abnormal (but highly ordered) alternative amyloid conformation, i.e. to form amyloid fibrils.[37]

ATTRwt amyloidosis

Wild-type transthyretin cardiac amyloidosis (formerly known as senile systemic amyloidosis or senile cardiac amyloidosis) is mainly a disease of elderly men. There is a 10-fold male predominance with the average age of presentation 70–80 years. Patients typically present with heart failure symptoms of dyspnoea and reduced exercise tolerance and 'right-sided' signs including peripheral oedema, elevated jugular venous pressure, pleural effusions, hepatomegaly (due to congestion), and ascites. In addition, the patient may describe anginal chest pain due to diffuse microvascular amyloid deposition. Atrial arrhythmias such as atrial flutter or atrial fibrillation are common and palpitations may be the presenting symptom.[23]

In most patients, the heart is the only organ affected but patients may describe carpal tunnel symptoms or indeed may have had previous surgery for carpal tunnel syndrome, sometimes many years before presentation with cardiac dysfunction.[38] Wild-type TTR amyloid deposits are found in a third of elderly people undergoing carpal tunnel decompression.[39]

A small proportion of patients present with haematuria and deposits of ATTR type are found in the bladder (3.9%).

The presence of an incidental plasma cell dyscrasia in patients with ATTRwt amyloidosis (found in a quarter of patients)[23] can complicate matters and may necessitate an endomyocardial biopsy to confirm the diagnosis.

Prognosis is much better than in patients with cardiac AL amyloidosis. Median survival is around 3–5 years.

Hereditary (variant) ATTR amyloidosis

Inheritance is autosomal dominant with variable penetrance. V30M is the commonest TTR variant worldwide. The most prevalent TTR variants in the UK population are V122I and T60A variants.

ATTR V122I amyloidosis

Three to four per cent of African-Americans carry the V122I variant. In a molecular epidemiological analysis, 66 transthyretin V122I alleles were found in DNA samples from 65 out of 1688 African-Americans.[40] The calculated allele frequency of 0.020 was similar for all geographic areas in the USA, equating to 3.9% of African-Americans (about 1.3 million) possessing the V122I allele. A subsequent study reviewing autopsy specimens supported the association with cardiac amyloidosis.[20] Penetrance, however, appears to be low with no significant difference detected in mortality over a 21-year follow-up between V122I carriers and non-carriers in one study. Although there was an increased risk of heart failure, overt cardiac abnormalities among V122I carriers was low (7%).[21]

The clinical phenotype of FAC associated with the V122I variant is very similar to ATTRwt amyloidosis. Patients usually present in their sixties. A history of carpal tunnel syndrome or atrial arrhythmia is common. In contrast to FAP associated with other TTR variants, neuropathy is rare. It is important that the diagnosis of FAC associated with the V122I variant is not overlooked in patients of African descent who present with heart failure. Often, increased left ventricular wall thickness is wrongly attributed to ethnicity or hypertension.

Large series of patients with this condition have not been described. One small US study of 11 patients suggests a more severe phenotype and a worse prognosis compared with ATTRwt amyloidosis.[41]

ATTR T60A amyloidosis

The TTR T60A variant is the commonest cause of FAP in the UK and the USA. Seven cases of FAP from seven different families originating from Donegal in the northwest of Ireland were described in 1987.[42] A further epidemiological study showed that 1.1% of this population carry the TTR T60A variant.[16] Patients typically present in their sixties.

The clinical phenotype is variable. The majority of patients have cardiac involvement with heart failure symptoms. It is the major determinant of prognosis. Median survival from diagnosis is 2.5–5.5 years. Some patients, despite having cardiac involvement, may have predominant symptoms from autonomic neuropathy with alternating diarrhoea and constipation and postural hypotension which are progressive and challenging to manage. Peripheral neuropathy is found in a quarter of patients and only a third of patients have a family history of amyloidosis.[43]

ATTR V30M amyloidosis

The TTR V30M variant is currently the commonest cause of hereditary amyloidosis in the world with Portugal, Sweden, Japan and Brazil all endemic countries. The condition was first described in 1952.[44] Of interest, the same mutation can cause a variety of phenotypes and is associated with a different age of onset depending on the geographical area of origin and whether inheritance is maternal or paternal. Early onset disease (with people in their 30s) is usually manifested by a combination of peripheral and autonomic neuropathy. These patients rarely have cardiac involvement. Late onset disease (with people presenting in their fifties or sixties) is more likely to have cardiac involvement.

Investigations

Blood and urine tests

Monoclonal whole immunoglobulin or free light chains (FLCs) are identifiable in the serum or urine of at least 95% of patients with AL amyloidosis using the most sensitive assays. Routine electrophoresis results are negative, however, in 50% cases. The lack of a measurable clone is a problem for diagnosis and for tracking response to treatment. The amount of plasma cell infiltrate identified on bone marrow biopsy is usually very modest (median: 10%).[5] In contrast to myeloma patients, there is a predominance of λ rather than κ light chain idiotype in patients with AL amyloidosis.[45]

It should also be borne in mind that incidental monoclonal gammopathy of undetermined significance (MGUS) occurs in >5% of persons aged >70 years.[46] Correct identification of ATTR amyloidosis is necessary to prevent inappropriate chemotherapy for systemic AL amyloidosis in people with a coincident MGUS. Lachmann et al. investigated 350 patients with an apparent diagnosis of AL amyloidosis and found an alternative genetic cause in 9.7%, including about 5% patients with hereditary ATTR amyloidosis.[47]

Electrocardiogram

Although small QRS complexes, particularly in the limb leads (<5 mm height), are seen on the electrocardiogram in the majority of patients with AL amyloidosis, this is not always the case for patients with TTR cardiac amyloidosis where conversely the criteria for left ventricular hypertrophy (LVH) can be met.[48] In a recent study of 64 patients with ATTR V122I amyloidosis, 44% of patients did not have low-voltage QRS complexes and in 26% of cases the ECG demonstrated LVH by standard criteria. Physicians should be made aware of this ECG finding in TTR amyloidosis, as its presence may lead to a delay in diagnosis (**Figures 9.1** and **9.2**).[49]

Conduction abnormalities are common in ATTRwt amyloidosis. First-degree AV block (10%), left bundle branch block (20%), and right bundle branch block (16%) have been reported.[23] In one study of 125 patients, 14% had a pacemaker in situ at presentation with a further 10% requiring a pacemaker during follow-up.[50] Other findings in cardiac AL amyloidosis include first-degree AV block (21%), non-specific intraventricular conduction delay (16%), second- or third-degree AV block (3%), atrial fibrillation/flutter (20%), and ventricular tachycardia (5%).[51]

A pseudoinfarct pattern and poor R wave progression is another common ECG finding, and atrial fibrillation is particularly common in wild-type ATTR, as previously mentioned.

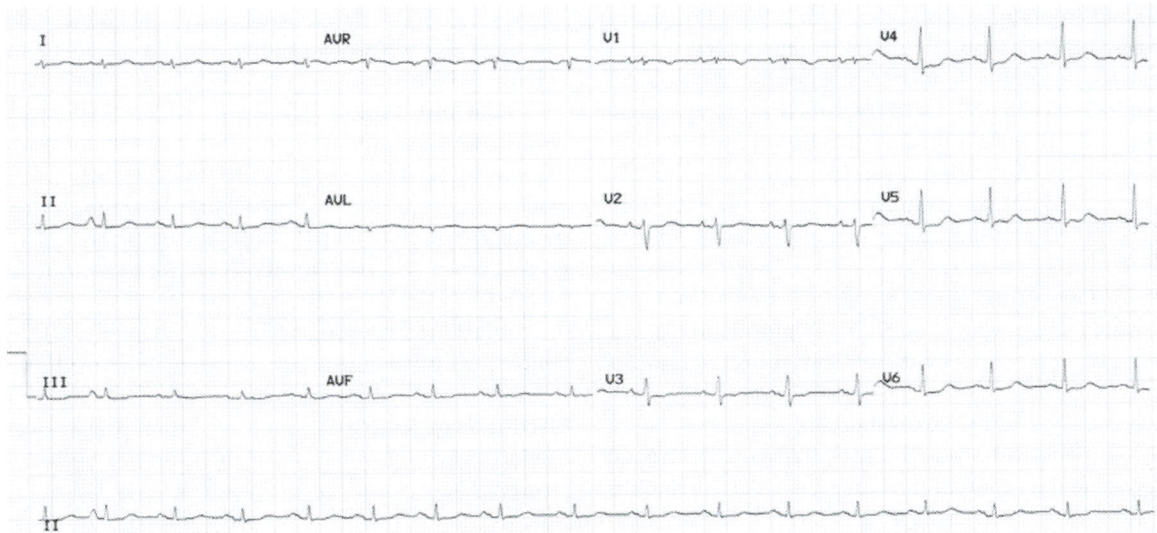

Figure 9.1 Typical ECG of patient with cardiac monoclonal immunoglobulin amyloidosis. Small QRS complexes (<5 mm) in the limb leads are evident.

Patients with advanced cardiac AL amyloidosis are at risk of developing complete heart block. In a study of 20 consecutive patients with Mayo stage III cardiac AL amyloidosis, implanted with a loop recorder for investigation of syncope or presyncope, 13 died, with a median follow-up of 300 days. In each of the eight evaluable cases, all had developed complete heart block prior to death followed by pulseless electrical activity.[52]

Cardiac catheterization

Although the diagnosis of cardiac amyloidosis may be made without invasive cardiac procedures, cardiac catheterization (**Figure 8.9**)

can play a role and shows a typical restrictive filling pattern in both ventricles with a dip-and-plateau pattern in diastole. In contrast to the pathophysiology of pericardial disease, the ventricular traces are often not identical.

Cardiac biomarkers and staging

Cardiac biomarkers may be helpful in raising the clinical suspicion of cardiac amyloidosis in a patient with known plasma cell dyscrasia and should prompt further investigation with ECG and echocardiography as initial assessment tools. The combination of elevated serum N-terminal pro B-type natriuretic peptide

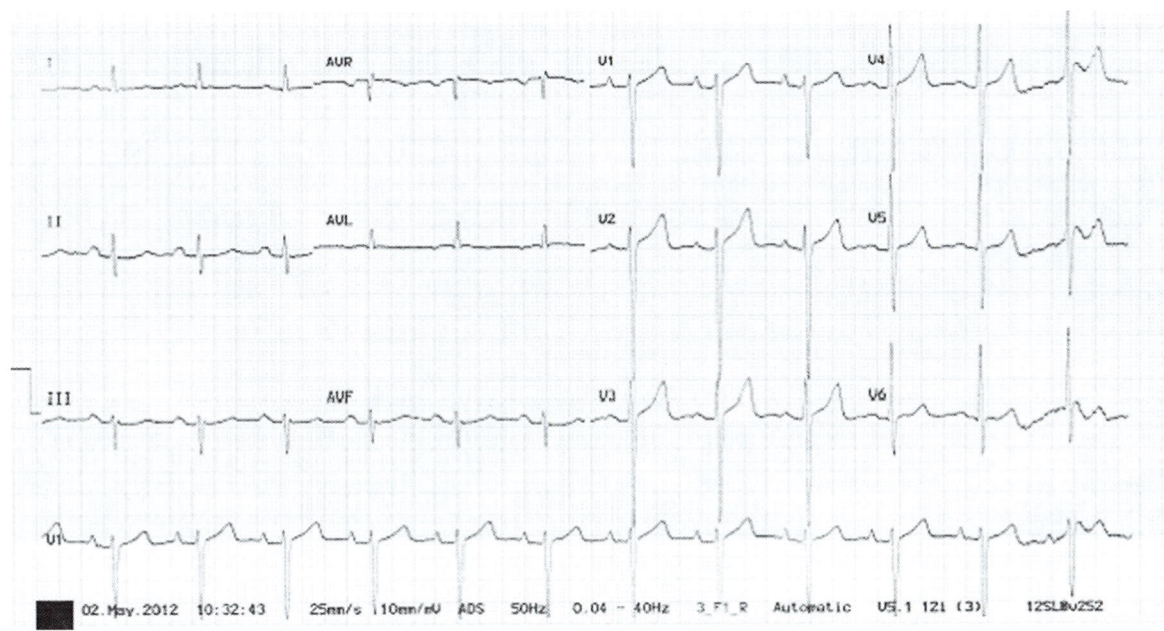

Figure 9.2 Typical ECG of patient with cardiac transthyretin amyloidosis. The voltage criteria for left ventricular hypertrophy are met.

(NT-proBNP) and troponin is associated with a poor prognosis. The Mayo staging system proposed in 2004 remains widely in clinical use:[53] stage I, with cardiac biomarkers below threshold values (cardiac troponin T <0.035 µg/L and NT-proBNP <332 ng/L) had the lowest risk of death with a median survival of 26.4 months; stage II, with either one of the biomarkers below threshold values, had a median survival of 10.5 months; and stage III, with both biomarkers above the threshold values, had a median survival of 3.5 months.

In 2012, the Mayo Clinic group produced an updated staging system which incorporated additional information about amyloidogenic FLC levels and used different cut-off values for cardiac biomarkers in order to try to better discriminate between groups.[54] More recently, a European collaborative work has analysed outcomes in 346 patients with stage III disease based on the original 2004 staging system and reported median survival of 7.1 months for patients diagnosed between 2001 and 2010.[55] Several variables are powerful clinical indicators, including poor performance status, severe postural hypotension, NYHA class ≥III, and low systolic blood pressure (BP; <100 mmHg). Patients with NT-proBNP >8500 ng/L (especially in the presence of systolic BP <100 mmHg) had median survival of 3 months in a historical series and can be called stage IIIb.[56] Patients with higher FLCs at diagnosis also have poorer outcomes.[57]

Patients with TTR cardiac amyloidosis have modestly elevated NT-proBNP with a median of 2681 ng/L and median troponin level 0.04 ng/mL in comparison to patients with AL amyloidosis (6040 ng/L and 0.05 ng/mL, respectively).[23]

Echocardiography

Echocardiography is an easily accessible investigation used to assess overall cardiac structure and function, and should be performed routinely in patients with suspected cardiac amyloidosis.[58]

There are many characteristic features of cardiac amyloidosis that can alert the ultrasonographer and physician to the diagnosis (Figure 9.3a, b).

Cardiac involvement in systemic AL amyloidosis is defined according to consensus opinion either by an endomyocardial biopsy demonstrating amyloidosis in the presence of clinical or laboratory evidence of involvement, or by echocardiographic evidence of amyloidosis (mean left ventricle wall thickness >12 mm with no other cardiac cause) in a patient with a positive result from a non-cardiac biopsy.[59]

Standard echocardiography with m-mode, 2D, pulse wave, continuous wave, and tissue Doppler may reveal all or some of the well-described abnormalities of cardiac amyloidosis such as biventricular concentric increased wall thickening, interatrial septal thickening, valve leaflet thickening, and biatrial dilatation ('owl's eye' appearance) with severely impaired diastolic ventricular function and a restrictive pattern of filling. The left ventricle (LV) and right ventricle (RV) cavities are nearly always normal or small in size and overall biventricular systolic function may be preserved. However, longitudinal function, assessed by tissue Doppler and speckle tracking, is reduced. Because the LV and RV rarely dilate, a reduced ejection fraction seen late in the disease is associated with a substantially reduced stroke volume. Pleural and pericardial effusions are common.

Rarely, in around 5% of patients with cardiac amyloidosis, left ventricular infiltration may mimic hypertrophic cardiomyopathy on the echocardiogram.[29] These patients often have normal or supranormal LV systolic function with normal voltage on the ECG.[34]

As the myocardial thickening is due to infiltration rather than hypertrophy, particularly in AL cardiac amyloidosis, the limb lead voltages decrease as the myocardium thickens, resulting in a decreased ratio of voltage to left ventricular mass. This is strongly

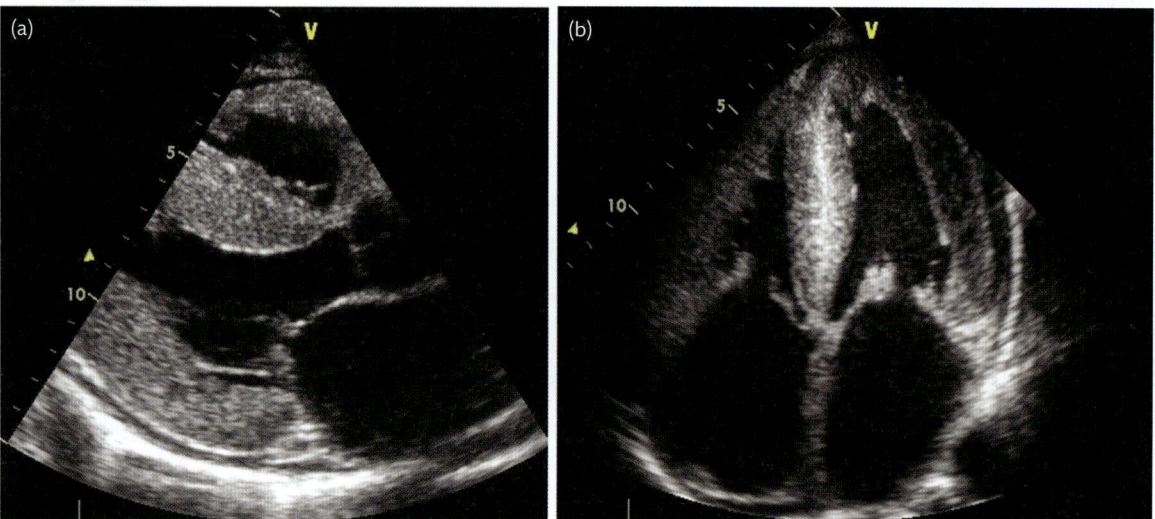

Figure 9.3 (a) Characteristic echocardiogram of patient with cardiac amyloidosis. Parasternal long-axis view. There is increased right ventricular (RV), interventricular (IVS) and left ventricular (LV) posterior wall thickness. The left atrium (LA) appears dilated and there is a small rim of pericardial fluid. (b) Characteristic echocardiogram of patient with cardiac amyloidosis. Four-chamber view. There is concentric increased left ventricular (LV) and right ventricular (RV) wall thickness, biatrial dilatation, increased thickness of the mitral and tricuspid valves and interatrial septum (IAS). A rim of pericardial fluid is evident.

suggestive of an infiltrative cardiomyopathy, of which amyloidosis is the commonest cause.[60] Usually, not all of the well-documented characteristic features are present, especially in early disease where differentiation from hypertensive disease, and other causes of increased LV wall thickness, is difficult. Partly for this reason, the diagnosis of cardiac amyloidosis is often delayed or not possible to make by standard echocardiography alone.

Myocardial strain imaging is a useful additional echocardiographic technique for cardiac amyloidosis (**Figure 9.4**).

Strain (deformation) is the percentage change in an object's dimension in comparison to the object's original dimension. Strain rate is the speed at which deformation occurs. Strain and strain rate imaging derived from tissue Doppler has been reported to be a more sensitive test than standard tissue Doppler for the detection of systolic impairment.[61] Two-dimensional (2D) speckle-tracking echocardiography uses automatic frame-by-frame tracking of natural acoustic markers in the myocardium (speckles) which move together with the tissue. It is a more reproducible technique than Doppler-derived strain imaging, and is reported to be an independent predictor of survival.[62] A 'relative apical sparing' pattern of longitudinal strain (bull's eye appearance) has been shown to be sensitive and specific for the diagnosis of cardiac amyloidosis in a study of 55 patients with cardiac amyloidosis and moderately increased LV wall thickness.[63]

Cardiac magnetic resonance imaging

Cardiac magnetic resonance (CMR) imaging is increasingly being recognized as an important tool in the evaluation of cardiac amyloidosis. Although the characteristic features of advanced cardiac amyloidosis can be diagnosed by echocardiography, these features are often not present in early disease. The ability of CMR to provide information regarding 'myocardial tissue characterization' is a major advantage over other imaging modalities. Also, CMR often provides more accurate measurements of volume, mass, and wall thickness which are of benefit in sequential assessment, for example in assessing response to treatment. The intrinsic signal (measured as the magnetic resonance parameters T1, T2, and T2*) from the myocardium without contrast agent can be used to distinguish normal from abnormal myocardium.

Alternatively, with an intravenous bolus of chelated gadolinium contrast (gadolinium diethylenetriamine penta-acetic acid (Gd-DPTA)), cardiac amyloidosis is associated with global

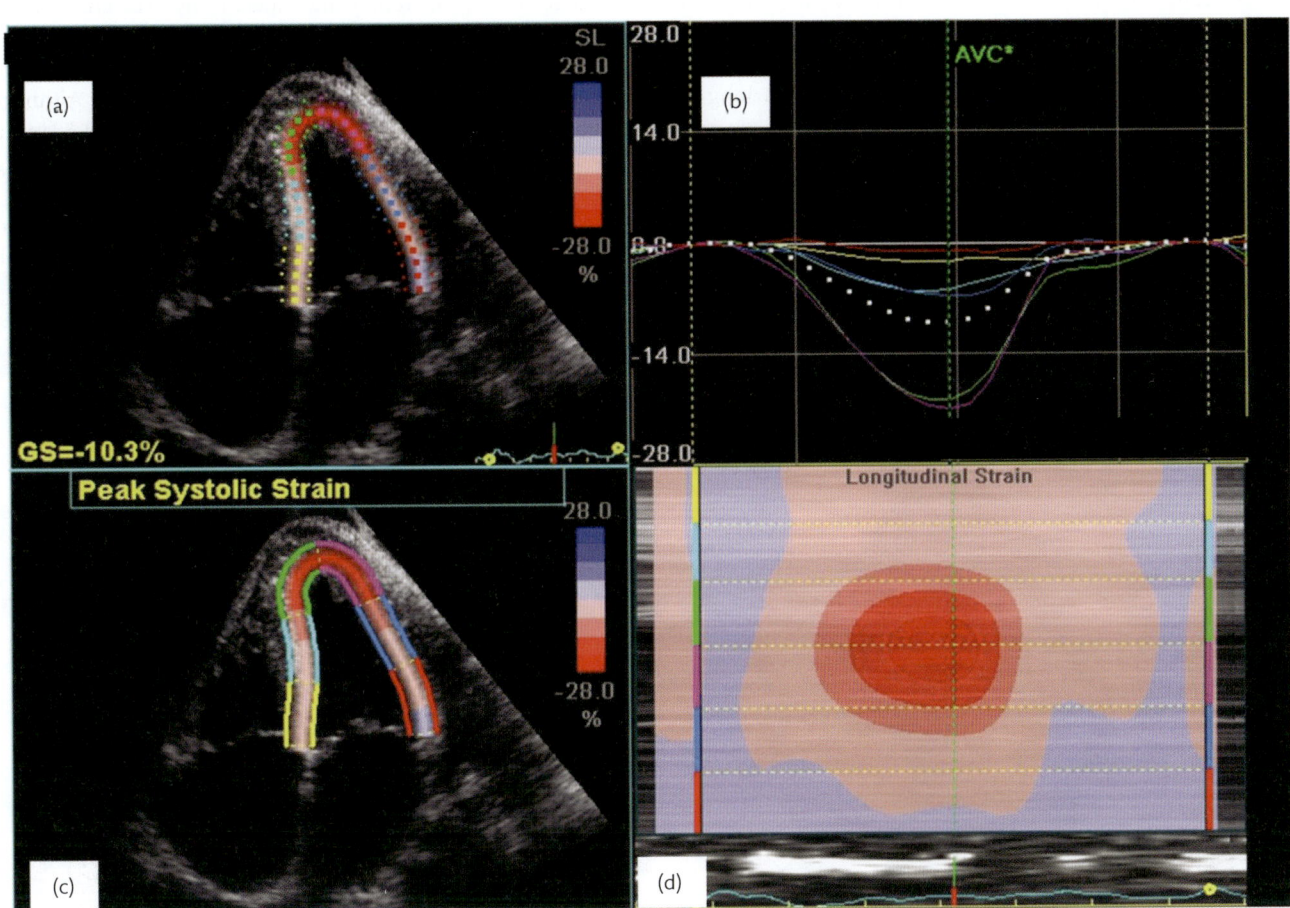

Figure 9.4 Two-dimensional strain with speckle tracking echocardiography of the left ventricle (LV) in the apical four-chamber view in a patient with cardiac amyloidosis. (a) LV segments and the GS (global longitudinal strain) is −10.3% in this case (normal: −20%). (b) Strain curves sampled in each of the LV segments, AVC (aortic valve closure). (c) Peak systolic strain for each LV segment. (d) Longitudinal strain processed as a colour map for each segment which demonstrates a longitudinal base to apex strain gradient i.e. reduced basal strain compared with apical strain giving rise to the typical 'bull's eye' appearance.

subendocardial late gadolinium enhancement (LGE) which, when 'classical', is almost pathognomonic of cardiac amyloidosis (particularly of AL type). The gadolinium accumulates in the gaps between cells with an increased volume of distribution in the 'scar' tissue or in areas of amyloid deposition (areas of interstitial expansion). This LGE can be evident even before there is increased LV or RV wall thickness and therefore potentially serves as a marker of early disease. The global LGE is in a non-coronary distribution. There is a dark blood pool resulting from similar myocardium and blood T1 values because of high myocardial uptake and fast blood washout.[64] In addition to the classical global subendocardial LGE pattern, other patterns of LGE in cardiac amyloidosis have been described. Some have found localized enhancement where others have found patchy or diffuse transmural LGE.[65] In TTR amyloidosis, there is usually RV as well as LV LGE and the pattern is often transmural.[66]

Transmural LGE has recently been described as an independent predictor of survival in cardiac amyloidosis.[67]

The use of gadolinium is relatively contraindicated in patients with severe renal impairment, (estimated glomerular filtration rate: <30 mL/min) which is quite common in patients with amyloidosis. The new T1 mapping technique in which a signal from the myocardium can be measured without contrast (native T1) may overcome the problem. The massive expansion of the extracellular compartment that occurs with amyloid can be quantified by T1 mapping: the native (non-contrast) myocardial longitudinal relaxation time of a tissue (T1: the time taken for recovery of

longitudinal magnetization), together with the post-contrast T1 and extracellular volume, are measured. Each pixel in the image is coded in colour, reflecting the absolute value of T1. Native myocardial T1 mapping measures myocardial intrinsic signal and is changed by pathology. Increases in native T1 occur in diffuse fibrosis and localized scar, but T1 is markedly elevated in the presence of cardiac amyloidosis and is helpful in differentiating increased LV wall thickness due to AL or TTR cardiac amyloidosis from other causes. The measurement of native T1 not only allows the detection of cardiac amyloidosis, but also shows promise in tracking change serially, in both cardiac AL and TTR amyloidosis.[68,69] It is therefore likely to be a helpful measurement in clinical trials of treatment for cardiac amyloidosis.

The extracellular volume (ECV) in the interstitium (which can be measured after Gd-DPTA contrast administration) is also greatly increased in cardiac amyloidosis compared with healthy subjects or other causes of increased LV wall thickness such as hypertrophic cardiomyopathy.[70,71] Both native T1 and ECV measurements predict prognosis in cardiac AL amyloidosis (**Figure 9.5**).[72]

Serum amyloid P component scintigraphy

All amyloid deposits contain serum amyloid P component (SAP), a normal plasma protein that binds specifically to all types of amyloid fibril. Radiolabelled SAP scintigraphy is a safe, non-invasive technique, developed at the NAC, which provides diagnostic images for the majority of patients with systemic amyloidosis.[73] Although the technique provides useful information regarding amyloid burden in

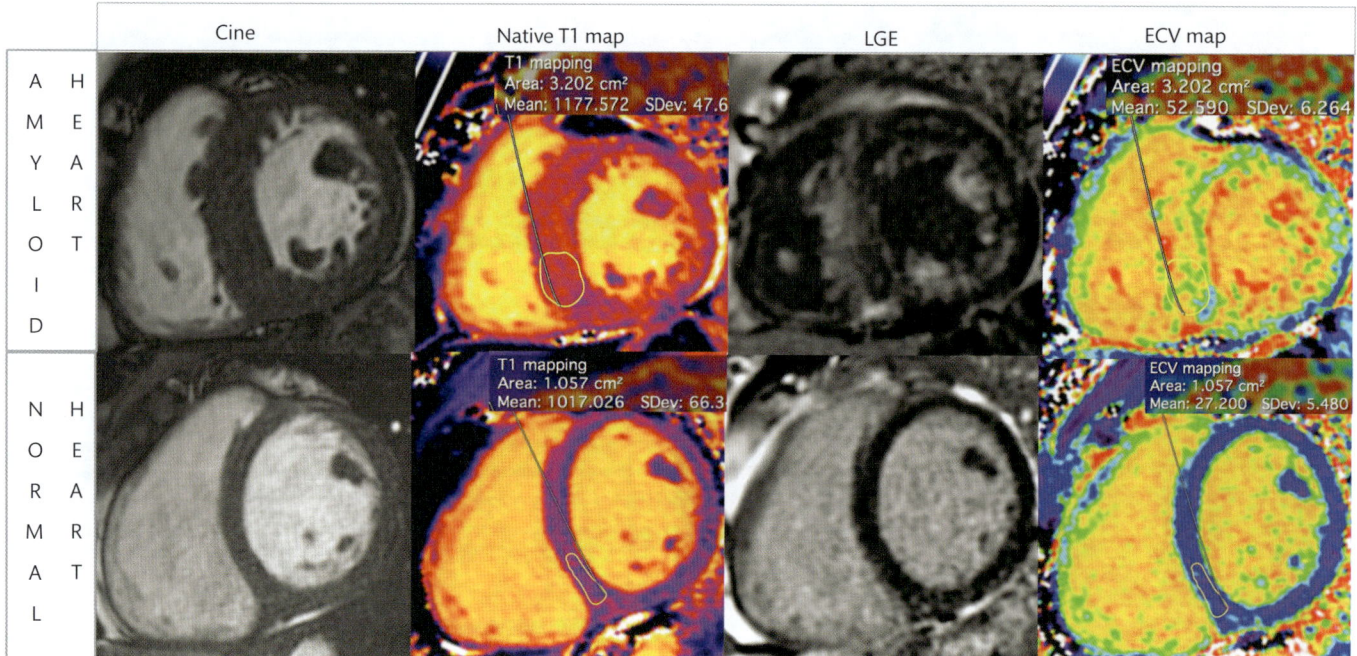

Figure 9.5 Cardiac magnetic resonance imaging of amyloid heart of transthyretin (TTR) type compared with normal heart (cross-sectional images). End-diastolic frames from cine (*left*), non-contrast (native) T1 maps (*middle left*), late gadolinium enhancement (*middle right*) and post-contrast ECV maps (*right*). In the upper panels there is increased left ventricular (LV) and right ventricular (RV) wall thickness (*left*); the native T1 value is elevated at 1177 ms (normal range: 950–1100 ms) (*middle left*); there is subendocardial LGE (*middle right*) and the extracellular volume (ECV) value (52) is elevated (normal: <35) (*right*). In the lower panels the LV and RV wall thickness is normal (*left*); the native T1 map value is normal (1017 ms) (*middle left*); there is no LGE (*middle right*) and the ECV value (27) is normal (*right*).

the liver, spleen, kidneys, bones, and adrenal glands, it cannot image amyloid burden in the heart.

99mTc-DPD scintigraphy

The bone-seeking radionuclide tracer 99m-technetium-3,3-diphosphono-1,2-propanodicarboxylic acid (^{99m}Tc-DPD) appears to localize with remarkable sensitivity in cardiac ATTR amyloid deposits.[74] The basis of the localization remains unknown. ^{99m}Tc-DPD is not available in the USA but similar results have been reported with the bone tracer ^{99m}Tc-pyrophosphate (^{99m}TcPYP).[75] Cardiac localization has been reported in a small proportion of patients with advanced systemic AL cardiac amyloidosis but the uptake is usually less than the uptake seen in ATTR cardiac amyloidosis. The results of ^{99m}Tc-DPD scintigraphy appear to be positive in all patients with clinically significant cardiac ATTR amyloidosis. The sensitivity of the techniques even allows detection of presymptomatic disease before detection by other imaging modalities (**Figure 9.6**).[76]

Histology

A biopsy of an organ in which amyloid is suspected may be required for a definitive diagnosis. If cardiac amyloidosis is suspected, then an endomyocardial biopsy may be indicated, particularly in a patient with a plasma cell dyscrasia, to differentiate between AL and ATTR types. However, due to the risk of bleeding, this should only be considered if other methods do not reveal amyloid deposits. In systemic forms of amyloidosis, microscopic deposits are very widespread. Abdominal fat aspiration is a simple, high-yield alternative method (to target organ biopsy) which can be performed in the clinic. A negative fat aspiration does not exclude amyloidosis. Rectal biopsy is another alternative with reasonable diagnostic sensitivity.[5]

Confirmation of the fibril type is crucial as this will guide therapy. Immunohistochemistry remains the most widely available method for fibril typing (**Figure 9.7**).[11]

Recently, non-biopsy guidelines have been developed for patients with ATTR cardiac amyloidosis who do not have a monoclonal gammopathy.[77] Results of bone scintigraphy (either using ^{99m}Tc-DPD or ^{99m}TcPYP) and biochemical investigations were analysed from 1217 patients with suspected cardiac amyloidosis referred for evaluation in specialist centres. Of 857 patients with histologically proven amyloid (374 with endomyocardial biopsies) and 360 patients subsequently confirmed to have non-amyloid cardiomyopathies, myocardial radiotracer uptake on bone scintigraphy was >99% sensitive and 86% specific for cardiac ATTR amyloid, with false positives almost exclusively from uptake in patients with cardiac AL amyloidosis. Importantly, the combined findings of grade 2 or 3 myocardial radiotracer uptake on bone scintigraphy and the absence of a monoclonal protein in serum or urine had a specificity and positive predictive value for cardiac ATTR amyloidosis of 100% (positive predictive value confidence interval: 98.0–100).

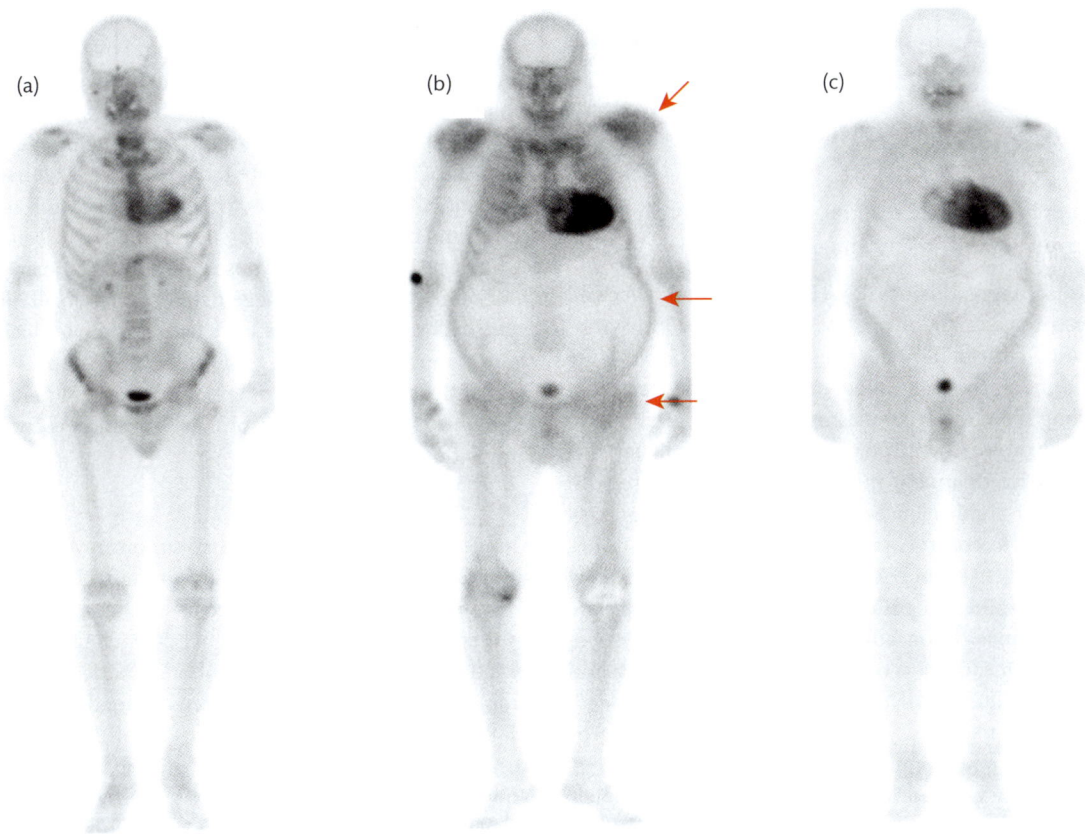

Figure 9.6 Cardiac and diffuse soft tissue uptake of ^{99m}Tc-DPD scintigraphy. (a) Patient with AL amyloidosis with grade 1 myocardial uptake and minimal uniform soft tissue deposition. (b) Grade 2 cardiac uptake in an ATTRwt patient with typical 'TTR pattern' of diffuse soft tissue uptake including deltoid, gluteal, and abdominal wall muscles (arrows). (c) Grade 3 cardiac uptake in ATTRwt patient with extensive soft tissue uptake (including abdominal wall) and no bony uptake.

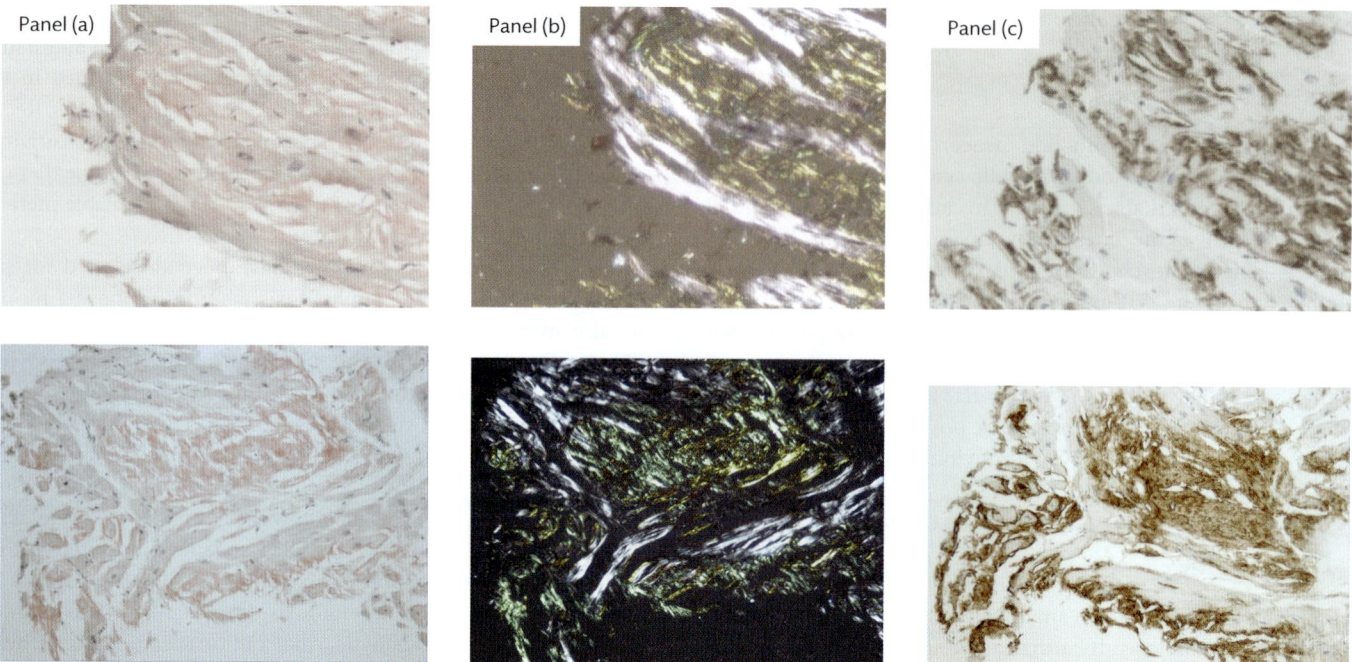

Panel (a)   Panel (b)   Panel (c)

Figure 9.7 Histology images from an endomyocardial biopsy. The presence of amyloid deposits is demonstrated throughout as a pink amorphous material when stained with Congo Red (a) with apple-green birefringence when viewed under high-intensity cross-polarized light (b). Immunohistochemical staining using monospecific antibodies reactive against transthyretin (TTR) shows the amyloid stains with antibodies against transthyretin (c), thereby confirming amyloidosis of ATTR amyloidosis.

Treatment of cardiac amyloidosis

Supportive

Treatment of all types of amyloidosis is currently based on the following principles:

- reducing the supply of amyloid forming precursor proteins;
- supporting the function of organs containing amyloid.

All types of cardiac amyloidosis (AL, ATTR (hereditary or wild type)) cause a restrictive cardiomyopathy which can lead to symptoms of heart failure. Heart failure in cardiac AL is generally rapidly progressive and difficult to treat, unless disease-specific treatment is effective in killing the underlying plasma cell clone. Heart failure in ATTRwt is usually more slowly progressive. However, all patients benefit from supportive treatment measures for heart failure with the need for meticulous fluid balance emphasized. Multidisciplinary involvement is crucial to control symptoms, maintain organ function, and manage toxic effects of treatment. Loop diuretics, usually in combination with mineralocorticoid receptor antagonists, are usually well tolerated. In addition, adherence to a daily fluid restriction of 1.5 L, daily weights to assess response to diuretic therapy, and salt restriction with adequate nutritional support is recommended. Specialist heart failure nurses are invaluable in the support they provide to help the patients maintain fluid balance.

Hypotension secondary to autonomic neuropathy can be challenging to manage. Midodrine, an α-agonist, can be added. Fludrocortisone is not usually particularly effective and may exacerbate fluid retention. In contrast to heart failure secondary to ischaemic cardiomyopathy, there is no evidence to support the use of angiotensin converting enzyme inhibitors or angiotensin II receptor blockers which may worsen hypotension. β-Blockers are often poorly tolerated due to hypotension and may exacerbate conduction abnormalities which are common in cardiac amyloidosis. There is no proven prognostic benefit for β-blockers in cardiac amyloidosis, so there should be a low threshold for reducing the dose or stopping them altogether. Historically, it has been advised that digoxin should be avoided. An in-vitro study reported digoxin binding to amyloid fibrils and cardiac amyloid tissue but the clinical significance of this is unclear. Digoxin in low doses may, in fact, be an alternative to β-blockers in the acute management of atrial fibrillation, with a rapid ventricular response in patients with AL amyloidosis due to the risk of profound hypotension with β-blocker therapy. Warfarin or novel oral anticoagulants should be prescribed in patients with atrial fibrillation, as intracardiac thrombus formation is common in cardiac amyloidosis.[26]

Device therapy

Conduction abnormalities are common in ATTRwt cardiac amyloidosis and patients often require pacemaker implantation during follow-up. Pacemaker at diagnosis has been shown to be to a poor prognostic marker in cardiac wild-type ATTR amyloidosis.[78] In practice, pacemaker implantation is guided by the current general guidelines. No specific recommendations exist for pacemaker, implantable cardioverter–defibrillator (ICD), or cardiac resynchronization therapy implantation in patients with cardiac amyloidosis in Europe. In contrast, the most recent US device implantation guidelines suggest consideration on a case-by-case basis for ICD implantation for primary and secondary prevention of sudden cardiac death,[79] an acknowledgement of case reports in the literature where benefit can be demonstrated but where the data are limited.[80]

Treatment of AL amyloidosis

Treatment of AL amyloidosis comprises chemotherapy that targets the underlying plasma cell dyscrasia (PCD), with the aim of rapidly reducing production of amyloidogenic light chains to limit progressive damage to amyloidotic organs. Most patients with AL amyloidosis have a PCD at the MGUS end of the spectrum but 10–15% patients have overt myeloma. Drugs for myeloma have been adapted for use in AL amyloidosis. With the progress in drugs over the last decade, median survival in AL amyloidosis has nearly doubled; but nearly one-quarter of all patients still die of disease-related complications within a few months of diagnosis.[5]

In current practice, most patients receive a cyclic combination of the alkylating agent cyclophosphamide, the proteasome inhibitor bortezemib and dexamethasone (CyBorD). If tolerated, this treatment regime is associated with high haematological response rates (>60%) with prolonged progression-free survival in a proportion of patients with Mayo stage III disease (which carries the poorest prognosis).[81]

Although effective in cardiac AL amyloidosis, CyBorD may lead to worsening heart failure symptoms with a fall in the ejection fraction, worsening fluid retention, and cardiac arrhythmias. High-risk patients (Mayo stage IIIb) should be closely monitored (including cardiac monitoring) during treatment.

Autologous stem cell transplant

Low-risk patients (around 15–20% of all cases) i.e. those with excellent performance status, low NT-proBNP and troponin levels, and good renal function are potential candidates for high-dose melphalan followed by autologous stem cell transplant (ASCT). Although one small randomized trial did not show superiority of ASCT over chemotherapy, data from non-randomized studies show excellent clonal response rates which translate into organ function improvement. There remains, however, significant treatment-related morbidity and mortality in those with cardiac involvement, making many patients unsuitable for ASCT. ASCT should only be undertaken in centres with experience in amyloidosis.

Treatment of ATTR amyloidosis

Transplantation

The liver is the major source of the precursor protein, transthyretin, and it may be transplanted to replace the amyloidogenic protein with normal, non-amyloidogenic, transthyretin. Liver transplantation is the treatment of choice in young patients with FAP associated with ATTR V30M variant, who do not have cardiac involvement, and early in the disease course.[82] FAP associated with variants such as T60A invariably has cardiac involvement. In these patients, liver transplantation unfortunately led to worsening cardiac amyloidosis due to deposition of wild-type TTR as amyloid on the pre-existing template of amyloid already in the heart.[43]

Cardiac disease is the dominant feature in patients with ATTR V122I amyloidosis and ATTRwt amyloidosis. Highly selected younger patients have been reported to do well following cardiac transplantation.[83,84] Since the average age of presentation is between 60 and 80 years, this is not an option for the majority of patients.

Novel therapies

Reduction of TTR production

RNA inhibitors (small interfering RNA: siRNA and antisense oligonucleotide (ASO) therapies) are two promising novel strategies which inhibit hepatic synthesis of both wild-type and variant TTR. The siRNA drug patisiran has been shown to reduce TTR production by >80%.[85] ASO therapy can also inhibit TTR production by 80%.[86] Both drugs are in phase III testing for FAP.

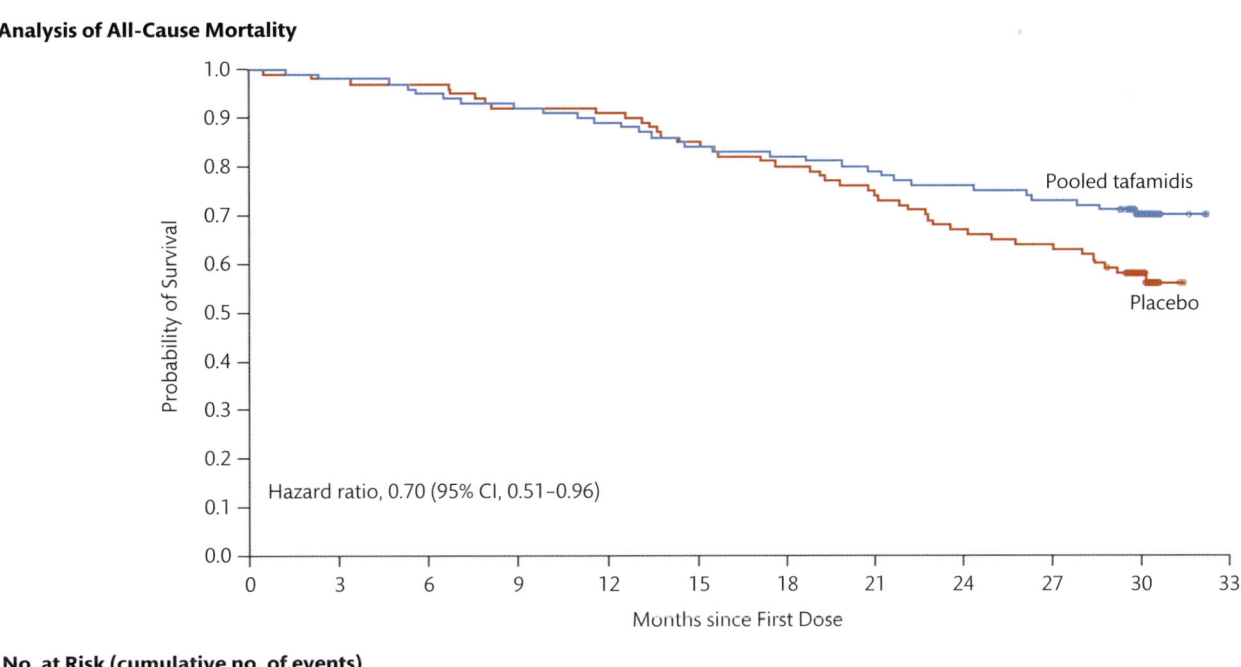

Figure 9.8 All-cause mortality in the ATTR-ACT trial. Patients were randomised to receive (in a 2:1:2 ratio) 80 mg or 20 mg of tafamidis, or placebo.

Source data from Maurer MS, Schwartz JH, Gundapaneni B, et al; ATTR-ACT Study Investigators. Tafamidis Treatment for Patients with Transthyretin Amyloid Cardiomyopathy. *N Engl J Med*. 2018 Sep 13;379(11):1007-1016. doi: 10.1056/NEJMoa1805689.

TTR stabilization

Diflunisal, an old fashioned, non-steroidal anti-inflammatory drug, has been shown *in vitro* to bind to wild-type and variant TTR. By maintaining the normal soluble TTR tetrameric structure, it inhibits the amyloidogenic misfolding of TTR. It has been found to reduce the rate of neurological progression and preserve quality of life at two years compared with placebo in patients with FAP.[87]

Tafamidis is a novel TTR stabilizer. It is licenced for use in the EU and Japan for the treatment of early FAP because neuropathic disease progressed at a slower rate with tafamidis compared with placebo over 18 months.[88] More recently, the ATTR-ACT study[89] compared tafamidis to placebo among 441 patients with ATTR (approximately 75% wild type). The primary endpoint of all-cause mortality followed by cardiovascular hospitalisations favoured tafamidis and was highly statistically significant (see Figure 9.8). There were much slower declines in 6 minute walk test distance and in Kansas City Cardiomyopathy Questionnaire score as well. The National Institute for Health and Care Excellence in England and Wales has not recommended it for use within the NHS despite its marketing authorisation.[90]

Immunotherapy

All amyloid deposits contain SAP, a normal plasma glycoprotein. The drug R-1-[6-[R-2-carboxy-pyrrolidin-1-yl]-6-oxo-hexanoyl] pyrrolidine-2-carboxylic acid (CPHPC) has been developed at the NAC. It cross-links pairs of SAP molecules *in vivo*[91] and triggers their prompt and virtual complete clearance from the blood.[92] CPHPC only leads to gradual depletion of SAP from amyloid deposits. However, antibodies to SAP can then target the SAP remaining on amyloid deposits. Since SAP is a universal component of all amyloid deposits, these antibodies will target all types of amyloid fibril proteins. Results of a phase 1 trial using this combined approach showed promising results with marked reduction in liver amyloid deposits.[93] Data on efficacy in cardiac disease are awaited.

Conclusion

Amyloidosis is not as rare as perceived and should be suspected early by clinicians in all specialties. Cardiac involvement is most common in ATTR and AL types of amyloidosis, and is a major determinant of prognosis. Confirmation of amyloid fibril type by immunohistochemistry, proteomics, and genetic sequencing is crucial as this will guide therapy. Several imaging modalities are available to aid the diagnosis of cardiac amyloidosis, with CMR and ^{99m}Tc-dicarboxypropane diphosphonate scintigraphy showing promise in detecting early disease. Promising novel treatments are now in clinical trials with the hope of halting organ disease progression and, indeed, of recovery and improved survival.

REFERENCES

1. Pepys MB. Amyloidosis. *Annu Rev Med* 2006;**57**:223–41.
2. Soma K, Takizawa MHU. A case of ST-elevated myocardial infarction resulting from obstructive intramural coronary amyloidosis. *Int Heart J* 2010;**51**(2):134–6.
3. Fonnescu C, Giovanale M, Verrecchia E, *et al.* Gastrointestinal amyloidosis: a case of chronic diarrhoea. *Eur Rev Med Pharmacol Sci* 2009;**13**:45–50.
4. Elli L, Falconieri G, Bardella MT, *et al.* Megaduodenum: an unusual presentation of amyloidosis? *Acta Gastroenterol Belg* 2010;**73**(2):287–91.
5. Wechalekar A, Gillmore JD, Hawkins PN. Systemic amyloidosis. *Lancet* 2016;**387**:2641–54.
6. Westermark P, Benson MD, Buxbaum JN, *et al.* A primer of amyloid nomenclature. *Amyloid* 2007;**14**:179–83.
7. Bonar L, Cohen AS, Skinner MM. Characterization of the amyloid fibril as a cross-beta protein. *Proc Soc Exp Biol Med* 1969;**131**:1373–75.
8. Pepys MB, Rademacher TW, Amatayakul-Chantler S, *et al.* Human serum amyloid P component is an invariant constituent of amyloid deposits and has a uniquely homogeneous glycostructure. *Proc Natl Acad Sci USA* 1994;**91**:5602–6.
9. Dember LM, Hawkins PN, Hazenberg BPC, *et al.* Eprodisate for the treatment of renal disease in AA amyloidosis. *N Engl J Med* 2007;**356**:2349–60.
10. Bodin K, Ellmerich S, Kahan MC, *et al.* Antibodies to human serum amyloid P component eliminate visceral amyloid deposits. *Nature* 2010;**468**:93–7.
11. Schonland SO, Hegenbart U, Bochtler T, *et al.* Immunohistochemistry in the classification of systemic forms of amyloidosis: a systematic investigation of 117 patients. *Blood* 2012;**119**:488–93.
12. Kyle RA, Linos A, Beard CM, *et al.* Incidence and natural history of primary systemic amyloidosis in Olmsted County, Minnesota, 1950 through 1989. *Blood* 1992;**79**:1817–22.
13. Pinney JH, Smith CJ, Taube JB, *et al.* Systemic amyloidosis in England: an epidemiological study. *Br J Haematol* 2013;**161**(4):525–32.
14. Tanskanen M, Peuralinna T, Polvikoski T, *et al.* Senile systemic amyloidosis affects 25% of the very aged and associates with genetic variation in alpha2-macroglobulin and tau: a population-based autopsy study. *Ann Med* 2008;**40**:232–9.
15. Wechalekar AD, Gillmore JD, Foard D, *et al.* 25 years of systemic amyloidosis. In: *Hazenberg PB ed International amyloidosis symposium Groningen: Netherlands* 2012.
16. Reilly MM, Staunton H, Harding AE. Familial amyloid polyneuropathy (TTR ala 60) in north west Ireland: a clinical, genetic, and epidemiological study. *J Neurol Neurosurg Psychiatry* 1995;**59**:45–9.
17. Sousa A, Coelho T, Barros J, Sequeiros J. Genetic epidemiology of familial amyloid polyneuropathy (FAP) type I in Povoa do Varzim and Vila do Conde (north of Portugal). *Am J Med Genet* 1995;**60**:512–21.
18. Holmgren G, Costa PM, Andersson C, *et al.* Geographical distribution of TTR met30 carriers in northern Sweden: discrepancy between carrier frequency and prevalence rate. *J Med Genet* 1994;**31**:351–4.
19. Hellman U, Alarcon F, Lundgren HE, Suhr OB, Bonaiti-Pellie C, Plante-Bordeneuve V. Heterogeneity of penetrance in familial amyloid polyneuropathy, ATTR Val30Met, in the Swedish population. *Amyloid* 2008;**15**:181–6.
20. Jacobson DR, Pastore RD, Yaghoubian R, *et al.* Variant-sequence transthyretin (isoleucine 122) in late-onset cardiac amyloidosis in black Americans. *N Engl J Med* 1997;**336**:466–73.
21. Quarta CC, Buxbaum JN, Shah AM, *et al.* The amyloidogenic V122I transthyretin variant in elderly black Americans. *N Engl J Med* 2015;**372**(1):21–9.
22. Falk RH. Diagnosis and management of the cardiac amyloidoses. *Circulation* 2005;**112**:2047–60.

23. Pinney JH, Whelan CJ, Petrie A, *et al*. Senile systemic amyloidosis: clinical features at presentation and outcome. *Journal of the American Heart Association* 2013;**2**(2).

24. Falk RH, Dubrey SW. Amyloid heart disease. *ProgCardiovasc Dis* 2010;**52**(4):347–61.

25. Navarro JF, Rivera M, Ortuno J. Cardiac tamponade as presentation of systemic amyloidosis. *Int J Cardiol* 1992;**36**:107–8.

26. Feng D, Edwards WD, Oh JK, *et al*. Intracardiac thrombus and embolism in patients with cardiac amyloidosis. *Circulation* 2007;**116**(21):2420–6.

27. Zubkov A, Rabinstein A, Dispenzieri A, Wijdicks E. Primary systemic amyloidosis with ischemic stroke as a presenting complication. *Neurology* 2007;**69**(11):1136–41.

28. Poels M, Ikram M, van der Lugt A, *et al*. Incidence of cerebral microbleeds in the general population: the Rotterdam Scan Study. *Stroke* 2011;**42**(3):656–61.

29. Dinwoodey D, Skinner M, Maron M, Davidoff R, Ruberg F. Light-chain amyloidosis with echocardiographic features of hypertrophic cardiomyopathy. *Am J Cardiol* 2008;**101**:674–6.

30. Chamarthi B, Dubrey SW, Cha K, Skinner M, Falk RH. Features and prognosis of exertional syncope in light-chain associated AL cardiac amyloidosis. *Am J Cardiol* 1997;**80**(9):1242–5.

31. Ridolfi R, Bulkley B, Hutchins G. The conduction system in cardiac amyloidosis. Clinical and pathological features in 23 patients. *Am J Med* 1977;**62**:677–86.

32. Al Suwaidi J, Velianou J, Gertz M, *et al*. Systemic amyloidosis presenting with angina pectoris. *Ann Intern Med* 1999;**131**:838–41.

33. Kyle RA, Greipp PR, O'Fallon WM. Primary systemic amyloidosis: multivariate analysis for prognostic factors in 168 cases. *Blood* 1986;**68**:220–4.

34. Dubrey SW, Cha K, Anderson J, *et al*. The clinical features of immunoglobulin light-chain (AL) amyloidosis with heart involvement. *Q J Med* 1998;**91**:141–57.

35. Liao R, Jain M, Teller P, *et al*. Infusion of light chains from patients with cardiac amyloidosis causes diastolic dysfunction in isolated mouse hearts. *Circulation* 2001;**104**:1594–7.

36. Benson MD, Kincaid JC. The molecular biology and clinical features of amyloid neuropathy. *Muscle Nerve* 2007;**36**:411–23.

37. Sacchettini JC, Kelly JW. Therapeutic strategies for human amyloid diseases. *Nat Rev Drug Discov* 2002;**1**:267–75.

38. Takei Y, Hattori T, Gono T, *et al*. Senile systemic amyloidosis presenting as bilateral carpal tunnel syndrome. *Amyloid* 2002;**9**:252–5.

39. Sekijima Y, Uchiyama S, Tojo K, *et al*. High prevalence of wild-type transthyretin deposition in patients with idiopathic carpal tunnel syndrome: a common cause of carpal tunnel syndrome in the elderly. *Hum Pathol* 2011;**42**(11):1785–91.

40. Jacobson DR, Pastore R, Pool S, *et al*. Revised transthyretin Ile 122 allele frequency in African-Americans. *Hum Genet* 1996;**98**:236–8.

41. Ruberg FL, Berk JL. Transthyretin (TTR) cardiac amyloidosis. *Circulation* 2012;**126**(10):1286–300.

42. Staunton H, Dervan P, Kale R, Linke RP, Kelly P. Hereditary amyloid polyneuropathy in north west Ireland. *Brain* 1987;**110** (Pt 5):1231–45.

43. Sattianayagam PT, Hahn AF, Whelan CJ, *et al*. Cardiac phenotype and clinical outcome of familial amyloid polyneuropathy associated with transthyretin alanine 60 variant. *Eur Heart J* 2012;**33**(9):1120–7.

44. Andrade C. A peculiar form of peripheral neuropathy;familiar atypical generalized amyloidosis with special involvement of the peripheral nerves. *Brain* 1952;**75**:408–27.

45. Kumar S, Dispenzieri A, Katzmann JA, *et al*. Serum immunoglobulin free light chain measurement in AL amyloidosis: prognostic value and correlations with clinical features. *Blood* 2010;**116**(24):5126–9.

46. Kyle RA, Therneau TM, Rajkumar SV, *et al*. Prevalence of monoclonal gammopathy of undetermined significance. *N Engl J Med* 2006;**354**(13):1362–9.

47. Lachmann HJ, Booth DR, Booth SE, *et al*. Misdiagnosis of hereditary amyloidosis as AL (primary) amyloidosis. *N Engl J Med* 2002;**346**:1786–91.

48. Rapezzi C, Merlini G, Quarta CC, *et al*. Systemic cardiac amyloidoses: disease profiles and clinical courses of the 3 main types. *Circulation* 2009;**120**:1203–12.

49. Dungu J, Sattianayagam PT, Whelan CJ, *et al*. The electrocardiographic features associated with cardiac amyloidosis of variant transthyretin isoleucine 122 type in Afro-Caribbean patients. *Am Heart J* 2012;**164**(1):72–9.

50. Patel K, Cavalla F, Fontana M, *et al*. The ECG features at presentation in patients with ATTRwt, ATTR T60A and ATTR V122I amyloidosis. *IXth International Symposium on Familial Amyloid Polyneuropathy, Brazil*, 2013.

51. Murtagh B, Hammill SC, Gertz MA, Kyle RA, Tajik AJ, Grogan M. Electrocardiographic findings in primary systemic amyloidosis and biopsy-proven cardiac involvement. *Am J Cardiol* 2005;**95**:535–7.

52. Sayed RH, Rogers D, Khan F, *et al*. A study of implanted cardiac rhythm recorders in advanced cardiac AL amyloidosis. *Eur Heart J* 2015;**36**(18):1098–105.

53. Dispenzieri A, Gertz M, Kyle R, *et al*. Serum cardiac troponins and N-terminal pro-brain natriuretic peptide: a staging system for primary systemic amyloidosis. *J Clin Oncol* 2004;**22**:3751–7.

54. Kumar S, Dispenzieri A, Lacy MQ, *et al*. Revised prognostic staging system for light chain amyloidosis incorporating cardiac biomarkers and serum free light chain measurements. *J Clin Oncol* 2012;**30**(9):989–95.

55. Wechalekar A, Schonland SO, Kastritis E, *et al*. European Collaborative Study of Treatment Outcomes in 347 Patients with Systemic AL Amyloidosis with Mayo Stage III Disease. *ASH Annual Meeting Abstracts* 2011;**118**(21):995.

56. Wechalekar AD, Schonland SO, Kastritis E, *et al*. A European collaborative study of treatment outcomes in 346 patients with cardiac stage III AL amyloidosis. *Blood* 2013;**121**(17):3420–7.

57. Wechalekar AD, Wassef N, Lachmann H, *et al*. High early mortality and poor outcomes for patients with AL amyloidosis presenting with high serum free light chains. *Haematologica* 2009;**94**:222.

58. Knight D, Patel K, Whelan C, *et al*. A guideline protocol for the assessment of restrictive cardiomyopathy—a protocol of the British Society of Echocardiography. *British Society of Echocardiography* 2014.

59. Gertz MA, Comenzo R, Falk RH, *et al*. Definition of organ involvement and treatment response in immunoglobulin light chain amyloidosis (AL): a consensus opinion from the 10th International Symposium on Amyloid and Amyloidosis. *Am J Hematol* 2005;**79**:319–28.

60. Carroll JD, Gaasch WH, McAdam KP. Amyloid cardiomyopathy: characterization by a distinctive voltage/mass relation. *Am J Cardiol* 1982;**49**:9–13.

61. Koyama J, Ray-Sequin PA, Falk RH. Longitudinal myocardial function assessed by tissue velocity, strain, and strain rate tissue Doppler echocardiography in patients with AL (primary) cardiac amyloidosis. *Circulation* 2003;**107**:2446–52.

62. Buss S, Emami M, Mereles D, *et al*. Longitudinal left ventricular function for prediction of survival in systemic light-chain amyloidosis: incremental value compared with clinical and biochemical markers. *J Am Coll Cardiol* 2012;**60**:1067–76.

63. Phelan D, Collier P, Thavendiranathan P, *et al*. Relative apical sparing of longitudinal strain using two-dimensional speckle-tracking echocardiography is both sensitive and specific for the diagnosis of cardiac amyloidosis. *Heart* 2012;**98**:1442–8.

64. Maceira AM, Joshi J, Prasad SK, *et al*. Cardiovascular magnetic resonance in cardiac amyloidosis. *Circulation* 2005;**111**:186–93.

65. Syed IS, Glockner JF, Feng D, *et al*. Role of cardiac magnetic resonance imaging in the detection of cardiac amyloidosis. *JACC Cardiovasc Imaging* 2010;**3**(2):155–64.

66. Dungu JN, Valencia O, Pinney JH, *et al*. CMR-based differentiation of AL and ATTR amyloidosis. *JACC Cardiovasc Imaging* 2014.

67. Fontana M, Pica S, Reant P, *et al*. Prognostic value of late gadolinium enhancement cardiovascular magnetic resonance in cardiac amyloidosis. *Circulation* 2015;**132**(16):1570–9.

68. Karamitsos TD, Piechnik SK, Banypersad SM, *et al*. Noncontrast T1 mapping for the diagnosis of cardiac amyloidosis. *JACC Cardiovascular imaging* 2013;**6**(4):488–97.

69. Fontana M, Banypersad SM, Treibel TA, *et al*. Native T1 mapping in transthyretin amyloidosis. *JACC Cardiovasc Imaging* 2014;**7**(2):157–65.

70. Sado DM, Flett AS, Banypersad SM, *et al*. Cardiovascular magnetic resonance measurement of myocardial extracellular volume in health and disease. *Heart* 2012;**98**(19):1436–41.

71. Banypersad SM, Sado DM, Flett AS, *et al*. Quantification of myocardial extracellular volume fraction in systemic AL amyloidosis: an equilibrium contrast cardiovascular magnetic resonance study. *Circ Cardiovasc Imaging* 2013;**6**(1):34–9.

72. Banypersad SM, Fontana M, Maestrini V, *et al*. T1 mapping and survival in systemic light-chain amyloidosis. *Eur Heart J* 2015;**36**(4):244–51.

73. Hawkins PN, Myers MJ, Lavender JP, Pepys MB. Diagnostic radionuclide imaging of amyloid: biological targeting by circulating human serum amyloid P component. *Lancet* 1988;**i**:1413–8.

74. Rapezzi C, Quarta CC, Guidalotti PL, *et al*. Usefulness and limitations of 99mTc-3,3-diphosphono-1,2-propanodicarboxylic acid scintigraphy in the aetiological diagnosis of amyloidotic cardiomyopathy. *Eur J Nucl Med Mol Imaging* 2011;**38**(3):470–8.

75. Bokhari S, Castano A, Pozniakoff T, Deslisle S, Latif F, Maurer MS. (99m)Tc-pyrophosphate scintigraphy for differentiating light-chain cardiac amyloidosis from the transthyretin-related familial and senile cardiac amyloidoses. *Circ Cardiovasc Imaging* 2013;**6**(2):195–201.

76. Hutt DF, Quigley AM, Page J, *et al*. Utility and limitations of 3,3-diphosphono-1,2-propanodicarboxylic acid scintigraphy in systemic amyloidosis. *Eur Heart J Cardiovasc Imaging* 2014;**15**(11):1289–98.

77. Gillmore J, Maurer M, Falk R *et al*. Nonbiopsy diagnosis of cardiac transthyretin amyloidosis. *Circulation* 2016;**133**(24):2404–12.

78. Pinney JH, Whelan CJ, Petrie A, *et al*. Senile systemic amyloidosis: clinical features at presentation and outcome. *J Am Heart Assoc* 2013;**2**(2):e000098.

79. Russo A, Stainback RF, Bailey SR, *et al*. ACCF/HRS/AHA/ASE/HFSA/SCAI/SCCT/SCMR 2013 appropriate use criteria for implantable cardioverter defibrillators and cardiac synchronisation therapy. *J Am Coll Cardiol* 2013;**61**:1318–68.

80. Patel K, Hawkins P, Whelan C, Gillmore JD. Life-saving implantable cardioverter defibrillator therapy in cardiac AL amyloidosis. *BMJ* 2014.

81. Venner CP, Lane T, Foard D, *et al*. Cyclophosphamide, bortezomib and dexamethasone therapy in AL amyloidosis is associated with high clonal response rates and prolonged progression free survival. *Blood* 2012;**119**(11):4387–90.

82. de Carvalho M, Conceicao I, Bentes C, Luis ML. Long-term quantitative evaluation of liver transplantation in familial amyloid polyneuropathy (Portugese V30M). *Amyloid* 2002;**9**:126–33.

83. Hamour IM, Lachmann HJ, Goodman HJ, *et al*. Heart transplantation for homozygous familial transthyretin (TTR) V122I cardiac amyloidosis. *Am J Transplant* 2008;**8**:1056–9.

84. Fuchs U, Zitterman A, Suhr O, *et al*. Heart transplantation in a 68 year old patient with senile systemic amyloidosis. *Am J Transplant* 2005;**5**:1159–62.

85. Coelho T, Adams D, Silva A, *et al*. Safety and efficacy of RNAi therapy for transthyretin amyloidosis. *N Engl J Med* 2013;**369**(9):819–29.

86. Adams D. Recent advances in the treatment of familial amyloid polyneuropathy. *Ther Adv Neurol Disord* 2013;**6**:129–39.

87. Berk JL, Suhr OB, Obici L, *et al*. Repurposing diflunisal for familial amyloid polyneuropathy: a randomized clinical trial. *JAMA* 2013;**310**(24):2658–67.

88. Coelho T, Maia LF, Martins da Silva A, *et al*. Tafamidis for transthyretin familial amyloid polyneuropathy: a randomized, controlled trial. *Neurology* 2012;79:785–92.

89. Maurer MS, Schwartz JH, Gundapaneni B, *et al*. ATTR-ACT Study Investigators. Tafamidis treatment for patients with transthyretin amyloid cardiomyopathy. *N Engl J Med* 2018;**379**:1007–16.

90. National Institute for Health and Care Excellence. Tafamidis for treating transthyretin amyloidosis with cardiomyopathy. Technology appraisal guidance [TA696] Published: 12 May 2021.

91. Pepys MB, Herbert J, Hutchinson WL, *et al*. Targeted pharmacological depletion of serum amyloid P component for treatment of human amyloidosis. *Nature* 2002;**417**:254–9.

92. Gillmore JD, Tennent GA, Hutchinson WL, *et al*. Sustained pharmacological depletion of serum amyloid P component in patients with systemic amyloidosis. *Br J Haematol* 2010;**148**(5):760–7.

93. Richards DB, Cookson LM, Berges AC, *et al*. Therapeutic clearance of amyloid by antibodies to serum amyloid P component. *N Engl J Med* 2015;**373**(12):1106–14.

RECOMMENDED READING

Falk RH. Diagnosis and management of the cardiac amyloidoses. *Circulation* 2005;**112**:2047–60.

Grogan M, Dispenzieri A. Natural history and therapy of AL cardiac amyloidosis. *Heart Fail Rev* 2015;**20**:155–62.

Knight D, Patel K, Whelan C, *et al*. A guideline protocol for the assessment of restrictive cardiomyopathy—a protocol of the British Society of Echocardiography. British Society of Echocardiography, 2014.

Pepys MB. Amyloidosis. *Annu Rev Med* 2006;**57**:223–41.

Rapezzi C, Merlini G, Quarta CC, *et al*. Systemic cardiac amyloidoses: disease profiles and clinical courses of the 3 main types. *Circulation* 2009;**120**:1203–12.

10

Acute viral myocarditis

Stephane Heymans

Introduction

The term 'myocarditis' was first introduced in the early nineteenth century by Corvisart, and initially included myocardial ischaemia. At the beginning of the twentieth century with the recognition of coronary artery disease as an important cause of heart disease, the term was refined.[1] It now applies to acute or chronic inflammatory responses of the heart to environmental or endogenous triggers, most commonly viruses, and less frequently to bacteria, fungi, and parasites. Important non-infectious causes include giant cell myocarditis, drug-induced hypersensitivity and cardiac manifestations of systemic autoimmunity such as sarcoidosis or systemic lupus erythematosus.[2–5]

Several reviews and position statements attempt to distinguish acute myocarditis more accurately from chronic 'inflammatory' cardiomyopathy, where detailed diagnostics including biopsies, molecular analysis, imaging, and clinical evaluation are required to refine the diagnosis and decide on targeted therapy.[6–10] The present chapter focuses on acute viral myocarditis (VM), its pathophysiology, diagnosis and specific treatment, and highlights where virus presence should be diagnosed and distinguished from the other infectious or non-infectious causes.

Epidemiology of acute myocarditis

The incidence of myocarditis as ascertained by the *International Classification of Diseases (ICD-9)* diagnoses was 22/100 000 or approximately 1.5 million cases in the 2013 world population.[11] The burden of myocarditis as a percentage of prevalent heart failure varies by age and region from approximately 0.5% to 4.0%.[12] Myocarditis is also responsible for sudden cardiovascular death in approximately 2% of infant cases, 5% of childhood cases, and 5–12% of cases of sudden death in young athletes.[13] The overall rate of myocarditis was 3% (six out of 200) in autopsies of patients experiencing sudden death in Japan.[14] It is estimated that around 70% of all cases of myocarditis are of viral origin.[6–10]

Acute viral myocarditis: pathophysiology

Acute VM typically presents with unexpected symptoms, raised blood biomarkers suggesting acute cardiomyocyte injury and a dynamic and changing electrocardiogram (ECG). Acute viral pericarditis is often accompanied by acute VM, increasingly diagnosed because of the increased sensitivity of myocyte injury biomarkers (troponins), and patients who might previously be diagnosed as having pericarditis are now classified as myopericarditis. Similar to other forms of heart disease, men are more often and severely affected than women, yet the mechanisms driving sex differences in myocarditis remain poorly understood.

Common cough viruses versus opportunistic ones

The most commonly identified pathogens in acute myocarditis are everyday cough viruses.[15] Enteroviruses (coxsackievirus, adenoviruses, and echovirus), human herpesvirus (HHV)-6, Epstein–Barr virus (EBV, also HHV4), and parvovirus-B19 (PVB19) are the most prevalent cardiotrophic viruses triggering acute cardiac inflammation in otherwise healthy individuals.[16–19] More than 70% of human beings—and their hearts—will contact these common viruses during their life without getting acute myocarditis. Only an 'unhappy few' develop symptoms of acute VM due to inappropriate cardiac inflammation, cardiac dysfunction, and/or arrhythmias. Those individuals must have a certain immune susceptibility, making them prone to exaggerated and harmful inflammation upon infection with specific cardiotrophic viruses.

This immune susceptibility—probably polygenetically defined—is different from immune deficiency. Other viruses, such as human immunodeficiency virus (HIV), cytomegalovirus (CMV), or hepatitis C virus, can endanger the heart only in immunosuppressed patients. Classical examples are CMV-myocarditis in immunosuppressed patients after cardiac transplantation, and HIV-myocarditis caused by loss of T-cell function induced by the virus itself.

Some viruses may persist in the heart, as seen in some subjects with a dilated cardiomyopathy (DCM) in whom there may (or may not) be ongoing increased inflammation. Parvovirus B-19[20–23] and human herpesvirus 6 (HHV-6) genomes[19] predominate as long-term viruses in the heart. The relevance of this virus persistence for the pathophysiology and treatment of heart failure is yet to be elucidated.

From virus infection to cardiac inflammation

The acute and first phase of VM (Figure 10.1) consists of both direct damage of the cardiomyocyte by the virus itself and damage from the inflammation directed against the virus-infected cardiomyocyte.

ACUTE PHASE	SUBACUTE PHASE	CHRONIC PHASE
• Viraemic dissemination • Viral replication • Cytokine responses • Cell death through virulence • Innate immunity	• Infiltration by innate, then adaptive immune cells • Auto-antibodies • Active viral elimination • Cell death mainly from inflammation	• Virus absent • Fibrotic replacement of dead cells • Auto antibodies OR • Persistence of virus and inflammation

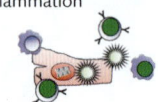 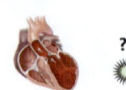

| Day 0 | Day 4-5 | Day 14-30 |

Figure 10.1 Pathogenesis of viral myocarditis. The acute phase consists of viral infection and replication in the heart, leading to cardiac cytokine expression, mainly interferons. Myocyte death may occur due to virus infection itself and/or the initial innate immunity. The second, subacute, phase develops as a result of immune dysregulation triggered by the initial cardiomyocyte infection. Innate and adaptive immunity will eliminate the virus. However, autoantibodies may develop. In the third, chronic, phase, a typical picture of dilated cardiomyopathy develops as a result of extensive myocardial injury and cardiac remodelling.

Direct destruction of the cardiomyocytes occurs by virus-mediated lysis, causing degradation of cell structures, which in turn facilitates entry of the virus into the cells with consequential myocyte injury and loss, and cardiac dilation.[24,25] Viral entry into cardiomyocytes may require specific cell-surface receptors such as the coxsackie-adenovirus receptor and decay-accelerating factor (DAF or CD55, for some coxsackie B virus strains).[26,27] Viral infection activates the innate immune response consisting of nitric oxide production, altered regulatory T-cell function, natural killer cells, and type I interferon release.[28–30] The immune response will itself also result in myocyte death through apoptosis and autophagy.[31] This initial phase frequently passes unnoticed since the initial damage is often limited or prevented by the innate immune response.

The initial cellular and humoral immune responses may improve outcome during phase 1 by eliminating the virus; conversely, when inappropriate, they are responsible for the harmful effect during phase 2. The second, subacute, phase develops as a result of immune dysregulation triggered by the initial cardiomyocyte infection and injury. This is in part induced by molecular mimicry,[32] which is caused by similarity between epitopes on viral and cardiac antigens. In genetically susceptible humans, a breakdown of T-cell tolerance to cardiac self-antigens will cause myocyte injury.

Finally, in the third phase, a typical picture of dilated cardiomyopathy (DCM) develops as a result of extensive myocardial injury. Progression from myocarditis to DCM seems to occur predominantly in patients with histologically confirmed persistent (chronic) inflammation. The inflammation either cannot eliminate the infective microbial agents or causes the development of pathogenic cardiac autoantibodies directed against myocardial structural, sarcoplasmic, or sarcolemmal proteins in stage 2.[33–35] This leads to a process of chronic autoantigen-driven inflammation, which can progress to dilated cardiomyopathy and end-stage heart failure.

The concept of the transition from acute viral infection through active inflammation to dilated cardiomyopathy also determines the opportunities for therapeutic intervention, which vary by stage of the disease.[6,36]

Sex differences

Men are diagnosed more often than women with myocarditis and have a worse prognosis.[37] Differences in innate immune responses to viral infection rather than increased viral replication may explain those sex differences.[36,38,39] Experimental models indicate that males have more aggressive cytotoxic T cells, pro-inflammatory macrophages type 1 (M1), and increased activation of toll-like receptor (TLR)-4-mediated inflammation than females.[40–42] The protective T cells (T-helper 2 response), B cells, and anti-inflammatory T-regulatory cells and macrophages type 2 (M2) dominate in females.[40–43]

Diagnosis of acute viral myocarditis

Clinical presentation

The initial evaluation of the patient with acute myocarditis includes a detailed history and a careful physical examination searching for any potential features that may provide clues to its aetiology, such as viral infection, toxic agents, or autoimmune diseases. Additional technical examination should include ECG, chest X-ray, blood studies, non-invasive imaging techniques, and endomyocardial biopsies.

Symptoms of acute VM vary, often starting with flu-like symptoms, either of the upper respiratory or gastrointestinal tracts, before any cardiac symptoms appear. Cardiac presentation may range from mild symptoms of chest pain, palpitations or dyspnoea, to ventricular arrhythmias or even life-threatening cardiogenic shock. Clinical scenarios highly suggestive of myocarditis include symptoms together with an abnormal and dynamic ECG, elevated troponins, and functional or structural abnormalities on cardiac imaging, typically myocardial oedema on cardiac magnetic resonance imaging. The ECG often mimics an acute myocardial infarction but with normal coronary arteries. In all cases of suspected myocarditis, it is therefore mandatory to exclude coronary artery disease and other cardiovascular (such as hypertension) or extracardiac non-inflammatory diseases that could explain the clinical presentation.

Other causes of acute myocarditis should appear in the differential diagnosis, most importantly autoimmune myocarditis. Giant cell myocarditis is the most aggressive of these, and the diagnosis is important since autoimmune myocarditis tends to be more chronic and require specific immunosupressive therapy, a treatment possibly deleterious in viral myocarditis.

ECG

The ECG in acute VM is usually abnormal and changing over time, but signs are neither specific nor sensitive. If present, ST-T segment elevation is typically concave in contrast to the convex elevation seen in myocardial ischaemia. Acute myocarditis may also result in 'idiopathic' atrial or ventricular arrhythmias, A-V delay, PQ-segment depression, or QRS prolongation. Despite the poor sensitivity and specificity, a standard 12-lead ECG should be performed in all patients with clinically suspected myocarditis.

Blood biomarkers

Myocyte injury enzymes are mainly elevated in the acute early stage of myocarditis and should be measured, with cardiac troponins being more sensitive than creatine kinase levels.[44] Their absence

does not exclude myocarditis, but rather suggests very mild myocarditis or chronic persistent myocarditis. Despite the differences in immune responses between acute myocardial ischaemia and acute VM, there are no specific blood biomarkers (or pattern of biomarkers) for acute myocarditis, resulting in many unwanted imaging procedures to exclude coronary artery disease. Increased C-reactive protein or sedimentation rate will confirm the presence of an inflammatory process, but will not help the further differential diagnosis.

The value of viral serology is low. Positive viral IgG serology does not imply acute VM but only indicates a patient's previous interaction with the virus. The prevalence of circulatory IgG antibodies to cardiotropic viruses in the general population is high—up to 70%—in the absence of any cardiac manifestation. Seroconversion (low IgG, raised IgM, and IgA) or increased viral PCR in blood at the time of the cardiac symptoms may indicate acute viral infection of the heart. Circumstances in which serological testing may be helpful include suspected hepatitis C, rickettsial phase 1 and phase 2, Lyme disease in endemic areas, and human immunodeficiency virus in high-risk patients.[6]

Autoantibodies may be involved in the pathophysiology of VM, at least in the more subacute or chronic stage, and during the long-term development of heart failure. Autoantibodies are not routinely determined in acute VM, since their diagnostic value and pathological role in the acute phase of VM is currently uncertain.[32]

Endomyocardial biopsy

The current indication for endomyocardial biopsy (EMB) is 'a strong reason to believe that the results will have a meaningful effect on subsequent therapeutic decisions', with the highest level of recommendation in life-threatening conditions.[45] More than 60% of patients with acute VM will spontaneously recover without cardiac dysfunction or chronic inflammation. EMBs should be obtained in those cases of acute myocarditis where initial cardiac systolic dysfunction or other clinical signs or blood biomarkers of cardiac injury do not show a trend to recovery within two to three days of the initial presentation. Recurrent myocarditis is another indication for EMB.

Analysis of the biopsies can identify the underlying cardiotrophic virus and its load, and/or the amount and type of inflammation (e.g. giant cell, eosinophilic myocarditis, sarcoidosis), leading to different treatments, either antiviral or immunosuppressants.

Immunohistochemical analysis of inflammation includes the quantification of CD3-staining T-cells and CD45 T-cells and monocytes. This increases the sensitivity for detecting cardiac inflammation, with the total number of CD3- and CD45-staining cells >15 per mm² being pathological (**Figure 10.2**). Other analyses include HLA-DR for autoimmune non-viral inflammation and CD68 macrophages as repair cells, but are not part of routine as their value is uncertain.[6]

Viral presence and quantification of viral load with reverse transcription–polymerase chain reaction (RT–PCR) is essential. In order to exclude systemic infection, peripheral blood should be investigated in parallel with EMB and determination of virus replication may add diagnostic value.[6] Sequencing of the amplified viral gene product may help to identify virus subtypes and recognize contaminations. Cardiotropic viruses include adenovirus,[16,17] hepatitis C,[46,47] CMV,[48] echovirus, EBV,[18] parvovirus B-19,[20–23] and HHV-6.[19] The latter three in the list predominate in subjects with more chronic symptoms and 'inflammatory cardiomyopathy'.

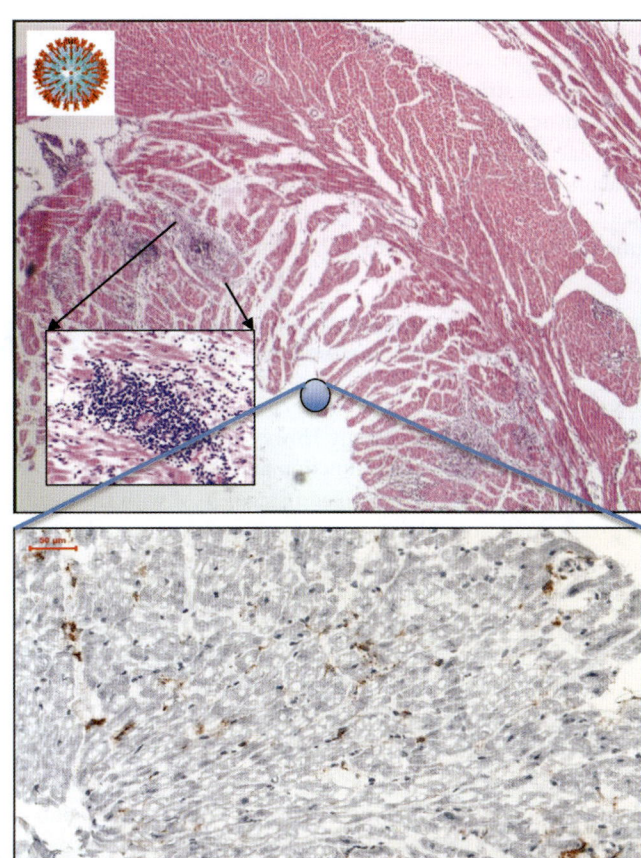

Figure 10.2 Haematoxylin and eosin (H&E) staining of acute myocarditis. Small (1 mm) subendomyocardial biopsies are not very sensitive for diagnosing myocarditis with H&E staining. Additional immunostaining of CD45 and CD3 lymphocytes is required to increase sensitivity (pathological if ≥15 per mm²) (*lower*: CD45-staining lymphocytes).

Imaging

Echocardiographic findings in acute VM are poorly sensitive and are non-specific. Marked LV dilation and systolic dysfunction, normal LV thickness, regional wall motion abnormalities, and diastolic dysfunction are all possible features. LV function may even be normal, thus limiting the utility of imaging for diagnosing myocarditis. Therefore, cardiac magnetic resonance (CMR) imaging is advised in addition to echocardiography.

CMR imaging is now the most important imaging tool in the diagnosis of myocardial oedema induced by inflammation. A combined CMR approach of T2-weighted imaging and early and late gadolinium enhancement provides high diagnostic accuracy and is the standard imaging approach in patients suspected of having acute myocarditis.[6,8,19] Increased late enhancement (LE) indicates myocardial injury, whereas T2-weighted images detect interstitial oedema and myocardial inflammation, with an increase in regional or global myocardial signal intensity. Increased global myocardial early gadolinium enhancement ratio between myocardium and skeletal muscle in T1-weighted images are suggestive of myocardial oedema.

The pattern of oedema distribution is different between acute myocarditis and ischaemia. Subendocardial or transmural enhancement

occurs in ischaemic heart disease, whereas acute VM has three distinct patterns, including: the absence of enhancement (59%); patchy or longitudinal striae of mid-wall enhancement (28%); and (in a minority) myocardial enhancement indistinguishable from patients with ischaemic cardiomyopathy (13%).[49] LE distributions in patients with acute MI are of a smaller number of areas in a segmental vascular distribution in contrast to a more diffuse, nodular or patchy, non-segmental vascular distribution in patients with acute myocarditis.[49]

Treatment of acute viral myocarditis

Acute VM will resolve in more than 70% of cases in the first days, not requiring any medical therapy. However, around a quarter of patients will develop cardiac dysfunction and some may present with cardiogenic shock or progress to end-stage DCM with the need for heart transplantation. If systolic dysfunction is present, the patient should receive standard heart failure treatment including β-blockers and angiotensin converting enzyme inhibitors or angiotensin II receptor blockers, and diuretics if indicated. Arrhythmias should be monitored and treated, but implantable cardioverter–defibrillator implantation should be deferred until resolution of the acute episode. Severe cases with haemodynamic instability should be managed in an intensive care unit which can offer mechanical cardiopulmonary assist devices as a bridge to recovery or to heart transplantation.

Non-steroidal anti-inflammatory drugs, notably colchicine and acetylsalicylic acid, are mandatory in the treatment of acute pericarditis, but their use in experimental models of myocarditis resulted in increased mortality.[10] Clinical data for their administration in myocarditis are inconclusive, and therefore they are not yet advised pending the results of further controlled trials. Their use in acute myopericarditis with a mild increase in troponins but no systolic dysfunction is still acceptable, but not based on evidence.

Patients with acute myocarditis should limit physical activity as long as the signs of myocardial inflammation and injury are present, as exercise during active viral infection may increase viral replication, facilitate arrhythmias, and shorten survival. Athletes should be advised to stop competitive sport for 2–6 months pending on the clinical presentation. Return to competition requires specialized evaluation during the first 6 months after the initial presentation.[50,51]

Antiviral therapies

There is no proof today that antiviral therapy is effective in acute VM. In patients with a high cardiac viral load of human herpesviruses, including HHV4 (also EBV) or HHV6, treatment with acyclovir, ganciclovir, and valacyclovir may be considered,[52,53] although its efficacy is unproven in myocarditis. In the future, therapies interfering with the innate immune response to viral infection, such as interferon-β, may emerge. However, until clinical trials are conclusive, antiviral therapies are only recommended in those patients with high viral load, and only with the involvement of an infectious disease specialist.

Intravenous immunoglobulin (IVIG) modulates innate immunity in a favourable way, and has antiviral properties. IVIG may be considered in myocarditis refractory to conventional heart failure therapy, both viral and autoimmune forms, particularly if autoantibody-mediated.[9] There are no firm recommendations for its use, since there is no evidence based on clinical trials.

Immunosuppression

Immune suppression is beneficial in patients with systemic disease-related or autoimmune myocarditis.[2,34] By contrast, in acute VM, immunosuppression may increase virus replication and worsen myocardial injury. The Myocarditis Treatment Trial failed to show any evidence to support the use of immunosuppressive therapy in patients with biopsy-proven myocarditis and reduced LV function: neither LV systolic function nor overall survival improved.[54] However, the diagnosis of myocarditis was made solely on the histological Dallas criteria, without the exclusion of viral presence.

Immunosuppression is thus not recommended in acute myocarditis unless significant viral presence has been excluded, or unless severe autoimmune myocarditis (particularly giant cell myocarditis or sarcoidosis with cardiac involvement) has been proven.

Follow-up of acute myocarditis

Patients who have had myocarditis should be followed for at least four years, as some patients may develop a subclinical dilated cardiomyopathy or clinical recurrence requiring EMB (and treatment in its own right). Cardiac enzymes (troponins) and function have to be reanalysed to look for persistent myocyte injury due to autoimmune processes with cardiac and/or skeletal muscle involvement.

Conclusion

Patients suspected of having acute myocarditis should undergo a complete cardiological work-up, including CMR. EMB is useful for both PCR and immunohistochemical analysis. Due to the lack of specific biomarkers able to distinguish myocarditis from ischaemic heart disease, coronary artery disease has to be excluded. A refined diagnostic process that includes molecular analysis of blood and EMBs is needed to prove viral presence and exclude autoimmune disease. The process is required to allow more targeted therapy, beside classical anti-heart failure treatment. A combined team of cardiologists, pathologists, microbiologists, immunologists and geneticists in specialized centres is required for this refined diagnosis and to improve understanding of the underlying pathological process in acute myocarditis. Multicentre randomized controlled trials of aetiology-driven treatment are required: a task for current and future generations.

REFERENCES

1. Mattingly TW. Changing concepts of myocardial diseases. *JAMA* 1965;**191**:33–37.
2. Sagar S, Liu PP, Cooper LT, Jr. Myocarditis. *Lancet* 2012;**379**:738–47.
3. Dennert R, Crijns HJ, Heymans S. Acute viral myocarditis. *Eur Heart J* 2008;**29**:2073–82.
4. Caforio AL, Pankuweit S, Arbustini E, *et al.* Current state of knowledge on aetiology, diagnosis, management, and therapy of myocarditis: a position statement of the European Society of Cardiology Working Group on Myocardial and Pericardial Diseases. *Eur Heart J* 2013;**34**:2636–48, 2648a–d.
5. Corsten MF, Schroen B, Heymans S. Inflammation in viral myocarditis: friend or foe? *Trends Mol Med* 2012;**18**:426–37.

6. Caforio AL, Pankuweit S, Arbustini E, *et al*. Current state of knowledge on aetiology, diagnosis, management, and therapy of myocarditis: a position statement of the European Society of Cardiology Working Group on Myocardial and Pericardial Diseases. *Eur Heart J* 2013;**34**:2636–48, 2648a–d.

7. Cooper LT, Jr. Myocarditis. *N Engl J Med* 2009;**360**:1526–38.

8. Dennert R, Crijns HJ, Heymans S. Acute viral myocarditis. *Eur Heart J* 2008;**29**:2073–82.

9. Kindermann I, Barth C, Mahfoud F, *et al*. Update on myocarditis. *J Am Coll Cardiol* 2012;**59**:779–92.

10. Liu PP, Mason JW. Advances in the understanding of myocarditis. *Circulation* 2001;**104**:1076–82.

11. Global Burden of Disease Study Collaborators. Global, regional, and national incidence, prevalence, and years lived with disability for 301 acute and chronic diseases and injuries in 188 countries, 1990–2013: a systematic analysis for the Global Burden of Disease Study 2013. *Lancet* 2015;**386**:743–800.

12. Cooper LT, Jr, Keren A, Sliwa K, Matsumori A, Mensah GA. The global burden of myocarditis: part 1: a systematic literature review for the Global Burden of Diseases, Injuries, and Risk Factors 2010 study. *Glob Heart* 2014;**9**:121–9.

13. Maron BJ, Udelson JE, Bonow RO, *et al*.; American Heart Association Electrocardiography and Arrhythmias Committee of Council on Clinical Cardiology, Council on Cardiovascular Disease in Young, Council on Cardiovascular and Stroke Nursing, Council on Functional Genomics and Translational Biology, and American College of Cardiology. Eligibility and Disqualification Recommendations for Competitive Athletes With Cardiovascular Abnormalities: Task Force 3: Hypertrophic Cardiomyopathy, Arrhythmogenic Right Ventricular Cardiomyopathy and Other Cardiomyopathies, and Myocarditis: A Scientific Statement From the American Heart Association and American College of Cardiology. *Circulation* 2015;**132**:e273–80.

14. Matoba R, Shikata I, Iwai K, *et al*. An epidemiologic and histopathological study of sudden cardiac death in Osaka Medical Examiner's Office. *Jpn Circ J* 1989;**53**:1581–8.

15. Schultheiss H-P, Kuhl U, Cooper LT. The management of myocarditis. *Eur Heart J* 2011;**32**:2616–25.

16. Bowles NE, Ni J, Kearney DL, *et al*. Detection of viruses in myocardial tissues by polymerase chain reaction. Evidence of adenovirus as a common cause of myocarditis in children and adults. *J Am Coll Cardiol* 2003;**42**:466–72.

17. Pauschinger M, Bowles NE, Fuentes-Garcia FJ, *et al*. Detection of adenoviral genome in the myocardium of adult patients with idiopathic left ventricular dysfunction. *Circulation* 1999;**99**:1348–54.

18. Chimenti C, Russo A, Pieroni M, *et al*. Intramyocyte detection of Epstein–Barr virus genome by laser capture microdissection in patients with inflammatory cardiomyopathy. *Circulation* 2004;**110**:3534–39.

19. Kuhl U, Pauschinger M, Noutsias M, *et al*. High prevalence of viral genomes and multiple viral infections in the myocardium of adults with 'idiopathic' left ventricular dysfunction. *Circulation* 2005;**111**:887–93.

20. Breinholt JP, Moulik M, Dreyer WJ, *et al*. Viral epidemiologic shift in inflammatory heart disease: the increasing involvement of parvovirus B19 in the myocardium of pediatric cardiac transplant patients. *J Heart Lung Transplant* 2010;**29**:739–46.

21. Bock CT, Klingel K, Kandolf R. Human parvovirus B19-associated myocarditis. *N Engl J Med* 2010;**362**:1248–9.

22. Pankuweit S, Moll R, Baandrup U, *et al*. Prevalence of the parvovirus B19 genome in endomyocardial biopsy specimens. *Hum Pathol* 2003;**34**:497–503.

23. Tschope C, Bock CT, Kasner M, *et al*. High prevalence of cardiac parvovirus B19 infection in patients with isolated left ventricular diastolic dysfunction. *Circulation* 2005;**111**:879–86.

24. McManus BM, Chow LH, Wilson JE, *et al*. Direct myocardial injury by enterovirus: a central role in the evolution of murine myocarditis. *Clin Immunol Immunopathol* 1993;**68**:159–69.

25. Maekawa Y, Ouzounian M, Opavsky MA, Liu PP. Connecting the missing link between dilated cardiomyopathy and viral myocarditis: virus, cytoskeleton, and innate immunity. *Circulation* 2007;**115**:5–8.

26. Bergelson JM, Cunningham JA, Droguett G, *et al*. Isolation of a common receptor for Coxsackie B viruses and adenoviruses 2 and 5. *Science* 1997;**275**:1320–3.

27. Martino TA, Petric M, Brown M, *et al*. Cardiovirulent coxsackieviruses and the decay-accelerating factor (CD55) receptor. *Virology* 1998;**244**:302–14.

28. Yuan J, Liu Z, Lim T, *et al*. CXCL10 inhibits viral replication through recruitment of natural killer cells in coxsackievirus B3-induced myocarditis. *Circ Res* 2009;**104**:628–38.

29. Jenke A, Holzhauser L, Löbel M, *et al*. Adiponectin promotes coxsackievirus B3 myocarditis by suppression of acute anti-viral immune responses. *Basic Res Cardiol* 2014;**109**:408.

30. Deonarain R, Cerullo D, Fuse K, Liu PP, Fish EN. Protective role for interferon-beta in coxsackievirus B3 infection. *Circulation* 2004;**110**:3540–3.

31. Kandolf R, Canu A, Hofschneider PH. Coxsackie B3 virus can replicate in cultured human foetal heart cells and is inhibited by interferon. *J Mol Cell Cardiol* 1985;**17**:167–81.

32. Lawson CM. Evidence for mimicry by viral antigens in animal models of autoimmune disease including myocarditis. *Cell Mol Life Sci* 2000;**57**:552–60.

33. Ciháková D, Sharma RB, Fairweather D, Afanasyeva M, Rose NR. Animal models for autoimmune myocarditis and autoimmune thyroiditis. *Methods Mol Med* 2004;**102**:175–93.

34. Caforio AL, Marcolongo R, Jahns R, *et al*. Immune-mediated and autoimmune myocarditis: clinical presentation, diagnosis and management. *Heart Fail Rev* 2013;**18**:715–32.

35. Fairweather D, Kaya Z, Shellam GR, Lawson CM, Rose NR. From infection to autoimmunity. *J Autoimmun* 2001;**16**:175–86.

36. Heymans S, Eriksson U, Lehtonen J, Cooper LT, Jr. The quest for new approaches in myocarditis and inflammatory cardiomyopathy. *J Am Coll Cardiol* 2016;**68**:2348–64.

37. Cocker MS, Abdel-Aty H, Strohm O, Friedrich MG. Age and gender effects on the extent of myocardial involvement in acute myocarditis: a cardiovascular magnetic resonance study. *Heart* 2009;**95**:1925–30.

38. Fairweather D, Cooper LT, Blauwet LA. Sex and gender differences in myocarditis and dilated cardiomyopathy. *Curr Probl Cardiol* 2013;**38**:7–46.

39. Frisancho-Kiss S, Nyland JF, Davis SE, *et al*. Sex differences in coxsackievirus B3-induced myocarditis: IL-12Rbeta1 signaling and IFN-gamma increase inflammation in males independent from STAT4. *Brain Res* 2006;**1126**:139–47.

40. Frisancho-Kiss S, Davis SE, Nyland JF, *et al*. Cutting edge: cross-regulation by TLR4 and T cell Ig mucin-3 determines sex differences in inflammatory heart disease. *J Immunol* 2007;**178**:6710–14.

41. Li K, Xu W, Guo Q, *et al*. Differential macrophage polarization in male and female BALB/c mice infected with coxsackievirus B3 defines susceptibility to viral myocarditis. *Circ Res* 2009;**105**:353–64.

42. Liu L, Yue Y, Xiong S. NK-derived IFN-γ/IL-4 triggers the sexually disparate polarization of macrophages in CVB3-induced myocarditis. *J Mol Cell Cardiol* 2014;**76**:15–25.

43. Frisancho-Kiss S, Nyland JF, Davis SE, *et al*. Cutting edge: T cell Ig mucin-3 reduces inflammatory heart disease by increasing CTLA-4 during innate immunity. *J Immunol* 2006;**176**:6411–15.

44. Lauer B, Niederau C, Kuhl U, *et al*. Cardiac troponin T in patients with clinically suspected myocarditis. *J Am Coll Cardiol* 1997;**30**:1354–9.

45. Cooper LT, Baughman KL, Feldman AM, *et al*., American Heart Association, American College of Cardiology, European Society of Cardiology, Heart Failure Society of America, Heart Failure Association of the European Society of Cardiology. The role of endomyocardial biopsy in the management of cardiovascular disease: a scientific statement from the American Heart Association, the American College of Cardiology, and the European Society of Cardiology. Endorsed by the Heart Failure Society of America and the Heart Failure Association of the European Society of Cardiology. *J Am Coll Cardiol* 2007;**50**:1914–31.

46. Matsumori A, Yutani C, Ikeda Y, Kawai S, Sasayama S. Hepatitis C virus from the hearts of patients with myocarditis and cardiomyopathy. *Lab Invest* 2000;**80**:1137–42.

47. Omura T, Yoshiyama M, Hayashi T, *et al*. Core protein of hepatitis C virus induces cardiomyopathy. *Circ Res* 2005;**96**:148–50.

48. Cohen JI, Corey GR. Cytomegalovirus infection in the normal host. *Medicine (Baltimore)* 1985;**64**:100–14.

49. McCrohon JA, Moon JC, Prasad SK, *et al*. Differentiation of heart failure related to dilated cardiomyopathy and coronary artery disease using gadolinium-enhanced cardiovascular magnetic resonance. *Circulation* 2003;**108**:54–9.

50. Basso C, Carturan E, Corrado D, Thiene G. Myocarditis and dilated cardiomyopathy in athletes: diagnosis, management, and recommendations for sport activity. *Cardiol Clin* 2007;**25**:423–9, vi.

51. Pelliccia A, Fagard R, Bjørnstad HH, *et al*., Study Group of Sports Cardiology of the Working Group of Cardiac Rehabilitation and Exercise Physiology; Working Group of Myocardial and Pericardial Diseases of the European Society of Cardiology. Recommendations for competitive sports participation in athletes with cardiovascular disease: a consensus document from the Study Group of Sports Cardiology of the Working Group of Cardiac Rehabilitation and Exercise Physiology and the Working Group of Myocardial and Pericardial Diseases of the European Society of Cardiology. *Eur Heart J* 2005;**26**:1422–45.

52. Kuhl U, Lassner D, Wallaschek N, *et al*. Chromosomally integrated human herpesvirus 6 in heart failure: prevalence and treatment. *Eur J Heart Fail* 2015;**17**:9–19.

53. Krueger GR, Ablashi DV. Human herpesvirus-6: a short review of its biological behavior. *Intervirology* 2003;**46**:257–69.

54. Mason JW, O'Connell JB, Herskowitz A, *et al*. A clinical trial of immunosuppressive therapy for myocarditis. The Myocarditis Treatment Trial Investigators. *N Engl J Med* 1995;**333**:269–75.

11

Iatrogenic heart failure

Stuart D. Rosen and Ahmad Khwanda

δύο, ὠφελέειν, ἢ μὴ βλάπτειν
[The physician has] two [objectives]: to help and do no harm.

Introduction

Hippocrates is credited with the succinct and timeless advice to the physician noted above and often referred to as 'first do no harm'. In this chapter we explore a number of areas in which the physician, albeit full of good intention, pursues a reasonable course of treatment, often for non-cardiological disease, and yet causes harm to the heart. We do not explore the issues of medical error, poor standards of care, or negligent practice.

There are a number of reasons why the heart might be more prone to adverse effects of treatment than some other organs. These include the fact that the heart has no 'let up'; it has to work continuously through life and its consumption of energy is prodigious, rendering it susceptible to particular stresses, such as the action of free radicals especially affecting processes involving cellular energetics. The heart is often subject to mechanical stresses and pressure overload[1] (for example, in hypertension) which evoke hypertrophic responses that, over time, prove maladaptive. There are also the reactions of the heart to metabolic stress[2] such as in diabetes (in addition to the accelerated vascular degeneration and increased risk of coronary heart disease in diabetes). Finally, a further fascinating expression of heart injury/acute dysfunction is that of takotsubo cardiomyopathy,[3] the precise mechanisms(s) for which are yet to be universally agreed, but which may include mediation through the unique and complex innervation that the heart receives from the brain.[4]

The definition of cardiotoxicity is itself controversial.[5] In the context of cancer treatment[6], an expert consensus statement defined cancer therapeutics-related cardiac dysfunction as a decrease in left ventricular ejection fraction (LVEF) of >10%, to an EF <53%, confirmed by repeat imaging. Further characterization was to be based on symptoms. For the purposes of this chapter, we are considering direct myocardial toxicity only, not indirect effects such as serotonin-mediated valve damage.

The overall incidence of serious, validated cases of drug-induced cardiomyopathy (DICM) is quite low, of the order of 180 cases per 100 000 cases of all adverse drug reaction cases reported to the French PharmacoVigilance Databases.[7] In Montastruc *et al.*'s series, most cases were attributable to drug categories that had DICM as a known potential side-effect, such as the anthracyclines or certain antivirals. More recently, a systematic review and pooled analysis by Albakri examined both the prevalence of drug-related cardiotoxicity and, significantly, the methods used to detect it.[8]

Acute heart failure

Iatrogenic acute heart failure typically occurs, even in the absence of pre-existing heart disease, in three scenarios:

Excessive intravenous fluid administration

Over-zealous administration of intravenous fluids remains an important problem and can seriously complicate the management of medical and surgical cases. Lack of attention to both the volume of fluids and their composition has been lamented by several authors. The UK's National Confidential Enquiry into Patient Outcome and Death, an independent group which maintains and improves standards of care by undertaking confidential surveys on patient management, found the prevalence of mismanagement in fluid administration to be up to 20% of all patients managed on surgical wards.[9-11] The National Institute for Health and Clinical Excellence in the UK has formulated guidelines on more thoughtful usage, emphasizing the '5 Rs': Resuscitation, Routine maintenance, Replacement, Redistribution, and Reassessment, as well as careful choice of fluid composition, to avoid, for example, hyperchloraemic acidosis.[12]

Use of cardio-depressant drugs

A large number of commonly prescribed drugs can depress cardiac function acutely, even in the absence of overt heart disease.[13] These include β-blockers, calcium channel blockers, anti-arrhythmic drugs (disopyramide, flecainide, amiodarone, and especially dronedarone), anaesthetic agents,[14] both local (quinidine, procainamide, lidocaine) and general (etomidate, propofol); analgesics (fentanyl); and centrally acting sympatholytic agents (clonidine, α-methyl-DOPA). In all these cases the effects are fairly predictable and will wear off with removal of the offending agent. In some instances, when the

drug is an antagonist of a particular receptor or ion channel, the effect can be reversed (e.g. by inotropes or intravenous calcium).

Chronic use of inotropic agents

A number of drugs can cause an unpredictable cardiomyopathy, sometimes presenting as an acute episode, with or without chest pain, but with patency of the epicardial coronary arteries at angiography. This is the so-called takotsubo cardiomyopathy (TCM), first described in 1991 by Dote and colleagues.[15] The condition was named after the shape of the affected left ventricle, which on imaging resembles a Japanese octopus trap, with a round bottom and a narrow neck. TCM is characterized by reversible impairment of systolic function, particularly the mid and apical segments of the left ventricle. Although symptoms typically have been reported in the context of emotional or physical stress, with sudden onset chest pain, ST segment elevation, and a rise in troponin, some cases are triggered by specific drugs.[16]

There seems to be a key role for catecholamines in the aetiology of TCM: some patients who present with this form of myocardial infarction have very high catecholamine levels, and ultrastructural changes seen in patients with TCM closely resemble those in animal models of cardiac tissue with prolonged exposure to elevated catecholamine levels (**Figure 11.1**).[17–19]

Adrenaline has a more pronounced effect than noradrenaline, perhaps related to a switch of the intracellular signalling cascade after adrenaline stimulation. Supraphysiological doses of adrenaline exert paradoxically negative inotropic effects, as the stimulating G_s protein second messenger is switched to an inhibiting G_i protein ('stimulus trafficking').

Most of the published papers on drug-related TCM are case reports rather than quantitative studies. However, three sets of circumstances are associated with TCM. Dobutamine infusion can cause clear-cut cases of TCM, assumed to be mediated directly through β_1 stimulation. In the case of adrenaline, the effect may or may not be compounded by microvascular constriction, adding ischaemia to the mix. A similar effect can be achieved by ephedrine and its derivatives.

Several drugs act *indirectly* to elicit a sympathomimetic response. Through withdrawal of parasympathetic input, atropine enhances sympathetic drive with consequences in terms of TCM. Duloxetine, nortriptyline and the major antidepressant venlafaxine block reuptake of catecholamines ('uptake-1'), thereby increasing the local concentration of adrenaline, noradrenaline, dopamine, and serotonin.

A third category of drug exerts more direct effects on cardiomyocytes, probably through a combination of positive inotropy and chronotropy, plus microvascular constriction. The phosphodiesterase III inhibitor anagrelide, used in the treatment of essential thrombocythaemia, is such a drug. Others are the anticancer drugs 5-fluorouracil, the pro-drug combretastatin, and pazopanib, discussed at greater length in the next section.

Chronic heart failure

Treatments for cancer

The presentation of cardiac injury can be considerably delayed after cancer treatment. With growing attention to 'survivorship',[20] the cruel irony of death from progressive heart failure is especially poignant after childhood cancers. This is one of several factors that has led to the rise of the relatively new interdisciplinary topic of cardio-oncology (www.BC-OS.org).

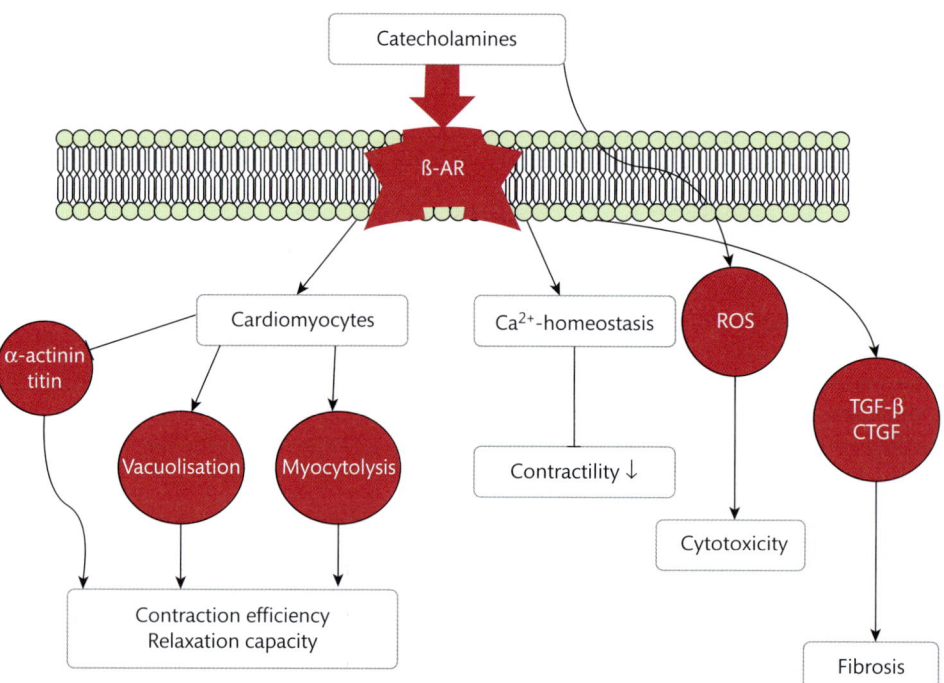

Figure 11.1 Catecholamine-mediated effects in the pathogenesis of stress cardiomyopathy. β-AR, β-adrenoceptors; ROS, reactive oxygen species; TGF-β, transforming growth factor-β; CTGF, connective tissue growth factor.

There are many mechanisms through which chemotheraputic agents can affect the heart; but within this chapter, the focus will be upon cardiomyopathy only. Reflecting the clinical importance and the scale of cardiomyopathic consequences, our discussion will start with anthracyclines and then continue with trastuzumab before a broader discussion.

Anthracyclines

The 1960s saw the introduction of anthracyclines, specifically daunorubicin and doxorubicin (Figure 11.2), for the treatment of range of solid and invasive tumours (breast, kidney, bladder, bone, ovary), leukaemias, and lymphomas. The anti-tumour activity of anthracyclines is achieved through several mechanisms. All anthracyclines undergo proteosome-mediated transport to the cell nucleus after entering the cell via the multidrug resistance pore. The drug then intercalates into nuclear DNA, impairing transcription and protein synthesis; there is inhibition of topoisomerase II, blocking repair of disrupted DNA strands; and promoting production of reactive oxygen species (ROS). ROS cause further oxidative injury to DNA, cell membranes, and mitochondria; and mediate activation of protein p53, which fixes to DNA and promotes transcription of the gene coding for Bax. The latter opens the mitochondrial pore, releasing cytochrome c which can initiate cellular apoptosis.[21,22]

Cardiotoxicity of anthracyclines

The efficacy of anthracyclines was rapidly apparent, but within less than a decade it was evident that patients could develop serious impairment of ventricular function, broadly in relation to the cumulative dose of anthracycline.[23] This is true for all the anthracyclines and anthracycline-like drugs (including daunorubicin, epirubicin, mitoxantrone, and others) and applies to all circumstances of administration of the drugs, whether neoadjuvant (e.g. pre-surgical treatment), adjuvant for the primary tumour, or for metastatic disease.

Molecular mechanisms of anthracycline-induced cardiomyopathy

Some of the processes that mediate the anti-tumour action of these drugs are the very cause of their cardiotoxicity. Cardiomyocytes are full of mitochondria and several mechanisms of action of anthracyclines impact on mitochondrial function, through direct and indirect routes.

In terms of direct toxicity, the induction of oxidative stress and apoptosis[24] are key. When anthracyclines bind with DNA, reactive

electrons are released which are ultimately transferred to generate superoxide ions by NAD(P)H oxidase. Superoxide and aglycone metabolites of anthracyclines bind to membranes, causing lipid peroxidation, with further ROS production. Cardiomyocytes are highly susceptible to the actions of ROS as they tend to lack ROS-detoxifying enzymes such as catalase. The importance of oxidative stress is supported by the observation that the mitochondria of transgenic mice that overexpress superoxide dismutase show enhanced resistance to anthracylines, as do mice that are knockouts for the NAD(P)H oxidase gene.[25]

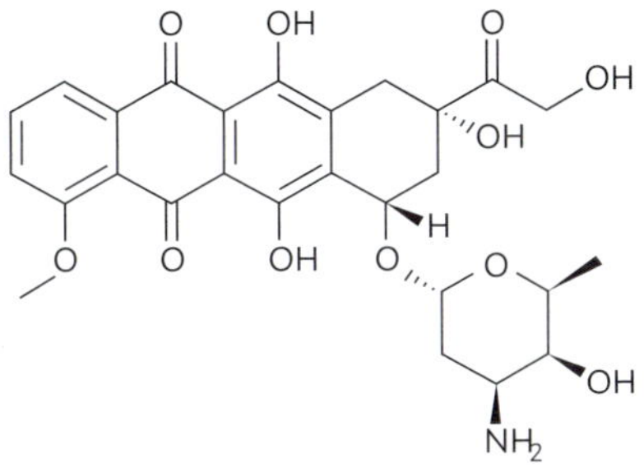

One of the consequences of oxidative stress is apoptosis. The superoxide generation stimulates the p53-mediated expression of Bax, which initiates apoptosis cascades. Preventing the cascades with pifithrin-α (an inhibitor of p53 and its receptor gene *Ba*) or GATA-4 (a transcriptional activator of Bcl-XL) protects cardiomyocytes from doxorubicin-induced apoptosis. These mechanisms are well summarized by Khouri *et al.*[26] (Figure 11.3).

Besides the above mechanisms, other processes, including Top2β-independent mechanisms of ROS production, are important, such as metabolic dysregulation (through anthracycline binding to cardiolipin; down-modulation of carnitine palmitoyl transferase leading to decreased β-oxidation and increased glycolysis); iron accumulation; calcium homeostasis dysregulation; and altered autophagy. These aspects have been excellently addressed by Muratibo *et al.*[27] (Figure 11.4).

In addition to apoptosis, other routes to cell death are highly significant, e.g. autophagy, necrosis, necroptosis, pyroptosis, and ferroptosis. These feature in discussions of pathophysiology of cardiotoxicity of several drugs but in general the categories have been most closely studied for anthracyclines.[28]

Ultrastructural changes after anthracyclines

A particular feature of anthracycline-induced cardiomyopathy is the intracellular ultrastructural changes including vacuolation, swelling, and fragmentation of mitochondrial cristae. A number of other ultrastructural changes typically occur in the myocyte, including loss of myofibrils, deformation of the nucleus, and dilation of the sarcoplasmic reticulum.[22]

Risk factors for anthracycline cardiomyopathy

Besides general risk factors for development of heart failure,[29] there are particular patients who are at increased risk of underlying anthracycline-induced cardiac toxicity (Box 11.1).[30]

Reducing the risk of anthracycline-induced chemotherapy

There are several models that can be used to compute risk; these are considered in detail elsewhere.[5]

In adults as well as children, the risk of cardiotoxicity may be higher than previously imagined, even at doses of anthracyclines that were previously considered safe, e.g. in the range 240–350 mg/m².

The method of administration may also be relevant to risk, with infusions of anthracyclines likely to be safer than boluses.[31] Enclosing the drug in liposomes may be advantageous.[32] The anthracyclines, such as epirubicin, may have a reduced risk of cardiomyopathy.[33] Several agents have been suggested as cardioprotective agents;[34] of these, dexrazoxane has shown the greatest promise.[35] The latter is

Figure 11.2 Molecular structure of doxorubicin.

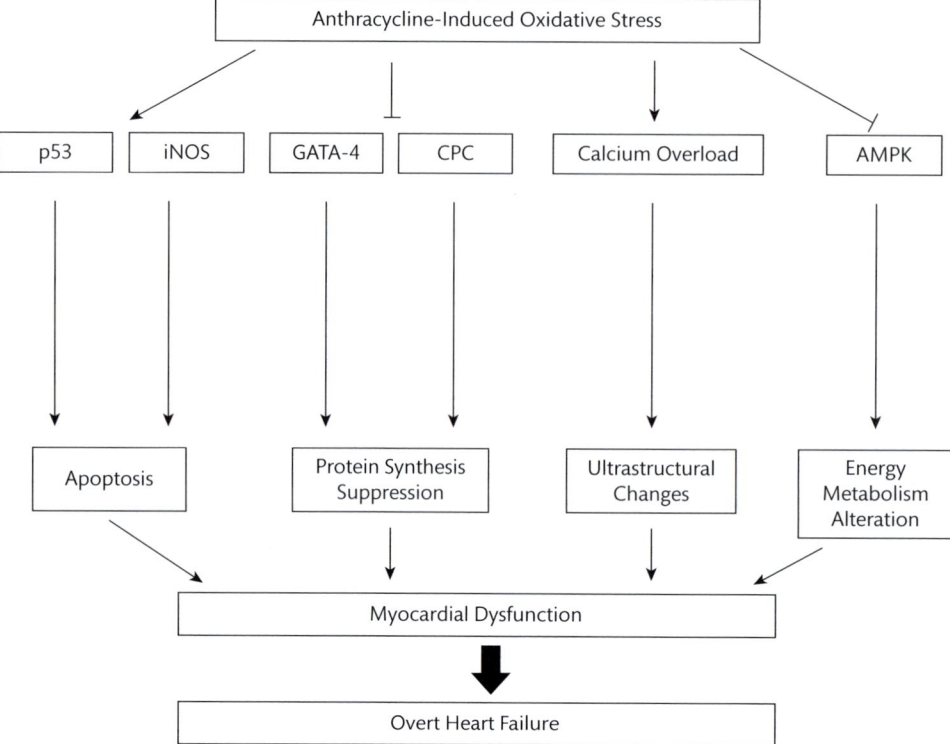

Figure 11.3 Mechanisms underlying anthracycline-induced cardiac toxicity.
Reproduced from Scott JM et al. Anthracycline-induced generation of oxidative stress is a central mediator of accelerated myofilament apoptosis via upregulation of the p53 pathway and inducible nitric oxide synthase (iNOS), suppression of myofilament protein synthesis via inhibition of cardiac progenitor cells (CPCs) and GATA-4, calcium overload resulting in ultrastructural changes to myocytes, and alterations in cardiac energy metabolism via downregulation of AMP-activated protein kinase (AMPK). These changes lead to myocardial dysfunction and ultimately heart failure. [Adapted from Scott et al.[141,142,143]].

licensed in the British National and European Formularies as an iron chelator but several other studies have examined its particular role with anthracyclines through, for example, its forming a tight complex with the ATPase domain of Top2α and Top2β (Figure 11.4).[27]

Cardiotoxicity of anthracyclines in childhood

Higher-dose anthracyclines (cumulative dose of up to 550 mg/m²) have increased the five-year survival in acute lymphoblastic leukaemia from <10% to >80% in the last three decades. However, several studies[36–38] of children treated for haematological malignancies have shown that, over the longer term, at least half develop systolic

and diastolic abnormalities, demonstrable by echocardiography or multi-gated radionuclide ventriculography (MUGA). It must be noted, though, that most of these data are derived from retrospective cross-sectional studies, with substantial variation in rates of subclinical cardiac impairment. For example, the incidence of overt heart failure varied from zero to 16% in 30 studies published between 1966 and 2000. In a single-site study, clinical congestive heart failure was reported in 8% of children after one year, in another 2.8% at six years, and a further 5% after 15 years for children treated between 1976 and 1997 with a cumulative dose of doxorubicin >300 mg/m². Even for the supposedly safe cumulative doxorubicin dose

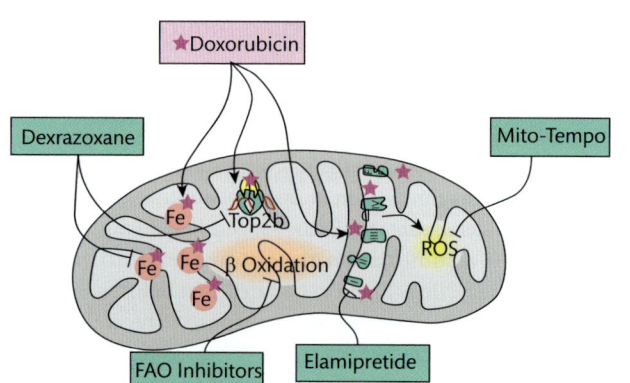

Figure 11.4 Effects of doxorubicin and of mitochondria-targeted drugs on mitochondrial function and metabolism.

of <300 mg/m², a study of 116 children followed up for a mean of 8.2 years after treatment for acute lymphoblastic leukaemia showed a substantial incidence of significantly reduced left ventricular wall thickness and increased left ventricular end-diastolic diameter compared with age-matched controls (**Figure 11.5**).

Clearly, as the numbers of children successfully treated for cancer rises steadily, the number at risk of heart failure will also increase and the need for prevention is very pressing.

Presentations of anthracycline cardiomyopathy in adults

The information on anthracycline-induced cardiomyopathy in adults is again mostly based on retrospective studies. However, apart from a very small number of cases of acute heart failure (which occur extremely early and are probably an idiosyncratic reaction), there are two particular clinical pictures of cardiotoxicity due to anthracyclines: early onset, chronic progressive, and late onset chronic progressive dysfunction. The former, which accounts for the majority of cases of anthracycline cardiotoxicity,[39] is an acute, dose-dependent form of cardiomyopathy occurring, in several historical series, in 1.6–2.1% of patients treated. The late onset presentation, which might not appear for several years, probably affects 1.6–5% of treated patients (**Figure 11.6**).

There is a wide range of effects of anthracyclines on the myocardium, from no detectable effect through subclinical diastolic dysfunction, asymptomatic LV systolic dysfunction and, finally, more severe expressions of symptomatic LV systolic dysfunction (ranging in turn from reversible heart failure to severe, irreversible dysfunction resulting in a death from heart failure) (**Figure 11.7**). In the first large prospective series of cases reported, Cardinale and colleagues followed a 'heterogeneous cohort' of 2625 patients receiving chemotherapy regimes that included anthracyclines, over a median five-year period.[39,40] The overall incidence of cardiotoxicity (defined as LVEF decrease >10 absolute points, and overall LVEF <50%), was 9% (n = 226). In 98% of these cases (n = 221), cardiotoxicity occurred within the first year, mean 3.5 months from the onset of treatment. Overall, end-chemotherapy LVEF and cumulative doxorubicin dose were independent correlates of cardiotoxicity. Of particular interest is the fact that recovery from cardiotoxicity was achieved in 25 (11%) patients who had full recovery and in 160 (71%) patients had partial recovery (LVEF increase >5 absolute points and to an overall LVEF >50%).

The prevalence of diastolic changes is substantial and prospective data to relate the changes in diastolic function to subsequent heart failure are starting to emerge.[41]

Overall, patients should be assessed before, during, and after chemotherapy with a combination of careful clinical assessment, sophisticated imaging,[42] and judicious application of biomarker results (especially troponin and B-type natriuretic peptide (BNP).

Trastuzumab cardiomyopathy

The monoclonal antibody trastuzumab (Herceptin) is an anti-growth factor agent and is usually used in patients who overexpress the *human epidermal growth factor receptor 2* (*HER2/ErbB2*) oncogene. The latter is a member of the ErbB-like oncogene family, which is amplified from 2- to 20-fold in 30% of patients with breast cancer.[43] HER2/ErbB2 has a protective role in myocardial stress.[44] Blocking

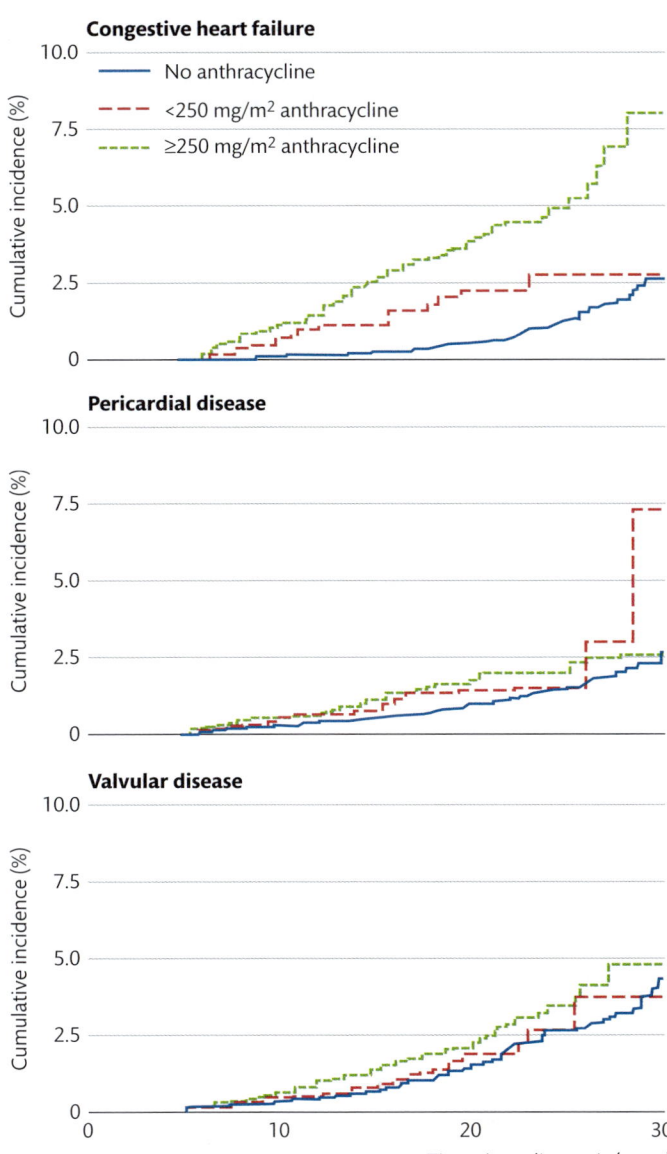

Figure 11.5 Cumulative incidence of cardiac disorder in children surviving cancers treated with anthracyclines, according to dose.
Source data from Mulrooney DA, Yeazel MW, Toana K, *et al.* Cardiac outcomes in a cohort of adult survivors of childhood and adolescent cancer: retrospective analysis of the Childhood Cancer Survivor Study cohort. *Br Med J* 2009;**339**:b4606.

the HER2 receptor increases the apoptotic response to cytotoxics. In practice,[45,46] trastuzumab is used in an adjuvant capacity, administered intravenously in cycles of therapy over a year.

In well-selected patients, there is an approximately 25% reduction in mortality with trastuzumab alone and yet greater effectiveness when trastuzumab is combined with an anthracycline or taxane. Besides trastuzumab's use in breast cancer—and about ten times as many patients are being treated now compared to a decade ago—there are potentially new indications for its use—for example, gastric stromal cell cancer.

Trastuzumab cardiotoxicity—molecular mechanisms

HER2 is essential for cardiomyocyte survival and stress adaptation.[47] The cardiomyocyte survival pathway is activated by

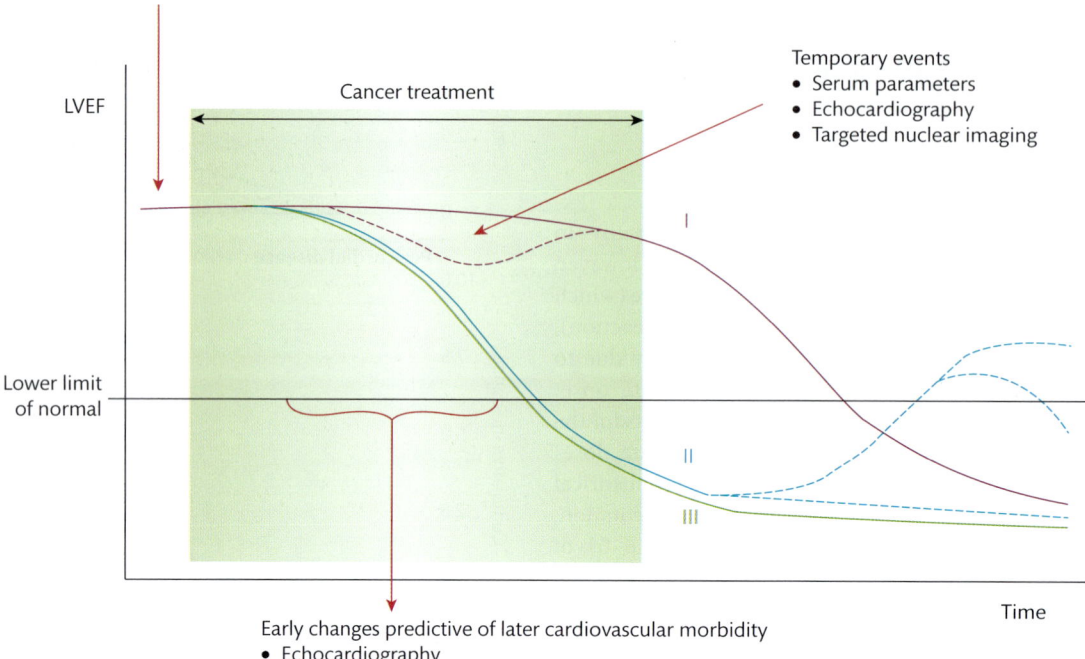

Baseline risk
- Genetic susceptibility
- Pre-existing risk factors for cardiovascular disease
- Factors associated with an increased risk for treatment-induced toxicity

Cancer treatment

LVEF

Temporary events
- Serum parameters
- Echocardiography
- Targeted nuclear imaging

Lower limit of normal

Time

Early changes predictive of later cardiovascular morbidity
- Echocardiography
- Targeted nuclear imaging
- Cardiac MRI

(I) Late onset cardiotoxicity (radiotherapy, anthracyclines);[16,17] (II) reversible cardiotoxicity (trastuzumab: dotted line indicates long-term consequences are still unknown);[18] (III) irreversible cardiotoxicity during treatment (anthracyclines);[16,19]

Figure 11.6 Left ventricular function and timing of detection of screening strategies during and after cancer treatment.
Reproduced from Altena R, Perik PJ, van Veldhuisen DJ, de Vries EG, Gietema JA. Cardiovascular toxicity caused by cancer treatment: strategies for early detection. *Lancet Oncol* 2009;10:391–399 with permission from Elsevier.

neuregulin, a paracrine peptide messenger that activates HER2, preventing death of the cardiomyocytes. Deletion or mutation of the *HER* gene is associated with dilated cardiomyopathy. Trastuzumab can thus cause cardiomyocyte toxicity via its effects on several signalling pathways—suppression of myofilament protein synthesis via the PI3K–Akt pathway, suppression of protein hypertrophy via the mitogen-activated protein kinase (MAPK) pathway, suppression of cell survival via the Src/Fak pathway, and upregulation of protein degradation via FOXO signalling (**Figure 11.8**).

Trastuzumab—clinical studies

The incidence of significant LV dysfunction associated with trastuzumab treatment ranges from 5.1%[48] to >15%,[49] although the incidence of later cardiac dysfunction is lower, of the order of 6%.[50]

The use of trastuzumab and anthracycline together causes impaired systolic function in a quarter of patients over three years. Trastuzumab therapy is associated with frequent (>40%), mild, mostly asymptomatic cardiac dysfunction which generally occurs after pretreatment with anthracyclines.[51] Overall, although the incidence of trastuzumab cardiomyopathy is substantially higher than that due to anthracyclines, it is generally reversible within months

on discontinuation of therapy, is not associated with ultrastructural changes, and carries a good prognosis.[52]

Anthracyclines plus trastuzumab

For many patients, especially those with metastatic breast disease, anthracycline therapy will already have been given, but the severity and/or extent of the underlying disease means that they will need to proceed to secondary treatment with trastuzumab, either as a direct treatment or in an adjuvant role. Treatments given in series in this way constitute a 'two hit' sequence in which anthracyclines induce the cardiac stress pathways, and then trastuzumab inhibits the HER2 receptor, interfering with this survival signalling pathway and promoting cardiotoxicity. In mice deficient in HER2 protein or its associated ligand, neuregulin, the induction of cardiac stress pathways by anthracycline promotes the onset of LV dysfunction.[40]

Anthracycline-type cardiomyopathy (type 1) thus differs from that associated with trastuzumab (type 2)[44,53] (**Figure 11.9**). However, clinical cases do not neatly divide into one of these two categories, with some cases of trastuzumab cardiomyopathy proving irreversible. In practice, few patients will have only been treated with only one category of drug, so there is a potential type 1/type 2 overlap,

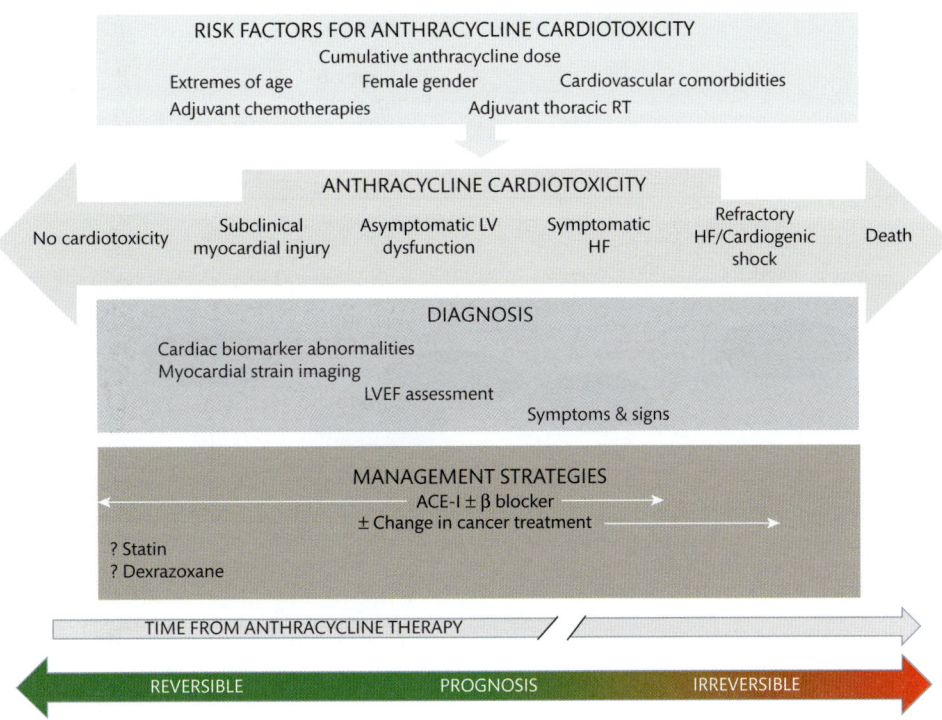

Figure 11.7 The continuum of myocardial response to anthracycline therapy.
Reproduced from Groarke JD, Nohria A. Anthacycline cardiotoxicity: A new paradigm for an old classic. *Circulation* 2015;**131**:1946–1949 with permission from Wolters Kluwer.

Other HER2-targeted anticancer therapies

Pertuzumab, in combination with trastuzumab and docetaxel, is licensed as a treatment of breast cancer (neoadjuvant or metastatic disease); it is a monoclonal antibody that inhibits dimerization of HER2 with other HER2 receptors. The combination of two anti-HER2 drugs appears to improve response rates without additional cardiotoxicity.[54] A conjugate drug, combining trastuzumab with the cytotoxic agent DM1, is effective in the neoadjuvant and metastatic disease settings, with an incidence of LV systolic dysfunction of 2–3%.[55]

Alkylating agents

Cyclophosphamide, a nitrogen mustard-type alkylating agent first synthesized in the 1950s, is frequently used in the treatment of lymphoma, leukaemia, some types of brain tumour, and a number of other solid tumours. As an alkylating agent, the drug attaches an alkyl group to the guanine base of DNA, interfering with DNA replication by forming DNA crosslinks. The latter are irreversible and lead to cell apoptosis. Cyclophosphamide also appears to induce immunomodulatory effects.[56]

Cyclophosphamide can cause cardiotoxicity via direct endothelial injury followed by extravasation of toxic metabolites, interstitial haemorrhage, and oedema, giving a histopathological appearance of haemorrhagic myocarditis.[48] The incidence of heart failure associated with the use of cyclophosphamide is between 7% and 28%. The cardiotoxicity risk appears, like that of anthracyclines, to be dose-related (being much higher after >150 mg/kg and 1.5 g/m^2/day), but to manifest itself early—within 10 days of the first dose. The risk of toxicity is greater with concomitant use of anthracyclines, mitoxantrone, or radiotherapy.[47,57]

Ifosfamide has a similar molecular structure and is of value in the treatment of testicular cancer, sarcomas (soft tissue and bone sarcomas), and some types of lymphoma. Its cardiotoxic effects seem similar to those of cyclophosphamide, although histopathological changes have not been reported. There is, though, a dose relationship for cardiotoxicity (>12.5 g/m^2).

Tyrosine kinase inhibitors and immunomodulatory therapies—targeted molecular therapy

Targeted molecular cancer therapy comprises a number of treatments employing molecules which, according to the National Cancer Institute *Dictionary of Cancer Terms*, operate via 'Interference with specific targeted molecules needed for carcinogenesis and tumour growth'. The term is often used synonymously with 'biological therapy' and includes immunomodulators. Among the numerous molecular pathways that are predicated upon a complex interacting set of kinases (termed the 'kinome' by Force[58,59] (**Figure 11.10**), several are involved in carcinogenesis through three phases: (i) mutation or overexpression of molecular factors leading to (ii) increased proliferation, angiogenesis, inhibition of apoptosis, generating (iii) a malignant phenotype.

Conversely, the therapeutic mechanisms of targeted molecular cancer drugs include inhibition of cell proliferation, inhibition of cell migration, reduction in cell survival (resistance to apoptosis), and inhibition of differentiation (e.g. angiogenesis).

However, as is also evident in **Figure 11.10**, several kinases are also signalling pathways intrinsic to cardiomyocyte function as well, such as:

- angiogenesis
- hypertrophy

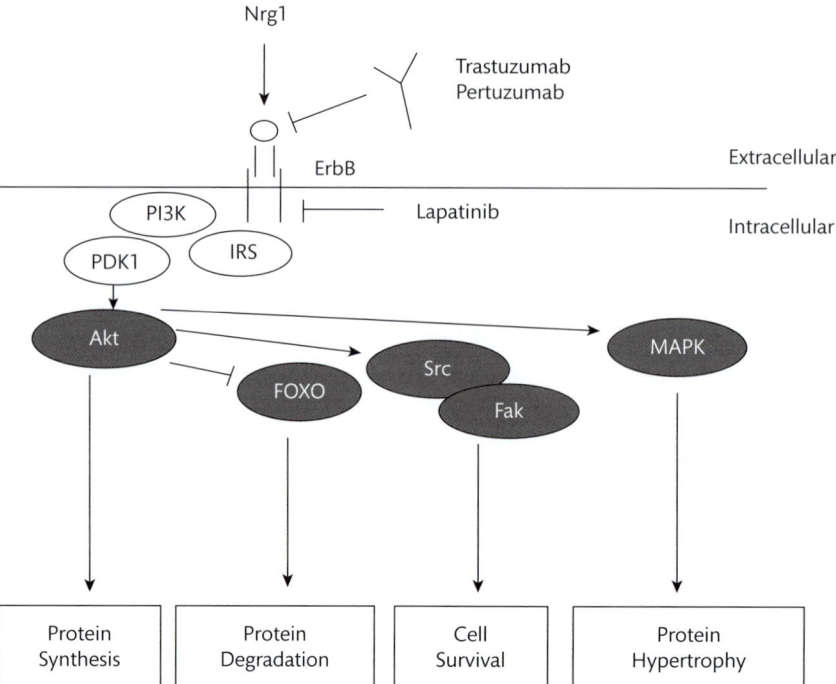

Figure 11.8 Mechanisms underlying molecularly targeted therapeutics-induced cardiac toxicity.
Reproduced from Khouri MG, Douglas PS, Mackey JR. Cancer therapy-induced cardiac toxicity in early breast cancer. *Circulation* 2012;**126**:2749–2763 with permission from Wolters Kluwer.

- energetics
- mitochondrial integrity
- cell survival
- migration
- apoptosis
- proliferation
- protein folding
- lipid synthesis
- calcium cycling.

Interference with these pathways may therefore have manifold effects on the cardiovascular system in general—especially in causing hypertension, the commonest adverse effect—but also causing asymptomatic and symptomatic ventricular dysfunction.

The risk factor profile for tyrosine kinase inhibitors is described in Table 11.1.

Immune checkpoint inhibitors

T lymphocytes include subsets which express checkpoint proteins including PD-1, that acts as an 'off switch' preventing the T cells from attacking other cells in the body. This is mediated by attachment to PD-L1, a protein expressed on some normal and malignant cells. Particular cancer cells express large amounts of PD-L1, assisting their avoidance of immune attack. Monoclonal antibodies that target either PD-1 or PD-L1 can block such binding and thereby boost the immune response against cancer cells.

PD-1 inhibitors include pembrolizumab and nivolumab; PD-L1 inhibitors include atezolizumab, avelumab, and durvalumab. CTLA-4 is another T-cell 'off switch', whose inhibitors include ipilimumab.

Table 11.1 Risk factors for cardiovascular complications with tyrosine kinase inhibitor therapy

Agent	Risk factors
Anti-HER2 compounds	

• Antibodies
  – Trastuzumab
  – Pertuzumab
  – T-DM1
• Tyrosine kinase inhibitor
  – Lapatinib
	• Previous or concomitant anthracycline treatment (short time between anthracycline and anti-HER 2 treatment)
	• Age (>65 years)
	• High BMI >30 kg/mg²
	• Previous LV dysfunction
	• Arterial hypertension
	• Previous radiation therapy

VEGF inhibitors	
• Antibodies • Bevacizumab • Ramucirumab	Pre-existing HF, significant CAD or left side VHD (e.g. mitral regurgitation), chronic ischaemic cardiomyopathy • Previous anthracycline
• Tyrosine kinase inhibitors • Sunitinib • Pazopanib • Axitinib • Neratinib • Afatinib • Sorafenib • Dasatinib	

BMI, body mass index; VEGF, vascular endothelial growth factor; HF, heart failure; CAD, coronary artery disease; VHD, valvular heart disease.

Reproduced from Zamorano JL, Lancellotti P, Rodriguez Muñoz D, *et al.*; ESC Scientific Document Group. 2016 ESC Position Paper on cancer treatments and cardiovascular toxicity developed under the auspices of the ESC Committee for Practice Guidelines: The Task Force for cancer treatments and cardiovascular toxicity of the European Society of Cardiology (ESC). *Eur Heart J* 2016 Sep 21;**37**(36):2768–2801. doi: 10.1093/eurheartj/ehw211. Epub 2016 Aug 26 with permission from Oxford University Press.

These drugs have been highly effective in the treatment of several cancers, especially melanoma, renal cell carcinoma and, to an extent, lung cancer.

There are important cases of cardiotoxicity associated with immune checkpoint inhibitors (ICIs). Several mechanisms may be involved—inflammatory cardiotoxicity; myocarditis; perimyocarditis; pericarditis; LV dysfunction without myocarditis; non-inflammation-mediated cardiotoxicity; asymptomatic non-inflammatory LV dysfunction; takotsubo-like syndrome with both basal and apical variants; coronary vasospasm; arrhythmias; and myocardial infarction. Of these, myocarditis is the most common cardiotoxic reaction and carries a high mortality.

Myocarditis in patients treated with immune checkpoint inhibitors has a prevalence of just over 1%; median time of onset 34 days (21–75) after starting ICI; there is a greater risk if drugs are used in combination.[60,61] There is a fourfold increase in risk if troponin T levels are >1.5 ng/mL. Significantly, high-dose steroids are effective; the key clinical issue is to recognize the diagnosis—cardiac magnetic resonance (CMR) imaging is hugely valuable in this regard—and move rapidly to treat. **Figure 11.11** summarizes the work-up.

CAR-T cell therapy

Among the most recent developments in cancer immunotherapy, the genetic engineering of chimeric antigen receptor T cells (CAR-T cells) holds tremendous promise in the treatment of some relapsing and refractory leukaemias and lymphomas. It is likely that despite the promise, a 'weather eye' will need to be kept on patients treated with CAR-T because of the small but crucial possibility of cardiotoxicity, either through direct immune-mediated injury to cardiomyocytes, or with the heart an innocent bystander to the effects of a cytokine storm.[62]

Other anticancer agents

Many other anticancer agents are associated with damage to the heart (**Table 11.2**) and there are several excellent references.[1,28]

Radiation and the heart

There are several cancers for which radiotherapy to the chest is key to treatment; these include Hodgkin's lymphoma, breast cancer, lung cancer, and oesophageal cancer.

Radiation-induced heart disease is mediated through direct and indirect routes, but the time-courses are long (**Figure 11.12**).

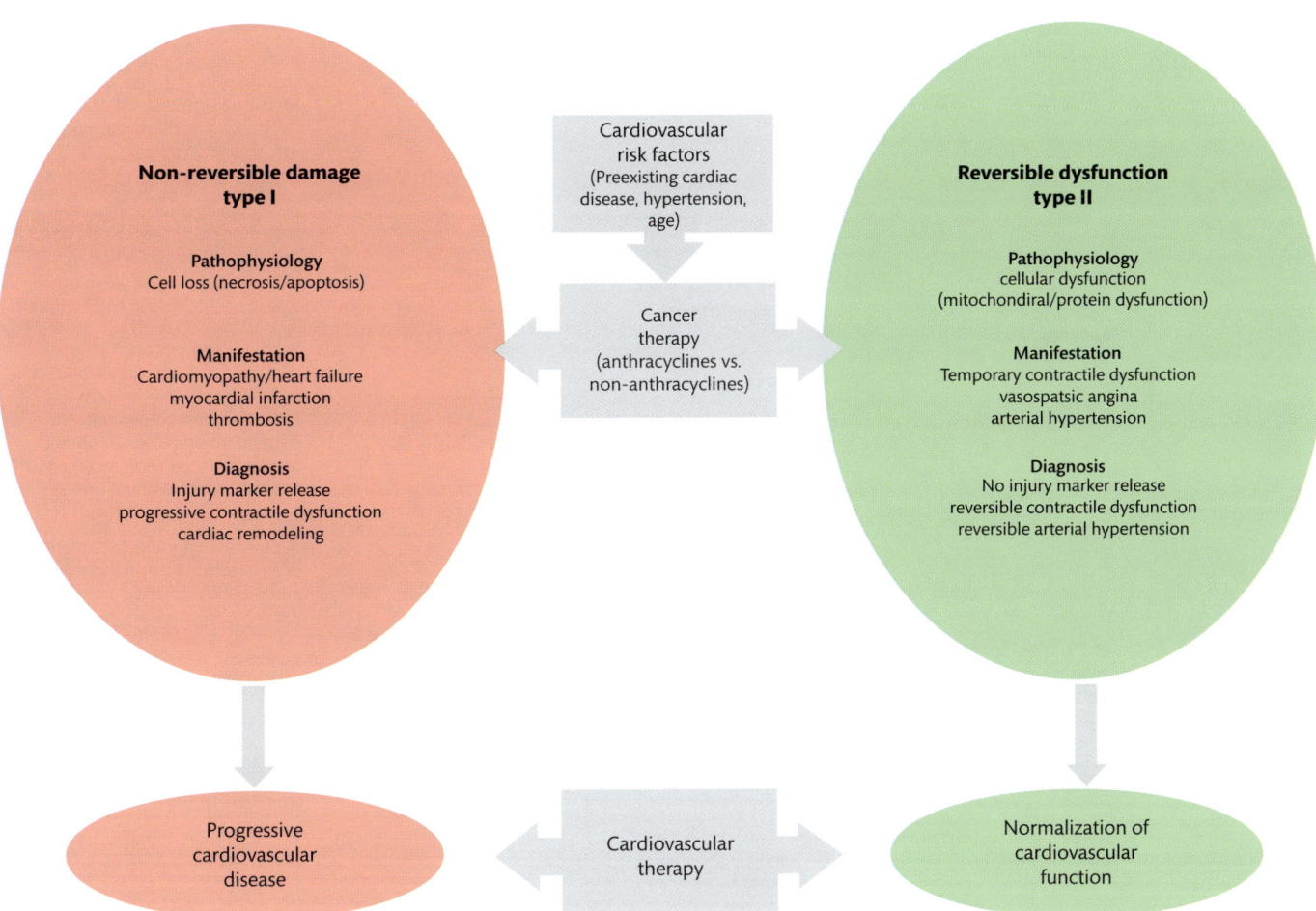

Figure 11.9 Type 1 vs type 2 cardiac response to chemotherapy.

Reproduced from Suter TM, Ewer MS. Cancer drugs and the heart: importance and management. *Eur Heart J* 2013;**34**:1102–1111 with permission from Oxford University Press.

Table 11.2 Other drugs with role in cancer therapy-related cardiomyopathy[a]

Drug	Mechanism of action on tumour	Usual tumour target	Incidence of cardiomyopathy	Mechanism of cardiomyopathy
Monoclonal antibody tyrosine kinase inhibitor (TKI) [1]				
Bevacizumab	Vascular endothelial growth factor (VEGF) inhibition	Breast (metastatic)	2.5–3.0%	'On' and 'Off target' effects of kinase inhibition
Small molecule TKIs [2–7]				
Dasatinib	Vascular endothelial growth factor (VEGF) inhibition	CML	2.0–4.0%	'On' and 'off target' effects of kinase inhibition
Imatinib	Vascular endothelial growth factor (VEGF) inhibition	Recurrent or resistant acute lymphoblastic leukaemia (ALL)	0.5%	'On' and 'off target' effects of kinase inhibition
Sunitinib	Vascular endothelial growth factor (VEGF) inhibition	Solid tumours, renal cell and gastrointestinal stromal tumour (GIST)	1.5–4.1% overt heart failure; up to 14% have >10% decline in LVEF	'On' and 'off target' effects of kinase inhibition
Sorafenib	VEGFR 2 and 3; c-kit; PDGFR-β; FLT3; RAF1, BRAF inhibition	Kidney, liver, thyroid	4–8%	Activation of the intrinsic apoptotic pathway and ATP depletion; deletion of RAF1 causing dilation, hypo-contractility, increased apoptosis and fibrosis
Lapatinib	Vascular endothelial growth factor (VEGF) inhibition; HER2 inhibition	Metastatic breast and solid tumours	1.5%	'On' and 'off target' effects of kinase inhibition
	Vascular endothelial growth factor (VEGF) inhibition	Advanced renal carcinoma and soft tissue sarcomas	Up to 7% but mild impairment of LV systolic function	'On' and 'off target' effects of kinase inhibition; catecholamine effects; modulation of NO
Dabrafenib/trametinib	BRAF/MEK inhibition	Melanoma; other solid tumours inc NSCLC	2–9%	Increase in mitochondrial permeability transition pore, increased sensitivity to calcium (Ca^{2+}) overload; overproduction of ROS; increased apoptosis.
Vemurafenib	BRAF/MEK inhibition	Melanoma; other solid tumours including NSCLC	~6%	Increase in mitochondrial permeability transition pore, increased sensitivity to calcium (Ca^{2+}) overload; overproduction of ROS; increased apoptosis
Mitoxantrone	DNA intercalation as for anthracyclines	Acute myeloid leukaemia, lymphomas, metastatic breast cancer, ovary, lung, hepatocellular	2.6%	As for anthracyclines
Bortezomib	Proteosome inhibitor	Multiple myeloma	1–5%	Inhibition of proteosomal-dependent ongoing sarcomeric protein turnover; enhancement of anthracycline toxicity
Carfilzomib	Proteosome inhibitor	Multiple myeloma	11–25%	Inhibition of proteasomal-dependent ongoing sarcomeric protein turnover; enhancement of anthracycline toxicity
Pomalidomide [8, 9,10]	Immunomodulation: inhibition of TNFα production, and enhancement of activity of T cells and natural killer cells, plus enhanced antibody-dependent cellular cytotoxicity	Relapsed/refractory myeloma Kaposi sarcoma	2% (when pre-treated with lenalidomide and bortezomib)	Off-target immunomodulatory effects
Clofarabine	Antimetabolite (purine)	Relapsed/refractory ALL in children	Transient LV dysfunction in up to 25%	Presumed off target effects on cardiomyocytes
5-Fluorouracil	Antimetabolite (thymidylate synthase inhibition)	Anal, breast, colorectal, oesophagus, stomach, pancreatic, skin and head and neck cancers	Anywhere from 1% to 68%	Vasospasm; TCM in few cases
Capecitabine	Antimetabolite	Solid tumours: breast, colon, rectum, stomach, oesophagus, pancreas	~2% for oral drug; 18% for high dose IV	Vasospasm; TCM in few cases

Table 11.2 *Continued*

Drug	Mechanism of action on tumour	Usual tumour target	Incidence of cardiomyopathy	Mechanism of cardiomyopathy
Cisplatin	Formation of DNA adducts, primarily intrastrand crosslinks that activate signal transduction pathways, involving ATR, p53, p73, MAPK, which can activate apoptosis	Solid tumours (testicular, ovarian, cervical, breast, bladder, head and neck, oesophageal, lung, mesothelioma, brain and neuroblastoma	2–8%	Oxidative and nitrosative stress
Arsenic trioxide	Down-regulation of the PML-RARα oncoprotein; induction of apoptosis	Acute promyelocytic leukaemia	1–2%	Generation of reactive oxygen species (ROS), calcium overload, inhibition of mitochondrial respiration, activation of caspase; induction of apoptosis
Lenalidomide	Direct anti-tumour effect, inhibition of angiogenesis, and immunomodulation	Multiple myeloma, lymphoma, myelodysplastic syndrome	<1%	Hypersensitivity myocarditis
Taxanes [11]				
Paclitaxel	Antimicrotubule	Metastatic breast cancer	1–2%	Direct cytotoxicity; increasing effective prevailing concentration of anthracyclines
Docetaxel	Antimicrotubule	Metastatic breast cancer	2.3–13%	Direct cytotoxicity; increasing effective prevailing concentration of anthracyclines
Vascular disrupting agents [11]				
Combretastatin [A-4 (CA-4) and A-1 (CA-1)]	Antimicrotubule	Head and neck cancers	Cases of TCM, especially with concomitant cisplatin use	Presumed off target effects on cardiomyocytes

[a] 5-Fluorouracil (5FU) and capecitabine are metabolized by dihydropyrimidine dehydrogenase (DPD). DPD deficiency is inherited as an autosomal recessive trait, although up to 8% of the population may have some degree of deficiency. People with DPD deficiency are at high risk of toxicity from 5FU and capecitabine which may manifest as severe cardiac toxicity. In clinical practice the mechanism most likely to cause cardiac symptoms is that of arterial vasoconstriction causing ischaemia and angina in 1–2% of cases.

References

[1] Valachis A, Nearchou A, Lind P, Mauri D. Lapatinib, trastuzumab or the combination added to preoperative chemotherapy for breast cancer: a meta-analysis of randomized evidence. *Breast Cancer Res Treat* 2012;**135**:655–62.

[2] Krop IE, Suter TM, Dang CT, *et al.* Feasibility and cardiac safety of trastuzumab emtansine after anthracycline-based chemotherapy as (neo)adjuvant therapy for human epidermal growth factor receptor 2-positive early-stage breast cancer. *J Clin Oncol* 2015;**33**:1136–42.

[3] Groarke JD, Choueiri TK, Slosky D, Cheng S, Moslehi J. Recognizing and managing left ventricular dysfunction associated with therapeutic inhibition of the vascular endothelial growth factor signaling pathway. *Curr Treat Options Cardiovasc Med* 2014;**16**:335.

[4] Motzer RJ, Hutson TE, Tomczak P. Sunitinib versus interferon alfa in metastatic renal-cell carcinoma. *N Engl J Med* 2007;**356**:115–24.

[5] Richards CJ, Je Y, Schutz FA. Incidence and risk of congestive heart failure in patients with renal and nonrenal cell carcinoma treated with sunitinib. *J Clin Oncol* 2011;**29**:3450–6.

[6] Hall PS, Harshman LC, Srinivas S, Witteles RM. The frequency and severity of cardiovascular toxicity from targeted therapy in advanced renal cell carcinoma patients. *J Am Coll Cardiol* 2013;**1**:72–8.

[7] Yeh ETH, Bickford CL. Cardiovascular complications of cancer therapy: Incidence pathogenesis, diagnosis and management. *J Am Coll Cardiol* 2009;**53**(24):2231–47.

[8] Tefferi A, Verstovsek S, Barosi G, *et al.* Pomalidomide is active in the treatment of anemia associated with myelofibrosis. *J Clin Oncol* 2009;**27**(27):4563–9.

[9] Miguel SL, Weisel K, Moreau P, *et al.* Pomalidomide plus low-dose dexamethasone versus high-dose dexamethasone alone for patients with relapsed and refractory multiple myeloma (MM-003): a randomised, open-label, phase 3 trial. *Lancet Oncol* 2013;**14**:1055–66.

[10] Vorinostat (Zolinza). Package Insert. Whitehouse Station, NJ: Merck & Co. Inc.

[11] Field JJ, Kanakkanthara A, Miller JH. Microtubule-targeting agents are clinically successful due to both mitotic and interphase impairment of microtubule function. *Bioorg Medicinal Chem* 2014;**22**:5050–9.

Radiation uncommonly causes heart failure. In a retrospective study of 14 358 five-year survivors of assorted cancers,[63] there was a hazard ratio of 5.9 for the development of heart failure in those receiving thoracic radiotherapy. The relative risk increased from two- to sixfold if the patients had exposure to both anthracyclines ≥250 mg/m² and radiation dose ≥1200 cGy to the heart (**Figure 11.13**). With cardiac radiation alone, there is usually a restrictive haemodynamic pattern of cardiac filling, associated with altered expression of collagen subtypes at the microscopic level, probably contributing to impaired diastolic function.[64] Interstitial fibrosis of the heart has been reported,[65] typically pericellular and perivascular, with infrequent replacement fibrosis.

Myocardial perfusion defects have frequently been reported in patients who have received mediastinal irradiation therapy, probably due to microvascular damage leading to myocardial fibrosis and diastolic dysfunction.

Over years, further remodelling can lead to progressive myocardial dysfunction and overt heart failure. It remains to be seen whether any particular drug pre-treatment could attenuate the effect on the human heart of some of the higher-intensity radiotherapy regimens, albeit animal studies suggest that this should be feasible.

Monitoring of effects of anticancer drugs

Electrocardiography

The 12-lead ECG is little used for the purpose, but could potentially be of value in screening for baseline cardiac disease before chemotherapy

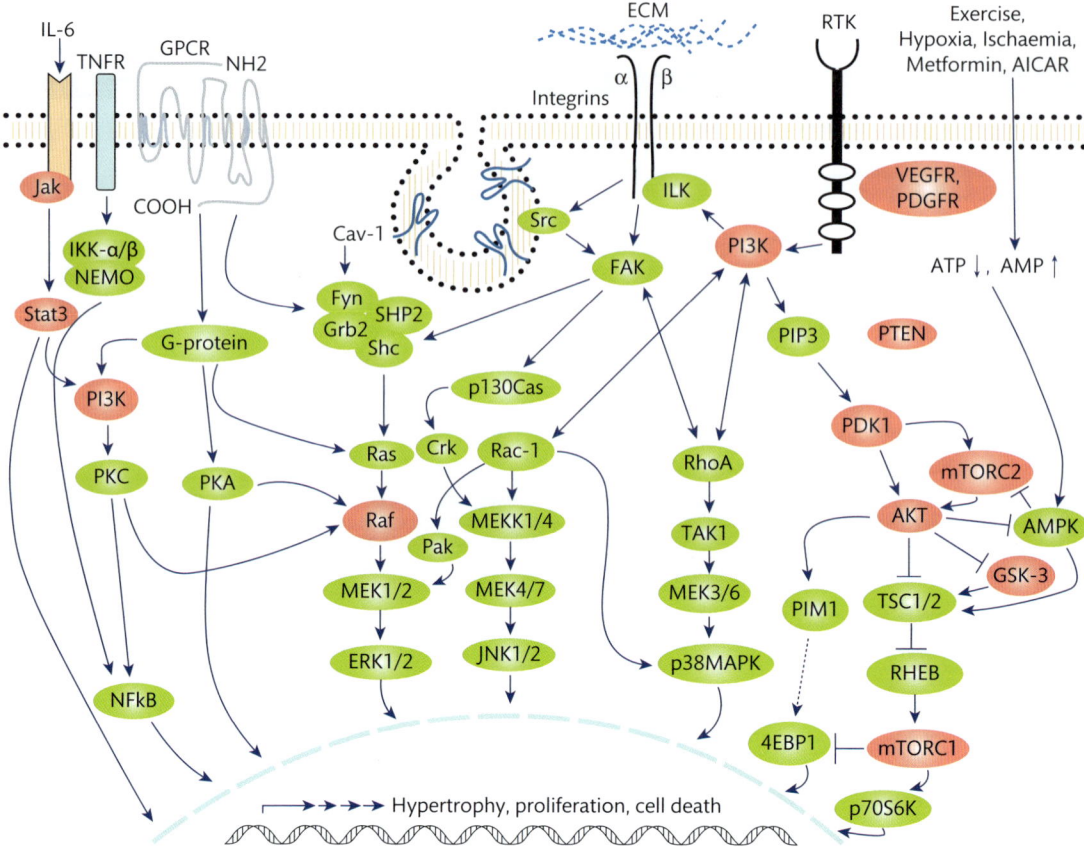

Figure 11.10 Key Signalling Pathways in the Heart and Cancer: Current drug targets (red).[58,59]

or monitoring for cardiotoxicity during treatment. Large-scale prospective studies are required before its value is definitely known.

Cardiac imaging

Imaging is vital in assessing patients before, during, and after cancer chemotherapy. Multigated acquisition (nuclear) scanning (MUGA)

has been used traditionally by oncologists and thus features in the largest historical series in the literature. Its strength is that it produces a reliable calculation of LVEF and there is low intraindividual and interobserver variation. The weaknesses of MUGA are: its insensitivity for early subtle changes, its limited diastolic information, and its use of radiation. Echocardiography has many strengths: there

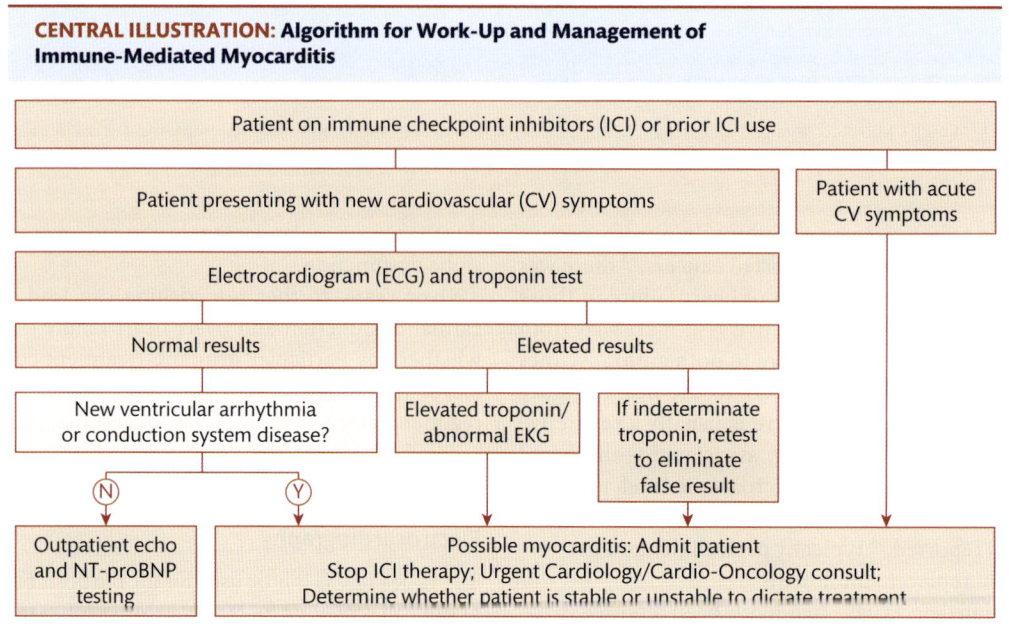

Figure 11.11 Management of Myocarditis in patients treated with immune checkpoint inhibitors

From: Mahmood SS, Fradley MG, Cohen JV, et al. Myocarditis in patients treated with immune checkpoint inhibitors. *J Am Coll Cardiol* 2018;71:1755–64

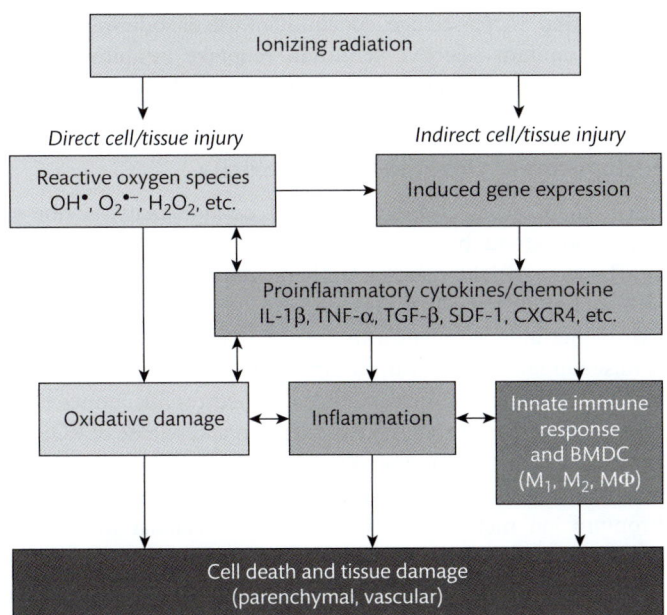

Figure 11.12 Mechanisms of radiation injury to the heart

From Kim JH, Jenrow KA, Brown SL. Mechanisms of radiation-induced normal tissue toxicity and implications for future clinical trials. Radiat Oncol J. 2014;32(3):103-115 doi :https://doi.org/10.3857/roj.2014.32.3.103.

arc no side-effects; the technique is non-invasive; it affords anatomical and functional data with high temporal and spatial resolution; and it gives information on systolic and diastolic function. CMR imaging gives detailed anatomy at high resolution and contrast, with reliable estimates of LV function and no radiation. CMR affords extra information from gadolinium enhancement, of particular value if myocarditis is suspected. Obvious limitations of CMR relate to availability, cost, suitability for detection of early changes, and the contraindication of any metal implants.

Changes in LVEF are late markers in the assessment of cardiac function. EF is a composite marker reflecting longitudinal, radial and circumferential myocardial contractility; and deterioration in contractility in any one of these can be compensated for by increased contractility in the other two directions. Recent recommendations

on imaging acknowledge that changes in myocardial deformation as measured through strain imaging occur earlier than changes in EF and at lower doses of anthracyclines.[35]

Whichever technique is employed, the key requirements are that the imaging is done before, during, and after chemotherapy; that a reliable technique is used and one with capacity for subtlety. Above all, use the same technique in an individual patient repeatedly, remembering that changes are more important than absolutes.

Biomarkers

Biomarkers of injury, especially troponin, are of value in pretreatment prediction of: vulnerability to chemotherapy; early identification of cardiac toxicity; monitoring of the anti-cancer treatment; and assessment of the effects of cardioprotective drug interventions.[66,67]

Biomarkers of load, particularly the natriuretic peptides, are helpful in defining the presence of heart failure, although the negative predictive value of BNP may be its greatest value. In addition, high-sensitivity C-reactive protein (CRP) has predicted cardiotoxicity in patients treated with trastuzumab, although this result is controversial.[68] Galectin-3, ST2, and growth differentiation factor-15 have been disappointing, but a rise in myeloperoxidase levels may indicate early toxicity. MicroRNAs are also under intense scrutiny in this regard.[69]

Cardio-oncological monitoring protocols and guidelines for treatment

Several statements and guidelines have now been published to guide the monitoring of cardiac function before, during and after cancer treatment[70,71] and they are coming into more widespread use. Following the earlier European Society for Medical Oncology (ESMO) guideline,[57] Hamo et al.[72] have summarized a practical algorithm for risk assessment, monitoring, and treatment of chemotherapy-induced cardiomyopathy, including advice as to when to discontinue the chemotherapy (Figure 11.8 and Table 11.3). A renewed position statement[73] has surveyed the topic broadly with recommendations for treatment and suggestions for future development. ESMO have recently updated their guidelines.[74]

The heart failure in this patient group should be treated with standard therapy; although there a few reports of the beneficial effects of these treatments specifically in chemotherapy-related

Table 11.3 Clinical algorithm for guiding management and monitoring of cardiac risk associated with use of anthracyclines

Clinical risk level a	Example	Total cumulative dose of doxonubicin		
		<300 mg/m²	300–450 mg/m²	> 450 mg/m²
Low	No cardiovascular history, middle aged, no previous anthracycline exposure	ECG and echo/MUGA at baseline	ECG and echo/MUGA at baseline + 3 months after completion of chemotherapy	ECG and Echo/MUGA at baseline and after every cycle of chemotherapy + 3 months after completion + yearly thereafter
Medium	Stable hypertension or ischaemic heart disease managed with medication	ECG and echo/MUGA at baseline + every 1–2 cycles of chemotherapy + 3 months after completion of chemotherapy	ECG and echo/MUGA at baseline and after every cycle of chemotherapy + 3 months after completion + yearly thereafter	Avoid anthracyclines
High	Previous anthracycline therapy, hypertension, elderly	ECG and echo/MUGA at baseline and after every cycle of chemotherapy + 3 months after completion + yearly thereafter	Avoid anthracyclines	Avoid anthracyclines

MUGA, multi-gated radionuclide ventriculography.

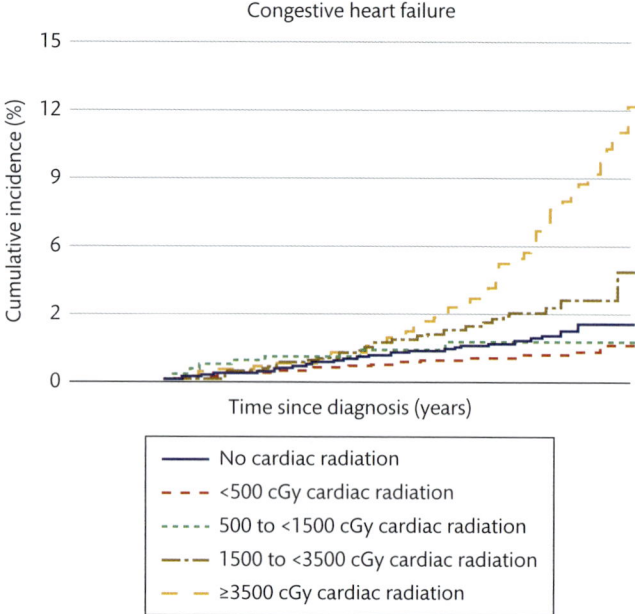

Figure 11.13 Cumulative incidence of heart failure among childhood cancer survivors by average cardiac radiation dose.
From Mulroony et al (BMJ2009; 339: b4606)

heart failure,[34,75] the situation has not yet been fully resolved (**Figure 11.14**).[76]

Standard drugs are also being studied as potential cardioprotective agents, which might allow one of the key objectives of the cardio-oncologist to be met: that is, the continuation of, or early reintroduction of, effective anticancer therapy.

Antipsychotics

Clozapine-induced myocarditis and cardiomyopathy

Clozapine is more effective than standard drugs in some patients with refractory schizophrenia, certainly with respect to 'positive' symptoms, but also probably for 'negative' symptoms. The improved efficacy is also associated with a far lower incidence of extrapyramidal and related adverse effects.[77] However, clozapine-induced cardiomyopathy is a concern, with an incidence ranging from 0.02% in the UK to 0.1% in Australia.[78,79] This statistic is based on reports to regulatory agencies and is thus almost certainly a considerable under-reporting of actual cases. An analysis of the French Pharmaco-Vigilance Database reported an odds ratio of 11.5 for developing cardiomyopathy with clozapine[7] and an Italian study suggested that a >5% decrease in LVEF occurred at one year in one-third of patients started on clozapine.[80]

Dose, risk factors, and duration of treatment

Clozapine-induced cardiomyopathy does not appear to be dose dependent.[81] The time to onset of clozapine-induced cardiomyopathy can vary between three weeks and four years, but most cases of cardiomyopathy appear within six to nine months of initiation,[82] whereas symptoms of myocarditis tend to occur within the first two months.[83]

There are no established risk factors for clozapine-induced cardiotoxicity; however, a few have been suggested, including rapid

dose titration, increased age, concomitant use of sodium valproate, and concomitant selective serotonin reuptake inhibitor use.[84,85] Another potential risk factor is the significant underlying cardiovascular risk present in patients with psychiatric issues.[86]

Mechanisms of clozapine cardiotoxicity

The mechanism of clozapine-induced cardiotoxicity is not yet clearly understood, but may be the result of a type I IgE-mediated acute hypersensitivity reaction.[67] There are peripheral eosinophilia and eosinophilic myocardial infiltrates in association with the onset of clozapine-induced myocarditis. Cardiac myeloperoxidase levels are raised in rats treated with clozapine, suggesting a role for oxidative stress. The activated eosinophils and neutrophils induce tissue injury and necrosis through the production and release of ROS and cytotoxic proteins.[87] The possible trigger is that clozapine undergoes bio-activation in myocardial tissue to a chemically reactive nitronium ion metabolite, which stimulates cellular injury, lipid peroxidation, and free radical production leading to the activation of pro-inflammatory cytokines including tumour necrosis factor-α (TNFα) and nuclear factor-κβ.[68]

Clozapine causes tachycardia at rest, perhaps due to decreased parasympathetic tone and increased adrenergic drive. Persistent inappropriate tachycardia causes impairment of left ventricular function both in animal models and in humans.[88] Furthermore, clozapine induces a rise in plasma catecholamines that correlates with the degree of myocardial inflammation.[89] Other potential mechanisms include cytochrome P450 1A2/1A3 enzyme deficiencies, blockade of calcium-dependent ion channels, increased production of inflammatory cytokines, and low serum selenium levels.[90]

Identification and screening

Tachycardia occurs in around 25% of users, especially during dose titration early in treatment.[91] When heart failure develops, 60% of patients present with breathlessness, 36% palpitations, and 4% fatigue.[92]

Cardiac biomarkers, including creatine kinase, troponin and BNP, are routinely measured in patients with clozapine-induced cardiac dysfunction although validation studies for BNP testing are awaited. No absolute diagnostic criteria exist for clozapine-induced cardiotoxicity and the diagnosis is usually made by a combination of clinical assessment and imaging. Transthoracic echocardiography is a primary and essential for pre-screening, initial diagnosis and serial assessment, often done six-monthly. However, CMR can provide a superior characterization, e.g. through detection of scar or oedema within myocardial tissues. However, to date, specific features of clozapine-induced cardiomyopathy on CMR are lacking because the condition is relatively rare.[93]

Prevention

Careful observation, monitoring for early adverse effects and early diagnosis are the mainstays of management in clozapine cardiotoxicity.

Several protocols for monitoring and treatment have been suggested, including an Australian protocol[94] which recommends active monitoring for four weeks, relying predominantly on troponin and CRP results. It encourages continuation of clozapine in the presence of mild illness, but defines a threshold for cessation. There has been one study in animals, which suggested that captopril protected against clozapine-induced myocarditis,[95] with a decrease in

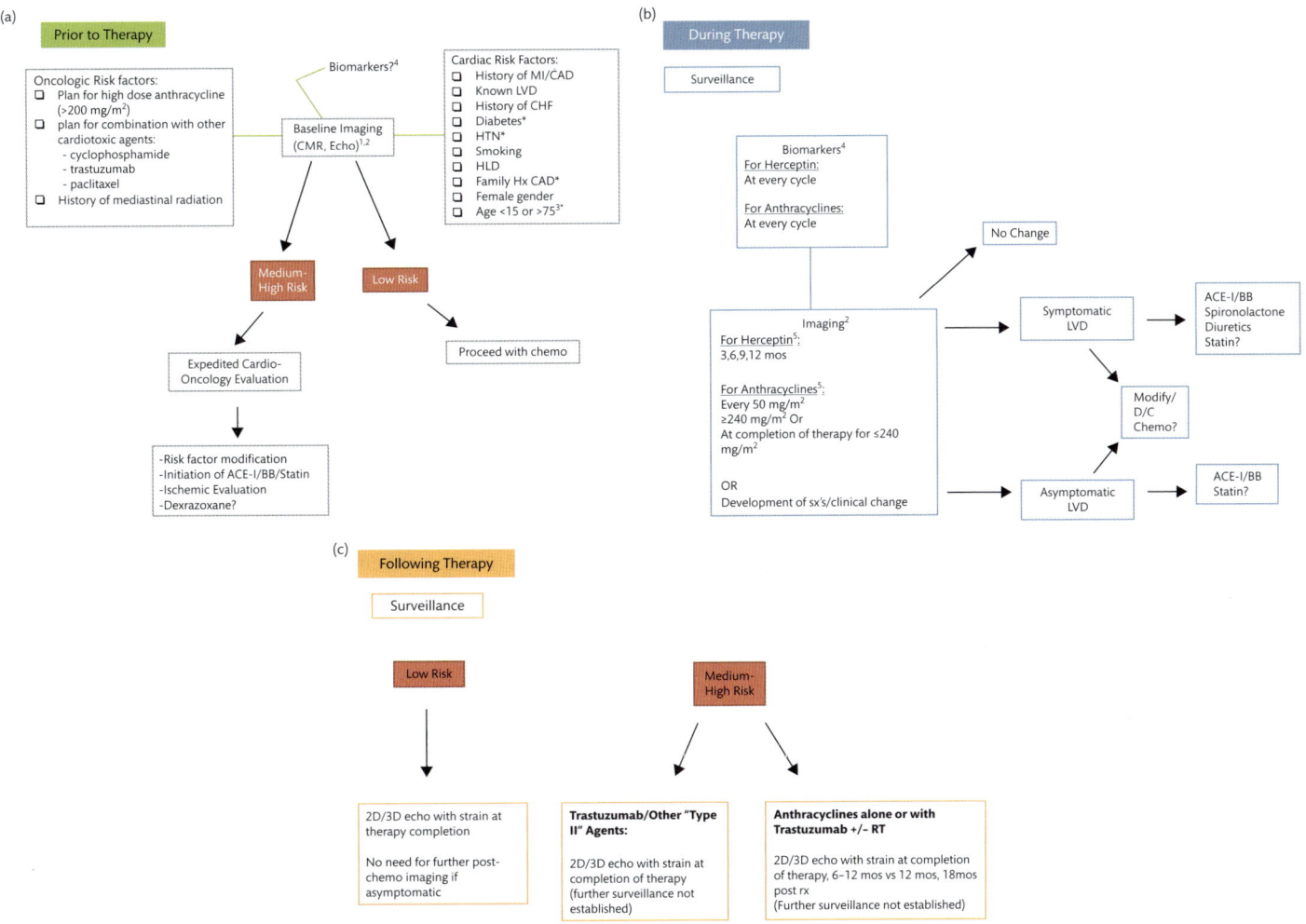

Figure 11.14 Cardiovascular treatment schedule before, during and after cancer therapy
Reproduced from Hamo CE, Bloom ME, Cardinale D, *et al.* Cancer-therapy related cardiac dysfunction and heart failure: Prevention, treatment guidelines and future directions. *Circ Heart Fail* 2016;**9**:e002843 with permission from Wolters Kluwer.

the histological hallmarks and biochemical markers of myocarditis in a dose-dependent manner. Larger, human studies are awaited to establish whether angiotensin converting enzyme inhibitors should be given as prophylaxis in patients who need clozapine.

Treatment and prognosis of established cases

Clozapine-induced myocarditis has a mortality rate ranging from 10% to 50%[96]. However, adoption of monitoring recommendations and early cessation of clozapine in the face of suspected adverse reaction improves clinical outcomes.[67,97] LV dysfunction caused by clozapine treatment is broadly reversible if clozapine therapy is discontinued.[98] Some patients present with fulminant myocarditis and may need management in intensive care.

Rechallenge with clozapine

This remains a controversial issue as some clinicians consider that a previous episode of clozapine-induced myocarditis is a firm contraindication. However, some data suggest that rechallenge could be a reasonable option for treatment-resistant patients.[99] In one small meta-analysis in 2018, 12 out of 19 patients (63%) were successfully rechallenged; time to rechallenge ranged from a few weeks to six

months post myocarditis.[100] It has been recommended that, should a rechallenge be attempted, the patient should be hospitalized while the dose is gradually increased slowly with routine and close monitoring.[101]

Lithium-induced cardiomyopathy

One case of takotsubo-type cardiomyopathy has been reported in a patient taking lithium on its own.[102] A similar case was reported in a patient taking a monoamine oxidase inhibitor together with lithium.[103] Basic science studies would suggest that the cardiotoxic effects of Li$^+$ were initiated from mitochondrial dysfunction and oxidative stress, which finally ends in cytochrome *c* release and cell-death-signalling heart cardiomyocytes.[104]

Electroconvulsive therapy

Electroconvulsive therapy (ECT) is still used in the treatment of intractable psychotic depression. ECT causes a marked hypertensive response and, less commonly, a severe bradycardia. There are cases of takotsubo cardiomyopathy following ECT, as well as of myocardial stunning and cardiogenic shock post ECT.[105] It is possible that β-blockade might help in the primary and secondary prevention of post-ECT takotsubo cardiomyopathy.

Antifungals

Amphotericin B

A few cases have been reported of cardiomyopathy between a week and several months of amphotericin (AmB) treatment.[106] In one case, myocardial biopsy showed myocyte hypertrophy with significant loss of myofibrils, reduction in the number of mitochondria and extensive intramitochondrial damage, suggesting direct toxicity of the drug on cardiac cells.

AmB may cause membrane permeability to increase with loss of ions and small molecules, altered ionic currents during the cardiac action potential[107] and/or effects on the sarcoplasmic reticular membrane ATPase system.[108] In all reported cases the cardiac function returned to normal after the cessation of AmB treatment.

Itraconazole

Between September 1992 and April 2001, the US Food and Drug Administration (FDA) received 58 reports of potential cases of congestive heart failure with itraconazole,[109] although most cases had other risk factors for heart failure. The time of onset of symptoms of heart failure ranged from one to 210 days with doses ranging between 100 and 800 mg/day with mean of 300 mg/day.

Itraconazole exerts a negative inotropic effect, but its mechanism of cardiotoxicity is uncertain. There may be an association with sodium channel blockade.[110] It is uncertain whether the heart damage is reversible.

Antiretrovirals—highly active antiretroviral therapy-associated cardiomyopathy

The reported incidence of all-cause dilated cardiomyopathy in HIV-infected patients is up to 8% in asymptomatic patients and up to 25% of autopsy cases.[111] However, although the introduction of highly active antiretroviral therapy (HAART) regimens has reduced the prevalence of human immunodeficiency virus (HIV)-associated cardiomyopathy by about 30% in developed countries,[112] specific antiretroviral therapy (ART) drugs are associated with myocardial damage and dysfunction. Cardiac effects have been noticed *in utero* and in the early postnatal period.[113] There is a high rate of abnormal echocardiographic findings in adult patients with HIV infection (75% on HAART) including 18% with LV systolic dysfunction, 6.5% with LV hypertrophy, 26% with diastolic dysfunction, and 57% with right ventricular pressure of >30 mmHg.[114]

Mechanism of HAART-related cardiomyopathy

Several animal studies report abnormal mitochondrial function in cardiomyocytes and depleted mitochondrial DNA as a result of exposure to nucleoside reverse transcriptase inhibitors, such as zidovudine and stavudine.[115,116]

HIV-1 protease inhibitors (PIs) may cause myocardial dysfunction by decreasing the uptake of glucose by GLUT4 blockade.[117] PIs might have effects at the mitochondrial level,[118] but the effects of PIs on the heart are uncertain. One meta-analysis by the FDA found no association between use of one PI (abacavir) and cardiovascular disease, but as patients with HIV have a higher prevalence of atherosclerotic cardiovascular disease, the results might be confounded. The inclusion of thymidine analogues along with PIs may also predispose to dilated cardiomyopathy.

In children, normal physiological myocardial hypertrophy appears to be blunted, especially after ART exposure during fetal and early postnatal life. HIV-negative infants exposed to ART and born to HIV-positive mothers have reduced LV mass, LV dimensions, and septal wall thickness. LV contractility improves but is still abnormal up to 2 years of age compared with unexposed infants.[92] The cardiac effects in these ART-exposed children are similar to those associated with the cardiotoxicity of anthracyclines.[119]

Nutritional deficiencies (common in HIV-infected subjects living in developing countries) may contribute to ventricular dysfunction independently of HAART such as selenium, vitamin B_{12}, and carnitine deficiencies.[120]

Exposed children with and without HIV infection are at risk for late cardiotoxicity. Raised cardiovascular biomarkers such as natriuretic peptides and troponins, as well as echocardiographic monitoring, may help identify at-risk individuals and prompt early treatment for heart failure.[97]

Rheumatological agents—the antimalarials

Chloroquine (CQ) and hydroxychloroquine (HCQ) are 4-aminoquinolines widely used in the treatment of rheumatoid arthritis, systemic lupus erythematosus, and other connective tissue disorders. Because of the small number of cases and the lack of systematic studies, it is impossible to calculate the incidence of CQ/HCQ cardiotoxicity; to date, reports have been published on 47 patients with biopsy-proven HCQ-induced cardiomyopathy. The duration of treatment ranged from 2 to 35 years. The mean cumulative dose for isolated CQ and HCQ cases were 1277 and 1843 g, respectively, and the overall pooled mean cumulative dose for all cases was 1612 g.[121]

HCQ is a cationic, weak amphiphilic base, capable of crossing cell membranes and preferentially binding to phospholipids. HCQ accumulates in lysosomes and causes direct inhibition of phospholipases, an alkaline shift in lysosomal pH, and a reduction in lysosomal hydrolase activity. There may be a role of autophagy in the pathophysiology of HCQ-induced cardiomyopathy.[122] There is pathological accumulation of metabolic products, such as glycogen and phospholipids, and lamellar inclusion bodies and curvilinear bodies in the cytoplasm, similar to what is seen in lysosomal storage disease. The cytoplasm becomes vacuolated with myofibrillar disorganization, contributing to the development of myocyte hypertrophy fibrosis.[123,124]

Macroscopically, the appearances of HCQ-induced cardiomyopathy are of concentric hypertrophy with restrictive features. A morphological classification of cardiomyopathy phenotypes including hypertrophic, dilated, restrictive, and/or biventricular endomyocardial fibrosis with conduction system abnormalities—including atrioventricular block and bundle branch block—are all possible, and progression to third-degree atrioventricular block is common.[100]

Clinical aspects

Risk factors for the development of HCQ-induced cardiotoxicity include older age, female sex, longer duration of therapy (>10 years), higher daily dose, pre-existing cardiac disease, and renal insufficiency.[125] However, it is unclear why only certain patients experience adverse events and why there is significant heterogeneity in the presentation of patients with CQ/HCQ-induced cardiomyopathy.[126] It is possible that some patients may possess a genetic predisposition such as α-galactosidase A polymorphism, the genetic basis for Fabry disease, with varying degrees of severity. CQ cardiomyopathy could

represent a phenocopy of Fabry disease as they are clinically and histologically similar.[127]

Like many other drug-induced cardiomyopathies, HCQ-induced cardiomyopathy can be partially reversed by stopping the offending drug.[128] There is a latent phase during which HCQ withdrawal can prevent progression to clinically significant cardiac disease. Because HCQ-induced cardiomyopathy is potentially reversible in its early stages, early identification of affected patients is particularly important.[129]

Screening in the setting of long-term HCQ use should include annual ECG, with early consideration of echocardiography. Follow-up with CMR and/or endomyocardial biopsy can follow an abnormal echo. Currently there is no defined role for cardiac-specific biomarkers.

Tumour necrosis factor-α inhibitors

Tumour necrosis factor-α inhibitors are widely used in the treatment of inflammatory bowel disease and other inflammatory conditions. Overall, studies of their effects on cardiovascular risk show mixed results.[130] In a case study based on the FDA's MedWatch programme, 47 cases of heart failure were identified after treatment with TNFα inhibitors (etanercept: 29 cases/infliximab: 18 cases).[131] By contrast, Wolfe et al. did not detect an increased risk of heart failure after these drugs.[132] For adalimumab, heart failure is a very rare side-effect.[133]

Interferon-induced cardiomyopathy

There are reports of dilated cardiomyopathy during interferon-α therapy, but the cardiomyopathy resolves rapidly with discontinuation of the drug.[134,135] The cardiac effects were not related to the daily dose, cumulative total dose, or period of therapy. Some of the patients in whom interferon caused cardiovascular sequelae had a history of coronary heart disease or had previously been given chemotherapy with drugs known to be cardiotoxic. Sonnenblick et al. suggest that cardiomyopathy was induced through impaired myocyte metabolism rather than through histological damage.[136]

Antidiabetic drugs

In placebo-controlled trials of adult patients with or at high risk for type 2 diabetes, thiazolidinedione therapy (e.g. rosiglitazone or pioglitazone) was found to be significantly and consistently associated with a higher risk of heart failure. The risk of serious/severe heart failure is also increased with the use of thiazolidinediones. Heart failure risks are similar to those of meta-analyses combining active- and placebo-controlled trials.[137]

Use of rosiglitazone was associated with higher odds of congestive heart failure, myocardial infarction, and death relative to pioglitazone in real world settings (odds ratio: 1.16; 95% confidence interval: 1.07–1.24; $P < 0.001$).[138]

Iron-overload cardiomyopathy

Patients with chronic anaemia are often treated with repeated blood transfusions. The spectrum of symptoms of iron-overload cardiomyopathy is varied, ranging from asymptomatic early in the disease process, up to terminal heart failure in severely overloaded patients.

In chronic iron overload, the toxicity is dose dependent and mediated through hydroxyl radicals, which are highly toxic; they damage the lipid-rich cell membrane, through peroxidation, which affects cellular organelles as well as the cell membrane.[139]

Biochemical markers and tissue biopsy were traditionally used to diagnose and guide therapy. However, newer diagnostic modalities such as T2*MRI can quantitate cardiac iron load from the early stage of cardiac iron deposition. The newer chelator, deferiprone, has been shown to be an effective treatment, especially when introduced early.[140]

Chromium/cobalt hip prostheses

One in eight of all total hip replacements requires revision within 10 years, 60% because of wear-related complications. The bearing surfaces may be made of cobalt/chromium, stainless steel, ceramic, or polyethylene. Friction between bearing surfaces and corrosion of non-moving parts can result in increased local and systemic metal concentrations. A recent systematic review[141] (11 cases of cardiomyopathy in 18 patients in 23 data papers) has shown that patients exposed to high circulating concentrations of cobalt from failed hip replacements can develop cardiomyopathy, which may not resolve completely even after removal of the prosthesis. Patients with ceramic components that fracture, and those with clinical or radiological features of local inflammation, appear to be at highest risk of developing cobalt-associated systemic effects.

Conclusion

It is a truism to say that almost all medications can cause side-effects. The number of drugs that have significant negative impact on the heart is small but important to know since the implications are great. Within the broader area of cardiac adverse reaction, impaired ventricular function and heart failure are highly prevalent, but the forewarned practitioner is forearmed!

REFERENCES

1. Katz AM. Cardiomyopathy of overload—a major determinant of prognosis in congestive heart failure. *N Engl J Med* 1990;**322**:100–10.
2. Wang TJ, Gupta, DK. Metabolic profiles in heart failure. *J Am Coll Cardiol* 2015;**65**:1521–3.
3. Szardien S, Möllman H, Willmer M, et al. Mechanisms of stress (takotsubo) cardiomyopathy. *Heart Fail Clin* 2013;**9**:197–205.
4. Rosen SD. From heart to brain: the genesis and processing of cardiac pain. *Can J Cardiol* 2012;**28**:S7–S19.
5. Bloom MW, Hamo CE, Cardinale C, et al. Cancer therapy-related cardiac dysfunction and heart failure. Part 1: Definitions, pathophysiology, risk factors and imaging. *Circ Heart Fail* 2016;**9**:e002661.
6. NCI Dictionary of Cancer Terms. Definition of cardiotoxicity. http://www.cancer.gov/dictionary?CdrID=44004%3E
7. Montastruc G, Favreliere S, Sommet A, et al. Drugs and dilated cardiomyopathies: a case/noncase study in the French PharmacoVigilance Database. *Br J Clin Pharm* 2010;**69**(3):287–94.
8. Albakri A. Drugs-related cardiomyopathy: a systematic review and pooled analysis of pathophysiology, diagnosis and clinical management. *Int Med Care* 2019;**3**:1–19.
9. National Confidential Enquiry into Patient Outcome and Death. *Knowing the risk: a review of the perioperative care of surgical patients.* NCEPOD, London, 2011, http://www.ncepod.org.uk/2011report2/downloads/POC_fullreport.pdf.

10. Lobo DN, Dube MG, Neal KR, et al. Problems with solutions: drowning in the brine of an inadequate knowledge base. *Clin Nutr* 2001;**20**:125–30.

11. Lobo DN, Bostock K, Neal KR, et al. The effect of postoperative salt and water restriction on recovery of gastrointestinal function and outcome in patients undergoing elective colonic resections: a prospective, randomised controlled study. *Br J Surg* 2001;**88**(S1):25–6.

12. https://www.nice.org.uk/guidance/cg174/chapter/1-recommendations.

13. Page RL, O'Bryant CL, Cheng D, et al. Drugs that may cause or exacerbate heart failure: a scientific statement from the American Heart Association. *Circulation* 2016;**134**(6):e32–69.

14. Zausig YA, Busse H, Lunz D, et al. Cardiac effects of induction agents in the septic rat heart. *Crit Care* 2009;**13**(5):R144–51.

15. Dote K, Sato H, Tateishi H, Uchida T, Ishihara M. Myocardial stunning due to simultaneous multivessel coronary spasms: a review of 5 cases. *J Cardiol* 1991;**21**:203–214.

16. Izumi Y. Drug-induced Takotsubo cardiomyopathy. *Heart Fail Clin* 2013;**9**:225–31.

17. Abraham J, Mudd JO, Kapur NK, Klein K, Champion HC, Wittstein IS. Stress cardiomyopathy after intravenous administration of catecholamines and beta-receptor agonists. *J Am Coll Cardiol* 2009;**53**(15):1320–5.

18. Lyon AR, Rees PS, Prasad S, Poole-Wilson PA, Harding SE. Stress (Takotsubo) cardiomyopathy—a novel pathophysiological hypothesis to explain catecholamine-induced acute myocardial stunning. *Nat Clin Pract Cardiovasc Med* 2008;**5**(1):22–9.

19. Ghadri JR, Wittstein IS, Prasad A, et al. on behalf of International Expert Consensus Document on Takotsubo Syndrome (Part I): clinical characteristics, diagnostic criteria, and pathophysiology. *Eur Heart J* 2018;**39**(22):2032–46.

20. http://www.cancer.gov/publications/dictionaries/cancer-terms?search=survivorship.

21. Minotti G, Menna P, Salvatorelli E, Cairo G, Gianni L. Anthracyclines: molecular advances and pharmacological developments in anti-tumor activity and cardiotoxicity. *Pharmacol Rev* 2004;**56**:185–229.

22. Van Dyke T. P53 and tumor suppression. *N Engl J Med* 2007;**356**:79–81.

23. Middleman E, Luce J, Frei E 3rd. Clinical trials with adriamycin. *Cancer* 1971;**28**:844–50.

24. Monsuez J-J, Charniot J-C, Vignat N, Artigou J-Y. Cardiac side-effects of cancer chemotherapy. *Int J Cardiol* 2010;**144**:3–15.

25. Wojnowski L, Kulle B, Schirmer M, et al. NAD(P)H oxidase and multidrug resistance protein genetic polymorphisms are associated with doxorubic-ininduced cardiomyopathy. *Circulation* 2005;**112**:3754–62.

26. Khouri MG, Douglas PS, Mackey JR. Cancer therapy-induced cardiac toxicity in early breast cancer. *Circulation* 2012;**126**:2749–63.

27. Murabito A, Hirsch E, Ghigo A. Mechanisms of anthracycline-induced cardiotoxicity: is mitochondrial dysfunction the answer? *Front Cardiovasc Med* 2020;**7**:1–12.

28. Ma W, Wei S, Zhang B, Li W. Molecular mechanisms of cardiomyocyte death in drug-induced cardiotoxicity. *Front Cell Dev Biol* 2020;**8**:1–17.

29. Kenchaiah S, Narula J, Vasan RS. Risk factors for heart failure. *Med Clin N Am* 2004;**88**:1145–72.

30. Zamorano JL, Lancellotti P, Rodriguez Muñoz D, et al. ESC Scientific Document Group, 2016 ESC Position Paper on cancer treatments and cardiovascular toxicity developed under the auspices of the ESC Committee for Practice Guidelines: The Task Force for cancer treatments and cardiovascular toxicity of the European Society of Cardiology (ESC). *Eur Heart J* 2016;**37**:2768–801.

31. Bryant J, Picot J, Baxter L, et al. Clinical and cost-effectiveness of cardioprotection against the toxic effects of anthracyclines given to children with cancer: a systematic review. *Br J Cancer* 2007;**96**:226–30.

32. Yamaguchi N, Fuji T, Aoi S, et al. Comparison of cardiac events associated with liposomal doxorubicin, epirubicin and doxorubicin in breast cancer: a Bayesian network meta-analysis. *Eur J Cancer* 2015;**51**:2314–20.

33. Fumoleau P, H Roche H, Kerbrat P, et al. Long-term cardiac toxicity after adjuvant epirubicin-based chemotherapy in early breast cancer: French Adjuvant Study Group Results. *Ann Oncol* 2006;**17**:85–92.

34. Wouters KA, Kremer LCM, Miller TI, Herman EH, Lipshultz SE. Protecting against anthracycline-induced myocardial damage: a review of the most promising strategies. *Br J Haematol* 2005;**131**:561–78.

35. Lipshultz SE, Scully RE, Lipsitz SR, et al. Assessment of dexrazoxane as a cardioprotectant in doxorubicin-treated children with high-risk acute lymphoblastic leukaemia: long-term follow-up of a prospective, randomised, multicentre trial. *Lancet Oncol* 2010;**11**:950–61.

36. Lipshultz SE, Colan SD, Gelber RD, et al. Late cardiac effects of doxorubicin therapy for acute lymphoblastic leukemia in childhood. *N Engl J Med* 1991;**324**(12):808–15.

37. Kremer LC, van Dalen EC, Offringa M, et al. Anthracycline-induced clinical heart failure in a cohort of 607 children: long-term follow-up study. *J Clin Oncol* 2001;**19**:191–6.

38. Rathe M, Carlsen NL, Oxhøj H, Nielsen G. Long-term cardiac follow-up of children treated with anthracycline doses of 300 mg/m or less for acute lymphoblastic leukemia. *Pediatr Blood Cancer* 2010;**54**(3):444–8.

39. Cardinale D, Colombo A, Bacchini G, et al. Early detection of anthracycline cardiotoxicity and improvement with heart failure therapy. *Circulation* 2015;**131**:1981–8.

40. Groarke JD, Nohria A. Anthracycline cardiotoxicity: a new paradigm for an old classic. *Circulation* 2015;**131**:1946–9.

41. Upshaw JN, Finkelman B, Hubbard RA, et al. Comprehensive assessment of changes in left ventricular diastolic function with contemporary breast cancer therapy. *J Am Coll Cardiol Imag* 2020;**13**:198–210.

42. Plana JC, Galderisi M, Barac A, et al. Expert consensus for multimodality imaging evaluation of adult patients during and after cancer therapy: a report from the American Society of Echocardiography and the European Association of Cardiovascular Imaging. *J Am Soc Echocardiogr* 2014;**9**:911–39.

43. Slamon DJ, Clark GM, Wong SG, et al. Human breast cancer: correlation of relapse and survival with amplification of the HER-2/neu oncogene. *Science* 1987;**235**:177–82.

44. Sawyer DB, Peng X, Chen B, Pentassuglia L, Lim CC. Mechanisms of anthracycline cardiac injury: can we identify strategies for cardio-protection? *Prog Cardiovasc Dis* 2010;**53**:105–13.

45. Romond EH, Perez EA, Bryant J, et al. Trastuzumab plus adjuvant chemotherapy for operable HER2-positive breast cancer. *N Engl J Med* 2005;**353**:1673–84.

46. Rayson D, Richel D, Chia S, et al. Anthracycline-trastuzumab regimens for HER2/neu-overexpressing breast cancer: current experience and future strategies. *Ann Oncol* 2008;**19**:1530–9.

47. Giraud M-N, Fluck M, Zuppinger C, Suter TM. Expressional reprogramming of survival pathways in rat cardiocytes by neuregulin-1β. *J Appl Physiol* 2005;**99**:313–22.

48. Procter M, Suter TM, de Azambuja E, *et al.* Longer-term assessment of trastuzumab-related cardiac adverse events in the Herceptin adjuvant (HERA) trial. *J Clin Oncol* 2010;**28**:3422–8.

49. Chen J, Long JB, Hurria A, *et al.* Incidence of heart failure or cardiomyopathy after adjuvant trastuzumab therapy for breast cancer. *J Am Coll Cardiol* 2012;**60**(24):2504–12.

50. Cameron D, Piccart-Gebhart MJ, Gelber RD, *et al.* 11 years' follow-up of trastuzumab after adjuvant chemotherapy in HER2-positive early breast cancer: final analysis of the HERceptin Adjuvant (HERA) trial. *Lancet* 2017;**389**(10075):1195–1205.

51. Ewer MS, Vooletich MT, Durand JB, *et al.* Reversibility of trastuzumab-related cardiotoxicity: new insights based on clinical course and response to medical treatment. *J Clin Oncol* 2005;**23**:7820–6.

52. Ewer MS, Lippman SM. Type II chemotherapy-related cardiac dysfunction: Time to recognise a new entity. *J Clin Oncol* 2005;**23**:2900–2.

53. Ewer MS, Ewer SM. Cardiotoxicity of anticancer treatments: what the cardiologist needs to know. *Nat Rev Cardiol* 2010;**7**:564–75.

54. Valachis A, Nearchou A, Lind P, Mauri D. Lapatinib, trastuzumab or the combination added to preoperative chemotherapy for breast cancer: a meta-analysis of randomized evidence. *Breast Cancer Res Treat* 2012;**135**:655–62.

55. Krop IE, Suter TM, Dang CT, *et al.* Feasibility and cardiac safety of trastuzumab emtansine after anthracycline-based chemotherapy as (neo)adjuvant therapy for human epidermal growth factor receptor 2-positive early-stage breast cancer. *J Clin Oncol* 2015;**33**:1136–42.

56. Sistigu A, Viaud S, Chaput N, *et al.* Immunomodulatory effects of cyclophosphamide and implementations for vaccine design. *Semin Immunopathol* 2011;**33**:369–83.

57. Goldberg MA, Antin JH, Guinan EC, Rappeport JM. Cyclophosphamide cardiotoxicity: an analysis of dosing as a risk factor. *Blood* 1986;**68**:1114–18.

58. Cheng H, Force T. Molecular mechanisms of cardiovascular toxicity of targeted cancer therapeutics. *Circ Res* 2010;**106**:21–34.

59. Lal H, Kolaja KL, Force T. Cancer genetics and the cardiotoxicity of the therapeutics. *J Am Coll Cardiol* 2013;**61**:267–74.

60. Tocchetti CG, Galdiero MR, Varricchi G. Cardiac toxicity in patients treated with immune checkpoint inhibitors. it is now time for cardio-immuno-oncology. *J Am Coll Cardiol* 2018;**71**:1765–7.

61. Escudier M. Clinical features, management, and outcomes of immune checkpoint inhibitor-related cardiotoxicity. *Circulation* 2017;**136**:2085–7.

62. Ghosh A, Chen DH, Guha A, Mackenzie S, Walker JM, Roddie C. CAR T cell therapy-related cardiovascular outcomes and management: systemic disease or direct cardiotoxicity *J Am Coll Cardiol CardioOnc* 2020;**2**:97–109.

63. Mulrooney DA, Yeazel MW, Toana K, *et al.* Cardiac outcomes in a cohort of adult survivors of childhood and adolescent cancer: retrospective analysis of the Childhood Cancer Survivor Study cohort. *Br Med J* 2009;**339**:b4606.

64. Chello M, Mastroroberto P, Zofrea RS, Bevacqua I, Marchese AR. Changes in the proportion of types I and III collagen in the left ventricular wall of patients with post-irradiative pericarditis. *Cardiovasc Surg* 1996;**4**:222–6.

65. Veinot JP, Edwards WD. Pathology of radiation-induced heart disease: a surgical and autopsy study of 27 cases. *Human Pathology* 1996;**27**:766–73.

66. Morandi P, Ruffini PA, Benvenuto GM, Raimondi R, Fosser V. Cardiac toxicity of high dose chemotherapy. *Bone Marrow Transpl* 2005;**35**:323–34.

67. Pai VB, Nahata MC. Cardiotoxicity of chemotherapeutic agents: incidence, treatment and prevention. *Drug Saf* 2000;**22**:263–302.

68. Onitilo AA, Engel JM, Stankowski RV, *et al.* High-sensitivity C-reactive protein (hs-CRP) as a biomarker for trastuzumab-induced cardiotoxicity in HER2-positive early-stage breast cancer: a pilot study. *Breast Cancer Res Treat* 2012;**134**:291–8.

69. Riddell E, Lenihan D. The role of cardiac biomarkers in cardio-oncology. Curr Prob Cancer 2018;**42**:375–85.

70. Eschenhagen T, Force T, Ewer MS, *et al.* Cardiovascular side effects of cancer therapies: a position statement from the Heart Failure Association of the European Society of Cardiology. *Eur J Heart Fail* 2010;**13**:1–10.

71. Curigliano G, Cardinale D, Suter T, *et al.* Cardiovascular toxicity induced by chemotherapy targeted agents and radiotherapy: ESMO Clinical Practice Guidelines. *Ann Oncol* 2012;**23** Suppl 7:vii155–vii166.

72. Hamo CE, Bloom ME, Cardinale D, *et al.* Cancer-therapy related cardiac dysfunction and heart failure: prevention, treatment guidelines and future directions. *Circ Heart Fail* 2016;**9**:e002843.

73. Task Force for cancer treatments and cardiovascular toxicity of the European Society of Cardiology (ESC). 2016 ESC Position Paper on cancer treatments and cardiovascular toxicity developed under the auspices of the ESC Committee for Practice Guidelines. *Eur Heart J* 2016;**37**(36):2768–801.

74. Curigliano G, Lenihan D, Fradley M, *et al.* on behalf of the ESMO Guidelines Committee. Management of cardiac disease in cancer patients throughout oncological treatment: ESMO consensus recommendations. *Ann Oncol* 2020;**31**(2):171–90.

75. Ponikowski P, Voors AA, Anker SD, *et al.* 2016 ESC Guidelines for the diagnosis and treatment of acute and chronic heart failure. *Eur Heart J* 2016;**37**:2129–200.

76. Vaduganathan M, Hirji SA, Qamar A, *et al.* Efficacy of neurohormonal therapies in preventing cardiotoxicity in patients with cancer undergoing chemotherapy. *J Am Coll Cardiol CardioOnc* 2019;**1**:54–65.

77. Rosenheck R, Cramer J, Xu W, *et al.* A comparison of clozapine and haloperidol in hospitalized patients with refractory schizophrenia. *N Engl J Med* 1997;**337**:809–15.

78. Kilian JG, Kerr K, Lawrence C, Celermajer DS. Myocarditis and cardiomyopathy associated with clozapine. *Lancet* 1999;**354**:1841–5.

79. Committee on Safety of Medicines. Myocarditis with antipsychotics: recent case with clozapine (Clozaril). *Curr Prob Pharmacovigil* 1993;**19**:9–10.

80. Rostagno C, Domenichetti S, Gensini GF. Does a subclinical cardiotoxic effect of clozapine exist? Results from a follow-up pilot study. *Cardiovasc Hematol Agents Med Chem* 2012;**10**(2):148–53.

81. Wheeler A, Hymerstone V, Robinson G. Outcomes for schizophrenia patients with clozapine treatment: how good does it get? *J Psychopharmacol* 2009;**23**:957–65.

82. Reinders J, Parsonage W, Lange D, *et al.* Clozapine-related myocarditis and cardiomyopathy in an Australian metropolitan psychiatric service. *Aust NZ J Psychiatry* 2004;**38**(11–12):915–22.

83. Frangogiannis NG, Smith CW, Entman ML. The inflammatory response in myocardial infarction. *Cardiovasc Res* 2002;**53**:31–47.

84. Ronaldson KJ, Fitzgerald PB, Taylor AJ, et al. Rapid clozapine dose titration and concomitant sodium valproate increase risk of myocarditis with clozapine: a case-control study. *Schizophr Res* 2012;**141**(2–3):173–8.

85. Youssef DL, Narayanan P, Gill N. Incidence and risk factors for clozapine-induced myocarditis and cardiomyopathy at a regional mental health service in Australia. *Austral Psychiatry* 2016;**24**(2):176–80.

86. Correll CU, Solmi M, Veronese N, et al. Prevalence, incidence and mortality from cardiovascular disease in patients with pooled specific severe mental illness: a large-scale meta-analysis of 3,211,768 patients and 113,383,368 controls. *World Psychiatry* 2017;**16**(2):163–80.

87. Williams, DP, O'Donnell CJ, Maggs JL, et al. Bioactivation of clozapine by murine cardiac tissue in vivo and in vitro. *Chem Res Toxicol* 2003;**16**:1359–64.

88. Leung JY, Barr AM, Procyshyn RM, Honer WG, Pang CC, Cardiovascular side effects of antipsychotic drugs: the role of the autonomic nervous system. *Pharmacol Ther* 2012;**135**:113–22.

89. Breier A, Buchanan RW, Waltrip RW, et al. The effect of clozapine on plasma norepinephrine: relationship to clinical efficacy. *Neuropsychopharmacology* 1994;**10**:1–7.

90. Layland JJ, Liew D, Prior DL. Clozapine-induced cardiotoxicity: a clinical update. *Med J Aust* 2009;**190**:190–2.

91. Meltzer HY, Alphs L, Green AI, et al. International Suicide Prevention Trial Study Group. Clozapine treatment for suicidality in schizophrenia: International Suicide Prevention Trial (InterSePT). *Arch Gen Psychiatry* 2003;**60**(1):82–91.

92. Alawami M, Wasywich C, Cicovic A, Kennedy C. A systematic review of clozapine induced cardiomyopathy. *Int J Cardiol* 2014;**176**:315–20.

93. Patel RK, Moore AM, Piper S, et al. Clozapine and cardiotoxicity—a guide for psychiatrists written by cardiologists. *Psychiatry Res* 2019;**282**:112491.

94. Ronaldson KJ, Fitzgerald PB, Taylor AJ, Topliss DJ, McNeil JJ. A new monitoring protocol for clozapine-induced myocarditis based on an analysis of 75 cases and 94 controls. *Aust NZ J Psychiatry* 2011;**45**:458–65.

95. Abdel-Wahab BA, Metwally ME, El-khawanki MM, Hashim AM. Protective effect of captopril against clozapine-induced myocarditis in rats: role of oxidative stress, proinflammatory cytokines and DNA damage. *Chemico-Biological Interact* 2014;**216**:43–52.

96. Bellissima BL, Tingle MD, Cicovic A, et al. A systematic review of clozapine-induced myocarditis. *Int J Cardiol* 2018;**259**:122–29.

97. Annamraju S, Sheitman B, Saik S, Stephenson A. Early recognition of clozapine-induced myocarditis. *J Clin Psychopharmacol* 2007;**27**:479–83.

98. Razminia M, Salem Y, Devaki S, et al. Clozapine induced myopericarditis: early recognition improves clinical outcome. *Am J Ther* 2006;**13**:274–6.

99. Manu P, Lapitskaya Y, Shaikh A, Nielsen J. Clozapine rechallenge after major adverse effects: clinical guidelines based on 259 cases. *Am J Ther* 2018;**25**(2):e218–e223.

100. Bellissima BL, Tingle MD, Cicovic A, et al. A systematic review of clozapine-induced myocarditis. *Int J Cardiol* 2018;**259**:122–9.

101. Cook SC, Ferguson BA, Cotes RO, et al. Clozapine-induced myocarditis: prevention and considerations in rechallenge. *Psychosomatics* 2015;**56**(6):685–90.

102. Kitami M. Oizumi H, Kish SJ, Furukawa Y. Takotsubo cardiomyopathy associated with lithium intoxication in bipolar disorder: a case report. *J Clin Psychopharm* 2014;**34**:410–11.

103. Nishaki KM, Aurigemma G, Rafeq Z, Starobin O. Reverse takotsubo after serotonin syndrome. *Tex Heart Inst J* 2011;**38**:568–72.

104. Salimi A, Gholamifar E, Naserzadeh P, Hosseini M-J, Pourahmad J. Toxicity of lithium on isolated heart mitochondria and cardiomyocyte: a justification for its cardiotoxic adverse effect. *J Biochem Mol Toxicol* 2017;**31**:e21836.

105. Sharp RP, Welch EB. Takotsubo cardiomyopathy as a complication of electroconvulsive therapy. *Ann Pharmacother* 2011;**45**:1559–65.

106. Soares JR, Nunes MC, Leite AF, et al. Reversible dilated cardiomyopathy associated with amphotericin B therapy. *J Clin Pharm Ther* 2014;**40**:333–35.

107. Schanne OF, Ruiz-Ceretti E, Deslauriers Y, et al. The effects of amphotericin B on the ionic currents of frog atrial trabeculae. *J Mol Cell Cardiol* 1977;**9**:907–20.

108. Rao MR, Hutcheson AE, Markov AK, et al. In vitro inhibition of rat heart sarcoplasmic reticular membrane ATPase activities by amphotericin B and their reversal by fructose-1,6-diphosphate. *Biochem Mol Biol Int* 1995;**37**:821–5.

109. Ahmad SR, Singer SJ, Leissa BG. Congestive heart failure associated with itraconazole. *Lancet* 2001;**357**:1766–7.

110. Qu Y, Fang M, Gao B, et al. Itraconazole decreases left ventricular contractility in isolated rabbit heart: mechanism of action. *Toxicol Appl Pharmacol* 2013;**268**:113–22.

111. Fisher SD, Kanda BS, Miller TL, Lipshultz SE. Cardiovascular disease and therapeutic drug-related cardiovascular consequences in HIV-infected patients. *Am J Cardiovasc Drugs* 2011;**11**:383–94.

112. Bijl M, Dieleman JP, Simoons M, Van Der Ende ME. Low prevalence of cardiac abnormalities in an HIV-seropositive population on antiretroviral combination therapy. *J AIDS* 2001;**27**:318–20.

113. Lipshultz SE, Shearer WT, Thompson B, et al. Cardiac effects of antiretroviral therapy in HIV-negative infants born to HIV-positive mothers. *J Am Coll Cardiol* 2011;**57**:76–85.

114. Mondy KE, Gottdiener J, Overton ET, et al. High prevalence of echocardiographic abnormalities among HIV-infected persons in the era of highly active antiretroviral therapy. *Antivir Ther* 2009;**14**(8):1195–208.

115. Torres SM, March TH, Carter MM, et al. In utero exposure of female CD-1 mice to AZT and/or 3TC: I. persistence of microscopic lesions in cardiac tissue. *Cardiovasc Toxicol* 2010;**10**:37–50.

116. Torres SM, Divi RL, Walker DM, et al. In utero exposure of female CD-1 mice to AZT and/or 3TC: II. Persistence of functional alterations in cardiac tissue. *Cardiovasc Toxicol* 2010;**10**:87–99.

117. Yan Q. Acute effects of HIV protease inhibitors on the failing heart. *Antiviral Ther* 2006;**11**:1051–1060.

118. Reyskens KMSE, Fisher T-L, Schisler JC, et al. Cardio-metabolic effects of HIV protease inhibitors (Lopinavir/Ritonavir). *PLoS One* 2013;**8**(9):e73347.

119. Lipshultz SE, Mas CM, Henkel JM, et al. HAART to heart: highly active antiretroviral therapy and the risk of cardiovascular disease in HIV-infected or exposed children and adults. *Expert Rev Anti Infect Ther* 2012;**10**:661–74.

120. Hoffman M, Lipshultz SE, Miller TL. Malnutrition and cardiac abnormalities in the HIV-infected patients. In: Miller TL, Gorbach S (eds), *Nutritional aspects of HIV infection*, pp. 33–9. Arnold, London, 1999.

121. Yogasundaram H, Putko BN, Tien J, *et al.* Hydroxychloroquine-induced cardiomyopathy: case report, pathophysiology, diagnosis, and treatment. *Can J Cardiol* 2014;**30**:1706–15.

122. Daniels BH, McComb RD, Mobley BC, *et al.* LC3 and p62 as diagnostic markers of drug-induced autophagic vacuolar cardiomyopathy: a study of 3 cases. *Am J Surg Pathol* 2013;**37**:1014–21.

123. Soong TR, Barouch LA, Champion HC, Wigley FM, Halushka MK. New clinical and ultrastructural findings in hydroxychloroquine-induced cardiomyopathy—a report of 2 cases. *Hum Pathol* 2007;**38**:1858–63.

124. Baguet JP, Tremel F, Fabre M. Chloroquine cardiomyopathy with conduction disorders. *Heart* 1999;**81**:221–3.

125. Nord JE, Shah PK, Rinaldi RZ, *et al.* Hydroxychloroquine cardiotoxicity in systemic lupus erythematosus: a report of 2 cases and review of the literature. *Semin Ann Rheum Dis* 2004;**33**:336–51.

126. Page RL, O'Bryant CL, Cheng D, Dow TJ, Ky B, Stein CM, Spencer AP, Trupp RJ, Lindenfeld J. Drugs that may cause or exacerbate heart failure. *Circulation* 2016;**134**:e32–e69.

127. Chatre C, Filippi N, Roubille F, Pers Y-M. Heart involvement in a woman treated with hydroxychloroquine for systemic lupus erythematosus revealing fabry disease. *J Rheumatol* 2016;**43**:997–8.

128. Yogasundaram H, Hung W, Paterson ID, Sergi C, Oudit GY. Chloroquine-induced cardiomyopathy: a reversible cause of heart failure. *ESC Hear Fail* 2018;**5**:372–5.

129. Tonnesmann T, Kandolf R, Lewalter T. Chloroquine cardiomyopathy—a review of the literature. *Immunopharmacol Immunotoxicol* 2013;**35**:434–42.

130. Schumacher SM, Prasad SVN. Tumor necrosis factor-α in heart failure: an updated review. *Curr Cardiol Rep* 2018;**20**(11):117.

131. Kwon HJ, Cote TR, Cuffe MS, Kramer JM, Braun MM. Case reports of heart failure after therapy with a tumor necrosis factor antagonist. *Ann Intern Med* 2003;**138**:807–11.

132. Wolfe F, Michaud K. Heart failure in rheumatoid arthritis: rates, predictors, and the effect of anti-tumor necrosis factor therapy. *Am J Med* 2004;**116**:305–11.

133. Emmert MY, Salzberg SP, Emmert LS, *et al.* Severe cardiomyopathy following treatment with the tumour necrosis factor-a inhibitor adalimumab for Crohn's disease. *Eur J Heart Fail* 2009;**11**:1106–9.

134. Cohen MC, Huberman MS, Nesto RW. Recombinant alpha-2 interferon-related cardiomyopathy. *Am J Med* 1988;**85**:549–51.

135. Deyton LR, Walker RE, Kovacs JA, *et al.* Reversible cardiac dysfunction associated with interferon alpha therapy in AIDS patients with Kaposi's sarcoma. *N Engl J Med* 1989;**321**:1246–9.

136. Sonnenblick M, Rosin A. Cardiotoxicity of interferon. A review of 44 cases. *Chest* 1991;**99**:557–61.

137. Hernandez AV, Usmani A, Rajamanickam A, Moheet A. Thiazolidinediones and risk of heart failure in patients with or at high risk of type 2 diabetes mellitus: a meta-analysis and meta-regression analysis of placebo-controlled randomized clinical trials. *Am J Cardiovasc Drugs* 2011;**11**:115–28.

138. Loke YK, Kwok CS, Singh S. Comparative cardiovascular effects of thiazolidinediones: systematic review and meta-analysis of observational studies. *BMJ* 2011;**342**:d1309.

139. Wood JC, Enriquez C, Ghugre N, *et al.* Physiology and pathophysiology of iron cardiomyopathy in thalassemia. *Ann NY Acad Sci* 2005;**1054**:386–95.

140. Gujja P, Rosing DR, Tripodi DJ, Shizukuda Y. Iron overload cardiomyopathy, better understanding of an increasing disorder. *J Am Coll Cardiol* 2010;**56**:1001–12.

141. Bradberry SM, Wilkinson JM, Ferner RE. Systemic toxicity related to metal hip prostheses. *Clin Toxicol (Phila)* 2014;**52**:837–47.

142. Scott JM, Khakoo A, Mackey JR, *et al.* Modulation of anthracycline-induced cardiotoxicity by aerobic exercise in breast cancer: current evidence and underlying mechanisms. *Circulation* 2011;**124**:642–50.

143. Altena R, Perik PJ, van Veldhuisen DJ, de Vries EG, Gietema JA. Cardiovascular toxicity caused by cancer treatment: strategies for early detection. *Lancet Oncol* 2009;**10**:391–9.

144. Suter TM, Ewer MS. Cancer drugs and the heart: importance and management. *Eur Heart J* 2013;**34**:1102–11.

12

Peripartum cardiomyopathy

Caroline Coats, Alice Jackson, and Mark Petrie

Introduction

Peripartum cardiomyopathy (PPCM) is an important cause of maternal and infant mortality worldwide. Although heart failure presenting in the puerperium is well recognized, PPCM is a distinct cardiomyopathy that requires a high index of suspicion for diagnosis. There are known risk factors, but the aetiology and natural history of this disorder are not fully understood. The past decade has seen an increase in knowledge about the epidemiology, pathophysiology, and genetics of this condition, leading to the first treatment trials, alongside international guidelines and registries.

Definition

Peripartum cardiomyopathy is currently defined by the European Society of Cardiology PPCM Working Group as 'an idiopathic cardiomyopathy presenting with heart failure secondary to left ventricular systolic dysfunction toward the end of pregnancy or in the months following delivery, where no other cause of heart failure is found. It is a diagnosis of exclusion. The left ventricle (LV) may not be dilated, but the ejection fraction (EF) is nearly always reduced below 45%'.[1] This definition is broader than previous ones which required that the condition manifested in the third trimester of pregnancy or the first five months postpartum.[2,3] Around 80% of patients present within four months postpartum; however, there is a small proportion of women who present earlier in pregnancy and of women who are diagnosed beyond five months postpartum.[4]

Epidemiology

On average, one in 1000 pregnancies is complicated by PPCM and the incidence, at least in the USA, appears to be increasing.[5,6] This may be because of increasing maternal age and multiple pregnancy, or just better recognition of the condition.

Geography

Women of African descent have a higher incidence of PPCM, with geographical hotspots in Nigeria (one in 100) and Haiti (one in 300).[7–9] There are a lack of prospective data from many parts of the world. The only population-based European estimate is from Denmark, where PPCM complicates one in 10 149 deliveries.[10] One other study from Sweden reported an incidence rate of one in 5719 deliveries, but may include other types of heart failure.[11] The variation in incidence reflects not only the population studied, but also the definition, era of the study, and methods used (**Figure 12.1**).

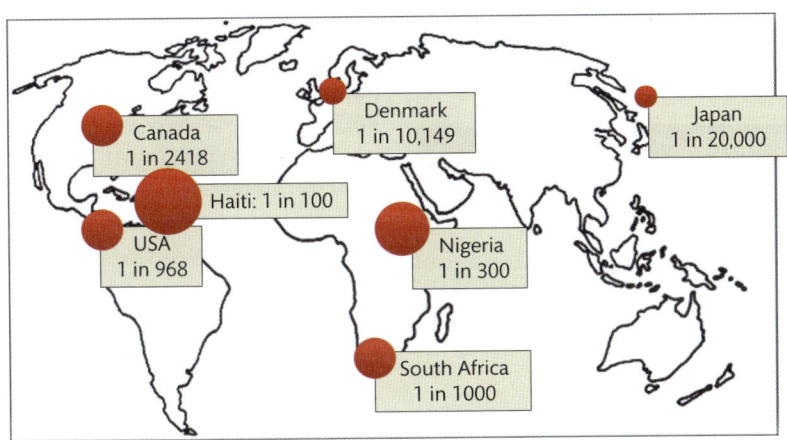

Figure 12.1 Incidence of peripartum cardiomyopathy worldwide.

Age

Although more prevalent in women aged >30 years, PPCM has been reported in individuals aged between 15 and 54 years.[6]

Ethnicity

According to hospital discharge data, the incidence of PPCM in the USA is lowest in Hispanics and highest in African-Americans, and this appears to be independent of socio-economic factors.[6,9,12]

Risk factors

In addition to age and ethnicity, several other risk factors for the development of PPCM have been identified (Box 12.1). PPCM is more common in multiparous women and those with multiple gestation. A higher incidence is observed in women with pre-eclampsia and eclampsia, as well as conventional cardiovascular risk factors including hypertension, obesity, diabetes, and smoking. The interaction between hypertension, pre-eclampsia, and PPCM is increasingly debated.

Environmental factors

A high salt intake and dietary deficiencies have been proposed as factors that increase the risk of PPCM. Whereas environmental factors may be important in some geographical regions, no causative links to diet have been established.

Genetic factors

Familial occurrence has been described and rare genetic variants have been found in women with PPCM.[13] A recent study of 172 patients with PPCM found that 15% of individuals had a pathogenic variant in the gene titin, *TTN*.[14] This is the same proportion as found in dilated cardiomyopathy (DCM), raising the possibility that PPCM may present as a *forme fruste* (atypical manifestation) of pre-existing DCM. Screening family members is advisable because 10–15% of family members will either have a sister or mother with PPCM or a brother with DCM.[15,16]

Pre-eclampsia

The prevalence of pre-eclampsia in women with PPCM is as high as 25%, compared to 3–5% in the general population.[17,18] Both conditions are associated with a lower serum oncotic pressure that can predispose to non-cardiogenic pulmonary oedema in the setting of other stressors. There is no universal consensus as to whether PPCM and pre-eclampsia are distinct entities.[19]

Box 12.1 Risk factors for peripartum cardiomyopathy

- Maternal age >30 years
- Multiparity
- Multigravida
- Geography
- Obesity
- Pregnancy-induced hypertension/eclampsia
- Tocolytics e.g. β_2 agonists
- Ethnic origin (e.g. African descent)
- Nutritional deficiencies

Aetiology

The aetiology of PPCM remains unknown. In normal pregnancy, the myocardium develops mild hypertrophy to accommodate the increased cardiac output that is necessary in pregnancy. In most women, the heart returns to normal via the activation of protective cardiac myocyte signalling pathways. In others, a failure of this defence mechanism leads to PPCM. In many women, cardiac function eventually returns to normal, but others can die or develop irreversible dysfunction.

Pathophysiology

Numerous hypotheses have been proposed, including viral antigen persistence, autoimmunity, stress-activated cytokines, myocyte apoptosis, and micronutrient deficiencies. Genetic factors and the role of prolactin are emerging as potentially causal factors.

Inflammation

Inflammation and apoptosis contribute to the pathogenesis of PPCM. Plasma markers of inflammation, including C-reactive protein (CRP), interleukin-6, tumour necrosis factor-α and the soluble death receptor, sFas/Apo1 are elevated in patients with PPCM, and correlate with increased LV dimension and lower LVEF at presentation.[20]

Viral persistence

Endomyocardial biopsies frequently show inflammatory infiltrates and viral genomes implicated in myocarditis.[21] Since immune defence is lowered in pregnancy, latent viral infections may become reactivated. The reported prevalence of myocarditis in patients with PPCM is highly variable, and, although it is possible that viral infection may trigger the condition, a causal role has not been established.

Vascular hormonal hypothesis

The concept that PPCM is a vascular disease triggered by hormonal changes during pregnancy comes from elegant mechanistic work carried out in mice.[22] The pituitary hormone, prolactin, is activated via a receptor on the cardiomyocyte which leads to an increased oxidative stress and an upregulation of cathepsin D. The cathepsin D protease is needed for the conversion of the normal 23 kDa prolactin into the abnormal 16 kDa prolactin subfragment. This cardiotoxic peptide is responsible for endothelial cell dissociation, prevention of capillary formation, and apoptosis.[23] Support for this mechanism is the observation that bromocriptine (a prolactin inhibitor) administration has been linked to recovery of LV function in patients with PPCM.[24,25] The second part to this hypothesis is the recognition that vascular endothelial growth factor signalling is inhibited by soluble FLT1.[26] This placental hormone, which is markedly elevated in pre-eclampsia and twin gestations, thus also provides support for the epidemiological link between PPCM and pre-eclampsia.[27]

Diagnosis

The clinical presentation of PPCM is highly variable and, because it is a rare condition, the diagnosis is often missed unless there is a high index of suspicion. Symptoms can be subtle and mimic those

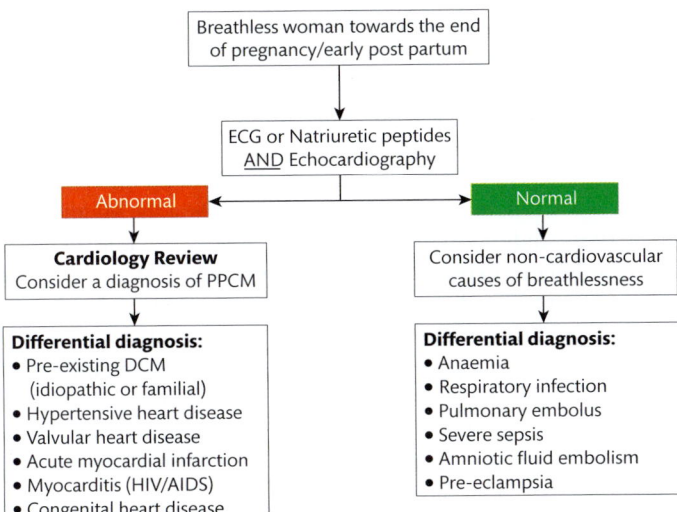

Figure 12.2 Approach to the breathless patient during or after pregnancy.

of normal pregnancy—the most frequent are dyspnoea, cough, and fatigue. Lower limb oedema, orthopnoea, paroxysmal nocturnal dyspnoea, palpitations, and dizziness can also occur. Less common are chest pain, right upper quadrant pain (due to hepatic congestion), nocturia, and postural hypotension. Sometimes the presentation can be very dramatic with acute pulmonary oedema, arrhythmias, or cardiogenic shock. Most women have severe symptoms (New York Heart Association class III or IV) by the time of diagnosis.[17] Foetal growth retardation can also be a sign that something is wrong with the mother's heart. A straightforward clinical approach to the breathless pregnant patient is illustrated in Figure 12.2. Physical examination may reveal abnormalities such as a gallop rhythm, jugular venous distension, and cardiomegaly.

Differential diagnosis

Not all heart failure during pregnancy is due to PPCM. Pre-existing cardiomyopathies as well as congenital and valvular heart diseases can be unmasked by pregnancy. Usually these present earlier than PPCM, and a history of hypertension, murmurs in childhood and any family history of cardiomyopathy or pre-eclampsia should be elicited.

Investigations

Basic laboratory and clinical investigations will usually be requested by a member of the obstetric team. Specific cardiovascular investigations may include:

- Electrocardiogram: an ECG is often non-specific and can be normal in PPCM, though most women have some sort of abnormality present. The presence of T-wave inversion, bundle branch block, and large voltage are abnormal in young women and should raise the possibility of a pre-existing cardiomyopathy. Any ECG abnormality in a pregnant or postpartum woman should prompt further investigation.
- Echocardiography: ultrasound imaging of the heart is fundamental to make a diagnosis of PPCM. Echocardiography can also quantify left ventricular function and estimate pulmonary pressures. Usually

all four cardiac chambers dilate—the left ventricle (LV) is always impaired. Mitral regurgitation is typically secondary to chamber dilation and is a marker of poor outcome. Careful evaluation of the right heart is important since a pulmonary embolus is an important differential diagnosis, but can also coexist in women with PPCM. Since pregnant women are more prone to clotting, assessment for LV thrombus should also be made.

- Chest X-ray: the foetal dose of radiation from a chest radiograph is small (<0.01 mGy) but should only be performed if other investigations fail to explain the cause of breathlessness.
- Cardiac magnetic resonance imaging: this has an evolving role and can complement the information provided by echocardiography.[28] It provides excellent anatomical definition and is safe in later stages of pregnancy. However, the use of gadolinium as a contrast agent is usually avoided as its safety in pregnancy is uncertain. Non-contrast mapping techniques can be useful to detect diffuse fibrosis and myocardial oedema but have not been widely applied in pregnancy. Women must be able to lie flat and perform breath-holds for the scan to be of diagnostic quality.
- Cardiac catheterization, higher-risk groups may have coronary disease. Women are more prone to coronary dissections during pregnancy. However, cardiac catheterization is usually avoided in pregnant women unless life-saving coronary intervention is anticipated.
- Endomyocardial biopsy: this may be performed to rule out fulminant myocarditis, but the yield is low, and, unless it will alter treatment, it should not be done.
- Biomarkers: levels of natriuretic peptides and cardiac troponins are typically elevated in PPCM but no specific cut-offs exist. Although not clinically available, recent work suggests that microRNA 146a may be a disease-specific biomarker and can distinguish PPCM from idiopathic dilated cardiomyopathy.[29] Markers of inflammation such as CRP may also be elevated.

Management

The management of PPCM is targeted at alleviating heart failure symptoms and improving prognosis with both drug and device therapies. Drug therapy should be carefully chosen to minimize risk to the foetus in pregnancy or infant during breastfeeding.

General pharmacotherapy

This includes preload reduction with diuretics and nitrates, and afterload reduction with hydralazine, nitrates, and amlodipine. β-blockers are frontline therapy. Although they can cause a degree of intrauterine growth retardation, their benefits outweigh their risks. Angiotensin converting enzyme inhibitors and angiotensin receptor blockers are contraindicated during pregnancy, but can be used during breastfeeding. Rigorous management of chronic heart failure includes fluid and salt restriction. Although diuretics have been said to reduce placental blood flow, they are frequently under-used during pregnancy. If fluid-overloaded, diuretic therapy usually results in improved cardiovascular status. Anticoagulation with heparin should be considered if LVEF <35%, if there is LV thrombus, or atrial fibrillation. The substantial rate of thromboembolism seen in PPCM[18,30] has led many to recommend anticoagulation for all patients with PPCM until 3–6 months postpartum.

Advanced heart failure therapies

In haemodynamically unstable patients, there may be a need to use inotropes (digoxin, dopamine, dobutamine), and mechanical circulatory support (intra-aortic balloon pump, extracorporeal membrane oxygenation, or LV assist device). Around 20% women with PPCM experience ventricular arrhythmias. A wearable or implantable cardioverter–defibrillator (ICD) should be considered.[31] A high threshold for ICD implantation is sensible as the high rate of recovery means that a patient might continue with an ICD in a heart with a normal ejection fraction. Cardiac resynchronization therapy is sometimes necessary.

Bromocriptine

Based on its key role in the pathophysiology of PPCM, pharmacological blockade of prolactin offers the possibility of a disease-specific therapy. One study from South Africa reported dramatic effects of bromocriptine. In a randomized trial of 20 patients, those given bromocriptine had a greater rate of recovery of cardiac function and lower mortality.[25] A recent German trial of one week versus eight weeks of bromocriptine found a high rate of cardiac recovery and very low mortality in both arms.[32] No placebo arm was included in this trial. No difference in outcomes of offspring has been reported to date.[33] Importantly, prolactin suppresses lactation, which is of concern, particularly in the developing world where unsafe water supplies and malnutrition make reliance on breast milk critical.[34] Large placebo-controlled clinical trials are needed to determine optimal dose, duration, and impact of treatment with bromocriptine therapy.[35]

Obstetric care

When a diagnosis of PPCM is being considered, escalation of obstetric care and involvement of cardiologists, anaesthetists, paediatricians, and the intensive care team is recommended. Spontaneous labour and vaginal deliveries are feasible in stable patients, whereas planned Caesarean section or early delivery is advised in unstable patients. In the European Society of Cardiology (ESC) PPCM registry, the mode of delivery was vaginal in 33% of women diagnosed prepartum and in 53% of women diagnosed postpartum.[18]

Breastfeeding

Whether a woman with PPCM should breastfeed has been controversial. If she is prescribed bromocriptine, lactation will be suppressed. If a patient is not prescribed bromocriptine, the risks associated with transmission of heart failure drugs to the baby should be considered.[36] Recent data from the prospective Investigations of Pregnancy-Associated Cardiomyopathy (IPAC) study of 100 women from North America demonstrated that breastfeeding was not associated with adverse outcomes or persistent myocardial dysfunction, indicating that it is not harmful.[37]

Prognosis

Mortality and morbidity

Mortality varies significantly according to ethnicity and geography. In the USA, in-hospital mortality for women with PPCM is 1.3% and has increased slightly over the past decade.[6] The overall frequency of

maternal adverse events (defined as mortality, cardiac arrest, heart transplant, mechanical circulatory support, acute pulmonary oedema, thromboembolism, or ICD or pacemaker) was 13.5%, with the commonest complication being thromboembolism, affecting 6.6% women.[6] This is similar to the rate of thromboembolism in the ESC PPCM registry (7%).[18] In this registry, overall six-month mortality was 6%, ranging from 4% in Europe to 10% in the Middle East. In the IPAC study, mortality at 12 months was 4%.[38] Little is known about the long-term prognosis for women with PPCM and there are only a handful of studies examining outcomes beyond five years; in studies from the USA, mortality ranged from 7% to 17%.[39–41]

Foetal outcomes (e.g. birth weight, neonatal morbidity, and infant mortality) are poorly characterized. Neonatal death occurred in 5% of live births in the ESC PPCM registry.[18] Studies that have compared PPCM and non-PPCM pregnancies with regards to neonatal mortality have produced conflicting results.[42,43]

Recovery and relapse

The overall prognosis of PPCM is variable, ranging from complete recovery to progressive heart failure and death. Complete normalization of LVEF occurs in around 50% of patients, but has been reported in up to 65% within six months of delivery.[44,45] The worst prognosis is seen in those aged >30 years, and in women with high parity and lower LVEF at presentation.[38] In those requiring transplantation, higher rates of rejection are observed compared to transplant recipients for other causes. The optimal duration of heart failure medication is not known.

Mechanical circulatory support and cardiac transplantation

In countries where advanced heart failure therapies are available, reported rates of cardiac transplantation in women with PPCM range from 0% to 11%.[1,46] Recent data from the Interagency Registry for Mechanically Assisted Circulatory Support (INTERMACS) registry showed that women with PPCM who receive mechanical circulatory support have a better survival than women with non-PPCM, with a two-year survival of 83% and a recovery rate of 6%.[47]

Contraception advice

Postnatal women and their partners need careful counselling about contraception.[48] Oestrogen and combined hormonal contraceptives should be avoided because oestrogen increases the risk of thromboembolism. Progestogen-releasing intrauterine devices (IUDs) or intramuscular, subcutaneous, and subdermal forms of progesterone-only contraception appear to be safe. Barrier methods have a high failure rate. Sterilization (e.g. tubal ligation or vasectomy) might be considered.

Risk of recurrence with a subsequent pregnancy

Women with PPCM should be counselled about relapse rate with future pregnancies. The extent of recovery determines the risks associated with another pregnancy. If the EF has normalized, there is a risk of recurrence (usually a decline in EF) affecting up to 20%. In those whose heart function has not recovered, the risk of recurrence is 30–50%. Persistently reduced LVEF before a subsequent pregnancy is associated with higher mortality and lower rate of full recovery at follow-up.[49]

Summary

Despite progress in understanding the pathophysiology of PPCM, it is still a rare and serious disorder that is often recognized late. The prior definitions of PPCM—emphasizing strict time-windows and echocardiograph cut-offs—are likely to have led to the condition being overlooked or misdiagnosed. Early diagnosis and multidisciplinary treatment are essential for better outcomes. Global efforts to support patient registries will help identify biomarkers to facilitate diagnosis and predict outcome. The clinical registry initiated by the Heart Failure Association of the European Society of Cardiology will be a rich source of longitudinal data on PPCM and will support the development of clinical guidelines. As we understand more about mechanisms that allow a heart to recover, our knowledge about PPCM will improve.

REFERENCES

1. Sliwa K, Hilfiker-Kleiner D, Petrie MC, et al. Current state of knowledge on aetiology, diagnosis, management, and therapy of peripartum cardiomyopathy: a position statement from the Heart Failure Association of the European Society of Cardiology Working Group on peripartum cardiomyopathy. Eur J Heart Fail 2010;12(8):767–78.

2. Maron BJ, Towbin JA, Thiene G, et al. Contemporary definitions and classification of the cardiomyopathies: an American Heart Association Scientific Statement from the Council on Clinical Cardiology, Heart Failure and Transplantation Committee; Quality of Care and Outcomes Research and Functional Genomics and Translational Biology Interdisciplinary Working Groups; and Council on Epidemiology and Prevention. Circulation 2006;113(14):1807–16.

3. Pearson GD, Veille JC, Rahimtoola S, et al. Peripartum cardiomyopathy: National Heart, Lung, and Blood Institute and Office of Rare Diseases (National Institutes of Health) workshop recommendations and review. JAMA 2000;283(9):1183–8.

4. Lampert MB, Lang RM. Peripartum cardiomyopathy. Am Heart J 1995;130(4):860–70.

5. Mielniczuk LM, Williams K, Davis DR, et al. Frequency of peripartum cardiomyopathy. Am J Cardiol 2006;97(12):1765–8.

6. Kolte D, Khera S, Aronow WS, et al. Temporal trends in incidence and outcomes of peripartum cardiomyopathy in the United States: a nationwide population-based study. J Am Heart Assoc 2014;3(3):e001056.

7. Sliwa K, Fett J, Elkayam U. Peripartum cardiomyopathy. Lancet 2006;368(9536):687–93.

8. Fett JD, Christie LG, Carraway RD, Murphy JG. Five-year prospective study of the incidence and prognosis of peripartum cardiomyopathy at a single institution. Mayo Clin Proc 2005;80(12):1602–6.

9. Gentry MB, Dias JK, Luis A, et al. African-American women have a higher risk for developing peripartum cardiomyopathy. J Am Coll Cardiol 2010;55(7):654–9.

10. Ersbøll AS, Johansen M, Damm P, et al. Peripartum cardiomyopathy in Denmark: a retrospective, population-based study of incidence, management and outcome. Eur J Heart Fail 2017;19(12):1712–20.

11. Barasa A, Rosengren A, Sandstrom TZ, Ladfors L, Schaufelberger M. Heart failure in late pregnancy and postpartum: incidence and long-term mortality in Sweden from 1997 to 2010. J Cardiac Fail 2017;23(5):370–8.

12. Brar SS, Khan SS, Sandhu GK, et al. Incidence, mortality, and racial differences in peripartum cardiomyopathy. Am J Cardiol 2007;100(2):302–4.

13. Cemin R, Janardhanan R, Donazzan L, Daves M. Peripartum cardiomyopathy: moving towards a more central role of genetics. Curr Cardiol Rev 2013;9(3):179–84.

14. Ware JS, Arany Z, Kealey A, Liu P, Cook SA, Safirstein J, et al. Shared Genetic Predisposition in Peripartum and Dilated Cardiomyopathies. N Engl J Med. 2016;374:233–41.

15. Morales A, Painter T, Li R, et al. Rare variant mutations in pregnancy-associated or peripartum cardiomyopathy. Circulation 2010;121(20):2176–82.

16. van Spaendonck-Zwarts KY, van Tintelen JP, van Veldhuisen DJ, et al. Peripartum cardiomyopathy as a part of familial dilated cardiomyopathy. Circulation 2010;121(20):2169–75.

17. Bello N, Rendon IS, Arany Z. The relationship between pre-eclampsia and peripartum cardiomyopathy: a systematic review and meta-analysis. J Am Coll Cardiol 2013;62(18):1715–23.

18. Sliwa K, Petrie MC, van der Meer P, et al. Clinical presentation, management and 6-month outcomes in women with peripartum cardiomyopathy: an ESC EORP registry. Eur Heart J 2020 Aug 25 [online ahead of print].

19. Bello NA, Arany Z. Molecular mechanisms of peripartum cardiomyopathy: a vascular/hormonal hypothesis. Trends Cardiovasc Med 2015;25(6):499–504.

20. Sliwa K, Forster O, Libhaber E, et al. Peripartum cardiomyopathy: inflammatory markers as predictors of outcome in 100 prospectively studied patients. Eur Heart J 2006;27(4):441–6.

21. Bultmann BD, Klingel K, Nabauer M, Wallwiener D, Kandolf R. High prevalence of viral genomes and inflammation in peripartum cardiomyopathy. Am J Obstet Gynecol 2005;193(2):363–5.

22. Hilfiker-Kleiner D, Kaminski K, Podewski E, et al. A cathepsin D-cleaved 16 kDa form of prolactin mediates postpartum cardiomyopathy. Cell 2007;128(3):589–600.

23. Bajou K, Herkenne S, Thijssen VL, et al. PAI-1 mediates the antiangiogenic and profibrinolytic effects of 16K prolactin. Nature Med 2014;20(7):741–7.

24. Hilfiker-Kleiner D, Meyer GP, Schieffer E, et al. Recovery from postpartum cardiomyopathy in 2 patients by blocking prolactin release with bromocriptine. J Am Coll Cardiol 2007;50(24):2354–5.

25. Sliwa K, Blauwet L, Tibazarwa K, et al. Evaluation of bromocriptine in the treatment of acute severe peripartum cardiomyopathy: a proof-of-concept pilot study. Circulation 2010;121(13):1465–73.

26. Damp J, Givertz MM, Semigran M, et al. Relaxin-2 and soluble Flt1 levels in peripartum cardiomyopathy: results of the multicenter IPAC study. JACC Heart Fail 2016;4(5):380–8.

27. Powe CE, Levine RJ, Karumanchi SA. Preeclampsia, a disease of the maternal endothelium: the role of antiangiogenic factors and implications for later cardiovascular disease. Circulation 2011;123(24):2856–69.

28. Arora NP, Mohamad T, Mahajan N, et al. Cardiac magnetic resonance imaging in peripartum cardiomyopathy. Am J Med Sci 2014;347(2):112–17.

29. Halkein J, Tabruyn SP, Ricke-Hoch M, et al. MicroRNA-146a is a therapeutic target and biomarker for peripartum cardiomyopathy. J Clin Invest 2013;123(5):2143–54.

30. Sliwa K, Mebazaa A, Hilfiker-Kleiner D, et al. Clinical characteristics of patients from the worldwide registry on peripartum cardiomyopathy (PPCM): EURObservational

Research Programme in conjunction with the Heart Failure Association of the European Society of Cardiology Study Group on PPCM. *Eur J Heart Fail* 2017;**19**(9):1131–41.

31. Duncker D, Haghikia A, Konig T, *et al.* Risk for ventricular fibrillation in peripartum cardiomyopathy with severely reduced left ventricular function-value of the wearable cardioverter/defibrillator. *Eur J Heart Fail* 2014;**16**(12):1331–6.

32. Hilfiker-Kleiner D, Haghikia A, Berliner D, *et al.* Bromocriptine for the treatment of peripartum cardiomyopathy: a multicentre randomized study. *Eur Heart J* 2017;**38**(35):2671–9.

33. Haghikia A, Podewski E, Libhaber E, *et al.* Phenotyping and outcome on contemporary management in a German cohort of patients with peripartum cardiomyopathy. *Basic Res Cardiol* 2013;**108**(4):366.

34. Black RE, Victora CG, Walker SP, *et al.* Maternal and child undernutrition and overweight in low-income and middle-income countries. *Lancet* 2013;**382**(9890):427–51.

35. Bauersachs J, Arrigo M, Hilfiker-Kleiner D, *et al.* Current management of patients with severe acute peripartum cardiomyopathy: practical guidance from the Heart Failure Association of the European Society of Cardiology Study Group on peripartum cardiomyopathy. *Eur J Heart Fail* 2016;**18**(9):1096–105.

36. European Society of Gynecology; Association for European Paediatric Cardiology; German Society for Gender Medicine; Regitz-Zagrosek V, Lundqvist CB, Borghi C, *et al.*, ESC Committee for Practice Guidelines *et al.* ESC Guidelines on the management of cardiovascular diseases during pregnancy: the Task Force on the Management of Cardiovascular Diseases during Pregnancy of the European Society of Cardiology (ESC). *Eur Heart J* 2011;**32**(24):3147–97.

37. Koczo A, Marino A, Jeyabalan A, *et al.* Breastfeeding, cellular immune activation, and myocardial recovery in peripartum cardiomyopathy. *J Am Coll Cardiol Basic Trans Sci* 2019;**4**:291–300.

38. McNamara DM, Elkayam U, Alharethi R, *et al.* Clinical outcomes for peripartum cardiomyopathy in North America: results of the IPAC Study (Investigations of Pregnancy-Associated Cardiomyopathy). *J Am Coll Cardiol* 2015;**66**(8):905–14.

39. Harper MA, Meyer RE, Berg CJ. Peripartum cardiomyopathy: population-based birth prevalence and 7-year mortality. *Obstet Gynecol* 2012;**120**(5):1013–19.

40. Pillarisetti J, Kondur A, Alani A, *et al.* Peripartum cardiomyopathy: predictors of recovery and current state of implantable cardioverter-defibrillator use. *J Am Coll Cardiol* 2014;**63**(25 Pt A):2831–9.

41. Felker GM, Thompson RE, Hare JM, *et al.* Underlying causes and long-term survival in patients with initially unexplained cardiomyopathy. *N Engl J Med* 2000;**342**(15):1077–84.

42. Gunderson EP, Croen LA, Chiang V, *et al.* Epidemiology of peripartum cardiomyopathy: incidence, predictors, and outcomes. *Obstet Gynecol* 2011;**118**(3):583–91.

43. Kao DP, Hsich E, Lindenfeld J. Characteristics, adverse events, and racial differences among delivering mothers with peripartum cardiomyopathy. *JACC Heart Fail* 2013;**1**(5):409–16.

44. Blauwet LA, Libhaber E, Forster O, *et al.* Predictors of outcome in 176 South African patients with peripartum cardiomyopathy. *Heart* 2013;**99**(5):308–13.

45. Fett JD. Peripartum cardiomyopathy: a puzzle closer to solution. *Wld J Cardiol* 2014;**6**(3):87–99.

46. Elkayam U. Clinical characteristics of peripartum cardiomyopathy in the United States: diagnosis, prognosis, and management. *J Am Coll Cardiol* 2011;**58**(7):659–70.

47. Loyaga-Rendon RY, Pamboukian SV, Tallaj JA, *et al.* Outcomes of patients with peripartum cardiomyopathy who received mechanical circulatory support. Data from the Interagency Registry for Mechanically Assisted Circulatory Support. *Circ Heart Fail* 2014;**7**(2):300–9.

48. Sliwa K, Petrie MC, Hilfiker-Kleiner D, *et al.* Long term prognosis, subsequent pregnancy, contraception and overall management of peripartum cardiomyopathy: practical guidance paper from the Heart Failure Association of the European Society of Cardiology Study Group on Peripartum Cardiomyopathy. *Eur J Heart Fail* 2018;**20**:951–62.

49. Hilfiker-Kleiner D, Haghikia A, Masuko D, *et al.* Outcome of subsequent pregnancies in patients with a history of peripartum cardiomyopathy. *Eur J Heart Fail* 2017;**19**(12):1723–8.

13

Takotsubo syndrome

Alexander R. Lyon

Introduction

Takotsubo syndrome (TTS) is an acute heart failure syndrome with a typical appearance of apical and midventricular dysfunction in the absence of culprit coronary artery disease, and is increasingly recognized since its first description by Sato and colleagues in Hiroshima in 1990 (see **Figure 13.1**).[1] Over the last 10 years there has been a rapid rise in the number of publications and reported incidence of TTS,[2] reflecting improved awareness, rapid access to diagnostic coronary angiography for patients presenting with acute chest pain and acute ECG changes, and advances in modern cardiac imaging. Studies of hospital coding of acute emergency admissions in the Nationwide Inpatient Sample from the USA reported initially 6837 cases of TTS in 2008,[3] rising to 24 701 cases in pooled 2008–2009 data, and to 21 748 cases in 2011 alone.[4] This corresponds to 100 cases per million population per annum.

Since the first description, a striking feature is the demographic skew, with 90% of cases in all major series (>100 cases) being postmenopausal women.[3] This raises the possibility that oestrogen exposure followed by withdrawal may be a factor in the pathophysiology, and this would be logical from the data showing that oestrogen has sympatholytic properties both centrally and directly on the myocardium. Ten per cent of cases are in men or younger women. It is often noted in these 'atypical cases' that they may have disruption of their sex hormone physiology, e.g. men taking androgen deprivation therapy, or younger women with anorexia.

Diagnostic criteria and triggers

Patients with TTS have a number of typical features which are important to identify in order to confirm the diagnosis. Various diagnostic strategies have been proposed, with the most recent and comprehensive being from the Takotsubo Syndrome Taskforce of the Heart Failure Association (HFA) of the European Society of Cardiology (see **Box 13.1**).[5]

The onset of TTS is characterized by symptoms similar to acute myocardial infarction, with central chest pain originating from the heart, breathlessness, sweating, and sometimes palpitations or blackouts. A classical feature is a stressful trigger, which is reported

in ~70% cases, although with careful history-taking the incidence of stressful triggers is probably higher. Fifty per cent of stressful triggers are emotional, and 50% reflect acute medical or surgical emergencies. Most patients with TTS require urgent coronary angiography to exclude ST-segment elevation myocardial infarction (STEMI) or non-(N)STEMI: in TTS the epicardial coronary arteries are typically normal, although given the predilection of the condition for older patients, bystander atherosclerotic coronary artery disease may be

(a)

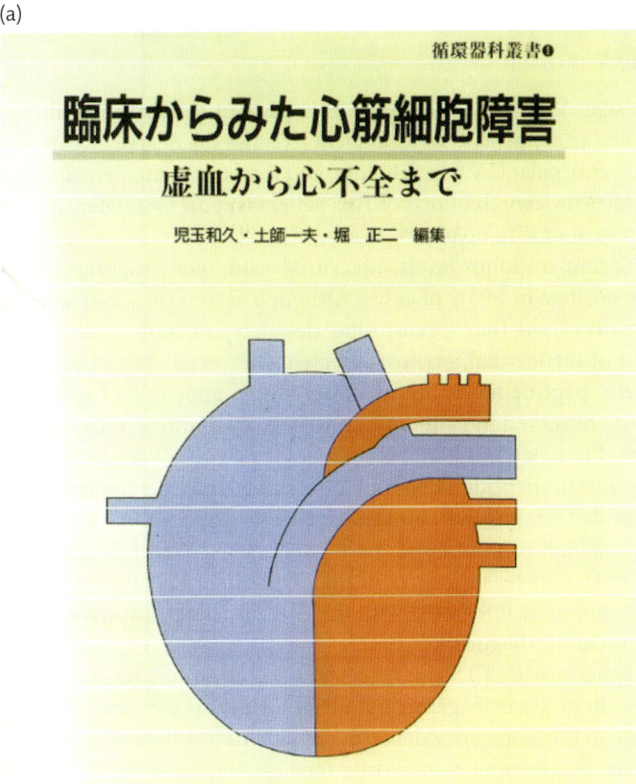

Figure 13.1 (a) Original description of takotsubo syndrome.
Reproduced from Sato H, Tateishi H, Uchida T, Dote K, Ishihara M. Tako-tsubo-like left ventricular dysfunction due to multivessel coronary spasm. In: Kodama K, Haze K, Hori M, editors. *Clinical aspect of myocardial injury: from ischemia to heart failure.* Tokyo: Kagakuhyoronsha Publishing Co.; 1990. p. 56–64 (in Japanese).

(b)

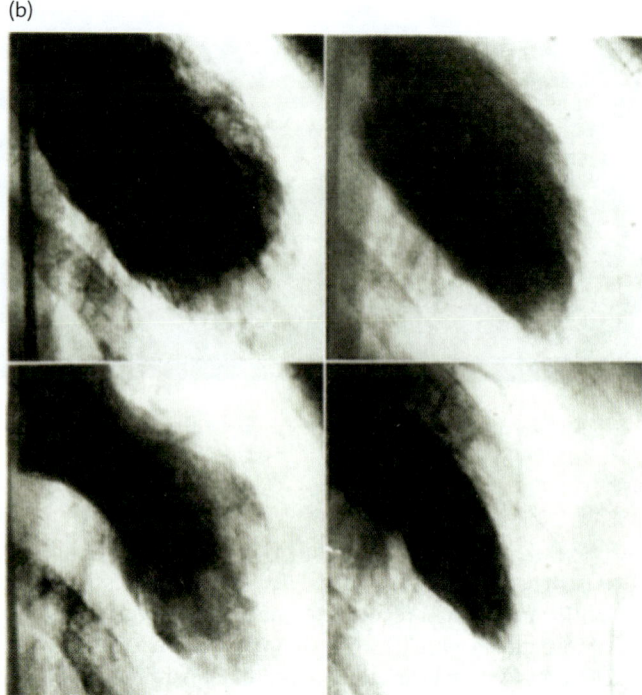

Figure 13.1 (b) The left ventriculography of case 1 at admission (*left*) and a week later (*right*). The left ventricle had a unique 'takotsubo shape' and it disappeared after a week.

Reproduced from Sato H, Tateishi H, Uchida T, Dote K, Ishihara M. Tako-tsubo-like left ventricular dysfunction due to multivessel coronary spasm. In: Kodama K, Haze K, Hori M, editors. *Clinical aspect of myocardial injury: from ischemia to heart failure.* Tokyo: Kagakuhyoronsha Publishing Co.; 1990. p. 56–64 (in Japanese).

Box 13.1 Heart Failure Association diagnostic criteria for takotsubo syndrome

1 Transient wall motion abnormalities of the left and/or right ventricular myocardium which are frequently, but not always, preceded by a stressful trigger (emotional or physical).

2 The regional wall motion abnormalities (RWMAs) usually[a] extend beyond a single epicardial vascular distribution, and often result in *circumferential dysfunction* of the ventricular segments involved (apical and/or mid-LV or basal segments).

3 The *absence of culprit atherosclerotic coronary artery disease* including acute plaque rupture, thrombus formation and coronary dissection or other pathological conditions to explain the pattern of temporary LV dysfunction observed (e.g. hypertrophic cardiomyopathy, viral myocarditis).

4 New and reversible electrocardiography (ECG) abnormalities (ST-segment elevation, ST depression, *left bundle branch block*[b], T-wave inversion and/or QTc prolongation) during the acute phase.

5 *Significantly elevated serum natriuretic peptide* (BNP or NT-proBNP) level during the acute phase.

6 Positive but relatively small elevation in cardiac troponin measured using a conventional assay (i.e. *disparity between the troponin level and the amount of the dysfunctional myocardium present*).[c]

7 Recovery of ventricular systolic function on cardiac imaging at follow-up.[d]

[a] Acute, reversible dysfunction of a single coronary territory has been reported.
[b] LBBB may be permanent. T-wave changes and QTc prolongation may take months to normalize.
[c] Troponin-negative cases have been reported, but are atypical.
[d] Small apical infarcts have been reported, but are atypical. Subendocardial infarcts have been reported, involving a small proportion of the acutely dysfunctional myocardium and are insufficient to explain the extent of acute RWMA observed.

Reproduced from Lyon AR, Bossone E, Schneider B, Sechtem U, Citro R, Underwood SR, *et al.* Current state of knowledge on Takotsubo syndrome: a Position Statement from the Taskforce on Takotsubo Syndrome of the Heart Failure Association of the European Society of Cardiology. *European Journal of Heart Failure.* 2016;**18**(1):8–27 with permission from John WIley and Sons.

present. Where it is present, it is important to clarify that the coronary artery disease is insufficient to cause the degree or pattern of left ventricular (LV) dysfunction, and therefore is incidental. Several studies reviewing cohorts of TTS patients report bystander coronary artery disease in up to 10% of cases.[6]

Serum troponin levels, measured using contemporary assays, are positive in >95% of cases. Although serum troponin levels are usually raised, they are disproportionately low compared to the extent of myocardial territory affected. Conversely the serum natriuretic peptide levels are extremely high, and much higher than those observed in acute myocardial infarction (see **Figure 13.2**).[7] The difference in biomarker phenotype, with a very high B-type natriuretic peptide (BNP) or N-terminal pro B-type natriuretic peptide (NT-proBNP) and relatively low troponin in cases of TTS versus high troponin and moderately raised BNP/NT-proBNP in STEMI, may be suggestive of the diagnosis prior to angiography,[8] but should be integrated with the clinical scenario and imaging to confirm the diagnosis.

Patients with TTS can be categorized according to presentation to help guide management strategies. Cases presenting usually *de novo* to the emergency department with TTS as their primary diagnosis, and without a coexisting medical condition which has triggered the syndrome, are defined as 'primary TTS'.[5] The physiological and emotional stress associated with a wide range of acute medical and surgical conditions can trigger catecholamine storms, and result in 'secondary TTS' as a secondary consequence of the pre-existing

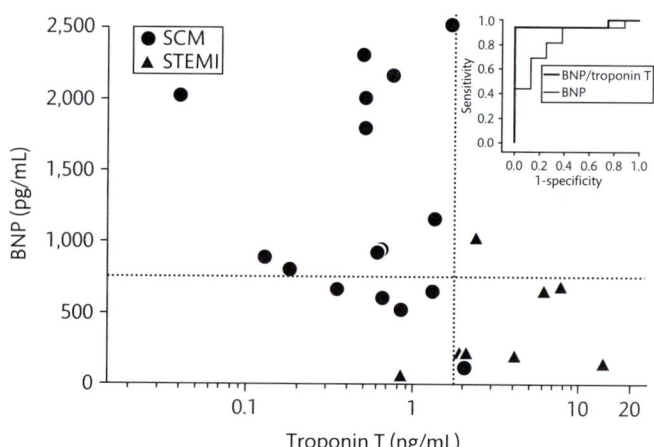

Figure 13.2 Cardiac biomarker profiles showing differences between takotsubo syndrome (SCM) and ST-segment elevation myocardial infarction (STEMI). BNP, B-type natriuretic peptide.

Reproduced from Madhavan M, Borlaug BA, Lerman A, Rihal CS, Prasad A. Stress hormone and circulating biomarker profile of apical ballooning syndrome (Takotsubo cardiomyopathy): insights into the clinical significance of B-type natriuretic peptide and troponin levels. *Heart* (British Cardiac Society) 2009;**95**(17):1436–41.

Box 13.2 Non-cardiac diseases, medical treatments, and other causes of secondary takotsubo syndrome

- Acute asthma and chronic obstructive pulmonary disease
- Thyrotoxicosis
- Addisonian crisis
- General anaesthetic induction
- Septic shock
- Myasthenic crisis
- Acute Guillain–Barré
- Acute systemic lupus erythematosus crisis
- Anaphylaxis
- Dobutamine stress echo
- Direct current cardioversion
- Exercise ECG testing
- Electroconvulsive therapy
- Acute cholecystitis
- Acute pancreatitis
- Pregnancy
- Near-drowning
- Attempted suicide (hanging)
- Taser stunning
- Restraint in custody
- Subarachnoid haemorrhage
- Head injury
- Stroke
- Cancer patients: high emotions/stress related to cancer scan results (clear, recurrence) and some cancer therapies, e.g. 5-flurouracil

medical condition (see **Box 13.2**).[5] Phaeochromocytoma and acute neurological emergencies such as subarachnoid haemorrhage are recognized triggers. There is also a growing number of cases triggered by drug administration (see **Box 13.3**). Secondary TTS can present in the acute respiratory, endocrinology, and neurology

Box 13.3 Drugs associated with triggering takotsubo syndrome

Catecholamines, and sympathomimetic and vagolytic drugs
- Epinephrine
- Dobutamine
- Metaraminol
- Ephedrine
- Ergonovine
- Oxymetazoline
- Atropine
- Venlafaxine
- Duloxetine
- Nortriptyline

Non-catecholaminergic and non-sympathomimetic drugs
- 5-Fluorouracil
- Combretastatin
- Cefotiam
- Pazopanib
- Anagrelide
- Levothyroxine
- Lumiracoxib
- Dipyridamole
- Potassium chloride

wards, acute surgical wards, the anaesthetic room and operating theatres, general and neurointensive care units, obstetric wards, and psychiatric departments.

Interestingly a stressful trigger is not essential and up to a third of cases have no overt stressful trigger, and appear to be 'spontaneous'.[6] Therefore the stressful trigger is not mandatory for the diagnosis.

Anatomical variants

The typical apical variant with apical and circumferential mid-ventricular hypokinesia, and basal hypercontractility, is present in around 80% cases. Other anatomical variants recognized include the inverted takotsubo or basal variant, with basal hypokinesia and apical hypercontractility, and the midventricular variant with circumferential midventricular hypokinesia, and both basal and apical hypercontractility (see **Figure 13.3**).

Clinical presenting features and complications

Patients presenting with primary TTS usually describe the sudden onset of acute chest pain, dyspnoea, and palpitations following a distinct stressful episode. Takotsubo syndrome can also be triggered by unexpected happy events including marriage proposals and winning the lottery.[9] Clinical examination and cardiac investigations depend upon the delay between onset of symptoms/stressful trigger and presentation to medical services, analogous to the evolving pattern of clinical features in patients with acute myocardial infarction. A diagnostic algorithm has been published which summarizes the pathway to aid investigation and diagnosis (see **Figure 13.4**).[5]

Patients presenting early (within 12 h of the stressful trigger) frequently have signs of sympathetic activation, with sinus tachycardia, hypertension, sweating, and anxiety, and in more severe cases acute pulmonary oedema, cardiogenic shock, and/or atrial or ventricular arrhythmias. During this phase they frequently have widespread ST elevation on their resting ECG (see **Figure 13.5**). After the initial catecholaminergic storm, patients with TTS develop a low cardiac output state with associated complications in the 24–72 h time window following the acute stress. This may be associated with relative bradycardia and possible peripheral vasodilatation. The ECG also evolves between 24 and 72 h with resolution of the ST elevation accompanied by widespread deep T-wave inversion and progressive prolongation of the QTc interval (see **Figure 13.5**), frequently to >500 ms with the associated risk of polymorphic ventricular tachycardia, *torsades de points* and ventricular fibrillation. Life-threatening ventricular tachyarrhythmias have been reported in up to 5% of cases.

Acute cardiovascular complications have been reported in up to 50% of patients with acute TTS (see **Box 13.4**). The new recommendation from the HFA Takotsubo Syndrome Taskforce is the implementation of risk stratification to ensure that patients at the highest risk are admitted to units with appropriate monitoring and resuscitation equipment (level 2 and level 3 care areas).[5] There are major and minor risk factors which can be simply identified at diagnosis to allow risk stratification (see **Table 13.1**).

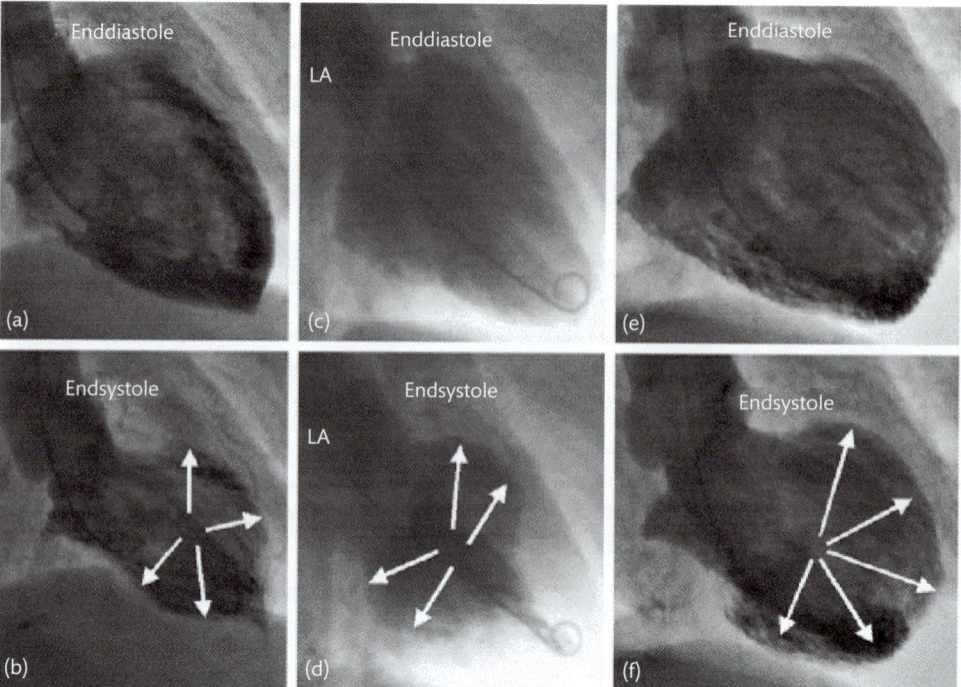

Figure 13.3 Anatomical variants of takotsubo syndrome. Midventricular (a, b), basal (c, d), and classical apical (e, f) anatomical variants during left ventriculography.

From Haghi D, Fluechter S, Suselbeck T, Kaden JJ, Borggrefe M, Papavassiliu T, et al. Cardiovascular magnetic resonance findings in typical versus atypical forms of the acute apical ballooning syndrome (takotsubo cardiomyopathy). *Int J Cardiol* 2007;**120**(2):205–11.

Cardiac imaging

Access to high-quality cardiac imaging is important to confirm the diagnosis and screen for acute complications.[10] Echocardiography is readily available in most cardiology units and aids diagnostic confirmation. Markedly reduced LV systolic function is the most prominent feature, alongside the characteristic pattern of wall motion abnormality, with an akinetic or markedly hypokinetic LV apex, and corresponding hypercontractility of the base. Citro and colleagues reported the distribution of regional wall motion abnormalities in 37 TTS patients compared with 37 matched anterior STEMI controls.[11] Using the standard 16-segment model of LV anatomy, they identified that the anterior basal segments (1 and 6) had preserved function in TTS patients compared to acute myocardial infaction (AMI) patients with anterior STEMI (see **Figure 13.6**). Conversely the inferior mid-LV and apical segments (8, 9, 10, 14; typically right coronary artery territory) were dysfunctional in TTS patients, consistent with circumferential hypokinesia of the apical and mid-LV myocardium, but preserved in the AMI cases (see **Figure 13.6**). More advanced echocardiographic techniques such as tissue Doppler and speckle-tracking demonstrate a significant loss of apical torsion and both ventricular systolic twist and twisting rate, which fully recovers at follow-up in patients with TTS, but remains perturbed in AMI controls.[12]

Echocardiography also has an important role to identify or exclude potential complications. Assessment for LV outflow tract obstruction is important in the presence of hypotension as this has important implications for further management. Contrast echocardiography may be helpful to exclude apical thrombosis.

Cardiac magnetic resonance (CMR) imaging in TTS patients during the acute phase is helpful to confirm the diagnosis in the 'non-echogenic' patients and in those where ventriculography was not performed. The use of late gadolinium enhancement (LGE) contrast imaging is very helpful to exclude AMI. In most cases LGE is completely absent both during the acute phase and at follow-up.[13] In a few cases patchy LGE during the acute phase has been reported, but was absent at follow-up.[14,15]

T2-weighted short-τ inversion recovery (T2w-STIR) studies are helpful during the acute phase, and show increased regional water content, probably due to acute myocardial oedema and inflammation.[16] The increased T2w-STIR signal matches the anatomical regions affected in the different variants (see **Figure 13.7**), though this is not specific for TTS: other forms of myocarditis should be considered and placed in the context of the clinical history.

In a small subgroup of patients, a pattern of small, transmural LGE persists, and is observed in the ventricular apex at follow-up. In the absence of coronary atherosclerosis, this may reflect pressure-induced ischaemia and myocardial necrosis due to the extremely high intraventricular pressures that can be generated during acute stress, with the thin-walled apex most susceptible, though histological confirmation of this LGE pattern is lacking. During the early phase of gadolinium contrast infusion the presence of LV apical thrombus can be evaluated.

Pathophysiology

The role of catecholamines appears central to the pathophysiology of TTS. This is supported by the frequent reports of a sudden,

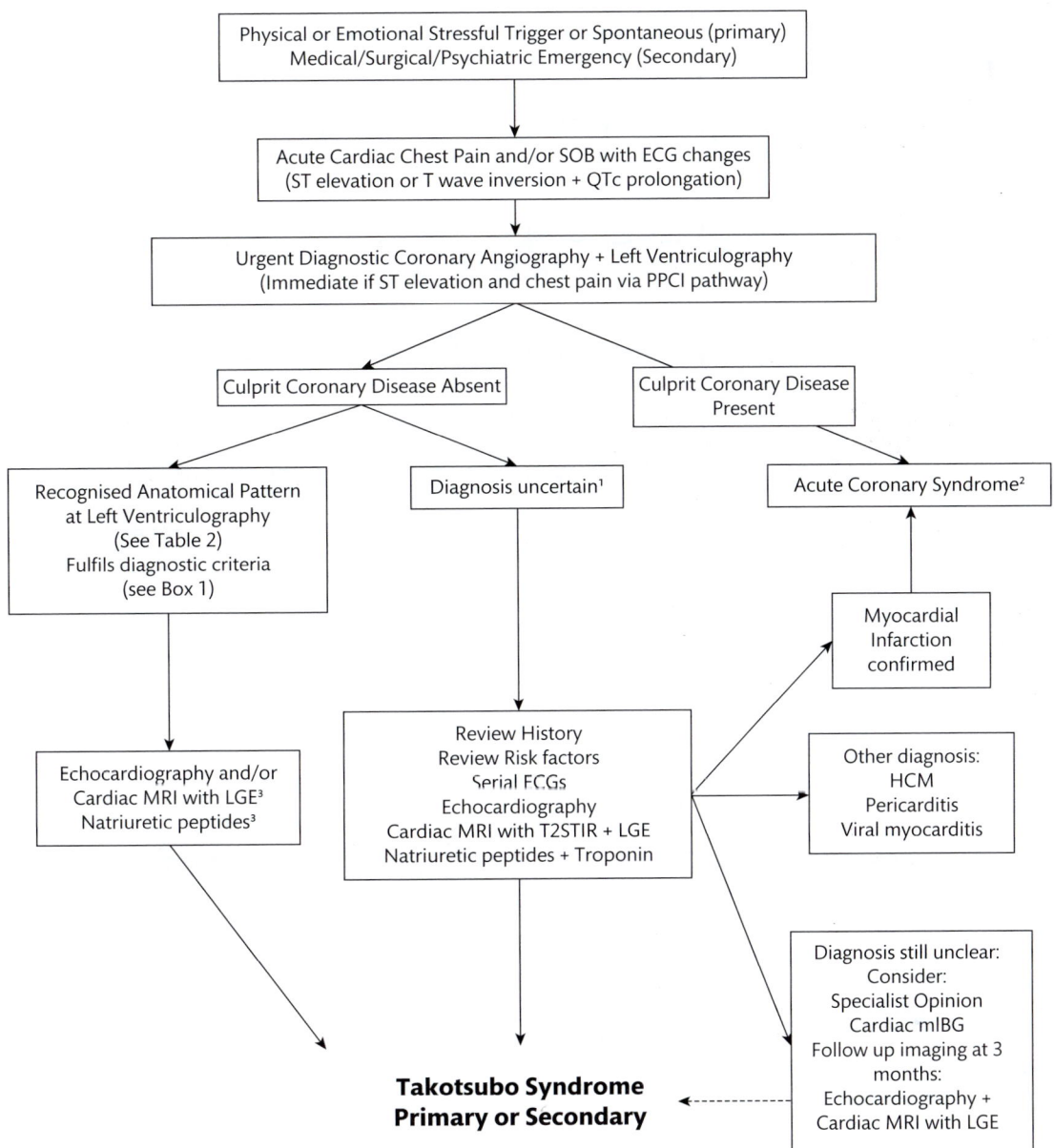

Figure 13.4 Takotsubo syndrome diagnostic algorithm.

Reproduced from Lyon AR, Bossone E, Schneider B, Sechtem U, Citro R, Underwood SR, *et al.* Current state of knowledge on Takotsubo syndrome: a Position Statement from the Taskforce on Takotsubo Syndrome of the Heart Failure Association of the European Society of Cardiology. *European Journal of Heart Failure* 2016;**18**(1):8–27 with permission from Wiley.

unexpected stressful precipitant, the signs of sympathetic activation at presentation, and secondary medical triggers including prescribed or self-administered catecholamines. Takotsubo syndrome has provided new insights into how the heart and cardiovascular system respond to sudden sympathetic activation and surge in catecholamines.[17]

Serum catecholamine serum levels, when measured at presentation, are significantly elevated compared both to resting levels in the same patient and to levels in comparable patients with acute heart failure secondary to AMI.[18] This may suggest that patients with TTS have the potential for excessive activation of their hypothalamic–pituitary–adrenal axis and epinephrine release in response to stress.

Several hypotheses have been proposed to explain TTS and the cardiac response to severe stress.[17] These can be broadly divided into vascular and myocardial causes, and may not be mutually exclusive, given that the entire cardiovascular system is exposed to the same 'catecholamine storm'.

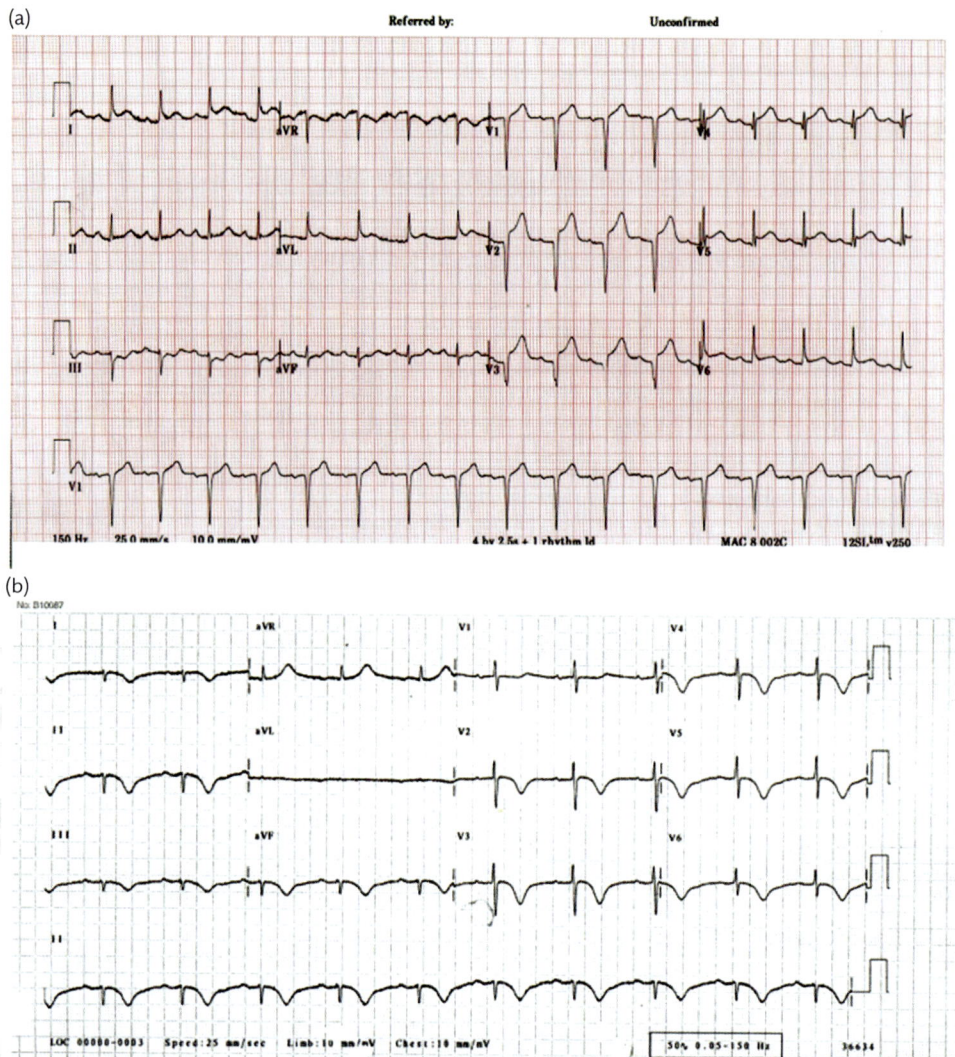

Figure 13.5 Typical electrocardiographic appearances from patients presenting with acute takotsubo syndrome. (a) Widespread ST elevation on the ECG from a lady presenting with takotsubo syndrome within 6 h of a stressful trigger. (b) Widespread T wave inversion with QT prolongation (QTc 505 ms) on the ECG from a lady presenting with Takotsubo syndrome 48 h after a stressful trigger.

Vascular hypotheses

Initially 'aborted' AMI was proposed, but several studies have refuted this explanation. Intracoronary ultrasound studies have not identified plaque rupture or thrombosis and CMR usually shows no

---

Box 13.4 Acute complications of takotsubo syndrome

- Acute mitral regurgitation
- Apical thrombus
- Left ventricular outflow tract obstruction may be present (16%)
- Ventricular wall rupture
- Pulmonary oedema (17.7%)
- Cardiogenic shock (4%)
- Pericarditis
- Left bundle branch block
- Atrial fibrillation (15%)
- Ventricular tachycardia, ventricular fibrillation (4.8%)
- Death 4–5%

---

evidence of LGE acutely or at follow-up.[19] A more conceivable vascular mechanism is multivessel coronary artery spasm, potentially with myocardial microcirculatory dysfunction, with TTS resulting from a form of ischaemic stunning with superimposed catecholamines. In one series, three out of 30 patients were observed to have spontaneous multivessel coronary vasospasm and 43% of patients tested had vasospasm as a result of pharmacological provocation with ergonovine or acetylcholine.[20] Another large case series revealed multivessel coronary spasm following acetylcholine provocation in 10% of patients.[21] However, the majority of patients do not have evidence of vasospasm at the time of diagnostic angiography, and it may be a modifier rather than an essential factor.

After any stress and high surges in catecholamines, generalized impairment of endothelial function is to be expected, and both coronary and peripheral arteries may be prone to vasospasm on provocation. It is important to distinguish between cause and association before all cases of TTS are attributed to multivessel vasospasm. Endomyocardial biopsies taken from patients with TTS show a pattern of myocardial abnormalities not associated with infarcted,

Table 13.1 Major and minor risk factors in takotsubo syndrome

Risk factor	Higher risk	Lower risk
Major risk factors		
Age (years)	≥75	<75
Systolic BP (mmHg)	<110	≥110
Acute pulmonary oedema	Present	Absent
Unexplained syncope, VT, or VF	Present	Absent
LVEF	<35%	≥35%
LVOTO (mmHg)	≥40	Absent/<40
Mitral regurgitation	Present	Absent
Apical thrombus	Present	Absent
New VSD or contained LV wall rupture	Present	Absent
Minor risk factors		
Age (years)	70–75	<70
ECG: QTc (ms)	≥500	<500
ECG: pathological Q waves	Present	Absent
ECG: persistent ST elevation	Present	Absent
LV ejection fraction	35–45%	≥45%
Physical stressor	Present	Absent
Natriuretic peptides (pg/mL)	BNP ≥600 NT-proBNP ≥2000	BNP <600 NT-proBNP <2000
Bystander obstructive coronary artery disease	Present	Absent
Biventricular involvement	Present	Absent

BP, blood pressure; VT, ventricular tachycardia; VF, ventricular fibrillation; LEVF, left ventricular ejection fraction; LVOTO, left ventricular outflow tract obstruction; VSD, ventricular septal defect.

Reproduced from Lyon AR, Bossone E, Schneider B, Sechtem U, Citro R, Underwood SR, et al. Current state of knowledge on Takotsubo syndrome: a Position Statement from the Taskforce on Takotsubo Syndrome of the Heart Failure Association of the European Society of Cardiology. European Journal of Heart Failure. 2016;**18**(1):8–27 with permission from John Wiley and Sons.

stunned, or hibernating myocardium, and the significant differences in histopathological features between TTS and acute infarction do not support a primary vascular cause for TTS.[21]

Myocardial hypotheses

Direct catecholamine-mediated stunning

One proposed mechanism for TTS is based on the negative inotropic effect of high-dose adrenaline on the LV myocardium (see Figure 13.8).[22] Studies in transgenic mice overexpressing the β_2-adrenoceptor in ventricular cardiomyocytes have previously demonstrated a differential response to low and high epinephrine concentrations.[23] Physiological β_2 stimulation causes G_s-mediated *positive* inotropy, but intense 'supraphysiological' stimulation alters the downstream effect to a G_i-mediated *negative* inotropy by a reversible process known as stimulus trafficking.[24] Stimulus trafficking is specific to adrenaline, as noradrenaline does not activate this pathway (see Figure 13.8).

A number of studies report that the mammalian heart has a higher density of β-adrenoceptors or β-adrenoceptor responsiveness in the apical myocardium compared to the basal myocardium. This β-adrenoceptor gradient is opposite to the sympathetic innervation

gradient, which is highest in the atria and basal ventricular myocardium, and falls towards the apical myocardium.[25] The sympathetic innervation gradient has been reported in normal human hearts, with the density of sympathetic nerve endings, as identified by tyrosine hydroxylase during autopsy, approximately 40% higher in the basal myocardium than in the apical myocardium.[25]

In the normal physiological setting, β-adrenoceptors but not the sympathetic nerve endings appear to determine the apical sensitivity to increases in catecholamines.

Several groups have developed in-vivo models of TTS, demonstrating acute, reversible apical and midventricular dysfunction in a 'takotsubo-like' pattern in response to exposure to high levels of adrenaline.[26–28] This acute adrenaline-dependent apical dysfunction could be inhibited by prior treatment with pertussis toxin, a selective G_i inhibitor, thus confirming a G_i-dependent mechanism.[26,27] Replicating features on isolated cardiomyocytes *in vitro*, acute adrenaline-mediated negative inotropy was shown to be β_2-G_i dependent, resulting from stimulus trafficking of the β_2-adrenoceptor from the normal 'stimulatory' G_s to the 'inhibitory' G_i pathway. Apical cardiomyocytes are more sensitive to catecholamines than basal cardiomyocytes isolated from the same ventricle, due to a higher density of β-adrenoceptors.

According to this hypothesis, the high serum adrenaline levels seen in patients with TTS would activate the myocardial β-adrenoceptors. Following an initial activation of $\beta_1 AR$-Gs and $\beta_2 AR$-G_s signalling, a negative feedback pathway via $\beta_2 AR$ phosphorylation switches the $\beta_2 AR$ to couple to G_i, activating negatively inotropic, antiapoptotic, and cardioprotective pathways to reduce the toxic effects of the sympathetic storm. The β_2-mediated negative inotropic action is greatest at the apex compared to basal myocardium, and is completely reversible on removal of the catecholamine stimulus.

There is evidence that these antiapoptotic pathways are activated in the hearts of patients with TTS from endomyocardial biopsies during the acute phase, but not at follow-up, consistent with a temporary cardioprotective effect during the stunning phase.[29] This would help to explain the full recovery and lack of permanent injury observed in most individuals with TTS. In addition, oestrogens have direct effects on expression of β-adrenoceptor genes in the ventricular myocardium that may account for the female preponderance. For more detailed discussion of the pathophysiology please see the following reviews.[17,30,31]

Genetic predisposition

Although the stressful trigger implies a strong environmental component to the pathophysiology, it is conceivable that some individuals may be predisposed to the development of TTS following a stressful trigger, because most individuals exposed to severe stress do not appear to develop TTS. Examples of several family members presenting with TTS have been published, e.g. mother and daughter, or the intriguing report of two sisters simultaneously developing TTS after being told of the death of their father, although at different locations.

Several groups have published small series applying genomic analysis to plausible targets including the cardiac β_1-, β_2- or α_1-adrenoceptors, as well as oestrogen receptors, but there have not been consistent results. Spinelli and colleagues reported a slightly

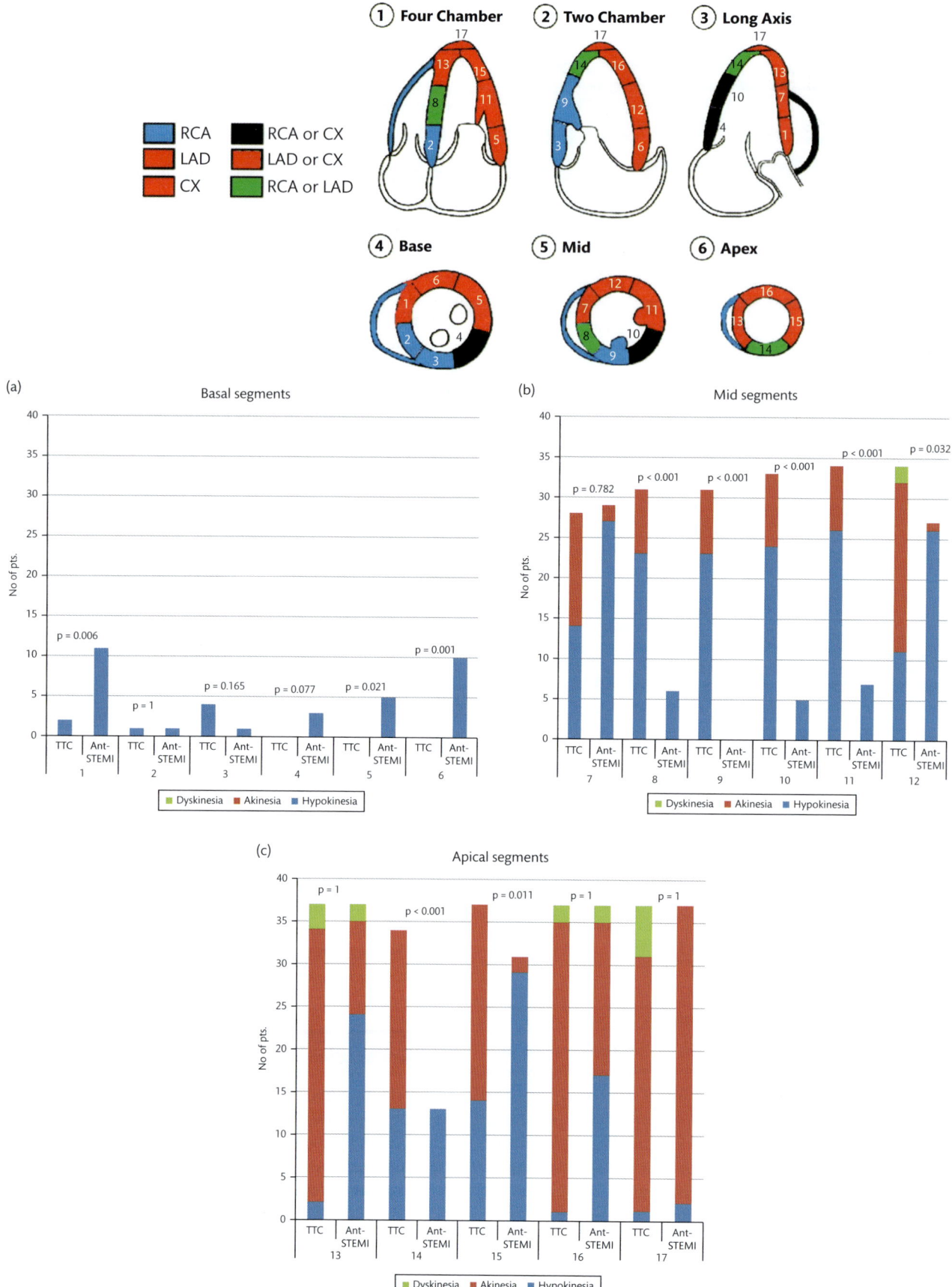

Figure 13.6 1 Left ventricular segmentation in apical (1, 2, 3) and short-axis (4, 5, 6) views according to typical coronary artery distribution (modified from Cerqueira et al.[9]).
2 Wall motion abnormalities of left ventricular segments in TTC vs. ant-STEMI patients: (a) basal; (b) mid; (c) apical. Ant-STEMI, anterior ST elevation myocardial infarction; TTC, takotsubo cardiomyopathy.

Source data from Citro R, Rigo F, Ciampi Q, D'Andrea A, Provenza G, Mirra M, et al. Echocardiographic assessment of regional left ventricular wall motion abnormalities in patients with tako-tsubo cardiomyopathy: comparison with anterior myocardial infarction. *European Journal of Echocardiography*. the Journal of the Working Group on Echocardiography of the European Society of Cardiology. 2011;**12**(7):542–9.

T2STIR   LGE

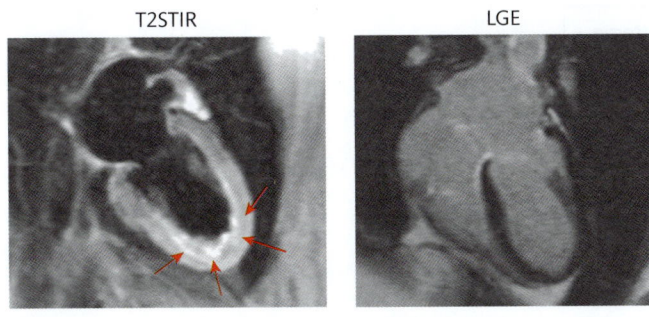

Figure 13.7 Example of cardiac magnetic resonance T2-STIR image (*left*) demonstrating increased signal (white) in the apical region of acute ventricular hypokinesia (see red arrows) from a patient with acute takotsubo syndrome. The late gadolinium enhancement (LGE) image from the same patient (*right*) shows no evidence of myocardial infarction or fibrosis.

higher prevalence of a 'gain-of-function' polymorphism of the enzyme G-protein-coupled receptor kinase 5 (GRK5L41Q) in their small cohort of Italian patients with TTS ($n = 22$) (GRK5L41Q 64 vs 44% in normal controls).[32] This is interesting as increased GRK5 activity would enhance stimulus trafficking of the β_2-adrenoceptors to the G_i pathway, and therefore link to the proposed hypothesis above. However, recently genetic analysis of an Australian cohort of 92 patients with TTS failed to replicate this finding, and also found no relevant polymorphisms in the oestrogen receptor α (*ERα*) and

catechol-*O*-methyl transferase (*COMT*) genes.[33] All these studies are limited by relatively small patient numbers compared to those usually required to demonstrate genetic causation in cardiovascular disease.

Treatment

The acute dysfunction observed in TTS is transient and reversible, and so the clinical strategy is to provide supportive care to sustain life and minimize complications until full recovery is achieved. Treatment strategies have been carefully reviewed and proposed by the HFA Takotsubo Syndrome Taskforce based on risk stratification and are summarized in **Figure 13.9**. In mild cases without complications and in low-risk cases, no treatment is necessary if recovery is rapid and uncomplicated, following the core medical principle of 'first do no harm'. Reviewing the multiple medications frequently initiated for patients with suspected acute coronary syndromes is helpful for all patients with TTS to ensure that they are not prescribed acute coronary syndrome drugs for which there is no evidence that they will derive benefit (such as antiplatelet agents, anticoagulants, and statins).

Cases of TTS with evidence of heart failure and more significant LV impairment may require a short course of medical therapy using 'standard' heart failure treatment (angiotensin converting enzyme inhibitors, β-blockers); in severe cases, consideration of mechanical support with LV assist devices (temporary percutaneous or surgical) or extracorporeal membrane oxygenation as a 'bridge to recovery' may be necessary. Unfortunately there is still little evidence on which

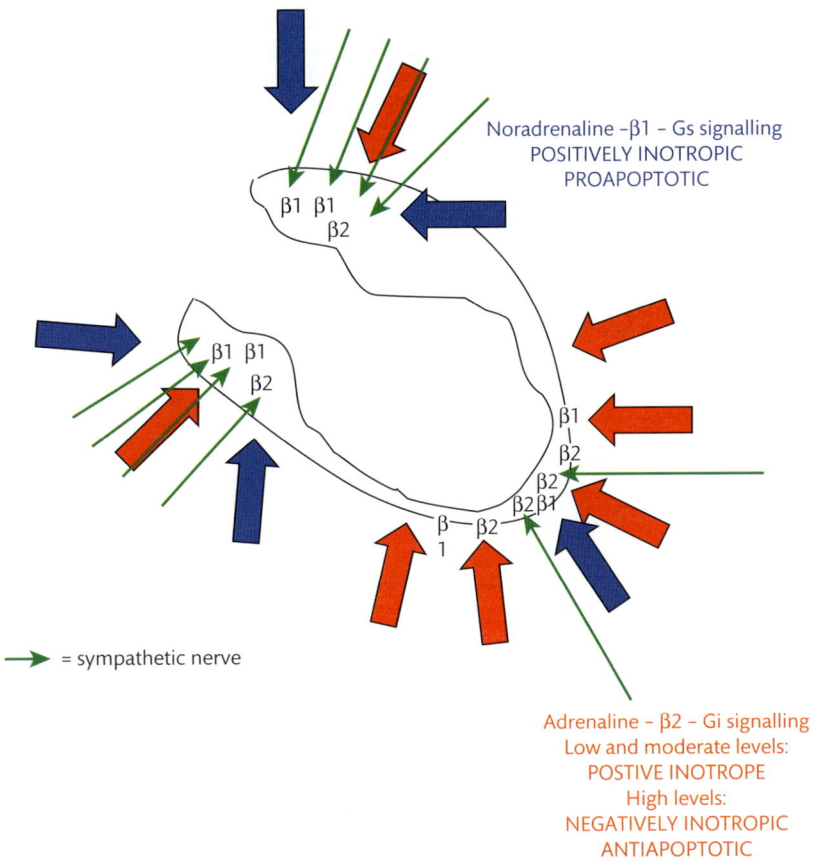

Figure 13.8 Schematic representation of the regional differences in response to high catecholamine doses explaining takotsubo syndrome.

Source data from Lyon AR, Rees PS, Prasad S, Poole-Wilson PA, Harding SE. Stress (Takotsubo) cardiomyopathy—a novel pathophysiological hypothesis to explain catecholamine-induced acute myocardial stunning. *Nature Clinical Practice Cardiovascular Medicine* 2008;**5**(1):22–9.

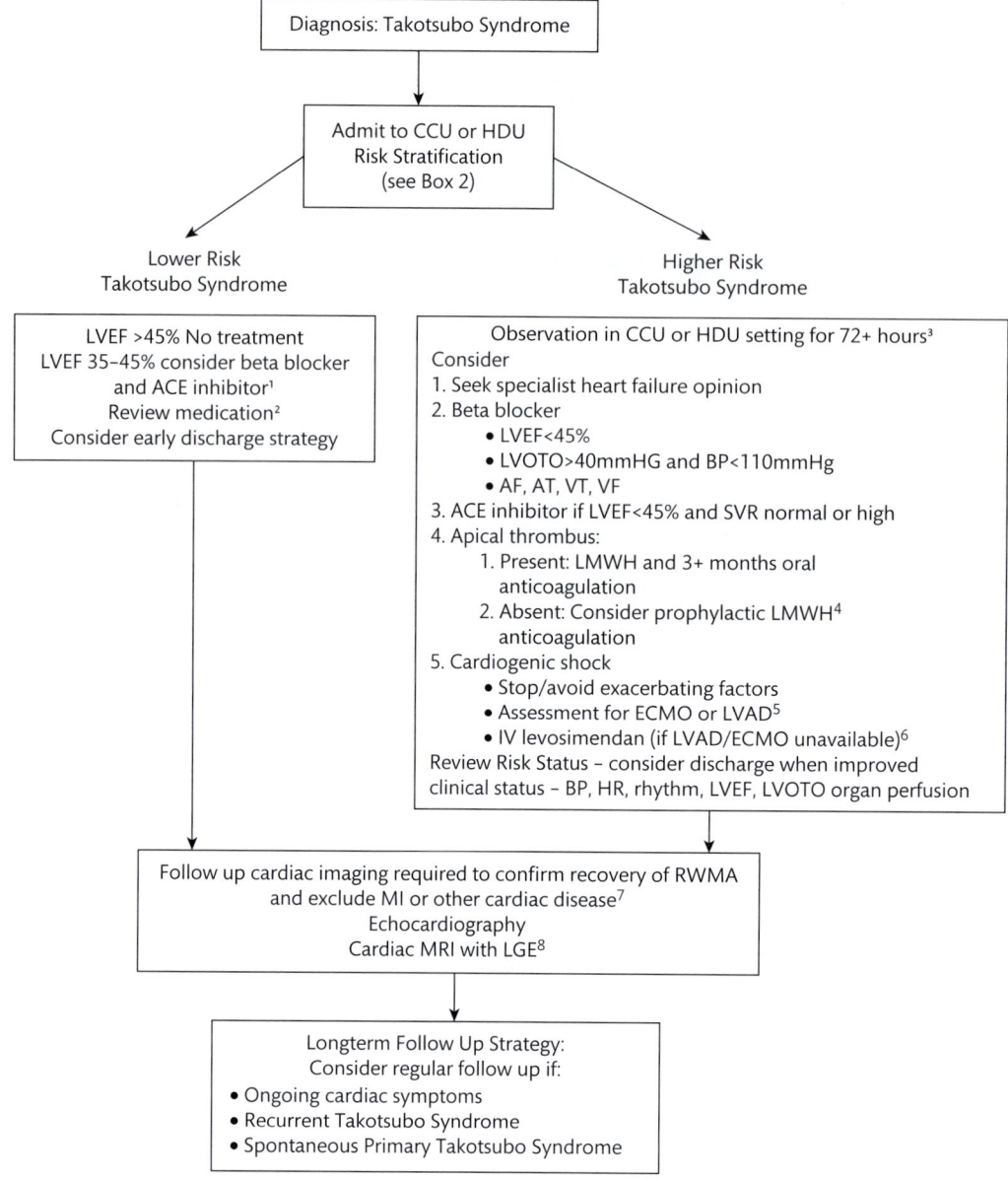

1. Consider carvedilol unless contraindicated.
2. Consider stopping statin and antiplatelet agents if started prior to coronary angiography unless otherwise indicated (e.g. coronary artery disease).
3. Continuous ECG monitoring with defibrillator and resuscitation equipment available.
4. Apical variants with a large apical akinetic zone.
5. Especially in primary Takotsubo syndrome with cardiogenic shock and progressive organ dysfunction.
6. Avoid loading dose, and levosimendan is contraindicated in patients with LVOTO or low SVR.
7. Consider repeat imaging 3–6 months following acute admission unless earlier imaging is indicated for other clinical reasons.
8. If available.

Figure 13.9 Takotsubo syndrome management algorithm.
Reproduced from Lyon AR, Bossone E, Schneider B, Sechtem U, Citro R, Underwood SR, *et al*. Current state of knowledge on Takotsubo syndrome: a Position Statement from the Taskforce on Takotsubo Syndrome of the Heart Failure Association of the European Society of Cardiology. *European Journal of Heart Failure* 2016;**18**(1):8–27 with permission from Wiley.

to base management strategies and the proposed management algorithms are based on expert opinion (level of evidence C).

Long-term outcome and prognosis

Patients who survive the acute TTS episode progressively recover, and macroscopic features of ventricular function, for example LV ejection fraction, normalize over the following days to weeks.[18] The timing depends upon the severity of the acute episode. The mildest cases may resolve within hours and may be missed. In contrast, the most severe cases may have ventricular wall motion abnormalities persisting for several weeks after the initial episode before finally resolving.

There is increasing evidence of permanent physiological abnormalities persisting beyond the timeframe when resting contractile

abnormalities have normalized 'macroscopically'.[34] A few studies have evaluated contractile reserve with cardiac stress at follow-up, revealing persisting abnormalities in the timeframe reported. It is not known whether the abnormalities were also present before the episode, reflecting the potential for inducible apical dysfunction in a susceptible individual, or are a result of injury and dysfunction following the acute episode. CMR studies have reported ongoing inflammation several months following the acute episode and persisting abnormalities of myocardial function on strain imaging.[35]

Clinically, most patients settle rapidly following the acute episode and become asymptomatic. However, approximately 10–15% of patients with TTS report new and persistent cardiac symptoms following the acute episode.[6] These include angina, exertional breathlessness, palpitations and/or a tremulous anxiety state, reflecting heightened sympathetic tone.

Anxiety is integrated in the physiological response to a catecholamine storm, and both anxiety and panic disorder may predispose to TTS, perhaps due to an altered threshold of catecholamine release for a given stress.[36,37] In the aftermath of TTS many patients are more aware of adrenaline and potentially sensitized. Some cases may develop a vicious cycle of anxiety-induced catecholamine storms with or without TTS episodes, catecholamine-induced cardiac symptoms, and further anxiety. Treatment strategies are designed to break the vicious cycle, and using both pharmacological (β-blockers) and psychological (cognitive behavioural therapy) therapeutic interventions can be helpful.

The prognosis of patients with TTS is complex. Whereas the patients do not have obstructive coronary artery disease or myocardial infarction, the prognosis in large cohorts is reported to be similar to that of matched cohorts with AMI.[6,38] However, several important differences exist. Long-term mortality in TTS is related to recurrence and to the complications of acute heart failure, and to the prognosis associated with the underlying disease in patients with secondary TTS. A new (limited) dataset suggests that patients with TTS have a higher incidence of cancer,[39] and thus the long-term mortality is driven equally by cardiovascular and non-cardiovascular causes of death, in contrast to the patients surviving myocardial infarction.

Conclusion

Takotsubo syndrome is a fascinating acute heart failure syndrome, now increasingly recognized by the medical community. Many facets of the condition remain to be understood or completely characterized, and current knowledge to guide optimal clinical practice is limited. National and international registries are collecting larger numbers of patients prospectively and should aid understanding of the epidemiology and natural history. Randomized trials are required to provide the scientific foundation for decision-making in the acute and long-term management due to the lack of current evidence-based treatments for patients with TTS.

REFERENCES

1. Sato H, Taiteishi H, Uchida T. Takotsubo-type cardiomyopathy due to multivessel spasm. In Kodama K, Haze K, Hon M (eds), *Clinical aspect of myocardial injury: from ischemia to heart failure*, pp. 56–64. Kagakuhyouronsya Co., Tokyo, 1990 [in Japanese].

2. Shao Y, Redfors B, Lyon AR, *et al*. Trends in publications on stress-induced cardiomyopathy. *Int J Cardiol* 2012;**157**(3):435–6.

3. Deshmukh A, Kumar G, Pant S, *et al*. Prevalence of Takotsubo cardiomyopathy in the United States. *Am Heart J* 2012;**164**(1):66–71.e1.

4. Minhas AS, Hughey AB, Kolias TJ. Nationwide Trends in Reported Incidence of Takotsubo Cardiomyopathy from 2006 to 2012. *Am J Cardiol* 2015;**116**(7):1128–31.

5. Lyon AR, Bossone E, Schneider B, *et al*. Current state of knowledge on Takotsubo syndrome: a Position Statement from the Taskforce on Takotsubo Syndrome of the Heart Failure Association of the European Society of Cardiology. *Eur J Heart Fail* 2016;**18**(1):8–27.

6. Templin C, Ghadri JR, Diekmann J, *et al*. Clinical Features and Outcomes of Takotsubo (Stress) Cardiomyopathy. *N Engl J Med* 2015;**373**(10):929–38.

7. Madhavan M, Borlaug BA, Lerman A, Rihal CS, Prasad A. Stress hormone and circulating biomarker profile of apical ballooning syndrome (Takotsubo cardiomyopathy): insights into the clinical significance of B-type natriuretic peptide and troponin levels. *Heart (Br Cardiac Soc)* 2009;**95**(17):1436–41.

8. Frohlich GM, Schoch B, Schmid F, *et al*. Takotsubo cardiomyopathy has a unique cardiac biomarker profile: NT-proBNP/myoglobin and NT-proBNP/troponin T ratios for the differential diagnosis of acute coronary syndromes and stress induced cardiomyopathy. *Int J Cardiol* 2012;**154**(3):328–32.

9. Ghadri JR, Sarcon A, Diekmann J, *et al*. Happy heart syndrome: role of positive emotional stress in takotsubo syndrome. *Eur Heart J* 2016;**37**(37):2823–9.

10. Bossone E, Lyon A, Citro R, *et al*. Takotsubo cardiomyopathy: an integrated multi-imaging approach. *Eur Heart J Cardiovasc Imag* 2014;**15**(4):366–77.

11. Citro R, Rigo F, Ciampi Q, *et al*. Echocardiographic assessment of regional left ventricular wall motion abnormalities in patients with tako-tsubo cardiomyopathy: comparison with anterior myocardial infarction. *Eur J Echocardiogr* 2011;**12**(7):542–9.

12. Meimoun P, Passos P, Benali T, *et al*. Assessment of left ventricular twist mechanics in Tako-tsubo cardiomyopathy by two-dimensional speckle-tracking echocardiography. *Eur J Echocardiogr* 2011;**12**(12):931–9.

13. Eitel I, von Knobelsdorff-Brenkenhoff F, Bernhardt P, *et al*. Clinical characteristics and cardiovascular magnetic resonance findings in stress (takotsubo) cardiomyopathy. *JAMA* 2011;**306**(3):277–86.

14. Naruse Y, Sato A, Kasahara K, *et al*. The clinical impact of late gadolinium enhancement in Takotsubo cardiomyopathy: serial analysis of cardiovascular magnetic resonance images. *J Cardiovasc Magn Reson* 2011;**13**:67.

15. Bruder O, Hunold P, Jochims M, *et al*. Reversible late gadolinium enhancement in a case of Takotsubo cardiomyopathy following high-dose dobutamine stress MRI. *Int J Cardiol* 2008;**127**(1):e22–4.

16. Iacucci I, Carbone I, Cannavale G, *et al*. Myocardial oedema as the sole marker of acute injury in Takotsubo cardiomyopathy: a cardiovascular magnetic resonance (CMR) study. *Radiol Med* 2013;**118**(8):1309–23.

17. Akashi YJ, Nef HM, Lyon AR. Epidemiology and pathophysiology of Takotsubo syndrome. *Nature Rev Cardiol* 2015;**12**(7):387–97.

18. Wittstein IS, Thiemann DR, Lima JA, *et al*. Neurohumoral features of myocardial stunning due to sudden emotional stress. *N Engl J Med* 2005;**352**(6):539–48.

19. Haghi D, Roehm S, Hamm K, *et al.* Takotsubo cardiomyopathy is not due to plaque rupture: an intravascular ultrasound study. *Clin Cardiol* 2010;**33**(5):307–10.

20. Kurisu S, Sato H, Kawagoe T, *et al.* Tako-tsubo-like left ventricular dysfunction with ST-segment elevation: a novel cardiac syndrome mimicking acute myocardial infarction. *Am Heart J* 2002;**143**(3):448–55.

21. Tsuchihashi K, Ueshima K, Uchida T, *et al.* Transient left ventricular apical ballooning without coronary artery stenosis: a novel heart syndrome mimicking acute myocardial infarction. Angina pectoris–myocardial infarction investigations in Japan. *J Am Coll Cardiol* 2001;**38**(1):11–18.

22. Lyon AR, Rees PS, Prasad S, Poole-Wilson PA, Harding SE. Stress (Takotsubo) cardiomyopathy—a novel pathophysiological hypothesis to explain catecholamine-induced acute myocardial stunning. *Nature Clin Pract Cardiovasc Med* 2008;**5**(1):22–9.

23. Heubach JF, Blaschke M, Harding SE, Ravens U, Kaumann AJ. Cardiostimulant and cardiodepressant effects through overexpressed human beta2-adrenoceptors in murine heart: regional differences and functional role of beta1-adrenoceptors. *Naunyn-Schmiedeberg's Arch Pharmacol* 2003;**367**(4):380–90.

24. Heubach JF, Ravens U, Kaumann AJ. Epinephrine activates both Gs and Gi pathways, but norepinephrine activates only the Gs pathway through human beta2-adrenoceptors overexpressed in mouse heart. *Mol Pharmacol* 2004;**65**(5):1313–22.

25. Kawano H, Okada R, Yano K. Histological study on the distribution of autonomic nerves in the human heart. *Heart Vessels* 2003;**18**(1):32–9.

26. Paur H, Wright PT, Sikkel MB, *et al.* High levels of circulating epinephrine trigger apical cardiodepression in a beta2-adrenergic receptor/Gi-dependent manner: a new model of Takotsubo cardiomyopathy. *Circulation* 2012;**126**(6):697–706.

27. Shao Y, Redfors B, Scharin Tang M, *et al.* Novel rat model reveals important roles of beta-adrenoceptors in stress-induced cardiomyopathy. *Int J Cardiol* 2013;**168**(3):1943–50.

28. Shao Y, Redfors B, Stahlman M, *et al.* A mouse model reveals an important role for catecholamine-induced lipotoxicity in the pathogenesis of stress-induced cardiomyopathy. *Eur J Heart Fail* 2013;**15**(1):9–22.

29. Nef HM, Mollmann H, Hilpert P, *et al.* Activated cell survival cascade protects cardiomyocytes from cell death in Tako-Tsubo cardiomyopathy. *Eur J Heart Fail* 2009;**11**(8):758–64.

30. Tranter MH, Wright PT, Sikkel MB, Lyon AR. Takotsubo cardiomyopathy: the pathophysiology. *Heart Fail Clin* 2013;**9**(2):187–96, viii–ix.

31. Gorelik J, Wright PT, Lyon AR, Harding SE. Spatial control of the betaAR system in heart failure: the transverse tubule and beyond. *Cardiovasc Res* 2013;**98**(2):216–24.

32. Spinelli L, Trimarco V, Di Marino S, *et al.* L41Q polymorphism of the G protein coupled receptor kinase 5 is associated with left ventricular apical ballooning syndrome. *Eur J Heart Fail* 2010;**12**(1):13–6.

33. Figtree GA, Bagnall RD, Abdulla I, *et al.* No association of G-protein-coupled receptor kinase 5 or beta-adrenergic receptor polymorphisms with takotsubo cardiomyopathy in a large Australian cohort. *Eur J Heart Fail* 2013;**15**(7):730–3.

34. Schwarz K, Ahearn T, Srinivasan J, *et al.* Alterations in cardiac deformation, timing of contraction and relaxation, and early myocardial fibrosis accompany the apparent recovery of acute stress-induced (takotsubo) cardiomyopathy: an end to the concept of transience. *J Am Soc Echocardiogr* 2017;**30**(8):745–5.

35. Neil CJ, Nguyen TH, Singh K, *et al.* Relation of delayed recovery of myocardial function after takotsubo cardiomyopathy to subsequent quality of life. *Am J Cardiol* 2015;**115**(8):1085–9.

36. Krishnamoorthy P, Garg J, Sharma A, *et al.* Gender differences and predictors of mortality in takotsubo cardiomyopathy: analysis from the National Inpatient Sample 2009–2010 Database. *Cardiology* 2015;**132**(2):131–6.

37. Delmas C, Lairez O, Mulin E, *et al.* Anxiodepressive disorders and chronic psychological stress are associated with Tako-Tsubo cardiomyopathy—new physiopathological hypothesis. *Circ J* 2013;**77**(1):175–80.

38. Redfors B, Vedad R, Angeras O, *et al.* Mortality in takotsubo syndrome is similar to mortality in myocardial infarction—a report from the SWEDEHEART registry. *Int J Cardiol* 2015;**185**:282–9.

39. Burgdorf C, Kurowski V, Radke PW. Long-term prognosis of transient left ventricular ballooning syndrome and cancer. *Heart Lung* 2011;**40**(5):472.

SECTION 4

Pathophysiology of heart failure
Cellular and molecular changes

14

The pathophysiology of heart failure

Theresa A. McDonagh and Henry J. Dargie

Introduction

The historic conception of heart failure was fundamentally a pathophysiological one: the 'inability of the heart to provide sufficient oxygen to the metabolizing tissues despite an adequate filling pressure'.[1] Initially the abnormalities found in the heart failure syndrome were described in terms of their haemodynamic effects. However, as the relationship between the pathophysiology of heart failure and its therapy has emerged over the last 20 years, it is now clear that the pathophysiology of heart failure is highly complex and also involves neurohormonal and inflammatory adaptations. These initially help the situation but chronically they contribute to progression of the syndrome and adversely affect the structure and function of the heart itself. This chapter reviews the pathophysiology of heart failure by outlining what is known about its key players: haemodynamic abnormalities, ventricular remodelling, neurohormonal activation and inflammatory responses.

While any type of cardiac pathology can ultimately lead to heart failure, most is known about the pathophysiology of heart failure due to myocardial contractile impairment leading to left ventricular systolic dysfunction. The majority of this chapter refers to such heart failure. We are now beginning to understand more about the pathophysiology of heart failure when it occurs in the presence of normal systolic function, but much more work needs to be done to unravel this syndrome further.

Haemodynamic responses

In response to a reduction in myocardial contractility and/or in the presence of an excessive haemodynamic load, the heart employs a number of adaptive mechanisms to maintain cardiac output. The most important of these is the Frank Starling mechanism, whereby an increase in preload is activated to help augment cardiac output (**Figure 14.1**).[2] Second, myocardial hypertrophy begins to provide greater contractility.[3] Activation of neurohormonal systems, in particular the renin angiotensin aldosterone system and sympathetic nervous system also stimulate contractility and increase preload by their effects on volume homeostasis and support of arterial pressure and perfusion.[4] These mechanisms initially improve cardiac performance, but chronically they become maladaptive.[1]

In heart failure with reduced ejection fraction (HFrEF), there is typically an increase in diastolic volume and a normal or low ratio of LV mass/LV end-diastolic volume. In contrast, in heart failure with normal ejection fraction (HFnEF), the LV volume is often normal but the LV is thickened, the myocardium is stiffer and ratio of LV mass/LV end-diastolic volume is increased.[5]

Cardiac contraction resulting from the interaction of actin and mysosin is trigerred by cytoplasmic calcium. The role of calcium and calcium cycling in HFrEF and HFnEF is covered in detail in Chapter x.

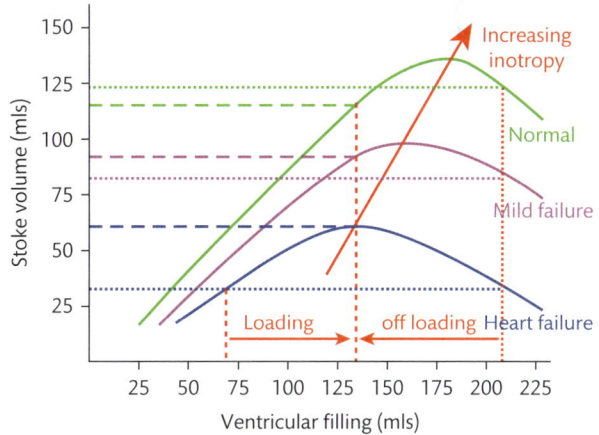

Figure 14.1 The relationship between preload (ventricular filling) and stroke volume in normal (green) and failing hearts (purple and blue). The Frank–Starling mechanism. With worsening heart failure, greater diastolic filling (preload) is needed to maintain a given cardiac output. The vertical red line illustrates that for a given filling pressure, the stroke volume falls with worsening heart failure. Beyond a peak preload, further increases result in a fall in stroke volume, and a therapeutic reduction in preload ('off loading') may result in increased stroke volume.

Adverse ventricular remodelling

This is the term that is most commonly used to describe the changes in size, shape and function of the left ventricle that occur as a result of the initial cardiac pathology and its subsequent progression with the activation of the neurohormonal systems described in more detail below. Pathology occurring at cellular, organ and systemic levels drives the process.[6]

The initial insult and its duration do determine the broad category of remodelling seen. Two distinct types are described. Firstly, concentric remodelling in which there is a generalized increase in LV wall thickness and mass. Ventricular dilation does not occur initially here but does subsequently over time. The second type of remodelling is often referred to as eccentric remodelling, a hallmark of which is dilatation of the ventricle, decreased systolic function, mitral, tricuspid and aortic valve regurgitation. This is classically seen following myocardial infarction, in states of volume overload, valve regurgitation and dilated cardiomyopathies.[6,7]

Cellular changes include myocyte hypertrophy, which can be triggered by increased load, neurohormonally driven signalling pathways, inflammation and oxidative stress. Ultimately these processes lead to post-translational modifications which result in a myocyte phenotype similar to that seen during foetal development, consequent upon activation of the 'foetal gene programme'. The changes seen include the generation of new sarcomeres, an increase in the size of myocytes and a change in their substrate preference from free fatty acids to glucose.[8] Whether these processes initially occur concentrically or eccentrically, they minimize ventricular wall stress, but over time they lead to progressive contractile dysfunction and dilation with a subsequent change in the shape of the LV from elliptical to spherical.[9]

Other events at cellular level are also occurring during ventricular remodelling. There is on-going cell death in all types of HF, by both necrosis and apoptosis (programmed cell death).[10] Myocardial necrosis is the predominant mode of cell death in myocardial infarction. It also occurs in anthracycline-induced and other toxic cardiomyopathies.[11] Apoptosis can be triggered by many of the same stimuli that lead to myocardial hypertrophy, i.e. load, neurohormonal driven signalling pathways, inflammation and oxidative stress.[12] Apoptosis also increases with ageing. Over time, the depletion of myocytes may lead to HF.[13]

Remodelling of the extracellular matrix (ECM) also occurs. The ECM is an important determinant of the architecture of the ventricles and, therefore, is a contributor to both systolic and diastolic function. Remodelling of the ECM can occur through replacement fibrosis following myocardial infarction. Necrosis leads to the release of growth factors in connective tissue and the formation of new fibroblasts. Synthesis of new ECM, which is also seen in pressure overload hypertrophy, increases myocardial stiffness, leading to a reduction in the rate of ventricular relaxation and emptying.[14] Fibrosis is augmented by chronic stimulation of the renin-angiotensin-aldosterone system, in particular by aldosterone.[15] In addition, there are changes in the interstitial matrix with an increase in fibrosis and collagen turnover.[16] There is an increase in the activity of matrix metalloproteinases (MMPs) and a decrease in their endogenous inhibitors, tissue inhibitors of metalloproteinases (TIMPS).[17] The net result is an increase in ventricular dilation. Fibrosis is covered in more detail in Chapter x.

The alteration in the geometry of the LV ultimately contributes to increased wall stress (by the law of Laplace). It leads to dilation of the mitral valve annulus and stretching and remodelling of the papillary muscles causing shortening of the posterior mitral valve leaflet, thereby causing functional (or 'ischaemic') mitral regurgitation. The mitral regurgitation exacerbates ventricular dilation by introducing an element of volume overload into the equation. The presence of mitral regurgitation in heart failure is therefore associated with an adverse prognosis.[18,19]

Adverse left ventricular remodelling is associated with increased mortality rates irrespective of the underlying cardiac pathology and is a target for many of the therapeutic advances in heart failure due to systolic dysfunction. In addition, the type of remodelling which occurs following myocardial infarction, where there is initial infarct expansion at the border zone between infarcted and normal myocardium, is a also a therapeutic target for re-perfusion strategies aimed at limiting infarct size. The afterload reducing effects of ACE inhibitors reduce wall stress post MI, which can also limit the remodelling process.[20-22] (**Figure 14.2**).

When coronary artery disease is the cause of the heart failure, further adverse remodelling can be exacerbated by intercurrent ischaemic events. LV dysfunction may have a component of hibernating myocardium in which myocytes in poorly perfused areas shut down their metabolic activities and cease to contract. Hibernation is potentially reversible by restoring perfusion.

The adverse remodelling process can lead to both electrical and mechanical dyssynchrony which then leads to a vicious cycle of a further reduction in cardiac output, augmented neurohormonal activation, reduction in LV function, more severe mitral incompetence and further ventricular remodelling. The dyssynchrony manifests as severe CHF and has a poor outlook: it is now the target of cardiac resynchronization therapy.[23-25]

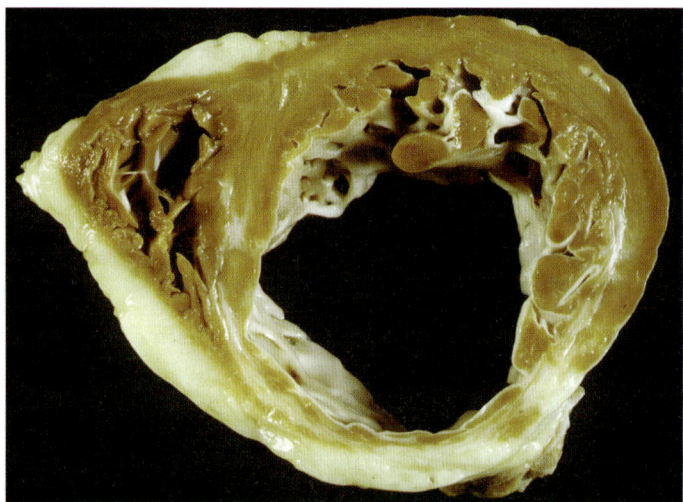

Figure 14.2 Pathological specimen of an adversely remodelled left ventricle showing LV hypertrophy, strands of fibrotic tissues and an inferior myocardial infarct scar. The LV shape is spherical.

Heart failure with normal systolic function

It seems logical to discuss heart failure with normal LV function (HFnEF) under the heading of remodelling as the main differences between predominantly systolic dysfunction and HFnEF seem to be related to the type of remodelling which the heart undergoes: in HFnEF, the LV hypertrophy phenotype predominates.

Up to 50% of patients who present with heart failure have normal LV systolic function. The syndrome has several other names: diastolic heart failure and HFnEF (see Chapter 30). The main abnormality occurs in diastole and is due to impaired relaxation or stiffness. This can be present at rest or may be induced by stress (e.g. exercise, tachycardia, or hypertension). Whilst the LVEF may be normal at rest, it does not increase with stress.[26]

Less is known about the pathophysiology of this form of heart failure. A lot of work has focussed on describing diastolic function in terms of haemodynamics by measuring LV pressure–volume loops and trying to quantify relaxation, filling abnormalities and chamber stiffness.[27]

HeFNEF can occur alone or in combination with systolic heart failure. In patients with isolated diastolic heart failure, the only abnormality in the LV pressure loops occurs in diastole, where the curve is shifted to the left (**Figure 14.3a**), indicating that at any given diastolic volume, there is an increase in diastolic pressure—even when the diastolic volume is normal. In patients with systolic heart failure (**Figure 14.3b**), there are changes in the pressure volume loop that include reduced LVEF and stroke volume. The diastolic portion is not normal either in that diastolic pressure is high. In mixed systolic and diastolic function (**Figure 14.3c**), there is usually a modest decrease in LVEF, and an increase in end diastolic volume and pressure, reflecting decreased chamber compliance.[27]

Endothelial dysfunction, arterial stiffening and increased ventricular stiffness also occur frequently in patients with HeFNEF, which can result in enhanced sensitivity to changes in load. This explains the rapid-onset pulmonary oedema seen in such patients with increases in load, and conversely, hypotension with decreases in load.[28] Exercise capacity is reduced for a number of reasons including impaired chronotropic response, reduced ventricular systolic and diastolic reserve, as well as impairment of oxygen uptake and utilization in peripheral muscles.[26,29,30]

Non-invasive ways of ascertaining the presence of diastolic dysfunction are covered in Chapter 23.

In HeFNEF, complex abnormalities occur at the level of the myofilaments, myocytes and matrix as well as at the level of the heart as a whole.[31] In the myofilaments, abnormal stiffness and relaxation can be due to changes of proteins within the contractile thick and thin filaments, myosin-binding protein C (MyBPC), and the linkage protein titin. Titin is a key player and changes in the PEVK domain of its isoforms can alter the stiffness and elastic recoil of the myocardium. At the myocyte level, calcium signalling and interaction with myofilaments plays an important role. Expression and post-translation modifications of the sarcoplasmic reticular channel (RyR), Ca^{2+} uptake proteins (PLB, SERCA), sarcolemma exchanger (NCX), and ion pumps can all occur. They are summarized in **Figure 14.4**.[32]

Importantly, the neurohormonal changes seen in systolic heart failure(discussed below) also occur in patients with HeFnEF, although to a lesser extent (**Figure 14.5**).[33]

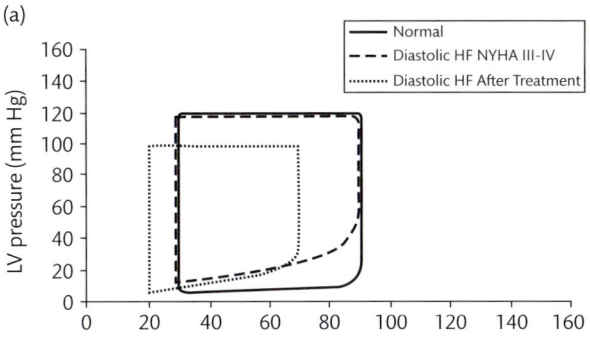

(a)

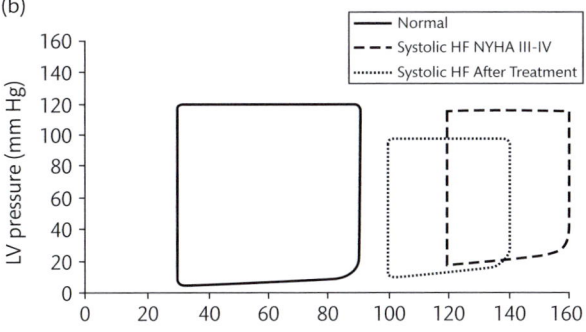

(b)

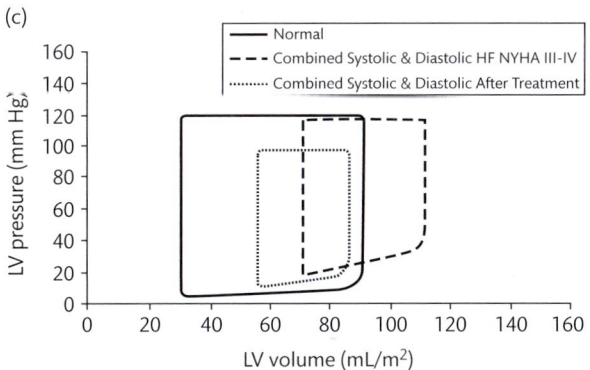

(c)

LV volume (mL/m²)

Figure 14.3 Pressure–volume loops contrasting isolated diastolic heart failure (a) with systolic heart failure (b) and combined systolic and diastolic heart failure (c). A normal patient subject (solid line) is compared with a patient with heart failure before (dashed line) and after (dotted line) treatment. HF, heart failure.

Reproduced from Zile MR, Brutsaert DL. New concepts in diastolic dysfunction and diastolic heart failure: Part II: causal mechanisms and treatment. *Circulation* 2002;**105**(12):1503–8 with permission from Wolters Kluwer.

Compared to patients with HFrEF, patients who develop heart failure with normal systolic function tend to be older, are more likely to be female and often have hypertension as the main aetiology, although CAD is a common finding as well.[34] It is, of course, the main type of heart failure found in hypertrophic cardiomyopathy and infiltrative cardiac diseases.

It is true to say that the fundamental physiological abnormality leading to HeFnEF is incompletely defined, but traditionally has been attributed to hypertensive remodelling. However, systemic microvascular endothelial inflammation associated with comorbidities is gaining credence as an additional mechanism. The combination leads to inflammation and fibrosis, increases in oxidative stress and alteration in cardiomyocyte signalling pathways. These then result in the cardiomyocyte remodelling and dysfunction.[35,36]

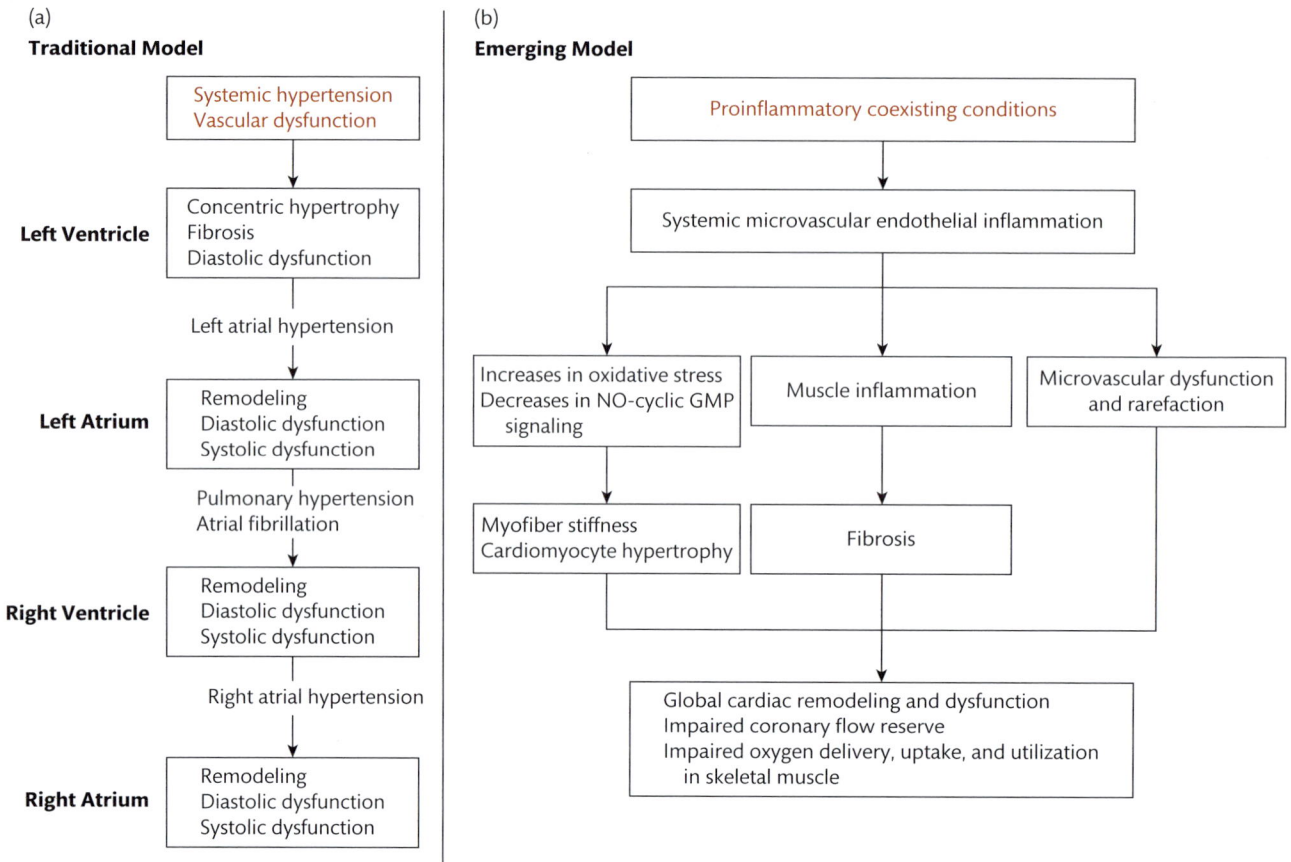

Figure 14.4 Traditional and emerging models for the pathophysiology pf HeFNEF.
Reproduced Redfield MM. Heart failure with preserved ejection fraction. *The New England Journal of Medicine* 2016;**375**(19):1868–77.

Neurhormonal activation

A variety of neurohormonal systems are activated in response to the alteration in cardiac function. These are well-developed evolutionary responses designed to protect against exsanguination. They therefore increase blood pressure and critical organ perfusion in the short term but ultimately also become maladaptive when chronically stimulated.

Sympathetic nervous system

Several mechanisms are involved in sympathetic nervous system activation, which occurs very early in heart failure, as soon as cardiac output drops. This is sensed by mechanoreceptors in the aortic arch, carotid sinus, left ventricular and renal afferents and leads to increased central sympathetic flow and raised circulating concentrations of noradrenaline. There is both increased neuronal release of noradrenaline and decreased synaptic re-uptake. Initially this supports the failing circulation by encouraging myocyte hypertrophy, an increased heart rate, vasoconstriction and lusitropy.[37,38] However, ultimately, the effects are deleterious. Both adrenaline and noradrenaline are directly toxic to the myocardium, promoting apoptosis and calcium overload.[39,40] Myocardial oxygen consumption is increased and further adverse remodelling takes place. Downregulation of β-1-adrenorecptors occurs which further inhibits the ability of the heart to respond to a catecholamine surge.[41,42]

The parasympathetic nervous system is also disturbed in heart failure. There is a reduction in vagal tone. The primary abnormality is thought to be a reduction in baroreceptor sensitivity.[43]

This link between sympathetic activation and heart failure was first described by Jay Cohn's group. They also noted that raised circulating concentrations of noradrenaline were associated with an adverse prognosis in heart failure.[38] The final endorsement of the deleterious effects of the SNS in heart failure came with the treatment trials that demonstrated improved outcomes for patients using β-blockers[44,45] (**Figure 14.6**).

Renin–angiotensin–aldosterone system

The drop in cardiac output also stimulates the renin–angiotensin–aldosterone system (RAAS). This does not have the immediate effects of SNS activation. Indeed, there is little activation of the RAAS in asymptomatic LV dysfunction and more profound activation as the syndrome progresses (**Figure 14.7**). The activation is also markedly increased by diuretic use.[46]

Release of renin from the juxtaglomerular apparatus in the kidney occurs through two main mechanisms: firstly, though adrenergic stimulation of β-receptors; and, secondly, through the decreased renal blood flow sensed by mechanoreceptors.[47] Renin circulates and converts angiotensinogen released by the liver into angiotensin I in the peripheral circulation. Angiotensin I is converted to angiotensin II (ang II) principally through the action of angiotensin converting enzyme (ACE) in the pulmonary circulation and other

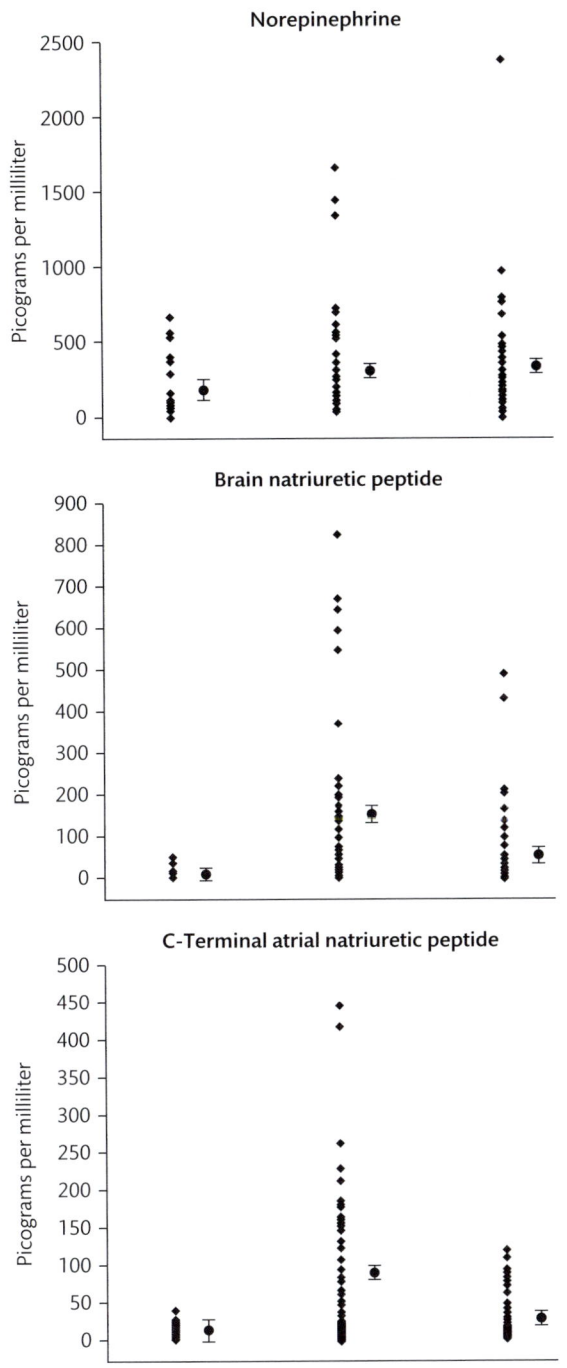

Figure 14.5 Concentrations of norepinephrine (noradrenaline), BNP and the C-terminal of ANP on the y axes. SHF, systolic heart failure; DHF, diastolic heart failure.

Source data from Kitzman DW, Little WC, Brubaker PH, *et al.* Pathophysiological characterization of isolated diastolic heart failure in comparison to systolic heart failure. *JAMA: the Journal of the American Medical Association* 2002;**288**(17):2144–50.

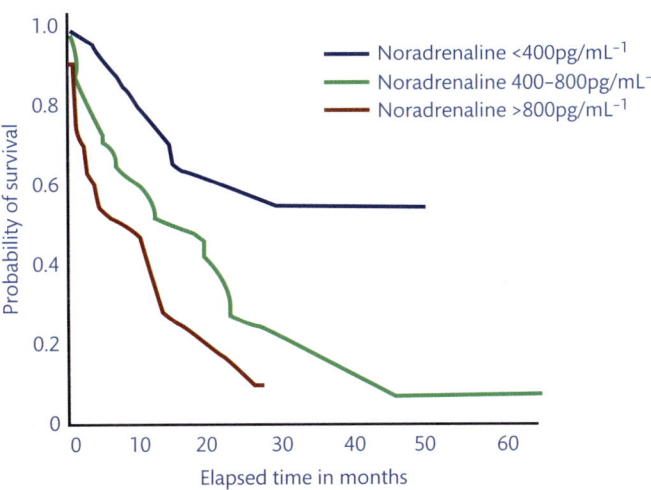

Figure 14.6 Plamsa norepinephrine (noradrenaline) concentrations above and below 600 pg/mL and survival.

Reproduced from Cohn JN, Levine TB, Olivari MT, *et al.* Plasma norepinephrine as a guide to prognosis in patients with chronic congestive heart failure. *The New England Journal of Medicine* 1984;**311**(13):819–23.

Angiotensin II is the principal effector hormone of the RAAS. It produces vasoconstriction, myocyte and vascular hypertrophy, and aldosterone release. In addition, it is responsible for the release of other neurohormones such as vasopressin, endothelin and catecholamines. It also causes thirst by a direct cerebral effect (**Figure 14.9**).

The effects are mediated by activation of two receptors. The ang II type I receptor (AT_1 receptor) is thought to be the one through which most of the deleterious effects occur. However, some adverse effects, such as apoptosis, can occur via stimulation of the type II receptor.

The importance of RAAS activation in the progression of heart failure has been greatly highlighted and further understood by the landmark treatment trials with ACE inhibitors, which were the first drugs to alter the mortality of the condition.[50–52] More recent trials with angiotensin receptor blockers have underscored this phenomenon.[53]

Aldosterone

Angiotensin II also causes release of the mineralocorticoid hormone, aldosterone. Under normal conditions aldosterone production is regulated via adrenocorticotrophin hormone and potassium concentrations. Aldosterone encourages sodium retention and potassium excretion. This potassium loss contributes to the arrhythmia burden in heart failure. Its release is also stimulated by endothelin, catecholamines and vasopressin. Plasma concentrations rise in proportion to the severity of heart failure.[54] More recently, aldosterone's role in causing fibrosis in the myocardium by promoting collagen turnover has been highlighted by trial results. In humans, aldosterone antagonists have beneficial effects on survival in patients with heart failure, and in both human and animal models there are reductions in fibrosis with treatment with aldosterone antagonists.[55–57]

Endothelin

In a similar fashion to angiotensin, endothelin is produced as a pre-pro peptide that is cleaved by a furin protease into big endothelin. Further cleavage by endothelin converting enzyme (a neutral

vascular beds. (**Figure 14.8**).[48] However, ang II is also produced in numerous tissues (including myocytes) by non-ACE-dependent pathways via proteases such as chymase, kallikrein, and cathepsin. These alternative pathways are thought to be the routes by which 'ACE and aldosterone escape' occur when patients are treated with ACE inhibitors.[49]

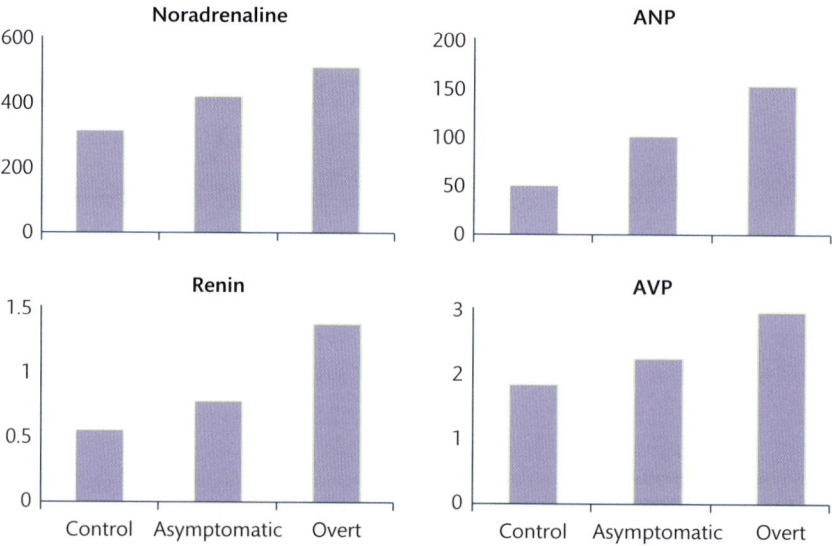

Figure 14.7 Plamsa norepinephrine (noradrenaline), renin, ANF (atrial natriuetic factor) and AVP (arginine vasopressin) concentrations in controls and from patients in the SOLVD (studies of left ventricular dysfunction) prevention and treatment arms. SOLVD prevention patients had asymptomatic LV systolic dysfunction. Those in the treatment trial had heart failure.

Source data from Francis GS, Cohn JN, Johnson G, Rector TS, Goldman S, Simon A. Plasma norepinephrine, plasma renin activity, and congestive heart failure. Relations to survival and the effects of therapy in V-HeFT II. The V-HeFT VA Cooperative Studies Group. *Circulation* 1993;**87**(6 Suppl):VI40–8.

endopeptidase) occurs to produce a family of three endothelins. Endothelin 1 is the predominant isoform expressed in man. It is mainly produced in endothelial cells. It acts via two receptors, A and B, which are G-protein coupled and activate phospholipase C, eventually leading to calcium release from the sarcoplasmic reticulum. Its principal effects are potent vasoconstriction, growth promotion, inotropy, and aldosterone and ang II release.[58–61]

Circulating concentrations of endothelin are elevated two- to three- fold in patients with heart failure in proportion to haemodynamic and functional disease severity (**Figure 14.10**).[61,62] Endothelin is thought to be a key player in the remodelling process. High plasma concentrations are independently associated with an adverse outcome, and track closely with the degree of pulmonary hypertension found.[63,64]

Despite early promise of endothelin A receptor blockade, which reduced hypertrophy, and mixed A and B receptor blockade with bosentan, which favourably altered haemodynamics, larger clinical trials with endothelin antagonists have been disappointing.[65–67]

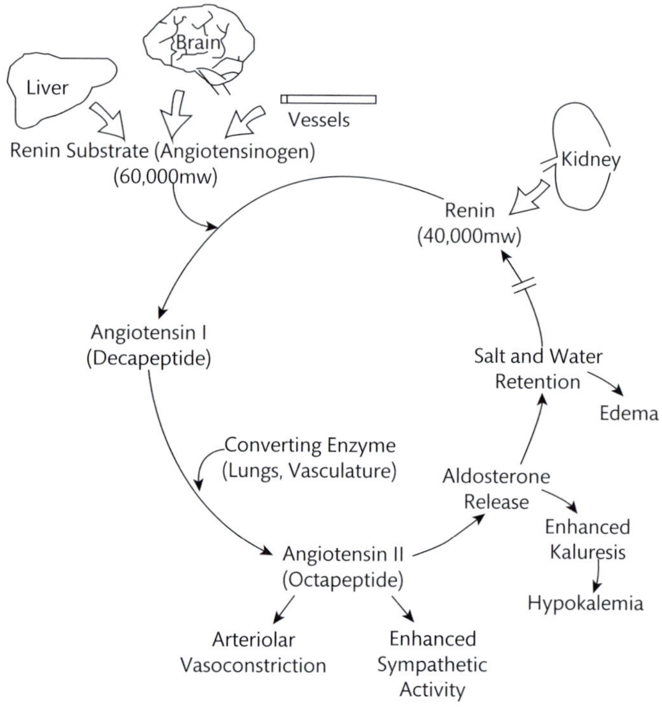

Figure 14.8 The renin–angiotensin–aldosterone system in heart failure.

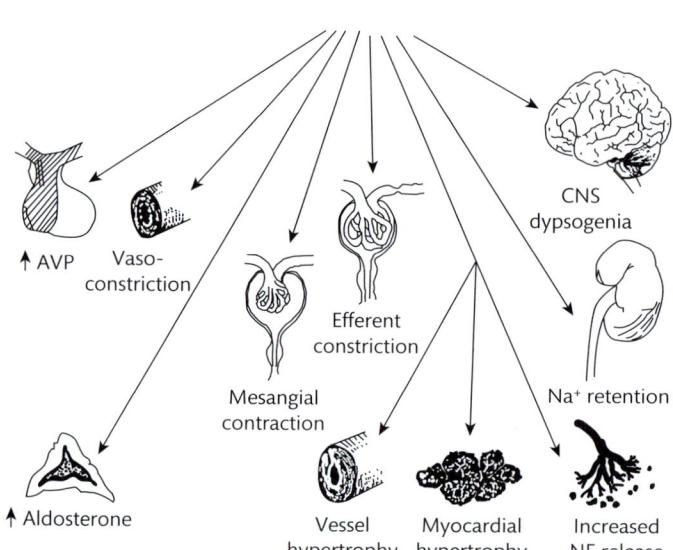

Figure 14.9 The actions of angiotensin II.

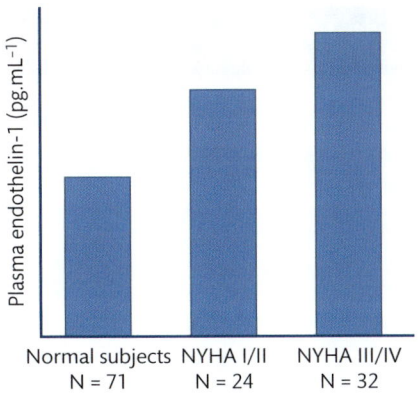

Figure 14.10 Plasma-soluble TNF receptors (tumour necrosis factor) and NYHA class and survival in heart failure.

Source data from Rodeheffer RJ, Lerman A, Heublein DM, Burnett JC, Jr. Increased plasma concentrations of endothelin in congestive heart failure in humans. *Mayo Clin Proc* 1992;**67**(8):719–24.

Vasopressin

Vasopressin, also known as antidiuretic hormone is a peptide released in response to a decrease in cardiac output, atrial stretch and a drop in plasma osmolality. Angiotensin II and noradrenaline also augment its release in heart failure. Vasopressin's main site of action is via its V2 receptor in the renal distal collecting tubule, where is increases both sodium and water absorption, thereby increasing intravascular volume. Vasopressin also acts via V1 and V2 receptors to cause vasoconstriction in the pulmonary and peripheral circulation. Short duration treatment with conivapatan and tolvaptan have demonstrated improvements in haemodynamics, fluid removal and electrolyte balance, but a recent long-term trial has not shown any conclusive effects on heart failure morbidity and mortality by antagonizing this system.[68,69]

Natriuretic peptides

The natriuretic peptide (NP) hormones produced by the heart are also activated in heart failure. The most important ones in heart failure are atrial natriuretic peptide (ANP) mainly produced in the atria and B-type natriuretic peptide (BNP), which is predominantly found in the ventricular myocardium.[70] Their release is stimulated by increased wall stress and stretch as well as by the circulating neurohormones, endothelin, angiotensin II, aldosterone, vasopressin and noradrenaline. The NPs act as counter-regulatory hormones and have a major role in controlling cardiovascular homeostasis via their key effector functions: natriuresis, diuresis and vasodilation. Plasma concentrations of the NPs are raised in proportion to the severity of heart failure and are powerful predictors of a poor prognosis in patients with heart failure.[71–74] While this counter-regulatory system is ultimately too weak to prevent progression of heart failure, the NPs have become very useful biomarkers to aid in the diagnosis, help in prognostication and as potential tools for therapy monitoring in heart failure (see Chapter 20).

Augmentation of the effects of NPs by use of intravenous recombinant BNP or urodilatin has not proved very successful to date.[75,76] However, NPs can be also augmented by reducing their breakdown by inhibiting the enzyme responsible, neprilysin. Neprilysin inhibition in combination with ACEI inhibition did not prove beneficial

in HF,[77] but the combination of an angiotensin receptor blocker with neprilysin inhibition resulted in very convincing improvements in mortality and morbidity in patients with HFrEF.[78] The findings underscore the importance of NPs in HFrEF. Further trials are underway in HeFnEF and in post MI LVSD. These trials may also shed light on the pathophysiological role of the NPs in other parts of the heart failure spectrum.

Inflammatory activation

Inflammation potentially has an important role in the pathophysiology of heart failure. As in other phases of cardiac pathology, we get a general indication of underlying generalized inflammation by the presence of a raised CRP concentration.[79]

The key players, to date, in the pathophysiology of heart failure, are inflammatory mediators, cytokines. Initial work in patients with advanced heart failure and cardiac cachexia showed that plasma concentrations of tumour necrosis factor-α (TNFα) were elevated.[80,81] Since then many studies have shown increases in other cytokines, such as interleukin-1β (IL-1β), IL-2, IL-6, Fas ligand, monocyte chemoattractant protein-1 (MCP-1) and macrophage inflammatory protein alpha (MIP-1α).[82] In a similar manner to neurohormonal activation, prolonged inflammatory activation with an imbalance between pro- and anti-inflammatory cytokines is ultimately deleterious in heart failure.

TNFα is the most studied cytokine, to date, in heart failure. It is predominantly released from macrophages; although neutrophils, lymphocytes, platelets, mast and endothelial cells can all produce it. In addition, it can be released by myocytes subject to stretch.

It is increased, as are its soluble receptors, in proportion to the severity of heart failure (**Figure 14.11**).[83] Increasing levels of both TNFα and IL-6 are independent predictors of a worse prognosis in heart failure.[84] The role of TNF-α in the progression of heart failure is attributed firstly to its negatively inotropic action, but also to its toxic effects on the myocardium which lead to apoptosis, myocyte hypertrophy and matrix remodelling, thereby contributing to progressive adverse ventricular remodelling. Similarly, both IL-1 and IL-6 are negatively inotropic in vitro and the circulating concentrations of both are increased in patients in proportion to the clinical and haemodynamic severity of their heart failure.[85,86]

Less is known about the role of chemokines in heart failure when compared to ischaemic heart disease. Monocyte chemoattractant protein-1 (MCP-1) production is stimulated by IL-1, IL-6, TNFα, and ang II. Levels of MCP-1 are increased in animal models of heart failure.[87] More recently MCP-1, MIP-1α and RANTES (regulated upon activation, normal T-cell expressed and secreted) have been shown to be elevated in patients and to correlate with traditional markers of disease severity such as NYHA class and ejection fraction.[88] Furthermore, chemokines and their receptors are found in biopsies taken from failing myocardium.[89] They may well play an important role in the pathogenesis of the condition.

To date, however, modulation of inflammatory mediators in heart failure by statins, TNFα receptors or monoclonal antibodies to TNFα has failed to demonstrate beneficial effects in large studies in patients with heart failure.[90,91]

(a)

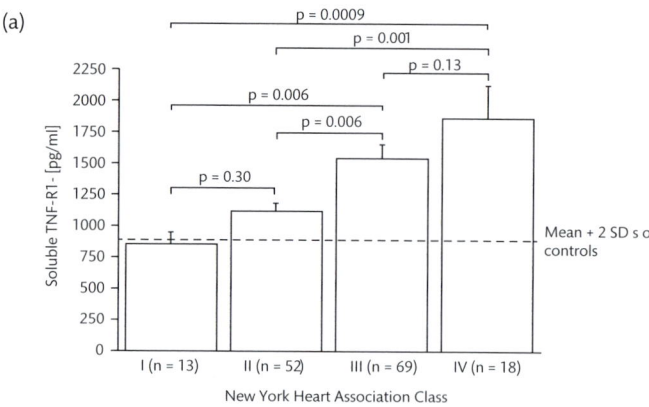

(b)

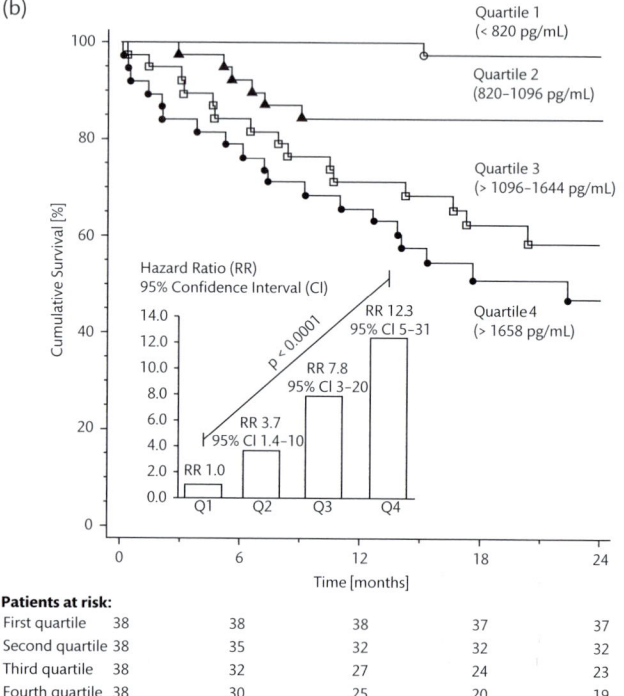

Box 14.1 Peptides, soluble receptors, cytokines, and chemokines with raised circulating concentrations in heart failure

- Novel biomarkers
- Matrix metalloproteinases
- Tissue inhibitors of metalloproteinases
- C-reactive protein
- Cystatin C
- Tenascin C
- Galectin 3
- Osteopontin
- PCIP (procollagen I C-terminal peptide)
- ICTP (carboxy-terminal telopeptide of type I collagen)
- ST2
- Adiponectin
- Copeptin
- Mid-regional natriuretic peptides
- Apelin
- Troponin
- Interleukin-6
- Tumour necrosis factor
- Endothelin
- Resistin
- RAGE
- Leptin
- Monocyte chemoattractant protein 1
- Growth/differentiation factor-15
- Myeloperoxidase
- Urocortin
- MicroRNAs

Figure 14.11 (a) Relationship between sTNF-R1 and NYHA functional class. Upper limit of normal concentrations of sTNF-R1 of healthy control subjects of similar age (mean + 2SD) is indicated, based on data published elsewhere. (b) Kaplan–Meier survival curves for sTNF-R1 quartiles at 24 months. Cut-off values and corresponding hazard ratios (small bar plots) are given. *P*-value refers to Cox proportional hazards analysis.

Reproduced from Rauchhaus M, Doehner W, Francis DP, *et al*. Plasma cytokine parameters and mortality in patients with chronic heart failure. *Circulation* 2000;**102**(25):3060–7 with permission from Wolters Kluwer.

Other novel biomarkers

Many other biomarkers have recently been shown to be elevated in patients with heart failure (**Box 14.1**). Whether these are mere epiphenomena or whether they are involved in the pathophysiology of the syndrome is as yet unclear. Some seem to be obvious candidates for a major role. Examples are ST2, the soluble receptor for IL-33, which seems linked to early fibrosis in the heart[92,93] and apelin, the endogenous ligand of the APJ receptor, which is a potent inodilator produced in the heart. Apelin is down regulated in heart failure and up-regulated in models of reverse remodelling.[94–96] Subsequent manipulation of these systems will unravel their roles.

Systemic consequences of heart failure

The heart failure syndrome does not just affect the heart. As a result of extensive compensatory activity, structural changes take place in vascular arterioles with increasing stiffness of vessels and endothelial dysfunction. Morphological and functional changes occur in skeletal muscle, and respiratory function is affected with an increase in physiological dead space and airways obstruction.[97–99]

Conclusions

The pathophysiological processes at play in the heart failure syndrome combine to produce a progressive state of reduced myocardial performance, a dilated and/or adversely remodelled heart, and ultimately death from progressive pump failure or ventricular arrhythmia. Except in cases where the myocardial function returns to normal or near normal, neurohormonal blockade leads to some reverse remodelling which does lead to an improved outlook for patients. However, the natural history of heart failure for many patients is that treatment merely serves to delay further deterioration in left ventricular function, which will eventually resume in association with co-morbidities—particularly renal dysfunction—and ultimately lead to progressive multi-organ failure and death.

REFERENCES

1. Braunwald E. Heart failure: pathophysiology and treatment. *Am Heart J* 1981;**102**(3 Pt 2):486–90.
2. Katz AM. The descending limb of the Starling curve and the failing heart. *Circulation* 1965;**32**(6):871–5.

3. Katz AM. Cellular mechanisms in congestive heart failure. *Am J Cardiol* 1988;**62**(2):3A–8A.

4. Francis GS, Cohn JN, Johnson G, *et al*. Plasma norepinephrine, plasma renin activity, and congestive heart failure. Relations to survival and the effects of therapy in V-HeFT II. The V-HeFT VA Cooperative Studies Group. *Circulation* 1993;**87**(6 Suppl):VI40–8.

5. Ohtani T, Mohammed SF, Yamamoto K, *et al*. Diastolic stiffness as assessed by diastolic wall strain is associated with adverse remodelling and poor outcomes in heart failure with preserved ejection fraction. *Eur Heart J* 2012;**33**(14):1742–9.

6. Mann DL. Basic mechanisms of left ventricular remodeling: the contribution of wall stress. *J Cardiac Fail* 2004;**10**(6 Suppl):S202–6.

7. Frey N, Olson EN. Cardiac hypertrophy: the good, the bad, and the ugly. *Annu Rev Physiol* 2003;**65**:45–79.

8. Opie LH, Commerford PJ, Gersh BJ, Pfeffer MA. Controversies in ventricular remodelling. *Lancet* 2006;**367**(9507):356–67.

9. St John Sutton M, Pfeffer MA, Moye L, *et al*. Cardiovascular death and left ventricular remodeling two years after myocardial infarction: baseline predictors and impact of long-term use of captopril: information from the Survival and Ventricular Enlargement (SAVE) trial. *Circulation* 1997;**96**(10):3294–9.

10. Narula J, Hajjar RJ, Dec GW. Apoptosis in the failing heart. *Cardiol Clin* 1998;**16**(4):691–710, ix.

11. Konstantinidis K, Whelan RS, Kitsis RN. Mechanisms of cell death in heart disease. *Arterioscler Thromb Vasc Biol* 2012;**32**(7):1552–62.

12. Kitsis RN, Mann DL. Apoptosis and the heart: a decade of progress. *J Mol Cell Cardiol* 2005;**38**(1):1–2.

13. Olivetti G, Abbi R, Quaini F, *et al*. Apoptosis in the failing human heart. *N Engl J Med* 1997;**336**(16):1131–41.

14. Katz AM, Zile MR. New molecular mechanism in diastolic heart failure. *Circulation* 2006;**113**(16):1922–5.

15. Creemers EE, Pinto YM. Molecular mechanisms that control interstitial fibrosis in the pressure-overloaded heart. *Cardiovasc Res* 2011;**89**(2):265–72.

16. Mann DL, Bristow MR. Mechanisms and models in heart failure: the biomechanical model and beyond. *Circulation* 2005;**111**(21):2837–49.

17. Polyakova V, Hein S, Kostin S, Ziegelhoeffer T, Schaper J. Matrix metalloproteinases and their tissue inhibitors in pressure-overloaded human myocardium during heart failure progression. *J Am Coll Cardiol* 2004;**44**(8):1609–18.

18. Mehra MR, Griffith BP. Is mitral regurgitation a viable treatment target in heart failure? The plot just thickened. *J Am Coll Cardiol* 2005;**45**(3):388–90.

19. Trichon BH, Felker GM, Shaw LK, Cabell CH, O'Connor CM. Relation of frequency and severity of mitral regurgitation to survival among patients with left ventricular systolic dysfunction and heart failure. *Am J Cardiol* 2003;**91**(5):538–43.

20. Pfeffer MA, Pfeffer JM. Ventricular enlargement following a myocardial infarction. *J Cardiovasc Pharmacol* 1987;**9** Suppl 2: S18–20.

21. Pfeffer MA, Pfeffer JM. Ventricular enlargement and reduced survival after myocardial infarction. *Circulation* 1987;**75**(5 Pt 2):IV93–7.

22. Pfeffer JM, Pfeffer MA. Angiotensin converting enzyme inhibition and ventricular remodeling in heart failure. *Am J Med* 1988;**84**(3A):37–44.

23. Spragg DD, Leclercq C, Loghmani M, *et al*. Regional alterations in protein expression in the dyssynchronous failing heart. *Circulation* 2003;**108**(8):929–32.

24. Spragg DD, Kass DA. Pathobiology of left ventricular dyssynchrony and resynchronization. *Prog Cardiovasc Dis* 2006;**49**(1):26–41.

25. Cleland JG, Daubert JC, Erdmann E, *et al*. The effect of cardiac resynchronization on morbidity and mortality in heart failure. *N Engl J Med* 2005;**352**(15):1539–49.

26. Borlaug BA. Mechanisms of exercise intolerance in heart failure with preserved ejection fraction. *Circ J* 2014;**78**(1):20–32.

27. Zile MR, Brutsaert DL. New concepts in diastolic dysfunction and diastolic heart failure: Part I: diagnosis, prognosis, and measurements of diastolic function. *Circulation* 2002;**105**(11):1387–93.

28. Gladden JD, Linke WA, Redfield MM. Heart failure with preserved ejection fraction. *Pflügers Arch* 2014;**466**(6):1037–53.

29. Borlaug BA, Lam CS, Roger VL, Rodeheffer RJ, Redfield MM. Contractility and ventricular systolic stiffening in hypertensive heart disease insights into the pathogenesis of heart failure with preserved ejection fraction. *J Am Coll Cardiol* 2009;**54**(5):410–18.

30. Dhakal BP, Malhotra R, Murphy RM, *et al*. Mechanisms of exercise intolerance in heart failure with preserved ejection fraction: the role of abnormal peripheral oxygen extraction. *Circ Heart fail* 2015;**8**(2):286–94.

31. Zile MR, Brutsaert DL. New concepts in diastolic dysfunction and diastolic heart failure: Part II: causal mechanisms and treatment. *Circulation* 2002;**105**(12):1503–8.

32. Kass DA, Bronzwaer JG, Paulus WJ. What mechanisms underlie diastolic dysfunction in heart failure? *Circ Res* 2004;**94**(12):1533–42.

33. Kitzman DW, Little WC, Brubaker PH, *et al*. Pathophysiological characterization of isolated diastolic heart failure in comparison to systolic heart failure. *JAMA* 2002;**288**(17):2144–50.

34. Zile MR, Baicu CF, Bonnema DD. Diastolic heart failure: definitions and terminology. *Prog Cardiovasc Dis* 2005;**47**(5):307–13.

35. Paulus WJ, Tschope C. A novel paradigm for heart failure with preserved ejection fraction: comorbidities drive myocardial dysfunction and remodeling through coronary microvascular endothelial inflammation. *J Am Coll Cardiol* 2013;**62**(4):263–71.

36. Shah SJ, Kitzman DW, Borlaug BA, *et al*. Phenotype-specific treatment of heart failure with preserved ejection fraction: a multiorgan roadmap. *Circulation* 2016;**134**(1):73–90.

37. Kaye DM, Lefkovits J, Jennings GL, *et al*. Adverse consequences of high sympathetic nervous activity in the failing human heart. *J Am Coll Cardiol* 1995;**26**(5):1257–63.

38. Cohn JN, Levine TB, Olivari MT, *et al*. Plasma norepinephrine as a guide to prognosis in patients with chronic congestive heart failure. *N Engl J Med* 1984;**311**(13):819–23.

39. Mann DL, Kent RL, Parsons B, Cooper GT. Adrenergic effects on the biology of the adult mammalian cardiocyte. *Circulation* 1992;**85**(2):790–804.

40. Singh K, Communal C, Sawyer DB, Colucci WS. Adrenergic regulation of myocardial apoptosis. *Cardiovasc Res* 2000;**45**(3):713–19.

41. Bristow MR. Myocardial beta-adrenergic receptor downregulation in heart failure. *Int J Cardiol* 1984;**5**(5):648–52.

42. Bristow MR. The adrenergic nervous system in heart failure. *N Engl J Med* 1984;**311**(13):850–1.

43. Binkley PF, Nunziata E, Haas GJ, Nelson SD, Cody RJ. Parasympathetic withdrawal is an integral component of autonomic imbalance in congestive heart failure: demonstration in human subjects and verification in a paced canine model of ventricular failure. *J Am Coll Cardiol* 1991;**18**(2):464–72.

44. Packer M, Bristow MR, Cohn JN, *et al*. The effect of carvedilol on morbidity and mortality in patients with chronic heart failure. U.S. Carvedilol Heart Failure Study Group. *N Engl J Med* 1996;**334**(21):1349–55.

45. Dargie HJ. Effect of carvedilol on outcome after myocardial infarction in patients with left-ventricular dysfunction: the CAPRICORN randomised trial. *Lancet* 2001;**357**(9266):1385–90.

46. Francis GS, Benedict C, Johnstone DE, *et al*. Comparison of neuroendocrine activation in patients with left ventricular dysfunction with and without congestive heart failure. A substudy of the Studies of Left Ventricular Dysfunction (SOLVD). *Circulation* 1990;**82**(5):1724–9.

47. Francis GS. The relationship of the sympathetic nervous system and the renin-angiotensin system in congestive heart failure. *Am Heart J* 1989;**118**(3):642–8.

48. Francis GS, Goldsmith SR, Levine TB, Olivari MT, Cohn JN. The neurohumoral axis in congestive heart failure. *Ann Intern Med* 1984;**101**(3):370–7.

49. Struthers AD. The clinical implications of aldosterone escape in congestive heart failure. *Eur J Heart Fail* 2004;**6**(5):539–45.

50. CONSENSUS Trial Study Group. Effects of enalapril on mortality in severe congestive heart failure. Results of the Cooperative North Scandinavian Enalapril Survival Study (CONSENSUS). *N Engl J Med* 1987;**316**(23):1429–35.

51. SOLVD Investigators. Effect of enalapril on survival in patients with reduced left ventricular ejection fractions and congestive heart failure. *N Engl J Med* 1991;**325**(5):293–302.

52. SOLVD Investigators. Effect of enalapril on mortality and the development of heart failure in asymptomatic patients with reduced left ventricular ejection fractions. *N Engl J Med* 1992;**327**(10):685–91.

53. Pfeffer MA, Swedberg K, Granger CB, *et al*. Effects of candesartan on mortality and morbidity in patients with chronic heart failure: the CHARM-Overall programme. *Lancet* 2003;**362**(9386):759–66.

54. Swedberg K, Eneroth P, Kjekshus J, Wilhelmsen L. Hormones regulating cardiovascular function in patients with severe congestive heart failure and their relation to mortality. CONSENSUS Trial Study Group. *Circulation* 1990;**82**(5):1730–6.

55. Struthers AD. Aldosterone: cardiovascular assault. *Am Heart J* 2002;**144**(5 Suppl):S2–7.

56. Weber KT. Aldosterone in congestive heart failure. *N Engl J Med* 2001;**345**(23):1689–97.

57. Pitt B, Zannad F, Remme WJ, *et al*. The effect of spironolactone on morbidity and mortality in patients with severe heart failure. Randomized Aldactone Evaluation Study Investigators. *N Engl J Med* 1999;**341**(10):709–17.

58. Miller WL, Redfield MM, Burnett JC, Jr. Integrated cardiac, renal, and endocrine actions of endothelin. *J Clin Invest* 1989;**83**(1):317–20.

59. Neubauer S, Ertl G, Haas U, Pulzer F, Kochsiek K. Effects of endothelin-1 in isolated perfused rat heart. *J Cardiovasc Pharmacol* 1990;**16**(1):1–8.

60. Cowburn PJ, Cleland JG, McArthur JD, *et al*. Pulmonary and systemic responses to exogenous endothelin-1 in patients with left ventricular dysfunction. *J Cardiovasc Pharmacol* 1998;**31** Suppl 1:S290–3.

61. Iwanaga Y, Kihara Y, Hasegawa K, *et al*. Cardiac endothelin-1 plays a critical role in the functional deterioration of left ventricles during the transition from compensatory hypertrophy to congestive heart failure in salt-sensitive hypertensive rats. *Circulation* 1998;**98**(19):2065–73.

62. McMurray JJ, Ray SG, Abdullah I, Dargie HJ, Morton JJ. Plasma endothelin in chronic heart failure. *Circulation* 1992;**85**(4):1374–9.

63. Pousset F, Isnard R, Lechat P, *et al*. Prognostic value of plasma endothelin-1 in patients with chronic heart failure. *Eur Heart J* 1997;**18**(2):254–8.

64. Pacher R, Bergler-Klein J, Globits S, *et al*. Plasma big endothelin-1 concentrations in congestive heart failure patients with or without systemic hypertension. *Am J Cardiol* 1993;**71**(15):1293–9.

65. Anand I, McMurray J, Cohn JN, *et al*. Long-term effects of darusentan on left-ventricular remodelling and clinical outcomes in the EndothelinA Receptor Antagonist Trial in Heart Failure (EARTH): randomised, double-blind, placebo-controlled trial. *Lancet* 2004;**364**(9431):347–54.

66. Torre-Amione G, Young JB, Colucci WS, *et al*. Hemodynamic and clinical effects of tezosentan, an intravenous dual endothelin receptor antagonist, in patients hospitalized for acute decompensated heart failure. *J Am Coll Cardiol* 2003;**42**(1):140–7.

67. McMurray JJ, Teerlink JR, Cotter G, *et al*. Effects of tezosentan on symptoms and clinical outcomes in patients with acute heart failure: the VERITAS randomized controlled trials. *JAMA* 2007;**298**(17):2009–19.

68. Udelson JE, Smith WB, Hendrix GH, *et al*. Acute hemodynamic effects of conivaptan, a dual V(1A) and V(2) vasopressin receptor antagonist, in patients with advanced heart failure. *Circulation* 2001;**104**(20):2417–23.

69. Konstam MA, Gheorghiade M, Burnett JC, Jr, *et al*. Effects of oral tolvaptan in patients hospitalized for worsening heart failure: the EVEREST Outcome Trial. *JAMA* 2007;**297**(12):1319–31.

70. Wei CM, Heublein DM, Perrella MA, *et al*. Natriuretic peptide system in human heart failure. *Circulation* 1993;**88**(3):1004–9.

71. Davis M, Espiner E, Richards G, *et al*. Plasma brain natriuretic peptide in assessment of acute dyspnoea. *Lancet* 1994;**343**(8895):440–4.

72. Maisel AS, Krishnaswamy P, Nowak RM, *et al*. Rapid measurement of B-type natriuretic peptide in the emergency diagnosis of heart failure. *N Engl J Med* 2002;**347**(3):161–7.

73. Tsutamoto T, Wada A, Maeda K, *et al*. Attenuation of compensation of endogenous cardiac natriuretic peptide system in chronic heart failure: prognostic role of plasma brain natriuretic peptide concentration in patients with chronic symptomatic left ventricular dysfunction. *Circulation* 1997;**96**(2):509–16.

74. Gardner RS, Ozalp F, Murday AJ, Robb SD, McDonagh TA. N-terminal pro-brain natriuretic peptide. A new gold standard in predicting mortality in patients with advanced heart failure. *Eur Heart J* 2003;**24**(19):1735–43.

75. O'Connor CM, Starling RC, Hernandez AF, *et al*. Effect of nesiritide in patients with acute decompensated heart failure. *N Engl J Med* 2011;**365**(1):32–43.

76. Packer M, O'Connor C, McMurray JJV, *et al*. Effect of ularitide on cardiovascular mortality in acute heart failure. *N Engl J Med* 2017;**376**(20):1956–64.

77. Packer M, Califf RM, Konstam MA, *et al*. Comparison of omapatrilat and enalapril in patients with chronic heart failure: the Omapatrilat Versus Enalapril Randomized Trial of Utility in Reducing Events (OVERTURE). *Circulation* 2002;**106**(8):920–6.

78. McMurray JJ, Packer M, Solomon SD. Neprilysin inhibition for heart failure. *N Engl J Med* 2014;**371**(24):2336–7.

79. Anand IS, Latini R, Florea VG, *et al*. C-reactive protein in heart failure: prognostic value and the effect of valsartan. *Circulation* 2005;**112**(10):1428–34.

80. Levine B, Kalman J, Mayer L, Fillit HM, Packer M. Elevated circulating levels of tumor necrosis factor in severe chronic heart failure. *N Engl J Med* 1990;**323**(4):236–41.

81. McMurray J, Abdullah I, Dargie HJ, Shapiro D. Increased concentrations of tumour necrosis factor in 'cachectic' patients with severe chronic heart failure. *Br Heart J* 1991;**66**(5):356–8.

82. Adamopoulos S, Parissis JT, Kremastinos DT. A glossary of circulating cytokines in chronic heart failure. *Eur J Heart Fail* 2001;**3**(5):517–26.

83. Rauchhaus M, Doehner W, Francis DP, *et al*. Plasma cytokine parameters and mortality in patients with chronic heart failure. *Circulation* 2000;**102**(25):3060–7.

84. Maeda K, Tsutamoto T, Wada A, *et al*. High levels of plasma brain natriuretic peptide and interleukin-6 after optimized treatment for heart failure are independent risk factors for morbidity and mortality in patients with congestive heart failure. *J Am Coll Cardiol* 2000;**36**(5):1587–93.

85. Torre-Amione G, Vooletich MT, Farmer JA. Role of tumour necrosis factor-alpha in the progression of heart failure: therapeutic implications. *Drugs* 2000;**59**(4):745–51.

86. MacGowan GA, Mann DL, Kormos RL, Feldman AM, Murali S. Circulating interleukin-6 in severe heart failure. *Am J Cardiol* 1997;**79**(8):1128–31.

87. Shioi T, Matsumori A, Kihara Y, et al. Increased expression of interleukin-1 beta and monocyte chemotactic and activating factor/monocyte chemoattractant protein-1 in the hypertrophied and failing heart with pressure overload. *Circ Res* 1997;**81**(5):664–71.

88. Aukrust P, Ueland T, Muller F, *et al*. Elevated circulating levels of C-C chemokines in patients with congestive heart failure. *Circulation* 1998;**97**(12):1136–43.

89. Damas JK, Eiken HG, Oie E, *et al*. Myocardial expression of CC- and CXC-chemokines and their receptors in human end-stage heart failure. *Cardiovasc Res* 2000;**47**(4):778–87.

90. Mann DL. Targeted anticytokine therapy and the failing heart. *Am J Cardiol* 2005;**95**(11A):9C–16C; discussion 38C–40C.

91. Mann DL, McMurray JJ, Packer M, *et al*. Targeted anticytokine therapy in patients with chronic heart failure: results of the Randomized Etanercept Worldwide Evaluation (RENEWAL). *Circulation* 2004;**109**(13):1594–602.

92. Januzzi JL, Jr., Peacock WF, Maisel AS, *et al*. Measurement of the interleukin family member ST2 in patients with acute dyspnea: results from the PRIDE (Pro-Brain Natriuretic Peptide Investigation of Dyspnea in the Emergency Department) study. *J Am Coll Cardiol* 2007;**50**(7):607–13.

93. Rehman SU, Mueller T, Januzzi JL, Jr. Characteristics of the novel interleukin family biomarker ST2 in patients with acute heart failure. *J Am Coll Cardiol* 2008;**52**(18):1458–65.

94. Chong KS, Gardner RS, Ashley EA, Dargie HJ, McDonagh TA. Emerging role of the apelin system in cardiovascular homeostasis. *Biomark Med* 2007;**1**(1):37–43.

95. Chong KS, Gardner RS, Morton JJ, Ashley EA, McDonagh TA. Plasma concentrations of the novel peptide apelin are decreased in patients with chronic heart failure. *Eur J Heart Fail* 2006;**8**(4):355–60.

96. Chen MM, Ashley EA, Deng DX, *et al*. Novel role for the potent endogenous inotrope apelin in human cardiac dysfunction. *Circulation* 2003;**108**(12):1432–9.

97. Mancini DM, Walter G, Reichek N, *et al*. Contribution of skeletal muscle atrophy to exercise intolerance and altered muscle metabolism in heart failure. *Circulation* 1992;**85**(4):1364–73.

98. Sullivan MJ, Higginbotham MB, Cobb FR. Increased exercise ventilation in patients with chronic heart failure: intact ventilatory control despite hemodynamic and pulmonary abnormalities. *Circulation* 1988;**77**(3):552–9.

99. Bank AJ, Lee PC, Kubo SH. Endothelial dysfunction in patients with heart failure: relationship to disease severity. *J Cardiac Fail* 2000;**6**(1):29–36.

15

Cytokines and inflammatory markers

Dimitrios Miliopoulos, Aggeliki Gkouziouta, Evangelos Leontiadis, and Stamatis Adamopoulos

Introduction

The expression of classic neurohormones, such as angiotensin II and noradrenaline, plays an important role in disease progression in chronic heart failure. This so-called neurohormonal activation seems to be involved in the cardiomyopathic process of adverse left ventricular remodelling and dysfunction, via both direct and indirect effects.[1,2] Therapies blocking the excessive activation of the renin–angiotensin system and the adrenergic system have become the mainstay of pharmacological treatment of chronic heart failure.[3]

Another important pathway in chronic heart failure progression is inflammatory activation.[4,5] Experimental studies have shown that proinflammatory cytokines may induce many aspects of the syndrome of chronic heart failure, such as left ventricular dysfunction, pulmonary oedema, and the process of left ventricular remodelling, including myocyte hypertrophy, progressive myocyte loss through either apoptosis or autophagy,[6] and endothelial dysfunction. Although the cause of the inflammation is unknown, both infectious (e.g. endotoxins) and non-infectious (e.g. oxidative stress, haemodynamic overload) events could be operating, including interaction with the neurohormone system. Inflammatory markers have emerged as potential indicators of the evolution of heart failure, ranging from their use for screening, diagnosis, determining prognosis, and guiding treatment.[7]

The emerging association of inflammatory mediators with the pathogenesis and progression of chronic heart failure has already resulted in the development of new anti-inflammatory strategies, which might be used as adjunctive therapy in patients with chronic heart failure.[8,9] Moreover, there is accumulating evidence that a critical network of interactions is formed by inflammatory and the classic neurohormonal mediators, and that many of the conventional therapies for heart failure may, at least partially, modulate the pro-inflammatory cytokine milieu. However, therapies tested so far have been largely disappointing.

The 'cytokine hypothesis'

In the early 1980s, cytokines were first characterized as a new group of peptides. They are secreted by different cell types and mediate cell-to-cell interactions via specific cell-surface receptors. They regulate key aspects of various cellular functions, such as activation, expansion, differentiation, and death.[10,11] The best-studied of these cytokines is tumour necrosis factor (TNF). Comparatively less is known about the interleukins (IL)-1, IL-2, IL-6, and interferon (IFN)-γ in the setting of chronic heart failure.

The chronic heart failure syndrome seems to progress, at least in part, as a result of the toxic effects exerted by endogenous cytokine cascades on the cardiac and skeletal muscle and on the peripheral circulation. So far, the origin of inflammatory mediators remains unclear and has been the subject of controversy. Several hypotheses have been described with respect to the source of proinflammatory cytokines in heart failure, which include:

- the 'infectious hypothesis'
- the 'tissue injury hypothesis'
- the 'neurohormonal hypothesis'.

The 'infectious hypothesis' proposes that endotoxin-induced immune activation happens secondary to bowel oedema (**Figure 15.1**). Persistent immunological stimulation by microbial antigens, which translocate into the body from the oedematous gastrointestinal tract, may lead to cytokine production by monocytes in the bloodstream and possibly other tissues.[12] Lipopolysaccharide is a bacterial endotoxin which strongly induces the production of TNFα and other proinflammatory mediators.[13,14] However, the hypothesis fails to account for several clinical and experimental observations. The beneficial effects of antimicrobial therapy are not clear so far. Patients with chronic heart failure and no peripheral oedema also have elevated plasma cytokines, whereas patients with right heart failure, although oedematous, do not have elevations of plasma cytokines.

Nevertheless, the cytokine explanation for disease progression in chronic heart failure (**Figure 15.2**) does not depend only on the infectious hypothesis. The 'tissue injury hypothesis' proposes that mechanical overload and shear stress induce the myocardial production of cytokines, growth factors, and stress proteins.[15,16] Hypoxia and ischaemia result in the expression of inflammatory cytokines such as TNFα, monocyte chemoattractant protein (MCP)-1, and IL-8 via activation of the transcription nuclear factor (NF)-κB.[15] Oxidized

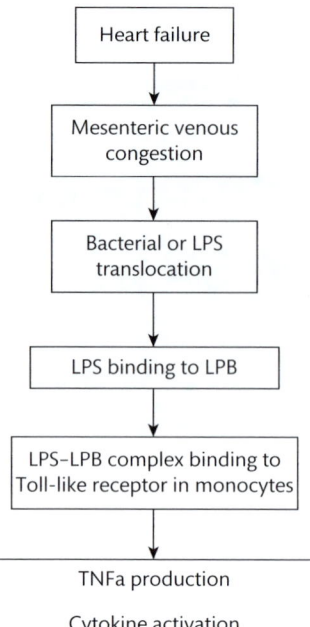

Figure 15.1 The 'infectious hypothesis' for cytokine activation in chronic heart failure. LPB, lipopolysaccharide-binding protein; LPS, lipopolysaccharide (endotoxin).

Source data from Niebauer J, Volk H-D, Kemp M, *et al*. Endotoxin and immune activation in chronic heart failure: a prospective cohort study. *Lancet* 1999;**353**:1838–42.

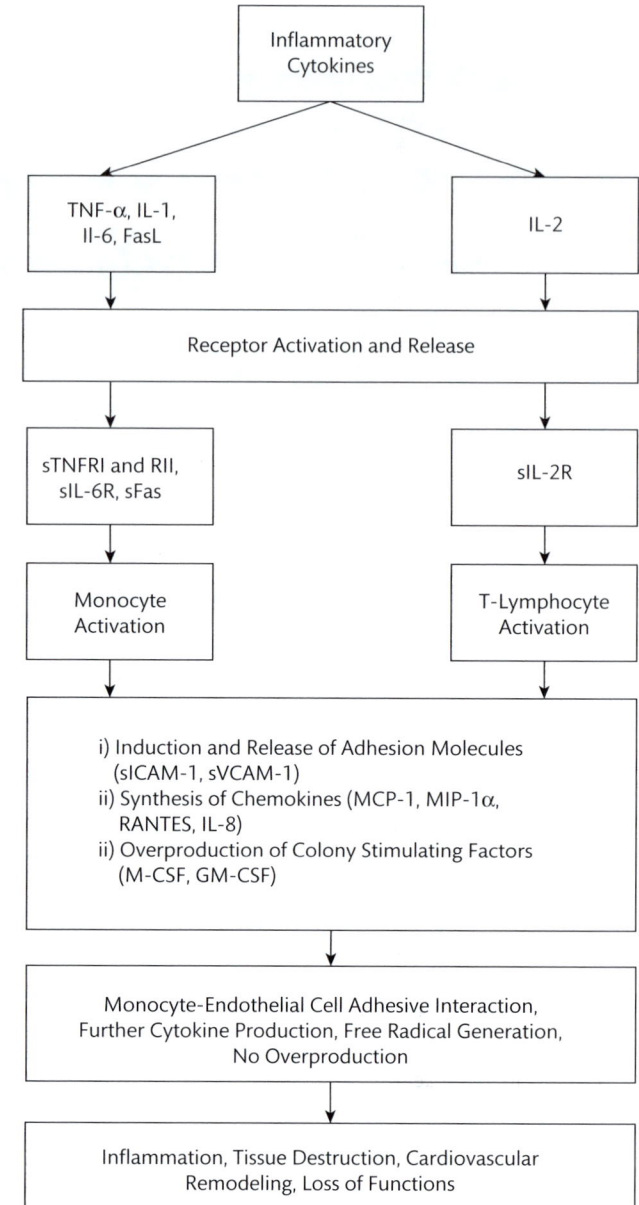

Figure 15.2 Schematic representation of the inflammatory cascade implicated in the pathophysiology of chronic heart failure.

Reproduced from Adamopoulos S, Parissis JT, Kremastinos DT. A glossary of circulating cytokines in chronic heart failure. *Eur J Heart Fail* 2001;**3**:517–26 with permission from John Wiley and Sons.

low-density lipoprotein cholesterol is a potent inducer of cytokine expression.

Recent studies have suggested that a group of receptors, named Toll-like receptors (TLRs), may be involved in immunological and inflammatory activation within the myocardium, not only in response to microbes but also to molecules released from injured and stressed cells. Ligand binding leads to the activation of several kinases and NF-κB.[16] Enhanced monocyte and macrophage expression of stimulatory molecules, including proinflammatory cytokines, follow as downstream effects. In this way, a powerful immune response is possible even in the absence of infection.

The chronic heart failure syndrome may cause tissue hypoxia and free-radical production, in turn leading to NF-κB-mediated production of cytokines. Elevated plasma cytokines further reduce impaired vasodilator reserve, triggering a vicious cycle of more severe tissue underperfusion.

The 'neurohormonal hypothesis' proposes that chronic β-adrenergic stimulation induces myocardial, but not systemic, elaboration of the major proinflammatory cytokines TNFα, IL-1β, and IL-6. There is thus a biological 'cross-talk' between the two cardinal neurohumoral systems in the myocardium.[17]

The deleterious effects of cytokines are mediated by causing reduced protein synthesis and increased protein degradation, in turn leading to muscle atrophy of the central (cardiac) and, perhaps more importantly, peripheral (skeletal) muscles. Proinflammatory cytokines and oxidative stress cause insulin resistance and downregulation of gene expression for the anabolic peptide insulin-like growth factor (IGF)-1 and reduce phosphorylation of the phosphatidylinositol-3-OH kinase (PI-3K), which in turn lowers the activation of the protein kinase B (Akt).[18,19] Reduced Akt activation in both skeletal muscle and heart decreases protein synthesis via

several mechanisms: first, reduced phosphorylation of the 'mammalian target of rapamycin' (known as mTOR) and glucogen synthase kinase;[20] and second, upregulation of activity of forkhead box 0 (FOXO) transcription factors, which in turn activate the ubiquitin–proteasome pathway, resulting in protein degradation.[21,22] In addition, both reduced tissue IGF-1 and insulin resistance activate caspase 3, resulting in further myofibrillar protein breakdown and degradation through the ubiquitin–proteasome pathway.[23]

Whether activated caspase 3 results in skeletal muscle apoptosis remains controversial.[24] 'Skeletal myopathy', resulting from the imbalance between increased muscle catabolism and attenuated muscle anabolism, plays a leading role in the genesis of symptoms of

exercise limitation and, through the exaggerated muscle ergoreflex,[25] dyspnoea.

Tumour necrosis factor-α

Tumour necrosis factor-α (TNFα) is one of the best-characterized proinflammatory mediators in chronic heart failure. It was first described in 1975 and named cachectin. TNFα is a pleiotropic cytokine which can be expressed by almost all nucleated cells and has multiple actions on both local and systemic inflammation.

TNFα is increased in relation to the severity of chronic heart failure and correlates with the degree of sympathetic and renin–angiotensin system activation.[26] TNFα is elevated not only in the circulation, but also in the myocardium of patients with chronic heart failure.[27] Recent research has shown that whereas TNFα rises in the serum of deteriorating patients who require left ventricular assist devices (LVADs), myocardial expression of TNFα falls after mechanical circulatory support.[28,29]

TNFα levels are particularly elevated in patients who are cachectic due to chronic heart failure and the levels have been found to be the strongest correlates of the degree of previous weight loss.[30]

TNFα may contribute directly to the evolution and progression of heart failure and is a predictor of worse outcome (**Figure 15.3**). In a substudy of the SOLVD study, patients with TNFα plasma levels >6.5 pg/mL had worse survival.[31] In a large population of advanced chronic heart failure patients, circulating TNFα was an independent predictor of mortality.[32]

Although TNFα is usually thought of as being harmful, some studies have suggested that TNFα has a protective, inotropic action on the failing heart as a stress response protein.[33] Further, injection of TNFα improves survival of TNFα knockout mice with viral myocarditis in a dose-dependent manner by increasing viral clearance.[34]

TNFα has been implicated in the development of left ventricular dysfunction and remodelling. It increases cardiac myocyte apoptosis, via activation of cytokine-induced nitric oxide (NO) synthase, ceramidase and sphingomyelin pathways, NF-κB activation, and the eventual uncoupling of β-adrenergic signalling[35] as well as via mitochondrial DNA damage. TNFα can mediate cardiac myocyte mitochondrial DNA damage and, therefore, dysfunction in cardiac myocytes via enhanced oxidative stress (overproduction of reactive oxygen species).[36] TNFα activation is regulated, among other factors, by the placental growth factor (PIGF), a vascular endothelial growth factor analogue. Specifically, PIGF acts as a regulator of the tissue inhibitor of metalloproteinases-3/TNFα converting enzyme axis, which is responsible for the TNFα activation. The above mechanism is recruited as an adaptive mechanism at first (as indicated by a ventricular pressure overload animal model) but eventually leads to the deleterious effects of the subsequent inflammatory response and cardiac remodelling.[37]

TNFα is capable of inducing endothelial dysfunction and skeletal muscle wasting, leading to 'skeletal myopathy' through chronic tissue underperfusion, enhanced muscle catabolism, and possibly myocyte apoptosis. Serum TNFα is inversely correlated with skeletal muscle blood flow and exercise capacity, in both stable and decompensated patients with chronic heart failure.[38] It may also contribute to elevated insulin and leptin levels and the development of anorexia and cachexia.[35]

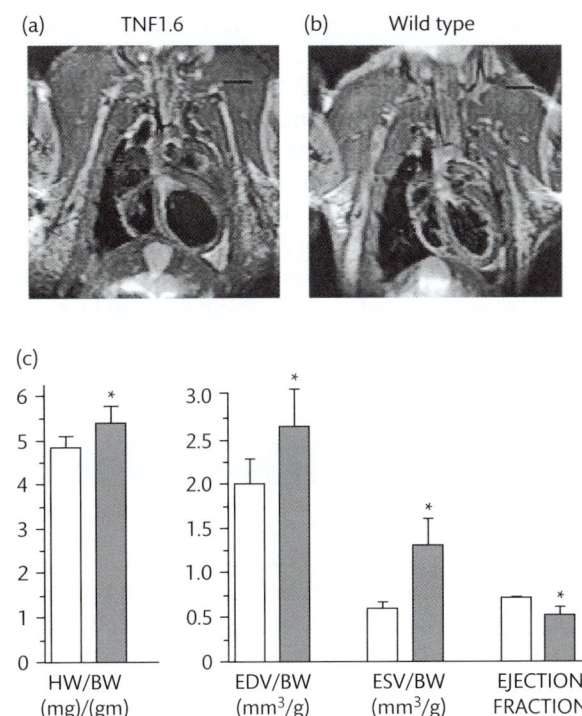

Figure 15.3 Transgenic mice with cardiac-specific overexpression of TNFα (TNF1.6) develop dilated cardiomyopathy. Representative magnetic resonance image (MRI, coronal view) from 24-week-old wild type (A) and TNF1.6 transgenic mice (B) at equivalent stage of cardiac cycle. (C) Transgenic animals demonstrate significant cardiac hypertrophy with chamber dilation and decreased ejection fraction as determined from MRI data (short-axis images). BW, body weight; EDV, end-diastolic volume; ESV, end-systolic volume; HW, heart weight. Open square, wild type; solid square, TNF1.6. $*P < 0.05$.
Reproduced from Feldman AM, Combes A, Wagner D, Kadakomi T, Kubota T, Li YY, McTiernan CJ, The role of tumor necrosis factor in the pathophysiology of heart failure. Am Coll Cardiol 2000;**35**:537–44 with permission from Elsevier.

TNF receptors

The effects of TNFα on the heart are initiated by two specific receptors on myocytes: a lower-affinity 55 kDa receptor (TNFR1) and a higher-affinity 75 kDa receptor (TNFR2).[10] TNFR1 is more abundant and appears to mediate the deleterious effects of TNFα, whereas TNFR2 appears to have a more protective role. Both receptors are cleaved from the cell membrane and subsequently converted to their soluble forms, sTNFR1 and sTNFR2. The soluble receptors may not only neutralize TNFα, inhibiting its highly cytotoxic activities, but perhaps also stabilize TNFα, potentiating its detrimental long-term actions in lower concentrations.[39]

Like TNFα itself, sTNF receptors are highest in patients with severe decompensated chronic heart failure and in cachectic chronic heart failure patients, but are also increased in stable patients with mild chronic heart failure. Plasma concentrations of sTNFR vary less than those of TNFα and are thought to indicate the history of inflammatory immune activation; therefore, they may be better markers of heart failure than serum levels of TNFα.

In patients with advanced chronic heart failure, sTNFR2 is a strong predictor of mortality, which may reflect its ability to act as

a 'slow-release reservoir' of bioactive TNF into the circulation.[31] In the setting of acute myocardial infarction, which is a powerful trigger for cytokine activation, sTNFR1 is a better short- and long-term predictor of death and chronic heart failure.[40] The reasons for the discrepancy may relate to differences in clinical settings, study population sizes, and demographics. It is not yet clear whether circulating sTNFR is an epiphenomenon, simply indicative of a generalized inflammatory state and not a true causal mediator of disease progression. Recent evidence suggests that signalling through both receptors is required to induce the inflammatory and remodelling responses to TNFα and that the overall balance between opposing receptor-specific effects determines the ultimate impact of TNFα.[41]

Interleukin-6

Circulating IL-6 is elevated in patients with chronic heart failure in relation to disease severity.[42] Like TNFα, IL-6 is a maladaptive protein, which participates in the development and progression of heart failure by exerting direct toxic effects on the heart and peripheral circulation. Its role is complex, as it has both proinflammatory and anti-inflammatory effects.[43] IL-6 may induce a hypertrophic response from myocytes and cause myocardial dysfunction by NO generation, but also appears to block cardiac myocyte apoptosis.[44] In the peripheral circulation, IL-6 production may contribute to abnormalities of endothelium-dependent vasodilation, vascular resistance, increased vascular permeability, or muscle wasting. IL-6 spillover in the peripheral circulation increases with the severity of chronic heart failure and is associated with sympathetic nervous system activity.[45]

Serum IL-6 is produced by many cell types, including leukocytes, endothelial cells, vascular smooth muscle cells, cardiomyocytes, and fibroblasts.[46] IL-6 may be more important in the development of chronic heart failure than other inflammatory markers, as it has effects on platelets, endothelium, the coagulation cascade, and metabolism factors. IL-6 is a central mediator of the acute-phase response and a primary determinant of the hepatic production of C-reactive protein (CRP) and TNFα. IL-6 concentrations, not surprisingly, correlate with TNFα and CRP levels.

IL-6 is a strong predictor of new-onset heart failure in healthy populations[47,48] and in older patients with acute ischaemic heart disease.[49] Its prognostic power in patients with established chronic heart failure is not clear. Increased concentrations of IL-6 are independently associated with a poorer prognosis in chronic heart failure patients, but concentrations of its soluble receptor (IL-6R) are not.[11,45] Other reports have not found significant prognostic value of IL-6.[50] Because of relatively high short-term variability and the non-normal distribution of IL-6 concentrations, interpretation of results may vary between studies.[51] In addition, episodes of myocardial ischaemia may trigger IL-6 production, making interpretation of prognostic data more difficult. Notably, a small subunit within the IL-6 receptor, named gp130, is a potent inducer of cardiomyocyte hypertrophy.[52,53] The gp130-signalling pathway seems to mediate the expression and activation of IL-6, IL-6/IL-6R complex, and other IL-6 related cytokines, such as leukaemia inhibitory factor and cardiotrophin-1, playing a critical role in both adaptive and maladaptive responses within the myocardium. Ventricular-restricted gp130 knockout mice develop dilated cardiomyopathy and profound

myocyte apoptosis.[53] However, the clinical significance of these findings in chronic heart failure remains uncertain.

Interleukin-1

The IL-1 cytokine family has four main members: IL-1α, IL-1β, IL-1 receptor antagonist (IL-1Ra), and IL-18. IL-1β is the major extracellular form in humans and a major proinflammatory cytokine.[54,55] The expression of IL-1β is increased in the coronary arteries and myocardium of patients with dilated cardiomyopathy when compared to those with ischaemic heart failure.[56] It has negative inotropic effects on the myocardium by uncoupling β-adrenergic signalling in a dose-dependent fashion, and it depresses myocardial contractility by stimulating NO synthase and ceramidase pathways.[57] IL-1β may also suppress cardiac function by increasing cyclooxygenase-2 and phospholipase A2 gene expression, and by phosphatidylinositol-3′ kinase activation, which results in NF-κB activation.[54,55] In addition, IL-1 is involved in myocyte apoptosis, hypertrophy, and arrhythmogenesis. IL-1β is raised in the myocardium of patients with heart failure and is increased in deteriorating patients.[58]

There is still little information about endogenous IL-1Ra, a naturally occurring cytokine, which blocks the action of IL-1, attenuating its effects. IL-1Ra is often considered a more sensitive marker of IL-1 system activation than IL-1 levels.[59] However, given that IL-1Ra is a specific antagonist of IL-1, elevated levels of IL-1Ra could represent an appropriate response to counteract the inflammatory process caused by IL-1.[59]

IL-18 is a more recently identified member of the IL-1 family, initially identified for its role in inducing IFNγ production.[60] IL-18 is produced by vascular endothelial cells and macrophages in the human heart. It is a proinflammatory cytokine with multiple biological functions and, like many cytokines, it acts synergistically with other similar proteins and mediators.[61] IL-18 is a strong predictor of future cardiovascular risk in stable and unstable angina[62] and is upregulated in the myocardium of patients with chronic heart failure. Although ischaemic insult is a major trigger of IL-18 expression, enhanced IL-18 processing is seen in patients with chronic heart failure of either ischaemic or non-ischaemic origin.[63] IL-18 may aggravate the inflammatory response via increased expression of endothelial cell adhesion molecules and secretion of proinflammatory mediators. It is a potent antiangiogenic cytokine and its inhibition might have beneficial effects on tissue remodelling.[60] IL-18 upregulates membrane Fas ligand expression and may therefore contribute to Fas-mediated apoptosis of Fas-expressing cardiomyocytes.

Granulocyte-macrophage colony-stimulating factor (GM-CSF)

The glycoprotein granulocyte-macrophage colony-stimulating factor (GM-CSF) stimulates the proliferation, differentiation, and activity of multiple myeloid cells including neutrophils, monocytes/macrophages, eosinophils, and dendritic cells. It belongs to the large family of haemopoietic cell colony-stimulating factors and stimulates a range of activities, including leukocyte adhesion, free-radical generation, and cytokine production.[46] It is implicated

in myelosuppressive disorders, drug-induced agranulocytosis, and immunodeficiency syndromes. In atherosclerosis, GM-CSF has angiogenic properties and confers some protective effects.[64] In human tissue from end-stage heart failure, GM-CSF is highly expressed. Elevated GM-CSF levels have been demonstrated in chronic heart failure, which were associated with both the neurohormonal activation and haemodynamic deterioration.[65]

Interleukin-10

Interleukin-10 was initially described as a cytokine synthesis inhibitory factor. It is produced by a variety of inflammatory cells, especially macrophages and T cells, and is found in advanced atherosclerotic plaques, where it confers a protective effect: IL-10 levels predict outcome in acute coronary syndromes.[66] IL-10 inhibits monocyte adherence to human aortic endothelial cells *in vitro*. The ability of IL-10 to suppress certain CD40/CD40L ligand-mediated monocyte responses may account for some of its antiatherogenic effects.[67]

IL-10 inhibits the production of matrix metalloproteinases (MMPs) and cytokines, activation of NF-κB, and apoptosis and cell death.[68] IL-10 downregulates the secretion of TNFα, IL-1, and IL-6 but enhances the release of sTNFR, contributing to the reduction of TNFα activity. IL-10 also attenuates the production of macrophage-derived NO and oxygen free radicals. Circulating IL-10 levels can be elevated in patients with dilated cardiomyopathy and IL-10 mRNA

can be detected in the failing myocardium, possibly as a counter-regulatory response.

One study indicated a differentiation in cytokine patterns with respect to heart failure aetiology; IL-10 was much lower in patients with dilated cardiomyopathy as compared to ischaemic cardiomyopathy.[69] On the other hand, other studies have shown decreased plasma levels of IL-10 with the lowest concentrations observed in advanced chronic heart failure. Administration of immunoglobulin to chronic heart failure patients increased plasma concentrations of IL-10 and improved left ventricular ejection fraction (LVEF) (**Figure 15.4**).[70,71]

Transforming growth factor-β

Transforming growth factor (TGF)-β deactivates macrophages by suppressing inducible NO synthase protein expression. It is a potent negative regulator of inflammation in vascular cells by downregulating cytokine-induced expression of adhesion molecules.[72] Members of the TGFβ superfamily are able to promote the differentiation of embryonic stem cells into cardiomyocytes.[73] Patients with idiopathic dilated cardiomyopathy have increased TGFβ₁ gene expression in macrophages associated with increased plasma concentrations. Excessive production of TGFβ₁ may reflect either an adaptive role of macrophages in tissue repair at the early stages of myocardial injury or impaired ventricular compliance with increased collagen deposition.[74]

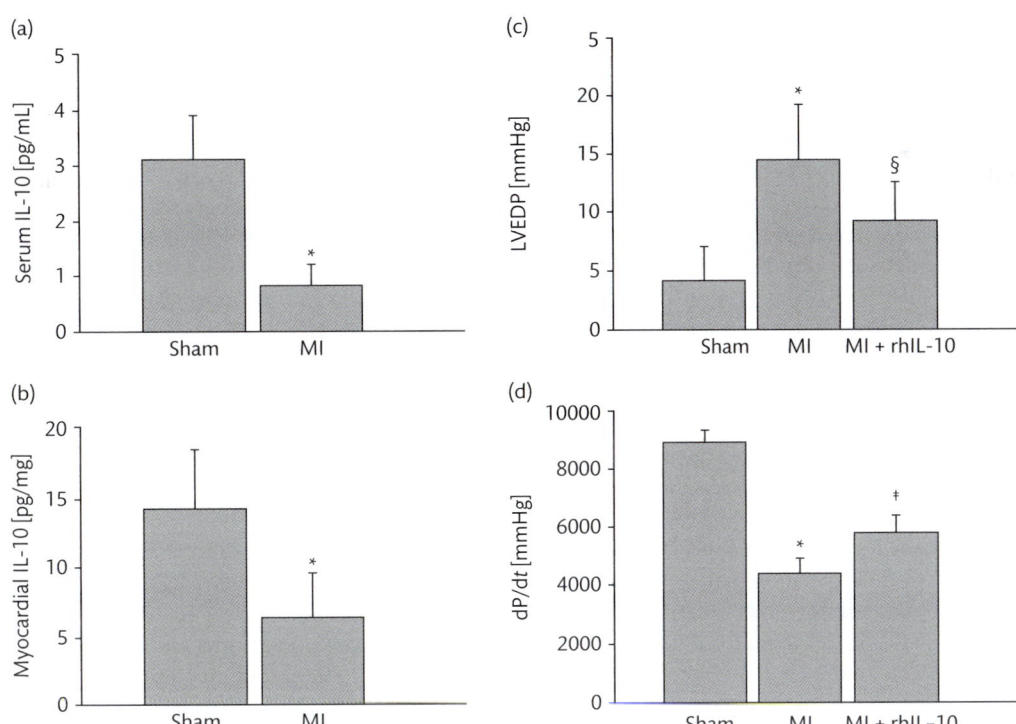

Figure 15.4 Soluble (a) and myocardial membrane-bound (b) IL-10 concentration in sham-operated rats and rats with myocardial infarction (MI). Data are expressed as mean ± SEM. *$P < 0.01$ vs sham rats. (c) Left ventricular end-diastolic pressure (LVEDP) and (d) dP/dt$_{max}$, parameter of systolic function, in sham-operated rats and rats with myocardial infarction (MI), untreated and treated with rhIL-10 for four weeks. Data are expressed as mean ± SEM. $P < 0.01$ vs sham; ‡$P < 0.05$ and §$P < 0.01$ rhIL-10 treatment vs untreated MI group.

Reproduced from Stumpf C, Seybold K, Petzi S, *et al*. Interleukin-10 improves left ventricular function in rats with heart failure subsequent to myocardial infarction. *Eur J Heart Fail* 2008;**10**:733–9 with permission from John Wiley and Sons.

Chemokines

Chemokines are a family of chemotactic cytokines and are important factors in the control and regulation of leukocyte trafficking into inflamed tissues.[75,76] The attraction of leukocytes is essential for inflammation and the host response to infection but may also play a critical role in the pathogenesis of chronic heart failure. Chemokines may promote myocardial failure both directly (e.g. modulation of apoptosis, fibrosis, and angiogenesis) and indirectly (e.g. recruitment and activation of infiltrating leukocytes). It is worth mentioning that fibroblasts themselves, activated by mechanical stretch sensed by integrins, may secrete chemokines attracting monocytes and promoting an inflammatory response which, in turn, leads to their transdifferentiation into myofibroblasts, thus participating actively in the pathophysiological process of the failing heart. Chemokines are classified into three distinct families on the basis of structure and function: C–C (e.g. monocyte chemoattractant protein-1), CXC (e.g. IL-8), and CX3C (e.g. fractalkine).

Monocyte chemoattractant protein-1

Monocyte chemoattractant protein-1 (MCP-1) belongs to the C–C subfamily, which lack an amino acid between the first two N-terminal cysteine residues.[76] It is produced by a variety of leukocytes, endothelial cells, and fibroblasts. MCP-1 is mainly characterized by its ability to induce directional migration of leukocytes, with a crucial role in controlling inflammation and immune responses. MCP-1 possesses chemotactic and activating effects for both monocytes and lymphocytes, and in particular, MCP-1 is a major signal for the accumulation of mononuclear leukocytes in disease.

The pathogenic role of MCP-1 (and its receptor CCR2) in atherosclerosis and its complications is via monocyte and neutrophil interactions with endothelium.[77] Raised levels of MCP-1 have been found in cardiac lymph and in the endothelium of small veins from ischaemic canine myocardium. Pressure overload induces myocardial expression of MCP-1, which attracts and activates monocytes and macrophages, and the recruited cells produce proinflammatory cytokines.[78,79] Hypoxia and ischaemia are also potent inducers of MCP-1, involving activation of NF-κB.

Myocardial overexpression of MCP-1 is associated with monocyte infiltration of the myocardium and cardiac hypertrophy, ventricular dilatation, and depressed contractile function. Serum MCP-1 correlates with the degree of left ventricular dysfunction and may also be involved in cardiomyocyte apoptosis in severe heart failure. Chronic exposure to MCP-1 favours myocardial apoptosis and ventricular dysfunction by inducing transcriptional factors: gene therapy directed against MCP-1 may slow the progression of heart failure.[80]

Its receptor is also useful in differentiating macrophage population in the myocardium. Cardiac macrophages can be divided into two generally distinct populations: CCR2+ and CCR2−. C–C chemokine receptor type 2 (CCR2) is a monocyte surface receptor and promotes monocyte migration to the site of inflammation after its activation. On one hand, CCR2+ macrophages are derived from these monocytes and are associated with persistent left ventricular systolic dysfunction and inflammation while being localized in scar and fibrotic areas of the myocardium. On the other hand, CCR2− macrophages can be found in viable myocardial areas and represent a tissue resident population that is not associated with adverse effects,[81] whereas their depletion is associated with worse outcomes

following myocardial infarction, namely increased infarct area and reduced left ventricular systolic function,[82] therefore suggesting a protective role of this macrophage population.

Macrophage inflammatory protein

Macrophage inflammatory protein (MIP)-1 is a C–C chemokine produced by various types of inflammatory cells, exerting chemotactic activity for both monocytes and lymphocytes. MIP-1 is high in patients with chronic heart failure, with particularly high levels in patients with the most severe heart failure.[80] Abundant expression of MIP-1 may be an important factor in mediating the infiltration and activation of mononuclear leukocytes into the myocardium of chronic heart failure patients but may also have other functions, such as generating reactive oxygen species and cytokine production.

Regulated on Activation Normal T-cell Expressed and Secreted (RANTES)

RANTES is a member of the C–C chemokine group, produced by a variety of cell types including platelets. It is a potent chemoattractant for T cells and monocytes, and is implicated in inflammatory diseases including atherosclerosis. RANTES may also modulate free-radical generation and the production of other cytokines.[83] It is highly expressed within atheroma and is upregulated (and has prognostic significance) in acute coronary syndromes.[46] RANTES is elevated in patients with advanced chronic heart failure and may have a role in disease progression via its effects on platelet–inflammatory cell interactions.[80] However, data on RANTES in chronic heart failure are sparse and further studies are needed.

Interleukin-8

Interleukin-8 is probably one of the best characterized neutrophil chemoattractants and degranulating agents. It is consistently found in macrophage-rich atherosclerotic plaques and it is thus implicated in early atherosclerotic progression.[84]

IL-8 is increased in patients with chronic heart failure with particularly high concentrations in those with the most both severe heart failure. Activated monocytes and platelets may contribute to increased levels of IL-8 in chronic heart failure.[75] IL-8 may be an important participant in both the systemic inflammatory response and the procoagulant activity in chronic heart failure. High IL-8 serum levels fall to near normal after haemodynamic recovery following ventricular assist device placement, suggesting that IL-8 may be a marker of tissue damage.[85]

Interleukin-17

Interleukin-17 is a proinflammatory cytokine and is secreted by a variety of immune cells including macrophages, dendritic cells, natural killer cells, and T cells.[86] IL-17 secretion results in the production of several other cytokines and the migration of neutrophils and macrophages to the site of inflammation.

IL-17 has been shown to be elevated in heart failure patients and its levels are associated with NYHA class.[87] Its deleterious effects in heart failure can be extrapolated from animal models. Specifically, IL-17 can increase inducible NO synthase synthesis causing endothelial and myocardial injury[88] while also stimulating the release of IL-6 and IL-1β whose effects have been described above.[89]

Finally it is important to note that a couple of polymorphisms in *IL-17* gene have been associated with heart failure development and

prognosis; rs8193037 in the *IL-17A* ligand gene has been associated with increased risk of heart failure while rs4819554 in the *IL-17RA* receptor gene has been associated with increased risk of mortality in heart failure patients.[90]

Adhesion molecules

Cell adhesion molecules (CAMs) are involved in the interactions between endothelial cells, leukocytes, and platelets. Thus, they have been implicated in a vast range of conditions including atherosclerosis, thrombosis, allograft rejection post transplantation, and restenosis following coronary angioplasty.[56] Three families of proteins have been described so far. The intracellular cell adhesion molecule-1 (ICAM-1) and vascular cell adhesion molecule-1 (VCAM-1) belong to the immunoglobulin superfamily. Integrins form the second subfamily. The selectins cause a typical 'rolling' of leukocytes on the endothelial surface, which is mainly mediated by leukocyte (L)-selectin and platelet (F)-selectin.

The significance of CAMs in chronic heart failure is unclear. The failing myocardium, and in particular the microvascular endothelium, gives signals to assist in leukocyte infiltration, via the upregulation and/or secretion of CAMs including P-selectin, E-selectin, L-selectin, ICAM-1, and VCAM-1. These molecules are important mediators of both endothelial–leukocyte adhesion and inflammatory responses.[91,92] Damage induced by oxygen free radicals and cytokine activation are stimulators of CAMs. The soluble forms of the adhesion molecules, generated by proteolytic cleavage of cell membrane-bound molecules, act as systemic activation signals for circulating cells.

There is increased endothelial production of adhesion molecules in chronic heart failure, increased expression of sICAM-1 and integrin CD11a/CD18 (lymphocyte function-associated antigen-1), and increased levels of soluble adhesion molecules. VCAM-1, E-selectin, and P-selectin are all also raised.[93,94] Soluble adhesion molecules (sVCAM-1 and sL-selectin) decrease after the implantation of mechanical circulatory support devices in patients with decompensated heart failure.

sICAM-1 increases with increasing severity of failure, which suggests that ICAM-1 may be associated with an adverse prognosis. High levels of sP-selectin or VCAM-1 are also independent predictors of outcome in patients with end-stage heart failure.[94] However, data regarding the prognostic value of CAMs are inconsistent. The limited sample size and the different immunological actions of the studied CAMs are all possible explanations for the inconsistency. Furthermore, the different sCAMs vary differently with time, heart failure treatment, and heart transplantation.[93]

Downstream signalling pathways

NF-κB is a transcription factor mainly involved in stress-induced, immune, and inflammatory responses. Activation of NF-κB can be triggered by multiple stimuli, such as angiotensin II, TLR, IgG, and reactive oxidant species (**Figure 15.5**). Functional NF-κB requires formation of heterodimers of the p50 and p65 subunits.[95] Activation of NF-κB involves the degradation of its inhibitory proteins by

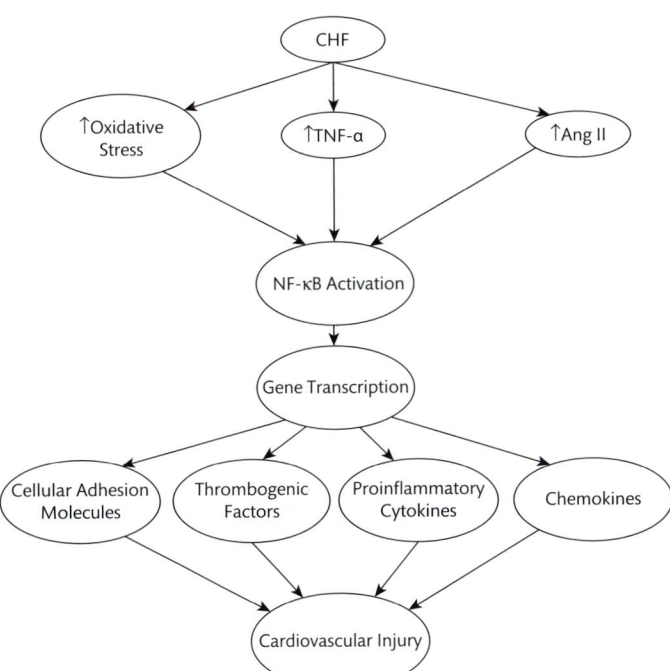

Figure 15.5 Biological stimuli for the production and effects of NF-κB on the cardiovascular system in chronic heart failure.
Source data from Adamopoulos S, Parissis JT, Kremastinos DT. A glossary of circulating cytokines in chronic heart failure. *Eur J Heart Fail* 2001;**3**:517–26.

specific kinases. The free NF-κB passes into the nucleus, where it binds to sites in the promoter regions of genes for inflammatory proteins such as TNFα, IL-1β, inducible NO synthase and adhesion molecules.[96] The activation of NF-κB leads to a coordinated increase in the expression of many genes, whose products are important mediators in the pathogenesis of chronic heart failure.

NF-κB is activated in myocardial tissue of the failing human heart.[5] Activation of NF-κB ameliorates myocardial hypertrophy and is involved in pro- and anti-apoptotic pathways in heart failure. Strategies targeting NF-κB improve the long-term prognosis in heart failure. In mice with targeted disruption of the NF-κB subunit p50, early survival after myocardial infarction is increased and ventricular dilatation is prevented, which is linked to decreased collagen production and deposition.[97]

Nitric oxide

The free-radical gas nitric oxide (NO) is enzymatically formed from L-arginine by three isoforms of NO synthase, which are all present in the heart:

- Endothelial NO synthase (eNOS) is expressed in endothelial cells of the coronary microvasculature and is also found in the subendocardial myocytes. eNOS is the source of vascular NO, acting as vasodilator.
- Neuronal NO synthase (nNOS) is found in the central and peripheral neuronal tissue as well as in cardiac myocytes.
- Inducible NO synthase (iNOS) can be expressed by many different cell types, including inflammatory cells, endothelial cells, and cardiac myocytes.[98]

NO inhibits platelet adherence and aggregation, induces vaso-dilatation, reduces the adherence of leukocytes to the endothelium, and suppresses the proliferation of vascular smooth muscle cells.[98]

iNOS produces large amounts of NO causing direct cytotoxic effects. iNOS expression is increased with increasing severity of heart failure. It is unclear whether wall stress or cytokine activation is the predominant stimulus for iNOS. TNFα is a potent inducer of iNOS expression in both endothelial and vascular smooth muscle cells resulting in enhanced NO production. These high levels of NO can exert both negative inotropic and apoptotic effects on cardiac myocytes. Therapy with LVADs normalizes iNOS expression in association with diminished cardiomyocyte apoptosis in the failing heart.[99]

C-reactive protein

C-reactive protein is a simple downstream marker of inflammation. IL-6 is the primary stimulus for the hepatic production of CRP within 6 h of stimulus.[100] CRP can also be produced from vascular walls, particularly in the atherosclerotic intima of human coronary arteries. Left ventricular dysfunction, systemic underperfusion by low cardiac output, hypoxia, and venous congestion may all be sources of increased IL-6 and, hence, CRP production.

CRP might worsen heart failure through multiple mechanisms. CRP is raised in chronic heart failure and higher plasma levels of CRP are associated with a worse haemodynamic and clinical profile; however, it is unclear whether the finding is related to active atherosclerosis.[101,102] Raised CRP is a predictor of future heart failure and adverse events in patients with vascular disease,[103] but its prognostic value in patients with established heart failure is less clear. There are no data in heart failure patients on the effects of treatment on CRP.

Novel inflammatory mediators

Leptin

Leptin is a major regulator of body mass and appetite.[104,105] In animal studies, it induces weight loss and anorexia and suppresses cardiac contractility through an NO-dependent pathway. Leptin is primarily produced by adipocytes, whereas its receptors are expressed in a variety of tissues, including the heart. Leptin is also related to fat mass in heart failure patients and therefore it should be interpreted having been corrected for fat mass.[106] Leptin can modulate other cytokines including interference with NF-κB effects. Leptin is increased in non-cachectic heart failure patients whereas it is normal or even inappropriately low in cachectic patients—a paradox which may be related to sympathetic nervous activation.

Activin A

Activin A is a member of the TGFβ superfamily involved in growth, differentiation, and survival. Activin A is raised in patients with chronic heart failure. Activin A is involved in ventricular remodelling by enhancing MCP-1 production, the generation of TGFβ₁ and MMPs, and specific gene expression associated with myocardial hypertrophy.[107]

TNF superfamily ligands

Fas and Fas ligand belong to the TNF receptor superfamily and might contribute to inflammation, apoptosis, and matrix degradation within the failing myocardium.[108]

The cross-linking of Fas with Fas ligand mediates apoptosis by triggering caspase activation. Soluble forms of Fas are raised in autoimmune diseases, myocarditis, and severe chronic heart failure. Fas/Fas ligand are associated with left ventricular remodelling and may have prognostic value in chronic heart failure.

The osteoprotegerin receptor activator for NF-κB (RANK)/RANK ligand (RANKL) axis is another member of the TNF receptor superfamily, which is a mediator in both experimental and clinical heart failure.[109]

Trimethylamine-N-oxide

The 'infectious hypothesis' of heart failure proposes that the intestinal oedema caused by the combination of increased venous pressure and perhaps intestinal injury caused by decreased blood perfusion leads to impairment in the barrier function of the intestinal epithelium, which then, in turn, allows the entry of proinflammatory factors into the body. The proinflammatory factors trigger the activation of several cytokines, the effects of which have been described above.[110]

Trimethylamine-N-oxide (TMAO) is a low molecular weight metabolite derived from the metabolism of choline, carnitine, creatinine, or lecithin by bacteria in the gut. Specifically, the gut microbes produce trimethylamine (TMA) which is then oxidized into TMAO by the hepatic flavin monooxygenase (FMO) or the bacterial trimethylamine monooxygenase (TMM) (**Figure 15.6**). TMAO is excreted by the kidneys.[111]

Several studies have reported a positive correlation between TMAO levels and mortality risk due to atherosclerosis and heart failure. One possible explanation of the association between TMAO and outcome is that because it is renally excreted, it may simply be

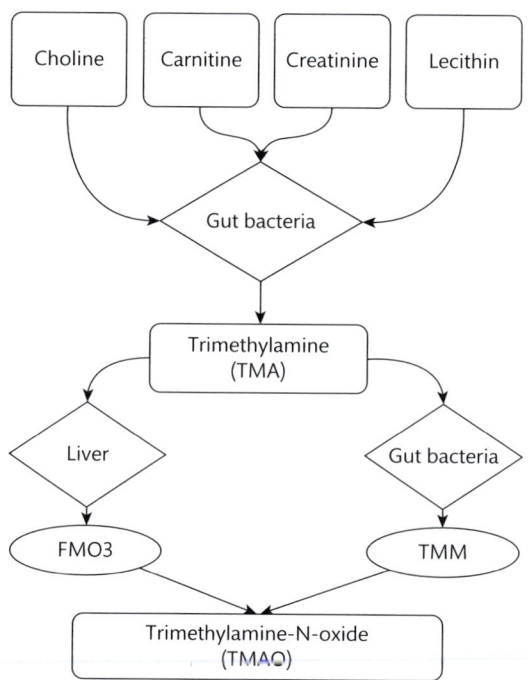

Figure 15.6 The TMAO synthesis pathway.

a marker of renal function:[111] however, other studies have reported that the correlation remains independently of the quality of renal function.[112,113]

Galectin-3

Galectin-3 is a soluble β-galactosidase-binding lectin secreted by activated cardiac macrophages. Its presence is necessary for normal macrophage function and is one of the stimuli for macrophage migration[114] (Figure 15.7b). In addition, galectin-3 binding sites can be found in the proliferating fibroblast nucleus. Both of these effects make galectin-3 an excellent biomarker of inflammation and subsequent fibrosis of the failing heart.

The potential role of galectin-3 in cardiac remodelling has been demonstrated in several studies.[115,116] The infusion of galectin-3 into the pericardial sack of wild type rats resulted in extensive myocardial fibrosis whereas the infusion of N-acetyl-seryl-aspartyl-lysyl-proline (Ac-SDKP) (an endogenous peptide that acts as an inhibitor to the effects of galectin-3) limits the extent of myocardial fibrosis and inflammation.[115] Moreover, there is upregulation of galectin-3 receptors in fibrotic tissues coming both from humans and animal models. This upregulation of galectin-3 receptors is regulated by osteopontin, a cytokine that is induced by tissue injury and participates in the pathophysiology of several diseases by promoting inflammation and fibrosis.[117]

Pentraxin-3

Pentraxins are a superfamily of soluble pattern-recognition proteins characterized by the presence of a cyclic multimeric structure in the carboxy-terminal region called the 'pentraxin domain'. They are divided into short and long pentraxins. The best-known short pentraxin is CRP. Pentraxin-3 (PTX3) is a long pentraxin which is induced primarily by IL-1 and TNFα in a variety of cell types, including endothelial cells, fibroblasts, and smooth muscle cells. PTX3 plasma levels increase during myocardial inflammation and damage at a higher rate than that of CRP. As a result, its role as a potent inflammation biomarker is worth studying.[118]

There have been two major trials studying the prognostic importance of PTX3 levels in heart failure patients: the CORONA and the GISSI-HF trials. In both trials, increasing PTX3 plasma levels was associated with increasing patient mortality (be it cardiovascular or all-cause), as well as heart-failure-related hospitalizations, independently of other biomarkers. In addition, PTX3 levels have been associated with left ventricular diastolic dysfunction and the severity of dilated cardiomyopathy.[119]

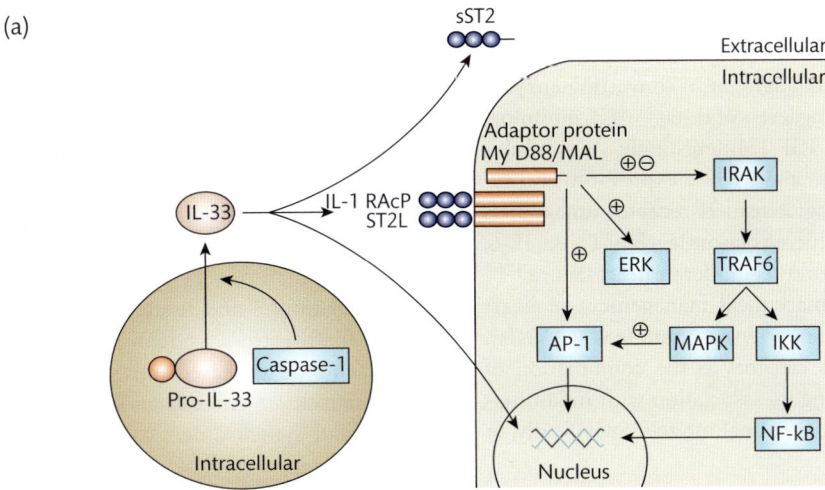

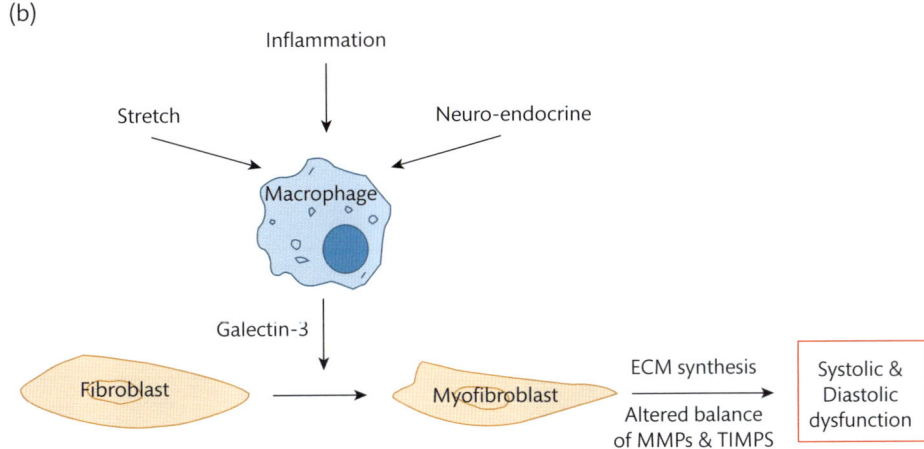

Figure 15.7 Pathophysiological processes of (a) sST2 and (b) galectin-3 in heart failure.

Reproduced from Meijers WC, van der Velde AR, de Boer RA. ST2 and Galectin-3: Ready for Prime Time? *EJIFCC* 2016;**27**:238–52.

ST2

ST2 is a member of the interleukin-1 receptor family and acts as a receptor for IL-33. It has two isoforms: a transmembrane one and a soluble one. The transmembrane ST2 is used for the expression of the effects of IL-33. IL-33 has cardioprotective functions; it reduces hypertrophy and fibrosis. The IL-33/ST2 pathway is activated following inflammation and cardiac stress. However, the soluble isoform acts as a decoy receptor for IL-33 in order to modulate its effects (**Figure 15.7a**). As a result, the soluble ST2 (sST2) can act as an excellent biomarker for myocardial inflammation.[114,120]

There have been several studies describing the role of sST2 in the prognosis of heart failure. Analysis of the HF-ACTION and PHFS studies showed a significant association between increasing sST2 levels and poor patient outcomes. Other studies have also shown that sST2 levels can predict short-term outcomes after discharge in patients with acute heart failure.[121,122]

Anti-inflammatory therapy

Immunomodulatory effects of traditional cardiovascular therapy

The beneficial effects of the traditional cardiovascular medications cannot be explained solely by their haemodynamic effects. Some drugs used in the treatment of chronic heart failure may also influence the persistent immune activation and inflammatory pathways. Treatment with high doses of angiotensin converting enzyme (ACE) inhibitors reduces circulating levels of IL-6.[123] ACE inhibitors may affect TNFα and can reduce IGF-1. Interestingly, ACE inhibitors may prevent NF-κB activation and MCP-1 expression, and reduce macrophage infiltration. Angiotensin II receptor antagonists downregulate inflammation by reducing plasma levels of TNFα, IL-6, and brain natriuretic peptides in mild-to-moderate heart failure.[124]

A novel addition to the pharmaceutical management of heart failure is angiotensin receptor–neprilysin inhibitors (ARNIs). Currently, the only agent of this category is the combination of sacubitril/valsartan. Data regarding its association with inflammation are scarce and most come from animal models. Specifically, in

a mouse model of treated aortic stenosis, ARNI treatment reduced inflammatory myocardial infiltration in addition to preserving cardiac function and reducing fibrosis.[125] Another study examined the effects of ARNI treatment on a mouse model of diabetic cardiomyopathy. It showed reduced intracellular levels of reactive oxygen species along with circulating levels of IL-1β, IL-6, and TNFα.[126]

Amlodipine reduces IL-6 levels, but with no effect on TNFα.[4] β-Adrenergic stimulation may modulate cytokine production from lymphocytes and monocytes. Carvedilol reduces IL-6.[127] On the other hand, long-term treatment with metoprolol has no significant effect on cytokine levels. The differential effects of α- and β-blockade on the cytokine network still need to be determined in more detail.

Statins may attenuate inflammatory responses and promote plaque stability independent of their cholesterol-lowering effects.[4,128] Statins reduce CRP levels and may be effective in preventing coronary events in patients with relatively low lipid levels but with elevated CRP.[128]

Apart from their short-term haemodynamic benefits, phosphodiesterase inhibitors can inhibit the production of TNFα and other cytokines in failing myocardium.[129] However, phosphodiesterase inhibitors are also related to an adverse outcome in chronic heart failure. Cardiac glycosides can also reduce levels of IL-6 and TNFα *in vivo*. Amiodarone causes a significant decrease in TNFα production by human mononuclear cells, suggesting a possible mechanism for a beneficial effect in heart failure.

However, some of the effects on the immune system may be secondary to improved left ventricular function and not a direct effect of the drugs. A non-pharmacological approach, physical training, induces beneficial changes in exercise capacity which are correlated with a reduction in inflammatory markers (**Figure 15.8**).[130] Exercise training restores, at least partially, abnormal immuno-inflammatory responses by depressing systemic inflammation with reduced proinflammatory cytokine (TNFα and IL-6) expression at both circulation[131] and tissue[132] level. In consequence, there is a fall in oxidative stress, as demonstrated by the reduced expression of iNOS and the increased activity of radical scavenger enzymes in skeletal muscle.[133] There is an inverse relation between iNOS expression and cytochrome *c* oxidase activity, suggesting that local

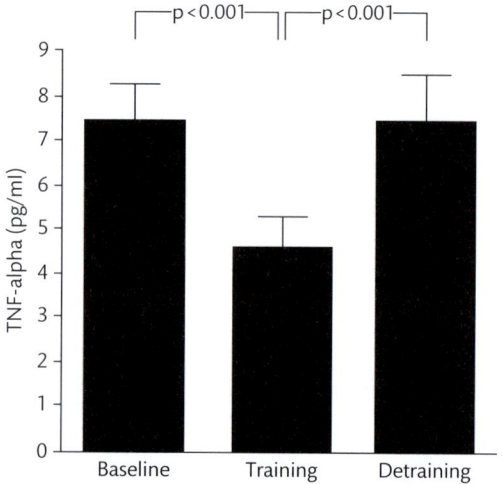
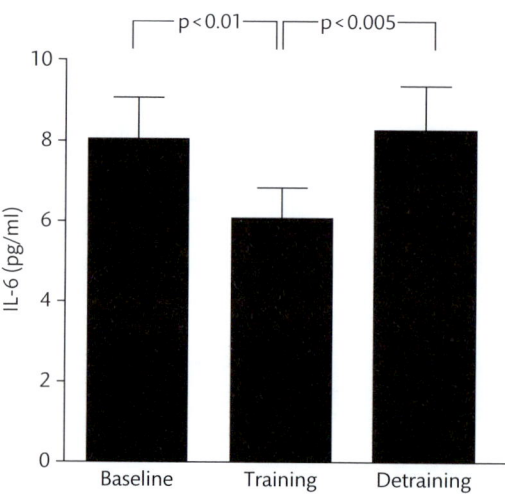

Figure 15.8 The anti-inflammatory effect of physical training in patients with chronic heart failure. The effects of a training programme on TNFα and IL-6 are shown.

Source data from Adamopoulos S, Parissis J, Karatzas D, *et al*. Physical training modulates proinflammatory cytokines and soluble Fas/soluble Fas ligand system in patients with chronic heart failure. *J Am Coll Cardiol* 2002;**39**:653–63.

anti-inflammatory effects may contribute to improved skeletal muscle oxidative metabolism with physical training.[134] The local anti-inflammatory effects of exercise may slow down or even reverse the catabolic wasting process associated with the progression of heart failure.

Anti-TNF studies: positive and negative results

Given the potential central role of TNFα, etanercept—a recombinant sTNFR type 2 protein, which functionally inactivates TNFα—has been tried as a treatment for chronic heart failure. An initial study showed beneficial effects on cardiac function and left ventricular remodelling in a small population with severe chronic heart failure. Subsequently, the long-term effects of etanercept were assessed by three large placebo-controlled trials: RENEWAL, RENAISSANCE, and RECOVER. The trials were terminated prematurely because of lack of evidence of beneficial effects.[135]

Infliximab is a chimeric monoclonal antibody which directly binds to the transmembrane form of TNF. Its use was associated with time- and dose-related increase in death and heart failure hospitalization in patients with moderate/severe heart failure.[136] The xanthine derivative pentoxifylline, which exerts peripheral vasodilatory effects and improves blood flow, also reduces TNFα. Treatment with pentoxifylline was associated with a significant improvement in functional class and LVEF, along with a decrease in circulating TNFα.[137] The observed changes did not correlate with each other, suggesting that the beneficial effects of pentoxifylline were independent of TNFα.

The failure of anti-TNFα therapy has led to much discussion. The intervention on a single cytokine may not be sufficient to have an impact on the progression of heart failure. TNFα is a pleiotropic cytokine, also implicated in cardioprotective pathways, at least early on in the disease process. It may be that immunomodulation is only or particularly valuable for those patients with strongly upregulated inflammatory status. Etanercept and infliximab may even have increased the biological half-life of TNFα, or it may be that the dose used was not sufficient to inhibit TNFα function. The future of anti-TNF therapy is very uncertain. Other agents that modulate the production of TNFα, such as inhibitors of lysophosphatidic acid acyltransferase, p38 MAP kinases, NF-κB, and TNFα converting enzyme may be treatments of the future.

Intravenous immunoglobulin or interferon

Intravenous immunoglobulin (IVIG) administration improves LVEF, haemodynamics, and exercise capacity in patients with chronic heart failure, independent of aetiology.[138] Others have found no impact of IVIG on recent-onset idiopathic dilated cardiomyopathy.[129] To add to the controversy, long-term therapy results in improved LVEF, associated with a marked elevation of IL-10, IL-1 receptor antagonist, and sTNFR. IVIG also reduced chemokines and their receptors in peripheral blood mononuclear cells, suggesting that direct blockade of the chemokine network may be an approach for future intervention.

A pilot study of INF-1β for the treatment of virus-related dilated cardiomyopathy showed improvement in symptoms and quality of life but no change in objective variables.[129]

Immunomodulation therapy: celacade

Celacade is an immunomodulation therapy designed to target chronic inflammation by activating the immune system's physiological anti-inflammatory response. A blood sample is rapidly exposed to a combination of physiochemical stressors *ex vivo* and then reinjected intramuscularly in an attempt to evoke beneficial immune responses. The physiological response of the immune system to the reinjected apoptotic cells is likely to increase inflammatory cytokine production, rather than impair it. Phase I and II clinical trials of celacade showed a low risk of side-effects and improved quality of life in heart failure patients.[139,140] ACCLAIM, a phase III trial, did not show any significant reduction in mortality or cardiovascular hospitalization,[141] but there was a benefit in some subgroups, particularly those with NYHA II class heart failure and those without a history of previous myocardial infarction.

Promising immunomodulation therapeutic options

Immunoadsorption allows the removal of circulating autoantibodies, such as those against the β₁-adrenergic and muscarinergic receptors or troponin I. It improves cardiac structure and function and decreases oxidative stress and myocardial inflammation.[109,129] It may only be effective in patients with cardiodepressant autoantibodies or only in combination with IVIG acting additively or synergistically.

Thalidomide has both anti-inflammatory and anti-oncogenic properties and has recently been evaluated on a limited number of patients. Other immunomodulatory treatments have the potential to improve myocardial function. Drugs targeting the kinase activity of PI3Kγ—a major component of signal transduction controlling leukocyte migration—can reduce cardiac inflammation. The MMP system is involved in ventricular remodelling: its inhibition may have beneficial effects, particularly in acute heart failure where MMP expression is related to acute dilatation and failure. Gene therapy with MCP-1 blocker attenuates the development of cardiac remodelling after myocardial infarction. IL-10 and IL-1R antagonist exert cardioprotective effects in viral myocarditis and against ischaemia reperfusion injury in mice.

Activators of peroxisome proliferator-activated receptors reduce endotoxin-stimulated TNFα expression and cardiac hypertrophy by inhibiting NF-κB activation, thereby decreasing inflammatory response. Tranilast is a mast-cell stabilizing agent, which has been found to modulate compensated hypertrophy, ventricular remodelling, and the production of anti-inflammatory cytokines such as IL-10.

Other emerging therapeutic targets include mannose-binding lectin, IL-18 and IL-6 antagonists, and T-cell and caspase inhibitors, which can tackle inflammation in the heart. More knowledge on inflammatory cytokines in heart failure and larger placebo-controlled randomized studies will allow the development of more effective therapeutic options. Finally, a promising approach suggests that there might be a role for standard immunosuppressant therapy, at least in selected patients. In the TIMIC study, 85 patients with biopsy-proven myocarditis but no evidence of myocardial viral genomes were randomized to receive prednisone and azathioprine for six months, in addition to conventional therapy for heart failure. The patients receiving active treatment had a significant increase in LVEF and a significant decrease in left ventricular dimensions and volumes compared with baseline (anti-remodelling effect). The study underlines the potential importance of endomyocardial biopsy in dilated cardiomyopathy.[142]

Interleukin-1 receptor antagonist: anakinra

As described above, IL-1 is a proinflammatory cytokine implicated in causing deteriorating systolic function, myocyte apoptosis, and hypertrophy in the failing heart. IL-1Ra is a naturally occurring IL-1 receptor antagonist that binds to the IL-1 receptor, ameliorating the effects of IL-1. Anakinra is a recombinant human IL-1 receptor antagonist, usually used as an anti-inflammatory drug in rheumatoid arthritis. Patients with rheumatoid arthritis often have impaired left ventricular diastolic function and treatment with anakinra results in normalization of the dysfunction, even within hours of treatment.[143] This observation has led to further studies in the role of anakinra in the treatment of heart failure.

There have been three major research studies of anakinra: (a) the VCU-ART and VCU-ART2 clinical trials studied the role of anakinra in preventing cardiac remodelling after myocardial infarction and (b) the D-HART pilot study studied the effects of anakinra treatment on the aerobic exercise capacity in patients with heart failure and preserved ejection fraction. All the studies showed evidence that treatment with anakinra positively affects cardiac remodelling and patients' clinical condition.[144,145] More research with the inclusion of more patients is needed for establishing the effect and safety of this novel treatment option.

Direct interleukin-1 antagonist: canakinumab

A more recent development is the emergence of direct IL-1 inhibition through a monoclonal antibody, canakinumab, specifically targeting IL-1β. Its efficacy in cardiovascular diseases was first demonstrated in the CANTOS trial where it was administered in patients with a recent myocardial infarction and elevated levels of CRP. Canakinumab reduced CRP levels as well as primary end-point events: non-fatal myocardial infarction, non-fatal stroke, and cardiovascular death.[146]

A subgroup analysis of CANTOS for heart failure patients demonstrated a dose-dependent reduction of both heart-failure-related mortality and hospitalization episodes.[147] In addition, another single-centre CANTOS substudy revealed that heart failure patients treated with canakinumab improved their exercise capacity (peak VO$_2$) and LVEF.[148]

Despite the above findings, these results come from a subgroup analysis and a small substudy (30 patients) without independent randomization, thus limiting their potential for generalization. Randomized clinical trials are now necessary for robust evidence of canakinumab benefit in heart failure.

Prophylactic effects of cytokines in heart failure

Despite the large volume of evidence supporting the importance of the 'cytokine hypothesis' in heart failure, there are also many studies supporting the notion that cytokines can have cardioprotective effects. The main anti-inflammatory cytokine studied in heart failure is IL-10; its levels are low in patients with heart failure, and higher levels predict better outcomes. Other anti-inflammatory cytokines include thrombospondin-1, which is released upon platelet activation, and TGFβ$_1$ in the early stages of heart failure.

Whereas the cardioprotective effects of specifically anti-inflammatory cytokines are clear, proinflammatory cytokines may paradoxically promote similar effects. Specifically, TNFα and IL-6, though they are both considered as typical proinflammatory cytokines, can activate the survivor activating factor enhancement (SAFE) pathway. The binding of TNFα and IL-6 to their corresponding receptors (TNFR2 and gp130) activates a common pathway, the JAK/STAT3 pathway. STAT3 (signal transducer and activator of transcription 3) is a transcription factor first described for its cardioprotective effects in myocardial infarction, since it is activated in ischaemic pre- and post-conditioning. The JAK/STAT3 pathway can also be activated by other stimuli, including erythropoietin, cannabinoid agonists, insulin, prostaglandins, high density lipoproteins, resveratrol, red wine, exercise training and melatonin.

The SAFE pathway is thus a potential therapeutic target in heart failure, but the route to safe activation of SAFE is complex. The activation of the TNF/JAK/STAT3 pathway requires the activation of TNFR2, though TNFα can also bind to TNFR1 resulting in myocardial remodelling and inflammation. In addition, overactivation of the pathway may also lead to the same effects. Thus, the SAFE pathway needs more investigation in order to promote its cardioprotective effects while minimizing its deleterious ones.[149]

REFERENCES

1. Mann DL. Mechanisms, models in HE: a combinatorial approach. *Circulation* 1999;**100**:999–1008.
2. Mann DL, Young JB. Basic mechanisms in congestive heart failure: recognizing the role of proinflammatory cytokines. *Chest* 1994;**105**:897–904.
3. Rouleau JL. Treatment of congestive heart failure: present and future. *Can J Cardiol* 2005;**21**:1084–8.
4. Damas JK, Gullestad L, Aukrust P. Cytokines as new treatment targets in chronic heart failure. *Curr Control Trials Cardiovasc Med* 2001;**2**:271–7.
5. Anker SD, von Haehling S. Inflammatory mediators in chronic heart failure: an overview. *Heart* 2004;**90**:464–70.
6. Knaapen MWM, Davies MJ, De Bie M, et al. Apoptotic versus autophagic cell death in heart failure. *Cardiovasc Res* 2001;**51**:304–12.
7. Pearson TA, Mensah GA, Alexander RW, et al. Markers of inflammation and cardiovascular disease: application to clinical and public health practice: a statement for healthcare professionals from the Centers for Disease Control and Prevention and the American Heart Association. *Circulation* 2003;**107**:499–511.
8. Murray DR, Dugan J. Overview of recent clinical trials in heart failure: what is the current standard of care? *Cardiol Rev* 2000;**8**:340–7.
9. Mann DL, Deswal A, Bozkurt B, Torre-Amione G. New therapeutics for chronic heart failure. *Annu Rev Med* 2002;**53**:59–74.
10. Dibbs Z, Kurrelmeyer K, Kalra D, et al. Cytokines in heart failure: pathogenetic mechanisms and potential treatment. *Proc Assoc Am Physns* 1999;**111**:423–8.
11. Anker SD, von Haehling S. Inflammatory mediators in chronic heart failure: an overview. *Heart* 2004;**90**:464–70.
12. Anker SD, Egerer KR, Volk HD, et al. Elevated soluble CD14 receptors and altered cytokines in chronic heart failure. *Am J Cardiol* 1997;**79**:1426–30.
13. Genth-Zotz S, von Haehling S, Bolger AP, et al. Pathophysiologic quantities of endotoxin-induced tumor necrosis factor-alpha

release in whole blood from patients with chronic heart failure. *Am J Cardiol* 2002;**90**:1226–30.

14. Niebauer J, Volk H-D, Kemp M, *et al.* Endotoxin and immune activation in chronic heart failure: a prospective cohort study. *Lancet* 1999;**353**:1838–42.

15. Paulus WJ. How are cytokines activated in heart failure? *Eur J Heart Fail* 1999;**1**:309–12.

16. Charalambous BM, Stephens RC, Feavers IM, Montgomery HE. Role of bacterial endotoxin in chronic heart failure: the gut of the matter. *Shock* 2007;**28**:15–23.

17. Murray DR, Prabhu SD, Chandrasekar B. Chronic beta-adrenergic stimulation induces myocardial proinflammatory cytokine expression. *Circulation* 2000;**101**:2338–41.

18. Schulze PC, Gielen S, Adams V, *et al.* Muscular levels of proinflammatory cytokines correlate with a reduced expression of insulinlike growth factor-I in chronic heart failure. *Basic Res Cardiol* 2003;**98**:267–74.

19. Hambrecht R, Schulze PC, Gielen S, *et al.* Reduction of insulin-like growth factor-I expression in the skeletal muscle of noncachectic patients with chronic heart failure. *J Am Coll Cardiol* 2002;**39**:1175–81.

20. Latres E, Amini AR, Amini AA, *et al.* Insulin-like growth factor-1 (IGF-l) inversely regulates atrophy-induced genes via the phosphatidylinositol 3-kinase/Akt/mammalian target of rapamycin (PI3K/Akt/mTOR) pathway. *J Biol Chem* 2005;**280**:2737–44.

21. Schulze PC, Fang J, Kassik KA, *et al.* Transgenic overexpression of locally acting IGF-1 inhibits ubiquitin-mediated muscle atrophy in chronic left ventricular dysfunction. *Circ Res* 2005;**97**:418–26.

22. Sandri M, Sandri C, Gilbert A, *et al.* Foxo transcription factors induce the atrophy-related ubiquitin ligase atrogin-1 and cause skeletal muscle atrophy. *Cell* 2004;**117**:399–412.

23. Du J, Wang X, Miereles C, Bailey JL, *et al.* Activation of caspase-3 is an initial step triggering accelerated muscle proteolysis in catabolic conditions. *J Clin Invest* 2004;**113**:115–23.

24. Conraads VM, Hoymans VY, Vermeulen T, *et al.* Exercise capacity in chronic heart failure patients is related to active gene transcription in skeletal muscle and not apoptosis. *Eur J Cardiovasc Prev Rehabil* 2009;**16**:325–32.

25. Piepoli M, Clark AL, Volterrani M, *et al.* Contribution of muscle afferents to the hemodynamic, autonomic, and ventilatory responses to exercise in patients with chronic heart failure: effects of physical training. *Circulation* 1996;**93**:940–52.

26. Levine B, Kalman J, Mayer L, Fillit HM, Packer M. Elevated circulating levels of tumor necrosis factor in severe chronic heart failure. *N Engl J Med* 1990;**323**:236–41.

27. Torre-Amione G, Kapadia S, Lee J, *et al.* Tumor necrosis factor-alpha and tumor necrosis factor receptors in the failing human heart. *Circulation* 1996;**93**:704–11.

28. Torre-Amione G, Stetson SJ, Youker KA, *et al.* Decreased expression of tumor necrosis factor-alpha in failing human myocardium after mechanical circulatory support: a potential mechanism for cardiac recovery. *Circulation* 1999;**100**:1189–93.

29. Birks EJ, Latif N, Owen V, *et al.* Quantitative myocardial cytokine expression and activation of the apoptotic pathway in patients who require left ventricular assist devices. *Circulation* 2001;**104**(12 Suppl 1):I233–40.

30. McMurray J, Abdullah I, Dargie HJ, Shapiro D. Increased concentrations of tumour necrosis factor in 'cachectic' patients with severe chronic heart failure. *Br Heart J* 1991;**66**:356–8.

31. Torre-Amione G, Kapadia S, Benedict C, *et al.* Proinflammatory cytokine levels in patients with depressed left ventricular ejection fraction: a report from the Studies Of Left Ventricular Dysfunction (SOLVD). *J Am Coll Cardiol* 1996;**27**:1201–6.

32. Deswal A, Petersen NJ, Feldman AM, *et al.* Cytokines and cytokine receptors in advanced heart failure: an analysis of the cytokine database from the Vesnarinone trial (VEST). *Circulation* 2001;**103**:2055–9.

33. Yokoyama T, Vaca L, Rossen RD, *et al.* Cellular basis for the negative inotropic effects of tumor necrosis factor-a in the mammalian heart. *J Clin Invest* 1993;**92**:2303–12.

34. Wada H, Saito K, Kanda T, *et al.* Tumor necrosis factor-alpha (TNF-alpha) plays a protective role in acute viral myocarditis in mice: a study using mice lacking TNF-alpha. *Circulation* 2001;**103**:743–9.

35. Bolger AP, Anker SD. Tumour necrosis factor in chronic heart failure: a peripheral view on pathogenesis, clinical manifestations and therapeutic implications. *Drugs* 2000;**60**:1245–57.

36. Suematsu N, Tsutsui H, Wen J, *et al.* Oxidative stress mediates tumor necrosis factor-alpha-induced mitochondrial DNA damage and dysfunction in cardiac myocytes. *Circulation* 2003;**107**:1418–23.

37. Carnevale D, Cifelli G, Mascio G, *et al.* Placental growth factor regulates cardiac inflammation through the tissue inhibitor of metalloproteinases-3/tumor necrosis factor-α-converting enzyme axis: crucial role for adaptive cardiac remodeling during cardiac pressure overload. *Circulation* 2011;**124**:1337–50.

38. Anker SD, Volterrani M, Egerer KR, *et al.* Tumour necrosis factor alpha as a predictor of impaired peak leg blood flow in patients with chronic heart failure. *Q J Med* 1998;**91**:199–203.

39. Ferrari R, Bachetti T, Confortini R, *et al.* Tumor necrosis factor soluble receptors in patients with various degrees of congestive failure. *Circulation* 1995;**92**:1479–86.

40. Valgimigli M, Ceconi C, Malagutti P, *et al.* Tumor necrosis factor-alpha receptor 1 is a major predictor of mortality and new-onset heart failure in patients with acute myocardial infarction: the Cytokine-Activation and Long-Term Prognosis in Myocardial Infarction (C-ALPHA) study. *Circulation* 2005;**111**:863–70.

41. Hamid T, Gu Y, Ortines RV, *et al.* Divergent tumor necrosis factor receptor-related remodeling responses in heart failure: role of nuclear factor-kappaB and inflammatory activation. *Circulation* 2009;**119**:1386–97.

42. MacGowan GA, Mann DL, Kormos RL, Feldman AM, Murali S. Circulating interleukin-6 in severe heart failure. *Am J Cardiol* 1997;**79**:1128–31.

43. Wollert KC, Drexler H. The role of interleukin-6 in the failing heart. *Heart Fail Rev* 2001;**6**:95–103.

44. Tsujinaka T, Fujita J, Ebisui C, *et al.* Interleukin 6 receptor antibody inhibits muscle atrophy and modulates proteolytic systems in interleukin 6 transgenic mice. *J Clin Invest* 1996;**97**:244–9.

45. Tsutamoto T, Hisanaga T, Wada A, *et al.* Interleukin-6 spillover in the peripheral circulation increases with the severity of heart failure, and the high plasma level of interleukin-6 is an important prognostic predictor in patients with congestive heart failure. *J Am Coll Cardiol* 1998;**31**:391–8.

46. Adamopoulos S, Parissis JT, Kremastinos DT. A glossary of circulating cytokines in chronic heart failure. *Eur J Heart Fail* 2001;**3**:517–26.

47. Vasan RS, Sullivan LM, Roubenoff R, *et al.* Inflammatory markers and risk of heart failure in elderly subjects without prior myocardial infarction: the Framingham Heart Study. *Circulation* 2003;**107**:1486–91.

48. Cesari M, Penninx BW, Newman AB, *et al.* Inflammatory markers and onset of cardiovascular events: results from the Health ABC study. *Circulation* 2003;**108**:2317–22.

49. Koukkunen H, Penttila K, Kemppainen A, *et al.* C-reactive protein, fibrinogen, interleukin-6 and tumor necrosis factor-alpha in the prognostic classification of unstable angina pectoris. *Ann Med* 2001;**33**:37–47.

50. Rauchhaus M, Doehner W, Francis DP, *et al.* Plasma cytokine parameters and mortality in patients with chronic heart failure. *Circulation* 2000;**102**:3060–7.

51. Dibbs Z, Thornby J, White BG, Mann DL. Natural variability of circulating levels of cytokines and cytokine receptors in patients with heart failure: implications for clinical trials. *J Am Coll Cardiol* 1999;**33**:1935–42.

52. Yamauchi-Takihara K. Gp130-mediated pathway and left ventricular remodeling. *J Card Fail* 2002;**8**(6 Suppl):S374–8.

53. Hirota H, Chen J, Betz UA, *et al.* Loss of a gp130 cardiac muscle cell survival pathway is a critical event in the onset of heart failure during biomechanical stress. *Cell* 1999;**97**:189–98.

54. Dinarello CA. Interleukin-1 and interleukin-1 antagonism. *Blood* 1991;**77**:1627–52.

55. Auron PE. The interleukin 1 receptor: ligand interactions and signal transduction. *Cytokine Growth Factor Rev* 1998;**9**:221–37.

56. Francis SE, Holden H, Holt CM, *et al.* Interleukin-1 in myocardium and coronary arteries of patients with dilated cardiomyopathy. *J Mol Cell Cardiol* 1998;**30**:215–23.

57. Cain BS, Meldrum DR, Dinarello CA, *et al.* Tumor necrosis factor-alpha and interleukin-1beta synergistically depress human myocardial function. *Crit Care Med* 1999;**27**:1309–18.

58. Testa M, Yeh M, Lee P, *et al.* Circulating levels of cytokines and their endogenous modulators in patients with mild to severe congestive heart failure due to coronary artery disease or hypertension. *J Am Coll Cardiol* 1996;**28**:964–71.

59. Thiele RI, Daniel V, Opelz G, *et al.* Circulating interleukin-1 receptor antagonist (IL-1RA) serum levels in patients undergoing orthotopic heart transplantation. *Transpl Int* 1998;**11**:443–8.

60. Dinarello CA. Interleukin-18, a proinflammatory cytokine. *Eur Cytokine Netw* 2000;**11**:483–6.

61. Puren AJ, Fantuzzi G, Gu Y, Su MS, Dinarello CA. Interleukin-18 (IFNgamma-inducing factor) induces IL-8 and IL-1beta via TNFalpha production from non- CD14+ human blood mononuclear cells. *J Clin Invest* 1998;**101**:711–21.

62. Blankenberg S, Tiret L, Bickel C, *et al.* Interleukin-18 is a strong predictor of cardiovascular death in stable and unstable angina. *Circulation* 2002;**106**:24–30.

63. Yamaoka-Tojo M, Tojo T, Inomata T, *et al.* Circulating levels of interleukin 18 reflect etiologies of heart failure: Th1/Th2 cytokine imbalance exaggerates the pathophysiology of advanced heart failure. *J Card Fail* 2002;**8**:21–7.

64. Seiler C, Pohl T, Wustmann K, *et al.* Promotion of collateral growth by granulocyte-macrophage colony-stimulating factor in patients with coronary artery disease: a randomized, double blind, placebo-controlled study. *Circulation* 2001;**104**:2012–17.

65. Parissis JT, Adamopoulos S, Venetsanou KF, *et al.* Clinical and neurohormonal correlates of circulating granulocyte-macrophage colony stimulating factor in severe heart failure secondary to ischemic or idiopathic dilated cardiomyopathy. *Am J Cardiol* 2000;**86**:707–10.

66. Heeschen C, Dimmeler S, Hamm CW, *et al.* Serum level of the antiinflammatory cytokine interleukin-10 is an important prognostic determinant in patients with acute coronary syndromes. *Circulation* 2003;**107**:2109–14.

67. Poe JC, Wagner DH Jr, Miller RW, Stout RD, Suttles J. IL-4 and IL-10 modulation of CD40-mediated signaling of monocyte IL-1beta synthesis and rescue from apoptosis. *J Immunol* 1997;**159**:846–52.

68. Silvestre JS, Mallat Z, Tamarat R, *et al.* Regulation of matrix metalloproteinase activity in ischemic tissue by interleukin-10: role in ischemia-induced angiogenesis. *Circ Res* 2001;**89**:259–264.

69. Stumpf C, Lehner C, Yilmaz A, Daniel WG, Garlichs CD. Decrease of serum levels of the anti-inflammatory cytokine interleukin-10 in patients with advanced chronic heart failure. *Clin Sci (Lond)* 2003;**105**:45–50.

70. Gullestad L, Aass H, Fjeld JG, *et al.* Immunomodulating therapy with intravenous immunoglobulin in patients with chronic heart failure. *Circulation* 2001;**103**:220–5.

71. Stumpf C, Seybold K, Petzi S, *et al.* Interleukin-10 improves left ventricular function in rats with heart failure subsequent to myocardial infarction. *Eur J Heart Fail* 2008;**10**:733–9.

72. Gamble JR, Khew-Goodall Y, Vadas MA. Transforming growth factor-beta inhibits E-selectin expression on human endothelial cells. *J Immunol* 1993;**150**:4494–503.

73. Tiedemann H, Asashima M, Grunz H, Knochel W. Pluripotent cells (stem cells) and their determination and differentiation in early vertebrate embryogenesis. *Dev Growth Differ* 2001;**43**:469–502.

74. Sanderson JE, Lai KB, Shum IO, Wei S, Chow LT. Transforming growth factor-beta expression in dilated cardiomyopathy. *Heart* 2001;**86**:701–8.

75. Damas JK, Gullestad L, Ueland T, *et al.* CXC-chemokines, a new group of cytokines in congestive heart failure-possible role of platelets and monocytes. *Cardiovasc Res* 2000;**45**:428–36.

76. Baggiolini M, Dewald B, Moser B. Interleukin-8 and related chemotactic cytokines: CXC and CC chemokines. *Adv Immunol* 1994;**55**:97–179.

77. Okada M, Matsumori A, Ono K, *et al.* Cyclic stretch upregulates production of interleukin-8 and monocyte chemotactic and activating factor/monocyte chemoattractant protein-1 in human endothelial cells. *Arterioscler Thromb Vasc Biol* 1998;**18**:894–901.

78. Shioi T, Matsumori A, Kihara Y, *et al.* Increased expression of interleukin-1 beta and monocyte chemotactic and activating factor/monocyte chemoattractant protein-1 in the hypertrophied and failing heart with pressure overload. *Circ Res* 1997;**81**:664–71.

79. Zhou L, Azfer A, Niu J, *et al.* Monocyte chemoattractant protein-1 induces a novel transcription factor that causes cardiac myocyte apoptosis and ventricular dysfunction. *Circ Res* 2006;**98**:1177–85.

80. Aukrust P, Veland T, Muller F, *et al.* Elevated circulating levels of C–C chemokines in patients with congestive heart failure. *Circulation* 1998;**97**:1136–43.

81. Bajpai G, Schneider C, Wong N, *et al.* The human heart contains distinct macrophage subsets with divergent origins and functions. *Nat Med* 2018;**24**:1234–45.

82. Bajpai G, Bredemeyer A, Li W, *et al.* Tissue resident CCR2⁻ and CCR2⁺ cardiac macrophages differentially orchestrate monocyte recruitment and fate specification following myocardial injury. *Circ Res* 2019;**124**:263–78.

83. Pattison J, Nelson PJ, Huie P, *et al.* RANTES chemokine expression in cell-mediated transplant rejection of the kidney. *Lancet* 1994;**343**:209–11.

84. Boisvert WA, Santiago R, Curtiss LK, Terkeltaub RA. A leukocyte homologue of the IL-8 receptor CXCR-2 mediates the accumulation of macrophages in atherosclerotic lesions of LDL receptor-deficient mice. *J Clin Invest* 1998;**101**:353–63.

85. Goldstein DJ, Moazami N, Seldomridge JA, *et al*. Circulatory resuscitation with left ventricular assist device support reduces interleukins 6 and 8 levels. *Ann Thorac Surg* 1997;**63**:971–4.

86. Onishi RM, Gaffen SL. Interleukin-17 and its target genes: mechanisms of interleukin-17 function in disease. *Immunology* 2010;**129**:311–21.

87. Li XF, Pan D, Zhang WL, *et al*. Association of NT-proBNP and interleukin-17 levels with heart failure in elderly patients. *Genet Mol Res* 2016;**15**(2).

88. Krstić J, Jauković A, Mojsilović S, *et al*. In vitro effects of IL-17 on angiogenic properties of endothelial cells in relation to oxygen levels. *Cell Biol Int* 2013;**37**:1162–70.

89. Lee J-H, Cho M-L, Kim J-I, *et al*. Interleukin 17 (IL-17) increases the expression of Toll-like receptor-2, 4, and 9 by increasing IL-1beta and IL-6 production in autoimmune arthritis. *J Rheumatol* 2009;**36**:684–92.

90. Sandip C, Tan L, Huang J, *et al*. Common variants in IL-17A/IL-17RA axis contribute to predisposition to and progression of congestive heart failure. *Medicine (Baltimore)* 2016;**95**:e4105.

91. Devaux B, Scholz D, Hirche A, Klovekorn WP, Schaper J. Upregulation of cell adhesion molecules and the presence of low grade inflammation in human chronic heart failure. *Eur Heart J* 1997;**18**:470–9.

92. Noutsias M, Seeberg B, Schultheiss HP, Kuhl U. Expression of cell adhesion molecules in dilated cardiomyopathy. *Circulation* 1999;**99**:2124–31.

93. Andreassen AK, Nordøy I, Simonsen S, *et al*. Levels of circulating adhesion molecules in congestive heart failure and after heart transplantation. *Am J Cardiol* 1998;**81**:604–8.

94. Yin WH, Chen JW, Ien HL, *et al*. The prognostic value of circulating soluble cell adhesion molecules in patients with chronic congestive heart failure. *Eur I Heart Fail* 2003;**5**:507–16.

95. Barnes PJ, Karin M. Nuclear factor-κB—a pivotal transcription factor in chronic inflammatory disease. *N Engl J Med* 1997;**336**:1066–71.

96. Satriano J, Schlondorff D. Activation and attenuation of transcription factor NF-κB in the mouse glomerular mesangial cells in response to tumour necrosis factor-alpha, immunoglobulin G, and adenosine 3′:5′-cyclic monophosphate. Evidence for involvement of reactive oxygen species. *J Clin Invest* 1994;**94**:1629–36.

97. Frantz S, Hu K, Bayer B, *et al*. Absence of NF-kappaB subunit p50 improves heart failure after myocardial infarction. *FASEB J* 2006;**20**:1918–20.

98. Paulus WJ, Frantz S, Kelly R. Nitric oxide and cardiac contractility in human heart failure: time for reappraisal. *Circulation* 2001;**104**:2260–2.

99. Patten RD, DeNofrio D, El-Zaru M, *et al*. Ventricular assist device therapy normalizes inducible nitric oxide synthase expression and reduces cardiomyocyte apoptosis in the failing human heart. *J Am Coll Cardiol* 2005;**45**:1419–24.

100. Baumann H, Gauldie J. Regulation of hepatic acute phase plasma protein genes by hepatocyte stimulating factors and other mediators of inflammation. *Mol Biol Med* 1990;**7**:147–59.

101. Anand IS, Latini R, Florea VG, *et al*. C-reactive protein in heart failure: prognostic value and the effect of valsartan. *Circulation* 2005;**112**:1428–34.

102. Kardys I, Knetsch AM, Bleumink GS, *et al*. C-reactive protein and risk of heart failure. The Rotterdam Study. *Am Heart J* 2006;**152**:514–20.

103. Yin WH, Chen JW, Ien HL, *et al*. Independent prognostic value of elevated high-sensitivity C-reactive protein in chronic heart failure. *Am Heart J* 2004;**147**:931–38.

104. Berry C, Clark AL. Catabolism in chronic heart failure. *Eur Heart J* 2000;**21**:521–32.

105. Kennedy A, Gettys TW, Watson P, *et al*. The metabolic significance of leptin in humans: gender based differences in relation to adiposity, insulin sensitivity, and energy expenditure. *J Clin Endocrinol Metab* 1997;**82**:1293–300.

106. Leyva F, Anker SD, Egerer K, *et al*. Hyperleptinaemia in chronic heart failure; relationships with insulin. *Eur Heart J* 1998;**19**:1547–51.

107. Yndestad A, Ueland T, Øie E, *et al*. Elevated levels of activin A in heart failure: potential role in myocardial remodeling. *Circulation* 2004;**109**:1379–85.

108. Yamaguchi S, Yamaoka M, Okuyarna M, *et al*. Elevated circulating levels and cardiac secretion of soluble Fas ligand in patients with congestive heart failure. *Am J Cardiol* 1999;**83**:1500–3.

109. Aukrust P, Gullestad L, Ueland T, Damas JK, Yndestad A. Inflammatory and anti-inflammatory cytokines in chronic heart failure: potential therapeutic implications. *Ann Med* 2005;**37**:74–85.

110. Tang WHW, Wang Z, Fan Y, *et al*. Prognostic value of elevated levels of intestinal microbe-generated metabolite trimethylamine-N-oxide in patients with heart failure: refining the gut hypothesis. *J Am Coll Cardiol* 2014;**64**:1908–14.

111. Cannon JA, McMurray JJ. Gut feelings about heart failure. *J Am Coll Cardiol* 2014;**64**:1915–16.

112. Tang WHW, Wang Z, Shrestha K, *et al*. Intestinal microbiota-dependent phosphatidylcholine metabolites, diastolic dysfunction, and adverse clinical outcomes in chronic systolic heart failure. *J Card Fail* 2015;**21**:91–6.

113. Suzuki T, Heaney LM, Bhandari SS, *et al*. Trimethylamine N-oxide and prognosis in acute heart failure. *Heart* 2016;**102**:841–8.

114. Meijers WC, van der Velde AR, de Boer RA. ST2 and galectin-3: ready for prime time? *Int Fed Clin Chem Lab Med* 2016;**27**:238–52.

115. Bošnjak I, Selthofer-Relatić K, Včev A. Prognostic value of galectin-3 in patients with heart failure. *Dis Markers* 2015;**2015**:1–6.

116. Felker GM, Fiuzat M, Shaw LK, *et al*. Galectin-3 in ambulatory patients with heart failure: results from the HF-ACTION study. *Circ Heart Fail* 2012;**5**:72–8.

117. Psarras S, Mavroidis M, Sanoudou D, *et al*. Regulation of adverse remodelling by osteopontin in a genetic heart failure model. *Eur Heart J* 2012;**33**:1954–63.

118. Bonacina F, Baragetti A, Catapano AL, *et al*. Long pentraxin 3: experimental and clinical relevance in cardiovascular diseases. *Mediators Inflamm* 2013;**2013**:725102.

119. Latini R, Gullestad L, Masson S, *et al*. Pentraxin-3 in chronic heart failure: the CORONA and GISSI-HF trials. *Eur J Heart Fail* 2012;**14**:992–9.

120. Felker GM, Fiuzat M, Thompson V, *et al*. Soluble ST2 in ambulatory patients with heart failure association with functional capacity and long-term outcomes. *Circ Hear Fail* 2013;**6**:1172–9.

121. Kim M-S, Jeong T-D, Han S-B, *et al*. Role of soluble ST2 as a prognostic marker in patients with acute heart failure and renal insufficiency. *J Korean Med Sci* 2015;**30**:569–75.

122. Dupuy AM, Curinier C, Kuster N, *et al*. Multi-marker strategy in heart failure: combination of ST2 and CRP predicts poor outcome. *PLoS One* 2016;**11**:e0157159.

123. Gullestad L, Aukrust P, Ueland T, *et al*. Effect of high- versus low-dose angiotensin converting enzyme inhibition on cytokine levels inchronic heart failure. *J Am Coll Cardiol* 1999;**34**:2061–7.

124. Tsutamoto T, Wada A, Maeda K, *et al*. Angiotensin II Type I receptor antagonist decreases plasma levels of tumor necrosis factor-alpha, interleukin-6 and soluble adhesion molecules in patients with chronic heart failure. *J Am Coll Cardiol* 2000;**35**:714–21.

125. Li X, Zhu Q, Wang Q, *et al*. Protection of sacubitril/valsartan against pathological cardiac remodeling by inhibiting the NLRP3 inflammasome after relief of pressure overload in mice. *Cardiovasc Drugs Ther* 2020;**34**(5):629–40.

126. Ge Q, Zhao L, Ren X-M, *et al*. LCZ696, an angiotensin receptor–neprilysin inhibitor, ameliorates diabetic cardiomyopathy by inhibiting inflammation, oxidative stress and apoptosis. *Exp Biol Med (Maywood)* 2019;**244**:1028–39.

127. Gullestad L, Ueland T, Brunsvig A, *et al*. Effect of metoprolol on cytokine levels in chronic heart failure—a substudy in the Metoprolol Controlled-Release Randomised Intervention Trial in Heart Failure (MERIT-HF). *Am Heart J* 2001;**141**:418–21.

128. von Haehling S, Anker SD. Statins for heart failure: at the crossroads between cholesterol reduction and pleiotropism? *Heart* 2005;**91**:1–2.

129. Heymans S, Hirsch E, Anker SD, *et al*. Inflammation as a therapeutic target in heart failure? A scientific statement from the Translational Research Committee of the Heart Failure Association of the European Society of Cardiology. *Eur J Heart Fail* 2009;**11**:119–29.

130. Adamopoulos S, Parissis J. Immunomodulatory effects of physical training in chronic heart failure. *Hellenic J Cardiol* 2003;**44**:49–55.

131. Adamopoulos S, Parissis J, Karatzas D, *et al*. Physical training modulates proinflammatory cytokines and soluble Fas/soluble Fas ligand system in patients with chronic heart failure. *J Am Coll Cardiol* 2002;**39**:653–63.

132. Gielen S, Adams V, Mobius-Winkler S, *et al*. Anti-inflammatory effects of exercise training in the skeletal muscle of patients with chronic heart failure. *J Am Coll Cardiol* 2003;**42**:861–8.

133. Linke A, Adams V, Schulze PC, *et al*. Antioxidative effects of exercise training in patients with chronic heart failure: increase in radical scavenger enzyme activity in skeletal muscle. *Circulation* 2005;**111**:1763–70.

134. Gielen S, Adams V, Linke A, *et al*. Exercise training in chronic heart failure: correlation between reduced local inflammation and improved oxidative capacity in the skeletal muscle. *Eur J Cardiovasc Prev Rehabil* 2005;**12**:393–400.

135. Mann DL, McMurray JJ, Packer M, *et al*. Targeted anticytokine therapy in patients with chronic heart failure: results of the Randomized Etanercept Worldwide Evaluation (RENEWAL). *Circulation* 2004;**109**:1594–602.

136. Chung ES, Packer M, Lo KH, Fasanmade AA, Willerson IT. Randomized, double-blind, placebo-controlled, pilot trial of infliximab, a chimeric monoclonal antibody to tumor necrosis factor-alpha, in patients with moderate-to-severe heart failure: results of the anti-TNF Therapy Against Congestive Heart failure (ATTACH) Trial. *Circulation* 2003;**107**:3133–40.

137. Bahrmann P, Hengst UM, Richartz BM, *et al*. Pentoxifylline in ischemic, hypertensive and idiopathic-dilated cardiomyopathy: effects on left-ventricular function, inflammatory cytokines and symptoms. *Eur J Heart Fail* 2004;**6**:195–201.

138. Gullestad L, Aass H, Fjeld JG, *et al*. Immunomodulating therapy with intravenous immunoglobulin in patients with chronic heart failure. *Circulation* 2001;**103**:220–5.

139. Torre-Amione G, Sestier F, Radovancevic B. Effects of a novel immune modulation therapy in patients with advanced chronic heart failure. Results of a randomized, controlled, phase II trial. *J Am Coll Cardiol* 2004;**44**:1181–6.

140. Torre-Amione G, Sestier F, Radovancevic B, Young J. Broad modulation of tissue responses (immune activation) by Celacade may favorably influence pathologic processes associated with heart failure progression. *Am J Cardiol* 2005;**95**:30–40C.

141. Torre-Amione G, Anker SD, Bourge RC, *et al*. Results of a non-specific immunomodulation therapy in chronic heart failure (ACCLAIM trial): a placebo-controlled randomised trial. *Lancet* 2008;**371**:228–36.

142. Frustaci A, Russo MA, Chimenti C. Randomized study on the efficacy of immunosuppressive therapy in patients with virus-negative inflammatory cardiomyopathy: the TIMIC study. *Eur Heart J* 2009;**30**:1995–2002.

143. Ikonomidis I, Lekakis JP, Nikolaou M, *et al*. Inhibition of interleukin-1 by anakinra improves vascular and left ventricular function in patients with rheumatoid arthritis. *Circulation* 2008;**117**:2662–9.

144. Abbate A, Van Tassell BW, Biondi-Zoccai G, *et al*. Effects of interleukin-1 blockade with anakinra on adverse cardiac remodeling and heart failure after acute myocardial infarction [from the Virginia Commonwealth University-Anakinra Remodeling Trial (2) (VCU-ART2) pilot study]. *Am J Cardiol* 2013;**111**:1394–400.

145. Van Tassell BW, Arena R, Biondi-Zoccai G, *et al*. Effects of interleukin-1 blockade with anakinra on aerobic exercise capacity in patients with heart failure and preserved ejection fraction (from the D-HART pilot study). *Am J Cardiol* 2014;**113**:321–7.

146. Ridker PM, Everett BM, Thuren T, *et al*. Antiinflammatory therapy with canakinumab for atherosclerotic disease. *N Engl J Med* 2017;**377**:1119–31.

147. Everett BM, Cornel JH, Lainscak M, *et al*. Anti-inflammatory therapy with canakinumab for the prevention of hospitalization for heart failure. *Circulation* 2019;**139**:1289–99.

148. Trankle CR, Canada JM, Cei L, *et al*. Usefulness of canakinumab to improve exercise capacity in patients with long-term systolic heart failure and elevated C-reactive protein. *Am J Cardiol* 2018;**122**:1366–70.

149. Lecour S, James RW. When are pro-inflammatory cytokines SAFE in heart failure? *Eur Heart J* 2011;**32**:680–5.

16

Calcium handling

Cherry Alexander, Godfrey Smith, and Rachel Myles

Introduction

Heart failure is a heterogeneous clinical syndrome accompanied by a variety of phenotypic changes, many of which have been linked to abnormalities in the intracellular calcium (Ca^{2+}) signal. These range from mechanical dysfunction, usually characterized by reduced systolic contractile function, to electrophysiological dysfunction including QT interval prolongation, an increased incidence of ventricular premature beats (VPBs), and arrhythmic sudden cardiac death (SCD). In ventricular myocardial cells, intracellular Ca^{2+} ion fluxes govern the translation of the depolarizing signal into mechanical contraction, a process termed excitation–contraction (E–C) coupling. Abnormalities of intracellular Ca^{2+} handling are thought to underlie both mechanical and electrophysiological dysfunction in failing myocardium. This chapter summarizes the events involved in normal E–C coupling and describes the changes observed in heart failure, with particular focus on the changes reported in remodelled ventricular myocardium. Changes in intracellular Ca^{2+} signalling in other cardiac cell types, such as atrial cardiomyocytes and Purkinje fibre cells, may also be crucial to the final heart failure phenotype, but less is known about pathological changes in these tissues, and therefore these are only mentioned briefly.

Cellular anatomy of the ventricular cardiomyocyte

Cellular dimensions

Ventricular myocardium is a functional syncytium of individual cardiomyocytes approximately 0.12 mm long, 0.02 mm wide, and 0.01 mm thick. A diagrammatic representation of a single cardiomyocyte is shown in **Figure 16.1**. The individual cellular dimensions do not change significantly across mammalian species (e.g. mice to whales); instead, the number of cells varies, with the human ventricles being made up of around 10^8 cardiomyocytes.

Intercalated discs

The structural integrity and electrical homogeneity of ventricular muscle is maintained by a specialized end-to-end connection between myocytes termed the intercalated disc. In adult hearts this consists of highly interdigitating membrane surfaces containing three types of functional links: the zona adherens, desmosomes, and gap junctions. Gap junctions provide the electrical link between myocytes by forming pore structures that produce a pathway of low electrical resistance, thus providing efficient electrical coupling between cells. In ventricular myocytes these pore structures are formed by two connexion units (connexin 43). The intercalated disc protein complex known as the zona adherens provides strong mechanical linkage between cells. It consists of two proteins, cadherin and catenin, which link the internal cytoskeleton of adjacent cells.

The near simultaneous activation of the large numbers of cardiomyocytes during each heartbeat occurs because the electrical signal that triggers contraction propagates from cell to cell via gap junctions at a relatively high velocity (~50 cm/s). The strong mechanical linkage between cells provided by the zona adherens and desmosomes ensures that the contraction of individual cardiomyocytes is summed to produce co-ordinated mechanical systole.

Transverse-axial tubular system

Ventricular myocytes have a sarcotubular system running transversely across the diameter of the cell, which is continuous with the surface membrane (sarcolemma). These invaginations of the surface membrane normally occur approximately every 2 μm (0.002 mm). Both electron and light microscopy have revealed that this transverse tubular system contains a considerable number of tubules running in the axial direction within the cell (see **Figure 16.1**), leading to the use of the more accurate description 'transverse-axial tubular' (TAT) system.[1,2] As in skeletal muscle, the major function of the TAT system in cardiac muscle is the rapid propagation of electrical excitation to the cell interior.[3] Recent studies have provided functional evidence that a number of proteins directly involved in E–C coupling are located in the TAT system.[4,5] The expression of L-type Ca^{2+} (LTCC) channels within the TAT system ensures that these extracellular Ca^{2+} channels in the surface membrane are brought into close proximity (10–20 nm) to the intracellular Ca^{2+} channels associated with the intracellular Ca^{2+} store, the sarcoplasmic reticulum (SR). The Na^{2+}/Ca^{2+} exchanger (NCX) is also located predominantly in the TAT system.[5] This protein is the main route of Ca^{2+} efflux from the cell, therefore its TAT system location ensures efficient Ca^{2+} efflux to

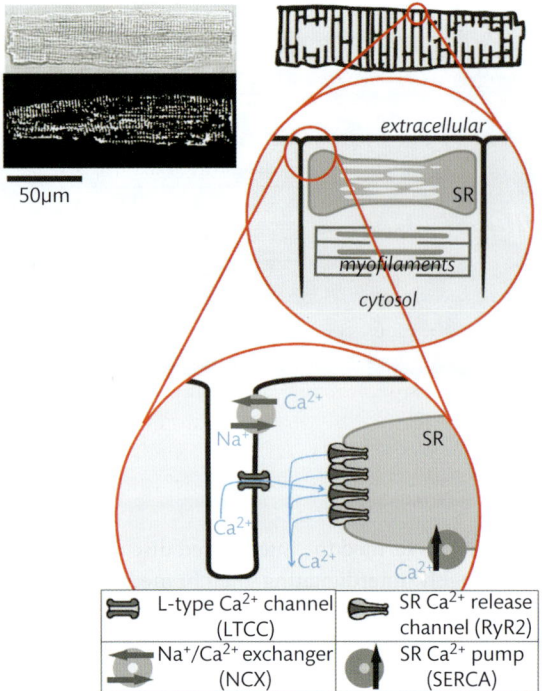

Figure 16.1 Diagrammatic representation of a single cardiomyocyte.

the extracellular space across the diameter of the myocyte. There is also functional and immunohistochemical evidence that the inward rectifying K$^+$ channel (I_{K1}) is expressed in the TAT system.[6] This channel plays an essential role in stabilizing the resting membrane potential and shaping the cardiac action potential and thus contributes to the overall cardiac excitability.[7]

Normal cardiac excitation–contraction coupling

Mechanism of systolic Ca^{2+} increase

Contraction of individual ventricular myocytes is initiated by the action potential (AP). Initial rapid depolarization, mediated by opening of sarcolemmal voltage-gated Na$^+$ channels, causes the opening of sarcolemmal voltage-gated LTCC. The resultant influx of Ca^{2+} triggers the release of a larger amount of Ca^{2+} from the SR by a process known an Ca^{2+}-induced Ca^{2+} release (CICR).[8] Ca^{2+} binding to the intracellular Ca^{2+} channel, the ryanodine receptor (RyR), causes it to open and enaable the route to release the Ca^{2+} stored within the SR. On the face of it, this mechanism would generate a positive feedback loop for intracellular Ca^{2+} release, resulting in an 'explosive' Ca^{2+} release event that emptied the SR on each beat. Yet E–C coupling is associated with an increase in intracellular Ca^{2+} concentration ([Ca^{2+}]$_i$) from approximately 100 nM during diastole to a peak that varies from around 700 nM to nearly 2000 nM during systole depending on various factors. The ability to generate this range of peak systolic Ca^{2+} values is a vital feature of normal cardiac function; it allows the strength of the heartbeat to vary, allowing the heart to respond to various challenges including altered mechanical load and heart rate. Fine control over the peak systolic Ca^{2+} and the subsequent force of contraction can be reconciled with an 'all-or-none' CICR mechanism as this type of release occurs only

in a limited volume of the cell, which acts as a functional Ca^{2+} release unit (CRU) and not the whole cytosol. Variable systolic Ca^{2+} can therefore be achieved by activation of variable numbers of independent CRUs within a single cell.[9] Evidence for CRUs emerged with the observation of discrete Ca^{2+} release events (Ca^{2+} sparks) occurring infrequently and asynchronously during diastole but occurring synchronously during systole.[10] Anatomical evidence for the existence of CRUs comes from electron micrography showing that surface membranes containing LTCCs come into close (10–20 nm) apposition to discrete clusters of RyRs in the intracellular SR membrane.[11,12] This is shown diagrammatically in **Figure 16.1**.

Regulation of sarcoplasmic reticulum Ca^{2+} release channel

As described above, the SR Ca^{2+} release channels are clustered into arrays on the junctional SR membrane, such that each channel contacts up to four of its neighbours. The size of these clusters is under debate, but estimates range from four to 30 channels.[13–15] In addition to cytosolic Ca^{2+}, other endogenous ions and small molecules (e.g. Mg^{2+}, ATP, and cADP-ribose) modulate the activity of RyR.[16,17] Phosphorylation of RyR via either Ca^{2+}-calmodulin-activated kinase (CaM kinase) or cAMP-activated kinase (A-kinase) are thought to alter the Ca^{2+} sensitivity of the channel.[18,19] CaM kinase especially has been found to play a significant part in the development of heart failure. Furthermore, auxiliary proteins are associated with the Ca^{2+} release channel and have been shown to modulate its activity. These include: FK506-binding protein,[19] sorcin,[20] calmodulin,[21] and S100A1[22] on the cytosolic side, and calsequestrin, junctin, and triadin on the luminal side.[23] Most of these regulatory pathways have been found to be altered in heart failure, making the overall picture of the activity of the RyR in heart failure complex.

Mechanism of diastolic Ca^{2+} decrease

Intracellular Ca^{2+} is restored to diastolic levels by several mechanisms. The dominant fraction of the intracellular Ca^{2+} (85–90%) is pumped back into the SR via the activity of the sarcoendoplasmic reticulum Ca^{2+}-ATPase (SERCA) pump. A significant proportion of Ca^{2+} (5–10%) is extruded across the plasma membrane by the sodium–calcium exchanger (NCX). Ca^{2+} is also removed from the cytosol by extrusion across the sarcolemma by the Ca^{2+}-ATPase, although its contribution on a beat-to-beat basis is thought to be quantitatively small (1–2%). The major flux pathways are illustrated in **Figure 16.1**. The rate at which diastolic Ca^{2+} is restored dictates the rate at which the heart relaxes during diastole and depends on the relative activity of these extrusion mechanisms. Another factor that influences the kinetics and final level of intracellular Ca^{2+} during diastole is the 'leak' of Ca^{2+} from the SR, which occurs mainly via the SR Ca^{2+} release channel. Normally the contribution of this mechanism to diastolic Ca^{2+} is minor, but a larger than normal Ca^{2+} SR leak may contribute to the heart failure phenotype. This leak can take two forms: (i) continuous loss of Ca^{2+} and (ii) spontaneous Ca^{2+} waves. Continuous loss of Ca^{2+} is assumed to occur across the complete SR network via dysfunctional RyR and may cause a limited increase in diastolic Ca^{2+} without local gradients of intracellular Ca^{2+}. As yet, although this pathway has been identified in animal models of heart failure,[24] the contribution that continuous Ca^{2+} leak makes to systolic and diastolic function in human heart failure is uncertain. Under some circumstances, local SR Ca^{2+} release within a region of

a heart cell can trigger a spontaneous wave (i.e. not dictated by an AP) of SR Ca²⁺ release that propagates throughout the cell at speeds of around 0.1 mm/s. At each point in the cell, as the wave occurs, the magnitude of SR Ca²⁺ release is comparable to that occurring during systole, but because propagation is much slower (up to 1 s for the wave to travel throughout the cell), the activation of the contractile proteins is asynchronous and therefore ineffective. The high $[Ca^{2+}]_i$ stimulates Ca²⁺ extrusion from the cell by the normal mechanisms, including SERCA and NCX. This spontaneous SR Ca²⁺ release tends to occur when cardiomyocytes experience higher than normal intracellular Ca²⁺, and the Ca²⁺ wave is an efficient mechanism of stimulation Ca²⁺ efflux from the cell.[25] However, the extrusion of this intracellular Ca²⁺ on the NCX generates a large inward current that can depolarize the membrane potential, causing so-called 'afterdepolarizations' which arise during the repolarization phase of the AP (early afterdepolarizations or EADs) or in diastole (delayed afterdepolarizations or DADs). These depolarizations may be of sufficient amplitude to trigger an AP, thus producing a VPB. This is not part of the normal E–C coupling process, and EADs and DADs are not common in healthy hearts. Changes in the SR function in heart failure may make spontaneous Ca²⁺ release more common and this may be the cellular basis for increased incidence of EADs, DADs, VPBs, and possibly arrhythmias in heart failure.

Changes in heart failure

Abnormal cell shape and structure in heart failure

Adult cardiac myocytes are incapable of mitosis, so the adaptive response to myocyte loss or mechanical stress in heart failure is hypertrophy of the surviving cells. In addition to gross changes in cell shape, recent work using confocal microscopy suggests that there is a relative loss of the TAT system in myocytes from animal models of heart failure,[26] and in human heart failure.[1] A reduction in the amount of functional TAT membrane is also indicated by a reduction in the ratio of membrane surface area to volume.[27,28] Disruption of the TAT system structure in such a way as to prevent a significant amount of expressed protein (e.g. LTCC, NCX, and I_{K1}) access to the surface membrane would have pronounced effects on cardiac excitability and E–C coupling, and may therefore be an important cause of the poor contractility observed in heart failure. This 'structural' hypothesis for dysfunction is in contrast to other studies that suggest altered expression of Ca²⁺ handling proteins as the primary cause of dysfunctional E–C coupling.[29] It is almost certainly the case that changes in cellular structure, the expression of the major Ca²⁺ handling proteins, and altered regulation of these channels, pumps, and exchangers all contribute to the complex heart failure phenotype.

Intracellular Ca²⁺ signals in failing hearts

Studies on human myocardium are difficult for a number of reasons including: (i) access to viable samples of normal and failing myocardium; (i) variation in age, medication, and underlying pathology in the available tissue which likely produces significant heterogeneity; and (i) selection bias meaning that samples are unlikely to be truly representative of human heart failure. Thus, animal models of heart failure are widely used to study subcellular changes. For technical reasons, most of these studies have been carried out in single isolated

ventricular myocardial cells, although confirmation in multicellular preparations and whole hearts is available in some cases. Human E–C coupling in heart failure has been studied in cells isolated from hearts explanted at the time of cardiac transplantation, and therefore reflects changes seen in end-stage heart failure, usually due either to ischaemic cardiomyopathy or to non-ischaemic dilated cardiomyopathy. It is important to note that experimental animal models are rarely allowed to develop end-stage heart failure and that the experimental techniques used to achieve a heart failure–life phenotype in animals (e.g. chronic rapid pacing or combined pressure and volume overload) are not the frequent causes of heart failure in humans. In addition, most experimental animals are smaller and have naturally higher resting heart rates than humans and many animals display significant differences from humans in their underlying cardiac electrophysiology, Ca²⁺ handling mechanisms, and contractile protein properties. These differences mean that extrapolation of data from animal models to the situation found in failing human myocardium should be undertaken with caution.

Changes in E–C coupling in heart failure

As suggested above, the changes in E–C coupling that accompany hypertrophy in failing hearts are complex and may depend on the duration, extent, and underlying aetiology of heart failure (e.g. dilated or ischaemic cardiomyopathy). The amplitude and time-course of intracellular Ca²⁺ transients are altered in both animal models of heart failure and in failing human myocardium. In general, systolic $[Ca^{2+}]_i$ is lower than normal, and the duration of the Ca²⁺ transient is prolonged in myocytes from failing myocardium (illustrated in **Figure 16.2**).[30–33] These changes are thought to be the predominant cause of the contractile dysfunction observed in heart failure. Despite pronounced electrophysiological changes in myocytes from failing hearts, changes in the amplitude and time-course of the L-type Ca²⁺ current are not commonly observed, indicating that, in general, the trigger for Ca²⁺ release from the SR is not altered in failing hearts.[29] Early studies suggested that the principal basis for reduced intracellular Ca²⁺ in heart failure was depressed SR function.[29] Whereas SERCA mRNA measurements in failing heats almost always show a significant reduction, a series of reports show no difference in SERCA protein expression or activity in heart failure.[22,34,35] In failing human hearts, a wide range of SERCA protein levels was measured, from 33% to 100% of normal values.[36] This variability may be related to differences in the underlying pathology, since a greater decrease in SR Ca²⁺ ATPase expression/activity was observed in myocardium from patients with ischaemic cardiomyopathy compared to dilated cardiomyopathy.[37] The functional impact of reduced SERCA expression is difficult to predict; in several studies involving animal models of heart failure, reduced systolic [Ca²⁺] was accompanied by unchanged SR Ca²⁺ content.[38–40] This has led to the suggestion that reduced ability of normal Ca²⁺ influx to trigger Ca²⁺ release from the SR is an important aspect of the pathology of heart failure. Direct evidence for this has been supplied by the technique of linescan confocal imaging. This technique allows rapid (every 1–2 ms) scanning of the $[Ca^{2+}]_i$ within a thin (~1 μm section) of a cardiac cell, indicating that, under normal circumstances, depolarization produces a synchronous Ca²⁺ release along the length of a ventricular myocyte.[41] However, measurements on myocytes from failing hearts indicate a heterogeneous activation pattern, suggesting that SR Ca²⁺ release does not occur to the same

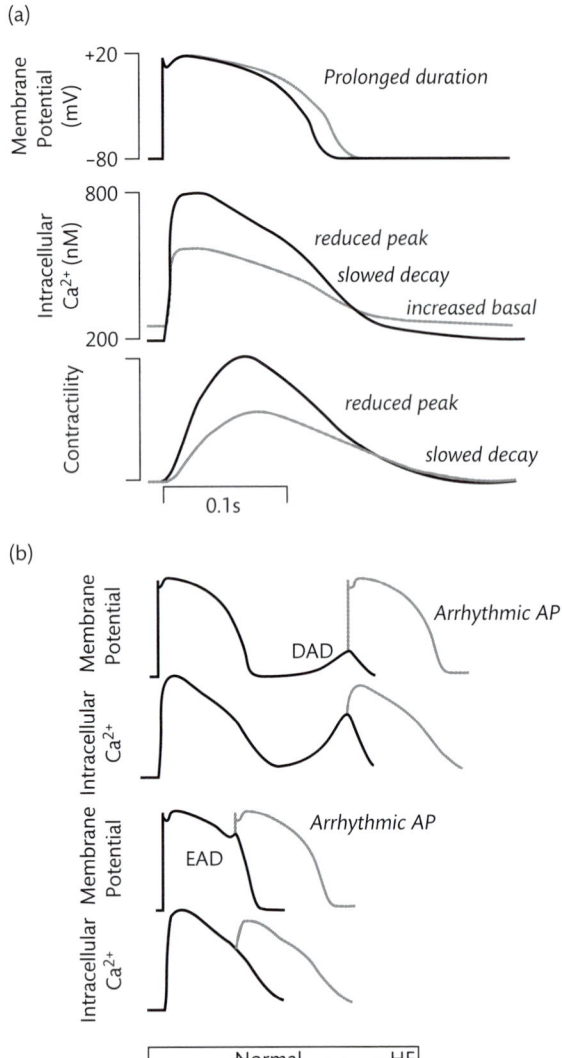

Figure 16.2 Duration of the Ca²⁺ transient is prolonged in myocytes from failing myocardium. HF, heart failure; DAD, delayed afterdepolarization; EAD, early afterdepolarization.

extent at every intracellular site.[38] One explanation for this result is a reduction in TAT system in failing cells diminishing the number of LTCC in close proximity to RyR.

Factors that alter ryanodine receptor function in heart failure

Recent work revealing the complex modulation of RyR function via association/dissociation of regulatory proteins or phosphorylation/dephosphorylation has led to the discovery that the pattern of regulation is significantly altered in heart failure. Initial work on human myocardium indicated that the 12.6 kDa member of the family of FK-506 binding proteins (FKBP12.6) was lost from RyR in failing hearts, and this altered RyR function in such a way as to increase the Ca²⁺ sensitivity of the RyR and increase leak of Ca²⁺ from the SR. Later work showed that the dissociation of FKBP12.6 from RyR in heart failure was the result of hyperphosphorylation of RyR by an associated A-kinase. However, the link between A-kinase, FKBP12.6, and RyR dysfunction in heart failure is not a universal finding, and other work suggests that RyR dysfunction in heart failure occurs independently

of A-kinase.[42] Other regulatory proteins, such as sorcin and S100A1, have been implicated,[43] as has CaM kinase. Increased CaM kinase activity is observed in heart failure and is associated with RyR dysfunction, increased leak from the SR and increased frequency of spontaneous Ca²⁺ release. Recent work has shown that CaM kinase in cardiomyocytes is implicated in EC coupling, gene transcription, and apoptosis.[44] Failing cardiomyocytes have an increased expression of CaMKII and it is thought that this disrupts normal Ca²⁺ homeostasis, increases SR Ca²⁺ leakage, and triggers EADs, creating pro-arrhythmic potential.[45–47] CaMKII has been shown to be associated with a transcriptional repressor gene called histone deacetylase 4 (HDAC4); once phosphorylated, HDAC4 has been shown to cause pathological remodelling of the heart.[48] Studies using transgenic CaMKII knockout mice prevented cardiac hypertrophy or remodelling in response to pressure overload, as well as a reduction in HDAC4 expression.[49] Further studies have shown that CaMKII inhibition prevents structural heart disease, cardiac dysfunction, and hypertrophy.[50] To this end, CaMKII inhibition could be used as a novel therapeutic target in the treatment of heart failure.

However, several studies have established that modification of the Ca²⁺ sensitivity of RyR alone cannot give rise to sustained effects on intracellular Ca²⁺ and contractility, as autoregulatory processes ensure that the Ca²⁺ transients are similar in amplitude despite large changes in RyR Ca²⁺ sensitivity.[51] Thus poor contractility cannot be simply addressed by a drug acting purely on the RyR, and it is likely that drugs with more than one intracellular action will be required for effective positive inotropy.

The link between intracellular Ca²⁺ and arrhythmias

Postulated mechanisms for arrhythmogenesis in heart failure have focused either on single-cell arrhythmic mechanisms, particularly triggered activity (due to early or later afterdepolarizations), or on heterogeneity of electrophysiological properties between cells (conduction velocity or refractoriness, predisposing to re-entry). EADs are defined as depolarizing potentials that occur before the AP repolarizes completely. EADs are facilitated by prolongation of AP duration, whether by delayed inactivation of either Na⁺ or Ca²⁺ currents or by reduction in repolarizing outward current. EADs may be caused by depolarizing current generated either by premature recovery from inactivation and reactivation of LTCC or by an inward current activated by a rise of intracellular Ca²⁺ (e.g. the forward mode NCX). However, there is no consensus as to whether EADs are triggered by, or are dependent upon, spontaneous SR Ca²⁺ release. Late EADs occur during phase 3 of the AP and are thought to be due to Ca²⁺-activated inward currents (NCX or the non-selective current or Ca²⁺ activated Cl⁻ current) generated by spontaneous Ca²⁺ SR release in a similar fashion to DADs.[52]

DADs are caused by spontaneous Ca²⁺ release from local regions of the SR which give rise to a transient inward current during the diastolic period. Conditions of intracellular Ca²⁺ overload, such as those produced by catecholamine administration or digitalis toxicity, predispose to DADs. Whereas early EADs are common during bradycardia, the amplitude and frequency of DADs increases with increasing heart rate. Interestingly, the changes in RyR function observed in heart failure are also thought to predispose the SR to spontaneous release and therefore to the generation of a late EAD or DAD. The increased incidence of these potential arrhythmic triggers manifests as increased VPBs and substantially increases the

Changes in sodium–calcium exchanger abundance and activity in heart failure

In cardiac muscle, sarcolemmal NCX plays an essential role in regulating $[Ca^{2+}]_i$. Changes in the activity of NCX modulate the force of contraction,[33,53] and may contribute to the poor mechanical function in heart failure. Furthermore, NCX activity is electrogenic and may generate pro-arrhythmic currents in normal and hypertrophic myocardium.[54] In many animal models of cardiac hypertrophy and heart failure, both NCX expression and activity are increased.[36,54–56] However, other studies have reported contrary findings.[57] The most difficult results to reconcile are those from a mouse aortic banding model of cardiac hypertrophy; in this study NCX protein and RNA levels were increased as NCX current was decreased.[58] When considering NCX expression pattern, these findings raise two interesting possibilities to explain the changes in NCX activity and abundance.

NCX expression pattern is altered in heart failure; the increased expression is the result of increases in NCX protein in the remaining TAT system and surface membrane. This NCX would be less effective at extruding Ca^{2+} since the disrupted TAT system would prevent Ca^{2+} within the centre of the cell having immediate access to the extracellular space.

NCX expression pattern is similar to normal, the increased NCX is within the TAT system, but a fraction of the TAT system has limited access to the extracellular space. A similar situation has been created experimentally by detubulating isolated rat cardiac myocytes.[5] This acute treatment markedly reduced the rate of Ca^{2+} extrusion but did not alter NCX expression levels. If a similar disconnection of the TAT system developed in the failing myocytes, the increased NCX expression would not be reflected in an increased Ca^{2+} extrusion from the cell.

Mitochondrial function in heart failure

Alongside remodelling of cellular structure and SR function, pathological hypertrophy is also associated with altered mitochondrial function that limits energy production of the cardiac cell and therefore inotropy. These studies suggest that major aspects of the pathophysiology of heart failure are linked to raised intracellular Na^+ and the subsequent lowering of mitochondrial Ca^{2+} level through the activity of mitochondrial NCX.[59–61] In the context of heart failure, the lower intramitochondrial Ca^{2+} and decreased NADP(H) redox potential increases oxidative stress within the cell. Inhibition of mitochondrial NCX with specific drugs abolishes the adverse effects of high intracellular Na^+ and, in doing so, reduces reactive oxygen species accumulation. This normalized mitochondrial function also prevented fibrosis and hypertrophic remodelling which, in a guinea-pig heart failure model, improved cardiac contractility and survival rates.[62] This suggests that modulation of mitochondrial NCX has the potential to become a novel target for heart failure treatment.

Contributions of non-ventricular tissue to the heart failure phenotype

Potentially, Ca^{2+} signalling disturbances in atrial cardiomyocytes and Purkinje cells may also contribute to the poor contractility and pro-arrhythmic status associated with heart failure.

Atrial cells are smaller in diameter (~0.01 mm) and length (~0.1 mm) than ventricular cardiomyocytes, and some measurements suggest that there is a less developed TAT system. The intracellular Ca^{2+} transients are smaller and slower in atrial myocytes from failing hearts in an analogous way to that observed in failing ventricular cardiomyocytes. Few human studies exist, but animal models of heart failure indicate that changes in Ca^{2+} signalling are associated with a reduction of the already poorly developed TAT system.[63] The E–C coupling process in atria is thought to rely more on propagation of the Ca^{2+} signal from the periphery to the central region of the cell rather than AP propagation into the cell diameter via the TAT system. Interestingly, several studies suggest that Ca^{2+} signalling within atrial cells is influenced by inositol-tris-phosphate-activated receptors (IP_3R) on the SR membrane as well as RyR.[64] The relative expression of IP_3R versus RyR channels is thought to be altered in failing hearts which may predispose the atrial cell to either initiate or sustain arrhythmic activity. In humans, heart failure is associated with an increased risk of atrial fibrillation (AF), but the cellular basis for this is unknown and further work is required to establish whether the modification of Ca^{2+} signalling may predispose to or sustain AF activity.

The Purkinje fibre network is made up of modified cardiomyocytes and is responsible for the rapid activation of the endocardial surface. The cells are wider (~0.03 mm) than ventricular cardiomyocytes with a less dense TAT system and fewer myofibrils and mitochondria. As with atrial cells, propagation of the surface depolarization to the centre of these cells is thought to occur via regenerative SR Ca^{2+} release. Complex patterns of Ca^{2+} release have been observed in Purkinje cells involving both central and peripheral sections of the SR network.[65] Analogous to atrial cells, IP_3R are thought to play a key role in regulating spontaneous Ca^{2+} release in Purkinje fibre cells. Several lines of evidence indicate that the trigger for sustained arrhythmias may arise within the Purkinje network, particularly those resulting from an ischaemia/reperfusion cycle.[66] The role of intracellular Ca^{2+} in the generation of EAD- or DAD-based arrhythmias in Purkinje cells is an active area of research. Surviving Purkinje cells within the infarct are more prone to spontaneous Ca^{2+} release and arrhythmic activity.[65] Modification of RyR is thought to contribute to this effect since this pro-arrhythmic activity can be normalized by the drug JTV 519,[65] lending support to the concept that Purkinje-fibre-based triggers for arrhythmic behaviour in heart failure may be amenable to specific pharmacological suppression by drugs acting to normalize intracellular Ca^{2+} handling.

Summary

Abnormalities of Ca^{2+} release and reuptake occur in the remodelled myocardium of failing hearts. These changes are thought to mediate both the poor inotropic and the pro-arrhythmic state of the failing heart. The molecular and structural basis for these changes appears to be multifactorial, and includes abnormal subcellular structure and altered regulation of Ca^{2+} signalling proteins. Basic research on failing human myocardium and animal models of the disease has suggested novel therapeutic approaches to normalize Ca^{2+} signalling in failing hearts, promising more effective pharmacological therapies in the near future.

REFERENCES

1. Soeller C, Cannell MB. Examination of the transverse tubular system in living cardiac rat myocytes by 2-photon microscopy and digital image-processing techniques. *Circ Res* 1999;**84**(3):266–75.

2. Forbes MS, Hawkey LA, Sperelakis N. The transverse-axial tubular system (TATS) of mouse myocardium: its morphology in the developing and adult animal. *Am J Anat* 1984;**170**(2):143–62.

3. Cheng H, Cannell MB, Lederer WJ. Propagation of excitation–contraction coupling into ventricular myocytes. *Pflügers* Archiv 1994;**428**(3):415–7.

4. Kawai M, Hussain M, Orchard CH. Excitation–contraction coupling in rat ventricular myocytes after formamide-induced detubulation. *Am J Physiol* 1999;**277**(2 Pt 2):H603–9.

5. Yang Z, Pascarel C, Steele DS, et al. Na+-Ca2+ exchange activity is localized in the T-tubules of rat ventricular myocytes. *Circ Res* 2002;**91**(4):315–22.

6. Gotoh Y, Imaizumi Y, Watanabe M, et al. Inhibition of transient outward K+ current by DHP Ca2+ antagonists and agonists in rabbit cardiac myocytes. *Am J Physiol* 1991;**260**(5 Pt 2):H1737–42.

7. McLerie M, Lopatin A. Dominant-negative suppression of IK1 in the mouse heart leads to altered cardiac excitability. *J Mol Cell Cardiol* 2003;**35**(4):367–78.

8. Fabiato A. Calcium-induced release of calcium from the cardiac sarcoplasmic reticulum. *Am J Physiol* 1983;**245**(1):1–14.

9. Stern MD. Theory of excitation–contraction coupling in cardiac muscle. *Biophys J* 1992;**63**(2):497–517.

10. Cannell MB, Cheng H, Lederer WJ. The control of calcium release in heart muscle. *Science* 1995;**268**(5213):1045–9.

11. Franzini-Armstrong C, Protasi F, Ramesh V. Shape, size, and distribution of Ca2+ release units and couplons in skeletal and cardiac muscles. *Biophys J* 1999;**77**(3):1528–39.

12. Gathercole DV, Colling DJ, Skepper JN, et al. Immunogold-labeled L-type calcium channels are clustered in the surface plasma membrane overlying junctional sarcoplasmic reticulum in guinea-pig myocytes—implications for excitation–contraction coupling in cardiac muscle. *J Mol Cell Cardiol* 2000;**32**(11):1981–94.

13. Keizer J, Smith GD, Ponce-Dawson S, Pearson JE. Saltatory propagation of Ca2+ waves by Ca2+ sparks. *Biophys J* 1998;**75**(2):595–600.

14. Izu LT, Mauban JRH, Balke CW, Wier WG. Large currents generate cardiac Ca2+ sparks. *Biophys J* 2001;**80**(1):88–102.

15. Cannell MB, Soeller C. Sparks of interest in cardiac excitation–contraction coupling. *Trends Pharmacol Sci* 2017;**19**(1):16–20.

16. Kermode H, Williams AJ, Sitsapesan R. The interactions of ATP, ADP, and inorganic phosphate with the sheep cardiac ryanodine receptor. *Biophys J* 1998;**74**(3):1296–304.

17. Rakovic S, Galione A, Ashamu GA, Potter BVL, Terrar DA. A specific cyclic ADP-ribose antagonist inhibits cardiac excitation–contraction coupling. *Curr Biol* 1996;**6**(8):989–96.

18. Bowling N, Walsh RA, Song G, et al. Increased protein kinase C activity and expression of Ca2+-sensitive isoforms in the failing human heart. *Circulation* 1999;**99**(3):384.

19. Marx SO, Reiken S, Hisamatsu Y, et al. PKA phosphorylation dissociates FKBP12.6 from the calcium release channel (ryanodine receptor). *Cell* 2000;**101**(4):365–76.

20. Lokuta AJ, Meyers MB, Sander PR, Fishman GI, Valdivia HH. Modulation of cardiac ryanodine receptors by sorcin. *J Biol Chem* 1997;**272**(40):25333–8.

21. Balshaw DM, Xu L, Yamaguchi N, Pasek DA, Meissner G. Calmodulin binding and inhibition of cardiac muscle calcium release channel (ryanodine receptor). *J Biol Chem* 2001;**276**(23):20144–53.

22. Naqvi RU, Tweedie D, MacLeod KT. Evidence for the action potential mediating the changes to contraction observed in cardiac hypertrophy in the rabbit. *Int J Cardiol* 2001;**77**(2):189–206.

23. Györke I, Hester N, Jones LR, Györke S. The role of calsequestrin, triadin, and junctin in conferring cardiac ryanodine receptor responsiveness to luminal calcium. *Biophys J* 2004;**86**(4):2121–8.

24. Shannon TR, Pogwizd SM, Bers DM. Elevated sarcoplasmic reticulum Ca2+ leak in intact ventricular myocytes from rabbits in heart failure. *Circ Res* 2003;**93**(7):592–4.

25. Diaz ME, Trafford AW, O'Neill SC, Eisner DA. Measurement of sarcoplasmic reticulum Ca2+ content and sarcolemmal Ca2+ fluxes in isolated rat ventricular myocytes during spontaneous Ca2+ release. *J Physiol (Lond)* 1997;**501**(Pt 1):3–16.

26. He J, Conklin MW, Foell JD, et al. Reduction in density of transverse tubules and L-type Ca2+ channels in canine tachycardia-induced heart failure. *Cardiovasc Res* 2001;**49**(2):298–307.

27. Gómez AM, Schwaller B, Porzig H, et al. Increased exchange current but normal Ca²⁺ transport via Na⁺-Ca²⁺ exchange during cardiac hypertrophy after myocardial infarction. *Circ Res* 2002;**91**(4):323.

28. Quinn FR, Currie S, Duncan AM, et al. Myocardial infarction causes increased expression but decreased activity of the myocardial Na+–Ca2+ exchanger in the rabbit. *J Physiol (Lond)* 2003;**553**(Pt 1):229–42.

29. Hasenfuss G, Meyer M, Schillinger W, et al. Calcium handling proteins in the failing human heart. *Basic Res Cardiol* 1997;**92**(1):87–93.

30. Gwathmey JK, Copelas L, MacKinnon R, et al. Abnormal intracellular calcium handling in myocardium from patients with end-stage heart failure. *Circ Res* 1987;**61**(1):70.

31. Beuckelmann DJ, Nabauer M, Erdmann E. Intracellular calcium handling in isolated ventricular myocytes from patients with terminal heart failure. *Circulation* 1992;**85**(3):1046–55.

32. Piacentino V, Weber CR, Chen X, et al. Cellular basis of abnormal calcium transients of failing human ventricular myocytes. *Circ Res* 2003;**92**(6):651.

33. Ranu HK, Terracciano CMN, Davia K, et al. Effects of Na+/Ca2+-exchanger overexpression on excitation–contraction coupling in adult rabbit ventricular myocytes. *J Mol Cell Cardiol* 2002;**34**(4):389–400.

34. Schwinger RHG, Böhm M, Schmidt U, et al. Unchanged protein levels of SERCA II and phospholamban but reduced Ca²⁺ uptake and Ca²⁺-ATPase activity of cardiac sarcoplasmic reticulum from dilated cardiomyopathy patients compared with patients with nonfailing hearts. *Circulation* 1995;**92**(11):3220.

35. Movsesian MA, Bristow MR, Krall J. Ca2+ uptake by cardiac sarcoplasmic reticulum from patients with idiopathic dilated cardiomyopathy. *Circ Res* 1989;**65**(4):1141.

36. Hasenfuss G, Schillinger W, Lehnart SE, et al. Relationship between Na⁺-Ca²⁺/exchanger protein levels and diastolic function of failing human myocardium. *Circulation* 1999;**99**(5):641.

37. Sen L, Cui G, Fonarow GC, Laks H. Differences in mechanisms of SR dysfunction in ischemic vs. idiopathic dilated cardiomyopathy. *Am J Physiol Heart Circ Physiol* 2000;**279**(2):H709.

38. Litwin SE, Zhang D, Bridge JHB. Dyssynchronous Ca²⁺ sparks in myocytes from infarcted hearts. *Circ Res* 2000;**87**(11):1040.

39. Pogwizd SM, Schlotthauer K, Li L, Yuan W, Bers DM. Arrhythmogenesis and contractile dysfunction in heart failure. *Circ Res* 2001;**88**(11):1159.

40. Gómez AM, Valdivia HH, Cheng H, *et al.* Defective excitation–contraction coupling in experimental cardiac hypertrophy and heart failure. *Science* 1997;**276**(5313):800.

41. Cheng H, Cannell M, Lederer W. Propagation of excitation–contraction coupling into ventricular myocytes. *Pflügers Archiv* 1994;**428**(3–4):415–17.

42. Yamamoto T, ElHayek R, Ikemoto N. Postulated role of interdomain interaction within the ryanodine receptor in Ca²⁺ channel regulation. *J Biol Chem* 2000;**275**(16):11618–25.

43. Most P, Bernotat J, Ehlermann P, *et al.* S100A1: a regulator of myocardial contractility. *Proc Natl Acad Sci USA* 2001;**98**(24):13889–94.

44. Grueter CE, Colbran RJ, Anderson ME. CaMKII, an emerging molecular driver for calcium homeostasis, arrhythmias, and cardiac dysfunction. *J Mol Med* 2007;**85**(1):5–14.

45. Koval OM, Guan X, Wu Y, *et al.* CaV1.2 β-subunit coordinates CaMKII-triggered cardiomyocyte death and afterdepolarizations. *Proc Natl Acad Sci USA* 2010;**107**(11):4996–5000.

46. Ai X, Curran JW, Shannon TR, Bers DM, Pogwizd SM. Ca²⁺/calmodulin-dependent protein kinase modulates cardiac ryanodine receptor phosphorylation and sarcoplasmic reticulum Ca²⁺ leak in heart failure. *Circ Res* 2005;**97**(12):1314.

47. Sag CM, Wadsack DP, Khabbazzadeh S, *et al.* Calcium/calmodulin-dependent protein kinase II contributes to cardiac arrhythmogenesis in heart failure. *Circ Heart Fail* 2009;**2**(6):664–75.

48. Kim Y, Phan D, van Rooij E, *et al.* The MEF2D transcription factor mediates stress-dependent cardiac remodeling in mice. *J Clin Invest* 2007;**118**(1):124–32.

49. Backs J, Backs T, Neef S, *et al.* The δ isoform of CaM kinase II is required for pathological cardiac hypertrophy and remodeling after pressure overload. *Proc Natl Acad Sci USA* 2009;**106**(7):2342–7.

50. Zhang R, Khoo MSC, Wu Y, *et al.* Calmodulin kinase II inhibition protects against structural heart disease. *Nat Med* 2005;**11**(4):409–17.

51. Eisner DA, Choi HS, Díaz ME, O'Neill SC, Trafford AW. Integrative analysis of calcium cycling in cardiac muscle. *Circ Res* 2000;**87**(12):1087.

52. Choi BR, Burton F, Salama G. Cytosolic Ca2+ triggers early afterdepolarizations and torsade de pointes in rabbit hearts with type 2 long QT syndrome. *J Physiol (Lond)* 2002;**543**(Pt 2):615–31.

53. Schillinger W, Janssen PML, Emami S, *et al.* Impaired contractile performance of cultured rabbit ventricular myocytes after adenoviral gene transfer of Na⁺–Ca²⁺ exchanger. *Circ Res* 2000;**87**(7):581.

54. Pogwizd SM, Qi M, Yuan W, Samarel AM, Bers DM. Upregulation of Na⁺/Ca²⁺ exchanger expression and function in an arrhythmogenic rabbit model of heart failure. *Circ Res* 1999;**85**(11):1009.

55. Hatem SN, Sham JS, Morad M. Enhanced Na(+)–Ca2+ exchange activity in cardiomyopathic syrian hamster. *Circ Res* 1994;**74**(2):253.

56. Hasenfuss G. Alterations of calcium-regulatory proteins in heart failure. *Cardiovasc Res* 1998;**37**(2):279–89.

57. Sipido KR, Volders PGA, Vos MA, Verdonck F. Altered Na/Ca exchange activity in cardiac hypertrophy and heart failure: a new target for therapy? *Cardiovasc Res* 2002;**53**(4):782–805.

58. Wang Z, Nolan B, Kutschke W, Hill JA. Na+–Ca2+ exchanger remodeling in pressure overload cardiac hypertrophy. *J Biol Chem* 2001;**276**(21):17706–11.

59. Marin-Garcia J, Goldenthal MJ. Mitochondrial centrality in heart failure. *Heart Fail Rev* 2008;**13**(2):137–50.

60. Rosca MG, Hoppel CL. Mitochondria in heart failure. *Cardiovasc Res* 2010;**88**(1):40–50.

61. Ventura-Clapier R, Garnier A, Veksler V, Joubert F. Bioenergetics of the failing heart. *Biochim Biophys Acta* 2011;**1813**(7):1360–72.

62. Liu T, Takimoto E, Dimaano VL, *et al.* Inhibiting mitochondrial Na+/Ca2+ exchange prevents sudden death in a guinea pig model of heart failure. *Circ Res* 2014;**115**(1):44–54.

63. Dibb KM, Clarke JD, Horn MA, *et al.* Characterization of an extensive transverse tubular network in sheep atrial myocytes and its depletion in heart failure. *Circ Heart Fail* 2009;**2**(5):482–9.

64. Berridge MJ, Bootman MD, Lipp P. Calcium—a life and death signal. *Nature* 1998;**395**(6703):645–8.

65. Boyden PA, Barbhaiya C, Lee T, ter Keurs HEDJ. Nonuniform Ca2+ transients in arrhythmogenic Purkinje cells that survive in the infarcted canine heart. *Cardiovasc Res* 2003;**57**(3):681–93.

66. Janse MJ, Wit AL. Electrophysiological mechanisms of ventricular arrhythmias resulting from myocardial ischemia and infarction. *Physiol Rev* 1989;**69**(4):1049–169.

17

Myocardial energetics

Julian O. M. Ormerod and Michael P. Frenneaux

Introduction

The heart requires very large amounts of energy, cycling many times its own weight in ATP daily, and uses a variable combination of carbohydrates, lipids, lactate, amino acids (and even ketones and alcohol) as fuel. A key feature of the healthy heart is 'metabolic flexibility', i.e. the ability to utilize different substrates according to circumstances. In the normal resting state, the majority of fuel is provided by lipids. Fatty acids provide the most ATP per gram of fuel but, when oxygen is limited (for example due to macro- or microvascular ischaemia as may be found in heart failure), glucose provides the most ATP per mole of oxygen consumed. From this point of view, a switch to glucose metabolism may be beneficial in various disease states. There is evidence that the metabolic switch occurs; it is often termed a 'reversion to a foetal programme of metabolism', as this metabolic profile mimics that seen in early life. The evidence is conflicting as to whether the metabolic switch is beneficial—both acutely, and perhaps especially in chronic disease states.

As the syndrome of heart failure progresses, a steady down-regulation of all aspects of cardiac metabolism may be seen. In extreme disease states, a severe deficiency in ATP can be demonstrated, but more subtle metabolic abnormalities are detectable at an earlier stage. Additionally, there are multiple downstream disturbances in mitochondrial function (including structural changes, changes in redox state and oxidative stress), in the transfer of high energy phosphates to the sites of utilisation and in excitation–contraction coupling.[1]

The detection of abnormalities of myocardial metabolism and energetics has spurred an interest in therapeutic modulation of metabolism in heart failure. This is attractive, as potentially such modulation would improve myocardial efficiency without the need for increased fuel delivery. Such therapies could have an additive effect to current heart failure management which generally relies on correction of the maladaptive neurohumoral consequences of the heart failure syndrome.

Normal cardiac metabolism

Cardiomyocytes are energy-hungry and have the highest mitochondrial content of any tissue in the body. Mitochondria make up fully one-third of the cellular volume.[2] In health in the fasting state, cardiomyocytes use fatty acids in greater amounts than glucose, in a ratio of approximately 70:30. Fatty acids and glucose are taken up into the mitochondria, where they undergo β-oxidation and glycolysis respectively, with the resulting acetyl-CoA feeding into the Krebs cycle. NADH (produced by the Krebs cycle) donates electrons to complex 1 of the electron transport chain and a series of electron transfers occurs along the respiratory chain complexes resulting in the extrusion of protons across the inner mitochondrial membrane, generating an electrochemical gradient that drives the phosphorylation of ADP to ATP by ATP synthase. This process is summarized in **Figure 17.1**.

Cardiomyocytes use a vast amount of ATP. Each heartbeat uses around 2% of the cellular store of ATP, and therefore the store turns over in its entirety every minute. This means the heart consumes approximately 6–30 kg of ATP per day. The relatively small energy store, compared to consumption, means that energy expenditure must be tightly coupled to ATP generation. Under normal circumstances, the heart is therefore very flexible in substrate utilization. For example, ketone bodies usually make up very little of the fuel used, but their use increases greatly in conditions of starvation. Equally, during intense exercise, myocardial uptake and metabolism of lactate produced in skeletal muscle increases at the expense of fatty acid oxidation. Most physiological measurements are taken in a fasting state when FFA are high; after a meal, insulin increases the uptake and oxidation of glucose as well as suppressing lipolysis in adipose tissue and reducing plasma FFA.

Metabolic changes in hypertrophy and heart failure

Evidence from animal models of heart failure (particularly in those resulting from hypertrophy), as well as from human patients, points to a relative increase in glycolysis. The increase mirrors the metabolism of the foetal heart, and has been viewed as an adaptive response to pathological hypertrophy. However, this is not necessarily the case. Although glucose oxidation may be increased relative to that of fatty acids, evidence from experimental models of heart failure suggests that carbohydrate oxidation is not correspondingly increased.

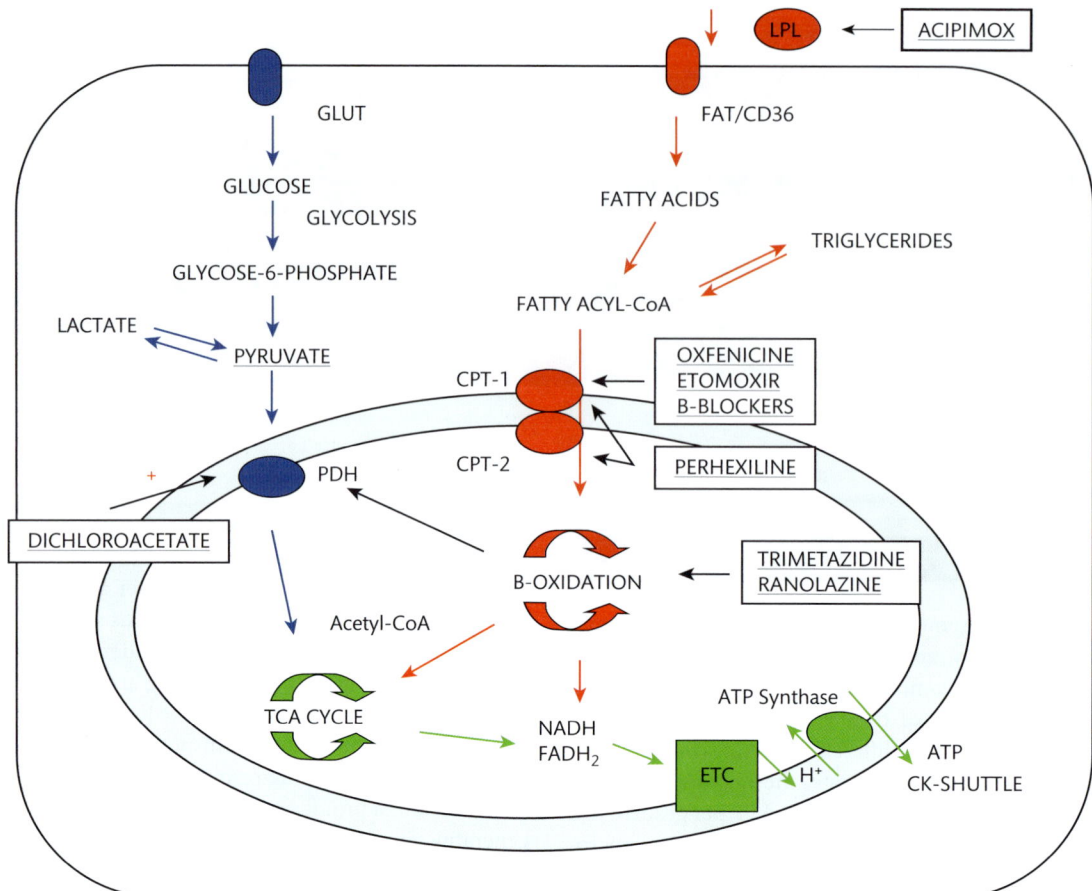

Figure 17.1 Summary of the basic metabolic pathways and the effect of metabolically active agents.

Reproduced from Ormerod JOM, Ashrafian H, Frenneaux MP. Impaired energetics in heart failure—a new therapeutic target. *Pharmacol Ther* 2008;**119**(3):264–274. doi:10.1016/j.pharmthera.2008.05.007.

This is because of reduced activity of the pyruvate dehydrogenase (PDH) enzyme complex that catalyses the conversion of pyruvate to acetyl-CoA. The result is a relative uncoupling of glycolysis from carbohydrate oxidation with incomplete compensation through anaplerotic pathways. Whilst the uncoupling reduces energy production, there may also be adaptive consequences—hypertrophy of heart muscle uses amino acid stores to build proteins, and because some amino acids are synthesized from Krebs cycle intermediates, the Krebs cycle may become depleted. Anaplerotic use of pyruvate (largely through carboxylation by pyruvate carboxylase) replenishes these vital intermediates. Hypertrophy is not only seen in pressure-overloaded systems; compensatory hypertrophy and increased cardiac weight is also a feature of dilated cardiomyopathy.

Later in the course of heart failure, uptake of free fatty acids into the mitochondria and β-oxidation within them decreases. Uptake into the cardiomyocyte, however, is unchanged or increased. The consequence is accumulation of free fatty acids in the cytosol of cardiomyocytes. These are stored as triacylglycerol in vesicles, but some are metabolized via alternative non-oxidative pathways, leading to the generation of ceramide and reactive oxygen species (ROS). The ROS may trigger cell death by necrosis or apoptosis. A further intermediate, diacylglycerol, contributes to insulin resistance in multiple organs including the heart. There is a correlation between lipid accumulation in the cardiomyocyte and progression

of disease, a condition termed 'lipotoxicity'. Lipotoxicity is not synonymous with increased fatty acid consumption, because when fatty acid oxidation *is* increased, lipid and ceramide accumulation and increased ROS generation do not occur and cell death is not a feature.

Significant lipid accumulation may also be seen in obesity and diabetes mellitus in the absence of heart failure; but both of these conditions may in themselves lead to cardiomyopathy. Cardiac dysfunction in these conditions shows a different metabolic profile to that seen in hypertrophy; fatty acid oxidation increases and glycolysis and glucose oxidation both decrease in the context of increased myocardial oxygen consumption, and with an increase in the O2 cost of energy production.[3]

The metabolic changes in the failing heart may be best viewed as a progressive loss of flexibility in substrate transport and metabolism, with a diminished ability to respond to changing circumstances such as the demands of exercise. It is clearly a more complex situation than a simple switch between two main sources of fuel, as maladaptive uncoupling of glucose metabolism and lipotoxicity demonstrate. The specific metabolic changes appear to be different in heart failure of different aetiologies: pressure- or volume-loading, ischaemia, or metabolic causes such as obesity and diabetes. The changes also vary through the course of disease progression, and the changes are at present incompletely understood. In the later

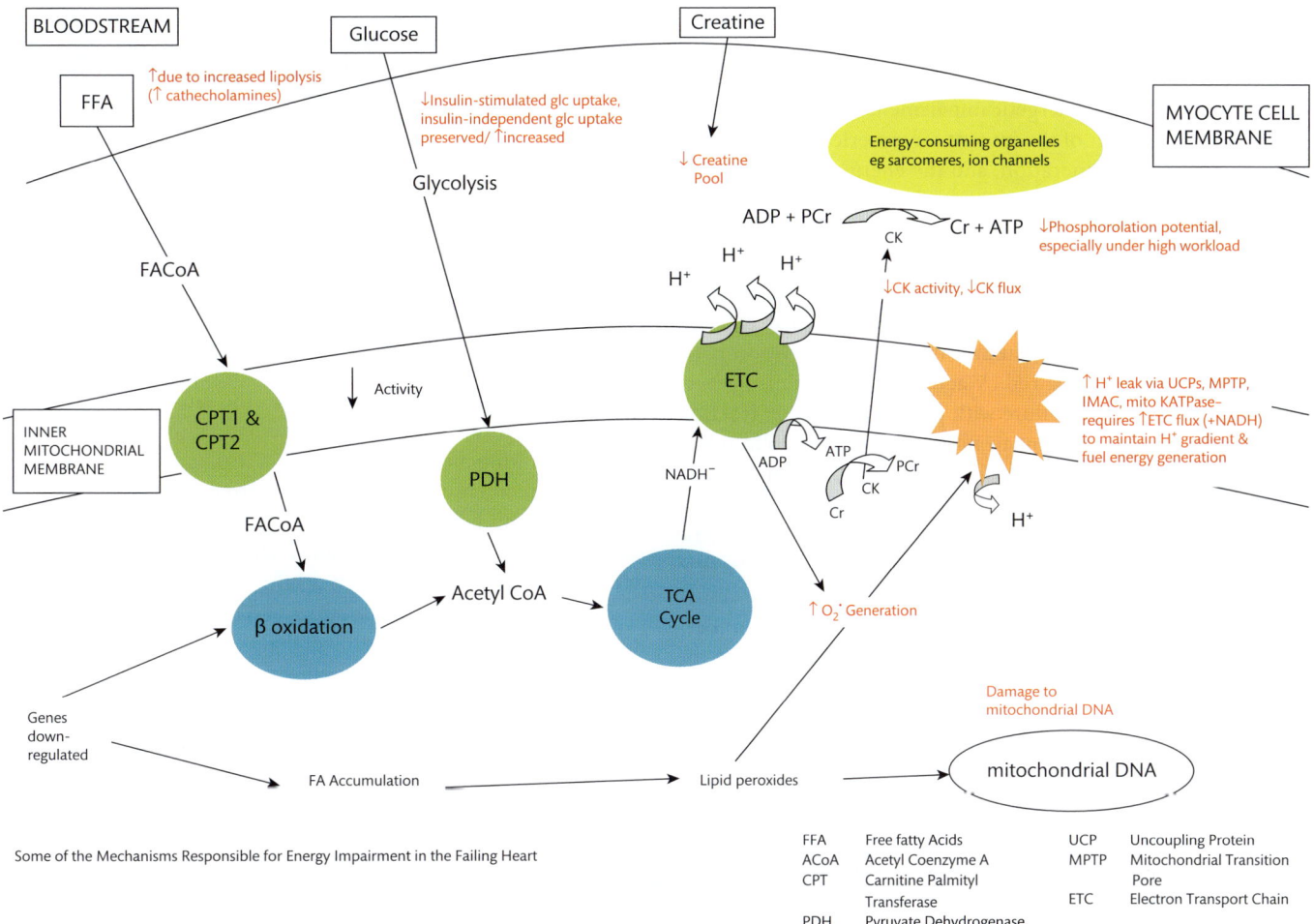

Figure 17.2 Summary of the various cellular changes underlying energetic insufficiency.

Reproduced from Siddiqi N, Singh S, Beadle R, Dawson D, Frenneaux M. Cardiac metabolism in hypertrophy and heart failure: implications for therapy. *Heart Fail Rev* 2013;**18**(5):595–606. doi:10.1007/s10741-012-9359-2 with permission from Springer.

stages of heart failure, additional abnormalities of energy generation (electron chain function), transport, storage and usage (excitation–contraction coupling) are of increasing importance in the maintenance and development of pathology. The changes are summarized in **Figure 17.2**.

Disturbed mitochondrial structure and function

As heart failure progresses, structural changes in mitochondrial size and shape, with abnormal cristae become more obvious.[4] Various enzymes, especially those involved in fatty acid oxidation, are downregulated in heart failure. Similar processes may be observed in other cardiomyopathies, such as hypertrophic cardiomyopathy (HCM). Mitophagy—the process by which senescent dysfunctional mitochondria and mitochondrial proteins are removed and the contents recycled to produce new mitochondria—is crucial in determining the response to cellular stress and there is evidence of impaired mitophagy in some models of heart failure. Furthermore, mice in genetic models of impaired mitophagy develop heart failure with age.

Reactive oxygen species are generated by 'slippage' at complexes I and III of the mitochondrial respiratory chain, and slippage

increases in heart failure. Increased ROS generation has a number of consequences including:

1. increased activity of mitochondrial uncoupling proteins which dissipates the electrochemical gradient across the mitochondrial membrane that drives ATP generation;

2. damaged mitochondrial DNA, resulting in reduced production of mitochondrial proteins and/or generation of abnormal/dysfunctional proteins, including respiratory chain complexes;

3. increased cardiolipin peroxidation; cardiolipin is crucial in organizing the respiratory chain complexes into functional units called 'respirasomes'. Dissociation of the respirasomes further increases ROS production and reduces ATP generation;

4. activation of kinases that are involved in both hypertrophic and apoptotic pathways. This may be an adaptive mechanism in ischaemic myocardium, protecting from ischaemia-reperfusion injury, but may reduce substrate availability and energetic efficiency in chronic heart failure.

Dysfunction of the electron transport chain might occur early in the course of disease,[3] and may in fact drive some of the changes in substrate utilization discussed above. The two aspects of disturbed metabolism are probably synergistic in the pathophysiology of

heart failure. Cardiac energetic impairment demonstrable by ³¹P magnetic resonance spectroscopy is a cardinal feature of most heart muscle diseases including dilated and hypertrophic cardiomyopathies. In HCM the energetic impairment is a consequence of an energy-wasting effect of the mutant sarcomeric proteins rather than impaired energy generation, and the energy-wasting plays a key role in impairing the highly energy-dependent process of left ventricle (LV) active relaxation during exercise, thereby contributing to exercise limitation. There is also evidence that the energetic impairment in HCM may be the primary stimulus for the development of hypertrophy by increasing intracellular calcium and thereby activating calmodulin. Similarly, energetic impairment plays a key role in impaired LV active relaxation during exercise in patients with heart failure with preserved ejection fraction (HFpEF). Also, it is important to note here that diastolic relaxation is a very energy-intensive process. Abnormalities in diastolic function often precede frank systolic dysfunction in heart failure with a reduced ejection fraction, and impaired energetics may be a primary abnormality in heart failure with preserved ejection fraction or early cardiomyopathy.[5,6] The frequency of heart failure in patients with genetic mitochondrial abnormalities also underscores the potential pathogenic role of energetic impairment in the pathogenesis of heart failure.

Energetic insufficiency and impaired excitation–contraction coupling

Mitochondria in the cardiomyocyte are closely associated with the sarcoplasmic reticulum, linking energy generation and expenditure. Structural remodelling of the cardiomyocyte may disrupt the close proximity of mitochondria. Abnormalities have been documented in various components of calcium cycling in heart failure (shown in **Figure 17.3**): L-type calcium channels are phosphorylated, which leads to a compensatory calcium leak from ryanodine-receptor calcium channels on the sarcoplasmic reticulum.[7] There is also downregulation of SERCA2A calcium transporters, which are responsible for reuptake of calcium into the sarcoplasmic reticulum. Increased cytosolic calcium also increases uptake into the mitochondrion. Mitochondrial calcium is a strong determinant of mitochondrial membrane potential; depolarized mitochondria produce more ROS and become ever more dysfunctional. Calcium leakage increases early afterdepolarizations, which increases the risk of ventricular arrhythmia and sudden death.

Phosphocreatine (PCr) is a buffer of ATP, allowing ATP to be rapidly regenerated as it is consumed. It also diffuses more rapidly than ATP through the cell, which means it can target ATP generation to

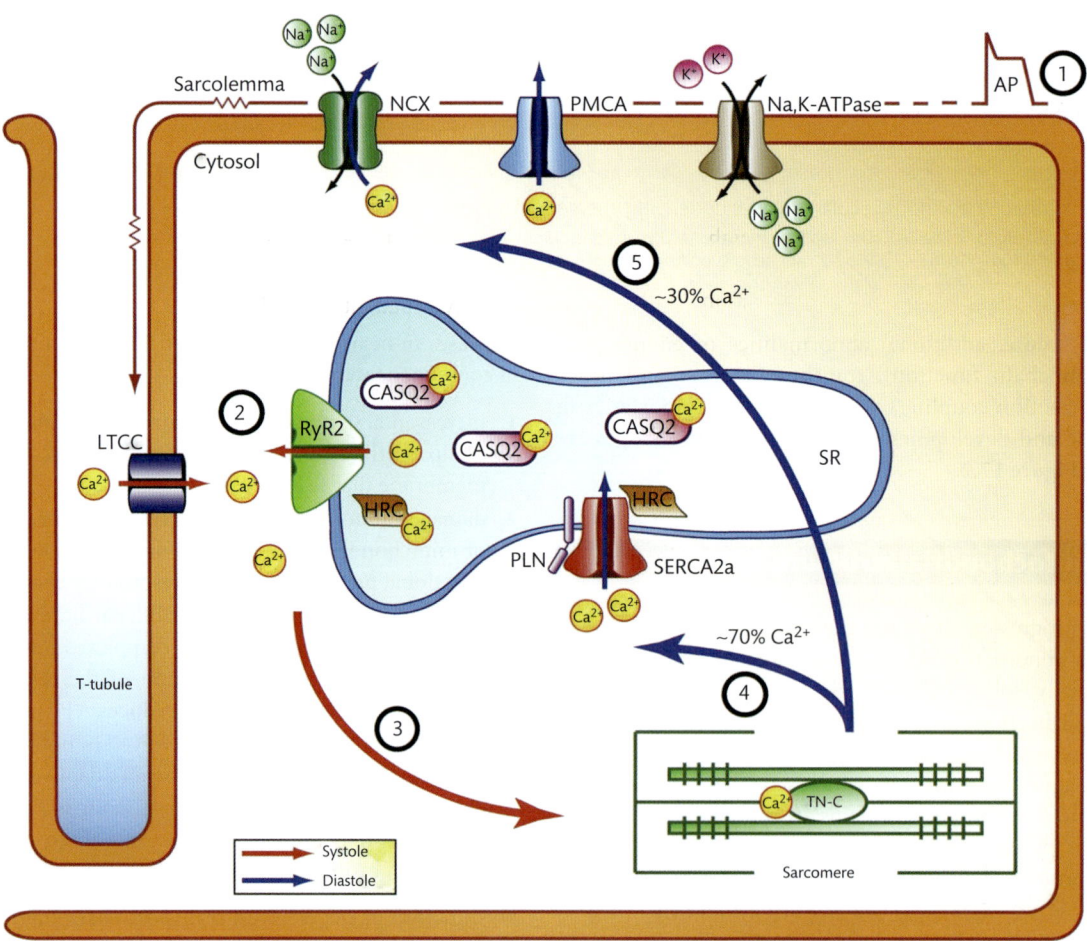

Figure 17.3 Multiple aspects of myocyte calcium cycling and excitation–contraction coupling are impaired in chronic heart failure.

Reproduced from Gorski PA, Ceholski DK, Hajjar RJ. Altered myocardial calcium cycling and energetics in heart failure—a rational approach for disease treatment. *Cell Metab* 2015;**21**(2):183–194. doi:10.1016/j.cmet.2015.01.005.

the most energetically active areas. PCr and (generally to a lesser extent) ATP levels are diminished in heart failure,[8] leading to a lower PCr:ATP ratio (measurable using ^{31}P magnetic resonance spectroscopy). A lower ratio predicts a worse outcome.[9] More challenging to measure *in vivo* is a decrease in flux through creatine kinase in patients with heart failure, and consequently knowledge is less developed. However, reduced creatine kinase (CK) flux may be present very early in the course of the disease and may, in fact, be an even better prognostic marker than PCr:ATP ratio.[10,11] Reduced CK flux is at least in part a consequence of ROS-mediated reduction in cytosolic CK activity. A major user of ATP in the cardiomyocyte is, of course, the actomyosin ATPase, which is the engine of myofibrillar contraction. However, SERCA2A and two membrane electrolyte transporters (PMCA and Na-K-ATPase) also use huge quantities of energy and so it is not surprising that energetic insufficiency causes both impaired excitation–contraction coupling and abnormalities in electrolyte shifts.

Therapeutic modulation of metabolism

Several widely used drugs have important effects on cardiac metabolism. Certain β-blockers, such as carvedilol, inhibit CPT-1 and reduce uptake of free fatty acids into the mitochondrion. Amiodarone has a similar effect *in vitro* which may be important clinically. The thiazolidinediones (such as pioglitazone) stimulate peroxisomal proliferator-activated receptor-γ, reducing circulating lipids and increasing glucose oxidation. Thiazolidinediones may improve myocardial energetics and efficiency, at least in the short term,[12] but they have important detrimental effects in chronic heart failure. It is unclear whether these are a consequence of metabolic modulation or off-target effects (particularly fluid retention). Metformin also affects myocardial metabolism, both through effects on the 'cellular thermostat', AMP-activated protein kinase (AMPK), and on AMPK-independent mechanisms.[13] Observational data suggest that metformin may reduce the risk of diabetic patients developing heart failure. A randomised trial has shown an improvement in myocardial efficiency in patients with heart failure on metformin.[14]

Dichloroacetate (DCA) increases the activity of the PDH enzyme complex by inhibiting the activity of the associated inhibitory kinase. It is used in the treatment of lactic acidosis (since activation of PDH directs pyruvate metabolism towards acetyl CoA production and away from lactate production). Studies in both experimental models of heart failure and in human heart failure have demonstrated that it increases left ventricular stroke work while reducing myocardial oxygen consumption, indicating a marked improvement in mechanical efficiency. However, long-term treatment with DCA has been associated with neurotoxicity.

The activity of PDH is reduced by acetyl-CoA, which is a product of both pyruvate metabolism through PDH (in glucose metabolism) and, separately, through fatty acid β-oxidation. Agents that inhibit β-oxidation therefore reduce total acetyl-CoA and remove part of the inhibition of PDH, so reciprocally increasing carbohydrate oxidation and increasing the efficiency of energy generation. Three potential routes to reducing fatty acid oxidation have been explored:

- Acipimox (a nicotinic acid derivative) reduces plasma fatty acid levels by inhibiting their release from fat stores. Acute administration of acipimox in patients with heart failure patients reduced myocardial fatty acid uptake and increased glucose uptake but surprisingly this was associated with a reduction in cardiac work and efficiency. In a randomized trial of acipimox given for 28 days to patients with heart failure, there was no improvement in cardiac function.

- Inhibition of fatty acid uptake into the mitochondrion may be achieved through inhibition of the transporter proteins, carnitine-palmitoyl transferase 1 and 2. Long-chain fatty acid CoA molecules undergo the addition of a carnitine group by the enzyme CPT1, facilitating their transport across the mitochondrial membrane. On the other side of the membrane the carnitine is removed by the enzyme CPT2. Oxfenacine and etomoxir are irreversible CPT 1 and 2 inhibitors and perhexiline is a reversible inhibitor. Perhexiline has the most encouraging data in heart failure, and there are safety concerns with the other two agents.[15,16] Originally an anti-anginal, perhexiline was withdrawn due to occasional unwanted effects (principally neuropathy and liver injury due to phospholipid accumulation). Around 5% of people are slow acetylators of the drug and they may be exposed to very high plasma levels. When serum levels are routinely measured, and appropriate dose adjustments made, perhexiline may be given safely.[17] A randomized placebo-controlled trial of short-term perhexiline in patients with chronic heart failure showed an improvement in VO$_{2max}$, skeletal muscle energetics, quality of life, and even LV ejection fraction both at rest and at peak dobutamine stress.[18] A subsequent randomized placebo-controlled trial in 50 patients with non-ischaemic cardiomyopathy showed an improvement in New York Heart Association (NYHA) class, which correlated with a 30% increase in PCr:ATP ratio.[19] Interestingly, cardiac substrate metabolism did not differ between groups, suggesting that change in substrate use is not the only mechanism of energetic improvement with perhexiline. Perhexiline also markedly improved cardiac energetics, symptoms and exercise capacity in patients with HCM.[20]

- The endogenous inhibitor of CPT1 is malonyl-CoA. Malonyl-CoA dehydrogenase (MCD) inhibitors increase malonyl-CoA levels and thereby inhibit CPT1 but their use in heart failure has not been investigated.

- Reduction of fatty acyl β-oxidation may be achieved directly through inhibition of the final enzyme in the pathway: long-chain 3 ketoacyl-CoA-thiolase. This is the likely target of trimetazidine.[21] Trimetazidine is likely to be cytoprotective,[22] which may be particularly beneficial in ischaemic heart disease; there is evidence that it also increases the activity of pyruvate dehydrogenase, thereby directly increasing glucose oxidation.[23] Early clinical investigations of trimetazidine centred on angina and ischaemic cardiomyopathy. An increase in ejection fraction was noted in a small early randomized controlled trial (RCT),[24] which was confirmed in a later small RCT, with an additional improvement in NYHA class.[25] A meta-analysis[26] and retrospective registry[27] have added to the weight of supporting evidence that trimetazidine may lead to an improvement in symptoms, echocardiographic measures, and even mortality.

- Ranolazine also inhibits fatty acid β-oxidation, although at therapeutic concentrations its effects are believed to be predominantly via inhibition of the slow inward sodium current. The effect on

the sodium current can improve myocardial energetics (by reducing/normalizing diastolic tension) and, through reduction of early afterdepolarisations, it appears to be anti-arrhythmic. There is less evidence for the use of ranolazine than trimetazidine in heart failure due to systolic dysfunction,[28] but there is a strong theoretical rationale for a role in HFpEF. There is some early clinical evidence of a benefit[29] and there is much interest in a potential role in hypertrophic cardiomyopathy, where diastolic impairment is near ubiquitous.[30]

- SGLT-2 inhibitors have recently been shown to have salutary effects on heart failure hospitalisation and mortality in patients with heart failure with or without diabetes. Whilst these agents have diuretic effects, these do not appear to explain their beneficial effects in heart failure fully. They also activate AMP kinase, the 'low-on-energy' sensor, which initiates complex metabolic changes augmenting cardiac energy production and inhibits mTOR, thereby enhancing autophagy. SGLT-2 inhibitors increase plasma ketones (an efficient substrate for cardiac energy production) and inhibit the cardiac sodium-hydrogen exchanger (which is activated in the failing heart, thereby increasing intracellular sodium and indirectly calcium, a potential cause of arrhythmia).[31]

Myocardial ROS generation is another potential therapeutic target. Coenzyme Q is a component of the respiratory chain with antioxidant properties. In one RCT of 420 patients (the Q Symbio study[32]), coenzyme Q supplementation significantly reduced the primary composite end-point of cardiovascular death, heart failure hospitalization, and need for mechanical support/urgent transplant. Recently interest has focused on novel antioxidants targeted to mitochondria. They are positively charged and lipophilic, and are therefore concentrated up to 1000-fold in the mitochondria. These include Mito Q, SS21, and SS31. Data in experimental models suggest a potential role in heart failure. Elamipretide is a mitochondrially targeted drug that reduces cardiolipin peroxidation, thereby maintaining respirasome integrity. In a recent study in a canine microembolization model, elamipretide reduced ROS generation, increased ATP generation and markedly improved cardiac function.[33] Studies are underway in patients with heart failure with reduced and preserved ejection fraction.

Future research

The vast majority of physiological research in humans is performed in the resting fasted state. The myocardial pool of ATP must be turned over every minute, or even more rapidly at greater levels of cardiac work, such as during exercise. The hallmark of cardiac metabolism is therefore flexibility in response to changing circumstances. Patients with heart failure frequently develop symptoms in the absence of resting systolic dysfunction (or at least reduced ejection fraction, as the two are not synonymous), and so future research should investigate dynamic changes in metabolism in health and disease. The development of new tracers for cardiac magnetic resonance imaging may make this possible.

The problem with current magnetic resonance spectroscopy techniques is low sensitivity, leading to very long acquisition times (an hour or more). Magnetic resonance techniques rely on the presence of polarizable nuclei, i.e. those with an odd atomic number and therefore an unpaired proton. Metabolic imaging uses nuclei

such as ^{13}C, which has a low natural abundance of around 1%, compared to the very abundant protons (^{1}H) used for standard imaging. Increasing ^{13}C can help metabolic imaging, but the most exciting recent innovation is technology to create hyperpolarized tracers for injection. These greatly improve signal-to-noise ratio and should lead to shorter acquisition times and more detailed assessment of cardiac metabolism and energetics in future.[34]

Conclusions

Normal cardiac metabolism is complex and adjusts depending on substrate availability and work rate, allowing the heart to perform at maximal efficiency in a variety of physiological states. Myocardial metabolism is disturbed in heart failure, with a shift towards glucose metabolism (which may have short-term benefits but be maladaptive in the long term) in the early stages of hypertrophy and then a progressive reduction in oxidation of both fatty acids and glucose in later stages. Lipid accumulates in the cytosol, leading to lipotoxicity and cell death. Some disease states (particularly obesity and diabetes mellitus) promote lipid accumulation at an earlier stage. Alongside these processes, mitochondria themselves become progressively impaired, oxidative metabolism becomes uncoupled from ATP generation, and the sarcomere uses ATP inefficiently. Myocardial energetics are progressively impaired, starting with a fall in PCr:ATP ratio, then eventually a reduction in total ATP, and the impaired energetics correlate with prognosis.

Various agents that affect cardiac metabolism and energetics have been evaluated, some in randomized placebo-controlled trials, with some very promising but overall mixed results.[35] The apparent discrepancy in efficacy may reflect pleiotropic effects of the drugs themselves, and the complexity of the metabolic changes seen in heart failure. The appropriate intervention needs to be targeted at the correct stage of disease and it may well be that one size does not fit all when it comes to metabolic modulation in heart failure. This is an exciting area of development for the management of heart failure, but has yet to enter the mainstream.

REFERENCES

1. Nickel A, Löffler J, Maack C. Myocardial energetics in heart failure. *Basic Res Cardiol* 2013;**108**(4):358.
2. Schaper J, Meiser E, Stämmler G. Ultrastructural morphometric analysis of myocardium from dogs, rats, hamsters, mice, and from human hearts. *Circ Res* 1985;**56**:377–91.
3. Fillmore N, Mori J, Lopaschuk GD. Mitochondrial fatty acid oxidation alterations in heart failure, ischaemic heart disease and diabetic cardiomyopathy. *Br J Pharmacol* 2014;**171**(8):2080–90.
4. Bugger H, Schwarzer M, Chen D, *et al*. Proteomic remodelling of mitochondrial oxidative pathways in pressure overload-induced heart failure. *Cardiovasc Res* 2010;**85**(2):376–84.
5. Rider OJ, Francis JM, Tyler D, *et al*. Effects of weight loss on myocardial energetics and diastolic function in obesity. *Int J Cardiovasc Imaging* 2013;**29**(5):1043–50.
6. Phan TT, Abozguia K, Nallur Shivu G, *et al*. Heart failure with preserved ejection fraction is characterized by dynamic impairment of active relaxation and contraction of the left

ventricle on exercise and associated with myocardial energy deficiency. *J Am Coll Cardiol* 2009;**54**(5):402–9.

7. Gorski PA, Ceholski DK, Hajjar RJ. Altered myocardial calcium cycling and energetics in heart failure—a rational approach for disease treatment. *Cell Metab* 2015;**21**(2):183–94.

8. Beer M, Seyfarth T, Sandstede J, *et al*. Absolute concentrations of high-energy phosphate metabolites in normal, hypertrophied, and failing human myocardium measured noninvasively with 31P-SLOOP magnetic resonance spectroscopy. *J Am Coll Cardiol* 2002;**40**(7):1267–74.

9. Neubauer S, Horn M, Cramer M, *et al*. Myocardial phosphocreatine-to-ATP ratio is a predictor of mortality in patients with dilated cardiomyopathy. *Circulation* 1997;**96**(7):2190–6.

10. Ingwall JS, Kramer MF, Fifer MA, *et al*. The creatine kinase system in normal and diseased human myocardium. *N Engl J Med* 1985;**313**(17):1050–4.

11. Bottomley PA, Panjrath GS, Lai S, *et al*. Metabolic rates of ATP transfer through creatine kinase (CK flux) predict clinical heart failure events and death. *Sci Transl Med* 2013;**5**(215):215re3.

12. Van Der Meer RW, Rijzewijk LJ, De Jong HWAM, *et al*. Pioglitazone improves cardiac function and alters myocardial substrate metabolism without affecting cardiac triglyceride accumulation and high-energy phosphate metabolism in patients with well-controlled type 2 diabetes mellitus. *Circulation* 2009;**119**(15):2069–77.

13. Saeedi R, Parsons HL, Wambolt RB, *et al*. Metabolic actions of metformin in the heart can occur by AMPK-independent mechanisms. *Am J Physiol Hear Circ Physiol* 2008;**294**(6):H2497–H2506.

14. Larsen AH, Jessen N, Helene Nørrelund H, *et al*. A randomised, double-blind, placebo-controlled trial of metformin on myocardial efficiency in insulin-resistant chronic heart failure patients without diabetes. *Eur J Heart Failure* 2020;**22**:1628–37.

15. Bachmann E, Weber E. Biochemical mechanisms of oxfenicine cardiotoxicity. *Pharmacology* 1988;**36**:238–48.

16. Cabrero A, Merlos M, Laguna JC, Carrera MV. Down-regulation of acyl-CoA oxidase gene expression and increased NF-kappaB activity in etomoxir-induced cardiac hypertrophy. *J Lipid Res* 2003;**44**(2):388–98.

17. Phuong H, Choi BY, Chong C-R, Raman B, Horowitz JD. Can perhexiline be utilized without long-term toxicity? A clinical practice audit. *Ther Drug Monit* 2016;**38**(1):73–78.

18. Lee L, Campbell R, Scheuermann-Freestone M, *et al*. Metabolic modulation with perhexiline in chronic heart failure: a randomized, controlled trial of short-term use of a novel treatment. *Circulation* 2005;**112**(21):3280–8.

19. Beadle RM, Williams LK, Kuehl M, *et al*. Improvement in cardiac energetics by perhexiline in heart failure due to dilated cardiomyopathy. *JACC Hear Fail* 2015;**3**(3):202–11.

20. Abozguia K, Elliott P, McKenna W, *et al*. Metabolic modulator perhexiline corrects energy deficiency and improves exercise capacity in symptomatic hypertrophic cardiomyopathy. *Circulation* 2010;**122**(16):1562–9.

21. Kantor PF, Lucien A, Kozak R, Lopaschuk GD. The antianginal drug trimetazidine shifts cardiac energy metabolism from fatty acid oxidation to glucose oxidation by inhibiting mitochondrial long-chain 3-ketoacyl coenzyme A thiolase. *Circ Res* 2000;**86**:580–8.

22. Yang Q, Yang K, Li AY. Trimetazidine protects against hypoxia-reperfusion-induced cardiomyocyte apoptosis by increasing microrna-21 expression. *Int J Clin Exp Pathol* 2015;**8**(4):3735–41.

23. Dyck JRB, Lopaschuk GD. Malonyl CoA control of fatty acid oxidation in the ischemic heart. *J Mol Cell Cardiol* 2002;**34**:1099–109.

24. Brottier L, Barat JL, Combe C, *et al*. Therapeutic value of a cardioprotective agent in patients with severe ischaemic cardiomyopathy. *Eur Heart J* 1990;**11**(3):207–12.

25. Fragasso G, Palloshi A, Puccetti P, *et al*. A randomized clinical trial of trimetazidine, a partial free fatty acid oxidation inhibitor, in patients with heart failure. *J Am Coll Cardiol* 2006;**48**(5):992–8.

26. Gao D, Ning N, Niu X, Hao G, Meng Z. Trimetazidine: a meta-analysis of randomised controlled trials in heart failure. *Heart* 2011;**97**(4):278–86.

27. Fragasso G, Rosano G, Baek SH, *et al*. Effect of partial fatty acid oxidation inhibition with trimetazidine on mortality and morbidity in heart failure: results from an international multicentre retrospective cohort study. *Int J Cardiol* 2013;**163**(3):320–5.

28. Murray GL, Colombo J. Ranolazine preserves and improves left ventricular ejection fraction and autonomic measures when added to guideline-driven therapy in chronic heart failure. *Heart Int* 2014;**9**(2):66–73.

29. Maier LS, Layug B, Karwatowska-Prokopczuk E, *et al*. RAnoLazINe for the treatment of diastolic heart failure in patients with preserved ejection fraction. The RALI-DHF proof-of-concept study. *JACC Hear Fail* 2013;**1**(2):115–122.

30. Ammirati E, Contri R, Coppini R, *et al*. Pharmacological treatment of hypertrophic cardiomyopathy: current practice and novel perspectives. *Eur J Heart Fail* 2016;**18**(9):1106–18.

31. Lopaschuk GD, Verma S. Mechanisms of Cardiovascular Benefits of Sodium Glucose Co-Transporter 2 (SGLT2) Inhibitors. A State-of-the-Art Review. *JACC Basic Transl Sci* 2020;**5**:632–44.

32. Mortensen SA, Rosenfeldt F, Kumar A, *et al*. The effect of coenzyme Q10 on morbidity and mortality in chronic heart failure. Results from Q-SYMBIO: a randomized double-blind trial. *JACC Hear Fail* 2014;**2**(6):641–9.

33. Sabbah HN, Gupta RC, Kohli S, *et al*. Chronic therapy with elamipretide (MTP-131), a novel mitochondria-targeting peptide, improves left ventricular and mitochondrial function in dogs with advanced heart failure. *Circ Hear Fail* 2016;**9**(2):e002206.

34. Rider OJ, Tyler DJ. Clinical implications of cardiac hyperpolarized magnetic resonance imaging. *J Cardiovasc Magn Reson* 2013;**15**(1):93.

35. Ormerod JOM, Ashrafian H, Frenneaux MP. Impaired energetics in heart failure—a new therapeutic target. *Pharmacol Ther* 2008;**119**(3):264–74.

18

The failing cardiomyocyte

Gábor Földes, Alexander R. Lyon, and Sian E. Harding

Introduction

The human myocardium consists of a variety of different cell types. The cell that has been most extensively studied is the cardiomyocyte, which represents the single contracting unit of the myocardium. It has been estimated that there are three billion cardiomyocytes in the human ventricular myocardium, organized into the complex three-dimensional architecture of the ventricular myocardial tissue. Conceptually there are two underlying pathophysiological problems at the level of the cardiomyocyte which drive the functional deterioration of the failing heart. The first is the numerical loss of cardiomyocytes, due both to the underlying aetiological disease process, for example acute myocardial infarction or chemotherapy and to further loss secondary to apoptosis and necrosis triggered by the neurohormonal and inflammatory activation in the failing myocardium irrespective of the initial injury. Second, the remaining viable cardiomyocytes are required to provide sufficient contractile force to maintain an adequate cardiac output, despite the loss of significant numbers and abnormal stress–strain relationships resulting from altered chamber geometry and extracellular matrix remodelling. The surviving cardiomyocytes compensate temporarily via transition to an adaptive hypertrophic state,[1,2] which is associated with activation of foetal gene expression patterns.[3] However, the persistent drive from the neurohormonal activation to maintain cardiac output, and activation of systemic inflammatory systems secondary to tissue hypoperfusion and congestion, combined with reduced metabolic efficiency in the hypertrophied cardiomyocytes, results in the development of contractile dysfunction of the hypertrophied cardiomyocyte.[4] Many of the changes are independent of the underlying cause, but there are specific factors that may also impair cardiomyocyte function further, for example, familial dilated cardiomyopathy due to mutations in the cytoskeletal or sarcomeric proteins.[5]

The communal endpoint for the failing heart, irrespective of underlying aetiology, is characterized at a cellular and molecular level by a distinctive failing signature. Cardiomyocytes isolated from failing human and animal hearts demonstrate impairment of both contraction (inotropy) and relaxation (lusitropy).[6] Mechanical dysfunction of failing cardiomyocytes is amplified at higher beating frequencies, increased calcium concentration or during catecholamine stimulation. The loss of the force–frequency response (the Treppe or Bowditch effect) is a hallmark characteristic of heart failure (see **Figure 18.1**).[6]

A variety of different pathophysiological factors have been proposed to underlie these mechanical alterations, including abnormal morphological, structural, and metabolic remodelling, and functional changes in signalling pathways, ionic fluxes, organelle function, and gene and protein expressions. It is becoming increasingly apparent that these are not independent processes, but rather that crosstalk and interplay between these different pathophysiological processes serves to amplify the abnormalities and drive the deterioration of the failing cardiomyocyte phenotype.

Morphological changes

Cardiomyocyte size and shape

Healthy human cardiomyocytes are elongated, rod-shaped structures, typically 20–30 μm wide, ~100 μm in length, and 20–30 μm in depth.[7] Studies using cell capacitance indicate a cell volume of ~100 pF, equating to ~30 pL.[8] A characteristic of failing cardiomyocytes is hypertrophy and enlargement (see **Figure 18.2**). The precise changes depend upon the underlying disease—for instance, cardiomyocytes from ventricles with pressure overload, e.g. left ventricular hypertrophy secondary to hypertension or aortic stenosis, exhibit increases in width and length, whereas cells from ventricles experiencing volume overload, e.g. mitral regurgitation or advanced dilated cardiomyopathy, demonstrate increases predominantly in length.[4] End-stage failing hearts explanted at transplantation contain myocytes exhibiting a decompensated failing phenotype. These cells are larger than normal myocytes but smaller than cells isolated from hearts with compensated left ventricular hypertrophy. Comparison of size changes with alteration in function concluded that the two were independent and that even those cells with normal dimensions from the hypertrophied heart were compromised.[9]

Sarcomere proteins

On the subcellular level, the contractile function of myocytes is dependent on the properties of actomyosin complex and associated regulatory proteins (troponin complex and myosin binding protein C).[10]

(a)

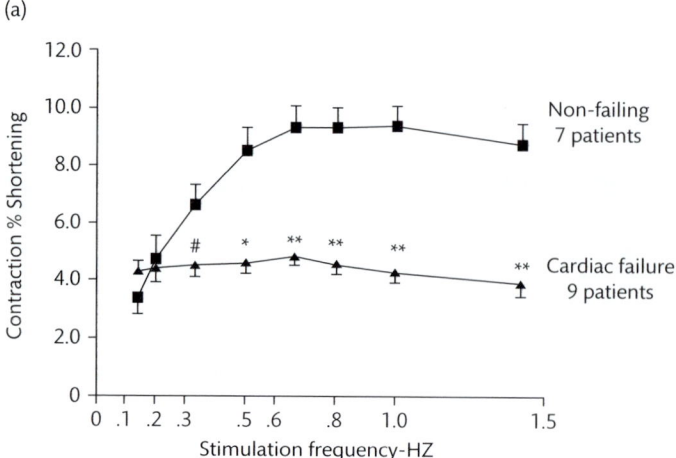

(b)

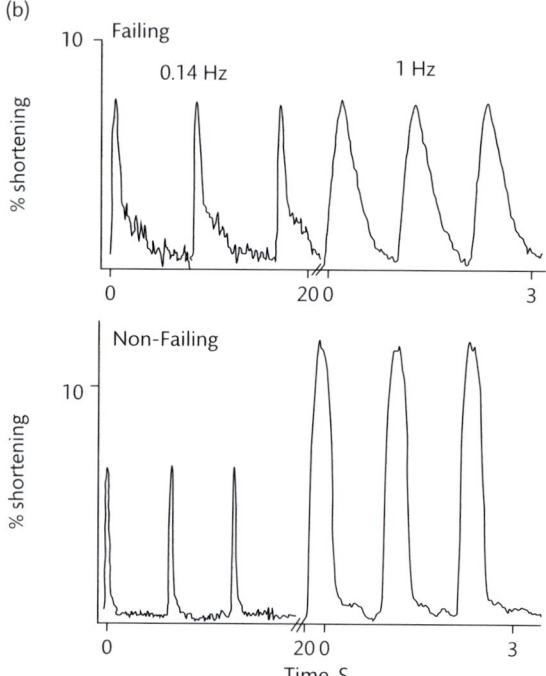

Time, S

Figure 18.1 Impaired force–frequency response and abnormal contraction and relaxation kinetics in failing human cardiomyocytes. (a) Plot of changes in cell length expressed in percentage shortening in response to increasing stimulation rate (maximally stimulating Ca^{2+} and 37°C). Analysis of covariance, failing vs non-failing hearts, $P < 0.001$. #$P < 0.05$, *$P < 0.01$, **$P < 0.001$, by t-test. (b) Tracings at high speed of cells from failing and non-failing hearts at 0.14 and 1.0 Hz in maximal Ca^{2+}. At 0.14 Hz, there is prolongation of relaxation in the myocyte from the failing heart (top) compared with the non-failing control heart (bottom). Although still evident at 1.0 Hz, this phenomenon becomes less prominent owing to an acceleration of relaxation in the myocyte from a failing heart.

Reproduced from Davies CH, Davia K, Bennett JG, et al. Reduced contraction and altered frequency response of isolated ventricular myocytes from patients with heart failure. *Circulation* 1995;**92** with permission from Wolters Kluwer.

Changed levels and disorganization in myofilament proteins can therefore largely contribute to systolic and diastolic dysfunction. For example, a shift of myosin heavy chain isoform from the fast α-myosin heavy chain (MHC) to a slower β-MHC is a well-known mechanism in altered myocyte contractile dynamics.[11] Similarly,

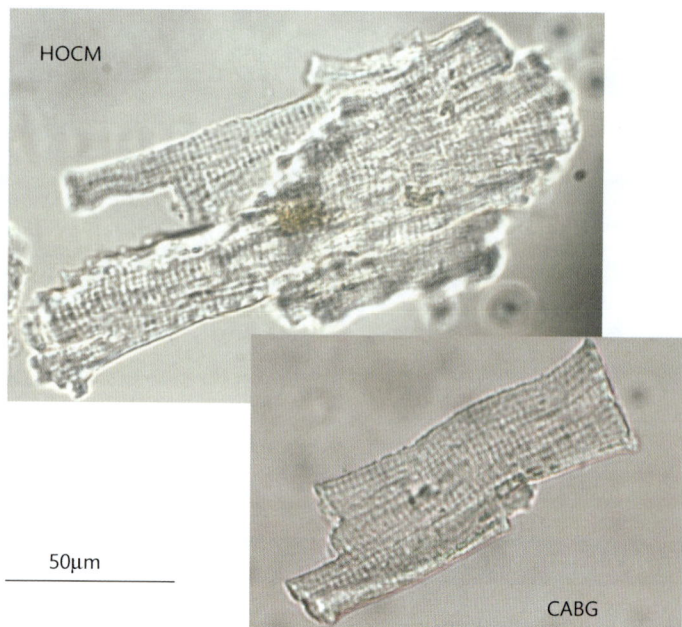

Figure 18.2 Brightfield images of human ventricular myocytes from a sample taken from a hypertrophic cardiomyopathy (HOCM) patient during cardiac transplantation and a biopsy of non-failing heart taken during the coronary artery bypass procedure. Both images show several rod-shaped striated ventricular cardiomyocytes attached via syncytial connections (multiple gap junctions not seen).

titin, a giant sarcomere protein responsible for the passive elasticity, shifts from a stiff N2B isoform to a compliant, high-molecular-weight N2BA isoform in failing myocytes. Pathological increase in N2BA:N2B ratio and parallel loss of titin is closely associated with deranged titin phosphorylation, overall resulting in lower passive stiffness.[12,13]

Surface topology

Normal ventricular cardiomyocytes are characterized by extremely organized surface architecture, reflecting the intracellular organization of the sarcomeric units for optimal excitation–contraction coupling. High-resolution scanning ion conductance microscopy and freeze–fracture electron microscopy revealed the regular pattern of indented grooves of the sarcolemma which overlie the Z-line of the myofilament sarcomere (see **Figure 18.3**).[14] These Z-grooves serve critical functional roles. Z-grooves form an anatomical restraint for sarcolemmal ion channels and receptors, allowing spatial compartmentalization of cell surface signalling.[15] Z-grooves also contain the origin of the transverse tubule (T-tubule) openings, which invaginate deep into the myocyte and underpin the spatial coupling of T-tubule and sarcoplasmic reticulum for efficient excitation–contraction coupling.[16] Between these surface Z-grooves lies the crest region of the cardiomyocyte. Normal cells are identified by the regular alternating architecture of Z-grooves and crest membrane.[14] In failing cardiomyocytes isolated from both end-stage failing human hearts at transplantation, and animal models of chronic heart failure, this surface topology is severely disrupted, with loss of Z-grooves, alteration of crest structures, and loss of T-tubule openings (see **Figure 18.3**).[17] As well as the invaginating, or transverse, tubules, there is a dense network of longitudinal connections between them maintained

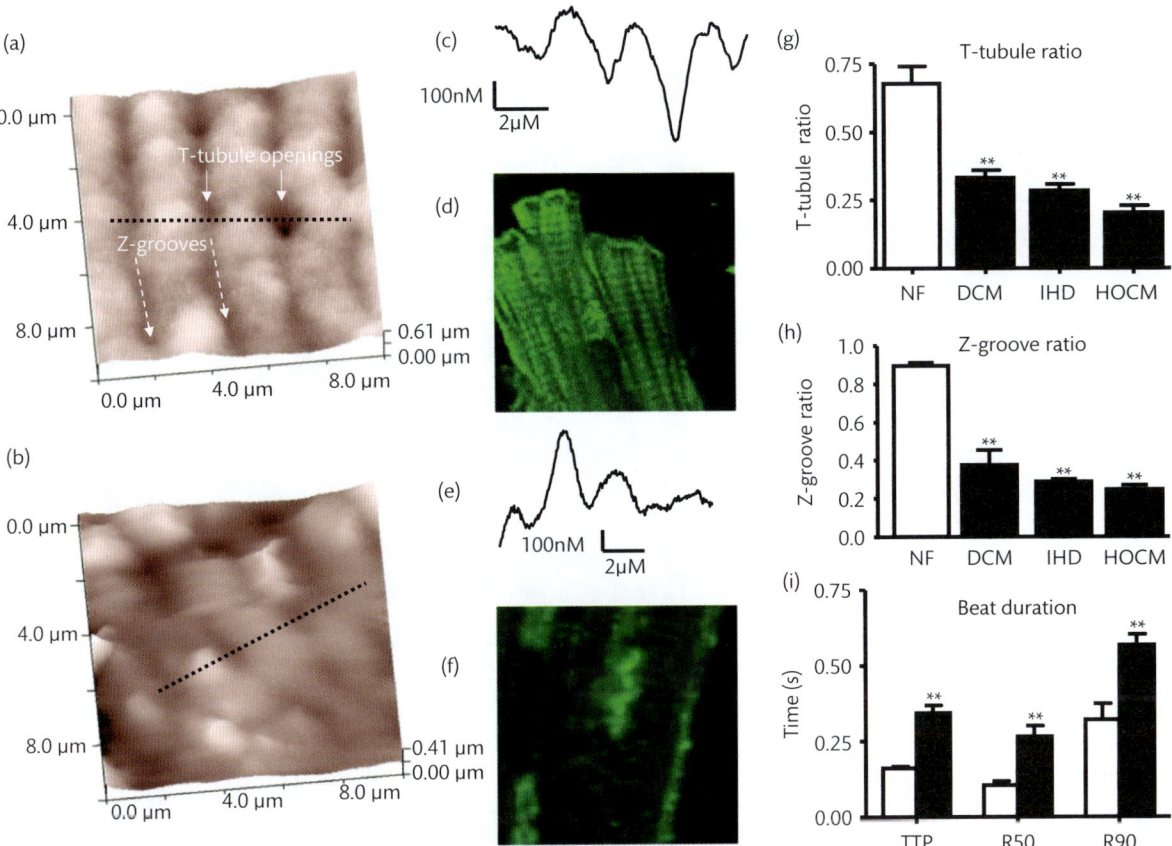

Figure 18.3 Scanning ion conductance microscopy images from the surface of cardiomyocytes isolated from non-failing (a) and failing (b) human hearts. The black dotted line represents the linear selection presented as a one-dimensional surface contour map from non-failing (c) and failing (e) human cardiomyocytes. Confocal images after staining with di-8-ANNEPPS in non-failing (d) and failing cardiomyocytes (f).
Reproduced from Lyon AR, MacLeod KT, Zhang Y, et al. Loss of T-tubules and other changes to surface topography in ventricular myocytes from failing human and rat heart. Proc Natl Acad Sci USA 2009;**106**(16).

by nexilin, and their disruption is also key to heart failure.[18] These changes have numerous functional consequences, such as spatial disruption and temporal delay in excitation–contraction coupling. Furthermore, heart failure progressively stiffens the cardiomyocyte membrane and displaces sub-sarcolemmal mitochondria. This can trigger localized mitochondrial-dependent Ca^{2+} release which initiates cell-wide Ca^{2+} wave propagation and could finally lead to arrhythmias on multicellular scales.[19] Interestingly these morphological changes appear independent of the underlying aetiology of the heart failure and reflect the part of the common phenotype of end-stage decompensated failing hearts.

Intercellular communication

Cardiomyocytes in healthy hearts are precisely integrated into the myocardial syncytium, with intercellular communication and passage of signalling molecules and electrical currents facilitated by gap junctions (GJs) located predominantly at intercalated discs. GJs are small macromolecular channels composed of channel-forming proteins known as connexins. One GJ is formed by two hemichannels, each consisting of six connexin molecules arranged in a hexagonal array around a central aqueous pore. These channels conduct ions between neighbouring cardiomyocytes, allowing current charge to flow between cells, and therefore are critical in determining the efficacy of electrical wavefront conduction across the heart.[20] The

transfer of charge between coupled cardiomyocytes depends upon the number of GJs, the location of GJs, and the conductivity of each GJ. GJ conductivity depends upon the connexin subtype, with connexin 43 (Cx43) the major connexin isoform expressed in ventricular cardiomyocytes.[21] Other important factors regulating GJ function include post-translational modifications such as phosphorylation (e.g. protein kinase C), local $[Ca^{2+}]_i$, and interaction with a variety of other structural and regulatory proteins which determine Cx43 delivery and location within the intercalated disc, e.g. zonula occludens, N-cadherin.[22]

Cx43 expression, phosphorylation and conductance are altered in ischaemic or failing human and animal myocardium, with Cx43 redistribution away from the intercalated discs and more even distribution across the cardiomyocyte surface (see **Figure 18.4**).[22–24] This impairs charge transfer between cardiomyocytes, reducing electrical and functional coupling, which may expose differences in action potential duration between uncoupled cardiomyocytes, and may predispose to conduction block. Animal heart failure models have provided further insights into the role of connexins in the development of both contractile and electrical dysfunction in the failing heart. A uniform reduction in connexin expression was demonstrated in the canine tachycardia–cardiomyopathy model, which amplified both the gradient for action potential duration (APD) dispersion and the conduction slowing in the subepicardial border with

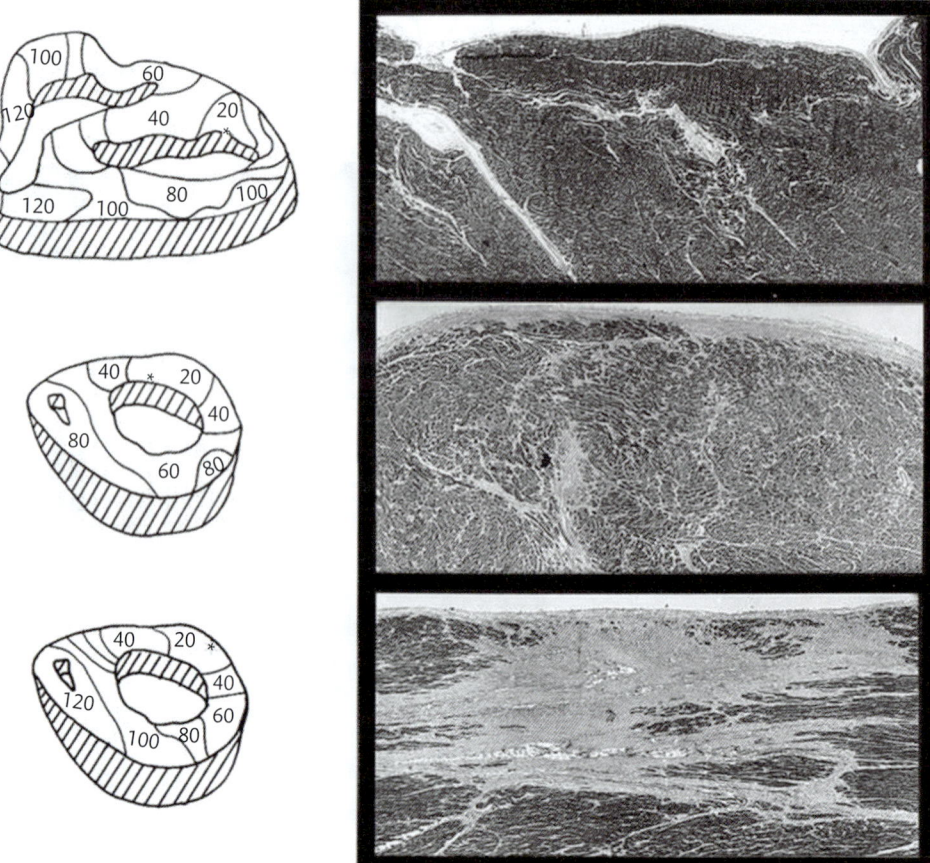

Figure 18.4 Regional fibrosis is located in areas of increased focal triggered activity within failing human hearts. *Left*, sections from activation maps showing sites of focal initiation of ventricular arrhythmias (*). Row 1, spontaneously occurring premature ventricular contraction (PVC) (level I) from a heart failure patient. Row 2, beat T1 (level IV) of three-beat ventral tachycardia (VT) from second heart failure patient. Row 3, beat T2 (level IV) of three-beat VT from first heart failure patient. *Right*, corresponding photomicrographs of trichrome-stained sections of myocardium in vicinity of focal initiation sites demonstrating minimal (*top*), moderate (*middle*), and extensive (*bottom*) fibrosis.
Reproduced from Pogwizd SM, McKenzie JP, Cain ME. Mechanisms underlying spontaneous and induced ventricular arrhythmias in patients with idiopathic dilated cardiomyopathy. *Circulation* 1998;**98**(22) with permission from Wolters Kluwer.

the M cells.[25] The reduction of Cx43 levels preceded the development of reduced conduction velocity, and a relative increase in the unphosphorylated connexin 43 correlated with the onset of significant left ventricular impairment in the pacing heart failure model.[26] The change in Cx43 phosphorylation status correlated with the shift in GJ distribution away from the intercalated discs and towards the lateral sarcolemmal membranes (see **Figure 18.4**). Alterations in cellular Cx43 distribution have also been reported in models of left ventricular dyssynchrony secondary to left bundle branch block with abnormal patterns of ventricular activation.[27] This compounds the mechanical and electrophysiological impairment resulting from dyssynchrony, and interestingly these changes in Cx43 distribution are normalized by biventricular pacing.

Extracellular factors

In the failing heart, in addition to gap junction uncoupling between cardiomyocytes, there are significant changes in the extracellular matrix (ECM) and architecture of the myocardium leading to cell slippage and increased resistance between cardiomyocytes,[28–30] microscopic and/or macroscopic scar formation, and altered perfusion with the generation of ischaemia.

Cardiac fibroblasts in failing hearts increase in number, demonstrate increased metabolic activity, and increase interstitial matrix synthesis and deposition.[31,32] The ECM includes interstitial collagens, proteoglycans, glycoproteins, cytokines, growth factors, matrikines, and proteases. Increased deposition of ECM in the failing heart has a number of important functional sequelae. At a cellular level, cardiomyocytes interact with the ECM via several adhesion proteins or anchors. In addition to providing structural support and transmitting mechanical forces from myofilament cross-bridging, these also serve to activate adverse intracellular secondary messenger pathways.[33] Interstitial matrix deposition also increases spatial uncoupling between adjacent cardiomyocytes. These changes reduce conduction velocity of the electrical depolarization wavefront, contributing to the arrhythmic substrate with focal points of conduction block.[34] Furthermore, fibroblasts within failing myocardium demonstrate increased connexin expression and may form gap junctions with cardiomyocytes. The functional chemical and metabolic sequelae of these de-novo cell–cell contacts remain to be explored, but the potential adverse effects upon myocardial electrical properties have been demonstrated.[35] The electrotonic coupling has been demonstrated between the cardiomyocytes and

fibroblasts via tunnelling nanotube connections between myocytes and non-myocytes in cardiac scar border tissue, which can modify the cardiac action potential.[36] Increased fibrosis is frequently noted around the arterioles and capillaries, and this contributes to the microvascular dysfunction and secondary myocardial ischaemia in the failing heart, irrespective of aetiology (see **Figure 18.4**).[6] Cardiac fibroblast and transformed myofibroblasts also secrete factors such as transforming growth factor-β, fibroblast growth factor-2, IL-6 family interleukins and endothelin-1, suggesting that there is a paracrine interplay between myocytes and fibroblasts.[37]

Functional and signalling changes

Impaired β-adrenoceptor signalling

Sympathetic stimulation of healthy ventricular muscle is predominantly achieved via activation of the β_1-adrenoceptor (AR) and β_2AR, located on the cardiomyocyte sarcolemma. β_1AR is the commonest receptor subtype, accounting for ~80% of βAR protein in healthy ventricular tissue. β_1AR and β_2AR are G-protein-coupled receptors and are targets for both noradrenaline, released from local sympathetic nerve endings, and circulating adrenaline, diffusing from the coronary circulation. Under normal physiological conditions, agonist binding to either receptor induces activation of G_s protein secondary messenger system. Gsα activates adenylyl cyclase, an enzyme which catalyses the production of cyclic 3′,5′-adenosine monophosphate (cAMP) and activation of protein kinase A (PKA). PKA phosphorylates many critical proteins involved in the excitation–contraction coupling system, including the L-type Ca^{2+} channel (LTCC) (increasing LTCC opening probability), the cardiac ryanodine receptor (RyR) (increases RyR opening probability and calcium release from the sarcoplasmic reticulum (SR) stores), troponin I (reducing the affinity of troponin I for troponin C), and phospholamban (PLB) (reducing PLB-mediated inhibition of the SR calcium ATPase channel (SERCA2a)).[38] These effects all increase the gain of the excitation–contraction coupling system during cardiomyocyte contraction and relaxation, leading to the positive inotropic and lusitropic response of ventricular myocardium to catecholamines after βAR activation.

Human myocytes from chronically failing hearts have a blunted contractile response to βAR stimulation, with a decreased β_1AR:β_2AR ratio[39] and an increased Gi:Gs ratio[40] (see **Figure 18.5**). The extent of this decrease correlates with the severity of cardiac impairment, and predominantly affects the β_1AR, whose levels can be reduced by up to 50%. β_2AR levels remain stable or are reduced only marginally and thus the β_1AR:β_2AR ratio is reduced from 4:1 towards 1:1 in failing hearts. Levels of Giα increase, with downregulation of Gsα, and this change in the Gs:Gi protein ratio is critical in the failing cardiomyocyte as β_2ARs (relatively increased in the failing myocardium) couple additionally to Gi proteins.[41] Inhibition of Gi activation using pertussis toxin can reverse functional βAR desensitization in ventricular myocytes from failing human hearts.[42] Increased β_2AR–Giα signalling in response to catecholamine stimulation results in a negative inotropic response.[43] The precise mechanism(s) underlying this negative inotropic response remain to be elucidated, but proposed mechanisms include Giα-mediated inhibition of adenylyl cyclase, activation of the Na^+/Ca^{2+} exchanger,

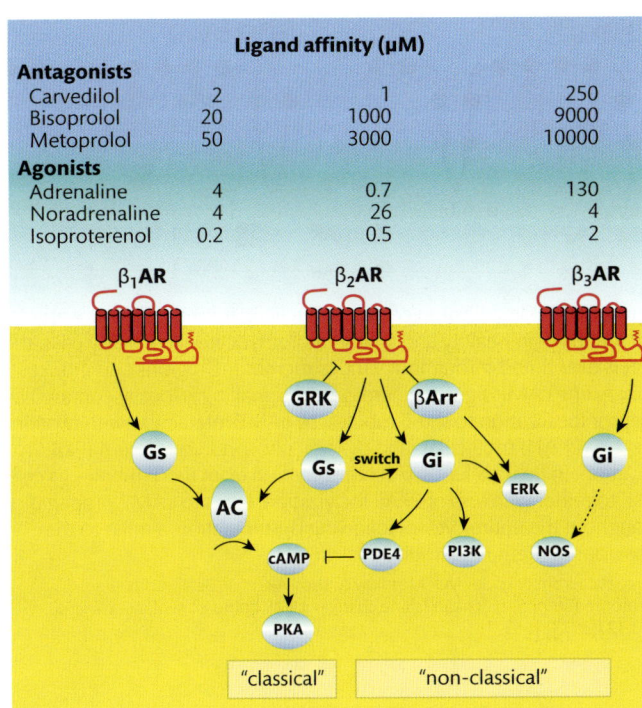

Ligand affinity (μM)			
Antagonists			
Carvedilol	2	1	250
Bisoprolol	20	1000	9000
Metoprolol	50	3000	10000
Agonists			
Adrenaline	4	0.7	130
Noradrenaline	4	26	4
Isoproterenol	0.2	0.5	2

Figure 18.5 Agonist activation and coupling/signalling properties of β-adrenergic receptor subtypes.
Reproduced from Lohse MJ, Engelhardt S, Eschenhagen T. What is the role of beta-adrenergic signaling in heart failure? *Circ Res* 2003;**93**(10) with permission from Wolters Kluwer.

competitive inhibition of β_2AR–Gs coupling, increased buffering of activated Gα by Gβγ released from activated Gi, and activation of the p38 mitogen-activated protein kinase (p38MAP kinase) pathway. It is of interest that certain β-blockers, including those used clinically, can activate the β_2AR–Gi-negative inotropic pathways.[44]

The location of βAR differs both between β_1AR and β_2AR subtypes in normal cardiomyocytes and between healthy and failing cardiomyocytes. In healthy ventricular myocytes, β_1ARs are located across the entire surface of the cell, and pharmacological receptor stimulation results in cell-wide propagating cAMP signals, independent of the origin of the β_1AR location.[45] By contrast, β_2ARs are restricted to the Z-groove and T-tubule openings, and have spatially restricted (compartmentalized) cAMP signals. In cardiomyocytes from failing hearts, where the organized Z-groove and T-tubule structure is altered (see surface topology), the β_2ARs were located across the entire cell surface, and agonist activation leads to cell-wide cAMP signals analogous to the β_1AR of the normal (and failing) myocytes (see **Figure 18.6**). This could be relevant as the G_i proteins are located in the intergroove crest membrane,[46] and therefore this physical β_2AR redistribution may contribute to increased βAR–Gi coupling and the failing cardiomyocyte phenotype. Differences in β_2AR compartmentalization have also been shown between apical and basal cardiomyocytes, where basal cardiomyocytes have more organized membranes (higher T-tubular and caveolar densities) and tighter spatial control of β_2AR–cAMP.[47]

Chronic βAR activation results in cardiomyocyte apoptosis and this contributes to myocardial dysfunction in heart failure.[48-50] However, evidence suggests that the β_1AR and β_2AR exert differing effects on cardiomyocyte survival pathways. Chronic β_1AR

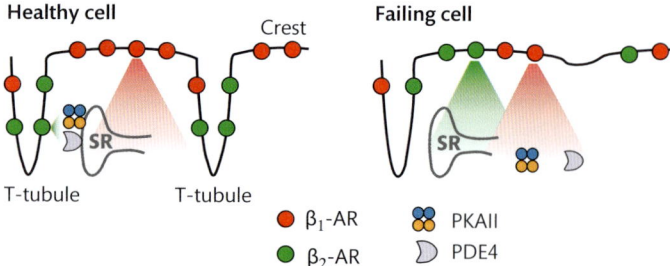

Figure 18.6 Organization of cAMP signalling from β₁-adrenoceptor (AR) and β₂AR in healthy and failing cardiomyocytes. In healthy cells, the β₁AR is distributed throughout various membrane regions and induces propagating cAMP signals, whereas β₂AR signalling is locally confined by receptor localization to the T-tubules, by cAMP interaction with protein kinase A (PKA) II molecules, and by local phosphodiesterase-4 (PDE4) activation. In heart failure, β₂AR redistribution from the T-tubules to cell crest, together with loss of PKAII localization, leads to cAMP propagation throughout the entire cytosol following β₂ stimulation, similar to the behaviour of the β₁AR stimulation.

Source data from Nikolaev VO, Moshkov A, Lyon AR, *et al.* Beta2-adrenergic receptor redistribution in heart failure changes cAMP compartmentation. *Science* 2010;**327**(5973):1653–1657.

activation is harmful to isolated cardiomyocytes, and in heart failure patients the increased sympathetic activation and noradrenaline levels correlate inversely with survival.[51] Activation of β₂AR–Gi-coupled pathway is protective via activation of anti-apoptotic pathways (Gβγi–PI3K–Akt pathway activation), but at the potential mechanical cost of negative inotropism. This may reflect an evolutionary response to protect the myocardium from the toxic effects of excessive catecholamine stimulation, particularly evident in the reversible takotsubo cardiomyopathy syndrome, where β₂AR–Gi coupling underlies apical cardiomyocyte hypocontractility.[52]

Calcium pathophysiology

The abnormalities of cardiomyocyte calcium physiology in the failing cardiomyocyte have been described in detail in Chapter 10. The major changes are listed below:

- decreased SR calcium reuptake;
- increased SR calcium leak with increased calcium spark and wave frequency during diastole;
- reduced SR calcium content;
- impaired trafficking of voltage-dependent L-type calcium channel to T-tubules. Reduced levels of BIN1 protein, which is needed to anchor microtubules for delivery;[53]
- increases extrusion by the sodium–calcium exchanger (NCX);
- elevated resting (baseline) calcium concentration;
- a reduction in peak amplitude of the stimulated calcium transient;
- increased time-to-peak amplitude;
- prolonged calcium transient decay kinetics: T_{50}, T_{90}, decay constant (tau);
- prolongation of action potential duration;
- increased calcium-dependent triggered activity (delayed afterdepolarizations);
- increased calcium sensor activity (calmodulin kinase II, calcineurin).

Sodium pathophysiology

There increasing evidence that cardiomyocyte sodium overload also develops in chronic heart failure resulting in abnormal mitochondrial function and potential to drive further diastolic calcium loading and pro-arrhythmia. In both hypertrophied and failing human and animal cardiomyocytes, $[Na^+]_i$ is elevated by ~3–6 mM.[54–56] The mechanisms underlying this are incompletely understood. This may be the result of reduced Na^+/K^+ ATPase gene expression[57–59] or activity,[60,61] increased sodium influx via the Na^+/H^+ exchanger (NHE)[62,63] and increased entry via the late Na^+ current.[64] Increased intracellular sodium ($[Na^+]_i$) has several deleterious sequelae that contribute to the development of the failing phenotype. First, the elevated $[Na^+]_i$ reduces the energy gradient for forward mode and stimulates an increase in NCX reverse mode activity. This effect is primarily during systole, when the higher $[Na^+]_i$, lower peak calcium levels, and prolonged APD promote reverse mode NCX function in the failing cardiomyocyte. This drives calcium entry into the failing cardiomyocyte and may be a compensatory mechanism to raise cell and SR calcium stores and increase contractile force. However, due to SERCA2a downregulation, the increased calcium entry via the NCX during the phases 1 and 2 of the action potential cannot be cleared into the SR. Instead the increased calcium influx must be balanced by increased forward mode NCX activity during phase,[4] which may contribute to the increased cellular triggered activity via afterdepolarizations.[65]

Second, NCX proteins are also present on the inner mitochondrial membrane. Increased $[Na^+]_i$ disrupts mitochondrial calcium uptake, and this contributes to energetic inefficiency of the failing cardiomyocyte via uncoupling of the calcium-sensitive energy supply–demand relationship.[66] Finally, increased $[Na^+]_i$ will potentially reduce the electrochemical gradient for clearance of H^+ ions by the NHE protein, impairing the buffering of intracellular acidosis in the failing cardiomyocyte.

Mitochondrial dysfunction and oxidative stress

Cardiomyocytes are highly metabolically active to meet the energy demands of cardiac contraction 60–100 times per minute for the lifetime of an individual. Cardiomyocytes are designed to perform highly efficient aerobic respiration co-ordinated by an organized lattice network of thousands of mitochondria in a single cardiomyocyte. Cardiomyocytes from failing hearts have impaired energetic efficiency (see Chapter 11).[67] This is reflected at both the cellular and intact organ level by the reduced phosphocreatine:ATP ratio, which has been demonstrated to directly correlate with severity of heart failure.[68] This is indicative of impaired mitochondrial function in failing cardiomyocytes, which is a reflection of the combined effects of cellular calcium and sodium overload and of increased oxidative stress. Oxidative stress is caused by mitochondrial dysfunction with increased production of reactive oxygen species (ROS). ROS levels are elevated in failing myocardium.[69,70] These are generated by a leak of superoxide anions from the electron transport chain or production of hydrogen peroxide. Oxidative stress is a driver of the spiralling deterioration of cardiomyocyte function in heart failure, as ROS interacts to accelerate several pathophysiological pathways. These include: increasing SR calcium leak via RyR2 oxidation;[71] impairing Na^+/K^+ ATPase and SERCA2a activity; mitochondrial membrane potential ($\Delta\psi m$) depolarization with uncoupling of ATP synthesis

from oxidative phosphorylation; and self-generation of further ROS generation and oxidative stress. A further critical outcome of increased mitochondrial oxidative stress is the predisposition to apoptosis.

Rearranged nuclear trafficking

Trafficking of signalling components between nucleus and cytoplasm is a key step in the transcriptional regulation of cardiomyocytes (see **Figure 18.7**). In failing cells, changes in nuclear transport machinery together with remodelling of the nuclear pore lead to increased nuclear export at the cost of nuclear import.[37,72] Given the central role of nuclear accumulation of specific signal transducers (e.g. HDAC kinases, NFATs) in hypertrophy and failure, this seems to be a key mechanism underlying the transcriptional changes. High nuclear export is also necessary for an increased de-novo protein synthesis

in hypertrophy. Thus, blockade of exportin-1-dependent traffic prevents or reverses nuclear and cellular remodelling responses (i.e. cell size and foetal gene expression).[73]

Abnormal gene regulation

Indeed, activation of foetal gene expression programmes is one of the hallmarks of the common final pathway of heart failure. This has been demonstrated in human heart failure samples, both with respect to foetal myocyte protein expression profiles.[74] The precise mechanisms underlying these switches are unknown, but it is clearly established that the adult failing heart undergoes a number of functional adaptive changes which generate cellular physiology reminiscent of the foetal ventricular myocardium. These include switches in metabolic pathways from fatty acid to carbohydrate metabolism, changes in T-tubule and SR physiology, altered sarcolemmal ion

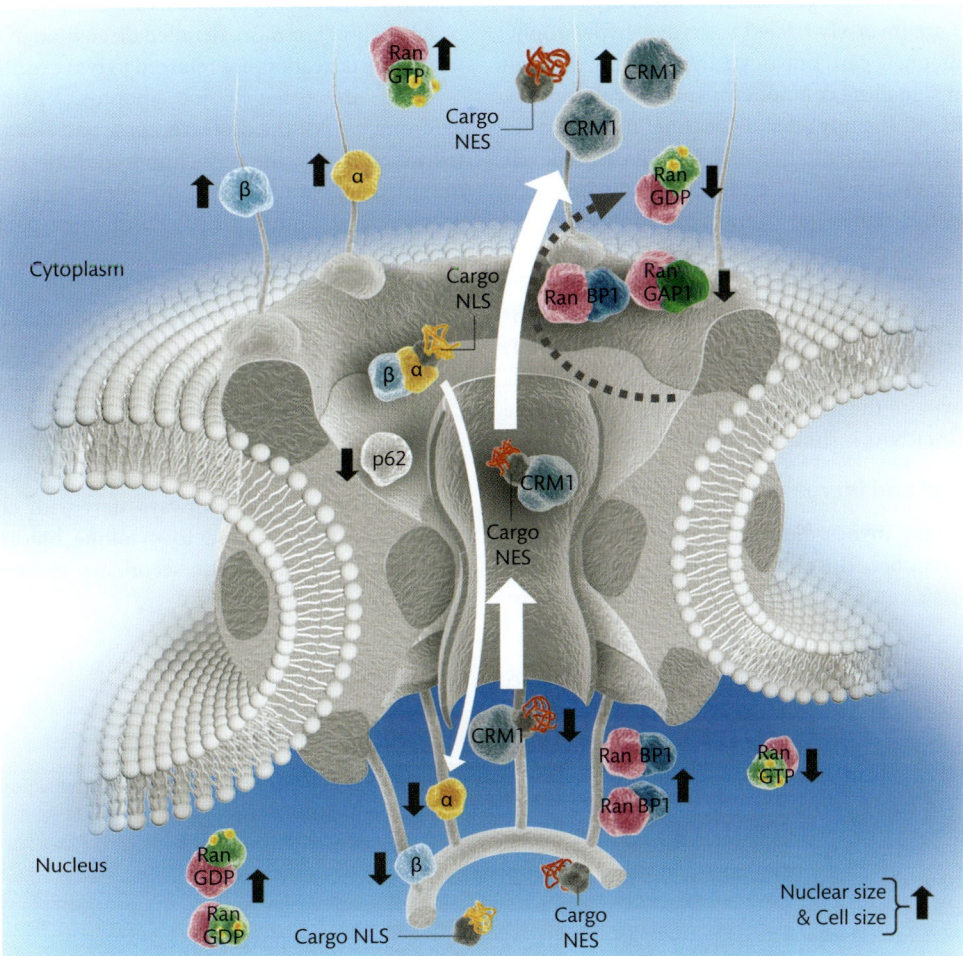

Figure 18.7 Hypothetical models of nuclear trafficking changes during cardiac hypertrophy. The balance between nuclear protein import and nuclear protein export is disrupted in (rat) cardiomyocyte exposed to phenylephrine for 48 h or with ischemic cardiomyopathy; under these hypertrophic stimuli, the demand for the nuclear export of transcription factors is exaggerated so that the export receptor (CRM1) is found to be constantly in the cytoplasm. Subsequently, RanBP1 (which facilitates GTP hydrolysis with RanGAP1) cannot be translocated into the cytoplasm by CRM1, and the other import transport receptors (importins α and β) are found sequestered in the cytoplasm with RanGTP. Thus, no importins are available in the nucleus to be recycled and released free in the cytoplasm for another import cycle. In hypertrophic conditions where nuclear and cell sizes are increased, CRM1 cytoplasmic translocation is increased, while cytoplasmic RanBP1, nucleoporin p62, and nuclear translocation of importins (α and β) are decreased. The size of the white arrow is proportional to the transport rate. An upward black arrow shows an increase while a downward black arrow shows a decrease.

Reproduced from Chahine MN, Mioulane M, Sikkel MB, *et al*. Nuclear pore rearrangements and nuclear trafficking in cardiomyocytes from rat and human failing hearts. *Cardiovasc Res* 2015;**105**(1):31–43 with permission from Oxford University Press.

channel expression, and alteration of myofilament myosin heavy chain isoforms. All these changes result in physiology characteristic of foetal ventricular myocardium.[3] The switch to foetal gene expression profiles may reflect the myocyte response to stress and the impaired oxygen supply–demand relationship in the failing heart in an attempt to optimize energy utilization and contractile function. Indeed foetal gene expression programmes are reactivated in chronically ischaemic hibernating myocardium.[75] Activation of foetal gene expression pathways has beneficial effects upon cell survival, at least initially. However, the changes from adult-to-foetal physiology introduce numerous inefficiencies in the adult heart, for example in excitation–contraction coupling, which may ultimately contribute to the vicious circle of decline begetting decline for cardiomyocytes within the failing myocardium.

Non-coding RNAs control cardiomyocyte growth, mRNA processing, and protein synthesis by regulating multiple genes in signalling pathways. The reactivation in a foetal profile of small non-coding RNA (microRNA, miR-) is a known process in heart failure.[76] Levels of miR-1 and miR-133 are inversely related to cardiac hypertrophy. High levels of miR-1 attenuate cardiomyocyte hypertrophy through modulation of calcium signalling components such as calmodulin. It was shown that SERCA2 therapy after myocardial infarction restored miR-1 levels in rats, leading to normalized expression levels of the sodium–calcium exchanger 1.[77] miR-133 modulates contractility by regulating the expression of multiple components of the β_1AR pathway.[78] Next-generation sequencing showed that long non-coding (lnc) RNA profile is also altered in heart failure. Notably, the expression profile of lncRNAs is better at distinguishing non-ischaemic from ischaemic failing myocardium than microRNA or mRNA. Alteration on ncRNA expressions directly influences cardiomyocyte phenotype in the failing heart;[79,80] the putative role of currently identified lncRNAs is shown in **Figure 18.8**.

Impaired cell survival and increased apoptosis

Another hallmark of failing myocardium is the progressive reduction in cardiomyocyte number. This may be the direct result of the causative disease, e.g. acute coronary occlusion with myocardial infarction, but also results from progressive activation of cell death pathways (apoptosis). Infarction and another acute myocardial injury initially cause acute cell necrosis resulting from a sudden depletion of ATP. Necrosis is characterized by cell swelling, membrane lysis, and release of intracellular contents into the interstitial space, resulting in inflammation and secondary injury. By contrast, apoptosis is an energy-consuming process of programmed cell death via protein and chromatin fragmentation which does not trigger an immune response.

Adult mammalian cardiomyocytes rarely undergo apoptosis within healthy hearts, with only one apoptotic cell visible per 10 000–100 000 cardiomyocytes.[81] By contrast, the rates of apoptosis, as measured using TUNEL (terminal deoxynucleotidyl transferase dUTP nick end labelling) staining for DNA condensation and fragmentation, are significantly increased in chronically failing hearts irrespective of aetiology (see **Figure 18.9**).[82] The biological pathways underlying apoptosis are complex and will be summarized briefly below. For more detailed discussion of the pathways involved in apoptosis, readers are referred to two excellent recent reviews.[83,84]

There are three major apoptotic pathways in ventricular cardiomyocytes: the death receptor pathway (also known as the extrinsic pathway), the mitochondrial death pathway (also known as the intrinsic pathway) and the endoplasmic reticulum (ER)-stress pathway (see **Figure 18.10**).[85] All three pathways converge upon a cascade of sequential activation of a family of 'suicide enzymes' known as caspases (cysteine and serine proteases).[86] These enzymes exist as prozymogens (inactive enzymes) and are cleaved by caspases upstream in the pathway to generate active enzymes, which catalyse the cleavage of the downstream prozymogen. The ultimate effector caspases (e.g. caspase 3) catalyse the breakdown of other target proteins in the cell which initiates irreversible protein degradation, DNA fragmentation, nuclear condensation, and cell death.

The death receptor pathways start with cell surface membrane receptors which respond to cytokine binding with activation of intracellular pro-apoptotic secondary messenger pathways. These

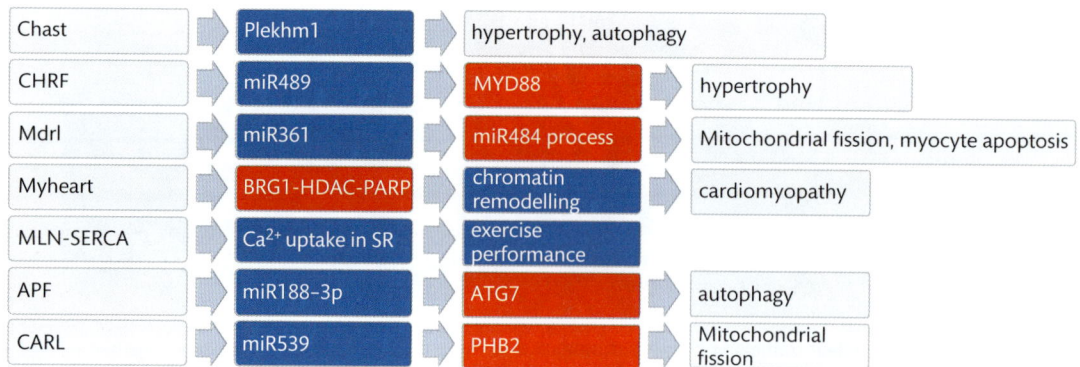

Figure 18.8 Examples of long non-coding RNAs in heart failure. LncRNAs regulate cardiac disease through various mechanisms. Chast (cardiac hypertrophy-associated transcript) lncRNA influences cardiomyocyte hypertrophy. Chrf functions as a sponge for miR489, which protects against heart failure and hypertrophy development by inhibiting MYD88. Mdrl inhibits miR361, which in turn blocks the miR484 process, thereby reducing mitochondrial fission and cardiomyocyte apoptosis. In cardiac stress, Reciprocal Myheart-BRG1/HDAC/PARP chromatin repressor complex inhibition constitutes a negative feedback circuit critical for maintaining cardiac function. MLN interacts with SERCA2A, thereby inhibiting Ca²⁺ uptake into the SR, and leading to reduced exercise performance. APF inhibits miR188-3p, leadings to increased ATG7 levels and autophagy. Cardiac apoptosis-related lncRNA (CARL) suppress mitochondrial fission by targeting miR539. Red boxes represent pro-apoptotic; blue boxes represent anti-apoptotic RNAs.

Source data from Lorenzen JM, Thum T. Long noncoding RNAs in kidney and cardiovascular diseases. *Nat Rev Nephrol* 2016;**12**(6):360–373 and Uchida S, Dimmeler S. Long noncoding RNAs in cardiovascular diseases. *Circ Res* 2015;**116**(4):737–750.

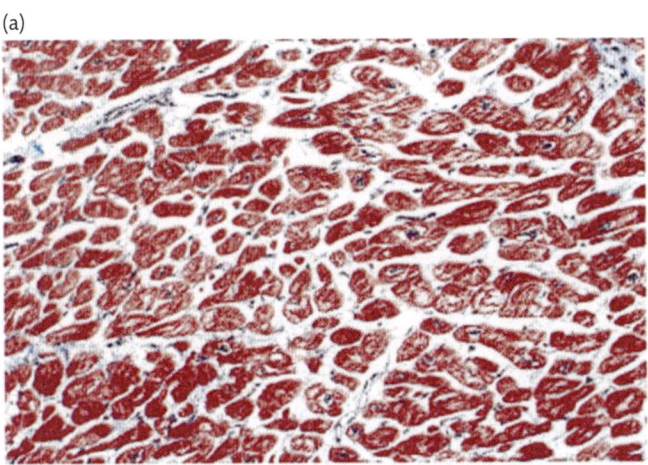

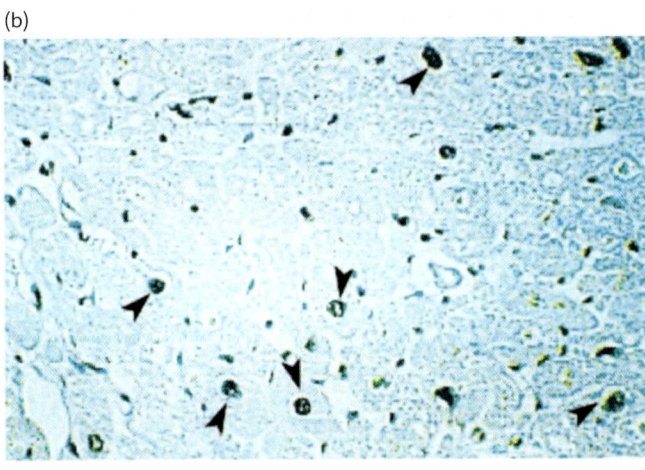

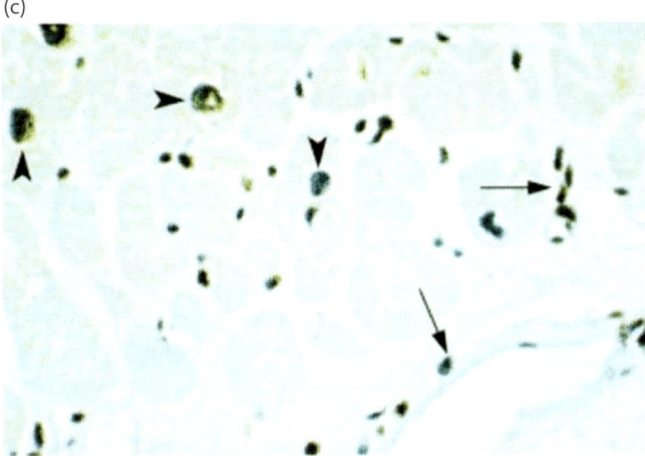

Figure 18.9 Evidence of apoptosis in end-stage idiopathic dilated cardiomyopathy. (a) Myocardial section from a patient with dilated cardiomyopathy contains normal myocytes and no interstitial fibrosis (Masson's trichrome staining, ×75). Extensive apoptosis can be seen in myocytes in (b) (arrowheads). Apoptosis usually occurs in groups of cells, and the severity varies from extensive (b) to mild (c) to absent in different regions of the myocardium. In addition to its presence in myocytes (arrowheads) in (c), apoptosis is also observed in vascular smooth muscle cells of an intramyocardial arteriole as well as in rare interstitial cells (arrows). (b, c): End-labelling for apoptotic nuclei and haematoxylin counterstaining, ×250.

are predominantly members of the TNF membrane receptor super-family, including the Fas receptors and tumour necrosis factor receptor 1 (TNFR1). Upon ligand binding, Fas receptors undergo oligomerization and recruit the Fas-associated death domain (FADD). The Fas–FADD complex binds to procaspase 8, activating this zymogen and promoting cleavage to the active caspase 8 enzyme. Caspase 8 initiates an intracellular cascade of caspase activation which culminates in the cleavage of DNA and degradation of critical homeostatic proteins, resulting in apoptosis. In fact, a transgenic mouse model with cardiac-restricted overexpression of caspase 8 developed dilated cardiomyopathy without need for any additional insult.[87]

The mitochondrial pathway is initiated by excessive oxidative stress and accumulation of mitochondrial ROS. Mitochondrial ROS accumulation occurs due to electron leak from various complexes of the inner mitochondrial membrane electron transport chain, resulting in superoxide anion generation. ROS are increased beyond levels that can be effectively buffered by the antioxidant systems in ischaemic myocardium, after reperfusion following acute ischaemia, and in chronically failing myocardium. This initiates increased permeability of the mitochondrial outer membrane via the assembly of the mitochondrial permeability transition pore (mPTP).[88] mPTP opening initiates an irreversible collapse of $\Delta\psi_m$ with cessation of ATP synthesis, mitochondrial swelling with focal rupture of the outer mitochondrial membrane, and release of several pro-apoptotic factors such as cytochrome *c*, apoptosis-inducing factor (AIF), endonuclease G (Endo G), and second mitochondria-derived activator of caspases (Smac/Diablo), resulting in the initiation of apoptosis. Cytochrome *c* binds to Apaf-1 and forms the apoptosome complex with activation of caspase 9. Caspase 9 cleaves and activates caspase 3, and the latter directly cleaves target proteins, including DNA polymerase, stimulating endonuclease activity and induction of apoptosis.

The mitochondrial death pathway has a number of regulatory systems, the most extensively investigated being the Bcl-2 protein family.[89] The Bcl-2 proteins are subdivided on structural classification into the 'multidomain' and 'BH3-only' subcategories. The pro-apoptotic multidomain Bcl-2 proteins Bax and Bak contribute to mPTP formation and activation of apoptosis. They are regulated by complementary anti-apoptotic multidomain proteins (prototypical Bcl-2 and Bcl-xl) which bind and competitively inhibit the pro-apoptotic Bax and Bak. The BH3-only proteins act as stress sensors, responding to increased levels of cellular stress including increased oxidative stress and growth factor deprivation. They mobilize to the mitochondria and regulate permeability transition. One example in cardiomyocytes is the Nix protein, where overexpression induces an apoptotic cardiomyopathy.[90] These may indirectly activate the Bcl-2 pathways via sequestration of the anti-apoptotic BH3-only proteins Bcl-2 and Bcl-xl. Therefore the balance of pro- and anti-apoptotic proteins is key to determining cardiomyocyte fate in the failing heart. For example, the ratio of Bax:Bcl-xl significantly increases during the transition from compensated hypertrophy to decompensated heart failure in a rodent model, correlating with the increase in cytoplasmic cytochrome *c* and caspase 3 activation.[91]

The third apoptotic pathway is activated by increased ER stress. The ER is the site of protein synthesis, including protein folding prior to export to the ultimate subcellular destination. Remodelling of the cardiomyocyte involves changes in protein synthesis and turnover as

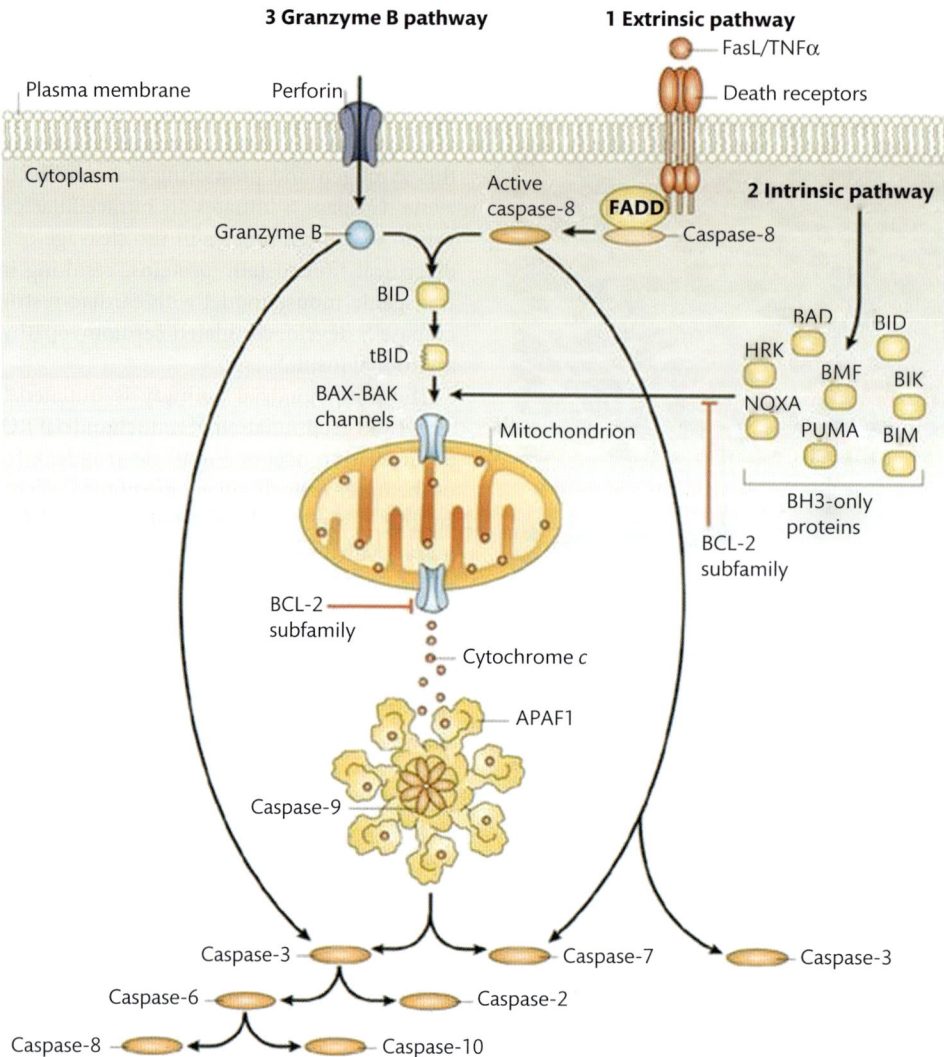

Figure 18.10 Pathways leading to intracellular caspase activation and initiation of apoptosis.
Reproduced from Taylor RC, Cullen SP, Martin SJ. Apoptosis: controlled demolition at the cellular level. *Nat Rev Mol Cell Biol* 2008;**9**(3) with permission from Springer Nature.

well as clearance of misfolded proteins and aggregates. Increased ER stress, secondary to abnormal calcium homeostasis, impaired energy utilization, hypoxia, oxidative stress, or abnormal ER protein transport, results in the accumulation of unfolded proteins in the ER lumen, and has been demonstrated in a variety of heart failure models and in end-stage human dilated cardiomyopathy.[92,93] This triggers a number homeostatic changes called the 'unfolded protein response' (UPR), involving ER-resident transmembrane proteins. The UPR detects the accumulation of misfolded proteins and initiates a transcriptional program to increase ER protein-folding capacity, degrade misfolded proteins, reduce basal protein synthesis rates, and inhibit ER overload. Whereas the UPR is compensatory, if prolonged, it also initiates apoptosis via activation of caspase 12 and upregulation of the transcription factor CHOP/GADD 153. Caspase 12 activates caspase 3 and apoptosis directly, whereas CHOP/GADD 153 increases expression of pro-apoptotic genes including the BH3-only protein Puma. Modulation of UPR by artificial chemical chaperones is a potential approach to control this

pathway.[94] Ubiquitin-proteasome system (UPS) is another regulator of protein degradation. Ubiquitinated proteins are accumulated in failing myocytes,[95] and this has been linked to reduced proteasomal activity in heart failure.[96] Accumulation of these protein aggregates is proteotoxic to the cells.

An additional homeostatic system which appears to interact with apoptosis is the autophagy pathways for recycling organelles and their proteins. The activity of autophagy pathways is dysregulated in heart failure models.[97] Examples of crosstalk between critical proteins in the regulation of autophagy and apoptosis have recently been reported.[98] For example, Atg5, an essential autophagy protein, activates apoptosis via both mitochondrial and death receptor pathways. UPR, UPS, and autophagy, along with other protein degradation systems, can regulate protein turnover.

In summary, apoptosis is a highly regulated cell death system which is increased in failing hearts due to activation of many different pro-apoptotic pathways, with the exhaustion of the counterbalancing anti-apoptotic systems.[99] The result is the progressive loss

of cardiomyocyte number after the initial insult, which insidiously increases the demands upon the remaining myocytes within the failing heart.

Summary

The biology of the failing cardiomyocyte is a complex interaction of a number of abnormal pathophysiological processes involving signalling pathways, intracellular ionic fluxes, intercellular communications, oxidative stress, impaired mitochondrial energetics, altered structural morphology, abnormal reactivation of foetal gene expression patterns, and activation of cell death pathways. The crosstalk between these pathways is complex, and positive feedback between these systems leads to the vicious cycle of deterioration of mechanical function and cell survival that characterize the phenotype of the failing cardiomyocyte. Identifying and targeting critical nodal points and master regulatory systems may identify novel therapeutic strategies which can recover multiple elements of the failing phenotype and translate into meaningful clinical benefits for patients with heart failure.

REFERENCES

1. Diez J, Gonzalez A, Lopez B, Querejeta R. Mechanisms of disease: pathologic structural remodeling is more than adaptive hypertrophy in hypertensive heart disease. *Nat Clin Pract Cardiovasc Med* 2005;**2**(4):209–16.
2. Dorn GW, Robbins J, Sugden PH. Phenotyping hypertrophy: eschew obfuscation. *Circ Res* 2003;**92**(11):1171–5.
3. Rajabi M, Kassiotis C, Razeghi P, Taegtmeyer H. Return to the fetal gene program protects the stressed heart: a strong hypothesis. *Heart Fail Rev* 2007;**12**(3–4):331–43.
4. Opie LH, Commerford PJ, Gersh BJ, Pfeffer MA. Controversies in ventricular remodelling. *Lancet* 2006;**367**(9507):356–67.
5. Davis J, Davis LC, Correll RN, et al. A tension-based model distinguishes hypertrophic versus dilated cardiomyopathy. *Cell* 2016;**165**(5):1147–59.
6. Davies CH, Davia K, Bennett JG, et al. Reduced contraction and altered frequency response of isolated ventricular myocytes from patients with heart failure. *Circulation* 1995;**92**(9):2540–9.
7. Severs NJ. The cardiac muscle cell. *Bioessays* 2000;**22**(2):188–99.
8. Terracciano CMN, Harding SE, Adamson DL, et al. Changes in sarcolemmal Ca entry and sarcoplasmic reticulum Ca content in ventricular myocytes from patients with end-stage heart failure following myocardial recovery after combined pharmacological and ventricular assist device therapy. *Eur Heart J* 2003;**24**(14):1329–39.
9. del Monte F, O'Gara P, Poole-Wilson PA, Yacoub MH, Harding SE. Cell geometry and contractile abnormalities of myocytes from failing human left ventricle. *Cardiovasc Res* 1995;**30**(2):281–90.
10. Hamdani N, Bishu KG, von Frieling-Salewsky M, Redfield MM, Linke WA. Deranged myofilament phosphorylation and function in experimental heart failure with preserved ejection fraction. *Cardiovasc Res* 2013;**97**(3):464–71.
11. Hamdani N, Kooij V, van DS, Merkus D, et al. Sarcomeric dysfunction in heart failure. *Cardiovasc Res* 2008;**77**(4):649–58.
12. Makarenko I, Opitz CA, Leake MC, et al. Passive stiffness changes caused by upregulation of compliant titin isoforms in human dilated cardiomyopathy hearts. *Circ Res* 2004;**95**(7):708–16.
13. Borbély A, Falcao-Pires I, van Heerebeek L, et al. Hypophosphorylation of the Stiff N2B titin isoform raises cardiomyocyte resting tension in failing human myocardium. *Circ Res* 2009;**104**(6):780–6.
14. Gorelik J, Yang LQ, Zhang Y, et al. A novel Z-groove index characterizing myocardial surface structure. *Cardiovasc Res* 2006;**72**(3):422–9.
15. Gorelik J, Gu Y, Spohr HA, et al. Ion channels in small cells and subcellular structures can be studied with a smart patch-clamp system. *Biophys J* 2002;**83**(6):3296–303.
16. Song LS, Sobie EA, McCulle S, et al. Orphaned ryanodine receptors in the failing heart. *Proc Natl Acad Sci USA* 2006;**103**(11):4305–10.
17. Lyon AR, MacLeod KT, Zhang Y, et al. Loss of T-tubules and other changes to surface topography in ventricular myocytes from failing human and rat heart. *Proc Natl Acad Sci USA* 2009;**106**(16):6854–9.
18. Spinozzi S, Liu C, Chen Z, et al. Nexilin is necessary for maintaining the transverse-axial tubular system in adult cardiomyocytes. *Circ Heart Fail* 2020;**13**(7):e006935.
19. Miragoli M, Sanchez-Alonso JL, Bhargava A, et al. Microtubule-dependent mitochondria alignment regulates calcium release in response to nanomechanical stimulus in heart myocytes. *Cell Rep* 2016;**14**(1):140–51.
20. Kleber AG, Rudy Y. Basic mechanisms of cardiac impulse propagation and associated arrhythmias. *Physiol Rev* 2004;**84**(2):431–88.
21. Peters NS, Green CR, Poole-Wilson PA, Severs NJ. Reduced content of connexin43 gap junctions in ventricular myocardium from hypertrophied and ischemic human hearts. *Circulation* 1993;**88**(3):864–75.
22. Giepmans BNG. Gap junctions and connexin-interacting proteins. *Cardiovasc Res* 2004;**62**(2):233–45.
23. Ai X, Pogwizd SM. Connexin 43 downregulation and dephosphorylation in nonischemic heart failure is associated with enhanced colocalized protein phosphatase type 2A. *Circ Res* 2005;**96**(1):54–63.
24. Akar FG, Spragg DD, Tunin RS, Kass DA, Tomaselli GF. Mechanisms underlying conduction slowing and arrhythmogenesis in nonischemic dilated cardiomyopathy. *Circ Res* 2004;**95**(7):717–25.
25. Poelzing S, Rosenbaum DS. Altered connexin43 expression produces arrhythmia substrate in heart failure. *Am J Physiol Heart Circ Physiol* 2004;**287**(4):H1762–70.
26. Akar FG, Nass RD, Hahn S, et al. Dynamic changes in conduction velocity and gap junction properties during development of pacing-induced heart failure. *Am J Physiol Heart Circ Physiol* 2007;**293**(2):H1223–30.
27. Spragg DD, Akar FG, Helm RH, et al. Abnormal conduction and repolarization in late-activated myocardium of dyssynchronously contracting hearts. *Cardiovasc Res* 2005;**67**(1):77–86.
28. Lindsey ML, Mann DL, Entman ML, Spinale FG. Extracellular matrix remodeling following myocardial injury. *Ann Med* 2003;**35**(5):316–26.
29. Olivetti G, Capasso JM, Sonnenblick EH, Anversa P. Side-to-side slippage of myocytes participates in ventricular wall remodeling acutely after myocardial infarction in rats. *Circ Res* 1990;**67**(1):23–34.

30. Beltrami CA, Finato N, Rocco M, et al. Structural basis of end-stage failure in ischemic cardiomyopathy in humans. *Circulation* 1994;**89**(1):151–63.

31. Hein S, Arnon E, Kostin S, et al. Progression from compensated hypertrophy to failure in the pressure-overloaded human heart: structural deterioration and compensatory mechanisms. *Circulation* 2003;**107**(7):984–91.

32. Souders CA, Bowers SL, Baudino TA. Cardiac fibroblast: the renaissance cell. *Circ Res* 2009;**105**(12):1164–76.

33. Kostin S, Hein S, Arnon E, Scholz D, Schaper J. The cytoskeleton and related proteins in the human failing heart. *Heart Fail Rev* 2000;**5**(3):271–80.

34. Pogwizd SM, McKenzie JP, Cain ME. Mechanisms underlying spontaneous and induced ventricular arrhythmias in patients with idiopathic dilated cardiomyopathy. *Circulation* 1998;**98**(22):2404–14.

35. Chilton L, Giles W, Smith GL. Evidence of intercellular coupling between co-cultured adult rabbit ventricular myocytes and myofibroblasts. *J Physiol* 2007;**583**(Pt 1):225–36.

36. Quinn TA, Camelliti P, Rog-Zielinska EA, et al. Electrotonic coupling of excitable and nonexcitable cells in the heart revealed by optogenetics. *Proc Natl Acad Sci USA* 2016;**113**(51):14852–7.

37. Molina-Navarro MM, Rosello-Lleti E, Tarazon E, et al. Heart failure entails significant changes in human nucleocytoplasmic transport gene expression. *Int J Cardiol* 2013;**168**(3):2837–43.

38. Lohse MJ, Engelhardt S, Eschenhagen T. What is the role of beta-adrenergic signaling in heart failure? *Circ Res* 2003;**93**(10):896–906.

39. Bristow MR, Ginsburg R, Umans V, et al. B1-and B2-adrenergic receptor subpopulations in nonfailing and failing human ventricular myocardium: Coupling of both receptor subtypes to muscle contraction and selective B1-receptor down-regulation in heart failure. *Circ Res* 1986;**59**(3):297–309.

40. Harding SE, Brown LA, Wynne DG, Davies CH, Poole-Wilson PA. Mechanisms of beta-adrenoceptor desensitisation in the failing human heart. *Cardiovasc Res* 1994;**28**(10):1451–60.

41. Davies CH, Davia K, Bennett JG, et al. Reduced contraction of isolated human ventricular myocytes in ischaemic cardiomyopathy. *Circulation* 1995;**92**(9):2540–9.

42. Brown LA, Harding SE. The effect of pertussis toxin on b-adrenoceptor responses in isolated cardiac myocytes from noradrenaline-treated guinea-pigs and patients with cardiac failure. *Br J Pharmacol* 1992;**106**(1):115–22.

43. Heubach JF, Ravens U, Kaumann AJ. Epinephrine activates both Gs and Gi pathways, but norepinephrine activates only the Gs pathway through human beta2-adrenoceptors overexpressed in mouse heart. *Mol Pharmacol* 2004;**65**(5):1313–22.

44. Gong H, Sun H, Koch WJ, et al. Specific β2AR Blocker ICI 118,551 actively decreases contraction through a Gi-coupled form of the β2AR in myocytes from failing human heart. *Circulation* 2002;**105**(21):2497–503.

45. Nikolaev VO, Moshkov A, Lyon AR, et al. Beta2-adrenergic receptor redistribution in heart failure changes cAMP compartmentation. *Science* 2010;**327**(5973):1653–7.

46. Head BP, Patel HH, Roth DM, et al. G-protein-coupled receptor signaling components localize in both sarcolemmal and intracellular caveolin-3-associated microdomains in adult cardiac myocytes. *J Biol Chem* 2005;**280**(35):31036–44.

47. Wright PT, Bhogal NK, Diakonov I, et al. Cardiomyocyte membrane structure and cAMP compartmentation produce anatomical variation in beta2AR-cAMP responsiveness in murine hearts. *Cell Rep* 2018;**23**(2):459–69.

48. Geng YJ, Ishikawa Y, Vatner DE, et al. Apoptosis of cardiac myocytes in Gsalpha transgenic mice. *Circ Res* 1999;**84**(1):34–42.

49. Communal C, Singh K, Pimental D, Colucci W. Norepinephrine stimulates apoptosis in adult rat ventricular myocytes of the b-adrenergic pathway. *Circ* 1998;**98**(13):1329–34.

50. Shizukuda Y, Buttrick PM, Geenen DL, et al. Beta-adrenergic stimulation causes cardiocyte apoptosis: influence of tachycardia and hypertrophy. *Am J Physiol* 1998;**275**(3):H961–8.

51. Packer M. Neurohormonal interactions and adaptations in congestive heart failure. *Circulation* 1988;**77**(4):721–30.

52. Lyon AR, Rees PS, Prasad S, et al. Stress (takotsubo) cardiomyopathy—a novel pathophysiological hypothesis to explain catecholamine-induced acute myocardial stunning. *Nat Clin Pract Cardiovasc Med* 2008;**5**(1):22–9.

53. Hong TT, Smyth JW, Chu KY, et al. BIN1 is reduced and Cav1.2 trafficking is impaired in human failing cardiomyocytes. *Heart Rhythm* 2012;**9**(5):812–20.

54. Pieske B, Maier LS, Piacentino V, III, et al. Rate dependence of [Na$^+$]i and contractility in nonfailing and failing human myocardium. *Circulation* 2002;**106**(4):447–53.

55. Despa S, Bossuyt J, Han F, et al. Phospholemman-phosphorylation mediates the beta-adrenergic effects on Na/K pump function in cardiac myocytes. *Circ Res* 2005;**97**(3):252–9.

56. Gray RP, McIntyre H, Sheridan DS, Fry CH. Intracellular sodium and contractile function in hypertrophied human and guinea-pig myocardium. *Pflügers Arch* 2001;**442**(1):117–23.

57. Dixon IM, Hata T, Dhalla NS. Sarcolemmal Na(+)-K(+)-ATPase activity in congestive heart failure due to myocardial infarction. *Am J Physiol* 1992;**262**(3 Pt 1):C664–71.

58. Kim CH, Fan TH, Kelly PF, et al. Isoform-specific regulation of myocardial Na,K-ATPase alpha-subunit in congestive heart failure. Role of norepinephrine. *Circulation* 1994;**89**(1):313–20.

59. Shamraj OL, Grupp IL, Grupp G, et al. Characterisation of Na/K-ATPase, its isoforms, and the inotropic response to ouabain in isolated failing human hearts. *Cardiovasc Res* 1993;**27**(12):2229–37.

60. Ove Semb S, Lunde PK, Holt E, et al. Reduced myocardial Na$^+$, K$^+$-pump capacity in congestive heart failure following myocardial infarction in rats. *J Mol Cell Cardiol* 1998;**30**(7):1311–28.

61. Bossuyt J, Ai X, Moorman JR, Pogwizd SM, Bers DM. Expression and phosphorylation of the Na-pump regulatory subunit phospholemman in heart failure. *Circ Res* 2005;**97**(6):558–65.

62. Baartscheer A, Schumacher CA, van Borren MMGJ, et al. Increased Na$^+$/H$^+$-exchange activity is the cause of increased [Na$^+$]i and underlies disturbed calcium handling in the rabbit pressure and volume overload heart failure model. *Cardiovasc Res* 2003;**57**(4):1015–24.

63. Yokoyama H, Gunasegaram S, Harding SE, Avkiran N. Sarcolemmal Na$^+$/H$^+$ exchanger activity and expression in human ventricular myocardium. *J Am Coll Cardiol* 2000;**36**(2):534–40.

64. Undrovinas AI, Maltsev VA, Kyle JW, Silverman N, Sabbah HN. Gating of the late Na$^+$ channel in normal and failing human myocardium. *J Mol Cell Cardiol* 2002;**34**(11):1477–89.

65. Pogwizd SM, Sipido KR, Verdonck F, Bers DM. Intracellular Na in animal models of hypertrophy and heart failure: contractile function and arrhythmogenesis. *Cardiovasc Res* 2003;**57**(4):887–96.

66. Maack C, Cortassa S, Aon MA, et al. Elevated cytosolic Na$^+$ decreases mitochondrial Ca^{2+} uptake during excitation–contraction coupling and impairs energetic adaptation in cardiac myocytes. *Circ Res* 2006;**99**(2):172–82.

67. Ingwall JS. The hypertrophied myocardium accumulates the MB creatine-kinase isoenzyme. *Eur Heart J* 1984;**5** Suppl F:129–39.

68. Beer M, Seyfarth T, Sandstede J, *et al.* Absolute concentrations of high-energy phosphate metabolites in normal, hypertrophied, and failing human myocardium measured noninvasively with (31)P-SLOOP magnetic resonance spectroscopy. *J Am Coll Cardiol* 2002;**40**(7):1267–74.

69. Ide T, Tsutsui H, Kinugawa S, *et al.* Direct evidence for increased hydroxyl radicals originating from superoxide in the failing myocardium. *Circ Res* 2000;**86**(2):152–7.

70. Ide T, Tsutsui H, Kinugawa S, *et al.* Mitochondrial electron transport complex I is a potential source of oxygen free radicals in the failing myocardium. *Circ Res* 1999;**85**(4):357–63.

71. Yan Y, Liu J, Wei C, *et al.* Bidirectional regulation of Ca2+ sparks by mitochondria-derived reactive oxygen species in cardiac myocytes. *Cardiovasc Res* 2008;**77**(2):432–41.

72. Tarazon E, Rivera M, Rosello-Lleti E, *et al.* Heart failure induces significant changes in nuclear pore complex of human cardiomyocytes. *PLoS One* 2012;**7**(11):e48957.

73. Chahine MN, Mioulane M, Sikkel MB, *et al.* Nuclear pore rearrangements and nuclear trafficking in cardiomyocytes from rat and human failing hearts. *Cardiovasc Res* 2015;**105**(1):31–43.

74. Razeghi P, Young ME, Alcorn JL, *et al.* Metabolic gene expression in fetal and failing human heart. *Circulation* 2001;**104**(24):2923–31.

75. Depre C, Kim SJ, John AS, *et al.* Program of cell survival underlying human and experimental hibernating myocardium. *Circ Res* 2004;**95**(4):433–40.

76. Thum T, Galuppo P, Wolf C, *et al.* MicroRNAs in the human heart: a clue to fetal gene reprogramming in heart failure. *Circulation* 2007;**116**(3):258–67.

77. Kumarswamy R, Lyon AR, Volkmann I, *et al.* SERCA2a gene therapy restores microRNA-1 expression in heart failure via an Akt/FoxO3A-dependent pathway. *Eur Heart J* 2012;**33**(9):1067–75.

78. Castaldi A, Zaglia T, Di M, *et al.* MicroRNA-133 modulates the beta1-adrenergic receptor transduction cascade. *Circ Res* 2014;**115**(2):273–83.

79. Lorenzen JM, Thum T. Long noncoding RNAs in kidney and cardiovascular diseases. *Nat Rev Nephrol* 2016;**12**(6):360–73.

80. Uchida S, Dimmeler S. Long noncoding RNAs in cardiovascular diseases. *Circ Res* 2015;**116**(4):737–50.

81. Soonpaa MH, Field LJ. Survey of studies examining mammalian cardiomyocyte DNA synthesis. *Circ Res* 1998;**83**(1):15–26.

82. Narula J, Haider N, Virmani R, *et al.* Apoptosis in myocytes in end-stage heart failure. *N Engl J Med* 1996;**335**(16):1182–9.

83. Diwan A, Krenz M, Syed FM, *et al.* Inhibition of ischemic cardiomyocyte apoptosis through targeted ablation of Bnip3 restrains postinfarction remodeling in mice. *J Clin Invest* 2007;**117**(10):2825–33.

84. Lee Y, Gustafsson AB. Role of apoptosis in cardiovascular disease. *Apoptosis* 2009;**14**(4):536–48.

85. Taylor RC, Cullen SP, Martin SJ. Apoptosis: controlled demolition at the cellular level. *Nat Rev Mol Cell Biol* 2008;**9**(3):231–41.

86. Communal C, Sumandea M, de Tombe P, *et al.* Functional consequences of caspase activation in cardiac myocytes. *Proc Natl Acad Sci USA* 2002;**99**(9):6252–6.

87. Wencker D, Chandra M, Nguyen K, *et al.* A mechanistic role for cardiac myocyte apoptosis in heart failure. *J Clin Invest* 2003;**111**(10):1497–504.

88. Halestrap AP. What is the mitochondrial permeability transition pore? *J Mol Cell Cardiol* 2009;**46**(6):821–31.

89. Kirshenbaum LA, de Moissac D. The bcl-2 gene product prevents programmed cell death of ventricular myocytes. *Circulation* 1997;**96**(5):1580–5.

90. Syed F, Odley A, Hahn HS, *et al.* Physiological growth synergizes with pathological genes in experimental cardiomyopathy. *Circ Res* 2004;**95**(12):1200–6.

91. Sharma PP, Greenlee RT, Anderson KP, *et al.* Prevalence and mortality of patients with myocardial infarction and reduced left ventricular ejection fraction in a defined community: relation to the second multicenter automatic defibrillator implantation trial. *J Interv Card Electrophysiol* 2007;**19**(3):157–64.

92. Okada K, Minamino T, Tsukamoto Y, *et al.* Prolonged endoplasmic reticulum stress in hypertrophic and failing heart after aortic constriction: possible contribution of endoplasmic reticulum stress to cardiac myocyte apoptosis. *Circulation* 2004;**110**(6):705–12.

93. Del Monte F, Hajjar RJ. Intracellular devastation in heart failure. *Heart Fail Rev* 2008;**13**(2):151–62.

94. Ozcan U, Yilmaz E, Ozcan L, *et al.* Chemical chaperones reduce ER stress and restore glucose homeostasis in a mouse model of type 2 diabetes. *Science* 2006;**313**(5790):1137–40.

95. Tsukamoto O, Minamino T, Okada K, *et al.* Depression of proteasome activities during the progression of cardiac dysfunction in pressure-overloaded heart of mice. *Biochem Biophys Res Commun* 2006;**340**(4):1125–33.

96. Predmore JM, Wang P, Davis F, *et al.* Ubiquitin proteasome dysfunction in human hypertrophic and dilated cardiomyopathies. *Circulation* 2010;**121**(8):997–1004.

97. Tannous P, Zhu H, Johnstone JL, *et al.* Autophagy is an adaptive response in desmin-related cardiomyopathy. *Proc Natl Acad Sci USA* 2008;**105**(28):9745–50.

98. Nishida K, Yamaguchi O, Otsu K. Crosstalk between autophagy and apoptosis in heart disease. *Circ Res* 2008;**103**(4):343–51.

99. Haider N, Arbustini E, Gupta S, *et al.* Concurrent upregulation of endogenous proapoptotic and antiapoptotic factors in failing human hearts. *Nat Clin Pract Cardiovasc Med* 2009;**6**(3):250–61.

RECOMMENDED READING LIST

Davis J, Davis LC, Correll RN, *et al.* A tension-based model distinguishes hypertrophic versus dilated cardiomyopathy. *Cell* 2016;**165**(5):1147–59.

Nikolaev VO, Moshkov A, Lyon AR, *et al.* Beta2-adrenergic receptor redistribution in heart failure changes cAMP compartmentation. *Science* 2010;**327**(5973):1653–7.

Severs NJ. The cardiac muscle cell. *Bioessays* 2000;**22**(2):188–99.

19

The interstitium and collagen in heart failure

Anne Pizard and Faiez Zannad

Introduction

By definition, the interstitium represents the space between the specialized cells of a tissue. The interstitial compartment is about four times the size of the plasma compartment in the human body and has the unique property of being in close proximity to active specialized cells (such as myocytes, hepatocytes, podocytes, and neurons). It is the site of constant exchanges of fluid, proteins, and electrolytes, which vary depending on the pathophysiological state of an individual. The composition and abundance of the interstitium is of major importance as it participates in the normal physiological function of every organ. In the heart, the cardiac interstitium plays an instrumental role in dynamic myocyte activity (particularly calcium flux) and the plasticity, elasticity, and turgor of the interstitium are vital to allow the cardiac chambers to reach their optimal contractile and relaxation states.

The interstitium is a very dynamic and malleable compartment. Its conformation is determined by the balance between the synthesis and degradation of its components as well as by its capacity for fluid retention. Its stiffness is dependent on the activity of extracellular matrix regulators. In physiological and pathological circumstances, the particular composition of the matrisome—defined as being *all* the components constituting the extracellular matrix (ECM) and all the factors associated with it—makes it a key player in the preservation of health and in the adaptation to various stresses.

Structure of the interstitium

The interstitium is a complex compartment in which interstitial fluid (ISF) and many different types of insoluble molecules (forming the ECM) undergo constant alterations to fulfil physiological needs. The boundary structure of the interstitium is delineated by the cell membrane—which is selectively permeable to specific ions and organic molecules—and the walls of blood vessels present in each organ. Both serve as attachment surfaces for the ECM and thus participate in the modelling of the geometry of the interstitium.

Interstitial fluid

The fluid of the interstitium bathes and surrounds specialized cells that use it as nutrient-supplying medium but also as a conduit for waste and as a biological compartment where electrical impulse conduction and propagation occur. It is formed by transcapillary filtration of plasma fluid and is drained by many lymphatic vessels. This aqueous medium contains ions, gaseous and organic molecules, as well as proteins (hormones, enzymes, and small peptides) and extracellular vesicles resulting from budding from cellular membranes.

This is a place of high and constant traffic where cells can communicate across the ISF by three modes: (i) free diffusion, where molecules disperse freely from one cell to another depending upon the concentration gradient of the signalling molecule; (ii) hindered diffusion, because of obstacles or transient binding interactions with components of the ECM; and (iii) facilitated diffusion, where regulators enhance the movement of specific signals.[1]

The flow of molecules through the ISF is greatly influenced by the balance between hydraulic conductance (defined as the flow of a fluid per unit pressure decrease across a unit area of the interstitial fluid) and the hydraulic resistance (the opposite of conductance). The size of the molecules being transported through the interstitial space is also a determinant of flow. Large molecules are slowed down by mechanical hindrance, the importance of which is very much dependent on the shape of the insoluble net-like component of the interstitium (that is, the ECM).[1] The fluid volume in the interstitial space is normally regulated within narrow limits by automatic readjustment of the interstitial hydrostatic and colloid osmotic pressures in response to perturbations in capillary filtration and by the lymphatics. This has been expertly reviewed elsewhere.[2]

The properties of the ISF responsible for the flow and transportation of molecules in the extracellular space are inextricably intertwined with the properties of components of the ECM. Importantly, ISF volume is also determined by the composition of the ECM in that proteoglycans and glycosaminoglycans have great capacity to bind water and form hydrated matrices resistant to compressive forces.[1]

Matrisome

The geometry of the interstitium undergoes alterations during the development, maturation, and ageing of the organism.[3] These changes are related to the organization and reorganization of an organ depending on the migration and differentiation of its specialized cells, adaptation to specific signalling, and composition of its matrisome. At any time in the myocardium, each cardiomyocyte contraction is accompanied with fine-tuned regulations of the volume and composition of the surrounding interstitium.

Core components of the extracellular matrix

The ECM is a fundamental insoluble component of the matrisome which provides architectural support and anchorage for the cells. The ECM consists of a complex meshwork of cross-linked structural and non-structural proteins. Although the insoluble nature of most of its constituents makes its biochemical characterization challenging, the completion of genome sequences allows a reasonably complete definition of the ECM proteins (Table 19.1).[4] The classification of the proteins is based on the inventory of shared functional domains. The resulting characteristic domain-based organization helps to define or exclude a protein from being categorized as an ECM protein. In mammals, the ECM comprises around 300 proteins, including 43 collagen subunits, 35 proteoglycans, and around 200 glycoproteins (Table 19.1).

Collagens are the main proteins of the ECM giving structural integrity to tissues. The fibrillar types of collagen (collagens I–III, IV and XI) provide tensile strength to the ECM that limits the distensibility of tissues. Of the total collagen protein in the heart, approximately 85% is of type I (forming thick fibres) and 11% of type III

collagen (forming thin fibers which maintain the elasticity of the matrix network).

Proteoglycans (aggrecan, versican, perlecan and decorin, Table 19.1) are proteins interspersed among collagen fibrils not only to fill the extracellular interstitial space but also to confer hydration by sequestering water within the tissue. Proteoglycans are both the major structural components of the ECM and the first endothelial layer (the endothelial glycocalyx). They are core proteins to which *glycosaminoglycan* (GAG) side chains are attached. GAGs are linear polymers of disaccharide units that are modified by sulfation and/or acetylation and/or deacetylation and have fixed negative charges. The polyanionic nature of the GAG network leads to electrostatic interactions with different molecules, particularly sodium ions. GAGs, especially heparin sulphates, also bind growth factors and sequester them in the ECM. GAGs create a high osmotic pressure environment.

When the interstitial GAG network is denser, *glycoproteins* (elastin, fibronectins, laminins, thrombospondins, and tenascins) not only participate in the assembly of the ECM but also contribute to the interactions between the ECM and cells, by acting as ligands for cell-surface receptors such as integrins. The latter transduce signals that regulate adhesion, migration, proliferation, differentiation, and apoptosis. Three useful databases provide information on the expression and distribution of various ECM proteins[5,6] and on interactions among ECM proteins.[7]

Matrisome-associated proteins

Table 19.1 summarizes a partial list of the matrisome-associated proteins.[8] The proteins can be classified as ECM-affiliated proteins,

Table 19.1 Matrisome composition

Core matrisome						
Glycoproteins (200[a])		GAGS	Proteoglycans (35[a])			
Prototypical matricellular proteins	Fibres	Hyaluronan	Hyalectans	Basement membrane proteoglycans	Small leucine-rich proteoglycans	
Fibronectin Laminin Thrombospondin SPARC Tenascin Osteopontin Periostin CCN Agrin Nidogen	Collagens (43a) Fibrillar col. III, col. V, col. XI Non-fibrillar elastins (not glysocylated) Fibulin Fibrillin EMILIN	Heparin sulfate, chondroitin sulfate, dermatan sulfate, keratin sulfate	Aggrecan Brevican Neurocan Versican	Perlecan Collagen XVIII Agrin	Class I: biglycan, decorin, asporin Class II: lumican, fibromodulin, PRELP, kerotocan, osteoadherin Class III: osteoglycin, epiphycan, optican Class IV: chondroadherin, nyctalopin, Tsukushi Class V: podocan, podocan-like protein 1	
Matrisome associated proteins						
ECM-affiliated proteins (176[a])		ECM regulators (250[a])			Secreted factors (352[a])	
Cell surface proteoglycans Syndecan, glypican, mucins, c-type lectins Secreted factors associated with solid phase complex Semaphorins and their homologous receptor, galectins, annexins		ECM cross-linking lysyl oxidases, transglutaminases, adamalysins (ADAMs and ADAMTS) ECM-modifying enzymes sulfatases, extracellular kinases, heparinises, serpins Proteases MMPs, cathepsins, serpins, etc., and their inhibitors TIMPs, cystatins			TGFβ Growth factors VEGF, FGF, HGF, PDGF, GDF BMPs Wnts Cytokines IL-1, IL-4, IL-6, IL-10, IL-13	

ADAMTS, desintegrin and metalloprotease with thrombospondin motifs; BMP, bone morphogenic protein; CCN, cellular communication network proteins; col., collagen; EMILIN, elastin microfibril interface-located protein; FGF, fibroblast growth factor; GAG, glycosaminoglycans; GDF, growth differentiation factor; HGF, hepatocyte growth factor; IL, interleukin; MMP, matrix metalloproteinase; PDGF, platelet-derived growth factor; PRELP, proline/arginine-rich end leucine-rich repeat protein; SPARC, secreted protein acidic and rich in cysteine; TGF, transforming growth factor; TIMPs, tissue inhibitor of metalloproteinases; VEGF, vascular endothelial growth factor.
[a]Gene count corrected for pseudo/non-coding genes in human.[8,10]

ECM regulators (such as proteases or cross-linking enzymes) and as secreted factors such as growth factors and cytokines. The net-like structure of the matrisome is based on the interaction of the matrisome proteins with each other and their interaction with affiliated proteins. The balance between synthesis, degradation, post-translational modifications, and cross-linking of ECM components is enabled by associated proteins, the activity of which undoubtedly contributes to the insolubility of ECM (Figure 19.1). Thus procollagen propeptidases are necessary to process collagens so that they can polymerize into mature collagen molecules.[9] Collagen fibrils, laminin, and other basement membrane proteins are cross-linked by disulfide bonding. Collagens and other core matrisome proteins are also substrates for matrix metalloproteases (MMPs), adamalysins, and transglutaminases.

Adamalysins are proteases, and many other proteolytic enzymes (including elastases and cathepsins) play a role.[10] Interestingly, the various proteolytic processes, by affecting ECM turnover, trigger the release of ECM-bound molecules including growth factors, cytokines, mucins, secreted C-type lectins, galectins, semaphorins, and plexins. Similarly, enzymes that degrade GAGs, such as heparanases and sulfatases, can also alter the properties of ECM proteoglycans. Thus the basal activity of the proteases and growth factors associated

with the matrisome participate in the maintenance of the ECM, while their activation following injury plays an important role in cardiac remodelling.

Associated cells

Although the functional specialized cells attract the most attention, the cardiac interstitium contains several distinct cell types. Interstitial cells are enmeshed in the matrisome and continuously sense the slightest alterations in their microenvironment (including pressure variations, sodium concentration variation, alteration of protease, and growth factor concentration and activation following injury) (Figure 19.2). Cardiac fibroblasts are the most abundant cell type in the mammalian heart and comprise approximately two-thirds of the total number of cardiac cells. During development, epicardial cells undergo epithelial–mesenchymal transition to generate cardiac fibroblasts which subsequently migrate into the developing myocardium to become resident cardiac fibroblasts.

In the adult heart under physiological conditions, cardiac fibroblasts remain quiescent with no significant inflammatory or proliferative activity, but they play an important role in forming and preserving the integrity of the matrix network. They are the predominant matrix-producing cells in the myocardium. Vascular cells (smooth muscle cells, endothelial cells, and pericytes) are also abundant in the cardiac interstitium, unlike immune cells (mast cells and macrophages), of which relatively small numbers reside in the mammalian heart under physiological conditions, usually localized around vessels.[11]

Pathological expansion of the interstitium

Whereas fluid overload has been associated with increased morbidity and mortality, here we focus on the pathological expansion of the interstitium due to the excessive accumulation of ECM proteins in the myocardium.

Myocardial fibrosis

Fibrosis is characterized by net accumulation of ECM and scleroderma represents its most severe form.[12] Myocardial fibrosis occurs spontaneously during ageing and its impact on myocardial structure and function has been extensively reviewed. Age positively correlates with the severity of atrial fibrosis and apoptosis, which provides the structural substrate facilitating the occurrence of atrial fibrillation through greater conduction disturbances.[13] Excessive myocardial fibrosis develops when collagen homeostasis becomes dysregulated secondary to alteration in the function and/or concentration of one or more of the players in the matrisome (Table 19.1). The impact of variables such as fibre diameter, fibre volume fraction, and organization (collagen cross-linking) become important factors in determining the trafficking of particles through the interstitium. Because it disrupts the exchanges within the interstitium,[1] the development of excessive fibrosis results in altered mechanical, electrical, and vasomotor properties that promote the development of heart failure, arrhythmias, and ischaemia. In the myocardium, ECM expansion via fibrosis results in many clinical features, including PR interval prolongation, bundle branch and heart block, atrial fibrillation, ventricular arrhythmia, as well as systolic and diastolic function.

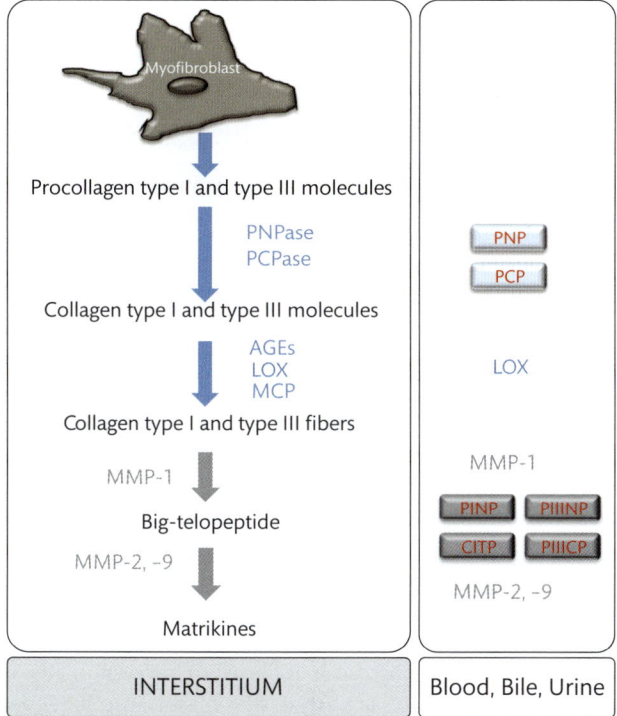

Figure 19.1 Schematic representation of the collagen homeostasis: synthesis and degradation of fibrillar collagen-derived peptides and associated biomarkers. PNPase and PCPase, procollagen N- and C-terminal proteinases; AGEs, advanced glycation end-products; LOX, lysyl oxidase; MCP, matricellular proteins; MMP, matrix metalloproteinase; PICP, procollagen type I carboxyterminal propeptide; PINP, procollagen type I amino-terminal propeptide; CITP, collagen type I cross-linked carboxy-terminal telopeptide; PIIICP, procollagen type III carboxy-terminal propeptide, PIIINP, procollagen type III amino-terminal propeptide. In blue: steps implicated in the synthesis of collagen I and III fibres. In grey: steps implicated in the degradation of collagen I and III fibres.

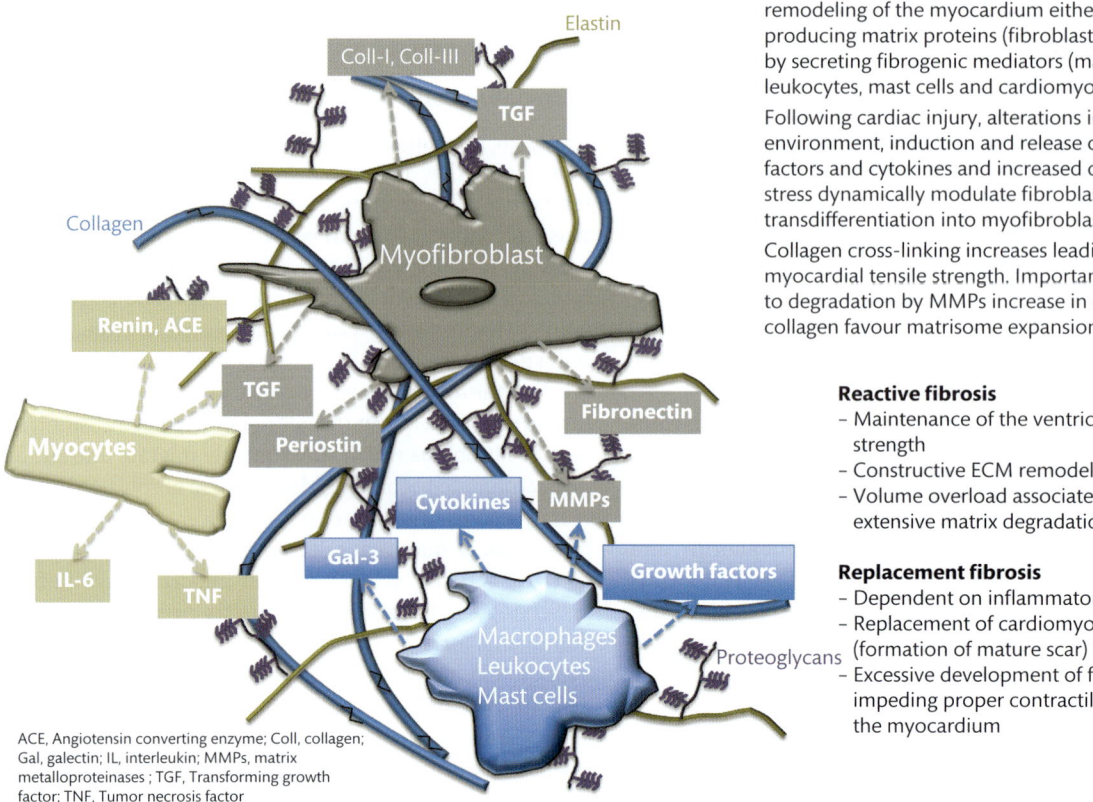

Several cell types are implicated in fibrotic remodeling of the myocardium either directly by producing matrix proteins (fibroblasts), or indirectly by secreting fibrogenic mediators (macrophages, leukocytes, mast cells and cardiomyocytes).

Following cardiac injury, alterations in the matrix environment, induction and release of growth factors and cytokines and increased of mechanical stress dynamically modulate fibroblast transdifferentiation into myofibroblasts.

Collagen cross-linking increases leading to increased myocardial tensile strength. Importantly by resisting to degradation by MMPs increase in cross-linked collagen favour matrisome expansion.

Reactive fibrosis
– Maintenance of the ventricule tensile strength
– Constructive ECM remodeling
– Volume overload associated with extensive matrix degradation

Replacement fibrosis
– Dependent on inflammatory reaction
– Replacement of cardiomyocyte loss (formation of mature scar)
– Excessive development of fibrosis impeding proper contractile function of the myocardium

ACE, Angiotensin converting enzyme; Coll, collagen; Gal, galectin; IL, interleukin; MMPs, matrix metalloproteinases ; TGF, Transforming growth factor; TNF, Tumor necrosis factor

Figure 19.2 Cardiac fibrosis development players.

Two distinct patterns of cardiac collagen tissue accumulation exist: reactive fibrosis and reparative fibrosis.

Reactive fibrosis develops progressively (as compared to reparative fibrosis) in the interstitial and perivascular space without notable cell loss. In ageing hearts,[14] cardiomyocyte loss is associated with cardiac fibrosis and therefore with expansion of the interstitium. Increased collagen deposition leads to progressive increase in ventricular stiffness. Diabetes and obesity are associated with acceleration and accentuation of fibrotic myocardial changes.[15] Stresses such as myocardial ischaemia, hypertensive heart disease, aortic valve stenosis, and hypertrophic cardiomyopathy can trigger its development.

Cardiac fibroblasts have long been viewed as the major producers of ECM during the fibrotic process. Several potential sources of cardiac myofibroblasts have been proposed (including circulating and resident fibroblasts, epicardial epithelial cells undergoing epithelial-to-mesenchymal transition, and endothelial-to-mesenchymal transdifferentiation).[11] All lead to cardiac myofibroblasts which are very sensitive to a wide variety of stimuli that affect their proliferative response depending on the pathological context. More recently, an important role for a population of bone marrow-derived cells—named fibrocytes—has been revealed in the control of cardiac fibrosis. Sharing the features of both monocytes and fibroblasts, fibrocytes contribute to tissue remodelling in response to pathological stress. Studies have demonstrated that age-related cardiac fibrosis and diastolic dysfunction coincide with accumulation of fibrocytes in the ventricular interstitial space.[16]

Reparative fibrosis, or replacement fibrosis, takes place in response to tissue injury to compensate for cardiomyocyte loss (after acute myocardial infarction, MI). Following MI, remodelling of the myocardium requires angiogenesis, myocyte hypertrophy, and fibroblast proliferation. Fibroblast activation and proliferation early after cardiac injury are necessary mechanisms critical for maintaining cardiac integrity and function, while the persistence of fibroblasts long after injury leads to chronic scarring and adverse ventricular remodelling. During MI with necrosis of myofibrils, there is stimulation of satellite cells (mostly macrophages), which can initiate tissue repair. The repair process appears to be highly dependent on the effects of transforming growth factor-β (TGFβ), interleukin-6 (IL-6), and fibroblast growth factor (FGF) (**Figure 19.2**).

The relative contribution of the various cell types is often dependent on the underlying cause of fibrosis. However, in all conditions associated with cardiac fibrosis, fibroblast transdifferentiation into secretory and contractile cells, termed myofibroblasts, is the key cellular event that drives the fibrotic response.[11] In any case where cardiac fibrosis develops, the integrity of the myocardium is maintained by the myofibroblasts[17] which accumulate at the site of the injury. They combine the expression of smooth muscle actin microfilaments characteristic of smooth muscle cells with the appearance of an extensive, synthetically active endoplasmic reticulum.[18]

Inflammatory cells and myofibroblasts are both involved in the initiation and formation of a secretome produced at the site of cardiomyocyte necrosis to regulate matrix turnover (**Figure 19.1**).

6

Myocardial fibrosis occurs when synthesis of fibrillar collagen types I and III predominates over their degradation (which is usually either unchanged or decreased). More specifically, an excess of highly cross-linked thick collagen type I fibres relative to poorly cross-linked thin collagen type III fibres is typical of adverse fibrosis. Recent studies have identified molecules involved in extracellular procollagen processing (such as procollagen proteinases) and collagen assembly (LOX and matricellular proteins) which determine the fibrotic response of the myocardium to an injury, along with changes in MMP type and activity that directly influence the myocardial collagen network.

Although cardiac myofibroblasts are the main effector cells, monocytes/macrophages, lymphocytes, mast cells, vascular cells, and cardiomyocytes may also contribute. Inflammatory cytokines and chemokines, reactive oxygen species (ROS), mast cell-derived proteases, hormones, and growth factors are some of the best-studied mediators of myocardial fibrosis.[11]

Detection of fibrosis

Direct histological assessment

So far, the reference standard methods for evaluating the distribution of myocardial fibrosis (that is, focal, interstitial or perivascular) and its quality remain the staining of biopsies from human tissue using histochemicals—particularly hydroxyproline, Sirius Red A—and immunohistochemistry. Although performing a biopsy of the myocardium is becoming technically easier with the improvement of minimally invasive endovascular instruments, it still puts the patient at risk. To avoid this, biomedical research is developing techniques that move away from biopsies with the aim of safely supporting clinical diagnostics.

Surrogate markers of fibrosis development

Given the importance of cardiac fibrosis in leading to myocardial dysfunction, non-invasive assessment of fibrosis would be a clinically useful tool. Two main options are available at present to assess the fibrosis non-invasively: imaging and measurement of circulating biomarkers both have advantages and disadvantages.

Cardiac magnetic resonance (CMR)[19,20] can identify focal irreversible replacement fibrosis with a high degree of accuracy and reproducibility as well as giving an assessment of cardiac structure and function. CMR is not yet as accurate in assessing the magnitude of diffuse interstitial fibrosis as histologic assessment.[21] It is, however, frequently promoted as a potential surrogate for cardiac fibrosis, potentially useful for stratifying the risk of sudden cardiac death. Ultrasound speckle-tracking and heart strain assessments are also being investigated as potential surrogates for cardiac fibrosis.[22]

Biomarkers from the ECM found in body fluids (most commonly in blood and urine[23]) are able to detect early changes in the structure and function of the heart and large vessels and the transition to heart failure: increased levels of the biomarkers are associated with worse outcome in patients with heart failure.[24] The measurement of various serum peptides arising from the metabolism of collagen types I and III may provide information on the extent of myocardial fibrosis.

Procollagen type I C-terminal propeptide (PICP), amino terminal propeptides of type-I procollagen (PINP), and N-terminal type III collagen peptide (PIIINP) are released with collagen I or III molecules in a stoichiometric manner during collagen biosynthesis, and so are markers of this process (Figure 19.1). Because fibrosis results from a reduction in the ratio of degradation to production of collagen fibre, the ratio of PICP to collagen type I carboxy-terminal telopeptide (CITP) in serum may serve as a marker of myocardial collagen accumulation.

Biomarkers of myofibroblast proliferation have been sought among their secretome; unfortunately those markers are not specific to the myocardium. Novel, more specific, biomarkers are needed to identify specific pathways of disease progression. Recent preclinical and clinical studies have discovered other molecules alongside TGFβ—inflammatory cytokines (such as IL-6), platelet-derived growth factor (PDGF) and connective tissue growth factor (CCN2, i.e. CTGF)—that could serve as surrogate biomarkers of cardiac fibrosis.[25,26] They include: CD28, CD69, tissue inhibitor of metalloproteinases (TIMP)-1, pentraxin-3, chitinase 3-like protein 3, as well as thrombospondin, cardiotrophin 1, galectin-3 (Gal-3), suppression of tumorigenicity 2 ST2, NADH oxidases, neutrophil gelatinase associates lipocalin, as well as microRNAs.[9]

Among them, Gal-3 seems particularly promising. It is a soluble β-galactoside-binding lectin which binds to and activates fibroblasts, thus leading to the deposition of collagen in the ECM and to progressive cardiac fibrosis. Because gal-3 expression is maximal at peak fibrosis and virtually absent after recovery, routine measurement in patients with heart failure may prove valuable in identifying those patients at highest risk for readmission or death, thus enabling physicians to tailor the level of care to individual patient needs.[27]

Similarly, cardiotrophin-1 may be a potential biomarker of myocardial fibrosis[9] in patients with heart failure as its cardiac level is associated with both excessive production of mature collagen I and III molecules and increased deposition of collagen I and III fibres.[28] ST2 is a member of the IL-1 receptor family, which was initially described in the context of cell proliferation, inflammatory states, and autoimmune diseases.[26] ST2 includes two forms: a membrane-bound (ST2L) and a soluble ST2 form (sST2) that share a common functional ligand, IL-33. The activation of ST2 by IL-33 mediates beneficial effects, including resistance to apoptosis and reduction in fibrosis.

Therapeutic opportunities for targeting fibrosis

Preclinical and clinical data suggest that mitigating or preventing ECM expansion may be important components of therapeutic success in patients with heart failure. Collagen regression occurs in humans after treatment with angiotensin converting enzyme (ACE) inhibitors,[24,29,30] angiotensin receptor antagonists, and mineralocorticoid receptor antagonists.[31-33] These agents, of course, improved outcomes in landmark large-scale trials with longer treatment duration. Renin–angiotensin–aldosterone system (RAAS) activation occurs in the myocardium, and RAAS modulators improve survival regardless of blood pressure-lowering effects, even in the absence of clinical heart failure. Patients with heart failure appear to benefit most from mineralocorticoid receptor antagonism if there is underlying myocardial fibrosis.[34,35]

Novel approaches targeting growth factors such as TGFβ, the ROS system or the endothelin system have been evaluated. However, these therapeutic approaches have effects (and unwanted side-effects)

other than simply preventing the development of fibrosis in the heart. Given the vital roles played by those pathways in homeostatic and reparative processes, long-term therapy may be challenging.

Novel biomarkers are required to act as a tool for therapeutic tailoring

There has been a dramatic improvement in treatment for heart failure with reduced ejection fraction, but heart failure is a clinically and pathophysiologically heterogeneous syndrome. Better biomarkers are still needed to improve screening, refine diagnosis, and guide molecularly targeted therapy, and, perhaps, eventually to help monitor therapeutic response. The term 'theragnostics' has been coined to describe formally a strategy that combines diagnostic tests with therapeutic interventions. Theragnostics covers a range of approaches such as pretreatment identification of subgroups of patient who are likely to respond to therapy or who are at higher risk of drug side-effects; and for monitoring drug efficacy and safety once treatment is commenced.

The ability of treatment to reduce myocardial fibrosis in patients with heart failure may be monitored by the measurement of various serum peptides arising from the metabolism of collagen types. Pharmacological agents may selectively influence biomarkers. Changes in biomarkers of collagen synthesis and degradation suggest that extracellular matrix remodelling is an active process in patients with congestive heart failure and left ventricular systolic dysfunction after acute myocardial infarction.[33]

Genetic disorders, toxin exposures, infections, inflammation, chronic metabolic diseases, and structural heart disease are all drivers of the development of interstitial heart disease.[17] It is appealing to dissect each and all of these pathways in order to find the most promising target molecules that sit at the nexus of multiple pro-fibrotic signalling networks.

Fibrosis pathways as potential biotargets

Novel potential targets for the treatment of cardiac fibrosis have been suggested or are currently under investigation.[9,36] Among them, an epigenetic approach targeting histone deacetylases (HDACs) is particularly promising. HDACs remove acetyl groups from lysine residues in thousands of proteins, thus placing them at a nexus of multiple pro-fibrotic signalling pathways.[37] Selective inhibitors of the zinc-dependent HDAC isoforms (using zinc chelators) suppress cardiac fibrosis, suggesting that they may be viable therapeutic options targeting cardiac fibrosis.[38]

Serelaxin is a recombinant form of the human ligand of relaxin receptor. Alone and in combination with an ACE inhibitor, it ameliorates fibrosis more effectively than ACE inhibition alone.[40]

Other emerging possibilities targeting myocardial fibrosis involve micro-ribonucleic acid (miRNA) antagonists and stem cells. The transcripts of matrisome molecules such as collagen, versican, and fibronectin are targeted by several miRNAs.[41] MiRNAs also regulate the levels of the transcript expression of matrisome-associated molecules as such TIMPs and MMPs.[41] Upregulation of specific miRNAs related to myocardial fibrosis has been found in animal models and in end-stage heart failure in humans.[42] Antagomir treatment using specific miRNA-21 antagonists has been successful in reducing myocardial fibrosis and heart failure in a murine pressure

overload model. MicroRNA manipulation should be developed further as a novel treatment strategy in the prevention of LV remodelling and heart failure.[43]

Yet to be proven effective for reducing fibrosis, stem cell therapy may be another option to improve the function of infarcted myocardium through the attenuation of the increase in cardiac expression of collagen types I and III and TGFβ. There is growing evidence supporting the hypothesis that paracrine mechanisms mediated by factors released by mesenchymal and bone marrow stem cells may contribute to infarct healing.[44] Using multiple cell lines in both animal and human validation experiments, cardiotrophin-1, apelin, non-structural ECM proteins, and several microRNAs have all been implicated in the development of myocardial interstitial fibrosis. These are all potential novel targets for the prevention or treatment of fibrosis.[9,20] Although these promising new options are either under evaluation or will be soon evaluated in humans, we need a better understanding of the underlying mechanisms triggered/targeted by their use to refine their specificity, to improve their mode of delivery and to give a clear understanding of their potential toxicity, both short and long term.

Conclusion and perspectives

From organogenesis to ageing, the myocardium undergoes remodelling of the interstitium that participates dynamically to myocardial compliance and performance. The abnormal expansion of the interstitium by fibrotic remodelling is an adaptive response to ageing and pathological stresses such as myocardial infarction. The development of non-invasive imaging together with biomarkers has improved the detection of alterations in the interstitium, resulting in better patient characterization. However, the mechanisms through which collagen accumulation and cross-linking increase need to be further elucidated to identify the origin of pathological alteration.

The 'omic' approaches have already refined our understanding of the players involved in the core matrisome associated-proteins, suggesting a list of potential targets for anti-fibrotic drugs. The better understanding of the pathologic processes will offer more therapeutic options. The ECM being ubiquitous, the ideal cardiovascular anti-fibrotic treatments should have an organ-specific mode of action and target specifically the unwanted fibrosis development without affecting the integrity of connective tissues and the reparative fibrosis needed for post-injury tissue healing.

The goal for biomarker research should be to provide clinicians with tools to stratify their patients according to the mechanisms of collagen accumulation and to the severity of the alteration.[45] Monitoring the efficacy of treatment using easily accessible circulating biomarkers/biotargets, supported by imaging to assess the impact on the heart, is a further target. Because fibrosis is a common consequence of both inflammation and endothelial dysfunction related to oxidative stress in ageing, hypertension, diabetes mellitus, obesity, ischaemia, and organ injury, it plays a key role in the pathophysiology of both heart and kidney. The search for novel biotargets should include antifibrotic targets for patients on the cardiorenal syndrome continuum.

REFERENCES

1. Fan D, Creemers EE, Kassiri Z. Matrix as an interstitial transport system. *Circ Res* 2014;**114**(5):889–902.
2. Reed RK, Rubin K. Transcapillary exchange: role and importance of the interstitial fluid pressure and the extracellular matrix. *Cardiovasc Res* 2010;**87**(2):211–17.
3. Bowers SL, Banerjee I, Baudino TA. The extracellular matrix: at the center of it all. *J Mol Cell Cardiol* 2010;**48**(3):474–82.
4. Hynes RO, Naba A. Overview of the matrisome—an inventory of extracellular matrix constituents and functions. *Cold Spring Harb Perspect Biol* 2012;**4**(1):a004903.
5. http://www.matrixome.com/bm/Home/home/home.asp
6. Human Protein Atlas; http://www.proteinatlas.org/
7. MatrixDB; http://matrixdb.ibcp.fr/
8. Naba A, Clauser KR, Hoersch S, et al. The matrisome: in silico definition and in vivo characterization by proteomics of normal and tumor extracellular matrices. *Mol Cell Proteomics* 2012;**11**(4):M111 014647.
9. Heymans S, Gonzalez A, Pizard A, et al. Searching for new mechanisms of myocardial fibrosis with diagnostic and/or therapeutic potential. *Eur J Heart Fail* 2015;**17**(8):764–71.
10. Bonnans C, Chou J, Werb Z. Remodelling the extracellular matrix in development and disease. *Nat Rev Mol Cell Biol* 2014;**15**(12):786–801.
11. Kong P, Christia P, Frangogiannis NG. The pathogenesis of cardiac fibrosis. *Cell Mol Life Sci* 2014;**71**(4):549–74.
12. Gasparovic H, Cikes M, Kopjar T, et al. Atrial apoptosis and fibrosis adversely affect atrial conduit, reservoir and contractile functions. *Interact Cardiovasc Thorac Surg* 2014;**19**(2):223–30; discussion 230.
13. Nicolosi PA, Tombetti E, Maugeri N, et al. Vascular remodelling and mesenchymal transition in systemic sclerosis. *Stem Cells Int* 2016;**2016**:4636859.
14. Horn MA, Trafford AW. Aging and the cardiac collagen matrix: novel mediators of fibrotic remodelling. *J Mol Cell Cardiol* 2016;**93**:175–85.
15. Cavalera M, Wang J, Frangogiannis NG. Obesity, metabolic dysfunction, and cardiac fibrosis: pathophysiological pathways, molecular mechanisms, and therapeutic opportunities. *Transl Res* 2014;**164**(4):323–35.
16. Cieslik KA, Trial J, Crawford JR, Taffet GE, Entman ML. Adverse fibrosis in the aging heart depends on signaling between myeloid and mesenchymal cells; role of inflammatory fibroblasts. *J Mol Cell Cardiol* 2014;**70**:56–63.
17. Schelbert EB, Fonarow GC, Bonow RO, Butler J, Gheorghiade M. Therapeutic targets in heart failure: refocusing on the myocardial interstitium. *J Am Coll Cardiol* 2014;**63**(21):2188–98.
18. Weber KT, Sun Y, Bhattacharya SK, Ahokas RA, Gerling IC. Myofibroblast-mediated mechanisms of pathological remodelling of the heart. *Nat Rev Cardiol* 2013;**10**(1):15–26.
19. Kanagala P, Cheng ASH, Singh A, et al. Relationship between focal and diffuse fibrosis assessed by CMR and clinical outcomes in heart failure with preserved ejection fraction. *JACC Cardiovasc Imag* 2019;**12**(11):2291–301.
20. Gyongyosi M, Winkler J, Ramos I, et al. Myocardial fibrosis: biomedical research from bench to bedside. *Eur J Heart Fail* 2017;**19**(2):177–91.
21. de Meester de Ravenstein C, Bouzin C, Lazam S, et al. Histological validation of measurement of diffuse interstitial myocardial fibrosis by myocardial extravascular volume fraction from Modified Look-Locker imaging (MOLLI) T1 mapping at 3 T. *J Cardiovasc Magn Reson* 2015;**17**:48.
22. Lisi M, Cameli M, Righini FM, et al. RV longitudinal deformation correlates with myocardial fibrosis in patients with end-stage heart failure. *JACC Cardiovasc Imag* 2015;**8**(5):514–22.
23. Zhang Z, Staessen JA, Thijs L, et al. Left ventricular diastolic function in relation to the urinary proteome: a proof-of-concept study in a general population. *Int J Cardiol* 2014;**176**(1):158–65.
24. Zannad F, Rossignol P, Iraqi W. Extracellular matrix fibrotic markers in heart failure. *Heart Fail Rev* 2010;**15**(4):319–29.
25. Jacobs L, Thijs L, Jin Y, et al. Heart 'omics' in AGEing (HOMAGE): design, research objectives and characteristics of the common database. *J Biomed Res* 2014;**28**(5):349–59.
26. Loncar G, Omersa D, Cvetinovic N, Arandjelovic A, Lainscak M. Emerging biomarkers in heart failure and cardiac cachexia. *Int J Mol Sci* 2014;**15**(12):23878–96.
27. de Boer RA, Voors AA, Muntendam P, van Gilst WH, van Veldhuisen DJ. Galectin-3: a novel mediator of heart failure development and progression. *Eur J Heart Fail* 2009;**11**(9):811–17.
28. Lopez B, Gonzalez A, Querejeta R, Larman M, Rabago G, Diez J. Association of cardiotrophin-1 with myocardial fibrosis in hypertensive patients with heart failure. *Hypertension* 2014;**63**(3):483–9.
29. Brilla CG, Funck RC, Rupp H. Lisinopril-mediated regression of myocardial fibrosis in patients with hypertensive heart disease. *Circulation* 2000;**102**(12):1388–93.
30. Macconi D, Remuzzi G, Benigni A. Key fibrogenic mediators: old players. Renin–angiotensin system. *Kidney Int Suppl* 2014;**4**(1):58–64.
31. Shinde AV, Frangogiannis NG. Fibroblasts in myocardial infarction: a role in inflammation and repair. *J Mol Cell Cardiol* 2014;**70**:74–82.
32. Hayashi M, Tsutamoto T, Wada A, et al. Immediate administration of mineralocorticoid receptor antagonist spironolactone prevents post-infarct left ventricular remodeling associated with suppression of a marker of myocardial collagen synthesis in patients with first anterior acute myocardial infarction. *Circulation* 2003;**107**(20):2559–65.
33. Iraqi W, Rossignol P, Angioi M, et al. Extracellular cardiac matrix biomarkers in patients with acute myocardial infarction complicated by left ventricular dysfunction and heart failure: insights from the Eplerenone Post-Acute Myocardial Infarction Heart Failure Efficacy and Survival Study (EPHESUS) study. *Circulation* 2009;**119**(18):2471–9.
34. Quilliot D, Alla F, Bohme P, et al. Myocardial collagen turnover in normotensive obese patients: relation to insulin resistance. *Int J Obes (Lond)* 2005;**29**(11):1321–8.
35. Olivier A, Pitt B, Girerd N, et al. Effect of eplerenone in patients with heart failure and reduced ejection fraction: potential effect modification by abdominal obesity. Insight from the EMPHASIS-HF trial. *Eur J Heart Fail* 2017;**19**(9):1186–97.
36. Ferreira JP, Machu JL, Girerd N, et al. Rationale of the FIBROTARGETS study designed to identify novel biomarkers of myocardial fibrosis. *ESC Heart Fail* 2018;**5**(1):139–48.
37. Schuetze KB, McKinsey TA, Long CS. Targeting cardiac fibroblasts to treat fibrosis of the heart: focus on HDACs. *J Mol Cell Cardiol* 2014;**70**:100–7.
38. Stratton MS, McKinsey TA. Epigenetic regulation of cardiac fibrosis. *J Mol Cell Cardiol* 2016;**92**:206–13.
39. Filippatos G, Teerlink JR, Farmakis D, et al. Serelaxin in acute heart failure patients with preserved left ventricular ejection fraction: results from the RELAX-AHF trial. *Eur Heart J* 2014;**35**(16):1041–50.

40. Samuel CS, Bodaragama H, Chew JY, *et al*. Serelaxin is a more efficacious antifibrotic than enalapril in an experimental model of heart disease. *Hypertension* 2014;**64**(2):315–22.

41. Rutnam ZJ, Wight TN, Yang BB. miRNAs regulate expression and function of extracellular matrix molecules. *Matrix Biol* 2013;**32**(2):74–85.

42. Piccoli MT, Bar C, Thum T. Non-coding RNAs as modulators of the cardiac fibroblast phenotype. *J Mol Cell Cardiol* 2016;**92**:75–81.

43. Gupta SK, Itagaki R, Zheng X, *et al*. miR-21 promotes fibrosis in an acute cardiac allograft transplantation model. *Cardiovasc Res* 2016;**110**(2):215–26.

44. Golpanian S, Wolf A, Hatzistergos KE, Hare JM. Rebuilding the damaged heart: mesenchymal stem cells, cell-based therapy, and engineered heart tissue. *Physiol Rev* 2016;**96**(3):1127–68.

45. Schelbert EB, Butler J, Diez J. Why clinicians should care about the cardiac interstitium. *JACC Cardiovasc Imag* 2019;**12**(11):2305–18.

20

Natriuretic peptides and novel biomarkers in heart failure

Theresa A. McDonagh

Introduction

Over the last 30 years there has been a proliferation in the number of potential heart failure biomarkers. Despite all this work, however, the only truly established biomarkers, i.e. those that have made it into routine clinical use for heart failure, are the natriuretic peptide (NP) hormones. Many other peptides, proteins, hormones, immune and inflammatory markers, and microRNAs have increased circulating concentrations in patients with heart failure, but their additional clinical value has yet to be established. This chapter concentrates on the NPs and their current clinical usage and then outlines the potential role of more novel biomarkers.

The natriuretic peptide system

The NP family, to date, consists of four structurally similar hormones, A, B, C, and D, each sharing a 17-amino acid disulfide ring structure (**Figure 20.1**). They are counter-regulatory hormones in heart failure and have a major role in controlling cardiovascular homeostasis via their key effector functions: natriuresis, diuresis, and vasodilatation.

The first to be discovered was atrial natriuretic peptide (ANP). Early experiments demonstrated that dilatation of the cardiac atria could induce natriuresis. Following this, secretory granules were then identified in the atria using electron microscopy. The significance of these became apparent when De Bold *et al.* subsequently injected atrial myocyte extracts into rats and observed both natriuresis and vasodilatation. The product of these secretory granules was therefore named ANP.[1,2]

Brain natriuretic peptide (BNP) was discovered in 1988. It was isolated first from porcine brain.[3] The active peptide of BNP is a 32-amino-acid structure. In contrast to ANP, in heart failure, it is mainly secreted from the left ventricle in response to increased left ventricle (LV) pressure, wall stress, and stretch.[4-8] Other stimuli also lead to its secretion, notably ischaemia, the neurohormone endothelin, and transforming growth factor (TGF)-β.

Figure 20.2 shows the main actions of ANP and BNP which include natriuresis, vasodilatation, antiproliferative effects, and inhibition of the sympathetic and renin–angiotensin systems, which are in overdrive in heart failure.[9-13]

Two further natriuretic peptides have since been identified: C-type natriuretic peptide (CNP) and D (dendroaspis)-type natriuretic peptide (DNP). CNP is principally found in the central

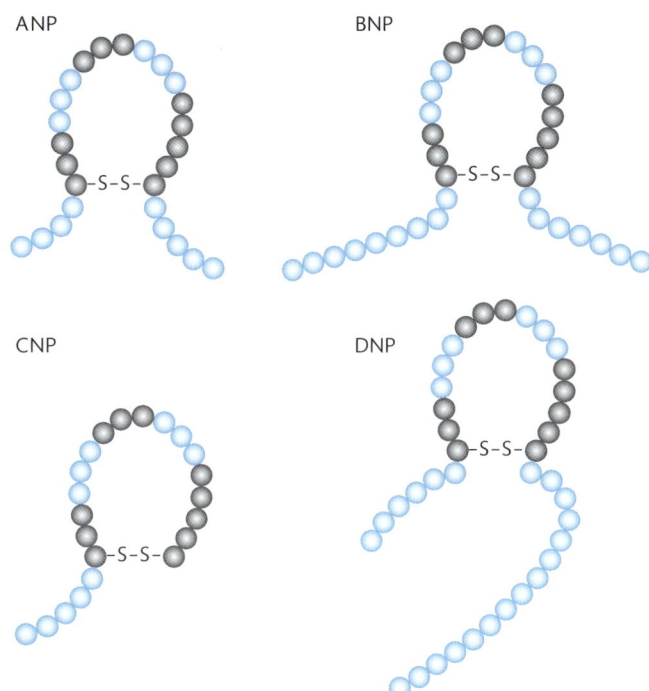

Figure 20.1 Schematic demonstrating the similar 17-amino-acid disulfide ring structure in the A-, B-, C-, and D-type natriuretic peptides. Identical amino acid sequences are marked in black.

Reproduced from Gardner RS, Chong KS, McDonagh TA. B-type natriuretic peptides in heart failure. *Biomark Med* 2007;**1**(2):243–50.

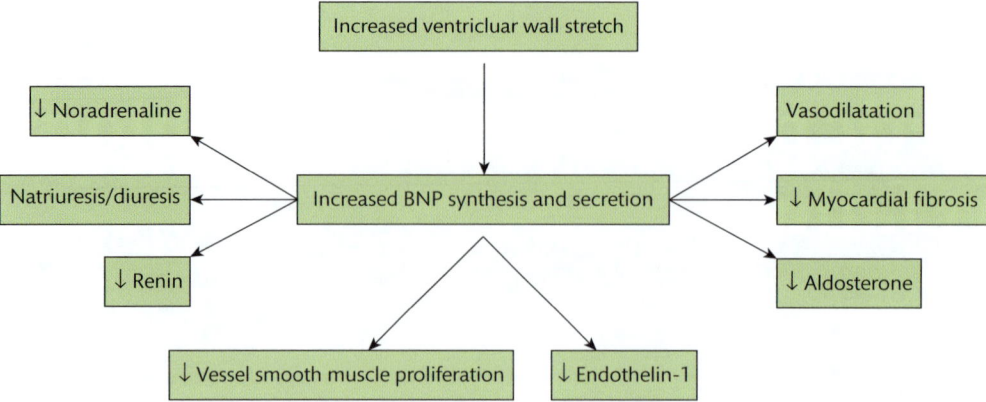

Figure 20.2 The action of B-type natriuretic peptides.
Reproduced from Gardner RS, Chong KS, McDonagh TA. B-type natriuretic peptides in heart failure. *Biomark Med* 2007;**1**(2):243–50.

nervous system (CNS) and vascular endothelium.[14] It has limited natriuretic and diuretic effects, but it is a potent vasodilator. DNP was initially isolated from the venom of the Green Mamba snake (*Dendroaspis augusticeps*) and has been shown to potently relax isolated precontracted rodent aorta and canine coronary arteries.[15] In addition, there is a renal NP, urodilatin, which is structurally similar to ANP.

The genes encoding human ANP and BNP are located on the short arm of chromosome 1. The BNP gene is a rapid response gene. BNP is synthesized *de novo* in response to stimuli. By contrast, ANP is stored in secretory granules and can be released into the circulation in response to an increase in left atrial pressure. The post-processing of both peptides is similar and is shown for BNP in **Figure 20.3**. B-type natriuretic peptide is produced as the pre-prohormone

BNP, processed to proBNP, and then cleaved by furin to mature, biologically active 32-amino-acid BNP and non-biologically active 76-amino-acid N-terminal (NT)-proBNP.[16] These are produced in a 1:1 ratio. ProBNP is synthesized by myocytes and fibroblasts principally in the ventricles (but also to a lesser degree in the atria) in response to an increase in LV filling pressure and wall stress. Picomolar concentrations are detectable in the plasma of normal subjects.[17]

The natriuretic peptides exert their action by binding to three different receptors: A, B, and C, which are located in the kidneys, vascular endothelium, adrenal glands and the CNS, as well as in the heart (**Figure 20.4**).[18] Interaction of natriuretic peptides with the A and B receptors leads to intracellular production of cGMP. The positive lusitropic effects of the hormones are thought to be

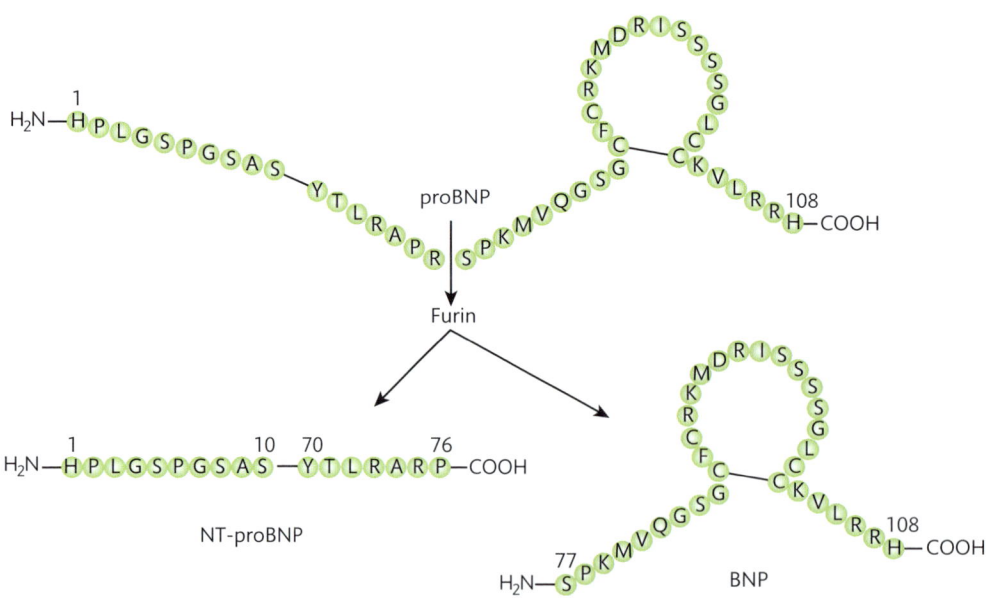

Figure 20.3 The enzymatic cleavage of proBNP into inactive NT-proBNP and biologically active BNP. A, alanine; BNP, B-type natriuretic peptide; C, cysteine; D, aspartic acid; F, phenylalanine; G, glycine; H, histidine; I, isoleucine; K, lysine; L, leucine; M, methionine; N, asparagine; NT-proBNP, N-terminal prohormone BNP; P, proline; ProBNP, prohormone BNP; Q, glutamine; R, arginine; S, serine; T, threonine; V, valine; Y, tyrosine.
Reproduced from Gardner RS, Chong KS, McDonagh TA. B-type natriuretic peptides in heart failure. *Biomark Med* 2007;**1**(2):243–50.

due to an increase in calcium entry into the myocytes. CNP acts via the NPR-B receptor, does not cause natriuresis or diuresis but does cause vasodilatation and exerts paracrine effects on vascular growth.

Clearance of the natriuretic peptides from the circulation is by two main mechanisms: first, via receptor-mediated endocytosis and lysosomal degradation; second, by enzymatic degradation by neprilysin, a neutral endopetidase (**Figure 20.4**).[19] The half-lives of the active hormones are shorter than those of the inactive N-terminal fragments, e.g. the mean half-life of BNP is 20 min, whereas NT-proBNP, which is cleared passively, in part by the kidneys, has a longer half-life of between 60 and 120 min.

Plasma concentrations of the natriuretic peptide hormones in humans are affected by several factors independent of the presence of cardiovascular pathology. They are higher in women than in men, are lower in obese subjects, and their values increase with age, a phenomenon which is thought to be associated with progressive nephron loss.[4,20–22]

The circulating concentrations of both ANP and BNP are raised in many cardiovascular conditions which affect both cardiac structure and function as well as renal dysfunction. Undoubtedly, the main focus of research interest for both ANP and BNP has been in heart failure.

There are four main areas in which measuring the plasma concentrations of NPs may be of use clinically, i.e. in diagnosis, screening for asymptomatic cardiac dysfunction, assigning prognosis, and in therapy monitoring for heart failure. A potential fifth use of NPs as therapeutic agents for heart failure is covered elsewhere in the book under therapies for heart failure with reduced ejection fraction (HFrEF) and acute heart failure.

Diagnosis

We have known for a considerable time that the circulating concentrations of the NPs are raised in patients with heart failure.[23–25] Importantly their concentrations are also elevated in the known precursor phase of heart failure—asymptomatic left ventricular systolic dysfunction (LVSD).[24,26] Natriuretic peptides are raised whether heart failure results from systolic dysfunction or whether it occurs in the presence of preserved systolic function.[27] They have also been shown to circulate in higher concentrations in patients with post myocardial infarction (MI) left ventricular dysfunction (LVD).[28–30] In considering their usefulness as diagnostic tests for heart failure we need to determine their sensitivity and specificity in determining the presence of heart failure as it presents clinically, e.g. in the acute setting, in primary care, and in the clinic setting for more chronic heart failure, and in the coronary care unit post myocardial infarction.

Acute heart failure

Davis *et al.* first reported on the usefulness of BNP in distinguishing whether breathlessness was due to heart failure or an exacerbation of chronic obstructive pulmonary disease in patients presenting acutely breathless to the accident and emergency department. A BNP concentration of ≥22 pg/mL predicted the presence of heart failure with a 93% sensitivity and 90% specificity.[31] This was subsequently confirmed in a much larger US study where the area under the curve for BNP diagnosing breathless due to heart failure in this setting was 0.97.[32] BNP is therefore an accurate means to diagnose heart failure presenting to the emergency department and to distinguish it reliably from other causes of acute breathlessness.

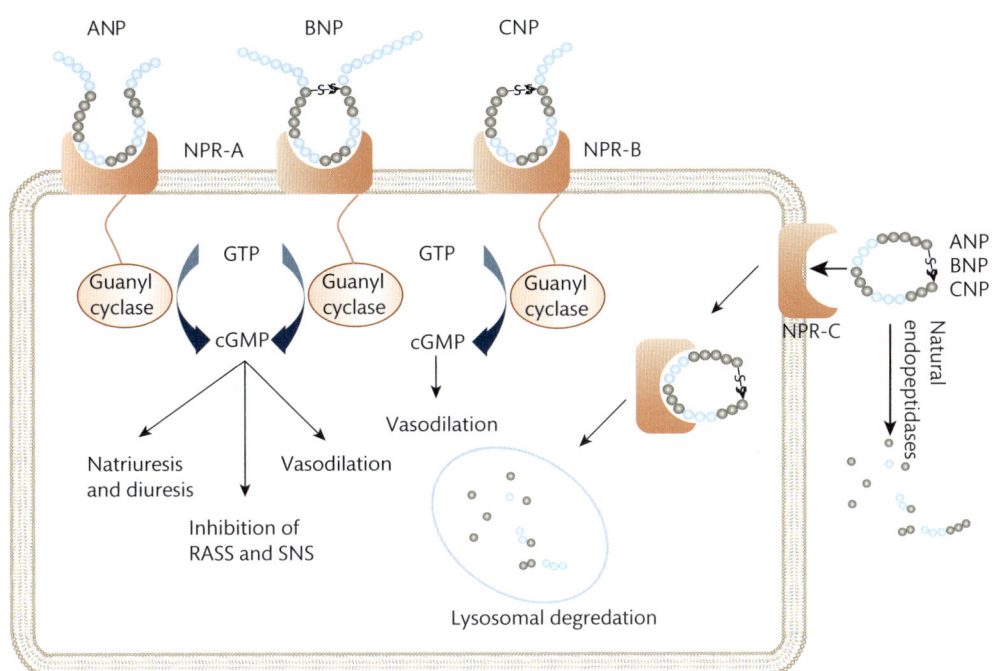

Figure 20.4 Action and clearance of natriuretic peptides. NP, natriuretic peptide; NPR, natriuretic peptide receptor.
Reproduced from Gardner RS, Chong KS, McDonagh TA. B-type natriuretic peptides in heart failure. *Biomark Med* 2007;**1**(2):243–50.

Chronic heart failure presenting in primary care and in outpatient clinics

Cowie *et al.* described the utility of the NP hormones in diagnosing incident heart failure cases assessed at a heart failure clinic in West London.[33] The reference standard diagnosis was a panel of three cardiologists reviewing the clinical and echocardiographic information. BNP was the most accurate of the peptides, superior to both ANP and N-ANP, in diagnosing heart failure: BNP concentration ≥22 pmol/L diagnosed heart failure with a sensitivity of 97%, specificity of 84%, a positive predictive accuracy of 70%, and a negative predictive accuracy of 97%. Interestingly in this study BNP was a far superior method for detecting heart failure than use of an increased cardiothoracic ratio on the chest X-ray. This work was later confirmed in a larger UK multicentre trial showing that both BNP and NT-proBNP have a similar diagnostic accuracy for the exclusion of heart failure in patients being referred from primary care suspected of having heart failure (see **Figure 20.5**).[34]

Post myocardial infarction

Struther's group first demonstrated that raised BNP concentration was the most sensitive method of detecting a left ventricular ejection fraction of ≤40% occurring post MI when compared to ANP, various clinical scoring systems, and to qualitative echocardiography.[35] Richards *et al.* subsequently compared many possible forms of the NPs in their ability to detect heart failure after a myocardial infarction. Both BNP and NT-proBNP were superior to the atrial peptides in terms of both their sensitivity and negative predictive accuracies. BNP was highly accurate at diagnosing heart failure with a sensitivity of 85% and a negative predictive accuracy of 93%.[28]

Therefore, NPs can diagnose heart failure accurately. Early studies used complex radioimmunoassays. More recent studies have employed more user-friendly enzyme-linked immunosorbent assays

Table 20.1 Suggested values of natriuretic peptides for the diagnosis of heart failure

Setting	BNP (pg/mL)	NT-proBNP (pg/mL)
Acute	≥100	≥300
Chronic	≥35	≥125

BNP, B-type natriuretic peptide; NT-proBNP, N-terminal B-type natriuretic peptide. Natriuretic peptide-guided therapy: individual patient data meta-analysis, n ≈ 2000. Source data from Ponikowski P, Voors AA, Anker SD, et al. 2016 ESC Guidelines for the diagnosis and treatment of acute and chronic heart failure: The Task Force for the diagnosis and treatment of acute and chronic heart failure of the European Society of Cardiology (ESC). Developed with the special contribution of the Heart Failure Association (HFA) of the ESC. European Journal of Heart Failure 2016;**18**(8): 891–975.

for BNP and NT-ProBNP, and point-of-care tests for BNP, which are now available in clinical practice.

Whereas the majority of published work demonstrates that the B-type peptides are superior to ANP in diagnosing heart failure, more recent work using assays directed at the mid region of the proANP molecule (which are more stable than previous assays to the C-terminal and N-terminal fragments of ANP) shows similar accuracy to the BNP studies.[36]

The striking feature of NPs diagnostically is their high negative predictive values—in other words if their concentrations are low, heart failure or LVD are highly unlikely. High concentrations are not, however, diagnostic of heart failure—they simply flag up the need for further detailed cardio-renal investigation to determine the cause of increase. As such, their most important diagnostic role is in helping to diagnose suspected heart failure in the breathless patients and allowing more cost-effective use of detailed cardiology imaging and expertise. Their diagnostic use is now well established in clinical practice and is underscored in both European and US clinical guidelines.[37,38] Simple cut-point concentrations have been described for the two most widely used assays and are shown in **Table 20.1**.

Screening

The second possible role for NPs in screening for asymptomatic disease is much less well studied. Screening lies under the diagnostic umbrella but refers to uncovering disease which is asymptomatic; heart failure, by definition, although difficult to diagnose, is a symptomatic condition. What is the evidence that NPs can screen for the most studied and treatable precursor phase of heart failure, asymptomatic LV systolic dysfunction (ASLVD)?

The first evidence to be published on this was from the North Glasgow MONICA study, where a population of 2000 men and women aged 25–74 years were screened by echocardiography: 3.1% had LVSD defined as a left ventricular ejection fraction (LVEF) ≤30%, and 1.4% of the population had ASLVD. BNP gave an area under the receiver operator characteristic (ROC) curve (AUC) of 0.884; this was superior to N-ANP.[26] The concentration of BNP used in this study was >17.9 pg/mL with the Peninsula radioimmunoassay. Recognizing that it would not be cost-effective to screen the entire population by this method but rather to target those most likely to have the disease—i.e. those >55 years with some manifestation of ischaemic heart disease—resulted in an AUC of 0.88. This compares very well with other established screening tests, e.g.

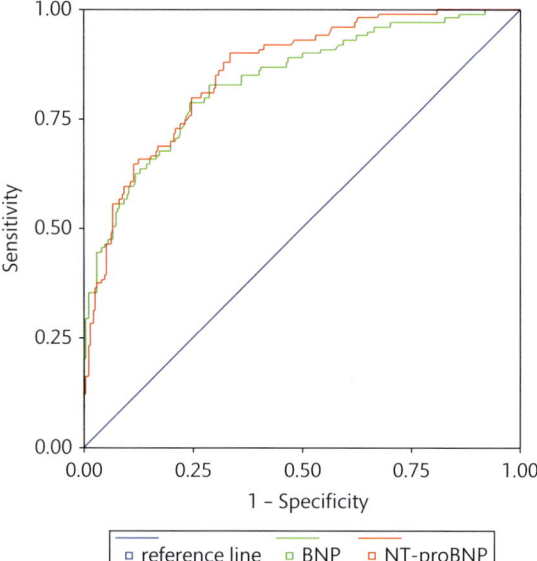

Figure 20.5 Receiver operating curves (ROC) for BNP and NT-proBNP. Reproduced from Zaphiriou A, Robb S, Murray-Thomas T, et al. The diagnostic accuracy of plasma BNP and NTproBNP in patients referred from primary care with suspected heart failure: results of the UK natriuretic peptide study. *Eur J Heart Fail* 2005;**7**(4):537–41 with permission from John Wiley and Sons.

prostate-specific antigen for prostatic cancer 0.92, mammography for breast cancer 0.85, and cervical cytology for cervical cancer 0.70.

A more recent study from the USA has screened for ASLVD in the Olmsted County population (1869 subjects aged >45 years) using the more modern, rapid assays for BNP and the N-terminal of BNP (NT-proBNP).[39] They have found similar results, this time for LVEF ≤40%. Interestingly BNP and NT-proBNP preformed similarly. The test was also effective in older individuals and females—there had been previous concerns that the normal rise in these peptides with age and the higher values in women might limit their usefulness as screening tools. The cut-point used for BNP in the total population was 66 pg/mL and was 228 pg/mL for NT-proBNP. This study also showed that LV systolic or diastolic function could be detected to similar degrees. Hobbs *et al.* have also compared these two peptides in an English population and report similar results.[40] BNP therefore seems to provide an accurate means of excluding LV dysfunction in the general population (with areas under the ROC curves of >0.85 and negative predictive values of >0.90).

Controversy exists as to whether BNP should be used alone or in combination with the ECG as a screening tool. Most groups have found in population-based studies of screening or in the detection of heart failure that the ECG does not add anything to the pick-up rate of LVD. However, in a large study of 1360 subjects, aged 45–80 years, Ng *et al.* reported that using a history of ischaemic heart disease and an ECG abnormality reduced the number of cases needing to be screened to detect one case of LVSD from 44 to seven with BNP alone.[41] Hedberg *et al.* also looked at screening with BNP/ECG or both in an elderly population of 407 subjects aged >75 years.[42] Both were highly efficient at excluding LVD; the ECG alone yielded fewer false positives, leading to their conclusion that in older individuals BNP added value only in those with an abnormal ECG. However, the argument about including the ECG with BNP as a screening test is largely academic, as in clinical practice both would be carried out. However, in general practice, where confidence in declaring an ECG truly normal is less than that in hospital practice, a BNP test would be easier to interpret as a first step in a screening strategy.

The vast majority of studies examining BNP as a screening test have measured plasma BNP. However, one study has reported on using urinary N-BNP and found that it gives similar AUCs to plasma N-BNP.[43] The accuracy of the diagnosis may also be improved by combining a blood and urinary strategy; however, further work is needed in this area before it could challenge a single blood value at present.[44]

Whereas the majority of studies using BNP to screen for ASLVD have been very positive, not all workers have found this. The Framingham study reported on their offspring cohort AUCs for 'any LVD' of 0.76 for men and 0.56 for women and for systolic dysfunction—an LVEF ≤40% and/or a fractional shortening <22% as an AUC for men of 0.79 and for women 0.85.[45] It is of note that in this study, LVEF was estimated visually rather than measured meticulously using Simpson's Bi-Plane Rule method employed in other population-based studies which have reported more favourable results.

An important question to be addressed under the heading of screening is whether screening would be cost-effective. Little work is available in this area. In a retrospective analysis from the North Glasgow MONICA study, Nielsen *et al.* reported that screening those at high risk (hypertensive and/or those with an abnormal

ECG) would reduce the cost per detected case of LVSD by 26% for the cost ratio of 1/20 (BNP/echocardiogram).[46] Heidenreich also addressed the issue in a meta-analysis of all population-based studies which have used BNP and echocardiography to detect LVSD in the general population.[47] He concluded that it would be cost-effective for populations with a prevalence of LVSD of at least 1%; screening with BNP followed by echocardiography increased outcome at a cost of $50 000 per quality-adjusted life-year gained.

In general, we can conclude that BNP can detect, with acceptable accuracy, ASLVD (systolic or otherwise) in the general population and in high-risk subgroups.

The question that therefore remains is why are we not screening in this manner? There are potentially several reasons. The first is economic and varies with differing health care systems, many of which are overwhelmed by detecting and treating the manifest stage of this condition, i.e. heart failure, never mind searching for asymptomatic disease. Another stated reason is that we do not yet have enough information about how to screen for ASLVD, what concentrations of BNP we should use, and whether age- and sex-specific cut-points are required. There is also the issue that in screening for ASLVD we will pick up other diseases, as an increased BNP concentration is a non-specific marker of cardiac structural and functional disease and of renal impairment, although the added value of BNP as a prognostic marker undoubtedly means that we would be uncovering important abnormalities by using this strategy. Lastly, however, the principal reason we are not doing this yet may be philosophical—perhaps we are not yet convinced that screening will really improve patient outcomes. Preliminary work on the effect of screening on outcomes is promising. McDonald *et al.* reported in the STOP-HF Trial that, among patients at risk of heart failure, BNP-based screening and collaborative care reduced the combined rates of LV systolic dysfunction, diastolic dysfunction, and heart failure.[48] We now await larger studies in this area before screening can be adopted more widely.

Prognosis

There is now a wealth of data that NPs are excellent prognostic markers in heart failure. Numerous studies confirm they are independent arbiters of a poor prognosis in all grades of heart failure ranging from ASLVD through to New York Heart Association (NYHA) class IV.[49-52] Indeed, they appear to be good single prognostic markers, when we examine studies that have used multivariable models including established and novel markers of poor outcome, including NYHA class, LVEF, peak VO_2, serum sodium concentration, QRS duration, plasma catecholamine, and endothelin.

In addition to their role in predicting all cause and cardiovascular mortality in heart failure, they also seem to be effective in determining sudden cardiac death—in a study by Berger *et al.*, an increased BNP concentration greater than the median was the only independent predictor of sudden death in 452 patients with LVSD.[53]

More recent work has also shown that midregional ANP has similar prognostic properties to the B-type NPs.[54]

The prognostic role of peptides has also been examined in patients being considered for cardiac transplantation. A recent study demonstrated that an NT-proBNP concentration greater than the median value at baseline was the single best predictor of mortality in these patients (**Figure 20.6**).[55] How we use the information gained from

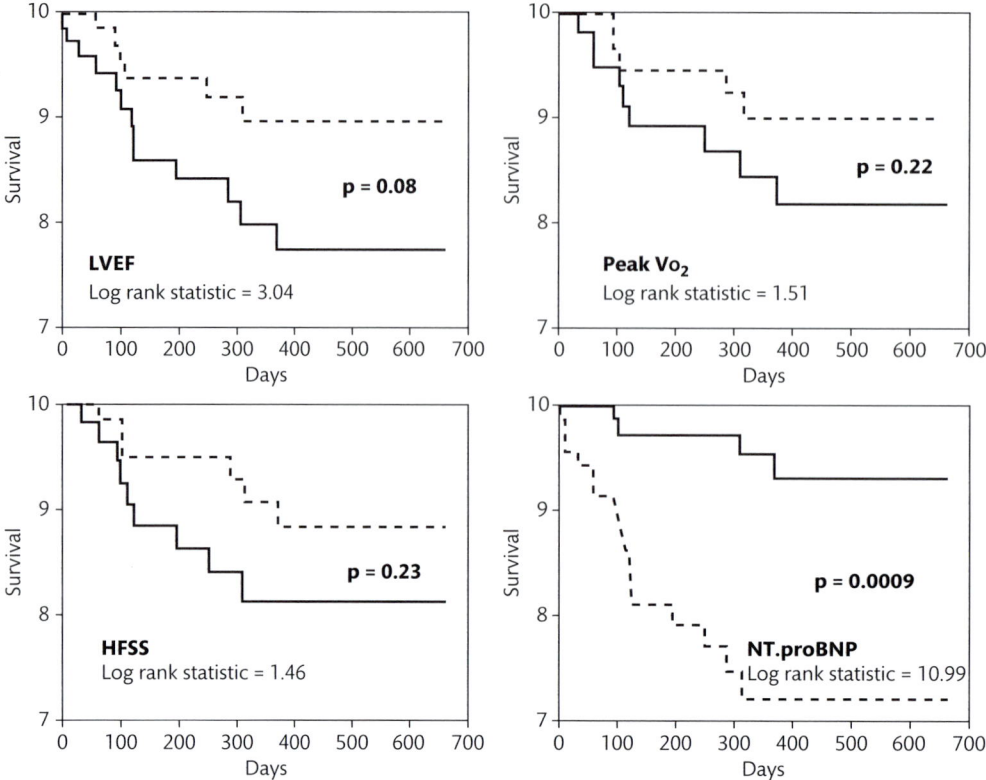

Figure 20.6 Kaplan–Meier survival curves for left ventricular ejection fraction (LVEF), maximum oxygen uptake (peak VO₂), heart failure survival score (HFSS), and NT-proBNP stratified above (broken line) and below (solid line) the median value against all-cause mortality.
Reproduced from Gardner RS, Chong V, Morton I, McDonagh TA. N-terminal brain natriuretic peptide is a more powerful predictor of mortality than endothelin-1, adrenomedullin and tumour necrosis factor-alpha in patients referred for consideration of cardiac transplantation. *Eur J Heart Fail* 2005;**7**(2):253–60 with permission from John Wiley and Sons.

this surrogate clinically is unclear, i.e. it remains to be determined whether we take a single baseline value or a concentration that fails to fall on follow-up or whether we need to incorporate BNP/NT-proBNP concentrations into our clinical scoring models for assessing prognosis in heart failure.

Therapy monitoring

The concept of monitoring patients using NPs arises out their prognostic ability and can be thought about in three different, yet related, ways. First, we could use BNP concentrations in a general sense to help us risk-stratify patients we are reviewing with the aim of trying to intensify the therapy of those we perceive to be at highest risk. Second, BNP could be used to aid discharge planning in patients admitted to hospital with decompensated heart failure. The third potential role concerns using BNP concentrations *per se* to serially monitor patients with heart failure and to use the values obtained in clinical decision-making, including the titration of therapy.

Studies in acute heart failure supplying further information about the usefulness of single or serial B-type NP measurements. Cheng *et al.* demonstrated in a study of 72 patients admitted to hospital with decompensated heart failure that the clinical end-points of death or readmission to hospital with heart failure occurred in those whose BNP concentrations increased during the admission.[56] There were no clinical end-points in those whose BNP concentrations fell. However, a single pre-discharge BNP concentration was

also an accurate determinant of readmission. Hence in the patient with decompensated heart failure, looking for a fall in BNP by serial monitoring is helpful clinically.

In an elegant study involving a derivation and validation cohort, in patients with decompensated heart failure, Logeart *et al.* reported that the pre-discharge BNP concentration was the best independent predictor of readmission, with a value of <300 pg/mL showing the lowest readmission rates.[57] However, those patients with the greatest decrease in BNP had a better outcome than those with a more modest reduction (hazard ratio (HR): 95% confidence interval (CI): 0.18 (0.07–0.48); $P = 0.001$). Hence in the decompensated situation, serially measuring BNP and aiming for a discharge BNP <300 pg/mL seems important for discharge planning. Serial BNP testing has also been shown to be of more value in this situation than repeated examination by Doppler echocardiography.[58]

In chronic heart failure (CHF), fewer data are available on serial measurements. In the Val-HeFT Study, those patients with the greatest reduction in their BNP concentration had the lowest mortality over the course of the study (**Figure 20.7**).[59] More recently the VAL-HeFT Group has published results using NT-proBNP from the placebo arm of the trial. A single determination of NT-proBNP showed higher prognostic discrimination than continuous changes of concentrations, expressed either as an absolute or percentage change. However, in the Cox proportional hazards model, stratification of patients into four categories according to NT-proBNP levels at two time-points four months apart with respect to a threshold concentration provided prognostic information in patients with

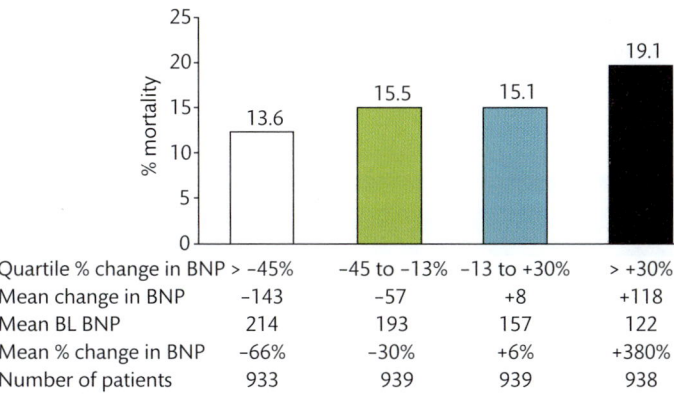

Quartile % change in BNP	> −45%	−45 to −13%	−13 to +30%	> +30%
Mean change in BNP	−143	−57	+8	+118
Mean BL BNP	214	193	157	122
Mean % change in BNP	−66%	−30%	+6%	+380%
Number of patients	933	939	939	938

Figure 20.7 Change in BNP concentrations and mortality.
Source data from Anand IS, Fisher LD, Chiang YT, et al. Changes in brain natriuretic peptide and norepinephrine over time and mortality and morbidity in the Valsartan Heart Failure Trial (Val-HeFT). *Circulation* 2003;**107**(9):1278–83.

CHF beyond that of a single determination.[60] Also, in chronic, but more advanced heart failure, Gardner *et al.* have shown that NT-proBNP concentrations greater than the median on follow-up also predict a poor outcome, as does an increase in NT-proBNP over four months of follow-up.[61] It would, therefore, appear that serially monitoring concentrations in CHF patients seems to give additional information to merely looking at baseline values.

Titration of therapy

This use of NPs as an HbA1c or biochemical Swan–Ganz catheter depends to some extent on what happens to their concentrations with the drug and device therapies we give for heart failure. Diuretics are known to reduce NP concentrations,[62,63] whereas there are reports suggesting that digoxin increases their levels.[64,65] However, it is the actions of the disease-modifying drugs which are perhaps the most interesting. There is good evidence that both angiotensin converting enzyme inhibitors (ACEi) and angiotensin II receptor blockers decrease BNP.[66,67] Tsutamoto has reported in 37 patients with CHF that treatment with spironolactone for four months significantly reduced BNP concentrations compared to placebo.[68] The information regarding β-adrenoreceptor antagonists and BNP is a little more confusing to date. Data from the RESOLVD study with metoprolol versus placebo treatment for 24 weeks reported a rise in BNP despite the expected improvement in LV function, reduction in mortality, and fall in angiotensin II and renin concentrations with metoprolol.[69] However, in a non-randomized Japanese study looking at 52 patients with CHF, again comparing metoprolol with placebo, both ANP and BNP concentrations fell with the β-blocker.[70] More recent work shows that they may increase BNP concentrations initially but chronically they seem to reduce it—this fits with their effects on long-term reverse remodelling.[71]

Hence at the moment two speculative schools of thought exist. The first presumes that initially the β-adrenoreceptor antagonists increase BNP due to their negatively inotropic and chronotropic properties and that as the beneficial effect of these drugs on LV function emerge the peptide concentrations fall. The second group proposes that the improvement seen with these drugs could be explained, at least in part, by their ability to increase NP levels.

Irrespective of the effect of β-blockade, evidence is now emerging to suggest that when we optimize therapy in patients with heart failure—be that increasing ACEi, adding spironolactone, or up-titrating β-adrenoreceptor antagonists (which is, after all, what we do when dealing clinically with heart failure patients)—BNP concentrations fall.[72]

Sacubutril valsartan, via its neprilysin inhibiting properties, will of course increase the circulating concentration of BNP, but not that of NT-proBNP.

Cardiac resynchronization therapy (biventricular pacing) also reduces BNP concentrations.[73] However, the real question is: can we use NP concentrations to target our drug and device therapies for heart failure?

There are many randomized studies of BNP-driven care versus usual care which address this question. Two small studies kick-started the work. Murdoch *et al.* randomized a small group of 20 patients attending a heart failure clinic to usual care or optimization of heart failure drugs according to BNP-driven care where the BNP target was to be within the normal range. The study showed a greater suppression of markers of the renin–angiotensin–aldosterone system in those receiving BNP-driven care.[74] Subsequently Richards' group published a small study of 69 patients attending a heart failure clinic.[75] They were randomized to care according to their NT-proBNP concentration/usual care. Those allocated to NT-proBNP-driven care had a significantly lower incidence of death or readmission to hospital at six months (*P* = 0.034), suggesting that this approach may give superior patient outcomes.

Since then, several larger studies have reported. In the STARS-BNP study, patients were randomized either to optimal medical therapy or to therapy guided to drive BNP below 100 pg/mL.[34] Mean doses of ACEi and β-adrenoreceptor antagonists were higher in the BNP-driven group, and the combined end-point of heart-failure-related death or hospitalization was significantly lower (24% vs 52%, *P* < 0.001) at the median follow-up of 15 months.

The multicentre TIME-HF study examined the use of NT-proBNP-guided therapy versus usual care in 499 patients with systolic heart failure. The primary end-point was survival free of any hospitalization and the secondary end-points included survival and survival free of heart failure hospitalization.

In the trial overall, the hazard ratio (95% confidence interval) for 18-month outcomes (standard therapy vs NT-proBNP-guided therapy) for the primary end-point was 0.92 (0.73–1.15), for survival 0.68 (0.46–1.01), both non-significant. Survival free of heart failure hospitalization was significantly reduced. The results were much more striking in those <75 years although the primary end-point was still not significantly reduced: 0.76 (0.53–1.09).[76]

The Battlescarred Study also reported similar results in a three-way randomization including NT-pro-BNP guided care, usual care and intensive medical care in 364 patients with heart failure. They enrolled both systolic and non-systolic heart failure patients. One-year mortality was less in both the hormone-guided (9.1%) and intensive clinically guided (9.1%) groups compared with usual care (18.9%; *P* = 0.03). However, three-year mortality was reduced in patients ≤75 years of age receiving hormone-guided treatment (15.5%) compared with their peers receiving either intensive clinically managed treatment (30.9%; *P* = 0.048) or usual care (31.3%; *P* = 0.021).[77]

Compared to the treatment trials for heart failure, these studies were small and probably underpowered to measure an effect on

mortality. Meta-analyses have subsequently followed. In an aggregate data meta-analysis, Felker *et al.* reported a significant mortality advantage for biomarker guided therapy (HR: 0.69; 95% CI: 0.55–0.86) compared to controls.[78] The most recent and the largest—an individual patient data meta-analysis on nearly 2000 patients—did report a small reduction in mortality, of borderline statistical significance (**Figure 20.8**).[79] However, there seemed to be no effect for those aged >75 years or in those with heart failure with preserved ejection fraction (HFpEF).[80]

Subsequent to this, a large multicentre trial, GUIDE-IT, was stopped early due to futility and reported no effect on using NP-guided approaches to optimizing treatment over guideline-directed usual care.[81]

So, to date, there is no convincing evidence that titrating heart failure therapies to try and drive down NP concentrations does consistently improve outcomes for patients.

However, it should also be pointed out that titrating therapy to reduce NP concentrations may be a bar too high. Lewin *et al.* compared using BNP concentrations to serial weight changes to try and determine clinical deterioration in patients attending a heart failure clinic.[83] They found that neither was accurate enough to predict clinical deterioration. They pointed out that we know little about the day-to-day, month-to-month variability of BNP in CHF patients to predict whether the changes we are looking for can be used. Wu recently showed that many short-term therapeutic studies of inpatients have largely resulted in statistically significant declines in BNP and NT-proBNP with clinical evidence of patient improvements.[84] In contrast, however, many therapeutic studies involving long-term outpatient monitoring have produced changes in BNP/

NT-proBNP that do not exceed the biological variance.[85] It may be that the reference change values—the changes in concentrations of BNP and NT-proBNP that detect a clinically meaningful change in patient status—are too large.[86]

Conclusions and the future for natriuretic peptides

The last 30 years have seen a huge transformation in the field of cardiac NP hormones from being merely of research interest to established biomarkers for heart failure. To date, they have a well-defined role in the diagnosis of heart failure and their prognostic abilities are beginning to be utilized. Under the diagnostic umbrella, their true role in screening for precursor phases of heart failure needs to be determined. Their prognostic utility requires further applied research to work out their role in risk stratification and treatment monitoring in heart failure. We need to study how they should be used to aid selection for more complex advanced heart failure therapies including cardiac resynchronization therapy defibrillator implantation and selection for cardiac transplantation. Of particular importance is any potential role they have in identifying those at risk of sudden death in heart failure to prioritize defibrillator therapy. We also have much to learn about any potential role in the emerging area of chemotherapy-induced cardiotoxicity as a cause of heart failure and monitoring for cancer therapies. In addition, we have to determine how NPs should be used with other more novel biomarkers which also predict an adverse outcome in heart failure.

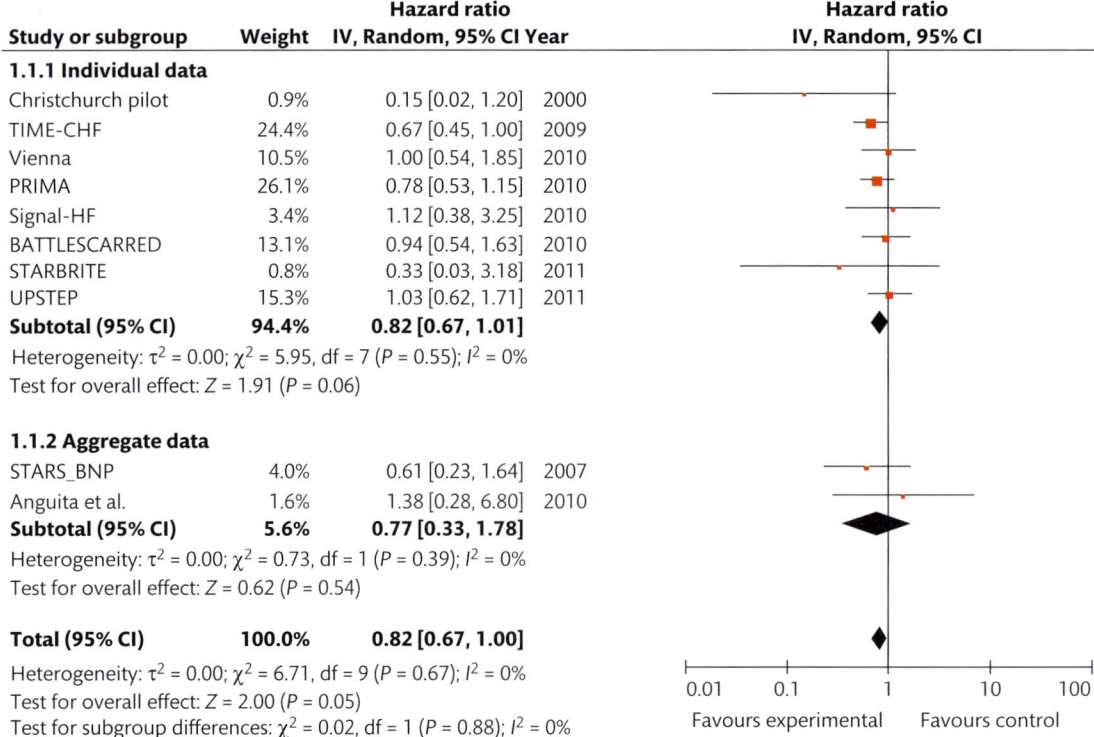

Figure 20.8 Natriuretic peptide-guided therapy: individual patient data meta-analysis.
Source data from Troughton R, Michael Felker G, Januzzi JL, Jr. Natriuretic peptide-guided heart failure management. *European Heart Journal* 2014;**35**(1):16–24.

Additional heart failure biomarkers

Many other putative biomarkers have now been described in heart failure. Myriad peptides, proteins, neurohormones, enzymes, and inflammatory markers are raised in circulating concentrations in heart failure patients (Box 20.1). Most of these are not routinely used clinically but are covered in other chapters in this book. The role of inflammatory markers such as C-reactive protein, tumour necrosis factor-α, and interleukin (IL)-6 is alluded to in Chapter 14, as are biomarkers associated with collagen turnover and fibrosis.

Troponin

The other most commonly used biomarker in cardiovascular disease, troponin (Tn), has now been widely studied in heart failure. Troponin is a marker of myocyte injury. Two cardiac specific proteins, cTnI and cTnT, exist in cardiac myocytes. They have become the reference standard markers of myocardial necrosis in patients with acute coronary syndromes.

Using standard assays, troponin concentrations are raised in about a quarter of patients with heart failure, irrespective of its aetiology.[87,88] With the newer high-sensitivity assays, Tn is detectable is nearly all patients with acute heart failure,[89] as well as in >90% of those with CHF.[90] They are independent predictors of prognosis in heart failure and add prognostic information to the NP hormones.[91,92]

ST2

ST2 is a member of the IL-1 receptor family. It exists in transmembrane (ST2L) and soluble (sST2) forms. The gene encoding ST2 resides on chromosome 2 and is upregulated in experimental models of heart failure. ST2 binds the ligand, IL-33, that is released by cardiomyocyte stretch. Interruption of the ST2 gene results in myocardial fibrosis and hypertrophy. ST2 concentrations are known to be increased after myocardial infarction.[93]

Rehman et al. measured ST2 in 346 patients with acute decompensated heart failure. The concentrations rose in proportion to disease severity. Whereas ST2 did correlate with traditional prognostic risk stratification markers such as NP, LVEF, and renal function, it was also associated with temperature and white blood cell count, reflecting its immunological function.[94] Januzzi et al. reported on the association between increased circulating concentrations of ST2 and higher mortality at one year, in patients with decompensated heart failure.[95] In that study, ST2 was inferior diagnostically to NT-proBNP but it did add value to it prognostically. ST2 was an independent predictor of prognosis in a multivariate model that included NT-proBNP. Patients with the worst outcomes had increased concentrations of both ST2 and NT-proBNP. Interestingly ST2 was equally predictive of death in those with HFrEF and HFpEF.[96] Several other studies have also confirmed the relationship between ST2 concentrations and adverse outcomes in acute decompensated heart failure[97,98] and in CHF.[99] Indeed, in a meta-analysis of studies in acute decompensated heart failure, ST2 was a stronger biomarker than B-type NP at predicting mortality (Figure 20.9).[100] It is also now evident that, in addition to single values, serial concentrations that rise or fail to fall in heart failure also predict poorer survival, both in the acute[101] and chronic[86] settings.

Unlike the B-type NPs, ST2 concentrations are less affected by obesity, age, atrial fibrillation, aetiology, or prior diagnosis of heart failure—making it an attractive candidate for monitoring. In addition the biological variability and reference change values for ST2 are less than for the natriuretic peptides.[102] Potentially they may be better for serial monitoring. However, large studies examining this are still awaited.

Galectin-3

Galectin-3, a soluble β-galactosidase-binding lectin, is the likely mediator of the known association between macrophage activation and myocardial fibrosis in the pathogenesis of heart failure.[103] Its circulating concentrations are raised across the spectrum of heart failure—acute and chronic, HFpEF and HFrEF—and they are strong and independent predictors of mortality.[104-106] Several studies have examined the use of serial plasma galectin-3 measurements in heart failure patients.[107-109] In the PROTECT trial, additional plasma galectin-3 sampling at six months provided significantly greater prognostic information than that of the baseline concentration alone.[108] Moreover, they demonstrated that an increase of ≥15% at any of the three-monthly review time-points conferred a worse prognosis, even after extensive clinical adjustments. In the Val-HeFT trial population, Anand et al. demonstrated that, over a four-month follow-up, for every 1 µg/L increase in galectin-3, there was an associated 2.9% increase in risk of mortality, 2.1% increased risk of first morbid event, and a 2.2% increased risk of heart failure hospitalization.[107] A small study in CHF found that serial monitoring with galectin-3 concentrations predicted cardiovascular admissions better than BNP.[110] We await further large-scale monitoring trials with galectin-3 to determine whether it can be used routinely for disease monitoring.

Box 20.1 Novel biomarkers in heart failure

- Matrix metalloproteinases
- Tissue inhibitors of metalloproteinases
- C-reactive protein
- Cystatin C
- Tenascin C
- Galectin-3
- Ghrelin
- Osteopontin
- Procollagen I C-terminal peptide (PCIP)
- Carboxyterminal-telopeptide of type I collagen (ICTP)
- ST2
- Adiponectin
- Copeptin
- Mid-regional natriuretic peptides
- Apelin
- Troponin
- Interleukin-6
- Tumour necrosis factor
- Endothelin
- Resistin
- Relaxin
- Receptor for advanced glycation end-products (RAGE)
- Leptin
- Monocyte chemoattractant protein-1
- Growth/differentiation factor-15
- Myeloperoxidase
- Urocortin
- MicroRNAs

Comparison to natruiretic peptides (NT-proBNP, MR-ADM, MR-proANP, BNP)
CRP and Troponins I and T in a Meta-analysis in Acute Decompensated Heart Failure

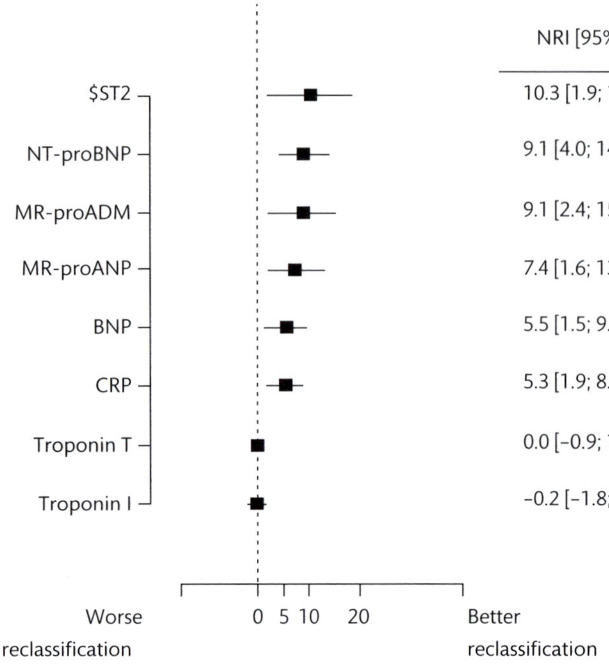

	NRI [95% CI]	IDI [95% CI]
$ST2	10.3 [1.9; 18.7]	0.048 [0.028; 0.067]
NT-proBNP	9.1 [4.0; 14.1]	0.025 [0.016; 0.034]
MR-proADM	9.1 [2.4; 15.8]	0.042 [0.028; 0.057]
MR-proANP	7.4 [1.6; 13.2]	0.028 [0.014; 0.041]
BNP	5.5 [1.5; 9.4]	0.020 [0.012; 0.027]
CRP	5.3 [1.9; 8.8]	0.011 [0.005; 0.016]
Troponin T	0.0 [−0.9; 1.0]	0.000 [−0.001; 0.002]
Troponin I	−0.2 [−1.8; 1.5]	0.000 [−0.001; 0.002]

Worse reclassification   0 5 10   20   Better reclassification

Figure 20.9 The prognostic potential of ST2.
Source data from Lassus J, Gayat E, Mueller C, *et al*. Incremental value of biomarkers to clinical variables for mortality prediction in acutely decompensated heart failure: the Multinational Observational Cohort on Acute Heart Failure (MOCA) study. *International Journal of Cardiology* 2013;**168**(3):2186–94.

Conclusions

The biomarker episode in heart failure history continues to evolve. To date, the NPs and troponins are the only ones being measured widely in clinical practice. However, we are moving beyond the diagnostic and prognostic potential of biomarkers into the arena of disease monitoring. Biomarkers that are integral to the complex pathophysiology of heart failure are likely to become more important, not only for their biomarker roles, but as novel therapeutic targets. As the sources of our biomarkers move from plasma and serum into the proteome, many more will emerge. The challenge for us clinically is how to integrate the profusion of information into pragmatic diagnostic, prognostic, and treatment algorithms.

REFERENCES

1. de Bold AJ, Borenstein HB, Veress AT, Sonnenberg H. A rapid and potent natriuretic response to intravenous injection of atrial myocardial extract in rats. *Life Sci* 1981;**28**(1):89–94.
2. de Bold AJ. Tissue fractionation studies on the relationship between an atrial natriuretic factor and specific atrial granules. *Can J Physiol Pharmacol* 1982;**60**(3):324–30.
3. Sudoh T, Kangawa K, Minamino N, Matsuo H. A new natriuretic peptide in porcine brain. *Nature* 1988;**332**(6159):78–81.
4. Wei CM, Heublein DM, Perrella MA, *et al.* Natriuretic peptide system in human heart failure. *Circulation* 1993;**88**(3):1004–9.
5. Yasue H, Yoshimura M, Sumida H, *et al.* Localization and mechanism of secretion of B-type natriuretic peptide in comparison with those of A-type natriuretic peptide in normal subjects and patients with heart failure. *Circulation* 1994;**90**(1):195–203.
6. Yoshimura M, Yasue H, Okumura K, *et al.* Different secretion patterns of atrial natriuretic peptide and brain natriuretic peptide in patients with congestive heart failure. *Circulation* 1993;**87**(2):464–9.
7. Edwards BS, Zimmerman RS, Schwab TR, Heublein DM, Burnett JC, Jr. Atrial stretch, not pressure, is the principal determinant controlling the acute release of atrial natriuretic factor. *Circ Res* 1988;**62**(2):191–5.
8. Kinnunen P, Vuolteenaho O, Ruskoaho H. Mechanisms of atrial and brain natriuretic peptide release from rat ventricular myocardium: effect of stretching. *Endocrinology* 1993;**132**(5):1961–70.
9. Kurtz A, Della BR, Pfeilschifter J, Taugner R, Bauer C. Atrial natriuretic peptide inhibits renin release from juxtaglomerular cells by a cGMP-mediated process. *Proc Natl Acad Sci USA* 1986;**83**(13):4769–73.
10. Kawaguchi H, Sawa H, Yasuda H. Effect of atrial natriuretic factor on angiotensin converting enzyme. *J Hypertens* 1990;**8**(8):749–53.
11. Oelkers W, Kleiner S, Bahr V. Effects of incremental infusions of atrial natriuretic factor on aldosterone, renin, and blood pressure in humans. *Hypertension* 1988;**12**(4):462–7.
12. Ebert TJ, Cowley AW, Jr. Atrial natriuretic factor attenuates carotid baroreflex-mediated cardioacceleration in humans. *Am J Physiol* 1988;**254**(4 Pt 2):R590–R594.
13. Kohno M, Yasunari K, Yokokawa K, *et al.* Inhibition by atrial and brain natriuretic peptides of endothelin-1 secretion after stimulation with angiotensin II and thrombin of cultured human endothelial cells. *J Clin Invest* 1991;**87**(6):1999–2004.

14. Hunt PJ, Richards AM, Espiner EA, Nicholls MG, Yandle TG. Bioactivity and metabolism of C-type natriuretic peptide in normal man. *J Clin Endocrinol Metab* 1994;**78**(6):1428–35.

15. Lee CY, Burnett JC, Jr. Natriuretic peptides and therapeutic applications. *Heart Fail Rev* 2007;**12**(2):131–42.

16. McKie PM, Burnett JC, Jr. B-type natriuretic peptide as a biomarker beyond heart failure: speculations and opportunities. *Mayo Clin Proc* 2005;**80**(8):1029–36.

17. Hunt PJ, Yandle TG, Nicholls MG, Richards AM, Espiner EA. The amino-terminal portion of pro-brain natriuretic peptide (Pro-BNP) circulates in human plasma. *Biochem Biophys Res Commun* 1995;**214**(3):1175–83.

18. Nakao K, Ogawa Y, Suga S, Imura H. Molecular biology and biochemistry of the natriuretic peptide system. I: Natriuretic peptides. *J Hypertens* 1992;**10**(9):907–12.

19. Kenny AJ, Bourne A, Ingram J. Hydrolysis of human and pig brain natriuretic peptides, urodilatin, C-type natriuretic peptide and some C-receptor ligands by endopeptidase-24.11. *Biochem J* 1993;**291**(Pt 1):83–8.

20. Redfield MM, Rodeheffer RJ, Jacobsen SJ, et al. Plasma brain natriuretic peptide concentration: impact of age and gender. *J Am Coll Cardiol* 2002;**40**(5):976–82.

21. McDonagh TA, Holmer S, Raymond I, et al. NT-proBNP and the diagnosis of heart failure: a pooled analysis of three European epidemiological studies. *Eur J Heart Fail* 2004;**6**(3):269–73.

22. McCullough PA, Duc P, Omland T, et al. B-type natriuretic peptide and renal function in the diagnosis of heart failure: an analysis from the Breathing Not Properly Multinational Study. *Am J Kidney Dis* 2003;**41**(3):571–9.

23. Francis GS, McDonald KM, Cohn JN. Neurohumoral activation in preclinical heart failure. Remodeling and the potential for intervention. *Circulation* 1993;**87**:IV90–6.

24. Lerman A, Gibbons RJ, Rodeheffer RJ, et al. Circulating N-terminal atrial natriuretic peptide as a marker for symptomless left-ventricular dysfunction [see comments]. *Lancet* 1993;**341**:1105–9.

25. Motwani JG, McAlpine H, Kennedy N, Struthers AD. Plasma brain natriuretic peptide as an indicator for angiotensin-converting-enzyme inhibition after myocardial infarction [see comments]. *Lancet* 1993;**341**:1109–13.

26. McDonagh TA, Robb SD, Murdoch DR, et al. Biochemical detection of left-ventricular systolic dysfunction. [see comments]. *Lancet* 1998;**351**(9095):9–13.

27. Lubien E, DeMaria A, Krishnaswamy P, et al. Utility of B-natriuretic peptide in detecting diastolic dysfunction: comparison with Doppler velocity recordings. *Circulation* 2002;**105**(5):595–601.

28. Richards AM, Nicholls G, Yandle TG, et al. Plasma N-terminal pro-brain natriuretic peptide and adrenomedullin: new neurohormonal predcitors of left ventricular function and prognosis after myocardial infarction. *Circulation* 1998;**97**:1921–29.

29. Talwar S, Squire IB, Downie PF, et al. Profile of plasma N-terminal proBNP following acute myocardial infarction;correlation with left ventricular systolic dysfunction. *Eur Heart J* 2000;**21**(18):1514–21.

30. Luchner A, Hengstenberg C, Lowel H, Trawinski J, Baumann M, Riegger GA et al. N-terminal pro-brain natriuretic peptide after myocardial infarction: a marker of cardio-renal function. *Hypertension* 2002;**39**(1):99–104.

31. Davis M, Espiner E, Richards G, et al. Plasma brain natriuretic peptide in assessment of acute dyspnoea. *Lancet* 1994;**343**:440–4.

32. Morrison LK, Harrison A, Krishnaswamy P, et al. Utility of a rapid B-natriuretic peptide assay in differentiating congestive heart failure from lung disease in patients presenting with dyspnea. *J Am Coll Cardiol* 2002;**39**(2):202–9.

33. Cowie MR, Struthers AD, Wood DA, et al. Value of natriuretic peptides in assessment of patients with possible new heart failure in primary care. *Lancet* 1997;**350**:1349–53.

34. Zaphiriou A, Robb S, Murray-Thomas T, et al. The diagnostic accuracy of plasma BNP and NTproBNP in patients referred from primary care with suspected heart failure: results of the UK natriuretic peptide study. *Eur J Heart Fail* 2005;**7**(4):537–41.

35. Choy AM, Darbar D, Lang CC, et al. Detection of left ventricular dysfunction after acute myocardial infarction: comparison of clinical, echocardiographic, and neurohormonal methods. *Br Heart J* 1994;**72**:16–22.

36. von Haehling S, Jankowska EA, Morgenthaler NG, et al. Comparison of midregional pro-atrial natriuretic peptide with N-terminal pro-B-type natriuretic peptide in predicting survival in patients with chronic heart failure. *J Am Coll Cardiol* 2007;**50**(20):1973–80.

37. Dickstein K, Cohen-Solal A, Filippatos G, et al. ESC Guidelines for the diagnosis and treatment of acute and chronic heart failure 2008: the Task Force for the Diagnosis and Treatment of Acute and Chronic Heart Failure 2008 of the European Society of Cardiology. Developed in collaboration with the Heart Failure Association of the ESC (HFA) and endorsed by the European Society of Intensive Care Medicine (ESICM). *Eur Heart J* 2008;**29**(19):2388–442.

38. Hunt SA, Abraham WT, Chin MH, et al. ACC/AHA 2005 Guideline Update for the Diagnosis and Management of Chronic Heart Failure in the Adult: a report of the American College of Cardiology/American Heart Association Task Force on Practice Guidelines (Writing Committee to Update the 2001 Guidelines for the Evaluation and Management of Heart Failure): developed in collaboration with the American College of Chest Physicians and the International Society for Heart and Lung Transplantation: endorsed by the Heart Rhythm Society. *Circulation* 2005;**112**(12):e154–e235.

39. Costello-Boerrigter LC, Boerrigter G, Redfield MM, et al. Amino-terminal pro-B-type natriuretic peptide and B-type natriuretic peptide in the general community: determinants and detection of left ventricular dysfunction. *J Am Coll Cardiol* 2006;**47**(2):345–53.

40. Hobbs FD, Davis RC, Roalfe AK, Hare R, Davies MK. Reliability of N-terminal proBNP assay in diagnosis of left ventricular systolic dysfunction within representative and high risk populations. *Heart* 2004;**90**(8):866–70.

41. Ng LL, Loke I, Davies JE, et al. Identification of previously undiagnosed left ventricular systolic dysfunction: community screening using natriuretic peptides and electrocardiography. *Eur J Heart Fail* 2003;**5**(6):775–82.

42. Hedberg P, Lonnberg I, Jonason T, Comparison of midregional pro-atrial natriuretic peptide with N-terminal pro-B-type natriuretic peptide in predicting survival in patients with chronic heart failure Electrocardiogram and B-type natriuretic peptide as screening tools for left ventricular systolic dysfunction in a population-based sample of 75-year-old men and women. *Am Heart J* 2004;**148**(3):524–9.

43. Vasan RS, Benjamin EJ, Larson MG, et al. Plasma natriuretic peptides for community screening for left ventricular hypertrophy and systolic dysfunction: the Framingham heart study. *JAMA* 2002;**288**(10):1252–9.

44. Ng LL, Loke IW, Davies JE, *et al.* Community screening for left ventricular systolic dysfunction using plasma and urinary natriuretic peptides. *J Am Coll Cardiol* 2005;**45**(7):1043–50.
45. Vasan RS, Benjamin EJ, Larson MG, *et al.* Plasma natriuretic peptides for community screening for left ventricular hypertrophy and systolic dysfunction: the Framingham heart study. *JAMA* 2002;**288**(10):1252–9.
46. Nielsen OW, McDonagh TA, Robb SD, Dargie HJ. Retrospective analysis of the cost-effectiveness of using plasma brain natriuretic peptide in screening for left ventricular systolic dysfunction in the general population. *J Am Coll Cardiol* 2003;**41**(1):113–20.
47. Heidenreich PA, Gubens MA, Fonarow GC, *et al.* Cost-effectiveness of screening with B-type natriuretic peptide to identify patients with reduced left ventricular ejection fraction. *J Am Coll Cardiol* 2004;**43**(6):1019–26.
48. Ledwidge M, Gallagher J, Conlon C, *et al.* Natriuretic peptide-based screening and collaborative care for heart failure: the STOP-HF randomized trial. *JAMA* 2013;**310**(1):66–74.
49. Tsutamoto T, Wada A, Maeda K, *et al.* Attenuation of compensation of endogenous cardiac natriuretic peptide system in chronic heart failure -Prognostic role of brain natriuretic peptide concentration in patients with chronic symptomatic left ventricular dysfunction. *Circulation* 1997;**96**:509–16.
50. McDonagh TA, Cunningham AD, Morrison CE, *et al.* Left ventricular dysfunction, natriuretic peptides, and mortality in an urban population. *Heart* 2001;**86**(1):21–6.
51. Gardner RS, Chong V, Morton I, McDonagh TA. N-terminal brain natriuretic peptide is a more powerful predictor of mortality than endothelin-1, adrenomedullin and tumour necrosis factor-alpha in patients referred for consideration of cardiac transplantation. *Eur J Heart Fail* 2005;**7**(2):253–60.
52. Gardner RS, Ozalp F, Murday AJ, Robb SD, McDonagh TA. N-terminal pro-brain natriuretic peptide. A new gold standard in predicting mortality in patients with advanced heart failure. *Eur Heart J* 2003;**24**(19):1735–43.
53. Berger R, Huelsmann M, Strecker K, *et al.* Neurohormonal risk stratification for sudden death and death owing to progressive heart failure in chronic heart failure. *Eur J Clin Invest* 2005;**35**(1):24–31.
54. Maisel A, Mueller C, Nowak R, *et al.* Mid-region pro-hormone markers for diagnosis and prognosis in acute dyspnea: results from the BACH (Biomarkers in Acute Heart Failure) trial. *J Am Coll Cardiol* 2010;**55**(19):2062–76.
55. Gardner RS, Chong V, Morton I, McDonagh TA. N-terminal brain natriuretic peptide is a more powerful predictor of mortality than endothelin-1, adrenomedullin and tumour necrosis factor-alpha in patients referred for consideration of cardiac transplantation. *Eur J Heart Fail* 2005;**7**(2):253–60.
56. Cheng V, Kazanagra R, Garcia A, *et al.* A rapid bedside test for B-type peptide predicts treatment outcomes in patients admitted for decompensated heart failure: a pilot study. *J Am Coll Cardiol* 2001;**37**(2):386–91.
57. Logeart D, Thabut G, Jourdain P, *et al.* Predischarge B-type natriuretic peptide assay for identifying patients at high risk of re-admission after decompensated heart failure. *J Am Coll Cardiol* 2004;**43**(4):635–41.
58. Gackowski A, Isnard R, Golmard JL, *et al.* Comparison of echocardiography and plasma B-type natriuretic peptide for monitoring the response to treatment in acute heart failure. *Eur Heart J* 2004;**25**(20):1788–96.
59. Anand IS, Fisher LD, Chiang YT, *et al.* Changes in brain natriuretic peptide and norepinephrine over time and mortality and morbidity in the Valsartan Heart Failure Trial (Val-HeFT). *Circulation* 2003;**107**(9):1278–83.
60. Masson S, Latini R, Anand IS, *et al.* Prognostic value of changes in N-terminal pro-brain natriuretic peptide in Val-HeFT (Valsartan Heart Failure Trial). *J Am Coll Cardiol* 2008;**52**(12):997–1003.
61. Gardner RS, Chong KS, Morton JJ, McDonagh TA. A change in N-terminal pro-brain natriuretic peptide is predictive of outcome in patients with advanced heart failure. *Eur J Heart Fail* 2007;**9**(3):266–71.
62. Anderson JV, Woodruff PW, Bloom SR. The effect of treatment of congestive heart failure on plasma atrial natriuretic peptide concentration: a longitudinal study. *Br Heart J* 1988;**59**(2):207–11.
63. Tsutsui T, Tsutamoto T, Maeda K, Kinoshita M. Comparison of neurohumoral effects of short-acting and long-acting loop diuretics in patients with chronic congestive heart failure. *J Cardiovasc Pharmacol* 2001;**38** Suppl 1:S81–S85.
64. Tsutamoto T, Wada A, Maeda K, *et al.* Digitalis increases brain natriuretic peptide in patients with severe congestive heart failure. *Am Heart J* 1997;**134**:910–16.
65. Kobusiak-Prokopowicz M, Swidnicka-Szuszkowska B, Mysiak A. [Effect of digoxin on atrial natriuretic peptide (ANP), brain natriuretic peptide (BNP) and cyclic 3′,5′-guanosine monophosphate (cGMP) in patients with chronic congestive heart failure]. *Pol Arch Med Wewn* 2001;**105**(6):475–82.
66. Yoshimura M, Yasue H, Tanaka H, *et al.* Responses of plasma concentrations of A type natriuretic peptide and B type natriuretic peptide to alacepril, an angiotensin-converting enzyme inhibitor, in patients with congestive heart failure. *Br Heart J* 1994;**72**:528–33.
67. Tsutamoto T, Wada A, Maeda K, *et al.* Relationship between plasma levels of cardiac natriuretic peptides and soluble Fas: plasma soluble Fas as a prognostic predictor in patients with congestive heart failure. *J Card Fail* 2001;**7**(4):322–8.
68. Tsutamoto T, Wada A, Maeda K, *et al.* Effect of spironolactone on plasma brain natriuretic peptide and left ventricular remodeling in patients with congestive heart failure. *J Am Coll Cardiol* 2001;**37**(5):1228–33.
69. The RESOLVD Investigators. Effect of metoprolol CR in patients with ischaemic and dilated cardiomyopathy. *Circulation* 2002;**101**:378–84.
70. Hara Y, Hamada M, Shigematsu Y, *et al.* Effect of beta-blocker on left ventricular function and natriuretic peptides in patients with chronic heart failure treated with angiotensin-converting enzyme inhibitor. *Jap Circ J* 2000;**64**(5):365–9.
71. Fung JW, Yu CM, Yip G, *et al.* Effect of beta blockade (carvedilol or metoprolol) on activation of the renin–angiotensin–aldosterone system and natriuretic peptides in chronic heart failure. *Am J Cardiol* 2003;**92**(4):406–10.
72. Maeda K, Tsutamoto T, Wada A, *et al.* High levels of plasma brain natriuretic peptide and interleukin-6 after optimized treatment for heart failure are independent risk factors for morbidity and mortality in patients with congestive heart failure. *J Am Coll Cardiol* 2000;**36**(5):1587–93.
73. Yu CM, Fung JW, Zhang Q, *et al.* Improvement of serum NT-ProBNP predicts improvement in cardiac function and favorable prognosis after cardiac resynchronization therapy for heart failure. *J Card Fail* 2005;**11**(5 Suppl):S42–S46.
74. Murdoch DR, McDonagh TA, Byrne J, *et al.* Titration of vasodilator therapy in chronic heart failure according to plasma brain natriuretic peptide concentration: randomized comparison

of the hemodynamic and neuroendocrine effects of tailored versus empirical therapy. *Am Heart J* 1999;**138**(6 Pt 1):1126–32.

75. Troughton RW, Frampton CM, Yandle TG, *et al*. Treatment of heart failure guided by plasma aminoterminal brain natriuretic peptide (N-BNP) concentrations. *Lancet* 2000;**355**(9210):1126–30.

76. Pfisterer M, Buser P, Rickli H, *et al*. BNP-guided vs symptom-guided heart failure therapy: the Trial of Intensified vs Standard Medical Therapy in Elderly Patients With Congestive Heart Failure (TIME-CHF) randomized trial. *JAMA* 2009;**301**(4):383–92.

77. Lainchbury JG, Troughton RW, Strangman KM, *et al*. N-terminal pro-B-type natriuretic peptide-guided treatment for chronic heart failure: results from the BATTLESCARRED (NT-proBNP-Assisted Treatment To Lessen Serial Cardiac Readmissions and Death) trial. *J Am Coll Cardiol* 2009;**55**(1):53–60.

78. Felker GM, Hasselblad V, Hernandez AF, O'Connor CM. Biomarker-guided therapy in chronic heart failure: a meta-analysis of randomized controlled trials. *Am Heart J* 2009;**158**(3):422–30.

79. Felker GM, Hasselblad V, Hernandez AF, O'Connor CM. Biomarker-guided therapy in chronic heart failure: a meta-analysis of randomized controlled trials. *Am Heart J* 2009;**158**(3):422–30.

80. Troughton RW, Frampton CM, Brunner-La Rocca HP, *et al*. Effect of B-type natriuretic peptide-guided treatment of chronic heart failure on total mortality and hospitalization: an individual patient meta-analysis. *Eur Heart J* 2014;**35**(23):1559–67.

81. Brunner-La Rocca HP, Eurlings L, Richards AM, *et al*. Which heart failure patients profit from natriuretic peptide guided therapy? A meta-analysis from individual patient data of randomized trials. *Eur J Heart Fail* 2015;**17**(12):1252–61.

82. Felker GM, Anstrom KJ, Adams KF, *et al*. Effect of natriuretic peptide-guided therapy on hospitalization or cardiovascular mortality in high-risk patients with heart failure and reduced ejection fraction: a randomized clinical trial. *JAMA* 2017;**318**(8):713–20.

83. Lewin J, Ledwidge M, O'Loughlin C, McNally C, McDonald K. Clinical deterioration in established heart failure: what is the value of BNP and weight gain in aiding diagnosis? *Eur J Heart Fail* 2005;**7**(6):953–7.

84. Wu AH. Serial testing of B-type natriuretic peptide and NTpro-BNP for monitoring therapy of heart failure: the role of biologic variation in the interpretation of results. *Am Heart J* 2006;**152**(5):828–34.

85. O'Hanlon R, O'Shea P, Ledwidge M, *et al*. The biologic variability of B-type natriuretic peptide and N-terminal pro-B-type natriuretic peptide in stable heart failure patients. *J Card Fail* 2007;**13**(1):50–5.

86. Piper SE, Sherwood RA, Amin-Youssef GF, Shah AM, McDonagh TA. Serial soluble ST2 for the monitoring of pharmacologically optimised chronic stable heart failure. *Int J Cardiol* 2015;**178**:284–91.

87. Missov E, Mair J. A novel biochemical approach to congestive heart failure: cardiac troponin T. *Am Heart J* 1999;**138**(1 Pt 1):95–9.

88. Braunwald E. Biomarkers in heart failure. *N Engl J Med* 2008;**358**(20):2148–59.

89. Felker GM, Hasselblad V, Tang WH, *et al*. Troponin I in acute decompensated heart failure: insights from the ASCEND-HF study. *Eur J Heart Fail* 2012;**14**(11):1257–64.

90. Masson S, Anand I, Favero C, *et al*. Serial measurement of cardiac troponin T using a highly sensitive assay in patients with chronic heart failure: data from 2 large randomized clinical trials. *Circulation* 2012;**125**(2):280–8.

91. Latini R, Masson S, Anand IS, *et al*. Prognostic value of very low plasma concentrations of troponin T in patients with stable chronic heart failure. *Circulation* 2007;**116**(11):1242–9.

92. Pascual-Figal DA, Casas T, Ordonez-Llanos J, *et al*. Highly sensitive troponin T for risk stratification of acutely destabilized heart failure. *Am Heart J* 2012;**163**(6):1002–10.

93. Daniels LB, Bayes-Genis A. Using ST2 in cardiovascular patients: a review. *Future Cardiol* 2014;**10**(4):525–39.

94. Rehman SU, Mueller T, Januzzi JL, Jr. Characteristics of the novel interleukin family biomarker ST2 in patients with acute heart failure. *J Am Coll Cardiol* 2008;**52**(18):1458–65.

95. Januzzi JL, Jr., Peacock WF, Maisel AS, *et al*. Measurement of the interleukin family member ST2 in patients with acute dyspnea: results from the PRIDE (Pro-Brain Natriuretic Peptide Investigation of Dyspnea in the Emergency Department) study. *J Am Coll Cardiol* 2007;**50**(7):607–13.

96. Manzano-Fernandez S, Mueller T, Pascual-Figal D, Truong QA, Januzzi JL. Usefulness of soluble concentrations of interleukin family member ST2 as predictor of mortality in patients with acutely decompensated heart failure relative to left ventricular ejection fraction. *Am J Cardiol* 2011;**107**(2):259–67.

97. Shah RV, Chen-Tournoux AA, Picard MH, van Kimmenade RR, Januzzi JL. Serum levels of the interleukin-1 receptor family member ST2, cardiac structure and function, and long-term mortality in patients with acute dyspnea. *Circ Heart Fail* 2009;**2**(4):311–19.

98. Boisot S, Beede J, Isakson S, *et al*. Serial sampling of ST2 predicts 90-day mortality following destabilized heart failure. *J Cardiac Fail* 2008;**14**(9):732–8.

99. Pascual-Figal DA, Ordonez-Llanos J, Tornel PL, *et al*. Soluble ST2 for predicting sudden cardiac death in patients with chronic heart failure and left ventricular systolic dysfunction. *J Am Coll Cardiol* 2009;**54**(23):2174–9.

100. Lassus J, Gayat E, Mueller C, *et al*. Incremental value of biomarkers to clinical variables for mortality prediction in acutely decompensated heart failure: the Multinational Observational Cohort on Acute Heart Failure (MOCA) study. *Int J Cardiol* 2013;**168**(3):2186–94.

101. Manzano-Fernandez S, Januzzi JL, Pastor-Perez FJ, *et al*. Serial monitoring of soluble interleukin family member ST2 in patients with acutely decompensated heart failure. *Cardiology* 2012;**122**(3):158–66.

102. Piper S, deCourcey J, Sherwood R, Amin-Youssef G, McDonagh T. Biologic variability of soluble ST2 in patients with stable chronic heart failure and implications for monitoring. *Am J Cardiol* 2016;**118**(1):95–8.

103. Sharma UC, Pokharel S, van Brakel TJ, *et al*. Galectin-3 marks activated macrophages in failure-prone hypertrophied hearts and contributes to cardiac dysfunction. *Circulation* 2004;**110**(19):3121–8.

104. Ho JE, Liu C, Lyass A, *et al*. Galectin-3, a marker of cardiac fibrosis, predicts incident heart failure in the community. *J Am Coll Cardiol* 2012;**60**(14):1249–56.

105. van Kimmenade RR, Januzzi JL, Jr. Emerging biomarkers in heart failure. *Clin Chem* 2012;**58**(1):127–38.

106. de Boer RA, Lok DJ, Jaarsma T, *et al*. Predictive value of plasma galectin-3 levels in heart failure with reduced and preserved ejection fraction. *Ann Med* 2011;**43**(1):60–8.

107. Anand IS, Rector TS, Kuskowski M, *et al.* Baseline and serial measurements of galectin-3 in patients with heart failure: relationship to prognosis and effect of treatment with valsartan in the Val-HeFT. *Eur J Heart Fail* 2013;**15**(5):511–18.

108. Motiwala SR, Szymonifka J, Belcher A, *et al.* Serial measurement of galectin-3 in patients with chronic heart failure: results from the ProBNP Outpatient Tailored Chronic Heart Failure Therapy (PROTECT) study. *Eur J Heart Fail* 2013;**15**(10):1157–63.

109. van der Velde AR, Gullestad L, Ueland T, *et al.* Prognostic value of changes in galectin-3 levels over time in patients with heart failure: data from CORONA and COACH. *Circ Heart fail* 2013;**6**(2):219–26.

110. Piper SE, de Courcey J, Sherwood RA, Amin-Youssef GF, McDonagh TA. Serial galectin-3 for the monitoring of optimally treated stable chronic heart failure: a pilot study. *Int J Cardiol* 2016;**207**:279–81.

SECTION 5
Diagnosis of heart failure

21

Diagnosing heart failure

Henry J. Dargie and Theresa A. McDonagh

It is often said that heart failure is not a diagnosis *per se* but a clinical syndrome consisting of a constellation of symptoms and signs, which are ultimately due to cardiac dysfunction. Nevertheless, it is important to diagnose accurately the presence of heart failure in order to facilitate the general and specific treatments that can modify its traditionally poor outlook.

The diagnosis of heart failure involves three distinct yet related phases. First, there is the confirmation that the patient has heart failure; second, the nature of the underlying cardiac dysfunction needs to be determined; and third, the actual aetiology of the cardiac dysfunction should be identified.

Following confirmation of the diagnosis of heart failure, some basic diagnostic tests must also be performed to determine the baseline status of key variables prior to initiation of therapy and to establish the presence of co-morbidities.

Unfortunately clinical symptoms and signs do not have sufficient accuracy to diagnose heart failure. They are often insensitive, or where they are sensitive they lack specificity (see Table 21.1). Relying on clinical acumen alone leads to wrongly diagnosing heart failure in up to half of cases.[1,2] This pertains in primary or secondary care. In the past, clinical scoring systems such as the Framingham or Boston criteria were used to try and improve the accuracy of clinical diagnosis.[3,4] However, these are not routinely used in clinical practice and are reserved for epidemiological studies, as other simpler and reproducible methods to infer the presence of heart failure have come into modern clinical practice.

Thus, symptoms and signs can be used to alert the clinician to the possible diagnosis of heart failure. The next stage is to improve the likelihood of cardiac dysfunction being detected. For this, two tests should be done—the measurement of natriuretic peptides (NPs) and a 12-lead ECG.

Figure 21.2 Di
Reproduced from Pc
and treatment of ac
ESC. *European Journ*

Diagnosing possible heart failure

The first phase of an accurate diagnosis of heart failure is to suspect it. This is where the cardinal symptoms and signs of heart failure have their place in the diagnostic algorithm. Patients with chronic heart failure may complain of breathlessness. This is usually on effort, but with severer disease they may describe orthopnoea and paroxysmal nocturnal dyspnoea. The presence of fluid retention often prompts patients to complain of ankle swelling. Frequently, tiredness can be a prominent symptom.

Many physical signs can be elicited on clinical examination. Traditionally more weight is given to diagnosing heart failure if the jugular venous pressure is elevated or if there are signs of peripheral oedema (Figure 21.1). This usually presents first of all as ankle oedema, but, as the disease progresses, sacral oedema, ascites, and pleural and pericardial effusions may all develop.

The pulse can be normal or there may be tachycardia, most commonly atrial fibrillation. The blood pressure may be low, normal, or high, depending on the stage of the disease and the underlying aetiology. Examination of the heart can also yield a number of abnormalities: a displaced apex beat, third and/or fourth heart sounds, and potentially a number of murmurs—most notably the pansystolic murmurs of mitral and tricuspid regurgitation.

The diagnosi
clear-cut than H
in diagnostic al
tural heart disea
left atrial volum
tients have 'diast
raised filling pre
(see Chapter x:
graphic abnorm
failure syndrom
according to the
with HFpEF or
heart failure, rai
terion reflecting
Echocardiogr
the aetiology of
disease.

(a)　　　　　　　　　　(b)

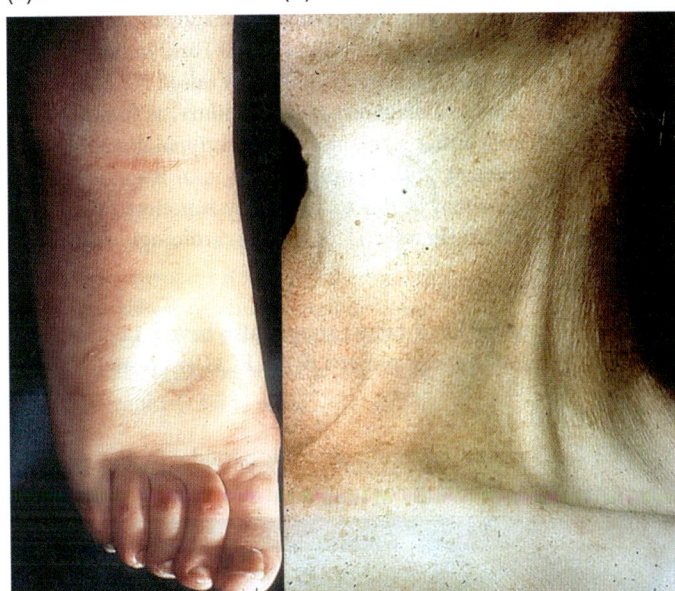

Figure 21.1 Signs of congestion in heart failure.

SECTION 5 266

Left column (partially cut off)

Table 21.1 Is

Clinical featur…
Breathlessness
Orthopnoea
Paroxysmal noc…
History of oede…
Tachycardia
Pulmonary crac…
Oedema on exa…
Third heart sou…
Raised jugular v…

Source data from S…

Natriuretic

Most work to
(BNP/NT-pro
emerged that
diagnostic cap
used for diag
hormones in t
failure.[5–9] Nur
acute heart fai
predictive acc
the patient's sy
work-up for p
able and their
guidelines.[10,11]
with the assay
acute or more
21.2.[12] In addi
as their conce
declining New
ejection fracti
type of cardia
are raised both
with preserved
tion does not e
specific marke
as of renal imp
symptoms and
centrations sho

Electrocardi…

Patients suspec
Heart failure i

Table 21.2 Su…
diagnosis of he…

Setting
Acute
Chronic

BNP, B-type natriure…

Main content

Table 21.3 Classification of heart failure according to the European Society of Cardiology 2016 Heart Failure Guideline

HFrEF	HFpEF	HFmrEF
Symptoms/signs	Symptoms/signs	Symptoms/signs
LVEF ≤40%	LVEF ≥50%	LVEF = 41–49%
–	1. Increased NP 2. At least one additional criterion of: relevant structural heart disease, e.g. LAE, LVH, or diastolic dysfunction[a]	1. Increased NP 2. At least one additional criterion of: relevant structural heart disease, e.g. LAE, LVH, or diastolic dysfunction[a]

HFrEF, heart failure with reduced ejection fraction; HFpEF, heart failure with preserved ejection fraction; HFmrEF, heart failure with mid-range ejection fraction; LVEF, left ventricular ejection fraction; NP, natriuretic peptide; LAE, left atrial enlargement; LVH, left ventricular hypertrophy.
See Chapter 23 for more detail.
[a]All patients require symptoms and/or signs and an LVEF category. Those with HFpEF and HFmrEF require to have elevated NP concentrations and additional evidence of structural heart disease or diastolic dysfunction.

Diagnosing the aetiology of heart failure

Once the presence of cardiac dysfunction has been confirmed, and its nature ascertained, the underlying cardiac pathology should be identified.

This usually involves further investigation; in western countries this is often aimed at diagnosing the presence of significant coronary artery disease. However, as there are many potential aetiologies, tests may also focus on arrhythmias, valve disease, specific myocardial diseases, genetics, metabolic, toxic, and infective causes.

Routine baseline investigations

Baseline haematology is required, as anaemia can both cause and exacerbate heart failure and is potentially treatable. Assessing renal function and electrolytes is mandatory before starting therapy. Glucose and HbA1c should be requested. Thyroid status should be measured—both hypo- and hyperthyroidism can cause heart failure and either is frequently found in patients being treated with amiodarone. Liver function tests and serum sodium are also useful, simple baseline prognostic markers. Ferritin should always be measured in the patient with diabetes and heart failure to exclude haemochromatosis and to screen for iron deficiency (along with the measurement of transferrin saturation). In addition, creatinine kinase measurement can alert clinicians to the presence of muscular dystrophy as a cause of heart failure.

Summary

Heart failure should be diagnosed by first having a high index of suspicion on clinical presentation. Second, the possibility of heart failure should be further refined by NP measurement, and, if possible, an ECG. If either of these are abnormal the patient needs to be referred for confirmation/exclusion of significant cardiac dysfunction as a cause of symptoms. The nature of the cardiac dysfunction

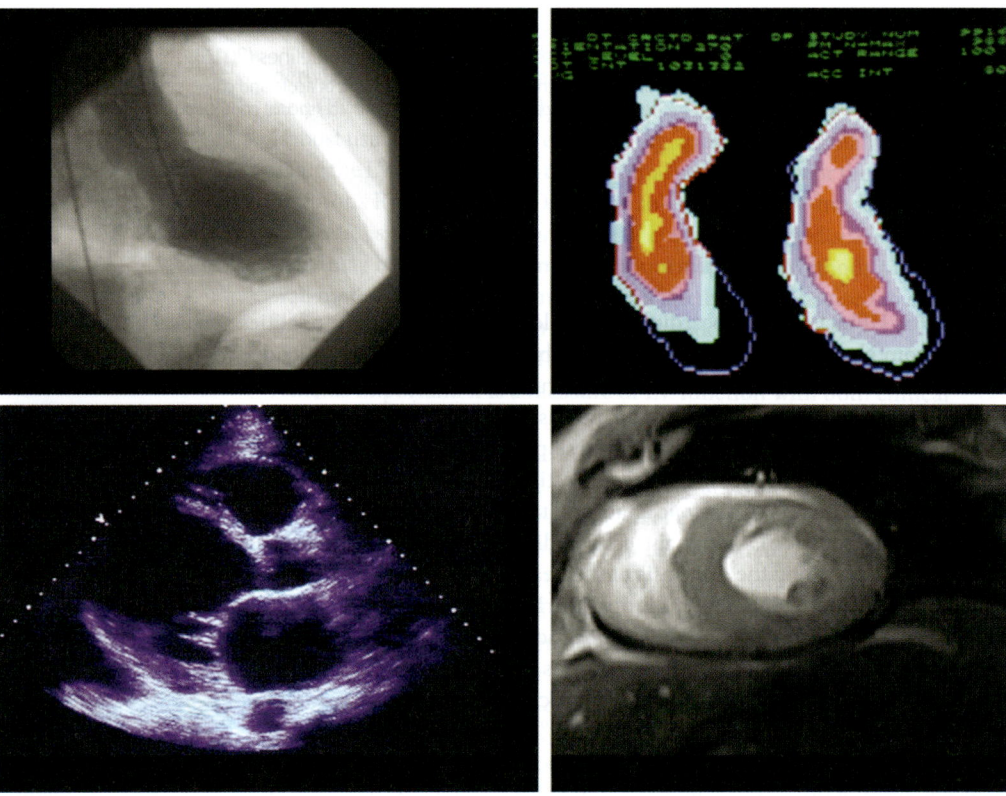

Figure 21.3 Cardiac dysfunction-imaging modalities.

should allow the patient to be broadly categorized into having heart failure with systolic dysfunction, HFrEF, *or* one of HFpEF and HFmrEF. The underlying aetiology of the heart disease should then be determined, if possible, and baseline assessments of renal function and tests for common co-morbidities should be performed.

This diagnostic process then sets the stage for the general pharmacotherapy of heart failure to begin, allows subgroups who will benefit from device therapy to be identified, defines the aetiology so that specific therapies aimed at targeting any potential reversal of the heart failure can be initiated, facilitates the treatment of co-morbidity, and aids in risk stratification.

Diagnosing heart failure is not yet perfect—it remains difficult and complex. In the future, the process will become more simple with the widespread use of NPs. Ideally, we should strive for a more streamlined definition of heart failure which, like its relation myocardial infarction, will comprise not only appropriate symptoms and the presence of cardiac dysfunction but also biomarkers with both diagnostic and prognostic accuracy. In the future, novel biomarkers may add incremental value to NPs for diagnosis, prognostication, and, perhaps, to allow treatment targeting to specific populations.

REFERENCES

1. Clarke KW, Gray D, Hampton JR. Evidence of inadequate investigation and treatment of patients with heart failure. *Br Heart J* 1994;**71**(6):584–7.
2. Hillis GS, Al-Mohammad A, Wood M, Jennings KP. Changing patterns of investigation and treatment of cardiac failure in hospital. *Heart* 1996;**76**(5):427–9.
3. Eriksson H, Svardsudd K, Caidahl K, *et al*. Early heart failure in the population. The study of men born in 1913. *Acta Med Scand* 1988;**223**(3):197–209.
4. McKee PA, Castelli WP, McNamara PM, Kannel WB. The natural history of congestive heart failure: the Framingham study. *N Engl J Med* 1971;**285**(26):1441–6.
5. Davis M, Espiner E, Richards G, *et al*. Plasma brain natriuretic peptide in assessment of acute dyspnoea. *Lancet* 1994;**343**(8895):440–4.
6. Cowie MR, Struthers AD, Wood DA, *et al*. Value of natriuretic peptides in assessment of patients with possible new heart failure in primary care. *Lancet* 1997;**350**(9088):1349–53.
7. McDonagh TA, Robb SD, Murdoch DR, *et al*. Biochemical detection of left-ventricular systolic dysfunction. *Lancet* 1998;**351**(9095):9–13.
8. Maisel AS, Krishnaswamy P, Nowak RM, *et al*. Rapid measurement of B-type natriuretic peptide in the emergency diagnosis of heart failure. *N Engl J Med* 2002;**347**(3):161–7.
9. Maisel A, Mueller C, Nowak R, *et al*. Mid-region pro-hormone markers for diagnosis and prognosis in acute dyspnea: results from the BACH (Biomarkers in Acute Heart Failure) trial. *J Am Coll Cardiol* 2010;**55**(19):2062–76.
10. Ponikowski P, Voors AA, Anker SD, *et al*. 2016 ESC Guidelines for the diagnosis and treatment of acute and chronic heart failure: The Task Force for the diagnosis and treatment of acute and chronic heart failure of the European Society of Cardiology (ESC). Developed with the special contribution of the Heart Failure Association (HFA) of the ESC. *Eur J Heart Fail* 2016;**18**(8):891–975.
11. Yancy CW, Jessup M, Bozkurt B, *et al*. 2013 ACCF/AHA guideline for the management of heart failure: a report of the American College of Cardiology Foundation/American Heart Association Task Force on Practice Guidelines. *J Am Coll Cardiol* 2013;**62**(16):e147–239.
12. Gardner RS, Ozalp F, Murday AJ, Robb SD, McDonagh TA. N-terminal pro-brain natriuretic peptide. A new gold standard in predicting mortality in patients with advanced heart failure. *Eur Heart J* 2003;**24**(19):1735–43.
13. Anand IS, Fisher LD, Chiang YT, *et al*. Changes in brain natriuretic peptide and norepinephrine over time and mortality and morbidity in the Valsartan Heart Failure Trial (Val-HeFT). *Circulation* 2003;**107**(9):1278–83.
14. Maisel A, Mueller C, Nowak RM, *et al*. Midregion prohormone adrenomedullin and prognosis in patients presenting with acute dyspnea: results from the BACH (Biomarkers in Acute Heart Failure) trial. *J Am Coll Cardiol* 2011;**58**(10):1057–67.
15. Parekh N, Maisel AS. Utility of B-natriuretic peptide in the evaluation of left ventricular diastolic function and diastolic heart failure. *Curr Opin Cardiol* 2009;**24**(2):155–60.
16. McDonagh TA, Holmer S, Raymond I, *et al*. NT-proBNP and the diagnosis of heart failure: a pooled analysis of three European epidemiological studies. *Eur J Heart Fail* 2004;**6**(3):269–73.
17. Davie AP, Francis CM, Love MP, *et al*. Value of the electrocardiogram in identifying heart failure due to left ventricular systolic dysfunction. *Br Med J* 1996;**312**(7025):222.
18. Zaphiriou A, Robb S, Murray-Thomas T, *et al*. The diagnostic accuracy of plasma BNP and NTproBNP in patients referred from primary care with suspected heart failure: results of the UK natriuretic peptide study. *Eur J Heart Fail* 2005;**7**(4):537–41.
19. Schiller NB, Shah PM, Crawford M, *et al*. Recommendations for quantitation of the left ventricle by two-dimensional echocardiography. American Society of Echocardiography Committee on Standards, Subcommittee on Quantitation of Two-Dimensional Echocardiograms. *J Am Soc Echocardiogr* 1989;**2**(5):358–67.
20. McGowan JH, Martin W, Burgess MI, *et al*. Validation of an echocardiographic wall motion index in heart failure due to ischaemic heart disease. *Eur J Heart Fail* 2001;**3**(6):731–7.
21. SOLVD Investigators. Effect of enalapril on survival in patients with reduced left ventricular ejection fractions and congestive heart failure. *N Engl J Med* 1991;**325**(5):293–302.
22. Cardiac Insufficiency Bisoprolol Study II (CIBIS-II): a randomised trial. *Lancet* 1999;**353**(9146):9–13.
23. Pitt B, Zannad F, Remme WJ, *et al*. The effect of spironolactone on morbidity and mortality in patients with severe heart failure. Randomized Aldactone Evaluation Study Investigators. *N Engl J Med* 1999;**341**(10):709–17.
24. Paulus WJ, Tschope C, Sanderson JE, *et al*. How to diagnose diastolic heart failure: a consensus statement on the diagnosis of heart failure with normal left ventricular ejection fraction by the Heart Failure and Echocardiography Associations of the European Society of Cardiology. *Eur Heart J* 2007;**28**(20):2539–50.
25. Ray SG, Metcalfe MJ, Oldroyd KG, *et al*. Do radionuclide and echocardiographic techniques give a universal cut off value for left ventricular ejection fraction that can be used to select patients for treatment with ACE inhibitors after myocardial infarction? *Br Heart J* 1995;**73**(5):466–9.

SECTION 6
Non-invasive investigation

22

Basic investigation of heart failure

Simon A. S. Beggs and Roy S. Gardner

Although the clinical history and examination may suggest a diagnosis of heart failure, objective evidence of cardiac dysfunction or a structural abnormality of the heart is also required. A number of diagnostic tests can be reliably employed to identify patients with left ventricular systolic dysfunction (LVSD). However, heart failure with preserved systolic function is less reliably pinpointed, particularly as the syndrome often represents a mixture of conditions rather than a specific entity.

As well as investigating patients to identify the presence and severity of cardiac dysfunction and any relevant co-morbidities, it is important to clarify the underlying aetiology. Some causes are potentially correctable and at least partial recovery of cardiac function should be possible. Appropriate investigations will also help to risk-stratify patients, identifying those suitable for advanced therapies such as device therapy (implantable cardioverter–defibrillator, cardiac resynchronization therapy (CRT), ventricular assist devices) and cardiac transplantation.

Although echocardiography is currently the principal diagnostic test for patients with heart failure, cardiac magnetic resonance imaging (CMR) is now considered to be the 'reference standard' method of assessing cardiac function. In addition, CMR is the most accurate non-invasive method by which to characterise myocardial tissue, which may provide a clue to the underlying aetiology. The investigations that should be performed, or at least considered, in the patient suspected of having heart failure are shown in Table 22.1. This chapter concentrates on the first-line investigations.

Electrocardiogram

The ECG is a simple, inexpensive, reproducible, and readily available investigation that should be performed in every patient suspected of having heart failure. The utility of this basic test is perhaps under-appreciated. ECG changes are very common in patients with heart failure, and a normal ECG is associated with a high negative predictive value (NPV) for heart failure (>90%): a patient with a completely normal ECG is most unlikely to have heart failure.

Conversely, although an abnormal ECG increases the likelihood of a patient having heart failure, it is a non-specific finding, and should prompt further investigation. In patients with heart failure, the ECG can be useful in helping to identify the underlying aetiology (e.g. prior myocardial infarction: Figure 22.1), but also which patients are likely to respond to therapies such as CRT (Figure 22.2). Finally, there are several other ECG features or abnormalities that may be relevant in a patient with heart failure and these are shown in Table 22.2 and Table 22.3.

Bundle branch block

Left bundle branch block (LBBB; Figure 22.2) is common in patients with heart failure. In the Italian Network chronic heart failure registry,[1] LBBB (diagnosed with a QRS duration >140 ms rather than the widely accepted duration of >120 ms) was found in 25.2% of individuals with chronic heart failure (CHF). LBBB was more prevalent in females and in patients with dilated cardiomyopathy, and found to be an independent predictor of all-cause death, as well as sudden death, in patients with CHF. LBBB was also shown to be an independent predictor of mortality in the CIBIS-2 study.[2] Further studies have since shown that accelerated QRS interval widening is independently associated with deterioration of cardiac function,[3] and death or need for urgent cardiac transplantation.[4] The crude rate of development of LBBB among stable ambulatory outpatients with CHF is nearly 11% per year.[5] However, it should be noted that the development of LBBB is occasionally reversible: usually this occurrence is in response to heart failure therapy.

Right bundle branch block (RBBB) is also seen in patients with heart failure. QRS ≥130 ms—whether secondary to LBBB or RBBB—can help to identify patients who may be suitable for CRT (see Chapter 58), although the evidence is greater for patients with LBBB.[6] CRT is contraindicated in patients with QRS <130 ms, where it may increase mortality.

Laboratory tests

Several laboratory tests should be considered mandatory in the assessment of the patient with suspected heart failure (see Table

Table 22.1 Basic investigations in conditions that may lead to heart failure

Aetiology	ECG	Bloods	Other investigations
Amyloid (see Chapter 9)	Atrial arrhythmia (particularly AF) P mitrale/pulmonale Abnormal axis Low precordial QRS amplitude	Serum and urine electrophoresis ESR	CMR Cardiac catheterization Endomyocardial biopsy
Cardiac sarcoidosis (see Chapter 8)	RBBB Conduction abnormalities Supraventricular and ventricular tachycardias	Serum ACE	Chest radiograph (bilateral hilar lymphadenopathy) Endomyocardial biopsy CMR
Haemochromatosis	Abnormalities are common	Ferritin Transferrin saturation	Genetic analysis (C282Y homozygosity) CMR (T2*) Endomyocardial biopsy
Dystrophinopathies (DMD and BMD)	Tall right precordial R waves ↑ R/S ratio Deep Q waves in lateral leads	Markedly elevated CK (10–20×) Dystrophin (↓ in DMD; abnormal molecular weight in BMD)	Genetic analysis
Myotonic dystrophy	Pathological Q waves (in the absence of CAD)	Mildly elevated CK	Genetic analysis Muscle biopsy EMG
Fabry disease	Conduction abnormalities	↓ α-Galactosidase A activity in males (may be normal in carriers)	Molecular studies
Pompe disease		Elevated CK Acid α-glucosidase	Muscle biopsy Genetic analysis
Chagas disease	Conduction abnormalities	Machado–Guerreiro complement fixation test	ELISA
Lyme disease	Conduction abnormalities Non-specific ST/T wave abnormalities	Lyme serology (ELISA and western blot analysis)	
Löffler endocarditis	Atrial fibrillation Non-specific T-wave abnormalities	Eosinophilia	
Myocarditis	Non-specific abnormalities ST/T abnormalities Arrhythmias	Raised WCC, CRP, and troponin	Cardiac MRI Endomyocardial biopsy Gallium scan

ACE, angiotensin converting enzyme; AF, atrial fibrillation; BMD, Becker muscular dystrophy; CAD, coronary artery disease; CK, creatine kinase; CMR, cardiac magnetic resonance imaging; CRP, C-reactive protein; DMD, Duchenne muscular dystrophy; ELISA, enzyme-linked immunosorbent assay; EMG, electromyography; ESR, erythrocyte sedimentation rate; RBBB, right bundle branch block; WCC, white cell count.

22.1), and in the monitoring of patients commenced on heart failure therapy. Other tests can be performed depending on the clinical context. The most relevant laboratory tests are expanded upon below.

Urea and electrolytes

The measurement of serum electrolytes and creatinine, and the estimation of glomerular filtration rate (eGFR) are important, both as a baseline and in the subsequent follow-up of the patient with heart failure.

Serum sodium

Hyponatraemia (Na^+ <135 mmol/L) is frequently seen in patients with heart failure and its presence is a powerful adverse prognostic sign. It is commonly caused by haemodilution, diuretic therapy (particularly where a thiazide is added to a loop diuretic), and release of arginine vasopressin (AVP). Hyponatraemia can also be caused by angiotensin converting enzyme inhibitor (ACE) inhibitors, angiotensin receptor blockers (ARBs), mineralocorticoid receptor antagonists (MRAs), angiotensin receptor–neprilysin antagonists (ARNIs), as well as proton pump inhibitors. It can often be improved by fluid restriction or avoidance of diuretic combinations

where possible. When these measures fail, AVP receptor antagonists (e.g. tolvaptan), used as aquaretics, are valuable in the treatment of resistant hyponatraemia. However, this class of medication does not improve long-term clinical outcomes.[7] Hypernatraemia (Na^+ >150 mmol/L) is occasionally seen in patients who have become dehydrated from overdiuresis.

Serum potassium

Hypokalaemia (K^+ <3.5 mmol/L) is commonly seen in patients on loop or thiazide diuretics, or those with secondary hyperaldosteronism. A hypokalaemic state increases the likelihood of arrhythmias, as well as the risk of side-effects from digoxin therapy. Serum potassium levels can be increased with the use of potassium supplements, potassium-sparing diuretics, MRAs, ACE inhibitors, ARBs, and ARNIs. Conversely, hyperkalaemia (K^+ >5.5 mmol/L) is often caused by such therapy, and may require either a reduction in dose or discontinuation of the offending drug.

The concomitant use of traditional potassium-binding resins to avoid such dose reductions has been limited by both their side-effect profile and undesirable sodium-loading effect. The emergence of a new generation of agents such as the potassium–calcium exchange polymer, patiromer, may lead to their increasing use. However, there

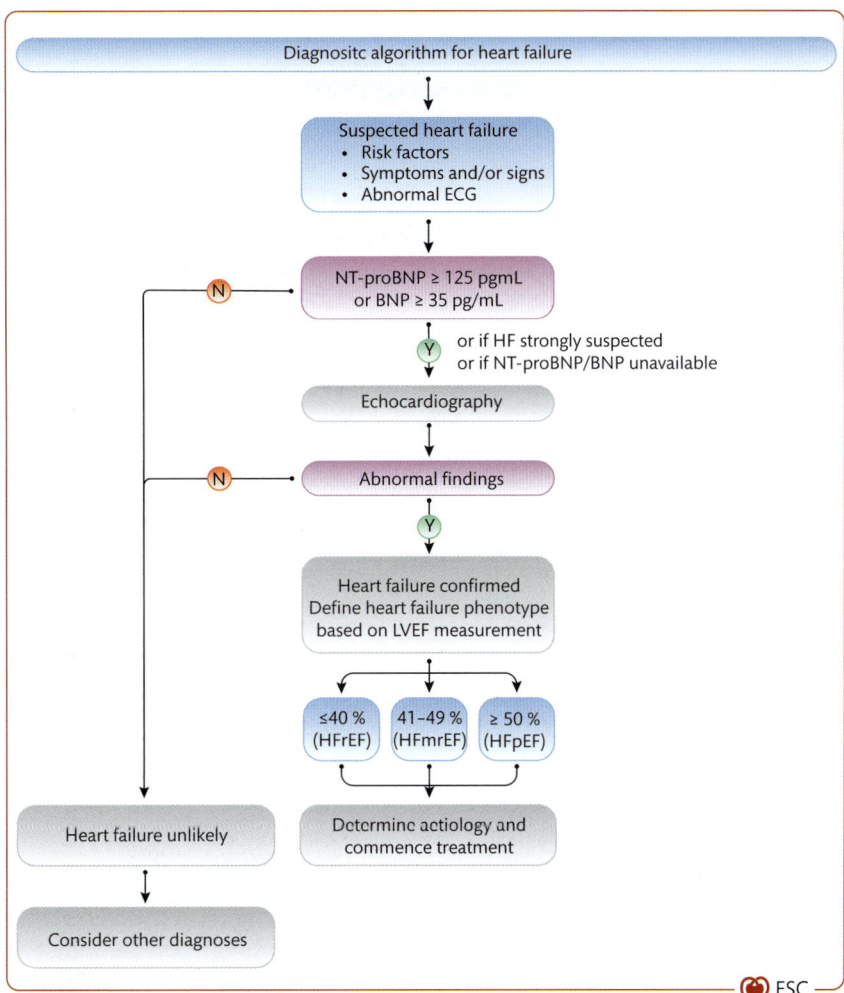

Figure 22.1 The diagnostic algorithm for chronic heart failure.

McDonagh TA, Metra M, Adamo M, Gardner RS, *et al*. ESC Scientific Document Group. 2021 ESC Guidelines for the diagnosis and treatment of acute and chronic heart failure. *Eur Heart J*. 2021 Aug 27:ehab368. doi: 10.1093/eurheartj/ehab36. © The European Society of Cardiology.

Reprinted by permission of Oxford University Press.

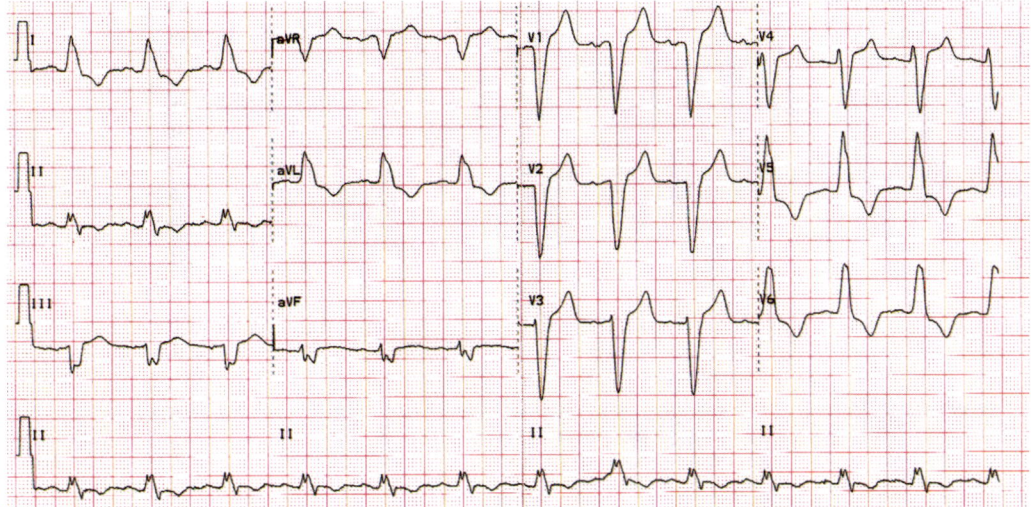

Figure 22.2 ECG demonstrating left bundle branch block.

Table 22.2 ECG features and potential causes

ECG feature	Potential cause	Investigations/therapy to be considered
Sinus tachycardia	Decompensated heart failure Thyrotoxicosis Sepsis Anaemia	Echo FBC TFT Infection screen
Sinus bradycardia	Drug related (β-blocker, digoxin, amiodarone, etc.) Hypothyroidism Sick sinus syndrome	If necessary remove or modify cause TFT
P mitrale	Causes of left atrial dilation: Mitral valve disease LVH Restrictive cardiomyopathy	Echo
P pulmonale	Causes of right atrial dilatation: Chronic lung disease Tricuspid regurgitation Atrial septal defect	Echo PFT CXR
Atrial fibrillation/flutter/tachycardia	Decompensated HF Ischaemia/infarction Mitral valve disease Hyperthyroidism HCM Restrictive cardiomyopathy Sepsis Drugs (digoxin toxicity may precipitate tachycardia)	Echo TFT Digoxin level Infection screen Consider rate vs rhythm control; radiofrequency ablation
Ventricular arrhythmias	Decompensated HF Acute ischaemia/infarction Previous myocardial infarction (i.e. scar-related)	Urea and electrolytes Mg Tn Coronary angiography CMR ICD
AV block	Drug toxicity (β-blocker, digoxin, amiodarone, etc) Ischaemia/infarction Sarcoidosis Myocarditis Lyme carditis Dystrophinopathies Laminopathies	Remove/treat cause Genetic testing CMR Lyme serology Pacemaker
Ischaemia/infarction	Coronary heart disease	Tn Echo Coronary angiography ± revascularization CMR
LBBB	Myocardial infarction Dilated cardiomyopathy Hypertension	Echo Tn Coronary angiography Consider CRT
RBBB	Acute or chronic lung disease Myocardial infarction	CXR PFTs Echo CMR Consider CRT
LVH	Hypertension Aortic stenosis Hypertrophic cardiomyopathy Coarctation	Echo CMR
Small voltage complexes	Obesity Obstructive lung disease Cardiac amyloid Pericardial effusion	CXR PFT Echo CMR

CMR, cardiac MRI; CRT, cardiac resynchronization therapy; CXR, chest radiograph; FBC, full blood count; LVH, left ventricular hypertrophy; ICD, implantable cardioverter–defibrillator; LBBB, left bundle branch block; PFT, pulmonary function tests; RBBB, right bundle branch block; TFT, thyroid function tests; Tn, troponin.

Table 22.3 Common ECG features of heart failure conditions

Condition	ECG features
Ischaemia	ST depression
Acute MI	Regional ST elevation (STEMI) or ST depression (NSTEMI/posterior MI) or new LBBB
Established MI	Regional Q waves and/or T-wave inversion
Dilated cardiomyopathy	Non-specific ST/T wave abnormalities
Restrictive cardiomyopathy	P mitrale/pulmonale; low precordial QRS amplitude; atrial arrhythmias
Hypertrophic cardiomyopathy	Usually abnormal (85%), with ST/T wave abnormalities and LVH particularly in the mid-precordial leads. Prominent inferior or precordial Q waves are also frequently seen (in up to 50%)
LV non-compaction	Usually abnormal with abnormalities that include LBBB or RBBB, fascicular block, atrial fibrillation, and ventricular tachycardia
Myocarditis	Non-specifically abnormal: ST/T abnormalities, arrhythmias; may mimic STEMI (particularly with pericardial involvement)
Arrhythmogenic RV cardiomyopathy	Epsilon waves or localized prolongation (>110 ms) of the QRS complex in right precordial leads (V1–V3) VT (usually of RV origin—LBBB morphology)
Dystrophinopathies	Tall right precordial R waves with an increased R/S ratio; deep Q waves in lateral leads; conduction disturbances
Cardiac sarcoid	Ventricular and supraventricular tachycardia; conduction disease
Cardiac amyloid	AF; small voltage QRS complexes
Lyme carditis	Conduction disease

AF, atrial fibrillation; LBBB, left bundle branch block; LV, left ventricular; MI, myocardial infarction; RV, right ventricular.

is no proof currently that using such agents along with ACE inhibitors/ARBs and MRAs maintains their efficacy. Where these strategies to manage hyperkalaemia fail, there is an increased likelihood of bradycardia or ventricular fibrillation, and on occasions may require correction with dialysis or ultrafiltration.

Serum creatinine and eGFR

Heart failure is not only a cardiac disorder, but rather a cardiorenal and neurohumoral syndrome, and a raised creatinine level is often a marker of coexisting renal dysfunction. Renal impairment is often associated with heart failure as a result of renal hypoperfusion, diuretic treatment, disease-modifying heart failure therapy (ACE inhibitors, ARBs, ARNIs, and MRAs), as well as other concomitant medication and comorbidities such as diabetes. Serum creatinine concentration, which is often quoted as a barometer of renal impairment, is actually a poor indicator of renal function.[8] Therefore, estimation of the glomerular filtration rate (eGFR: **Figure 22.3**) is preferred for the accurate assessment of renal function,[8] and the Modification of Diet in Renal Disease (MDRD) equations[9] have been validated in patients with severe CHF (**Figure 22.3**).[10] GFR <60 mL/min/1.73 m² is associated with complications of renal disease.[8] Moreover, GFR estimated by creatinine clearance (CrCl) is independently predictive of all-cause mortality in patients with asymptomatic[11] and symptomatic[11-14] LVSD.

Full blood count

Haemoglobin

Anaemia (Hb <13 g/dL in men, <12 g/dL in women) is common in patients with chronic heart failure,[15] and the proportion of patients with anaemia increases with worsening New York Heart Association functional class.[16] Anaemia is also associated with increased symptoms, more frequent hospitalizations, and, in some studies, with an increased mortality rate.[16-18] The cause of anaemia in CHF is likely

(1) MDRD-1 equation:

$$GFR = 170 \times [\text{plasma creatinine}]^{-0.999} \times [\text{age}]^{-0.176} \times [0.762 \text{ if patient is female}] \times [1.180 \text{ if patient is black}] \times [\text{SUN}]^{-0.170} \times [\text{albumin}]^{+0.318}$$

(2) MDRD-2 (abbreviated) equation:

$$GFR = 186 \times [\text{Pcr}]^{-1.154} [\text{age}]^{-0.203} \times [0.742 \text{ if patient is female}] \times [1.212 \text{ if patient is black}]$$

(3) Cockcroft–Gault formula normalized to a body surface area of 1.73m², (creatinine clearance, expressed in mL/minute/1.73m²):

$$GFR \text{ (males)} = \frac{1.23 \times \text{weight (kg)} \times [140 - \text{age}]}{\text{plasma creatinine (µmol/L)} \times 1.73/BSA}$$

$$GFR \text{ (females)} = \frac{1.03 \times \text{weight (kg)} \times [140 - \text{age}]}{\text{plasma creatinine (µmol/L)} \times 1.73/BSA}$$

where $BSA(m^2) = \sqrt{[\text{weight (kg)} \times \text{height (cm)}/3600]}$

Figure 22.3 Equations used in the estimation of glomerular filtration rate (eGFR; expressed in mL/min/1.73 m²).

to be multifactorial. It has often been put down to an 'anaemia of chronic disease', but other potential causes include haemodilution and erythropoietin suppression due to coexisting renal dysfunction,[18] proinflammatory effects of cytokines activated in patients with CHF, and a response to ACE inhibitors.[19] Iron deficiency is common in heart failure and is discussed below.

Liver function tests

Transaminases

Raised transaminases are frequently seen in heart failure patients with hepatic congestion. This can be associated with a rise in bilirubin, alkaline phosphatase, γ-glutamyl transferase and deranged

clotting—demonstrated by a prolonged prothrombin time. Deranged transaminases may also be a sign of drug toxicity (particularly from spironolactone or amiodarone).

Albumin

Low albumin (<30 g/L) is seen in patients with poor nutrition, those with chronic illness, and those with renal loss. A hypoalbuminaemic state may increase the difficulty of inducing diuresis in the volume-overloaded patient. Raised albumin (>45 g/L) can be seen in dehydrated/overdiuresed patients or those with myeloma. Nephrotic syndrome should be recalled as a differential diagnosis to heart failure in the setting of peripheral oedema and hypoalbuminaemia.

Thyroid function tests

Thyroid hormones have important effects on heart rate, cardiac contractility, the peripheral circulation, and the sympathetic nervous system. Concentrations of these hormones are frequently abnormal in patients with heart failure, particularly in those treated with amiodarone. Triiodothyronine (T_3) is low in patients with advanced heart failure, possibly due to a reduced conversion from thyroxine (T_4).

Both hypo- and hyperthyroidism can lead to the development of cardiac dysfunction. Hyperthyroidism initially induces a high-output state by an increase in heart rate and cardiac contractility, and the reduction in systemic vascular resistance. However, the incessant tachycardia and increased myocardial oxygen demand eventually may lead to left ventricular dilatation and a reduction in systolic function, resulting in a low-output state. The situation may be further exacerbated by the increased risk of atrial fibrillation. Thyrotoxicosis-induced heart failure may be reversed by treatment (e.g. by propylthiouracil). In one study, 85% had resolution of left ventricular dysfunction on achieving euthyroidism.[20]

Hypothyroidism causes a low-output state, mediated by reductions in heart rate and contractility. Cardiac function may worsen with coexisting heart failure and thyroxine replacement should be administered cautiously.

Natriuretic peptides

The B-type natriuretic peptides BNP and NT-proBNP (the inactive fragment of proBNP: **Figure 22.4**) are well known to be increased in patients with both asymptomatic and symptomatic LVSD,[21,22] increasing in proportion to the severity of CHF.[23] BNP is stable in whole blood for three days, can be measured by a rapid assay,[24] and increases only minimally following exercise.[25]

BNP can accurately detect LVSD in the general population,[26] but there is considerable debate about the potential role of BNP as a screening test for asymptomatic LVSD. The main role of BNP is currently as a 'rule-out' test to exclude heart failure due to its high NPV (up to 99%). One study has shown that BNP testing reduced the number of echocardiograms needed, and subsequent cost, in screening subjects for LVSD.[27]

Using a rapid point-of-care test for BNP, Dao *et al.* first demonstrated that BNP was both a sensitive and specific test to diagnose heart failure in patients presenting to the emergency department with dyspnoea.[28] Indeed, the NPV was 98% for BNP <80 pg/mL, and the availability of BNP measurements could have potentially corrected 96.7% of the diagnoses missed by the emergency department physician. These findings were confirmed in a larger prospective study of 1586 patients.[29] Again, BNP was found to have a high NPV (96% at BNP <50 pg/mL) and in multiple logistic regression analysis BNP added significant predictive power to other clinical variables in identifying which patients had acute heart failure (AHF).

The European Society of Cardiology has recommended a diagnostic algorithm using natriuretic peptides for untreated patients presenting with suspected heart failure of non-acute onset (**Figure 22.5**). Natriuretic peptides also exhibit high sensitivity among patients presenting with suspected AHF, and normal concentrations make the diagnosis unlikely (thresholds: BNP <100 pg/mL

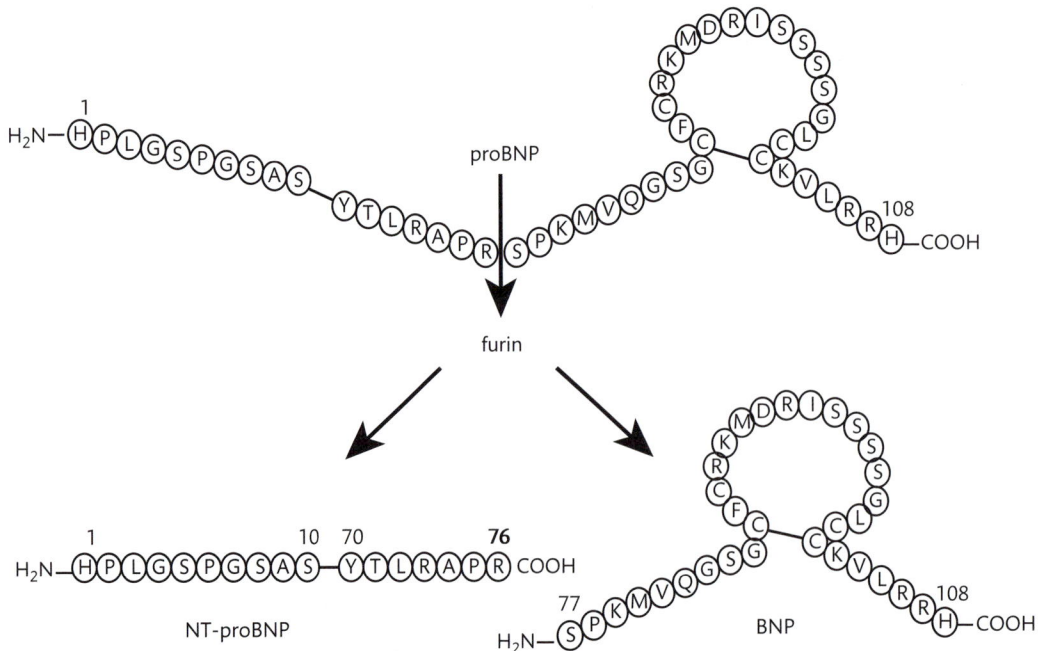

Figure 22.4 The cleavage of proBNP by furin into B-type natriuretic peptide (BNP) and the inactive fragment, NT-proBNP.

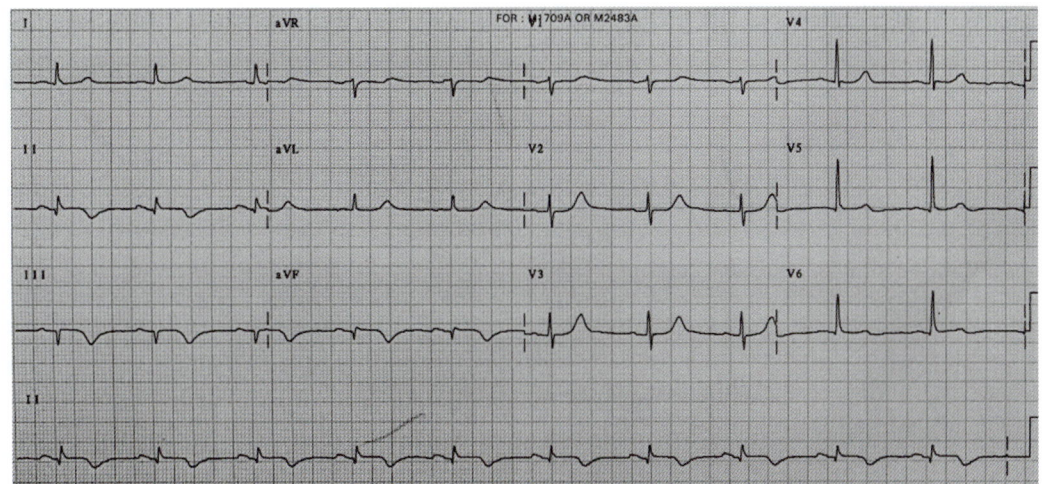

Figure 22.5 ECG evidence of an old inferior myocardial infarction, with Q waves and T wave inversion in leads II, III, and aVf.

or NT-proBNP <300 pg/mL).[30] Occasionally, NP concentrations may be unexpectedly low in patients presenting acutely with decompensated end-stage heart failure or right-sided heart failure.[30] Conversely, although BNP/NT-proBNP concentrations increase with age, and are normally higher in men than in women, increased values indicate either a cardiac functional/structural abnormality or renal dysfunction, and require further investigation. They are discussed further in Chapter 20.

Until recently, both BNP and NT-proBNP were felt to be equally useful. However, sacubitril–valsartan increases BNP (due to neprilysin antagonism, which induces the potentially beneficial effects of natriuresis and vasodilatation) but does not directly affect NT-proBNP, and so the latter has become more useful in contemporary practice.

Other laboratory tests

Glucose and glycated haemoglobin

Diabetes mellitus is commonly associated with coronary artery disease, and thus heart failure (see Chapter 35). Its presence is a strong independent predictor of mortality in patients with CHF.[31,32] The increased risk was later shown to be in patients with an ischaemic cardiomyopathy, rather than those with dilated cardiomyopathy.[33]

An elevated glycated haemoglobin (HbA1c) is an independent progressive risk factor for cardiovascular death, hospitalization for heart failure, and total mortality among both diabetic and non-diabetic patients with CHF.[34] Although intensification of hypoglycaemic therapy *per se* has not yet been shown to improve outcomes in heart failure patients, drugs that emerged as anti-diabetic agents have demonstrated clear benefits in this group. When added to optimal medical therapy in patients with heart failure, dapagliflozin (a sodium-glucose cotransporter 2 (SGLT2) inhibitor) reduces the risk of worsening heart failure or cardiovascular death; in fact, this is true regardless of the presence or absence of diabetes.[35] Empaglifozin—another SGLT2 inhibitor—is known to reduce heart failure hospitalizations and mortality in patients with type 2 diabetes.[36] At the time of writing, SGLT2 inhibitors (primarily dapagliflozin) are licenced for use in heart failure with or without concomitant diabetes

in the USA but not in the UK (where the presence of diabetes is mandated). An indication for use in heart failure without diabetes is likely to develop in the UK within the lifetime of this text; however, at present an elevated HbA1c remains the gateway to this important new medication.

Iron studies (ferritin and transferrin saturations ± C282Y genotyping)

Iron deficiency is common in heart failure patients with or without anaemia, and is associated with a worse prognosis in both.[37] The discovery of iron deficiency should prompt both deliberation on its aetiology and consideration of intravenous iron therapy. Intravenous ferric carboxymaltose is the preferred preparation, having been shown in two randomized trials to improve symptoms and functional capacity in iron-deficient patients (both anaemic and non-anaemic) with heart failure and reduced ejection fraction (HFrEF).[38,39] In both trials, iron deficiency was defined as serum ferritin <100 µg/L, or ferritin 100–299 µg/L and transferrin saturation <20%.

Conversely, the detection of iron overload is also important, as it can lead to conduction system disease or dilated cardiomyopathy. The chief cause is hereditary haemochromatosis (HH), an autosomal recessive disorder in which a mutation of the *HFE* gene (most commonly a C282Y mutation) causes increased intestinal iron absorption. The HH homozygous state has a prevalence of 0.45% in the USA,[18] with cardiac involvement being the presenting manifestation in 15% of individuals. Appropriate investigations include transferrin saturation, serum ferritin, and, where appropriate, C282Y *HFE* mutation analysis.

Troponin

An elevated troponin I or T indicates myocyte necrosis and is seen both in acute coronary syndrome (ACS) and in acute myocarditis. Minor increases in cardiac troponin are frequently seen in patients with advanced heart failure or during episodes of decompensation. Persistently elevated TnT concentrations have been shown to be associated with increasing left ventricular diastolic dimensions, decreasing left ventricular ejection fraction (LVEF), and increased risk of death.[40] Elevated troponin is an especially powerful

adverse prognostic marker in heart failure patients who also have elevated NPs.[41]

Caeruloplasmin

Wilson disease is an autosomal recessive defect in cellular copper transport which usually leads to hepatic cirrhosis, but rarely may also lead to cardiomyopathy. As the incorporation of copper into caeruloplasmin is also impaired, there is a reduction in serum caeruloplasmin concentrations present in most patients with Wilson's disease.

Urate

Serum uric acid is often raised in patients on diuretics, and may be a precursor for the development of gout. Raised uric acid concentrations have been shown to be strongly related to circulating markers of inflammation in patients with heart failure,[42] and are independently predictive of an adverse prognosis.[43,44]

Genetic screen

Genetic testing and counselling are important in cases of suspected familial cardiomyopathy, usually where there is a family history. Serum creatine kinase (CK) should also be checked as it can be raised in myotonic dystrophy or the dystrophinopathies. Genetic causes of heart failure are further considered in Chapter 5.

Further tests

Other tests that may be considered include urinalysis, a myeloma screen, autoantibodies (including antinuclear antibodies) where systemic lupus erythematosus is suspected, and urinary catecholamines for the investigation of phaeochromocytoma. Despite extensive research on heart failure biomarkers other than BNP/NT-proBNP (e.g. adrenomedullin, copeptin, galectin 3, ST2) none has yet emerged a test that can be recommended in clinical practice.

Chest radiograph

The chest radiograph is an important investigation in the diagnostic work-up of the breathless patient. However, a normal chest radiograph does not exclude a diagnosis of heart failure, as the cardiothoracic ratio (CTR) is normal (<0.5) in around 50% of cases. Indeed, there is a wealth of evidence from large heart failure trials showing that even patients with severe LVSD can have a normal heart size on chest radiograph (Table 22.4). Conversely, the chest radiograph may be suggestive of a cardiac abnormality when cardiomegaly (CTR >0.50) is present (Figure 22.6) or if there is evidence of pulmonary venous congestion, bilateral pleural effusions, or interstitial oedema. The chest radiograph can also help identify or exclude other causes of breathlessness, such as pericardial effusion (Figure 22.7), bronchial carcinoma (Figure 22.8), or emphysema.

Although an increased CTR may suggest cardiac abnormality, it need not reflect a reduced LVEF. Indeed, in the registry population of the Coronary Artery Surgery Study,[47] two-thirds of patients with CTR >0.50 had normal LVEF. In the absence of LV dilatation, other causes of radiographic cardiomegaly include pericardial fat, left ventricular hypertrophy, pericardial effusion (Figure 22.7), valvular dysfunction, and right heart dysfunction/dilatation.

Table 22.4 Cardiothoracic ratio in large heart failure trials

Trial	Mean CTR (SD) or [a](SEM)	Mean LVEF (%)	CTR ≤0.5 (%)
CIBIS[45]	0.55 ± 0.07	25.4	–
DIG[46]	0.53 ± 0.07	28.1	40
PRAISE	0.57 ± 0.01[a]	21	–
PROVED	0.50 ± 0.01[a]	29	–
RADIANCE	0.53 ± 0.01	27	–
SOLVD-P	0.50 ± 0.06	28	60
SOLVD-T	0.53 ± 0.07	25	53
VHeFT	0.53 ± 0.006	30	30[b]
VHeFT II	0.53 ± 0.006	29	29[b]

CTR, cardiothoracic ratio; LVEF, left ventricular ejection fraction; SD, standard deviation; SEM; standard error of the mean.
[b] <0.5.
Source data from Petrie MC, It cannot be cardiac failure because the heart is not enlarged on the chest X-ray, Eur J Heart Fail 2003;**5**:117–19.

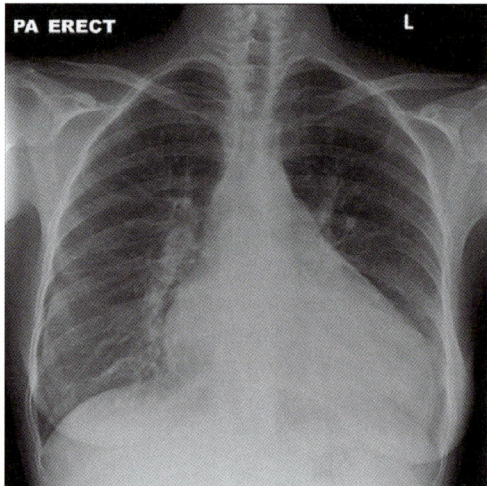

Figure 22.6 Posteroanterior chest radiograph of a 17-year-old girl with gross cardiomegaly. There is also evidence of fluid in the horizontal fissure and upper lobe venous diversion.

Thus, a normal heart size does not exclude significant, or even severe, LVSD in a patient with suspected heart failure, and cardiomegaly is not necessarily specific for LVSD. This is in contrast to the normal 12-lead ECG, which virtually rules out LVSD and, when abnormal, may point to an underlying aetiology. Although the CTR adds little additional diagnostic information to that obtained from the 12-lead ECG, other findings on the chest radiograph, such as pulmonary congestion or oedema, may support the diagnosis of cardiac dysfunction.

However, the CTR is of considerable prognostic value in patients with chronic heart failure and low LVEF. Higher CTR is predictive of the risk of worsening symptoms, hospitalization, and mortality. In addition, UK-HEART (UK heart failure evaluation and assessment of risk trial)—a multicentre prospective study designed to identify non-invasive markers of death and mode of death in patients with CHF—showed that a greater CTR was also predictive of sudden death (hazard ratio; 1.43 (95% confidence interval; 1.20–1.71), $P < 0.04$ for a 10% increase in CTR).[48]

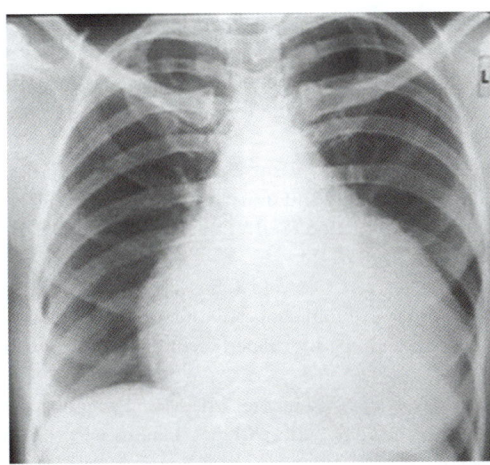

Figure 22.7 PA chest radiograph of a patient with pericardial effusion.

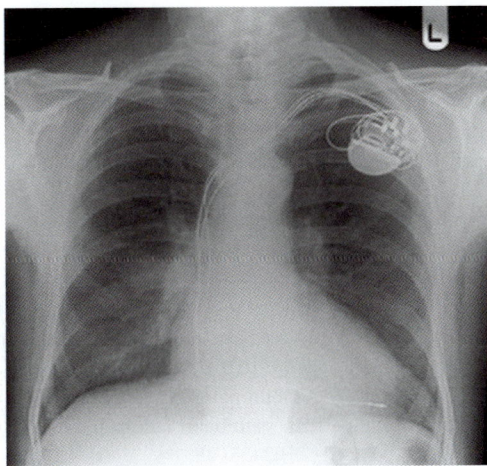

Figure 22.8 Chest radiograph showing two causes for breathlessness: (1) a right hilar mass was identified post-CRT-P implantation for congestive heart failure, and (2) subsequent biopsy revealed non-small-cell lung carcinoma.

Historically, a higher CTR may also help predict response to therapy. In the DIG trial, the benefit of digoxin appeared to be greater among patients at high risk.[49] Those who were more symptomatic, who had a lower ejection fraction, or who had greater CTR (>0.55) had a lower risk of experiencing death from, or hospitalization for, worsening CHF when randomized to digoxin compared to placebo.

Other investigations

Echocardiography (see Chapter 23) is a key investigation in the assessment of the patient suspected of having heart failure. It allows a very accessible and non-invasive assessment of myocardial and valvular function. However, CMR (see Chapter 24) is now the reference standard imaging modality for the assessment of myocardial function, allowing an accurate and reproducible measurement of cardiac volumes and left ventricular mass, as well as characterizing cardiac tissue and identifying areas of infarction or infiltration. Invasive investigations (Chapter 27) include right and left heart catheterization and endomyocardial biopsy. These investigations are considered in more detail in subsequent chapters.

Summary

Each investigation highlighted above is a piece of a diagnostic jigsaw and no single test can confirm the clinical syndrome of heart failure without the presence of symptoms. However, a normal BNP/NT-proBNP and ECG argue strongly against the presence of heart failure. Conversely, a raised BNP/NT-proBNP can have causes other than heart failure, and cardiomegaly on the chest radiograph is not a prerequisite for the diagnosis either, as a significant proportion of patients with LVSD have a normal CTR. Thus, the accurate assessment of the patient suspected of having heart failure requires a detailed history and examination, as well as objective evidence of cardiac dysfunction from careful investigation using echocardiography or CMR.

REFERENCES

1. Baldasseroni S, Opasich C, Gorini M, *et al.* Left bundle branch block is associated with increased 1-year sudden and total mortality rate in 5517 outpatients with congestive heart failure: a report from the Italian Network on Congestive Heart Failure. *Am Heart J* 2002;**143**:398–405.
2. Funck-Brentano C, Lancar R, Hansen S, *et al.* Predictors of medical events and of their competitive interactions in the Cardiac Insufficiency Bisoprolol Study 2 (CIBIS-2). *Am Heart J* 2001;**142**:989–97.
3. Shamim W, Yousufuddin M, Cicoria M, *et al.* Incremental changes in QRS duration in serial ECGs over time identify high risk elderly patients with heart failure. *Heart* 2002;**88**:47–52.
4. Grigioni F, Carinci V, Boriani G, *et al.* Accelerated QRS widening as an independent predictor of cardiac death or the need for heart transplantation in patients with congestive heart failure. *J Heart Lung Transplant* 2002;**21**:899–901.
5. Clark A, Goode K, Cleland JGF. The prevalence and incidence of left bundle branch block in ambulant patients with chronic heart failure. *Eur Heart J* 2008;**10**:696–702.
6. Cleland JG, Daubert JC, Erdmann E, *et al.* The effect of cardiac resynchronization on morbidity and mortality in heart failure. *N Engl J Med* 2005;**352**(15):1539–49.
7. Konstam MA, Gheorghiade M, Burnett JC Jr, *et al.* Effects of oral tolvaptan in patients hospitalized for worsening heart failure: the EVEREST Outcome Trial. *JAMA* 2007;**297**(12):1319–31.
8. Levey AS, Coresh J, Balk E. National Kidney Foundation practice guidelines for chronic kidney disease: evaluation, classification, and stratification. *Ann Intern Med* 2003;**139**:137–47.
9. Levey AS, Bosch JP, Lewis JB, *et al.* A more accurate method to estimate glomerular filtration rate from serum creatinine: a new prediction equation. *Ann Intern Med* 1999;**130**:461–70.
10. O'Meara E, Chong KS, Gardner RS, *et al.* The Modification of Diet in Renal Disease (MDRD) equations provide valid estimations of glomerular filtration rates in patients with advanced heart failure. *Eur J Heart Fail* 2006;**8**(1):63–7.
11. Dries DL, Exner DV, Domanski MJ, Greenberg B, Stevenson LW. The prognostic implications of renal insufficiency in asymptomatic and symptomatic patients with left ventricular systolic dysfunction. *J Am Coll Cardiol* 2000;**35**(3):681–9.

12. Mahon N, Blackstone EH, Francis GS, *et al.* The prognostic value of estimated creatinine clearance alongside functional capacity in ambulatory patients with chronic congestive heart failure. *J Am Coll Cardiol* 2002;**40**:1106–13.

13. Al-Ahmad A, Rand W, Manjunath G, *et al.* Reduced kidney function and anemia as risk factors for mortality in patients with left ventricular dysfunction. *J Am Coll Cardiol* 2001;**38**(4):955–62.

14. Hillege HL, Girbes ARJ, de Kam PJ, *et al.* Renal function, neurohormonal activation and survival in patients with chronic heart failure. *Circulation* 2000;**102**:203–10.

15. Ezekowitz JA, McAlister FA, Armstrong PW. Anemia is common in heart failure and is associated with a poor outcome. *Circulation* 2003;**107**:223–5.

16. Anand I, McMurray JJV, Whitmore J, *et al.* Anemia and its relationship to clinical outcome in heart failure. *Circulation* 2004;**110**:149–54.

17. Horwich TB, Fonarow GC, Hamilton MA, MacLellan WR, Borer JS. Anemia is associated with worse symptoms, greater impairment in functional capacity and a significant increase in mortality in patients with advanced heart failure. *J Am Coll Cardiol* 2002;**39**:1780–6.

18. Al Ahmad A, Rand W, Manjunath G, *et al.* Reduced kidney function and anemia as risk factors for mortality in patients with left ventricular dysfunction. *J Am Coll Cardiol* 2001;**38**(4):955–62.

19. Plata R, Cornejo A, Arratia C, *et al.* Angiotensin-converting-enzyme inhibition therapy in altitude polycythaemia: a prospective randomised trial. *Lancet* 2002;**359**:663–6.

20. Wong F, Siu S, Liu P, Blendis LM. Brain natriuretic peptide: is it a predictor of cardiomyopathy in cirrhosis? *Clin Sci (Lond)* 2001;**101**(6):621–8.

21. Lerman A, Gibbons RJ, Rodeheffer RJ, *et al.* Circulating N-terminal atrial natriuretic peptide as a marker for symptomless left-ventricular dysfunction. *Lancet* 1993;**341**:1105–9.

22. McDonagh TA, Cunningham AD, Morrison CE, *et al.* Left ventricular dysfunction, natriuretic peptides, and mortality in an urban population. *Heart* 2001;**86**:21–6.

23. Tsutamoto T, Wada A, Maeda K, *et al.* Attenuation of compensation of endogenous cardiac natriuretic peptide system in chronic heart failure—prognostic role of brain natriuretic peptide concentration in patients with chronic symptomatic left ventricular dysfunction. *Circulation* 1997;**96**:509–16.

24. Murdoch DR, Byrne J, Morton JJ, *et al.* Brain natriuretic peptide is stable in whole blood and can be measured using a simple rapid assay: implications for clinical practice. *Heart* 1997;**78**:594–7.

25. McNairy M, Gardetto N, Clopton P, *et al.* Stability of B-type natriuretic peptide levels during exercise in patients with congestive heart failure. *Am Heart J* 2002;**143**:406–11.

26. McDonagh TA, Robb SD, Murdoch DR, *et al.* Biochemical detection of left-ventricular systolic dysfunction. *Lancet* 1998; **351**(9095):9–13.

27. Nielsen OW, McDonagh TA, Robb SD, Dargie HJ. Retrospective analysis of the cost-effectiveness of using plasma brain natriuretic peptide in screening for left ventricular systolic dysfunction in the general population. *J Am Coll Cardiol* 2003;**41**:113–120.

28. Dao Q, Krishnaswamy P, Kazanegra R, *et al.* Utility of B-type natriuretic peptide in the diagnosis of congestive heart failure in an urgent-care setting. *J Am Coll Cardiol* 2001;**37**(2):379–85.

29. Maisel AS, Krishnaswamy P, Nowak R, *et al.* Rapid measurement of B-type natriuretic peptide in the emergency diagnosis of heart failure. *N Engl J Med* 2002;**347**(3):161–7.

30. Ponikowski P, Voors AA, Anker SD, *et al.* 2016 ESC Guidelines for the diagnosis and treatment of acute and chronic heart failure: The Task Force for the diagnosis and treatment of acute and chronic heart failure of the European Society of Cardiology (ESC). Developed with the special contribution of the Heart Failure Association (HFA) of the ESC. *Eur J Heart Fail* 2016;**18**(8):891–975.

31. Shindler DM, Kostis JB, Yusuf S, *et al.* Diabetes mellitus: a predictor of morbidity and mortality in the Studies Of Left Ventricular Dysfunction (SOLVD) trials and registry. *Am J Cardiol* 1996;**77**:1017–20.

32. Prazak P, Pfisterer M, Osswald S, Buser P, Burkart F. Differences of disease progression in congestive heart failure due to alcoholic as compared to idiopathic dilated cardiomyopathy. *Eur Heart J* 1996;**17**(2):251–7.

33. Dries DL, Sweitzer NK, Drazner MH, *et al.* Prognostic impact of diabetes mellitus in patients with heart failure according to the etiology of left ventricular systolic function. *J Am Coll Cardiol* 2001;**38**:421–8.

34. Gerstein HC, Swedberg K, Carlsson J, *et al.* The hemoglobin A1c level as a progressive risk factor for cardiovascular death, hospitalization for heart failure, or death in patients with chronic heart failure: an analysis of the Candesartan in Heart failure: Assessment of Reduction in Mortality and Morbidity (CHARM) program. *Arch Intern Med* 2008;**168**:1699–704.

35. McMurray JJV, Solomon SD, Inzucchi SE, *et al.* Dapagliflozin in patients with heart failure and reduced ejection fraction. *N Engl J Med* 2019;**381**:1995–2008.

36. Zinman B, Wanner C, Lachlin JM, *et al.* Empagliflozin, cardiovascular outcomes, and mortality in type 2 diabetes. *N Engl J Med* 2015; **373**:2117–28.

37. Cleland JGF, Zhang J, Pellicori P, *et al.* Prevalence and outcomes of anemia and hematinic deficiencies in patients with chronic heart failure. *JAMA Cardiol* 2016;**1**(5):539–47.

38. Anker SD, Comin Colet J, Filippatos G, *et al.* Ferric carboxymaltose in patients with heart failure and iron deficiency. *N Engl J Med* 2009;**361**(25):2436–48.

39. Ponikowski P, van Veldhuisen DJ, Comin-Colet J, *et al.* Beneficial effects of long-term intravenous iron therapy with ferric carboxymaltose in patients with symptomatic heart failure and iron deficiency. *Eur Heart J* 2015;**36**(11):657–68.

40. Sato Y, Yamada T, Taniguchi R, *et al.* Persistently increased serum concentrations of cardiac troponin T in patients with idiopathic dilated cardiomyopathy are predicitve of adverse outcomes. *Circulation* 2001;**103**:369–74.

41. Metra M, Nodari S, Parrinello G, *et al.* The role of plasma biomarkers in acute heart failure. Serial changes and independent prognostic value of NT-proBNP and cardiac troponin-T. *Eur J Heart Fail* 2007;**9**(8):776–86.

42. Leyva F, Anker SD, Godsland IF, *et al.* Uric acid in chronic heart failure: a marker of chronic inflammation. *Eur Heart J* 1998;**19**(12):1814–22.

43. Anker SD, Leyva F, Poole-Wilson P, Coats AJ. Uric acid as independent predictor of impaired prognosis in patients with chronic heart failure [abstract]. *J Am Coll Cardiol* 1998;**31**:154–5A.

44. Batin P, Wickens M, McEntegart D, Fullwood L, Cowley AJ. The importance of abnormalities of liver function tests in predicting mortality in chronic heart failure. *Eur Heart J* 1995;**16**(11):1613–18.

45. CIBIS Investigators and Committees. A randomised trial of beta-blockade in heart failure: the Cardiac Insufficiency Bisoprolol Study (CIBIS). *Circulation* 1994;**90**:1765–73.

46. Rathore SS, Curtis JP, Wang Y, Bristow MR, Krumholz HM. Association of serum digoxin concentration and outcomes in patients with heart failure. *JAMA* 2003;**289**(7):871–8.

47. Rihal CS, Davis KB, Kennedy JW, Gersh BJ. The utility of clinical, electrocardiographic, and roentgenographic variables in the prediction of left ventricular function. *Am J Cardiol* 1995;**75**(4):220–3.

48. Kearney MT, Fox KA, Lee AJ, *et al.* Predicting sudden death in patients with mild to moderate chronic heart failure. *Heart* 2004;**90**(10):1137–43.

49. Digitalis Investigation Group. The effect of digoxin on mortality and morbidity in patients with heart failure. *N Engl J Med* 1997;**336**(8):525–33.

23

Echocardiography

Alison Duncan

Introduction

Heart failure is a complex syndrome that can result from any structural or functional cardiac disorder that impairs the ability of the heart to function as a pump to support a physiological circulation. The most common cause of heart failure in the UK is coronary artery disease; other aetiologies include hypertension, atrial fibrillation, cardiomyopathies, valvular heart disease, pericardial disease, and intracardiac shunts.[1] Transthoracic echocardiography has a decisive role in the diagnosis, treatment, and follow-up of patients with heart failure.[2] Indeed, its importance was underscored in the UK 2010 National Institute for Health and Care Excellence (NICE) Guidelines for Heart Failure,[3] and in the 2013 American College of Cardiology/American Heart Association (ACC/AHA) guidelines for the diagnosis and management of heart failure.[4] Echocardiography utilizes ultrasound, which has no known adverse biological effects, is non-invasive, and is a relatively low-cost imaging modality. The use of echocardiography in the diagnosis, therapeutic management, and serial follow-up of the increasing number of patients with heart failure has therefore potentially large health benefits with relatively low patient cost.

Echocardiographic assessment of left ventricular function

Abnormalities of left ventricular (LV) function may be apparent even before clinical signs of heart failure are evident. Comprehensive echocardiographic assessment of LV function is therefore required. Table 23.1 outlines standard techniques for echo evaluation of LV function. The minimal requirements are an assessment of:

1. LV size and shape
2. global LV systolic function
3. regional systolic function
4. diastolic function
5. intracardiac haemodynamics
6. LV synchrony.

Assessment of left ventricular cavity size

Measurements of LV cavity size (end-diastolic dimension (EDD) and end-systolic dimension (ESD)) are made from M-mode or two-dimensional cross-sectional imaging of the LV at the level of the mitral valve tips at end diastole (Q wave of the preceding cardiac cycle) and at end systole (aortic valve closure) (Figure 23.1). Segmental wall thickness at end diastole (and thickening fraction from measurements at end systole) may also be determined using either method. Normal ranges for LV cavity size are presented in Table 23.2.[4]

Table 23.1 Assessment of left ventricular function

Echo variable	Assessment
LV cavity size	M-mode/2D measurements
Global LV systolic function	Qualitative evaluation of size, shape, and LVEF
	Quantification of LV dimensions, volumes, fractional shortening, EF (Simpson)
	Degree of LVH
	Doppler measurements (dP/dt in mitral regurgitation)
Regional systolic function	Qualitative evaluation (wall motion score index)
	Quantitative evaluation (M-mode or TDI)
	Newer techniques (strain, strain rate, tissue tracking)
Diastolic function	Transmitral flow velocities
	Annular tissue velocity (E:E′ ratio)
	Response to Valsalva manoeuvre
	Others (pulmonary vein flow, mitral flow propagation)
Synchrony	Doppler assessment of interventricular delay
	Intraventricular delay (M-mode, TDI, strain, 3D)
	Consequences of incoordination on global function

EF, ejection fraction; LV, left ventricular; LVH, left ventricular hypertrophy; TDI, tissue Doppler imaging.

LV cavity dimensions by M-mode

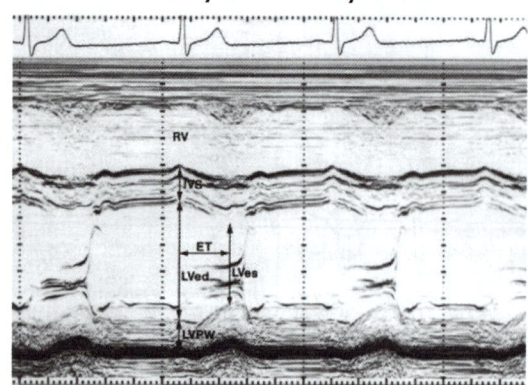

LV cavity dimensions by 2D

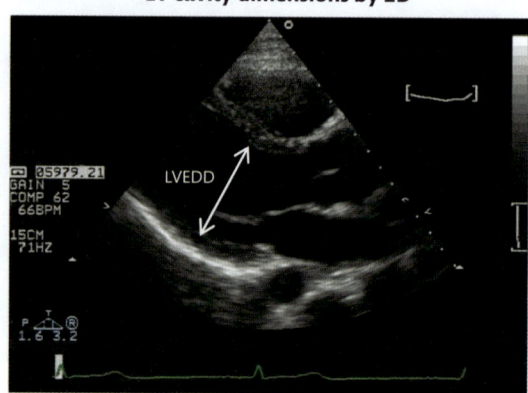

Figure 23.1 Measurement of left ventricular cavity size. *Left*: left ventricular M-mode taken from a parasternal long axis view at the level of the mitral valve tips. *Right*: still two-dimensional (2D) image from a parasternal long axis view. In 2D imaging, left ventricular cavity size is measured endocardial border to endocardial border in a line at right angles to each wall passing through the mitral valve tips. ET, ejection time; IVS, interventricular septum; LA, left atrium; LVed, left ventricular cavity size at end diastole; LVes, left ventricular cavity size at end systole; LVPW, left ventricular posterior wall; RV, right ventricle.

Table 23.2 Left ventricular size, mass, and function

Variable	Normal	Mild	Moderate	Severe
LV wall thickness				
IVSd/PW (cm)	0.6–1.2	1.3–1.5	1.6–1.9	≥2.0
LV dimension (women)				
LVIDd (cm)	3.9–5.3	5.4–5.7	5.8–6.1	≥6.2
LVIDd/BSA (cm/m²)	2.4–3.2	3.3–3.4	3.5–3.7	≥3.8
LV dimension (men)				
LVIDd (cm)	4.2–5.9	6.0–6.3	6.4–6.8	≥6.9
LVIDd/BSA (cm/m²)	2.2–3.1	3.2–3.4	3.5–3.6	≥3.7
LV volume (women)				
LV diastolic volume (mL)	56–104	105–117	118–130	≥131
LV systolic volume (mL)	19–49	50–59	60–69	≥70
LV volume (men)				
LV diastolic volume (mL)	67–155	156–178	179–201	≥202
LV systolic volume (mL)	22–58	59–70	71–82	≥83
LV volume index				
LV diastolic volume/BSA (mL/m²)	35–75	76–86	87–96	≥97
LV systolic volume/BSA (mL/m²)	12–30	31–36	37–42	≥43
LV function				
Fractional shortening (%)	25–43	20–24	15–19	<15
Ejection fraction (biplane Simpson)	>55	45–54	36–44	≤35
LV mass (women)				
LV mass (g)	66–150	151–171	172–182	≥182
LV mass/BSA (g/cm²)	44–88	89–100	101–112	≥112
LV mass (men)				
LV mass (g)	96–200	201–227	228–254	≥254
LV mass/BSA (g/cm²)	50–102	103–116	117–130	≥130

BSA, body surface area; LV, left ventricular.
Source data from Lang RM, Bierig M, Devereaux RB, et al. Recommendations for chamber quantification. J Am Soc Echocardiogr 2005;**18**:1440–63.

Assessment of global left ventricular function

Fractional shortening and ejection fraction

Fractional shortening may be calculated using measures of LV end-diastolic and end-systolic cavity size (as the percentage change in LV cavity dimension in systole with respect to diastole):

$$\text{Fractional shortening (\%)} = [(EDD - ESD)/EDD] \times 100$$

Although fractional shortening accurately quantifies basal LV function, it is reliable only in a symmetrically contracting heart without regional variability and thus is frequently inappropriate for the re-modelled ventricles of many heart failure patients. Assessment of LV systolic function thus depends more on values of LV ejection fraction (LVEF). Calculation of LVEF is based on guidelines from the American Society of Echocardiography using the principle of slicing the LV from mitral valve annulus to apex into a series of 20 discs.[5] The volume of each disc is calculated (using the diameter and thickness of the slice) and then all the discs are summated to provide LV volumes at end diastole and end systole (**Figure 23.2**). LVEF (%) is calculated as:

$$[(EDV - ESV)/EDV] \times 100$$

Accuracy is improved by using diameters in two perpendicular planes (apical four- and two-chamber). Normal ranges for LV fractional shortening and LVEF are presented in **Table 23.2**. The ASE guidelines define an abnormal LVEF as <55%, with the cut-offs for moderately and severely reduced LVEF as 36–44% and <35% respectively.

The 'summation of discs' method assumes that the imaging planes are orthogonal and is absolutely dependent on detection of the endocardial border and therefore image quality of the echocardiogram. Interobserver variability and beat-to-beat variability may be significant if image quality is suboptimal. Real-time three-dimensional echo imaging has the advantage of taking into account variation in ventricular shape in all directions rather than just the two biplane measurements (**Figure 23.3**a), with good correlation

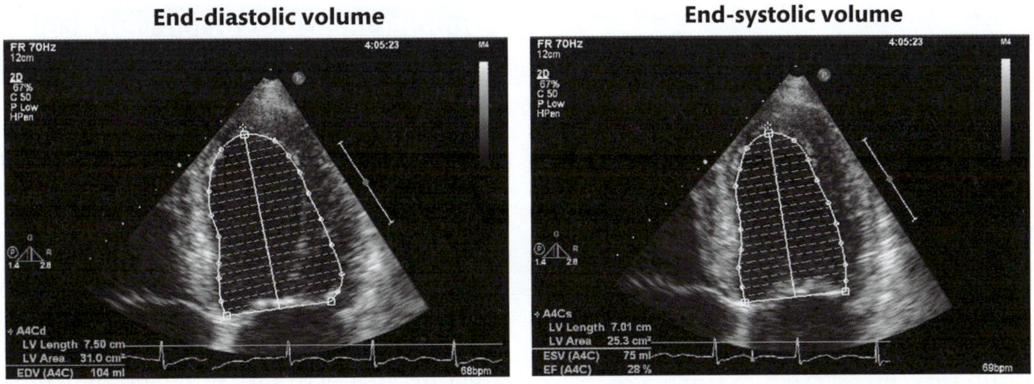

End-diastolic volume

End-systolic volume

Figure 23.2 Calculation of Simpson's biplane left ventricular ejection fraction. Left: still end-diastolic frame in apical four-chamber view calculating end-diastolic volume (EDV); right: still end-systolic frame in apical four-chamber view calculating end-systolic volume (ESV).

with cardiac volumes obtained from cardiac magnetic resonance imaging (CMR). However, good-quality endocardial border definition is still required.[6]

Despite the historical use of LVEF as 'a measure of LV systolic function', its use has distinct disadvantages. As an ejection-phase index, LVEF is highly load-dependent; thus, a change in LVEF over time may not necessarily be due to a change in the intrinsic contractility of the myocardium (a true measure of systolic function), but may merely reflect a change in the loading conditions. Nevertheless, LVEF and 'systolic function' continue to be used interchangeably in the literature. Moreover, since LVEF is affected by preload and afterload, it can give misleading information in several clinical situations; for example, the falsely high LVEF in severe mitral regurgitation when underlying LV systolic function is abnormal, the low LVEF in severe aortic stenosis which can increase markedly after valve replacement, and the variable LVEF in atrial fibrillation. Furthermore, LVEF does not correlate with heart failure symptoms, exercise capacity, or myocardial oxygen consumption.[7] Despite these major limitations, echo measurement of LVEF continues to be standard practice, providing, as it does, not only the standard entry criterion for many heart failure clinical trials,[8–10] but guidance for therapeutic intervention such as defibrillator device therapy and timing of surgery for valve disease,[11,12] and affording prognostic information (predicting major adverse cardiac events, cardiovascular mortality, and sudden death) in the heart failure population.[13,14]

Left ventricular thickness and mass

The clinical importance of LV mass relates to the identification of pathological LV hypertrophy (LVH). In the echocardiographic

(a)
3D calculation of LV volumes and LVEF

(b)
3D calculation of LV Mass

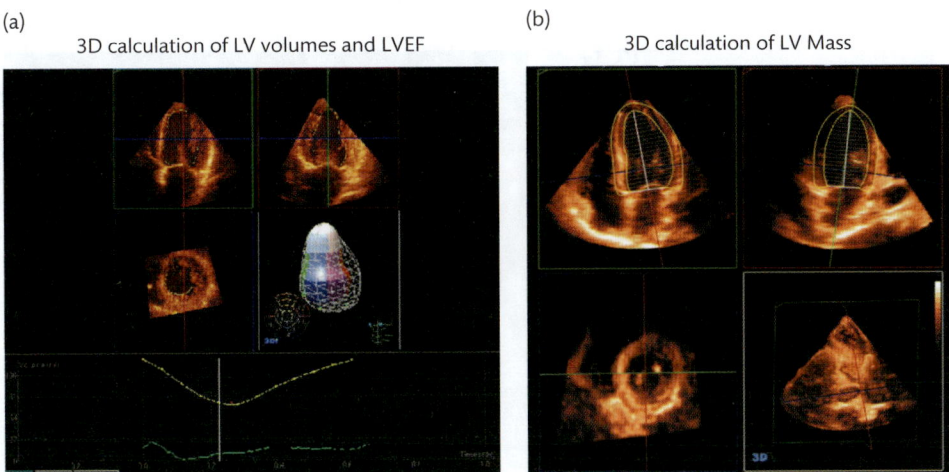

Figure 23.3 Calculation of left ventricular volumes using transthoracic three-dimensional (3D) echo. (a) Calculation of left ventricular volumes and ejection fraction. A 3D image set is acquired from the apex, the left ventricular border is traced in two planes, and the rest of the left ventricular border is tracked automatically to create a volume-rendered outline of the left ventricular throughout the cardiac cycle. From this, a mathematical model or 'cast' of the left ventricular is created using all 3D data points. Calculated left ventricular volume may be plotted against time during one cardiac cycle. End-diastolic and end-systolic volumes plus ejection fraction and sphericity index can be derived from these data. (b) Example of left ventricular mass calculation where apical four- and two-chamber sections have been created from a full volume dataset of the left ventricular, endocardial and epicardial borders of the left ventricular myocardium is identified and a biplane Simpson's rule calculation applied to derive both left ventricular and myocardial volumes. The latter is multiplied by the specific gravity of heart muscle to obtain the displayed mass.

substudy of the SOLVD trial, increased LV mass was associated with high mortality and rate of cardiovascular hospital stays, independent of LVEF.[14] LVH may be secondary to other pathology (aortic valve disease or hypertension) or it may be a primary myocardial problem (hypertrophic cardiomyopathy, infiltrative cardiomyopathy). Physiological hypertrophy (in athletes or during pregnancy) is usually reversible. In elderly people, there is sometimes septal angulation and thickening that creates the impression of septal hypertrophy but the LV mass is usually unchanged. LV mass may be calculated using M-mode techniques and the formula:

$$LV\ mass = 1.04\big([LVID+PWT+LVST]-LVID\big)-14g$$

where LVID is the LV internal dimension during diastole, PWT is the posterior wall thickness, and IVST is the interventricular septal thickness.[15] Two-dimensional methods, including the truncated ellipsoid and the area–length formula, might be more appropriate for distorted ventricles with regional wall motion abnormalities. Both methods, however, rely heavily on geometric assumptions and are therefore subject to inaccuracies from foreshortening. These limitations may be partially overcome using three-dimensional echocardiographic techniques (Figure 23.3b).

Normal ranges for left ventricular mass are presented in Table 23.2. LVH may be graded by reporting relative wall thickness (calculated as $(2\times PWT)/LVEDD$) and overall LV mass, and reported as (1) normal; (2) concentric LVH (increased relative wall thickness with increased mass); (3) eccentric LVH (increased mass with normal relative wall thickness); (4) concentric remodelling (normal mass with increased relative wall thickness). Concentric changes suggest pressure overload (due to aortic stenosis or hypertension), whereas eccentric changes suggest volume overload (e.g. due to aortic regurgitation).

Doppler measures of left ventricular systolic function

Doppler echocardiography can evaluate indices of the isovolumic contraction phases of the cardiac cycle, which may be more representative of the LV contractile state. The change in LV pressure over time (dP/dt) is closely related to the mitral regurgitation trace obtained using echocardiography using continuous wave Doppler across the mitral valve (**Figure 23.4**). Assuming any change in left atrial pressure during systole has negligible effect on this pressure difference, a plot of LV dP/dt can be generated from the first derivative of the pressure difference plot.[16] The faster the rise in LV pressure, the more co-ordinated the LV systolic function.[17]

Alternatively, stroke distance can be calculated from the velocity–time integral (VTI) of the LV outflow tract using pulse-wave Doppler from an apical five-chamber view. The product of stroke distance (normally 18–22 cm) and LV outflow tract area provides quantitative Doppler assessment of LV stroke volume. Cardiac output may be subsequently calculated as the product of stroke volume and heart rate.

Assessment of regional left ventricular systolic function

Two-dimensional regional wall motion abnormalities

Regional wall motion abnormalities may occur in any dilated cardiomyopathy but are most commonly associated with coronary artery disease. Echocardiography is an extremely useful tool for identifying LV wall motion abnormalities, assessed subjectively, and attributed to specific coronary territories. The right coronary artery usually

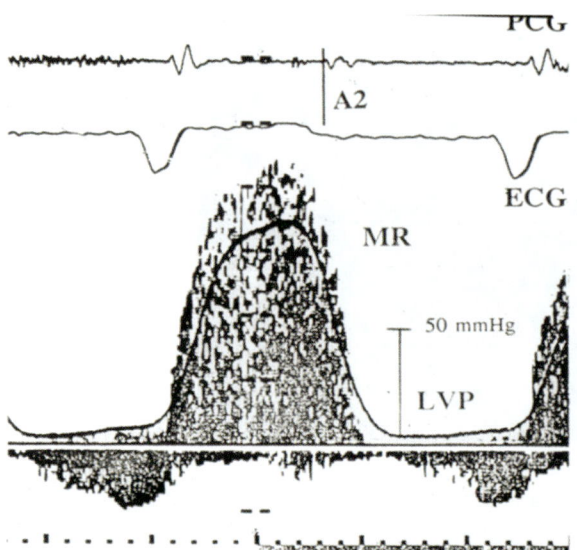
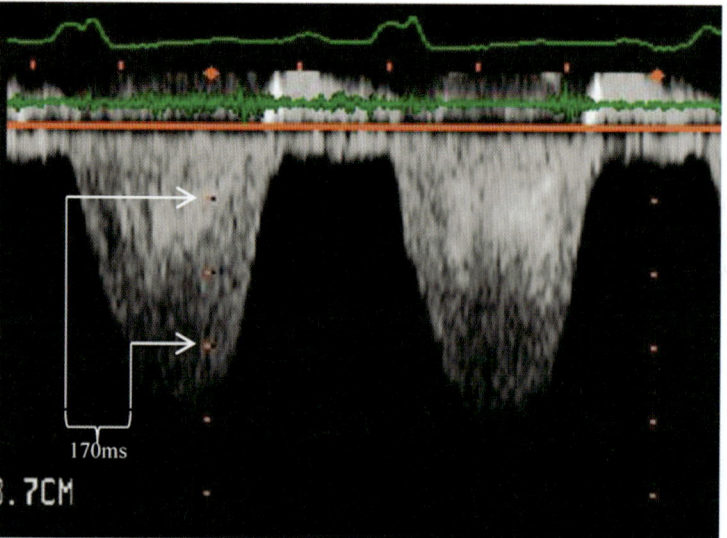

Figure 23.4 Measurement of dP/dt. *Left*: change in left ventricular pressure (LVP, measured by tip manometer) is closely associated with mitral regurgitation (MR) trace obtained using transoesophageal echocardiography. *Right*: measurement of dP/dt: record MR at 100 mm/s and measure the time for the MR velocity jet to rise from 1 to 4 m/s (i.e. from 4 to 36 mmHg). dP/dt >1200 mmHg/s (<27 ms between points) relates to normally timed left ventricular contraction whereas values <800 mmHg/s (>40 ms) suggest severely prolonged contractile state.

supplies the right ventricle and LV inferioseptal segments; the left anterior descending artery supplies the LV anterior, anteroseptal, and apical segments; and the circumflex artery supplies the LV lateral wall. However, there may be considerable variation and/or overlap between individual patients.

Qualitative assessment

A standard 16-segment model of the LV (lateral, septal, inferior, anterior segments at the apex, midpapillary, and basal levels, and anteroseptal and posterior segments at the midpapillary and basal levels)[18] or, more recently, a 17-segment model that includes a true apical segment,[19] is used to assess regional function. Each region is given a score where 1 is normal, 2 is hypokinetic (endocardial excursion <5 mm), 3 is akinetic (endocardial excursion <2 mm), and 4 is dyskinetic (endocardium moves outwards in systole). The overall wall motion score index, calculated by averaging the scores of all individual segments, is related to prognosis.[20] The technique is subjective, with variable reproducibility between centres, although its accuracy may be improved with the use of contrast agents that opacify the left ventricular cavity and enhance endocardial border delineation.

Quantitative assessment

Quantitation of regional function has been performed with a number of echocardiographic and Doppler modalities with increasingly reliable reproducibility (Table 23.3). Some techniques, such as M-mode and tissue Doppler imaging (TDI), are in routine clinical practice, while others are emerging as possible measures of regional function that can detect subclinical disease in a similar fashion.

Longitudinal regional left ventricular systolic function

Assessment of annular longitudinal function by measurement of amplitude (M-mode) or velocity (tissue Doppler) is a clinically useful tool for assessing systolic LV function. Normal LV contraction depends on the coordinate function of longitudinally and circumferentially directed muscle fibres (twisting and untwisting with accompanying longitudinal shortening and lengthening), and loss of these interactions, evident early in LV disease, are readily detected using echocardiography (Figure 23.5). Abnormalities of the mitral annular motion have been described in a variety of conditions. Patients with acute myocardial infarction have reduced displacement more marked at the region of the annulus related to the site

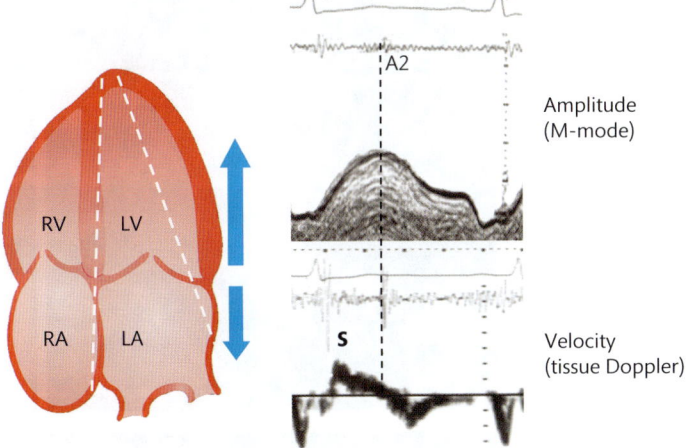

Figure 23.5 Quantification of longitudinal cardiac motion. *Left*: schematic diagram of the motion of the lateral and septal long axis, which moves upwards towards the left ventricular apex during systole, returns to its original position in mid-diastole, and moves further away from away from the left ventricular apex during atrial contraction. *Right top*: corresponding M-mode of lateral M-mode long-axis motion at the lateral wall. Note that in a co-ordinate segment, the long-axis motion peaks at aortic valve closure (A2), and amplitude is measured on the vertical scale. *Right bottom*: corresponding tissue Doppler velocity trace of the lateral wall (vertical scale). Note that the peak systolic velocity (S) corresponds with the peak rate of change of the systolic long-axis amplitude, and the peak early diastolic velocity (E) corresponds to the peak rate of change of early backward motion of the lateral wall. LA, left atrium; LV left ventricle; RA, right atrium; RV, right ventricle.

of infarct;[21] systolic long-axis abnormalities may occur in 38–52% of heart failure patients with normal LVEF;[22,23] and reductions in long-axis amplitude and velocity can be detected before reduction in LVEF or symptoms develop in hypertension, diabetes, 'diastolic heart failure', and hypertrophic cardiomyopathy among others.[24–26] Moreover, long-axis amplitude is strongly related to LVEF,[27] and is a useful predictor of prognosis in a variety of clinical conditions.[28]

From digitally recorded tissue Doppler loops of one or more heart beats containing velocity data from the entire myocardium, two alternative tissue Doppler entities can be derived: (1) strain rate (the rate of deformation between two points a predefined distance apart)[29] and (2) speckle (tissue) tracking (echo software detects frame-to-frame migration of two-dimensional speckle signals from the myocardium from high-resolution two-dimensional imaging and then calculates myocardial strain independent of the angle of incidence) (Figure 23.6).[30] From a 16-segment LV model, the average motion amplitude toward the apex in systole for each segment can be measured and a 'global systolic contraction amplitude index' calculated.[31] These newer techniques may be useful in the early detection of subclinical heart disease, and in the identification and measurement of left ventricular dyssynchrony, but disadvantages include a large signal-to-noise ratio and wide inter- and intraobserver measurement variability.[32]

Assessment of left ventricular diastolic function

A large proportion of patients who present with symptoms of heart failure have LVEF within the normal range; these patients

Table 23.3 Quantitative assessment of regional systolic function

Function	Radial	Longitudinal
Displacement and thickening	Colour kinesis	Annular M-mode
	Anatomical M-mode	Tissue tracking
Velocity	Speckle strain	TDI or speckle strain
Deformation	Speckle strain	TDI or speckle strain
Timing	TDI (time to peak systole or onset of diastole)	TDI (time to peak systole or onset of diastole)

TDI, tissue Doppler imaging.

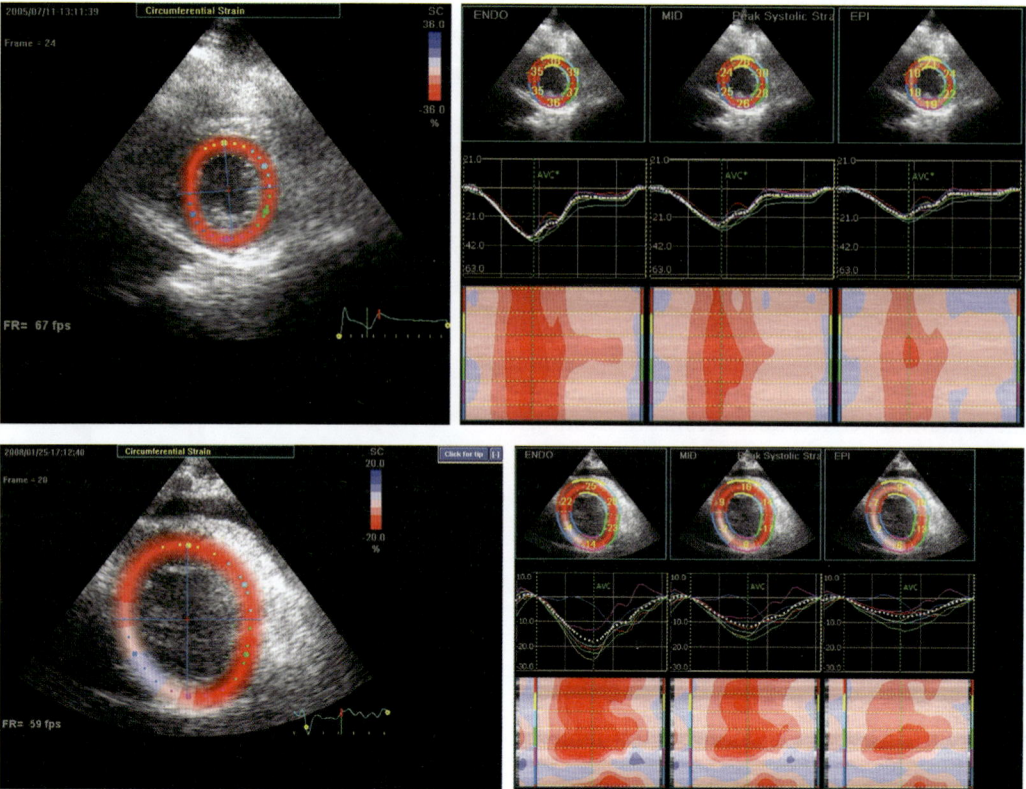

Figure 23.6 Use of speckle tracking in assessment of left ventricular disease. *Top*: Short-axis end-systolic colour-coded radial strain image at the level of the papillary muscle of a subject with normal left ventricular function (*left*). The related strain curves for the endocardial, mid-myocardial, and epicardial layer of one cardiac cycle for the six segments within the short-axis view are given (*right*). There is a gradual decline in circumferential strain from the endocardial to epicardial layers in all the segments. *Bottom*: Short-axis end-systolic colour-coded radial strain image at the level of the papillary muscle of a subject with prior posterior wall myocardial infarction (*left*). The related strain curves for the endocardial, mid-myocardial, and epicardial layers of one cardiac cycle of the six segments within the short-axis view are given (*right*). There is considerable reduction of strain of each of the layers of the posterior segment.

Reproduced from Adamu U, Schmitz F, Becker M, Kelm M, Hoffmann R. Advanced speckle tracking echocardiography allowing a three-myocardial layer-specific analysis of deformation parameters. *Eur J Echocardiogr* 2009;**10**:303–8 with permission from Oxford University Press.

are frequently referred to as having 'diastolic heart failure.' The use of such a term is troublesome, not least because no simple definition of diastolic disease itself has emerged, but also because it presumes an understanding of the mechanisms leading to the disorder and therefore justification of the substitution of a mechanistic term for a descriptive phrase. 'Increased resistance to filling' has been suggested. However, whereas the resistance of a valve orifice or circulation can be readily identified in terms of pressure decrease and flow, resistance to filling involves neither and so is poorly defined. This lack of reference standards by which discrete mechanisms can be assessed in individual patients is a major impediment to identifying and quantifying disturbances in disease—so is the reality that LV filling is totally load dependent. Nevertheless, a variety of echocardiographic techniques are frequently used to determine a series of abnormalities of diastolic function, the cornerstone of which is the measurement of transmitral flow (LV filling) (**Figure 23.7**). Pulmonary venous flow, left atrial size, and TDI of the mitral annulus are also considered. These measurements have demonstrated considerable prognostic value in symptomatic and asymptomatic patients with either preserved or abnormal LV systolic function.[33]

Diastole has traditionally been defined as the period in the cardiac cycle from the end of aortic ejection to the onset of ventricular tension development of the succeeding beat. It has four distinct phases:

- Isovolumic relaxation: between aortic valve closure and mitral valve opening.

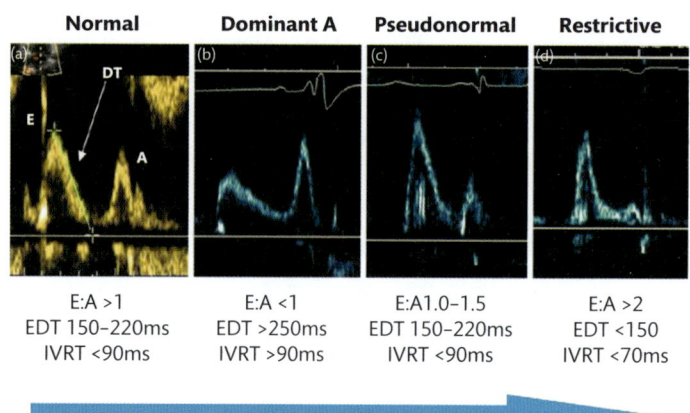

Normal	Dominant A	Pseudonormal	Restrictive
E:A >1	E:A <1	E:A1.0–1.5	E:A >2
EDT 150–220ms	EDT >250ms	EDT 150–220ms	EDT <150
IVRT <90ms	IVRT >90ms	IVRT <90ms	IVRT <70ms

Increasing left atrial pressure

Figure 23.7 A range of left ventricular filling patterns: normal, late diastolic (dominant A), pseudonormal, early diastolic (restrictive filling). EDT, E-wave deceleration time; IVRT, isovolumetric relaxation time.

- Early filling: accounting for 80% of ventricular filling in normal young subjects.
- Diastasis: as LA and LV pressures equalize.
- Atrial systole: accounting for the remainder of ventricular filling.

Dominant A wave

Diastolic function is traditionally characterized in the literature according to severity. So-called 'mild diastolic dysfunction', usually present early in disease development (ischaemia, aortic stenosis, hypertension, hypertrophy), is detected as prolongation of age-related isovolumic relaxation time (IVRT: time between aortic valve closure and mitral valve opening), decrease in early diastolic flow velocity (E wave) and a greater reliance on atrial contraction (A wave) to fill the left ventricle (E:A ratio <1). This pattern of LV filling is usually attributed to 'impaired relaxation', although the exact meaning of the term is rarely specified in the literature (i.e. slow, delayed, or incomplete). In practice, it is nearly always associated with early diastolic incoordination (continued inward long-axis shortening after the end of ejection, associated with outward motion elsewhere),[34] causing an abnormal shape change in early diastole which prevents the LV from becoming spherical (Figure 23.8). Such delayed contraction prolongs the fall in LV pressure and profoundly

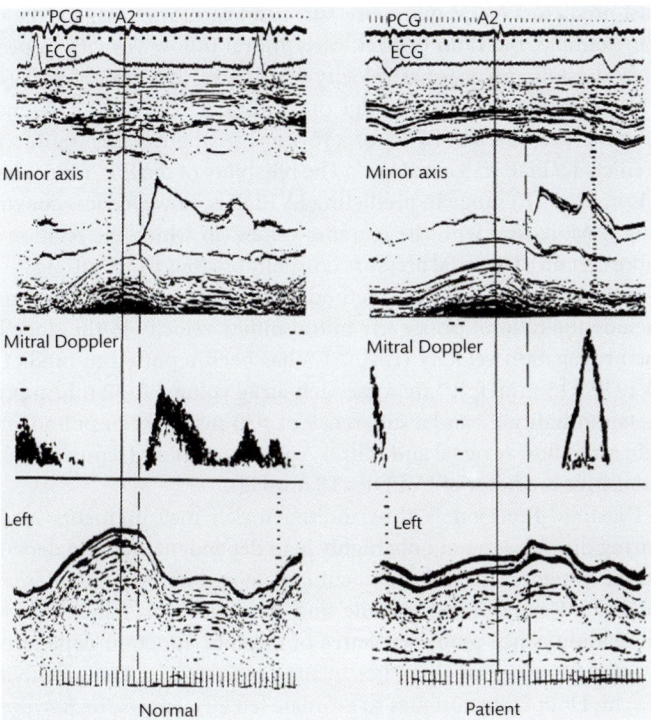

Figure 23.8 Interaction between long-axis incoordination and left ventricular filling. Long isovolumic relaxation time and isolated A wave would support a diagnosis of diastolic disease in the patient above. Prolonged isovolumic relaxation time is associated with increased tension in the left ventricle due to continued inward movement of the lateral long axis after the aortic valve has closed (A2), due in part to reduced long-axis amplitude during systole and in part to delayed activation (patient has left bundle branch block (LBBB) on ECG). LBBB results in a delay in the onset, and therefore a delay in the offset, of long-axis amplitude.
Reproduced with permission from Henein MY, Gibson DG. Suppression of left ventricular early diastolic filling by long axis asynchrony. *Br Heart J* 1995;**73**(2):151–7.

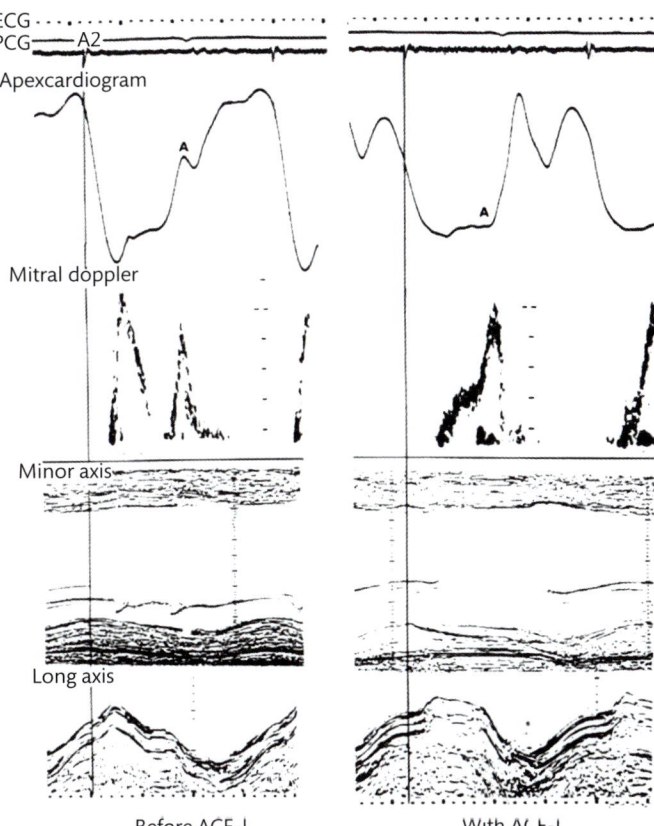

Figure 23.9 Effect of angiotensin converting enzyme (ACE) inhibition on left atrial pressure and left ventricular filling. Left ventricular filling and apexcardiogram from a patient with dilated cardiomyopathy and raised left atrial pressure (*left*) and response to ACE inhibition (*right*). Note the significant fall in end-diastolic pressure with treatment and reversal of left ventricular filling pattern, despite appearance of marked early diastolic long axis incoordination. ACEi, ACE inhibitor.
Reproduced with permission from Henein MY, Das SK, O'Sullivan C, Kakkar VV, Gillbe CE, Gibson DG. ACE inhibitors unmask incoordinate diastolic wall motion in restrictive left ventricular disease. *Heart* 1996;**75**:151–8.

affects early diastolic filling, reducing its peak velocity or suppressing it altogether. Clinically, this pattern is associated with the combination of LV disease and a low or normal filling pressure. It may thus be unmasked by a Valsalva manoeuvre. It is also common in patients initially presenting with restrictive filling who have responded favourably to treatment with diuretic and angiotensin converting enzyme (ACE) inhibitor (Figure 23.9).[35] This sequence of events illustrates how a patient may improve clinically at the same time that diastolic measurements become more abnormal. Moreover, filling with a dominant A is common in inducible ischaemia, during angioplasty[36] or dobutamine stress.[37] It is even associated with activation abnormalities.[38] Thus echocardiographic disturbances occurring during diastole, which result in abnormalities of 'diastolic' function, may in fact have their origins much earlier in the cardiac cycle, during systole, or even earlier, during activation.

Restrictive filling pattern

With disease progression, LV fibrosis develops and chamber compliance decreases. Often referred to as 'severe diastolic dysfunction' in the literature, this form of LV disease relates to the passive

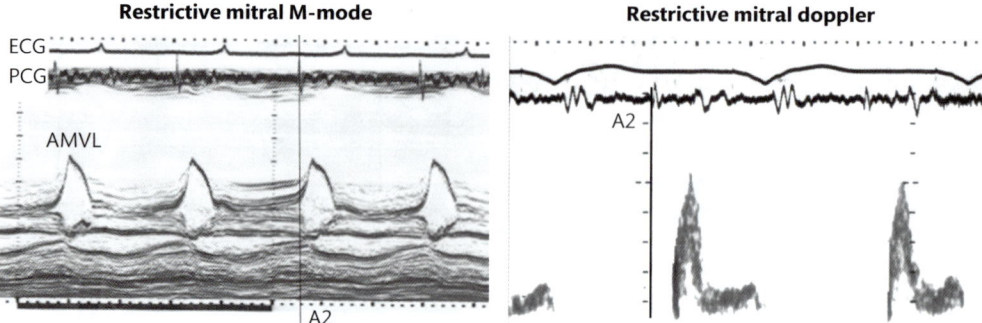

Figure 23.10 Restrictive left ventricular filling. *Left*: mitral valve leaflets open before the aortic valve has closed (A2), suggesting that left atrial pressure is significantly raised. *Right*: restrictive filling with associated third heart sound on a phonocardiogram.

properties of the ventricle. It occurs when left atrial pressure is elevated such that early diastolic flow is extremely rapid, and left atrial and LV pressures equalize quickly during early diastole. It is detected echocardiographically as a short (<40 ms) isovolumic relaxation time, an increased E:A ratio (>2) and a short E-wave deceleration time (<150 ms), which is often accompanied by a third heart sound (Figure 23.10). Acceleration and deceleration rates of the E wave are both increased, implying high pressure gradients, both forward and reversed. Reduced A-wave amplitude is not usually caused by failure of left atrial contraction, since mechanical function can still be demonstrated either by direct measurement of left atrial pressure, by its indirect effect on the apexcardiogram, or by detecting retrograde blood flow into the pulmonary veins. The combination of an increased atrial pressure wave with no flow across the mitral valve demonstrates increased end-diastolic LV stiffness. Such 'restrictive filling' is good evidence of raised left atrial pressure, which overrides any relaxation abnormality. It gives no direct information about the cause of the underlying diastolic disease. It may be specific, as occurs in amyloid or eosinophilic heart disease, or non-specific (a combination of LV cavity dilation, hypertrophy, or diabetes), or even the simple result of fluid overload distending an otherwise normal ventricle. Whatever the underlying aetiology, a restrictive filling pattern should be regarded as the result of a combination of diastolic disease and a high filling pressure, and it identifies patients with a poor prognosis when detected at rest[39] or during stress.[40] Since a raised left atrial pressure is an important component of the clinical syndrome of heart failure, estimation of filling pressure should be an integral part of echocardiographic evaluation in these patients.

'Normal' filling pattern

Just as with isovolumic relaxation time, raised left atrial pressure and diastolic disease have opposite effects on the E:A ratio, and so the combination of the two leads to a ratio between 1.0 and 2.0, often referred to by the unsatisfactory term 'pseudonormalization'.[41] The LV filling pattern should not, however, be considered in isolation, so that recognizing pseudonormality is less of a problem than the literature might suggest. The majority of patients in whom the question arises are elderly people, in whom an E:A ratio >1 would be unusual anyway. They also have clear evidence of structural LV disease, either cavity dilatation or LVH. In a minority, pressure termination of forward atrial flow can be demonstrated, showing near restrictive filling. The ratio E:E' (peak early diastolic velocity to peak ring velocity) may

be useful in these circumstances. When this ratio is increased, then left atrial pressure is likely to be high. However, since a low value of E' may be the result of reduced systolic amplitude, it may simply be a surrogate marker of LV disease. A dominant E wave in an elderly patient with LV disease should suggest a raised LV filling pressure. Recognizing pseudonormality in young patients, in whom a dominant E wave would in fact be normal, has received little attention in the literature. Other measures of diastolic function include TDI, early LV filling flow propagation slope (V_p), left atrial volumes, and pulmonary venous inflow. These measures are less dependent on loading conditions and heart rate and have been reported to be robust predictors of LV filling pressures and cardiovascular mortality. For example, the ratio of peak early mitral inflow velocity to peak early diastolic myocardial velocity (E:E' ratio) has been correlated with pulmonary capillary wedge pressure (E:E' ≤8 predicts LV end-diastolic pressure (LVEDP) of <15 mmHg whereas E:E' ratio >15 predicts LVEDP ≥15 mm Hg).[42] The reliability of the E:E' ratio when it is in the 8–15 range in predicting LVEDP is, however, less convincing.[43] Moreover, with the extreme values (in which the relation is more certain), left atrial pressure is usually obvious from mitral filling pattern anyway. Alternative methods of estimating left atrial pressure include the ratio of peak early mitral inflow velocity to the slope of the propagation velocity (E:V_p ≥1.5 has been reported to predict a LVEDP >15 mmHg);[44] increased left atrial volume (>32 mL/m predicts morbidity);[45] and a difference of >30 ms between pulmonary vein atrial flow reversal and mitral A-wave durations (reported to be a sensitive predictor of LVEDP >18 mmHg).[46]

Diastolic function is thus multifactorial; measurements made during diastole are not only highly load dependent, but also depend on the patient's age and therapeutic drug regime. Absolute demarcation between isolated 'systolic' and 'diastolic' heart failure may be misleading, since many measures of diastolic function depend on events occurring much earlier in the cardiac cycle. The sensitivity of echo Doppler techniques to estimate left atrial pressure, however, has had real clinical significance in patients with the clinical syndrome of heart failure.

Use of echo Doppler in assessment of intracardiac haemodynamics

Intracardiac pressure measurements have traditionally required invasive methods. This limitation, which also precludes serial measurements except in the intensive care context, can be circumvented with

the use of echocardiographic techniques, which convert regurgitant velocity measurements into pressure decreases using the Bernoulli equation, modified to give the formula $4V^2$ (where V = velocity recorded across a regurgitant jet). **Figure 23.11** illustrates the use of echo Doppler in the estimation of right atrial pressure (from the properties of the inferior vena cava), right ventricular/pulmonary artery systolic pressure (from the tricuspid regurgitant trace), and pulmonary artery mean and diastolic pressures (from the pulmonary regurgitation trace).[47] As discussed earlier, a combination of long axis

and echo Doppler can be used to estimate elevated left and right end-diastolic pressures.

Left ventricular synchrony

Maximal energy transfer from the myocardium to the circulation is dependent on the co-ordinated, though non-uniform, action of both circumferentially and longitudinally directed myocardial

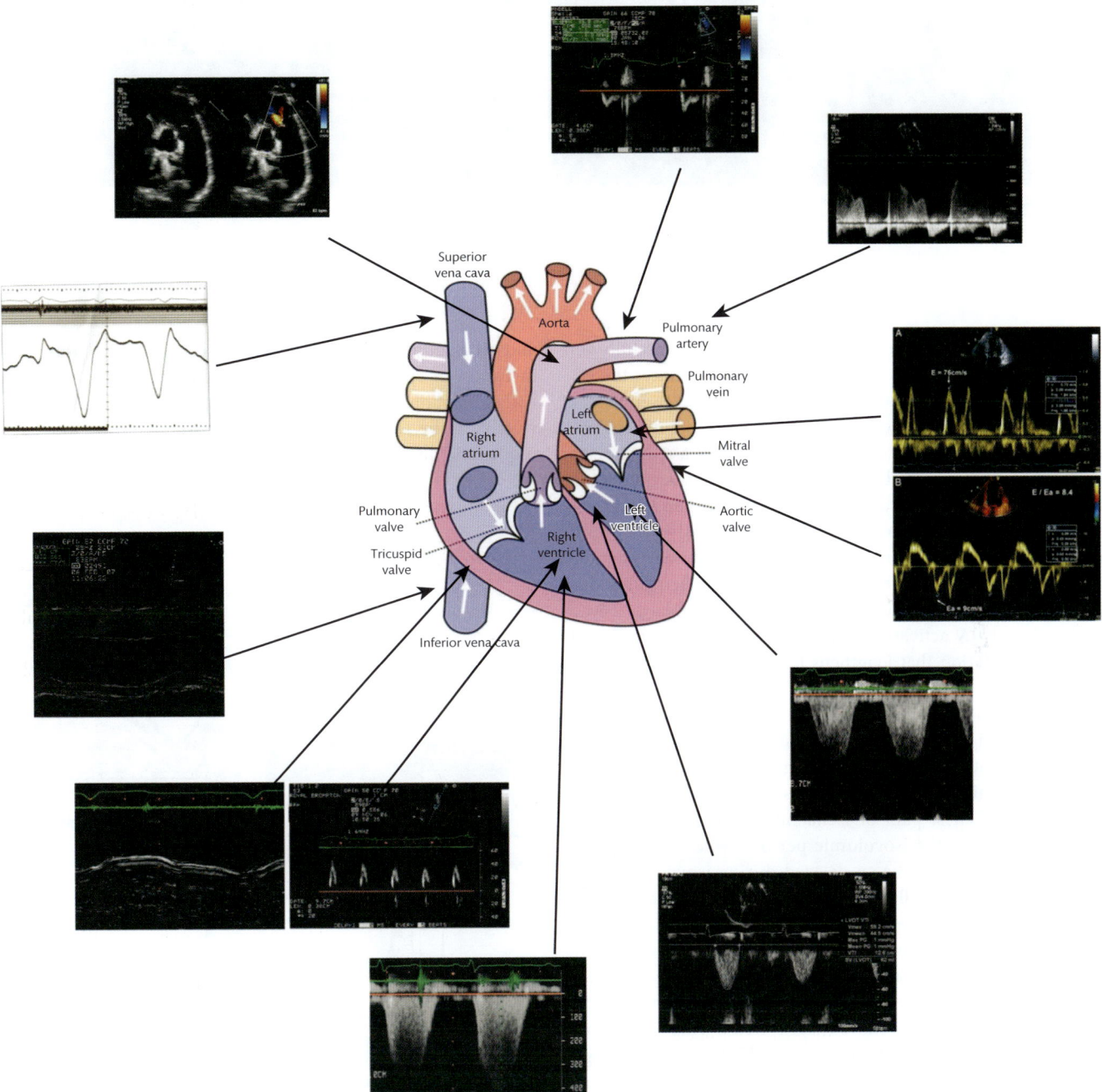

Figure 23.11 Non-invasive haemodynamic assessment using echo. Right atrial pressure is estimated from inferior vena cava size and collapsibility, right ventricular systolic pressure from the peak tricuspid regurgitation velocity, right ventricular mean and end-diastolic pressure from pulmonary regurgitation velocity trace, and pulmonary vascular resistance from pulmonary acceleration time. Restrictive right ventricular function is determined from analysis of right ventricular long-axis function, right ventricular filling pattern, hepatic vein flow, and jugular venous pressure trace. Restrictive left ventricular filling may be determined from analysis of left ventricular long-axis function, left ventricular filling pattern, E:E' ratio, and pulmonary venous flow. Mitral regurgitation (peak dP/dt) and stroke volume provide an estimate of left ventricular systolic function.

Pre-systolic MR   **Post-systolic MR**

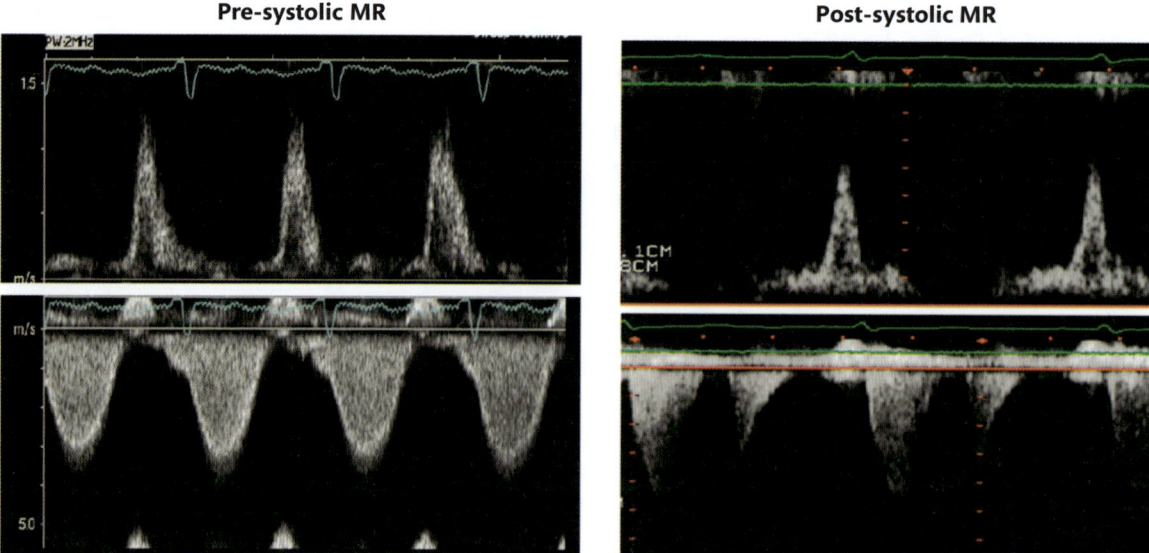

Figure 23.12 Limitation of left ventricular filling time by long duration of mitral regurgitation (MR). *Left*: long mitral regurgitation with a presystolic component that shortens available left ventricular filling time. *Right*: local incoordination in the left ventricular posterior wall in early diastole results in long postejection mitral regurgitation that limits left ventricular filling to late diastole.

fibres. Loss of this interaction leads to LV dyssynchrony, usefully defined as 'incoordinate ventricular wall motion that reduces the extent of intrinsic energy transfer from myocardium to useful work on the circulation'. Its functional consequences are significant impairment of maximal cardiac function as a result of a reduction in the proportion of myocardial energy transmitted to the circulation (cycle efficiency). Activation abnormalities are common in patients with heart failure and are a major contributor to LV dyssynchrony. Patients with the combination of a long PR interval and left bundle branch block may have very early and prolonged LV activation due to low action potentials that are not detected on a standard 12-lead ECG.[48] Such early LV activation results in a 'presystolic' component of mitral regurgitation that lengthens the total duration of mitral regurgitation and significantly shortens available LV filling time (**Figure 23.12**, *left*).

Dyssynchrony is also a major manifestation of coronary artery disease. Indeed, it has long been recognized that patients with chronic stable angina have asynchronous wall motion at rest, even in the absence of chest pain or ischaemic ECG changes. This is most obvious during the isovolumic periods, when the onset of long-axis shortening may be so delayed during isovolumic contraction that it not only follows that of minor axis shortening, but results in long-axis shortening during isovolumic relaxation.[36] Such continued inward movement is associated with 'postejection' mitral regurgitation and consequent shortening of left ventricular filling time at rest (**Figure 23.12**, *right*).[33] This local mechanical dyssynchrony becomes even more exaggerated during pharmacological stress,[37] so that further shortening of LV filling time at high heart rates (**Figure 23.13**) may be enough to limit the normal increase in stroke volume during stress.

Measuring well-defined intervals in the cardiac cycle is a noninvasive means of assessing LV function. The Tei index, described as 'a Doppler index of combined systolic and diastolic performance' is one such measure. It represents the sum of isovolumic contraction

and relaxation times normalized to ejection time.[49] However, the inclusion of ejection time introduces noise and limits its applicability. A more sensitive measure is total isovolumic time (t_{IVT}), which can be readily measured using simple echo Doppler techniques and derived as (60 − (total ejection time + total filling time))

No CAD   **CAD**

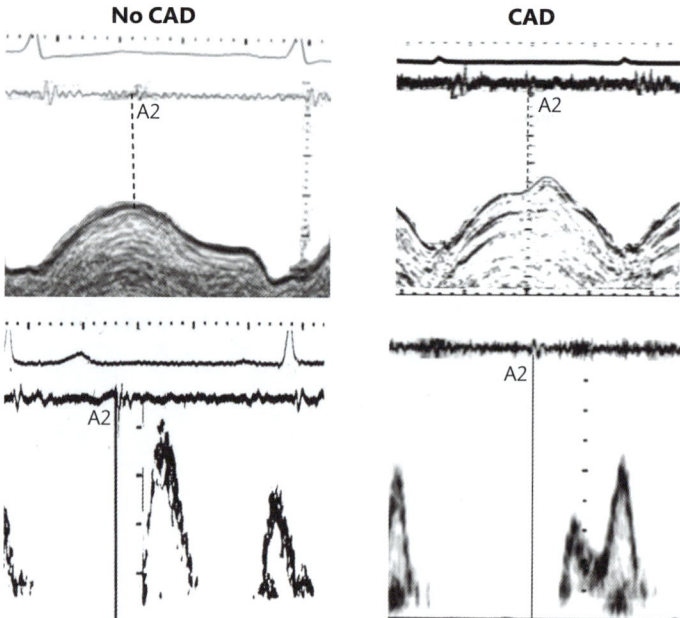

Figure 23.13 Effect of regional dyssynchrony on left ventricular filling. *Left*: in a control subject, normal timing of retraction of the mitral annulus coincides with early diastolic filling (E wave). *Right*: in a patient with coronary artery disease (CAD), continued inward movement of the long axis during early diastole at rest prolongs isovolumic relaxation time and delays early diastolic filling with overall limitation of filling time with respect to RR interval.

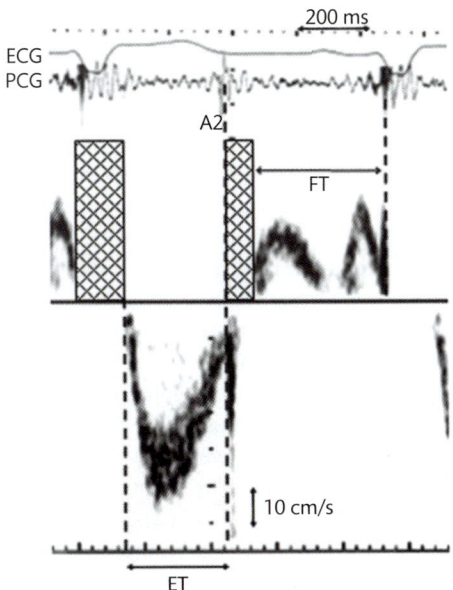

HR = 64bpm

Ejection time 300 ms, total ejection time per minute (0.30*64) = 19.2 s/min
Filling time 400 ms, total filling time per minute (0.40*64) = 26.6 s/min

t-IVT = 60 − (19.2 + 26.6) = 14.6 s/min

Figure 23.14 Effect of regional dyssynchrony on left ventricular filling. *Left*: in a control subject, normal timing of retraction of the mitral annulus coincides with early diastolic filling (E wave). *Right*: in a patient with coronary artery disease (CAD), continued inward movement of the long axis during early diastole at rest prolongs isovolumic relaxation time and delays early diastolic filling with overall limitation of filling time with respect to RR interval.

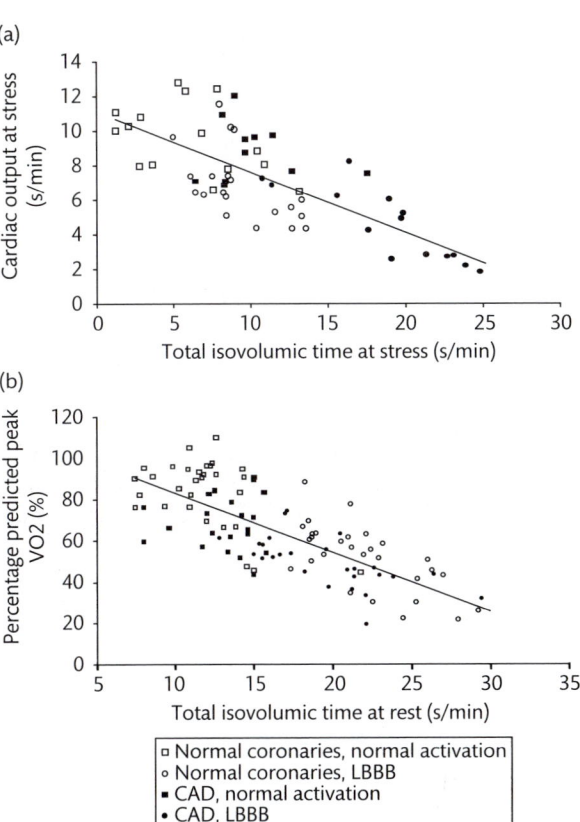

Figure 23.15 Correlation between total isovolumic time, peak stress cardiac output, and exercise capacity. *Top*: Correlation between total isovolumic time and peak stress cardiac output. Patients with left bundle branch block (LBBB) and coronary artery disease (CAD) had the lowest cardiac output at peak stress. *Bottom*: Correlation between total isovolumic time and percentage predicted peak exercise capacity (VO₂). Patients with (LBBB) had the longest total isovolumic time at rest and the lowest % predicted peak VO₂, irrespective of whether CAD was present.

Source data from Duncan AM, Francis DP, Henein MY, Gibson DG. Limitation of cardiac output by total isovolumic time during pharmacologic stress in patients with dilated cardiomyopathy: activation-mediated effects of left bundle branch block and coronary artery disease. *J Am Coll Cardiol* 2003;**41**:121–8, and Duncan A, Francis D, Gibson D, Henein M. Limitation of exercise tolerance in chronic heart failure: distinct effects of left bundle branch block and coronary artery disease. *J Am Coll Cardiol* 2004;**43**:1524–31.

(Figure 23.14).[50] The durations of LV ejection and filling times provide an indication of the effectiveness of global cardiac synchrony. Its reciprocal, the time in the cardiac cycle when the ventricle is neither ejecting nor filling (the isovolumic time or 'wasted' time), provides a useful method of expressing the effects of regional dyssynchrony on global cardiac function.[51] When total isovolumic time is expressed in terms of seconds per minute, it is independent of heart rate, which is an advantage when comparing changes in global dyssynchrony with time (i.e. between rest and stress, or between baseline assessment and follow-up).

Unlike many echo measures including ejection fraction, total isovolumic time is related to the amount of ventricular dyssynchrony, peak stress cardiac output, and exercise capacity. Patients with the longest total isovolumic times are those with the most LV dyssynchrony,[52] the lowest cardiac output at peak stress (Figure 23.15a),[53] and the lowest peak oxygen consumption during cardiopulmonary exercise testing (Figure 23.15b).[54] Patients with the longest total isovolumic time (i.e. most global dyssynchrony) are potentially those most likely to benefit from cardiac resynchronization therapy (CRT).[55]

Thus, simple echo Doppler measures of global cardiac dyssynchrony may have benefit in the expanding field of predicting responders to CRT, quantifying the degree of response, and optimizing pacemaker settings.

Use of echo in therapeutic management of patients with heart failure

Echocardiography not only provides clinical measures and prognostic assessments in patients with heart failure but can also supply information to guide application of heart failure therapies.

Medical therapy

Echocardiographic LVEF is an entry criterion in many clinical trials designed to assess the therapeutic effect of various medical therapies in heart failure, including ACE inhibitors, β-blockers, and aldosterone antagonists.[8–10] A reduction in LVEF may highlight the detrimental effects on LV function of cardiotoxic medications, including anthracycline chemotherapeutic agents.[56] A more detailed echocardiographic examination, assessing specifically LV filling pattern and segmental incoordination, may demonstrate the beneficial

effect of ACE inhibitors in off-loading the LV, particularly in patients with raised left atrial pressure (restrictive filling pattern), reducing LVEDP, and unmasking segmental incoordination.[35]

Implantable cardioverter–defibrillators

Strategies for implantable cardioverter–defibrillators (ICDs) rely on LVEF for selecting patients for the devices.[11] Repeat LVEF assessment at 30–40 days after myocardial infarction and after initiation of optimal heart failure medical therapy is necessary to determine candidacy for ICD.

Cardiac resynchronization therapy

CRT reduces mortality, improves functional status, and increases LVEF in patients with severe left ventricle disease.[57–59] Current recommendations advocate that patients with LVEF ≤35%, moderate-to-severe heart failure symptoms, and QRS duration >130 ms should undergo CRT. Debate continues as to whether existing echo methods of assessing LV dysschrony provide additional predictive value in determining those patients most likely to benefit from resynchronization.[59] The difficulty may lie in the type of echo measurement that is being used. In order for CRT to be successful, the baseline abnormality (regional dyssynchrony) not only needs to be present, but such regional dyssynchrony should also be haemodynamically limiting (i.e. result in global dyssynchrony). Patients with the most global dyssynchrony (long total isovolumic time >15 s/min and/or long interventricular delay >40 ms) have been shown to demonstrate significant clinical response to CRT.[55,59] Most studies, however, have concentrated on regional assessment of intraventricular dyssynchrony.

Echo markers of intraventricular dyssynchrony

Intraventricular dyssynchrony may be measured using a variety of echo techniques (M-mode, tissue Doppler, tissue tracking, and three-dimensional imaging). Although the assessment of regional dyssynchrony gained great impetus in the literature in recent years, the relation between specific areas of regional dyssynchrony and their effect on global dyssynchrony, particularly during exercise, remains undefined. Moreover, since the publication of the PROSPECT trial, the reproducibility of various echo techniques for quantifying intraventricular dyssynchrony across different echo institutions has been seriously questioned.[60,61] Multiple methods for assessing intraventricular dyssynchrony are quoted in the literature, including:

- septal–posterior delay >130 ms, as measured by M-mode;[62]
- septal–posterior wall delay >65 ms, as measured by tissue Doppler (**Figure 23.16a**);[63]
- systolic dyssynchrony index >33 ms, as measured by tissue Doppler (Figure 23.16b);[64]
- anterior–septal to posterior wall peak strain >130 ms, as measured by tissue tracking;[65]
- systolic dyssynchrony index >5%, as measured by three-dimensional endocardial border detection and segmental volume analysis.[66]

Reported difficulties with the reproducibility of assessment of regional LV-dyssynchrony-using techniques have limited their use in clinical practice, and echo indices of dyssynchrony will only become credible and applicable after they have been shown to be predictive in large prospective randomized trials.

Pacing optimization

Continued presystolic mitral regurgitation in patients after implantation of a DDD or CRT pacing device is associated with little or no clinical improvement. Echo Doppler techniques may be used to optimize the delay between pacing the right atrium and right ventricle (AV delay) in order to shorten or remove presystolic mitral regurgitation and thereby increase LV filling time (**Figure 23.17**).

The aim is to choose the shortest AV delay that maximizes LV filling, using either the iterative method (whereby a long AV delay (e.g. 150 ms) is programmed on the pacemaker, the AV delay is then shortened in 20 ms stages until the A wave starts to be truncated, then the AV delay is gradually extended by 10 ms steps until the A wave is just complete) or the Ritter method (whereby a short AV delay (e.g. 50 ms) is programmed and the time from start QRS to end of A wave is measured (QA_{short}), then a long AV delay (e.g. 150 ms) is programmed and the time from start QRS to end of A wave (QA_{long}) is measured; the optimal delay is then calculated as $AV_{long\,delay} + QA_{long} - QA_{short}$). In theory, optimization of delay between pacing left and right ventricles (VV delay) with atriobiventricular pacemakers is possible, but no morbidity or mortality benefit has been documented for any of this. Moreover, optimization of pacemaker settings at rest takes no account of haemodynamic changes that occur during exercise or stress, which remains a major limitation of this technique.

Revascularization (viable myocardium)

Stunned or hibernating myocardium denotes viable but dysfunctional tissue. Increasing myocardial oxygen demand by stressing the heart with pharmacological agents (dobutamine or dipyridamole) can identify segments that are viable and potentially functional by inducing them to contract. Traditionally this requires qualitative assessment of wall motion score (whereby an akinetic segment becomes hypokinetic, or a hypokinetic segment thickens normally during low dose stress and then deteriorates again at high dose (biphasic response);[67] similar abnormalities may be quantitatively demonstrated using M-mode techniques.[68]

Transcatheter aortic and mitral valve intervention

The role of transoesophageal echocardiography is mandatory in transcatheter mitral valve techniques (MitraClip, transventricular artificial neochordae, mitral valve-in-valve, mitral valve implantation, and paravalvular leak closure) (**Figure 23.18**), and is useful in transcatheter aortic valve implantation to visualize correct device implantation and monitor for complications (device migration, paravalvular leak, pericardial collection, new wall motion abnormalities), but a full description of the use of echocardiography is beyond the scope of this chapter.

Mitral valve surgery

'Functional' mitral regurgitation is multifactorial in patients with heart failure, and may be due to dilatation of the mitral annulus, malcoaptation of the mitral valve leaflets, and/or tethering of the mitral valve leaflets from remodelling-induced displacement of one

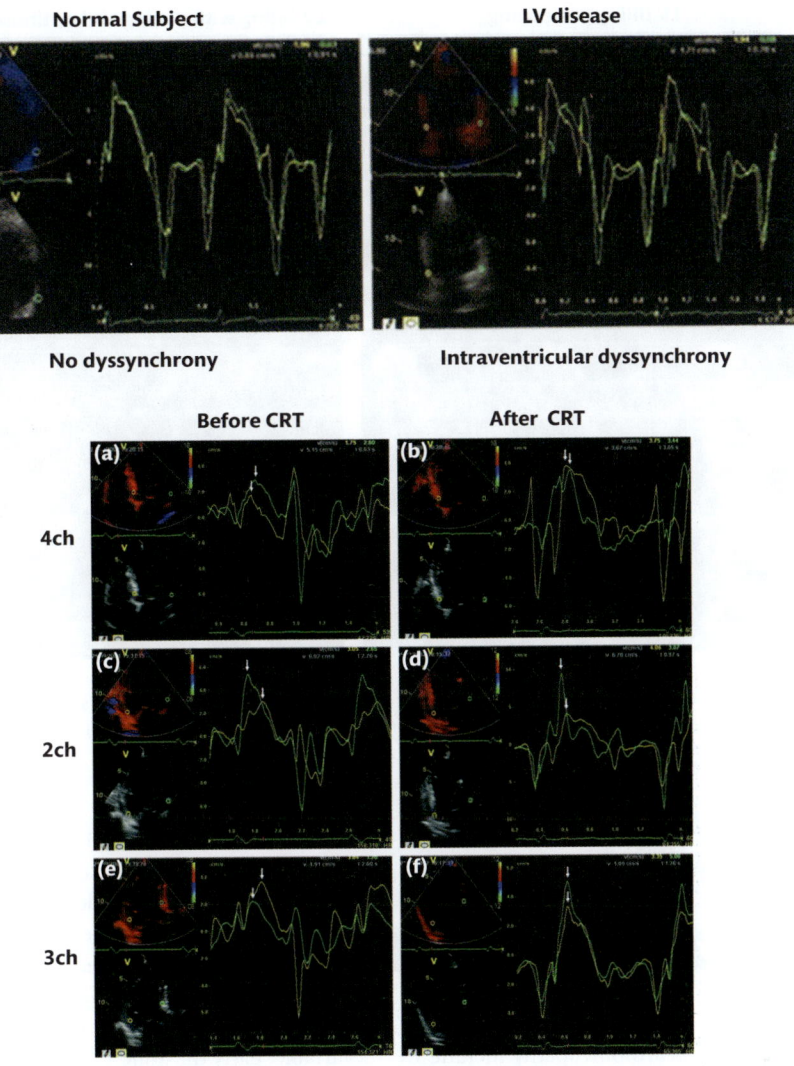

Figure 23.16 Use of tissue Doppler in assessment of dyssynchrony. (A) Septal–lateral delay >65 ms. *Left:* Normal subject with no intraventricular dyssynchrony between septum (yellow curve) and lateral wall (green curve). *Right:* Severe intraventricular dyssynchrony between the septum and lateral wall. (B) Dyssynchrony index from 12 segments >33 ms. A patient with left ventricular mechanical dyssynchrony in multiple segments before (a, c, e) and after (b, d, f) cardiac resynchronization therapy (CRT). Before CRT, the apical four-chamber view (a) shows only mild delay of basal lateral segment over the basal septal segment of 30 ms. In the apical two-chamber view (c), there was severe delay in the basal inferior wall over the basal anterior wall of 130 ms which was significantly improved after CRT (d). In the apical long-axis view (e), the basal posterior wall was delayed over the basal anteroseptal wall of 90 ms which was totally abolished after CRT (f). The peak systolic velocity during the ejection phase in each view is shown by the arrows.

(A) Reproduced from Bax JJ, Ansalone G, Breithardt OA, *et al.* Echocardiographic evaluation of cardiac resynchronization therapy: ready for routine clinical use? A critical appraisal. *J Am Coll Cardiol* 2004;**44**:1–9, with permission; (B) Reproduced from Yu CM, Bax JJ, Monaghan M, Nihoyannopoulos P. Echocardiographic evaluation of cardiac dyssynchrony for predicting a favourable response to cardiac resynchronisation therapy. *Heart* 2004;**90**:17–22.

or both papillary muscles. Physiological stress echo may be useful in planning mitral valve repair, particularly when combined with three-dimensional assessment during stress, since surgery has demonstrated efficacy even in advanced heart failure.[69]

Ventricular assist devices

Ventricular assist devices (a left ventricular assist device, LVAD or biventricular assist device, bi-VAD) are commonly used as bridges to heart transplantation or ventricular recovery. The pump sucks from the ventricle and ejects directly into the aorta, thus reducing wall stress and allowing the myocardium to recover. Echo can detect significant valvular disease, intracardiac shunts, significant right

ventricular disease, or pulmonary hypertension preoperatively, and thrombus formation within the VAD or other causes of inflow cannula obstruction postoperatively.

Cardiac transplantation

Many attempts have been made to assess the echocardiographic predictors of acute rejection, as the non-invasive diagnosis of episodes of rejection might obviate the need for repeated myocardial biopsy. Echocardiographic changes associated with rejection after cardiac transplantation include an increase in posterior wall thickness, an increase in left ventricular mass, and a decrease in diastolic compliance, with associated development of a restrictive mitral inflow

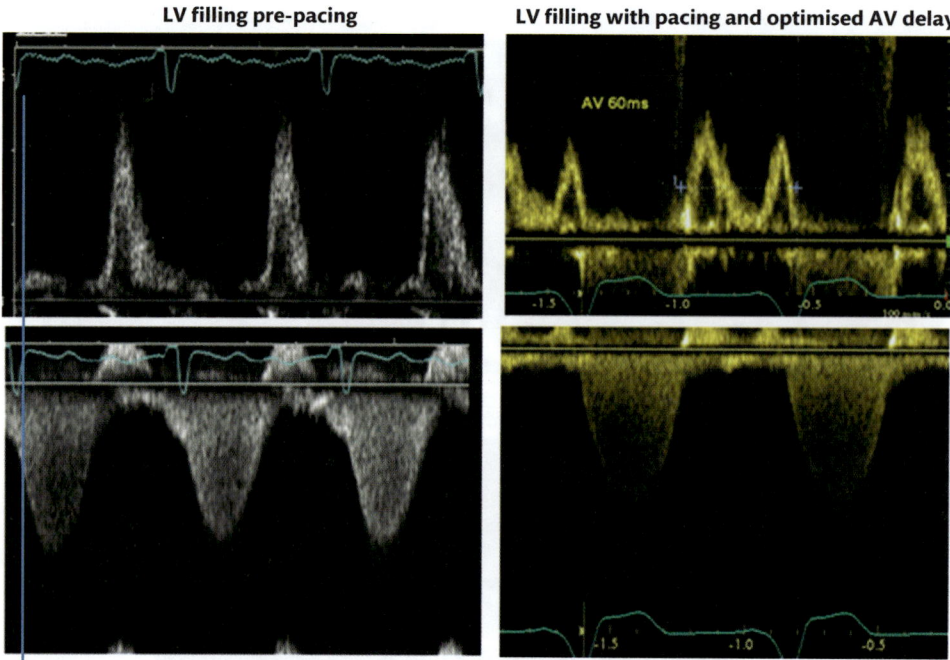

Figure 23.17 Effect of pacing on left ventricular filling time when left ventricular filling is limited by presystolic mitral regurgitation. *Left*: short left ventricular filling time before pacing due to presystolic mitral regurgitation. *Right*: after pacing and shortening the atrioventricular delay, the presystolic component of mitral regurgitation is removed, allowing significant increase in left ventricular filling time.

pattern. Unfortunately, most of these changes indicate advanced rejection and therefore are of limited use as screening tools.

Specific echo findings in cardiomyopathies

Dilated cardiomyopathy

Echocardiographic findings in dilated cardiomyopathy include LV dilatation, increased LV volumes, LVEF <40%, functional mitral regurgitation to varying degrees (**Figure 23.19**), reduced LV long-axis amplitude, global and regional dyssynchrony, and pulmonary hypertension. There is no definite echocardiographic picture that differentiates different stages, but as the LV dilates, wall stress increases (Laplace's law), resulting in both increased sphericity and

myocardial oxygen consumption. Regional wall motion abnormalities are not non-specific, and may be present in ischaemic and idiopathic cardiomyopathy; dobutamine stress echo may be useful in differentiating between the two.[68]

The presence of right ventricular enlargement and dysfunction is variable but a poor prognostic sign if present. Tricuspid regurgitation is common and varies in severity. The LV filling pattern is highly variable; early diastolic E wave is often dominant, and is associated with a short isovolumic relaxation time and a third heart sound which strongly suggests elevated LVEDP. Alternatively, ventricular filling may occur entirely during atrial systole, and be associated with a long isovolumic relaxation time and a fourth heart sound, which strongly suggests low or normal LVEDP. Finally, with sinus tachycardia, filling time at rest may be so short that only a single

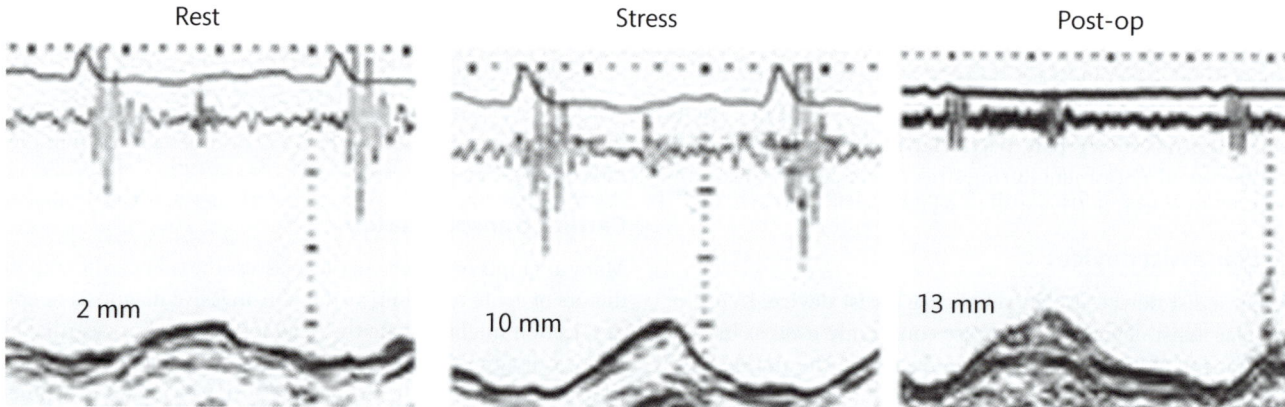

Figure 23.18 Improved left ventricular long-axis amplitude with stress predicts viable myocardium. Long axis M-mode recordings of lateral wall. There is a 30% increase in systolic amplitude with stress, suggesting the presence of viable myocardium, which was confirmed by significant increase in long-axis amplitude at rest after revascularization.

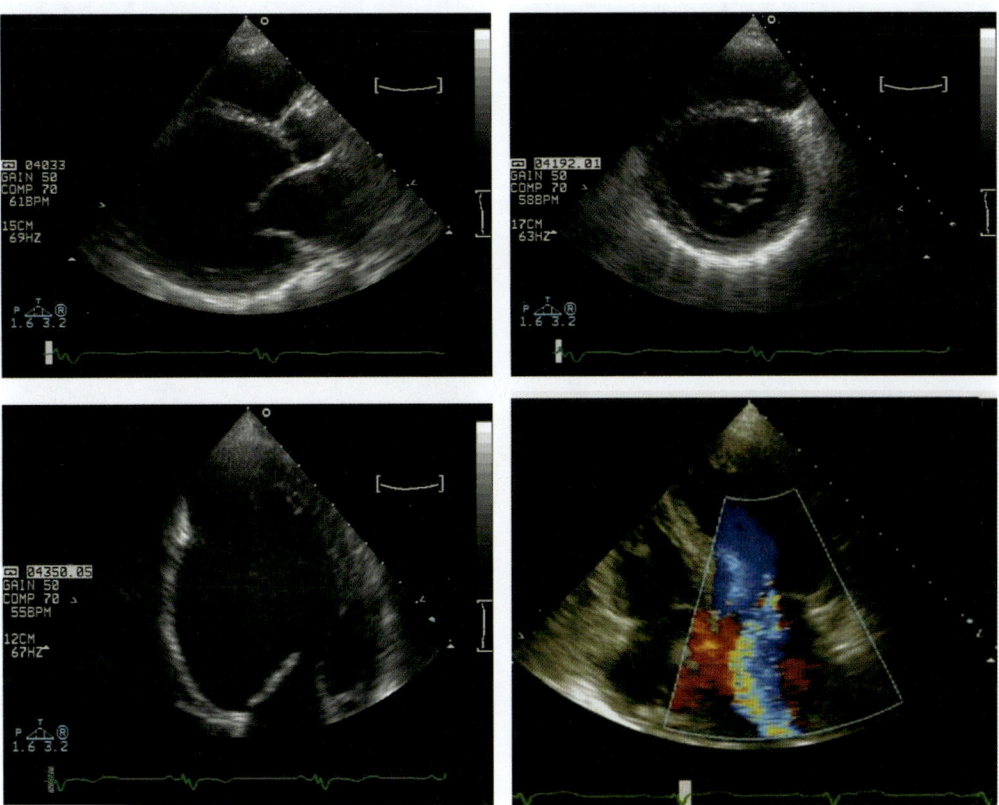

Figure 23.19 Echo features of dilated cardiomyopathy. *Top left*: parasternal long-axis view showing dilated left ventricular cavity size and tenting of mitral valve. *Top right*: parasternal short axis view. *Bottom left*: spherical left ventricular with hypokinetic septum and dilated right ventricle. *Bottom right*: significant mitral and tricuspid regurgitation.

filling peak is recorded, consisting of superimposed E and A waves, and accompanied by a summation gallop. As discussed above, LV filling time may shorten even further during stress, and may become the rate-limiting step during exercise.

Hypertrophic cardiomyopathy

The echo pattern in hypertrophic cardiomyopathy is highly variable; there may be disproportionate septal hypertrophy in relation to the LV posterior wall (ratio >1.3:1.0), concentric LVH, in which the septal and posterior walls are equal in thickness, or hypertrophy confirmed to the apical segments. Significant LV outflow tract obstruction is usual if asymmetric septal hypertrophy and systolic anterior motion of the mitral valve (SAM) are present (**Figure 23.20**), but midcavity obstruction is also common, particularly when there is concentric LVH and the patient is hypovolaemic or on inotropes. Colour Doppler is useful for identifying the level of obstruction.

Left ventricular non-compaction

This is an inherited condition characterized by marked trabeculation, usually within the LV apex. LVEF may be reduced, and areas of non-compaction may become substrates for left-sided thrombi and arrhythmias. To identify non-compaction, left-sided contrast agents are usually required. In apical views the trabeculation is usually seen

as a partially contrast-filled layer. A ratio of >2:1 non-compacted (trabeculations) myocardium to compacted (normal) myocardium at end systole suggests LV non-compaction.

Restrictive cardiomyopathy

Restrictive cardiomyopathy is a group of disorders characterized by limitation of LV filling caused by increased LV stiffness (decreased LV compliance) during mid and late diastole. Amyloid infiltration is present in about half of these cases, and the aetiology is often undefined in the remainder. LV cavity size is usually normal, although LVEF may be significantly reduced. Biatrial enlargement is usually present and peak inflow velocity during early diastole is often normal, but its duration is short, so acceleration and deceleration times are reduced, reflecting the combined effects of increased myocardial stiffness and a high left atrial pressure.[45] Restrictive filling does not represent a specific diagnosis, as patients with dilated cardiomyopathy or severe LVH may show restrictive physiology.

Right ventricular function

Right ventricular function has significant clinical relevance since it is highly related to prognosis[70] and has an important role in determining exercise capacity.[71] Assessing the size of the right ventricle may be difficult, because of its complex shape, but measuring

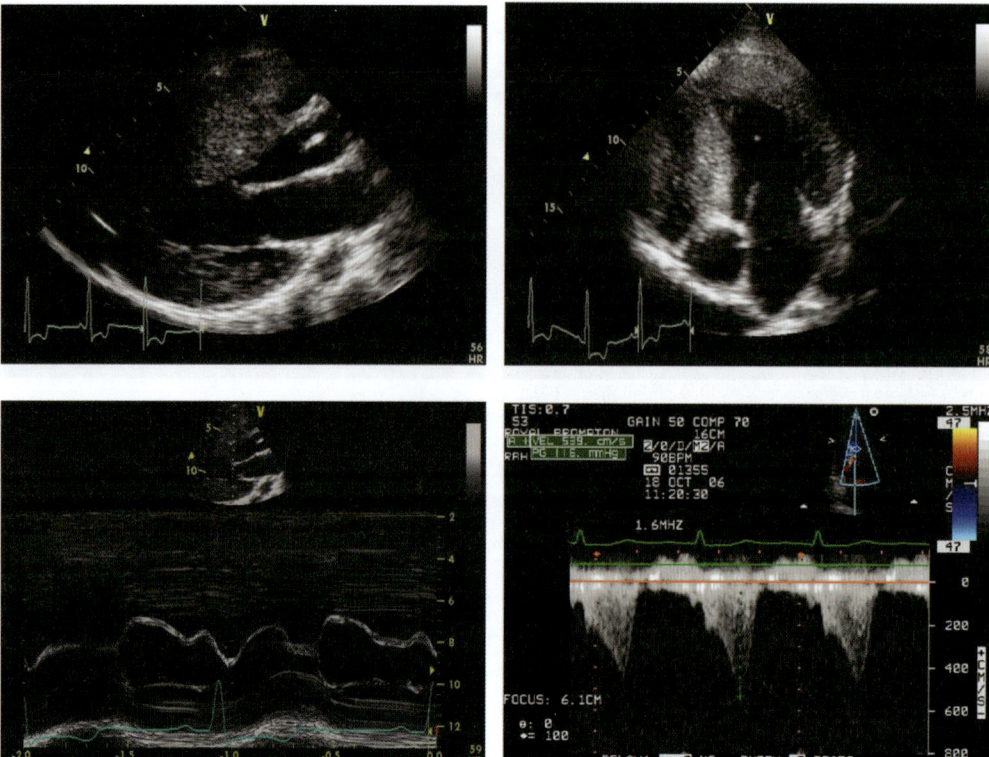

Figure 23.20 Echo features of hypertrophic cardiomyopathy. *Top left*: concentric left ventricular hypertrophy, with narrowing of left ventricular outflow tract. *Top right*: biventricular hypertrophy. *Bottom left*: systolic anterior motion of the mitral valve (SAM) detected readily by M-mode. Bottom right: significant left ventricular outflow tract obstruction, with velocity reaching 6 m/s. Symptoms of breathlessness may be due to dynamic left ventricular outflow tract obstruction or abnormal left ventricular diastolic function (usually prolonged isovolumic relation time, decrease in the rate of early diastolic filling, and increase in the atrial component of left ventricular filling).

end-diastolic length, the diameter at midcavity, and the diameter of the tricuspid annulus usually suffice (the latter should be <40 mm). Right ventricular function is assessed qualitatively and quantitatively, the latter by measuring tricuspid annular motion using M-mode (normal right ventricular amplitude is 15–20 mm in the absence of severe tricuspid regurgitation or pulmonary hypertension).

Identifying right ventricular pressure or volume overload can aid clinical assessment of right heart function. Although often considered together, they usually represent two different initial pathologies; right ventricular volume overload suggests right-sided valvular regurgitation or a right-to-left shunt. Pressure overload suggests pulmonary hypertension or pulmonary stenosis. Pressure overload can develop from volume overload, and occasionally vice versa, in which case features of both will be present. Assessing right ventricular size, free wall thickness, and septal motion are key since volume overload usually leads to increased cavity size and pressure overload usually leads to increased wall thickness (though the two findings may coexist), and volume overload is related to a flattened septum in diastole, whereas pressure overload is associated with a flattened septum in both systole and diastole.

Severe tricuspid regurgitation may be present in late left ventricular disease or if the primary pathology involves the right ventricle. In this case, the right atrium and right ventricle are usually both dilated, the right atrial pressure is increased, and the peak right AV pressure decrease declines. The decline in pressure decrease

should not be taken as a sign of reduction in pulmonary artery pressure, particularly in patients who show clinical deterioration, but as a sign of increasing right atrial pressure. Restrictive right ventricular filling physiology is associated with poor prognosis in a fashion similar to left ventricular haemodynamics.

Chronic constrictive pericarditis

A rare, but clinically important, cause of heart failure is pericardial disease, and chronic constrictive pericarditis is an example of pure diastolic heart failure with a low cardiac output state. It is characterized by a thickened, adherent pericardium (Figure 23.21) that restricts ventricular filling and limits chamber expansion and maximal diastolic volumes. Elevated filling pressures are required to maintain adequate cardiac output. End-diastolic pressures in all heart chambers are usually elevated and equalized. Compensatory mechanisms are activated but may ultimately fail, leading to elevated venous pressure, salt and water retention, and reduced cardiac output. The clinical similarity between constrictive pericarditis and restrictive cardiomyopathy may make the differential diagnosis difficult in some cases, since both have stiff and incompliant left ventricle in late diastole and the LV is unable to fill without a significant rise in LVEDP. However, constrictive pericarditis is an extracardiac constraint whereas restrictive cardiomyopathy is an intrinsic disease of the myocardium. Thus motion of the ventricular long axes and

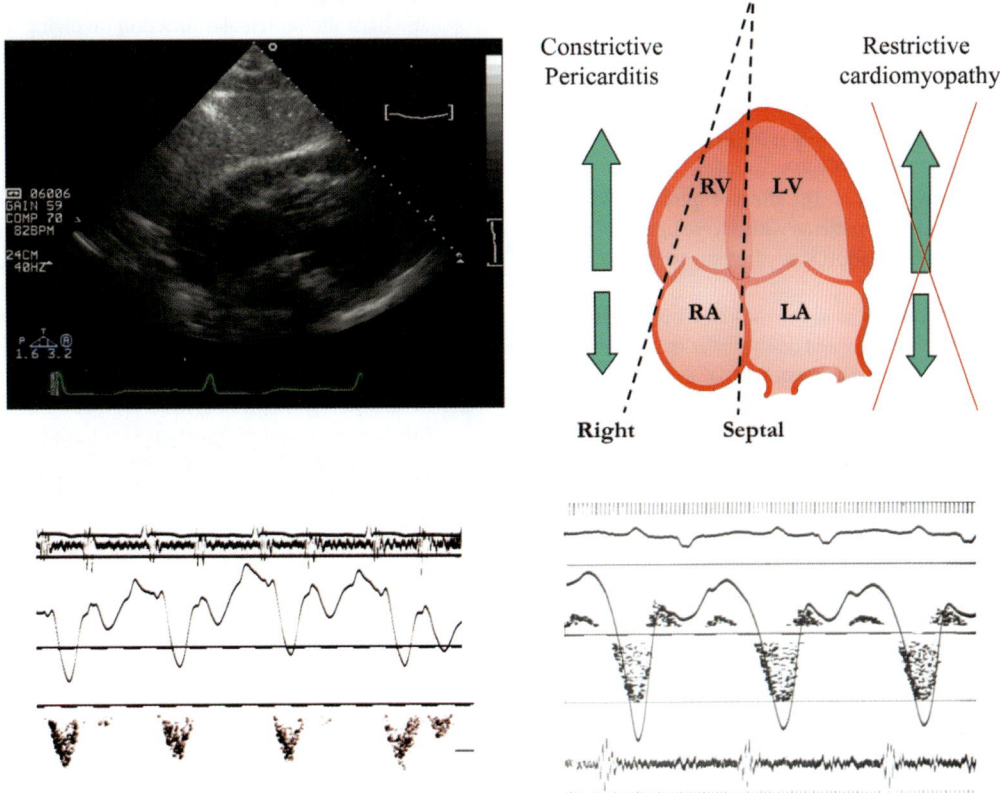

Figure 23.21 Pathophysiology of pericardial constriction. *Top left*: subcostal view of pericardial adhesions between right ventricular/right atrial free wall and the visceral pericardium. *Top right*: in constrictive pericarditis, long-axis function is maintained but is reduced in restrictive cardiomyopathy. *Bottom left*: apical systolic movement of right ventricular long axis corresponds to deep X descent in constrictive pericarditis (corresponding to systolic descent on superior vena cava flow). *Bottom right*: lack of apical systolic movement of right ventricular long axis reduces X descent on jugular venous pressure and produces dominant Y descent (corresponding to diastolic descent on superior vena cava flow).

associated influence on vena caval flow help differentiate between the two conditions.

a central role in the diagnosis and management of patients with heart failure.

Conclusion

Echocardiography is the single most useful non-invasive imaging tool in the heart failure population. It readily identifies patterns of disease, rapidly differentiating myocardial from structural or pericardial heart disease, and the dilated left ventricle from the hypertrophied left ventricle in a widely available clinical setting. More subtle echo techniques quantify the degree of left ventricular impairment, determine the presence of RWMA, differentiate restrictive left ventricular physiology from reduced early diastolic filling rates, quantify the degree of functional mitral regurgitation and pulmonary hypertension, identify occult right ventricular disease, and define the effects of abnormal activation on ventricular function. Echocardiography not only provides insights into the pathophysiological mechanisms underlying the various aetiologies of heart failure, but also identifies patients at high risk for cardiovascular morbidity and mortality and provides important data for therapeutic decision-making, including defining candidacy for medications, implantable cardiac devices, surgical procedures, and resynchronization. Thus, echocardiography continues to play

REFERENCES

1. Cowie MR, Wood DA, Coats AJ, *et al.* Incidence, aetiology of heart failure; a population-based study. *Eur Heart J* 1999;**20**:421–8.
2. Senni M, Rodeheffer RJ, Tribouilloy CM, *et al.* Use of echocardiography in the management of congestive heart failure in the community. *J Am Coll Cardiol* 1999;**33**:164–70.
3. National Institute for Health and Care Excellence. Management of chronic heart failure in adults in primary and secondary care. NICE Guidelines August 2010. http://www.nice.org.uk
4. Yancy CY, Jessup M, Boskurt B, *et al.* 2013 ACCF/AHA Guideline for the Management of Heart Failure. *J Am Coll Cardiol* 2013;**62**:1495–539.
5. Lang RM, Bierig M, Devereaux RB, *et al.* Recommendations for chamber quantification. *J Am Soc Echocardiogr* 2005;**18**:1440–63.
6. Jacobs LD, Salgo IS, Goonewardena S, *et al.* Rapid online quantification of left ventricular volume from real-time three-dimensional echocardiographic data. *Eur Heart J* 2006;**27**:460–8.
7. Franciosa JA, Park M, Levine TB. Lack of correlation between exercise capacity and indexes of resting left ventricular performance in heart failure. *Am J Cardiol* 1981;**47**:33–9.

8. Edner M, Bonarjee VV, Nilsen DW, et al. Effect of enalapril initiated early after acute myocardial infarction on heart failure parameters, with reference to clinical class and echocardiographic determinants. CONSENSUS II Multi-Echo Study Group. *Clin Cardiol* 1996;**19**:543–8.

9. Cardiac Insufficiency Bisoprolol Study II (CIBIS-II): a randomised trial. *Lancet* 1999;**353**:9–13.

10. Pitt B, Zannad F, Remme WJ, et al. The effect of spironolactone on morbidity and mortality in patients with severe heart failure. Randomized Aldactone Evaluation Study Investigators. *N Engl J Med* 1999;**341**:709–17.

11. Moss AJ, Hall WJ, Cannom DS, et al. and MADIT Investigators. Improved survival with an implanted defibrillator in patients with coronary disease at high risk for ventricular arrhythmia. *N Engl J Med* 1996;**335**:1933–40.

12. Lee R, Marwick TH. Assessment of subclinical left ventricular dysfunction in asymptomatic mitral regurgitation. *Eur J Echocardiogr* 2007;**8**:175–84.

13. Sutton MSJ, Pfeffer MA, Plappert T, et al., for the SAVE Investigators. Quantitative two-dimensional echocardiographic measurements are major predictors of adverse cardiovascular events after acute myocardial infarction. The protective effects of captopril. *Circulation* 1994;**89**:68–75.

14. Quinones MA, Breenberg BH, Kopelen HA, et al., for the SOLVD Investigators. Echocardiographic predictors of clinical outcomes in patients with left ventricular dysfunction enrolled in the SOLVD registry and trials: significance of left ventricular hypertrophy. *J Am Coll Cardiol* 2005;**35**:1237–44.

15. Devereux R, Reichek N. Echocardiographic determination of left ventricular mass in man. *Circulation* 1977;**55**:613–18.

16. Chen C, Rodriguez L, Lethor JP, et al. Continuous wave Doppler echocardiography for non-invasive assessment of left ventricular dP/dt and relaxation time constant from mitral regurgitant spectra in patients. *J Am Coll Cardiol* 1994;**23**:970–76.

17. Xiao HB, Brecker SJ, Gibson DG. Effects of abnormal activation on the time course of the left ventricular pressure pulse in dilated cardiomopathy. *Br Heart J* 1992;**68**:403–7.

18. Schiller NB, Shah PM, Crawford M, et al. Recommendations for quantitation of the left ventricle by two-dimensional echocardiography. *J Am Soc Echocardiogr* 1989;**2**:258–67.

19. Lang RM, Bierig M, Devereux RB, et al. American Society of Echocardiography's Nomenclature and Standards Committee; Task Force on Chamber Quantification; American College of Cardiology Echocardiography Committee; American Heart Association; European Association of Echocardiography, European Society of Cardiology. Recommendations for chamber quantification. *Eur J Echocardiogr* 2006;**7**:79–108.

20. Nishimura RA, Tajik AJ, Shub C, et al. Role of two-dimensional echocardiography in the prediction of inhospital complications after acute myocardial infarction. *J Am Coll Cardiol* 1984;**4**:1080–7.

21. O'Sullivan CA, Ramzy IS, Li W, et al. The effect of the localization of Q wave myocardial infarction on ventricular electromechanics. *Int J Cardiol* 2002;**84**:241–7.

22. Yip G, Wang M, Zhang Y, et al. Left ventricular long axis function in diastolic heart failure is reduced in both diastole and systole: time for a redefinition? *Heart* 2002;**87**:121–5.

23. Yu CM, Lin H, Yang H, et al. Progression of systolic abnormalities in patients with 'isolated' diastolic heart failure and diastolic dysfunction. *Circulation* 2002;**105**:1195–201.

24. Tan YT, Wenzelburger F, Lee E, et al. The pathophysiology of heart failure with normal ejection fraction: exercise echocardiography reveals complex abnormalities of both systolic and diastolic ventricular function involving torsion, untwist, and longitudinal motion. *J Am Coll Cardiol* 2009;**54**:36–46.

25. Nishikage T, Nakai H, Lang RM, Takeuchi M. Subclinical left ventricular longitudinal systolic dysfunction in hypertension with no evidence of heart failure. *Circ J* 2008;**72**:189–94.

26. Ha JW, Lee HC, Kang ES, et al. Abnormal left ventricular longitudinal functional reserve in patients with diabetes mellitus: implication for detecting subclinical myocardial dysfunction using exercise tissue Doppler echocardiography. *Heart* 2007;**93**:1571–6.

27. Pai RG, Bodenheimer MM, Pai SM, Koss JH, Adamick RD. Usefulness of systolic excursion of the mitral anulus as an index of left ventricular systolic function. *Am J Cardiol* 1991;**67**:222–4.

28. Sveälv BG, Olofsson EL, Andersson B. Ventricular long-axis function is of major importance for long-term survival in patients with heart failure. *Heart* 2008;**94**:284–9.

29. Artis NJ, Oxborough DL, Williams G, Pepper CB, Tan LB. Two dimensional strain imaging: a new echocardiographic advance with research and clinical applications. *Int J Cardiol* 2008;**123**:240–8.

30. Adamu U, Schmitz F, Becker M, Kelm M, Hoffmann R. Advanced speckle tracking echocardiography allowing a three-myocardial layer specific analysis of deformation parameters. *Eur J Echocardiogr* 2009;**10**:303–8.

31. Søgaard P, Egeblad H, Kim WY, et al. Tissue Doppler imaging predicts improved systolic performance and reversed left ventricular remodeling during long-term cardiac resynchronization therapy. *J Am Coll Cardiol* 2002;**40**:723–30.

32. Panaich S, Briasoulis A, Cardozo S, Afonso L. Incremental value of two dimensional speckle tracking echocardiography in the functional assessment and characterization of subclinical left ventricular dysfunction. *Curr Cardiol Rev* 2017;**13**:32–40.

33. Franklin KM, Aurigemma GP. Prognosis in diastolic heart failure. *Prog Cardiovasc Dis* 2005;**47**:333–9.

34. Henein MY, Gibson DG. Suppression of left ventricular early diastolic filling by long axis asynchrony. *Br Heart J* 1995;**73**:151–7.

35. Henein MY, Das SK, O'Sullivan C, et al. ACE inhibitors unmask incoordinate diastolic wall motion in restrictive left ventricular disease. *Heart* 1696;**75**:151–8.

36. Henein MY, Priestley K, Davarashvili T, Buller N, Gibson DG. Early changes in left ventricular subendocardial function after successful coronary angioplasty. *Br Heart J* 1993;**69**:501–6.

37. Duncan AM, O'Sullivan CA, Carr-White GS, Gibson DG, Henein MY. Long axis electromechanics during dobutamine stress in patients with coronary artery disease and left ventricular dysfunction. *Heart* 2001;**86**:397–404.

38. Xiao HB, Lee CH, Gibson DG. Effect of left bundle branch block on diastolic function in dilated cardiomyopathy. *Br Heart J* 1991;**66**:443–7.

39. Pinamonti B, Zecchin M, Di Lenarda A, et al. Persistence of restrictive left ventricular filling pattern in dilated cardiomyopathy: an ominous prognostic sign. *J Am Coll Cardiol* 1997;**29**:604–12.

40. Duncan AM, Lim E, Gibson DG, Henein MY. Effect of dobutamine stress on left ventricular filling in ischemic dilated cardiomyopathy: pathophysiology and prognostic implications. *J Am Coll Cardiol* 2005;**46**:488–96.

41. Ommen SR, Nishimura RA, Appleton CP, et al. Clinical utility of Doppler echocardiography and tissue Doppler imaging in the estimation of left ventricular filling pressures: a comparative

simultaneous Doppler catheterization study. *Circulation* 2000;**102**:1788–94.

42. Garcia MJ, Ares MA, Asher C, *et al.* An index of early left ventricular filling that combined with pulsed Doppler peak E velocity may estimate capillary wedge pressure. *J Am Coll Cardiol* 1997;**29**:448–54.

43. Mullens W, Borowski AG, Curtin RJ, Thomas JD, Tang WH. Tissue Doppler imaging in the estimation of intracardiac filling pressure in decompensated patients with advanced systolic heart failure. *Circulation* 2009;**119**:62–70.

44. Garcia MJ, Smedira NG, Greenberg NL, *et al.* Color M-mode Doppler flow propagation velocity is a preload insensitive index of left ventricular relaxation: animal and human validation. *J Am Coll Cardiol* 2000;**35**:201–8.

45. Takemoto Y, Barnes ME, Seward JB, *et al.* Usefulness of left atrial volume in predicting first congestive heart failure in patients ≥65 years of age with well-preserved left ventricular systolic function. *Am J Cardiol* 2005;**96**:832–6.

46. Rossi A, Loredana L, Cicoira M, *et al.* Additional value of pulmonary vein parameters in defining pseudonormalization of mitral inflow pattern. *Echocardiography* 2001;**18**:673–9.

47. Sorrell VL, Reeves WC. Noninvasive right and left heart catheterization. *Echocardiography* 2001;**18**:31–41.

48. Xiao HB, Brecker SJ, Gibson DG. Effects of abnormal activation on the time course of the left ventricular pressure pulse in dilated cardiomyopathy. *Br Heart J* 1992;**68**:403–7.

49. Tei C. New non-invasive index for combined systolic and diastolic ventricular function. *J Cardiol* 1995;**26**:135–6.

50. Duncan A, Francis D, Henein Y, Gibson D. Importance of left ventricular activation in determining myocardial performance (Tei) index: comparison with total isovolumic time. *Int J Cardiol* 2004;**95**:211–17.

51. Duncan A, O'Sullivan C, Gibson D, Henein M. Electromechanical interrelations during dobutamine stress in normal subjects and patients with coronary disease: comparison of changes in activation and inotropic state. *Heart* 2001;**85**:411–16.

52. Duncan A, Wait D, Gibson D, Daubert J. Left ventricular remodelling and haemodynamic effects of multisite biventricular pacing in patients with congestive heart failure and activation disturbances. *Eur Heart J* 2003;**24**:430–41.

53. Duncan AM, Francis DP, Henein MY, Gibson DG. Limitation of cardiac output by total isovolumic time during pharmacologic stress in patients with dilated cardiomyopathy: activation-mediated effects of left bundle branch block and coronary artery disease. *J Am Coll Cardiol* 2003;**41**:121–8.

54. Duncan A, Francis D, Gibson D, Henein M. Limitation of exercise tolerance in chronic heart failure: distinct effects of left bundle branch block and coronary artery disease. *J Am Coll Cardiol* 2004;**43**:1524–31.

55. Duncan AM, Lim E, Clague J, Gibson D, Henein M. Predicting response to cardiac resynchronization therapy: comparison of segmental and global markers of dyssynchrony. *Eur Heart J* 2006;**27**:2426–32.

56. Youssef G, Links M. The prevention and management of cardiovascular complications of chemotherapy in patients with cancer. *Am J Cardiovasc Drugs* 2005;**5**:233–43.

57. Cazeau S, Leclercq M, Lavergne T, *et al.* for the MUltisite STimulation In Cardiomyopathies (MUSTIC) Study Investigators. Effects of multisite biventricular pacing in patients with heart failure and intraventricular conduction delay. *N Engl J Med* 2001;**344**:873–80.

58. Abraham WT, Fisher WG, Smith AL, *et al.* for the MIRACLE Study Group. Cardiac resynchronization in chronic heart failure. *N Engl J Med* 2002;**346**:1845–53.

59. Cleland JG, Daubert JC, Erdmann E, *et al.* Cardiac Resynchronization Heart Failure (CARE-HF) Study Investigators. The effect of cardiac resynchronization on morbidity and mortality in heart failure. *N Engl J Med* 2005;**352**:1539–49.

60. Hawkins NM, Petrie MC, MacDonald MR, Hogg KJ, McMurray JV. Selecting patients for cardiac resynchronization therapy: electrical or mechanical dyssynchrony? *Eur Heart J* 2006;**27**:1270–81.

61. Chung ES, Leon AR, Tavazzi L, *et al.* Results of the Predictors of Response to CRT (PROSPECT) trial. *Circulation* 2008;**117**:2608–16.

62. Pitzalis MV, Iacoviello M, Romito R, *et al.* Ventricular asynchrony predicts a better outcome in patients with chronic heart failure receiving cardiac resynchronization therapy. *J Am Coll Cardiol* 2005;**45**:65–9.

63. Bax JJ, Ansalone G, Breithardt OA, *et al.* Echocardiographic evaluation of cardiac resynchronization therapy: ready for routine clinical use? A critical appraisal. *J Am Coll Cardiol* 2004;**44**:1–9.

64. Yu CM, Bax JJ, Monaghan M, Nihoyannopoulos P. Echocardiographic evaluation of cardiac dyssynchrony for predicting a favourable response to cardiac resynchronisation therapy. *Heart* 2004;**90**:17–22.

65. Suffoletto MS, Dohi K, Cannesson M, Saba S, Gorcsan J 3rd. Novel speckle-tracking radial strain from routine black-and-white echocardiographic images to quantify dyssynchrony and predict response to cardiac resynchronization therapy. *Circulation* 2006;**113**:960–8.

66. Kapetanakis S, Kearney MT, Siva A, *et al.* Real-time three-dimensional echocardiography: a novel technique to quantify global left ventricular mechanical dyssynchrony. *Circulation* 2005;**112**:992–1000.

67. Picano E, Sicari R, Landi P, *et al.* Prognostic value of myocardial viability in medically treated patients with global left ventricular dysfunction early after an acute uncomplicated myocardial infarction: a dobutamine stress echocardiographic study. *Circulation* 1998;**98**:1078–84.

68. Duncan AM, Francis DP, Gibson DG, Henein MY. Differentiation of ischemic from nonischemic cardiomyopathy during dobutamine stress by left ventricular long-axis function: additional effect of left bundle-branch block. *Circulation* 2003;**108**:1214–20.

69. Bolling SF, Pagani FD, Deeb GM, Bach DS. Intermediate-term outcome of mitral reconstruction in cardiomyopathy. *J Thorac Cardiovasc Surg* 1998;**115**:381–6.

70. Ghio S, Gavazzi A, Campana C, *et al.* Independent and additive prognostic value of right ventricular systolic function and pulmonary artery pressure in patients with chronic heart failure. *J Am Coll Cardiol* 2001;**37**:183–8.

71. Webb-Peploe KM, Henein MY, Coats AJ, Gibson DG. Echo derived variables predicting exercise tolerance in patients with dilated and poorly functioning left ventricle. *Heart* 1998;**80**:565–9.

24

Nuclear medicine in heart failure

Pushan Bharadwaj and S. Richard Underwood

Introduction

Nuclear medicine, sometimes known as molecular imaging, involves the characterization and measurement of biological processes *in vivo* using small amounts of radiolabelled tracers. It is the most sensitive imaging technique in routine use, providing images of nano- or even of picomolar concentrations of the tracer. In patients with heart failure, biological processes such as myocardial perfusion, metabolism (both fatty acid and glucose), injury (including necrosis and apoptosis), and innervation are relevant and can be imaged.

The ideal tracer is a biological molecule labelled with an isotope of one of its constituent elements (carbon, oxygen, nitrogen, etc.), since the tracer will have biological properties identical to those of the natural compound. Such isotopes are positron emitters and are imaged by positron emission tomography (PET), which relies on detecting the synchronous 511 keV photons emitted in opposite directions when the positron annihilates with an electron in the surrounding tissue.

More common tracers use foreign elements such as iodine or technetium bound to a pharmaceutical that provides useful biological properties. These radiopharmaceuticals usually emit single gamma photons that are imaged by a gamma camera, often using single-photon emission computed tomography (SPECT) to produce tomograms or three-dimensional images.

PET has some inherent advantages over SPECT, such as higher resolution and more reliable attenuation correction that simplifies quantification of the biological process being imaged. However, PET is more expensive and, with the exception of fluorine-18, the very short-lived radionuclides have to be generated on site, requiring the additional expense of a cyclotron.

There are several areas in the management of chronic heart failure where radionuclide imaging is now routine, including diagnosis of the underlying cause in newly presenting heart failure, assessment of myocardial viability and hibernation in ischaemic heart disease, identifying the subtype of cardiac amyloidosis, diagnosis of cardiac sarcoidosis, and investigation before resynchronization pacing and defibrillator implantation.

Ischaemic heart disease

Myocardial perfusion scintigraphy (MPS) is an established technique for the diagnosis of coronary artery disease.[1] There are fewer studies of its diagnostic accuracy in patients with left ventricular dysfunction but the sensitivity in this setting is high.[2] However, the specificity of the technique is not as high because non-ischaemic myocardial scarring and inducible perfusion abnormalities can also occur in primary and secondary muscle disorders.[3,4] Features that suggest ischaemic heart disease are large areas of either transmural scarring or inducible ischaemia in a coronary distribution, impaired ventricular function in proportion to the loss of viable muscle, and predominant involvement of the left ventricle.

Viability and hibernation

It is important to distinguish between myocardial viability and hibernation. Although these terms are sometimes used interchangeably, they are different entities. Viable myocytes are alive, irrespective of their ability to function, and viable myocardium contains viable myocytes. Viability is not a dichotomy and there is a continuum from fully viable myocardium with no scarring, through partial thickness scarring to transmural scarring.

Hibernation is an ischaemic syndrome whereby viable myocardium loses its ability to contract but is able to recover contractile function once the ischaemia is abolished.[5] Hibernation was initially thought to be the result of reduced resting perfusion with contractile function being reduced in order to rematch oxygen supply and demand.[6] It is now thought to be the result of repetitive episodes of ischaemia and stunning that mimic chronic reduction of function.[7] It is likely that early hibernation is the same phenomenon as repetitive stunning but that changes in myocyte and myocardial structure later develop that may or may not be reversible. Hence, prolonged hibernating myocardium may lose its ability to recover and ultimately its viability through myocyte loss by apoptosis or necrosis.[8,9]

In order to detect hibernating myocardium, all imaging techniques rely upon detecting a triad of signs: viability, function, and ischaemia (**Figure 24.1**). The imaging definition of hibernation is therefore muscle that is viable but akinetic and where inducible ischaemia can be demonstrated. Without all three of these signs, even an area of viable but akinetic myocardium may not be hibernating. It could for instance simply be an area of partial thickness scarring without hibernation where the scarring is sufficient to abolish function.

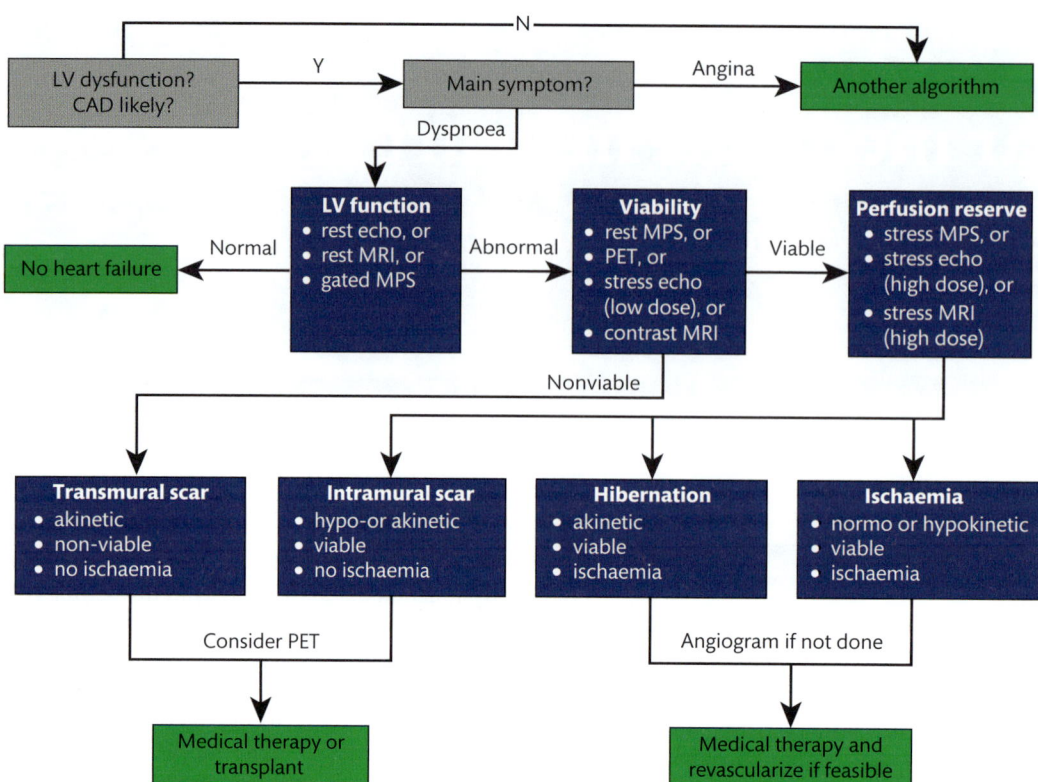

Figure 24.1 Algorithm for the investigation of patients presenting with possible ischaemic heart disease and heart failure.
Reproduced from Underwood SR, Bax JJ, vom Dahl J, *et al*. Imaging techniques for the assessment of myocardial hibernation. *Eur Heart J* 2004;**25**:815–36 with permission from Oxford University Press.

Several radionuclide techniques can be used to detect myocardial viability and hibernation.[10–12] They rely on the fact that all myocardial tracers are taken up only by viable cells, irrespective of the uptake mechanism. Hence, myocardial uptake reflects myocardial viability. In addition, tracers such as thallium-201, technetium-99m MIBI and tetrofosmin, nitrogen-13 ammonia, oxygen-15 water, and rubidium-82 have relatively high extraction and are fixed in the myocyte in proportion to delivery, hence they are dual tracers of viability and perfusion. When perfusion is less than $0.25 \, \text{mL min}^{-1} \, \text{g}^{-1}$ or less than 30% of the blood flow in normal myocardium, recovery of function is unlikely after revascularization.[13] Preserved resting perfusion in an area of dysfunction after an episode of ischaemia indicates stunning.

Perfusion imaging

Thallium-201

Thallium-201, injected as thallous chloride, is a potassium analogue and its retention is an energy-dependent process reflecting myocyte viability and perfusion.[14] Conventional imaging for the detection of myocardial ischaemia involves injection during stress (dynamic exercise or pharmacological). Imaging within 30 min of this stress injection reflects a combination of myocardial viability and perfusion. After this time, the thallium equilibrates between the intra- and extracellular spaces and takes up a distribution that reflects viability alone, irrespective of perfusion. Defects in the stress images that improve after redistribution, therefore, indicate hypoperfusion at the time of injection, or areas with inducible hypoperfusion, commonly referred to as 'inducible ischaemia' although ischaemia may not actually have been present. Redistribution imaging is normally performed 4 h after the stress injection, although imaging up to 24 h allows even better detection of viable myocardium at the expense of lower-quality images as the thallium is excreted.

Using conventional stress-redistribution imaging, areas of dysfunctional viable muscle with inducible hypoperfusion are likely to be hibernating.[15] However, redistribution may be slow and the simple stress-redistribution technique can underestimate myocardial viability.[16] More sensitive techniques involve a further injection of thallium at rest after stress-redistribution imaging (the reinjection technique)[17] or a separate day resting injection of thallium with early and delayed imaging (rest-redistribution) (Figure 24.2).[18] Resting injections are best given under nitrate cover (e.g. after sublingual glyceryl trinitrate) in order to abolish resting hypoperfusion and to give the best chance of thallium reaching any viable myocyte.

Technetium-99m perfusion tracers

The technetium-based tracers sesta-methoxyisobutylisonitrile (MIBI) and tetrofosmin have similar physiological properties to thallium although they have less avid extraction and are trapped within the myocyte, preventing redistribution. Separate stress and

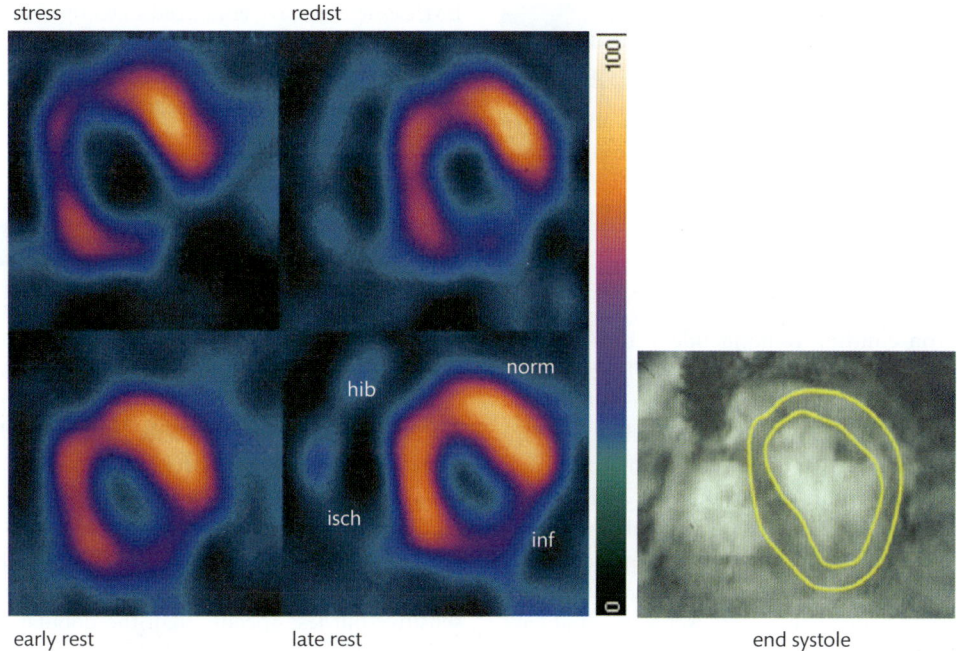

Figure 24.2 Midventricular short-axis tomograms from a thallium-201 myocardial perfusion scan (MPS) (left) and end-systolic ciné gradient echo MRI with endo- and epicardial contours superimposed (right). The MPS images were acquired immediately after stress injection of thallium (stress), following redistribution of this injection (redist), and then on a separate day early (early rest) and late (late rest) after a resting injection of thallium. The combined images show: (1) normal antero-lateral perfusion in viable and thickening muscle (norm); (2) partial-thickness inferolateral infarction with reduced thickening and some inducible ischaemia superimposed (inf); (3) inferoseptal ischaemia in fully viable and thickening myocardium (isch); (4) anteroseptal ischaemia in fully viable myocardium that does not thicken, in other words, hibernation (hib).

rest injections are therefore required to detect inducible perfusion abnormalities. In contrast, technetium-99m has better imaging characteristics with a higher energy gamma emission (140 keV) and a shorter half-life (6 h). This leads to higher-resolution images, higher injected doses without excessive radiation exposure, and hence easier ECG gating for information on ventricular function.[19] The lack of redistribution means that viable but hypoperfused myocardium can be underestimated[20] and resting injections of MIBI and tetrofosmin should be injected under nitrate cover when assessing viability (**Figure 24.3**).[21-24] Clinically relevant viability has been defined as resting MIBI or tetrofosmin uptake of more than 50–60% of maximum but attenuation in regions such as the inferior wall means that a lower threshold may be relevant.[25]

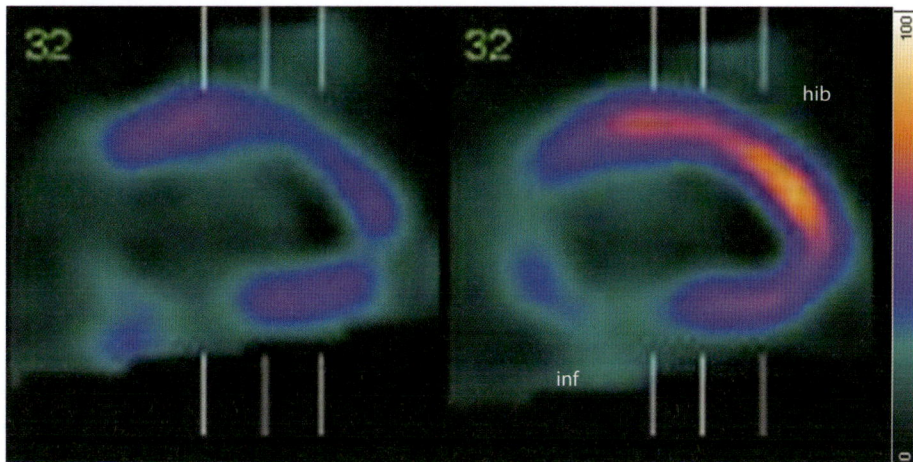

Figure 24.3 Vertical long-axis tomograms after stress (*left*) and rest (*right*) injection of MIBI. The resting injection was given after sublingual glyceryl trinitrate. There is almost transmural infarction of the basal inferior wall (inf) and this area did not thicken on ECG-gated imaging, in keeping with the infarction. There is inducible ischaemia in fully viable myocardium in the apical anterior wall that also failed to thicken on ECG-gated imaging, indicating hibernation (hib).

Metabolic imaging

The myocardium is very flexible in choice of substrates for energy production, but β-oxidation of fatty acids and glycolysis are the two main mechanisms of ATP production.[26] Under aerobic conditions fatty acid oxidation is the pathway of choice, but under hypoxic conditions glucose metabolism predominates because of its greater efficiency.[27]

2-Fluorodeoxyglucose

Fluorine-18 is a positron-emitting radionuclide with a half-life of 110 min and it can therefore be imaged by PET without the need for on-site production. As 2-deoxy-2-[18F]fluoro-d-glucose (FDG) it is widely used in oncology because of the affinity of rapidly dividing cells for the tracer. Uptake depends upon glucose transport, metabolism and trapping within the cell, and so FDG is a marker of glucose metabolism. Because normal myocardial metabolism uses fatty acids, if FDG is injected and imaged under fasting conditions there is no myocardial uptake but areas of glucose uptake indicate areas of current or recent ischaemia that have switched to glucose metabolism.[28] Alternatively, if FDG is injected after a glucose meal or during insulin and glucose infusion, myocardial uptake is normal and defects indicate areas of scarring (**Figures 24.4** and **24.5**).

Fatty acids

Straight-chain fatty acids can be labelled with radionuclides but their rapid metabolism complicates imaging. The β-methyl branched fatty acids are more suitable and the most widely used has been β-methyl-*p*-[123I]iodophenyl-pentadecanoic acid (BMIPP), although the tracer is currently only available commercially in Japan. When BMIPP is injected under fasting conditions it is extracted by the myocytes and converted into BMIPP-CoA, but it is not metabolized further. This results in high uptake and slow washout, making it very suitable for imaging.[29]

Images are usually compared with thallium or technetium images. Concordant defects are scar, whereas discordant defects with a larger metabolic defect are likely to be hibernating.[30,31] Discordant BMIPP defects have enhanced FDG uptake as a result of the metabolic shift[32] and have little fibrosis.[33] In a pooled study of 103 patients, 84% of segments with discordant BMIPP defects improved in function after revascularization but only 11% of those with concordant defects did so.[34]

Detection of hibernation

There are few large-scale studies of the accuracy of imaging techniques for predicting recovery of ventricular function after revascularization. Meta-analyses are confounded by different populations recruited, techniques used and imaging definitions of hibernation. For what it is worth, the weighted mean sensitivity and specificity for recovery of regional function after revascularization have been estimated as 92% and 63% for FDG PET, 87% and 54% for thallium MPS, 83% and 65% for technetium MPS, and 80% and 78% for dobutamine stress echocardiography. In general, all of the radionuclide techniques have similar accuracy and are said to be more sensitive but less specific than the dobutamine wall motion techniques.[35] In reality, though, the radionuclide techniques are more specific if the triad of signs referred to above is required before hibernation is diagnosed.

Fewer studies have looked at the improvement of global left ventricular function after revascularization but a similar trend is apparent in meta-analyses.[35] Fewer studies still have looked at more important measures such as symptoms and hard coronary events, but in non-randomized observational studies patients with hibernation who are revascularized have better clinical outcome than those without hibernation, and the worst outcome is in patients with hibernation who are not revascularized. These observations can, however, only be hypothesis-generating; randomized studies are needed to support the use of imaging in selecting patients with heart failure who will benefit from revascularization. The role of radionuclide imaging for detecting hibernating myocardium and improving clinical outcome has now been evaluated in several trials that are reviewed below.

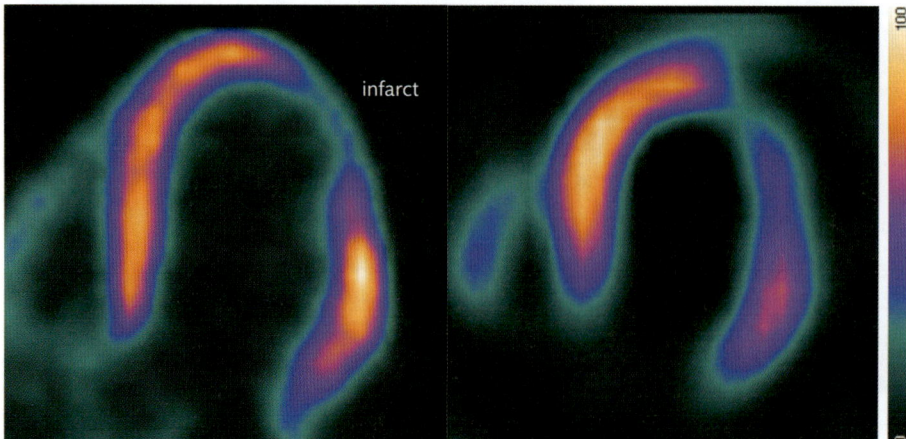

Figure 24.4   Horizontal long-axis tomograms acquired using FDG PET (*left*) and tetrofosmin SPECT (*right*). The FDG was injected after a glucose load and acipimox. The tetrofosmin was injected after sublingual glyceryl trinitrate. There is partial thickness infarction of the apical lateral wall (infarct). The PET images have higher resolution but the pattern of tracer uptake is very similar indicating that both tracers can be used successfully to assess myocardial viability.

^{13}N ammonia

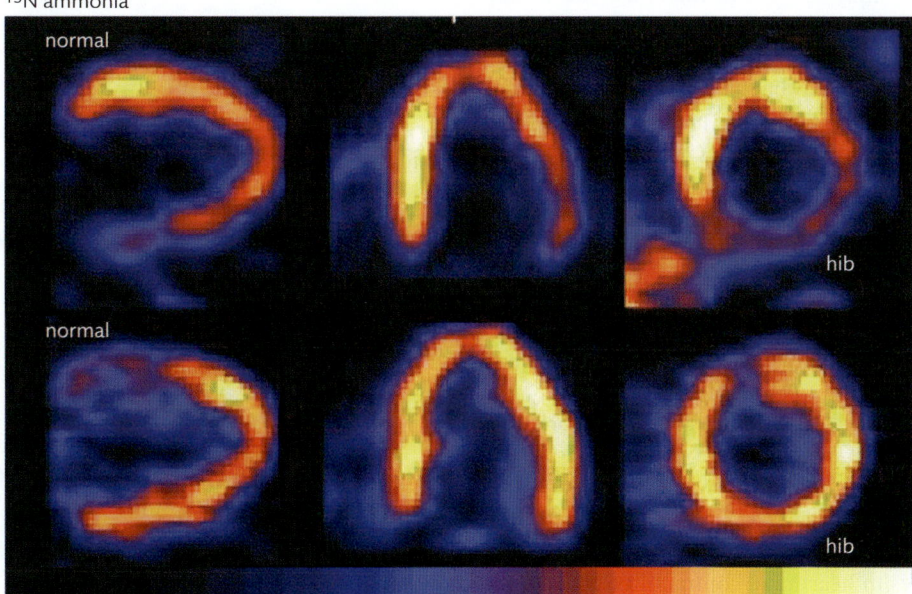

^{18}F 2-fluorodeoxyglucose

Figure 24.5 Positron emission tomograms in vertical long-axis (*left*), horizontal long-axis (*centre*), and short-axis planes (*right*), acquired after resting injections of nitrogen-13 ammonia (*top*) and fluorine-18 2-fluorodeoxyglucose (FDG) with glucose loading (*bottom*). The inferolateral myocardium (hib) has normal viability (FDG uptake) but reduced resting perfusion (ammonia), which is the typical mismatched pattern of hibernation. The basal anterior wall (normal) has a reversed mismatch with normal resting perfusion (ammonia) and hence viability but reduced glucose metabolism (FDG). This emphasizes the importance of adequate glucose loading when FDG is used to assess viability
Images courtesy of Professor Marcus Schwaiger, Munich.

Clinical trials of radionuclide imaging in heart failure

CHRISTMAS (Carvedilol Hibernation Reversible Ischemia Trial: Marker of Success) was a double-blind, randomized trial of medical therapy in chronic left ventricular (LV) dysfunction.[36] The efficacy of carvedilol for improving LV function was tested in patients with hibernation or ischaemia using both radionuclide and echocardiographic techniques. The total burden of hibernation and ischaemia was a predictor of improved LV ejection fraction (LVEF) and there was little or no increase in LVEF in the absence of hibernation. The role of revascularization was not addressed.

The PARR-1 (Positron Emission Tomography and Recovery Following Revascularization) study[37] was a prospective multicentre cohort study showing that the extent of scar was an independent predictor of recovery of LV function after revascularization; the smaller the scar, the greater the improvement in LVEF. However, small numbers (82 patients) and the absence of parameters such as ventricular volume and stress-induced ischaemia limited this pilot study.

The PARR-2 study[38] was designed to assess the effectiveness of PET-assisted management in patients with severe LV dysfunction and suspected CAD compared with standard care. A total of 430 patients were randomized to receive PET assessment of hibernation (ammonia-FDG imaging) (218 patients) or standard care (212 patients). The PET findings were used to recommend appropriate management depending upon the presence or absence of hibernation. The primary outcome measure of hospital admission for congestive heart failure, myocardial infarction, or cardiac death was achieved in 30% of the PET patients and 36% of those with standard care (hazard ratio 0.78) but this was not statistically significant. There was no reduction in cardiac events in the PET arm compared with the standard care. However, almost 25% of the FDG-PET study group were not managed according to imaging recommendations at the discretion of the treating clinician. In a separate analysis including only those who adhered to the PET-guided recommendations, there was a significant benefit for FDG PET. A substudy of the PARR-2 trial confirmed that patients with larger amounts of perfusion–metabolism mismatch have improved outcome with revascularization.[39] Viability in >7% of the LV myocardium predicted benefit from revascularization with regard to a composite end-point of cardiac death, myocardial infarction, or repeat hospital admission at one year.

The Ottawa-FIVE substudy[40] of the PARR-2 trial was a post-hoc analysis of the utility of PET-assisted management of patients with severe LV dysfunction and suspected CAD. This substudy also showed significant benefit of the FDG-PET-assisted approach. Among the non-Ottawa-FIVE patients of the PARR-2 study, there was no significant difference in the primary end-point based on an FDG-PET versus standard-of-therapy approach. This emphasized the importance of institutional expertise when these imaging techniques are used.

STICH (Surgical Treatment for Ischemic Heart Failure)[41] was designed to examine the outcome of patients with CAD and LV dysfunction randomized either to OMT alone or OMT plus coronary artery bypass grafting (CABG). There was no significant difference between the two groups with respect to the primary end-point of death of any cause; however, patients assigned to CABG had significantly lower mortality. Ten years later, the mortality by any cause was reduced by 8% in patients who underwent CABG.[42]

A non-randomized substudy of STICH examined the role of myocardial viability in identifying patients who might have a survival benefit with CABG.[43] Viability tests included SPECT and dobutamine stress echocardiography but not FDG-PET and cardiac magnetic resonance imaging, and these were performed in only half of enrolled patients without randomization. Viability assessment did not confer any survival benefit, but this finding has been criticized for several reasons:

1. Viability testing was at physician discretion after randomization to treatment group and hence was susceptible to bias.
2. There was significant crossover between the randomized groups.
3. The imaging definition of viability was that patients with small amounts of scar were deemed to be viable and those with large scar to be non-viable without any consideration of the presence of inducible ischaemia that might benefit from revascularization.

Cardiac innervation imaging

In mild heart failure, increased sympathetic tone is helpful because it leads to increases in heart rate, contractility, and venous return. As the syndrome worsens, this overactivity becomes unfavourable because of downregulation of β-adrenoceptors, leading to progressive LV dysfunction.[44] The sympathetic overactivity also increases the risk of arrhythmia mainly around focal areas of denervation.

Myocardial innervation can be imaged in a number of ways. [^{11}C] Meta-hydroxyephedrine (HED) is an analogue of noradrenaline that concentrates in the presynaptic nerve terminal by the uptake-1 mechanism, providing high-quality PET images capable of quantification.[45] Meta-[^{123}I]iodobenzylguanidine (mIBG) is a guanethidine analogue with a similar mechanism of uptake that is suitable for both planar and SPECT imaging. Initial mIBG uptake corresponds with the density of sympathetic innervation and washout rate thereafter with the frequency of nerve terminal firing and hence sympathetic activity. Uptake is quantified from the ratio of myocardial to mediastinal uptake, and washout is measured from changes between 15 min and 4 h images (**Figure 24.6**).[46]

Low myocardial uptake and rapid washout are associated with poor prognosis in both ischaemic heart failure and dilated cardiomyopathy,[47,48] and myocardial uptake appears to be at least equal to left ventricular ejection fraction (LVEF) for predicting death and other major cardiac events.[49,50]

Other applications of mIBG imaging may be the prediction of life-threatening arrhythmias and hence the need for an implanted defibrillator, since ventricular arrhythmias may arise from the border of an area of scarring with viable muscle that is denervated (**Figure 24.7**).[51] In a study, of 50 patients with previous myocardial infarction and left ventricular dysfunction, significant abnormality on semiquantitative mIBG SPECT, was 77% sensitive and 75% specific for predicting ventricular arrhythmias on provocation testing.[52] Patients with appropriate defibrillator discharges have lower myocardial mIBG uptake than those without.[53,54]

The widest experience of the role of mIBG imaging for risk assessment in heart failure comes from the multicentre ADMIRE-HF study.[55,56] In this study, 964 patients with NYHA class II and III heart failure were studied with primary end-points of heart failure progression, life-threatening arrhythmia, and cardiac death. There

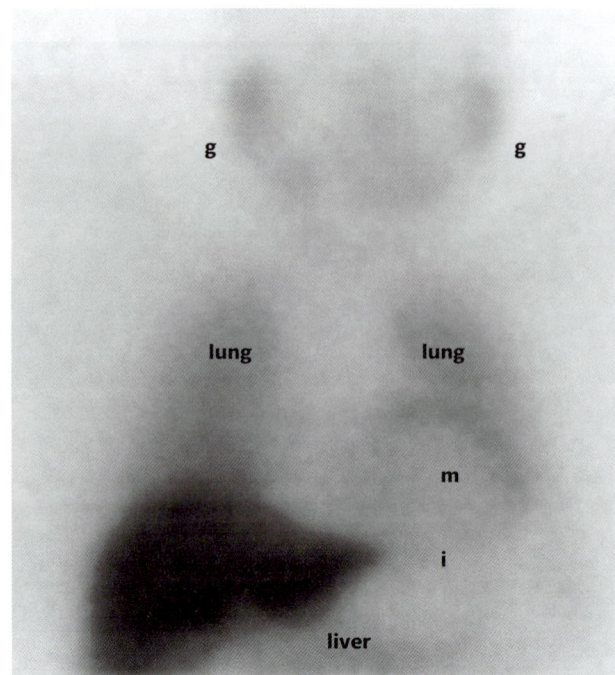

Figure 24.6 Anterior projection image 4 h after injection of [^{123}I]*meta*-iodobenzyl guanidine (mIBG). Myocardial uptake (m) is a measure of sympathetic innervation and tone. The patient had previous inferior infarction (i) with HF (NYHA 3). There is normal liver, lung and salivary gland (g) uptake. The heart to mediastinal ratio of mIBG uptake was 1.56, suggesting annual mortality in the region of 7% (see ADMIRE-HF study[58]).

were 51 cardiac deaths in patients with heart-to-mediastinal ratio (HMR) of mIBG <1.6 compared with 2 in the high-uptake group, and 37% of patients with HMR <1.6 developed one of the end-points compared with 15% with HMR >1.6 ($P < 0.0001$). The negative predictive value of high HMR for cardiac death within two years was 98.8%. Heart failure death was more common in the lowest group but arrhythmias were more common with intermediate HMR (1.2–1.6), suggesting that focal as opposed to global denervation is more likely to cause arrhythmias and sudden cardiac death.

Radionuclide ventriculography

Radionuclide ventriculography (RNV) is an accurate and reproducible method of assessing ventricular function. It is sometimes referred to as MUGA (multigated acquisition) but the acronym is not sufficiently descriptive and RNV is preferred. Injections of technetium-99 pertechnetate and a stannous agent label the blood pool with the tracer. Images are acquired after the tracer is in equilibrium with the blood pool (the equilibrium technique) and/or during its first pass through the central circulation (the first pass technique). The former mainly provides information on left ventricular function but the latter can also be used to assess right ventricular function and left-to-right shunting. Traditionally, image acquisition is planar in the left anterior oblique projection that best separates the left and right ventricles but emission tomographic

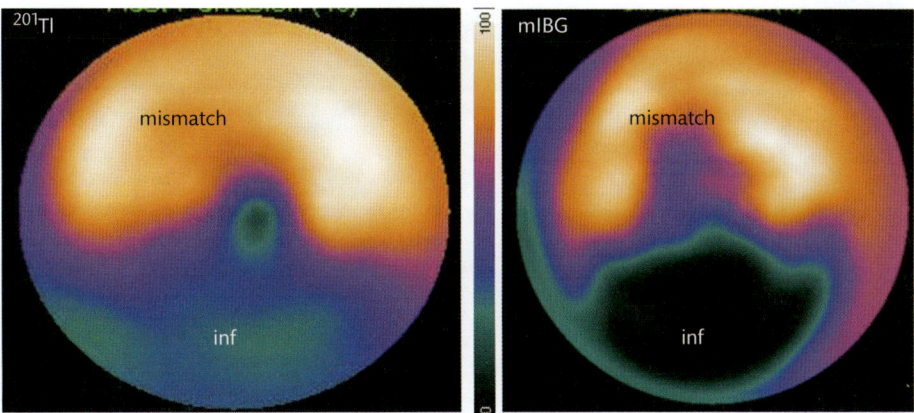

Figure 24.7 Polar plots of thallium uptake (*left*) indicating myocardial viability, and mIBG uptake (*right*) indicating sympathetic innervation. There is almost transmural inferior infarction (inf), and a neighbouring area anteroapically of reduced innervation in viable myocardium (mismatch). The mismatch may be a substrate for arrhythmia.

imaging is used increasingly. ECG-gated acquisition provides 16–32 frames over the cardiac cycle, with each frame containing counts from an average cycle over what is typically a 10 min acquisition for planar imaging.

In the planar equilibrium technique, left ventricular count changes over the cardiac cycle are used to calculate ejection fraction and other parameters of both global and regional function, including diastolic function. Ejection fraction measurements require the subtraction of counts from structures in front of and behind the left ventricle and these are usually estimated from a region of interest lateral to the left ventricle. The estimation of background is a source of inter- and intraobserver variability but the technique is otherwise accurate and reproducible because it makes no assumptions about ventricular geometry. In the tomographic technique, ventricular volumes can be measured either geometrically or by summing counts within the ventricles.[57,58]

Assessment of ventricular synchrony

Gated SPECT imaging has been used to assess scar burden, LV function and dyssynchrony. Regional ventricular function is also possible by Fourier analysis of count changes derived either from RNV or from MPS, since myocardial count changes in MPS are related to myocardial thickening. Using either technique, Fourier analysis can be applied to changes in geometry, such as the distance between the centre of the ventricle and the endocardium. Fourier analysis provides the parameters of phase and amplitude, which define the fundamental harmonic of contraction. Phase approximates to the time of end systole and can be expressed in milliseconds or more commonly as degrees or fraction of the cardiac cycle. Amplitude approximates to the magnitude of count changes through the cardiac cycle and hence to the extent of regional motion. Both parameters can be derived from whole ventricular counts, from regions, or from individual image pixels. The histogram of phase values provides a simple method of displaying the mean and standard deviation of phase from any of these regions, and hence both inter- and intraventricular synchrony.

The combination of low LVEF and significant interventricular dyssynchrony measured by RNV predicts improved systolic function six months after cardiac resynchronization therapy (CRT) (Figure 24.8).[59] Similar analyses of MPS have shown a sensitivity and specificity of 70% and 74%, respectively, for predicting clinical improvement after CRT.[60,61]

Sarcoidosis

Sarcoidosis is a chronic inflammatory disorder, characterized by the presence of non-caseating granulomas and most frequently involving the lungs and thoracic lymph nodes.[62] Cardiac involvement is less common although it can be asymptomatic and is often underestimated. In patients with advanced heart failure cardiac sarcoidosis is present in >3% of patients on myocardial biopsy at the time of LVAD implantation,[63] possibly more due to the inherent lack of sensitivity of biopsy for a patchy condition. Multiple imaging techniques are usually required for the diagnosis and assessment of cardiac involvement including echocardiography, X-ray computed tomography, magnetic resonance imaging (MRI), and scintigraphy.

Gallium-67 citrate scintigraphy has long been used as a non-specific marker of inflammation and its presence was a major diagnostic factor in the Japanese Ministry of Health diagnostic criteria.[64] The technique can be insensitive,[65] albeit improved by SPECT-CT.[66] More recently the sensitivity of FDG-PET for the detection of inflammation has led to it becoming an essential investigation for the assessment of cardiac sarcoidosis, and it is among the criteria for the diagnosis of cardiac sarcoidosis recommended by the Heart Rhythm Society alongside gallium-67 scintigraphy, and MRI for the assessment of myocardial scar.[67] Given the higher resolution of MRI than PET, it is more sensitive for small areas of scar, whereas FDG-PET is more sensitive for the inflammatory component of the disease.[68]

A meta-analysis has shown overall sensitivity and specificity of FDG-PET for the detection of cardiac sarcoidosis of 90% and 81%, respectively, although the true specificity is likely to be higher because the studies used the Japanese Ministry of Health criteria as the diagnostic standard and it is likely that FDG-PET is more sensitive than the criteria.[69] FDG-PET also has prognostic relevance

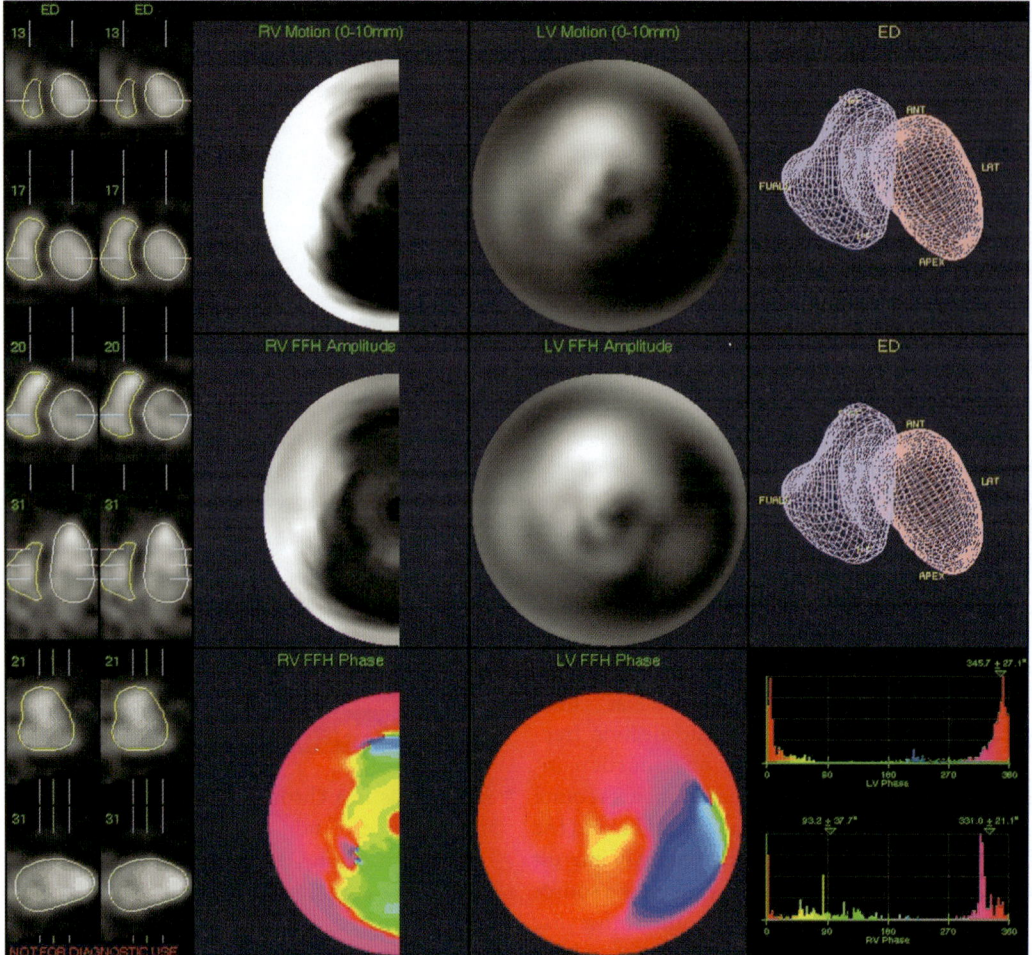

Figure 24.8 ECG-gated blood pool SPECT for the assessment of ventricular function in a 76-year-old woman with alcoholic cardiomyopathy and heart failure. The polar plots of ventricular phase (*bottom centre*) show an area of almost paradoxical motion in the left ventricle inferolaterally (blue) and interventricular dyssynchrony (green in the right ventricle). After resynchronization pacing, NYHA class improved from III to I, left ventricular end-diastolic volume fell from 205 to 122 mL and left ventricular ejection fraction improved from 15% to 36%.

in cardiac sarcoidosis with abnormal scans significantly related to ventricular arrhythmia or death over 1.5 years, and patients with evidence of both myocardial inflammation and scar having a hazard ratio of 3.9 for adverse events.[70] When monitoring treatment of cardiac sarcoidosis there is an association between suppression of myocardial inflammation and improvement in LV function,[71] but it is not yet established whether suppression of inflammation reduces event rates or might even avoid the need for implanted defibrillator therapy, since arrhythmias can be related as much to scar as to inflammation.

Several other radiopharmaceuticals have been used to image sarcoid-related inflammation including ^{111}In-octreotide and pentetreotide using SPECT,[72] and gallium-68 citrate using PET. ^{68}Ga-citrate has the same biological characteristics as ^{67}Ga-citrate but is a generator-produced positron emitter providing better quality images than the SPECT tracer, although possibly hampered by early blood pool activity due to its shorter half-life of 68 min.[73] ^{68}Ga-Dotatate is a somatostatin receptor type-2 analogue that is well established in the imaging of neuroendocrine tumours. Somatostatin is a neurotransmitter, a regulator of endocrine and exocrine secretion

and a modulator of inflammation. Dotatate therefore highlights the myocardial inflammation of sarcoidosis and has the advantage that metabolic preparation to abolish normal myocardial glucose metabolism is not required.[74]

Amyloidosis

Amyloidosis is an abnormality of protein secondary, tertiary, and/or quaternary structure in which native proteins become misfolded in response to genetic or other factors, aggregate and deposit as amyloid tissue in various organs including the myocardium, kidneys, nerves, gastrointestinal tract, liver, and soft tissues.[75,76] There are about 30 different types of amyloidosis, each due to a specific protein misfolding. They are grouped into localized and systemic forms but the two that most commonly affect the heart are amyloid light-chain (AL amyloidosis) and transthyretin-related amyloidosis (TTR), which can either be hereditary (autosomal dominant) or senile, so-called 'wild type'.

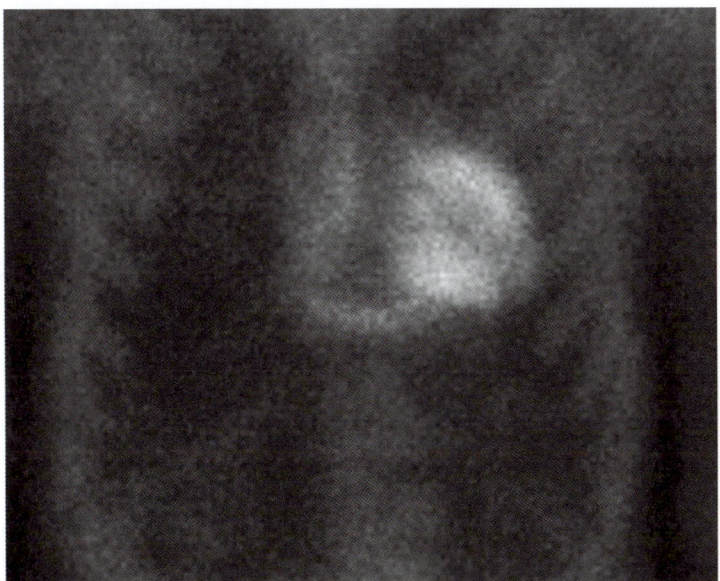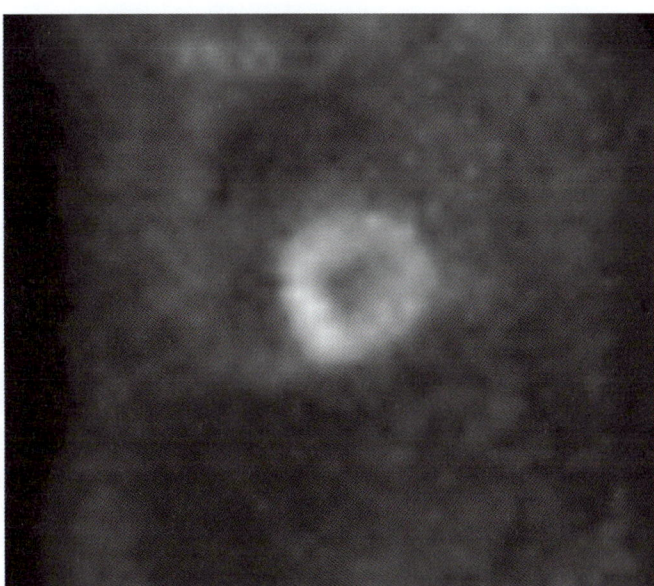

Figure 24.9 [99m]Technetium- labelled 3,3- diphosphono- 1,2- propanodicarboxylic acid (DPD) in a patient with transthyretin amyloidosis, showing uptake in both ventricles. *Left*, antero-posterior view; *right*, left anterior oblique view.

The prevalence of cardiac amyloidosis is not clear, but it is underrecognized and it is a cause of significant morbidity and mortality. A quarter of deaths of those aged >80 years have transthyretin amyloid deposits in the myocardium,[77] and it is present in 15% of patients with severe aortic stenosis undergoing transcatheter aortic valve replacement[78] and in 13% with heart failure but preserved ejection fraction.[79] In a cohort of 1034 patients with TTR cardiac amyloidosis there was substantial delay in diagnosis of more than four years in 42% of patents with wild-type disease and the patients used hospital services a median of 17 times in the three years before diagnosis, by which time quality of life was poor.[80]

When myocardial involvement is suspected, echocardiography has some characteristic features but is usually unable to distinguish between different causes of myocardial hypertrophy or AL from TTR amyloidosis. Magnetic resonance imaging also has characteristic features, particularly the kinetics of myocardial gadolinium contrast, native T1 imaging and imaging of extracellular volume, but it is also unable to distinguish between AL and TTR amyloidosis. By contrast, many different radionuclide tracers have been used to image the distribution of amyloid.

It has been known for many years that occasional myocardial activity of bone-seeking tracers can occur,[81] but only more recently has diphosphonate or pyrophosphate imaging been studied more systematically. Perugini first described a system of grading myocardial activity by comparison with bone and showed that more intense activity (grades 2 and 3) perfectly distinguished between AL and TTR cardiac amyloidosis.[82] A meta-analysis of studies showed 92% sensitivity and 95% specificity for TTR provided that AL was excluded by plasma or urine testing.[83]

It is less clear whether scintigraphy can be used to assess prognosis in cardiac amyloidosis or to monitor the effect of treatment. A large UK study of 602 patients did not show a statistically significant relationship between Perugini grade and mortality (although there was a trend), whereas a multicentre study of 229 patients in the USA did show a relationship between quantification of myocardial activity and outcome.[84] It is likely that Perugini grading may be too 'coarse' to be used to assess prognosis.

Conclusion

- Radionuclide imaging is a widely available method of obtaining information on the pathophysiology, extent, prognosis, and treatment options in patients with heart failure. It provides information non-invasively on myocardial perfusion, metabolism, innervation, or injury through necrosis and apoptosis.

- Perfusion imaging can aid the diagnosis of the cause of heart failure, as well as providing information on myocardial viability and hibernation.

- Radionuclide ventriculography is an accurate and reproducible technique for assessing left ventricular function.

- Assessment of interventricular dyssynchrony by radionuclide techniques has the potential to assist selection of patients who will benefit from resynchronization pacing.

- Metabolic imaging with FDG under fasting conditions can identify areas of sarcoid-mediated myocardial inflammation and is now an important component of the diagnosis and monitoring of cardiac sarcoidosis.

- In suspected amyloidosis, the presence or absence of transthyretin-related cardiac involvement can be diagnosed by ^{99m}Tc-labelled bone-seeking tracers.

REFERENCES

1. Underwood SR, Anagnostopoulos C, Cerqueira M, *et al.* Myocardial perfusion scintigraphy: the evidence. *Eur J Nucl Med Mol Imaging* 2004;31:261–91.

2. Klocke FJ, Baird MG, Lorell BH, *et al.* ACC/AHA/ASNC guidelines for the clinical use of cardiac radionuclide imaging. *Circulation* 2003;**108**:1404–18.

3. Pasternac A, Noble J, Streulens Y, *et al.* Pathophysiology of chest pain in patients with cardiomyopathies and normal coronary arteries. *Circulation* 1982;**65**:778–89.

4. Miller WL, Hodge DO, Tointon SK, *et al.* Relationship of myocardial perfusion imaging findings to outcome of patients with heart failure and suspected ischemic heart disease. *Am Heart J* 2004;**147**:714–20.

5. Rahimtoola SH. The hibernating myocardium. *Am Heart J* 1982;**117**:211–21.

6. Schwarz ER, Speakman MT, vom Dahl J, Kloner RA. Hibernating myocardium: is there evidence for chronic flow reduction? *Heart Dis* 1999;**1**:155–62.

7. Braunwald E, Kloner RA. The stunned myocardium: prolonged, post-ischaemic ventricular dysfunction. *Circulation* 1982;**66**:1146–9.

8. Canty JM Jr, Fallavollita JA. Chronic hibernation and chronic stunning: a continuum. *J Nucl Cardiol* 2000;**7**:509–27.

9. Maes A, Flameng W, Nuyts J, *et al.* Histological alterations in chronically hypoperfused myocardium. Correlation with PET findings. *Circulation* 1994;**90**:735–45.

10. Bax JJ, Wijns W, Cornel JH, *et al.* Accuracy of currently available techniques for prediction of functional recovery after revascularization in patients with left ventricular dysfunction due to chronic coronary artery disease: comparison of pooled data. *J Am Coll Cardiol* 1997;**30**:1451–60.

11. Allman KC, Shaw LJ, Hachamovitch R, Udelson JE. Myocardial viability testing and impact of revascularization on prognosis in patients with coronary artery disease and left ventricular dysfunction: a meta-analysis. *J Am Coll Cardiol* 2002;**39**:1151–8.

12. Underwood SR, Bax JJ, vom Dahl J, *et al.* Imaging techniques for the assessment of myocardial hibernation. *Eur Heart J* 2004;**25**:815–36.

13. Gewirtz H, Fischman AJ, Abraham S, *et al.* Positron emission tomographic measurements of absolute regional myocardial blood flow permits identification of nonviable myocardium in patients with chronic myocardial infarction. *J Am Coll Cardiol* 1994;**23**:851–9.

14. Bonow RO, Dilsizian V. Thallium-201 for assessment of myocardial viability. *Semin Nucl Med* 1991;**21**:230–41.

15. Rozanski A, Berman DS, Gray R, *et al.* Use of thallium-201 redistribution scintigraphy in the preoperative differentiation of reversible and nonreversible myocardial asynergy. *Circulation* 1981;**64**:936–44.

16. Liu P, Kiess MC, Okada RD, *et al.* The persistent defect on exercise thallium imaging and its fate after myocardial revascularisation: does it represent scar or ischaemia? *Am Heart J* 1985;**110**:996–1001.

17. Dilsizian V, Bonow RO. Current diagnostic techniques for assessing myocardial viability in patients with hibernating and stunned myocardium. *Circulation* 1993;**87**:1–20.

18. Sivaratnam DA, Bonow RO, Kalff V. Assessment of myocardial viability in dysfunctional myocardium. In: Ell PJ, Gambhir SS (eds), *Nuclear medicine: clinical diagnosis and treatment*, pp. 1159–70. Churchill Livingstone, London, 1994.

19. Bonow RO, Dilsizian V. Thallium-201 and technetium-99m-sestamibi for assessing viable myocardium. *J Nucl Med* 1992;**33**:815–18.

20. Cuocolo A, Pace L, Ricciardelli B, *et al.* Identification of viable myocardium in patients with chronic coronary artery disease: comparison of thallium-201 scintigraphy with reinjection and technetium 99m-methoxyisobutylisonitrile. *J Nucl Med* 1992;**33**:505–11.

21. Bisi G, Sciagra R, Santoro GM, Rossi V, Fazzini PF. Technetium-99m-sestamibi imaging with nitrate infusion to detect viable hibernating myocardium and predict post revascularization recovery. *J Nucl Med* 1995;**36**:1994–2000.

22. Maurea S, Cuocolo A, Soricelli A, *et al.* Myocardial viability index in chronic coronary artery disease: technetium-99m-methoxy isobutyl isonitrile redistribution. *J Nucl Med* 1995;**36**:1953–60.

23. Udelson JE, Coleman PS, Metherall JA, *et al.* Predicting recovery of severe regional ventricular dysfunction: comparison of resting scintigraphy with 201Tl and 99mTc-sestamibi. *Circulation* 1994;**89**:2552–61.

24. Levine MG, McGill CC, Ahlberg AW, *et al.* Functional assessment with electrocardiographic gated single-photon emission computed tomography improves the ability of technetium-99 m sestamibi myocardial perfusion imaging to predict myocardial viability in patients undergoing revascularization. *Am J Cardiol* 1999;**83**:1–5.

25. Sciagra R, Pellegri M, Pupi A, *et al.* Prognostic implications of Tc-99 m sestamibi viability imaging and subsequent therapeutic strategy in patients with chronic coronary artery disease and left ventricular dysfunction. *J Am Coll Cardiol* 2000;**36**:739–45.

26. Neubauer S. The failing heart: an engine out of fuel. *New Engl J Med* 2007;**356**:1140–51.

27. Liedke AJ. Alterations of carbohydrate and lipid metabolism in the acutely ischemic heart. *Prog Cardiovasc Dis* 1981;**23**:321–36.

28. Schelbert HR. 18F-deoxyglucose and the assessment of myocardial viability. *Semin Nucl Med* 2002;**32**:60–9.

29. Knapp FF, Kropp J. Iodine-123-labelled fatty acids for myocardial single-photon emission tomography: current status and future perspectives. *Eur J Nucl Med* 1995;**22**:361–81.

30. Taki J, Nakajima K, Matsunari I, *et al.* Impairment of regional fatty acid uptake in relation to wall motion and thallium-201 uptake in ischaemic but viable myocardium, assessment with iodine-123-labelled beta-methyl-branched fatty acid. *Eur J Nucl Med* 1995;**22**:1385–92.

31. Kawamoto M, Tamaki N, Yonekura Y, *et al.* Combined study with I-123 fatty acid and thallium-201 to assess ischemic myocardium. *Ann Nucl Med* 1994;**8**:47–54.

32. Tamaki N, Tadamura E, Kawamoto M, *et al.* Decreased uptake of iodinated branched fatty acid analog indicates metabolic alterations in ischemic myocardium. *J Nucl Med* 1995;**36**:1974–80.

33. Kudoh T, Tadamura E, Tamaki N, *et al.* Iodinated free fatty acid and 201Tl uptake in chronically hypoperfused myocardium: histological correlation study. *J Nucl Med* 2000;**41**:293–6.

34. Tamaki N, Morita K, Kawai Y. The Japanese experience with metabolic imaging in the clinical setting. *J Nucl Cardiol* 2007;**14**(Suppl 3):S145–52.

35. Schinkel AF, Bax JJ, Poldermans D, *et al.* Hibernating myocardium: diagnosis and patient outcomes. *Curr Probl Cardiol* 2007;**32**:375–410.

36. Cleland JGF, Pennell DJ, Ray SG, *et al.* Myocardial viability as a determinant of the ejection fraction response to carvedilol in patients with heart failure (CHRISTMAS trial): randomised controlled trial. *Lancet* 2003;**362**:14–21.

37. Beanlands RSB, Ruddy TD, deKemp RA, *et al.* Positron emission tomography and recovery following revascularization (PARR-1): the importance of scar and the development of a prediction rule for the degree of recovery of left ventricular function. *J Am Coll Cardiol* 2002;**40**:1735–43.

38. Beanlands RSB, Nichol G, Huszti E, *et al.* F-18-fluorodeoxyglucose positron emission tomography imaging-assisted management of patients with severe left ventricular dysfunction and suspected coronary disease: a randomized, controlled trial (PARR-2). *J Am Coll Cardiol* 2007;**50**:2002–12.

39. D'Egidio G, Nichol G, Williams KA, *et al.* Increasing benefit from revascularization is associated with increasing amounts of myocardial hibernation: a substudy of the PARR-2 trial. *J Am Coll Cardiol Imag* 2009;**2**:1060–8.

40. Abraham A, Nichol G, Williams KA, *et al.* ^{18}F-FDG PET imaging of myocardial viability in an experienced center with access to ^{18}F-FDG and integration with clinical management teams: the Ottawa-FIVE substudy of the PARR 2 trial. *J Nucl Med* 2010;**51**:567–74.

41. Velazquez EJ, Lee KL, Deja Marek A, *et al.* Coronary-artery bypass surgery in patients with left ventricular dysfunction. *N Engl J Med* 2011;**364**:1607–16.

42. Velazquez EJ, Lee KL, Jones RH, *et al.* Coronary-artery bypass surgery in patients with ischemic cardiomyopathy. *N Engl J Med* 2016;**374**:1511–20.

43. Bonow RO, Maurer G, Lee KL, *et al.* Myocardial viability and survival in ischemic left ventricular dysfunction. *N Engl J Med* 2011;**364**:1617–25.

44. Ungerer M, Böhm M, Elce JS, Erdmann E, Lohse MJ. Altered expression of beta-adrenergic receptor kinase and beta-adrenergic receptors in the failing human heart. *Circulation* 1993;**87**:454–63.

45. Bengel FM, Schwaiger M. Assessment of cardiac sympathetic neuronal function using PET imaging. *J Nucl Cardiol* 2004;**11**:603–16.

46. Carrio I. Cardiac neurotransmission imaging. *J Nucl Med* 2001;**42**:1062–76.

47. Merlet P, Benvenuti C, Moyse D, *et al.* Prognostic value of MIBG imaging in idiopathic dilated cardiomyopathy. *J Nucl Med* 1999;**40**:917–23.

48. Arimoto T, Takeishi Y, Niizeki T, *et al.* Cardiac sympathetic denervation and ongoing myocardial damage for prognosis in early stages of heart failure. *J Card Fail* 2007;**13**:34–41.

49. Merlet P, Valette H, Dubois-Rande J, *et al.* Prognostic value of cardiac metaiodo-benzylguanidine in patients with heart failure. *J Nucl Med* 1992;**33**:471–7.

50. Agostini D, Verberne HJ, Burchert W, *et al.* I-123-mIBG myocardial imaging for assessment of risk for a major cardiac event in heart failure patients: insights from a retrospective European multicenter study. *Eur J Nucl Med Mol Imaging* 2008;**35**:535–46.

51. Bax JJ, Boogers MM, Schuijf JD. Nuclear imaging in heart failure. *Cardiol Clin* 2009;**27**:265–76.

52. Bax JJ, Kraft O, Buxton AE, *et al.* 123-I-MIBG scintigraphy to predict inducibility of ventricular arrhythmias on cardiac electrophysiology testing. *Circ Cardiovasc Imaging* 2008;**1**:131–40.

53. Nagahara D, Nakata T, Hashimoto A, *et al.* Predicting the need for an implantable cardioverter defibrillator using cardiac metaiodobenzylguanidine activity together with plasma natriuretic peptide concentration or left ventricular function. *J Nucl Med* 2008;**49**:225–33.

54. Arora R, Ferrick KJ, Nakata T, *et al.* I-123 MIBG imaging and heart rate variability analysis to predict the need for an implantable cardioverter defibrillator. *J Nucl Cardiol* 2003;**10**:121–31.

55. Jacobson AF, Lombard J, Banerjee G, Camici P. 123I-mIBG scintigraphy to predict risk for adverse cardiac outcomes in heart failure patients: design of two prospective multicenter international trials. *J Nucl Cardiol* 2009;**16**:113–21.

56. Jacobson AF, Senior R, Cerqueira M, *et al.* Myocardial iodine-123 meta-iodobenzylguanidine imaging and cardiac events in heart failure: results of the prospective ADMIRE-HF (AdreView Myocardial Imaging for Risk Evaluation in Heart Failure) study. *J Am Coll Cardiol* 2010;**55**:2212–21.

57. Botvinick EH, O'Connell JW, Kadkade PP, *et al.* Potential added value of three-dimensional reconstruction and display of single photon emission computed tomographic gated blood pool images. *J Nucl Cardiol* 1998;**5**:245–55.

58. Harel F, Finnerty V, Gregoire J, *et al.* Comparison of left ventricular contraction homogeneity index using SPECT gated blood pool imaging and planar phase analysis. *J Nucl Cardiol* 2008;**15**:80–5.

59. Toussaint JF, Lavergne T, Kerrou K, *et al.* Basal asynchrony and resynchronization with biventricular pacing predict long-term improvement of LV function in heart failure patients. *Pacing Clin Electrophysiol* 2003;**26**:1815–23.

60. Henneman MM, Chen J, Dibbets-Schneider P, *et al.* Can LV dyssynchrony as assessed with phase analysis on gated myocardial perfusion SPECT predict response to CRT? *J Nucl Med* 2007;**48**:1104–11.

61. Adelstein EC, Saba S. Scar burden by myocardial perfusion imaging predicts echocardiographic response to cardiac resynchronization therapy in ischemic cardiomyopathy. *Am Heart J* 2007;**153**:105–12.

62. Statement on sarcoidosis. Joint statement of the American Thoracic Society (ATS), the European Respiratory Society (ERS) and the World Association of Sarcoidosis and Other Granulomatous Disorders (WASOG) adopted by the ATS Board of Directors and by the ERS Executive Committee, February 1999. *Am J Respir Crit Care Med* 1999;**160**:736–55.

63. Segura AM, Radovancevic R, Demirozu ZT, Frazier OH, Buja LM. Granulomatous myocarditis in severe heart failure patients undergoing implantation of a left ventricular assist device. *Cardiovasc Pathol* 2014;**23**:17–20.

64. Hiraga H, Yuwai K, Hiroe M. Diagnostic standard and guidelines for sarcoidosis. *Jpn J Sarcoidosis Granulomatous Disord* 2007;**27**:89–102.

65. Okayama K, Kurata C, Tawarahara K, *et al.* Diagnostic and prognostic value of myocardial scintigraphy with thallium-201 and gallium-67 in cardiac sarcoidosis. *Chest* 1995;**107**:330–4.

66. Nakazawa A, Ikeda K, Ito Y, *et al.* Usefulness of dual ^{67}Ga and ^{99m}Tc-sestamibi single-photon-emission CT scanning in the diagnosis of cardiac sarcoidosis. *Chest* 2004;**126**:1372–6.

67. Birnie DH, Sauer WH, Bogun F, *et al.* HRS expert consensus statement on the diagnosis and management of arrhythmias associated with cardiac sarcoidosis. *Heart Rhythm* 2014;**11**:1305–24.

68. Youssef G, Leung E, Mylonas I, *et al.* The use of 18F-FDG PET in the diagnosis of cardiac sarcoidosis: a systematic review and metaanalysis including the Ontario experience. *J Nucl Med* 2012;**53**:241–8.

69. Ohira H, Tsujino I, Ishimaru S, *et al.* Myocardial imaging with ^{18}F-fluoro-2-deoxyglucose positron emission tomography and magnetic resonance imaging in sarcoidosis. *Eur J Nucl Med Mol Imaging* 2008;**35**:933–41.

70. Blankstein R, Osborne M, Naya M, *et al.* Cardiac positron emission tomography enhances prognostic assessments of patients with suspected cardiac sarcoidosis. *J Am Coll Cardiol* 2014;**63**:329–36.

71. Osborne MT, Hulten EA, Singh A, *et al.* Reduction in ^{18}F-fluorodeoxyglucose uptake on serial cardiac positron emission tomography is associated with improved left ventricular ejection fraction in patients with cardiac sarcoidosis. *J Nucl Cardiol* 2014;**21**:166–74.

72. Bombardieri E, Ambrosini V, Aktolun C, *et al.* ^{111}In-pentetreotide scintigraphy: procedure guidelines for tumour imaging. *Eur J Nucl Med Mol Imaging* 2010;**37**:1441–8.

73. Segard T, Morandeau LMJA, Dunne ML, *et al.* Comparison between gallium-68 citrate positron emission tomography-computed tomography and gallium-67 citrate scintigraphy for infection imaging. *Intern Med J* 2019;**49**:1016–22.

74. Bravo PE, Singh A, di Carli MF, Blankstein R. Advanced cardiovascular imaging for the evaluation of cardiac sarcoidosis. *J Nucl Cardiol* 2019;**26**:188–99.

75. Dorbala S, Ando Y, Bokhari S, *et al.* ASNC/AHA/ASE/EANM/ HFSA/ISA/SCMR/SNMMI expert consensus recommendations for multimodality imaging in cardiac amyloidosis: part 1 of 2—evidence base and standardized methods of imaging. *J Nucl Cardiol* 2019;**26**:2065–123.

76. Dorbala S, Ando Y, Bokhari S, *et al.* ASNC/AHA/ASE/EANM/ HFSA/ISA/SCMR/SNMMI expert consensus recommendations for multimodality imaging in cardiac amyloidosis: part 2 of 2—diagnostic criteria and appropriate utilization. *J Nucl Cardiol* 2019. https://doi.org/10.1007/s12350-019-01761-5

77. Tanskanen M, Peuralinna T, Polvikoski T, *et al.* Senile systemic amyloidosis affects 25% of the very aged and associates with genetic variation in alpha-2-macroglobulin and tau: a population-based autopsy study. *Ann Med* 2008;**40**:232–99.

78. Scully PR, Treibel TA, Fontana M, *et al.* Prevalence of cardiac amyloidosis in patients referred for transcatheter aortic valve replacement. *J Am Coll Cardiol* 2018;**71**:463–4.

79. González-López E, Gallego-Delgado M, Guzzo-Merello G, *et al.* Wild-type transthyretin amyloidosis as a cause of heart failure with preserved ejection fraction. *Eur Heart J* 2015;**36**:2585–94.

80. Lane T, Fontana M, Martinez-Naharro A, *et al.* Natural history, quality of life, and outcome in cardiac transthyretin amyloidosis. *Circulation* 2019;**140**:16–26.

81. van Antwerp JD, O'Mara RE, Pitt MJ, Walsh S. Technetium-99m diphosphonate accumulation in amyloid. *J Nucl Med* 1975;**16**:238–40.

82. Perugini E, Guidalotti PL, Salvi F, *et al.* Noninvasive etiologic diagnosis of cardiac amyloidosis using ^{99m}Tc-3,3-diphosphono-1,2-propanodicarboxylic acid scintigraphy. *J Am Coll Cardiol* 2005;**46**:1076–84.

83. Treglia G, Glaudemans AWJM, Bertagna F, *et al.* Diagnostic accuracy of bone scintigraphy in the assessment of cardiac transthyretin-related amyloidosis: a bivariate meta-analysis. *Eur J Nucl Med Mol Imaging* 2018;**45**:1945–55.

84. Castano A, Haq M, Narotsky DL, *et al.* Multicenter study of planar technetium-99m pyrophosphate cardiac imaging: predicting survival for patients with ATTR cardiac amyloidosis. *JAMA Cardiol* 2016;**1**:880–9.

25

Cardiovascular magnetic resonance in heart failure

Brian P. Halliday and Sanjay K. Prasad

Cardiovascular magnetic resonance in heart failure

Cardiovascular magnetic resonance (CMR) has an increasingly important role in the assessment of patients with heart failure. One major advantage of this modality is the ability to perform tissue characterization without exposure to ionizing radiation, enabling accurate diagnosis and improved prognostication. Given the high spatial resolution and the ability to image in any plane, it also provides reference-standard quantification of chamber size and function. Accurate assessment of left ventricular ejection fraction is fundamental to current decision-making in the contemporary management of heart failure. This chapter covers the basics of magnetic resonance imaging, including the components of a typical scan performed to evaluate a patient with heart failure, and discusses the major benefits CMR offers in the assessment of patients with heart failure with reduced ejection fraction (HFrEF) and those with preserved ejection fraction (HFpEF).

Basics of magnetic resonance imaging

CMR uses radiofrequency energy to excite hydrogen nuclei within the heart, blood vessels and surrounding structures to produce magnetic resonance signal, whilst the patient lies within a strong, static magnetic field. As the patient enters the scanner, the hydrogen nuclei align with or against the static magnetic field ($B0$) (**Figure 25.1**). In steady state, there is a small excess of hydrogen nuclei aligning with $B0$, creating a small net magnetization in the longitudinal direction (Z). Radiofrequency pulses are then used to flip the net magnetization vector away from the 'Z' direction, into the 'XY' direction. The hydrogen nuclei subsequently return to their original state of equilibrium in a process known as relaxation. Relaxation generates the magnetic resonance signal which is detected by receiver coils close to the patient. The signal is then converted into an image by the Fourier transformation.

Relaxation is composed of two components: longitudinal and transverse relaxation. Longitudinal relaxation, also known as T1 relaxation, refers to the recovery of net magnetization in the 'Z' direction. Transverse relaxation refers to the decay of magnetization in the 'XY' direction. This process is influenced by T2 relaxation. Hydrogen nuclei are surrounded by different molecular environments in different tissues. The interaction with the surrounding environment affects the time it takes for T1 and T2 relaxation to occur. The extent to which the overall signal relies on T1 and T2 relaxation is influenced by the type and timing of the pulses used. Images produced by sequences with different properties can therefore be 'weighted' towards the T1 or T2 relaxation. Considering the variation in T1 and T2 relaxation times in different tissues, specific sequences can be used to generate different contrasts between tissues. T1-weighted images are useful for identifying myocardial fat, whereas T2 images are helpful in detecting an increase in the water content of a tissue and evaluating myocardial inflammation.

Assessment of morphology and function

A major component of CMR for the investigation of heart failure is the acquisition of high-spatial-resolution cine imaging which enables the accurate assessment of cardiac morphology and function. Cine imaging is produced by creating an image of the heart at multiple time-points throughout the cardiac cycle. Typically, data are acquired continuously throughout multiple cardiac cycles

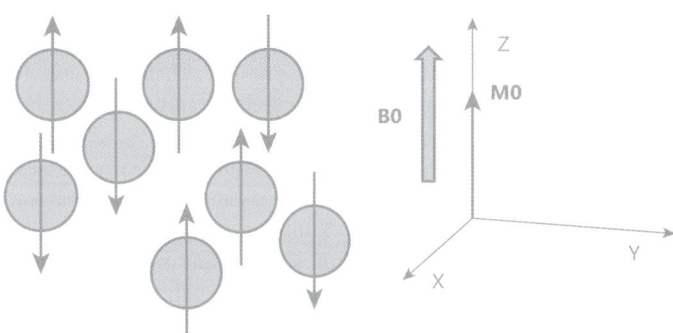

Figure 25.1 (*Left*) Hydrogen nuclei arrangement in a static magnetic field (*B0*). (*Right*) At rest, there is a small net magnetization in the longitudinal direction (*Z*) due to a slight excess of hydrogen nuclei aligning with the field.

as patients holds their breath. The data are then divided into the relevant phase of the cardiac cycle using the ECG signal. In certain circumstances, such as patients with marked heart rate variability, 'prospective gating' may be used. Prospective gating acquires data for a specific length of time after a pre-specified point following each R wave. This technique has the disadvantage of not imaging the entire cardiac cycle.

Cine images can be acquired in any anatomical plane and this is one of the major advantages of CMR over other imaging modalities. Using localizer images as landmarks, long axis images are typically acquired in two-, three- and four-chamber planes followed by images of the right ventricular outflow tract and the right ventricular long axis. Consecutive short axis images are acquired from the atrio-ventricular ring to the apex. These images enable reference-standard quantitative assessment of left and right ventricular size and function without geometrical assumptions. Available software packages track the cardiac valves during the cardiac cycle, ensuring the exclusion of atrial and arterial blood from the ventricular volume analyses. Accurate assessment of right ventricular function with other imaging modalities can be challenging due to its variable and complex shape. The three-dimensional capability of CMR provides a major advantage in this setting. Given the accuracy and reproducibility of CMR in determining chamber size and function, use of this modality may avoid repeated studies which are often requested with less precise methods. It has also been demonstrated that CMR-determined left ventricular ejection fraction is a better predictor of adverse arrhythmic events compared to the same measure determined by echocardiography.[1] There may be advantages to using CMR-determined left ventricular ejection fraction in the selection of patients for implantable cardioverter–defibrillators (ICDs). Given the reproducibility, it is also the ideal method to use when examining changes of cardiac function following an intervention as part of clinical trials.

Qualitative assessment of left and right ventricular wall motion is aided by high spatial resolution and enables the detection of abnormalities secondary to infarction, myocardial scar, or fatty infiltration. If specific pathology such as arrhythmogenic cardiomyopathy is suspected, a stack of long axis images through the right ventricle may also be acquired.

Myocardial strain is now considered a more sensitive marker of pathology than left ventricular ejection fraction and is increasingly being used to detect early disease. Regional and global longitudinal, radial, and circumferential strain can be assessed using tissue tracking, feature tracking, or displacement encoding with stimulated echoes. Increased atrial size and volume are important markers of chronically raised ventricular filling pressure. The latter is readily assessed using the biplane area length method and remains robust in atrial fibrillation.[2]

The multiplanar ability of CMR also enables the accurate assessment of valve disease, including the interrogation of individual leaflets and the valvular apparatus. Functional mitral regurgitation, secondary to annular dilatation and leaflet tethering, is a common feature of heart failure. A stack of images through the mitral valve enables the assessment of individual scallops, the chordae, and papillary muscles. Mitral regurgitation is accurately assessed using phase-contrast velocity mapping. Mitral regurgitant volume can be estimated by subtracting the aortic forward flow volume, measured using phase-contrast mapping, from the total left ventricular

stroke volume. Primary valvular disease may also be the cause of heart failure. Organic mitral regurgitation is assessed in a similar fashion to functional disease. Data have suggested that CMR is more accurate at identifying high-risk patients with organic mitral regurgitation compared to echocardiography.[3] Similarly, the cause and severity of aortic regurgitation is accurately assessed using cine imaging and flow mapping. Regurgitant volume and CMR-derived left ventricular end-diastolic volume have been shown to be strong predictors of adverse outcome without surgery.[4] Aortic stenosis may be accurately evaluated using valve planimetry and by estimating the maximal jet velocity using flow mapping.

Tissue characterization

Tissue characterization forms the second main component of the CMR exam in heart failure. Gadolinium contrast, an agent which dramatically shortens T1 relaxation, is frequently used to produce tissue contrast and demonstrate pathology. Following injection, gadolinium passes through the vascular tree followed by tissues with an adequate blood supply. Imaging performed at the point of transit through a specific blood vessel forms the basis of angiography. Early cardiac imaging, when the contrast remains in the blood pool, may be used to detect avascular structures within the heart, such as thrombi, which appear dark (**Figure 25.2a**). Imaging during the first pass of gadolinium through the myocardium forms the basis of perfusion imaging. This is typically performed in three short axis slices and images are acquired at the same time-point in the cardiac cycle across several consecutive heart beats. Regional perfusion defects present during vasodilator stress and absent at rest suggest the presence of epicardial coronary stenoses (**Figure 25.2b**). CMR has excellent diagnostic accuracy for the diagnosis of coronary disease and is superior to single-photon emission computed tomography.[5]

Gadolinium subsequently reaches steady state around 10 min after injection and accumulates in tissues with expanded extracellular space and disrupted cell membranes. Areas of myocardial scar or acute injury will have a relatively high concentration of gadolinium and short T1 relaxation times compared to healthy myocardium. The aim of late gadolinium enhancement (LGE) imaging is to capture the signal at the time when the longitudinal magnetization of healthy tissue is zero (**Figure 25.3**). Healthy tissues therefore appear black or 'nulled'. At the same time-point, given the relative differences in T1 relaxation, areas of myocardium where gadolinium has accumulated will produce a strong signal and appear bright. This enables the detection of myocardial scar, as in cases of chronic myocardial infarction (**Figure 25.2c**), dilated cardiomyopathy or cardiac sarcoidosis or acute myocardial injury, as in cases of acute myocardial infarction or myocarditis.

T2-weighted sequences are used to image oedema. Water-bound hydrogen nuclei have long T2 relaxation times and this property is manipulated by specific sequences to produce high signal in oedematous tissues. The short tau inversion recovery (STIR) sequence is most frequently used and incorporates radiofrequency preparation pulses to suppress signal from blood and fat. This enables the detection of active inflammation in cases of acute injury, such as myocardial infarction or myocarditis or chronic injury such as that seen in cardiac sarcoidosis (**Figure 25.2d**).

Parametric mapping is a contemporary quantitative CMR technique that takes serial images throughout T1 or T2 relaxation.

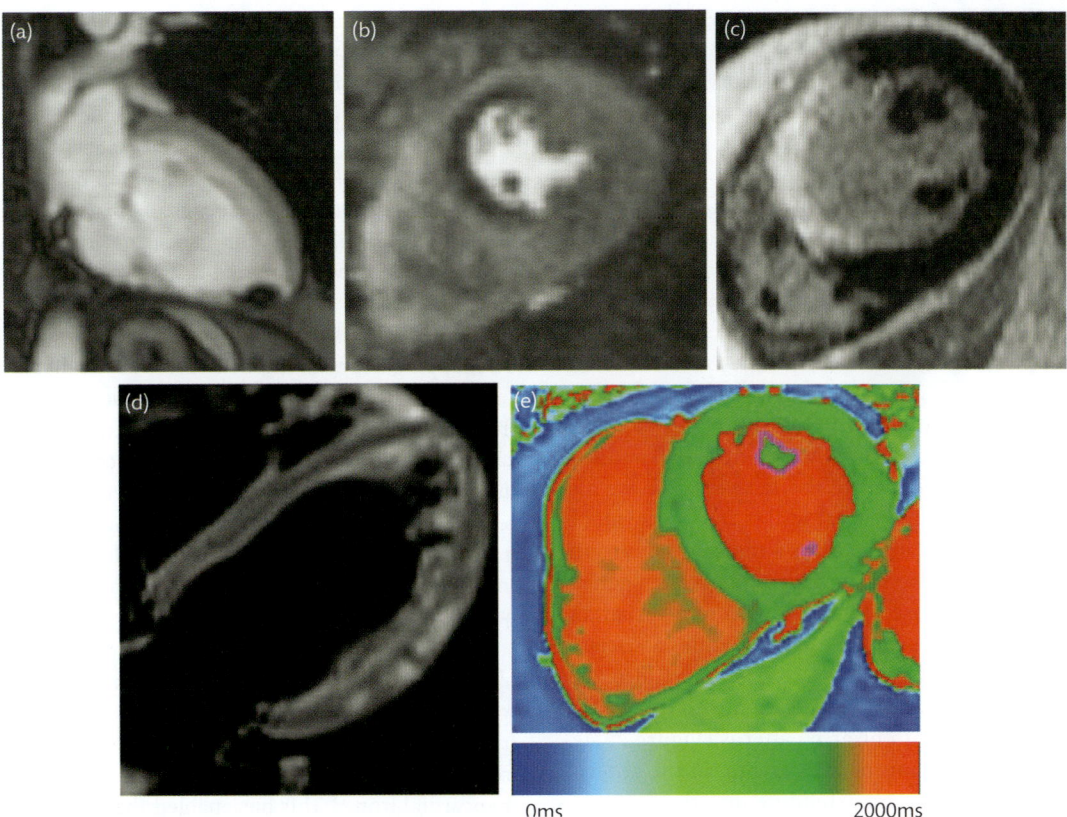

Figure 25.2 CMR techniques used to evaluate a patient presenting with heart failure. (a) Early gadolinium image of the left ventricle in a two-chamber plane demonstrating thrombus adjacent to the inferior wall at apical level. The inferior wall appears thinned, consistent with an inferior myocardial infarction. (b) First-pass perfusion imaging in a short-axis plane at mid-ventricular, performed following the administration of adenosine demonstrating a perfusion defect in the anterior and septal walls. (c) Late gadolinium enhancement imaging in a short-axis plane at mid-ventricular level demonstrating transmural enhancement of the anteroseptum and anterior wall, in keeping with mycoardial infarction. (d) STIR imaging of the left ventricle in a horizontal long-axis plane demonstrating increased signal in the basal and mid anterolateral wall, in keeping with myocardial oedema. There is also increased signal around the apical trabeculation; this is due to poor 'nulling' of the blood pool signal associated with vascular stasis rather than oedema. (e) Native T1 map of the left and right ventricle in a mid-ventricular short-axis plane. The colour of each voxel of the myocardium represents its T1 value.

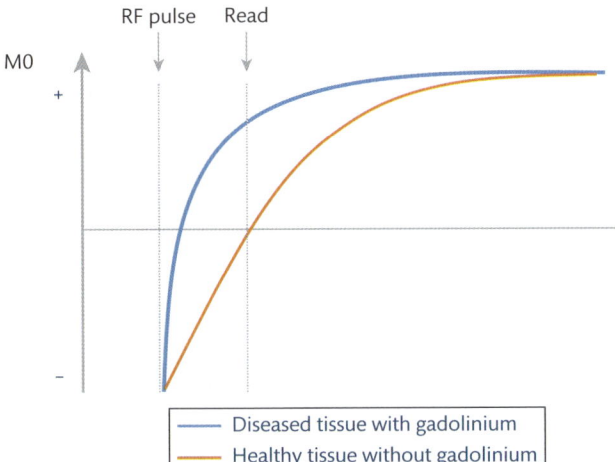

Figure 25.3 Recovery of longitudinal magnetization in late gadolinium enhancement imaging. The aim of LGE imaging is to acquire the data at the point where the signal from healthy tissue is 'nulled'. At the same time-point, there has been greater recovery of longitudinal magnetization in tissues where gadolinium has accumulated and therefore greater signal. RF, radiofrequency.

Images are typically acquired when the heart is static in diastole during breath-holding. The specific T1 or T2 time of each voxel within the image is quantified and a visual map can be constructed where the signal intensity of each voxel corresponds to the specific T1 or T2 value (**Figure 25.2e**). T1 mapping can be performed before and after the administration of gadolinium. The extracellular volume fraction of the myocardium can be derived from the pre- and post-contrast T1 values by estimating the volume of gadolinium in the extracellular space relative to the blood pool. Pre-contrast or native T1 values and the extracellular volume fraction have been shown to correlate with the degree of interstitial fibrosis in diseases such as dilated cardiomyopathy and hypertrophic cardiomyopathy.[6,7] This technique has the ability to identify global changes that may be missed by LGE, which relies on a reference area of normal myocardium. It is important to emphasize, however, that elevation of T1 values is not specific to interstitial fibrosis. This may also occur with oedema and protein deposition, whereas iron overload and intracellular storage disorders are associated with a reduction in values. T2 mapping is typically used for the detection and quantification of oedema, which is associated with elevation in T2 values.

CMR in the evaluation of heart failure with reduced ejection fraction

Diagnosis

The ability to distinguish between ischaemic and non-ischaemic causes of HFrEF using LGE imaging in a radiation-free test is one of the major strengths of CMR. Previous myocardial infarction is evidenced by LGE arising in the subendocardium, becoming transmural to varying degrees depending on the severity and duration of ischaemia (**Figure 25.4a**). LGE imaging of non-ischaemic dilated cardiomyopathy (DCM) demonstrates mid-wall LGE sparing the subendocardium in around 30–40% of cases.[8] The remaining cases have no evidence of LGE. Mid-wall LGE classically occurs in the septum (**Figure 25.4b**); however, mid-wall and sub-epicardial patterns in the free-wall of the left ventricle are also recognized. Whereas LGE in the lateral wall is frequently attributed to a previous episode of myocarditis—the cause of around one-third of DCM—it may also be seen in patients with genetic cardiomyopathies, such as those associated with rare variants in *LMNA* and desmosomal genes and cardiomyopathies associated with muscular dystrophies. Cardiac sarcoidosis may also present with HFrEF. LGE may occur in any location with this disease and is frequently associated with bizarre patterns (**Figure 25.4c**). A 'Shepherd's crook' distribution of LGE arising in the anterior free-wall of the right ventricle and extending into the septum is recognized.

Before the increase in CMR availability, patients presenting with HFrEF typically underwent echocardiography to determine the degree of left ventricular dysfunction and an invasive coronary angiogram to investigate a possible ischaemic cause. One study, however, demonstrated that 13% of patients diagnosed with a non-ischaemic aetiology following echocardiography and angiography had previous asymptomatic myocardial infarction as evidenced by subendocardial or transmural LGE.[9] Large general population studies have confirmed a relatively high prevalence of asymptomatic myocardial infarction.[10] Cases with unobstructed coronary arteries on angiography and evidence of previous infarction on CMR appear likely to have had secondary-to-embolic events or plaque rupture with subsequent recanalization. A further study investigating patients with new-onset HFrEF demonstrated that CMR was at least as accurate as coronary angiography in determining the aetiology of disease. Compared to a reference standard combination of CMR and angiography, CMR alone had 97% accuracy for the diagnosis compared to 95% for coronary angiography.[11] It has been proposed that CMR can act as a gatekeeper to coronary angiography for patients with HFrEF. The authors estimated that this approach was more cost-effective compared to one where all patients underwent angiography.

The use of T2-weighted imaging, including STIR sequences and T2 mapping, plays an important role in the diagnosis of acute myocarditis. Whereas an 'infarct-like' presentation may be the most frequent, acute myocarditis may present with heart failure and is occasionally associated with a malignant course. Accurate and prompt diagnosis may be made using CMR with endomyocardial biopsy reserved for cases of progressive heart failure that may require immunosuppression. Oedema imaging also plays an important role in the identification of patients with active cardiac sarcoidosis, requiring treatment.

Heart failure secondary to myocardial iron overload related to blood transfusions is the most common cause of death in patients with thalassaemia major.[12] Myocardial T2* is a variable related to transverse relaxation and dramatically shortens in the presence of iron. Measurement of T2* can reproducibly quantify the degree of myocardial iron.[13] This has enabled the early diagnosis of myocardial iron overload using a simple and rapid non-invasive test and has transformed the management and outcome of patients. Cardiac dysfunction is reversible if identified and treated early with iron chelation. This has become the standard of care.

Risk stratification and treatment selection in ischaemic cardiomyopathy

In cases of ischaemic cardiomyopathy, it has been demonstrated that the degree of scar transmurality determines the likelihood of functional improvement following revascularization. A landmark paper established that 70% of segments with scar that occupied ≤25% of wall thickness demonstrated functional recovery following revascularization compared to 2% of those with a scar

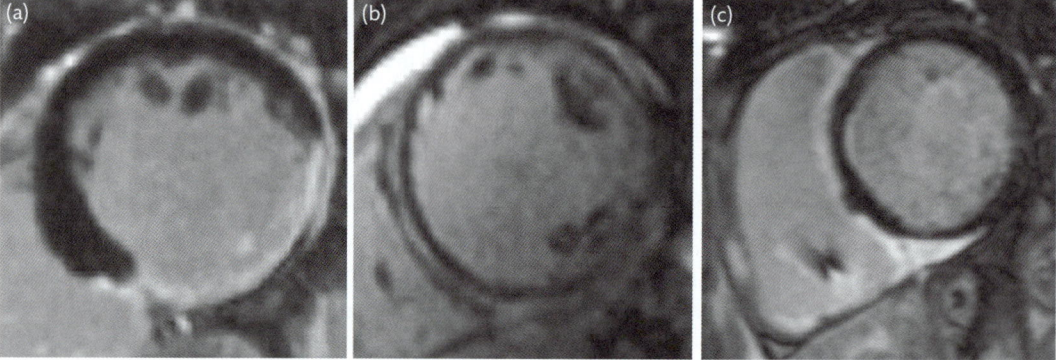

Figure 25.4 (a) Transmural enhancement of the inferior and inferolateral wall extending into the inferoseptum, characteristic of myocardial infarction in the territory supplied by the right coronary artery. (b) Mid-wall enhancement of the septum characteristic of the pattern commonly seen with non-ischaemic dilated cardiomyopathy. (c) Bizarre pattern of enhancement involving the septum secondary to cardiac sarcoidosis. The enhancement is most marked on the right ventricular side of the septum and spares the subendocardium of the left ventricle. There is also artefact produced by a right ventricular pacing lead following previous episodes of atrioventricular block.

thickness >75%.[14] LGE transmurality is now an established method of determining myocardial viability and some clinicians use this technique to select patients for revascularization. It has also been demonstrated that assessing contractile reserve using low-dose dobutamine CMR may increase the accuracy of predicting functional recovery in patients with intermediate scar thickness.[15] The use of contrast-free T1 mapping to determine myocardial viability is also an exciting area of research that offers potential to improve precision and remove the need for gadolinium. It is important to emphasize, however, that the benefit of revascularization in heart failure remains uncertain.[16] Studies investigating the benefit of revascularization in heart failure patients with evidence of myocardial ischaemia are ongoing and aim to provide further evidence.

The presence and extent of LGE have been associated with the occurrence of adverse outcomes in patients with ischaemic cardiomyopathy.[17,18] Patients with these features may therefore benefit from more intensive follow-up and medical therapy. There is also particular interest in using the presence, size, and type of scar to select patients who are most likely to benefit from ICDs. A major cause of sudden cardiac death in patients with ischaemic cardiomyopathy is scar re-entry ventricular tachycardia.[19] Several studies have demonstrated an association between sudden cardiac death and major arrhythmic events and the presence of scar.[20-22] The interaction of surviving areas of conducting myocardium within peripheral areas of scar is thought to be particularly important in arrhythmia generation. There has therefore been interest in identifying the size of the heterogeneous 'grey zone', which may be linked with the greatest risk. Studies using semi-automated techniques to identify this zone have suggested that the size of this area is a better predictor of arrhythmic events compared to overall scar mass.[21,22] The benefit of using a CMR-guided approach to ICD selection is under investigation in randomized trials.

It has also been suggested CMR may be used to guide left ventricular lead position in patients receiving cardiac resynchronization. One study demonstrated lower rates of reverse remodelling in patients for whom the left ventricular lead was positioned over areas of scarred myocardium.[23] Avoiding large areas of scar identified on pre-implant scans may therefore prove beneficial.

Other CMR features, including the presence of microvascular obstruction and intramyocardial haemorrhage, are associated with adverse outcomes in patients following myocardial infarction.[18] Additional treatments that prevent or slow ventricular remodelling and reduce the incidence of heart failure in these patients are awaited.

Given the association between native T1 and diffuse myocardial changes such as interstitial fibrosis, there is also interest in the use of native T1 mapping to risk-stratify patients with ischaemic cardiomyopathy. This avoids the need for contrast and has the potential to detect diffuse changes in non-infarcted myocardium that are not detected by LGE. A recent study demonstrated that native T1 value of non-infarcted myocardium was the sole independent predictor of all-cause mortality in patients with CAD.[24] Whether elevation in native T1 values in these patients is driven solely by interstitial fibrosis and whether the underlying processes are reversible with treatment remain unclear. However, it is possible that this technique may be used to identify patients who would benefit from novel anti-fibrotic therapies.[24]

Risk stratification and treatment selection in non-ischaemic cardiomyopathy

There is a wealth of data demonstrating a strong association between the presence of mid-wall LGE and adverse outcomes in DCM. Multiple studies and meta-analyses have linked LGE with increased rates of death, sudden cardiac death, major arrhythmic events, and heart failure events.[8,20] The largest study to date demonstrated a three-fold increase in death and a five-fold increase in the rate of sudden cardiac death and aborted sudden cardiac death in patients with mid-wall LGE.[8] Given the results of the recent DANISH trial, which failed to demonstrate a reduction in mortality with primary prevention ICDs in patients with non-ischaemic HFrEF, additional methods that identify patients with the highest risk of SCD who may be most likely to gain benefit are required.[25] Similar to ischaemic cardiomyopathy, a proportion of SCD in DCM is secondary to scar re-entry ventricular tachycardia. It is therefore plausible that the detection of mid-wall scar using CMR may be able to improve our current approach to selection. This is supported by observations from electrophysiological studies in DCM patients.[26] In this study, operators were only able to induce arrhythmia in those with LGE. Furthermore, in each of these cases the origin of the arrhythmia was mapped to the location corresponding to the enhancement on CMR.

Building on these observations, a recent study investigating DCM patients referred for cardiac resynchronization therapy demonstrated that, of those with mid-wall LGE, patients who received a defibrillator had lower mortality compared to those who received a pacing device. There was no difference in outcome between patients without mid-wall LGE who received defibrillators compared to pacing devices.[27] Further work has also demonstrated a nine-fold increase in the rate of sudden cardiac death events associated with the presence of mid-wall LGE among patients with DCM and a left ventricular ejection fraction >40%.[28] Patients with mild and moderate degrees of left ventricular impairment currently represent a large proportion of those who suffer SCD, yet current guidelines for ICDs do not account for this. Whether these patients with lower competing risks of death from non-sudden causes gain longevity from ICD implantation requires confirmation in ongoing randomized trials.

Additional features from CMR may also be able to identify patients at risk of adverse heart failure outcomes. It is possible that intensive medical management, novel therapies, and close follow-up will reduce the risk of adverse events in these individuals. Left atrial volume, right ventricular impairment, and reduced longitudinal strain have all been associated with adverse heart failure outcomes.[29-31] Native T1 values have also been associated with increased all-cause mortality and adverse heart failure events.[32] It is possible that identifying patients with the most severe interstitial changes using parametric mapping may enable the identification of patients most likely to benefit from targeted anti-fibrotic therapies.

Heart failure with preserved ejection fraction

Diagnosis

HFpEF is a heterogeneous syndrome characterized by concentric remodelling, left ventricular diastolic dysfunction and myocardial fibrosis. The overall prognosis of patients with the disease is poor. Currently, there is an absence of evidence-based treatments for this

(a)   (b)

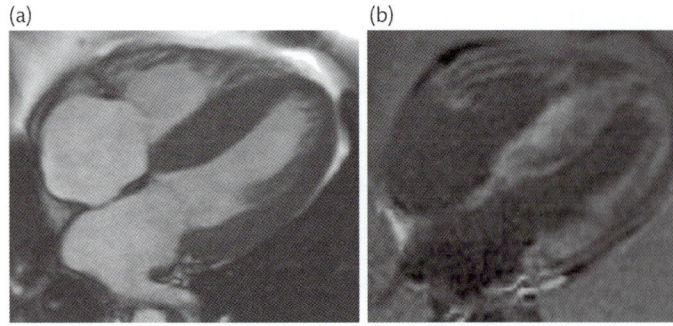

Figure 25.5 CMR features of cardiac amyloidosis. (a) Steady-state free precession image in end diastole in the horizontal long-axis plane demonstrating severe concentric left ventricular hypertrophy. (b) Phase-sensitive inversion recovery late gadolinium enhancement image in the horizontal long-axis plane demonstrating diffuse transmural late enhancement with rapid 'wash-out' of gadolinium from the blood pool.

disease phenotype which accounts for 50% of all heart failure.[33] Precise characterization of the substrate and research into novel therapies are required. The disease is typically associated with advanced age, hypertension, obesity, diabetes mellitus and renal impairment. However, less commonly, it may be the result of specific pathologies such as cardiac amyloidosis, hypertrophic cardiomyopathy, or constrictive pericarditis. These conditions have diverse disease courses and different implications for the investigation of associated diseases and family screening. Disease-specific treatments are now available for amyloidosis and constrictive pericarditis and are on the horizon for hypertrophic cardiomyopathy. Accurate and prompt diagnosis is therefore important. CMR plays an important role in the diagnosis of the specific phenocopies that may present as HFpEF. A single-centre study of patients with HFpEF, excluding those with suspected cardiomyopathy or constrictive pericarditis, found that CMR diagnosed previously undetected pathology in 27% of patients.[34] This included previously undiagnosed myocardial infarction, hypertrophic cardiomyopathy, and constrictive pericarditis.

CMR is a sensitive method of detecting transthyretin and light-chain cardiac amyloidosis. LGE imaging characteristically demonstrates abnormal gadolinium kinetics with difficulty in finding the correct inversion time to 'null' the myocardium. Phase sensitive inversion recovery (PSIR) sequences are less susceptible to operator error in selecting the correct inversion time and now enable more reliable and reproducible assessment (**Figure 25.5**). Early

in the disease course, LGE may be subtle or absent, becoming subendocardial and then transmural in more extensive disease.[35] Native T1 times and extracellular volume fraction rise early in the disease course. These techniques therefore appear to be a sensitive way of detecting mild disease and instituting early treatment.[36] Both variables rise as the disease advances and have been shown to correlate with the burden of amyloid. Regression of light-chain disease following chemotherapy has also been demonstrated using CMR.[37] This suggests that parametric mapping can play an important role in the non-invasive monitoring of disease progression.

The diagnosis of hypertrophic cardiomyopathy may be suspected in patients presenting with HFpEF who have a positive family history, electrocardiogram abnormalities or left ventricular hypertrophy that is disproportionate to the degree of any hypertension. CMR enables the assessment of the pattern of hypertrophy, the degree of any asymmetry and accurate measurement of wall thickness. LGE is typically patchy and diffuse, involving the ventricular insertion points and the areas with greatest wall thickness. Other supporting evidence includes the presence of multiple myocardial crypts, systolic anterior motion of the mitral valve and left ventricular outflow tract obstruction.[38] Elongation of the mitral valve leaflets and hypertrophy of the papillary muscles may also be seen.[39] Detection of apical patterns of hypertrophy that may be missed by echocardiography is also reliably performed. Non-contrast myocardial T1 mapping also plays an important role in the diagnosis of Anderson–Fabry disease, another phenocopy which may present with HFpEF.[40] Early diagnosis is essential due to the availability of disease-specific treatment. In this condition, native T1 values reduce in the presence of intracellular lipid storage and this can be used to distinguish the disease process from hypertrophic cardiomyopathy and cardiac amyloid.[40]

Constrictive pericarditis is another uncommon cause of heart failure in patients with preserved ejection fraction. Prompt diagnosis can be notoriously difficult and a multi-modality approach including CMR is often required, providing many complementary elements to echocardiography. Pericardial thickness can be accurately measured on T1-weighted turbo spin echo images (**Figure 25.6**). An increase in pericardial thickness beyond 4 mm raises suspicion of the diagnosis, although this may not be increased in some patients with the condition. The presence of constrictive physiology may be indicated by the presence of a diastolic septal bounce and marked leftward septal motion during inspiration on free-breathing imaging. Distension of the inferior vena cava

(a)   (b)   (c)

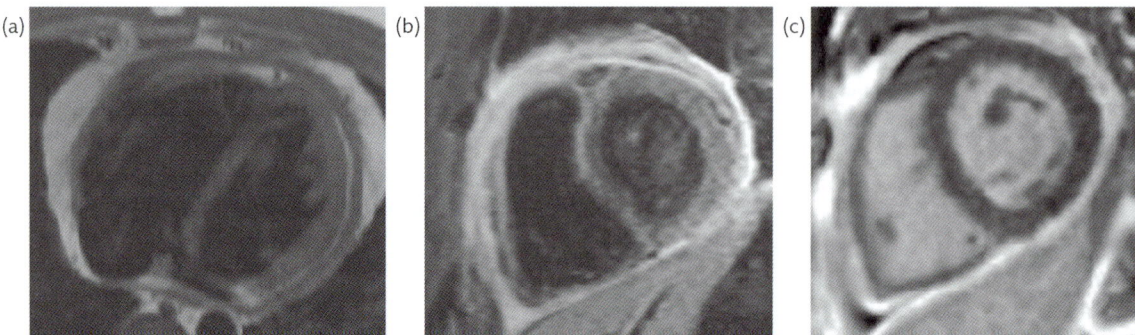

Figure 25.6 Imaging of pericarditis with features of constriction. (a) T1-weighted turbo spin echo in a trans-axial plane demonstrating thickening of the pericardium. (b) STIR image in a short-axis plane demonstrating high signal intensity throughout the pericardium, consistent with oedema. (c) Late gadolinium enhancement image in a short-axis plane demonstrating global enhancement of the pericardium.

can also be confirmed. Pericardial oedema may be observed with STIR images and indicates active pericarditis (**Figure 25.6**). In the absence of disease, the pericardium does not enhance following gadolinium due to its avascular nature. LGE therefore indicates neovascularization as part of an inflammatory process and may be used to confirm the diagnosis of pericarditis. Patients with large amounts of pericardial LGE are more likely to have resolution of constrictive physiology with anti-inflammatory therapy compared to those with smaller amounts.[41] It is therefore possible that CMR may be used to guide therapy.

Risk stratification and treatment selection in HFpEF

Trials of therapy have been disappointing in patients with HFpEF. Currently, there is an absence of evidence-based therapies that improve outcomes. One explanation for this may be heterogeneity of patients in the studies due to the absence of robust definitions. Precise definitions and improved disease and substrate characterization may enable the identification of patients who benefit from specific therapies. For example, whereas spironolactone failed to improve overall outcomes among patients with HFpEF in one trial, post-hoc analysis suggested that patients with the most severe disease and worst outcome may have gained benefit.[42] Spironolactone has anti-fibrotic properties and interstitial fibrosis is a common feature of HFpEF, which correlates with the severity of disease. It is plausible that those with the greatest fibrotic burden are most likely to gain overall benefit. A study of patients with HFpEF and those with elevated natriuretic peptide level who were deemed to be at risk of developing the condition demonstrated that extracellular volume fraction correlated well with disease severity and was associated with death and heart failure hospitalization.[43] Therefore, not only may it possible to risk-stratify HFpEF patients with CMR, it may also be possible to select specific patients who are most likely to gain outcome benefit from specific therapies.

As discussed, CMR plays an important role in the investigation and diagnosis of transthyretin and light-chain amyloidosis. There is growing evidence that CMR data can risk-stratify both groups of patients. In a study of transthyretin disease, extracellular volume fraction was associated with death, independently of other prognostic variables such as natriuretic peptide level and age.[36] Similarly, an extracellular volume fraction >0.45 was associated with mortality, independently of markers of systolic and diastolic function and natriuretic peptide level in patients with light-chain associated disease.[44] CMR may therefore be able to improve diagnosis and disease monitoring, and to select patients with severe disease who require the most intensive treatment and, in addition, those with such advanced disease that aggressive treatment is no longer beneficial.

Conclusion

CMR enables precise characterization of disease substrate and offers incremental value in risk stratification for patients presenting with all forms of heart failure. Accurate and prompt diagnosis enabling the prescription of evidence-based therapies appears key to improving outcomes. As we move further into an era of precision and personalized medicine, deep phenotyping of disease using advanced non-invasive techniques is likely to play a greater role in decision-making regarding novel therapeutics. Evidence from ongoing trials is awaited to confirm that CMR-guided approaches are associated with improved outcomes for our patients.

REFERENCES

1. Pontone G, Guaricci AI, Andreini D, et al. Prognostic benefit of cardiac magnetic resonance over transthoracic echocardiography for the assessment of ischemic and nonischemic dilated cardiomyopathy patients referred for the evaluation of primary prevention implantable cardioverter–defibrillator therapy. *Circ Cardiovasc Imaging* 2016;**9**(10):e004956.
2. Anderson JL, Horne BD, Pennell DJ. Atrial dimensions in health and left ventricular disease using cardiovascular magnetic resonance. *J Cardiovasc Magn Reson* 2005;**7**:671–5.
3. Penicka M, Vecera J, Mirica DC, et al. Prognostic implications of magnetic resonance-derived quantification in asymptomatic patients with organic mitral regurgitation: comparison with doppler echocardiography-derived integrative approach. *Circulation* 2018;**137**:1349–60.
4. Myerson SG, d'Arcy J, Mohiaddin R, et al. Aortic regurgitation quantification using cardiovascular magnetic resonance: Association with clinical outcome. *Circulation* 2012;**126**:1452–60.
5. Greenwood JP, Maredia N, Younger JF, et al. Cardiovascular magnetic resonance and single-photon emission computed tomography for diagnosis of coronary heart disease (CE-MARC): a prospective trial. *Lancet* 2012;**379**:453–60.
6. Nakamori S, Dohi K, Ishida M, et al. Native T1 mapping and extracellular volume mapping for the assessment of diffuse myocardial fibrosis in dilated cardiomyopathy. *JACC Cardiovasc Imaging* 2017;**11**:48–59.
7. Iles L, Pfluger H, Phrommintikul A, et al. Evaluation of diffuse myocardial fibrosis in heart failure with cardiac magnetic resonance contrast-enhanced T1 mapping. *J Am Coll Cardiol* 2008;**52**:1574–80.
8. Gulati A, Jabbour A, Ismail TF, et al. Association of fibrosis with mortality and sudden cardiac death in patients with nonischemic dilated cardiomyopathy. *JAMA* 2013;**309**:896–908.
9. McCrohon JA, Moon JC, Prasad SK, et al. Differentiation of heart failure related to dilated cardiomyopathy and coronary artery disease using gadolinium-enhanced cardiovascular magnetic resonance. *Circulation* 2003;**108**:54–9.
10. Schelbert EB, Cao JJ, Sigurdsson S, et al. Prevalence and prognosis of unrecognized myocardial infarction determined by cardiac magnetic resonance in older adults. *JAMA* 2012;**308**:890–6.
11. Assomull RG, Shakespeare C, Kalra PR, et al. Role of cardiovascular magnetic resonance as a gatekeeper to invasive coronary angiography in patients presenting with heart failure of unknown etiology. *Circulation* 2011;**124**:1351–60.
12. Zurlo MG, De Stefano P, Borgna-Pignatti C, et al. Survival and causes of death in thalassaemia major. *Lancet* 1989;**2**:27–30.
13. Anderson LJ, Holden S, Davis B, et al. Cardiovascular T2-star (T2*) magnetic resonance for the early diagnosis of myocardial iron overload. *Eur Heart J* 2001;**22**:2171–9.
14. Kim RJ, Wu E, Rafael A, et al. The use of contrast-enhanced magnetic resonance imaging to identify reversible myocardial dysfunction. *N Engl J Med* 2000;**343**:1445–53.
15. Glaveckaite S, Valevicienc N, Palionis D, et al. Value of scar imaging and inotropic reserve combination for the prediction of

segmental and global left ventricular functional recovery after revascularisation. *J Cardiovasc Magn Reson* 2011;**13**:35.

16. Velazquez EJ, Lee KL, Deja MA, *et al.* Coronary-artery bypass surgery in patients with left ventricular dysfunction. *N Engl J Med* 2011;**364**:1607–16.

17. Kelle S, Roes SD, Klein C, *et al.* Prognostic value of myocardial infarct size and contractile reserve using magnetic resonance imaging. *J Am Coll Cardiol* 2009;**54**:1770–7.

18. Eitel I, de Waha S, Wohrle J, *et al.* Comprehensive prognosis assessment by CMR imaging after st-segment elevation myocardial infarction. *J Am Coll Cardiol* 2014;**64**:1217–26.

19. de Bakker JM, van Capelle FJ, Janse MJ, *et al.* Reentry as a cause of ventricular tachycardia in patients with chronic ischemic heart disease: electrophysiologic and anatomic correlation. *Circulation* 1988;**77**:589–606.

20. Disertori M, Rigoni M, Pace N, *et al.* Myocardial fibrosis assessment by LGE is a powerful predictor of ventricular tachyarrhythmias in ischemic and nonischemic LV dysfunction: a meta-analysis. *JACC Cardiovasc Imaging* 2016;**9**:1046–55.

21. Yan AT, Shayne AJ, Brown KA, *et al.* Characterization of the peri-infarct zone by contrast-enhanced cardiac magnetic resonance imaging is a powerful predictor of post-myocardial infarction mortality. *Circulation* 2006;**114**:32–9.

22. Roes SD, Borleffs CJ, van der Geest RJ, *et al.* Infarct tissue heterogeneity assessed with contrast-enhanced MRI predicts spontaneous ventricular arrhythmia in patients with ischemic cardiomyopathy and implantable cardioverter–defibrillator. *Circ Cardiovasc Imaging* 2009;**2**:183–90.

23. Taylor RJ, Umar F, Panting JR, Stegemann B, Leyva F. Left ventricular lead position, mechanical activation, and myocardial scar in relation to left ventricular reverse remodeling and clinical outcomes after cardiac resynchronization therapy: a feature-tracking and contrast-enhanced cardiovascular magnetic resonance study. *Heart Rhythm* 2016;**13**:481–9.

24. Puntmann VO, Carr-White G, Jabbour A, *et al.* Native T1 and ECV of noninfarcted myocardium and outcome in patients with coronary artery disease. *J Am Coll Cardiol* 2018;**71**:766–778.

25. Kober L, Thune JJ, Nielsen JC, *et al.* Defibrillator implantation in patients with nonischemic systolic heart failure. *N Engl J Med* 2016;**375**:1221–30.

26. Bogun FM, Desjardins B, Good E, *et al.* Delayed-enhanced magnetic resonance imaging in nonischemic cardiomyopathy: utility for identifying the ventricular arrhythmia substrate. *J Am Coll Cardiol* 2009;**53**:1138–45.

27. Leyva F, Zegard A, Acquaye E, *et al.* Outcomes of cardiac resynchronization therapy with or without defibrillation in patients with nonischemic cardiomyopathy. *J Am Coll Cardiol* 2017;**70**:1216–27.

28. Halliday BP, Gulati A, Ali A, *et al.* Association between midwall late gadolinium enhancement and sudden cardiac death in patients with dilated cardiomyopathy and mild and moderate left ventricular systolic dysfunction. *Circulation* 2017;**135**:2106–15.

29. Gulati A, Ismail TF, Jabbour A, *et al.* Clinical utility and prognostic value of left atrial volume assessment by cardiovascular magnetic resonance in non-ischaemic dilated cardiomyopathy. *Eur J Heart Fail* 2013;**15**:660–70.

30. Gulati A, Ismail TF, Jabbour A, *et al.* The prevalence and prognostic significance of right ventricular systolic dysfunction in nonischemic dilated cardiomyopathy. *Circulation* 2013;**128**:1623–33.

31. Romano S, Judd RM, Kim RJ, *et al.* Feature-tracking global longitudinal strain predicts death in a multicenter population of patients with ischemic and nonischemic dilated cardiomyopathy incremental to ejection fraction and late gadolinium enhancement. *JACC Cardiovasc Imaging* 2018;**11**(10):1419–29.

32. Puntmann VO, Carr-White G, Jabbour A, *et al.* T1-mapping and outcome in nonischemic cardiomyopathy: all-cause mortality and heart failure. *JACC Cardiovasc Imaging* 2016;**9**:40–50.

33. Redfield MM, Jacobsen SJ, Burnett JC, Jr, *et al.* Burden of systolic and diastolic ventricular dysfunction in the community: appreciating the scope of the heart failure epidemic. *JAMA* 2003;**289**:194–202.

34. Kanagala P, Cheng ASH, Singh A, *et al.* Diagnostic and prognostic utility of cardiovascular magnetic resonance imaging in heart failure with preserved ejection fraction—implications for clinical trials. *J Cardiovasc Magn Reson* 2018;**20**:4.

35. Fontana M, Pica S, Reant P, *et al.* Prognostic value of late gadolinium enhancement cardiovascular magnetic resonance in cardiac amyloidosis. *Circulation* 2015;**132**:1570–9.

36. Martinez-Naharro A, Treibel TA, Abdel-Gadir A, *et al.* Magnetic resonance in transthyretin cardiac amyloidosis. *J Am Coll Cardiol* 2017;**70**:466–77.

37. Martinez-Naharro A, Abdel-Gadir A, Treibel TA, *et al.* CMR-verified regression of cardiac al amyloid after chemotherapy. *JACC Cardiovasc Imaging* 2018;**11**:152–4.

38. Captur G, Lopes LR, Patel V, *et al.* Abnormal cardiac formation in hypertrophic cardiomyopathy: fractal analysis of trabeculae and preclinical gene expression. *Circ Cardiovasc Genet* 2014;**7**:241–8.

39. Maron MS, Olivotto I, Harrigan C, *et al.* Mitral valve abnormalities identified by cardiovascular magnetic resonance represent a primary phenotypic expression of hypertrophic cardiomyopathy. *Circulation* 2011;**124**:40–7.

40. Sado DM, White SK, Piechnik SK, *et al.* Identification and assessment of Anderson–Fabry disease by cardiovascular magnetic resonance noncontrast myocardial T1 mapping. *Circ Cardiovasc Imaging* 2013;**6**:392–8.

41. Feng D, Glockner J, Kim K, *et al.* Cardiac magnetic resonance imaging pericardial late gadolinium enhancement and elevated inflammatory markers can predict the reversibility of constrictive pericarditis after antiinflammatory medical therapy: a pilot study. *Circulation* 2011;**124**:1830–7.

42. Pfeffer MA, Claggett B, Assmann SF, *et al.* Regional variation in patients and outcomes in the treatment of preserved cardiac function heart failure with an aldosterone antagonist (topcat) trial. *Circulation* 2015;**131**:34–42.

43. Schelbert EB, Fridman Y, Wong TC, *et al.* Temporal relation between myocardial fibrosis and heart failure with preserved ejection fraction: association with baseline disease severity and subsequent outcome. *JAMA Cardiol* 2017;**2**:995–1006.

44. Banypersad SM, Fontana M, Maestrini V, *et al.* T1 mapping and survival in systemic light-chain amyloidosis. *Eur Heart J* 2015;**36**:244–51.

26

Computed tomography imaging techniques

Laurens F. Tops, Michiel A. de Graaf, Victoria Delgado, and Jeroen J. Bax

Computed tomography techniques

Acquisition protocols

For the acquisition of cardiac computed tomography (CT), a gantry containing an X-ray tube and a detector system rotates around the patient to acquire multiple images during a single rotation. Whereas the earliest systems allowed acquisition of four slices per rotation, current systems consist of up to 320 detector rows with sub-millimetre slice thickness. In addition, temporal resolution has been improved by faster rotation times as well as the introduction of dual-source CT systems. Nevertheless, most systems still require a low and stable heart rate (preferably <65 beats/min) to obtain good image quality. The reduced cardiac and coronary movement in heart failure patients may have a beneficial effect on the interpretability of cardiac CT. Moreover, heart failure patients receiving β-blockers often present with relatively low heart rates.[1] To further reduce the heart rate, β-blocking medication can be administered prior to coronary CT angiography (CTA) imaging. However, in patients with severe heart failure and low blood pressure (<100 mmHg), this is contraindicated because of the risk of decompensated heart failure.

In addition, sublingual nitroglycerine is administered and the resulting vasodilatation improves the interpretation of the small coronary arteries. During the administration of a bolus of iodinated contrast agent, a three-dimensional dataset of the entire heart is obtained within a single breath-hold of <10 s. Data acquisition is synchronized to the ECG to allow reconstruction of motion-free images. At present, several acquisition techniques are available, which are specified in Table 26.1.

During ECG-gated spiral acquisition, the patient is moved continuously through the gantry at a slow speed while images are continuously acquired. This approach allows retrospective reconstruction of high-resolution datasets at any desired interval of the cardiac cycle. To reduce radiation exposure, dose modulation can be applied. During dose modulation, the tube current is lowered during the phases that are expected not to be used for reconstruction of the coronary arteries. Although the images during these phases contain more noise and are of lower image quality, evaluation of non-coronary structures remains possible.

For sequential scanning, or step-and-shoot protocols, several heart beats are scanned and the table is moved in steps between the acquired heartbeats. The resulting images can be fused to create one image. Newer CT scanners with a large number of detectors (i.e. 256 or 320 rows) provide sufficient coverage to visualize the entire heart in one heartbeat. For step-and-shoot protocols, prospective ECG-triggering is often used. With this method, data acquisition is triggered by the ECG at a pre-selected phase. Most often, the end-diastolic phase (around 75% of the R–R interval) is selected, since this is the phase in the cardiac cycle with the least coronary movement. Because imaging is performed during a small proportion of the cardiac cycle, considerable reduction in radiation dose has been achieved using this scanning mode. However, heart rate needs to be stable and low, as no other phases can be reconstructed retrospectively. Moreover, since there is

Table 26.1 Different acquisition protocols for coronary computed tomography angiography

Table movement	ECG timing	Assessment of LV function	Radiation dose
Continuous movement (spiral)	Retrospective ECG gating	Yes	High
Continuous movement (spiral)	ECG-tube modulation	Yes	Moderate
Sequential movement[a] (step-and-shoot)	ECG-tube modulation	Yes	Low–moderate
Sequential movement[a] (step-and-shoot)	Prospective ECG, triggering	No	Low
High-pitch spiral	Prospective ECG, triggering	No	Very low

[a] Wide-volume CT scanners have a coverage of 16 cm and do not require table movement.

no acquisition of data during the full cardiac cycles, assessment of myocardial function is not possible. Therefore with the sequential scanning methods, full-beat scanning with tube modulation is also available. With this method, data from the entire cardiac cycle are obtained with moderate–low motion radiation exposure, facilitating assessment of myocardial dimensions, function and wall motion. Newer dual-source CT scanners are equipped with two sets of X-ray tubes and detector systems at a 90° angle which rotate simultaneously. With these scanners, data can be acquired in 50% of the time needed with conventional CT scanners. This results in excellent temporal resolution with very low radiation exposure. The improved temporal resolution also facilitates acquisition of data at higher heart rates.

When cardiac CT was introduced, radiation doses were relatively high, with average radiation exposure of 12 mSv and maximum doses up to 30 mSv.[2] With current radiation reduction protocols, radiation exposure has become less than 1 mSv.

Assessment of coronary atherosclerosis

The most simple and quickest assessment of CAD on cardiac CT is the coronary artery calcium (CAC) score based on non-contrast CT. The presence of calcium in the coronary arteries is an accurate marker for CAD, as coronary calcifications occur exclusively in the presence of atherosclerosis.[3] Moreover, coronary calcifications have high X-ray attenuation values (Hounsfield Units), and are therefore easily recognized during CT imaging without contrast. The traditional method to quantify coronary calcifications is the Agatston score.[4] Using this method, a CAC score that can vary from 0 to >1000 is obtained. This score provides an estimate of the total atherosclerotic burden in the coronary arteries. However, the CAC score shows poor correlation with the presence of significant CAD.[5] Therefore, additional contrast-enhanced coronary CTA is often performed. As compared to CAC scoring, contrast-enhanced coronary CTA has several important advantages, including assessment of stenosis severity as well as the detection of non-calcified plaque, providing a more detailed assessment of the presence and severity of CAD. Traditionally, stenosis severity is visually quantified into categories. The absence of coronary atherosclerosis is defined as normal. Wall irregularities with <30% luminal narrowing is considered mild CAD, and lesions with 30–50% stenosis are defined as non-significant CAD. Luminal narrowing of ≥50% is considered a significant stenosis and a stenosis of ≥70% is defined as severe stenosis. In addition, coronary plaque composition is graded as non-calcified plaque (defined by the absence of coronary calcium), calcified plaque or partially calcified plaque. For the interpretation of coronary CTA, dedicated workstations are typically used. These workstations allow, in addition to manual scrolling through the axial images, interactive manipulation of the dataset, including processing of three-dimensional reconstructions, including curved multiplanar reformations. Moreover, these workstations facilitate (automatic) analysis of left ventricular (LV) dimensions and function.

Diagnosis of heart failure

Aetiology of heart failure

Coronary artery calcium score

The absence of any calcium implies a very low likelihood of clinically relevant CAD. Presumably, CAC scoring may therefore allow rapid differentiation between ischaemic and non-ischaemic aetiology in patients presenting with heart failure of unknown origin. This concept was explored by Abunassar et al.[6] In their study, 153 patients with heart failure were identified from a cohort of patients in whom CAC scoring was performed. All patients with ischaemic heart failure presented with a positive CAC score, whereas 30% of patients with non-ischaemic heart failure demonstrated absence of calcium. An Agatston score of 0 accurately identified patients with non-ischaemic heart failure with a specificity of 100% and a positive predictive value of 100%. However, as expected, both sensitivity and negative predictive value were relatively low (32% and 34%, respectively). Thus, the absence of calcium in patients with heart failure strongly supports the diagnosis of non-ischaemic heart failure. However, the presence of calcium provides little incremental clinical diagnostic value. Indeed, despite the close correlation between the Agatston score and total atherosclerotic burden, the technique does not permit direct evaluation of the stenosis severity. High CAC scores reflecting extensive calcifications can be observed in the absence of any luminal narrowing, whereas severe stenosis can be present at sites with minimal calcium. Nonetheless, despite this limitation, CAC scoring may represent a practicable initial screening approach to determine whether an ischaemic origin is likely or not, thereby allowing more appropriate selection of further (invasive) analysis.

Computed tomography coronary angiography

In the general population, the diagnostic accuracy of coronary CTA to detect significant stenosis has been studied extensively against invasive coronary angiography. A meta-analysis on pooled data from 15 studies, including 960 patients with stable angina, demonstrated excellent diagnostic accuracy with a sensitivity of 100% and a specificity of 89%. Notably, the high negative predictive value of 99% enables CAD to be conclusively ruled out in these patients.[7] For this reason, coronary CTA is considered an attractive tool to exclude significant CAD and thus avoid invasive coronary angiography in patients with a low to intermediate likelihood of CAD.[8] However, particularly in the presence of extensive calcifications or motion artefacts, detected lesions are frequently overestimated on coronary CTA. Thus, somewhat lower positive predictive values have been reported (64–89%).[9,10] In addition, the information obtained by coronary CTA is restricted to coronary anatomy and provides no information on coronary function. The technique therefore cannot differentiate between lesions that are haemodynamically relevant and those that are not. Consequently, the clinical value of coronary CTA is limited in patients with a high clinical suspicion of having significant CAD.

There are fewer data available on the diagnostic accuracy of coronary CTA for patients with heart failure. Andreini et al. studied 61 consecutive patients admitted with heart failure of unknown aetiology using 16-slice CT.[1] For comparative purposes, 139 patients undergoing invasive coronary angiography for other clinical indications were also investigated with coronary CTA. Overall, the technical success rate of the procedure was 97%. On a segmental level, diagnostic accuracy in heart failure patients was high, with a sensitivity and specificity of 99% and 96%, respectively. Interestingly, sensitivity and negative predictive values to detect significant CAD were higher in the heart failure population than in the control population, probably because of the lower prevalence of CAD in this

population (27.8% in the heart failure group vs 70.5% in the control group). Importantly, coronary CTA allowed correct classification of ischaemic versus non-ischaemic cardiomyopathy in all patients.

Other studies have identified the presence of extensive calcifications as a major cause of reduced image quality and incorrect diagnosis.[11] In this regard, a stepwise approach incorporating CAC scoring and coronary CTA, as proposed by Cornily et al., may be attractive.[12] In their algorithm, coronary evaluation consisted of initial CAC scoring followed by coronary CTA in selected cases. Patients with a CAC score of ≥1000 were referred directly to invasive coronary angiography, based on the rationale not only that the performance of coronary CTA will be lower but also that many patients will have abnormal studies requiring further evaluation anyway. In the majority of patients, however, CAC scores of <1000 were obtained. In these patients, coronary CTA was shown accurately to rule out CAD as the underlying cause of heart failure and thus avoid invasive coronary angiography in 21 out of 27 (78%) patients.

Recently the concept of coronary CTA as gatekeeper for invasive coronary angiography in heart failure patients was further explored by Ten Kate et al.[13] For this purpose, 93 patients with reduced LV ejection fraction (LVEF) were included. A stepwise protocol was used in which all patients were assessed for CAC score. The 43 patients with absence of calcium (CAC score 0) were classified as non-ischaemic heart failure without additional imaging tests. All 50 patients with CAC score >0 underwent coronary CTA. Of these patients, 38 (41%) presented with a negative coronary CTA and 12 (13%) with a positive coronary CTA (>50% luminal narrowing in left main, proximal left anterior descending coronary artery or multi-vessel disease). This algorithm, including the CAC score and coronary CTA, demonstrated a sensitivity of 100%, specificity of 93%, negative predictive value of 100%, and positive predictive value of 67% to distinguish between ischaemic and non-ischaemic heart failure. Most importantly, using the this algorithm, almost 80% of patients could be refrained from further (invasive) imaging. It should, however, be noted that this was a small, single-centre population with relatively young patients. Recently published guidelines for the diagnosis and treatment of patients with heart failure indicate that coronary CTA may indeed be considered to rule out underlying CAD non-invasively in patients with low to intermediate likelihood of significant CAD.[8] A clinical example of a patient presenting with heart failure and evaluated by coronary CTA is shown in Figure 26.1.

Recently, coronary CTA has been complemented by functional measurements, in order to combine the anatomical stenosis severity with the haemodynamic (functional) consequences of the stenosis. This includes CTA-derived fractional flow reserve (FFRct), which is based on computational fluid dynamics,[14] and has been demonstrated to correlate well with invasive FFR assessments.[15] Another approach to determine the haemodynamic significance of a coronary stenosis is CT myocardial perfusion, which enables (similar to nuclear perfusion imaging) assessment of the myocardial perfusion at stress and rest, in order to detect myocardial ischaemia.[16]

Assessment of left ventricular size and function

In addition to assessment of CAD, cardiac CT can also provide detailed information on cardiac chamber morphology, dimensions, and function. Importantly, after acquisition, cardiac CT datasets can be reformatted in any desired plane and, depending on the acquisition technique (see Table 26.1), reconstructed at multiple phases

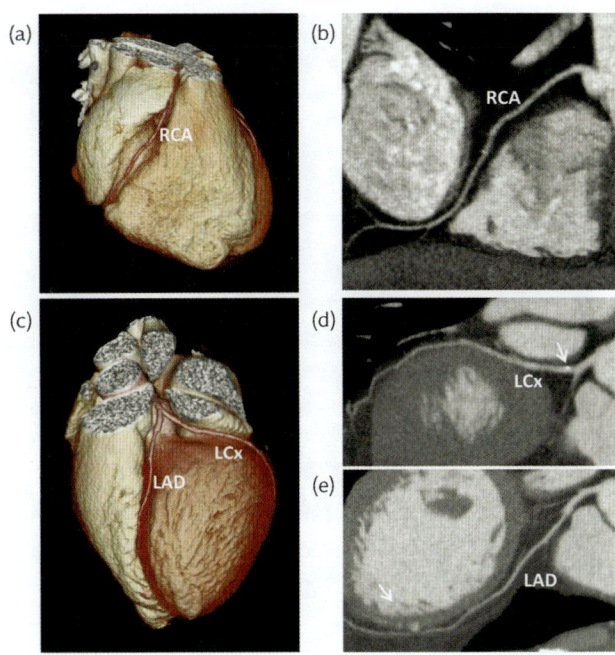

Figure 26.1 Patient example of non-invasive coronary angiography with cardiac CT. In this 49-year old patient presenting with LV dilatation and reduced LVEF (32% on two-dimensional echocardiography), prospectively triggered 320-row coronary CTA was performed to rule out CAD. (a Three-dimensional volume-rendered reconstruction showing the course of the right coronary artery (RCA). (b) The curved multiplanar reconstruction of the RCA illustrates patency of the artery without significant atherosclerosis. (c) Three-dimensional volume-rendered reconstruction showing the left coronary system and the curved multiplanar reconstructions of the left circumflex coronary (LCx) and left anterior descending coronary arteries (LAD) are shown in (d) and (e) respectively. Only minor wall irregularities with non-obstructive plaque in the LAD (arrow) and minimal calcification in the LCx (arrow) were observed, thereby excluding ischaemic origin of HF.

of the cardiac cycle. Typically, to assess LV volumes and function, datasets are reformatted in the short- and long-axis orientation, as illustrated in Figure 26.2. Subsequently, end-systolic and end-diastolic phases are determined by selecting the smallest and largest cross-sectional LV cavity areas.

The high contrast between the LV cavity and the myocardium has facilitated the development of dedicated software algorithms that automatically detect endo- and epicardial borders. Consequently, end-diastolic and end-systolic volumes are derived to obtain LVEF. Displaying the images in cine-loop format allows evaluation of segmental wall motion in addition to global function.

Myocardial dimension and function

Numerous studies have shown excellent correlations between cardiac CT and other imaging methods for assessment of myocardial function. A recent meta-analysis by Pickett et al. compared the accuracy of cardiac CT for the assessment of LVEF and right ventricular ejection fraction (RVEF) compared to magnetic resonance imaging (MRI) based on data from 206 studies, including 7047 patients.[17] For the assessment of LVEF, a slight overestimation of cardiac CT was observed (bias: 1.1%). The correlation between LVEF on cardiac CT compared to MRI was as good as three-dimensional echocardiography compared to MRI ($r = 0.855$ and $r = 0.888$ respectively).

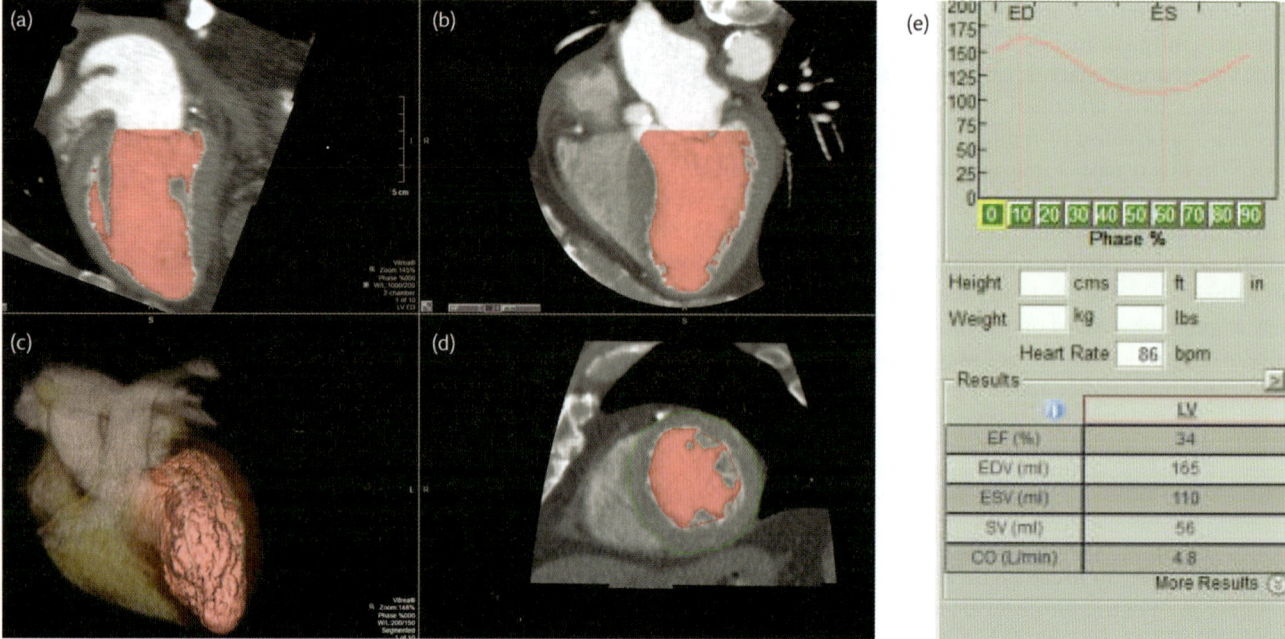

Figure 26.2 Evaluation of left ventricular function with cardiac CT. In (a) and (b), respectively, the reconstructed two- and four-chamber views of the LV are shown. (c) Three-dimensional volume rendering of the LV and (d) the short axis views. The two- and four-chamber views and the short axis view reconstructed throughout the cardiac cycle are provided, showing a dilated LV with severely reduced wall motion. Using automated software (e) LV volumes were calculated at 110 mL in end diastole and 165 mL in end systole, resulting in an LVEF of 34%.

Similar results were reported for the assessment of RVEF; cardiac CT showed a slight overestimation (bias: 4.7%) and correlation with MRI was similar as compared to three-dimensional echocardiography ($r = 0.75$ and $r = 0.79$, respectively). For both parameters, cardiac CT was superior compared to standard two-dimensional echocardiography. Also for end-diastolic and end-systolic volumes, assessment with cardiac CT does not differ significantly from MRI.[18]

Myocardial wall motion

Comparison against two-dimensional echocardiography and MRI has revealed high accuracy of cardiac CT for detection of regional wall motion abnormalities.[19,20] Using 64-slice CT technology, Henneman et al. showed that 96% of segments were scored identically on 64-slice CT and two-dimensional echocardiography ($\kappa = 0.82$).[20] Although patients with reduced LVEF were included in these investigations, only few studies have specifically focused on patients with heart failure. Butler et al. studied 25 patients with LVEF <45% with two-dimensional echocardiography and cardiac CT.[19] In this cohort with reduced LVEF (average 36 ± 8% on two-dimensional echocardiography), cardiac CT was shown to provide similar results as with two-dimensional echocardiography for both global and regional function. This is confirmed in a recent meta-analysis of 53 studies and 1814 patients; the sensitivity of cardiac CT for detection of wall motion abnormalities was 90% and specificity was 97%.[21]

Although cardiac CT allows reliable assessment of LV function and wall motion, routine use of cardiac CT for this purpose is not recommended considering the risk of radiation and contrast agents.

Assessment of myocardial scar

For assessment of infarcted myocardium, MRI is currently considered the reference standard. However, cardiac CT can also assess the presence and extent of myocardial infarction and viability. Left ventricular end-diastolic wall thickness can easily be determined on cardiac CT, and end-diastolic wall thickness <6 mm correlates with the presence of larger, transmural myocardial infarction.[22] Moreover, several studies have demonstrated that LV hypoenhancement reflects scar tissue. This concept, which dates back to experimental animal studies in the 1970s, is based on the kinetics of the contrast agent used for cardiac CT. Similar to MRI, cardiac CT is performed during the administration of contrast agents, reflecting first-pass perfusion. In both chronic and acute settings, the presence of hypoperfused areas on cardiac CT has been shown to correlate with delayed enhancement MRI and gated single-photon emission computed tomography.[23–25] An example of early hypoenhancement on cardiac CT is shown in **Figure 26.3**.

However, areas of decreased myocardial perfusion can represent either microvascular obstruction or areas of myocardial necrosis. Delayed enhancement imaging, which results in regional hyperenhancement of scar tissue similar to MRI, may possibly provide more accurate evaluation of myocardial infarction (see **Figure 26.3**). Gerber et al. showed that a combined cardiac CT protocol of early hypoenhancement and delayed enhancement MRI 10 min after contrast injection allowed characterization of myocardial infarction with contrast patterns highly similar to MRI.[23] Between cardiac CT and MRI, areas of early hypoenhancement and late hyperenhancement showed good agreement on a segmental basis (92% and 82%, respectively). Importantly, absolute sizes of early hypoenhanced and late hyperenhanced myocardium were also highly correlated without significant differences between the two techniques. Similarly, Nieman et al. included 28 patients who underwent both cardiac CT (first pass and delayed enhancement) and MRI.[25] Eleven of the 15 patients with delayed enhancement on

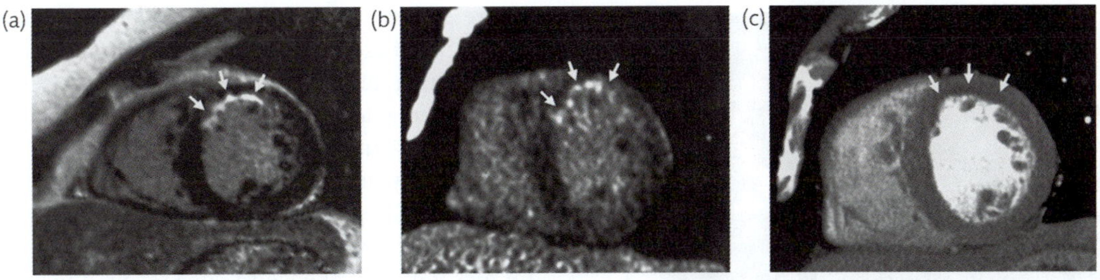

Figure 26.3 Short axis views obtained with cardiac CT (b and c) and MRI (a) in a patient with anterior myocardial infarction. In (b) and (c), a region with, respectively late hyperenhancement and early hypoenhancement, is indicated by the arrows. Especially for the late hyperenhancement, correlation with delayed enhancement MRI (a) was excellent.

Reproduced from Mahnken AH, Koos R, Katoh M, et al. Assessment of myocardial viability in reperfused acute myocardial infarction using 16-slice computed tomography in comparison to magnetic resonance imaging. *J Am Coll Cardiol* 2005;45(12):2042–7 with permission Elsevier.

MRI also displayed delayed enhancement on cardiac CT. Moreover, the percentage of myocardium showing delayed enhancement was similar on cardiac CT and delayed enhancement MRI. The contrast-to-noise ratio for cardiac CT was significantly inferior to MRI.

Le Polain de Waroux *et al.* applied a combination of coronary CTA and delayed enhancement CT to determine the underlying aetiology of heart failure in 71 patients.[26] Coronary CTA correctly identified all patients with significant CAD on invasive coronary angiography, and delayed enhancement CT identified 28 out of 29 (96%) patients with either subendocardial or transmural infarction on delayed enhancement MRI.

Valvular heart disease

Valvular heart disease is an important cause of heart failure. Especially at older ages, the prevalence of severe aortic stenosis increases, resulting in more heart failure hospitalizations.[27] In addition, LV remodelling in patients with heart failure may also result in significant secondary mitral and tricuspid regurgitation.[28,29] Although echocardiography is the cornerstone of imaging in valvular heart disease, CT may provide important additional information for correct evaluation and treatment of valvular heart disease in patients with heart failure. The advent of transcatheter valve interventions has provided alternative therapeutic options to heart failure patients with significant valvular heart disease and contraindications or high risk for surgery. The role of cardiac CT in the diagnosis and (percutaneous) treatment of valvular heart disease will be reviewed in the following paragraphs.

Aortic valve

Because of the high spatial resolution, cardiac CT can provide important information for the diagnosis of the severity of aortic stenosis and for guidance of therapy in patients with heart failure and severe aortic stenosis.

The evaluation of aortic stenosis severity may be challenging in this subgroup of patients. In the presence of impaired LV systolic function (LVEF ≤40%), aortic valve area may be reduced (≤1.0 cm²) in combination with a relatively low mean transvalvular gradient (<40 mmHg), the so-called low-flow, low-gradient, severe aortic stenosis.[30] It is essential to investigate whether the reduced LV function is due to the severe aortic stenosis ('true severe aortic stenosis')

or due to an underlying cardiomyopathy ('pseudo-severe aortic stenosis'). Whereas in true severe aortic stenosis LV function may improve after valve replacement, this may not be the case in patients with pseudo-severe aortic stenosis. In general, stress echocardiography is used to differentiate between true and pseudo-severe aortic stenosis. If stress echocardiography is not conclusive, CT has been shown to identify accurately patients with severe aortic stenosis based on the aortic valve calcification burden using a modified Agatston score (**Figure 26.4**).

In 49 patients with at least mild aortic stenosis and reduced LVEF (<40%), an aortic valve calcium score threshold of 1651 arbitrary units provided a high sensitivity (95%) and specificity (89%) for identification of severe aortic stenosis.[31] In addition, underestimation of the cross-sectional area of the LV outflow tract may result in significant underestimation of the aortic valve area based on the continuity equation. With two-dimensional transthoracic echocardiography (the imaging technique of first choice to estimate the aortic valve area) the LV outflow tract is assumed to be perfectly circular and its area is derived from the diameter of this circle. However, CT has demonstrated that the LV outflow tract is rather elliptical and the planimetered area of the LV outflow tract on CT is larger than the area derived from two-dimensional measurements. By introducing the CT-derived cross-sectional area of the LV outflow tract into the continuity equation, the aortic valve area may be larger, leading to reclassification of severe aortic stenosis to moderate aortic stenosis. In 191 patients with severe aortic stenosis (46% with low gradient), Kamperidis *et al.* demonstrated that the integration of CT-derived LV outflow tract area and echocardiography-derived transvalvular gradients resulted in a reclassification of 33% of patients with low-gradient severe aortic stenosis to moderate aortic stenosis.[32]

Furthermore, CT is currently an important imaging modality in the selection of patients for transcatheter aortic valve implantation. It provides essential information on the feasibility of peripheral vascular access: the dimensions, tortuosity, as well as the presence and extent of calcifications of the femoral arteries and thoracic aorta can be accurately assessed with CT (**Figure 26.4**). In addition, CT can be used to evaluate the anatomy of the aortic valve and aortic root.[33,34] It enables exact measurement of the dimensions and eccentricity of the aortic annulus, which may impact on the incidence of postprocedural paravalvular aortic regurgitation.[35] Furthermore, the relation between the aortic annulus and the ostia of the coronary

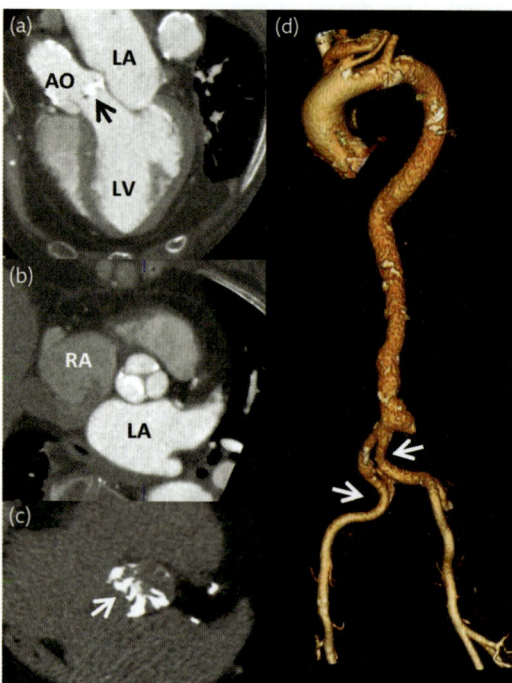

Figure 26.4 Assessment of aortic valve, peripheral arteries, and aorta with CT prior to transcatheter aortic valve implantation. (a) Reconstructed three-chamber view in systole, with dilated LV, and calcified aortic valve with restrictive cusp (arrow) and reduced valve opening. On the short axis view of the aortic valve (b), the tricuspid anatomy of the aortic valve can be appreciated. On non-contrast enhanced CT, the calcification burden of the aortic valve (arrow) can be measured and has been correlated with the severity of aortic valve stenosis. (d) CT data from the aorta and peripheral arteries. The arrows point to the pronounced angulation of the iliac arteries but without significant calcification. AO, aorta; LA, left atrium; LV, left ventricle; RA, right atrium.

arteries can be assessed with CT, with potential impact on the procedural feasibility.

Mitral valve

Mitral valve regurgitation is prevalent in patients with heart failure. Left ventricular dilatation and remodelling may result in geometrical distortion of the subvalvular apparatus of the mitral valve and LV systolic dysfunction may result in reduced closing forces of the mitral valve, leading to secondary or 'functional' mitral regurgitation. Since the presence and severity of mitral regurgitation negatively affect prognosis, additional mitral valve surgery during coronary bypass grafting should be considered in patients with ischaemic cardiomyopathy and secondary mitral regurgitation. For optimal planning of the surgical procedure, detailed information of the LV shape, the geometry of the valve, and the severity of mitral regurgitation is needed. Echocardiography remains the preferred technique, but CT may provide important additional information. CT enables detailed visualization of the subvalvular apparatus, including the anatomy of the papillary muscles.[36] In addition, the dimensions and shape of the mitral valve annulus and mitral leaflet characteristics (e.g. tenting height, tethering angles in relation to the mitral annulus) can be assessed. With the use of CT, it has been demonstrated that remodelling of the mitral valve may occur in heart

failure patients and moderate to severe secondary mitral regurgitation.[36] In these patients, posterior mitral leaflet angles and mitral valve tenting height were significantly increased at the central and posteromedial levels, as compared to heart failure patients without mitral regurgitation.[36]

In recent years, several strategies for percutaneous treatment of severe mitral regurgitation targeting different aspects of the mitral valve have become available. Mitral valve repair with the MitraClip mimics the surgical edge-to-edge repair. The procedural safety has been demonstrated, with a low adverse-event rate. Moreover, a significant reduction in mitral regurgitation and improvement of functional status have been shown.[37] Although echocardiography is the imaging technique of choice to evaluate the feasibility for MitraClip, CT may provide additional information regarding the anatomy of the inter-atrial septum and mitral valve (calcifications). Also, with recently developed techniques, the integration of pre-procedural acquired CT and fluoroscopy may facilitate MitraClip implantation.[38]

Another percutaneous approach to treat severe mitral regurgitation is the (in)direct annuloplasty which aims to re-shape the mitral valve annulus. Using a transvenous approach, a device is positioned in the coronary sinus in order to approximate the different parts of the mitral valve, resulting in better leaflet coaptation. The procedural feasibility depends on the distance between the coronary sinus and the mitral annulus, and remodelling of the mitral annulus may be inefficient when the coronary sinus courses along the left atrial wall rather than along the mitral annulus. In addition, the course of the left circumflex coronary artery between the coronary sinus and the mitral valve annulus may be associated with risk of compression of the coronary artery and subsequent myocardial infarction (**Figure 26.5**). With the use of cardiac CT, the relation between the coronary sinus, the mitral valve annulus and the circumflex coronary artery can be well visualized. Importantly, it has been demonstrated that in a large proportion of patients the circumflex coronary artery courses between the mitral valve annulus and the coronary sinus.[39] Therefore, cardiac CT can provide important information for selection of patients with severe mitral regurgitation for percutaneous annuloplasty.

Finally, several percutaneous mitral valve replacement devices have recently become available.[40] These devices are typically delivered via a transapical approach and contain a self-expanding frame with a prosthetic valve of bovine pericardial tissue. To determine procedural feasibility, the mitral valve anatomy (most especially annulus dimensions) and calcifications, papillary muscle, and chordae anatomy and configuration of the LV outflow tract should be assessed (**Figure 26.5**). The struts of the stent of current transcatheter mitral valve replacement devices are covered by pericardial or fabric sealing cuff that may protrude into the LV cavity, push the anterior mitral leaflet towards the interventricular septum and cause LV outflow tract obstruction. A perpendicular orientation of the mitral annulus trajectory relative to the longitudinal axis of the LV outflow tract and pronounced sigmoid basal interventricular septum increase the risk of LV outflow tract obstruction.

Tricuspid valve

Symptomatic severe tricuspid regurgitation is common in patients with heart failure. Right ventricular dilatation and presence of pacemaker leads are important causes of tricuspid regurgitation, which is associated with increased mortality at long-term follow-up. Novel

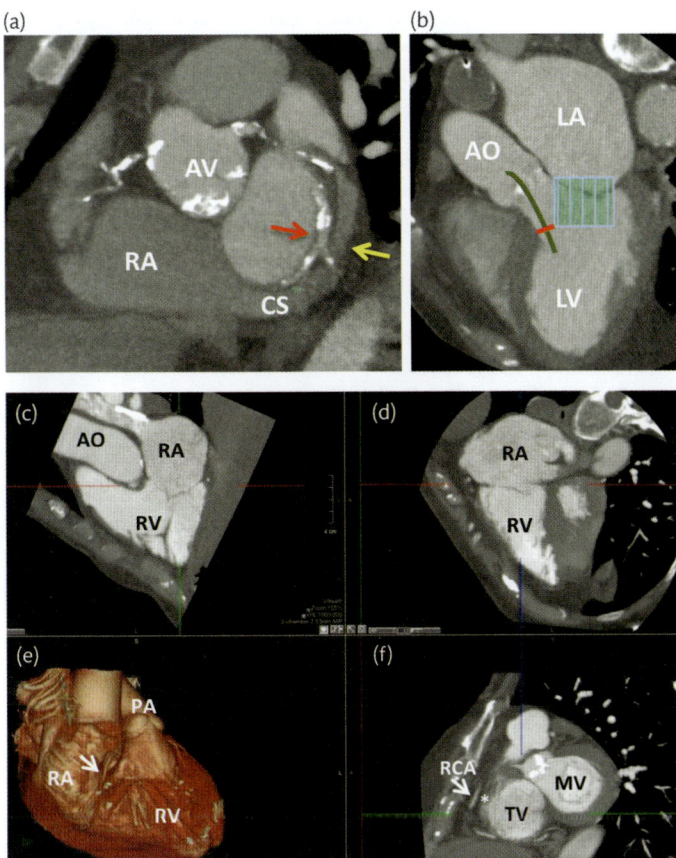

Figure 26.5 CT assessment of the mitral valve. In transcatheter mitral valve annuloplasty, the spatial relationship between the coronary sinus and the left circumflex coronary artery is important. (a) Double oblique short axis view of the mitral annulus shows the course of the left circumflex coronary artery (red arrow) internally to the coronary sinus (CS, yellow arrow) indicating the risk of coronary artery impingement. In transcatheter mitral valve implantation techniques, the position of the transcatheter valve is overlaid onto the mitral valve and LV, potentially compromising the flow through the left ventricular outflow tract (red line). (c–f) Multiplanar reformation planes of the tricuspid valve (TV) with the reconstructed apical right ventricular outflow tract view (c), the apical four-chamber view (d), the short axis view (f) and the three-dimensional volume rendering of the heart (e). From panels c and d, two orthogonal diameters of the tricuspid annulus and the longitudinal diameter of the right ventricle (RV) can be measured. From the short-axis view the spatial relationship of the right coronary artery (RCA) and the tricuspid valve annulus can be assessed (asterisk). The three-dimensional volume rendering also shows the course of the RCA along the tricuspid annulus (arrow). AO, aorta; CS, coronary sinus; LA, left atrium; LV, left ventricle; MV, mitral valve; PA, pulmonary artery; RA, right atrium; RCA, right coronary artery; TV, tricuspid valve.

transcatheter valve technologies have been developed to treat patients with symptomatic severe secondary tricuspid regurgitation and can be classified according to the target mechanism. Cardiac CT plays a central role in the selection of patients for these therapies (**Figure 26.5**). In heterotopic implantation of transcatheter valves into the caval veins, accurate assessment of the dimensions of the inferior and superior vena cava and the distance between the entrance of inferior vena cava into the right atrium and the hepatic veins should be assessed to select or customize the prosthesis size.[41] When using transcatheter techniques that target the tricuspid

annulus, accurate assessment of the annulus geometry and the spatial relationship of the right coronary artery and the tricuspid annulus should be assessed to prevent impingement of this coronary artery.[41] Transcatheter systems that are implanted in the tricuspid valve to fill the regurgitant orifice area are usually anchored in the right ventricular apex, and therefore accurate assessment of the right ventricular dimensions and geometry is important.[41]

Device therapies

Cardiac resynchronization therapy

In symptomatic heart failure patients with wide QRS complex and depressed LV function, cardiac resynchronization therapy (CRT) is a well-established treatment option that can provide symptomatic benefit and reduce mortality. Nevertheless, a substantial proportion of patients do not experience clinical benefit from CRT.[42] It has been demonstrated that accurate positioning of the LV pacing lead is essential for a good response to CRT. However, cardiac venous anatomy is highly variable and may challenge optimal LV lead positioning in a number of patients. CT enables detailed visualization of the coronary sinus and its tributaries before the implantation.[43] The non-invasive assessment of venous anatomy with CT may have significant impact on the implantation strategy and procedural outcome (**Figure 26.6**).

Giraldi *et al.* demonstrated in 40 patients with unfavourable venous anatomy assessed with CT that changing the treatment strategy from a conventional transvenous approach to surgical epicardial LV lead placement resulted in a significant improvement in LVEF, New York Heart Association functional class, and exercise capacity.[44] In addition, a recent randomized trial demonstrated that image-guided position of the LV lead reduces the proportion of non-responders to CRT.[45] With the use of cardiac CT, echocardiography and nuclear imaging, the optimal cardiac vein for positioning the LV lead was determined in 89 patients, whereas routine LV lead placement was performed in 93 patients. In the image-guided group, fewer patients reached the primary end-point (death, heart failure hospitalization, no improvement in functional capacity) as compared to the conventional group (26% vs 42%, $P < 0.05$). However, no differences in LV reverse remodelling were noted between the two groups.[45]

Assessment of cardiac venous anatomy with CT prior to CRT implantation may be relevant in the subgroup of patients with history of myocardial infarction since it has been demonstrated that in this group of patients the left marginal vein may be less frequently observed, as compared with control patients and patients with CAD (27% vs 71% and 61%, respectively, $P < 0.001$).[43]

Left ventricular assist device

Left ventricular assist device has become a feasible treatment option for patients with symptomatic heart failure despite optimal medical (including CRT) treatment. Left ventricular assist devices can be used as a bridge to heart transplantation, as destination therapy for those ineligible for transplantation, or as a bridge to myocardial recovery. At present, both pulsatile flow and continuous flow devices are available. For the selection of patients for LV assist device, echocardiography remains the imaging technique of choice since it can provide a comprehensive evaluation of cardiac structure and function.[46] In addition, CT is used to evaluate vascular anatomy before the operation, similar to percutaneous aortic valve procedures.

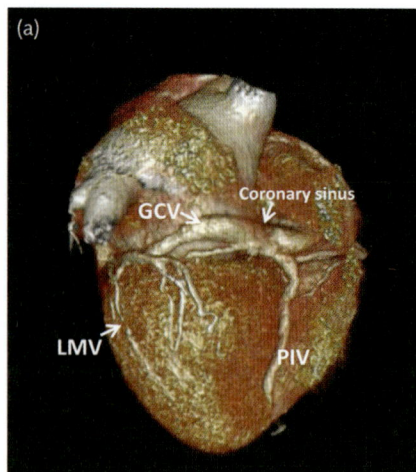
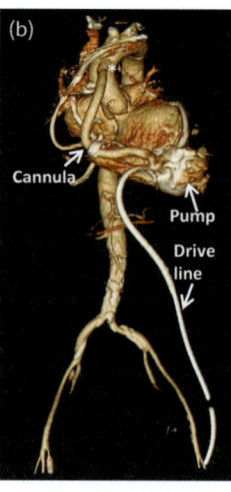

Figure 26.6 CT assessment for heart failure device therapies. For implantation of cardiac resynchronization therapy, the cardiac venous anatomy can be assessed with computed tomography. (a) Coronary sinus and its tributaries, the posterior interventricular vein (PIV), the great cardiac vein (GCV), and the left marginal vein (LVM), which is the preferred target for LV lead placement. (b) Three-dimensional volume rendering of the heart, aorta, and iliac arteries of a patient with a left ventricular assist device. The outflow cannula connecting the pump and the ascending aorta can be visualized. The asterisk indicates the anastomosis of the outflow cannula with the aorta.

During follow-up, CT may be a valuable tool for the assessment of LV assist device outflow cannula thrombosis when clinical and echocardiographic parameters are inconclusive. In addition, kinking or malposition of the outflow cannula can be assessed with CT (**Figure 26.6**). In 28 LV assist device patients with suspected cannula thrombosis or inflow cannula malposition who underwent surgical inspection, Raman *et al.* demonstrated that CT could detect these complications with a sensitivity and specificity of 85% and 100%, respectively.[47] Finally, CT may be helpful for detection of complications such as cardiac tamponade, aortic root thrombi or infection after implantation.[48] The present chapter is an update of the chapter in the previous edition.[49]

REFERENCES

1. Andreini D, Pontone G, Pepi M, *et al.* Diagnostic accuracy of multidetector computed tomography coronary angiography in patients with dilated cardiomyopathy. *J Am Coll Cardiol* 2007;**49**(20):2044–50.
2. Hausleiter J, Meyer T, Hermann F, *et al.* Estimated radiation dose associated with cardiac CT angiography. *JAMA* 2009;**301**(5):500–7.
3. Margolis JR, Chen JT, Kong Y, *et al.* The diagnostic and prognostic significance of coronary artery calcification. A report of 800 cases. *Radiology* 1980;**137**(3):609–16.
4. Agatston AS, Janowitz WR, Hildner FJ, *et al.* Quantification of coronary artery calcium using ultrafast computed tomography. *J Am Coll Cardiol* 1990;**15**(4):827–32.
5. Haberl R, Becker A, Leber A, *et al.* Correlation of coronary calcification and angiographically documented stenoses in patients with suspected coronary artery disease: results of 1,764 patients. *J Am Coll Cardiol* 2001;**37**(2):451–7.
6. Abunassar JG, Yam Y, Chen L, D'Mello N, Chow BJ. Usefulness of the Agatston score = 0 to exclude ischemic cardiomyopathy in patients with heart failure. *Am J Cardiol* 2011;**107**(3):428–32.
7. von Ballmoos MW, Haring B, Juillerat P, Alkadhi H. Meta-analysis: diagnostic performance of low-radiation-dose coronary computed tomography angiography. *Ann Intern Med* 2011;**154**(6):413–20.
8. Montalescot G, Sechtem U, Achenbach S, *et al.* 2013 ESC guidelines on the management of stable coronary artery disease: the Task Force on the management of stable coronary artery disease of the European Society of Cardiology. *Eur Heart J* 2013;**34**(38):2949–3003.
9. Budoff MJ, Dowe D, Jollis JG, *et al.* Diagnostic performance of 64-multidetector row coronary computed tomographic angiography for evaluation of coronary artery stenosis in individuals without known coronary artery disease: results from the prospective multicenter ACCURACY (Assessment by Coronary Computed Tomographic Angiography of Individuals Undergoing Invasive Coronary Angiography) trial. *J Am Coll Cardiol* 2008;**52**(21):1724–32.
10. Miller JM, Rochitte CE, Dewey M, *et al.* Diagnostic performance of coronary angiography by 64-row CT. *N Engl J Med* 2008;**359**(22):2324–36.
11. Ghostine S, Caussin C, Habis M, *et al.* Non-invasive diagnosis of ischaemic heart failure using 64-slice computed tomography. *Eur Heart J* 2008;**29**(17):2133–40.
12. Cornily JC, Gilard M, Le GG, *et al.* Accuracy of 16-detector multislice spiral computed tomography in the initial evaluation of dilated cardiomyopathy. *Eur J Radiol* 2007;**61**(1):84–90.
13. ten Kate GJ, Caliskan K, Dedic A, *et al.* Computed tomography coronary imaging as a gatekeeper for invasive coronary angiography in patients with newly diagnosed heart failure of unknown aetiology. *Eur J Heart Fail* 2013;**15**(9):1028–34.
14. Min JK, Leipsic J, Pencina MJ, *et al.* Diagnostic accuracy of fractional flow reserve from anatomic CT angiography. *JAMA* 2012;**308**(12):1237–45.
15. Koo BK, Erglis A, Doh JH, *et al.* Diagnosis of ischemia-causing coronary stenoses by noninvasive fractional flow reserve computed from coronary computed tomographic angiograms. Results from the prospective multicenter DISCOVER-FLOW (Diagnosis of Ischemia-Causing Stenoses Obtained Via Noninvasive Fractional Flow Reserve) study. *J Am Coll Cardiol* 2011;**58**(19):1989–97.
16. Rochitte CE, George RT, Chen MY, *et al.* Computed tomography angiography and perfusion to assess coronary artery stenosis causing perfusion defects by single photon emission computed tomography: the CORE320 study. *Eur Heart J* 2014;**35**(17):1120–30.
17. Pickett CA, Cheezum MK, Kassop D, Villines TC, Hulten EA. Accuracy of cardiac CT, radionucleotide and invasive ventriculography, two- and three-dimensional echocardiography, and SPECT for left and right ventricular ejection fraction compared with cardiac MRI: a meta-analysis. *Eur Heart J Cardiovasc Imaging* 2015;**16**(8):848–52.
18. Greupner J, Zimmermann E, Grohmann A, *et al.* Head-to-head comparison of left ventricular function assessment with 64-row computed tomography, biplane left cineventriculography, and both 2- and 3-dimensional transthoracic echocardiography: comparison with magnetic resonance imaging as the reference standard. *J Am Coll Cardiol* 2012;**59**(21):1897–907.

19. Butler J, Shapiro MD, Jassal DS, *et al*. Comparison of multidetector computed tomography and two-dimensional transthoracic echocardiography for left ventricular assessment in patients with heart failure. *Am J Cardiol* 2007;**99**(2):247–9.

20. Henneman MM, Schuijf JD, Jukema JW, *et al*. Assessment of global and regional left ventricular function and volumes with 64-slice MSCT: a comparison with 2D echocardiography. *J Nucl Cardiol* 2006;**13**(4):480–7.

21. Kaniewska M, Schuetz GM, Willun S, Schlattmann P, Dewey M. Noninvasive evaluation of global and regional left ventricular function using computed tomography and magnetic resonance imaging: a meta-analysis. *Eur Radiol* 2017;**27**(4):1640–59.

22. Henneman MM, Schuijf JD, Dibbets-Schneider P, *et al*. Comparison of multislice computed tomography to gated single-photon emission computed tomography for imaging of healed myocardial infarcts. *Am J Cardiol* 2008;**101**(2):144–8.

23. Gerber BL, Belge B, Legros GJ, *et al*. Characterization of acute and chronic myocardial infarcts by multidetector computed tomography: comparison with contrast-enhanced magnetic resonance. *Circulation* 2006;**113**(6):823–33.

24. Mahnken AH, Koos R, Katoh M, *et al*. Assessment of myocardial viability in reperfused acute myocardial infarction using 16-slice computed tomography in comparison to magnetic resonance imaging. *J Am Coll Cardiol* 2005;**45**(12):2042–7.

25. Nieman K, Shapiro MD, Ferencik M, *et al*. Reperfused myocardial infarction: contrast-enhanced 64-Section CT in comparison to MR imaging. *Radiology* 2008;**247**(1):49–56.

26. le Polain de Waroux JB, Pouleur AC, Goffinet C, *et al*. Combined coronary and late-enhanced multidetector-computed tomography for delineation of the etiology of left ventricular dysfunction: comparison with coronary angiography and contrast-enhanced cardiac magnetic resonance imaging. *Eur Heart J* 2008;**29**(20):2544–51.

27. Kamperidis V, Delgado V, van Mieghem NM, *et al*. Diagnosis and management of aortic valve stenosis in patients with heart failure. *Eur J Heart Fail* 2016;**18**(5):469–81.

28. Arsalan M, Walther T, Smith RL, Grayburn PA. Tricuspid regurgitation diagnosis and treatment. *Eur Heart J* 2017;**38**(9):634–8.

29. Rossi A, Dini FL, Faggiano P, *et al*. Independent prognostic value of functional mitral regurgitation in patients with heart failure. A quantitative analysis of 1256 patients with ischaemic and non-ischaemic dilated cardiomyopathy. *Heart* 2011;**97**(20):1675–80.

30. Pibarot P, Dumesnil JG. Low-flow, low-gradient aortic stenosis with normal and depressed left ventricular ejection fraction. *J Am Coll Cardiol* 2012;**60**(19):1845–53.

31. Cueff C, Serfaty JM, Cimadevilla C, *et al*. Measurement of aortic valve calcification using multislice computed tomography: correlation with haemodynamic severity of aortic stenosis and clinical implication for patients with low ejection fraction. *Heart* 2011;**97**(9):721–6.

32. Kamperidis V, van Rosendael PJ, Katsanos S, *et al*. Low gradient severe aortic stenosis with preserved ejection fraction: reclassification of severity by fusion of Doppler and computed tomographic data. *Eur Heart J* 2015;**36**(31):2087–96.

33. Delgado V, Schuijf JD, Bax JJ. Pre-operative aortic valve implantation evaluation: multimodality imaging. *EuroIntervention* 2010;**6** Suppl G:G38–G47.

34. Tops LF, Wood DA, Delgado V, *et al*. Noninvasive evaluation of the aortic root with multislice computed tomography implications for transcatheter aortic valve replacement. *JACC Cardiovasc Imaging* 2008;**1**(3):321–30.

35. Jilaihawi H, Kashif M, Fontana G, *et al*. Cross-sectional computed tomographic assessment improves accuracy of aortic annular sizing for transcatheter aortic valve replacement and reduces the incidence of paravalvular aortic regurgitation. *J Am Coll Cardiol* 2012;**59**(14):1275–86.

36. Delgado V, Tops LF, Schuijf JD, *et al*. Assessment of mitral valve anatomy and geometry with multislice computed tomography. *JACC Cardiovasc Imaging* 2009;**2**(5):556–65.

37. Maisano F, Franzen O, Baldus S, *et al*. Percutaneous mitral valve interventions in the real world: early and 1-year results from the ACCESS-EU, a prospective, multicenter, nonrandomized post-approval study of the MitraClip therapy in Europe. *J Am Coll Cardiol* 2013;**62**(12):1052–61.

38. van Mieghem NM, Rodriguez-Olivares R, Ren BC, *et al*. Computed tomography optimised fluoroscopy guidance for transcatheter mitral therapies. *EuroIntervention* 2016;**11**(12):1428–31.

39. Tops LF, Van de Veire NR, Schuijf JD, *et al*. Noninvasive evaluation of coronary sinus anatomy and its relation to the mitral valve annulus: implications for percutaneous mitral annuloplasty. *Circulation* 2007;**115**(11):1426–32.

40. Blanke P, Naoum C, Webb J, *et al*. Multimodality imaging in the context of transcatheter mitral valve replacement: establishing consensus among modalities and disciplines. *JACC Cardiovasc Imaging* 2015;**8**(10):1191–208.

41. van Rosendael PJ, Kamperidis V, Kong WFK, *et al*. Computed tomography for planning transcatheter tricuspid valve therapy. *Eur Heart J* 2017;**38**(9):665–74.

42. Shanks M, Delgado V, Ng AC, *et al*. Clinical and echocardiographic predictors of nonresponse to cardiac resynchronization therapy. *Am Heart J* 2011;**161**(3):552–7.

43. Van de Veire NR, Schuijf JD, De Sutter J, *et al*. Non-invasive visualization of the cardiac venous system in coronary artery disease patients using 64-slice computed tomography. *J Am Coll Cardiol* 2006;**48**(9):1832–8.

44. Giraldi F, Cattadori G, Roberto M, *et al*. Long-term effectiveness of cardiac resynchronization therapy in heart failure patients with unfavorable cardiac veins anatomy comparison of surgical versus hemodynamic procedure. *J Am Coll Cardiol* 2011;**58**(5):483–90.

45. Sommer A, Kronborg MB, Nørgaard BL, *et al*. Multimodality imaging-guided left ventricular lead placement in cardiac resynchronization therapy: a randomized controlled trial. *Eur J Heart Fail* 2016;**18**(11):1365–74.

46. Estep JD, Stainback RF, Little SH, Torre G, Zoghbi WA. The role of echocardiography and other imaging modalities in patients with left ventricular assist devices. *JACC Cardiovasc Imaging* 2010;**3**(10):1049–64.

47. Raman SV, Sahu A, Merchant AZ, *et al*. Noninvasive assessment of left ventricular assist devices with cardiovascular computed tomography and impact on management. *J Heart Lung Transplant* 2010;**29**(1):79–85.

48. Vivo RP, Kassi M, Estep JD, *et al*. MDCT assessment of mechanical circulatory support device complications. *JACC Cardiovasc Imaging* 2015;**8**(1):100–2.

49. Schuijf JD, Tops LF, Bax JJ. CT imaging techniques. In: McDonagh TA, Gardner RS, Clark A, Dargie H, eds. *Oxford Textbook of Heart Failure*. 2011.

RECOMMENDED READING

Andreini D, Pontone G, Pepi M, *et al*. Diagnostic accuracy of multidetector computed tomography coronary angiography

in patients with dilated cardiomyopathy. *J Am Coll Cardiol* 2007;**49**(20):2044–50.

Ballmoos MW von, Haring B, Juillerat P, Alkadhi H. Meta-analysis: diagnostic performance of low-radiation-dose coronary computed tomography angiography. *Ann Intern Med* 2011;**154**(6):413–20.

Blanke P, Naoum C, Webb J, *et al.* Multimodality imaging in the context of transcatheter mitral valve replacement: establishing consensus among modalities and disciplines. *JACC Cardiovasc Imaging* 2015;**8**(10):1191–208.

Henneman MM, Schuijf JD, Dibbets-Schneider P, *et al.* Comparison of multislice computed tomography to gated single-photon emission computed tomography for imaging of healed myocardial infarcts. *Am J Cardiol* 2008;**101**(2):144–8.

Kamperidis V, van Rosendael PJ, Katsanos S, *et al.* Low gradient severe aortic stenosis with preserved ejection fraction: reclassification of severity by fusion of Doppler and computed tomographic data. *Eur Heart J* 2015;**36**(31):2087–96.

Miller JM, Rochitte CE, Dewey M, *et al.* Diagnostic performance of coronary angiography by 64-row CT. *N Engl J Med* 2008;**359**(22):2324–36.

Min JK, Leipsic J, Pencina MJ, *et al.* Diagnostic accuracy of fractional flow reserve from anatomic CT angiography. *JAMA* 2012;**308**(12):1237–45.

Pickett CA, Cheezum MK, Kassop D, Villines TC, Hulten EA. Accuracy of cardiac CT, radionucleotide and invasive ventriculography, two- and three-dimensional echocardiography, and SPECT for left and right ventricular ejection fraction compared with cardiac MRI: a meta-analysis. *Eur Heart J Cardiovasc Imaging* 2015;**16**(8):848–52.

Raman SV, Sahu A, Merchant AZ, *et al.* Noninvasive assessment of left ventricular assist devices with cardiovascular computed tomography and impact on management. *J Heart Lung Transplant* 2010;**29**(1):79–85.

Rochitte CE, George RT, Chen MY, *et al.* Computed tomography angiography and perfusion to assess coronary artery stenosis causing perfusion defects by single photon emission computed tomography: the CORE320 study. *Eur Heart J* 2014;**35**(17):1120–30.

Sommer A, Kronborg MB, Nørgaard BL, *et al.* Multimodality imaging-guided left ventricular lead placement in cardiac resynchronization therapy: a randomized controlled trial. *Eur J Heart Fail* 2016;**18**(11):1365–74.

Tops LF, Wood DA, Delgado V, *et al.* Noninvasive evaluation of the aortic root with multislice computed tomography implications for transcatheter aortic valve replacement. *JACC Cardiovasc Imaging* 2008;**1**(3):321–30.

27

Cardiopulmonary exercise testing in chronic heart failure

Carrie Ferguson and Klaus K. Witte

Introduction

Chronic heart failure (CHF) is characterized by exercise intolerance, usually due to breathlessness or fatigue in the presence of cardiac dysfunction. Hence when assessing a patient with such symptoms, in addition to appropriate cardiac imaging, some form of standardized exercise testing is important to measure objectively the degree and nature of the symptoms and to confirm their aetiology. In addition, exercise capacity (measured as peak oxygen uptake) is a powerful predictor of mortality and is used as a marker of the need for cardiac transplantation. Although useful data can be gained from a standard treadmill/cycle ergometer-based exercise test,[1] or a corridor walk test, additional and independent information is available when the test is performed while measuring pulmonary gas exchange.[2]

Definitions and variables

In patients with CHF, an exercise test with or without pulmonary gas analysis yields important information about ischaemia, inducible arrhythmias, and prognosis.[3-6] Pulmonary gas exchange measurements made during exercise are accurate and reproducible[7] as well as robust predictors of outcomes.[8-11]

During an incremental exercise test, patients exercise to intolerance while wearing a tight-fitting mask or mouthpiece with nose-clip, with respired gas concentrations and volumes sampled to determine pulmonary gas exchange variables. This can either be done by sampling from a large bag at intervals (Douglas bag method) or more commonly on a breath-by-breath basis. The rate of oxygen uptake ($\dot{V}O_2$), minute ventilation (as a product of tidal volume and frequency of breathing), and carbon dioxide output ($\dot{V}CO_2$) can be measured (**Figure 27.1**). Exercise duration, heart rate, blood pressure changes, and peak heart rate are often quoted, but the variables most commonly used to describe the exercise response are peak oxygen uptake ($p\dot{V}O_2$), anaerobic threshold (AT), the derived variables of the relationship of ventilation to carbon dioxide output ($\dot{V}E/\dot{V}CO_2$ slope), and the ratio of $\dot{V}CO_2$ to $\dot{V}O_2$ (respiratory exchange ratio or RER).

Anaerobic and aerobic metabolism

Skeletal muscle cellular activity requires energy, which is stored in skeletal muscle myocytes in the form of creatine phosphate and glycogen. Creatine phosphate is rapidly accessible, but stores are sufficient for only a few seconds of work. The currency of energy transfer is in the breaking and reformation of the terminal phosphate bond of adenosine triphosphate (ATP). The energy released when this bond is broken is used for a cycle of linking and releasing of the two elements of their contractile structure, actin and myosin. The linking and subsequent release leads to conformational

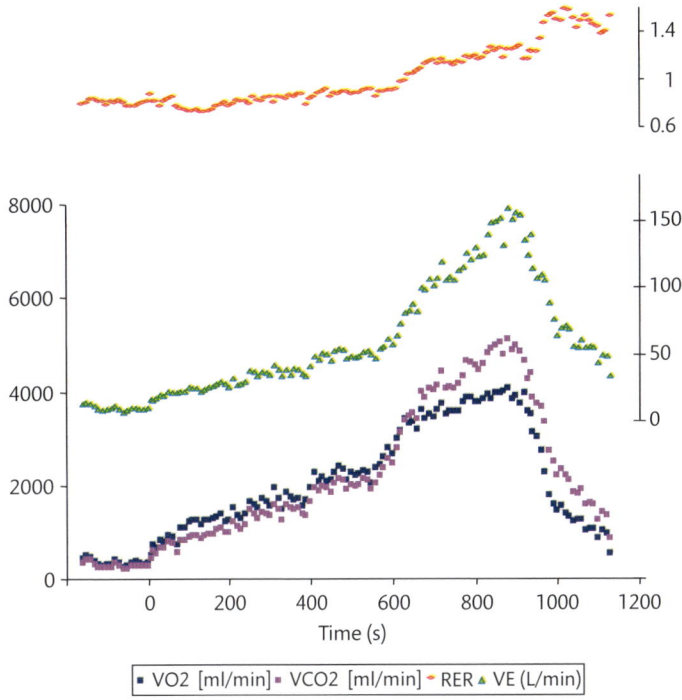

Figure 27.1 Cardiopulmonary dataset from a control participant showing increases in oxygen uptake (VO_2), carbon dioxide output (VCO_2), ventilation (VE), and respiratory exchange ratio (RER) during a ramp incremental exercise test. HF, heart failure.

changes in the cell. If neighbouring cells perform this activity in a controlled and co-ordinated manner, contraction of the muscle can take place. Other cellular activities such as biosynthesis and active transport are also supported by the energy released from the hydrolysis of the ATP.

Aerobic metabolism

The production of units of ATP, which must continuously be regenerated at the appropriate rate to allow cellular work to continue, depends largely upon the oxidation in the mitochondria of carbohydrates, fatty acids, and, in conditions of starvation, protein. Carbohydrate sources (such as glycogen) are converted initially to pyruvate, and then enter the tricarboxylic acid cycle (TCA or the Krebs cycle), as acetyl-CoA, eventually forming carbon dioxide, high-energy electrons, and hydrogen ions. On the other hand, fatty acids undergo β-oxidation but then also enter the Krebs cycle as acetyl CoA units. The release of the protons and the entry of the electrons into the electron-transport chain is dependent upon the consumption of oxygen and leads to the production of water and the regeneration of ATP (**Figure 27.2**). An important part of the process is the reduction of nicotinamide adenine dinucleotide (NAD^+) to NADH. NADH is the route through which electrons enter the electron transport chain, in the process being oxidized again to NAD^+.

Anaerobic metabolism

In situations where the rate of glycolytic flux leads to an accumulation of pyruvate, there is an increase in the cytosolic NADH/NAD^+ ratio. Thus, in order to allow for the re-oxidization of NADH to NAD^+, pyruvate is instead converted to lactate. This is termed anaerobic metabolism and leads to the production of fewer ATP molecules for each molecule of substrate than aerobic metabolism. The

metabolic acidosis that occurs due to performing high rates of anaerobic glycolysis is also associated with the development of muscle fatigue.

In most circumstances, both aerobic and anaerobic metabolism occur simultaneously in all cells, but in skeletal muscle cells, particularly at high workloads, anaerobic metabolism provides a greater proportion of the energy than at rest.

Energy substrates

The ratio of the rate of oxygen consumption ($\dot{Q}_{O_2}$) to carbon dioxide production ($\dot{Q}_{CO_2}$) in the tissues is a consequence of the substrate used. When using glucose, each molecule of oxygen used leads to the formation of one molecule of carbon dioxide.

$$C_6H_{12}O_6 + 6O_2 \rightarrow 6H_2O + 6CO_2 + 36ATP$$

This leads to a respiratory quotient (RQ: $\dot{Q}_{CO_2}/\dot{Q}_{O_2}$) of one. Lipids are much more reduced than carbohydrate, and so when fatty acids are oxidized, $\dot{Q}_{CO_2}$ is lower than the $\dot{Q}_{O_2}$ with a correspondingly lower RQ of ~0.7:

$$C_{16}H_{32}O_2 + 23O_2 \rightarrow 16H_2O + 16CO_2 + 130ATP$$

where $C_{16}H_{32}O_2$ is palmitic acid, a commonly used fatty acid.

In humans at rest, there is a preponderance of fatty acid metabolism, so the CO_2 production is lower than O_2 consumption and the RQ is ~0.85. The higher the proportion of carbohydrate used, the greater the ventilatory requirement to eliminate the CO_2 produced.

With metabolic gas exchange measurements, 'whole body' gas exchange is measured from the difference between inspired and expired oxygen and carbon dioxide at the mouth and is not a direct measure of cellular metabolism. As with RQ, $\dot{V}_{O_2}$ and $\dot{V}_{CO_2}$

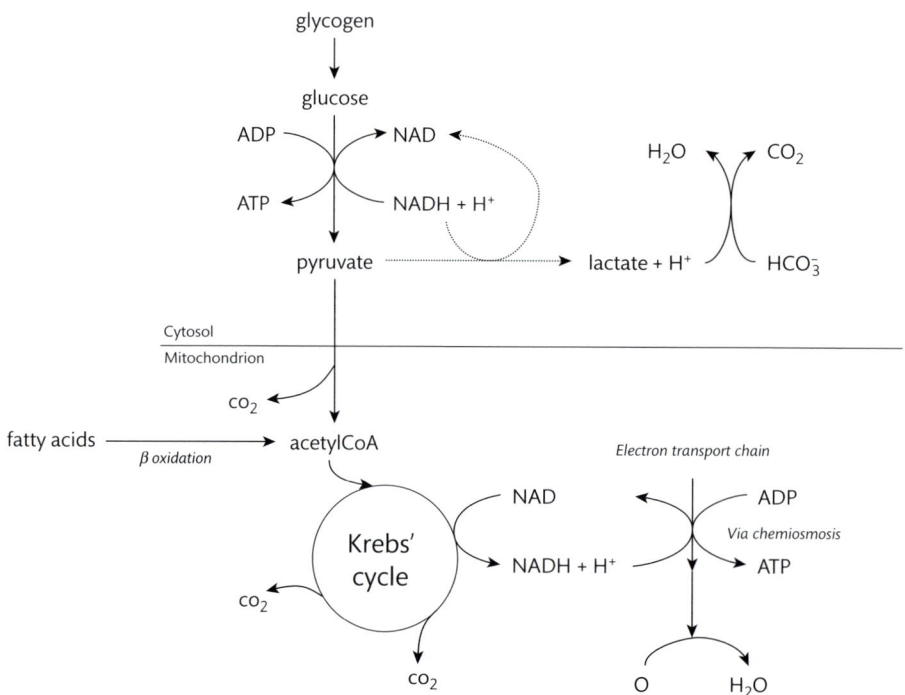

Figure 27.2 Aerobic and anaerobic metabolism (dashed lines show the passage of protons into the electron transport chain).

measured at the mouth can be expressed as a ratio: the respiratory exchange ratio (RER).

Oxygen uptake

During exercise there is a several-fold increase in oxygen consumption by skeletal muscle cells. The physiological adaptations to exercise include increased cardiac output from a resting level of 3.5 L/min to typically 20 L/min, with local arterial vasodilation to increase oxygen delivery to exercising muscles. There is a rightward shift of the oxyhaemoglobin dissociation curve, encouraging unloading of oxygen in areas of acidosis, and there is increased ventilation up to 150 L/min.

The body's upper limit of oxygen utilization is determined by the maximal cardiac output,[12] arterial O_2 content, the fractional distribution of cardiac output to the exercising muscle,[13] and the ability of the muscle to extract O_2.[14] Ventilation is a limiting factor only when the ventilatory requirement to eliminate the CO_2 produced by aerobic metabolism and the bicarbonate buffering of lactic acid[15] are in excess of the maximum voluntary ventilation (MVV).

The measurement of $\dot{V}O_2$ at the mouth is used as a surrogate measure of oxygen consumption ($\dot{Q}O_2$) in the skeletal muscles. Oxygen *consumption* at the cellular level is only a small percentage of resting oxygen uptake. However, during exercise, most of the increase in oxygen uptake at the mouth reflects increased oxygen consumption in the skeletal muscles. Hence oxygen uptake at the mouth and oxygen consumption are assumed to be equivalent. The value is presented either as an absolute (mL/min) or referenced to body weight (mL/kg/min).

Physiologists refer to the concept of maximal oxygen uptake ('$\dot{V}O_2$ max') as the oxygen uptake plateau reached where an increase in imposed workload no longer elicits an increase in $\dot{V}O_2$. However, during continuous ramp–incremental tests in normal subjects, a plateau in $\dot{V}O_2$ is rarely seen (incidence often <50%), and in patients with heart failure $\dot{V}O_2$ is often limited by symptoms meaning that they are almost never able to exercise to such a plateau. A flattening of the $\dot{V}O_2$–work rate relationship is therefore not seen. In the absence of any confirmatory evidence that $\dot{V}O_2$ max has been achieved, the term 'peak $\dot{V}O_2$' should be used when a plateau is not seen, and is used as an index of peak exercise capacity.

Carbon dioxide output

Metabolic activity produces carbon dioxide and water as waste products. The amount of carbon dioxide produced for a given energy release is determined by the substrate and how it is metabolized. As with oxygen consumption, the carbon dioxide production occurs in the metabolizing tissues but is measured at the mouth. During high-intensity exercise there is also additional CO_2 production from bicarbonate buffering of lactic acid, and a further contribution to the CO_2 output from 'compensatory' hyperventilation that reduces stored CO_2.

Ventilation

Ventilation (in L/min) is a product of frequency (*f*) and tidal volume (V_T) at the mouth. The relationship between oxygen uptake and workload during submaximal exercise is linear.[16] However, the ventilatory response is not related linearly to $\dot{V}O_2$. Instead, there is a close relationship between the $\dot{V}CO_2$ and minute ventilation ($\dot{V}E$)

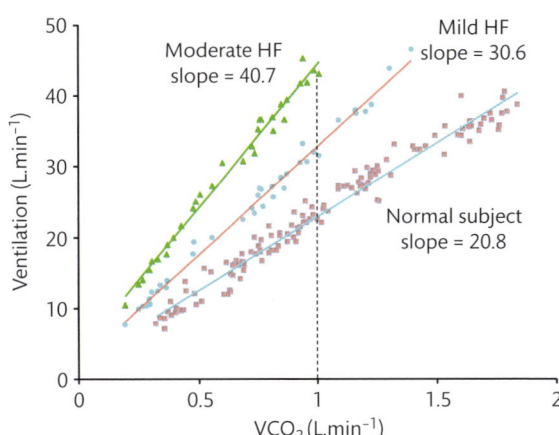

Figure 27.3 The ventilation/carbon dioxide output (VE/VCO$_2$) slope in two patients with chronic heart failure and a control subject.

(**Figure 27.3**).[17–19] This relationship, termed the $\dot{V}E/\dot{V}CO_2$ slope, becomes steeper above the point of respiratory compensation.[18]

The relation between ventilation and carbon dioxide output is given by

$$VE/VCO_2 = 863/PaCO_2 \times (1 - V_D / V_T) \qquad (27.1)$$

where 863 is a constant to standardize volume measurements, $PaCO_2$ is the arterial tension of carbon dioxide and V_D/V_T is dead space as a fraction of tidal volume. A consequence is that, in the short term at least, $\dot{V}CO_2$ is determined by ventilation: if a subject hyperventilates with respect to carbon dioxide production, $\dot{V}CO_2$ increases as the carbon dioxide passing through the lungs is blown off, and $PaCO_2$ will fall.[20]

The equation above includes a calculation for dead space: lung tissue that is ventilated but not perfused, including bronchi, trachea, and underperfused alveoli. As a result of perfusion changes and the increased frequency of ventilation,[21] dead space ventilation as a fraction of tidal volume is greater in patients with CHF than in control subjects. This might contribute to exercise limitation and symptoms in patients with CHF, hence estimated V_D/V_T is frequently presented within a cardiopulmonary exercise report.

Derived variables

Several variables are commonly derived from the basic measurements. It must be borne in mind that derived variables especially suffer from a multiplication of errors when calculated from poorly performed tests.

Ventilatory equivalents

The ventilatory equivalents for oxygen ($V_{eq}O_2$ or $\dot{V}E/\dot{V}O_2$) and carbon dioxide ($V_{eq}CO_2$ or $\dot{V}E/\dot{V}CO_2$) give an impression of the instantaneous ventilation required at a particular time-point for the metabolic gas in question and are usually plotted against work rate or time in a progressive test. Both decline early on during progressive exercise until the anaerobic threshold (AT) at which point $V_{eq}O_2$ increases, followed (after a delay) by an increase in $V_{eq}CO_2$ at the point of respiratory compensation. Both ventilatory equivalents for oxygen and carbon dioxide are higher in patients with CHF than in

controls throughout exercise. Both a high $V_{eq}CO_2$ and $\dot{V}E/\dot{V}CO_2$ slope >34 carry adverse prognostic significance in CHF.[22]

Respiratory exchange ratio

A problem with incremental testing in a population of subjects unused to maximal exercise tests is determining whether a maximum has been reached, or whether exercise is 'submaximal'. Where a genuine plateau in oxygen uptake is reached, then a maximum test can be inferred confidently. For most patients with heart failure, the respiratory exchange ratio (RER: $\dot{V}CO_2/\dot{V}O_2$) is usually used as confirmatory evidence of maximal effort in the absence of a plateau.

When glucose is the metabolic substrate used, the RER is 1.0 (one mole of CO_2 is produced for each mole of O_2 consumed). The RER for lipid metabolism is ~0.7 as lipid is more highly reduced than glucose. At rest in patients and normal subjects alike, the ratio is around 0.85, representing the balance between fatty acid and glucose metabolism. However, as exercise progresses, ATP is generated, increasingly from anaerobic metabolism. This shift away from aerobic metabolism leads to an increase in lactate + H^+ production, with the H^+ ions buffered in the blood stream by HCO_3^- ions, generating additional CO_2. Thus, as a result of this blood buffering creating an additional source of carbon dioxide output, the RER gradually rises. A test is usually taken to be maximal when the RER is >1.1; in practice in heart failure populations, an RER of ≥1.0 is often accepted. Higher RER levels improve the prognostic information of the data collected,[23] whereas those with low RER levels are much less informative.[24]

The anaerobic threshold

At low workloads, aerobic metabolism is able to support energy production completely, and the requirement for anaerobic metabolism is low. During incremental exercise, there comes a point at which aerobic energy provision must be progressively supplemented from anaerobic metabolism to meet the ATP demands of the exercise. At this point, lactate accumulates above resting levels, and the accompanying H^+ is buffered by bicarbonate in the blood. Bicarbonate in turn is converted to water and CO_2, which is added to the metabolic CO_2 production and blown off at the lungs in order to maintain plasma pH at physiological levels. The result is a non-linear increase in $\dot{V}CO_2$ relative to $\dot{V}O_2$, detectable from the pulmonary gas exchange data.[25] The point at which this occurs is termed the anaerobic threshold (AT) and can be identified by plotting $\dot{V}O_2$ against $\dot{V}CO_2$, known as the V-slope method (**Figure 27.4**).[27] AT is recorded as the oxygen uptake at this point.

The identification of a discrete breakpoint in the $\dot{V}O_2$ vs $\dot{V}CO_2$ relationship is arbitrary as the increase in CO_2 output is progressive,[26] but it can nevertheless be reasonably reliably estimated by pulmonary gas exchange analysis.[27]

There is a high correlation between the AT and $p\dot{V}O_2$,[28] making the anaerobic threshold a potentially useful submaximal measure of exercise capacity that is independent of patient motivation.[29]

There are also supplementary criteria that can support the identification of the AT; additional criteria depend upon the changing ventilatory response to $\dot{V}O_2$ during exercise.[30,31] At the AT, due to the additional CO_2 from blood buffering increasing the ventilatory requirements, there is hyperventilation with respect to $\dot{V}O_2$, as $\dot{V}E$ remains proportional to the $\dot{V}CO_2$. The equal increases in $\dot{V}CO_2$ and

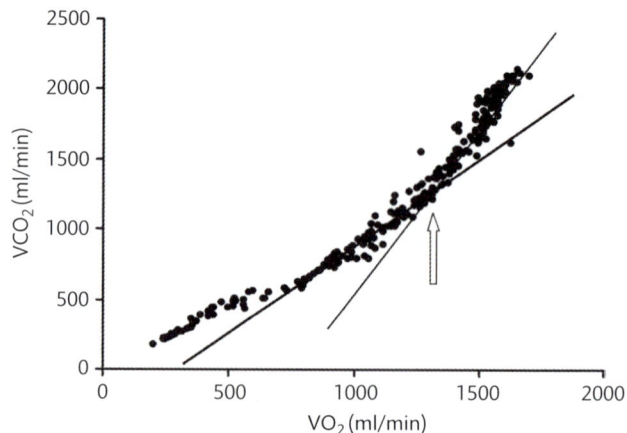

Figure 27.4 The V-slope method for estimating the anaerobic threshold (AT) in a patient with chronic heart failure. The arrow indicates the estimated AT.

$\dot{V}E$ above the AT lead to the arterial tension of carbon dioxide remaining relatively stable, although this is only maintained for a short period (~2 min), known as 'isocapnic buffering'. After this short period, $\dot{V}E$ then increases out of proportion to the $\dot{V}CO_2$, with this 'compensatory' hyperventilation helping to limit the fall in pH associated with high rates of anaerobic metabolism by decreasing the arterial tension of carbon dioxide.[32]

$\dot{V}E/\dot{V}CO_2$ slope

During ramp incremental exercise the relationship of ventilation to oxygen and carbon dioxide is linear throughout exercise below the AT. In patients with heart failure, the slope of the $\dot{V}E/\dot{V}CO_2$ relationship is increased (the slope is steeper) throughout a ramp incremental exercise test, so that for a given carbon dioxide output, there is more $\dot{V}E$ (**Figure 27.3**).[33] The $\dot{V}E/\dot{V}CO_2$ slope is directly related to both mortality and morbidity.[34] Peak $\dot{V}O_2$ and the $\dot{V}E/\dot{V}CO_2$ slope are inversely related to each other,[34,35] so that the more reduced the exercise capacity, the greater the ventilatory response to exercise (**Figure 27.5**).

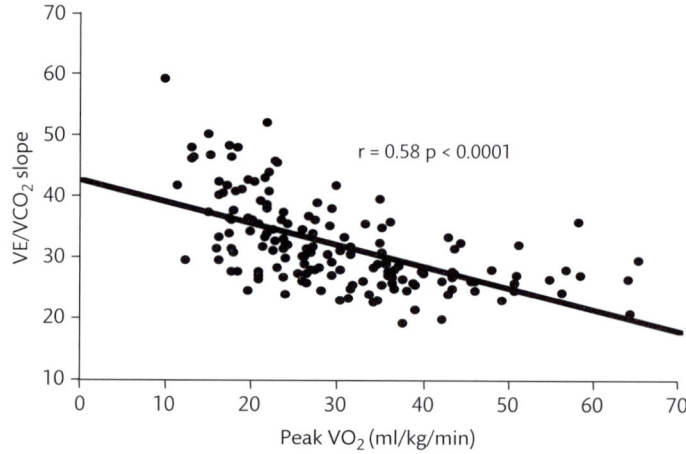

Figure 27.5 The inverse relationship between the ventilation/carbon dioxide output (VE/VCO₂) slope and peak oxygen uptake (pVO₂).

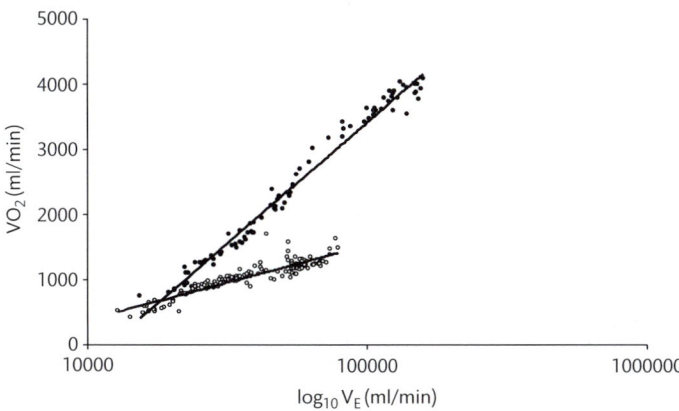

Figure 27.6 The oxygen uptake efficiency slope in a patient (open circles) and a control subject (filled circles). The slope of this relationship is steeper in the control subject.

Other variables

Additional variables can contribute further information. Cyclic fluctuations in ventilation, known as exercise-induced oscillatory breathing (EOV), are exacerbated in patients with CHF both at rest and during exercise.[36,37] There are at least two definitions of cyclical breathing, but patients with EOV by either definition have a worse prognosis.[38]

The oxygen uptake efficiency slope (OUES) is derived by plotting $\dot{V}O_2$ as a function of $\log_{10} \dot{V}E$, which is an approximately linear relation.[39] The steeper the slope, the more oxygen is taken up for a given unit ventilation (Figure 27.6). OUES is reduced in CHF in proportion to disease severity, and is lower in those with atrial fibrillation (AF) compared to sinus rhythm.[40,41] It increases with physical training. One advantage of the OUES as a measure is that it can be measured from submaximal data and does not depend upon reaching peak exertion. The OUES is predictive of prognosis even when derived from submaximal tests.[42]

Combining peak variables occasionally offers greater prognostic power. For example, peak cardiac power output—the product of cardiac output and mean arterial blood pressure at peak exercise—relates to exercise capacity and outcomes.[43] However, not all combinations of peak variables are of greater predictive value than their constituent measurements.[44]

Can the cause of exercise intolerance in CHF be determined from peak variables?

The cause of exercise intolerance and the abnormal physiology during exercise in CHF (such as the increased $\dot{V}E/\dot{V}CO_2$ slope), and the relative contributions of central haemodynamics, peripheral vasculature, and skeletal muscle adaptations, are incompletely understood. Variables such as ventilation, cardiac (power) output, pulmonary gas exchange kinetics[45] and heart rate increase can all be measured during an incremental exercise test as a function of exercise load. Thus, the exercise measures and derived variables will all correlate highly with each other, and all will correlate to some degree with prognosis.[46] Which is the most 'powerful' predictor will vary from dataset to dataset by random chance. There is a temptation to plot one variable as a function of another, and assume that the

mathematically dependent variable plotted on the *y*-axis is somehow determined by the variable on the *x*-axis: this is certainly not the case. Correlation does not imply cause and effect. An absurd example is the observation that hair length (if measured accurately) will also increase as a function of duration of an exercise test, and would correlate closely with peak $\dot{V}O_2$: however, increase in hair length is clearly not the determinant of peak $\dot{V}O_2$! A more controversial example is the influence of chronotropic incompetence and whether it is a limitation of heart rate increase that determines exercise capacity. Chronotropic incompetence is more frequent and more severe in patients taking β-blockers than in those not taking these agents, yet they do not induce a reduction in peak $\dot{V}O_2$.[47–49] It cannot be assumed, therefore, that any variable derived from an exercise test determines exercise capacity. It makes as much sense to state that exercise capacity, for example, determines peak cardiac power output or peak heart rate.

Methods of pulmonary gas exchange measurement

The measurement of peak oxygen uptake (p$\dot{V}O_2$) requires a form of exercise equipment, usually either a programmable treadmill or a stationary electromagnetically braked cycle, and a metabolic gas analyser. A 12-lead electrocardiograph (ECG) monitor is used for safety and to determine heart rate. Ideally, the laboratory should be air-conditioned to achieve a stable temperature and humidity. Repeated exercise tests on subjects should take place at about the same time in the day, and not within 3 h of a main meal. Caffeine should be avoided for 3 h before a test. Participants should be advised to wear comfortable shoes, and wear a loose shirt or vest under which the ECG electrodes can be applied to the skin.

All metabolic gas analysis systems must measure ventilation and analyse the concentrations of oxygen and carbon dioxide in expired air. In a typical system, subjects wear a mask or breathe through a mouthpiece (with a nose-clip) attached to a flow meter which allows for the measurement of tidal volume (V_T) and frequency of ventilation (*f*). These are then used to derive total minute ventilation ($\dot{V}E$ in L/min). Connected to the flow meter is a sample tube which continuously samples a small proportion of the inspired and expired air to measure the concentrations of oxygen and carbon dioxide. By knowing $\dot{V}E$ and the concentrations of oxygen and carbon dioxide, the rates of $\dot{V}O_2$ and $\dot{V}CO_2$ can be derived.

Gas analysers

Mass spectrometry is the reference standard form of gas analysis. It provides rapid and reliable online breath-by-breath assessment of oxygen and carbon dioxide concentrations but the equipment is expensive, and requires regular maintenance. Sampled gases are subjected to an electron beam and thereby converted to charged ions. These are then accelerated in an electric field and their direction altered by a magnetic field. Detectors produce an output according to the numbers of ions striking them per unit time. Alternatives to mass spectrometry include paramagnetic analysers or gas chromatography linked to thermal conductivity detectors for oxygen analysis and infra-red absorption detectors for carbon dioxide.

Flow-sensing devices

The most common and maintenance-free devices for measuring flow are low-resistance turbines, which are less affected by ambient temperature and humidity than alternative devices, but resistance and inertia of the vane may reduce sensitivity. Alternatives include pneumotachometers which measure a pressure fall across two capillary tubes, and anemometers which calculate air flow based upon the temperature change in a thin electrified wire stretched across the tube.

Although initial work was performed using intermittent Douglas bag collections of expired air, most equipment now measures ventilatory and pulmonary gas exchange variables on a breath-by-breath basis. This requires a temporal adjustment of the gas analysis, which takes longer than the flow assessment, to maintain accuracy.[50]

Calibration

Small errors in sampling are magnified by the calculations performed during and subsequent to the test. The equipment should therefore be calibrated before each test. Typically, the flow signal is calibrated by passing a fixed volume (e.g. 3 L) through the sensor at different flow rates, while the gas analysers are calibrated using two different gas mixtures that span the expected inspired and expired O_2 and CO_2 concentrations. Exercise tests should be carried out and interpreted by experienced personnel, with appropriate support from equipment manufacturers. Equipment should be serviced regularly.

Preparation of the subject

The procedure must be explained in full to each participant. When a maximal test is being undertaken, it should be made clear before the test starts that the aim is to assess peak exercise capacity and that the participant will be encouraged to exercise to their limit. During the test, they should be asked to score their symptoms of breathlessness or fatigue according to a recognized rating of perceived exertion scale (such as the Borg score, Table 27.1),[51] and they should be discouraged from talking during the test, as this affects the quality of the pulmonary gas exchange measures and derived responses.

Table 27.1 The Borg scale of perceived exertion

0	Nothing at all
0.5	Very, very slight
1	Very slight
2	Slight
3	Moderate
4	Somewhat severe
5	Severe
6	
7	Very severe
8	
9	Very, very severe
10	Maximal

Source data from Borg G. Subjective effort and physical activities. Scand J Rehab 1978;**6**:108–13.

Simple signals should be agreed upon, such as raising of the left hand to stop the test. The participant should receive standardized encouragement at the mid-point of each stage such as 'you're doing well', 'keep it up'.

Participants respond differently to the mask or the mouthpiece. The mouthpiece commonly causes distress and hypersalivation, but is associated with fewer gas leaks. By contrast, masks are more comfortable but have a higher incidence of leaks and a larger dead space volume. Both options should be available.

Haemodynamic assessment

Throughout the test, a 12-lead electrocardiograph should be monitored, and a hard copy is usually printed with each exercise stage or at appropriate intervals. Blood pressure and heart rate should also be recorded at these time-points. Some devices allow intermittent determination of cardiac output by inert gas dilution. It is important to explain and demonstrate the procedure before the test.

Spirometry

Basic assessment of pulmonary function can be performed routinely on any participant undergoing an exercise test. Using the software within the gas exchange system, a maximal flow-volume loop can be measured, from which forced expiratory volume in one second (FEV_1) and forced vital capacity (FVC) and inspiratory volumes can be calculated. The FEV_1 can be used to calculate predicted maximum voluntary ventilation (MVV):[52] $MVV = FEV_1 \times 35$.

Resting data

Three to five minutes of resting data should be collected before exercise begins. This allows the subject to become familiar with the mouthpiece or mask, and the investigators to identify leaks and analyser problems. Baseline oxygen uptake should be between 3 and 5 mL/kg/min and the respiratory exchange ratio <0.9. Baseline heart rate and blood pressure should be measured at the end of this phase.

Exercise protocols

Protocols for both stationary cycle and treadmill exercise are available and the choice of equipment is often dictated by the experience of the personnel and the space available in the laboratory. Treadmill-based exercise is more natural and often leads to a higher peak $\dot{V}O_2$ since participants also carry their own body weight. By contrast, cycle exercise allows for improved haemodynamic monitoring (reduced movement artifacts) and more gradual increments in workload. During incremental exercise tests the rate of increase in work must be selected with the aim that exercise time is between 6 and 12 min as this maximizes peak $\dot{V}O_2$.[53]

Treadmill exercise

The Bruce protocol,[54] modified by the addition of a 'stage 0' at onset consisting of 3 min of exercise at 1.61 km/h (1 mile/h) with a 5% gradient, is often used (Table 27.2). However, the steps between each stage are large, such that many subjects stop exercise immediately after a stage begins. Alternatives are the Balke protocol,[55] which has a constant speed and gradual increase in incline (1% per minute), and the Naughton[56] protocol which has shorter stages with smaller increments in both speed and incline, and 3 min rest periods between exercise phases. Each of these has been criticized for excessive

Table 27.2 The Bruce protocol

Stage	Duration (s)	Speed (mph)	Grade (%)
0	180	1.0	5
1	180	1.7	10
2	180	2.5	12
3	180	3.4	14
4	180	4.2	16
5	180	5.0	18
6	180	5.5	20
7	180	6.0	22
8	180	6.5	22

An additional 'stage 0' is added to allow patients with severe exercise limitation to perform some exercise.
Source data from Bruce PA, McDonough IR. Stress testing in screening for cardiovascular disease. Bull NY Acad Med 1969;**45**:1288–1305.

duration of exercise, hence other treadmill protocols that result in a linear increase in work rate, and the attainment of peak $\dot{V}O_2$ within 6–12 min have been proposed.[57] During the test, the subject should be encouraged not to use the handrails except as a guide and for balance. Dependence on handrails alters the work being performed and the reliability of the $\dot{V}O_2$ data.[58]

Cycle exercise

Subject preparation for exercise on the stationary cycle proceeds as for treadmill exercise. The work rate against which the subject pedals is increased gradually until intolerance. The ramp protocol is the most commonly employed and consists of continuous increments of work rate, aiming for 10 min of exercise.

Peak exercise and recovery

Exercise tests should be symptom-limited maximal tests. At peak exercise, heart rate and blood pressure should be measured and an ECG printed. The rating of perceived exertion and the reason for stopping should be noted. Once the subject has signalled intolerance, cycle resistance should be reduced to zero or the treadmill should be slowed to minimum with no incline, and cycling or walking should continue for a further few minutes or so. Monitoring should continue until heart rate and gas exchange have returned to resting values.

What is peak exercise?

The point at which an increased work rate does not lead to an increase in $\dot{V}O_2$ is defined as '$\dot{V}O_2$max'. In most untrained subjects (and especially patients with heart failure), $\dot{V}O_2$max is rarely reached before exercise is discontinued due to symptoms of fatigue or dyspnoea.[59] In the absence of any confirmatory evidence that $\dot{V}O_2$max has been attained,[60] the oxygen uptake at termination of exercise is peak $\dot{V}O_2$ (p$\dot{V}O_2$). RER <1 is regarded as a sign of submaximal test and the data must be interpreted in light of this.[59]

RER consistently >1.0 at the end of exercise suggests that close to peak exercise has been performed.[61] The prognostic value of p$\dot{V}O_2$ depends largely on the RER at peak.[24,62] The anaerobic threshold can be used to extrapolate $\dot{V}O_2$max, but, although useful, extrapolated $\dot{V}O_2$max is less reliable than peak $\dot{V}O_2$.[63]

Box 27.1 Variables to be reported from an exercise test with metabolic gas exchange

- Indication
- Demographics: age, height, weight, BMI
- Baseline findings
- Exercise modality
- Exercise protocol
- Collection method—mask vs mouthpiece
- Reasons for stopping exercise
- Complications
- Rating of perceived exertion (max score)
- Resting and peak heart rate and blood pressure
- Resting and peak $\dot{V}O_2$ and anaerobic threshold
- $\dot{V}E/\dot{V}CO_2$ slope
- Electrocardiogram changes—ischaemia
- Possible aetiology of exercise impairment

Analysis and interpretation

The data from the last 20 to 30 s of exercise are averaged to give peak ventilation ($\dot{V}E$), oxygen uptake ($\dot{V}O_2$), and carbon dioxide output ($\dot{V}CO_2$). The anaerobic threshold (AT) is also estimated and reported from gas exchange data (**Box 27.1**).

Safety of cardiopulmonary exercise testing and contraindications

Peak symptom-limited exercise testing using either a treadmill or cycle in a controlled setting is safe. In the largest published series of exercise testing in >6000 men assessed for possible ischaemic heart disease, there were no deaths and the incidence of ventricular tachycardia, defined as three or more consecutive beats, was 1.1%.[64] In another series of 289 patients with severe left ventricular dysfunction (<35%), only one resuscitated cardiac arrest with ventricular fibrillation occurred, and non-sustained ventricular tachycardia occurred in 20%, with hypotension in 5%.[65] In a larger population of 2037 heart failure patients in whom 4411 exercise tests were performed (HF-ACTION study), the death rate was zero per 1000 exercise tests and the major cardiac event rate was 0.45 per 1000 exercise tests, this being the result of one episode of ventricular fibrillation and one episode of sustained ventricular tachycardia.[66]

Abnormalities of pulmonary gas exchange in chronic heart failure patients

Patients with CHF typically have a reduced exercise time, lower than predicted peak $\dot{V}O_2$, and a higher than normal slope of the relationship between $\dot{V}E$ and $\dot{V}CO_2$ (**Figure 27.3**). The $\dot{V}E/\dot{V}CO_2$ slope and peak $\dot{V}O_2$ are inversely related to each other and both are independently related to prognosis (**Figures 27.5** and **27.7**).

Reduced oxygen uptake—cardiac or peripheral

The aetiology of the impaired exercise capacity in patients with CHF remains incompletely understood. The haemodynamic hypothesis suggests that in certain individuals there is a single dominant pathology, either increased pulmonary fluid leading to breathlessness or poor skeletal muscle perfusion causing fatigue. However, regardless of the limiting symptom experienced during an exercise test,

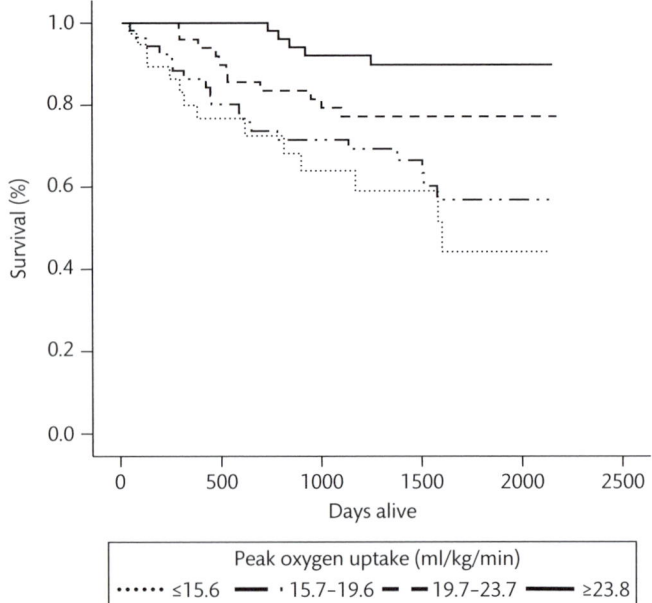

Figure 27.7 The prognostic information from peak oxygen uptake by quartiles.

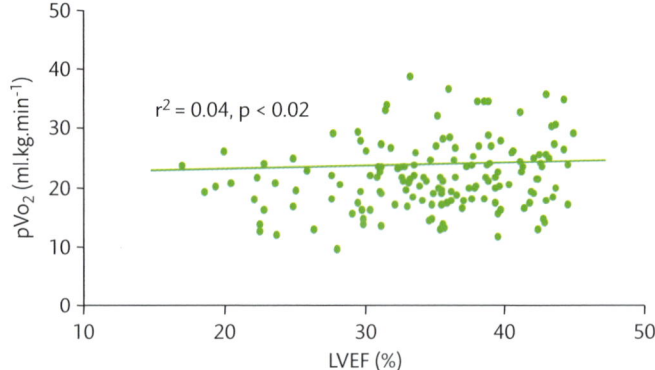

Figure 27.8 The poor relationship between left ventricular function (left ventricular ejection fraction; LVEF) and peak oxygen uptake.

objective measures of exercise tolerance are similar in patient cohorts whichever symptom is dominant,[67] and the prognosis is related to the peak $\dot{V}o_2$ achieved and not the nature of the symptoms experienced.[68] Furthermore, the type of exercise performed seems to influence whether individuals suffer breathlessness or fatigue. Slowly incrementing tests and cycle exercise are more likely to lead to fatigue;[69] in contrast, rapidly incremental exercise tests more frequently lead to breathlessness. Cycle exercise is more often stopped by fatigue than breathlessness compared with treadmill exercise, even when the same level of exercise is performed.[70,71] These findings suggest that there is a common underlying pathology resulting in symptoms; and that the symptoms are variably reported by patients depending upon context.

Central haemodynamics

Many studies have failed to show a significant link between exercise performance and left ventricular performance (**Figure 27.8**).[72–78] Furthermore, acute increases in resting cardiac contractility through inotropes[79–80] or cardiac transplantation,[81,82] increased cardiac output following mitral valvuloplasty,[83] and conversely, reductions in contractility and heart rate rise with β-blockers,[47] have no immediate impact on exercise capacity. By contrast, although exercise training can lead to impressive increases in exercise capacity which appear after a prolonged period of training, it has no effect on cardiac function.[84,85]

Chronotropic incompetence

Patients with CHF have a lower heart rate rise during exercise. This has been suggested as an aetiological factor for the exercise intolerance in CHF. However, heart rate limitation seems not to reduce peak $\dot{V}o_2$ in CHF patients,[47,48] and increasing heart rate during exercise also has no beneficial effect.[49,86] It is therefore unlikely that chronotropic incompetence is a mediator, but rather a marker of impaired exercise capacity.[87,88] As such, however, it is of course related to outcome in the same manner as other peak variables.

Lung function

Many investigators have described abnormalities of pulmonary function in patients with CHF. Spirometric variables are variously reported to be abnormal in heart failure,[89] although large numbers of patients have normal spirometry.[90,91] Nevertheless, some spirometric indices do correlate with exercise capacity,[92] especially in patients with more modest symptoms.[93]

Large airways function is abnormal in some patients with CHF,[94] but although there was some reversibility of airways obstruction with nebulized β-agonists, this had no effect on exercise capacity.[95]

Bronchoconstriction is a major component of acute pulmonary oedema.[96,97] Cabanes *et al.* suggested that there was an increase in bronchial reactivity in patients with heart failure.[98] The effect could be partially reversed with albuterol, a β-stimulant and, paradoxically, with inhaled methoxamine, a bronchoconstrictor.[99] The hypothesis here was that if left atrial pressure increased as a result of exercise, the veins draining the distal bronchi into the left atrium might become congested, and methoxamine would improve exercise capacity by constricting these vessels. However, others have found no increase in bronchial hyperresponsiveness to stimulation with methacholine or sodium metabisulphite, no change in cough responsiveness to capsaicin, and no evidence for exercise-induced bronchospasm.[100]

Patients with CHF also have impaired transalveolar diffusion as measured by transcapillary carbon monoxide diffusion (DLco).[101] DLco is directly related to exercise capacity,[102] and the increased ventilatory response during exercise,[103] and hence is a prognostic marker.[104] It can be improved by angiotensin converting enzyme inhibitors (an effect countered by aspirin),[105] exercise training,[106] and sildenafil,[107] but not by ultrafiltration,[108] suggesting that the cause of the impaired diffusion is vascular, possibly endothelial, rather than being related to lung blood volume or haemodynamic status.

Diaphragmatic weakness has been implicated in the symptomatology of CHF. The histological abnormalities seen in the skeletal muscle of heart failure patients (see below), are also seen in the diaphragm.[109] The ability to generate negative intrathoracic pressure is slightly reduced in heart failure patients when compared with controls.[110] This weakness, combined with reduced lung compliance leading to increased diaphragmatic work, especially in the supine position,[111] suggests that respiratory muscle dysfunction could contribute to exercise limitation. However, overall diaphragmatic strength at rest appears to be well preserved,[112,113] and contractile

diaphragmatic fatigue is uncommon in CHF patients during an exercise test.[114]

Finally, patients ventilate at the same proportion of their maximum ventilatory volume at peak exercise as control subjects, further refuting the suggestion that ventilatory capacity limits exercise in CHF.[115] However, as is discussed generally in relation to skeletal muscle, diaphragmatic fatigue, when present, causes sympathetic activation and reduction in leg blood flow.[116,117] These changes could potentially contribute to the cycle of impaired muscle perfusion, worsening of the skeletal myopathy, and the abnormal ventilatory response to exercise.

Ventilation–perfusion mismatching

Ventilation–perfusion matching in the lung is commonly abnormal in patients with CHF. Ventilation, V, and perfusion, Q, are ideally equal, leading to a V/Q ratio of 1.0 in an idealized lung unit. Where perfusion is greater than ventilation ($V/Q < 1.0$), there is effectively shunting of venous blood; where ventilation is greater than perfusion ($V/Q > 1.0$), there is 'wasted ventilation', or dead space. At rest in upright normal subjects, for example, there is a gradient of V/Q ratios from apex to base of the lung leading to dead space in the apices.

Increased dead space may be a cause of the elevated $\dot{V}E/\dot{V}CO_2$ slope. Equation (27.1) suggests that when $\dot{V}E/\dot{V}CO_2$ is increased, if $PaCO_2$ is constant, then V_D/V_T must be increased. However, whilst this may be true, it does not imply that increased dead space ventilation is the cause of the increased $\dot{V}E/\dot{V}CO_2$ slope. Several lines of evidence suggest that it may not be. First, the exercise hyperventilation seen during exercise in CHF patients is present from the outset of exercise[118,119] whereas any abnormalities in blood chemistry and increases in dead space ventilation would worsen as exercise progresses. Secondly, although during submaximal exercise V_D/V_T is higher in patients than in controls, at peak exercise controls have a higher absolute dead space ventilation than patients.[91] Furthermore, some data suggest that apical lung perfusion is increased in heart failure patients at rest compared with controls[120] (which leads to better V/Q matching) and it does not deteriorate during exercise.[120] Third, β-blockade with carvedilol reduces hyperventilation without changing V_D/V_T.[20] Finally, correcting for the increased dead space ventilation due to breathing frequency in CHF patients does not weaken the correlation between the increased ventilatory response to exercise and peak $\dot{V}O_2$,[33] and increasing anatomical dead space in normal subjects does not cause an increase in the $\dot{V}E/\dot{V}CO_2$ slope.[121]

A conceptual problem with all hypotheses for the origin of the increased $\dot{V}E/\dot{V}CO_2$ in heart failure that rely on pulmonary pathology is the absence of a physiological signal. Arterial blood gas tensions are normal or supranormal during exercise in patients with heart failure with a higher PaO_2 and lower $PaCO_2$ than in normal subjects.[122,123] Indeed, where blood gas tensions are abnormal, there is usually another explanation for the symptoms of breathlessness.[123] There is no dead space ventilation detector, and how increased dead space ventilation would be communicated to the respiratory centres in order to stimulate 'compensatory' hyperventilation is unclear. On the other hand, if there were a stimulus to excess ventilation arising outside the lungs, there would be a tendency for an excessive fall in arterial CO_2. Increasing dead space ventilation might thus be a physiological response to prevent even greater reductions in $PaCO_2$.

Peripheral haemodynamics

In CHF, despite impaired ventricular function, the blood pressure response to exercise is not usually abnormal (particularly at submaximal work rates),[124] as a consequence of increased peripheral resistance.[125,126] The increased peripheral vascular resistance is a result of chronically increased sympathetic tone and renin–angiotensin system activation. There is arterial smooth muscle hypertrophy and activation of fibroblasts with hyalinosis of the vascular wall.[127] These changes lead to reduced arterial compliance[128] and hence to poor vasodilation in skeletal muscle arterioles during exercise.[129]

In addition, there is a reduced response to endogenous vasodilatory stimuli,[130,131] to infused hyperosmolar solutions,[132] and to pharmacological agents.[133] There are also increased in levels of endothelin, a powerful vasoconstrictor.[134]

Skeletal muscles

The skeletal muscles are abnormal in patients with CHF. There is a general reduction in muscle bulk early in the course of heart failure,[135] and there is a shift from type I (slow twitch) to type IIb (fast twitch) fibres within skeletal muscles.[136] Type IIb fibres are more easily fatiguable and have less aerobic capacity than type I fibres. Capillary density is also reduced.[137] Hence there is an earlier need for anaerobic metabolism during exercise than normal. It is also becoming clear that perfusion within muscles and fibre recruitment may be impaired in CHF,[138] and muscle strength is also reduced,[139] as is endurance.[135] Exercise capacity in heart failure patients is related to both muscle strength and bulk,[140-142] and the reduction in endurance correlates with exercise performance.[143]

From a patient's point of view, the ability to perform repeated submaximal exercise (endurance) may be more important than peak force generation (strength), and early quadriceps fatiguability has been reported.[135,144] Fatigue is independent of acute changes in blood flow[145,146] and of central factors.[147] Fatiguability has been shown in a very small muscle group[148] in which blood flow is unlikely to be limited by cardiac reserve, suggesting that intrinsic muscle factors mediate fatiguability. It is not difficult to imagine how such abnormal muscles might lead to fatigue, but it is less clear how they might lead to breathlessness.

Ergoreceptors are muscle receptors sensitive to work. Stimulation of the receptors during exercise leads to ventilation and sympathetic activation—the ergoreflex. The degree of activation is in part related to the work performed per unit of muscle mass and to the metabolic state of the muscle. In normal subjects, for example, the ventilatory response to a given work rate is much greater if the work is performed by arms rather than legs.[149] Furthermore, when normal subjects exercise with cuffs inflated to suprasystolic pressure, thus preventing the washout of the metabolic products of exercise, the ventilatory response to exercise is greater than in the control situation.[149]

The ergoreflex can be quantified by experiments involving cuff inflation around an exercising limb. During exercise in a normal subject, ventilation progressively increases with an increase in vascular resistance in the non-exercising limbs. There is a swift return to normal at the end of exercise. If a cuff is inflated at peak exercise proximal to the exercising muscle, the muscle is 'frozen' in its exercising state.[150] The consequent persisting increase in ventilation compared with the control response is the ergoreflex response.[151] In heart failure patients, presumably due to skeletal muscle abnormalities, the ergoreflex response

generated by post-exercise regional circulatory occlusion is much greater, both in terms of haemodynamic responses and in terms of the ventilatory response.[152,153] The reflex is sensitive to metabolic stimulation rather than movement.[154] The increased ventilatory response to exercise is proportional to the increased ergoreflex activity,[152] and a training programme can reduce the contribution of the ergoreflex to ventilation,[152] presumably due to physiological adaptations within the skeletal muscles that increase aerobic capacity.

The precise exercise stimulus responsible for triggering the ergoreflex is not clear. Possibilities include potassium, particularly as arterial potassium rises on exercise,[155,156] mirroring closely the increase in ventilation.[157] However, potassium rises during exercise do not demonstrate an inflection similar to that seen in the rise in ventilation during heavy exercise.[158] Furthermore, β-blockers lead to a greater rise in arterial potassium for a given workload, but do not increase minute ventilation.[159] Another possible contributor is prostaglandin production, as local prostaglandin levels in exercising muscle correlate with the ventilatory response.[160] However, patients taking regular aspirin, a powerful inhibitor of inflammatory prostaglandin production, do not demonstrate a clinically significant difference in ventilatory response to exercise compared with those not taking aspirin.[161]

In addition to a metabolic response to exercise, there are suggestions that nerve fibres sensitive to stretch might be involved in the response to ventilation. Muscle sympathetic nerve activity (MSNA) is related to the $\dot{V}E/\dot{V}CO_2$ slope in CHF patients,[162] and passive limb movement leads to an increase in MSNA in CHF patients but not controls,[163] proportional to heart failure severity.[164] This suggests the existence of a mechanoreflex in addition to the metaboreflex.

The concept that peripheral muscle receptors sensitive to work, whether they be metabo- or mechanoreceptors, contribute to ventilation, and that this reflex is abnormal in patients with CHF, provides an elegant and unifying hypothesis explaining both breathlessness and fatigue in these patients.[165] Patients with heart failure have weak, structurally abnormal skeletal muscles, which are performing more work per unit muscle volume than normal muscle. In turn, this results in greater production of the metabolic products of exercise in the context of impaired perfusion. This leads to an increased stimulation of ergoreceptors sensitive to metabolic products, which stimulate increased ventilation relative to carbon dioxide output, thus increasing the $\dot{V}E/\dot{V}CO_2$ slope and reducing $P_{a}CO_2$.

Sympathetic activation and ventilation

The increased sympathetic activation of CHF may also contribute to the ventilatory response to exercise. Acute and chronic β-blockade, although having little effect on maximal[166] or submaximal exercise capacity,[167,168] reduces submaximal and maximal ventilation during exercise, and also reduces the $\dot{V}E/\dot{V}CO_2$ slope.[47,48] On the other hand, increasing presynaptic catecholamine levels leads to an increase in ventilation in normal subjects, perhaps by sensitizing the ergoreceptors.[169]

Use of data from pulmonary gas exchange variables

Diagnosis, prognosis, and transplant assessment

In subjects referred for investigation of symptoms of breathlessness and fatigue, a carefully performed exercise test provides an objective measure of exercise capacity. Cardiopulmonary exercise testing gives an overall assessment of the severity of the pathophysiology of CHF, integrating skeletal muscle, lung, endothelial, and cardiac function.

Perhaps more than other single clinical measures, peak $\dot{V}O_2$ is a sensitive predictor of morbidity and mortality.[88,170] Peak $\dot{V}O_2$ of <14 mL/kg/min has been used as a functional criterion for selecting patients for cardiac transplantation.[148] However, since the incorporation of β-blockers into routine management, patients have a better outlook for a given exercise capacity, and a peak $\dot{V}O_2$ of around 10–12 mL/kg/min is increasingly used as the cut-off for identifying patients at especially high risk who might therefore benefit from transplantation.[145] Nevertheless, the value of peak $\dot{V}O_2$ as a risk assessment tool remains in the presence of optimal medical therapy,[147,171,172] and referral for transplant assessment can safely be deferred in patients with peak $\dot{V}O_2$ >18 mL/kg/min.

More recently, it has become clear that an elevated $\dot{V}E/\dot{V}CO_2$ slope provides additional and independent prognostic information, and unlike peak $\dot{V}O_2$ does not require maximal effort.[173] Combining peak $\dot{V}O_2$ and $\dot{V}E/\dot{V}CO_2$ slope improves risk assessment in some[174] but not all studies.[44]

Differential diagnosis

Cardiopulmonary exercise (CPX) testing not only may aid with prognostic assessment but also may assist in establishing the cause of symptoms of exercise intolerance in an individual. The most common differential diagnoses are chronic obstructive pulmonary disease, obesity, psychogenic hyperventilation, and poor effort. Data collected during a routine CPX test can add to clinical information and data from non-invasive imaging. Table 27.3 shows the CPX variables seen with important differential diagnoses.

Response to therapy

With aggressive neurohormonal blockade, appropriate device therapy and careful hospital and community-based management programmes, mortality rates of <10% and hospitalization rates of <20% per annum can be achieved for many patients with CHF. Contemporary randomized, placebo-controlled studies exploring the effects of new therapies on mortality and morbidity therefore require ever-increasing numbers of subjects. As a non-invasive, reproducible, and repeatable surrogate for outcome and an objective measure of heart failure severity, exercise testing with or without pulmonary gas exchange is increasingly used as an end-point in studies in CHF. Improvements in exercise capacity in smaller studies can also help plan larger mortality studies. So, for example, early studies of cardiac resynchronization therapy showed improvements in exercise capacity,[175-177] allowing better planning of the CARE-HF study using the earlier studies as a guide.[178]

Conclusions

In addition to helping with diagnosis in patients presenting with symptoms of exercise intolerance, CPX testing provides reliable and objective information on prognosis in patients with CHF and can be used to stratify patients requiring transplant assessment. Exercise testing is non-invasive and low risk and can be

Table 27.3 Results from cardiopulmonary exercise testing in patients with differential diagnoses

Variable	Chronic heart failure	Chronic obstructive airways disease	Obesity	Hyperventilation	Poor effort
$p\dot{V}O_2$	↓	↓	↓	↓	↓
AT	↓	↔/↓	↓	↔	Often impossible to determine or normal
RER at peak	↔	↔	↔	↓ at peak	↓
$\dot{V}E/\dot{V}CO_2$	↑	↑	↑/↔	↑/↔	↑/↔
Breathing reserve	↔/↑	↓	↑	↑	↓
Vital capacity	↓	↑	↓	↔	↑
$P_{et}CO_2$	↑	↑	↔	↓	↔
Comments	Reduced $\Delta \dot{V}O_2/\Delta WR$, oscillatory breathing	Increased dead space, FEV_1 low	Physical examination confirms obesity	RER and ventilation ↑ prior to exercise, abrupt further increase in ventilation at onset of exercise	

$p\dot{V}O_2$, peak oxygen uptake; RER, respiratory exchange ratio; $\dot{V}E/\dot{V}CO_2$, relationship between ventilation and carbon dioxide output; $P_{et}CO_2$, end tidal carbon dioxide; $\Delta\dot{V}O_2/\Delta WR$, ratio between change in oxygen uptake and change in work rate.

easily repeated in order to monitor responses to therapy, in both daily clinical practice and research settings. However, the test must be carried out and interpreted in a controlled manner by experienced staff.

REFERENCES

1. Myers J, Prakash M, Froelicher V, *et al*. Exercise capacity and mortality among men referred for exercise testing. *N Engl J Med* 2002;**346**:793–801.
2. Clark AL, Coats AJS. Exercise endpoints in chronic heart failure. *Int J Cardiol* 2000;**73**:61–6.
3. Willens HJ, Blevins RD, Wrisley D, *et al*. The prognostic value of functional capacity in patients with mild to moderate heart failure. *Am Heart J* 1987;**114**:377–82.
4. Cohn JN, Johnson GR, Shabetai R, *et al*. Ejection fraction, peak exercise oxygen consumption, cardiothoracic ratio, ventricular arrhythmias, and plasma norepinephrine as determinants of prognosis in heart failure. The V-HeFT VA Cooperative Studies Group. *Circulation* 1993;**87**(6 Suppl):VI5–16.
5. Francis GS, Goldsmith SR, Cohn JN. Relationship of exercise capacity to resting left ventricular performance and basal plasma norepinephrine levels in patients with congestive heart failure. *Am Heart J* 1982;**104**(4 Pt 1):725–31.
6. Hsich E, Gorodeski EZ, Starling RC, *et al*. Importance of treadmill exercise time as an initial prognostic screening tool in patients with systolic left ventricular dysfunction. *Circulation* 2009;**119**:3189–97.
7. Myers J. *Essential of cardiopulmonary exercise testing*. Human Kinetics, Champaign, IL, 1996.
8. Stelken AM, Younis LT, Jennison SH, *et al*. Prognostic value of cardiopulmonary exercise testing using percent achieved of predicted peak oxygen uptake for patients with ischemic and dilated cardiomyopathy. *J Am Coll Cardiol* 1996;**27**:345–52.
9. Myers J, Gullestad L, Vagelos R, *et al*. Clinical, hemodynamic, and cardiopulmonary exercise test determinants of survival in patients referred for evaluation of heart failure. *Ann Intern Med* 1998;**129**(4):286–93.
10. Keteyian SJ, Patel M, Kraus WE, *et al*.; HF-ACTION Investigators. Variables measured during cardiopulmonary

exercise testing as predictors of mortality in chronic systolic heart failure. *J Am Coll Cardiol* 2016;**67**:780–9.
11. Shafiq A, Brawner CA, Aldred HA, *et al*. Prognostic value of cardiopulmonary exercise testing in heart failure with preserved ejection fraction. The Henry Ford HospITal CardioPulmonary EXercise Testing (FIT-CPX) project. *Am Heart J* 2016;**174**:167–72.
12. Taylor HL, Buskirk E, Henschel A. Maximal oxygen intake as an objective measure of cardiorespiratory performance. *J Appl Physiol* 1955;**8**:73–80.
13. Andersen P. Saltin B. Maximal perfusion of skeletal muscle in man. *J Appl Physiol* 1985;**366**:233–49.
14. Vogel JA, Gleser MA. Effect of carbon monoxide on oxygen transport during exercise. *J Appl Physiol* 1972;**32**:234–9.
15. Whipp BJ, Ward SA. Coupling of ventilation to pulmonary gas axchange during exercise. In Whipp BJ, Wasserman K (eds), *Exercise: pulmonary physiology and pathophysiology*, p. 275. Marcel Dekker, New York, 1991.
16. Whipp BJ. Ventilatory control during exercise in humans. *Annu Rev Physiol* 1983;**45**:393–412.
17. Brown SE, Wiener S, Brown RA, Maratelli PA, Light RW. Exercise performance following a carbohydrate load in chronic airflow obstruction. *Am J Appl Physiol* 1985;**58**:1340–6.
18. Wasserman K, Van Kessel AL, Burton GB. Interaction of physiological mechanisms during exercise. *J Appl Physiol* 1967;**22**:71–85.
19. Cassaburi R, Whipp BJ, Wasserman K, Beaver WL, Koyal SN. Ventilatory and gas exchange dynamics in response to sinusoidal work. *J Appl Physiol Respir Environ Exercise Physiol* 1977;**42**:300–11.
20. Agostoni P, Contini M, Magini A, *et al*. Carvedilol reduces exercise-induced hyperventilation: a benefit in normoxia and a problem with hypoxia. *Eur J Heart Fail* 2006;**8**:729–35.
21. Witte KK, Thackray SD, Nikitin NP, Cleland JG, Clark AL. Pattern of ventilation during exercise in chronic heart failure. *Heart* 2003;**89**:610–14.
22. Arena R, Myers J, Aslam SS, Varughese EB, Peberdy MA. Peak VO2 and VE/VCO2 slope in patients with heart failure: a prognostic comparison. *Am Heart J* 2004;**147**:354–60.
23. Mezzani A, Corra U, Bosimini E, Giordano A, Giannuzzi P. Contribution of peak respiratory exchange ratio to peak VO2

prognostic reliability in patients with chronic heart failure and severely reduced exercise capacity. *Am Heart J* 2003;**145**:1102–7.

24. Ingle L, Witte KK, Cleland JG, Clark AL. The prognostic value of cardiopulmonary exercise testing with a peak respiratory exchange ratio of <1.0 in patients with chronic heart failure. *Int J Cardiol* 2008;**127**:88–92.

25. Stringer W, Wasserman K, Casaburi R. The VCO2/VO2 relationship during heavy, constant work rate exercise reflects the rate of lactic acid accumulation. *Eur J Appl Physiol Occup Physiol* 1995;**72**:25–31.

26. Hughson RH, Weisiger KW, Swanson GD. Blood lactate concentration increases as a continuous function in progressive exercise. *J Appl Physiol* 1987;**62**:1975–81.

27. Simonton CA, Higginbotham MB, Cobb FR. The ventilatory threshold: quantitative analysis of reproducibility and relation to arterial lactate concentration in normal subjects and in patients with chronic congestive heart failure. *Am J Cardiol* 1988;**62**:100–7.

28. Hoh H, Taniguchi K, Koike A, Doi M. Evaluation of severity of heart failure using ventilatory gas analysis. *Circulation* 1990;**81**(1 Suppl 2):II31–II37.

29. Lipkin DP, Bayliss J, Poole-Wilson PA. The ability of a submaximal exercise test to predict maximal exercise capacity in patients with heart failure. *Eur Heart J* 1985;**6**:829–33.

30. Cohen-Solal A, Zannad F, Kayanakis JG, *et al*. Multicentre study of the determination of peak oxygen uptake and ventilatory threshold during bicycle exercise in chronic heart failure. Comparison of graphical methods, interobserver variability and influence of the exercise protocol. The VO2 French Study Group. *Eur Heart J* 1991;**12**:1055–63.

31. Whipp BJ, Ward SA, Wasserman K. Respiratory markers of the anaerobic threshold. *Adv Cardiol* 1986;**35**:47–64.

32. Wasserman K, Hansen J, Sue D, Stringer W, Whipp B (eds). *Principles of exercise testing and interpretation: including pathophysiology and clinical applications*, 5th edn, pp. 71–107. Lippincott Williams & Wilkins, Philadelphia, 2011.

33. Buller NP, Poole-Wilson PA. Mechanism of the increased ventilatory response to exercise in patients with chronic heart failure. *Br Heart J* 1990;**63**:281–3.

34. Francis DP, Shamim W, Davies LC, *et al*. Cardiopulmonary exercise testing for prognosis in chronic heart failure: continuous and independent prognostic value from VE/VCO2 slope and peak VO2. *Eur Heart J* 2000;**21**:154–61.

35. Davies SW, Emery TM, Watling MIL, Wannamethee G, Lipkin DP. A critical threshold of exercise capacity in the ventilatory response to exercise in heart failure. *Br Heart J* 1991;**65**:179–83.

36. Corrà U, Giordano A, Bosimini E, *et al*. Oscillatory ventilation during exercise in patients with chronic heart failure: clinical correlates and prognostic implications. *Chest* 2002;**121**(5):1572–80.

37. Leite JJ, Mansur AJ, de Freitas HF, *et al*. Periodic breathing during incremental exercise predicts mortality in patients with chronic heart failure evaluated for cardiac transplantation. *J Am Coll Cardiol* 2003;**41**(12):2175–81.

38. Ingle L, Isted A, Witte KK, Cleland JG, Clark AL. Impact of different diagnostic criteria on the prevalence and prognostic significance of exertional oscillatory ventilation in patients with chronic heart failure. *Eur J Cardiovasc Prev Rehabil* 2009;**16**(4):451–6.

39. Baba R, Nagashima M, Goto M, *et al*. Oxygen uptake efficiency slope: a new index of cardiorespiratory functional reserve derived from the relation between oxygen uptake and minute ventilation during incremental exercise. *J Am Coll Cardiol* 1996;**28**:1567–72.

40. Ueshima K, Myers J, Ribisl PM, *et al*. Hemodynamic determinants of exercise capacity in chronic atrial fibrillation. *Am Heart J* 1993;**125**:1301–5.

41. Defoor J, Schepers D, Reybrouck T, Fagard R, Vanhees L. Oxygen uptake efficiency slope in coronary artery disease: clinical use and response to training. *Int J Sports Med* 2006;**27**:730–7.

42. Davies LC, Wensel R, Georgiadou P, *et al*. Enhanced prognostic value from cardiopulmonary exercise testing in chronic heart failure by non-linear analysis: oxygen uptake efficiency slope. *Eur Heart J* 2006;**27**(6):684–90.

43. Williams SG, Cooke GA, Wright DJ, *et al*. Peak exercise cardiac power output; a direct indicator of cardiac function strongly predictive of prognosis in chronic heart failure. *Eur Heart J* 2001;**22**:1496–503.

44. Ingle L, Witte KK, Cleland JG, Clark AL. Combining the ventilatory response to exercise and peak oxygen consumption is no better than peak oxygen consumption alone in predicting mortality in chronic heart failure. *Eur J Heart Fail* 2008;**10**:85–8.

45. Witte KK, Thackray SD, Lindsay KA, Cleland JG, Clark AL. Metabolic gas kinetics depend upon the level of exercise performed. *Eur J Heart Fail* 2005;**7**:991–6.

46. Samejima H, Omiya K, Uno M, *et al*. Relationship between impaired chronotropic response, cardiac output during exercise, and exercise tolerance in patients with chronic heart failure. *Jpn Heart J* 2003;**44**:515–25.

47. Witte KKA, Thackray SDR, Nikitin NP, Cleland JGF, Clark AL. The effects of α- and β-blockade on ventilatory responses to exercise in chronic heart failure. *Heart* 2003;**89**:1169–73.

48. Witte KKA, Nikitin NP, Cleland JGF, Clark AL. The effects of long-term β-blockade on the ventilatory responses to exercise in chronic heart failure. *Eur J Heart Fail* 2005;**4**:612–17.

49. Jamil HA, Gierula J, Paton MF, *et al*. Chronotropic incompetence does not limit exercise capacity in chronic heart failure. *J Am Coll Cardiol* 2016;**67**:1885–96.

50. Proctor DN, Beck KC. Delay time adjustments to minimize errors in breath-by-breath measurement of VO_2 during exercise. *J Appl Physiol* 1996;**81**(6):2495–9.

51. Borg G. Subjective effort and physical activities. *Scand J Rehab* 1978;**6**:108–13.

52. Jones RS, Buston MH, Wharton MJ. The effect of exercise on ventilatory function in the child with asthma. *Br J Dis Chest* 1962;**56**:78–86.

53. Buchfuhrer MJ, Hansen JE, Robinson TE, *et al*. Optimizing the exercise protocol for cardiopulmonary assessment. *J Appl Physiol* 1983;**55**:1558–64.

54. Bruce PA, McDonough IR. Stress testing in screening for cardiovascular disease. *Bull NY Acad Med* 1969;**45**:1288–1305.

55. Balke B, Ware RW. An experimental study of physical fitness of Air Force personnel. *US Armed Forces Med J* 1959;**10**:675–88.

56. Nagle FJ, Balke B, Naughton JP. Gradational step tests for assessing work capacity. *J Appl Physiol* 1965;**20**:745–8.

57. Porszasz J, Casaburi R, Somfay A, Woodhouse LJ, Whipp BJ. A treadmill ramp protocol using simultaneous changes in speed and grade. *Med Sci Sports Exerc* 2003;**35**:1596–603.

58. McConnell TR, Clark BA III. Prediction of maximal oxygen consumption during handrail-supported treadmill exercise. *J Cardiopulm Rehabil* 1987;**7**:324–31.

59. Ramos-Barbon D, Fitchett D, Gibbons WJ, Latter DA, Levy RD. Maximal exercise testing for the selection of heart transplantation

candidates: limitation of peak oxygen consumption. *Chest* 1999;**115**:410–17.

60. Bowen TS, Cannon DT, Begg G, *et al*. A novel cardiopulmonary exercise test protocol and criterion to determine maximal oxygen uptake in chronic heart failure. *J Appl Physiol* 2012;**113**(3):451–8.

61. Dickstein K, Aarsland T, Svanes H, Barvik S. A respiratory exchange ratio equal to 1 provides a reproducible index of submaximal cardiopulmonary exercise performance. *Am J Cardiol* 1993;**71**:1367–9.

62. Mezzani A, Corra U, Bosimini E, Giordano A, Giannuzzi P. Contribution of peak respiratory exchange ratio to peak VO2 prognostic reliability in patients with chronic heart failure and severely reduced exercise capacity. *Am Heart J* 2003;**145**:1102–7.

63. Butler NP, Poole-Wilson PA. Extrapolated maximal oxygen consumption. A new method for the objective analysis of respiratory gas exchange during exercise. *B Heart J* 1988;**59**:212–17.

64. Myers J, Prakash M, Froelicher V, *et al*. Exercise capacity and mortality among men referred for exercise testing. *N Engl J Med* 2002;**346**:793–801.

65. Squires RW, Allison TG, Johnson BD, Gau GT. Non-physician supervision of cardiopulmonary exercise testing in chronic heart failure: safety and results of a preliminary investigation. *J Cardiopulm Rehabil* 1999;**19**:249–53.

66. Keteyian SJ, Isaac D, Thadani U, *et al*.; HF-ACTION Investigators. Safety of symptom-limited cardiopulmonary exercise testing in patients with chronic heart failure due to severe left ventricular systolic dysfunction. *Am Heart J* 2009;**158**(4 Suppl):S72 7.

67. Clark AL, Sparrow JL, Coats AJ. Muscle fatigue and dyspnoea in chronic heart failure: two sides of the same coin? *Eur Heart J* 1995;**16**:49–52.

68. Witte KK, Clark AL. Dyspnoea versus fatigue: additional prognostic information from symptoms in chronic heart failure? *Eur J Heart Fail* 2008;**10**:1224–8.

69. Lipkin DP, Canepa-Anson R, Stephens MR, Poole-Wilson PA. Factors determining symptoms in heart failure: comparison of fast and slow exercise tests. *Br Heart J* 1986;**55**:439–45.

70. Fink LI, Wilson JR, Ferraro N. Exercise ventilation and pulmonary artery wedge pressure in chronic stable congestive heart failure. *Am J Cardiol* 1986;**57**:249–53.

71. Witte KKA, Clark AL. Cycle exercise causes a lower ventilatory response to exercise in chronic heart failure. *Heart* 2005;**91**:225–6.

72. Witte KK, Nikitin NP, De Silva R, Cleland JG, Clark AL. Exercise capacity and cardiac function assessed by tissue Doppler imaging in chronic heart failure. *Heart* 2004;**90**:1144–50.

73. Clark AL, Swan JW, Laney R, *et al*. The role of right and left ventricular function in the ventilatory response to exercise in chronic heart failure. *Circulation* 1994;**89**:2062–9.

74. Chandrashekhar Y, Anand IS. Relation between major indices of prognosis in patients with chronic congestive heart failure: studies of maximal exercise oxygen consumption, neurohormones and ventricular function. *Indian Heart J* 1992;**44**:213–16.

75. Carell ES, Murali S, Schulman DS, Estrada-Quintero T, Uretsky BF. Maximal exercise tolerance in chronic congestive heart failure. Relationship to resting left ventricular function. *Chest* 1994;**106**:1746–52.

76. Davies SW, Fussell AL, Jordan SL, Poole-Wilson PA, Lipkin DP. Abnormal diastolic filling patterns in chronic heart failure—relationship to exercise capacity. *Eur Heart J* 1992;**13**:749–57.

77. Higginbotham MB, Morris KG, Conn EH, Coleman RE, Cobb FR. Determinants of variable exercise performance among patients with severe left ventricular dysfunction. *Am J Cardiol* 1983;**51**:52–60.

78. Benge W, Litchfield RL, Marcus ML. Exercise capacity in patients with severe left ventricular dysfunction. *Circulation* 1980;**61**:955–9.

79. Ribeiro JP, White HD, Arnold JM, Hartley LH, Colucci WS. Exercise responses before and after long-term treatment with oral milrinone in patients with severe heart failure. *Am J Med* 1986;**81**:759–64.

80. Petein M, Levine TB, Cohn JN. Persistent hemodynamic effects without long-term clinical benefits in response to oral piroximone (MDL 19,205) in patients with congestive heart failure. *Circulation* 1986;**73**(3 Pt 2):III230–6.

81. Leung TC, Ballman KV, Allison TG, *et al*. Clinical predictors of exercise capacity 1 year after cardiac transplantation. *J Heart Lung Transplant* 2003;**22**:16–27.

82. Douard H, Parrens E, Billes MA, *et al*. Predictive factors of maximal aerobic capacity after cardiac transplantation. *Eur Heart J* 1997;**18**:1823–8.

83. Marzo K, Herrmann HA, Rein A, Mancini D. Acute effect of balloon mitral valvuloplasty on exercise capacity ventilation and skeletal muscle oxygenation. *Circulation* 1991;**84** (Suppl II):11–72.

84. Smart N, Haluska B, Jeffriess L, Case C, Marwick TH. Cardiac contributions to exercise training responses in patients with chronic heart failure: a strain imaging study. *Echocardiography* 2006;**23**:376–82.

85. Jonsdottir S, Andersen KK, Sigurosson AF, Sigurosson SB. The effect of physical training in chronic heart failure. *Eur J Heart Fail* 2006;**8**:97–101.

86. Van Thielen G, Paelinck BP, Beckers P, Vrints CJ, Conraads VM. Rate response and cardiac resynchronisation therapy in chronic heart failure: higher cardiac output does not acutely improve exercise performance: a pilot trial. *Eur J Cardiovasc Prev Rehabil* 2008;**15**(2):197–202.

87. Witte KK, Clark AL. Chronotropic incompetence does not contribute to submaximal exercise limitation in patients with chronic heart failure. *Int J Cardiol* 2009;**134**:342–4.

88. Witte KK, Cleland JG, Clark AL. Chronic heart failure, chronotropic incompetence, and the effects of beta blockade. *Heart* 2006;**92**:481–6.

89. Moore DP, Weston AR, Hughes JMB, Oakley CM, Cleland JGF. Effects of increased inspired oxygen concentrations on exercise performance in chronic heart failure. *Lancet* 1992;**339**:850–3.

90. RS Wright, MS Levine, PE Bellamy, *et al*. Ventilatory and diffusion abnormalities in potential heart transplant recipients. *Chest* 1990;**98**:816–20.

91. Clark AL, Volterrani M, Swan JW, Coats AJS. Increased ventilatory response to exercise in chronic heart failure: relation to pulmonary pathology. *Heart* 1997;**77**:138–46.

92. Kraemer MD, Kubo SH, Rector TS, Brunsvold N, Bank AJ. Pulmonary and peripheral vascular factors are important determinants of peak exercise oxygen uptake in patients with heart failure. *J Am Coll Cardiol* 1993;**21**:641–8.

93. Ingle L, Shelton RJ, Cleland JG, Clark AL. Poor relationship between exercise capacity and spirometric measurements in patients with more symptomatic heart failure. *J Card Fail* 2005;**11**:619–23.

94. Witte KKA, Morice A, Clark AL, Cleland JGF. Airways resistance in chronic heart failure measured by impulse oscillometry. *J Cardiac Fail*. 2002;**8**:225–31.

95. Witte KKA, Morice A, Clark AL, Cleland JGF. The reversibility of airways resistance in chronic heart failure. *J Cardiac Fail* 2004;**10**:149–54.

96. Light RM, George RB. Serial pulmonary function in patients with acute heart failure. *Arch Intern Med* 1983;**143**:429–33.

97. Peterman W, Barth J, Entzian P. Heart failure and airways obstruction. *Int J Cardiol* 1987;**17**:207–9.

98. Cabanes LR, Weber SN, Matran R, *et al*. Bronchial hyperresponsiveness to methacholine in patients with impaired left ventricular function. *N Engl J Med* 1989;**320**:1317–22.

99. Cabanes L, Costes F, Weber S, *et al*. Improvement in exercise performance by inhalation of methoxamine in patients with impaired left ventricular function. *N Engl J Med* 1992;**326**:1661–5.

100. Chua TP, Lalloo UG, Worsdell MY, *et al*. Airway and cough responsiveness and exhaled nitric oxide in non-smoking patients with stable chronic heart failure. *Heart* 1996;**76**:144–49.

101. Puri S, Baker BL, Oakley CM, Hughes JM, Cleland JG. Increased alveolar/capillary membrane resistance to gas transfer in patients with chronic heart failure. *Br Heart J* 1994;**72**:140–4.

102. Puri S, Baker BL, Dutka DP, *et al*. Reduced alveolar-capillary membrane diffusing capacity in chronic heart failure. Its pathophysiological relevance and relationship to exercise performance. *Circulation* 1995;**91**:2769–74.

103. Smith AA, Cowburn PJ, Parker ME, *et al*. Impaired pulmonary diffusion during exercise in patients with chronic heart failure. *Circulation* 1999;**100**:1406–10.

104. Guazzi M, Pontone G, Brambilla R, Agostoni P, Reina G. Alveolar-capillary membrane gas conductance: a novel prognostic indicator in chronic heart failure. *Eur Heart J* 2002;**23**:467–76.

105. Guazzi M, Marenzi G, Alimento M, Contini M, Agostoni P. Improvement of alveolar-capillary membrane diffusing capacity with enalapril in chronic heart failure and counteracting effect of aspirin. *Circulation* 1997;**95**:1930–6.

106. Guazzi M, Reina G, Tumminello G, Guazzi MD. Improvement of alveolar-capillary membrane diffusing capacity with exercise training in chronic heart failure. *J Appl Physiol* 2004;**97**:1866–73.

107. Guazzi M, Tumminello G, Di Marco F, Fiorentini C, Guazzi MD. The effects of phosphodiesterase-5 inhibition with sildenafil on pulmonary hemodynamics and diffusion capacity, exercise ventilatory efficiency, and oxygen uptake kinetics in chronic heart failure. *J Am Coll Cardiol* 2004;**44**:2339–48.

108. Agostoni PG, Guazzi M, Bussotti M, *et al*. Lack of improvement of lung diffusing capacity following fluid withdrawal by ultrafiltration in chronic heart failure. *J Am Coll Cardiol* 2000;**36**:1600–4.

109. Lindsay DC, Lovegrove CA, Dunn MJ, *et al*. Histological abnormalities of muscle from limb, thorax and diaphragm in chronic heart failure. *Eur Heart J* 1996;**17**:1239–50.

110. Carmo MM, Barbara C, Ferreira T, *et al*. Diaphragmatic function in patients with chronic left ventricular failure. *Pathophysiology* 2001;**8**:55–60.

111. Nava S, Larovere MT, Fanfulla F, *et al*. Orthopnea and inspiratory effort in chronic heart failure patients. *Respir Med* 2003;**97**:647–53.

112. Hughes PD, Polkey MI, Harrus ML, *et al*. Diaphragm strength in chronic heart failure. *Am J Respir Crit Care Med* 1999;**160**:529–34.

113. Dayer MJ, Hopkinson NS, Ross ET, *et al*. Does symptom-limited cycle exercise cause low frequency diaphragm fatigue in patients with heart failure? *Eur J Heart Fail* 2006;**8**:68–73.

114. Kufel TJ, Pineda LA, Junega RG, Hathwar R, Mador MJ. Diaphragmatic function after intense exercise in congestive heart failure patients. *Eur Respir J* 2002;**20**:1399–405.

115. Clark AL, Davies LC, Francis DP, Coats AJ. Ventilatory capacity and exercise tolerance in patients with chronic stable heart failure. *Eur J Heart Fail* 2000;**2**:47–51.

116. St Croix CM, Morgan BJ, Wetter TJ, Dempsey JA. Reflex effects from a fatiguing diaphragm increase sympathetic efferent activity (MSNA) to limb muscle in humans. *J Physiol* 2000;**529**:493–504.

117. Sheel AW, Derchak PA, Morgan BJ, *et al*. Fatiguing inspiratory muscle work causes reflex reduction in resting leg blood flow in humans. *J Physiol* 2001;**537**(Pt 1):277–89.

118. Metra M, Dei Cas L, Panina G, Visioli O. Exercise hyperventilation chronic congestive heart failure, and its relation to functional capacity and hemodynamics. *Am J Cardiol* 1992;**70**:622–8.

119. Clark AL, Coats AJ. Relationship between ventilation and carbon dioxide production in normal subjects with induced changes in anatomical dead space. *Eur J Clin Invest* 1993;**23**:428–32.

120. Mohsenifar Z, Amin DK, Shah PK. Regional distribution of lung perfusion and ventilation in patients with chronic congestive heart failure and its relationship to cardiopulmonary hemodynamics. *Am Heart J* 1989;**117**:887–91.

121. Clark AL, Volterrani M, Piepoli M, Coats AJS. Factors which alter the relationship between ventilation and carbon dioxide production during exercise: implications for the understanding of the increased ventilatory response to exercise in chronic heart failure. *Eur J Appl Physiol* 1996;**73**:144–8.

122. Rubin SA, Brown HV. Ventilation and gas exchange during exercise in severe chronic heart failure. *Am Rev Respir Dis* 1984;**129**(2 Pt 2):S63–4.

123. Clark AL, Coats AJ. Usefulness of arterial blood gas estimations during exercise in patients with chronic heart failure. *Br Heart J* 1994;**71**:528–30.

124. Sullivan MJ, Knight JD, Higginbotham MB, Cobb FR. Relation between central and peripheral haemodynamics during exercise in patients with chronic heart failure. Muscle blood flow is reduced with maintenance of arterial perfusion pressure. *Circulation* 1989;**80**:769–81.

125. LeJemtal TH, Maskin CS, Chadwick B, Sinoway L. Near maximal oxygen extraction by exercising muscles in patients with severe heart failure: a limitation to the benefits of training. *J Am Coll Cardiol* 1983;**1**:662A.

126. LeJemtel TH, Maskin CS, Lucido D, Chadwick BJ. Failure to augment maximal limb blood flow in response to one-leg versus two-leg exercise in patients with severe heart failure. *Circulation* 1986;**74**:245–51.

127. Wroblewski H, Kastrup J, Norgaard T, Mortensen S-A, Haunso S. Evidence of increased microvascular resistance and arteriolar hyalinosis in skin in congestive heart failure secondary to idiopathic dilated cardiomyopathy. *Am J Cardiol* 1992;**69**:769–74.

128. Arnold JMO, Marchiori GE, Imrie JR, *et al*. Large artery function in patients with chronic heart failure. Studies of brachial artery diameter and haemodynamics. *Circulation* 1991;**84**:2418–25.

129. Zelis R, Nellis SH, Longhurst J, Lee G, Mason DT. Abnormalities in the regional circulations accompanying congestive heart failure. *Prog Cardiovasc Dis* 1975;**18**:181–99.

130. Kubo SH, Rector TS, Bank AJ, Williams RE, Heifetz SM. Endothelium-dependent vasodilation is attenuated in patients with heart failure. *Circulation* 1991;**84**:1589–96.

131. Katz SD, Biasucci L, Sabba C, et al. Impaired endothelium-mediated vasodilation in the peripheral vasculature of patients with congestive heart failure. *J Am Coll Cardiol* 1992;**19**:918–25.

132. Bank AJ, Rector TS, Burke MN, Tschumperlin LK, Kubo SH. Impaired forearm vasodilation to hyperosmolal stimuli in patients with congestive heart failure secondary to idiopathic dilated cardiomyopathy or to ischemic cardiomyopathy. *Am J Cardiol* 1992;**70**:1315–19.

133. Franciosa JA, Goldsmith SR, Cohn JN. Contrasting immediate and long-term effects of isosorbide dinitrate on exercise capacity in congestive heart failure. *Am J Med* 1980;**69**:559–66.

134. McMurray JJ, Ray SG, Abdullah I, Dargie HJ, Morton JJ. Plasma endothelin in chronic heart failure. *Circulation* 1992;**85**:1374–9.

135. Minotti JR, Pillay P, Chang L, Wells L, Massie BM. Neurophysiological assessment of skeletal muscle fatigue in patients with congestive heart failure. *Circulation* 1992;**86**:903–8.

136. Lipkin DP, Jones DA, Round JM, Poole-Wilson PA. Abnormalities of skeletal muscle in patients with chronic heart failure. *Int J Cardiol* 1988;**18**:187–95.

137. Schaufelberger M, Eriksson BO, Grimby G, Held P, Swedberg K. Skeletal muscle alterations in patients with chronic heart failure. *Eur Heart J* 1997;**18**:971–80.

138. Mancini DM, Walter G, Reichnek N, et al. Contribution of skeletal muscle atrophy to exercise intolerance and altered muscle metabolism in heart failure. *Circulation* 1992;**85**:1364–73.

139. Buller NP, Jones D, Poole-Wilson PA. Direct measurements of skeletal muscle fatigue in patients with chronic heart failure. *Br Heart J* 1991;**65**:20–4.

140. Volterrani M, Clark AL, Ludman PF, et al. Determinants of exercise capacity in chronic heart failure. *Eur Heart J* 1994;**15**:801–9.

141. Clark A, Coats A. Mechanisms of exercise intolerance in cardiac failure: abnormalities of skeletal muscle and pulmonary function. *Curr Opin Cardiol* 1994;**9**:305–14.

142. Minotti JR, Pillay P, Oka R, et al. Skeletal muscle size: relationship to muscle function in heart failure. *J Appl Physiol* 1993;**75**:373–81.

143. Wilson JR, Mancini DM, Simson M. Detection of skeletal muscle fatigue in patients with heart failure using electromyography. *Am J Cardiol* 1992;**70**:488–93.

144. Lipkin DP, Jones DA, Round JM, Poole-Wilson PA. Abnormalities of skeletal muscle in patients with chronic heart failure. *Int J Cardiol* 1988;**18**:187–95.

145. Zugck C, Haunstetter A, Krüger C, et al. Impact of beta-blocker treatment on the prognostic value of currently used risk predictors in congestive heart failure. *J Am Coll Cardiol* 2002;**39**(10):1615–22.

146. Minotti JR, Christoph I, Oka R, et al. Impaired skeletal muscle function in patients with congestive heart failure. Relationship to systemic exercise performance. *J Clin Invest* 1991;**88**:2077–82.

147. Butler J, Khadim G, Paul KM, et al. Selection of patients for heart transplantation in the current era of heart failure therapy. *J Am Coll Cardiol* 2004;**43**:787–93.

148. Mancini DM, Eisen H, Kussmaul W, et al. Value of peak exercise oxygen consumption for optimal timing of cardiac transplantation in ambulatory patients with heart failure. *Circulation* 1991;**83**:778–86.

149. Clark AL, Piepoli M, Coats AJ. Skeletal muscle and the control of ventilation on exercise: evidence for metabolic receptors. *Eur J Clin Invest* 1995;**25**:299–305.

150. Arnolda L, Conway M, Dolecki M, et al. Skeletal muscle metabolism in heart failure:a 31P nuclear magnetic resonance spectroscopy study of leg muscle. *Clin Sci* 1990;**79**:583–9.

151. Piepoli M, Clark AL, Coats AJS. Muscle metaboreceptors in the hemodynamic, autonomic and ventilatory responses to exercise in man. *Am J Physiol* 1995;**269**:H1428–36.

152. Piepoli M, Clark AL, Volterrani M, et al. Contribution of muscle afferents to the hemodynamic, autonomic, and ventilatory responses to exercise in patients with chronic heart failure: effects of physical training. *Circulation* 1996;**93**:940–52.

153. Grieve DAA, Clark AL, McCann GP, Hillis WS. The Ergoreflex in patients with chronic stable heart failure. *Int J Cardiol* 1999;**68**:157–64.

154. Scott AC, Francis DP, Davies LC, et al. Contribution of skeletal muscle 'ergoreceptors' in the human leg to respiratory control in chronic heart failure. *J Physiol* 2000;**529** Pt 3:863–70.

155. Sjoggard G, Adams RA, Saltin B. Water and ion shifts in skeletal muscle of humans with intense dynamic knee extension. *Am J Physiol* 1985;**248**:R190–6.

156. Linton RAF, Band DM. The effects of potassium on carotid body chemoreceptor activity and ventilation in the cat. *Respir Physiol* 1985;**59**:65–70.

157. Paterson DJ, Robbins PA, Conway J. Changes in arterial plasma potassium and ventilation during exercise in man. *Respir Physiol* 1989;**78**:323–30.

158. McLoughlin P, Popham P, Bruce RCH, Linton RAF, Band DM. Plasma potassium and the ventilatory threshold in man. *J Physiol* 1990;**427**:44P.

159. Lim M, Linton RAF, Wolff CB, Band DM. Propranolol, exercise and arterial potassium. *Lancet* 1981;**ii**:591.

160. Scott AC, Wensel R, Davos CH, et al. Chemical mediators of the muscle ergoreflex in chronic heart failure: a putative role for prostaglandins in reflex ventilatory control. *Circulation* 2002;**106**:214–20.

161. Witte KK, Clark AL. The effect of aspirin on the ventilatory response to exercise in chronic heart failure. *Eur J Heart Fail* 2004;**6**:745–8.

162. Witte KK, Notarius CF, Ivanov J, Floras JS. Muscle sympathetic nerve activity and ventilation during exercise in subjects with and without chronic heart failure. *Can J Cardiol* 2008;**24**:275–8.

163. Middlekauff HR, Chiu J, Hamilton MA, et al. Muscle mechanoreceptor sensitivity in heart failure. *Am J Physiol Heart Circ Physiol* 2004;**287**:H1937–43.

164. Negrão CE, Rondon MU, Tinucci T, et al. Abnormal neurovascular control during exercise is linked to heart failure severity. *Am J Physiol Heart Circ Physiol* 2001;**280**:H1286–92.

165. Clark AL, Poole-Wilson PA, Coats AJ. Exercise limitation in chronic heart failure: central role of the periphery. *J Am Coll Cardiol* 1996;**28**:1092–102.

166. Australia/New Zealand Heart Failure Research Collaborative Group. Randomised, placebo-controlled trial of carvedilol in patients with congestive heart failure due to ischaemic heart disease. *Lancet* 1997;**349**:375–80.

167. US Carvedilol Heart Failure Study Group. Carvedilol inhibits clinical progression in patients with mild symptoms of heart failure. *Circulation* 1996;**94**:2800–6.

168. Cohn JN, Fowler MB, Bristow MR, *et al.*, for the US Carvedilol Heart failure Study Group. Safety and efficacy of carvedilol in severe heart failure. *J Cardiac Fail* 1997;**3**:173–9.

169. Clark AL, Galloway S, MacFarlane N, *et al.* Catecholamines contribute to exertional dyspnoea and to the ventilatory response to exercise in normal humans. *Eur Heart J* 1997;**18**:1829–33.

170. Francis DP, Shamim W, Davies LC, *et al.* Cardiopulmonary exercise testing for prognosis in chronic heart failure: continuous and independent prognostic value from VE/VCO(2)slope and peak VO(2). *Eur Heart J* 2000;**21**:154–61.

171. Koelling TM, Joseph S, Aaronson KD. Heart failure survival score continues to predict clinical outcomes in patients with heart failure receiving beta-blockers. *J Heart Lung Transplant* 2004;**23**:1414–22.

172. Geisberg C, Goring J, Listerman J, *et al.* Impact of optimal heart failure medical therapy on heart transplant listing. *Transplant Proc* 2006;**38**:1493–5.

173. Chua TP, Ponikowski P, Harrington D, *et al.* Clinical correlates and prognostic significance of the ventilatory response to exercise in chronic heart failure. *J Am Coll Cardiol* 1997;**29**:1585–90.

174. Corrà U, Mezzani A, Bosimini E, *et al.* Ventilatory response to exercise improves risk stratification in patients with chronic heart failure and intermediate functional capacity. *Am Heart J* 2002;**143**:418–26.

175. Cazeau S, Leclercq C, Lavergne T, *et al.*; Multisite Stimulation in Cardiomyopathies (MUSTIC) Study Investigators. Effects of multisite biventricular pacing in patients with heart failure and intraventricular conduction delay. *N Engl J Med* 2001;**344**:873–80.

176. Varma C, Sharma S, Firoozi S, McKenna WJ, Daubert JC; Multisite Stimulation in Cardiomyopathy (MUSTIC) Study Group. Atriobiventricular pacing improves exercise capacity in patients with heart failure and intraventricular conduction delay. *J Am Coll Cardiol* 2003;**41**:582–8.

177. Auricchio A, Stellbrink C, Sack S, *et al.*; Pacing Therapies in Congestive Heart Failure (PATH-CHF) Study Group. Long-term clinical effect of hemodynamically optimized cardiac resynchronization therapy in patients with heart failure and ventricular conduction delay. *J Am Coll Cardiol* 2002;**39**:2026–33.

178. Cleland JG, Daubert JC, Erdmann E, *et al.*; Cardiac Resynchronization–Heart Failure (CARE-HF) Study Investigators. The effect of cardiac resynchronization on morbidity and mortality in heart failure. *N Engl J Med* 2005;**352**:1539–49.

28

Invasive investigation

Simon A. S. Beggs and Roy S. Gardner

Catheter studies

The technique for human cardiac catheterization was first developed by Werner Forssmann. In 1929, he inserted a cannula into his own antecubital vein, through which he passed a catheter for 65 cm and then walked to the X-ray department, where a photograph was taken of the catheter lying in his right atrium. His approach was frowned upon and he was forced to give up cardiology for a career in urology. However, he was subsequently awarded the Nobel Prize in Physiology or Medicine in 1956, along with André Frédéric Cournand and Dickinson W. Richards who developed ways of applying his technique to heart disease diagnosis and research.

Despite advances in non-invasive imaging, there are frequent occasions when invasive investigation is required. This chapter aims to summarize these techniques and demonstrate how both right and left heart catheterization can offer valuable information about the patient.

Seldinger technique

The Seldinger technique (Figure 28.1) was introduced by Dr Sven-Ivar Seldinger (1921–1998), a Swedish radiologist, in 1953.[1] Although originally described for percutaneous arteriography, the technique is now used to place catheters in a variety of locations including veins, arteries, or body cavities such as pleural or pericardial spaces.

Central venous cannulation

Obtaining central venous access is a key skill in the management of an ill patient, allowing invasive pressure monitoring, infusion of therapy, and access for procedures such as temporary pacing, pulmonary artery catheterization, and endomyocardial biopsy. The three routes commonly employed are the internal jugular vein, the subclavian vein, and the femoral vein.

The use of ultrasound to guide cannulation of the internal jugular vein significantly improves the success rate (100% compared to 88%, $P < 0.001$), decreases access time (mean of 9.8 s vs 44.5 s, $P < 0.001$), and reduces the complication rate ($P < 0.001$) compared to cannulation using anatomical landmarks in more than 600 patients.[2] In 2002, a technology appraisal from the UK National Institute for Health and Care Excellence (NICE) recommended that central venous cannulation (CVC) should be performed using direct vision where possible (e.g. Bard° Site-Rite° ultrasound system; Figure 28.2).[3] However, NICE acknowledged that CVC using anatomical landmarks was a skill that should be maintained, particularly in emergency situations when direct vision equipment is not immediately available.

Internal jugular vein access

The internal jugular vein is most often used as it allows the catheter to be inserted under direct ultrasound guidance, thus reducing the potential for complications such as carotid artery puncture or pneumothorax. Compared to a femoral approach, the site can be kept sterile. Indeed, a critical aspect in any invasive procedure is

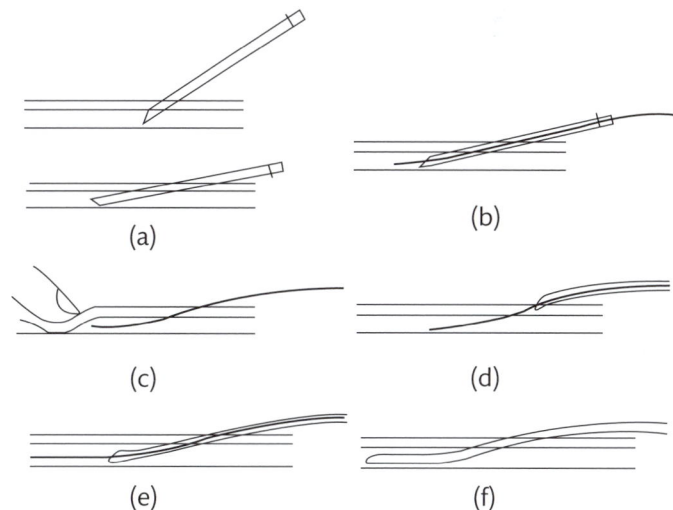

Figure 28.1 The Seldinger technique: (a) The artery punctured. The needle pushed upwards. (b) The guidewire inserted. (c) The needle withdrawn and the artery compressed. (d) The catheter threaded onto the guide wire. (e) The catheter inserted into the artery. (f) The guide wire withdrawn.

Reproduced from Seldinger SI. Catheter replacement of the needle in percutaneous arteriography; a new technique. *Acta Radiol* 1953;**39**:368–76.

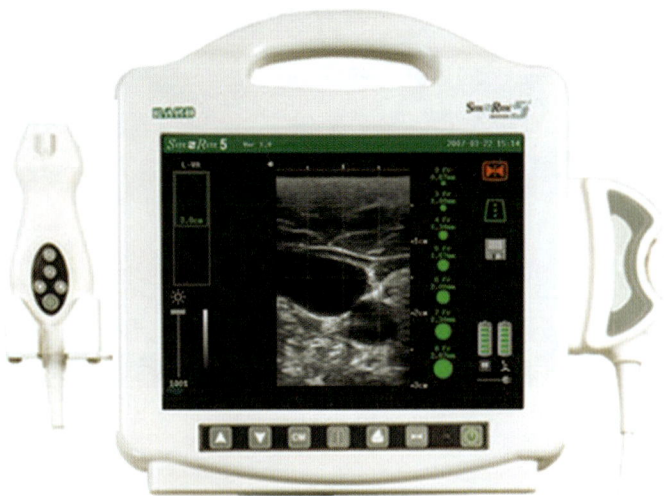

Figure 28.2 An example of a portable ultrasound to facilitate central venous cannulation.

Copyright © C. R. Bard, Inc. used with permission. Bard and SiteRite are registered trademarks of C. R. Bard, Inc.

scrupulous attention to aseptic technique. The skin should be prepared and draped and local anaesthetic should be infiltrated into the skin and subcutaneous tissues. The catheter is flushed in preparation for insertion.

Place the patient supine in a head-down tilt. For a right internal jugular approach, rotate the head 30–45° to the left to open up the anterior triangle, which is formed by the sternal and clavicular heads of the sternomastoid muscle. The carotid artery can be palpated with the left hand, thus reducing the risk of an inadvertent arterial puncture. After making an incision in the skin, insert a 20-gauge needle at 45° to the skin lateral to the carotid artery, aiming for the right nipple in men and the right anterior superior iliac spine in women (**Figure 28.3**). Once the vein is found, using the Seldinger technique, a J-tipped wire is advanced through the needle into the vein. It is important never to advance the wire against resistance and always to ensure that control and sight of the guide wire is maintained.

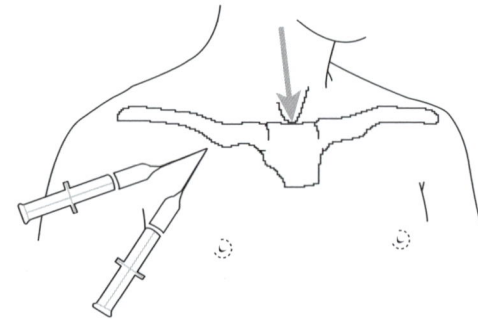

Figure 28.4 Approach for cannulation of the right subclavian vein.

Reproduced from Myerson SG, Choudhury RP, Mitchell A. *Emergencies in cardiology*, pp. 291–293, Oxford University Press, Oxford, 2005, with permission from Oxford University Press.

The needle is then removed, leaving the wire in place over which is inserted a dilator. On removing the dilator, the catheter can then be gently twisted into position and the guide wire removed. The catheter is then sutured and the site covered with a sterile dressing. A check chest radiograph should be performed.

Subclavian vein access

The subclavian vein route can be more comfortable for patients, particularly if the catheter is expected to be *in situ* for a few days. However, this approach exposes the patient to a greater risk of pneumothorax and arterial puncture. The right subclavian vein is the preferred side for endomyocardial biopsy and temporary pacing (to avoid the side most commonly used for permanent systems). Again, the approach uses the Seldinger technique as described above using anatomical markings (**Figure 28.4**).

Femoral vein access

The femoral approach is largely used for emergency access. Although it has a low rate of immediate complications, it is the site that is most prone to line infections. The vein lies medial to the femoral artery (**Figure 28.5**). Again, this approach uses the Seldinger technique as described above.

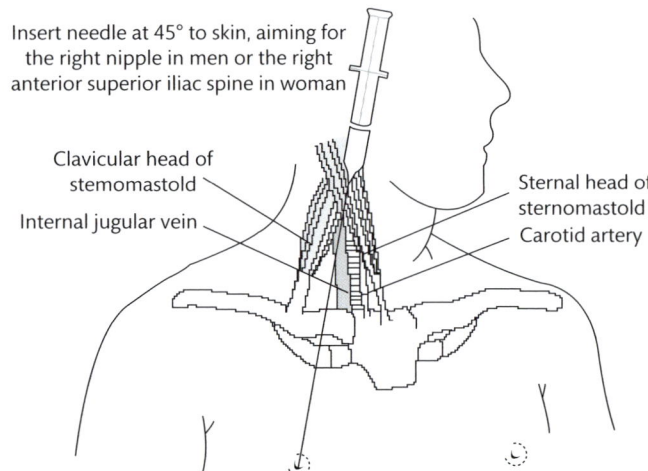

Figure 28.3 Anatomy of right internal jugular vein.

Reproduced from Myerson SG, Choudhury RP, Mitchell A. *Emergencies in cardiology*, pp. 291–293, Oxford University Press, Oxford, 2005, with permission from Oxford University Press.

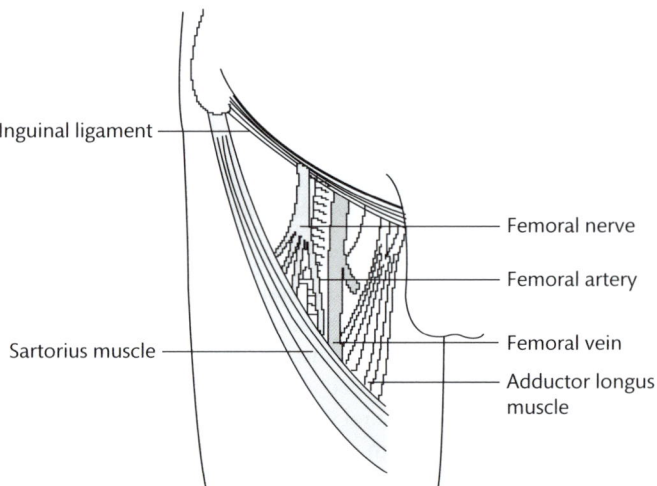

Figure 28.5 The anatomy of the right femoral vein.

Reproduced from Myerson SG, Choudhury RP, Mitchell A. *Emergencies in cardiology*, pp. 291–293, Oxford University Press, Oxford, 2005, with permission from Oxford University Press.

Complications of central venous cannulation

As with any invasive procedure, there are well-recognized complications that may result from CVC. These include bleeding, inadvertent arterial puncture, vascular damage including late vessel stenosis, pneumothorax (particularly with subclavian access), infection (especially femoral vein access), arrhythmia, and air embolism.

Central venous pressure

The central venous pressure (CVP) is usually measured from a catheter with its tip in the superior vena cava or from the proximal port of a pulmonary artery catheter lying in the right atrium.

The normal CVP waveform (Figure 28.6) consists of three peaks (a, c, and v) and two descents (x and y). The a wave is the result of atrial contraction and immediately follows the p wave on the ECG, occurring at the end of diastole. As the atrium relaxes and pressure falls, there is a transient increase in atrial pressure (c wave) following the R wave on the surface ECG, produced by isovolumic right ventricular contraction causing closure of the tricuspid valve, displacing the valve into the right atrium.

The x descent represents the fall in atrial pressure during ventricular systole that occurs due to the effect of ventricular contraction on atrial geometry, and ongoing atrial relaxation. The v wave is caused by venous filling of the atrium during late ventricular systole (peaking just after the T wave on the ECG) when the tricuspid valve is still closed. When the valve opens, blood flows from the right atrium into the right ventricle, leading to a decrease in atrial pressure, represented by the y descent.

Following insertion of a central venous catheter into either the subclavian or internal jugular vein, central venous (i.e. right atrial) pressure can be measured by connecting the distal port of the catheter to pressure-monitoring equipment. The patient should be lying flat, and the pressure transducer placed and zeroed by opening to atmospheric pressure at the level of the patient's right atrium (fourth intercostal space in the midaxillary line). CVP should be measured at end expiration. A normal CVP is between 0 and 7 mmHg (10–15 cmH$_2$O). Causes of an elevated right atrial pressure include right ventricular infarction/failure, fluid overload, pulmonary hypertension, tricuspid stenosis or regurgitation, pulmonary stenosis, and left-to-right shunts (e.g. ventricular septal defect, VSD). There are also several classical abnormalities of the right atrial waveform, listed in Table 28.1.

Right heart catheterization

The pulmonary artery flotation catheter (PAC) was first invented by Jeremy Swan and William Ganz, from the Cedars–Sinai Medical Centre, Los Angeles, USA, the idea coming from the observation of sailing boats in the water.[4] A PAC can be used to measure pressures

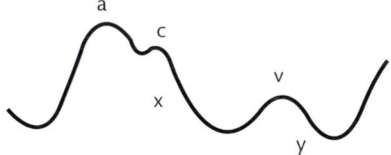

Figure 28.6 The right atrial pressure wave form.

Table 28.1 Abnormalities of the right atrial waveform

Feature	Cause
Canon 'a' waves	Atrioventricular dissociation (e.g. ventricular tachycardia, ventricular pacing, complete heart block)
Tall 'a' waves	Tricuspid stenosis
Tall 'v' waves	Tricuspid regurgitation
Brisk x descent	Pericardial tamponade
Brisk y (and x) descents	Pericardial constriction; myocardial restriction

in the right heart (right atrium, right ventricle, pulmonary artery, and pulmonary capillary wedge pressure), cardiac output (using thermodilution), and to assess pulmonary and systemic vascular resistance. It can also be used to detect intracardiac shunts (e.g. VSDs), as well as to measure mixed venous oxygen saturation.

The Swan–Ganz catheter for the measurement of cardiac output has four ports: balloon tip, proximal port, distal port that sits in the pulmonary artery, and a thermistor located at the distal end of the catheter. The basic PAC has a balloon for flotation and a single lumen at the catheter tip. The catheters are ideally suited to be floated from the neck, rather than the femoral route.

Trials to study the benefits of PACs have been difficult to perform because of the extreme heterogeneity of the patient population. However, two recent multicentre prospective trials have been published that may radically reduce the use of PACs. The ESCAPE trial (Evaluation Study of Congestive Heart Failure and Pulmonary Artery Catheterization Effectiveness) looked specifically at the use of PACs in guiding the management of patients with decompensated chronic heart failure and concluded that there was no indication for the routine use of PACs.[5] In an intensive care population that included patients with acute myocardial infarction, the FACTT trial concluded that PACs did not improve survival or organ function but were associated with more catheter-related complications, mainly arrhythmias.[6] Furthermore, a meta-analysis of 13 randomized controlled studies involving more than 5000 patients concluded that the use of the PAC neither increased overall mortality or days in hospital nor conferred benefit in critically ill patients.[7]

Thus PACs should be reserved for patients being assessed for cardiac transplantation, those in whom there is clinical uncertainty as to their haemodynamic status (e.g. right ventricular infarction), or those with established left ventricular dysfunction and acute change in fluid status, e.g. bleeding, sepsis, or renal failure. Normal values for PAC measurements are shown in Table 28.2.

Technique

The PAC is most easily manoeuvred via the superior vena cava from the internal jugular vein or the subclavian vein, but can be introduced through the inferior vena cava from the femoral vein. Because of the potential for ventricular arrhythmias—particularly on crossing the tricuspid valve and in the right ventricular outflow tract—the patient should be monitored and full resuscitation equipment should be available during manipulation of the PAC. In many centres, the PAC is manipulated according to pressure waveform (Figure 28.7). However, it is good practice to use fluoroscopy in order to minimize complications.

Table 28.2 Findings on right heart catheterization

(a) Normal values

Variable	Abbreviation	Normal range
Stroke volume	SV	70–100 mL
Cardiac output	CO	4–6 L/min
Right atrial pressure	RAP	0–5 mmHg
Right ventricular pressure	RVP	20–25/0–5 mmHg
Pulmonary artery pressure	PAP	20–25/10–15 mmHg
Pulmonary capillary wedge pressure	PCWP	6–12 mmHg
Mixed venous oxygen saturation	SVO_2	70–75%

(b) Derived variables

Variable	Abbreviation	Calculation	Normal range
Cardiac index	CI	Cardiac output/BSA	2.5–3.5 L/min/m³
Stroke index	SI or SVI	Stroke volume/BSA	40–60 mL/m²
Systemic vascular resistance	SVR	(MAP – RAP × 79.9)/CO	900–1100 dyne/s/cm⁵
SVR index		(MAP – RAP × 79.9)/CI	1740–2400 dyne/s/m²
Pulmonary vascular resistance	PVR	(PAP – PCWP × 79.9)/CO	25–125 dyne/s/cm⁵
Right ventricular stroke work index	RVSWI	SVI × (mPAP – mRAP) × 0.0136	7.9–9.7 g/m²/beat

(c) Findings in cardiac conditions

Hypovolaemia	Sepsis	LV failure	RV failure	Tamponade	Acquired VSD
CVP ↓	↑	↑	↑	↑	↑
PCWP ↓	↑	↑	↓	↑	↑
CO ↓	↓	↓	↓	↓	↓
SVR ↑	↑	↑	↑	↑	↑
A–V SaO₂ ↑	↑	↑	↑	↑	↓

A–V SaO₂, difference in arterial and mixed venous oxygen saturations; LV, left ventricular; RV, right ventricular; VSD, ventricular septal defect.

Before use, all the lumens of the catheter should be flushed and the balloon inflated with 1.5 mL of air to test its integrity. The pressure line should then be connected to the distal port of the PAC and the transducer zeroed at the level of the right atrium. Insert the catheter into the central venous cannula until its tip lies in the right atrium (15–20 cm from the right internal jugular or subclavian route). The characteristic right atrial tracing should be obtained (see Central venous pressure). To assist with transit through the right heart, the balloon is then inflated with 1.5 mL of air. On advancing the catheter, record the waveforms in the right ventricle (25–35 cm) and pulmonary artery (40–50 cm) in end expiration (**Figure 28.7**). The right ventricular waveform is identified by an increase in systolic pressure and low diastolic pressure, which approximates right atrial pressure (RAP). The right ventricular end-diastolic pressure is measured at the R wave of the ECG.

When the pulmonary capillary wedge pressure (PCWP) trace appears, the catheter should not be advanced further and the balloon should be deflated. If the pulmonary artery trace does not reappear, the catheter should be withdrawn by 2 cm and the balloon gently reinflated once the pulmonary artery trace does appear. A stable wedge position allows the catheter to be left in position with a pulmonary artery trace that then shows a PCWP trace on balloon inflation. It is important not to inflate the balloon if resistance is felt, or to leave the

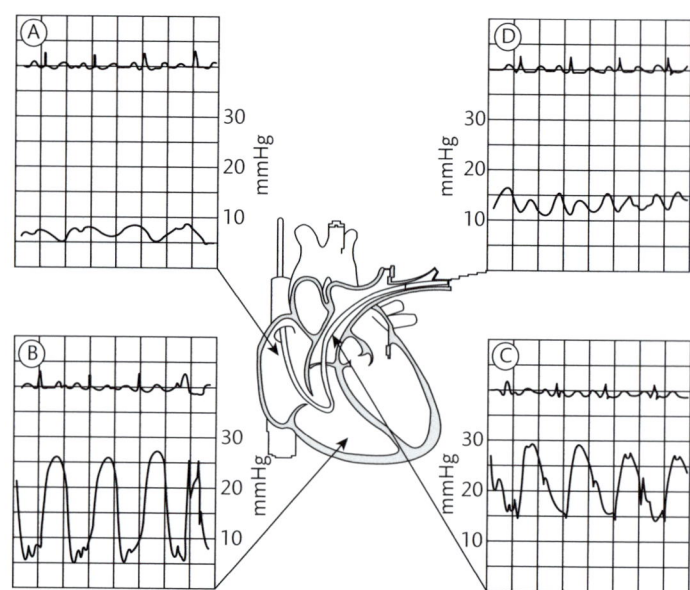

Figure 28.7 Picture of waveforms in the right heart.

Reproduced from Myerson SG, Choudhury RP, Mitchell A, *Emergencies in cardiology*, pp. 291–293, Oxford University Press, Oxford, 2005, with permission from Oxford University Press.

balloon inflated, because of the potential for trauma or pulmonary artery rupture. If the pressure trace continues to rise on balloon inflation, it suggests 'over-wedging' and the balloon should be deflated and the catheter withdrawn by 2 cm before reinflation. If the trace is damped, the catheter may be kinked or the lumen partially occluded with thrombus or affected by the presence of air bubbles.

Pulmonary capillary wedge pressure

The PCWP is a damped and delayed reflection of left atrial pressure. Although a good wedge trace has a left atrial waveform with a and v waves, the c wave is often difficult to discern. In a normal individual, the pulmonary artery diastolic pressure is similar to the mean PCWP (6–12 mmHg), because of low pulmonary vascular resistance. The mean PCWP cannot be higher than the mean pulmonary artery pressure. The optimal left atrial filling pressure (PCWP) in the presence of left ventricular systolic dysfunction is higher (~14 mmHg).

There are several conditions in which the PCWP does not give a fair representation of left atrial or left ventricular end-diastolic pressure. Where there is an elevation of pulmonary vascular resistance (e.g. with pulmonary hypertension, chronic obstructive airways disease, pulmonary embolism, hypoxaemia), the PCWP may exaggerate the actual left atrial pressure. Severe mitral regurgitation results in a prominent systolic (v) wave that may cause the PCWP trace to resemble the pulmonary artery trace (Figure 28.8). In this situation, the a and v waves and mean PCWP pressures should all be recorded, with the left ventricular end-diastolic pressure (LVEDP) best approximated by measuring pressure prior to the regurgitant v wave. Another important example is mitral stenosis, where there is a pressure gradient caused by obstruction to blood flow between left atrium and left ventricle. As a result, left atrial pressure (estimated by PCWP) will exceed LVEDP.

Cardiac output measurement–thermodilution technique

This technique uses a modification of the Fick principle. A fixed volume (such as 10 mL) of ice-cold saline is rapidly injected into the proximal port of the PAC. The rate of temperature change is detected by the thermistor at the catheter tip, 30 cm distal to the site of injection. The volume and temperature of injected saline are entered into a cardiac output computer which then derives the cardiac output from the change in temperature at the catheter tip. At least five measurements should be taken and averaged—more if the patient has atrial fibrillation or an unstable rhythm. The readings should fall within 10% of each other and those with irregular traces should be discarded. An important potential cause of error is significant tricuspid regurgitation, where some of the bolus falls back into the right atrium, rendering the technique meaningless. Septal defects have a similar effect.

Vascular resistance

Vascular resistance (R) describes the resistance to flow offered by a circulation (primarily small arterioles—'resistance vessels'), and is calculated by the fraction of pressure gradient and mean flow (i.e. cardiac output). Although pulmonary vascular resistance (PVR) is commonly quoted in Wood units, systemic vascular resistance (SVR) is usually measured in absolute units (dyne s^{-1} cm^{-5}), by multiplying by a factor of 79.9. The normal ranges are shown in Table 28.2.

PVR is the resistance to flow offered by the pulmonary vasculature, and relies on the transpulmonary gradient (TPG: the pressure difference between the mean pulmonary artery pressure (PA_m) and mean left atrial pressure (LA_m)) and cardiac output (CO, in L/min), calculated using the following equations:

$$TPG = PA_m - LA_m (or PA_m - PCWP_m)$$

$$PVR = \frac{TPG}{CO} (Wood\ units), or$$

$$PVR = \frac{79.9 \times TPG}{CO} (dyne\ /s/\ cm^{-5})$$

Mean PCWP is often used in lieu of LAP, accepting the limitations of PCWP in the estimation of LAP.

The calculation of PVR is particularly important in the assessment of patients for cardiac transplantation, because an elevated PVR is a risk factor for premature death after transplantation.[8,9] An elevated PVR is commonly found in patients with chronic heart failure, particularly in the presence of valvular heart disease, and it may or may not be reversible. Irreversible pulmonary hypertension is an absolute contraindication to cardiac transplantation.[9] It is defined as:

- PVR >5 Wood units, or
- PVR index (PVRI) >6, or
- TPG >16 mmHg, or
- Pulmonary artery systolic pressure >60 mmHg in addition to one of the three criteria above.

If the PVR is elevated (but <5), reversibility can be assessed with the use of oxygen and vasodilator therapy (such as with glyceryl trinitrate or sodium nitroprusside) while maintaining systolic blood pressure to >85 mmHg. If this is unsuccessful, or hypotension precludes the use of vasodilators, an infusion of dobutamine or insertion of an intra-aortic balloon pump can be tried. If the PVR does fall, then the successful regime should be recorded in the notes and the PVR reassessed at least every six months. If the PVR can be reduced to <2.5 but at the cost of a fall in systolic blood pressure to

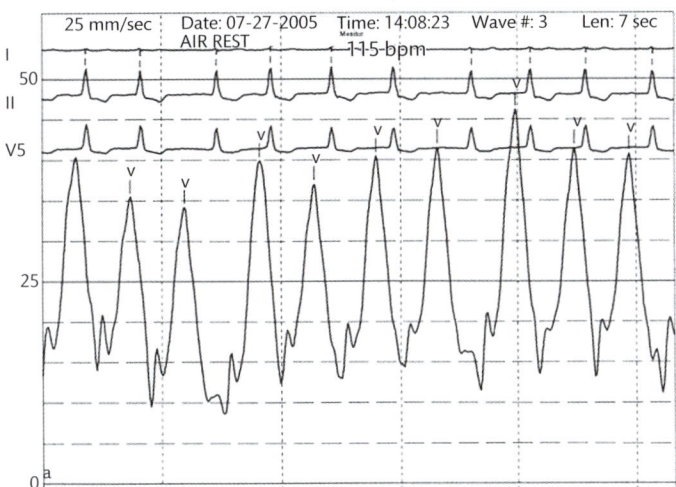

Figure 28.8 Pulmonary capillary wedge pressure tracing from a patient with acute mitral regurgitation showing giant V waves. The rhythm is atrial fibrillation.

<85 mmHg, the patient remains at high risk of right ventricular failure and death following cardiac transplantation.

SVR is the resistance offered by the peripheral circulation and is almost invariably raised in patients with chronic heart failure, due to the activation of the renin–angiotensin–aldosterone and sympathetic nervous systems, as well as the endogenous release of vasoconstrictors such as endothelin. SVR is calculated using the mean aortic and right atrial (RA) pressures, and CO in the following equation:

$$SVR = \frac{79.9 \text{ (mean aortic pressure} - \text{mean RA pressure)}}{\text{Cardiac output (dyne.scm}^{-5})}$$

Mixed venous oxygen saturation

Assuming that there is no intracardiac shunt, mixed venous oxygen saturation can be measured from a pulmonary artery blood sample which should be taken slowly to avoid 'arterialization', i.e. pulmonary venous sampling. The normal mixed venous oxygen saturation is 70–75%. Low-output states result in increased tissue oxygen extraction, and therefore low mixed venous saturation. High mixed venous saturations occur in high-output states including septic shock or in low-output states where there is a left-to-right shunt, such as ventricular septal rupture.

Plasma lactate

In shock, tissue hypoxia prevents the aerobic metabolism of pyruvate into water and carbon dioxide. Instead, lactate is formed, which can be measured, offering useful data regarding tissue perfusion. A sample of either venous or arterial blood is collected into a heparin fluoride tube for analysis, although many arterial blood gas analysers now measure lactate as standard. A normal plasma lactate is 0.3–1.3 mmol/L. An initial rise in lactate may be seen after improving tissue perfusion, reflecting the washout from previously hypoperfused tissue.

Shunt calculation

Left-to-right shunts can be calculated by measuring oxygen saturations during cardiac catheterization ('a shunt run') with the chamber or vessel in which there is a step up in oxygen saturation indicating the level of the shunt. The ratio of pulmonary flow to systemic flow is given by:

$$\frac{\text{Pulmonary flow}}{\text{Systemic flow}} = \frac{\text{Aortic SaO}_2 - \text{mean venous Sao}_2}{98 - \text{PASao}_2}$$

where PF is pulmonary flow, SF is systemic flow, 98 is the assumed percentage oxygen saturation in the pulmonary veins, and mixed venous saturation is

$$\frac{3 \times \text{SVC saturation} + \text{IVC saturation}}{4}$$

Right ventricular stroke work index

Mechanical support of a failing left ventricle utilizing a left ventricular assist device (LVAD) has the important effect of placing the patient's right ventricle under increased haemodynamic strain. In the setting of insufficient contractile reserve, RV failure will

ensue—the consequences of which may be catastrophic. A preoperative assessment of RV function can be made via the right ventricular stroke work index (RVSWI), which is calculated with PAC data (see Table 28.2). Over recent years, several studies have demonstrated that a low preoperative RVSWI predicts the subsequent development of RV failure and adverse clinical outcomes in LVAD recipients.[10,11] This technique has become standard practice in many transplant centres to determine the suitability of candidates for LVAD implantation.

Difficulty in placing the PAC

The commonest difficulty experienced with PACs is in steering the catheter into the pulmonary artery. There are several techniques that can aid successful positioning. With the balloon inflated, the catheter will float more readily through the tricuspid valve with the patient in the head-down position. Conversely, the head-up position can be used to aid flotation out of the right ventricle. Deep inspiration will increase right ventricular output transiently due to increased venous return, which may also help with catheter passage, particularly in patients with a low CO.

The catheter can also be stiffened or guided with the use of a long 0.25″ (0.64 mm) J-tipped wire introduced via the distal lumen to steer the wire up into the right ventricular outflow tract. A guide wire can be particularly useful from the femoral route when the catheter may point downward into the right ventricular apex. To avoid myocardial perforation in this situation, force should never be applied.

Complications of PACs

As well as the complications of CVC, there are several recognized adverse sequelae from the use of a PAC. These include:

- Arrhythmias—PACs may induce arrhythmias from their passage through the right heart. The arrhythmias are predominantly ventricular in origin, due to irritation of the right ventricular outflow tract. However, complete heart block can also occur secondary to stunning of the right bundle branch in patients who already have left bundle branch block. Atrial arrhythmias are less common.
- Pulmonary artery rupture—the risk of pulmonary artery trauma can be minimized by ensuring that the PAC is not pushed, nor the balloon inflated, against resistance.
- Pulmonary infarction—the risk of pulmonary infarction can be greatly reduced by avoiding the PAC balloon being inflated for prolonged periods of time.
- Valvular trauma—manipulation of the PAC can cause either tricuspid or pulmonary valve trauma. It is of particular importance to deflate the PAC balloon before withdrawing the catheter.
- Infection—potentially endocarditis.
- Catheter knotting—this is less likely with the use of fluoroscopy and the avoidance of excessive catheter loops. Where the catheter is seen to loop, it should not be pulled tight. Rather, advancing the catheter and manipulating it with a guide wire may untie the knot. Where this is not possible, the knot can often be snared from the femoral vein and should not be pulled through the internal jugular vein. However, rarely, vascular surgery may be required.

Left heart catheterization

Measurement of left ventricular end-diastolic pressure

The measurement of LVEDP (**Figures 28.9** and **28.10**) contributes to the assessment of left ventricular filling pressures. The traces are recorded as part of a left heart catheterization study, where a catheter is placed directly into the left ventricle. The LVEDP is measured at the onset of isovolumic contraction (occasionally termed the C- or Z-point: see **Figures 28.9 and 28.10**). This usually coincides with the R wave of the ECG, and is best recorded after the a wave in an LAP tracing. The normal LVEDP is <12 mmHg: it may be elevated in the presence of mitral or aortic incompetence, left ventricular systolic dysfunction, VSD, tamponade, or pericardial constriction. The LVEDP may also be elevated if there is myocardial hypertrophy (e.g. hypertensive heart disease) or myocardial infiltration (e.g. amyloid). Conversely, a low LVEDP is seen in hypovolaemia and mitral stenosis.

Pressure gradients

An assessment of aortic stenosis can be made during cardiac catheterization by measuring the peak-to-peak (pullback) gradient, peak instantaneous gradient, mean gradient and, where the CO is known,

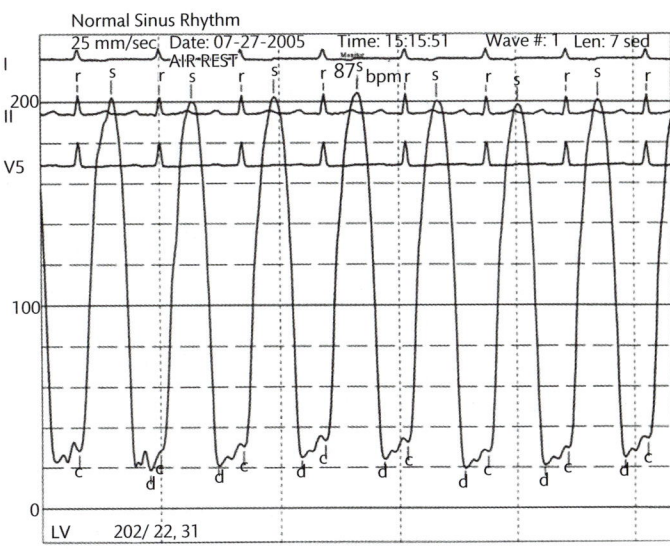

Figure 28.10 Left ventricular pressure trace in patient with chronic heart failure and hypertension. The left ventricular systolic pressure reaches over 200 mmHg, with an end-diastolic pressure of 31 mmHg measured at the c-point.

the valve orifice area (**Figure 28.11**). Indeed, until advances in echocardiography, pullback gradients were routinely performed in the assessment of patients with aortic stenosis.

In aortic stenosis, the peak-to-peak (pullback) gradient is obtained by the careful withdrawal of a catheter from the left ventricle into the aorta while constantly recording pressure. The gradient is generally lower, and is a less accurate reflection of valve area, than the peak instantaneous gradient obtained by simultaneous recording of ventricular and ascending aortic pressure with either two catheters or a double lumen catheter (or, indeed, echocardiography) (**Figure 28.12**). An alternative method of calculating an aortic gradient involves the simultaneous recording of ventricular and femoral arterial pressure, although this method has the

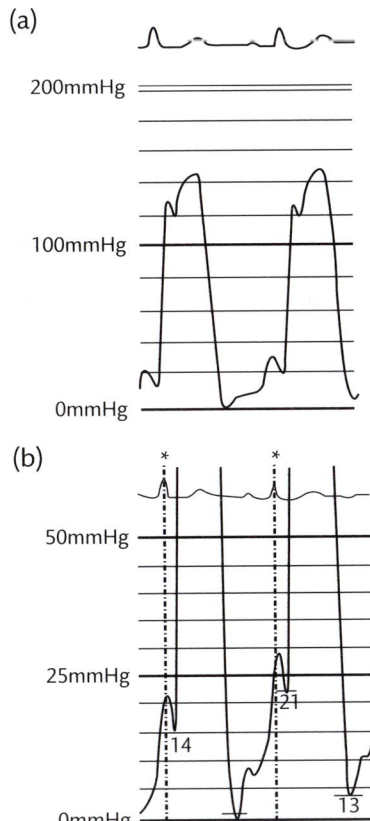

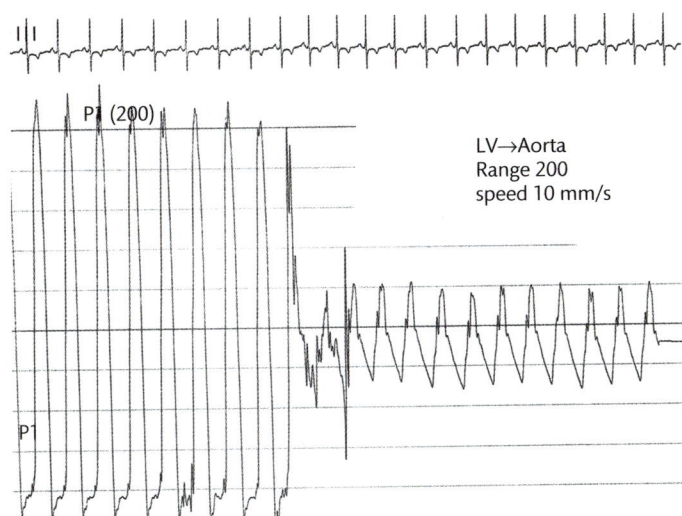

Figure 28.9 (a) The left ventricular pressure trace is shown with a close-up view (b) of the left ventricular end-doastolic pressure (LVEDP). The point to assess the LVEDP equates to the peak of the R wave, indicated by (*). The mean of several traces should be taken (three if sinus rhythm, five if atrial fibrillation).

Source data from Gardner, R., McDonagh, T., and Walker, N., *Oxford Specialist Handbook Heart Failure 2e*, Oxford University Press, Oxford, 2014.

Figure 28.11 Pressure trace from a pigtail catheter pulled back from the left ventricle into the ascending aorta illustrates an aortic valve gradient of 80 mmHg.

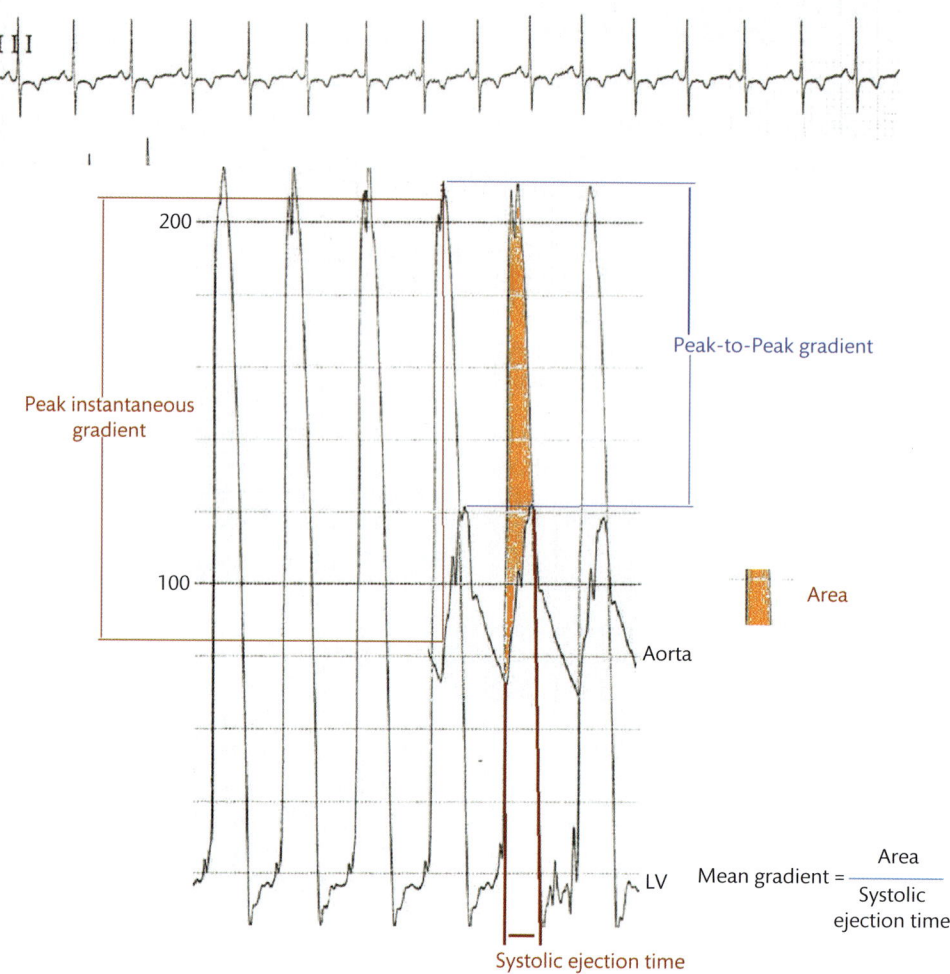

Figure 28.12 Simultaneous left ventricular and aortic pressure tracing in a patient with aortic stenosis demonstrating three different measures of severity of stenosis. Mean gradient = area/systolic ejection time.

potential for error due to the delay in pressure transmission and the alteration of the pressure waveform.

The Gorlin formula can be used to assess aortic valve area:

$$\text{aortic valve area (cm}^2\text{)}$$

$$= \frac{\text{Cardiac output }(\frac{1}{\text{min}})}{44.3 \times \text{SEP} \times \text{HR}\sqrt{\text{Mean aortic gradient(mmHg)}}}$$

where SEP is systolic ejection period, i.e. the length of time where left ventricular pressure is greater than aortic pressure) and HR is the heart rate. In a similar way to simultaneous pressure recording in the assessment of aortic stenosis, mitral stenosis can be evaluated by simultaneous left ventricular pressure and PCWP (or left atrial pressure) measurement.

Constriction versus restriction

Despite very different underlying pathological processes, the clinical and haemodynamic findings in constriction and restriction are similar and may be difficult to differentiate. Both conditions present with enlarged atria, normal-sized ventricles, and normal systolic function. However, non-compliance of the ventricular myocardium (restriction) or pericardium (constriction) results in diastolic dysfunction.

The diagnosis of constriction may be suggested by thickening and/or calcification of the pericardium—best seen on cardiac computed tomography. Pulsus paradoxus—the exaggeration of the normal reduction in blood pressure with inspiration—is often present in constriction, but rarely with restriction. There are some haemodynamic differences that may differentiate between the two conditions. The classical finding in constrictive pericarditis is the equalization of diastolic pressures (within 5 mmHg in the majority of cases) on simultaneous left and right heart catheterization. Furthermore, the right ventricular systolic pressure is nearly always <60 mmHg (and usually <40 mmHg) in constriction, whereas it is frequently >40 mmHg in restriction (**Figure 28.13**). Table 8.7 (p. 109) highlights the main differences between the two conditions.

Coronary angiography

Although coronary angiography is often unnecessary for the routine management of a patient with heart failure, it can help to clarify the underlying aetiology, and offer useful prognostic information (an ischaemic aetiology is associated with a higher risk of morbidity and mortality). Moreover, it should be considered in patients who suffer from angina recalcitrant to medical therapy, in suspected ischaemic

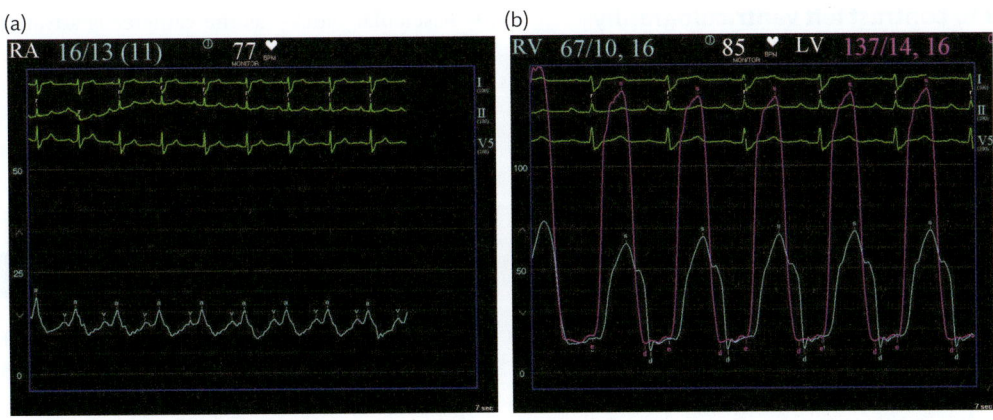

Figure 28.13 (a) Right atrial pressure and (b) simultaneous right and left ventricular pressure tracings in a patient with restrictive cardiomyopathy.

cardiomyopathy, or in patients with a history of symptomatic ventricular arrhythmia or aborted cardiac arrest.[12]

Coronary revascularization for the relief of heart failure symptoms in patients with ischaemic cardiomyopathy remains an area of continuing interest and uncertainty. This was the issue under investigation in the Surgical Treatment for Ischemic Heart Failure (STICH) trial, which demonstrated a benefit of CABG compared with medical therapy in terms of all-cause mortality, cardiovascular (CV) mortality, and CV hospitalizations after extended follow-up (10 years).[13] This is a potentially seminal finding but, surprisingly, the presence or absence of viable myocardium did not identify patients with more or less to gain from surgical revascularization. Whether a similar benefit from revascularization can be attained via percutaneous coronary intervention is being evaluated in the REVascularisation for Ischaemic VEntricular Dysfunction (REVIVED) trial (NCT01920048), which is currently recruiting in the UK.

Finally, coronary angiography may help predict whether a patient with heart failure is likely to benefit from a primary prevention implantable cardioverter–defibrillator (ICD). The recent large Defibrillator Implantation in Patients with Non-ischemic Systolic Heart Failure (DANISH) trial found no reduction in all-cause mortality with an ICD in patients with non-ischaemic cardiomyopathy.[14] Although no guideline amendments have yet filtered through, this finding at least exacerbates existing differences between the recommendations for primary prevention ICDs in patients with ischaemic and non-ischaemic cardiomyopathy. There was rigorous case ascertainment in DANISH, with non-ischaemic cardiomyopathy status usually determined by coronary angiography. It is feasible that invasive assessment of the coronary arteries may thus become more popular as part of the decision-making process about who will benefit from an ICD.

Contrast left ventriculography

Contrast left ventriculography can provide important information regarding global and regional cardiac function and mitral regurgitation (Figure 28.14), as well as the size and position of VSDs. It is an invasive procedure and is now infrequently performed in the routine investigation of heart failure patients, as the quality of non-invasive imaging has greatly improved.

In order to achieve an adequate contrast injection, it is necessary to inject a relatively large volume of contrast over a short period of time. Typical settings are 30–45 mL of contrast at a rate of 10–15 mL/ s, achieved by passing a catheter with multiple side-holes into the mid-left ventricular cavity and using a power injector to deliver contrast. An angled pigtail catheter is often used to minimize the catheter entanglement in the mitral valve apparatus, and hence reduce ectopy. It is of paramount importance that precautions are taken to prevent air embolism.

Images are best acquired in the 30° RAO projection (viewing the high lateral, anterior, apical, and inferior walls) and 45–60° LAO with 20° cranial tilt (viewing the lateral and septal walls: a useful view to assess for a VSD). Measurements can be obtained of ventricular volumes, and hence LVEF, and regional wall motion. LVEF can be calculated from the following equation:

$$LVEF(\%) = \frac{(End\text{-}diastolic\ volume - End\text{-}systolic\ volume)}{End\text{-}diastolic\ volume \times 100}$$

The severity of mitral regurgitation is assessed from the degree of opacification of the left atrium during contrast left ventriculography (Figure 28.14).

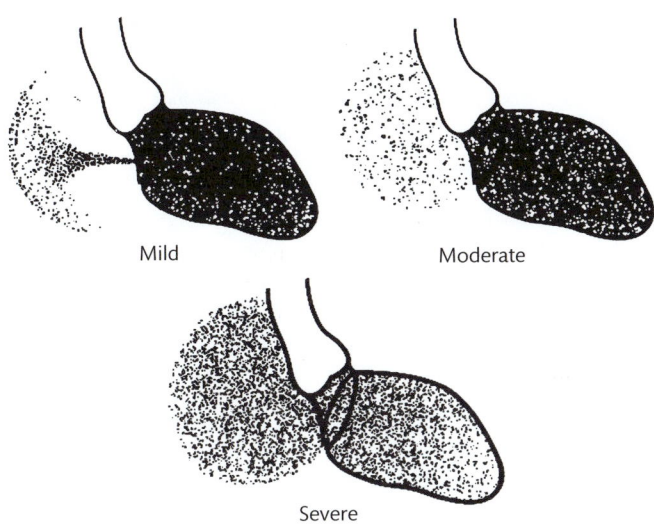

Figure 28.14 Assessment of severity of mitral regurgitation from contrast left ventriculography.

Reproduced from Mitchell A, West N, Leeson P, Banning, A. *Oxford Specialist Handbook Cardiac Catheterization and Coronary Intervention*, Figure 4.23, Oxford University Press, Oxford, 2008, with permission from Oxford University Press.

Contraindications to contrast left ventriculography

When considering left ventricular contrast ventriculography, it is important to consider whether a non-invasive means of assessing ventricular or valvular function might be preferable. This is particularly true in patients with a significant left main coronary artery stenosis or aortic valve stenosis, mural thrombus, renal impairment, and in those with left ventricular systolic pressure ≥180 mmHg, or LVEDP ≥25 mmHg.

Complications of contrast left ventriculography

There are a number of complications of contrast left ventriculography:

- Cardiac arrhythmias—ventricular extrasystoles are common, and usually result from stimulation of the ventricular endocardium by the catheter or jet of contrast medium. They can be minimized by repositioning the catheter. Short runs of ventricular tachycardia can also occur, but usually resolve on removal of the catheter from the ventricle.
- Embolism—the embolization of air or thrombus during contrast injection can have catastrophic results. The risk of embolism should be minimized by meticulous technique in ensuring that the injector system is free of bubbles or thrombus. Contrast ventriculography should also be avoided in patients with known left ventricular thrombus.
- Intramyocardial staining—usually caused by improper positioning of the catheter so that it lies underneath a papillary muscle or one of the side holes abuts the endocardium. Small stains are of limited significance, but larger stains may be associated with refractory ventricular arrhythmias or perforation and the development of cardiac tamponade.
- Contrast reactions—allergies to contrast media are reasonably common. However, it is more common to have powerful flushing sensations caused by vasodilatation.

- Fascicular block—as the catheter is advanced into the left ventricle, transient left anterior fascicular block may occur as the anterior fascicle of the left bundle lies close to the left ventricular outflow tract. Patients who already have right bundle branch block and left posterior fascicular block may develop transient complete heart block.

Endomyocardial biopsy

In 1962, Sakakibara and Konno first reported their experience with transvascular cardiac biopsy. Eleven years later, Caves described transvenous endomyocardial biopsy to diagnose cardiac allograft rejection.

Right ventricular endomyocardial biopsies are commonly taken after heart transplantation to assess allograft rejection. Only in very rare instances is a left ventricular biopsy indicated (e.g. due to multiple previous right ventricular biopsies) because of the risk of systemic embolization. There are few occasions when an endomyocardial biopsy is necessary in patients with chronic heart failure, and there remains considerable controversy surrounding the use of this procedure to evaluate the cause of dilated cardiomyopathy. Current guidelines state that endomyocardial biopsy should not be performed in the routine evaluation of patients with heart failure.[12] Rare exceptions are when an infiltrative cardiac condition is suspected and the result would influence therapy, although diagnostic information can often be obtained by other methods (**Table 28.3**). In an acute presentation of new heart failure, endomyocardial biopsy is indicated if giant cell myocarditis is suspected, as the condition often progresses rapidly, and these patients should be considered for circulatory support and urgent listing for cardiac transplantation. Biopsies of intracardiac masses can also be undertaken, where the result is necessary prior to surgery (**Figure 28.15**).[15] An example of normal histology is shown in **Figure 28.16**.

Table 28.3 Interpretation of biopsy data

Condition	Tissue biopsied	Stain(s)	Features
Amyloid (Figure 28.17, Figure 28.18)	Heart Buccal mucosa Rectum, kidney	Congo Red Sirius Red	Apple-green birefringence. Myocytes are ringed by pink-staining extracellular deposits of amyloid
Sarcoidosis (Figure 8.4, p. 110)	Heart Hilar lymph nodes Lung, skin	H&E	Non-caseating granuloma with myocyte destruction and replacement fibrosis
Haemochromatosis (Figure 8.5, p. 111)	Heart Liver	Perls stain (Prussian blue)	Granular intracellular cardiac myocyte deposits of haemosiderin are stained blue with both Perls stain
Endomyocardial fibrosis	Endomyocardium	H&E	
Viral myocarditis (Figure 8.1, p. 103)	Endomyocardium	H&E	Sensitivity as low as 35% due to transient and patchy myocardial involvement
Giant cell myocarditis (Figure 8.2, p. 104)	Endomyocardium	H&E	Widespread necrosis and inflammation with the presence of lymphocytes, histiocytes, eosinophils, as well as the characteristic multinucleated giant cells
Chagas disease	Endomyocardium	H&E	Parasitization of myofibres by trypanosomes, accompanied by an inflammatory infiltrate
Heart transplant rejection (Figure 24.19, Figure 24.20)	Endomyocardium	H&E	Histological features include interstitial oedema, inflammatory infiltration and immunoglobulin deposition. More severe rejection is marked by myocyte death and occasionally interstitial haemorrhage.

H&E, haematoxylin and eosin.

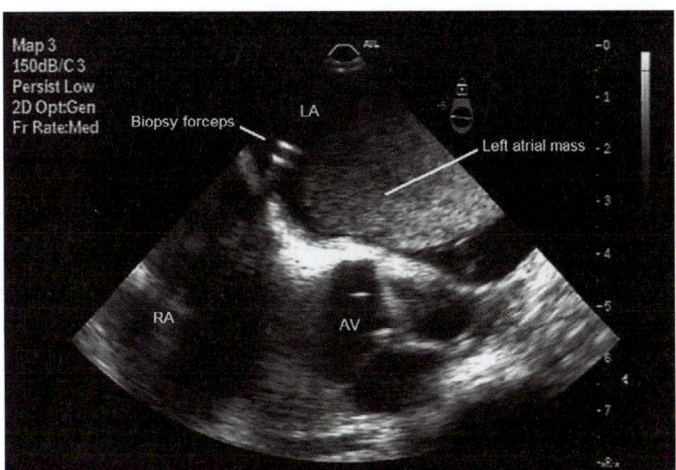

Figure 28.15 Transoesophageal echocardiogram illustrating a transseptal biopsy of a left atrial mass. RA, right atrium; LA, left atrium; AV, aortic valve.

Reproduced from Jackson CE, Gardner RS, Connelly DT. A novel approach for a novel combination: a trans-septal biopsy of left atrial mass in recurrent phyllodes tumour. *Eur J Echocardiogr* 2009;10:171–2 with permission from Oxford University Press.

Procedure

The patient should be adequately monitored by continuous ECG, pulse oximetry, and blood pressure. The following equipment should be immediately available in the event of a complication (see below): resuscitation trolley, temporary pacing line, pericardiocentesis tray, and chest drain kit.

Right ventricular endomyocardial biopsies are generally undertaken via the right internal jugular vein using a using an 8–9 F sheath with haemostasis valve, through which a 50 cm disposable bioptome is passed. Biopsies can also be taken from the femoral or subclavian veins, although the femoral route requires a long sheath

and a 104 cm bioptome. The subclavian approach may be technically challenging, and for this reason is generally reserved for occasions when endomyocardial biopsy cannot be performed from other routes (e.g. jugular venous thrombosis), as the angle between the subclavian vein and superior vena cava angle is often too acute for the relatively stiff bioptome to negotiate easily. Often, by taking a more lateral approach, or by using a longer sheath, this difficulty can be overcome. In the unusual circumstance where left ventricular biopsy is necessary, this is invariably performed via the femoral artery.

Before use, the bioptome must first be checked to ensure that the jaws approximate tightly and that the 90° bend lines up with the bioptome handle. It is advisable to ask the patient to stop breathing when putting the bioptome into the sheath (and again when removing) in order to reduce the risk of air embolism.

Right ventricular biopsy

Using fluoroscopy, the bioptome is directed laterally along the superior vena cava into the mid-right atrium, at which point it is rotated anteriorly (anticlockwise) through the tricuspid valve, and advanced into the RV gradually rotating posteriorly to the interventricular septum. The position can be confirmed using 30° RAO and 60° LAO projections. At this point, the tip is withdrawn slightly when it abuts the endocardium (seen fluoroscopically and felt as slight resistance). The bioptome jaws are then opened and advanced on to the endocardial surface. The jaws are then closed and the bioptome withdrawn briskly but smoothly. Tissue is then gently removed from the jaws and placed in an appropriate preservative. In view of the various histopathological techniques, it is best to discuss preservative solutions with the pathologist prior to the procedure. Typically, 10% neutral buffered formalin is used. For the assessment of cardiac allograft rejection, five or six biopsy specimens are required because of the multifocal nature of rejection. In cases of suspected infiltrative disease, a cardiac magnetic resonance imaging beforehand can reduce false-negative results by identifying areas of interest.

Histology specimens from a patient with cardiac amyloidosis are shown in **Figures 28.17** and **28.18**. Illustrations of biopsy samples of

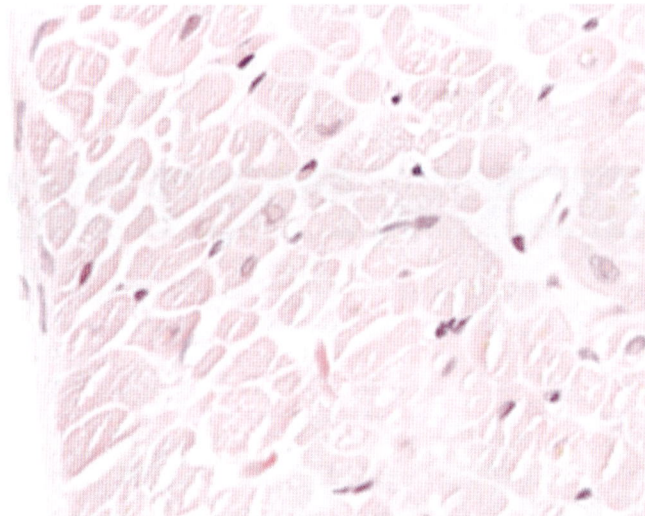

Figure 28.16 Normal myocardium stained with haematoxylin and eosin (×400). The endocardium on the left is a thin uniform layer with underlying myocardium that comprises cardiac myocytes that are closely applied to one another with little intervening stroma that includes small blood vessels.

Courtesy of Dr Allan McPhaden, Glasgow Royal Infirmary.

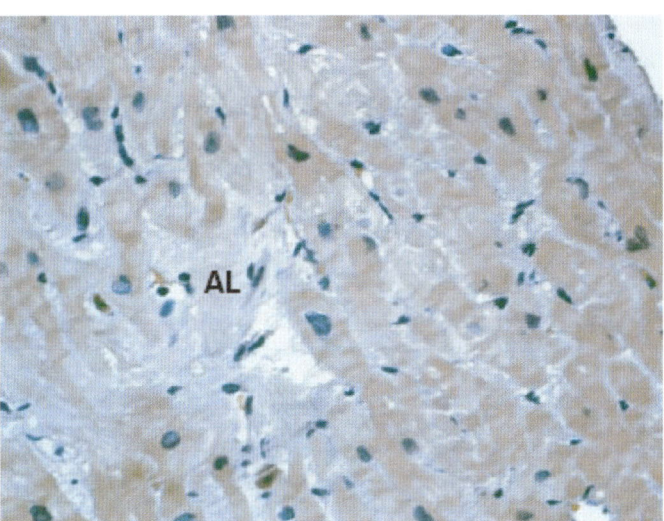

Figure 28.17 Histopathology of cardiac amyloid, demonstrating apple green birefringence with polarized light. Congo Red, ×200.

Courtesy of Dr Allan McPhaden, Glasgow Royal Infirmary.

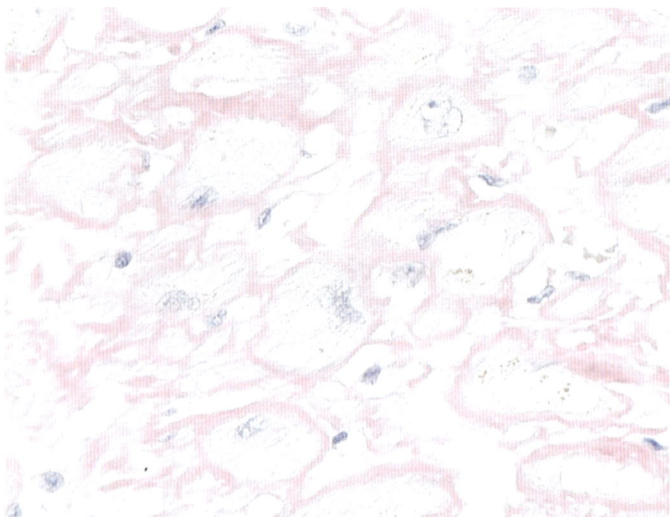

Figure 28.18 Amyloidosis. Individual myocytes are ringed by pink-staining extracellular deposits of amyloid in a case of primary amyloidosis. Sirius Red, ×400.
Courtesy of Dr Allan McPhaden, Glasgow Royal Infirmary.

patients with sarcoidosis, iron deposition, viral and giant cell myocarditis are shown in Figures 8.1–8.4 (pp. 00–00).

Heart transplant rejection surveillance

Despite much research in the pursuit of a surrogate marker of heart transplant rejection, nothing has been found to date that has successfully avoided the need for endomyocardial biopsy. Although rejection episodes are less frequent with advances in immunosuppressive regimes, endomyocardial biopsy remains the cornerstone investigation for the monitoring of rejection. Surveillance biopsies are generally performed weekly for the first six weeks, then fortnightly to three months, and then every six weeks for the remainder of the first postoperative year, because of the high incidence of rejection episodes during this time.

Acute cellular rejection

On light microscopy, histological features of acute cellular rejection (ACR) include interstitial oedema, inflammatory infiltration, and immunoglobulin deposition (Table 28.4). More severe rejection is marked by myocyte death and occasionally interstitial haemorrhage.

Antibody-mediated rejection

Evolving immunopathologic and serologic techniques have in recent years permitted the characterization of an entity whose very existence was previously a matter of some controversy. Antibody-mediated rejection (AMR) describes B-cell-initiated damage to the transplanted heart, the treatment for which differs from that given for more commonplace T-cell-mediated ACR. AMR is responsible for a number of clinical, histological, immunopathological, and serological sequelae (Table 28.5). The severity of AMR is classified according to working criteria defined by the International Society for Heart and Lung Transplantation (Table 28.6).

Ischaemic injury

Despite technical advances in the transportation and preservation of donor organs, varying degrees of ischaemic injury remain inevitable in the perioperative period. Histological evidence of early ischaemic injury is a frequent finding up to six weeks following transplant, and the finding of multicellular infiltrate accompanying myocyte necrosis may be challenging to differentiate from acute cellular rejection. As a general rule, the inflammatory infiltrate is a more pronounced finding than myocyte damage in acute rejection, whereas the reverse is true in early ischaemic injury.[17]

Late ischaemic injury occurs as a result of allograft coronary disease, and secondary histological evidence of this process (Table 28.7) may prompt further investigation, up to and including invasive coronary angiography.

Quilty effect

The Quilty effect—an infiltration of B-cell and T-cell lymphocytes detected at endomyocardial biopsy—is a phenomenon found

Table 28.4 Grades of acute cellular rejection on endomyocardial biopsy (2004) ISHLT scale with previous 1990 ISHLT scale for comparison

2004 ISHLT grading		1990 ISHLT grading	
Grade 0 R	No rejection	Grade 0	No rejection
Grade 1 R (mild)	Interstitial and/or perivascular infiltrate with up to 1 focus of myocyte damage (Figure 28.19)	Grade 1 (mild) A: focal	Focal perivascular and/or interstitial infiltrate without myocyte damage
		B: diffuse	Diffuse infiltrate without myocyte damage
		Grade 2 (moderate, focal)	One focus of infiltrate with associated myocyte damage
Grade 2 R (moderate)	≥2 foci of infiltrate with associated myocyte damage	Grade 3 (moderate) A: focal	Multifocal infiltrate with myocyte damage
Grade 3 R (severe)	Diffuse infiltrate with multifocal myocyte damage ± oedema ± haemorrhage ± vasculitis (Figure 28.20)	B: diffuse	Diffuse infiltrate with myocyte damage
		Grade 4 (severe)	Diffuse, polymorphous infiltrate with extensive myocyte damage ± oedema ± haemorrhage ± vasculitis

ISHLT, International Society for Heart and Lung Transplantation.

Source data from Stewart S, Winters GL, Fishbein MC et al. Revision of the 1990 Working Formulation for the Standardization of Nomenclature in the Diagnosis of Heart Rejection. J Heart Lung Transplant. 2005 Nov;**24**(11):1710–20.

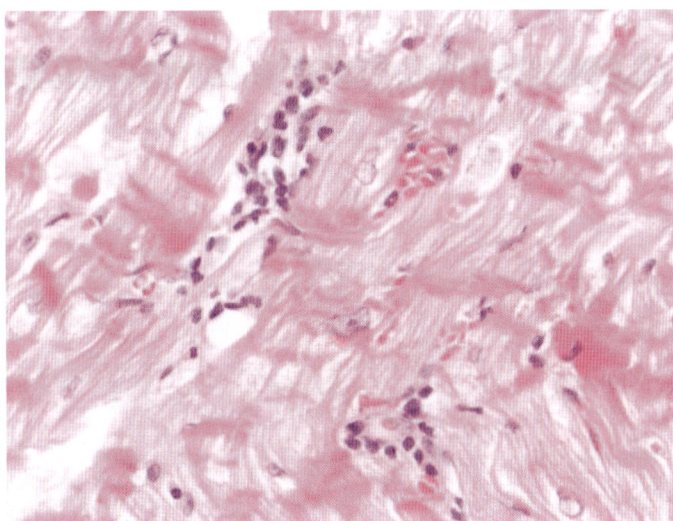

Figure 28.19 Low grade cardiac allograft rejection. The myocardium contains small perivascular aggregates of mononuclear cells (ISHLT Grade 1R). Haematoxylin and eosin, ×400.
Courtesy of Dr Allan McPhaden, Glasgow Royal Infirmary.

exclusively in transplanted hearts. The significance of Quilty remains a matter of debate because, despite the suspicion that it may represent subclinical rejection, until now the relationship of Quilty to rejection has remained unclear. In general, a diagnosis of Quilty does not mandate intensification of immunosuppression therapy. Differentiation from acute rejection is thus important, and this is thankfully of relative simplicity when the Quilty infiltrate is confined to the endocardium. Although the biopsy prevalence of Quilty is low (~10%), the lifetime incidence in cardiac transplant patients is high, with 50–74% of patients having at least one instance of Quilty during their post-transplant follow-up.

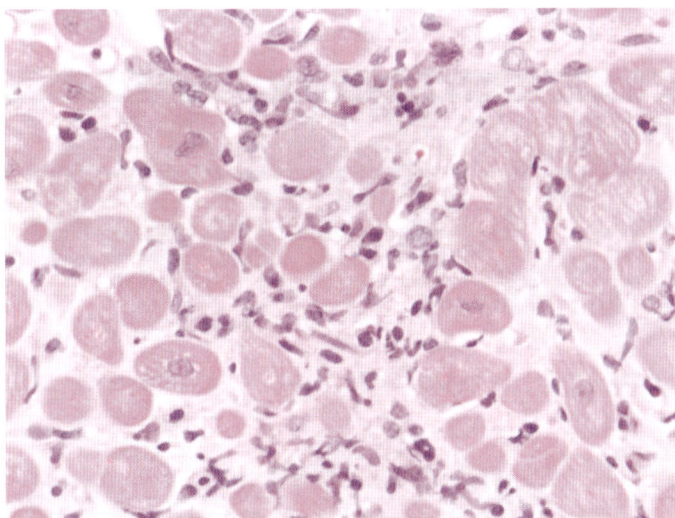

Figure 28.20 High-grade cardiac allograft rejection. The myocardium contains perivascular aggregates of mononuclear cells with extension into the interstitium associated with multiple foci of cardiac myocyte degeneration. Haematoxylin and eosin, ×400.
Courtesy of Dr Allan McPhaden, Glasgow Royal Infirmary.

Complications

In order to minimize the risk to patients, endomyocardial biopsies should be performed by expert operators in experienced centres. The risk of serious complication from endomyocardial biopsy is <1%. Nevertheless, the procedure should still only be performed when there is strong reason to believe that the results will have a significant impact on subsequent therapeutic decisions or prognosis.

Myocardial perforation

The most significant complication from endomyocardial biopsy is perforation—usually of the right ventricular free wall, which is only 1–2 mm in thickness. Perforation can lead quickly to cardiac tamponade, and is often heralded by the patient experiencing sharp chest pain (less likely after cardiac transplantation), followed by an exaggerated vagal response (bradycardia and hypotension) that is frequently unresponsive to atropine administration. If a perforation is suspected, an echocardiogram should be performed without delay, before taking any further biopsies. Because of the risks of tamponade, a pericardiocentesis kit should always be immediately available in the biopsy room.

Arrhythmias

Although the presence of premature ventricular contractions is often an indication that the bioptome has crossed into the ventricle, and therefore to be expected, ventricular tachycardia can occur. This often responds to the bioptome (or sheath) being removed from the ventricular cavity. Sustained ventricular tachycardia may rarely result, requiring overdrive pacing, anti-arrhythmic drugs, or electrical cardioversion.

Supraventricular arrhythmias may also occur as the bioptome, sheath, or guide wire stimulates the right atrium, particularly in cases where there are increased filling pressures. These are invariably transient.

Pneumothorax

A pneumothorax can be caused by puncture of the lung pleura, particularly when using a subclavian or a low internal jugular vein approach. The risk can be minimized by using direct vision (e.g. Site-Rite®) and a mid-high internal jugular approach, or avoided altogether by using a femoral approach. If a pneumothorax is suspected, fluoroscopy of the lung edge or chest radiograph should be carried out without delay. A chest drain kit should always be available in the biopsy room.

Conduction disturbance

Pressure against the septum around the tricuspid valve apparatus from the bioptome or sheath can transiently induce right bundle branch block which is of particular concern in the third of heart failure patients who already have a left bundle branch block, when complete heart block or asystole can ensue. Removal of the insult usually resolves this problem, although occasionally a temporary pacing line may be required, and this should be immediately available.

Lead displacement

In the current era of advanced heart failure management, many patients have either an ICD or cardiac resynchronization therapy

Table 28.5 Findings in acute antibody-mediated rejection (AMR)

		Required findings	Optional
1	Clinical evidence of acute graft dysfunction		Recommended in combination with other evidence to support diagnosis of AMR
2	Histological evidence of acute capillary injury (a + b required)	(a) Capillary endothelial changes (b) Macrophages in capillaries	(c) Neutrophils in capillaries (d) Interstitial oedema/haemorrhage
3	Immunopathologic evidence for antibody-mediated injury (a or b or c required)	(a) IgG, IgM, and/or IgA + C3d and/or C4d or C1q (2–3+) by IF (b) CD 68 for macrophages in capillaries (CD31 or CD34) and/or C4d (2–3+ intensity) in capillaries by paraffin IH (c) Fibrin in vessels (severe)	
4	Serological evidence of anti-HLA or anti-donor antibodies		Anti-HLA class I and/or class II or other anti-donor antibody at time of biopsy (supportive of clinical and/or morphological findings)

Source data from Colvin MM, Cook JL, Chang P et al. Antibody-mediated rejection in cardiac transplantation: emerging knowledge in diagnosis and management. A scientific statement from the American Heart Association. Circulation. 2015;131:00–00.

pacemaker or defibrillator *in situ*. Where possible, right heart catheterization or right ventricular endomyocardial biopsy should be avoided until device leads have had the opportunity to bed down. This is especially true of passive fix leads and coronary sinus left ventricle leads.

Other complications

Other complications that may result are air embolism or thromboembolism, nerve palsy, haematoma, inadvertent arterial puncture, arteriovenous fistula.

Implantable haemodynamic monitors

The pathophysiologic phenomenon common to all acute heart failure decompensations is a rise in intracardiac filling pressures and/or pulmonary vascular pressures. The recent emergence of novel implantable haemodynamic monitors is an attempt to capitalize on this concept, with the ambition of providing 'early warning' systems that might guide therapeutic interventions and thus reduce adverse events.

Several implantable haemodynamic monitors have been examined in randomized controlled trials enrolling patients with heart failure, including the HeartPOD system (which permits direct measurement of left atrial pressure)[18] and Chronicle system (which utilizes a transvenous right ventricular pressure sensor similar to a pacemaker lead).[19] To date, the only study that could be considered pivotal in this field is the CHAMPION trial (CardioMEMS Heart Sensor Allows Monitoring of Pressure to Improve Outcomes in NYHA Class III Heart Failure Patients), which utilized the CardioMEMS device—a wireless, implantable, battery-free pulmonary artery pressure sensor.[20] CHAMPION randomized patients into two groups: one in which clinicians were armed with daily CardioMEMS pulmonary artery pressure readings to help guide treatment decisions, or the other in which they were not. The primary end-point was the rate of heart failure hospitalization at six months, which was significantly reduced in the active treatment group (hazard ratio: 0.70; 95% confidence interval: 0.60–0.84;

Table 28.6 ISHLT working formulation for the pathological diagnosis of antibody-mediated rejection (AMR)[17]

Category	Description
pAMR 0: negative for pathological AMR	Negative histology and immunopathology
pAMR 1 (H+): histopathological AMR only	Histological findings positive; immunopathological findings negative
pAMR 1 (I+): immunopathological AMR only	Histological findings negative; immunopathological findings positive
pAMR 2: pathological AMR	Histological and immunopathological findings both positive
pAMR 3: severe pathological AMR	Histopathological findings include interstitial haemorrhage, capillary fragmentation, mixed inflammatory infiltrates and marked oedema

ISHLT, International Society for Heart and Lung Transplantation.
Source data from Colvin MM, Cook JL, Chang P et al. Antibody-mediated rejection in cardiac transplantation: emerging knowledge in diagnosis and management. A scientific statement from the American Heart Association. Circulation. 2015;131:1608–39.

Table 28.7 Non-rejection biopsy findings

Ischaemic injury	Findings
Early	Initial histological findings include contraction band necrosis and/or myocyte necrosis that may extend to endocardium, evolving to mixed inflammatory infiltrate as healing progresses.
Late	Secondary myocardial changes indicative of coronary ischaemia include vacuolization of myocytes and presence of microinfarcts.
Quilty effect	An infiltration of B-cell and T-cell lymphocytes unique to the transplanted heart.
Infection	Viruses are the predominant infectious cause of post-transplant myocarditis (typically cytomegalovirus infection). Lymphocytic infiltrate may be accompanied by intranuclear inclusion bodies on routine light microscopy.
Post-transplant lymphoproliferative disorder (PLTD)	A relatively rare finding at endomyocardial biopsy, PLTD includes a large group of lymphoid proliferations from reactive lymphoid hyperplasia to frank lymphoma. EBV infection is closely associated.

Source data from Stewart S, Winters GL, Fishbein MC et al. Revision of the 1990 Working Formulation for the Standardization of Nomenclature in the Diagnosis of Heart Rejection. J Heart Lung Transplant. 2005 Nov;24(11):1710–20.

$P < 0.0001$). The results of the CHAMPION trial must be treated with a sliver of caution given that it was a single trial conducted in a single country (the USA); however, the powerfully intuitive mechanism by which CardioMEMS appears efficacious hints tantalizingly that a new generation of diagnostic tools may soon move from the development phase to clinical practice.

REFERENCES

1. Seldinger SI. Catheter replacement of the needle in percutaneous arteriography; a new technique. *Acta Radiol* 1953;**39**:368–76.
2. Denys BG, Uretsky BF, Reddy PS. Ultrasound-assisted cannulation of the internal jugular vein. A prospective comparison to the external landmark-guided technique. *Circulation* 1993;**87**:1557–62.
3. National Institute for Health and Care Excellence. *Guidance on the use of ultrasound locating devices for placing central venous catheters.* London: NICE, 2002. http://www.nice.org.uk/nicemedia/pdf/Ultrasound_49_GUIDANCE.pdf.
4. Swan HJ, Ganz W, Forrester J, et al. Catheterization of the heart in man with use of a flow-directed balloon-tipped catheter. *N Engl J Med* 1970;**283**:447–51.
5. Binanay C, Califf RM, Hasselblad V, et al. Evaluation study of congestive heart failure and pulmonary artery catheterization effectiveness: the ESCAPE trial. *JAMA* 2005;**294**:1625–33.
6. Wheeler AP, Bernard GR, Thompson BT, et al. Pulmonary-artery versus central venous catheter to guide treatment of acute lung injury. *N Engl J Med* 2006;**354**:2213–24.
7. Shah MR, Hasselblad V, Stevenson LW, et al. Impact of the pulmonary artery catheter in critically ill patients: meta-analysis of randomized clinical trials. *JAMA* 2005;**294**:1664–70.
8. Kirklin JK, Naftel DC, Kirklin JW. Pulmonary vascular resistance and the risk of heart transplantation. *J Heart Lung Transplant* 1988;**7**:331–6.
9. Mehra MR, Canter CE, Hannan MM, et al. The 2016 International Society for Heart Lung Transplantation listing criteria for heart transplantation: a 10-year update. *J Heart Lung Transplant* 2016;**35**(1):1–23.
10. Ochiai Y, McCarthy PM, Smedira NG, et al. Predictors of severe right ventricular failure after implantable left ventricular assist device insertion: analysis of 245 patients. *Circulation* 2002;**106**:I-198–I-202.
11. Schenk S, McCarthy PM, Blackstone EH, et al. Duration of inotropic support after left ventricular assist device implantation: risk factors and impact on outcome. *J Thorac Cardiovasc Surg* 2006;**131**(2):447–54.
12. Ponikowski P, Voors AA, Anker SD, et al. 2016 ESC Guidelines for the diagnosis and treatment of acute and chronic heart failure: the Task Force for the diagnosis and treatment of acute and chronic heart failure of the European Society of Cardiology (ESC). Developed with the special contribution of the Heart Failure Association (HFA) of the ESC. *Eur J Heart Fail* 2016;**18**(8):891–975.
13. Velazquez EJ, Lee KL, Jones RH, et al. Coronary-artery bypass surgery in patients with ischemic cardiomyopathy. *N Engl J Med* 2016;**374**:1511–20.
14. Køber L, Thune JJ, Nielsen JC, et al. Defibrillator implantation in patients with nonischemic systolic heart failure. *N Engl J Med* 2016;**375**(13):1221–30.
15. Jackson CE, Gardner RS, Connelly DT. A novel approach for a novel combination: a trans-septal biopsy of left atrial mass in recurrent phyllodes tumour. *Eur J Echocardiogr* 2009;**10**:171–2.
16. Stewart S, Winters GL, Fishbein MC, et al. Revision of the 1990 Working Formulation for the Standardization of Nomenclature in the Diagnosis of Heart Rejection. *J Heart Lung Transplant* 2005;**24**(11):1710–20.
17. Colvin MM, Cook JL, Chang P, et al. Antibody-mediated rejection in cardiac transplantation: emerging knowledge in diagnosis and management. A scientific statement from the American Heart Association. *Circulation* 2015;**131**:1608–39.
18. Abraham WT, Adamson PB, Costanzo MR, et al. Hemodynamic monitoring in advanced heart failure: results from the LAPTOP-HF trial. *J Card Fail* 2016;**22**:940.
19. Bourge RC, Abraham WT, Adamson PB, et al. Randomized controlled trial of an implantable continuous hemodynamic monitor in patients with advanced heart failure: the COMPASS-HF study. *J Am Coll Cardiol* 2008;**51**(11):1073–9.
20. Abraham WT, Adamson PB, Bourge RC, et al. Wireless pulmonary artery haemodynamic monitoring in chronic heart failure: a randomised controlled trial. *Lancet* 2011;**377**:658–66.

SECTION 8
Prognostication

29

Prognostication

Joanne Simpson and Roy S. Gardner

Introduction

Recent advances in pharmacological and device therapy for the management of heart failure have resulted in improvements in survival in clinical trials. However, heart failure continues to reduce the quality and quantity of life for many patients,[1] and once a patient is hospitalized with heart failure, mortality rates at 30 days, 1 year and 5 years can be as high as 6.2%, 27.7% and 45.5%, respectively.[2]

Heart failure is a frequently progressive condition, although after commencing treatment patients usually reach a period of clinical 'stability', the duration of which varies between individuals. Most patients, if they do not suffer from sudden death, will ultimately deteriorate with refractory heart failure symptoms leading up to their death. Identifying such patients is one of the great challenges of heart failure management. Decisions regarding appropriateness and timing of scarce treatments (such as cardiac transplantation or mechanical circulatory support), or the need for end of life care can be aided by repeated prognostic assessment. As the 1-year mortality following cardiac transplantation is ~15.5%,[3] the selection of candidates for cardiac transplantation is therefore determined by identifying those patients whose annual mortality from heart failure exceeds this rate and who might therefore benefit prognostically from advanced therapy.

Prognostic assessment of chronic heart failure (CHF) can be made by a number of methods including evaluation of univariable predictors, and multivariable clinical models, and the most relevant of these are summarized in this chapter.

Univariable predictors of heart failure

There are more than 300 prognostic markers described in patients with heart failure, the most significant of which are shown in Table 29.1. Many studies have examined clinical, haemodynamic, and neurohormonal variables to assist with risk stratification, although it is important to look at such data in the context of the latest disease-modifying therapy. The traditional markers, including left ventricular ejection fraction (LVEF) and the peak oxygen uptake (pVo_2), consistently offer useful prognostic information. More recently, neurohormones have been shown to demonstrate the greatest prognostic potential in identifying patients at the greatest risk of an adverse outcome.

Risk according to demographics

Age

The Framingham Heart Study showed that mortality increased with advancing age, with a 27% increase in mortality per decade in men and 61% increase per decade in women.[4] This is confirmed by other studies which have shown that increasing age is an independent risk factor for all-cause mortality and heart failure hospitalization.[5-10] Advancing age is consistently a predictor of adverse outcome in modern therapeutic trials.[11-14] However, despite the increased risk that elderly heart failure patients currently face, their fate is substantially better than that it was 50 years ago. Further data from the Framingham study demonstrated a 5-year mortality of 54% in men and 40% in women in the period 1990–1999, compared to 65% and 66% in 1950–1969, in patients surviving at least 30 days after the onset of heart failure.[15]

Sex

Despite occasional conflicting reports, the majority of previous studies have found that women with heart failure have better survival than men.[4,16] The Framingham study showed that between 1948 and 1988, women had a median survival time after diagnosis of 3.2 years compared to 1.7 years for men; after 5 years, 38% of women and 25% of men with CHF were alive.[4] Whereas improvements in survival have been demonstrated overall, the differences in survival between men and women remain.

Women also have lower risk in modern therapeutic trials.[17-21] However, in the Italian Network on Congestive Heart Failure Registry,[22] there was no difference in outcome between men and women, and in the Studies of Left Ventricular Dysfunction (SOLVD) trial,[11] where an ischaemic aetiology was more common, women had a poorer prognosis than men. Heart failure pharmacological trials are not powered to show differences in outcomes by sex, and frequently women only represent 20–30% of included participants, which may account for the conflicting findings. Moreover, there are reported differences in underlying aetiology, pathophysiology,

Table 29.1 Powerful markers of an adverse outcome in patients with heart failure

Category	Prognostic marker	Relationship
Demographics	Age	Direct
Aetiology	Ischaemic heart disease	Direct
Co-morbidity	Chronic renal failure	Direct
	Diabetes mellitus	Direct
	Body mass index	Inverse
Symptoms and signs	Pulse	Direct
	Blood pressure	Inverse
	NYHA class	Direct
	S3	Adverse
Therapy	ARNI	Beneficial
	ACE inhibitors/ARBs	Beneficial
	β-Blocker	Beneficial
	Aldosterone antagonist	Beneficial
Laboratory tests	Sodium	Inverse
	Troponin	Direct
	Creatinine	Direct
	Haemoglobin	Inverse
	hsCRP	Direct
ECG	QRS duration	Direct
	Non-sustained VT	Direct
Imaging	Left ventricular end-diastolic dimension	Direct
	Left atrial volume	Direct
	Left ventricular ejection fraction	Inverse
Haemodynamics	Peak VO$_2$	Inverse
	6 min walk	Inverse
	Pulmonary capillary wedge pressure	Direct
	Cardiac output	Inverse
Neurohormones	B-type natriuretic peptide/NT-proBNP	Direct
	Atrial natriuretic peptide	Direct
	Noradrenaline	Direct
	Adrenomedullin	Direct
	Endothelin-1	Direct

and use of evidence-based therapies between women and men. Nevertheless, the majority of studies have found that men have poorer outcomes than women. A further observational study of 5491 consecutive patients admitted to hospital with heart failure followed for 5–8 years found that males had an increased risk of death when compared with females, after adjusting for age.[23]

The sex differences in outcome vary with aetiology and appear to be more marked in patients with non-ischaemic heart failure. Adams *et al.* found that women with non-ischaemic heart failure had a significantly better outcome than men (male relative risk: 3.08).[24] By contrast, ischaemic heart failure had a similar outcome in both men and women. A similar finding was also shown in a pooled analysis

of more than 11 000 patients from five modern therapeutic randomized trials in patients with reduced LVEF (MERIT HF, PRAISE, PRAISE II, PROMISE, and VEST).[16] In multivariable analysis, male sex was associated with significantly worse prognosis, particularly for those with a non-ischaemic aetiology of heart failure. There were similar findings in a comparison of outcomes in 2400 women and 5199 men in the CHARM trial, which included patients with both reduced and normal LVEF.[19] Women had lower risks of most fatal and non-fatal outcomes; these differences were not explained by LVEF or the cause of heart failure.

Race

In a prospective study of patients admitted with decompensated heart failure, African-Americans had a similar mortality but greater functional decline and were around 8 years younger on presentation than White Americans.[25] In the SOLVD registry,[26] Black patients with CHF were also at a greater risk of death and worsening heart failure, but had a higher prevalence of diabetes, prior stroke, and left ventricular dysfunction of a non-ischaemic aetiology, making interpretation difficult. Physiological differences in the renin–angiotensin–aldosterone and neuroendocrine systems could account for any difference in outcome, with angiotensin converting enzyme (ACE) inhibitors thought to be less effective at modifying disease progression in Black compared to White patients.[27] Additional pre-existing differences include the underlying aetiology of heart failure, genetics, and reported adherence to heart failure medications.

Region

Recent requirements for an increase in sample size in heart failure randomized controlled trials to show treatment effect has resulted in globalization of heart failure trials. Regional differences have been described in baseline characteristics, medical care, trial practice, outcomes and even treatment effect. The most notable of these was described in the sub-analysis of Treatment of Preserved Cardiac Function of Heart Failure With an Aldosterone Antagonist (TOPCAT) where patients in Russia and Georgia had lower event rates by a factor of four when compared to those from the USA, Argentina, Brazil, and Canada.[28] This difference in treatment effect has not been observed in trials of patients with CHF with reduced ejection fraction. Analyses of the ATLAS trial revealed significant variations in use of heart failure medications, a higher prevalence of diabetes in North America, greater use of coronary revascularization in USA and Canada, and lower incidence of ischaemic cardiomyopathy in southern and western Europe.[29] Similarly, analyses of PARADIGM-HF by region found significant differences in baseline characteristics and background heart failure therapy where North American patients were most likely to have an implantable cardioverter–defibrillator but less likely to be prescribed a mineralocorticoid receptor antagonist when compared with other regions.[30] There were also differences observed in outcomes with patients in North America having the highest rate of the primary composite end-point of cardiovascular death or heart failure hospitalization, whereas patients from Western Europe had the lowest rates. Two further trials in patients with acute heart failure have described similar differences in long term outcomes by region.[31,32]

Risk by aetiology

Chronic heart failure of ischaemic aetiology carries a greater risk of morbidity and mortality than that of a non-ischaemic aetiology.[17] Exceptions to this rule are infiltrative causes of myocardial disease, such as amyloidosis and haemochromatosis.[33] Although an ischaemic aetiology is an independent predictor of mortality in patients with a reduced ejection fraction, patients with mild coronary artery disease appear to have a similar 5-year survival to those with a non-ischaemic cardiomyopathy.[9] There is some evidence that revascularization of ischaemic myocardium may improve prognosis,[34,35] although in the STICH trial, patients undergoing surgical revascularization had a three-fold risk of death at 30 days when compared to those randomized to medical therapy alone.

Risk according to coexisting disease

Chronic renal impairment

Renal impairment is often associated with heart failure due to renal hypoperfusion, and the use of diuretics, ACE inhibitors, angiotensin receptor antagonists, aldosterone antagonists, angiotensin receptor–neprilysin inhibitors (ARNI), and other concomitant medication. Serum creatinine concentration, which is often quoted as a barometer of renal impairment, is actually a poor indicator of renal function.[36] An estimation of the glomerular filtration rate (GFR) is better for the accurate assessment of renal function,[36] and the Modification of Diet in Renal Disease (MDRD) equations[37] have recently been validated in patients with severe CHF.[38] GFR <60 mL/min/1.73 m^2 is associated with complications of renal disease.[36] Moreover, reduced GFR is independently predictive of all-cause mortality in asymptomatic[39] and symptomatic[39–42] left ventricular systolic dysfunction. In advanced heart failure, however, N-terminal pro B-type natriuretic peptide (NT-proBNP) appears to be a superior marker of prognosis.[43] Elevated levels of blood urea nitrogen (BUN) also predict morbidity and mortality.[44,45] BUN levels are affected by protein catabolism and tubular reabsorption and are therefore thought to reflect disease severity, not solely renal function. In addition to being an independent predictor of adverse outcome, an increase in BUN levels during hospital admission, as shown in the PROTECT study, were the strongest predictor of all-cause mortality at 180 days.[46]

Diabetes mellitus

Diabetes mellitus is a strong independent predictor of increased mortality in patients with heart failure[47] and this increased risk was later shown to be more marked in patients with an ischaemic cardiomyopathy, rather than those with a dilated cardiomyopathy.[48] One large population-based study of 48 858 patients with diabetes showed that a 1% increase in HbA1c levels was associated with 12% increase risk of death or hospitalization for heart failure, after adjusting for age and sex.[49] Pre-diabetes mellitus (defined as HbA1c of 6.0–6.4 mmol/L) is also related to increased morbidity and mortality when compared to normoglycaemia in patients with heart failure with reduced ejection fraction.[50]

Alcohol abuse

Excessive intake of alcohol is also a strong independent predictor of mortality.[51] Importantly, with total abstinence from alcohol, patients with an alcoholic cardiomyopathy can have a significant improvement in LVEF and functional status.[52] However, the prognosis for those who continue to consume excess alcohol is poor.[53]

Psychosocial

Heart failure patients with major depression are at increased risk of death as well as hospitalization.[54] Social isolation is also a significant predictor of mortality.[55] Better marital quality, as assessed by the marital satisfaction scale, is associated with better 4-year survival independent of New York Heart Association (NYHA) class.[56]

Risk according to clinical variables

Symptoms

NYHA class

A higher NYHA class has frequently been shown to be an independent predictor of mortality.[9,21,22,57]

Quality of life

In a cohort of patients with mild–moderate CHF, worsening quality of life as measured by the Minnesota Living with Heart Failure Questionnaire (MLHFQ) was an independent predictor of increasing 1-year mortality or worsening heart failure.[58] However, there is no correlation between MLHFQ and traditional prognostic indicators, such as LVEF and peak Vo_2.[59] Another health-related quality-of-life (HRQL) questionnaire has also been shown to predict mortality and CHF-related hospitalization.[60]

Syncope

Syncope in CHF, whether cardiac in origin or not, is independently predictive of sudden death.[61]

Signs

Cardiac signs

Heart rate >86/min and systolic blood pressure <119 mmHg are independently associated with poorer outcome in CHF.[21,22,57] The prognostic importance of raised jugular venous pressure and a third heart sound in patients with heart failure was evaluated in a retrospective analysis of the SOLVD treatment trial.[62] Both signs were associated with a significantly poorer NYHA class, but each was independently associated with an adverse outcome. A third heart sound was also an independent predictor of 1-year mortality in the Italian Network on Congestive Heart Failure Registry.[22]

Clinical profile

In a prospective analysis of 452 patients, subjects were classified by clinical assessment into four profiles: dry–warm, wet–warm, wet–cold, and dry–cold, on the basis of the absence/presence of signs of congestion, and evidence suggesting adequate or inadequate perfusion. Patients who were either wet–cold or wet–warm had an increased risk of death or urgent transplantation on multivariate analysis.[63]

Body weight

Obesity, as defined by a body mass index (BMI) >31 kg/m², is not associated with increased mortality in patients with advanced CHF after 5 years of follow-up.[64] Paradoxically, high BMI is an independent predictor of better survival. This could be partly explained by higher blood pressure in the overweight and obese patients, allowing a significantly greater use of disease-modifying therapy. However, low body weight and significant weight loss predict increased mortality, possibly reflecting a higher degree of cytokine activation.[65,66]

Exercise

Although a meta-analysis of small-scale trials of rehabilitation suggested that there may have been a survival benefit from exercise training,[67] the near-definitive HF-ACTION trial showed no effect of a formal training programme on survival. Training was associated with better quality of life.[68,69] An updated Cochrane review supports these findings: in a review of 33 trials with nearly 5000 patients, exercise-based rehabilitation did not alter all-cause mortality but did improve quality of life and reduce the risk of hospital admissions.[70]

Risk according to drug therapy

There is compelling evidence that ARNIs,[71] ACE inhibitors,[72–76] β-blockers,[77–79] mineralocorticoid receptor antagonists[80,81] and the SGLT2 inhibitor, dapagliflozin,[82] are associated with better survival. The association between some other drugs and prognosis is less clear-cut.

Diuretics

In a retrospective study, high doses of diuretic (>80 mg furosemide or equivalent per day) were independently associated with greater total mortality, sudden death, and pump failure death.[83] However, although diuretic dose relates to mortality, in multivariable models congestion is strongly associated with an adverse outcome but not the use, or dose, of loop diuretics.[84]

HMG-CoA reductase inhibitors (statins)

Statin therapy is beneficial for the primary and secondary prevention of ischaemic heart disease.[85,86] However, two studies have shown that rosuvastatin does not alter prognosis in patients with heart failure, whether or not it is due to coronary heart disease.[87,88]

Amiodarone

Although it appears to be a relatively safe anti-arrhythmic agent in CHF, there is conflicting information about the effect of amiodarone on mortality. In the GESICA study,[89] there was a 28% relative risk reduction in mortality with amiodarone, but the mortality reduction was not confirmed in the larger, placebo-controlled CHF-STAT study.[90] Furthermore, in SCD-HeFT—the largest clinical trial of amiodarone in heart failure—amiodarone was not associated with an improved prognosis.[91]

Digoxin

Although digoxin improves symptoms and reduces hospitalization in CHF, it has a neutral effect on mortality.[92,93] However, a post-hoc analysis of the DIG trial suggests that male subjects with higher serum digoxin concentrations (>1.2 ng/mL) have a higher mortality than patients receiving placebo.[94]

Hydralazine/isosorbide dinitrate

The combination of hydralazine and isosorbide dinitrate is associated with a lower mortality than placebo,[95] but is less effective than enalapril.[96] However, the A-HeFT study was stopped early because it showed that the addition of hydralazine and isosorbide dinitrate to standard care (including 69% on ACE inhibitors and 74% on β-blockers) in African-American patients was superior to placebo (43% relative risk reduction in all-cause mortality).[97]

Risk according to biochemistry and haematology

Electrolytes

Several studies have shown hyponatraemia to be an independent predictor of increasing mortality[98–102] and hypokalaemia to be an independent predictor of sudden cardiac death.[98] Serum magnesium is not an independent risk factor for death in patients with moderate–severe CHF.[103] More recently, hypochloraemia has been found to be a predictor for adverse outcome.[104,105]

Troponin

Over the past decade, an increasing number of studies has demonstrated that a significant proportion of patients with CHF (10–49%) have detectable circulating troponin (Tn).[106] Persistently elevated Tn concentrations are associated with an adverse prognosis regardless of the aetiology of heart failure. Raised Tn on high sensitivity assays is also predictive of adverse outcome in univariable and multivariable analyses in patients whose troponin was undetectable on older assays.[107,108] Raised Tn level is also associated with an adverse outcome in acute, and acute decompensated, heart failure.[106,109]

Urate

Increasing serum uric acid is strongly related to raised circulating markers of inflammation in patients with heart failure.[110] Several studies have shown that raised uric acid concentration is independently predictive of a worse prognosis.[84,111] Interestingly, a retrospective study has suggested that long-term use of high-dose allopurinol could be associated with reduced mortality, possibly by negating the adverse effect of raised urate concentration.[112]

Liver function tests

Abnormalities in liver function tests are associated with an adverse prognosis in CHF, most notably increasing aspartate transaminase and bilirubin.[84]

C-reactive protein

Inflammatory markers such as C-reactive protein (CRP), as well as the interleukins IL-4 and IL-6, increase during episodes of acute decompensation, returning to baseline once patients become compensated.[113] Patients admitted with decompensated heart failure who subsequently die or require readmission following discharge have a higher baseline CRP concentration than those who remain event-free.[114] In the Val-HeFT trial, the cumulative likelihood of death or

a first morbid event increased progressively with quartiles of serum CRP.[115]

Haemoglobin

Anaemia is an independent predictor of mortality in patients with new-onset heart failure,[116] mild–moderate CHF,[43] and advanced CHF.[117] Indeed, in the latter study, patients in the lowest haemoglobin (Hb) quartile were 86% more likely to die at 1 year than those in the highest Hb quartile. In ambulatory patients with CHF, lower haemoglobin and lower serum iron were independent predictors of a worse outcome.[118] Hb is a significant predictor of progressive pump failure but not sudden death. Although the treatment of anaemia in CHF with subcutaneous erythropoietin and intravenous iron improves some aspects of the condition, the randomized control trial of darbepoetin alfa (RED-HF) in anaemic heart failure patients was neutral.[119]

Red cell distribution width

Red cell distribution width is a readily available measure of the variation in erythrocyte volume. As well as offering prognostic information in CHF,[120] it is also a marker of adverse outcome in patients with acute heart failure, regardless of anaemia status.[121] It has prognostic value additional to that of B-type natriuretic peptide.[122]

White cell count

In a retrospective analysis of the SOLVD study, white cell count >7000/mm^3 was an independent predictor of worse all-cause and cardiovascular mortality in patients with left ventricular systolic dysfunction of ischaemic aetiology, but not in those with a dilated cardiomyopathy.[123]

Platelet function

Although platelet activity is increased in 22% of patients with stable CHF (vs 7% in normal controls), the degree of activation is similar in CHF of ischaemic and non-ischaemic aetiologies, and platelet activation is not related to NYHA class or to subsequent outcome.[124]

Erythrocyte sedimentation rate

An erythrocyte sedimentation rate above the median value (14 mm/h) is associated with a poor survival, independent of age, NYHA class, LVEF, and peak Vo_2.[125]

Risk according to ECG

Atrial fibrillation

Atrial fibrillation (AF) is much more common in patients with CHF than in normal individuals, with prevalence ranging from 10% to 50%. Data assessing the outcome of AF in patients with CHF have been conflicting, with most showing no impact on survival.

In the V-HeFT study, AF did not increase major morbidity or mortality in mild–moderate heart failure.[126] A follow-up of patients in the SOLVD trials with asymptomatic left ventricular dysfunction or NYHA class II–III heart failure found that AF (present in only 6.4%) was a significant predictor of increased all-cause mortality,[127] primarily due to pump failure, as there was no increase in mortality from arrhythmia. Around 18% of patients in the CHARM series had AF at baseline which was independently linked to increased mortality, both in patients with low or preserved LVEF.[128]

One study noted an improvement in the prognosis of patients with AF and CHF with the use of ACE inhibitor therapy, amiodarone, and avoidance of class Ia antiarrhythmic drugs.[129]

Heart rate variability

In a prospective study, a standard deviation of R–R interval of <100 ms identified patients at increased risk of death due to progressive pump failure but not sudden cardiac death.[98] However, conversely, a retrospective analysis of data from the Veterans Affairs' Survival Trial of Anti-arrhythmic Therapy in Congestive Heart Failure, the lowest quartile of the standard deviation of R–R intervals was an independent predictor of sudden death, as well as total mortality.[130]

PR interval

Around one in five patients with CHF have a long PR interval. Increasing PR interval is associated with worse survival in patients with CHF in univariable analysis, but is not an independent predictor of an adverse prognosis.[131]

QRS duration

QRS prolongation (>120 ms) is an independent predictor of both total mortality and sudden death in patients with severe CHF (LVEF <30%).[132] In moderate CHF (LVEF 30–40%), however, QRS duration is associated only with increased mortality but not sudden death. Right bundle branch block is not associated with excess mortality.

In the Italian Network on Congestive Heart Failure Registry,[133] left bundle branch block (LBBB)—diagnosed with QRS duration >140 ms—was found in 25.2% of individuals with CHF. LBBB was more common in women and in patients with dilated cardiomyopathy, and was an independent predictor of all-cause death and sudden death in patients with CHF. LBBB was also an independent predictor of mortality in the CIBIS-2 study.[21]

In two subsequent studies, progressive QRS-interval widening was independently associated with deterioration of cardiac function,[134] and death[135] or need for urgent cardiac transplantation.[136,137] CRT should be considered in patients with severe LVSD, and prolonged QRS (>130 ms), particularly when of an LBBB morphology.[138]

QT dispersion

In a substudy of Diamond-CHF,[139] QT dispersion was not a predictor of outcome and in another study QT dispersion and maximum QT interval were found to be univariable but not independent predictors of all-cause mortality and sudden death.[140]

Ventricular tachycardia

Patients with moderate–severe CHF who have evidence of non-sustained ventricular tachycardia on 24 h Holter monitoring have an increased risk of total mortality and sudden death.[98,141]

Risk according to imaging

Chest radiograph

A higher cardiothoracic ratio (CTR) is predictive of the risk of worsening symptoms, hospitalization, and mortality,[142] particularly

in the patient with CHF and low LVEF. In addition, UK-HEART (United Kingdom—Heart Failure Evaluation and Assessment of Risk Trial)—a multicentre prospective study designed to identify non-invasive markers of death and mode of death in patients with CHF—showed that a higher CTR was also predictive of sudden death.[143]

Echocardiography

Greater left ventricular dimensions (end-systolic and end-diastolic) independently predict all-cause mortality and sudden cardiac death.[98,144] Furthermore, patients with heart failure with severe mitral or tricuspid regurgitation on echocardiography are also at increased risk of death.[145]

In a study using dobutamine echocardiography, patients with moderate–severe left ventricular dysfunction and viable or ischaemic myocardium had a worse prognosis, independent of age and LVEF.[146]

Cardiac magnetic resonance imaging

There are few prognostic data from studies of cardiac magnetic resonance imaging (CMR) in patients with CHF. However, in a study of 279 patients with poor-quality echocardiograms, the presence of reduced left ventricular function (<40%) on CMR stress-testing was independently associated with all-cause mortality.[147] Further tissue characterization with the volume of late gadolinium enhancement is directly proportional to risk of death.[148,149] A study randomizing patients with mild–moderate left ventricular systolic dysfunction and left ventricular scar or fibrosis detected on CMR to receive either implantable cardioverter–defibrillator therapy or an implantable loop recorder is in progress.[150]

Risk according to haemodynamics

Left ventricular ejection fraction

A lower ejection fraction is associated with a poorer outcome in patients with CHF.[21,142,151] Patients with mild CHF whose LVEF increases during exercise radionuclide ventriculography have much better survival than those who do not.[152]

Right ventricular ejection fraction

In a small study by Di Salvo et al.,[153] a right ventricular ejection fraction of ≥35% during exercise was an independent predictor of better survival and was a stronger predictor of outcome than either peak VO_2 or percentage of predicted VO_2 achieved.

Peak VO_2

Peak oxygen consumption (pVo_2) of <10 mL/kg/min is associated with a 1-year mortality of 77% compared with 21% for those patients who achieved a pVo_2 of 10–18 mL/kg/min.[154] pVo_2 has become widely accepted as a marker of prognosis,[8,142,155–158] as well as a marker for the timing of transplantation.[159] Initially, those patients with pVo_2 <14 mL/kg/min were identified as a high-risk cohort of patients, with a 1-year mortality of 30% compared with those with a value >14 mL/kg/min who had a 1-year mortality of 6%. However, with widespread use of β-blockade, the cut-off has fallen to 12 mL/kg/min.[160]

Many studies have since attempted to 'fine-tune' the predictive power of pVo_2. As pVo_2 is affected by age, sex, body composition, and body conditioning, the percentage of predicted pVo_2 actually achieved might be a better marker, but adds minimal precision to pVo_2 alone.[161] As oxygen consumption is corrected for total body weight, and body fat consumes very little oxygen, body-fat-adjusted pVo_2 (pVo_2 lean) may provide greater prognostic precision, especially in women and in those who are obese.[162]

Six-minute walk test

The six-minute walk test is simple and non-invasive. The distance covered during a test is inversely related to morbidity and mortality in patients with mild–moderate[163] as well as advanced[164] CHF, and in those of advanced age.[165]

However, in other studies, the six-minute walk test distance was only able to predict mortality in univariable analysis, and was not an independent predictor of survival.[166,167]

Invasive haemodynamic variables

There are inconsistent reports of the predictive power of right heart catheter data in patients with CHF. No single variable consistently predicts outcome, although many studies have found that increasing pulmonary capillary wedge pressure (PCWP) is independently predictive of increasing mortality.[168,169] Other studies have found other right heart pressure measurements to be similarly predictive of outcome,[170,171] and increasing right atrial pressure measured non-invasively is associated with a worse prognosis,[172] as is increasing pulmonary artery pressure.[173] However, there is also a role for right heart catheterization in patient selection for cardiac transplantation, since an increased pulmonary vascular resistance has consistently been shown to increase the risk of early graft failure.[174,175]

Risk according to neurohormones

Adrenomedullin

This 52-amino-acid peptide is almost ubiquitously expressed throughout the human cardiovascular system. It has potent vasodilating and natriuretic effects, and is raised in heart failure in proportion to the severity of the disease.[176] Although increasing adrenomedullin is an independent predictor of death or urgent cardiac transplantation in patients with mild–moderate CHF,[177] it is not as powerful a predictor of prognosis as endothelin-1 or NT-proBNP.[178,179] As plasma levels of adrenomedullin may be inaccurate because of its short half-life, an assay has been developed for the more stable mid-regional portion of the pro-peptide (MR-proADM) which may offer further prognostic information.[180]

Catecholamines

A high plasma noradrenaline level is an independent predictor of worse morbidity and mortality in patients with LVSD and NYHA class I and II symptoms.[181] In a sub-study of the Val-HeFT trial, noradrenaline level above the median at baseline was an independent predictor of mortality, although not as powerful as increasing B-type natriuretic peptide.[182]

Endothelin

Endothelin-1 is a 21-amino-acid polypeptide with potent and long-lasting vasoconstricting properties. It is raised in patients with CHF. Higher levels independently predict mortality, clinical deterioration, and the need for cardiac transplantation in patients with CHF.[183–187] However, one study showed that there was no difference in endothelin-1 concentrations between patients with mild CHF and healthy controls.[188] Endothelin also correlates positively with pulmonary artery pressure in CHF:[189] increasing PAP is itself related to a worse prognosis.[190]

Natriuretic peptides

Atrial and B-type natriuretic peptides (ANP and BNP) are polypeptides produced in response to cardiac stretch. They stimulate natriuresis, induce vasodilation, and are antiproliferative. They also inhibit the renin–angiotensin–aldosterone and sympathetic nervous systems.

Atrial natriuretic peptides

ANP and NT-proANP are raised in patients with CHF,[191,192] correlating closely with the severity of CHF, and are associated with increased mortality.[193] The mid-regional segment of the pro-atrial natriuretic peptide molecule (MR-proANP) is more stable in plasma than either proANP or mature ANP and is emerging as a promising biomarker. Raised MR-proANP is an independent predictor of increasing mortality in acutely decompensated heart failure,[194] and may be a better marker than BNP and its variants in patients with CHF.[195,196]

B-type natriuretic peptide

BNP and its N-terminal inactive fragment (NT-proBNP) are increased in both symptomatic and asymptomatic LVSD,[191] increasing in proportion to the severity of CHF.[197] Currently, they appear to be the most potent prognostic markers available in heart failure, and are predictive of morbidity and mortality in asymptomatic or minimally symptomatic LVSD,[191] in mild–moderate CHF,[166] and in patients with advanced heart failure referred for consideration of cardiac transplantation.[198]

Cytokines

Tumour necrosis factor

Tumour necrosis factor-α (TNFα) is a proinflammatory cytokine and is increased in patients with severe CHF, particularly in those with cachexia.[199,200] Although TNFα has not been shown to be an independent marker of prognosis, TNF soluble receptor-1 has.[201]

Interleukin-6

IL-6 is a proinflammatory and vasodepressor cytokine that mediates both inflammatory and immune responses: like TNFα, it is increased in patients with heart failure. In a study of NYHA class III patients, IL-6 was an independent predictor of mortality at 1 year, and was as least as predictive as LVEF.[202] By contrast, there were no significant differences in the plasma concentrations of IL-1, IL-10, IL-12, and TNFα between survivors and non-survivors. Plasma concentrations of IL-6 follow a circadian rhythm, peaking at midnight.

Novel biomarkers

Several emerging biomarkers have shown promise as predictors in heart failure, and are currently being investigated (Table 29.2).[203] Many of them arise from our greater understanding of the pathophysiological processes in heart failure, in particular the components of novel neurohormonal pathways with possible roles—both protective and deleterious.

Risk according to composite scoring systems

A number of multivariable models have been used to develop composite scoring systems as predictive models with the aim of generating a much more accurate and individual estimate of prognosis than is possible with single variables.[101,204–211] As with the single-variable studies, however, the scoring systems quickly become out of date with the development of new therapies. Two systematic reviews to date have described the deficiencies in current available prognostic models, suggesting reasons why they have not been widely used in clinical practice by the heart failure community.[212,213] The main reasons include: the models are generated from patients selected for randomized control trials rather than 'real-world' heart failure populations; lack of external validation; and moderate performance as measured by the C-statistic.

EFFECT model

The EFFECT model was retrospectively derived and tested, and was intended for use in patients hospitalized for heart failure.[205] The derivation cohort included patients from the EFFECT study who presented with heart failure between 1999 and 2001. The model was then validated in a separate cohort presenting between 1997 and 1999. Multiple clinical characteristics (age, respiratory rate, systolic pressure, blood urea nitrogen, and serum sodium concentration) and co-morbidities were included and the resultant scores correlated with 30-day and 1-year mortality. However, no information was given on background therapy, and the model was created prior to the routine use of natriuretic peptides. An online calculator is available at www.ccort.ca/CHFriskmodel.aspx.

Heart Failure Survival Score

One commonly used scoring system is the Heart Failure Survival Score (HFSS),[101] which was developed and validated in patients with advanced heart failure (NYHA class III and IV symptoms). The score stratifies patients by risk—low, medium, and high (equating to a 1-year survival rate of 88%, 60%, and 35%, respectively)—of death or urgent transplantation and incorporates seven variables (heart rate, mean blood pressure, serum sodium, ejection fraction, pV_{O_2}, presence of ischaemic heart disease, and conduction delay on electrocardiography; Figure 29.1). In an invasive version of the HFSS, PCWP was included as an eighth variable. Unfortunately, due to the timing of the original model, only a small percentage of patients involved in the initial HFSS study were established on current standards of medical or device therapy. In particular, the use of β-blockers and spironolactone was very low, and both can alter some of the variables used in the scoring system, as well as the prognosis of CHF. However, a later study validated the HFSS

Table 29.2 Summary of novel biomarkers in acute and chronic heart failure

Biomarker	Plasma levels in ADHF	Independent prognostic information?	Levels altered with therapy?	Plasma levels in CHF	Independent prognostic information?	Levels altered with therapy?
MR-proANP	↑	Yes	U	↑	Yes	U
MR-proADM	U	U	U	↑	Yes	U
Copeptin	↑	Yes	U	↑	Yes	U
Apelin	↔	No	No	↓	U	Yes
Urocortin	U	U	U	↑	U	U
CgA	↑	Yes	U	↑	Yes	No
CoQ₁₀	U	U	U	↓	Yes	U
Adiponectin	↑	Yes	U	↑	Yes	U
H-FABP	U	U	U	↑	Yes	Yes
MLC-1	U	U	U	↑	Yes	U
Osteopontin	U	U	U	↑	Yes	U
GDF-15	U	U	U	↑	Yes	U
Pentraxin-3	U	U	U	↑	Yes	U
Secretory sphingomyelinase	U	U	U	↑	Yes	U
CT-1	U	U	U	↑	Yes	U
Gal-3	↑	Yes	U	↑	U	No
ST2	↑	Yes	U	↑	Yes	U
Cystatin C	↑	Yes	U	↑	Yes	U
SP-B	↑	U	Yes	↑	U	Yes

ADHF, acutely decompensated heart failure; CHF, congestive heart failure; ↑, raised; ↓, reduced; ↔, no change; U, unknown.
Reproduced from Dalzell JR, Jackson CE, McDonagh TA, Gardner RS. Novel biomarkers in heart failure: an overview. Biomark Med 2009;**3**(5):483–93.

in patients on current therapy.[214] A conflicting study found that a simplified risk stratification model with only two variables—LVEF and either V_{O_2} or six-minute walk test distance—was superior to the HFSS.[215]

The Seattle Heart Failure Model

The Seattle Heart Failure Model (SHFM) was derived from the PRAISE-1 database of 1125 heart failure patients with the use of a multivariable Cox model. It was subsequently prospectively validated in five additional cohorts: ELITE-2, Val-HeFT, UW, RENAISSANCE, and INCHF involving 9942 heart failure patients with 17 307 person-years of follow-up.[204] Although no patients in the derivation cohort were on β-blockers, up to 72% of the validation

population were. Importantly, the validation cohorts also included patients with a wide range of ages (14–100 years), ejection fractions (1–75%), and heart failure symptoms (NYHA class I–IV).

The SHFM accurately predicts survival of heart failure patients (**Figure 29.2**) with the use of commonly obtained clinical characteristics (NYHA class, ischaemic aetiology, diuretic dose,

Coronary artery disease (yes = 1; no = 0)	(. . . . . . . × 0.6931) =	+
Intraventricular conduction delay (y = 1; n = 0)	(. . . . . . . × 0.6083) =	+
Left ventricular ejection fraction (%)	(. . . . . . . × –0.0464) =	+
Heart rate (bpm)	(. . . . . . . × 0.0216) =	+
Na⁺ concentration (mmol/L)	(. . . . . . . × –0.0470) =	+
Mean arterial pressure (mmHg)	(. . . . . . . × –0.0255) =	+
Peak VO₂ (mL/minute/kg)	(. . . . . . . × –0.0546) =	
	HFSS = ...	

- High risk   <7.19   35% 1-year survival.
- Medium risk   7.20–8.09   60% 1-year survival.
- Low risk   >8.10   88% 1-year survival.

Figure 29.1 The Heart Failure Survival Score.

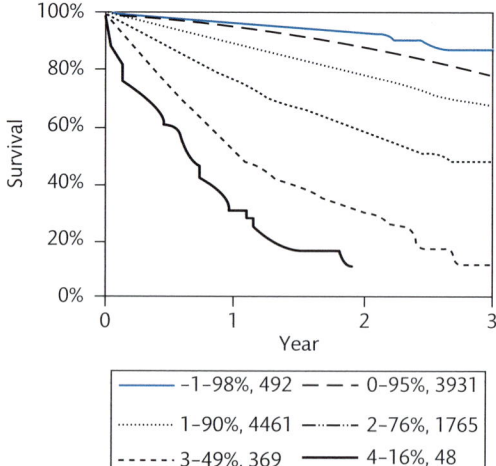

Legend:
- –1–98%, 492
- 0–95%, 3931
- 1–90%, 4461
- 2–76%, 1765
- 3–49%, 369
- 4–16%, 48

Figure 29.2 The combined dataset of the derivation and five validation cohorts for a Seattle Heart Failure Score rounded to –1 to 4. The score. the predicted 1-year survival for the score, and the number of patients with that score are shown.

Reproduced from Levy WC, *et al*. The Seattle Heart Failure Model: prediction of survival in heart failure. *Circulation* 2006;113:1424–33, with permission from Wolters Kluwer.

LVEF, systolic blood pressure, serum sodium, haemoglobin, percentage lymphocytes, uric acid, and serum cholesterol). It has a distinct advantage over the HFSS which relies on pV_{O_2} to calculate a score. The Seattle model also provides information about the likely mode of death. In an analysis of 10 538 ambulatory patients with predominantly systolic heart failure (NYHA class II–IV), the score was predictive of the risk of sudden death and of pump failure.[216]

Interestingly, renal function was not an independent predictor in the SHFM, and two extremely powerful prognostic markers—V_{O_2} and BNP/NT-proBNP—were not included in the development of the model, as the data were available in fewer than 1% of the patients in the six data sets.

An online calculator is available at www.SeattleHeartFailure Model.org.

MAGGIC risk score

The Meta-analysis Global Group in Chronic Heart Failure (MAGGIC) performed a large meta-analysis using individual patient-level data with the primary aim of comparing mortality rates in patients with heart failure and reduced or normal left ventricular ejection fraction.[206] The MAGGIC risk score was derived from 39 372 patients from 30 clinical and cohort studies from the MAGGIC meta-analysis. Of these, 15 851 (40.2%) died during a median follow-up of 2.5 (interquartile range: 1.0–3.9) years. Overall in MAGGIC only 67% of patients were treated with an ACE inhibitor/ARB, 34% with a β-blocker and 21% with a MRA.

There were 13 independent predictors. Increasing all-cause mortality was associated with: increasing age (per 10 years), NYHA class, and creatinine (per 10 µmol/L up to 350 µmol/L); male sex; current smoking; diabetes; chronic obstructive pulmonary disease; and heart failure duration >18 months. Conversely, decreasing all-cause mortality was associated with: BMI (per 1 kg/m² increase up to 30 kg/m²), systolic blood pressure (per 10 mmHg increase), LVEF (per 5% increase up to 40%), ACE inhibitor/ARB use, and β-blocker use. There were significant interactions between LVEF and age and LVEF and systolic blood pressure. A simple integer score was derived with a maximum score of 57 where a high score conferred a poorer prognosis. An online risk calculator is available at http://www.heartfailurerisk.org/. The MAGGIC score was not prospectively validated, however. It has since been validated in the Swedish Heart Failure Registry with only moderate results.[217]

BIOSTAT-HF

BIOSTAT-CHF was a large European study designed to develop and prospectively validate risk models in heart failure.[210] The models were designed for all-cause mortality, heart failure hospitalizations, and the composite of all-cause mortality and heart failure hospitalization and were derived from 2516 patients recruited from 2010 to 2014. The mean follow-up was 21 months. The model was prospectively externally validated in 1738 patients. The prediction models for mortality, hospitalization owing to heart failure, and the combined outcome had C-statistic values of 0.73, 0.69, and 0.71, respectively. The strongest predictors of mortality were increasing age, higher blood urea nitrogen, NT-proBNP, lower haemoglobin, and absence of β-blocker therapy.

Summary

In clinical trials, the 1-year mortality of patients with severe CHF may be as low as 7.6%.[71] The real challenge is identifying those patients at greatest risk of death, and therefore those who would benefit most from triaged resources (such as heart failure liaison nurse input). Furthermore, prognostication may help identify individuals who stand to benefit from advanced therapies such as mechanical circulatory support and cardiac transplantation, or end-of-life care. Targeting patients at higher risk of adverse outcome can lead to the 'personalized medicine' approach recommended in the treatment algorithm in the latest edition of the European Society for Cardiology guidelines.[138] In addition to guiding future management, helping inform patients and their families, accurate predictive models could have a wider use in identifying high-risk patients for clinical trials.

The ideal prognostic tool would be cost-effective, readily available, reproducible, minimally invasive, and both sensitive and specific. However, the heterogeneous nature of heart failure, varying modes of death, and the diverse populations in which potential predictive variables have been studied are just some of the reasons why the performance of individual variables in predicting adverse outcome is inconsistent. Whereas multivariable modelling in heart failure provides a more accurate prediction of risk, the models derived to date have had limitations. Patients included were not receiving contemporary evidence-based guideline recommended therapies; few of the studies are prospectively validated in external populations, and even fewer contain natriuretic peptides, the most powerful univariable predictors of outcome identified so far in heart failure.

Large prospective studies of patients on currently recommended therapies, with natriuretic peptides, and with appropriate statistical validation are therefore required in order to improve prognostication in heart failure.

REFERENCES

1. Gerber Y, Weston SA, Redfield MM, *et al.* A contemporary appraisal of the heart failure epidemic in Olmsted County, Minnesota, 2000 to 2010. *JAMA Intern Med* 2015;**175**:996–1004.
2. National Heart Failure Audit April 2015–March 2016. http://www.ucl.ac.uk/nicor/audits/heartfailure/documents/annualreports/annual-report-2015-6-v8.pdf.
3. Lund LH, Edwards LB, Kucheryavaya AY, *et al.* The registry of the International Society for Heart and Lung Transplantation: thirty-first official adult heart transplant report—2014; focus theme: retransplantation. *J Heart Lung Transplant* 2014;**33**:996–1008.
4. Ho KK, Anderson KM, Kannel WB, *et al.* Survival after the onset of congestive heart failure in Framingham heart study subjects. *Circulation* 1993;**88**:107–15.
5. van Veldhuisen DJ, Boomsma F, de Kam PJ, *et al.* Influence of age on neurohormonal activation and prognosis in patients with chronic heart failure. *Eur Heart J* 1998;**19**:753–60.
6. Adams KF, Dunlap SH, Sueta CA, *et al.* Relation between gender, etiology and survival in patients with symptomatic heart failure. *J Am Coll Cardiol* 1996;**28**:1781–8.
7. Rich MW, Beckham V, Wittenberg C, *et al.* A multidisciplinary intervention to prevent the readmission of elderly patients with congestive heart failure. *N Engl J Med* 1995;**333**:1190–5.

8. Myers J, Gullestad L, Vagelos R, *et al.* Clinical, hemodynamic, and cardiopulmonary exercise test determinants of survival in patients referred for evaluation of heart failure. *Ann Intern Med* 1998;**129**:286–293.

9. Bart BA, Shaw LK, McCants CB, *et al.* Clinical determinants of mortality in patients with angiographically diagnosed ischemic or nonischemic cardiomyopathy. *J Am Coll Cardiol* 1997;**30**:1002–1008.

10. Rich MW, McSherry F, Williford WO, *et al.* Effect of age on mortality, hospitalizations and response to digoxin in patients with heart failure: The DIG study. *J Am Coll Cardiol* 2001;**38**:806–813.

11. Bourassa MG, Gurne O, Bangdiwala SI, *et al.* Natural history and patterns of current practice in heart failure. *J Am Coll Cardiol* 1993;**22**:A14–A19.

12. Cohen-Solal A, McMurray JJ, Swedberg K, *et al.* Benefits and safety of candesartan treatment in heart failure are independent of age: insights from the Candesartan in Heart failure – Assessment of Reduction in Mortality and morbidity programme. *Eur Heart J* 2008;**29**:3022–3028.

13. Tavazzi L, Swedberg K, Komajda M, *et al.* Efficacy and safety of ivabradine in chronic heart failure across the age spectrum: insights from the SHIFT study. *Eur J Heart Fail* 2013;**15**:1296–1230

14. Jhund PS, Fu M, Bayram E, *et al.* Efficacy and safety of LCZ696 (sacubitril valsartan) according to age: insights from PARADIGM-HF. *Eur Heart J* 2015;**36**:2576–84.

15. Levy D, Kenchaiah S, Larson MG, *et al.* Long-term trends in the incidence of and survival with heart failure. *N Engl J Med* 2002;**347**:1397–402.

16. Frazier CG, Alexander KP, Newby LK, *et al.* Associations of gender and etiology with outcomes in heart failure with systolic dysfunction: a pooled analysis of 5 randomized control trials. *J Am Coll Cardiol* 2007;**49**:1450–8.

17. Simon T, Mary-Krause M, Funck-Brentano C. Sex differences in the prognosis of congestive heart failure; results from the cardiac insufficiency bisoprolol study (CIBIS II). *Circulation* 2001;**103**:375–80.

18. Ghali JK, Pina IL, Gottlieb SS, Deedwania PC, Wikstrand JC. Metoprolol CR/XL in female patients with heart failure: analysis of the experience in Metoprolol Extended-Release Randomized Intervention Trial in Heart Failure (MERIT-HF). *Circulation* 2002;**105**:1585–91.

19. O'Meara E, Clayton T, McEntegart MB, *et al.* Sex differences in clinical characteristics and prognosis in a broad spectrum of patients with heart failure: results of the Candesartan in Heart failure: Assessment of Reduction in Mortality and morbidity (CHARM) program. *Circulation* 2007;**115**:3111–20.

20. Adams KF Jr, Sueta CA, Gheorghiade M, *et al.* Gender differences in survival in advanced heart failure. Insights from the FIRST study. *Circulation* 1999;**99**:1816–21.

21. Funck-Brentano C, Lancar R, Hansen S, *et al.* Predictors of medical events and of their competitive interactions in the Cardiac Insufficiency Bisoprolol Study 2 (CIBIS-2). *Am Heart J* 2001;**142**:989–97.

22. Opasich C, Tavazzi L, Lucci D, *et al.* Comparison of one-year outcome in women versus men with chronic congestive heart failure. *Am J Cardiol* 2000;**86**:353–57.

23. Gustafsson F, Torp-Pederson C, Burchardt H, *et al.* Female sex is associated with a better long-term survival in patients hospitalized with congestive heart failure. *Eur Heart J* 2004;**25**:129–35.

24. Adams KF, Dunlap SH, Sueta CA, *et al.* Relation between gender, etiology and survival in patients with symptomatic heart failure. *J Am Coll Cardiol* 1996;**28**:1781–8.

25. Vaccarino V, Gahbauer E, Kasl SV, *et al.* Differences between African Americans and whites in the outcome of heart failure: evidence for a greater functional decline in African Americans. *Am Heart J* 2002;**143**:1058–67.

26. Dries DL, Exner DV, Gersh BJ, *et al.* Racial differences in the outcome of left ventricular dysfunction. *N Engl J Med* 1999;**340**:609–16.

27. Exner DV, Dries DL, Domanski MJ, Cohn JN. Lesser response to angiotensin-converting-enzyme inhibitor therapy in black as compared with white patients with left ventricular dysfunction. *N Engl J Med* 2001;**344**:1351–7.

28. Pfeffer MA, Claggett B; Assmann SF, *et al.* Regional variation in patients and outcomes in the Treatment of Preserved Cardiac Function Heart Failure With an Aldosterone Antagonist (TOPCAT) Trial. *Circulation* 2015;**131**(1):34–42.

29. Massie BM, Cleland JG, Armstrong PW, *et al.* Regional differences in the characteristics and treatment of patients participating in an international heart failure trial. The Assessment of Treatment with Lisinopril and Survival (ATLAS) Trial Investigators. *J Card Fail* 1998;**4**:3–8.

30. Kristensen SL, Martinez F, Jhund PS, *et al.* Geographic variations in the PARADIGM-HF heart failure trial. *Eur Heart J* 2016;**37**(41):3167–74.

31. Blair JE, Zannad F, Konstam MA, *et al.* Continental differences in clinical characteristics, management, and outcomes in patients hospitalized with worsening heart failure results from the EVEREST (Efficacy of Vasopressin Antagonism in Heart Failure: Outcome Study with Tolvaptan) program. *J Am Coll Cardiol* 2008;**52**:1640–8.

32. Greene SJ, Fonarow GC, Solomon SD, *et al.* Global variation in clinical profile, management, and post-discharge outcomes among patients hospitalized for worsening chronic heart failure: findings from the ASTRONAUT trial. *Eur J Heart Fail* 2015;**17**:591–600.

33. Felker GM, Thompson RE, Hare JM, *et al.* Underlying causes and long-term survival in patients with initially unexplained cardiomyopathy. *N Engl J Med* 2000;**342**:1077–84.

34. Di CM, Asgarzadie F, Schelbert HR, *et al.* Quantitative relation between myocardial viability and improvement in heart failure symptoms after revascularization in patients with ischemic cardiomyopathy. *Circulation* 1995;**92**:3436–44.

35. Velazquez EJ, Lee KL, Jones RH, *et al.* Coronary-artery bypass surgery in patients with ischemic cardiomyopathy. *N Engl J Med* 2016 **374**:1511–20.

36. Levey AS, Coresh J, Balk E. National Kidney Foundation practice guidelines for chronic kidney disease: evaluation, classification, and stratification. *Ann Intern Med* 2003;**139**:137–47.

37. Levey AS, Bosch JP, Lewis JB, *et al.* A more accurate method to estimate glomerular filtration rate from serum creatinine: a new prediction equation. *Ann Intern Med* 1999;**130**:461–70.

38. O'Meara E, Chong KS, Gardner RS, *et al.* The Modification of Diet in Renal Disease (MDRD) equations provide valid estimations of glomerular filtration rates in patients with advanced heart failure. *Eur J Heart Fail* 2006;**8**:63–7.

39. Dries DL, Exner DV, Domanski MJ, Greenberg B, Stevenson LW. The prognostic implications of renal insufficiency in asymptomatic and symptomatic patients with left ventricular systolic dysfunction. *J Am Coll Cardiol* 2000;**35**:681–9.

40. Mahon N, Blackstone EH, Francis GS, *et al.* The prognostic value of estimated creatinine clearance alongside functional capacity in ambulatory patients with chronic congestive heart failure. *J Am Coll Cardiol* 2002;**40**:1106–13.

41. Al-Ahmad A, Rand W, Manjunath G, *et al.* Reduced kidney function and anemia as risk factors for mortality in patients with left ventricular dysfunction. *J Am Coll Cardiol* 2001;**38**(4):955–62.

42. Hillege HL, Girbes ARJ, de Kam PJ, *et al.* Renal function, neurohormonal activation and survival in patients with chronic heart failure. *Circulation* 2000;**102**:203–10.

43. Gardner RS, Chong KS, O'Meara E, *et al.* Renal dysfunction, as measured by the modification of diet in renal disease equations, and outcome in patients with advanced heart failure. *Eur Heart J* 2007;**28**:3027–33.

44. Klein L, Massie BM, Leimberger JD, *et al.* Admission or changes in renal function during hospitalization for worsening heart failure predict postdischarge survival: results from the outcomes of a prospective trial of intravenous milrinone for exacerbations of chronic heart failure (OPTIME-CHF). *Circ Heart Fail* 2008;**1**:25–33.

45. Filippatos G, Rossi J, Lloyd-Jones DM, *et al.* Prognostic value of blood urea nitrogen in patients hospitalized with worsening heart failure: insights from the Acute and Chronic Therapeutic Impact of a Vasopressin Antagonist in Chronic Heart Failure (ACTIV in CHF) Study. *J Card Fail* 2007;**13**:360–364.

46. Cleland JG, Chiswell K, Teerlink JR, *et al.* Predictors of postdischarge outcomes from information acquired shortly after admission for acute heart failure: a report from the Placebo-Controlled Randomized Study of the Selective A1 Adenosine Receptor Antagonist Rolofylline for Patients Hospitalized With Acute Decompensated Heart Failure and Volume Overload to Assess Treatment Effect on Congestion and Renal Function (PROTECT) Study. *Circ Heart Fail* 2014;**7**:76–87.

47. Shindler DM, Kostis JB, Yusuf S, *et al.* Diabetes mellitus: a predictor of morbidity and mortality in the Studies Of Left Ventricular Dysfunction (SOLVD) trials and registry. *Am J Cardiol* 1996;**77**:1017–20.

48. Dries DL, Sweitzer NK, Drazner MH, *et al.* Prognostic impact of diabetes mellitus in patients with heart failure according to the etiology of left ventricular systolic function. *J Am Coll Cardiol* 2001;**38**:421–8.

49. Iribarren C, Karter AJ, Go AS, *et al.* Glycemic control and heart failure among adult patients with diabetes. *Circulation* 2001;**103**:2668–2673.

50. Kristensen SL, Preiss D, Jhund PS, *et al.*; PARADIGM-HF Investigators and Committees. Risk related to pre-diabetes mellitus and diabetes mellitus in heart failure with reduced ejection fraction: insights from prospective comparison of ARNI With ACEI to determine impact on global mortality and morbidity in heart failure trial. *Circ Heart Fail* 2016;**9**(1). pii: e002560.

51. Prazak P, Pfisterer M, Osswald S, Buser P, Burkart F. Differences of disease progression in congestive heart failure due to alcoholic as compared to idiopathic dilated cardiomyopathy. *Eur Heart J* 1996;**17**:251–7.

52. Guillo P, Mansourati J, Maheu B, *et al.* Long-term prognosis in patients with alcoholic cardiomyopathy and severe heart failure after total abstinence. *Am J Cardiol* 1997;**79**:1276–8.

53. Lazarevic AM, Nakatani S, Neskovic AN, *et al.* Early changes in left ventricular function in chronic asymptomatic alcoholics: relation to the duration of heavy drinking. *J Am Coll Cardiol* 2000;**35**:1599–606.

54. Jiang W, Alexander J, Christopher E, *et al.* Relationship of depression to increased risk of mortality and rehospitalization in patients with congestive heart failure. *Arch Intern Med* 2001;**161**:1849–56.

55. Murberg TA, Bru E. Social relationships and mortality in patients with congestive heart failure. *J Psychosomatic Res* 2001;**151**:521–7.

56. Coyne JC, Rohrbaugh MJ, Shoham V, *et al.* Prognostic importance of marital quality for survival of congestive heart failure. *Am J Cardiol* 2001;**88**:526–9.

57. Pernenkil R, Vinson JM, Shah AS, *et al.* Course and prognosis in patients > or = 70 years of age with congestive heart failure and normal versus abnormal left ventricular ejection fraction. *Am J Cardiol* 1997;**79**:216–19.

58. Hulsmann M, Berger R, Sturm B, *et al.* Prediction of outcome by neurohumoral activation, the six-minute walk test and the Minnesota Living with Heart Failure Questionnaire in an outpatient cohort with congestive heart failure. *Eur Heart J* 2002;**23**:886–91.

59. Ben-Gal T, Zafrir N, Berman M, *et al.* Self-assessed quality of life in patients evaluated for heart transplantation: correlation with prognostic indicators. *Transplant Proc* 2001;**33**:2904–5.

60. Konstam V, Salem D, Pouleur H, *et al.* Baseline quality of life as a predictor of mortality and hospitalization in 5,025 patients with congestive heart failure. SOLVD Investigations. Studies of Left Ventricular Dysfunction Investigators. *Am J Cardiol* 1996;**78**:890–5.

61. Middlekauff HR, Stevenson WG, Stevenson LW, Saxon LA. Syncope in advanced heart failure: high risk of sudden death regardless of origin of syncope. *J Am Coll Cardiol* 1993;**21**:110–16.

62. Drazner MH, Rame JE, Stevenson LW, *et al.* Prognostic importance of elevated jugular venous pressure and a third heart sound in patients with heart failure. *N Engl J Med* 2001;**345**:574–81.

63. Nohria A, Tsang SW, Fang JC, *et al.* Clinical assessment identifies hemodynamic profile that predict outcomes in patients admitted with heart failure. *J Am Coll Cardiol* 2003;**41**:1797–804.

64. Horwich TB, Fonarow GC, Hamilton MA, *et al.* The relationship between obesity and mortality in patients with heart failure. *J Am Coll Cardiol* 2001;**38**:789–95.

65. Anker SD, Ponikowski PP, Clark AL, *et al.* Cytokines and neurohormones relating to body composition alterations in the wasting syndrome of chronic heart failure. *Eur Heart J* 1999;**20**:683–93.

66. Anker SD, Ponikowski P, Varney S, *et al.* Wasting as independent risk factor for mortality in chronic heart failure. *Lancet* 1997;**349**:1050–3 [erratum appears in *Lancet* 1997;**349**(9060):1258].

67. Piepoli MF, Davos C, Francis DP, Coats AJ. Exercise training meta-analysis of trials in patients with chronic heart failure (ExTraMATCH). *BMJ* 2004;**328**:189.

68. O'Connor CM, Whellan DJ, Lee KL, *et al.* Efficacy and safety of exercise training in patients with chronic heart failure: HF-ACTION randomized controlled trial. *JAMA* 2009;**301**:1439–50.

69. Flynn KE, Pina IL, Whellan DJ, *et al.* Effects of exercise training on health status in patients with chronic heart failure: HF-ACTION randomized controlled trial. *JAMA* 2009;**301**:1451–9.

70. Taylor RS, Sagar VA, Davies EJ, *et al.* Exercise-based rehabilitation for heart failure. *Cochrane Database Syst Rev* 2014;(4):CD003331.

71. McMurray JJ, Packer M, Desai AS, *et al.* Angiotensin-neprilysin inhibition versus enalapril in heart failure. *N Engl J Med* 2014;**371**:993–1004.

72. SOLVD Investigators. Effect of enalapril on survival in patients with reduced left ventricular ejection fractions and congestive heart failure. *N Engl J Med* 1991;**325**:293–302.

73. SOLVD Investigators. Effect of enalapril on mortality and the development of heart failure in asymptomatic patients with reduced left ventricular ejection fractions. *N Engl J Med* 1992;**327**:685–91.

74. Garg R, Yusuf S. Overview of randomized trials of angiotensin-converting enzyme inhibitors on mortality and morbidity in patients with heart failure. Collaborative Group on ACE Inhibitor Trials. *JAMA* 1995;**273**:1450–6 [erratum appears in *JAMA* 1995;**274**:462].

75. Pfeffer MA, Braunwald E, Moye LA, *et al.* Effect of captopril on mortality and morbidity in patients with left ventricular dysfunction after myocardial infarction. Results of the survival and ventricular enlargement trial. The SAVE Investigators. *N Engl J Med* 1992;**327**:669–77.

76. Acute Infarction Ramipril Efficacy (AIRE) Study Investigators. Effect of ramipril on mortality and morbidity of survivors of acute myocardial infarction with clinical evidence of heart failure. *Lancet* 1993;**342**:821–8.

77. Cleland PJ, McGowan J, Clark A. The evidence for beta-blockers in heart failure. *Br Med J* 1999;**318**:824–5.

78. Packer M, Coats AJ, Fowler MB, *et al.* Effect of carvedilol on survival in severe chronic heart failure. *N Engl J Med* 2001;**344**:1651–8.

79. CAPRICORN Investigators. Effect of carvedilol on outcome after myocardial infarction in patients with left ventricular dysfunction:the CAPRICORN randomised trial. *Lancet* 2001;**357**:1385–90.

80. Pitt B, Zannad F, Remme WJ, *et al.* The effect of spironolactone on morbidity and mortality in patients with severe heart failure. Randomized Aldactone Evaluation Study Investigators. *N Engl J Med* 1999;**341**:709–17.

81. Zannad F, McMurray JJV, Krum H, *et al.* Eplerenone in patients with systolic heart failure and mild symptoms. *N Engl J Med* 2011;**364**:11–21.

82. McMurray JJ, Solomon SD, Inzucchi SE, *et al.*, on behalf of the DAPA-HF Trial Committees and Investigators. Dapagliflozin in patients with heart failure and reduced ejection fraction. *N Engl J Med* 2019;**381**:1995–2008.

83. Neuberg GW, Miller AB, O'Connor CM, *et al.* Diuretic resistance predicts mortality in patients with advanced heart failure. *Am Heart J* 2002;**144**:31–8.

84. Pellicori P, Cleland JG, Zhang J, *et al.* Cardiac dysfunction, congestion and loop diuretics: their relationship to prognosis in heart failure. *Cardiovasc Drugs Ther* 2016;**30**:599–609.

85. Shepherd J, Cobbe SM, Ford I, *et al.* Prevention of coronary heart disease with pravastatin in men with hypercholesterolaemia. *N Engl J Med* 1995;**333**:1301–7.

86. Scandinavian Simvastatin Survival Study group. Randomised trial of cholesterol lowering in 4444 patients with coronary heart disease: The Scandinavian Simvastatin Survival Study. *Lancet* 1994;**344**:1383–9.

87. Kjekshus J, Apetrei E, Barrios V, *et al.* Rosuvastatin in older patients with systolic heart failure. *N Engl J Med* 2007;**357**:2248–61.

88. Tavazzi L, Maggioni AP, Marchioli R, *et al.* Effect of rosuvastatin in patients with chronic heart failure (the GISSI-HF trial): a randomised, double-blind, placebo-controlled trial. *Lancet* 2008;**372**:1231–9.

89. Doval HC, Nul DR, Grancelli HO, *et al.* Randomised trial of low-dose amiodarone in severe congestive heart failure. *Lancet* 1994;**344**:493–8.

90. Singh SN, Fletcher RD, Fisher SG, *et al.* Amiodarone in patients with congestive heart failure and asymptomatic ventricular arrhythmia. Survival Trial of Antiarrhythmic Therapy in Congestive Heart Failure. *N Engl J Med* 1995;**333**:77–82.

91. Bardy G, Lee KL, Mark DB, *et al.* Amiodarone or an implantable cardioverter–defibrillator for congestive heart failure. *N Engl J Med* 2005;**352**:225–37.

92. Digitalis Investigation Group. The effect of digoxin on mortality and morbidity in patients with heart failure. *N Engl J Med* 1997;**336**:525–33.

93. Packer M, Gheorghiade M, Young JB, *et al.* Withdrawal of digoxin from patients with chronic heart failure treated with angiotensin-converting-enzyme inhibitors. RADIANCE Study. *N Engl J Med* 1993;**329**:1–7.

94. Rathore SS, Curtis JP, Wang Y, Bristow MR, Krumholz HM. Association of serum digoxin concentration and outcomes in patients with heart failure. *JAMA* 2003;**289**:871–8.

95. Cohn JN, Archibald DG, Ziesche S, *et al.* Effect of vasodilator therapy on mortality in chronic congestive heart failure: results of a Veterans Administration Cooperative study. *N Engl J Med* 1986;**314**:1547–52.

96. Cohn JN, Johnson G, Ziesche S, *et al.* A comparison of enalapril with hydralazine–isosorbide dinitrate in the treatment of patients with chronic congestive heart failure. *N Engl J Med* 1991;**325**(5):303–10.

97. Taylor AL, Ziesche S, Yancy C, *et al.* Combination of isosorbide dinitrate and hydralazine in blacks with heart failure. *N Engl J Med* 2004;**351**:2049–57.

98. Nolan J, Batin PD, Andrews R, *et al.* Prospective study of heart rate variability and mortality in chronic heart failure. *Circulation* 1998;**98**:1510–16.

99. Lee WH, Packer M. Prognostic importance of serum sodium concentration and its modification by converting-enzyme inhibition in patients with severe chronic heart failure. *Circulation* 1986;**73**:257–67.

100. Parameshwar J, Keegan J, Sparrow J, *et al.* Predictors of prognosis in severe chronic heart failure. *Am Heart J* 1992;**123**:421–6.

101. Aaronson KD, Schwartz JS, Chen TM, *et al.* Development and prospective validation of a clinical index to predict survival in ambulatory patients referred for cardiac transplant evaluation. *Circulation* 1997;**95**:2660–7.

102. Cleland JGF, Dargie HJ, Ford I. Mortality in heart failure: clinical variables of prognostic value. *Br Heart J* 1987;**58**:572–82.

103. Eichhorn EJ, Tandon PK, DiBianco R, *et al.* Clinical and prognostic significance of serum magnesium concentration in patients with severe chronic congestive heart failure: the PROMISE Study. *J Am Coll Cardiol* 1993;**21**(3):634–40.

104. Grodin JL, Verbrugge FH, Ellis SG, *et al.* Importance of abnormal chloride homeostasis in stable chronic heart failure. *Circ Heart Fail* **2016**;**9**:e002453.

105. Testani JM, Hanberg JS, Arroyo JP, *et al.* Hypochloraemia is strongly and independently associated with mortality in patients with chronic heart failure. *Eur J Heart Fail* 2016;**18**:660–8.

106. Jackson CE, Dalzell JR, Gardner RS. Prognostic utility of cardiac troponin in heart failure: a novel role for an established biomarker. *Biomark Med* 2009;**3**(5):483–93.

107. Sato Y, Yamada T, Taniguchi R, *et al.* Persistently increased serum concentrations of cardiac troponin T in patients with

idiopathic dilated cardiomyopathy are predicitve of adverse outcomes. *Circulation* 2001;**103**:369–74.

108. Latini R, Masson S, Inder S, et al. Prognostic value of very low plasma concentrations of troponin T in patients with stable chronic heart failure. *Circulation* 2007;**116**:1242–9.

109. Fonarow GC, Peacock WF, Horwich TB, et al. Usefulness of B-type natriuretic peptide and cardiac troponin levels to predict in-hospital mortality from ADHERE. *Am J Cardiol* 2008;**101**:231–7.

110. Leyva F, Anker SD, Godsland IF, et al. Uric acid in chronic heart failure: a marker of chronic inflammation. *Eur Heart J* 1998;**19**:1814–22.

111. Anker SD, Leyva F, Poole-Wilson P, Coats AJ. Uric acid as independent predictor of impaired prognosis in patients with chronic heart failure [Abstract]. *J Am Coll Cardiol* 1998;**31**:154–55A.

112. Struthers AD, Donnan PT, Lindsay P, et al. Effect of allopurinol on mortality and hospitalisations in chronic heart failure: a retrospective cohort study. *Heart* 2002;**87**:229–34.

113. Sato Y, Takatsu Y, Yamada T, et al. Serial circulating concentrations of C-reactive protein, interleukin (Il)-4 and Il-6 in patients with acute left heart decompensation. *Clin Cardiol* 1999;**22**(12):811–13.

114. Alonso-Martinez JL, Llorente-Diez B, Echegaray-Agara M, et al. C-reactive protein as a predictor of improvement and readmission in heart failure. *Eur J Heart Fail* 2002;**4**:331–6.

115. Anand IS, Latini R, Florea VG, et al. C-reactive protein in heart failure: prognostic value and the effect of valsartan. *Circulation* 2005;**112**:1428–34.

116. Ezekowitz JA, McAlister FA, Armstrong PW. Anemia is common in heart failure and is associated with poor outcomes: insights from a cohort of 12065 patients with new-onset heart failure. *Circulation* 2003;**107**:223–5.

117. Horwich TB, Fonarow GC, Hamilton MA et al. Anemia is associated with worse symptoms, greater impairment in functional capacity and a significant increase in mortality in patients with advanced heart failure. *J Am Coll Cardiol* 2002;**39**:1780–6.

118. Cleland JG, Zhang J, Pellicori P, et al. Prevalence and outcomes of anemia and hematinic deficiencies in patients with chronic heart failure. *JAMA Cardiol* 2016;**1**:539–47.

119. Swedberg K, Young JB, Anand IS, et al. Treatment of anemia with darbepoetin alfa in systolic heart failure. *N Engl J Med* 2013;**368**:1210–19.

120. Al Najjar Y, Goode KM, Zhang J, Cleland JG, Clark AL. Red cell distribution width: an inexpensive and powerful prognostic marker in heart failure. *Eur J Heart Fail* 2009;**11**:1155–62.

121. Pascual-Figal DA, Bonaque JC, Redondo B, et al. Red blood cell distribution width predicts long-term outcome regardless of anaemia status in acute heart failure patients. *Eur J Heart Fail* 2009;**11**:840–6.

122. Jackson CE, Dalzell JR, Bezlyak V, et al. Red cell distribution width has incremental prognostic value to B-type natriuretic peptide in acute heart failure. *Eur J Heart Fail* 2009;**11**:1152–4.

123. Cooper HA, Exner DV, Waclawiw MA, Domanski MJ. White blood cell count and mortality in patients with ischemic and nonischemic left ventricular systolic dysfunction (an analysis of the Studies of Left Ventricular Dysfunction [SOLVD]). *Am J Cardiol* 1999;**84**:252–7.

124. Gurbel PA, Gattis WA, Fuzaylov SY, et al. Evaluation of platelets in heart failure: is platelet activity related to etiology, functional class, or clinical outcomes? *Am Heart J* 2002;**143**:1068–75.

125. Sharma R, Rauchhaus M, Ponikowski PP, et al. The relationship of the erythrocyte sedimentation rate to inflammatory cytokines and survival in patients with chronic heart failure treated with angiotensin-converting enzyme inhibitors. *J Am Coll Cardiol* 2000;**36**:523–8.

126. Carson PE, Johnson GR, Dunkman WB, et al. The influence of atrial fibrillation on prognosis in mild to moderate heart failure. The V-HeFT Studies. The V-HeFT VA Cooperative Studies Group. *Circulation* 1993;**87**:VI102–10.

127. Dries DL, Exner DV, Gersh BJ, et al. Atrial fibrillation is associated with an increased risk for mortality and heart failure progression in patients with asymptomatic and symptomatic left ventricular systolic dysfunction: a retrospective analysis of the SOLVD trials. *J Am Coll Cardiol* 1998;**32**:695–703.

128. Olsson LG, Swedberg K, Ducharme A, et al. Atrial fibrillation and risk of clinical events in chronic heart failure with and without left ventricular systolic dysfunction: results from the Candesartan in Heart failure-Assessment of Reduction in Mortality and morbidity (CHARM) program. *J Am Coll Cardiol* 2006;**47**:1997–2004.

129. Stevenson WG, Stevenson LW, Middlekauff HR, et al. Improving survival for patients with atrial fibrillation and advanced heart failure. *J Am Coll Cardiol* 1996;**28**:1458–63.

130. Bilchick KC, Fetics B, Djoukeng R, et al. Prognostic value of heart rate variability in chronic congestive heart failure (Veterans Affairs' Survival Trial of Antiarrhythmic Therapy in Congestive Heart Failure). *Am Heart J* 2002;**90**:24–8.

131. Nikolaidou T, Pellicori P, Zhang J, et al. Prevalence, predictors, and prognostic implications of PR interval prolongation in patients with heart failure. *Clin Res Cardiol* 2018;**107**:108–19.

132. Iuliano S, Fisher SG, Karasik PE, et al. QRS duration and mortality in patients with congestive heart failure. *Am Heart J* 2002;**143**:1085–91.

133. Baldasseroni S, Opasich C, Gorini M, et al. Left bundle branch block is associated with increased 1-year sudden and total mortality rate in 5517 outpatients with congestive heart failure: a report from the Italian Network on Congestive Heart Failure. *Am Heart J* 2002;**143**:398–405.

134. Shamim W, Yousufuddin M, Cicoria M, et al. Incremental changes in QRS duration in serial ECGs over time identify high risk elderly patients with heart failure. *Heart* 2002;**88**:47–52.

135. Clark AL, Goode K, Cleland JG. The prevalence and incidence of left bundle branch block in ambulant patients with chronic heart failure. *Eur J Heart Fail* 2008;**10**:696–702.

136. Grigioni F, Carinci V, Boriani G, et al. Accelerated QRS widening as an independent predictor of cardiac death or the need for heart transplantation in patients with congestive heart failure. *J Heart Lung Transplant* 2002;**21**:899–901.

137. Kristensen SL, et al. Prevalence and incidence of intraventricular conduction delays and outcomes in patients with heart failure and reduced ejection fraction: insights from PARADIGM-HF and ATMOSPHERE. *Eur J Heart Fail* 2020 July 28 (online ahead of print).

138. Ponikowski P, Voors AA, Anker SD, et al. 2016 ESC Guidelines for the diagnosis and treatment of acute and chronic heart failure: The Task Force for the diagnosis and treatment of acute and chronic heart failure of the European Society of Cardiology (ESC). *Eur J Heart Fail*;**18**:891–975.

139. Brendorp B, Elming H, Jun L, et al. QT dispersion has no prognostic information for patients with advanced congestive heart failure and reduced left ventricular systolic function. *Circulation* 2001;**103**:831–5.

140. Brooksby P, Batin PD, Nolan J, *et al*. The relationship between QT intervals and mortality in ambulant patients with chronic heart failure. The United Kingdom Heart Failure Evaluation and Assessment of Risk Trial (UK-HEART). *Eur Heart J* 1999;**20**:1335–41.

141. Doval HC, Nul DR, Grancelli HO, *et al*. Nonsustained ventricular tachycardia in severe heart failure. Independent marker of increased mortality due to sudden death. GESICA-GEMA Investigators. *Circulation* 1996;**94**:3198–203.

142. Cohn J, Johnson G, Shabetai R, *et al*. for the V-HEFT VA Cooperative studies group. Ejection fraction, peak exercise consumption, cardiothoracic ratio and plasma norepinephrine as determinates of prognosis in heart failure. *Circulation* 1993;**87**(6 Suppl):VI5–16.

143. Kearney MT, Fox KA, Lee AJ, *et al*. Predicting sudden death in patients with mild to moderate chronic heart failure. *Heart* 2004;**90**:1137–43.

144. Baker BJ, Leddy C, Galie N, *et al*. Predictive value of M-mode echocardiography in patients with congestive heart failure. *Am Heart J* 1986;**111**:697–702.

145. Koelling TM, Aaronson KD, Cody RJ, Bach DS, Armstrong WF. Prognostic significance of mitral regurgitation and tricuspid regurgitation in patients with left ventricular systolic dysfunction. *Am Heart J* 2002;**144**, 524–9.

146. Williams MJ, Odabashian J, Lauer MS, Thomas JD, Marwick TH. Prognostic value of dobutamine echocardiography in patients with left ventricular dysfunction. *J Am Coll Cardiol* 1996;**27**:132–9.

147. Hundley WG, Morgan TM, Neagle, *et al*. Magnetic resonance imaging determination of cardiac prognosis. *Circulation* 2002;**106**:2328–33.

148. Cheong BY, Muthupillai R, Wilson JM, *et al*. Prognostic significance of delayed-enhancement magnetic resonance imaging: survival of 857 patients with and without left ventricular dysfunction. *Circulation* 2009;**120**:2069–76.

149. Mordi I, Jhund PS, Gardner RS, *et al*. Late Gadolinium enhancement and NT-proBNP identify low risk of death or arrhythmic events in patients with primary prevention implantable cardioverter defibrillators. *J Am Coll Cardiol Imaging* 2014;**7**:561–9.

150. Selvanayagam JB. Cardiac Magnetic Resonance GUIDEd Management of Mild–moderate Left Ventricular Systolic Dysfunction. (CMR_GUIDE.) ClinicalTrials.gov Identifier: NCT01918215.

151. Cohn JN. Prognosis in congestive heart failure. [Review] *J Cardiac Fail* 1996;**2**:S225–9.

152. Nagaoka H, Isobe N, Kubota S, *et al*. Myocardial contractile reserve as prognostic determinant in patients with idiopathic dilated cardiomyopathy without overt heart failure. *Chest* 1997;**111**:344–50.

153. Di ST, Mathier M, Semigran MJ, Dec GW. Preserved right ventricular ejection fraction predicts exercise capacity and survival in advanced heart failure. *J Am Coll Cardiol* 1995;**25**:1143–53.

154. Szlachcic J, Massie B, Kramer B, *et al*. Correlates and prognostic implication of exercise capacity in chronic congestive heart failure. *Am J Cardiol* 1985;**55**:1037–42.

155. Likoff MJ, Chandler SL, Kay HR. Clinical determinants of mortality in chronic congestive heart failure secondary to idiopathic or dilated cardiomyopathy. *Am J Cardiol* 1987;**59**:634–8.

156. Cicoira M, Davos C, Florea V, *et al*. Chronic heart failure in the very elderly: clinical status, survival, and prognostic factors in 188 patients more than 70 years old. *Am Heart J* 2001;**142**:174–80.

157. Myers J, Gullestad L, Vagelos R, *et al*. Cardiopulmonary exercise testing and prognosis in severe heart failure: 14 mL/kg/min revisited. *Am Heart J* 2000;**139**:78–84.

158. Mejhert M, Linder-Klingsell E, Edner M, Kahan T, Persson H. Ventilatory variables are strong prognostic markers in elderly patients with heart failure. *Heart* 2002;**88**:239–43.

159. Mancini DM, Eisen H, Kussmaul W, *et al*. Value of peak exercise consumption for optimal timing of cardiac transplantation in ambulatory patients with heart failure. *Circulation* 1991;**83**:778–86.

160. O'Neill JO, Young JB, Pothier CE, Lauer MS. Peak oxygen consumption as a predictor of death in patients with heart failure receiving beta-blockers. *Circulation* 2005;**111**:2313–18.

161. Aaronson KD, Mancini DM. Is percentage of predicted maximal exercise oxygen consumption a better predictor of survival than peak exercise oxygen consumption for patients with severe heart failure? *J Heart Lung Transplant* 1995;**14**:981–9.

162. Osman AF, Mehra MR, Lavie CJ, *et al*. The incremental prognostic importance of body fat adjusted peak oxygen consumption in chronic heart failure. *J Am Coll Cardiol* 2000;**36**:2126–31.

163. Bittner V, Weiner DH, Yusuf S, *et al*. Prediction of mortality and morbidity with a six-minute walk test in patients with left ventricular dysfunction. *JAMA* 1993;**270**:1702–7.

164. Shah MR, Hasselblad V, Gheorghiade M, *et al*. Prognostic usefullness of the six-minute walk in patients with advanced congestive heart failure secondary to ischemic or nonischaemic cardiomyopathy. *Am J Cardiol* 2001;**88**:987–93.

165. Ingle L, Rigby AS, Carroll S, *et al*. Prognostic value of the 6 min walk test and self-perceived symptom severity in older patients with chronic heart failure. *Eur Heart J* 2007;**28**:560–8.

166. Hüllsmann M, Berger R, Sturm B, *et al*. Prediction of outcome by neurohumoral activation, the six-minute walk test and the Minnesota Living with Heart Failure Questionnaire in an outpatient cohort with congestive heart failure. *Eur Heart J* 2002;**23**:886–91.

167. Opasich C, Pinna GD, Mazza A, *et al*. Six-minute walking performance in patients with moderate-to-severe heart failure. *Eur Heart J* 2001;**22**:488–96.

168. Keogh AM, Baron DW, Hickie JB. Prognostic guides in patients with idiopathic or ischemic dilated cardiomyopathy assessed for cardiac transplantation. *Am J Cardiol* 1990;**65**:903–8.

169. Griffin BP, Shah PK, Ferguson J, Rubin SA. Incremental prognostic value of exercise hemodynamic variables in chronic congestive heart failure secondary to coronary artery disease or dilated cardiomyopathy. *Am J Cardiol* 1991;**67**:848–53.

170. Morley D, Brozena S. Assessing risk by hemodynamic profile in patients awaiting cardiac transplantation. *Am J Cardiol* 1994;**73**:379–83.

171. Komajda M, Jais P, Reeves F, Goldfarb B, Bouhour JB. Factors predicting mortality in idiopathic dilated cardiomyopathy. *Eur Heart J* 1990;**11**:824–31.

172. Pellicori P, Clark AL, Kallvikbacka-Bennett A, *et al*. Non-invasive measurement of right atrial pressure by near-infrared spectroscopy: preliminary experience. A report from the SICA-HF study. *Eur J Heart Fail* 2017;**19**:883–92.

173. Damy T, Goode KM, Kallvikbacka-Bennett A, *et al*. Determinants and prognostic value of pulmonary arterial

pressure in patients with chronic heart failure. *Eur Heart J* 2010;**18**:2280–90.

174. Kirklin JK, Naftel DC, Kirklin JW, *et al.* Pulmonary vascular resistance and the risk of heart transplantation. *J Heart Lung Transplant* 1988;**7**:331–6.

175. Erickson KW, Constanzo-Nordin MR, O'Sullivan EJ, *et al.* Influence of preoperative transpulmonary gradient on late mortality after orthotopic heart transplantation. *J Heart Lung Transplant* 1990;**9**:526–37.

176. Jougasaki M, Wei C, McKinley LJ. Elevation of circulating and ventricular adrenomedullin in human congestive heart failure. *Circulation* 1995;**92**:286–9.

177. Pousset F, Masson F, Chavirovskaia O, *et al.* Plasma adrenomedullin, a new independant predictor of prognosis in patients with chronic heart failure. *Eur Heart J* 2000;**21**:1009–14.

178. Gardner RS, Chong V, Morton I, McDonagh TA. N-terminal brain natriuretic peptide is a more powerful predictor of mortality than endothelin-1, adrenomedullin and tumour necrosis factor-alpha in patients referred for consideration of cardiac transplantation. *Eur J Heart Fail* 2005;**7**:253–60.

179. Richards AM, Nicholls G, Yandle TG, *et al.* Plasma N-terminal pro-brain natriuretic peptide and adrenomedullin: new neurohormonal predcitors of left ventricular function and prognosis after myocardial infarction. *Circulation* 1998;**97**:1921–9.

180. Adlbrecht C, Hulsmann M, Strunk G, *et al.* Prognostic value of plasma midregional pro-adrenomedullin and C-terminal-pro-endothelin 1 in chronic heart failure outpatients. *Eur J Heart Fail* 2009;**11**:361–6.

181. Tsutamoto T, Wada A, Maeda K, *et al.* Plasma brain natriuretic peptide level as a biochemical marker of morbidity and mortality in patients with asymptomatic or minimally symptomatic left ventricular dysfunction. *Eur Heart J* 1999;**20**:1799–807.

182. Anand IS, Fisher LD, Chiang YT, *et al.* Changes in brain natriuretic peptide and norepinephrine over time and mortality and morbidity in the valsartan heart failure trial (Val-HeFT). *Circulation* 2003;**107**:1278–83.

183. McMurray JJ, Ray SG, Abdullah I, Dargie HJ, Morton JJ. Plasma endothelin in chronic heart failure. *Circulation* 1992;**85**:1374–9.

184. Pousset F, Isnard R, Lechat P, *et al.* Prognostic value of plasma endothelin-1 in patients with chronic heart failure. *Eur Heart J* 1997;**18**:254–8.

185. Pacher R, Stanek B, Hülsmann M, *et al.* Prognostic impact of big endothelin-1 plasma concentrations compared with invasive haemodynamic evaluation in severe heart failure. *J Am Coll Cardiol* 1996;**27**:633–41.

186. Stanek B, Frey B, Hülsmann M, *et al.* Validation of big endothelin plasma levels compared with established neurohormonal markers in patients with severe chronic heart failure. *Transplant Proc* 1997;**29**:595–6.

187. Hülsmann M, Stanek B, Frey B, Sturm B, *et al.* Value of cardiopulmonary exercise testing and big endothelin plasma levels to predict short-term prognosis os patients with chronic heart failure. *J Am Coll Cardiol* 1998;**32**:1695–700.

188. Daggubati S, Parks JR, Overton RM. Adrenomedullin, endothelin, neuropeptide Y, atrial, brain, and C-natriuretic prohormone peptides compared as early heart failure indicators. *Cardiovasc Res* 1997;**36**:246–55.

189. Cody RJ, Haas GJ, Binkley PF, *et al.* Plasma endothelin correlates with the extent of pulmonary hypertension in patients with chronic congestive heart failure. *Circulation* 1992;**85**:504–9.

190. Rickenbacher PR, Trindade PT, Haywood GA, *et al.* Transplant candidates with severe left ventricular dysfunction managed with medical treatment: characteristic and survival. *J Am Coll Cardiol* 1996;**27**:1192–7.

191. Lerman A, Gibbons RJ, Rodeheffer RJ, *et al.* Circulating N-terminal atrial natriuretic peptide as a marker for symptomless left-ventricular dysfunction. *Lancet* 1993;**341**:1105–9.

192. Francis GS, Benedict C, Johnstone DE, *et al.* Comparison of neuroendocrine activation in patients with left ventricular dysfunction with and without congestive heart failure: a substudy of the Studies of Left Ventricular Dysfunction (SOLVD). *Circulation* 1990;**82**:1724–9.

193. McDonagh TA, Cunningham AD, Morrison CE, *et al.* Left ventricular dysfunction, natriuretic peptides, and mortality in an urban population. *Heart* 2001;**86**:21–6.

194. Gegenhuber A, Struck J, Dieplinger B, *et al.* Comparative evaluation of B-type natriuretic peptide, mid-regional pro-A-type natriuretic peptide, mid-regional pro-adrenomedullin, and Copeptin to predict 1-year mortality in patients with acute destabilized heart failure. *J Card Fail* 2007;**13**:42–9.

195. von Haehling S, Jankowska EA, Morgenthaler NG, *et al.* Comparison of midregional pro-atrial natriuretic peptide with N-terminal pro-B-type natriuretic peptide in predicting survival in patients with chronic heart failure. *J Am Coll Cardiol* 2007;**50**:1973–80.

196. Moertl D, Berger R, Struck J, *et al.* Comparison of midregional pro-atrial and B-type natriuretic peptides in chronic heart failure: influencing factors, detection of left ventricular systolic dysfunction, and prediction of death. *J Am Coll Cardiol* 2009;**53**:1783–90.

197. Tsutamoto T, Wada A, Maeda K, *et al.* Attenuation of compensation of endogenous cardiac natriuretic peptide system in chronic heart failure: prognostic role of plasma brain natriuretic peptide concentration in patients with chronic symptomatic left ventricular dysfunction. *Circulation* 1997;**96**:509–16.

198. Gardner RS, Ozalp F, Murday AJ, Robb SD, McDonagh TA. N-terminal pro-brain natriuretic peptide. A new gold standard in predicting mortality in patients with advanced heart failure. *Eur Heart J* 2003;**24**:1735–43.

199. Levine B, Kalman J, Mayer L, *et al.* Elevated circulating levels of tumour necrosis factor in severe chronic heart failure. *N Engl J Med* 1990;**323**:236–41.

200. McMurray JJ, Abdullah I, Dargie HJ, *et al.* Increased concentrations of tumour necrosis factor in 'cachectic' patients with severe chronic heart failure. *Br Heart J* 1991;**66**:356–8.

201. Rauchhaus M, Doehner W, Francis DP. Plasma cytokine parameters and mortality in patients with chronic heart failure. *Circulation* 2000;**102**:3060–7.

202. Kell R, Haunstetter A, Dengler TJ. Do cytokines enable risk stratification to be improved in NYHA functional class III patients? *Eur Heart J* 2002;**23**:70–8.

203. Dalzell JR, Jackson CE, McDonagh TA, Gardner RS. Novel biomarkers in heart failure: an overview. *Biomark Med* 2009;**3**(5):483–93.

204. Levy WC, Mozaffarian D, Linker DT, *et al.* The Seattle Heart Failure Model: prediction of survival in heart failure. *Circulation* 2006;**113**:1424–33.

205. Lee DS, Austin PC, Rouleau JL, Liu PP, Naimark D, Tu JV. Predicting mortality among patients hospitalized for heart failure: derivation and validation of a clinical model. *JAMA* 2003;**290**:2581–7.

206. Pocock SJ, Ariti CA, McMurray JJ, *et al.* Predicting survival in heart failure: a risk score based on 39 372 patients from 30 studies. *Eur Heart J* 2013;**34**:1404–13.

207. Pocock SJ, Wang D, Pfeffer MA, *et al.* Predictors of mortality and morbidity in patients with chronic heart failure. *Eur Heart J* 2006;**27**:65–75.

208. Senni M, Parrella P, De Maria R, *et al.* Predicting heart failure outcome from cardiac and comorbid conditions: the 3C-HF score. *Int J Cardiol* 2013;**163**:206–11.

209. Barlera S, Tavazzi L, Franzosi MG, *et al.* Predictors of mortality in 6975 patients with chronic heart failure in the Gruppo Italiano per lo Studio della Streptochinasi nell'Infarto Miocardico-Heart Failure trial: proposal for a nomogram. *Circ Heart Fail* 2013;**6**:31–9.

210. Voors AA, Ouwerkerk W, Zannad F, *et al.* Development and validation of multivariable models to predict mortality and hospitalization in patients with heart failure. *Eur J Heart Fail* 2017;**19**:627–34.

211. Alba AC, Agoritsas T, Jankowski M, *et al.* Risk prediction models for mortality in ambulatory patients with heartfailure: a systematic review. *Circ Heart Fail* 2013;**6**:881–9.

212. Rahimi K, Bennett D, Conrad N, *et al.* Risk prediction in patients with heart failure: a systematic review and analysis. *JACC Heart Fail* 2014;**2**:440–6.

213. Koelling TM, Joseph S, Aaronson KD. Heart failure survival score continues to predict clinical outcomes in patients with heart failure receiving beta-blockers. *J Heart Lung Transplant* 2004;**23**:1414–22.

214. Zugck C, Kruger C, Kell R, *et al.* Risk stratification in middle-aged patients with congestive heart failure: prospective comparison with the heart failure survival score (HFSS) and a simplified two-variable model. *Eur J Heart Fail* 2001;**3**:577–85.

215. Mozaffarian D, Anker SD, Anand I, *et al.* Prediction of mode of death in heart failure: the Seattle Heart Failure Model. *Circulation* 2007;**116**:392–8.

216. Sartipy U, Dahlström U, Edner M, Lund LH. Predicting survival in heart failure: validation of the MAGGIC heart failure risk score in 51,043 patients from the Swedish heart failure registry. *Eur J Heart Fail* 2014;**16**:173–9.

Introduction

The treatment now available for people with heart failure is based on large, robust randomized trials of medical and device therapy. The consequence is the remarkable increase in quality of life and prognosis for patients. However, a major feature shared by most of the trials is that they have recruited patients who were, apart from their heart failure, otherwise reasonably well. Those with malignant disease, severe renal dysfunction, significant anaemia, significant chronic lung disease, or other co-morbidity are usually excluded from trials by design. Older patients are often poorly represented in trials. Quite why older people are not included is difficult to assess: it may be because investigators view a trial as being potentially burdensome for older people; it may be because older people themselves are less likely to consent.

One of the great challenges of caring for individual patients in clinical practice is thus that they may not be very similar to the people included in trials. They are likely to be at least a decade older (trial populations are frequently aged around 60–65 years); more likely to be female (≥75% of patients in trials are men); more likely to have 'heart failure with normal ejection fraction' (only trials of heart failure and reduced ejection fraction have been

unequivocally positive); and they are far more likely to have important co-morbidities.

The prevalence of co-morbidities in an unselected population with heart failure is very high. Among Medicare beneficiaries in the USA, for example, only 4% of patients have no co-morbidities (see Table S9.1 and Figures S9.1 and S9.2).[1,2] The number of co-morbidities an individual patient is likely to have (as well as the number of medications he or she is likely to be taking) is slowly increasing (see Figure S9.3).[3,4] The more co-morbidities the patient has, the more likely he or she is to be admitted to hospital and the worse the prognosis.[5] Recent work on patients with *incident* heart failure in Olmstead County, Minnesota, USA, showed that the mean number of co-morbidities per patient was more than four, and that the presence of co-morbidities again strongly predicted an increased risk of hospitalization or death.[6] Although the presence of co-morbidities has an important impact on the risks a patient faces, and although admission to hospital is very common following a heart failure diagnosis, the reason for admission is more likely to be non-cardiovascular than cardiovascular.[7]

A related issue is that of frailty. However it is measured, frailty is common in both patients with acute presentations to hospital[8] and those with chronic heart failure.[9] Associated with frailty is malnutrition,[10] and both frailty and malnutrition are strongly associated both with co-morbidity and worsening prognosis. Co-morbidities are important for patients with heart failure. A practical consequence is that far removed from the particulars of a clinical trial, it can be difficult for physicians to know exactly what condition their patient has: for patients presenting acutely with breathlessness, for example, a huge proportion is treated for more than one condition.[11] Among older people in the community, breathlessness is very common,[12,13] even in the absence of cardiovascular disease. Making the diagnosis of heart failure can be extremely difficult in, say, an obese patient with anaemia and a long history of smoking.

Table S9.1 Twenty most common non-cardiac chronic disease conditions for patients aged ≥65 years with chronic heart failure (*n* = 122 630)

Chronic disease defined by CCS code	Prevalence (%)
Essential hypertension	55
Diabetes mellitus	31
COPD and bronchiectasis	26
Ocular disorders (retinopathy, macular disease, cataract, glaucoma)	24
Hypercholesterolaemia	21
Peripheral and visceral atherosclerosis	16
Osteoarthritis	16
Chronic respiratory failure/insufficiency/arrest or other lower respiratory disease excluding COPD/bronchiectasis	14
Thyroid disorders	14
Hypertension with complications and secondary hypertension	11
Alzheimer disease/dementia	9
Depression/affective disorders	8
Chronic renal failure	7
Prostatic hyperplasia	7
Intravertebral injury, spondylosis, or other chronic back disorders	7
Asthma	5
Osteoporosis	5
Renal insufficiency (acute and unspecified renal failure)	4
Anxiety, somatoform disorders, and personality disorders	3
Cerebrovascular disease, late effects	3

CCS, Clinical Classification System, from *International Classification of Diseases*; COPD, chronic obstructive pulmonary disease.
Data taken from *J Am Coll Cardiol* 2003;**42**:1226.

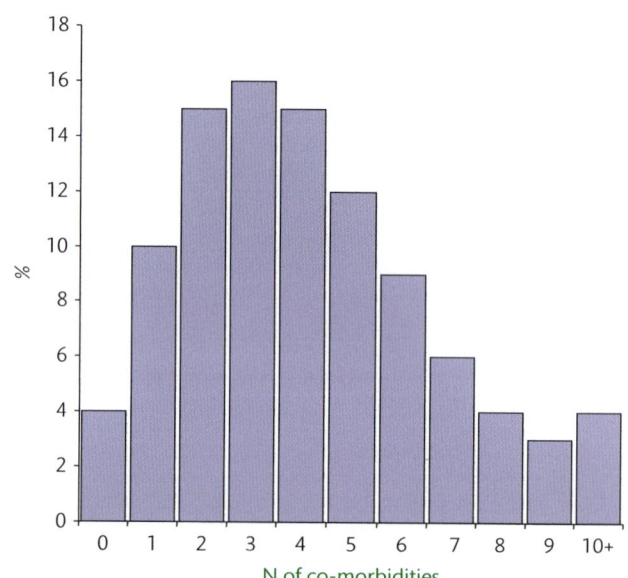

Figure S9.1 Number of different co-morbidities among a cross-sectional sample of 122 630 US Medicare beneficiaries aged ≥65 years. Table from Braunstein *et al.*[1]

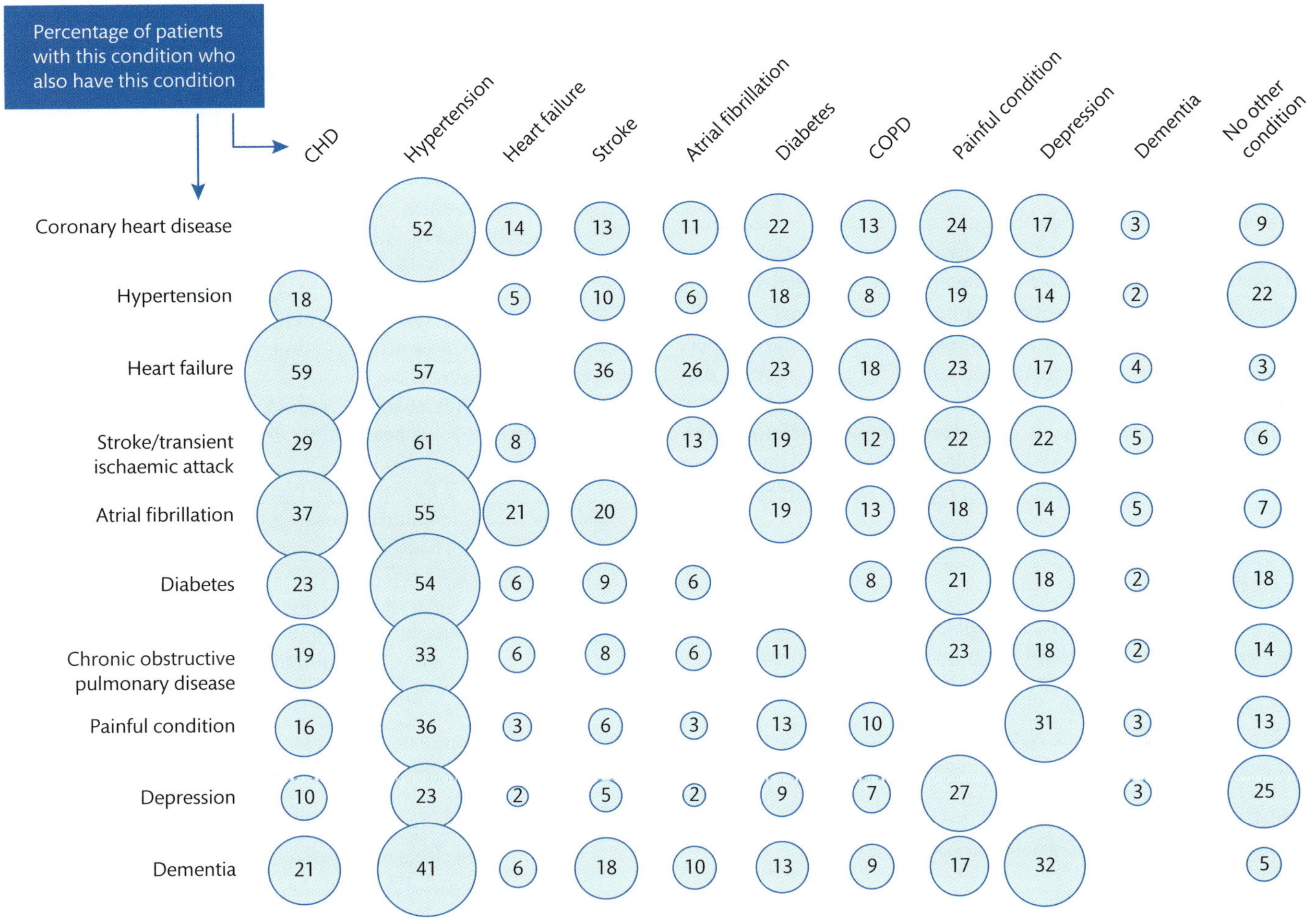

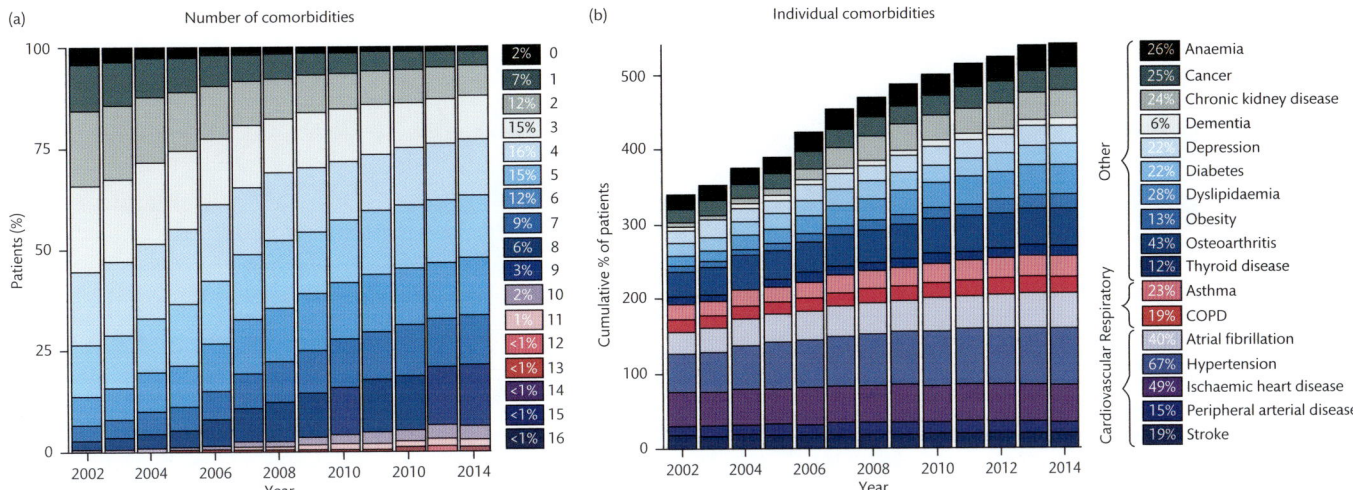

Figure S9.2 Infographic showing the relations between common co-morbidities.
Data from Farmer et al.[2]

Figure S9.3 The increasing number of co-morbidities among patients at diagnosis. (a) the proportion of the total number of patients with any given number of co-morbidities. (b) the rising number of patients affected by specific co-morbidities.

Conrad N, Judge A, Tran J, Mohseni H, Hedgecott D, Crespillo AP, Allison M, Hemingway H, Cleland JG, McMurray JJV, Rahimi K. Temporal trends and patterns in heart failure incidence: a population-based study of 4 million individuals. *Lancet* 2018;391:572–580.

Even once a firm diagnosis of heart failure has been made, treatment is more complex. The treatment of the heart failure may have impacts on the co-morbidities, and vice versa. Whether treatments that might affect long-term prognosis from heart failure are appropriate in patients with other life-limiting conditions is another challenge: patients' priorities may very well differ from those of their treating physician. The National Institute for Health and Care Excellence has recently published guidance on these issues,[14] particularly emphasizing the need for individualized patient care.

As well as the clinical problem of determining the relative contributions of cardiac co-morbidities to a patient's symptoms (diastolic dysfunction, valvular disease, arrhythmias, and pulmonary hypertension) there are the particular problems of treating airways disease, renal dysfunction, and arthritis. As diabetes becomes ever more common (and its management ever more complex), treating both conditions in the same patient is especially problematic. In this section we consider common co-morbidities of patients with heart failure.

REFERENCES

1. Braunstein JB, Anderson GF, Gerstenblith G, *et al.* Noncardiac comorbidity increases preventable hospitalizations and mortality among Medicare beneficiaries with chronic heart failure. *J Am Coll Cardiol* 2003;**42**:1226–33.
2. Farmer C, Fenu E, O'Flynn N, Guthrie B. Clinical assessment and management of multimorbidity: summary of NICE guidance. *Br Med J* 2016;**354**:i4843.
3. Wong CY, Chaudhry SI, Desai MM, Krumholz HM. Trends in comorbidity, disability, and polypharmacy in heart failure. *Am J Med* 2011;**124**:136–43.
4. Conrad N, Judge A, Tran J, *et al.* Temporal trends and patterns in heart failure incidence: a population-based study of 4 million individuals. *Lancet* 2018;**391**(10120):572–80.
5. Böhm M, Pogue J, Kindermann I, *et al.* Effect of co-morbidities on outcomes and angiotensin converting enzyme inhibitor effects in patients with predominantly left ventricular dysfunction and heart failure. *Eur J Heart Fail* 2014;**16**:325–33.
6. Manemann SM, Chamberlain AM, Boyd CM, *et al.* Multimorbidity in heart failure: effect on outcomes. *J Am Geriatr Soc* 2016;**64**:1469–74.
7. Dunlay SM, Redfield MM, Weston SA, *et al.* Hospitalizations after heart failure diagnosis a community perspective. *J Am Coll Cardiol* 2009;**54**:1695–702.
8. Sze S, Zhang J, Pellicori P, *et al.* Prognostic value of simple frailty and malnutrition screening tools in patients with acute heart failure due to left ventricular systolic dysfunction. *Clin Res Cardiol* 2017;**106**:533–41.
9. Sze S, Pellicori P, Zhang J, Weston J, Clark AL. Identification of frailty in chronic heart failure. *JACC Heart Fail* 2019;**7**:291–302.
10. Sze S, Pellicori P, Kazmi S, *et al.* Prevalence and prognostic significance of malnutrition using 3 scoring systems among outpatients with heart failure: a comparison with body mass index. *JACC Heart Fail* 2018;**6**:476–86.
11. Dharmarajan K, Strait KM, Tinetti ME, *et al.* Treatment for multiple acute cardiopulmonary conditions in older adults hospitalized with pneumonia, chronic obstructive pulmonary disease, or heart failure. *J Am Geriatr Soc* 2016;**64**:1574–82.
12. Ho SF, O'Mahony MS, Steward JA, *et al.* Dyspnoea and quality of life in older people at home. *Age Ageing* 2001;**30**:155–9.
13. Miner B, Tinetti ME, Van Ness PH, *et al.* Dyspnea in community-dwelling older persons: a multifactorial geriatric health condition. *J Am Geriatr Soc* 2016;**64**:2042–50.
14. National Institute for Health and Care Excellence. *Multimorbidity: clinical assessment and management* (NICE clinical guideline 56). London: NICE; 2016.

Heart failure with preserved ejection fraction
Pathophysiology and treatment

L. van Heerebeek and Walter J. Paulus

Introduction

Heart failure with preserved ejection fraction (HFpEF) accounts for 50% of all cases of heart failure, and its prevalence relative to heart failure with reduced EF (HFrEF) continues to rise at a rate of 1% per year. Patients with HFpEF have only slightly lower mortality rates than patients with HFrEF.[1] By 2020, the prevalence of HFpEF is projected to exceed 8% of people aged >65 years and the relative prevalences of HFpEF and HFrEF are predicted to be 69 and 31%, turning HFpEF into the most prevalent heart failure phenotype.[1]

HFpEF is diagnosed in the presence of heart failure signs and/or symptoms, preserved (or normal) left ventricular (LV) systolic function, with a left ventricular ejection fraction (LVEF) >50% and LV end-diastolic volume index (LVEDVI) <97 mL/m² together with evidence of diastolic LV dysfunction (**Figure 30.1**).[2] By contrast with the situation in HFrEF, large trials testing neurohumoral inhibition in patients with HFpEF have consistently failed to reach a positive primary outcome either individually or on meta-analysis.[3] The failure of neurohumoral inhibition in the large HFpEF outcome trials is due to incomplete understanding of HFpEF pathophysiology, suboptimal study designs, inadequate diagnostic criteria or statistical power, patient heterogeneity, and poor matching of therapeutic mechanisms and primary pathophysiological processes.[3,4] The conceptual framework for HFpEF treatment needs to change from a 'one size fits all' strategy to placing the emphasis on an individualized approach based on phenotypic patient characterization and diagnostic and pathophysiological stratification of myocardial disease processes.[3,4]

Normal diastolic function allows adequate filling of the heart without an excessive increase in diastolic filling pressure both at rest and with exercise. The term diastolic dysfunction indicates an abnormality of diastolic distensibility, filling or relaxation of the LV, regardless of whether the EF is normal or abnormal and regardless of whether the patient is symptomatic or asymptomatic. The term HFpEF refers to a clinical syndrome characterized by symptoms or signs of heart failure, preserved LVEF and diastolic LV dysfunction.[2]

Diagnosis of HFpEF

According to recent recommendations, three obligatory conditions need to be satisfied for the diagnosis of HFpEF: (i) presence of signs or symptoms of congestive heart failure; (ii) presence of preserved LV systolic function, defined as LVEF >50% and LVEDVI <97 mL/m², and (iii) evidence of diastolic LV dysfunction determined either by invasive measurements or by echocardiography alone or by echocardiography in conjunction with biomarkers (**Figure 30.1**).[2]

HFpEF: high diastolic LV stiffness

Diastolic LV dysfunction in HFpEF is evident from slow LV relaxation and elevated diastolic LV stiffness, which lead to an increase in diastolic filling pressures and limit cardiac performance at rest, during atrial pacing and exercise.[5,6] In the absence of endocardial or pericardial disease, high diastolic LV stiffness results from increased myocardial stiffness, which is regulated by the extracellular matrix (ECM) and the cardiomyocytes (**Figure 30.2**).[7]

Regulation of diastolic stiffness by the ECM

The ECM contributes to passive stiffness in diastole and prevents overstretch, myocyte slippage and tissue deformation during ventricular filling, while components of the ECM also serve as modulators of growth and tissue differentiation.[8] Collagen importantly determines ECM-based stiffness, through regulation of its total amount, expression of collagen type I, and degree of collagen crosslinking, which are increased and linked to diastolic LV dysfunction[9] and outcome[10] in patients with HFpEF. Myocardial collagen turnover is dynamically modulated by: the local renin–angiotensin–aldosterone system (RAAS) and transforming growth factor-β (TGFβ); and through modulation of the balance between collagen synthesis and degradation (by matrix metalloproteinases (MMPs) and tissue inhibitors of MMPs (TIMPs)).[8]

In HFpEF, fibroblasts are presumed to convert to myofibroblasts because of exposure to TGFβ as a result of monocyte/macrophage

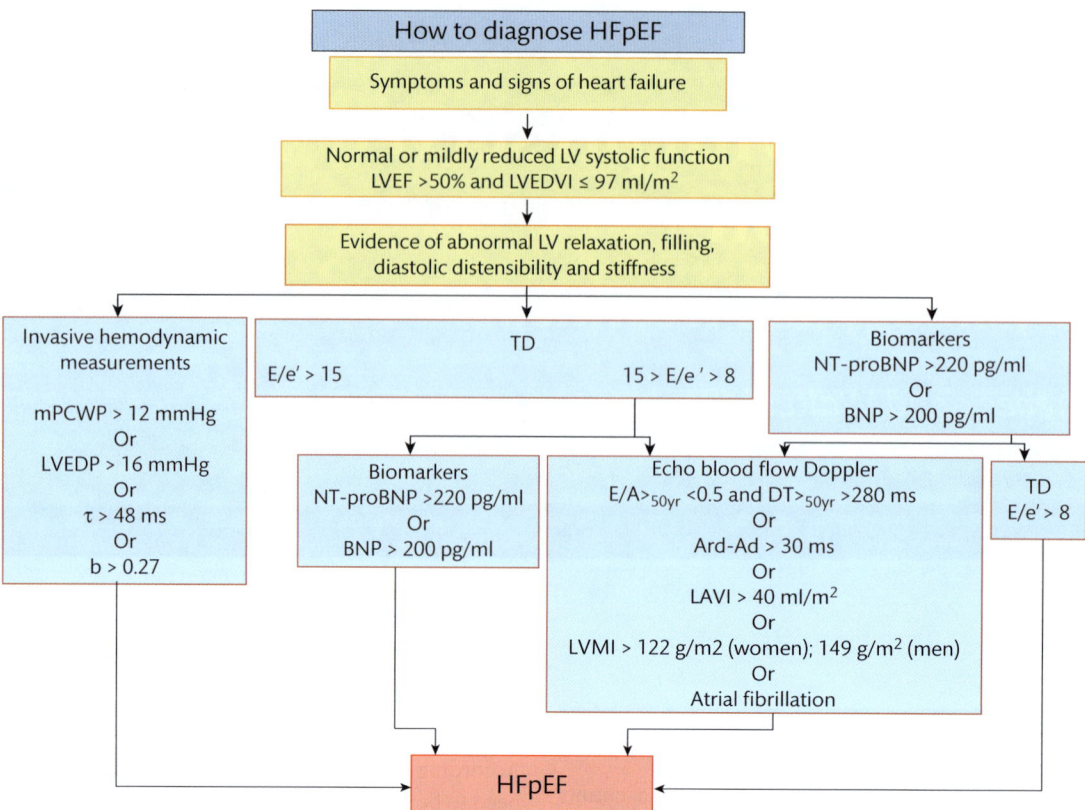

Figure 30.1 Diagnostic flowchart on 'How to diagnose HFpEF' in a patient suspected of having HFpEF. LVEDVI, left ventricular end-diastolic volume index; mPCWP, mean pulmonary capillary wedge pressure; LVEDP, left ventricular end-diastolic pressure; τ, time constant of left ventricular relaxation; b, constant of left ventricular chamber stiffness; TD, tissue Doppler; E, early mitral valve flow velocity; e', velocity of mitral annulus early diastolic motion; NT-proBNP, N-terminal-pro B-type natriuretic peptide; BNP, B-type natriuretic peptide; E/A, ratio of early (E) to late (A) mitral valve flow velocity; DT, deceleration time; LVMI, left ventricular mass index; LAVI, left atrial volume index; Ard, duration of reverse pulmonary vein atrial systole flow; Ad, duration of mitral valve trial wave flow.

myocardial infiltration, while matrix degradation is decreased because of altered expression of MMPs and upregulation of TIMPs.[11] Distinct expression profiles of MMPs and TIMPs also correspond to unequal patterns of myocardial collagen deposition: in HFpEF, there is mainly interstitial fibrosis, whereas in dilated cardiomyopathy, there is both replacement and interstitial fibrosis.[12] Interestingly, LV endomyocardial biopsy studies demonstrate that one-third of HFpEF patients have a normal myocardial collagen volume fraction (CVF), despite similarly elevated LV end-systolic wall stress and LV stiffness modulus when compared to HFpEF patients with raised CVF.[13] In such patients, high diastolic LV stiffness must be due to elevated intrinsic cardiomyocyte passive stiffness.[13]

Regulation of myocardial stiffness by the cardiomyocytes

In addition to myocardial fibrosis, increased cardiomyocyte stiffness also contributes to high diastolic LV stiffness in HFpEF.[12–15] Cardiomyocyte stiffness is mainly determined by the elastic sarcomeric protein titin, which functions as a bidirectional spring, responsible for early diastolic recoil and late diastolic distensibility (**Figure 30.2**).[16] Titin is the largest protein in the human body and can be considered the backbone of the (half-) sarcomere, with its NH₂ terminus anchored at the Z-disk, the elastic spring segment running through the I-band, and its longest

portion bound to the thick filament, reaching all the way to the M-band.[16] Titin-based cardiomyocyte stiffness results from dynamic changes in expression of stiff (N2B) and compliant (N2BA) isoforms and from post-translational modifications including titin isoform phosphorylation and oxidative changes of the N2B segment.[16] Phosphorylation of titin at its N2B segment by protein kinase A (PKA) and protein kinase G (PKG) increase its compliance, thereby acutely lowering cardiomyocyte stiffness (**Figure 30.2**).[16] By contrast, phosphorylation of titin's PEVK segment by protein kinase C (PKC)-α and oxidative stress-induced formation of disulfide bridges in the stiff N2B segment increase titin-based stiffness (**Figure 30.2**).[16]

Studies of endomyocardial tissue from patients with HFpEF, HFrEF, and aortic stenosis have demonstrated significantly stiffer cardiomyocytes in HFpEF than in HFrEF and aortic stenosis.[12–15] This increased cardiomyocyte stiffness is related to increased expression of the stiff titin N2B isoform in HFpEF relative to HFrEF,[12] and to reduced phosphorylation of titin.[14] Hypophosphorylation of titin resulted from lower myocardial PKG activity and reduced myocardial cGMP concentration in HFpEF compared to HFrEF and aortic stenosis.[15]

The generation of the second messenger molecule cGMP results from activation of soluble guanylate cyclase (sGC) by nitric oxide (NO) and from activation of particulate GC (pGC) by natriuretic peptides (NPs) (**Figure 30.2**).[17] Once generated, cGMP activates

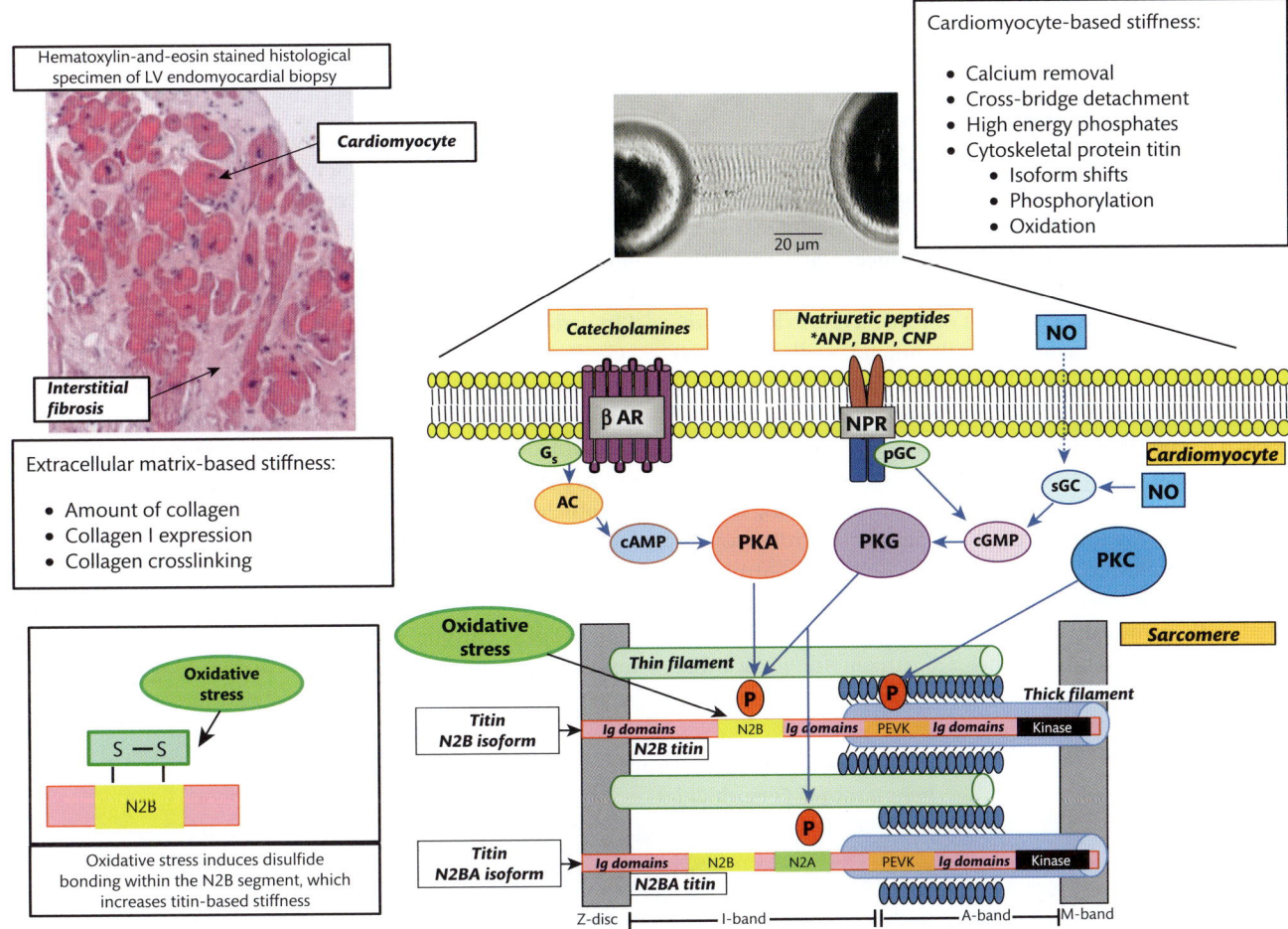

Figure 30.2 Extracellular matrix and cardiomyocytes determine myocardial stiffness. Extracellular matrix-based stiffness is predominantly regulated by collagen. Cardiomyocyte-based stiffness is predominantly regulated by the giant elastic sarcomeric protein titin (see text). Cardiomyocyte signalling pathways involved in regulating cardiac titin stiffness. Titin-based stiffness can be modulated by reversible phosphorylation of the N2B segment by both PKA and PKG. Activation of PKA results from stimulation by signaling through the β-adrenergic pathway, which is coupled to the second messenger cAMP. Activation of PKG results from stimulation by the second messenger cGMP. Generation of cGMP results from either activation of sGC by NO or from activation of pGC by NPs. PKC-mediated phosphorylation of the PEVK segment of titin increases cardiomyocyte stiffness. Oxidative stress-mediated formation of disulphide bonds in the N2B segment of titin increases cardiomyocyte stiffness. Circled Ps indicate phosphorylatable sites. AC, adenylyl cyclase; ANP, atrial natriuretic peptide; βAR, β-adrenergic receptor; BNP, brain-type natriuretic peptide; cAMP, cyclic adenosine monophosphate; cGMP, cyclic guanosine monophosphate; CNP, C-type natriuretic peptide; G, G-stimulatory protein; PDE5, phosphodiesterase type 5; Ig, immunoglobulin domains; NO, nitric oxide; NPR, natriuretic peptide receptor; PEVK, unique sequence rich in proline, glutamic acid, valine and lysine; PDE5, phosphodiesterase type 5; pGC, particulate guanylate cyclase; sGC, soluble guanylate cyclase.

PKG, allowing PKG-mediated phosphorylation of a vast number of target proteins, exerting a wide range of downstream effects such as enhanced re-uptake of calcium (Ca^{2+}) into the sarcoplasmic reticulum, inhibition of Ca^{2+} influx, suppression of hypertrophic signalling through inhibition of G-protein-coupled receptors and the transient receptor potential canonical channel; inhibition of ischaemia–reperfusion injury through phosphorylation of the ATP-sensitive potassium channel; and stimulation of LV relaxation and LV distensibility by phosphorylation of troponin I and the stiff titin N2B segment.[17] The downregulation of myocardial cGMP–PKG signalling seen in HFpEF is related to reduced myocardial BNP expression and increased microvascular inflammation and oxidative stress, which impair both the NP–cGMP and NO–cGMP axes.[15]

Reduced myocardial BNP expression in HFpEF could result from a number of factors. Obesity and insulin resistance lower myocardial BNP expression and induce concentric LV remodelling and hypertrophy, which lowers both systolic and diastolic LV wall stress.[18,19] In addition, increased expression of phosphodiesterase (PDE) type 9 breaks down cGMP specifically generated through the NP–pGC axis.[20] Impaired NO–cGMP signalling could result from the increased inflammation and oxidative stress observed in HFpEF, which was inferred from the high prevalence of co-morbidities such as hypertension, obesity and diabetes mellitus type 2 (DM2).[15]

Patients with HFpEF are generally older, more likely to be female and have a high prevalence of atrial fibrillation (AF) and non-cardiac co-morbidities, such as obesity, metabolic syndrome, type 2 diabetes, salt-sensitive hypertension, chronic obstructive pulmonary disease, anaemia, and renal dysfunction.[1,21] Highly prevalent co-morbidities in HFpEF share systemic inflammation and endothelial dysfunction as common and unifying factors, while

inflammation and endothelial dysfunction have been unequivocally demonstrated to play an important pathophysiological role in patients with HFpEF.

Inflammation and endothelial dysfunction

Myocardial inflammation contributes to ECM changes and diastolic dysfunction in HFpEF.[11] In an endomyocardial biopsy study, when compared with controls, HFpEF patients had increased inflammatory cell TGFβ expression, which induces transdifferentiation of fibroblasts into myofibroblasts, with increased production of collagen and decreased expression of MMP type 1. Both myocardial collagen and the quantity of inflammatory cells correlated with diastolic LV dysfunction.[11] Endothelial dysfunction is widely prevalent in HFpEF, and is associated with worse outcome.[22,23] Microvascular endothelial inflammation is also associated with myocardial capillary rarefaction, which has recently been demonstrated in HFpEF myocardium.[24] Compared to controls, HFpEF patients had lower myocardial capillary density regardless of the severity of epicardial coronary disease.[24] In both control and HFpEF subjects, the severity of myocardial fibrosis was inversely associated with myocardial vascular density. Group differences in LV fibrosis were attenuated after adjustment for myocardial vascular density, suggesting that reduced myocardial vascular density contributes to myocardial fibrosis.[24]

The new paradigm for HFpEF

The new HFpEF paradigm proposes that co-morbidities (and especially obesity) drive structural and functional remodelling in HFpEF through induction of systemic endothelial inflammation (**Figure 30.3**).[25] Because of this proinflammatory state, coronary microvascular endothelial cells produce reactive oxygen species, which limits NO bioavailability for adjacent cardiomyocytes. Limited NO bioavailability decreases sGC activity, thereby lowering cGMP generation, leading to reduced PKG activity. Reduced cardiomyocyte cGMP–PKG signalling augments cardiomyocyte stiffness through hypophosphorylation of titin and increases cardiomyocyte hypertrophy because of impaired PKG-mediated antihypertrophic activity.[25] Furthermore, coronary microvascular endothelial inflammation favours subendothelial migration of leucocytes, which stimulates myofibroblast formation and interstitial collagen deposition. Both increased cardiomyocyte stiffness and interstitial fibrosis induce diastolic LV dysfunction.[25]

In HFpEF, chronic systemic inflammation affects not only the myocardium but also other organs such as lungs, skeletal muscles,

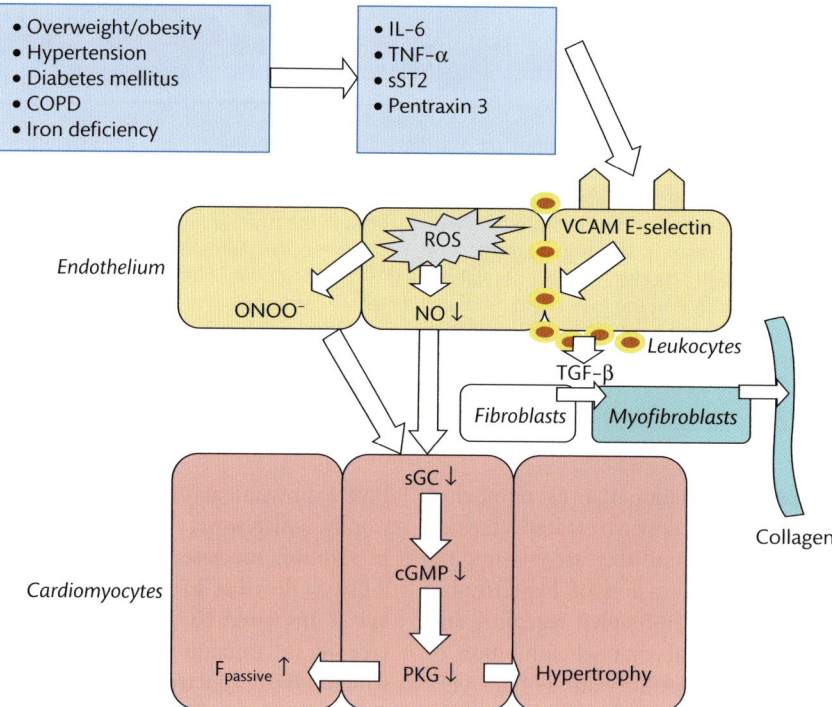

Figure 30.3 Co-morbidities induce a systemic proinflammatory state with elevated plasma levels of in IL-6, TNF-α, sST2 and pentraxin 3. Coronary microvascular endothelial cells reactively produce reactive oxygen species (ROS), VCAM and E-selectin. Production of ROS leads to formation of peroxynitrite (ONOO⁻) and reduced NO bioavailability, both of which lower soluble guanylate cyclase (sGC) activity in adjacent cardiomyocytes. Lower sGC activity decreases cGMP concentration and protein kinase G (PKG) activity. Low PKG activity raises cardiomyocyte stiffness (F_passive) because of hypophosphorylation of titin and removes the brake on prohypertrophic stimuli inducing cardiomyocyte hypertrophy. VCAM and E-selectin expression in endothelial cells favours migration into the subendothelium of monocytes. These monocytes release TGFβ. The latter stimulates conversion of fibroblasts to myofibroblasts, which deposit collagen in the interstitial space. IL-6, interleukin-6; sST2, soluble ST2; TGF-β, transforming growth factor-β; TNF-α, tumour necrosis factor-α; VCAM, vascular cell adhesion molecule.

Reproduced from Paulus WJ, Tschöpe C. A novel paradigm for heart failure with preserved ejection fraction: comorbidities drive myocardial dysfunction and remodeling through coronary microvascular endothelial inflammation. *J Am Coll Cardiol* 2013;**62**:263–71 with permission from Elsevier.

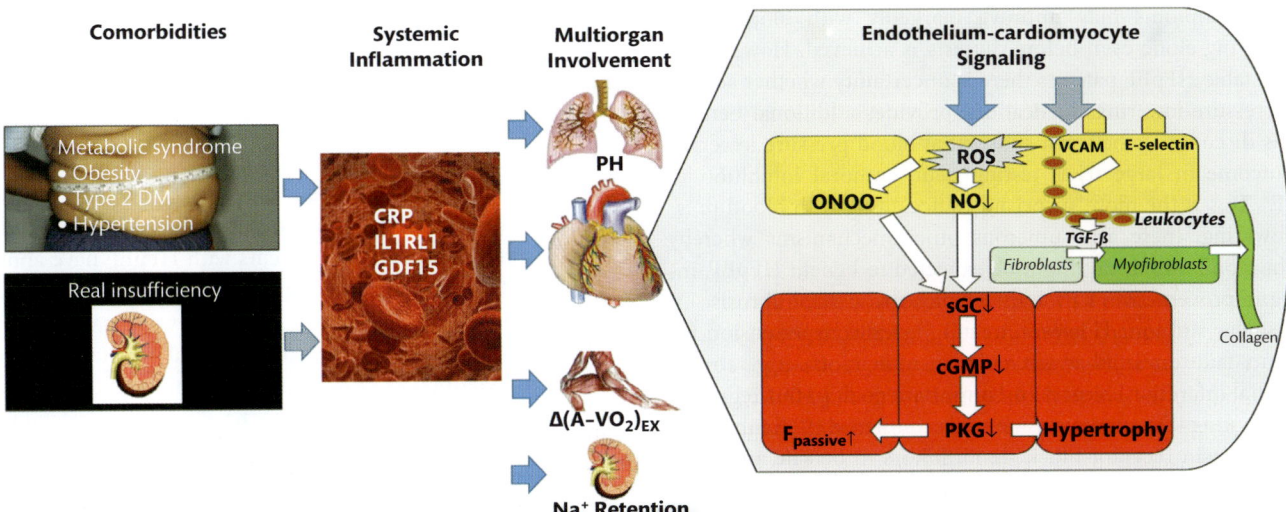

Figure 30.4 Systemic and myocardial signalling in HFPEF. Co-morbidities induce systemic inflammation, evident from elevated plasma levels of inflammatory biomarkers such as soluble interleukin 1 receptor-like 1 (IL1RL1), C-reactive protein (CRP), and growth differentiation factor 15 (GDF15). Chronic inflammation affects the lungs, myocardium, skeletal muscle and kidneys leading to diverse HFpEF phenotypes with variable involvement of pulmonary hypertension (PH), myocardial remodelling, deficient skeletal muscle oxygen extraction ($\Delta A - VO_2$) during exercise (Ex) and renal Na^+ retention. Myocardial remodelling and dysfunction begins with coronary endothelial microvascular inflammation manifest from endothelial expression of adhesion molecules such as vascular cell adhesion molecule (VCAM) and E-selectin. Expression of adhesion molecules attracts infiltrating leukocytes secreting transforming growth factor-β (TGF- β), which converts fibroblasts to myofibroblasts with enhanced interstitial collagen deposition. Endothelial inflammation also results in presence of reactive oxygen species (ROS), reduced nitric oxide (NO) bioavailability, and production of peroxynitrite ($ONOO^-$). This reduces soluble guanylate cyclase (sGC) activity, cyclic guanosine monophosphate (cGMP) content and the favourable effects of protein kinase G (PKG) on cardiomyocyte stiffness and hypertrophy.

Reproduced from Shah SJ, Kitzman DW, Borlaug BA, *et al*. Phenotype specific treatment of heart failure with preserved ejection fraction: a multi-organ roadmap. *Circulation* 2016;**134**:73–90 with permission from Wolters Kluwer.

and kidneys (Figure 30.4). Although HFpEF patients may stop exercising because of a rapid and brisk rise in LV filling pressures,[26] in a substantial subset of patients effort tolerance is limited by inappropriate pulmonary vasoconstriction (as shown by the development of pulmonary hypertension), or by inadequate peripheral skeletal muscle vasodilation, perfusion, and oxygen utilization (as shown by the absence of the widening of the arteriovenous oxygen difference which usually accompanies exercise).[27–29] Systemic inflammation also affects the renal microcirculation and the ability of the kidneys to excrete a sodium load. Inability to excrete a sodium load contributes to the progressive volume expansion observed during transition from chronic compensated to acute decompensated HFpEF[30] and explains the efficacy of diuretics as they restore the pressure–natriuresis relationship.

Treatment of HFpEF: shift from 'one size fits all' strategy to phenotype-specific treatment

Although diastolic LV dysfunction represents the dominant abnormality in HFpEF, ancillary mechanisms also contribute, such as LV systolic dysfunction, ventricular–vascular stiffening, impaired systemic vasodilatory reserve, chronotropic incompetence, pulmonary hypertension, and right ventricular (RV) dysfunction.[3,4] HFpEF therefore represents a complex and heterogeneous clinical syndrome, where multiple cardiac and vascular abnormalities, cardiovascular risk factors, and overlapping extracardiac co-morbidities may be present in various combinations.[3,4]

Treatment for HFrEF largely follows a 'one size fits all' paradigm, with most patients offered treatment with β-blockers, angiotensin converting enzyme (ACE) inhibitors, and mineralocorticoid

receptor antagonists. By contrast, we propose a paradigm shift toward phenotype-specific treatment for patients with HFpEF: the numerous steps of the HFpEF signalling cascade, which range from systemic inflammation to myocardial titin elasticity, are potential targets for a HFpEF treatment strategy.[30]

Co-morbidities

Metabolic risk is increasingly recognized as an important contributor to HFpEF. Recent longitudinal non-invasive studies over a four-year time interval show close correlations between diastolic LV stiffness and body mass index (BMI) and conclude that central adiposity predisposes to HFpEF.[31] These findings are consistent with the high prevalence of overweight/obesity in large HFpEF outcome trials, registries, and population studies, which almost uniformly report a median BMI >30 kg/m². As increased body adiposity promotes inflammation and impairs cardiac, arterial, renal, and skeletal muscle function, weight loss should be included in HFpEF treatment strategies for the majority of those who are obese.

Recently, a trial of 20-week caloric restriction diet was feasible and appeared safe in older, obese HFpEF patients, and it significantly improved symptoms, peak oxygen consumption (Vo_2) and quality-of-life scores.[32] The combination of weight loss diet with endurance exercise training was additive and produced a large (2.5 mL/kg/min) increase in peak Vo_2. The increase in peak Vo_2 was strongly correlated with reduced body fat mass, increased percentage lean body mass, higher thigh muscle/intermuscular fat ratio, and lower biomarkers of inflammation.[32]

Arterial hypertension is found in ≥80% of patients with HFpEF. In patients with acutely decompensated HFpEF and high blood

pressure, symptoms may improve markedly with blood pressure lowering alone even before diuresis is achieved. However, in chronic stable HFpEF patients there is uncertainty whether adding blood-pressure-lowering medications provides additional benefit. There is discordance between substantial blood pressure lowering and outcome in large trials testing neurohumoral inhibition in HFpEF.[3] This is the more surprising, since along with blood pressure lowering, there are numerous other mechanisms whereby neurohumoral inhibition might be expected to benefit HFpEF, including improvements in LV hypertrophy, myocardial fibrosis, LV and vascular stiffness. However, treating arterial hypertension for non-heart-failure-related macrovascular indications (e.g. stroke, myocardial infarction) remains an important goal. In this regard, it is worth noting that large outcome trials confirmed ACE inhibitors and angiotensin receptor blockade inhibitors to be safe and well-tolerated as antihypertensives.[3]

Systemic inflammation

The presence of systemic inflammation supports the use of statins in HFpEF. Statins exert rapid and direct effects on endothelial redox balance, which are independent of low-density lipoprotein lowering and consist of reduced superoxide anion production and restored NO bioavailability.[33] Analysis of endomyocardial biopsy material shows that statin-treated HFpEF patients have less myocardial nitrotyrosine, higher myocardial PKG activity, less cardiomyocyte hypertrophy and lower cardiomyocyte resting tension.[25] These findings are in line with the positive outcome in several observational studies showing that statin use is associated with lower mortality in patients with HFpEF.[34] A randomized trial testing statins in HFpEF is urgently needed and it remains to be explored whether other novel approaches to treat systemic inflammation might be effective in HFpEF.

Pulmonary hypertension

The right ventricle in HFpEF displays heightened afterload-sensitivity, suggesting that reduction in pulmonary pressures is likely to be beneficial. An early single-centre trial reported salutary effects on haemodynamics and right ventricular function following treatment with the phosphodiesterase 5 inhibitor (PDE5-I) sildenafil.[35] A large randomized controlled trial, however, failed to corroborate this finding.[36] A recent trial reported significant improvement in pulmonary vascular function in response to dobutamine in HFpEF patients, greatly exceeding the pulmonary vasodilatory response seen in non-heart failure controls.[37] Improved right ventricular–pulmonary artery coupling in this study was achieved predominantly through reduction in afterload rather than through enhanced right ventricular function, highlighting the importance of controlling pulmonary hypertension in HFpEF. Several trials are currently testing the effects of pulmonary vasodilators targeting cGMP, NO, and endothelin systems in subjects with HFpEF.

Skeletal muscle function

Skeletal muscle oxygen extraction

Exercise intolerance can be objectively measured as a fall in peak Vo_2. By the Fick equation, Vo_2 is the product of cardiac output and arteriovenous oxygen difference ($\Delta A - VO_2$). Many studies show that peak exercise $\Delta A - VO_2$ is significantly reduced in HFpEF and accounts for ≥50% of patients' severely reduced peak VO_2.[27–29,38]

Patients with HFpEF have abnormalities in skeletal muscle mass, composition, vascularization, and oxidative metabolism which are similar to those in patients with HFrEF (see Chapter XX).

- Haykowsky *et al.* showed that compared to age-matched healthy controls, older patients with HFpEF have significantly reduced percent total lean body mass and percent leg lean mass.[38] However, peak Vo_2 indexed to total lean body mass or leg lean mass remains significantly reduced. Thus patients with HFpEF have abnormal O_2 utilization that is independent of (and in addition to) their reduced muscle mass.
- HFpEF patients also have impaired skeletal muscle oxidative metabolism. Kitzman *et al.* showed that compared to healthy age-matched controls, HFpEF patients have a shift in skeletal muscle fibre type distribution from oxidative, slow type 1 fibres to glycolytic, fast type 2 fibres, resulting in a lower type1/type 2 fibre ratio. These alterations are associated with their severely reduced peak exercise Vo_2.[27]

These extensive skeletal muscle abnormalities in HFpEF confirm that HFpEF is a systemic disorder involving not only the heart but other organ systems. Skeletal muscle and cardiac abnormalities are incited by common, circulating factors such as proinflammatory cytokines originating from multiple co-morbidities.[25]

Unlike the myocardium, which is terminally differentiated and has minimal capacity for regeneration, skeletal muscle has robust capacity for rapid repair, regeneration, and growth, which can be exploited by participation in an exercise training programme. Exercise training improves endothelial dysfunction, systemic inflammation and metabolic syndrome. In the randomized Ex-DHF trial, patients with HFpEF randomized to endurance/resistance training had improved exercise capacity and quality of life.[39] Furthermore, exercise training and caloric restriction both significantly improved symptoms, peak oxygen consumption and quality-of-life scores in older, obese HFpEF patients.[32] The combination of weight loss diet and endurance training was additive and produced a large increase in peak VO_2.

Renal dysfunction

HFpEF and renal dysfunction are mutually promoting.[40] HFpEF promotes renal dysfunction by a number of mechanisms, including:

- elevated central venous pressure, which results from pulmonary hypertension and RV dysfunction;
- inability to raise cardiac output following arterial vasodilation because of chronotropic incompetence and fixed LV stroke volume; and
- systemic inflammation, endothelial dysfunction, and low NO bioavailability (partially because of renal-specific paracrine and pro-inflammatory mediators),[40] which reduce renal blood flow and sodium excretion.[30,40]

Limited tolerability of systemic vasodilation and impaired sodium excretion are of therapeutic importance.[41] Impaired sodium excretion implies that the arterial pressure–natriuresis relationship is shifted to the right (**Figure 30.5**). Under these conditions, a fall in arterial pressure induced by systemic vasodilation without an increase in cardiac output is especially deleterious as it leads to additional sodium retention and extracellular volume expansion, which wipes out any direct beneficial effect of vasodilation on LV filling pressures.[41] Rightward

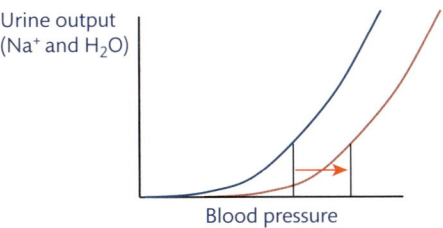

Figure 30.5 The relationship between blood pressure and natriuresis. In HFpEF, the curve moves to the right, meaning that higher blood pressure is needed to achieve a given natriuresis.

displacement of the arterial pressure–natriuresis relation is corrected by diuretics, which are central to the HFpEF treatment strategy.

Myocardial NO bioavailability

In the HFpEF signalling cascade, cardiomyocytes are deprived of NO and cGMP because of altered paracrine communication between inflamed microvascular endothelial cells and cardiomyocytes.[25,42] However, replacing NO with isosorbide mononitrate tended to reduce activity levels in patients with HFpEF.[43] Organic nitrates may produce greater than expected hypotensive effects in HFpEF patients or potentially impair cardiac output through excessive preload reduction.[41] Organic nitrates tonically increase local NO levels and require bioactivation in the tissues. Exogenous nitrates cause pharmacologic tolerance, and preload reduction can chronically lower renal perfusion pressure, which is countered by renal sodium retention. This may override any beneficial reduction in filling pressures.

In contrast to organic nitrates, the inorganic nitrate–nitrite pathway represents an important alternative route to restore NO signalling in HFpEF.[44] Formerly considered as an inert by-product of NO metabolism, nitrite is now known to function as an important in-vivo NO reservoir. Nitrite is preferentially reduced to NO in the presence of hypoxia and acidosis, which occurs during physical exercise, thus delivering NO at the time and locations (i.e. skeletal and cardiac muscles) of greatest need. In a placebo-controlled trial of patients with HFpEF, acute infusion of sodium nitrite preferentially reduces diastolic LV and pulmonary artery pressures during exercise while restoring cardiac output reserve toward normal.[44] Part of the benefit is mediated by vasodilation, but evidence for a direct myocardial benefit such as increased stroke work was also observed.

Myocardial cGMP content

A substantial number of patients with HFpEF have pathological ventricular hypertrophy with interstitial fibrosis and diastolic chamber stiffening. This has encouraged efforts to block key activators and to stimulate intrinsic suppressors of fibrosis. Among the attractive pathways which might stimulate suppression of fibrosis are those coupled to cGMP and its effector kinase PKG.

PKG stimulation has potent anti-fibrotic and anti-hypertrophic effects in cultured myocytes and fibroblasts, and has been protective in a wide array of experimental cardiac disease models including pressure-overload hypertrophy.[45] There are many approaches to stimulating PKG activity already in clinical use or under active investigation (Figure 30.6). Stimulation of PKG requires cGMP, which is either synthesized by sGC activated by NO or by pGC linked to

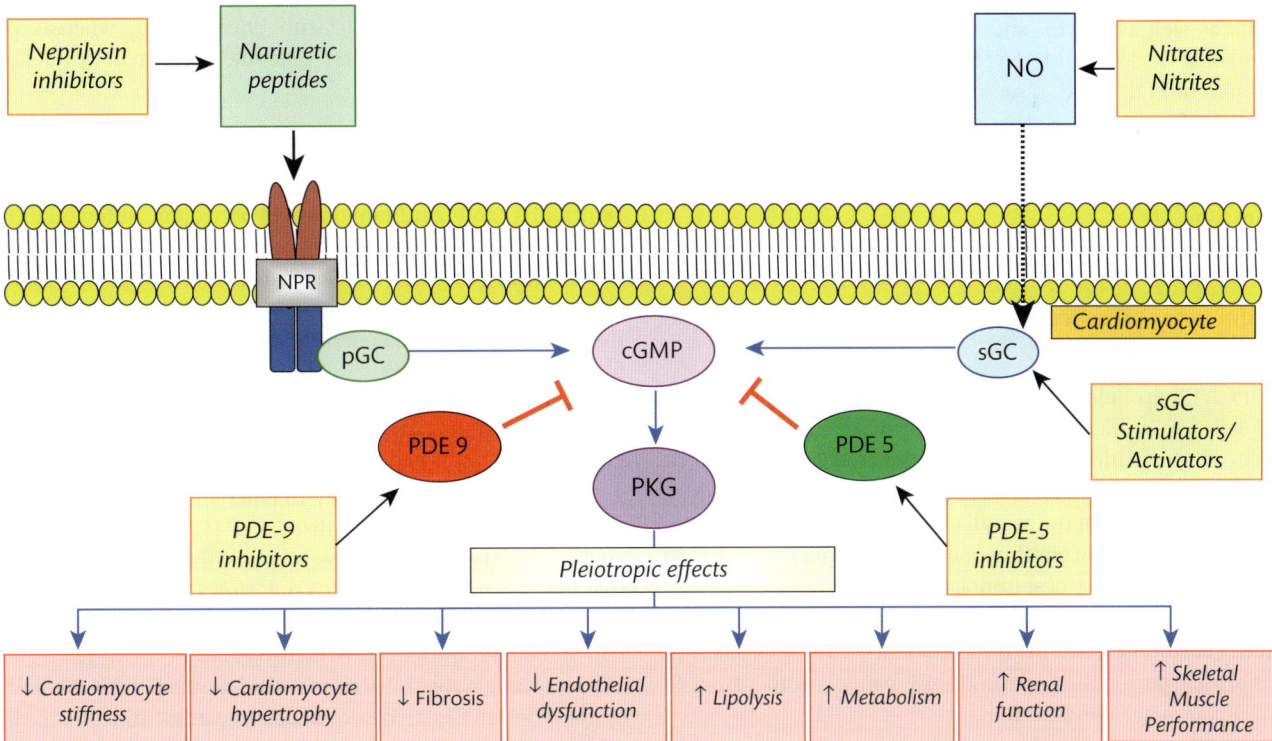

Figure 30.6 Therapeutic strategies to upregulate myocardial cGMP–PKG signalling. NO, nitric oxide; sGC, soluble guanylate cyclase; NEP, neutral endopeptidase; pGC, particulate guanylate cyclase; PKG, protein kinase G; PDE5, phosphodiesterase-5; cGMP, cyclic guanylate monophosphate. Phenotype specific HFpEF treatment strategy using a matrix of predisposition phenotypes and clinical presentation phenotypes. Only therapeutic measures indicated in bold are currently established. All other therapeutic measures require further testing in specific phenotype.

the NP receptor.[17,45] This is in turn counterbalanced by hydrolysis of cGMP back to GMP by select members of the phosphodiesterase (PDE) superfamily. Inhibition of specific PDEs, which leads to increased cGMP, can also increase PKG activity.

Four members of the PDE superfamily (PDE1, PDE2, PDE 5, and PDE9) regulate cGMP in the heart. PDE5 and PDE9 are selective for cGMP. PDE5 largely affects cGMP derived from NO–sGC, while PDE9 regulates cGMP derived from NP–pGC.[17,20] These local pools impact different intracellular compartments of PKG as detected by differences in net phosphokinomes and effects on transcriptional regulation.[17,20]

Administration of sGC activators or stimulators could provide downstream correction for the low myocardial NO bioavailability seen in HFpEF.

- The sGC stimulator, vericiguat, is currently being tested in the SOCRATES-PRESERVED trial.
- Because of concentric LV remodelling, natriuretic peptide (NP) stimulation is less marked in HFpEF than in HFrEF, a finding that may limit counter-stimulation via this pathway. NPs are degraded by circulating neprilysin. Inhibition of this peptidase could augment deficient NP–pGC signalling and therefore be beneficial in HFpEF, as suggested by the fall in NP following administration of valsartan/sacubitril in the phase 2 PARAMOUNT study.[46] Use of valsartan/sacubitril is currently being tested in the multicentre PARAGON-HF trial.
- Another approach is to block PDEs to increase cGMP levels and hence PKG activity. Because PDE5 inhibition was neutral in a large randomized controlled trial,[36] inhibiting PDE9 may therefore be an alternative. A recent study found marked upregulation of PDE9 protein in human LV biopsies from HFpEF patients as well as HFrEF and aortic stenosis patients.[20] This suggests that the low cGMP levels might be related to enhanced expression of PDE9, and, if so, inhibiting this PDE should have beneficial effects. In mice subjected to sustained pressure-overload, blocking PDE9 by gene deletion or selective pharmacological inhibition suppressed hypertrophy, fibrosis, and chamber dysfunction.[20]

Extracellular matrix

To date, three pharmaceutical agents that affect the extracellular matrix have been tested in HFpEF.

- In TOPCAT, spironolactone (a mineralocorticoid receptor antagonist) failed to reduce the composite primary end-point in the overall trial population[47] but not in patients with elevated BNP, which was a marker of enrolment in the Americas ($P = 0.003$).[48] The neutral outcome in the overall population may have been related to aberrant patient enrolment in Russia/Republic of Georgia rather than to inefficacy of spironolactone.
- In PARAMOUNT, valsartan/sacubitril lowered NT-proBNP and reduced LA volume index in HFpEF patients.[46] These effects support fibrosis-specific therapy for HFpEF patients with advanced extracellular matrix modification.[30]
- The loop diuretic torasemide affects collagen crosslinking and its use has been shown to improve diastolic LV dysfunction in patients with hypertensive heart disease.[49]

Therapeutic strategy based on phenotypic characterization and pathophysiological stratification

HFpEF is a diverse syndrome initiated by a variety of co-morbidities and inflammatory mediators with extracardiac manifestations and cardiac abnormalities.[3,4,25] The underlying phenotypic heterogeneity is far greater in HFpEF than in HFrEF and may be an important reason for the failure of HFpEF clinical trials.[3,4] According to a recent expert panel, HFpEF treatment should be individualized taking the phenotypic diversity of patients into account, which results in a treatment matrix covering both clinical presentation phenotypes and predisposition-related phenotypic features (**Figure 30.7**).[30]

Phenotypic characterization

In a recent study, phenomapping analysis using statistical learning algorithms demonstrated that patients with HFpEF recruited according to uniform diagnostic criteria could be divided into three main distinct subgroups, which differed markedly in clinical characteristics, cardiac structure and function, invasive haemodynamics and outcome, despite similar end-systolic and end-diastolic elastances on LV pressure–volume analysis.[4] In this study, the following subgroups were identified:

- younger patients with moderate diastolic LV dysfunction and relatively low BNP;
- obese, diabetic patients with high prevalence of obstructive sleep apnoea who had the worst LV relaxation; and
- older patients with significant chronic kidney disease, electric and myocardial remodelling, pulmonary hypertension, and right ventricular dysfunction.

Survival free of cardiovascular hospitalization or death was compromised most in patients with phenotype 3, whereas patients in phenotype 2 had a worse outcome compared to phenotype 1 patients.[4]

Pathophysiological stratification

Clinical and translational studies have shown varying degrees of ventricular and cardiomyocyte hypertrophy, interstitial fibrosis and capillary rarefaction,[12–15] suggesting distinct (and possibly evolutionary) stages of myocardial disease progression. Although neurohumoral inhibition did not improve primary end-points in the large HFpEF trials, many of them reached statistical significance for secondary end-points, subgroups or post-hoc analyses.[3,48] The involvement of RAAS in HFpEF thus appears more subtle than in HFrEF, probably requiring up-front identification of pathophysiological subgroups of HFpEF patients.

The presence of AF is likely to emerge as an indicator of an advanced stage of myocardial disease in HFpEF. A recent subgroup analysis of HFpEF patients recruited in the RELAX trial suggested that the presence of AF was an indicator of longstanding HFpEF.[50] HFpEF patients with AF were older than those in sinus rhythm, but had similar symptom severity, co-morbidities, and renal function. Despite comparable LV size and mass, patients with AF had worse systolic (lower EF, stroke volume, and cardiac index) and diastolic (shorter deceleration time and larger left atria) function compared to those in sinus rhythm. Patients with AF had higher pulmonary artery systolic pressure and higher NT-proBNP, aldosterone,

| HFpEF Clinical Presentation Phenotypes | | | | | |
	Lung Congestion	+ Chronotropic Incompetence	+ Pulmonary Hypertension (CpcPH)	+ Skeletal Muscle weakness	+ Atrial Fibrillation
Overweight/obesity/ metabolic syndrome/ type 2 DM	• Diuretics (loop diuretic in DM) • Caloric restriction • Statins • Inorganic nitrite/nitrate • Sacubitril • Spironolactone	+ Rate adaptive atrial pacing	+ Pulmonary vasodilators (e.g. PDE5I)	+ Exercise training programme	+ Cardioversion + Rate Control + Anticoagulation
+Arterial hypertension	+ ACEI/ARB	+ ACEI/ARB + Rate adaptive atrial pacing	+ ACEI/ARB + Pulmonary vasodilators (e.g. PDE5I)	+ ACEI/ARB + Exercise training programme	+ ACEI/ARB + Cardioversion + Rate Control + Anticoagulation
+Renal dysfunction	+ Ultrafiltration if needed	+ Ultrafiltration if needed + Rate adaptive atrial pacing	+ Ultrafiltration if needed + Pulmonary vasodilators (e.g. PDE5I)	+ Ultrafiltration if needed + Exercise training programme	+ Ultrafiltration if needed + Cardioversion + Rate Control + Anticoagulation
+CAD	+ ACEI + Revascularization	+ ACEI + Revascularization + Rate adaptive atrial pacing	+ ACEI + Revascularization + Pulmonary vasodilators (e.g. PDE5I)	+ ACEI + Revascularization + Exercise training programme	+ ACEI + Revascularization + Cardioversion + Rate Control + Anticoagulation

(Left axis label: HFpEF Predisposition Phenotypes)

Figure 30.7 Phenotype specific HFpEF treatment strategy using a matrix of predisposition phenotypes and clinical presentation phenotypes. Only therapeutic measures indicated in bold are currently established. All other therapeutic measures require further testing in specific phenotype.
Source data from Shah SJ, Kitzman DW, Borlaug BA, *et al.* Phenotype-specific treatment of heart failure with preserved ejection fraction: a multi-organ roadmap. *Circulation* 2016;**134**:73–90.

endothelin-1, troponin I, and C-telopeptide for type I collagen levels, suggesting more severe neurohumoral activation, myocyte necrosis, and fibrosis.[50]

Conclusion

HFpEF represents a complex disorder with a heterogeneous constellation of co-morbidities and underlying pathogenic mechanisms. The lack of effective treatment poses a formidable challenge for clinicians and translational researchers. Over the past decade, significant progress has been made in understanding HFpEF pathophysiology and recognizing the importance of co-morbidities and disease heterogeneity. However, numerous issues regarding underlying pathophysiological mechanisms remain unresolved. For instance, patients with substantial diastolic dysfunction with or without structural heart disease in the setting of hypertensive heart disease may behave differently from those with chronotropic incompetence or from those with normal blood pressure but inflammatory activation in the setting of metabolic risk factors.

Pathogenic mechanisms vary during the course of the HFpEF disease trajectory and there are thus different abnormalities (and potential therapeutic targets) at different time-points in the disease. The additive role of pre-existing or newly developing non-cardiac co-morbidities on structural and functional remodelling in HFpEF is incompletely understood.

Important future goals in enhancing our understanding of HFpEF pathophysiology and improving the subclassification of patients with HFpEF include increasing acquisition of HFpEF myocardial tissue, for instance through LV endomyocardial biopsies;

and improvement in experimental HFpEF models. Stimulation of crosstalk and the formation of collaborative networks between translational researchers and clinicians is fundamental to improve insight into structural and functional cardiovascular dysfunction in the setting of coexisting variable pathogenic mechanisms and co-morbidities in HFpEF patients.

The conceptual framework of HFpEF treatment needs to recognize the heterogeneity of HFpEF and to shift from a 'one size fits all' strategy to an individualized approach based on phenotypic patient characterization leading to personalized therapy for patients with HFpEF.

REFERENCES

1. Steinberg BA, Zhao X, Heidenreich PA, *et al.*; Get with the Guidelines Scientific Advisory Committee and Investigators. Trends in patients hospitalized with heart failure and preserved left ventricular ejection fraction: prevalence, therapies, and outcomes. *Circulation* 2012;**126**:65–75.
2. Paulus WJ, Tschöpe C, Sanderson JE, *et al.* How to diagnose diastolic heart failure: a consensus statement on the diagnosis of heart failure with normal left ventricular ejection fraction by the Heart Failure and Echocardiography Associations of the European Society of Cardiology. *Eur Heart J* 2007;**28**:2539–50.
3. Senni M, Paulus WJ, Gavazzi A, *et al.* New strategies for heart failure with preserved ejection fraction: the importance of targeted therapies for heart failure phenotypes. *Eur Heart J* 2014;**35**:2797–811.
4. Shah SJ, Katz DH, Selvaraj S, *et al.* Phenomapping for novel classification of heart failure with preserved ejection fraction. *Circulation* 2015;**131**:269–79.

5. Zile MR, Baicu CF, Gaasch WH. Diastolic heart failure—abnormalities in active relaxation and passive stiffness of the left ventricle. *N Engl J Med* 2004;**350**:1953–59.

6. Westermann D, Kasner M, Steendijk P, et al. Role of left ventricular stiffness in heart failure with normal ejection fraction. *Circulation* 2008;**117**:2051–60.

7. Borlaug BA, Paulus WJ. Heart failure with preserved ejection fraction: pathophysiology, diagnosis and treatment. *Eur Heart J* 2011;**32**:670–9.

8. Spinale FG. Myocardial matrix remodeling and the matrix metalloproteinases: influence on cardiac form and function. *Physiol Rev* 2007;**87**:949–62.

9. Kasner M, Westermann D, Lopez B, et al. Diastolic tissue Doppler indexes correlate with the degree of collagen expression and cross-linking in heart failure and normal ejection fraction. *J Am Coll Cardiol* 2011;**57**:977–85.

10. López B, Ravassa S, González A, et al. Myocardial collagen cross-linking is associated with heart failure hospitalization in patients with hypertensive heart failure. *J Am Coll Cardiol* 2016;**67**:251–60.

11. Westermann D, Lindner D, Kasner M, et al. Cardiac inflammation contributes to changes in the extracellular matrix in patients with heart failure and normal ejection fraction. *Circ Heart Fail* 2011;**4**:44–52.

12. van Heerebeek L, Borbely A, Niessen HWM, et al. Myocardial structure and function differ in systolic and diastolic heart failure. *Circulation* 2006;**113**:1966–73.

13. Borbely A, van der Velden J, Papp Z, et al. Cardiomyocyte stiffness in diastolic heart failure. *Circulation* 2005;**111**:774–81.

14. Borbely A, Falcao-Pires I, van Heerebeek, et al. Hypophosphorylation of the stiff N2B titin isoform raises cardiomyocyte resting tension in failing human myocardium. *Circ Res* 2009;**104**:780–6.

15. van Heerebeek L, Hamdani N, Falcao-Pires I, et al. Low myocardial protein kinase G activity in heart failure with preserved ejection fraction. *Circulation* 2012;**126**:830–9.

16. Linke WA, Hamdani N. Gigantic business: titin properties and function through thick and thin. *Circ Res* 2014;**114**:1052–68.

17. Lee DI, Kass DA. Phosphodiesterases and cyclic GMP regulation in heart muscle. *Physiology (Bethesda)* 2012;**27**:248–58.

18. Madamanchi C, Alhosaini H, Sumida A, Runge MS. Obesity and natriuretic peptides, BNP and NT-proBNP: mechanisms and diagnostic implications for heart failure. *Int J Cardiol* 2014;**176**:611–17.

19. Iwanaga Y, Nishi I, Furuichi S, et al. B-type natriuretic peptide strongly reflects diastolic wall stress in patients with chronic heart failure: comparison between systolic and diastolic heart failure. *J Am Coll Cardiol* 2006;**47**:742–8.

20. Lee DI, Zhu G, Sasaki T, et al. Phosphodiesterase 9A controls nitric-oxide-independent cGMP and hypertrophic heart disease. *Nature* 2015;**519**:472–6.

21. Ather S, Chan W, Bozkurt B, et al. Impact of noncardiac comorbidities on morbidity and mortality in a predominantly male population with heart failure and preserved versus reduced ejection fraction. *J Am Coll Cardiol* 2012;**59**:998–1005.

22. Lam CS, Brutsaert DL. Endothelial dysfunction: a pathophysiologic factor in heart failure with preserved ejection fraction. *J Am Coll Cardiol* 2012;**60**:1787–89.

23. Akiyama E, Sugiyama S, Matsuzawa Y, et al. Incremental prognostic significance of peripheral endothelial dysfunction in patients with heart failure with normal left ventricular ejection fraction. *J Am Coll Cardiol* 2012;**60**:1778–86.

24. Mohammed SF, Hussain S, Mirzoyev SA, et al. Coronary microvascular rarefaction and myocardial fibrosis in heart failure with preserved ejection fraction. *Circulation* 2015;**131**:550–9.

25. Paulus WJ, Tschöpe C. A novel paradigm for heart failure with preserved ejection fraction: comorbidities drive myocardial dysfunction and remodeling through coronary microvascular endothelial inflammation. *J Am Coll Cardiol* 2013;**62**:263–71.

26. Borlaug BA. Mechanisms of exercise intolerance in heart failure with preserved ejection fraction. *Circ J* 2014;**78**:20–32.

27. Kitzman DW, Nicklas B, Kraus WE, et al. Skeletal muscle abnormalities and exercise intolerance in older patients with heart failure and preserved ejection fraction. *Am J Physiol Heart Circ Physiol* 2014;**306**:H1364–70.

28. Santos M, Opotowsky AR, Shah AM, et al. Central cardiac limit to aerobic capacity in patients with exertional pulmonary venous hypertension: implications for heart failure with preserved ejection fraction. *Circ Heart Fail* 2015;**8**:278–85.

29. Dhakal BP, Malhotra R, Murphy RM, et al. Mechanisms of exercise intolerance in heart failure with preserved ejection fraction: the role of abnormal peripheral oxygen extraction. *Circ Heart Fail* 2015;**8**:286–94.

30. Shah SJ, Kitzman DW, Borlaug BA, et al. Phenotype-specific treatment of heart failure with preserved ejection fraction: a multi-organ roadmap. *Circulation* 2016;**134**:73–90.

31. Wohlfahrt P, Redfield MM, Lopez-Jimenez F, et al. Impact of general and central adiposity on ventricular–arterial aging in women and men. *JACC Heart Fail* 2014;**2**:489–99.

32. Kitzman DW, Brubaker P, Morgan T, et al. Effect of caloric restriction or aerobic exercise training on peak oxygen consumption and quality of life in obese older patients with heart failure with preserved ejection fraction: a randomized clinical trial. *JAMA* 2016;**315**:36–46.

33. Ramasubbu K, Estep J, White DL, Deswal A, Mann DL. Experimental and clinical basis for the use of statins in patients with ischemic and nonischemic cardiomyopathy. *J Am Coll Cardiol* 2008;**51**:415–26.

34. Alehagen U, Benson L, Edner M, Dahlström U, Lund LH. Association between use of statins and mortality in patients with heart failure and ejection fraction of ≥50. *Circ Heart Fail* 2015;**8**:862–70.

35. Guazzi M, Vicenzi M, Arena R, Guazzi MD. Pulmonary hypertension in heart failure with preserved ejection fraction: a target of phosphodiesterase-5 inhibition in a 1-year study. *Circulation* 2011;**124**:164–74.

36. Redfield MM, Chen HH, Borlaug BA, et al.; RELAX Trial. Effect of phosphodiesterase-5 inhibition on exercise capacity and clinical status in heart failure with preserved ejection fraction: a randomized clinical trial. *JAMA* 2013;**309**:1268–77.

37. Andersen MJ, Hwang SJ, Kane GC, et al. Enhanced pulmonary vasodilator reserve and abnormal right ventricular: pulmonary artery coupling in heart failure with preserved ejection fraction. *Circ Heart Fail* 2015;**8**:542–50.

38. Haykowsky M, Brubaker P, Morgan T, et al. Impaired aerobic capacity and physical functional performance in older heart failure patients with preserved ejection fraction: role of lean body mass. *J Gerontol A Biol Sci Med Sci* 2013;**68**:968–75.

39. Edelmann F, Gelbrich G, Düngen HD, et al. Exercise training improves exercise capacity and diastolic function in patients with heart failure with preserved ejection fraction: results of the Ex-DHF (Exercise training in Diastolic Heart Failure) Pilot Study. *J Am Coll Cardiol* 2011;**58**:1780–91.

40. Ter Maaten JM, Damman K, Verhaar MC, et al. Connecting heart failure with preserved ejection fraction and renal dysfunction: the role of endothelial dysfunction and inflammation. Eur J Heart Fail 2016;**18**:588–98.

41. Schwartzenberg S, Redfield MM, From AM, et al. Effects of vasodilation in heart failure with preserved or reduced ejection fraction implications of distinct pathophysiologies on response to therapy. J Am Coll Cardiol 2012;**59**:442–51.

42. Franssen C, Chen S, Unger A, et al. Myocardial microvascular inflammatory endothelial activation in heart failure with preserved ejection fraction. JACC Heart Fail 2016;**4**:312–24.

43. Redfield MM, Anstrom KJ, Levine JA, et al. Isosorbide mononitrate in heart failure with preserved ejection fraction. N Engl J Med 2015;**373**:2314–24.

44. Borlaug BA, Koepp KE, Melenovsky V. Sodium nitrite improves exercise hemodynamics and ventricular performance in heart failure with preserved ejection fraction. J Am Coll Cardiol 2015;**66**:1672–82.

45. Greene SJ, Gheorghiade M, Borlaug BA, et al. The cGMP signaling pathway as a therapeutic target in heart failure with preserved ejection fraction. J Am Heart Assoc 2013;**2**:e000536.

46. Solomon SD, Zile M, Pieske B, et al.; Prospective comparison of ARNI with ARB on Management Of heart failUre with preserved ejectioN fracTion (PARAMOUNT) Investigators. The angiotensin receptor neprilysin inhibitor LCZ696 in heart failure with preserved ejection fraction: a phase 2 double-blind randomised controlled trial. Lancet 2012;**380**:1387–95.

47. Pitt B, Pfeffer MA, Assmann SF, et al.; TOPCAT Investigators. Spironolactone for heart failure with preserved ejection fraction. N Engl J Med 2014;**370**:1383–92.

48. Pfeffer MA, Claggett B, Assmann SF, et al. Regional variation in patients and outcomes in the Treatment of Preserved Cardiac Function Heart Failure With an Aldosterone Antagonist (TOPCAT) trial. Circulation 2015;**131**:34–42.

49. López B, Querejeta R, González A, et al. Impact of treatment on myocardial lysyl oxidase expression and collagen cross-linking in patients with heart failure. Hypertension 2009;**53**:236–42.

50. Zakeri R, Borlaug BA, McNulty SE, et al. Impact of atrial fibrillation on exercise capacity in heart failure with preserved ejection fraction: a RELAX trial ancillary study. Circ Heart Fail 2014;**7**:123–30.

RECOMMENDED READING

Abel ED, Litwin ES, Sweeney G. Cardiac remodelling in obesity. Physiol Rev 2008;**88**:389–419.

Berry C, Poppe KK, Gamble GD, et al.; MAGGIC Collaborative Group. Prognostic significance of anaemia in patients with heart failure with preserved and reduced ejection fraction: results from the MAGGIC individual patient data meta-analysis. Q J Med 2016;**109**:377–82.

Borlaug BA, Kass DA. Ventricular–vascular interaction in heart failure. Heart Fail Clin 2008;**4**:23–36.

Borlaug BA, Lam CS, Roger VL, et al. Contractility and ventricular systolic stiffening in hypertensive heart disease insights into the pathogenesis of heart failure with preserved ejection fraction. J Am Coll Cardiol 2009;**54**:410–18.

Borlaug BA, Redfield MM, Melenovsky V, et al. Longitudinal changes in left ventricular stiffness: a community-based study. Circ Heart Fail 2013;**6**:944–52.

Boudina S, Abel ED. Diabetic cardiomyopathy revisited. Circulation 2007;**115**:3213–23.

Campbell DJ, Somaratne JB, Prior DL, et al. Obesity is associated with lower coronary microvascular density. PLoS One 2013;**8**:e81798.

Cheng JM, Akkerhuis KM, Battes LC, et al. Biomarkers of heart failure with normal ejection fraction: a systematic review. Eur J Heart Fail 2013;**15**:1350–62.

Collier P, Watson CJ, Voon V, et al. Can emerging biomarkers of myocardial remodelling identify asymptomatic hypertensive patients at risk for diastolic dysfunction and diastolic heart failure? Eur J Heart Fail 2011;**13**:1087–95.

Damkjaer M, Vafaee M, Moller ML, et al. Renal cortical and medullary blood flow responses to altered NO availability in humans. Am J Physiol Regul Integr Comp Physiol 2010;**299**:R1449–55.

de Boer RA, Lok DJ, Jaarsma T, et al. Predictive value of plasma galectin-3 levels in heart failure with reduced and preserved ejection fraction. Ann Med 2011;**43**:60–8.

Dorfs S, Zeh W, Hochholzer W, et al. Pulmonary capillary wedge pressure during exercise and long-term mortality in patients with suspected heart failure with preserved ejection fraction. Eur Heart J 2014;**35**:3103–12.

Eggebeen J, Kim-Shapiro DB, Haykowsky M, et al. One week of daily dosing with beetroot juice improves submaximal endurance and blood pressure in older patients with heart failure and preserved ejection fraction. JACC Heart Fail 2016;**4**:428–37.

Falcao-Pires I, Leite-Moreira AF. Diabetic cardiomyopathy: understanding the molecular and cellular basis to progress in diagnosis and treatment. Heart Fail Rev 2012;**17**:325–344.

Flachskampf FA, Biering-Sørensen T, Solomon SD, et al. Cardiac imaging to evaluate left ventricular diastolic function. JACC Cardiovasc Imaging 2015;**8**:1071–93.

Fonorow GC, Stough WG, Abraham WT, et al.; OPTIMIZE-HF Investigators and Hospitals. Characteristics, treatments and outcomes of patients with preserved systolic function hospitalized for heart failure: a report from the OPTIMIZE-HF Registry. J Am Coll Cardiol 2007;**50**:768–77.

Greene SJ, Gheorghiade M, Borlaug BA, et al. The cGMP signaling pathway as a therapeutic target in heart failure with preserved ejection fraction. J Am Heart Assoc 2013;**2**(6):e000536.

Guazzi M. Pulmonary hypertension in heart failure preserved ejection fraction: prevalence, pathophysiology, and clinical perspectives. Circ Heart Fail 2014;**7**:367–77.

Hillege HL, Nitsch D, Pfeffer MA, et al.; Candesartan in Heart Failure: Assessment of Reduction in Mortality and Morbidity (CHARM) Investigators. Renal function as a predictor of outcome in a broad spectrum of patients with heart failure. Circulation 2006;**113**:671–8.

Hoendermis ES, Liu LC, Hummel YM, et al. Effects of sildenafil on invasive haemodynamics and exercise capacity in heart failure patients with preserved ejection fraction and pulmonary hypertension: a randomized controlled trial. Eur Heart J 2015;**36**:2565–2573.

Hoenig MR, Bianchi C, Rosenzweig A, et al. The cardiac microvasculature in hypertension, cardiac hypertrophy and diastolic heart failure. Curr Vasc Pharmacol 2008;**6**:292–300.

Kalogeropoulos A, Georgiopoulou V, Psaty BM, et al.; Health ABC Study Investigators. Inflammatory markers and incident heart failure risk in older adults: the Health ABC (Health, Aging, and Body Composition) study. J Am Coll Cardiol 2010;**55**:2129–2137.

Kao DP, Lewsey JD, Anand IS, et al. Characterization of subgroups of heart failure patients with preserved ejection fraction with possible implications for prognosis and treatment response. Eur J Heart Fail 2015;**17**:925–35.

Kawaguchi M, Hay I, Tetics B, et al. Combined ventricular systolic and arterial stiffening in patients with heart failure and preserved

ejection fraction: implications for systolic and diastolic reserve limitations. *Circulation* 2003;**107**:714–20.

Kitzman DW, Haykowsky MJ. Mechanisms of exercise training in heart failure with preserved ejection fraction: central disappointment and peripheral promise. *Am Heart J* 2012;**164**:807–9.

Lam CS, Roger VL, Rodeheffer RJ, *et al.* Cardiac structure and ventricular–vascular function in persons with heart failure and preserved ejection fraction from Olmsted County, Minnesota. *Circulation* 2007;**115**:1982–90.

Leite-Moreira AF. Current perspectives in diastolic dysfunction and diastolic heart failure. *Heart* 2006;**92**:712–18.

López B, González A, Querejeta R, *et al.* Galectin-3 and histological, molecular and biochemical aspects of myocardial fibrosis in heart failure of hypertensive origin. *Eur J Heart Fail* 2015;**17**:385–392.

Melenovsky V, Hwang SJ, Lin G, *et al.* Right heart dysfunction in heart failure with preserved ejection fraction. *Eur Heart J* 2014;**35**:3452–62.

Mohammed SF, Hussain I, AbouEzzeddine OF, *et al.* Right ventricular function in heart failure with preserved ejection fraction: a community-based study. *Circulation* 2014;**130**:2310–20.

Nochioka K, Sakata Y, Miyata S, *et al.*; CHART-2 Investigators. Prognostic impact of statin use in patients with heart failure and preserved ejection fraction. *Circ J* 2015;**79**:574–82.

Owan TE, Hodge DO, Herges RM, *et al.* Trends in prevalence and outcome of heart failure with preserved ejection fraction. *N Engl J Med* 2006;**355**:251–9.

Redfield MM, Jacobsen SJ, Burnett JC JR, *et al.* Burden of systolic and diastolic ventricular dysfunction in the community: appreciating the scope of the heart failure epidemic. *JAMA* 2003;**289**:194–202.

Regitz-Zagrosek V, Brokat S, Tschope C. Role of gender in heart failure with normal left ventricular ejection fraction. *Prog Cardiovasc Dis* 2007;**49**:241–51.

Rusinaru D, Houpe D, Szymanski C, *et al.* Coronary artery disease and 10-year outcome after hospital admission for heart failure with preserved and with reduced ejection fraction. *Eur J Heart Fail* 2014;**16**:967–76.

Senni M, Paulus WJ, Gavazzi A, *et al.* New strategies for heart failure with preserved ejection fraction: the importance of targeted therapies for heart failure phenotypes. *Eur Heart J* 2014;**35**:2797–811.

Vanderpool R, Gladwin MT. Harnessing the nitrate-nitrite-nitric oxide pathway for therapy of heart failure with preserved ejection fraction. *Circulation* 2015;**131**:334–6.

van der Velde AR, Gullestad L, Ueland T, *et al.* Prognostic value of changes in galectin-3 levels over time in patients with heart failure: data from CORONA and COACH. *Circ Heart Fail* 2013;**6**:219–26.

van Empel VP, Mariani J, Borlaug BA, Kaye DM. Impaired myocardial oxygen availability contributes to abnormal exercise hemodynamics in heart failure with preserved ejection fraction. *J Am Heart Assoc* 2014;**3**:e001293.

Witteles RM, Fowler MB. Insulin-resistant cardiomyopathy. *J Am Coll Cardiol* 2008;**51**:93–102.

Yancy CW, Lopatin M, Stevenson LW, *et al.* for the ADHERE Scientific Advisory Committee and Investigators. Clinical presentation, management, and in-hospital outcomes of patients admitted with acute decompensated heart failure with preserved systolic function. A Report from the Acute Decompensated Heart Failure National Registry (ADHERE). *J Am Coll Cardiol* 2006;**47**:76–84.

Zile MR, Gottdiener JS, Hetzel SJ, *et al.*; I-PRESERVE Investigators. Prevalence and significance of alterations in cardiac structure and function in patients with heart failure and a preserved ejection fraction. *Circulation* 2011;**124**:2491–501.

31

Right heart failure

Andrew L. Clark

Most discussions of heart failure focus on the left ventricle and its dysfunction. The right heart is, of course, commonly affected in patients with heart failure: both by the same disease processes that affect the left heart, or as a consequence of left heart disease. The right heart itself is much less commonly affected in isolation, but patients with heart disease do commonly present with 'right heart failure'.

Anatomy and physiology

The right heart is the low pressure segment of the circulation responsible for pumping blood to the lungs. In contrast to the left ventricle, the right ventricle is more coarsely trabeculated, and usually has a prominent moderator band. There is a papillary muscle arising from the interventricular septum attached to the tricuspid valve, but no septal papillary muscle in the left heart. The aortic and mitral valves are in continuity with each other, but the pulmonary valve is a separate structure arising from the infundibulum of the right ventricle. The inflow and outflow portion of the right ventricle are thus separated.

The arrangement of muscle fibres is different between the ventricles: there is no middle layer of circumferential fibres in the right unlike the left ventricle, with the result that the right ventricle is more reliant on longitudinally aligned fibres.[1] A key difference between right and left ventricles is that the right is working against a very much lower impedance,[2] and the right heart is very sensitive to changes in afterload.[3] A final physiological consideration is that the left ventricle contributes very importantly to right ventricular function:[4] in a dog model, even if the right ventricular free wall was removed altogether, the right ventricle still generated near-normal pressure.[5] The right ventricle is subject to the same haemodynamic mechanisms as the left: as the right heart fails, so a higher filling pressure, the central venous pressure, is required to maintain right heart output. Typically, in health, the central venous pressure is around zero.

The filling pressure required is, of course, the haemostatic pressure tending to drive fluid out of the systemic veins. With worsening of right heart function, the haemostatic pressure will ultimately exceed the forces tending to retain fluid in the vasculature (principally the colloid osmotic pressure and the resistance provided by the basement membrane) and/or the rate at which that fluid can be drained away (the lymphatic drainage). As this point is reached, so oedema fluid starts to form in the tissues.

Although abrupt damage to the right ventricle in adult life can be catastrophic, normal exercise capacity in the absence of the right heart from the circulation is possible, and in some studies there is little direct relation between right ventricular function and exercise capacity.[6]

Assessment of right ventricular function

The complex shape of the right ventricle has historically made it difficult to assess its size, shape, and function.

Echocardiography is much more readily available than other techniques for assessing right heart function. Although the right ventricle is the part of the heart lying closest to the transthoracic echo probe, its function can be difficult to assess. It is not possible to measure the right ventricular ejection fraction accurately due to its shape. Various indices have been derived;[7] perhaps the most useful is the tricuspid annular plane systolic excursion (TAPSE) which is easy to measure and is reproducible: an M-mode cursor is placed across the lateral tricuspid valve annulus from the apical four-chamber view and is used to measure the movement of the tricuspid valve plane during right ventricular systole (see **Figure 31.1**). Fractional area change, again measured from the apical view, is also used but is less reproducible.

Doppler echocardiography is very widely used to estimate the pulmonary artery pressure as some degree of tricuspid regurgitation (TR) is very common. It is important to remember that the velocity of TR recorded gives an estimate of the pressure fall between right ventricle and right atrium: an estimate of right atrial pressure has to be added to give the pulmonary artery pressure, and the assumption is made that there is no significant pulmonary stenosis. In severe tricuspid regurgitation, the velocity of the jet may be low even when the pulmonary artery pressure is high: the right atrial pressure is also high and has to be added to the estimate (see **Figure 31.2**).

Nuclear techniques can be used to determine right ventricular ejection fraction without the complex geometry of the right

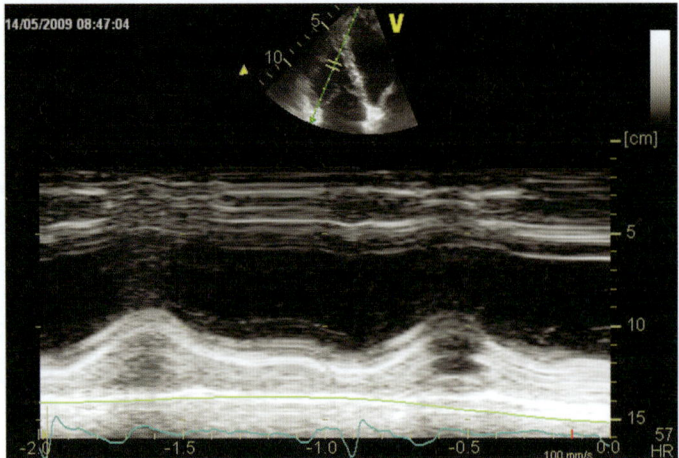

Figure 31.1 Tricuspid annular plane systolic excursion (TAPSE) measured in a normal heart.

ventricle mattering too much, but the best measures of right ventricular function come from computed tomography (CT) and magnetic resonance imaging (MRI). Both techniques give comparable data including right (and left) ventricular volumes and ejection fractions, myocardial mass measurements and morphological information. MR imaging is now the standard technique, and much more accurate than echocardiographic measurements.[8]

Syndrome of right heart failure

Older textbooks of cardiology often referred to heart failure in terms of pairings: forward vs backward failure; acute vs chronic; right vs left, and so on. The syndrome of right heart failure is characterized by fluid retention and manifests most commonly as ankle oedema.

The fluid excess has to be in the order of 5 L before it is clinically noticeable; individual patients may tolerate volumes in excess of 20 L before seeking help. Because the fluid collects under the influence of gravity, the ankles are usually first affected, extending up to the thighs and abdominal walls. The sacrum is a common collection site in a bed-bound patient. Oedema affecting the external genitalia is common in men. Ultimately, pleural and pericardial effusions form, as does ascites. The old-fashioned terms, anasarca (Gk: ανα- throughout; σάρξ flesh) and dropsy are sometimes applied to the clinical syndrome.

Fluid retention as a manifestation of right heart failure is usually accompanied by raised neck veins, but occasionally, right heart failure may be suspected in the presence of raised neck veins alone. Many patients have tricuspid regurgitation, giving rise to giant CV waves in the jugular venous wave form (**Figure 31.2**). Superior vena cava obstruction or more localized venous obstruction (such as subclavian vein obstruction) will not result in ankle swelling (see **Figure 31.3**). As the right atrium is usually dilated in people with right heart failure, atrial fibrillation is common. There is usually a right ventricular (parasternal) heave and a murmur of tricuspid regurgitations is often heard.

Differential diagnosis and investigations

Peripheral oedema is not diagnostic of right heart failure. The most common cause is dependent oedema, followed by impaired venous drainage (see **Table 31.1**). It is vital to consider the differential diagnosis before starting treatment with loop diuretic: the cycle of elderly patient with hypertension–calcium antagonist–ankle oedema–loop diuretic–gout is all too common. Obesity is increasingly common, and fat legs are treated with diuretic to little effect!

An outline of the differential diagnosis of right heart failure is shown in **Table 31.2**. Any patient presenting with ankle oedema should have a urine dipstick test, and a biochemical profile to assess renal and hepatic synthetic function.

A 12-lead electrocardiogram gives invaluable clues as to the cause of right heart failure (see **Figures 31.4** and **31.5**). Simple spirometry is helpful in suggesting whether cor pulmonale is likely, and a chest X-ray is vital (see **Figure 31.6**). The first step in imaging the heart is echocardiography, and a transoesophageal echocardiogram (TOE) can be very helpful where the patient has unexplained pulmonary hypertension or suspected congenital heart disease.

CT and MRI may be necessary, and MRI especially is helpful in cases where right ventricular cardiomyopathy is suspected.

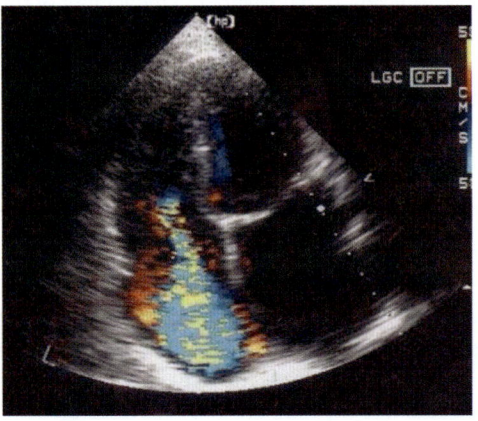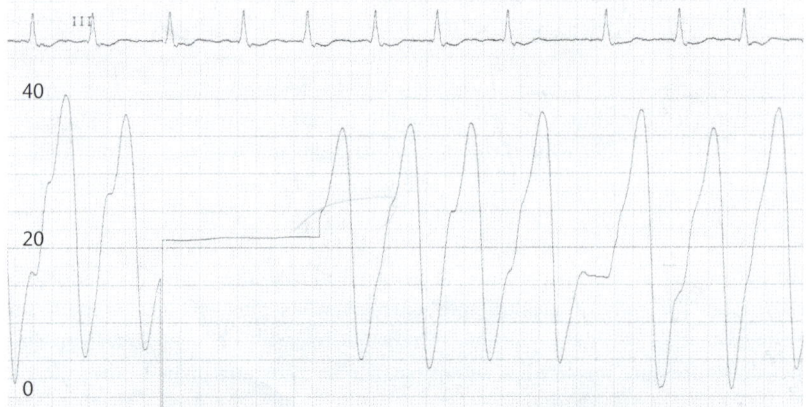

Figure 31.2 Severe tricuspid regurgitation (TR) seen in the echocardiographic frame on the left (colour jet). The velocity of the TR was 2.3 m/s leading to an estimate of pulmonary artery pressure of 21 mmHg. *Right*: right atrial pressure (measured directly during right heart catheterization), which, at around 40 mmHg, should be added to get a good estimate of pulmonary artery pressure.

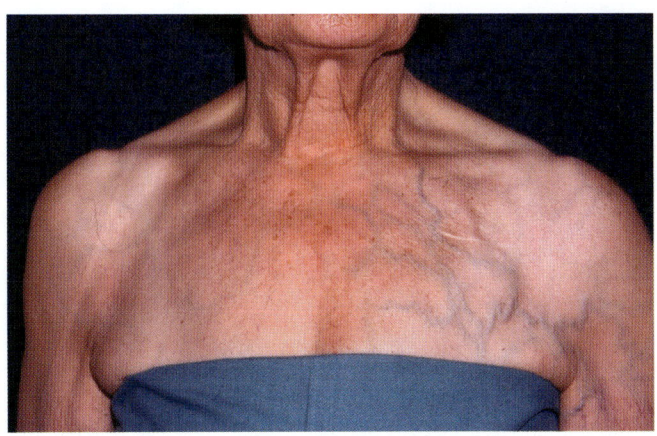

Figure 31.3 Dilated veins on the left-hand side of a patient's chest. The cause is subclavian vein obstruction caused by pacemaker leads, not heart failure.

Cardiac catheterization is vital in giving direct haemodynamic information: notably, it is the only way to measure the pulmonary artery pressure with certainty, and the pressure changes of constrictive pericarditis can only be obtained this way.

Specific syndromes of right heart failure

Acute ischaemic heart disease

Patients with acute myocardial infarction frequently have right ventricular involvement. In patients with anterior infarction, there is an association between the degrees of left and right ventricular dysfunction reflecting damage to the shared interventricular septum.[9] The clinical picture is usually dominated by left ventricular damage.

After an inferior myocardial infarction, usually caused by obstruction to the right coronary artery, there is little relation between right and left ventricular dysfunction. Predominant damage of the right ventricular free wall may lead to a picture of cardiogenic shock (hypotension and oliguria) in the presence of a clear chest X-ray and normal, or near-normal, left ventricular function on

Table 31.1 Differential diagnosis of ankle oedema[a]

Cause	Comments
Dependent oedema	Sedentary lifestyle
Venous insufficiency	Past history of deep vein thrombosis; iron staining; varicose veins
Drugs	Dihydropyridine calcium antagonists
Hypoalbuminaemia	Nephrotic syndrome
Lymphoedema	High protein fluid; woody swelling
Fat	Generalized obesity
Venous obstruction	Inferior vena cava obstruction; retroperitoneal fibrosis
Fluid overload	Pregnancy; iatrogenic
Arthritis	Pain and stiffness common
Cardiac	

[a] Common causes are listed.

Table 31.2 Outline of differential diagnosis of right heart failure

Cause	Examples
Left-sided heart failure	Left ventricular failure Mitral valve disease
Congenital heart disease	Atrial septal defect Right ventricle as systemic ventricle
Pulmonary hypertension	Primary Cor pulmonale Thromboembolic
Pericardial disease	Constrictive pericarditis
Primary right heart disease	Ischaemia Valvular disease (e.g. carcinoid) Specific cardiomyopathy

echocardiography. The echo will often demonstrate impaired right ventricular function, although bedside images in coronary care units are often of indifferent quality, and the right ventricle can be difficult to assess. ST segment elevation in lead V4R is sensitive and specific for right ventricular infarction.[10]

Other useful bedside investigations include pulmonary artery catheterization. As a general guide to the management of patients in intensive care, the pulmonary artery catheter has fallen into disrepute:[11,12] but it remains extremely helpful in guiding treatment in specific situations. Where right ventricular infarction is the cause of acute heart failure, the central venous pressure will be high and pulmonary capillary wedge pressure will be low.

The diagnosis is important to make: orthodox treatment of acute heart failure aimed at reducing left ventricular filling pressure with diuretic and vasodilators will make the situation worse. Diuretics and vasodilators should be stopped; and large volumes of fluid may be necessary to keep the right ventricular filling pressure high enough to maintain cardiac output. Percutaneous coronary intervention may be helpful in restoring some right ventricular function.

Pulmonary arterial hypertension

Pulmonary arterial hypertension (see Chapter 35)—often still called primary pulmonary hypertension)—should be suspected in a young woman presenting with apparent right heart failure. As pulmonary hypertension advances, cardiac output becomes fixed as the right ventricle is generating its maximal amount of work at rest. Any exertion leads to breathlessness as the extra oxygen demand of the exercising muscles can only be met by increasing oxygen extraction. The mixed venous oxygen saturation may fall to extremely low levels, and reflects right heart function.

Pulmonary thromboembolic disease

Acute large pulmonary emboli may be confused with heart failure on occasion, and may result in acute right heart failure. The acute pulmonary obstruction results in an abrupt increase in right ventricular afterload, to which the right ventricle is very sensitive. The right ventricle dilates and pulmonary artery pressure rises rapidly.

Left ventricular function becomes compromised as it becomes underfilled, and hypoxia develops due to ventilation–perfusion mismatching. At first sight, hypoxia seems an odd development as vascular obstruction should simply lead to an increase in dead space, but generalized ventilation/perfusion mismatching occurs, leading to right-to-left shunting.[13]

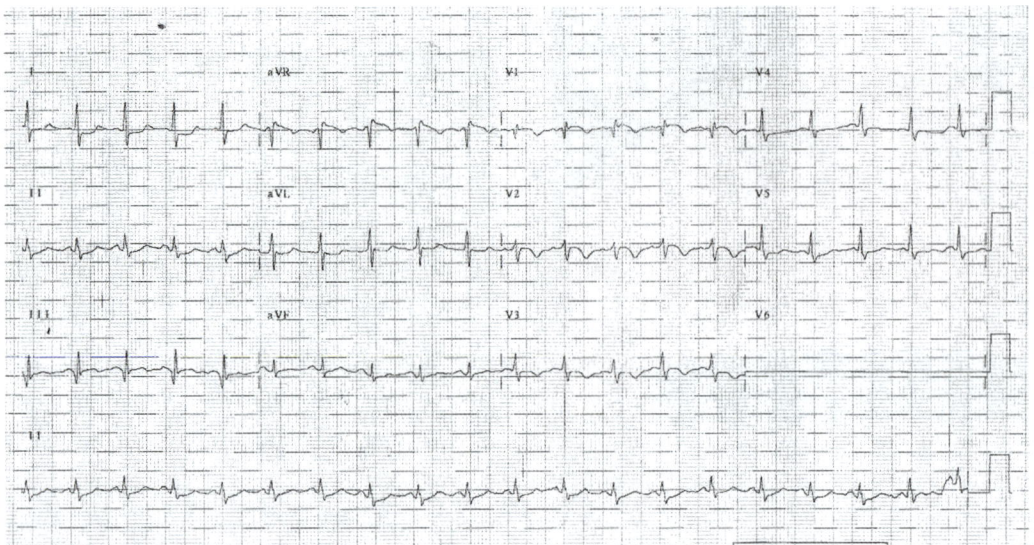

Figure 31.4 Twelve-lead ECG from a 39-year-old man with acute right heart failure 72 h after weight reduction surgery. Note the sinus tachycardia, the S1Q3T3 pattern, and changes in the right-sided chest leads (lead 6 not recorded). The diagnosis was acute pulmonary embolism.

The most important part of the management of pulmonary emboli is to think of the diagnosis in the first place. Various scoring schemes are reported that help estimate the risk that a pulmonary embolus is present,[14] but these can only be used once the diagnosis is considered.

Repeated pulmonary emboli may rarely lead to chronic pulmonary hypertension (Chapter 35). Chronic embolic occlusion of the pulmonary circulation appears to result from incomplete re-absorption and removal of initial emboli. Contrast CT scanning is helpful in establishing the diagnosis. It is a very important diagnosis to reach in a patient presenting with right heart failure and pulmonary hypertension because the surgical treatment, pulmonary thrombendarterectomy, although dangerous, is potentially curative.[15]

Cor pulmonale

Chronic cor pulmonale is the long-term consequence of lung disease in patients with chronic airways disease. The most potent stimulus

to generating pulmonary hypertension in such patients is hypoxia: chronic hypoxia results in pulmonary vascular re-modelling following hypoxic vasoconstriction.[16] The increased pulmonary vascular resistance in turn leads to pulmonary hypertension, right ventricular hypertrophy, and right ventricular failure.

The clinical features are of right heart failure: marked fluid retention with dependent oedema and raised jugular venous pressure in a patient with chronic productive cough and breathlessness. Patients are frequently cyanosed. Examination of the heart is usually limited by chest hyperinflation. The key investigation is spirometry: most patients have marked reductions in forced expiratory volume in 1 s (FEV$_1$) and forced vital capacity (FVC).

The echocardiogram is often unhelpful (and challenging) due to the overinflated lungs: it will, however, usually show good left ventricular function, and may show evidence of right ventricular hypertrophy and pulmonary arterial hypertension.

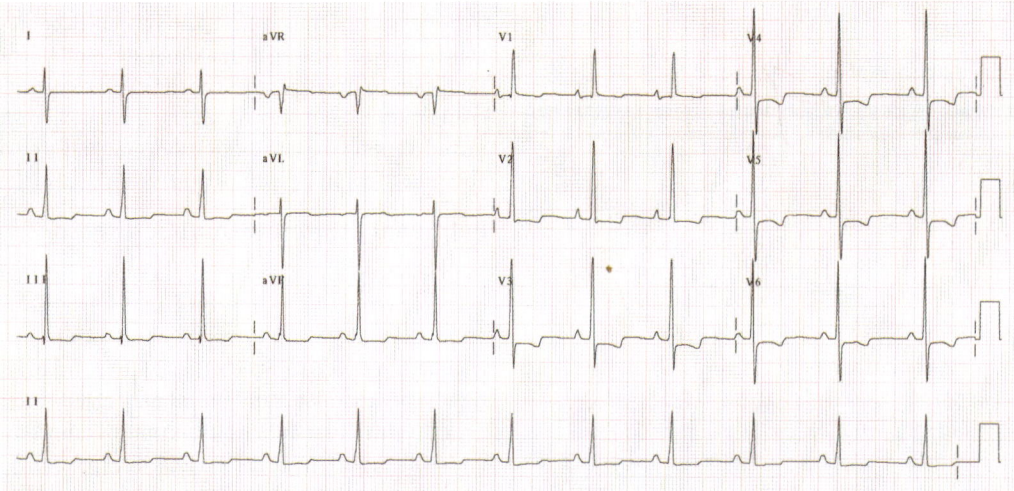

Figure 31.5 Twelve-lead ECG from a 17-year-old woman with chronic ankle oedema and breathlessness on exertion, diagnosed as asthma. There is right axis deviation and changes in the chest leads, consistent with right ventricular hypertrophy. The diagnosis was primary pulmonary hypertension.

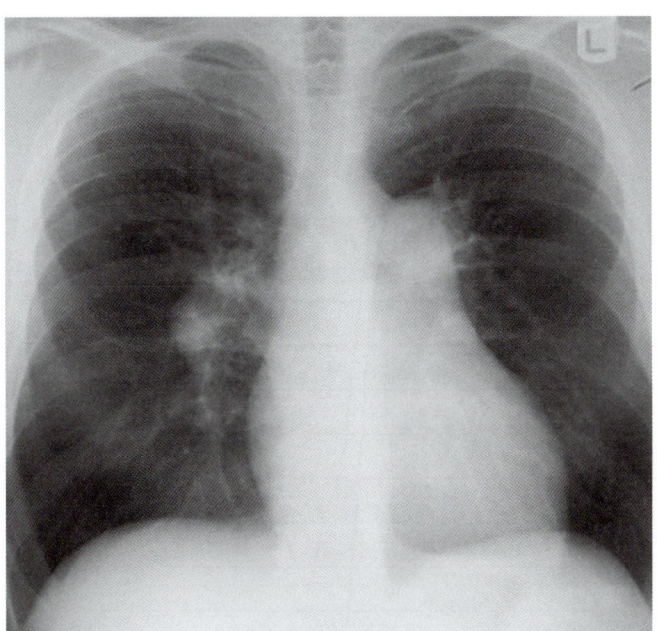

Figure 31.6 Plain chest X-ray of the same patient as in Figure 30.3 showing a dilated pulmonary artery with peripheral pruning suggestive of pulmonary hypertension.

Patients with cor pulmonale should be assessed for long-term oxygen therapy, the only intervention to have a marked impact on survival.[17] It should be considered for patients with an arterial oxygen tension <55 mmHg or saturation <88%. Oxygen therapy has to be given for at least 19 h per day to be effective.[18]

Chronic rheumatic heart disease

The right-sided heart valves are almost never affected by rheumatic disease on their own,[19] but some involvement of the tricuspid valve is common in patients who have other valves affected.[20,21] Tricuspid stenosis causes right heart failure with predominant fluid retention and anasarca. Giant A waves in the jugular venous pulse and very slow y descent are important clinical clues. Tricuspid stenosis will protect the patient with mitral stenosis from pulmonary oedema by reducing right heart output.

Although tricuspid regurgitation can be caused by the rheumatic process itself, secondary regurgitation due to dilation of the right ventricle and tricuspid valve ring is more common. Prominent clinical features of tricuspid regurgitation are abdominal bloating and discomfort from the swollen liver; and fullness in the neck due to the giant cV waves of tricuspid regurgitation in the jugular veins. Tricuspid valve surgery is often necessary at the time of valve surgery for rheumatic mitral valve disease, often in the form of a tricuspid valve ring.

An increasingly frequent clinical problem is that of chronic right heart failure and tricuspid regurgitation some time after surgery for left-sided valvular disease. Up to two-thirds of patients undergoing isolated mitral valve replacement will have significant tricuspid regurgitation after 10 years.[22] Significant tricuspid regurgitation is associated with a worse long-term prognosis.[23] There is some evidence to suggest that an aggressive approach to the tricuspid valve at the time of initial mitral valve surgery reduces the risk of long-term

tricuspid regurgitation,[24] but selection of patients for repeat surgery many years after an initial valve replacement is difficult.

Other valvular heart disease

The tricuspid valve can be affected by other pathologies. For instance, endocarditis affecting the tricuspid valve, especially when associated with intravenous drug use, may result in severe tricuspid regurgitation either due to destruction of the valve itself or to surgical removal of the valve. Although in the short term most individuals can tolerate tricuspid valve removal, some patients develop intractable right heart failure later. The decision to replace the valve is difficult: it is vital to be certain that the patient no longer uses intravenous drugs. Long-term anticoagulation is often needed.

Carcinoid tumours are rare gastrointestinal tumours that produce 5-hydroxytryptamine (5HT, serotonin). If a carcinoid tumour should metastasize to the liver, then the 5HT is no longer cleared by the liver from the circulation and it will reach the heart. Serotonin causes fibrosis of the tricuspid valve, sometimes with involvement of the pulmonary valve.

The diagnosis of a carcinoid tumour has usually been made by the time the patient presents to a cardiologist, but should be suspected in a patient with unexplained tricuspid regurgitation, especially if there are systemic symptoms such as flushing, diarrhoea, and bronchospasm. Tricuspid regurgitation is typically the dominant cardiac lesion, although tricuspid stenosis also occurs (**Figure 31.7**). Although the outcome is bleak once carcinoid heart disease has developed,[25] patients often die from the consequences of tricuspid regurgitation rather than carcinomatosis, and therefore surgery should be offered to selected patients.[26]

Atrial septal defect

Unoperated atrial septal defects (ASDs) frequently present late in life, often presenting as right heart failure with apparently normal left ventricular function. It used to be said that approximately half of patients with unoperated ASDs died by the age of 50 years, but this observation is based on ASDs large enough to have been detected on chest X-rays. Smaller defects are compatible with normal life expectancy.

Obvious clues to the diagnosis are the physical signs of a right ventricular heave and pulmonary flow murmur. The fixed splitting of the second heart sound may not be very clear. The ECG will show evidence of right ventricular hypertrophy or right bundle branch block, and may show right axis deviation in a secundum defect or left axis deviation if the defect is a primum one.

The echocardiogram will very often confirm the diagnosis, although the inter-atrial septum is frequently poorly seen. Some flow across the inter-atrial septum will usually be detectable, and the right heart appears dilated and overloaded. Transoesophageal echocardiography usually allows a definitive diagnosis and allows assessment of the defect for percutaneous closure.

Coronary angiography will determine closure technique: if the patient has normal coronary arteries, percutaneous closure is usually possible for all but very large defects. Surgical closure may be needed for those with non-secundum defects, very large defects, and those needing revascularization.

Special mention should be made of sinus venosus ASDs. These are mal-alignment defects higher in the atrial septum than secundum

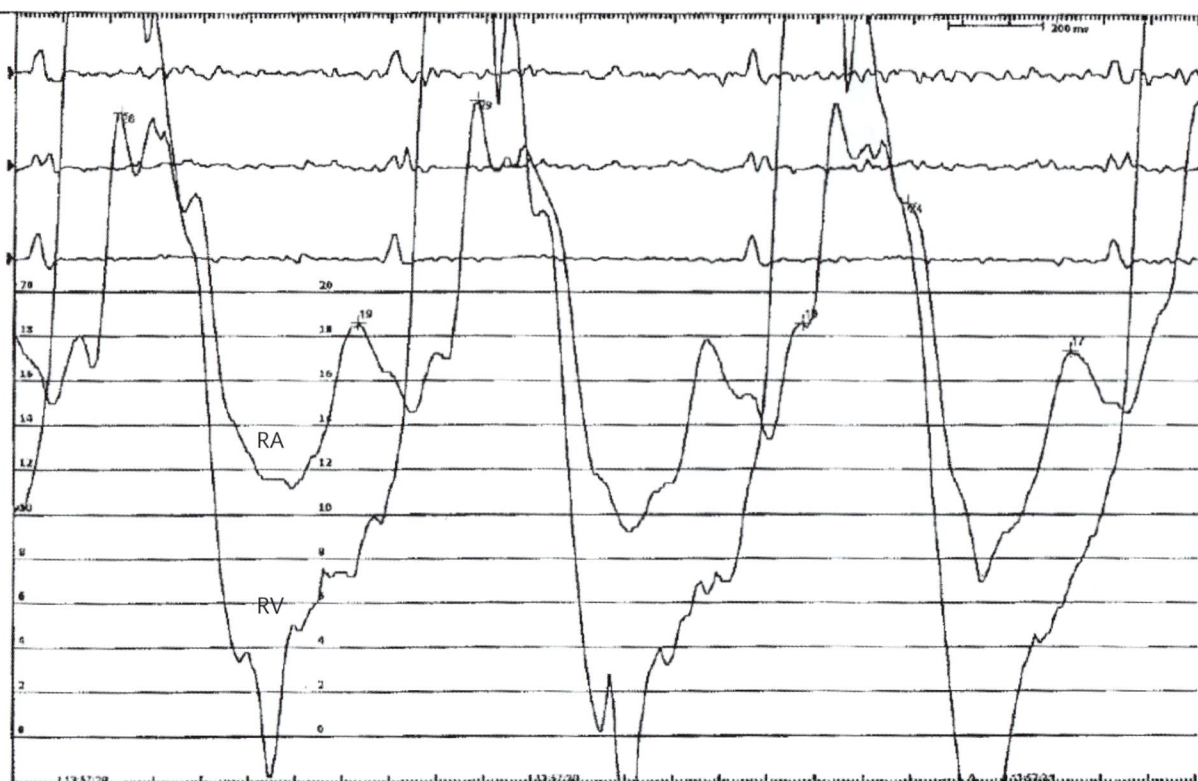

Figure 31.7 Tricuspid stenosis is a patient with carcinoid heart disease. Simultaneous recordings from the right atrium (RA) and right ventricle (RV) are shown. The difference between the two in diastole represents the gradient across the valve.

defects (see **Figure 31.8**). The superior vena cava enters the right atrium over-riding the defect, usually at the same point as the right upper pulmonary vein. The defect is easily missed on echocardiography, and even on TOE if it is not specifically sought. Any patient thought to have primary pulmonary hypertension should have TOE performed by an experienced operator to exclude this possible treatable lesion.

Congenital heart disease

An unusual problem discussed in more detail in Chapter 5 is that of failure of a systemic right ventricle. Older patients born with transposition of the great vessels who have been palliated with a Mustard or Senning procedure have a right ventricle supporting the systemic

circulation. Patients with congenitally corrected transposition have similar physiology. The systemic right ventricle is likely to fail in early middle-age.

Pericardial constriction

Constrictive pericarditis can be a difficult diagnosis to make clinically, and it is common for a patient to wait several years with recurring symptoms before being diagnosed.

Pathology

Constriction can develop as the consequence of any inflammatory process affecting the pericardium. Tuberculosis was once the

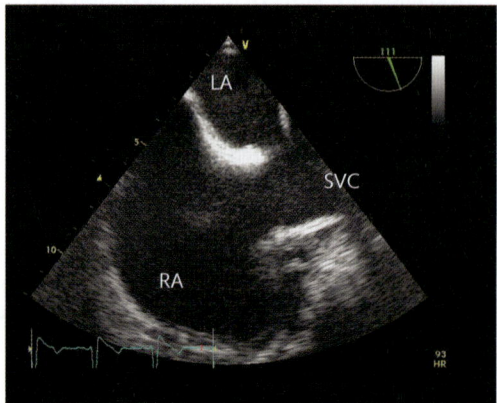
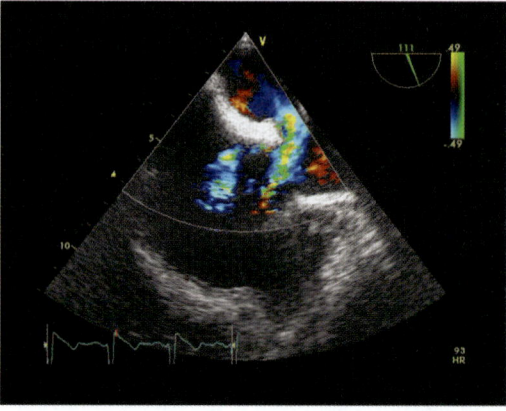

Figure 31.8 Two frames from a transoesophageal echocardiogram. The inter-atrial septum is shown with a defect high in the septum highlighted by the colour flow image. RA, right atrium; LA, left atrium; SVC, superior vena cava.

commonest cause in industrialized societies, but has become rare. Trauma (particularly post-cardiac surgery), previous acute pericarditis, uraemia, and connective tissue diseases are causes, although many patients have no known specific cause.

The pericardium gradually thickens with the two layers becoming adherent and densely fibrosed. Calcification is common, and may extend into the myocardium, making eventual surgical therapy difficult.

Clinical picture

Constrictive pericarditis may take years to develop. The clinical picture is dominated by right heart failure with apparently normal or near-normal left ventricular function. Peripheral oedema develops together with symptoms of liver congestion and ascites. The ascites can be very striking and may be confused with end-stage liver disease, particularly as 'cardiac cirrhosis' may develop.

Fatigue, muscle wasting and frank cachexia are common as the disease progresses, together with atrial fibrillation.

Pathophysiology

The pericardium in constrictive pericarditis acts to restrain filling of the heart, with the maximum volumes of the different chambers essentially individually fixed. In consequence of impaired ventricular filling in diastole, atrial pressure rises, and thus the moment the atrioventricular valves open in diastole, there is a sudden rush of blood from atria to ventricles that is abruptly halted as soon as the maximum volume of the ventricles is reached. These phenomena result in a raised jugular venous pressure, abrupt y descent (the x descent is preserved, giving a prominent M- or W-shaped wave form to the JVP) and loud third heart sound; and a 'dip-and-plateau' pressure trace is recorded from the ventricles. As the constriction usually affects all cardiac chambers, there is equalization of the diastolic pressure in all cardiac chambers (see **Figure 31.9**).

Diagnosis

The key to diagnosing constrictive pericarditis is to suspect it in the first place. The chest X-ray may demonstrate pericardial constriction, and CT or MRI of the heart may demonstrate the thickened pericardium (**Figure 31.10**).

The echocardiogram may sometimes show pericardial thickening, but the key echocardiographic feature is abnormal transmitral and tricuspid diastolic blood flow with respiration. There is a great exaggeration of the normal pattern: during inspiration, there is an increase in trans-tricuspid flow and marked reduction in transmitral flow, which is reversed in expiration.[27] The interventricular septum is often seen to bounce early in diastole as a consequence of the rapid filling, and may be seen to move markedly from side to side during the respiratory cycle.

Cardiac catheterization with careful simultaneous measurement of pressures in the different cardiac chambers (particularly right and left ventricles; and right atrium and left ventricle) will confirm the haemodynamics of constriction. Occasionally the signs may be missed in a patient who has been treated with high doses of diuretic. If there is a strong clinical suspicion of constriction, an acute fluid load of 500 mL saline can bring out the haemodynamic features.[28] The cardinal features of constriction on cardiac catheterization are: raised right and left heart end-diastolic pressures equal within 5 mmHg; mean right atrial pressure >15 mmHg; and right ventricular end-diastolic pressure greater than one-third of right ventricular systolic pressure. The positive predictive value is >90% if all three criteria are fulfilled.[29]

The major differential diagnosis is restrictive cardiomyopathy. The two conditions can be similar clinically, and distinguishing between the two is vital. Restriction is usually caused by some infiltrative process such as amyloidosis; the result is a small voltage ECG and thickened myocardium on echocardiography. The septal bounce is not seen in restriction, nor is pericardial calcification.

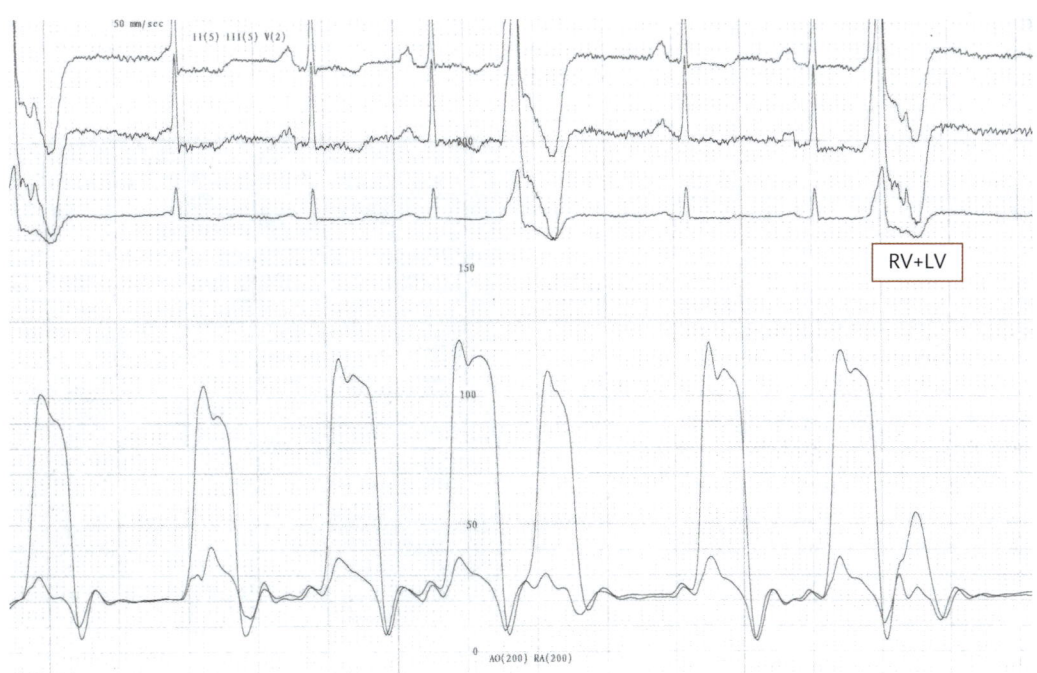

Figure 31.9 Simultaneous recordings of pressures from left and right ventricles. The patient is in sinus rhythm with ectopics. The diastolic pressures are identical with a 'dip-and-plateau' wave form strongly suggestive of constrictive pericarditis.

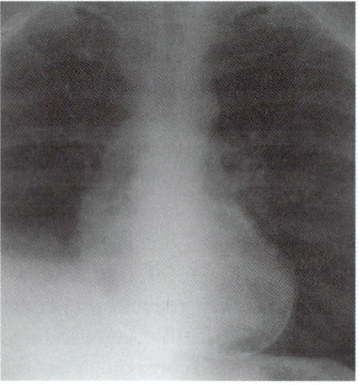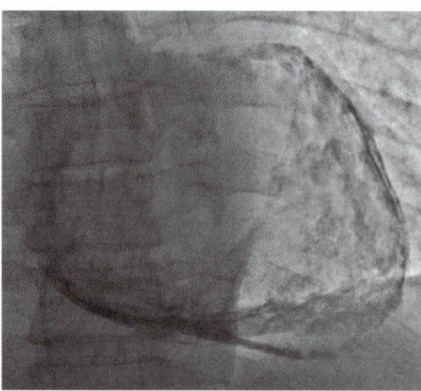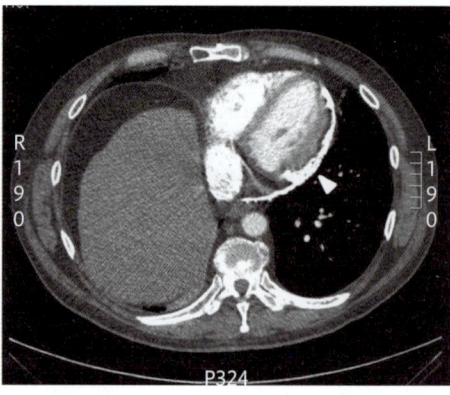

Figure 31.10 Imaging from three patients with constrictive pericarditis. *Left*: plain chest X-ray showing pericardial calcification inferiorly and extending around the apex in a patient with tuberculous pericarditis. *Middle*: fluoroscopic frame during cardiac catheterization showing diffuse calcification throughout the pericardium. *Right*: slice from a CT scan showing dense pericardial calcification around the free wall of the left ventricle (white arrow head).

The haemodynamics of restriction are also subtly different: the left-sided filling pressures are typically higher than the right (whereas they are identical in constriction), and pulmonary hypertension is frequent (whereas pulmonary artery pressure is rarely significantly raised in constrictive pericarditis).

Treatment

Although constrictive pericarditis is a potentially 'curable' cause of right heart failure, pericardectomy is a difficult and dangerous operation with a mortality rate of up to 15%.[30] The difficulty lies with the visceral pericardium's dense adherence to the myocardium and difficulty identifying a tissue plane between peri- and myocardium. In many patients, the pericardium is incompletely excised and recurrence of constriction is common. Fewer than half of patients are free of symptoms 10 years postoperatively.[31] Perhaps the most important prognostic indicator is the extent of left ventricular damage preoperatively;[32] the left ventricle may become damaged by the combination of extension of fibrosis from the pericardium and atrophy. It is important to make the diagnosis of constrictive pericarditis and operate as quickly as possible to maximize the chances of recovery.

Arrhythmogenic right ventricular cardiomyopathy (or dysplasia)

Arrhythmogenic right ventricular cardiomyopathy (or dysplasia: ARVC or ARVD) is a rare cardiomyopathy specifically affecting the right ventricle. There is gradual loss of right ventricular myocytes, probably by apoptosis, and their replacement by fibrous and fatty tissue. Involvement of the right ventricle is often patchy, but the inflow area, apex, and infundibulum are most usually affected and form the so-called 'triangle of dysplasia'.[33] Late in the course of the disease, the left ventricle may also be involved.

ARVC is genetically determined and inherited as an autosomal dominant with variable penetrance. Most genes that have been identified so far code for a desmosomal protein, commonly desmin, but other abnormal genes (such as that coding for the cardiac ryanodine receptor) have been described.[34]

The dominant clinical feature is ventricular tachycardia of right ventricular origin (so the 12-lead ECG shows a left bundle branch block pattern). In some patients, symptoms of right heart failure may dominate. The diagnosis can be difficult to reach: echocardiographic imaging is often normal early in the course of the disease. Myocardial biopsy may miss patches of involvement. MRI is particularly helpful in detecting areas of fatty replacement of right ventricular myocardium.

Management is usually dominated by the need to control arrhythmias, with β-blockers being helpful, and many patients require consideration of an implantable cardioverter–defibrillator. Heart transplantation may be needed for uncontrollable heart failure or arrhythmia.

Uhl anomaly has some similarity to ARVC, but is characterized by failure of right ventricular myocardium to develop in foetal life.[35,36] The anomaly presents with severe right heart failure in early life.

Miscellaneous

Other rare pathologies can cause right heart failure, such as right atrial tumours and traumatic damage to the tricuspid valve.

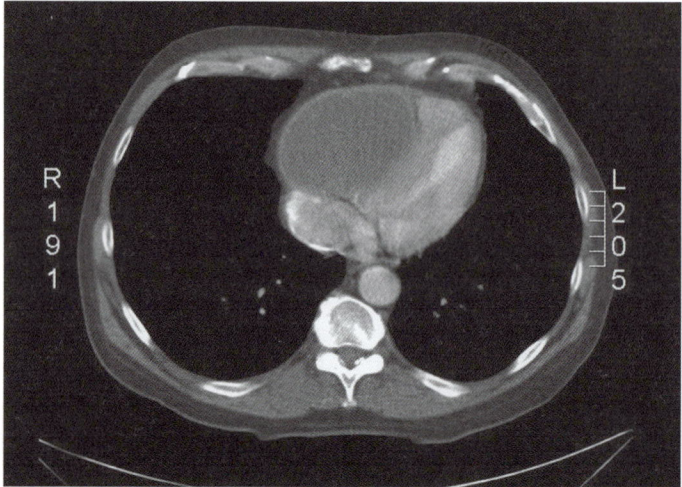

Figure 31.11 Computed tomography from a 57-year-old man presenting with right heart failure. A large pericardial cyst (arrowed) was causing compression of the right heart.

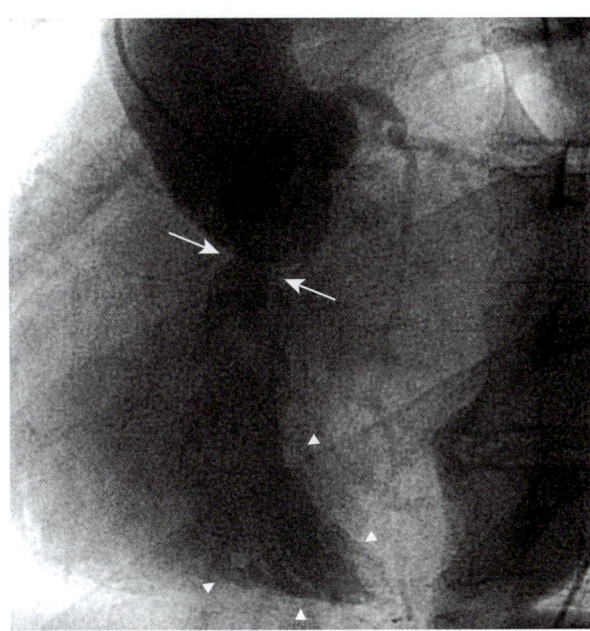

Figure 31.12 Aortogram from a 27-year-old woman who presented with right heart failure. She had a continuous murmur, and the aortogram shows a ruptured sinus of Valsalva aneurysm (arrows) with the right ventricular cavity outlined (arrow heads).

Pacemaker leads can cause thrombosis, infection or tricuspid valve damage leading to right heart failure. External compression of the heart may cause right heart failure (**Figure 31.7**). An occasional patient with an acquired intracardiac shunt may present with right heart failure (**Figure 31.8**).

REFERENCES

1. Sanchez-Guintana D, Anderson RH, Ho SY. Ventricular myoarchitecture in tetralogy of Fallot. *Heart* 1996;**76**:280–6.
2. Redington AN, Rigby ML, Shinebourne EA, *et al.* Changes in the pressure–volume relation of the right ventricle when its loading conditions are modified. *Br Heart J* 1990;**63**:45–9.
3. Shekerdemian LS, Bush A, Lincoln C, *et al.* Cardiopulmonary interactions in healthy children and children after simple cardiac surgery: the effects of positive and negative pressure ventilation. *Heart* 1997;**78**:587–93.
4. Damiano RJ Jr, La Follette P Jr, Cox JL, Lowe JE, Santamore WP. Significant left ventricular contribution to right ventricular systolic function. *Am J Physiol* 1991;**261**(5 Pt 2):H1514–24.
5. Hoffman D, Sisto D, Frater RW, Nikolic SD. Left-to-right ventricular interaction with a noncontracting right ventricle. *J Thorac Cardiovasc Surg* 1994;**107**:1496–502.
6. Clark AL, Swan JW, Laney R, *et al.* The role of right and left ventricular function in the ventilatory response to exercise in chronic heart failure. *Circulation* 1994;**89**:2062–9.
7. Lee KS, Abbas AE, Khandheria BK, Lester SJ. Echocardiographic assessment of right heart hemodynamic parameters. *J Am Soc Echocardiogr* 2007;**20**:773–82.
8. Helbing WA, Bosch HG, Maliepaard C, *et al.* Comparison of echocardiographic methods with magnetic resonance imaging for assessment of right ventricular function in children. *Am J Cardiol* 1995;**76**:589–94.
9. Caplin JL, Dymond DS, Flatman WD, Spurrell RA. Global and regional right ventricular function after acute myocardial infarction: dependence upon site of left ventricular infarction. *Br Heart J* 1987;**58**:101–9.
10. Lopez-Sendon J, Coma-Canella I, Alcasena S, Seoane J, Gamello C. Electrocardiographic findings in acute right ventricular infarction: sensitivity and specificity of electrocardiographic alterations in right precordial leads V4R, V3R, VI, V2 and V3. *J Am Coll Cardiol* 1985;**6**:1273–9.
11. Harvey S, Harrison DA, Singer M, *et al.*; PAC-Man study collaboration. Assessment of the clinical effectiveness of pulmonary artery catheters in management of patients in intensive care (PAC-Man): a randomised controlled trial. *Lancet* 2005;**366**:472–7.
12. Binanay C, Califf RM, Hasselblad V, *et al.*; ESCAPE Investigators and ESCAPE Study Coordinators. Evaluation study of congestive heart failure and pulmonary artery catheterization effectiveness: the ESCAPE trial. *JAMA* 2005;**294**:1625–33.
13. Altemeier WA, Robertson HT, McKinney S, Glenny RW. Pulmonary embolization causes hypoxemia by redistributing regional blood flow without changing ventilation. *J Appl Physiol* 1998;**85**:2337–43.
14. Wells PS, Anderson DR, Rodger M, *et al.* Derivation of a simple clinical model to categorize patients probability of pulmonary embolism: increasing the models utility with the SimpliRED D-dimer. *Thromb Haemost* 2000;**83**:416–20.
15. Thistlethwaite PA, Kaneko K, Madani MM, Jamieson SW. Technique and outcomes of pulmonary endarterectomy surgery. *Ann Thorac Cardiovasc Surg* 2008;**14**:274–82.
16. Burger CD. Pulmonary hypertension in COPD: a review and consideration of the role of arterial vasodilators. *COPD* 2009;**6**:137–44.
17. Medical Research Council Working Party. Long term domiciliary oxygen therapy in chronic hypoxic cor pulmonale complicating chronic bronchitis and emphysema. Report of the Medical Research Council Working Party. *Lancet* 1981;**1**:681–6.
18. Nocturnal Oxygen Therapy Trial Group. Continuous or nocturnal oxygen therapy in hypoxemic chronic obstructive lung disease: a clinical trial. *Ann Intern Med* 1980;**93**:391–8.
19. Finnegan P, Abrams LD. Isolated tricuspid stenosis. *Heart* 1973;**35**:1207–10.
20. Yousof AM, Shafei MZ, Endrys G, *et al.* Tricuspid stenosis and regurgitation in rheumatic heart disease: a prospective cardiac catheterization study in 525 patients. *Am Heart J* 1985;**110**:60–4.
21. Henein MY, O'Sullivan CA, Li W, *et al.* Evidence for rheumatic valve disease in patients with severe tricuspid regurgitation long after mitral valve surgery: the role of 3D echo reconstruction. *J Heart Valve Dis* 2003;**12**:566–72.
22. Porter A, Shapira Y, Wurzel M, *et al.* Tricuspid regurgitation late after mitral valve replacement: clinical and echocardiographic evaluation. *J Heart Valve Dis* 1999;**8**:57–62.
23. Song H, Kim MJ, Chung CH, *et al.* Factors associated with development of late significant tricuspid regurgitation after successful left-sided valve surgery. *Heart* 2009;**95**:931–6.
24. Dreyfus GD, Corbi PJ, Chan KM, Bahrami T. Secondary tricuspid regurgitation or dilatation: which should be the criteria for surgical repair? *Ann Thorac Surg* 2005;**79**:127–32.
25. Pellikka PA, Tajik AJ, Khandheria BK, *et al.* Carcinoid heart disease. Clinical and echocardiographic spectrum in 74 patients. *Circulation* 1993;**87**:1188–96.

26. Connolly HM, Nishimura RA, Smith HC, *et al.* Outcome of cardiac surgery for carcinoid heart disease. *J Am Coll Cardiol* 1995;**25**:410–16.

27. Oh JK, Hatle LK, Seward JB, *et al.* Diagnostic role of Doppler echocardiography in constrictive pericarditis. *J Am Coll Cardiol* 1994;**23**:154–62.

28. Bush C, Stang J, Wooley C. Occult constrictive pericardial disease. Diagnosis by rapid volume expansion and correction by pericardiectomy. *Circulation* 1977;**56**:924–30.

29. Vaitkus P, Kussmaul W. Constrictive pericarditis versus restrictive cardiomyopathy: a reappraisal and update of diagnostic criteria. *Am Heart J* 1991;**122**:1431–41.

30. Trotter MC, Chung KC, Ochsner JL, McFadden PM. Pericardiectomy for pericardial constriction. *Am Surg* 1996;**62**:304–7.

31. Ling LH, Oh JK, Schaff HV, *et al.* Constrictive pericarditis in the modern era: evolving clinical spectrum and impact on outcome after pericardiectomy. *Circulation* 1999;**100**:1380–6.

32. Ha JW, Oh JK, Schaff HV, *et al.* Impact of left ventricular function on immediate and long-term outcomes after pericardiectomy in constrictive pericarditis. *J Thorac Cardiovasc Surg* 2008;**136**:1136–41.

33. McKenna WJ, Thiene G, Nava A, *et al.* Diagnosis of arrhythmogenic right ventricular dysplasia/cardiomyopathy. Task Force of the Working Group Myocardial and Pericardial Disease of the European Society of Cardiology and of the Scientific Council on Cardiomyopathies of the International Society and Federation of Cardiology. *Br Heart J* 1994;**71**:215–18.

34. Basso C, Corrado D, Marcus FI, Nava A, Thiene G. Arrhythmogenic right ventricular cardiomyopathy. *Lancet* 2009;**373**:1289–300.

35. Uhl HS. A previously undescribed congenital malformation of the heart: almost total absence of the myocardium of the right ventricle. *Bull Johns Hopkins Hosp* 1952;**91**:197–209.

36. Gerlis LM, Schmidt-Ott SC, Ho SY, Anderson RH. Dysplastic conditions of the right ventricular myocardium: Uhl's anomaly vs arrhythmogenic right ventricular dysplasia. *Br Heart J* 1993;**69**:142–50.

32

Anaemia and iron deficiency

Paul R. Kalra and Michael Pope

Anaemia

Prevalence

Anaemia is a common comorbidity recognized in numerous chronic conditions including rheumatological diseases, renal dysfunction, and diabetes mellitus, many of which have inflammation as part of their underlying pathophysiology.[1] Anaemia is also frequently observed in the elderly, with a variety of causes including nutritional deficiency, malabsorption, excess blood loss, and chronic disease.[2] Bearing in mind that chronic heart failure (CHF) is more prevalent in the elderly and frequently coexists with multiple conditions, it is unsurprising that anaemia is commonly associated with CHF.

Several studies have sought to identify both the prevalence of anaemia in CHF and to delineate the nature of the relationship between the two conditions. Although the World Health Organization criteria for anaemia has been the most used (haemoglobin <13 g/dL in men and <12 g/dL in women), definitions have varied considerably, as have the demographics of the populations evaluated especially in respect of the severity of heart failure.[3] Estimates of prevalence therefore range between 4% and 61%.[4] A large meta-analysis by Groenveld *et al.* in 2008 analysed 34 studies with a combined total of 153 180 patients with CHF: 37.2% were anaemic.[5] This is consistent with a recently published study of 4456 patients referred to a single centre heart failure clinic which identified anaemia in 33.3% of those with a diagnosis of CHF (**Figure 32.1**).[6]

Clinical consequences of anaemia

Low haemoglobin is consistently associated with greater symptom limitation and higher New York Heart Association (NYHA) functional class in patients with CHF.[7,8] There is a positive correlation between increasing haemoglobin and greater peak oxygen consumption (VO_2) during exercise testing: conversely, the lower the

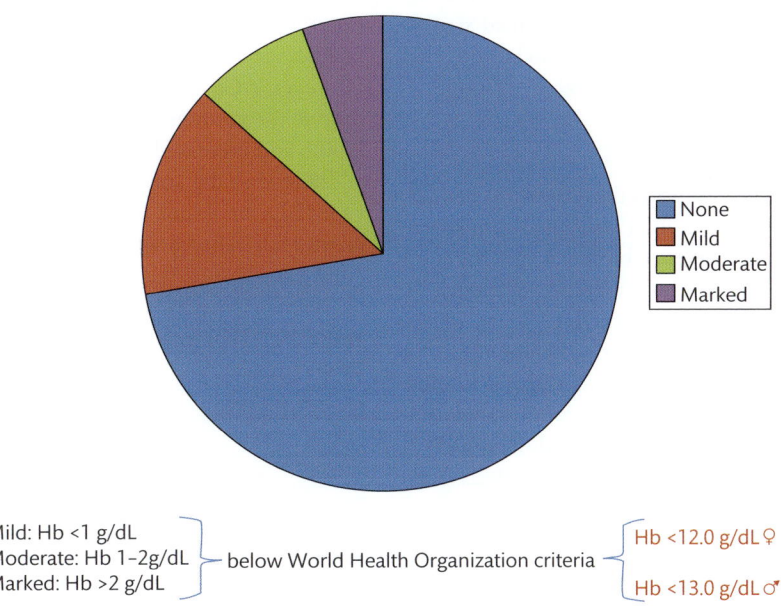

Mild: Hb <1 g/dL
Moderate: Hb 1–2g/dL — below World Health Organization criteria
Marked: Hb >2 g/dL

Hb <12.0 g/dL ♀
Hb <13.0 g/dL ♂

Figure 32.1 Severity of anaemia among 4456 patients presenting with suspected heart failure to a single centre.

Source data from Cleland JG, Zhang J, Pellicori P, Dicken B, Dierckx R, Shoaib A, *et al.* Prevalence and outcomes of anemia and hematinic deficiencies in patients with chronic heart failure. *JAMA Cardiol* 2016;**1**(5):539–47.

haemoglobin, the lower the peak VO_2.[7,9] This could be a direct consequence of the lower oxygen delivery to metabolizing tissues that is likely seen with anaemia, but it might also reflect the fact that anaemia is merely a marker of the underlying severity of heart failure and/or any co-morbidities.

A strong independent relationship is also seen between anaemia and clinical outcomes in patients with CHF. The large volume of data collected from diverse CHF populations has demonstrated consistent findings with a clear inverse association between lower haemoglobin and increased all-cause mortality.[4,10–14] There is, however, a number of confounding factors that complicate the association, and in many studies anaemia is also associated with more severe heart failure as measured by NYHA functional class, increasing age, worse renal function, lower body mass index, lower albumin, female sex, and lower blood pressure.

The association between anaemia and clinical outcomes is present regardless of left ventricular systolic function and is closely related to functional class (as outlined above) rather than to ejection fraction.[11,12] Indeed, in one analysis there seemed to be an inverse relationship between haemoglobin and ejection fraction, with higher haemoglobin levels observed in those with lower ejection fractions. The authors postulated that low haemoglobin induces cytokine production leading to exaggerated nitric oxide-mediated vasodilatation and thus a reduction in afterload and a subsequent increase in ejection fraction and cardiac output.[11]

Renal dysfunction is extremely common in CHF and is consistently associated with adverse outcomes.[15,16] Renal dysfunction is a well-recognized cause of anaemia and the complex relationships in the cardio–renal–anaemia syndrome, as it has come to be termed,[17] are implicated in many of the pathophysiological changes observed in heart failure, including left ventricular remodelling, renal hypoperfusion, neurohormonal activation and altered erythropoietin production.[16–18] However, numerous studies have confirmed the prognostic importance of anaemia independent of renal function.[3,7,11,14,18] Groenveld's meta-analysis reported an unadjusted odds ratio for mortality in those with anaemia of 1.96 (95% confidence interval (CI): 1.74–2.21; $P < 0.001$) which remained significant after adjusting for multiple confounding factors including renal function (hazard ratio (HR) 1.46; 95% CI: 1.26–1.69; $P < 0.001$).[5]

Erythropoietin

The use of recombinant human erythropoietin (rHuEPO) has become routine in the management of anaemia associated with severe chronic kidney disease and some evidence of beneficial effects on cardiac remodelling in this population led to interest in the use of erythropoietins in patients with anaemia and CHF.[3] Many of the early small trials with relatively short study periods using rHuEPO in combination with intravenous or oral iron in a regimen similar to that used in end-stage renal disease suggested that the approach might improve symptoms and reduce hospital admissions.[19–21] Subsequent trials using darbepoietin-α and a meta-analysis published in 2009 seemed to support these findings, without effect on mortality.[22,23]

In light of these encouraging early results, a large, randomized, double-blind, placebo-controlled trial (RED-HF) involving 2278 patients with haemoglobin 9–12 g/dL, NYHA functional class II–IV and left ventricular ejection fraction (LVEF) <40% aimed to

determine whether therapy with darbepoietin-α improved clinical outcomes. There was no significant difference in the primary outcome of death or hospitalization for worsening heart failure between the groups, but more strokes and significantly more thromboembolic events were seen in the darbepoietin-α group. This study has therefore conclusively eliminated erythropoietin as a routine therapeutic strategy for patients with CHF.[24]

Further aetiological considerations

The lack of success with the use of rHuEPO in large outcome trials highlights the complexity of the relationship between anaemia and heart failure. Although renal dysfunction is likely to be an important factor, there are multiple potential mechanisms that could contribute to anaemia. These include haemodilution, drug therapy, chronic inflammation, and haematinic deficiency, particularly iron (Table 32.1).[3]

Given the magnitude of neurohormonal activation and subsequent expansion of plasma volume that characterizes heart failure, haemodilution as opposed to a genuine reduction in red cell mass might be responsible for anaemia.[25] Although haemodilution may have some impact, Androne et al. used ^{131}I-tagged albumin to measure red blood cell mass and plasma volume and demonstrated that anaemia, whether with or without haemodilution, was associated with an adverse prognosis.[25] Further trials using haemodynamic monitoring to adjust for volume status in patients with advanced heart failure still found that anaemia independently predicted a poor outcome.[7] How common or important haemodilution might be is still not clear.

The renin–angiotensin–aldosterone system is the key pathophysiological target for drug therapy in CHF. There is also evidence of the involvement of this neurohormonal pathway in haematopoiesis. Angiotensin II causes a fall in renal glomerular perfusion, reducing peritubular oxygen tension and stimulating erythropoietin secretion. It may have some direct effect on marrow erythrocyte precursors.[4] This is consistent with the observation of increased levels of erythropoietin in heart failure. Angiotensin converting enzyme (ACE) inhibitors and angiotensin II receptor antagonists (ARB) cause a fall in haemoglobin level by blocking this pathway.[6,26] However, ACE inhibitors and ARBs are clearly beneficial in CHF despite the counterintuitive association between the fall in haemoglobin and increased survival.

There may be some impact of β-blockade on anaemia too. In COMET, carvedilol was associated with a better outcome, but a greater fall in haemoglobin.[27]

Table 32.1 Potential causes of anaemia in patients with heart failure

Haematinic deficiency	Iron, B_{12} folate
Renal impairment	Impaired erythropoietin production, 'anaemia of chronic disease'
Pharmacological treatment	Angiotensin converting enzyme inhibitors, angiotensin II receptor antagonists, β-blockers, antiplatelets, anticoagulation
Haemodilution	
'Anaemia of chronic disease'	Inflammation, impaired iron utilization, impaired erythropoietin production and response

Iron status

Physiological significance

Iron has a critical role in erythropoiesis and haemoglobin synthesis but its physiological significance extends well beyond. The unique biochemical properties enabling iron to transition between bivalent (ferrous, Fe^{2+}) and trivalent (ferric, Fe^{3+}) oxidative states make it an important cofactor in the enzymatic catalysis of a number of biochemical reactions. As an important component of haemoglobin, iron plays a key role in oxygen transport, but is also involved in oxygen storage as a component of myoglobin. Furthermore, iron is a major cofactor for oxidative enzymes and is an integral component of respiratory chain proteins and thus has a vital role in mitochondrial function. This is of particular importance in tissues with a high energy demand such as skeletal and cardiac muscle.[28]

Iron metabolism

Iron is absorbed from the gut via duodenal and jejunal enterocytes. Whilst there is no specific pathway for iron excretion, homeostasis is maintained by the loss of iron during the continuous turnover of gut and skin epithelium, bleeding, and the tight regulation of iron absorption and distribution. Dietary iron exists in both organic and inorganic forms absorbed via a system of luminal transmembrane transport proteins, oxidative and reducing enzymes, and regulatory proteins. Iron then enters the circulation across the basolateral cell membrane through the transmembrane channel ferroportin in a process involving enzymatic oxidation of ferrous to ferric iron as shown in **Figure 32.2**.[28]

Absorbed iron exists in either utilized or stored forms. Utilized iron includes both the circulating ferric form bound to transferrin, and intracellular iron found predominantly in erythrocyte and reticulocyte haemoglobin. Iron is stored bound to ferritin and is found

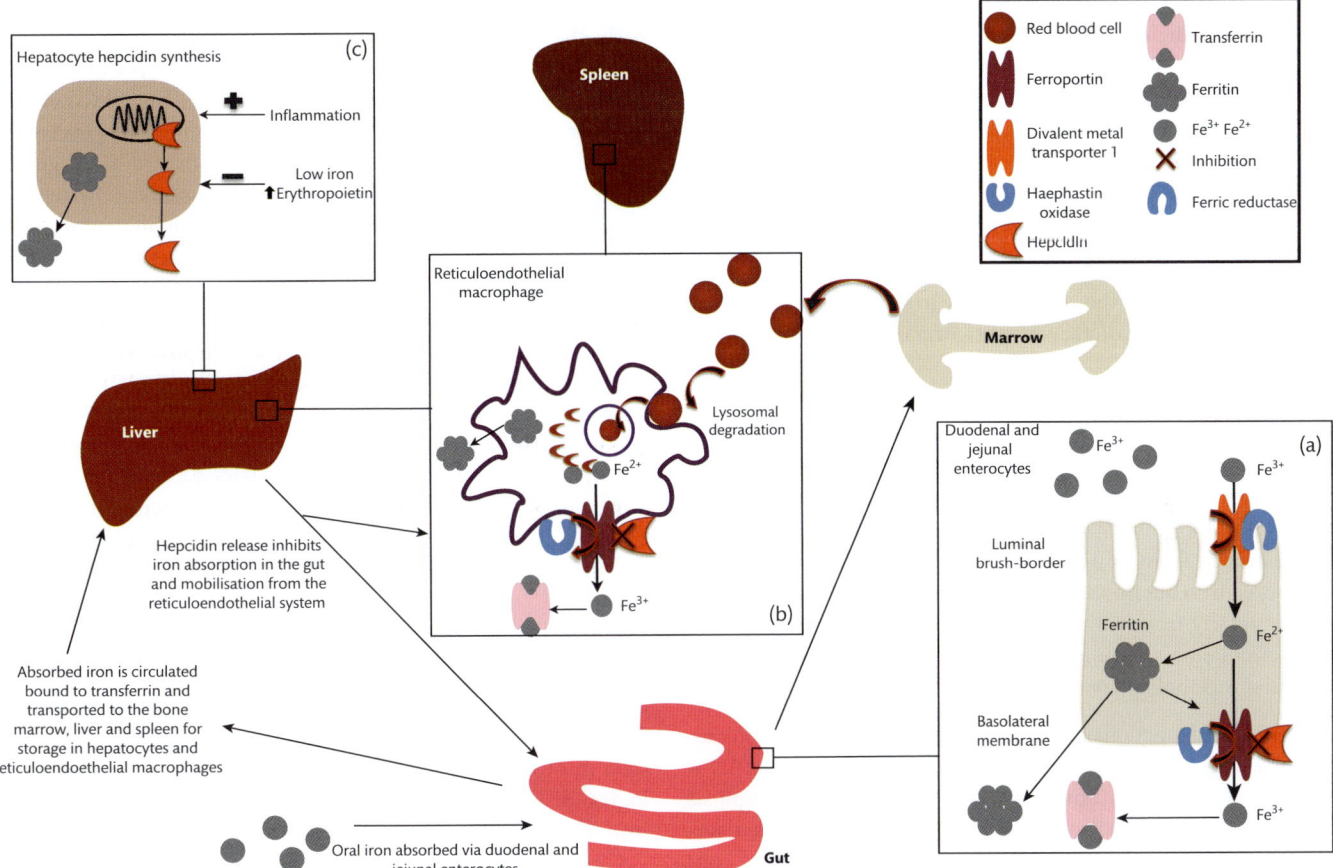

Figure 32.2 Iron absorption, distribution, metabolism, and regulation. Oral iron is absorbed in the gut across the luminal brush border membrane of duodenal and jejunal enterocytes. Box A outlines the absorption of iron in the gut lumen via the Divalent Metal Transporter 1 (DMT1) on the brush border membrane. Ferric iron (Fe^{3+}) is reduced to its ferrous form (Fe^{2+}) by ferric reductase. Absorbed iron can either be stored within the cytoplasm packaged as ferritin, a proportion of which enters the circulation, or transported across the basolateral membrane. Iron absorbed across the basolateral membrane is oxidized to its ferric form (Fe^{3+}) by haephastin oxidase and is transported via ferroportin iron channels and packaged with transferrin for transport within the circulation. Circulating iron bound to transferrin reaches the bone marrow, liver, and spleen. In bone marrow, iron is used for haematopoiesis or stored as ferritin. Iron is also taken up and stored as ferritin within hepatocytes and splenic cells. Stored iron can then be released into the circulation from stored ferritin pools or through recycling of senescent erythrocytes by reticuloendothelial macrophages within the liver and spleen (box B). Erythrocytes are engulfed and broken down by lysosomal degradation to release iron from haem which is then either converted to ferritin or exported via ferroportin channels and haephastin oxidase-mediated oxidation. Box C illustrates the role of hepatocytes which hold iron stored as ferritin and regulate iron metabolism. Inflammation results in the upregulation and release of the small peptide hormone hepcidin. This inhibits the expression of proteins involved in the absorption of iron across the basolateral membrane of enterocytes and causes the internalization of ferroportin channels. The end result is reduced absorption and trapping of iron within iron stores in hepatocytes and reticuloendothelial cells.

predominantly in hepatocytes, marrow and splenic cells, and can be released into the circulation either directly from hepatocytes or through macrophage-mediated recycling of senescent erythrocytes. Serum ferritin levels therefore serve as a useful surrogate measure of stored iron levels in patients without chronic disease. Ferritin is, however, potentially unreliable as an index of iron stores in CHF as CHF is an inflammatory state.[6]

The absorption and subsequent transfer of iron between stored and utilized forms is tightly regulated. Although not fully understood, the small peptide hormone hepcidin is thought to play a crucial role.[29,30] Hepcidin is secreted predominantly by hepatocytes and interacts with the cell surface protein ferroportin. The result is reduced expression of proteins involved in transmembrane iron transport across the basolateral membrane of duodenal and jejunal enterocytes and the internalization of ferroportin channels in the gut, hepatocytes, and reticuloendothelial cells. The final consequence is a reduction in both absorption of iron and the export of intracellular iron stores into the circulation. Iron (absorbed or following degradation of erythrocytes) also becomes trapped within the reticuloendothelial system. Whereas hepcidin expression and release from hepatocytes is reduced by conditions such as low iron stores, hypoxia, and impaired erythropoiesis, it is promoted by systemic inflammation.[28–30]

Iron deficiency: classification and diagnosis

Bearing in mind the distinction between utilized and stored iron, iron deficiency (ID) can be classified as both absolute and functional.

- Absolute ID reflects the depletion of iron stores caused most commonly by poor dietary intake, impaired absorption, and blood loss.
- Functional ID can be further subdivided.
  - ID can be brought about by enhanced erythropoiesis, either due to anaemia of another aetiology or due to excess endogenous erythropoietin. There is then an insufficient iron supply to meet the demands of increasing erythropoiesis.
  - ID can arise from iron sequestration.[31] There are normal levels of stored iron but impaired mobilization from intracellular sites (particularly from within the reticuloendothelial system) into the circulation. There is then a reduction of iron available for cellular metabolism, particularly.[1,28,32]

Both absolute and functional ID result in iron-restricted erythropoiesis.

Routine use of the reference standard for the diagnosis of ID—bone marrow biopsy—is limited by its invasive nature. Diagnosis therefore relies on analysis of serum biomarkers. Ferritin is a surrogate marker of stored iron and, under normal physiological conditions, a value of <30 μg/L can be used to diagnose absolute ID. Ferritin is an acute phase reactant, released primarily from hepatocytes in response to systemic inflammation and in chronic conditions (such as CHF) a higher cut-off value of 100 μg/L might be considered more appropriate. However, there is increasing evidence that ferritin levels bear little or no relation to iron status in heart failure.[6,28,31]

Whereas absolute ID is diagnosed by quantification of iron stores, functional iron deficiency is identified by estimation of circulating iron bound to transferrin and thus available for cell metabolism. Measurements of either circulating iron or transferrin

alone are unreliable, but rather the percentage of circulating transferrin that has iron bound to it is used (transferrin saturation, T_{SAT}). A level of <20% represents insufficient availability of iron to metabolizing cells.[28,31]

Traditionally, both ferritin and T_{SAT} have been considered important in the context of CHF. However, the association between inflammation and ferritin levels makes it difficult to interpret. A single-centre study evaluated iron status in patients with CHF using bone marrow analysis to define ID, and demonstrated serum ferritin to be a poor marker of ID.[33] On this basis, it had been suggested that in patients with CHF absolute ID is seen with a ferritin of <100 μg/L, and functional ID when ferritin is 100–300 μg/L and T_{SAT} <20%. However, in light of further evidence demonstrating weak correlation between ferritin and iron status in heart failure, T_{SAT} remains the most clinically important measurement.[6]

In CHF it is thought that functional ID occurs earlier in the course of the disease, and that, as CHF progresses, iron stores gradually become depleted.[34] Clinically, therefore, especially when considering the limitations of current laboratory markers, methods to detect early changes associated with iron-restricted erythropoiesis would be highly attractive. There has been some success by identifying newly formed iron-deficient reticulocytes using flow-cytometric analysis to measure either haemoglobin content or percentage of hypochromic reticulocytes.[31] These methods are also capable of distinguishing between functional ID associated with enhanced erythropoiesis from iron sequestration and can be used to track response to iron therapy. However, they are not yet in routine clinical use. Among the last indices to be affected by ID are the basic haematological values including haemoglobin, mean cell volume (MCV), mean corpuscular haemoglobin, mean corpuscular haemoglobin concentration, and red cell distribution width (RDW). RDW is also a strong marker of adverse outcomes in heart failure with prognostic power similar to that of N-terminal pro-B-type natriuretic peptide (NT-proBNP).[35] This may be explained by the correlation between elevated RDW and increased levels of interleukin (IL)-6 and reduced T_{SAT}, reflecting a state of inflammation and impaired iron metabolism.[36]

Mechanisms of iron deficiency in CHF

Inflammation in CHF is associated with increased secretion of circulating pro-inflammatory cytokines including IL-1, IL-6, and tumour necrosis factor-α (TNFα).[37,38] The process is similar to that seen in other chronic inflammatory conditions such as rheumatological diseases, where it is intimately related to the mechanisms of iron metabolism.[1,39]

Circulating inflammatory mediators, particularly IL-6, potently stimulate hepcidin production. In mouse models, hepcidin overexpression results in anaemia resistant to erythropoiesis-stimulating agents (ESA).

The importance of hepcidin in CHF, either as part of the pathophysiology of heart failure itself or associated co-morbidities such as renal dysfunction, is not clear and the evidence is contradictory. Jankowska et al. examined a number of biochemical indices in a broad cohort of 321 patients with stable heart failure and LVEF <45%.[40] Those in NYHA class I had higher levels of serum ferritin and hepcidin, and the levels of both fell with increasing heart failure severity. By contrast, markers of inflammation (such as

high-sensitivity C-reactive protein (hs-CRP) and IL-6) increased with worsening functional class. There was no association between serum ferritin or hepcidin and hs-CRP either across or within functional classes, and both ferritin and hepcidin were inversely related to levels of IL-6. Furthermore, although ID and iron-restricted erythropoiesis (as measured by T_{SAT} and soluble transferrin receptors) became more common with increasing severity of heart failure, neither hepcidin nor ferritin correlated with the presence of anaemia or level of haemoglobin at any severity of heart failure and was accompanied by markedly lower circulating hepcidin.[40]

Most of the evidence discussed so far relates to iron-sequestration and functional ID. However, functional ID can be caused by enhanced erythropoiesis where iron pools are unable to meet the increased demands. Circulating erythropoietin (EPO) is raised in heart failure, becoming higher with worsening functional class, and associated with worse prognosis.[32] EPO powerfully suppresses hepcidin production and may therefore be related to the lower hepcidin levels seen in patients with worse symptoms. Ongoing studies are evaluating this complex relationship.

Prevalence and prognosis of iron deficiency in CHF

Earlier studies evaluating the prevalence of ID in CHF focused on patients with anaemia and used different definitions of ID. A large Canadian cohort study used hospital discharge and coding data from 12 065 patients with newly diagnosed heart failure. Of the 17% diagnosed as anaemic, 21% had ID and 58% 'anaemia of chronic disease'.[41] The only study conducted using bone marrow aspirations examined 37 anaemic patients with advanced severe heart failure and identified ID in 73%.[33] A study of 296 patients with both reduced and preserved systolic function identified ID in 13%. Although the definition used in this study was purely a serum ferritin <30 µg/L, ID was equally prevalent in patients with and without anaemia.[42]

The increasing recognition of the presence of functional ID in the absence of anaemia led to studies in a more general CHF population. Jankowska et al. examined 546 patients with stable CHF and LVEF ≤45%. Defining ID as a ferritin <100 µg/L, or ferritin 100–300 µg/L with T_{SAT} <20%, 37% of patients had ID. This included 32% of those with normal haemoglobin, and 57% of those with anaemia.[43] A further study in 157 patients using the same definition identified ID in 69%, 78%, and 65% of all, anaemic, and non-anaemic patients respectively.[44] Recent data included 4456 patients referred to a single outpatient clinic for a period of nine years and identified ID in 43–68% of those with anaemia and 14–35% of those with normal haemoglobin levels, depending on definition used.[6]

There is a strong relation between ID and prognosis. ID is associated with both high levels of NT-proBNP and more advanced NYHA functional class.[43] ID is an independent predictor of poor outcome: in a study of 546 patients, three-year event-free survival was 54% in patients with ID and 67% in those without (where an event was all-cause death and heart transplantation) (Figure 32.3).[43]

Klip et al. analysed a pooled cohort of 1506 patients with both reduced and preserved ejection fraction over a mean follow-up of 2.5 years.[45] ID was present in 50% whereas 28.3% were anaemic. Although ID was more prevalent among those with anaemia (61.2%), it was common in those without anaemia (45.6%). Both frequency of anaemia and ID increased with higher NYHA class.

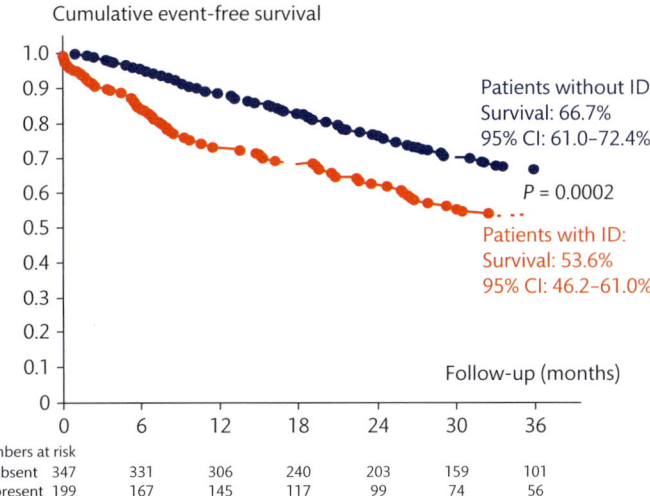

Cumulative event-free survival

Patients without ID:
Survival: 66.7%
95% CI: 61.0–72.4%

P = 0.0002

Patients with ID:
Survival: 53.6%
95% CI: 46.2–61.0%

Follow-up (months)

Numbers at risk							
ID absent	347	331	306	240	203	159	101
ID present	199	167	145	117	99	74	56

Figure 32.3 Three-year event-free survival Kaplan–Meier curves in 546 patients with systolic heart failure with versus without iron deficiency.
Reproduced from Jankowska EA, Rozentryt P, Witkowska A, Nowak J, Hartmann O, Ponikowska B, et al. Iron deficiency: an ominous sign in patients with systolic chronic heart failure. Eur Heart J 2010;31(15):1872–80 with permission of Oxford University Press.

Mortality was higher in those with ID versus those without, and ID was an independent predictor of mortality in both anaemic and non-anaemic patients (Figure 32.4).[45] Other factors associated with ID included female sex, elevated NT proBNP, and low MCV.[45] In the cohort studied by Cleland et al., univariable analyses demonstrated strong associations between lower haemoglobin, serum iron, and T_{SAT} with all-cause and cardiovascular mortality.[6]

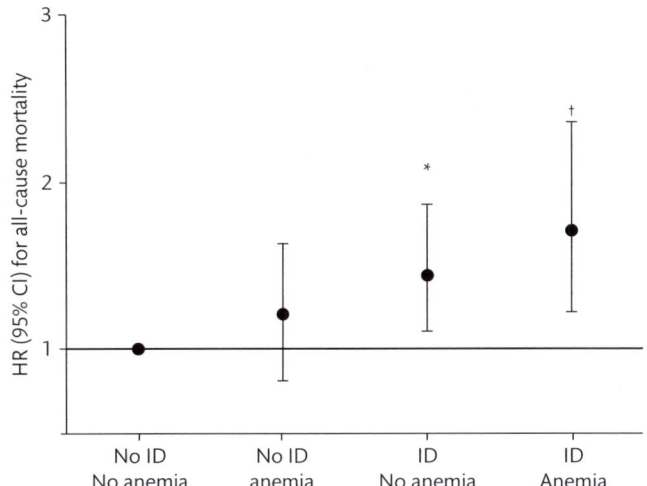

Figure 32.4 Hazard ratios for mortality among patients with/without anaemia and with/without iron deficiency (ID). Following adjustment for all variables associated with mortality in univariate analysis, ID remained an independent predictor of mortality in anaemic (P < 0.001) and non-anaemic patients (P < 0.01). ID with anaemia was associated with higher mortality (HR: 1.71; 95% CI: 1.24–2.36; P = 0.001) as was ID without anaemia (HR: 1.44; 95% CI: 1.11–1.87; P = 0.006).
Reproduced from Klip IT, Comin-Colet J, Voors AA, Ponikowski P, Enjuanes C, Banasiak W, et al. Iron deficiency in chronic heart failure: an international pooled analysis. Am Heart J 2013;165(4):575–82.e3 with permission from Elsevier.

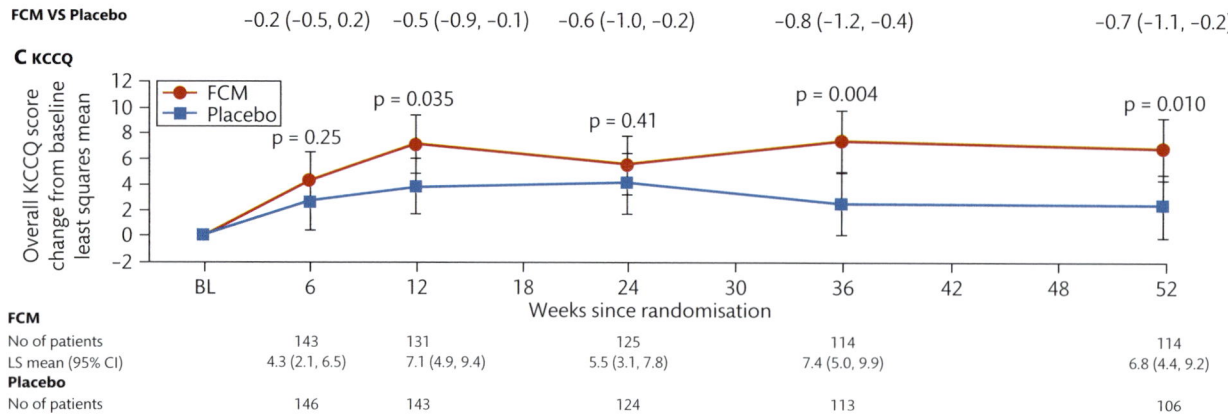

Figure 32.5 Beneficial impact of intravenous ferric carboxymaltose on six-minute walk test assessed at six months as compared with placebo in the CONFIRM-HF study.

Reproduced from Ponikowski P, van Veldhuisen DJ, Comin-Colet J, Ertl G, Komajda M, Mareev V, *et al.* Beneficial effects of long-term intravenous iron therapy with ferric carboxymaltose in patients with symptomatic heart failure and iron deficiency. *Eur Heart J* 2015;**36**(11):657–68 with permission from Oxford University Press.

Therapeutic strategies

Intravenous iron

Oral iron is poorly absorbed, especially in patients with inflammatory conditions as a result of the alteration in iron metabolism discussed above. In trials in patients with renal disease, oral iron is inferior to intravenous preparations in correcting anaemia.[32] IRONOUT evaluated the impact of oral iron polysaccharide versus placebo in 225 participants with CHF and iron deficiency.[46] Oral iron did not influence the primary end-point of change in exercise capacity as measured by change in peak oxygen consumption between baseline and 16 weeks. Elevated baseline hepcidin predicted refractoriness to oral iron therapy. These data suggest that oral iron is unlikely to be of value to the general heart failure population.

A number of small studies has evaluated intravenous iron (iron sucrose) in patients with heart failure due to left ventricular systolic dysfunction and anaemia. Intravenous iron leads to an increase in haemoglobin, T_{SAT}, and ferritin levels and is also associated with improvements in quality of life, LVEF, exercise capacity and functional class.[47–50] One study suggested that there was benefit irrespective of the presence of anaemia.[49]

Two large trials, FAIR-HF and CONFIRM-HF, recruited 459 and 304 patients respectively.[51,52] FAIR-HF was a randomized, double-blind, placebo-controlled trial evaluating the use of intravenous ferric carboxymaltose in patients with heart failure and ejection fraction <40% (in NYHA II) or ≤45% (in NYHA III). Patients had to have iron deficiency (defined as ferritin <100 µg/L, or ferritin 100–300 µg/L with T_{SAT} <20%) regardless of the presence of anaemia. Iron therapy was administered weekly until the iron deficit was corrected, followed by monthly maintenance dosing for a follow-up period of 24 weeks. Fifty per cent of patients in the intervention group had improvement in self-reported Patient Global Assessment score versus 28% in the placebo group and there were significant improvements in NYHA class and 6 min walk distance. The beneficial effects were seen irrespective of the presence of anaemia. There was no evidence of harmful effects including anaphylaxis or excess infection in the therapy arm.[51]

The findings were supported by the subsequent CONFIRM-HF trial conducted in a similar patient group. This double-blind, randomized, placebo-controlled study enrolled patients with symptomatic CHF (NYHA II–III), LVEF ≤45%, elevated BNP or NT-proBNP and haemoglobin ≤15 g/dL with the same definition of ID as in FAIR-HF. Intravenous ferric carboxymaltose was administered according to body weight, haemoglobin value, and iron indices. There was a significant improvement in the primary outcome measure of 6 min walk distance at 24 weeks in the treatment group of 33 ± 11 min ($P = 0.002$), which was sustained at 52 weeks (**Figure 32.5**).[52] Although the study was not powered to evaluate harder outcomes, treatment with intravenous iron was associated with a reduction in the risk of hospitalization for worsening heart failure (HR: 0.39; 95% CI: 0.19–0.82; $P = 0.009$) (**Figure 32.6**).[52] The EFFECT-HF study ($n = 174$) demonstrated a significant improvement in peak

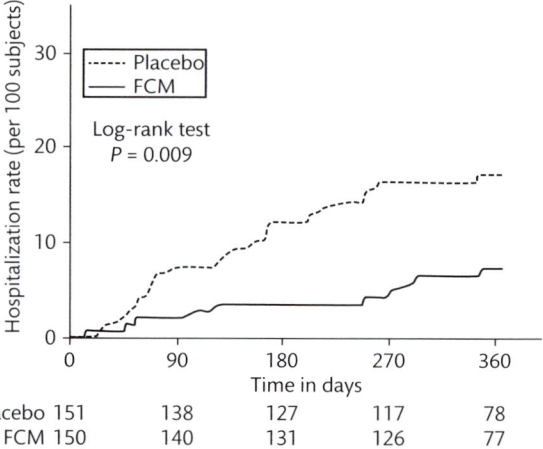

Figure 32.6 Kaplan–Meier analysis demonstrating a reduction in the time to hospitalization for worsening heart failure in patients in the CONFIRM-HF study treated with intravenous iron (FCM) as compared with placebo.

Reproduced from Ponikowski P, van Veldhuisen DJ, Comin-Colet J, Ertl G, Komajda M, Mareev V, *et al.* Beneficial effects of long-term intravenous iron therapy with ferric carboxymaltose in patients with symptomatic heart failure and iron deficiency[†]. *Eur Heart J* 2015;**36**(11):657–68 with permission from Oxford University Press.

oxygen consumption over six months with intravenous ferric carboxymaltose as compared with standard care.[53]

These important studies have been extremely challenging to deliver due to the difficulties with the double-blinding: intravenous iron is dark brown, thereby necessitating blinded and unblinded teams at each centre. However, strict blinding is imperative for studies with primary end-points that relate to functional outcomes or quality of life.

A meta-analysis published in 2016 combined the data then available, including 851 patients (the vast majority from the FAIR-HF and CONFIRM studies),[54] confirmed the benefits of intravenous iron on symptoms, with significant improvements in 6 min walk test and reduction in NYHA functional class. Of particular interest, the analysis suggested that intravenous iron led to a significant reduction in the combined end-point of all-cause death or cardiovascular hospitalization, the risk of the combined end-point of cardiovascular

death or hospitalization for worsening HF, and the risk of HF hospitalization (**Figure 32.7**).[54]

Some caution needs to be exercised when interpreting data from studies not powered to detect hard end-points (as seen previously with rHuEPO). AFFIRM-AHF randomised 1132 patients with LVEF<50% following an admission with acute heart failure to intravenous ferrix carboxymaltose versus placebo. Over 52 weeks, intravenous iron appeared safe and was associated with a significant reduction in heart failure hospitalization with no effect on cardiovascular death. However, there still remain unknowns, including the long-term efficacy and safety of intravenous iron treatment. Further data from ongoing studies, including IRONMAN (EudraCT reference 2015-004196-73), that are also powered on the end-point of cardiovascular death and heart failure hospitalization, will help establish the precise role of intravenous iron therapy in clinical practice.

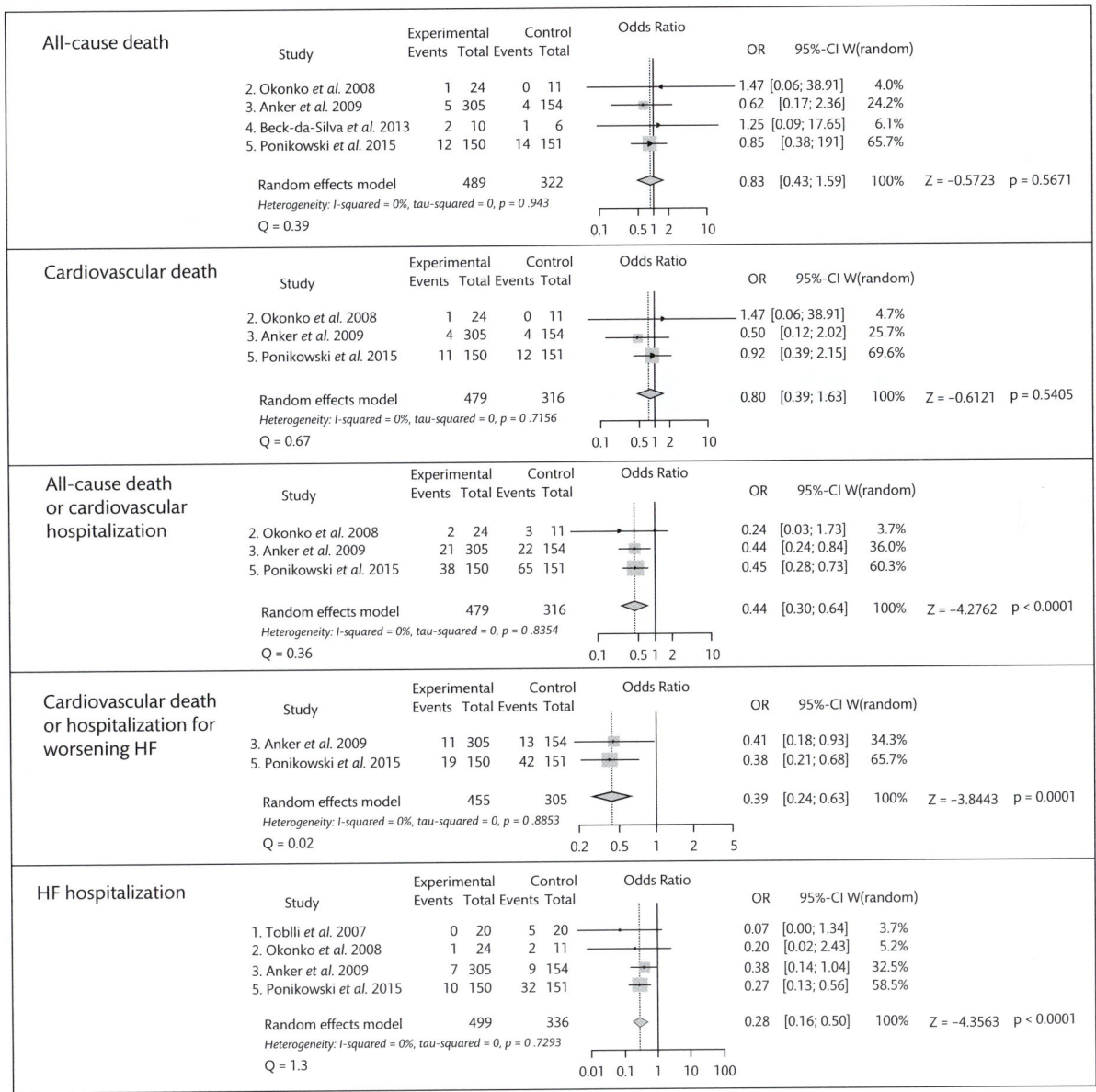

Figure 32.7 Meta-analysis of data from 851 patients suggesting a beneficial effect of intravenous iron therapy on outcomes in iron deficient patients with heart failure and reduced ejection fraction.

Reproduced from Jankowska EA, Tkaczyszyn M, Suchocki T, Drozd M, von Haehling S, Doehner W, et al. Effects of intravenous iron therapy in iron-deficient patients with systolic heart failure: a meta-analysis of randomized controlled trials. Eur J Heart Fail 2016;**18**(7):786–95 with permission from John Wiley and Sons

Table 32.2 Available intravenous iron preparations

	Cosmofer®	Venofer®	Monofer®	Ferinject®	Diafer®
Generic name	LMW iron dextran	Iron sucrose	Iron isomaltoside 1000 (10%)	Ferric carboxymaltose	Iron isomaltoside 1000 (5%)
Manufacturer	Pharmacosmos	Vifor	Pharmacosmos	Vifor	Pharmacosmos
License	Iron deficiency	Iron deficiency	Iron deficiency	Iron deficiency	Iron deficiency (CKD dialysis)
Maximum single dose	20 mg/kg	200 mg	20 mg/kg	1000 mg	200 mg
Administration time	Infusion: 4–6 h Bolus: slow IV injection (0.2 mL/min)	Infusion: 100 mg: 15 min 200 mg: 30 min Bolus: slow IV injection (1 mL/min)	Infusion: ≤1000 mg: >15 min >1000 mg: ≥30 min Bolus: 250 mg/min (up to 500 mg)	Infusion: 15 min Bolus: 100 mg/min (>200–500 mg) 15 min (>500–1000 mg)	Bolus: no minimum injection time (fast push IV injection)

LMW, low molecular weight; CKD, chronic kidney disease; IV, intravenous.

Current guidelines

The European Society of Cardiology published updated guidelines on the management of CHF in 2016.[55] These acknowledge the association between ID and a worse prognosis and base recommendations primarily on the results of the FAIR-HF and CONFIRM-HF studies. They recommend consideration of the use of intravenous ferric carboxymaltose in symptomatic patients with reduced ejection fraction and ID (defined as serum ferritin <100 μg/L, or 100–299 μg/L with T_{SAT} <20%) in order to improve symptoms, exercise capacity, and quality of life. However, they also acknowledge the paucity of data on major outcomes and the long-term safety of intravenous iron therapy.

Challenges

The identification of iron deficiency remains a challenge. Bone marrow biopsy is recognized as the reference standard, and several combinations of serum biomarkers are widely used. All of these methods have significant weaknesses and no single, or combination, blood test reliably identifies ID in patients with heart failure. Ferritin is the most widely used surrogate marker of iron stores but is of limited value in heart failure (low ferritin still does represent iron deficiency). Whereas a consensus definition has been adopted for clinical trials, further work is needed to identify an accurate, quick, and cost-efficient measurement that can be routinely used in clinical practice.

Although ID is frequently related to the pathophysiology of heart failure, it may also be a sign of further underlying disease. Patients with heart failure are often elderly, in whom other conditions, including malignancy, are common. Distinguishing ID associated with CHF from ID resulting from occult blood loss on the basis of serum markers alone is very difficult. Should detection of ID therefore trigger investigations for alternative causes in all patients? Some physicians would advocate investigation only in the presence of symptoms of underlying disease. However, this also lacks sensitivity and there is little consensus on the most appropriate approach.

Various intravenous iron preparations have been used in clinical trials and clinical practice. These have subtle differences in formulation and administration with no data on direct comparisons of clinical efficacy. These are summarized in Table 32.2.

Conclusions and future perspectives

Anaemia is a frequent comorbidity in patients with CHF and is associated with a poorer prognosis. Whereas numerous factors contribute to the aetiology of anaemia, ID has emerged as perhaps the most important and has been widely evaluated. Serum biomarkers have some limitations in diagnosing ID, and the mechanisms of iron metabolism in CHF are both complex and poorly understood. It is clear, however, that both absolute and functional ID are associated with an adverse prognosis in CHF that is independent of the presence of anaemia or LVEF. To date, trials of intravenous iron in patients with CHF and reduced ejection fraction have shown that iron replacement leads to improvement in symptoms, quality of life, and functional class for up to a year. An ongoing study in the UK is evaluating the effect of intravenous iron in patients with CHF and reduced ejection fraction (LVEF <45%) on cardiovascular mortality and recurrent hospitalization for worsening heart failure.

REFERENCES

1. Weiss G, Goodnough LT. Anemia of chronic disease. *N Engl J Med* 2005;**352**(10):1011–23.
2. Joosten E, Pelemans W, Hiele M, *et al.* Prevalence and causes of anaemia in a geriatric hospitalized population. *Gerontology* 1992;**38**(1–2):111–17.
3. Felker GM, Adams KF, Gattis WA, O'Connor CM. Anemia as a risk factor and therapeutic target in heart failure. *J Am Coll Cardiol* 2004;**44**(5):959–66.
4. Tang YD, Katz SD. Anemia in chronic heart failure: prevalence, etiology, clinical correlates, and treatment options. *Circulation* 2006;**113**(20):2454–61.
5. Groenveld HF, Januzzi JL, Damman K, *et al.* Anemia and mortality in heart failure patients a systematic review and meta-analysis. *J Am Coll Cardiol* 2008;**52**(10):818–27.
6. Cleland JG, Zhang J, Pellicori P, *et al.* Prevalence and outcomes of anemia and hematinic deficiencies in patients with chronic heart failure. *JAMA Cardiol* 2016;**1**(5):539–47.
7. Horwich TB, Fonarow GC, Hamilton MA, MacLellan WR, Borenstein J. Anemia is associated with worse symptoms, greater impairment in functional capacity and a significant increase in

mortality in patients with advanced heart failure. *J Am Coll Cardiol* 2002;**39**(11):1780–6.

8. Anand I, McMurray JJ, Whitmore J, *et al.* Anemia and its relationship to clinical outcome in heart failure. *Circulation* 2004;**110**(2):149–54.

9. Kalra PR, Bolger AP, Francis DP, *et al.* Effect of anemia on exercise tolerance in chronic heart failure in men. *Am J Cardiol* 2003;**91**(7):888–91.

10. Sharma R, Francis DP, Pitt B, *et al.* Haemoglobin predicts survival in patients with chronic heart failure: a substudy of the ELITE II trial. *Eur Heart J* 2004;**25**(12):1021–8.

11. O'Meara E, Clayton T, McEntegart MB, *et al.* Clinical correlates and consequences of anemia in a broad spectrum of patients with heart failure: results of the Candesartan in Heart Failure: Assessment of Reduction in Mortality and Morbidity (CHARM) Program. *Circulation* 2006;**113**(7):986–94.

12. von Haehling S, van Veldhuisen DJ, Roughton M, *et al.* Anaemia among patients with heart failure and preserved or reduced ejection fraction: results from the SENIORS study. *Eur J Heart Fail* 2011;**13**(6):656–63.

13. Anand IS, Kuskowski MA, Rector TS, *et al.* Anemia and change in hemoglobin over time related to mortality and morbidity in patients with chronic heart failure: results from Val-HeFT. *Circulation* 2005;**112**(8):1121–7.

14. Go AS, Yang J, Ackerson LM, *et al.* Hemoglobin level, chronic kidney disease, and the risks of death and hospitalization in adults with chronic heart failure: the Anemia in Chronic Heart Failure: Outcomes and Resource Utilization (ANCHOR) Study. *Circulation* 2006;**113**(23):2713–23.

15. Mahon NG, Blackstone EH, Francis GS, *et al.* The prognostic value of estimated creatinine clearance alongside functional capacity in ambulatory patients with chronic congestive heart failure. *J Am Coll Cardiol* 2002;**40**(6):1106–13.

16. Dries DL, Exner DV, Domanski MJ, Greenberg B, Stevenson LW. The prognostic implications of renal insufficiency in asymptomatic and symptomatic patients with left ventricular systolic dysfunction. *J Am Coll Cardiol* 2000;**35**(3):681–9.

17. Silverberg DS, Wexler D, Iaina A, *et al.* Anemia, chronic renal disease and congestive heart failure—the cardio renal anemia syndrome: the need for cooperation between cardiologists and nephrologists. *Int Urol Nephrol* 2006;**38**(2):295–310.

18. de Silva R, Rigby AS, Witte KK, *et al.* Anemia, renal dysfunction, and their interaction in patients with chronic heart failure. *Am J Cardiol* 2006;**98**(3):391–8.

19. Silverberg DS, Wexler D, Blum M, *et al.* The use of subcutaneous erythropoietin and intravenous iron for the treatment of the anemia of severe, resistant congestive heart failure improves cardiac and renal function and functional cardiac class, and markedly reduces hospitalizations. *J Am Coll Cardiol* 2000;**35**(7):1737–44.

20. Silverberg DS, Wexler D, Sheps D, *et al.* The effect of correction of mild anemia in severe, resistant congestive heart failure using subcutaneous erythropoietin and intravenous iron: a randomized controlled study. *J Am Coll Cardiol* 2001;**37**(7):1775–80.

21. Mancini DM, Katz SD, Lang CC, *et al.* Effect of erythropoietin on exercise capacity in patients with moderate to severe chronic heart failure. *Circulation* 2003;**107**(2):294–9.

22. van der Meer P, Groenveld HF, Januzzi JL, van Veldhuisen DJ. Erythropoietin treatment in patients with chronic heart failure: a meta-analysis. *Heart* 2009;**95**(16):1309–14.

23. Ponikowski P, Anker SD, Szachniewicz J, *et al.* Effect of darbepoetin alfa on exercise tolerance in anemic patients with symptomatic chronic heart failure: a randomized, double-blind, placebo-controlled trial. *J Am Coll Cardiol* 2007;**49**(7):753–62.

24. Swedberg K, Young JB, Anand IS, *et al.* Treatment of anemia with darbepoetin alfa in systolic heart failure. *N Engl J Med* 2013;**368**(13):1210–19.

25. Androne AS, Katz SD, Lund L, *et al.* Hemodilution is common in patients with advanced heart failure. *Circulation* 2003;**107**(2):226–9.

26. Volpe M, Tritto C, Testa U, *et al.* Blood levels of erythropoietin in congestive heart failure and correlation with clinical, hemodynamic, and hormonal profiles. *Am J Cardiol* 1994;**74**(5):468–73.

27. Komajda M, Anker SD, Charlesworth A, *et al.* The impact of new onset anaemia on morbidity and mortality in chronic heart failure: results from COMET. *Eur Heart J* 2006;**27**(12):1440–6.

28. Jankowska EA, von Haehling S, Anker SD, Macdougall IC, Ponikowski P. Iron deficiency and heart failure: diagnostic dilemmas and therapeutic perspectives. *Eur Heart J* 2013;**34**(11):816–29.

29. Ganz T, Nemeth E. Hepcidin and disorders of iron metabolism. *Annu Rev Med* 2011;**62**:347–60.

30. Nemeth E, Tuttle MS, Powelson J, *et al.* Hepcidin regulates cellular iron efflux by binding to ferroportin and inducing its internalization. *Science* 2004;**306**(5704):2090–3.

31. Goodnough LT, Nemeth E, Ganz T. Detection, evaluation, and management of iron-restricted erythropoiesis. *Blood* 2010;**116**(23):4754–61.

32. van Veldhuisen DJ, Anker SD, Ponikowski P, Macdougall IC. Anemia and iron deficiency in heart failure: mechanisms and therapeutic approaches. *Nat Rev Cardiol* 2011;**8**(9):485–93.

33. Nanas JN, Matsouka C, Karageorgopoulos D, *et al.* Etiology of anemia in patients with advanced heart failure. *J Am Coll Cardiol* 2006;**48**(12):2485–9.

34. von Haehling S, Jankowska EA, van Veldhuisen DJ, Ponikowski P, Anker SD. Iron deficiency and cardiovascular disease. *Nat Rev Cardiol* 2015;**12**(11):659–69.

35. Al-Najjar Y, Goode KM, Zhang J, Cleland JG, Clark AL. Red cell distribution width: an inexpensive and powerful prognostic marker in heart failure. *Eur J Heart Fail* 2009;**11**(12):1155–62.

36. Allen LA, Felker GM, Mehra MR, *et al.* Validation and potential mechanisms of red cell distribution width as a prognostic marker in heart failure. *J Card Fail* 2010;**16**(3):230–8.

37. Anker SD, von Haehling S. Inflammatory mediators in chronic heart failure: an overview. *Heart* 2004;**90**(4):464–70.

38. Oikonomou E, Tousoulis D, Siasos G, *et al.* The role of inflammation in heart failure: new therapeutic approaches. *Hellenic J Cardiol* 2011;**52**(1):30–40.

39. Weiss G. Modification of iron regulation by the inflammatory response. *Best Pract Res Clin Haematol* 2005;**18**(2):183–201.

40. Jankowska EA, Malyszko J, Ardehali H, *et al.* Iron status in patients with chronic heart failure. *Eur Heart J* 2013;**34**(11):827–34.

41. Ezekowitz JA, McAlister FA, Armstrong PW. Anemia is common in heart failure and is associated with poor outcomes: insights from a cohort of 12 065 patients with new-onset heart failure. *Circulation* 2003;**107**(2):223–5.

42. Witte KK, Desilva R, Chattopadhyay S, *et al.* Are hematinic deficiencies the cause of anemia in chronic heart failure? *Am Heart J* 2004;**147**(5):924–30.

43. Jankowska EA, Rozentryt P, Witkowska A, *et al.* Iron deficiency: an ominous sign in patients with systolic chronic heart failure. *Eur Heart J* 2010;**31**(15):1872–80.

44. Okonko DO, Mandal AK, Missouris CG, Poole-Wilson PA. Disordered iron homeostasis in chronic heart failure: prevalence, predictors, and relation to anemia, exercise capacity, and survival. *J Am Coll Cardiol* 2011;**58**(12):1241–51.

45. Klip IT, Comin-Colet J, Voors AA, *et al.* Iron deficiency in chronic heart failure: an international pooled analysis. *Am Heart J* 2013;**165**(4):575–82.e3.

46. Lewis GD, Malhotra R, Hernandez AF, *et al.* Effect of oral iron repletion on exercise capacity in patients with heart failure with reduced ejection fraction and iron deficiency: the IRONOUT HF randomized clinical trial. *JAMA* 2017;**317**:1958–1966.

47. Bolger AP, Bartlett FR, Penston HS, *et al.* Intravenous iron alone for the treatment of anemia in patients with chronic heart failure. *J Am Coll Cardiol* 2006;**48**(6):1225–7.

48. Toblli JE, Lombraña A, Duarte P, Di Gennaro F. Intravenous iron reduces NT-pro-brain natriuretic peptide in anemic patients with chronic heart failure and renal insufficiency. *J Am Coll Cardiol* 2007;**50**(17):1657–65.

49. Okonko DO, Grzeslo A, Witkowski T, *et al.* Effect of intravenous iron sucrose on exercise tolerance in anemic and nonanemic patients with symptomatic chronic heart failure and iron deficiency FERRIC-HF: a randomized, controlled, observer-blinded trial. *J Am Coll Cardiol* 2008;**51**(2):103–12.

50. Usmanov RI, Zueva EB, Silverberg DS, Shaked M. Intravenous iron without erythropoietin for the treatment of iron deficiency anemia in patients with moderate to severe congestive heart failure and chronic kidney insufficiency. *J Nephrol* 2008;**21**(2):236–42.

51. Anker SD, Comin Colet J, Filippatos G, *et al.* Ferric carboxymaltose in patients with heart failure and iron deficiency. *N Engl J Med* 2009;**361**(25):2436–48.

52. Ponikowski P, van Veldhuisen DJ, Comin-Colet J, *et al.* Beneficial effects of long-term intravenous iron therapy with ferric carboxymaltose in patients with symptomatic heart failure and iron deficiency. *Eur Heart J* 2015;**36**(11):657–68.

53. van Veldhuisen DJ, Ponikowski P, van der Meer P, *et al.*; EFFECT-HF Investigators. Effect of ferric carboxymaltose on exercise capacity in patients with chronic heart failure and iron deficiency. *Circulation* 2017;**136**:1374–1383.

54. Jankowska EA, Tkaczyszyn M, Suchocki T, *et al.* Effects of intravenous iron therapy in iron-deficient patients with systolic heart failure: a meta-analysis of randomized controlled trials. *Eur J Heart Fail* 2016;**18**(7):786–95.

55. Ponikowski P, Voors AA, Anker SD, *et al.* 2016 ESC Guidelines for the diagnosis and treatment of acute and chronic heart failure: The Task Force for the diagnosis and treatment of acute and chronic heart failure of the European Society of Cardiology (ESC). Developed with the special contribution of the Heart Failure Association (HFA) of the ESC. *Eur J Heart Fail* 2016;**18**(8):891–975.

RECOMMENDED READING

Anker SD, Comin Colet J, Filippatos G, *et al.* Ferric carboxymaltose in patients with heart failure and iron deficiency. *N Engl J Med* 2009;**361**(25):2436–48.

Cleland JG, Zhang J, Pellicori P, *et al.* Prevalence and outcomes of anemia and hematinic deficiencies in patients with chronic heart failure. *JAMA Cardiol* 2016;**1**(5):539–47.

Groenveld HF, Januzzi JL, Damman K, *et al.* Anemia and mortality in heart failure patients a systematic review and meta-analysis. *J Am Coll Cardiol* 2008;**52**(10):818–27.

Jankowska EA, Rozentryt P, Witkowska A, *et al.* Iron deficiency: an ominous sign in patients with systolic chronic heart failure. *Eur Heart J* 2010;**31**(15):1872–80.

Jankowska EA, Tkaczyszyn M, Suchocki T, *et al.* Effects of intravenous iron therapy in iron-deficient patients with systolic heart failure: a meta-analysis of randomized controlled trials. *Eur J Heart Fail* 2016;**18**(7):786–95.

Jankowska EA, von Haehling S, Anker SD, Macdougall IC, Ponikowski P. Iron deficiency and heart failure: diagnostic dilemmas and therapeutic perspectives. *Eur Heart J* 2013;**34**(11):816–29.

van Veldhuisen DJ, Anker SD, Ponikowski P, Macdougall IC. Anemia and iron deficiency in heart failure: mechanisms and therapeutic approaches. *Nat Rev Cardiol* 2011;**8**(9):485–93.

von Haehling S, Jankowska EA, van Veldhuisen DJ, Ponikowski P, Anker SD. Iron deficiency and cardiovascular disease. *Nat Rev Cardiol* 2015;**12**(11):659–69.

Nanas JN, Matsouka C, Karageorgopoulos D, *et al.* Etiology of anemia in patients with advanced heart failure. *J Am Coll Cardiol* 2006;**48**(12):2485–9.

Ponikowski P, Kirwan BA, Anker SD, McDonagh T, Dorobantu M, Drozdz J, et al. Ferric carboxymaltose for iron deficiency at discharge after acute heart failure: a multicentre, double-blind, randomised, controlled trial. *Lancet.* 2020;**396**(10266):1895–904.

Ponikowski P, van Veldhuisen DJ, Comin-Colet J, *et al.* Beneficial effects of long-term intravenous iron therapy with ferric carboxymaltose in patients with symptomatic heart failure and iron deficiency. *Eur Heart J* 2015;**36**(11):657–68.

Swedberg K, Young JB, Anand IS, *et al.* Treatment of anemia with darbepoetin alfa in systolic heart failure. *N Engl J Med* 2013;**368**(13):1210–19.

33

Renal dysfunction

Darren Green and Philip A. Kalra

Introduction

Up to 55% of patients with heart failure have evidence of chronic kidney disease (CKD) stages 3–5 (estimated glomerular filtration rate (eGFR) of 15–59 mL/min; see Table 33.1), and mortality rises in proportion to fall in GFR (see Figure 33.1).[1] In patients with heart failure, advanced CKD is as prognostically important as low left ventricular ejection fraction (LVEF).[2] Heart failure and its treatment may also play an important role in the pathophysiology of acute kidney injury (AKI), with a further associated risk of adverse outcome. Cardiovascular disease is the leading cause of death in patients with CKD, and structural cardiac abnormalities are highly prevalent in dialysis patients.

Epidemiology

Mortality in patients who have both renal and cardiovascular disease is much higher than in the general population. The difficulty in defining a precise epidemiologic association between heart failure and CKD is that much of the available data are derived from clinical trials and studies that have strict inclusion and exclusion criteria. These selection criteria limit the understanding of how renal disease impacts on other medical conditions—not just heart failure—as patients with advanced CKD are typically excluded from clinical trials. However, the majority of elderly patients with heart failure will have some degree of CKD, as may many younger patients. A prospective cohort study of all-comers to a heart failure clinic found that fewer than 17% of patients had normal renal function.[2] The presence of renal impairment in patients with heart failure confers a major detrimental impact upon survival. For patients with advanced CKD, mortality increases by ~1% for each 1 mL/min fall in creatinine clearance.[2]

Heart failure is likely to develop and progress in patients of all ages with end-stage kidney disease (ESKD). Many factors contribute, including hypertension (found in >90% of patients with ESKD), anaemia, and fluid overload. Of patients starting renal replacement therapy (RRT), 74% have echocardiographic evidence of left ventricular hypertrophy (LVH), indicating that the cardiac structural changes associated with ESKD are already present during progression of CKD rather than being a specific effect of dialysis therapy. At the initiation of RRT, 36% of patients have left ventricular dilation, and 15% severe LV systolic dysfunction. Indeed, 4.5% of patients having dialysis fulfil ACC/ASA/ESC criteria for implantable cardioverter–defibrillator therapy based on primary and secondary prevention studies of patients with heart failure.[3–5] Foley *et al.* followed a cohort of 259 patients from the time of starting dialysis for a mean of 41 months. They assessed baseline and follow-up echocardiography. Seventy per cent of patients had an increase in left ventricular mass index (LVMI) and 50% an increase in LV cavity volume between scans. Thirty-three per cent of patients developed heart failure, with half of the heart failure episodes being *de novo*. Furthermore, each 10 mmHg rise in mean arterial pressure was associated with a relative risk of de-novo heart failure of 1.44.[6]

Table 33.2 shows the relative annual mortality figures for patients with anaemia, CKD, and heart failure, or with combinations of these conditions[7] in a study of a random cohort of 5% of Medicare database patients (1 321 156 subjects). The patients were subdivided according to the presence or absence of anaemia, CKD (excluding ESKD), and heart failure, identified as co-morbidities on Medicare claims. The relative risk of death in the presence of these conditions, matched for age and other co-morbidities, against the remainder of the cohort is shown. The annual mortality for patients with no history of anaemia, CKD, or heart failure was 4%, for patients with CKD it was 8%, and for patients with all three co-morbidities, 23%.

As a general rule, all-cause mortality rises significantly as GFR falls. The excess mortality includes a disproportionate number of deaths due to left ventricular pump failure[8] and the mortality risk is equally high in patients with both systolic and diastolic

Table 33.1 Stages of chronic kidney disease based on eGFR

Stage	eGFR (mL/min/1.73 m²)
1	≥90
2	60–89
3a	45–59
3b	30–44
4	15–29
5	<15 or RRT

eGFR, estimated glomerular filtration rate; RRT, renal replacement therapy.

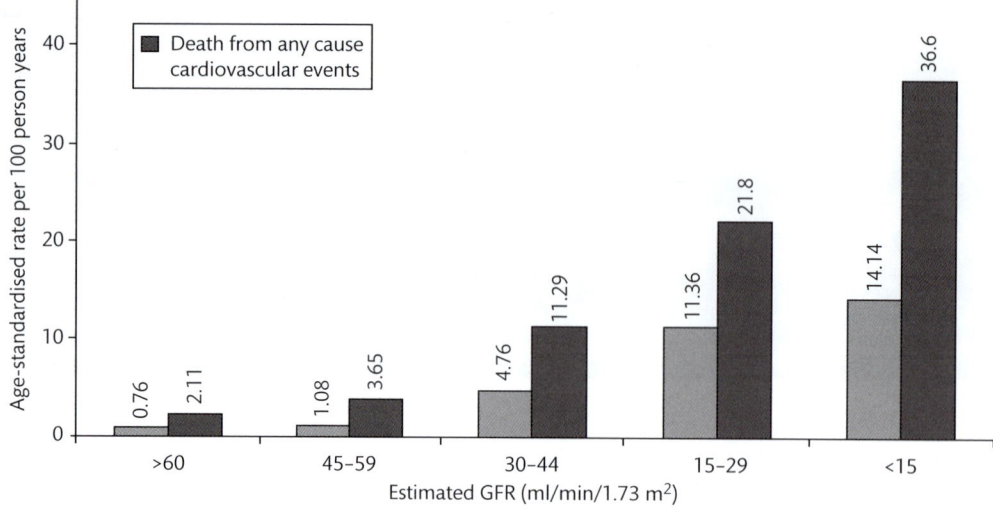

Figure 33.1 Rates of death and cardiovascular events by estimated glomerular filtration rate (eGFR).
Reproduced from Go AS, Chertow GM, Fan D, McCulloch CE, Hsu C. Chronic kidney disease and the risks of death, cardiovascular events, and hospitalization. *N Engl J Med* 2004;**351**(13):1296–305.

dysfunction.[9] Data from the US Renal Data System show that cardiomyopathy, congestive heart failure or pulmonary oedema is the primary cause of death in dialysis patients with a rate of 11.4 events per 1000 patient-years.[10]

The cardiorenal syndrome

The term 'cardiorenal syndrome' was first used to describe the common finding of AKI in patients admitted to hospital with decompensated heart failure. The term evolved to include worsening of renal function in response to heart failure treatment, and the barrier to management that it may cause. Ronco *et al.* then classified chronic as well as acute cardiorenal disease into five types of cardiorenal syndrome.[11] Decompensated heart failure as a cause or effect of AKI are types 1 and 3 respectively; CHF as a cause and effect of CKD are types 2 and 4. Type 5 was classed as cardiac and renal end-organ damage from a common underlying pathology, most often diabetes mellitus, atherosclerosis, and/or hypertension.

Table 33.2 Relative annual mortality figures for patients who have had inpatient hospital visits relating to anaemia, CKD, and heart failure

Risk factor	Hazard ratio
No anemia, CHF, or CKD	1.00
Anemia only	1.60
CKD only	1.64
CHF only	2.25
CHF and CKD	3.30
Anemia, CHF, and CKD	3.63

CHF, chronic heart failure; CKD, chronic kidney disease.
The baseline annual mortality for patients with no history of anaemia, CKD, or heart failure is 4%.
Source data from C. Herzog, H. Muster, S. Li, Collins A. Impact of congestive heart failure, chronic kidney disease, and anemia on survival in the Medicare population. *Journal of Cardiac Failure*, vol. **10**, 2004, pp. 467–472.

The recognition that pathological cardiorenal interaction may manifest in or result from cardiac pathologies other than heart failure has yielded the Acute Dialysis Quality Initiative cardiorenal classification system. This system acknowledges the wider spectrum of cardiac disease that may be precipitated by renal impairment, such as sudden cardiac death, and the wider impact of heart disease on CKD as well as AKI. However, neither the Ronco classification of cardiorenal syndrome nor the broader ADQI classification have any practical use in their current incarnations. They provide no mechanistic, therapeutic, or prognostic guidance, and do not accommodate the complex interactions of coexisting acute and chronic illnesses. For this reason, terms and definitions relating to cardiorenal syndrome are likely to continue to change in response to evolving understanding.

Cardiorenal pathophysiology in heart failure

Heart failure and renal disease may be caused by the same underlying disease or be precipitants of one another, often with bidirectional worsening of disease. For example, CKD is an independent risk factor for developing cardiovascular disease, particularly coronary artery disease (CAD), hypertension, and LVH. CAD is responsible for more than half of incident cases of heart failure,[12] and hypertension is the leading cause of heart failure in older patients. Arterial disease and hypertension are also major causes of renal disease.

Common underlying disease

Hypertension

Hypertension is extremely common in patients with CKD and is associated with a high rate of de-novo cardiac failure and ischaemic heart disease, especially in those on dialysis. Although even modestly elevated blood pressure is associated with LVH and cardiomyopathy, in the study of dialysis patients by Foley *et al.* discussed above, only a mean arterial pressure of ≥106 mmHg was independently

associated with de-novo heart failure. Tight control of hypertension is fundamental to the renal physician's practice. However, in ESKD mortality is most strongly associated with low blood pressure,[6] and systolic pump failure will lead to low blood pressure irrespective of renal function. Hence, if a dialysis patient develops significant heart failure, their anti-hypertensive therapy may need to be reduced.

Three-quarters of all dialysis patients have echocardiographic evidence of LVH. The presence of LVH in ESKD is associated with an adjusted relative risk of cardiac death of 2.7 (95% confidence interval: 0.9–8.2).[13] LVH develops early in CKD; in a study of 175 consecutive patients attending a pre-dialysis clinic, LVMI increased as creatinine clearance fell, and LVH was independently associated with age and systolic hypertension.[14] Aggressive management of hypertension in such patients can cause LVH to regress to the level seen in their non-hypertensive counterparts,[15] thereby potentially improving outcome. **Figure 33.2** demonstrates that there is a link between LVMI and eGFR even in the early stages of CKD.[16]

Cardiac magnetic resonance imaging has improved our understanding of the morphological changes seen in ESKD. An emerging body of evidence indicates that cardiac fibrosis rather than LV mass is a more sensitive marker of adverse outcome in ESKD. Postmortem LV histological analysis in haemodialysis patients demonstrates a disordered, fibrotic, and hypertrophic remodelling pattern to explain this. Fibrotic cardiac remodelling also leads to aberrant conduction and this finding may also explain the high rate of arrhythmia seen in ESKD, where 26% of patients suffer sudden cardiac death compared to 11% in the general population.

Atherosclerosis

Atherosclerosis is a multi-system disease. CAD is the most common cause of heart failure, and 40% of patients with CKD have evidence of CAD.[17] CKD is a pro-atherosclerotic condition and, in turn, atherosclerosis can lead to and exacerbate CKD. Vascular damage occurs at a microvascular level in the kidney and is very often independent of renal artery stenosis (RAS). The association of RAS with heart failure is discussed separately below. Intra-renal arterial disease will lead to chronic glomerular damage. Smoking is independently associated with the development and risk of progression of CKD and the pathway is likely to involve the same atheromatous processes that contribute to CAD. The mechanisms by which CKD may exacerbate coronary artery atherosclerosis are also discussed in more detail below.

Diabetes mellitus, proteinuria, and the metabolic syndrome

Diabetic nephropathy is responsible for 20% of all new dialysis cases in the UK.[18] Worldwide, this rises to as much as 40% in the USA and 55% in parts of the Indian subcontinent.[19] In addition, up to 7.5% of the prevalent dialysis population will have type 2 diabetes mellitus that developed after RRT was started.[20] Insulin resistance and chronic hyperglycaemia both lead to endothelial dysfunction, in which the usual anti-atheromatous properties of vascular endothelium are disrupted. Subsequent macrovascular disease manifests most often as CAD and CKD. Microvascular disease is responsible for diabetic autonomic neuropathy, and early endothelial disruption in the kidneys produces proteinuria, which is a reliable early marker of progressive CKD.[21] Patients with a urine albumin/creatinine ratio of 30–299 mg/g, a range termed 'microalbuminuria', have a 9.2-fold risk of progression to established diabetic nephropathy compared to a control group of patients with no microalbuminuria.[22]

Microalbuminuria is independently associated with a relative risk of cardiovascular mortality of 1.87 in diabetic patients (compared to those without albuminuria), and, in a 10-year follow-up of diabetic patients with microalbuminuria, 9% of all-cause mortality was attributed to heart failure.[23] In the Heart Outcomes Prevention Evaluation (HOPE) trial, microalbuminuria was associated with an adjusted relative risk of 3.23 for hospitalization for heart failure. Importantly, this was similar for diabetic and non-diabetic patients, indicating a significant risk of heart failure for patients with other illnesses causing proteinuria (see **Table 33.3**).[24]

Diabetes mellitus is often part of the metabolic syndrome, in which there is coexistent obesity, hypertension, high triglycerides, and low-density-lipid cholesterol, and high circulating levels of prothrombotic and proinflammatory markers. These are all risk factors for cardiovascular and renal vascular damage, which emphasizes why diabetes is associated with such a high cardiorenal morbidity and mortality.

Renal disease as precipitant to cardiovascular disease

The renin–angiotensin pathway

CKD can contribute to overactivation of the renin–angiotensin–aldosterone system (RAAS), which in turn both contributes to the development of cardiovascular disease and further exacerbates CKD, thereby initiating a pathway of progressive cardiorenal disease.

One of the primary purposes of the RAAS is to adapt to a fall in blood pressure in order to maintain vital organ blood flow. Angiotensin II causes sodium retention, expansion of the extracellular compartment, vasoconstriction, and restoration of organ

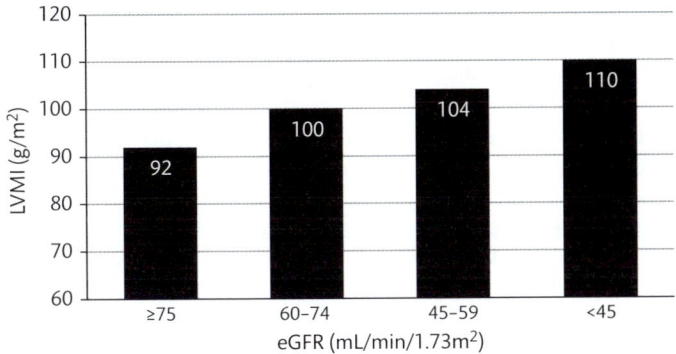

Figure 33.2 The correlation of left ventricular mass index (LVMI) and estimated glomerular filtration rate (eGFR).

Table 33.3 Relative risk of hospitalization due to heart failure according to degree of albuminuria, measured by albumin/creatinine ratio (ACR), listed by quartiles

ACR (mg/mmol)	<0.22	0.22–0.57	0.58–1.62	>1.62
All patients	1	1.19	1.95	3.79
Diabetic patients	1	0.72	1.83	3.65
Non-diabetic patients	1	1.45	1.86	2.93

Source data from Gerstein HC, Mann J, Yi Q, *et al.* Albuminuria and risk of cardiovascular events, death, and heart failure in diabetic and non-diabetic individuals. *JAMA: The Journal of the American Medical Association* 2001;**286**(4):421–426.

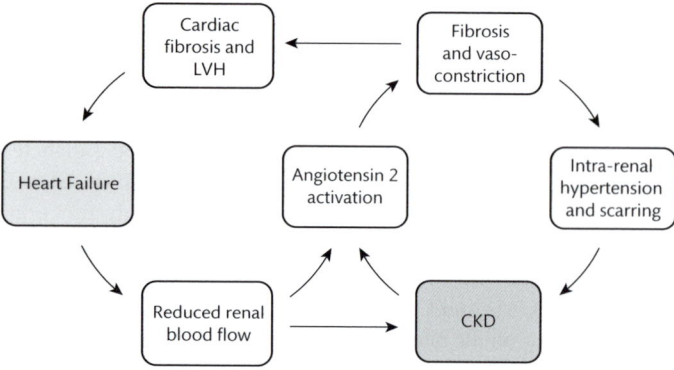

Figure 33.3 Simplified schematic diagram showing the central role of renin–angiotensin–aldosterone system (RAAS) activation in the pathogenesis of the cardiorenal syndrome in patients with heart failure and chronic kidney disease (CKD).

perfusion. CKD causes chronic overactivation of the RAAS, and this appears to play a prominent pathophysiological role in the subsequent progression and exacerbation of intra-renal and cardiac damage.

Angiotensin II causes postglomerular arteriolar vasoconstriction, leading to intra-renal hypertension and glomerular damage. Its systemic vasoconstrictive activity also leads to LVH. Angiotensin II and aldosterone upregulate the activity of proinflammatory cytokines such as fibroblast growth factor, platelet-derived growth factor and transforming growth factor-β_1. These cytokines contribute to endothelial dysfunction, thereby promoting CAD and renal vascular disease, and are associated with intra-renal and myocyte fibrosis. Progression of CKD and heart failure may follow, ultimately resulting in an ever-worsening cycle of progressive cardiorenal organ damage (**Figure 33.3**).

Arterial calcification and vascular stiffness

There is a five-fold increase in vascular calcification of the coronary arteries in dialysis patients compared to other patients with coronary atheroma.[25] Indeed, there are fundamental differences between the coronary calcification associated with renal disease and the arterial calcification found in CAD, which is typically focal and affects the intimal layer of the arterial wall. In CKD, however, there is evidence of more widespread calcification affecting the medial layer of the arterial wall driven by osteoblastic transformation of smooth muscle cells. This is again associated with an excess of mortality.[26] The calcification starts developing in the early stages of CKD and is present in >50% of patients at the time of starting dialysis.[27] Calcification is often progressive, but may be halted by renal transplantation.[28]

The pathophysiology of calcification is complex and involves an interplay between many predisposing factors including hyperphosphataemia, hypercalcaemia and hyperparathyroidism, all of which can stimulate calcification of vascular smooth muscle cells and within the vascular matrix; CKD also leads to a reduction in endogenous inhibitors of calcification, such as fetuin A. Vascular calcification and renal bone abnormalities are both encompassed by the term 'chronic kidney disease–mineral bone disorder' (CKD-MBD).

The clinical manifestation of calcification within the larger 'conduit' arteries is an increase in vascular stiffness which can be measured non-invasively with pulse wave velocity (PWV). An increase in PWV is associated with increased LVMI and with reduced coronary filling. These may eventually predispose to heart failure.[29] In some small studies increased PWV, and thus vascular stiffness, has been shown to be more important than hypertension in the development of LVH.

That CKD-MBD represents a major cardiovascular risk highlights the importance of strict adherence to a 'renal' diet and appropriate use of phosphate binders at an early stage of CKD. There are possible risks of calcification associated with long-term use of high doses of oral calcium, as used in phosphate binders. However, this proposed risk is not based on findings from randomized studies.

Endothelial dysfunction and Inflammation

Endothelial dysfunction plays an important role in heart failure. It leads to a loss of the usual endothelium-mediated vasodilatory response to nitric oxide which is in turn an independent predictor of cardiovascular mortality in patients with heart failure. RAAS activation, mediated by CKD, exacerbates endothelial dysfunction by increasing the production of reactive oxygen species.[30] Patients are less able to reduce afterload (which is increased by the vascular stiffness discussed above). Endothelial dysfunction has also been linked with abnormal myocardial remodelling and CAD.

CKD is a major contributor to endothelial dysfunction. Although an elevated serum creatinine—and its mathematical transformation into eGFR—is used to signify CKD, there is a host of other metabolites that are not routinely measured in CKD, many of which contribute to the oxidative stress that in turn leads to end-organ damage. Further, some circulating proinflammatory cytokines, such as interleukin-6, are normally excreted via the kidneys but cannot be removed by dialysis. These accumulate in advanced CKD and contribute to the endothelial dysfunction.[31] CRP is a surrogate marker of in-vivo inflammation and is often chronically raised in CKD, especially in patients with tunnelled venous catheters as access for haemodialysis.[32] Chronically elevated CRP in dialysis patients is associated with increased cardiovascular mortality, although not specifically from heart failure.[33]

Salt and water retention

AKI as a primary event may lead to acute decompensated heart failure, even in patients with previously normal cardiac function. Retention of sodium and fluid occur due to renal injury and to attempts to resuscitate the unwell patient with intravenous fluid. When AKI supervenes, patients with underlying cardiovascular disease may also find that their medication, particularly diuretics and angiotensin converting enzyme (ACE) inhibitors, are stopped on admission to hospital. This increases the likelihood of a secondary episode of heart failure. Furthermore, electrolyte and metabolite disorders may develop, which may further exacerbate decline in cardiac function. Specifically, renal acidosis is associated with pulmonary hypertension and right heart failure, and electrolyte disturbances leave patients at risk of arrhythmia and loss of effective atrial activity.

Patients with AKI and heart failure are difficult to manage. If oliguric AKI occurs and does not respond to early resuscitation, patients are at particular risk if acute pulmonary oedema or significant hyperkalaemia occur. They are unlikely to respond to diuretics, and so haemodialysis or haemofiltration is often necessary and should be considered early in the clinical course.

Chronic salt and water retention in advanced CKD can contribute to hypertension and ventricular dilation. In one study, Kayikcioglu *et al.* managed hypertension in haemodialysis patients using dietary salt restriction and modification of dialysis target weight to control blood pressure, with no antihypertensive drugs. They achieved a target blood pressure of <140/90 mmHg in 90% of patients.[34] Symptomatic hypotension was common but fell to 7% of cases at 12 months. There was a reduction in LVMI from 164 ± 64 to 112 ± 36 g/m² during follow-up.[35]

Anaemia

Anaemia is a risk factor for both the development of, and poor outcome in, heart failure, independent of concurrent or causative CKD. Given the high incidence of anaemia associated with CKD, the contributory importance and treatment of anaemia has to be considered when managing the patient with CKD and heart failure. Figure 33.2 outlines the additive effect on mortality of coexistent anaemia, CKD, and heart failure.

Arteriovenous fistula formation

An arteriovenous fistula (AVF) is the preferred access for haemodialysis. It carries a three-fold lower risk of infection than tunnelled central venous catheters and there is a lower all-cause mortality in patients who dialyse via a fistula.[36] However, the creation of a shunt from the high-pressure arterial circulation into the lower-pressure venous system leads to circulatory changes and, ultimately, cardiac remodelling, which may cause high-output cardiac failure in a few individuals.

As little as one week after fistula formation, cardiac output may increase by up to 15%. There is an increased venous return and sympathetic activation with resultant resting tachycardia, and an increase in left ventricular end-diastolic volume, indicative of a greater circulating volume. The changes are thought in part to be a consequence of neurohormonal responses to the reduced vascular resistance that follows AVF formation, and patients with high-flow fistulae have higher circulating levels of natriuretic peptides because of the high-volume state. There is also eccentric hypertrophy of the left ventricle in response to dilation.[37] Although the majority of haemodialysis patients tolerate their fistula without any clinical circulatory problems, a few patients are at risk of high-output cardiac failure. In such cases, ligation of the fistula must be considered as a therapeutic option. Male sex and use of proximal vessels for fistulae formation are independent risk factors for the need for fistula ligation.

Renal artery stenosis

Atherosclerotic renovascular disease (ARVD) is common, and it is frequently seen in association with other cardiovascular diseases such as CAD, peripheral vascular disease, and stroke.[38] ARVD is detectable in approximately one-third of elderly patients presenting acutely to hospital with heart failure.[39] In addition, 54% of a UK outpatient secondary-care heart failure population had atherosclerotic renal artery stenosis of >50%.[40] Similarly, heart failure is present in 38% of elderly US patients with ARVD,[41] and heart failure leads to an almost three-fold increase in mortality risk compared to patients with ARVD but without heart failure.[42] In many patients with ARVD and heart failure, there is preserved LVEF, but patients with heart failure have higher filling pressures, higher LVMI and a greater prevalence of diastolic dysfunction than patients without

heart failure.[42] Systematic echocardiographic studies of cardiac structure and function in ARVD have shown that only 5% of patients had normal hearts, that the prevalence of LVH was twice as great as in CKD patients without ARVD, and that changes progress over time.[43,44]

Heart failure as a cause of kidney disease

Patients admitted with decompensated heart failure have a worse outcome if there is associated AKI. A rise in serum creatinine of as little as 9 μmol/L is associated with both a prolonged inpatient stay and increased mortality.[45] The amount of change in creatinine is of more prognostic significance than the baseline creatinine.[46] In one study of 1004 patients admitted to hospital with decompensated heart failure, 25% had a rise in serum creatinine of >26.5 μmol/L (0.3 mg/dL). The presence of diabetes mellitus, hypertension, or CKD was an independent predictor of post-admission AKI.[47] Anaemia, age, and the use of drugs blocking the renin–angiotensin system and diuretics are predictors of AKI in the setting of acute hospitalization for heart failure. However, the precise pattern of risk is difficult to define because the definition of AKI varies from study to study. A 0.3 mg/dL rise in creatinine was defined as 'worsening renal function' (WRF) in the POSH study (the Prospective Outcomes Study in Heart failure). WRF was independently associated with higher serum creatinine levels on admission (odds ratio (OR): 3.02), pulmonary oedema (OR: 3.35), and atrial fibrillation (OR: 0.35). WRF was associated with an increase in average length of inpatient stay of two days but readmission rates—and, importantly, mortality—were not affected.[48]

The fact that AKI usually occurs very soon after hospital admission for heart failure suggests that low-output cardiac failure is important in its pathogenesis. Drugs blocking the renin–angiotensin system lead to reduced renal perfusion and have a deleterious effect upon renal function, due to actions on glomerular haemodynamics (that are beneficial when perfusion is better). However, hypotension and a low-cardiac output state are not present in all patients who develop renal dysfunction. Other factors are important and there is an association between higher right atrial pressures and lower GFR.[49] Thus venous congestion and volume overload appear to contribute to AKI, a pathogenetic theory supported by experimental models in which temporary occlusion of renal veins leads to a temporary decline in GFR.[49] Similar pathological mechanisms may also account for the evolution of CKD in chronic heart failure given that lower ejection fraction does not correlate closely with the likelihood of progression of CKD, and CKD may occur in cases where there is normal LVEF.

Heart failure therapy in patients with CKD

Improving heart failure prognosis in CKD

Drugs that act on the renin–angiotensin–aldosterone pathway

The use of RAAS blockade, particularly ACE inhibitors, is associated with improved survival in heart failure. ACE inhibitors also affect glomerular filtration and may lead to AKI during decompensated heart failure with resultant uncertainty as to how these drugs may be best managed during the episode. However, the extent to which ACE inhibitors are implicated in AKI may be overstated. In the Studies of

Left Ventricular Dysfunction (SOLVD) trial, 16% of patients treated with enalapril (mean daily dose: 16.6 mg) developed a rise in serum creatinine >44 µmol/L. However, the proportion for the placebo arm was 12%.[50] Also, such studies do not usually report improvements in GFR but it is estimated that 10% may have comparable improvements in renal function due to improved cardiac output. Furthermore, RAAS overactivation may lead to acute worsening of both cardiac and renal function, and so cessation of ACE inhibitors is of possible detriment in such cases. Hence, although suspension of ACE inhibitors during acute illness is often the safest action, their timely reintroduction is also necessary.

Fear of deteriorating renal function is often a reason for underprescribing ACE inhibitors for long-term cardioprotection in CKD patients. However, ACE inhibition is protective against renal deterioration even in CKD stage 4 and deterioration in the presence of renovascular disease is much less common than anticipated at ~11%. A rise in creatinine with the introduction of ACE inhibitors in patients with heart failure of up to 50% above baseline or to a creatinine of 200 µmol/L is accepted in some guidelines, provided renal function subsequently stabilizes. A rise in creatinine of up to 30% followed by stable renal function should be accepted and should not lead to stopping the drug or further investigation, whereas a greater rise raises the possibility of ARVD: renal imaging may be indicated in selected cases. A caveat to the above may be in advanced CKD, where a 30% change in renal function may be the difference between requiring maintenance dialysis and not. Such decisions must be taken on a case-by-case basis until the clinical trial evidence is available.

What may be required is a different approach to ACE inhibitor dosing for heart failure where CKD is present. The ATLAS trial compared high- versus low-dose lisinopril in 3164 patients with heart failure (>30 mg per day versus 2.5–5 mg). Overall, there was a reduction in mortality (12%) and heart failure hospitalization (24%) in the high-dose arm. However, in a post-hoc analysis of study patients with advanced CKD (n = 988) there was no difference in mortality or heart failure outcomes, but the high-dose arm did suffer significantly more adverse effects in respect of hypotension, hyperkalaemia, and decline in renal function.[51] These findings support the administering of ACE inhibitors to heart failure patients with advanced CKD, but favouring a low-dose approach.

Long-term monitoring of renal function in patients with CKD on ACE inhibitors is vital, as is adequate counselling about the risk of AKI and the importance of seeking medical advice in the event of a dehydrating illness such as diarrhoea.

Angiotensin II receptor blockers (ARBs) have a similar profile of adverse effects compared to ACE inhibitors, so that converting from ACE inhibitor to ARB in cases of hyperkalaemia is unlikely to improve matters. However, a change may be indicated in cases of ACE inhibitor-related cough.

Spironolactone, a mineralocorticoid receptor antagonist (MRA), improves survival in heart failure[52] but at the expense of increasing risk of hyperkalaemia, and its use in patients with CKD is thus potentially limited. The RALES trial excluded patients with significant renal impairment.[52] Dual blockade of the RAAS using an MRA and either an ACE inhibitor or an ARB is commonplace and is generally considered safe for treatment of heart failure,[53] provided appropriate monitoring of the risk for hyperkalaemia is in place. The combined use of ACE inhibitor and ARB is not routinely advised, and triple RAAS blockade should be avoided completely.

The evidence for ACE inhibitor and ARB use in dialysis patients is conflicting. The Fosinopril in Dialysis Trial (FOSIDIAL, n = 397) compared fosinopril with placebo during two years of treatment. The relative risk of cardiovascular events in patients on ACE inhibitor was 0.93 (95% CI: 0.68–1.26) (P = 0.35).[54] The change in systolic blood pressure in the treatment arm was 146–141 vs 145–143 mmHg in placebo. By contrast, a small open trial of candesartan vs placebo (n = 80) demonstrated statistically better outcome in the treatment arm during 19 ± 1 months of follow-up (cardiovascular events: 16% vs 46%; mortality: 0% vs 19%).[55]

Limited data also exist for the use of MRA in ESKD. These drugs are generally avoided because of the expected high risk of hyperkalaemia. However, a meta-analysis of studies of spironolactone in ESKD showed no increased risk of adverse events due to hyperkalaemia in 7051 patients.[56] It is therefore difficult to provide robust advice on the use of drugs acting on the RAAS in ESKD, except to say that close monitoring of possible adverse effects is vital if they are used.

β-Blockers

β-Blockade confers significant survival benefit in patients with stage 3 CKD, CAD, and heart failure (OR 0.75 vs matched patients not on beta-blockade).[57] Dialysis patients with heart failure (LVEF <35%) also benefit (two-year all-cause mortality, carvedilol vs placebo: 51.7% vs 73.2%; P < 0.001)[58] and are less likely to develop de-novo heart failure if pre-emptively prescribed a β-blocker (OR: 0.69 vs matched patients not on β-blocker).[59] However, β-blockers appear to be under-used in patients with CKD and on dialysis compared to matched patients without renal impairment,[57] despite the fact that poor renal function has little adverse effect on the efficacy of β-blockade in treatment of heart failure. There is no evidence for significantly increased rate of adverse effects (such as bradycardia, hyperkalaemia, and hypotension) with β-blockers in patients with advanced CKD. The exception is in elderly patients with a low GFR where there is a modest tendency to bradyarrhythmias necessitating drug discontinuation (2.3% vs 0.8% in placebo).[60] For these reasons, β-blockers are increasingly being used for pre-emptive cardioprotection in advanced CKD and ESKD.

Digoxin

As is the case with β-blockers, the efficacy of digoxin is not affected by CKD and efficacy does not correlate with GFR.[61] However, digoxin toxicity is more common in patients with CKD as the drug is partially eliminated by the kidney; for those patients with ESRD, the drug is not removed by dialysis. Digoxin can also contribute to hyperkalaemia and drugs such as calcium gluconate, used in the management of hyperkalaemia, can exacerbate the arrhythmic risk of digoxin toxicity. As digoxin does not confer the same survival benefit as β-blockers in heart failure, it should not be considered a first-line therapy for heart failure in patients with CKD.

Peritoneal dialysis

The principle of removing ascites to treat heart failure was first demonstrated 60 years ago. The possibility of using peritoneal dialysis as a management strategy for chronic heart failure in patients with

and without CKD is now also gaining support. In one small study ($n = 17$, mean age 64 ± 9 years), patients with refractory heart failure who were started on peritoneal dialysis had a significant survival benefit (82% 12-month survival) and fewer hospital admissions (reduction from 62 ± 16 to 11 ± 5 days/patient/year).[62] In refractory heart failure, the ability of the kidneys to generate a diuresis is blunted. Off-loading fluid from the circulation by removal during peritoneal dialysis will improve haemodynamics—for example, by reducing right atrial pressure—so improving cardiac function and renal perfusion. There is a trend towards offering peritoneal dialysis rather than haemodialysis to patients with CKD stage 5 and coexistent heart failure. The theory is that patients with markedly impaired ventricular function will benefit from gradual fluid removal and so be less likely to suffer collapse relating to hypotension, and/or serious arrhythmias that might result from haemodialysis. However, the evidence to support this practice is conflicting and derived from small, non-randomized studies.

One drawback that may prevent more widespread use of peritoneal dialysis in patients with heart failure and earlier stages of CKD is that patients need to be mobile and quite physically able to manage the technique; even where assisted PD programmes are available, patients will be expected to manage all or some of their therapy. A 5 L bag of dialysis fluid weighs 5 kg and carrying two or more of these to a peritoneal dialysis machine is an effort for any dialysis patient.

Anaemia management

The CONFIRM-HF trial of 304 patients with systolic heart failure (LVEF $\leq$45%), compared the effect of intravenous iron using ferric carboxymaltose against placebo on functional status. Importantly, patients were not specifically required to be anaemic. The inclusion criteria allowed for haemoglobin values up to 135 g/L. From 24 weeks after initiation of treatment, and up to the study end at 52 weeks, patients receiving intravenous iron demonstrated greater improvement in 6 min walk test, a reduction in New York Heart Association score, and reduced risk of hospitalization for heart failure (hazard ratio: 0.39 (95% CI: 0.19–0.82); $P = 0.009$) than patients receiving placebo. This study excluded patients with CKD. The mean eGFR in patients receiving iron was 66 ± 22 mL/min/1.73 m^2.[63]

Importantly, the volume of administration of dose-equivalent ferric carboxymaltose (and iron isomaltoside) is much lower than for iron dextran. The latter is typically diluted to 500 mL using 0.9% NaCl for administration, compared with 100 mL for the others. This is important for heart failure and CKD patients alike in whom fluid restriction is of particular importance. This, alongside cost, should be considered when deciding which intravenous iron preparation to use in heart failure.

The landmark trial in anaemia management in CKD was TREAT (Trial to Reduce Cardiovascular Endpoints with Aranesp Therapy). This aimed to show a benefit in using erythropoiesis stimulating agents (ESAs) to achieve a higher than usual target haemoglobin (130 g/L) in diabetic pre-dialysis CKD patients. However, there was an excess of thromboembolic events and cerebrovascular events in the ESA arm compared to placebo.[64] Despite these specific findings, there was no difference between treatment and placebo arms in respect of the primary composite end-point of death or cardiovascular event. This has led to lower target haemoglobin in CKD anaemia treatment, typically of 100–120 g/L.

Revascularization of renal artery stenosis

As demonstrated by the high prevalence of preserved systolic function in patients with heart failure and RAS, RAS is likely to be causative in many cases of heart failure rather than simply representing coexistent atheroma in another arterial tree. The heart failure is by way of RAAS overactivation, accelerated hypertension, and CKD.

There have been two randomized controlled trials (RCTs) of more than 800 patients with ARVD which failed to show a benefit of using endovascular intervention (angioplasty and stenting) as first-line therapy for ARVD compared to medical therapy alone. These were the Angioplasty and Stenting for Renal Artery Lesions (ASTRAL) trial and the Cardiovascular Outcomes in Renal Atherosclerotic Lesions (CORAL) trial.[65,66] However, these studies excluded patients with a previously recommended indication for intervention, particularly flash pulmonary oedema. Given that flash pulmonary oedema generally represents decompensation of heart failure in ARVD patients, very few heart failure patients were recruited to ASTRAL and CORAL. This means that there are presently no data from randomized studies to guide the use of renal artery revascularization specifically within the heart failure population.

Observational studies do suggest that heart failure patients represent the clinical phenotype most likely to improve after renal revascularization. Indeed, 'flash pulmonary oedema' is already recognized as an indication for revascularization. A case report using cardiac magnetic resonance imaging quantified a reduction in left ventricular mass from 161 g before revascularization to 108 g one year after, and in left ventricular end-diastolic volume from 193 to 124 mL.[67]

On a broader scale, in a case–control study of 100 patients with ARVD and heart failure, revascularization was associated with a five-fold reduction in heart failure hospitalization compared to medical management alone. A further study, also of 100 patients, has shown that patients with ARVD and chronic heart failure who have never previously suffered acute pulmonary oedema may also benefit from revascularization. Here, the hazard ratio for death in the revascularization group was 0.76 (0.58–0.99; $P = 0.04$) compared to medically managed patients.[68]

Management of the acute admission with heart failure

Diuretics

The potential for nephrotoxicity and decline in renal function with diuretic usage may cause a therapeutic dilemma. Patients with decompensated heart failure with either associated AKI or underlying CKD are more likely to suffer further AKI due to diuretic drugs, and the adverse effect is even more pronounced in patients receiving RAAS blockade.

Patients with AKI or CKD are less responsive to diuretics than patients without renal impairment but there is a reluctance to prescribe high-dose loop diuretics in patients with renal disease. This is based on a fear of renal toxicity and pre-renal failure due to intravascular volume depletion. It is frequently not appreciated that in fluid-overloaded patients with heart failure the adverse effects on renal function due to an elevated right atrial pressure and renal congestion are greater than the impact of reduced cardiac output. Inducing a significant diuresis with high-dose diuretics in this situation may result in a significant improvement rather than deterioration in

renal function. Key to the assessment of the likely impact of diuretic therapy on renal function in these patients is a careful assessment of the intravascular volume status of the patient.

It is true that the use of high doses of diuretics is correlated with poor outcome in heart failure,[69] but this association is most likely due to the diuretic resistance seen in patients with the more severe forms of the cardiorenal syndrome, and in those with very poor haemodynamic status, also a marker of more severe heart failure.

It is important to note that using diuretics purely to improve urine output in acutely unwell oliguric patients will not improve renal function (in fact it may worsen it in those with hypovol-aemia), and so diuretics should only be used when the removal of excesses of fluid is clinically required. Therapeutic B-type natriuretic peptide (nesiritide) does not reduce the need for diur-etic, nor increase urine output in patients admitted acutely with heart failure.[70] Nitrates and hydralazine are useful alternatives to blockade of the renin–angiotensin system when heart failure ex-acerbations are complicated by AKI. However, hypotension may preclude their use.

In the acute setting, if nitrates are unable to stabilize a patient with severe heart failure coupled with AKI and diuretic resist-ance, the treatment options become quite limited, at which point haemofiltration may need to be considered.

Inotropes

Positive inotropic agents were once regularly used for treating pa-tients with decompensated heart failure, but this practice has now fallen from favour. Low doses of dopamine interact with specific receptors in the kidney leading to an increase in renal blood flow without apparent significant inotropic effect, and hence dopa-mine continues to be used by some at a 'renal dose', with the aim of improving the response to diuretics, and reducing the incidence and progression of AKI.[71] Unfortunately, any data showing the bene-fits of low-dose dopamine regimes have derived from small-scale selected non-randomized studies.

Haemofiltration

Haemofiltration is the ultrafiltration of fluid from the body via an extracorporeal machine. It uses the same principle as that used to off-load fluid from haemodialysis patients, and it can now be achieved with portable machines designed specifically for ultrafiltration only. Ultrafiltration has the advantage over diuretic therapy in that more rapid fluid and sodium removal is possible during the early phase of an admission with decompensated heart failure, minimizing the tendency to deterioration of renal function or hypotension that might accompany high-dose diuretic therapy. The controlled nature of the haemofiltration process may thus benefit patients with labile blood-pressure response during treatment. Studies have shown a short-term improvement in outcome with ultrafiltration instead of intravenous diuresis as first-line therapy for patients with an acute admission with heart failure,[72] but longer-term outcome results are still awaited. There is little evidence to support the use of peritoneal dialysis in the management of acute heart failure. The logistics and safety of inserting a peritoneal dialysis catheter in an acutely unwell patient, followed by its immediate use, are likely to preclude its be-coming a standard therapy.

Diagnostic and therapeutic use of B-type natriuretic peptide

In the general population, N-terminal pro-B-type natriuric peptide (NT-proBNP) is a first-line test for primary care clinicians in ruling out or diagnosing heart failure. Guidelines generally concur that levels >400 pg/mL suggest the presence of prognostically signifi-cant heart failure which warrants referral to secondary care services. However, the evidence behind the use of NT-proBNP as a diagnostic tool has come from studies that either excluded patients with signifi-cant CKD, or studies that showed reduced clinical efficacy of NT-proBNP in the context of coexistent CKD.

Difficulties in interpretation of NT-proBNP in the setting of CKD arise because levels may be elevated in CKD in the absence of heart failure. NT-proBNP correlates strongly with LVH, LV dilation, and extracellular fluid accumulation, and is partly metabolized in the renal parenchyma. Hence, levels will often be elevated in patients with reduced renal function regardless of the presence or absence of heart failure. It is not removed by dialysis, but post-haemodialysis BNP levels show a fall that correlates with ultrafiltration volume. Elevated BNP is less likely to occur in patients using peritoneal dialysis.

Due to the prevalence of kidney disease in the heart failure popu-lation and vice versa, it is vital to have better understanding of NT-proBNP in such scenarios. NT-proBNP is probably still useful in diagnosing heart failure in ESKD, but only if higher diagnostic cut-offs are used, which reduces the sensitivity of the test. Its use should not replace clinical judgement in these patients.[70,73,74]

Although BNP increases renal perfusion, its therapeutic use does not reduce the occurrence of AKI in decompensated heart failure in patients with pre-existent CKD.[75] BNP reduces distal tubular reabsorption of sodium leading to diuresis, an effect which is lost in CKD where glomerular or tubular disease predominates. The blunting of the diuretic effect of BNP may contribute to the high occurrence of heart failure in CKD patients, as such patients are less able to mount an effective response to fluid overload.

Acute pulmonary oedema and renal artery stenosis

Thirty-four per cent of older patients requiring hospital admission for decompensation of heart failure will have RAS, and more than half of patients seen in secondary care heart failure clinics have RAS. Patients with CAD are very likely to have RAS, and so this renal diagnosis should be considered in patients admitted to hospital with heart failure decompensation as revascularization may be appro-priate in selected cases. Screening all patients with heart failure for RAS using renal angiography is not clinically practical, but it should be considered in high-risk phenotypes such as those admitted with acute pulmonary oedema who have CKD, LVH, and hypertension.

Conclusion

Heart failure in CKD carries an excess mortality through a het-erogeneous series of pathophysiological interactions. Prevention of LVH through blood pressure management and volume control, and early modification of risk factors for CAD, are vital. Proteinuria and change in eGFR are early indicators of adverse cardiovascular outcome and indicate the need for early therapeutic intervention. Simple medical therapy, such as β-blockers and ACE inhibitors, are

effective but probably under-used in patients with heart failure and renal impairment. These agents are safe provided that patients are appropriately monitored. Management of heart failure in the setting of acute or chronic kidney disease is complicated by the potentially nephrotoxic effect of many current therapies. Peritoneal dialysis and haemofiltration are measures that may yet improve the outcome of cardiorenal disease but there is a current lack of randomized clinical trial data in this regard.

REFERENCES

1. Go AS, Chertow GM, Fan D, McCulloch CE, Hsu C. Chronic kidney disease and the risks of death, cardiovascular events, and hospitalization. *N Engl J Med* 2004;**351**(13):1296–305.
2. McAlister FA, Ezekowitz J, Tonelli M, Armstrong PW. Renal insufficiency and heart failure: prognostic and therapeutic implications from a prospective cohort study. *Circulation* 2004;**109**(8):1004–9.
3. Foley RN, Parfrey PS, Harnett JD, Kent GM. The prognostic importance of left ventricular geometry in uremic cardiomyopathy. *J Am Coll Cardiol* 1995;**5**(12):2024–2031.
4. Parfrey PS, Foley RN. The clinical epidemiology of cardiac disease in chronic renal failure. *Am J Kidney Dis* 1999;**10**:1606–15.
5. Saravanan P, Freeman G, Davidson NC. Risk assessment for sudden cardiac death in dialysis patients: how relevant are conventional cardiac risk factors? *Int J Cardiol* 2010;**144**(3):431–2.
6. Foley RN, Parfrey PS, Harnett JD, *et al.* Impact of hypertension on cardiomyopathy, morbidity and mortality in end-stage renal disease. *Kidney Int* 1996;**49**(5):1379–85.
7. Herzog C, Muster H, Li S, Collins A. Impact of congestive heart failure, chronic kidney disease, and anemia on survival in the Medicare population. *J Card Fail* 2004;**10**(6):467–72.
8. Dries DL, Exner DV, Domanski MJ, Greenberg B, Stevenson LW. The prognostic implications of renal insufficiency in asymptomatic and symptomatic patients with left ventricular systolic dysfunction. *J Am Coll Cardiol* 2000;**35**(3):681–9.
9. Campbell RC, Sui X, Filippatos G, *et al.* Association of chronic kidney disease with outcomes in chronic heart failure: a propensity-matched study. *Nephrol Dial Transplant* 2009;**24**(1):186–93.
10. Anonymous. Section H—Mortality and causes of death. In: *USRDS 2008 Annual Data Report*. 2008. p. 619–70.
11. Ronco C, Haapio M, House AA, Anavekar N, Bellomo R. Cardiorenal syndrome. *J Am Coll Cardiol* 2008;**52**(19):1527–39.
12. Fox KF, Cowie MR, Wood DA, *et al.* Coronary artery disease as the cause of incident heart failure in the population. *Heart* 2001;**22**(3):228–36.
13. Silberberg JS, Barre PE, Prichard SS, Sniderman AD. Impact of left ventricular hypertrophy on survival in end-stage renal disease. *Kidney Int* 1989;**36**(2):286–90.
14. Levin A, Singer J, Thompson C, Ross H, Lewis M. Prevalent left ventricular hypertrophy in the predialysis population: identifying opportunities for intervention. *Am J Kidney Dis* 1996;**27**(3):347–54.
15. Cannella G, Paoletti E, Delfino R, *et al.* Regression of left ventricular hypertrophy in hypertensive dialyzed uremic patients on long-term antihypertensive therapy. *Kidney Int* 1993;**44**(4):881–6.

16. Verma A, Anavekar NS, Meris A, *et al.* The relationship between renal function and cardiac structure, function, and prognosis after myocardial infarction: the VALIANT *Echo Study. J Am Coll Cardiol* 2007;**50**(13):1238–45.
17. Stack AG, Bloembergen WE. Prevalence and clinical correlates of coronary artery disease among new dialysis patients in the United States: a cross-sectional study. *Jo Am Soc Nephrol* 2001;**12**(7):1516–23.
18. Farrington K, Hodsman A, Casula A, Ansell D, Feehally J. ESRD prevalent rates in 2007 in the UK: national and centre-specific analyses. In: *UK Renal Registry 11th Annual Report* 2007, Chapter 4, pp. 43–68.
19. Ritz E, Rychlík I, Locatelli F, Halimi S. End-stage renal failure in type 2 diabetes: a medical catastrophe of worldwide dimensions. *Am J Kidney Dis* 1999;**34**(5):795–808.
20. Catalano C. De novo diabetes in dialysis patients: when diabetes is not diabetic nephropathy. *Nephrol Dial Transplant* 1996;**11**(6):938–41.
21. Hadi HA, Suwaidi JA. Endothelial dysfunction in diabetes mellitus. *Vasc Health Risk Manag* 2007;**3**(6):853–76.
22. Nelson RG, Knowler WC, Pettitt DJ, *et al.* Assessment of risk of overt nephropathy in diabetic patients from albumin excretion in untimed urine specimen. *Arch Intern Med* 1991;**151**(9):1761–5.
23. Rossing P, Hougaard P, Borch-Johnsen K, Parving H. Predictors of mortality in insulin dependent diabetes: 10 year observational follow up study. *BMJ* 1996;**31**(3):779–84.
24. Gerstein HC, Mann J, Yi Q, *et al.* Albuminuria and risk of cardiovascular events, death, and heart failure in diabetic and nondiabetic individuals. *JAMA* 2001;**286**(4):421–6.
25. Braun J, Oldendor FM, Moshage W, *et al.* Electron beam computed tomography in the evaluation of cardiac calcification in chronic dialysis patients. *Am J Kidney Dis* 1996;**27**(3):394–401.
26. London GM. Arterial media calcification in end-stage renal disease: impact on all-cause and cardiovascular mortality. *Nephrol Dial Transplant* 2003;**18**(9):1731–40.
27. Hujairi NM, Afzali B, Goldsmith DJ. Cardiac calcification in renal patients: what we do and don't know. *Am J Kidney Dis* 2003;**43**(2):234–43.
28. Moe SM, O'Neill KD, Reslerova M, *et al.* Natural history of vascular calcification in dialysis and transplant patients. *Nephrol Dial Transplant* 2004;**19**(9):2387–93.
29. Wang M, Tsai W, Chen J, Cheng M, Huang J. Arterial stiffness correlated with cardiac remodelling in patients with chronic kidney disease. *Nephrology* 2007;**12**(6):591–7.
30. Bongartz LG, Cramer MJ, Doevendans PA, Joles JA, Braam B. The severe cardiorenal syndrome: 'Guyton revisited'. *Eur Heart J* 2005;**26**(1):11–17.
31. Tripepi G, Mallamaci F, Zoccali C. Inflammation markers, adhesion molecules, and all-cause and cardiovascular mortality in patients with ESRD: searching for the best risk marker by multivariate modeling. *J Am Soc Nephrol* 2005;**16**:s83–88.
32. Hung AM, Ikizler TA. Hemodialysis central venous catheters as a source of inflammation and its implications. *Sem Dial* 2008;**21**(5):401–4.
33. Apple FS, Murakami MM, Pearce LA, Herzog CA. Multi-biomarker risk stratification of N-terminal pro-B-type natriuretic peptide, high-sensitivity C-reactive protein, and cardiac troponin T and I in end-stage renal disease for all-cause death. *Clin Chem* 2004;**50**:2279–85.
34. Kayikcioglu M, Tumuklu M, Ozkahya M, *et al.* The benefit of salt restriction in the treatment of end-stage renal disease by haemodialysis. *Nephrol Dial Transplant* 2009;**24**(3):956–62.

35. Ozkahya M, Toz H, Qzerkan F, *et al.* Impact of volume control on left ventricular hypertrophy in dialysis patients. *J Nephrol* 2002;**15**(6):655–60.

36. Fluck R, Rao R, van Schalkwyk D, Ansell D, Feest T. The UK Vascular Access Survey—follow-up data and repeat survey (chapter 5). *Nephrol Dial Transplant* 2007;**22**(Suppl 7):vii51–7.

37. MacRae JM. Vascular access and cardiac disease: is there a relationship? *Curr Opin Nephrol Hyperten* 2006;**15**(6):577–82.

38. Shurrab A, MacDowall P, Wright J, Mamtora H, Kalra P. The importance of associated extra-renal vascular disease on the outcome of patients with atherosclerotic renovascular disease. *Nephron Clin Prac* 2003;**93**(2):51–7.

39. MacDowall P, Kalra Pa, O'Donoghue DJ, *et al.* Risk of morbidity from renovascular disease in elderly patients with congestive cardiac failure. *Lancet* 1998;**352**(9121):13–16.

40. de Silva R, Loh H, Rigby AS, *et al.* Epidemiology, associated factors, and prognostic outcomes of renal artery stenosis in chronic heart failure assessed by magnetic resonance angiography. *Am J Cardiol* 2007;**100**(2):273–9.

41. Kalra PA, Guo H, Kausz AT, *et al.* Atherosclerotic renovascular disease in United States patients aged 67 years or older: risk factors, revascularisation, and prognosis. *Kidney Int* 2005;**68**(1):293–301.

42. Kane GC, Xu N, Mistrik E, *et al.* Renal artery revascularisation improves heart failure control in patients with atherosclerotic renal artery stenosis. *Nephrol Dial Transplant* 2010;**25**(3):813–20.

43. Wright JR, Shurrab AE, Cooper A, *et al.* Progression of cardiac dysfunction in patients with atherosclerotic renovascular disease. *Q J Med* 2009;**102**(10):695–704.

44. Wright JR, Shurrab AE, Cooper A, *et al.* Left ventricular morphology and function in patients with atherosclerotic renovascular disease. *J Am Soc Nephrol* 2005;**16**(9):2746–53.

45. Gottlieb S. The prognostic importance of different definitions of worsening renal function in congestive heart failure. *J Card Fail* 2002;**8**(3):136–41.

46. Smith GL, Vaccarino V, Kosiborod M, *et al.* Worsening renal function: what is a clinically meaningful change in creatinine during hospitalization with heart failure? *J Card Fail* 2003;**9**(1):13–25.

47. Forman DE, Butler J, Wang Y, *et al.* Incidence, predictors at admission, and impact of worsening renal function among patients hospitalized with heart failure. *J Am Coll Cardiol* 2004;**43**(1):61–7.

48. Cowie MR, Komajda M, Murray-Thomas T, Underwood J, Ticho B. Prevalence and impact of worsening renal function in patients hospitalized with decompensated heart failure: results of the prospective outcomes study in heart failure (POSH). *Eur Heart J* 2006;**27**(10):1216–22.

49. Ljungman S, Laragh J, Cody R. Role of the kidney in congestive heart failure. Relationship of cardiac index to kidney function. *Drugs* 1990;**39**(Suppl 4):10–21.

50. SOLVD Investigators, Yusuf S, Pitt B, Davis CE, *et al.* Effect of enalapril on survival in patients with reduced left ventricular ejection fractions and congestive heart failure. *New Eng J Med* 1990;**325**(5):293–302.

51. Packer M, Poole-Wilson PA, Armstrong PW, *et al.* Comparative effects of low and high doses of the angiotenisin-converting enzyme inhibitor, lisinopril, on morbidity and mortality in chronic heart failure. *Circulation* 1999;**100**:2312–18.

52. RALES Investigators. Effectiveness of spironolactone added to an angiotensin-converting enzyme inhibitor and a loop diuretic for severe chronic congestive heart failure (the Randomized Aldactone Evaluation Study [RALES]. *Am J Cardiol* 1996;**78**(8):902–7.

53. Young JB, Dunlap ME, Pfeffer MA, *et al.* Mortality and morbidity reduction with candesartan in patients with chronic heart failure and left ventricular systolic dysfunction: results of the CHARM low-left ventricular ejection fraction trials. *Circulation* 2004;**110**(17):2618–26.

54. Zannad F, Kessler M, Lehert P, *et al.* Prevention of cardiovascular events in end-stage renal disease: results of a randomized trial of fosinopril and implications for future studies. *Kidney Int* 2006;**70**(7):1318–24.

55. Takahashi A, Takase H, Toriyama T, *et al.* Candesartan, an angiotensin II type-1 receptor blocker, reduces cardiovascular events in patients on chronic haemodialysis—a randomized study. *Nephrol Dial Transplant* 2006;**21**(9):2507–12.

56. Chua D, Lo A, Lo C. Spironolactone use in heart failure patients with end-stage renal disease on hemodialysis: is it safe? *Clin Cardiol* 2010;**33**(10):604–8.

57. Ezekowitz J, McAlister FA, Humphries KH, *et al.* The association among renal insufficiency, pharmacotherapy, and outcomes in 6,427 patients with heart failure and coronary artery disease. *J Am Coll Cardiol* 2004;**44**(8):1587–92.

58. Cice G, Ferrara L, D'Andrea A, D'Isa S. Carvedilol increases two-year survival in dialysis patients with dilated cardiomyopathy—a prospective, placebo-controlled trial. *J Am Coll Cardiol* 2003;**43**:1438–44.

59. Abbott K, Trespalacios F, Agodoa L, Taylor A, Bakris G. Beta-blocker use in long-term dialysis patients. *Arch Intern Med* 2004;**164**:2465–71.

60. Cohen-Solal A, Kotecha D, van Veldhuisen DJ, *et al.* Efficacy and safety of nebivolol in elderly heart failure patients with impaired renal function: insights from the SENIORS trial. *Eur J Heart Fail* 2009;**11**(9):872–80.

61. Shlipak MG, Smith GL, Rathore SS, Massie BM, Krumholz HM. Renal function, digoxin therapy, and heart failure outcomes: evidence from the digoxin intervention group trial. *J Am Soc Nephrol* 2004;**15**(8):2195–203.

62. Sánchez J, Ortega T, Rodríguez C, *et al.* Efficacy of peritoneal ultrafiltration in the treatment of refractory congestive heart failure. *Nephrol Dial Transplant* 2010;**25**(2):605–61.

63. Ponikowski P, van Veldhuisen DJ, Comin-Colet J, *et al.* Beneficial effects of long-term intravenous iron therapy with ferric carboxymaltose in patients with symptomatic heart failure and iron deficiency. *Eur Heart J* 2015;**36**(11):657–68.

64. Pfeffer M, Burdmann E, Chen C, *et al.* A trial of darbepoetin alfa in type 2 diabetes and chronic kidney disease. *N Engl J Med* 2009;**361**(21):2019–32.

65. Wheatley K, Ives N, Gray R, *et al.* Revascularization versus medical therapy for renal-artery stenosis. *N Engl J Med* 2009;**361**:1953–62.

66. Cooper CJ Murphy TP, Cutlip DE, *et al.* Stenting and medical therapy for atherosclerotic renal-artery stenosis. *N Engl J Med* 2014;**370**:13–22.

67. Chrysochou C, Schmitt M, Siddals K, *et al.* Reverse cardiac remodelling and renal functional improvement following bilateral renal artery stenting for flash pulmonary oedema. *Nephrol Dial Transplant* 2013;**28**(2):479–83.

68. Green D, Ritchie JP, Chrysochou C, Kalra PA. Revascularisation of atherosclerotic renal artery stenosis for chronic heart failure versus acute pulmonary oedema. *Nephrology (Carlton)* 2018;**23**(5):411–17.

69. Pellicori P, Cleland JG, Zhang J, *et al.* Cardiac dysfunction, congestion and loop diuretics: their relationship to prognosis in heart failure. *Cardiovasc Drugs Ther* 2016;**30**:599–609.

70. Dhar S, Pressman GS, Subramanian S, *et al.* Natriuretic peptides and heart failure in the patient with chronic kidney disease: a review of current evidence. *Postgrad Med J* 2009;**85**(1004):299–302.

71. Elkayam U, Ng TM, Hatamizadeh P, Janmohamed M, Mehra A. Renal vasodilatory action of dopamine in patients with heart failure: magnitude of effect and site of action. *Circulation* 2008;**117**(2):200–5.

72. Bart BA, Boyle A, Bank AJ, *et al.* Ultrafiltration versus usual care for hospitalized patients with heart failure: the Relief for Acutely Fluid-Overloaded Patients With Decompensated Congestive Heart Failure (RAPID-CHF) trial. *J Am Coll Cardiol* 2005;**46**(11):2043–6.

73. McCullough PA, Sandberg KR. B-type natriuretic peptide and renal disease. *Heart Fail Rev* 2003;**8**(4):355–8.

74. Cataliott A, Malatino L, Jougasak IM, *et al.* Circulating natriuretic peptide concentrations in patients with end-stage renal disease: role of brain natriuretic peptide as a biomarker for ventricular remodeling. *Mayo Clin Proc* 2001;**76**(11):1111–19.

75. Witteles RM, Kao D, Christopherson D, *et al.* Impact of nesiritide on renal function in patients with acute decompensated heart failure and pre-existing renal dysfunction a randomized, double-blind, placebo-controlled clinical trial. *J Am Coll Cardiol* 2007;**50**(19):1835–40.

34

Chronic lung disease

Sara Roversi, Michael Greenstone, Simon P. Hart, and Nathaniel M. Hawkins

Introduction and epidemiology

Chronic obstructive pulmonary disease (COPD) is a worldwide epidemic, characterized by persistent respiratory symptoms and airflow limitation due to airway and/or alveolar abnormalities, usually caused by significant exposure to noxious particles or gases (mostly cigarette smoke).[1] This disease is commonly associated with cardiac disease, including heart failure, and the presence of one will affect the prognosis, diagnosis, and treatment of the other.[2]

Prevalence estimates vary greatly across studies investigating COPD and heart failure, due to significant differences in cohort selection, population characteristics, diagnostic criteria and measurement methods. In many cohorts, the diagnosis of COPD was based on self-report rather than on spirometry and is thus inaccurate. Nevertheless, 17–35% of patients with heart failure are estimated to have COPD,[3] while 7–31% of patients with COPD have concurrent heart failure.[4] Not surprisingly, studies investigating elderly and/or hospitalized patients usually report the highest prevalence rates.[5,6] Moreover, a significant number of patients remain undiagnosed: for example, a recent study documented that in an outpatient heart failure population, 34% of the patients had airflow obstruction, of whom 78% at least moderate, but only one in three had previously been diagnosed with COPD (Table 34.1).[7] Spirometry is constantly reported to be under-used in patients with heart failure, even in contemporary practice.[8] Interestingly, reported COPD prevalence has a trend towards higher rates in more recent studies, perhaps reflecting the co-morbidities of an ageing population, or a growing awareness regarding COPD.[9] Further, the occurrence of COPD is similar in patients with heart failure with reduced ejection fraction (HFrEF) and preserved ejection fraction (HFpEF), perhaps with a slightly higher prevalence in the latter group.[10]

Not surprisingly, prognosis is generally worse in patients with both diseases. In the heart failure population, COPD has been reported as an independent predictor of all-cause hospitalization, heart failure hospitalization, and all-cause mortality,[11] while the relationship with events such as acute myocardial infarction or arrhythmic death is not as clear.[12] For example, the risk of sudden cardiac death is almost two-fold higher in patients with a diagnosis of COPD compared to the general population, but the presence of heart failure does not seem to affect significantly the association between COPD and sudden cardiac death.[13]

Table 34.1 Prospective studies reporting the prevalence of spirometry-diagnosed airflow obstruction in patients with heart failure, with and without a previous clinical diagnosis of COPD

Study	Setting	N	Confirmed airflow obstruction (%)		History of COPD without confirmed airflow obstruction (%)
			overall	previously undiagnosed	
Arnaudis [1]	inpatient	348	132 (38)	107 (31)	8 (4)
Apostolovic[2]	outpatient	174	48 (28)*	48 (28)	-
Bektas [3]	outpatient	199	68 (34)	43 (22)	3 (2)
Boschetto [4]	outpatient	118	36 (30)	23 (64)	
Dalsgaard[5]	outpatient	590	225 (38)	178 (30)	24 (4)
Iversen[6]	inpatient	489	169 (35)	97 (20)	35 (7)
Steinacher[7]	outpatient	89	22 (24)	15 (17)	4 (5)
Valk [8]	primary care	106	30 (28)	21 (20)	
Wada [9]	outpatient	753	79 (10)*	79 (10)	-

* only patients without a previous clinical diagnosis of COPD were included.

On the other hand, cardiovascular disease is the most important cause of both morbidity and mortality in patients with mild or moderate COPD and is the leading cause of hospitalization.[23] At first, it was thought that patients with COPD died primarily from respiratory failure rather than cardiovascular disease. However, the attribution was usually made from chart review rather than autopsy. Subsequent data, derived from the autopsy reports of deceased patients hospitalized for severe exacerbation of COPD, suggested that the leading cause of death was heart failure, followed by pneumonia and thromboembolic events, all more common than respiratory failure.[24] Further, in the large TORCH (Towards a Revolution in COPD Health) trial, cardiovascular causes and malignancy were as common as acute exacerbations as a cause of death.[25] Thus, current research is underlining the importance of cardiac diseases in contributing to increased mortality in patients with COPD.[26]

Pathogenic mechanisms

Cardiac disease and respiratory function are strongly correlated, with reduced lung function being described as a putative risk factor for cardiovascular disorders. There is a strong body of evidence linking lung function, COPD and vascular events. For example, in the National Health and Nutrition Examination Survey, the risk of cardiovascular death was five-fold greater in those in the lowest quintile of forced expiratory volume in the 1st second (FEV_1) compared to the highest.[27] Similar studies have documented an increased risk of incident heart disease with declining FEV_1, including higher risk of ischaemic heart disease,[28] atrial fibrillation,[29] and heart failure.[30,31] More specifically, a monotonic increase in the rate of incident heart failure with decreasing quartiles of FEV_1 was documented in 13 360 participants in the Atherosclerosis Risk in Communities (ARIC) study, and the adjusted hazard ratio (HR) was 2.23 (95% confidence interval (CI): 1.69–2.93) for male patients in the lowest quartile of FEV_1, compared to the highest.[2] The explanation of this association is still debated, the greater question being whether reduced lung function (expressed as FEV_1) is purely a marker of increased risk for cardiac disease, or if there is a causal relationship.

The COPD–heart failure association may simply reflect shared common risk factors (e.g. smoking, inflammation, physical inactivity, obesity, and diabetes), although most epidemiologic studies do not seem to support this hypothesis. Accordingly, the correlation between reduced lung function and increased incidence of heart failure stands after adjustment for confounders such as age, smoke, blood glucose levels, blood pressure, cholesterol, body mass index, antihypertensive treatment, systolic blood pressure, and left ventricular mass.[31] Further, the increased risk associated with low FEV_1 remains even when cardiac and inflammatory markers are included in the model, i.e. C-reactive protein (CRP), troponin, and natriuretic peptides.[31] These data suggest that the established risk factors for heart failure do not explain the increased risk associated with reduced FEV_1, and that altered lung function may cause or worsen heart failure.

The pathogenic mechanisms by which lung dysfunction promotes cardiac dysfunction have been widely debated, but remain unclear. Distortions of the lung structure, hypoxia, hypercapnia, acidosis, and abnormal inflammatory response have all been described as potential causes. For example, it has been suggested that emphysema and lung hyperinflation may hinder venous return, due to raised intrathoracic pressure, reducing left ventricular (LV) filling and inducing ventricular dysfunction.[32]

Pulmonary hypertension is a known and well-documented co-morbidity of COPD. Pulmonary hypertension is secondary to intimal thickening and medial hypertrophy of the pulmonary arteries, hypoxic pulmonary vasoconstriction, and endothelial dysfunction.[33] Pulmonary hypertension, in turn, increases chronically the right ventricular afterload, resulting in right ventricular hypertrophy and dilatation, progressing to systolic and diastolic dysfunction, and leading to the clinical syndrome of right heart failure with systemic congestion.[34] Pulmonary hypertension in COPD carries a poor prognosis, but the pressure is rarely markedly elevated at rest. Pulmonary artery pressure may become quite abnormal on exercise, during sleep, or at the time of an exacerbation, and contribute to disability over and above that due to the airflow obstruction alone.[35] Moreover, it has been suggested that an increase in the end-diastolic pressure of the right ventricle (RVEDP) on exercise stretches the right atrium, thereby increasing sympathetic activation and activating the renin–angiotensin–aldosterone system, promoting salt and water retention. The increase in RVEDP also leads to abnormal interventricular septal motion, thereby impairing left ventricular function and further contributing to left heart involvement. Eventually, the left heart is affected, resulting in global heart failure.[36]

To compound matters, COPD patients often present with a persistent and partially unexplained autonomic dysfunction, including altered chemoreceptor regulation due to hypoxaemia and hypercapnia, and neurohormonal activation due to systemic inflammation, resulting in loss of parasympathetic tone, increased sympathetic tone, and altered baroreceptor sensitivity.[37] Decline in FEV_1 correlates with raised inflammatory markers such as CRP and fibrinogen, with inflammation connected to many of the systemic manifestations, such as muscle weakness and weight loss.[38] Moreover, patients with COPD exhibit increased arterial stiffness compared with appropriately matched normal subjects.[39] Taken together, these alterations are linked to higher risk of cardiac stress and myocardial injury, well-known risk factors for heart failure.

Various clinical studies have tested these hypotheses. Some degree of systolic and/or diastolic dysfunction, or structural heart alterations are commonly reported in patients with COPD.[40] For example, a significant linear association was observed between pulmonary hyperinflation and LV mass in participants of the Multi-Ethnic Study of Atherosclerosis (MESA) COPD Study, suggesting an adaptive response to the COPD-induced intrathoracic pressure changes.[41] In the same cohort, percent emphysema and COPD were associated with significant reduction in total pulmonary vein area, suggesting reduced LV filling.[42]

Finally, it should be noted that both COPD and heart failure are diseases of advancing age. Multi-morbidity increases with age, with clear disease clusters described.[43] For example, elderly patients with heart failure present high single prevalence of arrhythmias, coronary artery disease, or COPD (i.e. >25%), but when disease patterns are analysed, cardiac disease and lung disease seem to cluster: patients with a diagnosis of heart failure and COPD have a seven-fold higher risk of being diagnosed also with arrhythmia, or a five-fold higher risk of associated coronary artery disease, as compared with control groups without heart failure or COPD.[43]

Effect of COPD co-morbidity on heart failure outcomes

Patients with heart failure and COPD suffer more than patients with either condition alone. Symptom burden, hospitalization, and mortality are all increased, in both the stable and acute settings.[44] Heart failure studies and registries concur on the detrimental impact of COPD on survival,[3,45] although this association is weakened (sometimes to non-significant) when adjusting for confounders such as co-morbidities and medications.[46] Similarly, a concomitant diagnosis of COPD at the time of heart failure hospitalization/ambulatory visit conveys an almost 30% increased risk of hospitalization in the subsequent year.[8] Several explanations have been proposed, including lower prescription of heart failure medications, worse haemodynamics, higher inflammatory status, and clustering of co-morbidities.[47] Further, lung infections and exacerbations of COPD may worsen heart failure symptoms, and, according to some reports, account for up to 20% of heart failure exacerbations.[48,49]

The diagnosis of COPD

Definition

The Global Initiative for Chronic Obstructive Lung Disease (GOLD) defines COPD as 'a common, preventable, and treatable disease characterized by persistent respiratory symptoms and airflow limitation that is due to airway and/or alveolar abnormalities, usually caused by significant exposure to noxious particles or gases'.[1] The definition is important because it emphasizes the need for an objective demonstration of airflow limitation, and spirometry is required to make the diagnosis. Persistent symptoms (e.g. chronic dyspnoea, cough, sputum, wheezing, and chest tightness) and history of exposure to noxious stimuli such

as cigarette smoke are similarly important. Although most COPD patients have a 20 pack-year smoking history, the condition is increasingly recognized in non-smokers, especially in the developing world where environmental smoke and other toxins may be important.[50]

Spirometry is a physiological, non-invasive test, which assesses lung function by measuring the volume of air that the patient can expel after a maximal inspiration.[51] The measured values are then compared with predicted normal values determined on the basis of age, height, sex, and ethnicity. Several indices can be derived from spirometry, the most relevant being FEV_1, forced vital capacity (FVC), and the FEV_1/FVC ratio. Values of FEV_1 and FVC are measured in litres and expressed as a percentage of the predicted normal values. Values are measured at baseline and after a single dose of short-acting bronchodilator, to assess reversibility.[51]

According to the 2017 GOLD document, post-bronchodilator FEV_1/FVC <0.70 confirms persistent airflow limitation and identifies COPD in patients with appropriate symptoms and predisposing risks.[1] To assess COPD severity, three different aspects must be considered separately, i.e. the severity of airflow limitation (FEV_1 and % predicted), the magnitude of symptoms measured with specific questionnaires, and the frequency of exacerbations (Table 34.2). The requirement to demonstrate airflow obstruction ensures that individuals with chronic respiratory symptoms such as dyspnoea, recurrent cough, and sputum are not misdiagnosed as having COPD.

The diagnosis of asthma (differential diagnosis with COPD)

According to the 2017 update of the Global Strategy for Asthma Management and Prevention,[52] asthma is 'a heterogeneous disease, usually characterized by chronic airway inflammation, defined by the history of respiratory symptoms such as wheeze, shortness of

Table 34.2 COPD assessment according to the 2017 GOLD report [104]

Severity of airflow limitation		Symptoms and exacerbation		
STAGE	FEV_1 (% predicted)	STAGE	symptoms	exacerbation history
GOLD 1 (mild)	≥ 80	A	less symptoms*	non-frequent#
GOLD 2 (moderate)	50 – 79	B	more symptoms*	non-frequent#
GOLD 3 (severe)	30 – 49	C	less symptoms*	frequent#
GOLD 4 (very severe)	< 30	D	more symptoms*	frequent#

Aim of spirometric assessment	Aim of ABCD assessment tool
- confirm diagnosis and assess prognosis	-consider patient-reported outcomes and highlight the importance of exacerbation prevention
-selected therapeutic decisions (e.g. interventional procedures)	-therapeutic recommendations (pharmacologic treatment algorithms is based on ABCD)
- identification of rapid decline	

* symptoms are measured with standardized questionnaire; less symptoms are defined as mMRC 0-1 or CAT <10; more symptoms are defined as mMRC ≥ 2 or CAT ≥ 10.

non-frequent exacerbation are defined as 0 -1 exacerbation per year, not leading to hospital admission; frequent exacerbations are defined as ≥ 2 exacerbations per year, or at least 1 exacerbation leading to hospital admission.

CAT = COPD Assessment Test; COPD = chronic obstructive pulmonary disease; GOLD = Global Initiative for Chronic Obstructive Lung Disease; FEV_1= forced expiratory volume in the 1st second; mMRC= modified British Medical Research Council questionnaire.

breath, chest tightness and cough that vary over time and in intensity, together with variable expiratory airflow limitation'. As symptoms characteristically vary over time, it is not unusual for asthmatic patients to be completely asymptomatic for weeks or months at a time, and then experience episodic flare-ups, triggered by factors such as allergen exposure, cold air, respiratory infections, and exercise.[53] Similarly, bronchial obstruction is reversible, and may not always be present, which differs significantly from COPD where airflow obstruction is persistent.[54] Thus, normal spirometry does not exclude the diagnosis of asthma, while it excludes the diagnosis of COPD. Furthermore, in patients with a baseline obstructive pattern, a change in FEV_1 >12% and >200 mL in response to inhaled bronchodilators favours the diagnosis of asthma rather than COPD. Finally, although asthma can start at any age, the first symptoms such as wheezing and bronchial hyper-responsiveness are generally detected during childhood,[55,56] whereas COPD is a disease of adulthood.[57] However, some patients may have clinical features of both asthma and COPD, and the term asthma–COPD overlap syndrome has been recently introduced to describe this clinical entity.[58] The differential diagnosis between asthma and COPD is relevant also in the setting of heart failure, since management strategy may differ (e.g. stronger caution to β-blockers in asthmatic patients).

Clinical assessment of the patient with chronic lung disease

The clinical history and examination provide important clues for identifying patients whose predominating problem is chronic lung disease. Patients with COPD have a history of exposure to noxious stimuli (mostly cigarette smoke), complain of persistent and progressive dyspnoea, often coupled with chronic cough and sputum; they report more frequent or prolonged 'winter colds,' or seek consultations for 'chest infections', which are usually mild exacerbations.[59]

Cough is usually the first symptom to develop, at first intermittently and sometimes unproductive. Regular production of sputum for at least three months in two consecutive years is indicative of chronic bronchitis, and possibly underlying bronchiectasis. However, this pattern is not typical of COPD, where sputum production is variable.[60] The pattern of breathlessness is unhelpful in distinguishing respiratory from cardiac disease, but prominent wheeze is more suggestive of COPD. Orthopnoea is seen with advanced COPD, and is also a prominent symptom in patients with diaphragmatic weakness due to neuromuscular disease. Paroxysmal nocturnal dyspnoea is typically considered a feature of heart failure, but may occur in patients with asthma, and less commonly in patients with very advanced COPD. Chest tightness is a frequent complaint of patients with COPD, but usually associated with new infective symptoms or bouts of prolonged coughing.

The physical examination is rarely diagnostic in COPD, since the most typical signs usually occur in advanced disease.[1] Lung auscultation may be normal, although in more severe patients wheezing and prolonged expiration are often present.[61] Early inspiratory crackles at the lung bases are sometimes heard and may be misinterpreted as indicating pulmonary oedema if the patient has a cardiac history. Signs of hyperinflation (a barrel chest, pursed lip breathing, and the use of accessory muscles of respiration) correlate with emphysema and indicate severe COPD. With severe disease, weight loss and anorexia are also common.

Imaging of the lung

Chest radiography is often the first test in patients with respiratory symptoms, as it is rapid, inexpensive and readily available. The presence of bullae and the indirect signs of hyperinflation and vascular alterations suggest pulmonary emphysema, whereas bronchial wall thickening and increased lung markings indicate chronic bronchitis, both common in COPD patients.[62] Other signs indicating COPD are lung hyperinflation with flattened diaphragm and increased retrosternal volume, hyperlucency of the lungs, and rapid tapering of the vascular markings. However, sensitivity and specificity are low in mild disease, and a chest X-ray is recommended mostly to exclude other diseases. Similarly, computed tomography (CT) of the chest is not routinely recommended, except in patients with additional indication, e.g. to exclude other lung disease (**Figures 33.1** and **33.2**).

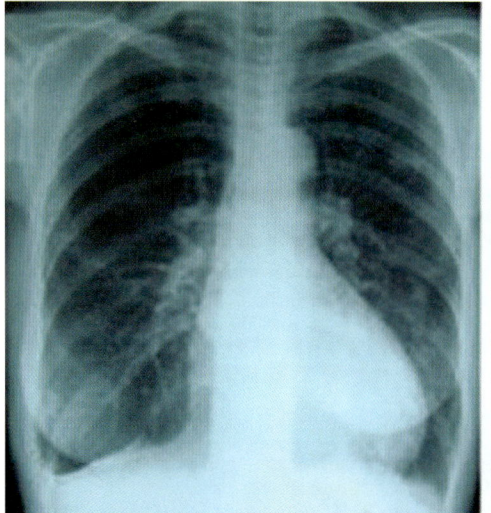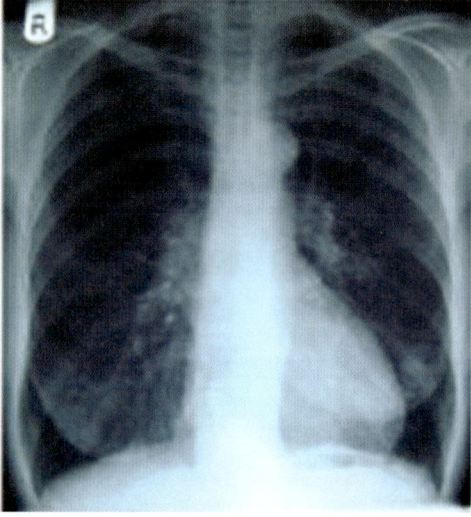

Figure 34.1 A 60-year-old woman with severe chronic obstructive pulmonary disorder and cardiac failure secondary to mitral valve disease and impaired left ventricular systolic function. (a) There are small bilateral pleural effusions, Kerley B lines at the right base, and pulmonary venous distension in the left upper lobe. There is no venous diversion to the right upper lobe because of her severe emphysema. (b) Following treatment the costophrenic angles are preserved and the subtle changes in the left upper lobe have resolved.

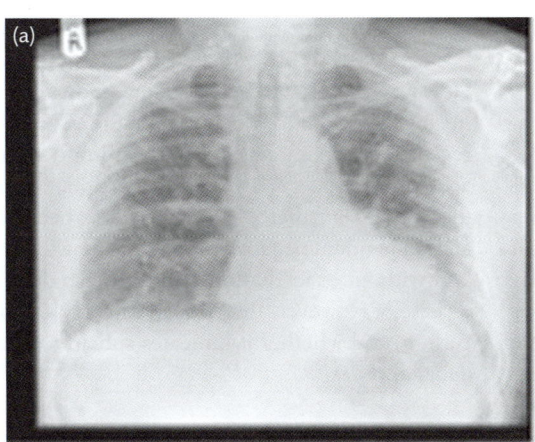
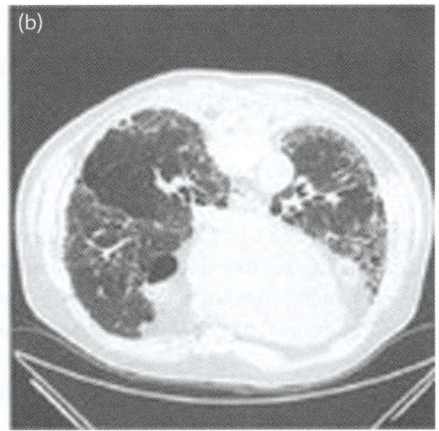

Figure 34.2 A 74-year-old man with previous coronary artery surgery and hypertension with a three-month history of progressive dyspnoea. (a) Plain chest radiograph shows borderline cardiomegaly and 'congested' lung fields with interstitial shadowing. (b) Prone high-resolution computed tomography shows bilateral lower lobe fibrosis with predominantly subpleural reticulation and honeycombing suggestive of idiopathic pulmonary fibrosis.

Lung ultrasound has increased in contemporary practice, especially in the hospital setting, with the ability to identify pleural effusions, pneumothoraces, alveolar consolidation, and interstitial syndrome. It is particularly useful in the patient with acute severe respiratory symptoms, to separate the differential diagnosis between acute exacerbation of COPD, acute heart failure, and other diseases.[63] For example, lung sliding with posterior B-lines usually indicates haemodynamic pulmonary oedema; abolished lung sliding is suggestive of pneumothorax; and anterior lung consolidation or unilateral lung signs suggest pneumonia.[64]

Imaging of the heart in COPD

Echocardiography is often unsatisfactory in patients with COPD due to poor acoustic windows, usually related to air trapping. In about 10% of COPD patients from a primary care study echocardiographic images were unsatisfactory, and this prevalence may increase to 50% in COPD patients with very severe airflow obstruction.[65]

Nevertheless, echocardiography remains the cornerstone of heart failure assessment. Although the diagnosis of HFrEF is straightforward (left ventricular ejection fraction <40%),[66] that of HFpEF is challenging in the context of pulmonary disease. Recent guidelines

have attempted to simplify the multitude of diastolic parameters,[66,67] many of which require good-quality echocardiographic images. Moreover, the aforementioned alterations in thoracic pressure and ventricular filling undoubtedly influence those diastolic measures which are volume dependent. Accordingly, estimates of the prevalence of HFpEF and diastolic dysfunction vary widely, and prospective studies including echocardiographic parameters are scarce and small (Table 34.3). Important questions are whether these alterations truly represent 'heart failure', impact symptoms and outcomes, or are amenable to treatment.

Similarly, echocardiography is central to assessing right heart dysfunction. The classic paradigm of right heart failure due to COPD indicates that the right ventricle becomes hypertrophic and/or dilated in response to pulmonary hypertension. Interestingly, increased right ventricle wall thickness and altered right ventricular systolic function have been reported also in COPD patients without pulmonary hypertension at rest, suggesting that right heart disease may begin long before clinically evident pulmonary hypertension.[68]

Cardiac magnetic resonance imaging is the best alternative for patients with non-diagnostic echocardiographic studies, although

Table 34.3 Prospective studies reporting the prevalence of echocardiographic findings indicating HFpEF and/or diastolic dysfunction in patients with COPD

Study	COPD N	Setting	Age, mean (SD)	HFpEF n (%)	LVDD n (%)	Poor echographic window n (%)
Adler [105]	78	Inpatient	69 (9)	44%	NA	NA
Abrough [106]	238	Inpatient	68 (15)	NA	48 (20)	12 (5)
Boussuges [107]	52	Outpatient	60 (10)	NA	26 (50)	18 (35)
Huang [108]	75	Inpatient	83 (6)	38 (50)	48 (64)	NA
Kwon [109]	184[a]	Outpatient	74 (8)	98 (53)	NA	NA
Lopez-Sanchez [110]	71	Outpatient	65 (7)	NA	64 (90)	NA
Marcun [111]	127	Inpatient	70 (10)	22 (17)	NA	NA
Rutten [112]	405	Outpatient	73 (5)	41 (10)	NA	42 (10)

HFpEF, heart failure with preserved ejection fraction; COPD, chronic obstructive pulmonary disease; LVDD, left ventricle diastolic dysfunction; NA, not available; SD, standard deviation.
[a] Study population included patients with known COPD and heart failure.

Note: Table 34.3 references are present in the end of this chapter

its use may be limited by contraindications, higher costs, and lower availability as compared to echocardiography.[69]

Lung function testing for the diagnosis of COPD

As stated previously, only simple spirometry is necessary to detect airflow obstruction and diagnose COPD. Post-bronchodilator fixed ratio of $FEV_1/FVC <0.70$ is usually the spirometric criterion for significant airflow limitation, due to its simplicity. However, it may result in incorrect diagnoses, i.e. overdiagnosis in the elderly and underdiagnosis <45 years; therefore a cut-off based on the lower limit of normal values, or on z-scores, has been suggested in these patients.[1]

Spirometry also defines the severity of airflow limitation, according to percentage predicted FEV_1. However, sometimes more detailed tests are required, particularly if the degree of the airflow obstruction seems at variance with the clinical picture. Since measurements of absolute lung volumes, such as residual volume and total lung capacity (TLC), are not obtained with a simple spirometry, different techniques have been developed, such as body plethysmography, nitrogen washout, and gas dilution.[70] COPD patients typically exhibit gas trapping, manifesting as a rise in residual volume, and static hyperinflation in more severe disease, increasing TLC.

Peak expiratory flow meters may be useful for recognizing changes in airway calibre, especially in asthmatic patients, but are inadequate for making a new diagnosis of COPD and are therefore not currently recommended, due to low specificity.[1]

Lung function testing in cardiac disease

In the setting of heart failure, spirometry should be performed only when the patient is stable and euvolaemic.[71] In patients with acute congestion, interstitial and submucosal oedema compress and obstruct the airways, and induce bronchial hyper-responsiveness, thus leading to an overestimation of airflow obstruction and of COPD severity.[72] FEV_1 consistently improves by 15–20% after treatment with diuretics. There is also a measurable reduction in vital capacity, which may take several weeks to return to normal.[73]

Furthermore, even stable patients with chronic heart failure may present an altered spirometry, usually exhibiting a restrictive pattern, reflecting cardiomegaly, respiratory muscle weakness, and interstitial fibrosis.[65] Therefore, in some heart failure patients with concomitant lung disease, the spirometric pattern may be mixed, or difficult to interpret. In these circumstances adjunctive tests with measurements of lung volumes may uncover hyperinflation and gas trapping, thus confirming the presence of COPD.[74]

Natriuretic peptides

Natriuretic peptides (NPs) are a useful diagnostic tool in patients with suspected heart failure thanks to their high negative predictive value, which practically rules-off the diagnosis in patients with low blood concentrations.

In patients with lung disease the diagnostic accuracy is reduced since concentrations may be elevated in the presence of acute and stable COPD, pulmonary hypertension, pulmonary emboli, and concurrent cardiac disease.[75] In patients with stable COPD, levels typically overlap with compensated heart failure, thus increasing the rate of false-positive results. While negative predictive values remain high, the specificity and positive predictive value are thus reduced.[76]

The picture during acute events is even more complex. NPs have been extensively investigated in undifferentiated acute dyspnoea. However, there have been very few studies examining utility in diagnosing heart failure during an acute exacerbation of COPD. In a recent systematic review, NP elevation occurred in 16–60% of exacerbations and persisted in approximately one-half of patients at discharge.[77] Further, NP elevation has been repeatedly reported as an independent negative prognostic marker in COPD patients, with and without exacerbations, and independent of associated cardiac disease.[78] However, the clinical interpretation of these data is uncertain, and whether it indicates subclinical cardiac involvement is debated.

General consideration on treatment

The central message when treating patients with heart failure and concomitant COPD is that the management of both conditions should not deviate from international guidelines. However, there are a few caveats to keep in mind.

β-Blockers in patients with heart failure and COPD: β-adrenoceptor blockade

The β-adrenoreceptors are G-protein-linked cell-surface receptors, which mediate different effects in different tissues, responding to catecholamine stimulation, especially adrenaline and noradrenaline. In the heart, β_1-receptors increase rate and contractility. β_1-Adrenoreceptor antagonism leads to left ventricular reverse remodelling, improving symptoms, morbidity, and mortality in landmark clinical trials. In the lungs, activation of β_2-receptors induces relaxation of bronchial smooth muscle and bronchodilation. Therefore, stimulating this mechanism has positive effects in patients with airflow obstruction.

This is the basis for one of the most relevant concerns regarding management of patients with concomitant heart failure and COPD, since β-antagonists are indicated for the first, and β-agonists are indicated for the latter. This apparent conflict has led to endless discussions on putative cardiac side-effects of COPD drugs, as well as concerns for bronchospasms with β-blocker use.[79]

Recent published data support an overall good safety profile of these drug regimens in co-morbid patients.

Under-use of β-blockers in patients with heart failure and COPD

In contrast to asthma, the airflow obstruction that characterizes COPD is largely irreversible post-bronchodilators, including β_2-agonists. Thus, there is no strict contraindication to β-blocker use, although β_1-selective drugs should be preferred.[66] Nevertheless, evidence from several studies suggests that β-blockers are under-used in patients with both heart failure and COPD. For example, in the 2003 Euro Heart Failure Survey, 'pulmonary disease' was the most powerful independent predictor of β-blocker under-use.[80] Similarly, in a large primary care survey in Scotland, only 18% of patients with heart failure and COPD were prescribed β-blockers compared with 41% for those without COPD.[9] Recently, there seems to be a positive trend: in the 2013 QUALIFY international survey on HFrEF, only 13% of all patients did not receive β-blockers, and only 28% of those due to concomitant lung disease.[81]

Do β-blockers make lung function worse in patients with COPD?

Putative negative effects of β-blockers on lung function include increased airflow obstruction, reduced FEV_1, and increased breathlessness. A few small studies have described a reduction in FEV_1 with β-blocker use, but without significant clinical implications.[82] Caution may be advised in patients with very severe impairment of lung function, such as COPD patients requiring long-term oxygen therapy, where β-blockers may not be beneficial, and could even be harmful.[83]

Cardioselective β-blockers such as bisoprolol and nebivolol exhibit much greater affinity for $β_1$-receptors than for β-receptors, and thus exert less effect on lung function. Carvedilol is the only non-cardioselective β-blocker indicated in heart failure. A few small prospective studies have addressed the topic of cardioselectivity in COPD, reporting that FEV_1 was lower with carvedilol and higher with bisoprolol, but 6 min walk distance and New York Heart Association functional class were not significantly different, and that switching between a $β_1$-selective to a non-selective β-blocker was well tolerated.[84] Similarly, a retrospective analysis from the OPTIMIZE-HF registry found no significant association between heart failure outcomes and β-blocker selectivity.[85] Again, this may be different in COPD patients with more severe disease, as β-blocker titration was better with bisoprolol than carvedilol in moderate/severe COPD.[86]

Finally, β-blockers are associated with improved outcomes, including all-cause mortality, in patients with COPD and concomitant heart disease, consistent with the landmark trials in the general heart failure population.[87] Therefore, β-blocker therapy is strongly indicated in heart failure patients with COPD, although cardioselective β-blockers are preferred.[66]

Other cardiovascular drugs

Concomitant lung disease does not pose specific concerns to drug treatments with medications such as angiotensin converting enzyme inhibitors, mineralocorticoid receptor antagonists, angiotensin receptor neprilysin inhibitor, or ivabradine, which should be prescribed according to usual indications.[88]

Cardiovascular effects of bronchodilators

The cardiac safety of bronchodilators has been broadly discussed, and questions have been raised on putative pro-arrhythmic effects and increased risk of adverse cardiac events including mortality.[89] Published data suggest an overall good safety profile of drugs such as long-acting muscarinic antagonists (LAMA) and long-acting $β_2$-agonists (LABA),[90] although safety information specifically in heart failure patients is limited.

Early observational studies demonstrated a dose–response relationship between risk of heart failure hospitalization/death and use of inhaled β-agonists in HFrEF, although mostly referring to short-acting β-agonist compounds,[91] though clinical trials suggested reasonable cardiac safety.[90] More recent evidence is still contradictory. In a retrospective analysis from the Ontario population-based COPD registry of elderly patients ($n = 191\,005$), new users of LABA or tiotropium were at higher risk of hospitalization or emergency department visit for heart failure, especially in the first two to three weeks (adjusted odds ratio: 1.31 (95% CI: 1.12–1.52) and

1.14 (1.01–1.28)).[92] Conversely, no significant correlation between LABA and mortality was reported in 1294 elderly patients enrolled in a longitudinal, retrospective, single centre Irish heart failure registry.[93] Likewise, no significant differences in cardiac events, including heart failure, were observed in a retrospective analysis of new users of LABA compared to tiotropium from a UK primary care database ($n = 463\,899$).[94]

The cardiac safety of LAMA has been similarly debated, again with conflicting results. Short-acting bronchodilators, such as ipratropium, may slightly increase the risk of heart failure, whereas there appears no additional risk of heart failure with LAMA such as tiotropium. Accordingly, two large randomized clinical trials examining tiotropium in patients with COPD reported no excess mortality, exacerbation, or major cardiovascular adverse events, including no additional risk of incident heart failure.[93,95,96]

Conclusively, the recent SUMMIT trial[97] evaluated the combined treatment with inhaled corticosteroid (fluticasone furoate) and LABA (vilanterol) in 16 485 patients with moderate COPD and a history, or increased risk, of cardiovascular disease. This trial, the largest survival study to date in the setting of heightened cardiovascular risk, confirmed the cardiovascular safety of these drugs. However, heart failure patients with severely reduced ejection fraction were excluded, and no heart-failure-specific analysis has been published to date.

Amiodarone pulmonary toxicity

Lung disease in patients treated with amiodarone was first described when used as an investigational drug in the USA in the early 1980s.[98] At the time, amiodarone was widely prescribed in the UK and continental Europe, with >500 000 patient-years of experience, but an association between amiodarone and pulmonary toxicity had never been reported.

Subsequent reports indicated that the risk of amiodarone pulmonary toxicity (APT) was likely dose-related (generally ≥400 mg/day) and that clinical manifestations usually appeared within a few weeks or months of initiating treatment.[99] Current estimates indicate a 2–5% incidence rate of APT, more frequent in older patients, with higher doses, and with longer duration of therapy.[100]

APT may be asymptomatic, or manifest as cough, progressive breathlessness, occasionally fever and chest pain, sometimes with crackles on lung auscultation. The clinical presentation is generally diffuse interstitial lung disease or a hypersensitivity syndrome, which may mimic infection. Less commonly, patients may manifest acute respiratory distress syndrome, pulmonary nodules, or pleural effusions. CT generally shows diffuse ground glass and reticular abnormalities, indicating ongoing inflammatory and fibrotic changes. Pathologic findings include interstitial pneumonitis, organizing pneumonia, focal foamy alveolar macrophages, or diffuse alveolar damage (Figure 34.3). None of these clinical or radiological features are specific, and other diagnoses need to be considered and excluded.[101]

The mechanism of APT seems to be directly related to the pharmacokinetics of amiodarone. Following absorption from the gastrointestinal tract, lipid-soluble amiodarone is distributed to fat and many other tissues, including lung, thyroid, kidney, and liver. It has a long half-life (~30 days) and a slow release from the tissues. Macrophages, including pulmonary macrophages, show lipidosis and a characteristic foamy appearance with multilamellar lysosomal

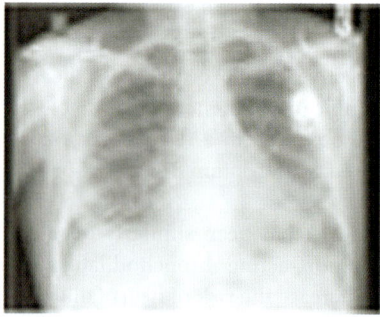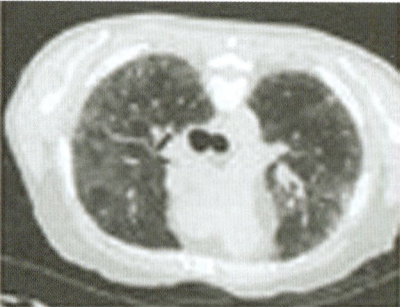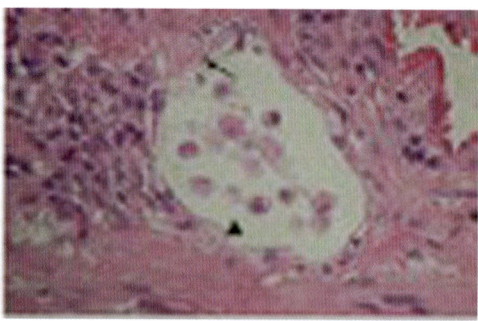

Figure 34.3 Amiodarone pulmonary toxicity. (a) Chest radiograph demonstrating bilateral interstitial shadowing. The patient has a ventricular pacemaker and has had previous coronary artery bypass surgery. (b) High-resolution computed tomography, performed with the patient lying prone, showing bilateral fibrosis and ground-glass change. (c) Histology of a video-assisted thoracoscopic lung biopsy demonstrating foamy type II alveolar epithelial cells (arrow) and alveolar spaces filled with macrophages (arrowhead). Other areas of the biopsy showed interstitial chronic inflammation and fibrosis, and scattered areas of organizing pneumonia.

inclusions. The tissue accumulation mirrors sites of toxic effects of amiodarone, so drug sequestration is probably the main determinant of toxicity, acting likely through an enhanced and abnormal inflammatory response.[102] However, the precise mechanism of amiodarone-induced tissue injury remains unknown.

Periodic follow-up of patients treated with amiodarone, with baseline and yearly chest X-ray, and possibly serial pulmonary function testing has been repeatedly suggested, although the true clinical utility remains unproven.[100] Further testing, such as CT, bronchoscopy with bronchoalveolar lavage, or lung biopsy may be useful in selected cases of suspected APT, to exclude other diagnosis.

Treatment of APT consists of discontinuing amiodarone and, in severe cases, administration of corticosteroids. Usually, 40–60 mg/day of prednisone is prescribed. The dose can be decreased after 4–8 weeks to minimize side-effects, although prolonged therapy may be required. Mortality rates reach 10% in severely ill patients, but are substantially lower in the general population, especially when the diagnosis is made early.[103]

REFERENCES

1. Vogelmeier CF, Criner GJ, Martinez FJ, *et al.* Global Strategy for the Diagnosis, Management, and Prevention of Chronic Obstructive Lung Disease 2017 Report: GOLD Executive Summary. *Eur Respir J* 2017;**195**(5):557–82.
2. Roversi S, Fabbri LM, Sin DD, Hawkins NM, Agustí A. Chronic obstructive pulmonary disease and cardiac diseases: an urgent need for integrated care. *Am J Respir Crit Care Med* 2016;**194**(11):1319–36.
3. Rushton CA, Satchithananda DK, Jones PW, *et al.* Non-cardiovascular comorbidity, severity and prognosis in non-selected heart failure populations: a systematic review and meta-analysis. *Int J Cardiol* 2015;**196**:98–106.
4. Müllerova H, Agusti A, Erqou S, *et al.* Cardiovascular comorbidity in COPD. Systematic literature review. *Chest* 2013;**144**:1163–78.
5. Konecny T, Park JY, Somers KR, *et al.* Relation of chronic obstructive pulmonary disease to atrial and ventricular arrhythmias. *Am J Cardiol* 2014;**114**:272–7.
6. Chen W, Thomas J, Sadatsafavi M, *et al.* Risk of cardiovascular comorbidity in patients with chronic obstructive pulmonary disease: a systematic review and meta-analysis. *Lancet Respir Med* 2015;**3**:631–9.

7. Dalsgaard M, Plesner LL, Schou M, *et al.* Prevalence of airflow obstruction in patients with stable systolic heart failure. *BMC Pulm Med* 2017;**17**:6.
8. Canepa M, Straburzynska-Migaj E, Drozdz J, *et al.* Characteristics, treatments and 1-year prognosis of hospitalized and ambulatory heart failure patients with chronic obstructive pulmonary disease in the European Society of Cardiology Heart Failure Long-Term Registry. *Eur J Heart Fail* 2018;**20**(1):100–10.
9. Hawkins NM, Jhund PS, Simpson CR, *et al.* Primary care burden and treatment of patients with heart failure and chronic obstructive pulmonary disease in Scotland. *Eur J Heart Fail* 2010;**12**:17–24.
10. Mentz RJ, Kelly JP, von Lueder TG, *et al.* Noncardiac comorbidities in heart failure with reduced versus preserved ejection fraction. *J Am Coll Cardiol* 2014;**64**:2281–93.
11. Rusinaru D, Saaidi I, Godard S, *et al.* Impact of chronic obstructive pulmonary disease on long-term outcome of patients hospitalized for heart failure. *Am J Cardiol* 2008;**101**:353–8.
12. Hawkins NM, Huang Z, Pieper KS, *et al.* Chronic obstructive pulmonary disease is an independent predictor of death but not atherosclerotic events in patients with myocardial infarction: analysis of the Valsartan in Acute Myocardial Infarction Trial (VALIANT). *Eur J Heart Fail* 2009;**11**:292–8.
13. Lahousse L, Niemeijer MN, van den Berg ME, *et al.* Chronic obstructive pulmonary disease and sudden cardiac death: the Rotterdam study. *Eur Heart J* 2015;**36**:1754–61.
14. Arnaudis B, Lairez O, Escamilla R, Fouilloux A, Fournier P, Monteil B, et al. Impact of chronic obstructive pulmonary disease severity on symptoms and prognosis in patients with systolic heart failure. *Clin Res Cardiol Off J Ger Card Soc.* 2012 Sep;**101**(9):717–26.
15. Apostolovic S, Jankovic-Tomasevic R, Salinger-Martinovic S, Djordjevic-Radojkovic D, Stanojevic D, Pavlovic M, et al. Frequency and significance of unrecognized chronic obstructive pulmonary disease in elderly patients with stable heart failure. *Aging Clin Exp Res.* 2011 Dec;**23**(5-6):337–42.
16. Bektas S, Franssen FME, van Empel V, Uszko-Lencer N, Boyne J, Knackstedt C, et al. Impact of airflow limitation in chronic heart failure. *Neth Heart J Mon J Neth Soc Cardiol Neth Heart Found.* 2017 May;**25**(5):335–42.
17. Boschetto P, Fucili A, Stendardo M, Malagù M, Parrinello G, Casimirri E, et al. Occurrence and impact of chronic obstructive pulmonary disease in elderly patients with stable heart failure. *Respirol Carlton Vic.* 2013 Jan;**18**(1):125–30.

18. Dalsgaard M, Plesner LL, Schou M, Kjøller E, Vestbo J, Iversen K. Prevalence of airflow obstruction in patients with stable systolic heart failure. *BMC Pulm Med.* 2017 Jan 6;**17**(1):6.

19. Iversen KK, Kjaergaard J, Akkan D, Kober L, Torp-Pedersen C, Hassager C, et al. Chronic obstructive pulmonary disease in patients admitted with heart failure. *J Intern Med.* 2008 Oct;**264**(4):361–9.

20. Steinacher R, Parissis JT, Strohmer B, Eichinger J, Rottlaender D, Hoppe UC, et al. Comparison between ATS/ERS age- and gender-adjusted criteria and GOLD criteria for the detection of irreversible airway obstruction in chronic heart failure. *Clin Res Cardiol Off J Ger Card Soc.* 2012 Aug;**101**(8):637–45.

21. Valk MJ, Broekhuizen BD, Mosterd A, Zuithoff NP, Hoes AW, Rutten FH. COPD in patients with stable heart failure in the primary care setting. *Int J Chron Obstruct Pulmon Dis.* 2015;**10**:1219–24.

22. Wada H, Nakano Y, Nagao T, Osawa M, Yamada H, Sakaguchi C, et al. Detection and prevalence of chronic obstructive pulmonary disease in a cardiovascular clinic: evaluation using a hand held FEV_1/FEV_6 meter and questionnaire. *Respirol Carlton Vic.* 2010 Nov;**15**(8):1252–8.

23. Rodríguez LAG, Wallander M-A, Martín-Merino E, *et al.* Heart failure, myocardial infarction, lung cancer and death in COPD patients: a UK primary care study. *Respir Med* 2010;**104**:1691–9.

24. Zvezdin B, Milutinov S, Kojicic M, *et al.* A postmortem analysis of major causes of early death in patients hospitalized with COPD exacerbation. *Chest* 2009;**136**:376–80.

25. McGarvey LP, John M, Anderson JA, *et al.* Ascertainment of cause-specific mortality in COPD: operations of the TORCH Clinical Endpoint Committee. *Thorax* 2007;**62**:411–15.

26. Rothnie KJ, Yan R, Smeeth L, *et al.* Risk of myocardial infarction (MI) and death following MI in people with chronic obstructive pulmonary disease (COPD): a systematic review and meta-analysis. *BMJ Open* 2015;**5**:e007824.

27. Sin DD, Wu L, Man SFP. The relationship between reduced lung function and cardiovascular mortality: a population-based study and a systematic review of the literature. *Chest* 2005;**127**:1952–9.

28. Tockman MS, Pearson JD, Fleg JL, *et al.* Rapid decline in FEV1. A new risk factor for coronary heart disease mortality. *Am J Respir Crit Care Med* 1995;**151**:390–8.

29. Li J, Agarwal SK, Alonso A, *et al.* Airflow obstruction, lung function, and incidence of atrial fibrillation: the Atherosclerosis Risk in Communities (ARIC) study. *Circulation* 2014;**129**:971–80.

30. Agarwal SK, Heiss G, Barr RG, *et al.* Airflow obstruction, lung function, and risk of incident heart failure: the Atherosclerosis Risk in Communities (ARIC) study. *Eur J Heart Fail* 2012;**14**:414–22.

31. Wannamethee SG, Shaper AG, Papacosta O, *et al.* Lung function and airway obstruction: associations with circulating markers of cardiac function and incident heart failure in older men—the British Regional Heart Study. *Thorax* 2016;**71**:526–34.

32. Boussuges A, Pinet C, Molenat F, *et al.* Left atrial and ventricular filling in chronic obstructive pulmonary disease. An echocardiographic and Doppler study. *Am J Respir Crit Care Med* 2000;**162**:670–5.

33. Seeger W, Adir Y, Barberà JA, *et al.* Pulmonary hypertension in chronic lung diseases. *J Am Coll Cardiol* 2013;**62**:D109–16.

34. Han MK, McLaughlin VV, Criner GJ, *et al.* Pulmonary diseases and the heart. *Circulation* 2007;**116**:2992–3005.

35. Naeije R. Pulmonary hypertension and right heart failure in chronic obstructive pulmonary disease. *Proc Am Thorac Soc* 2005;**2**:20–2.

36. Weitzenblum E. Chronic cor pulmonale. *Heart* 2003;**89**:225–30.

37. Van Gestel AJR, Steier J. Autonomic dysfunction in patients with chronic obstructive pulmonary disease (COPD). *J Thorac Dis* 2010;**2**:215–22.

38. Maclay J, MacNee W. Cardiovascular disease in COPD—mechanisms. *Chest* 2013;**143**:789–807.

39. Patel ARC, Kowlessar BS, Donaldson GC, *et al.* Cardiovascular risk, myocardial injury, and exacerbations of chronic obstructive pulmonary disease. *Am J Respir Crit Care Med* 2013;**188**:1091–9.

40. Sabit R, Bolton CE, Fraser AG, *et al.* Sub-clinical left and right ventricular dysfunction in patients with COPD. *Respir Med* 2010;**104**:1171–8.

41. Smith BM, Kawut SM, Bluemke DA, *et al.* Pulmonary hyperinflation and left ventricular mass: the Multi-Ethnic Study of Atherosclerosis COPD Study. *Circulation* 2013;**127**:1503–11, 1511e1–6.

42. Smith BM, Prince MR, Hoffman EA, *et al.* Impaired left ventricular filling in COPD and emphysema: is it the heart or the lungs? The Multi-Ethnic Study of Atherosclerosis COPD Study. *Chest* 2013;**144**:1143–51.

43. Sinnige J, Korevaar JC, Westert GP, *et al.* Multimorbidity patterns in a primary care population aged 55 years and over. *Fam Pract* 2015;**32**:505–13.

44. Mentz RJ, Fiuzat M, Wojdyla DM, *et al.* Clinical characteristics and outcomes of hospitalized heart failure patients with systolic dysfunction and chronic obstructive pulmonary disease: findings from OPTIMIZE-HF. *Eur J Heart Fail* 2012;**14**:395–403.

45. De Blois J, Simard S, Atar D, *et al.* COPD predicts mortality in HF: the Norwegian Heart Failure Registry. *J Card Fail* 2010;**16**:225–9.

46. Van Deursen VM, Urso R, Laroche C, *et al.* Co-morbidities in patients with heart failure: an analysis of the European Heart Failure Pilot Survey. *Eur J Heart Fail* 2014;**16**:103–11.

47. Hawkins NM. Chronic obstructive pulmonary disease and heart failure in Europe—further evidence of the need for integrated care. *Eur J Heart Fail* 2018;**20**:111–13.

48. Mosterd A, Hoes AW. Reducing hospitalizations for heart failure. *Eur Heart J* 2002;**23**:842–5.

49. Macchia A, Monte S, Romero M, *et al.* The prognostic influence of chronic obstructive pulmonary disease in patients hospitalised for chronic heart failure. *Eur J Heart Fail* 2007;**9**:942–8.

50. Drost EM, Skwarski KM, Sauleda J, *et al.* Oxidative stress and airway inflammation in severe exacerbations of COPD. *Thorax* 2005;**60**:293–300.

51. Miller MR, Hankinson J, Brusasco V, *et al.* Standardisation of spirometry. *Eur Respir J* 2005;**26**:319–38. doi:10.1183/09031936.05.00034805

52. GINA Report, Global Strategy for Asthma Management and Prevention | Documents/Resources | GINA. http://www.ginasthma.org/documents/4

53. Fabbri LM, Romagnoli M, Corbetta L, *et al.* Differences in airway inflammation in patients with fixed airflow obstruction due to asthma or chronic obstructive pulmonary disease. *Am J Respir Crit Care Med* 2003;**167**:418–24. doi:10.1164/rccm.200203-183OC

54. Martinez FD, Vercelli D. Asthma. *The Lancet* 2013;**382**:1360–72. doi:10.1016/S0140-6736(13)61536-6

55. Eder W, Ege MJ, von Mutius E. The asthma epidemic. *N Engl J Med* 2006;**355**:2226–35. doi:10.1056/NEJMra054308

56. British Thoracic Society Scottish Intercollegiate Guidelines Network. British Guideline on the Management of Asthma. *Thorax* 2008;**63 Suppl 4**:iv1–121. doi:10.1136/thx.2008.097741

57. Kabra SK, Lodha R, Singhal T. Chronic obstructive pulmonary disease in children. *Indian J Pediatr* 2001;**68 Suppl 2**:S50–4.

58. Bateman ED, Reddel HK, Zyl-Smit RN van, *et al.* The asthma–COPD overlap syndrome: towards a revised taxonomy of chronic airways diseases? *Lancet Respir Med* 2015;**3**:719–28. doi:10.1016/S2213-2600(15)00254-4

59. Miravitlles M, Worth H, Soler Cataluña JJ, *et al.* Observational study to characterise 24-hour COPD symptoms and their relationship with patient-reported outcomes: results from the ASSESS study. *Respir Res* 2014;**15**:122. doi:10.1186/s12931-014-0122-1

60. Pauwels RA, Rabe KF. Burden and clinical features of chronic obstructive pulmonary disease (COPD). *Lancet Lond Engl* 2004;**364**:613–20. doi:10.1016/S0140-6736(04)16855-4

61. Brockhuizen BD, Sachs AP, Oostvogels R, *et al.* The diagnostic value of history and physical examination for COPD in suspected or known cases: a systematic review. *Fam Pract* 2009;**26**:260–8. doi:10.1093/fampra/cmp026

62. Muller N, Coxson H. Chronic obstructive pulmonary disease • 4: Imaging the lungs in patients with chronic obstructive pulmonary disease. *Thorax* 2002;**57**:982–5. doi:10.1136/thorax.57.11.982

63. Trovato GM, Sperandeo M. Sounds, ultrasounds, and artifacts: which clinical role for lung imaging? *Am J Respir Crit Care Med* 2013;**187**:780–1. doi:10.1164/ajrccm.187.7.780

64. Lichtenstein DA. BLUE-protocol and FALLS-protocol: two applications of lung ultrasound in the critically ill. *Chest* 2015;**147**:1659–70. doi:10.1378/chest.14-1313

65. Hawkins NM, Petrie MC, Jhund PS, *et al.* Heart failure and chronic obstructive pulmonary disease: diagnostic pitfalls and epidemiology. *Eur J Heart Fail* 2009;**11**:130–9. doi:10.1093/eurjhf/hfn013

66. Ponikowski P, Voors AA, Anker SD, *et al.* 2016 ESC Guidelines for the diagnosis and treatment of acute and chronic heart failure. *Eur Heart J* 2016;[**Epub ahead of print**]. doi:10.1093/eurheartj/ehw128

67. Nagueh SF, Smiseth OA, Appleton CP, *et al.* Recommendations for the evaluation of left ventricular diastolic function by echocardiography: an update from the American Society of Echocardiography and the European Association of Cardiovascular Imaging. *J Am Soc Echocardiogr Off Publ Am Soc Echocardiogr* 2016;**29**:277–314. doi:10.1016/j.echo.2016.01.011

68. Rubin LJ. Cor pulmonale revisited. *J Am Coll Cardiol* 2013;**62**:1112–3. doi:10.1016/j.jacc.2013.06.034

69. Kawut SM, Poor HD, Parikh MA, *et al.* Cor pulmonale parvus in chronic obstructive pulmonary disease and emphysema: the MESA COPD study. *J Am Coll Cardiol* 2014;**64**:2000–9. doi:10.1016/j.jacc.2014.07.991

70. Wanger J, Clausen JL, Coates A, *et al.* Standardisation of the measurement of lung volumes. *Eur Respir J* 2005;**26**:511–22. doi:10.1183/09031936.05.00035005

71. Light RW, George RB. Serial pulmonary function in patients with acute heart failure. *Arch Intern Med* 1983;**143**:429–33.

72. Puri S, Dutka DP, Baker BL, *et al.* Acute saline infusion reduces alveolar-capillary membrane conductance and increases airflow obstruction in patients with left ventricular dysfunction. *Circulation* 1999;**99**:1190–6.

73. Snashall PD, Chung KF. Airway obstruction and bronchial hyperresponsiveness in left ventricular failure and mitral stenosis. *Am Rev Respir Dis* 1991;**144**:945–56. doi:10.1164/ajrccm/144.4.945

74. Brenner S, Güder G, Berliner D, *et al.* Airway obstruction in systolic heart failure--COPD or congestion? *Int J Cardiol* 2013;**168**:1910–6. doi:10.1016/j.ijcard.2012.12.083

75. Bozkanat E, Tozkoparan E, Baysan O, *et al.* The significance of elevated brain natriuretic peptide levels in chronic obstructive pulmonary disease. *J Int Med Res* 2005;**33**:537–44.

76. Rutten FH, Cramer M-JM, Zuithoff NPA, *et al.* Comparison of B-type natriuretic peptide assays for identifying heart failure in stable elderly patients with a clinical diagnosis of chronic obstructive pulmonary disease. *Eur J Heart Fail* 2007;**9**:651–9. doi:10.1016/j.ejheart.2007.01.010

77. Hawkins NM, Khosla A, Virani SA, *et al.* B-type natriuretic peptides in chronic obstructive pulmonary disease: a systematic review. *BMC Pulm Med* 2017;**17**:11. doi:10.1186/s12890-016-0345-7

78. Pavasini R, Tavazzi G, Biscaglia S, *et al.* Amino terminal pro brain natriuretic peptide predicts all-cause mortality in patients with chronic obstructive pulmonary disease: Systematic review and meta-analysis. *Chron Respir Dis* 2017;**14**:117–26. doi:10.1177/1479972316674393

79. Hawkins NM, Petrie MC, Macdonald MR, *et al.* Heart failure and chronic obstructive pulmonary disease the quandary of beta-blockers and beta-agonists. *J Am Coll Cardiol* 2011;**57**:2127–38. doi:10.1016/j.jacc.2011.02.020

80. Komajda M, Follath F, Swedberg K, *et al.* The EuroHeart Failure Survey programme—a survey on the quality of care among patients with heart failure in Europe. Part 2: treatment. *Eur Heart J* 2003;**24**:464–74.

81. Komajda M, Anker SD, Cowie MR, *et al.* Physicians' adherence to guideline-recommended medications in heart failure with reduced ejection fraction: data from the QUALIFY global survey. *Eur J Heart Fail* 2016;**18**:514–22.

82. Key A, Parry M, West MA, *et al.* Effect of β-blockade on lung function, exercise performance and dynamic hyperinflation in people with arterial vascular disease with and without COPD. *BMJ Open Respir Res* 2017;**4**:e000164.

83. Ekström MP, Hermansson AB, Ström KE. Effects of cardiovascular drugs on mortality in severe chronic obstructive pulmonary disease. *Am J Respir Crit Care Med* 2013;**187**:715–20.

84. Jabbour A, Macdonald PS, Keogh AM, *et al.* Differences between beta-blockers in patients with chronic heart failure and chronic obstructive pulmonary disease: a randomized crossover trial. *J Am Coll Cardiol* 2010;**55**:1780–7.

85. Mentz RJ, Wojdyla D, Fiuzat M, *et al.* Association of beta-blocker use and selectivity with outcomes in patients with heart failure and chronic obstructive pulmonary disease (from OPTIMIZE-HF). *Am J Cardiol* 2013;**111**:582–7.

86. Lainscak M, Podbregar M, Kovacic D, *et al.* Differences between bisoprolol and carvedilol in patients with chronic heart failure and chronic obstructive pulmonary disease: a randomized trial. *Respir Med* 2011;**105**:S44–9.

87. Stefan MS, Rothberg MB, Priya A, *et al.* Association between β-blocker therapy and outcomes in patients hospitalised with acute exacerbations of chronic obstructive lung disease with underlying ischaemic heart disease, heart failure or hypertension. *Thorax* 2012;**67**:977–84.

88. Böhm M, Robertson M, Ford I, *et al.* Influence of cardiovascular and noncardiovascular co-morbidities on outcomes and treatment effect of heart rate reduction with ivabradine in stable heart failure (from the SHIFT Trial). *Am J Cardiol* 2015;**116**:1890–7.

89. Singh S, Loke YK, Enright P, *et al*. Pro-arrhythmic and pro-ischaemic effects of inhaled anticholinergic medications. *Thorax* 2013;**68**:114–16.

90. Lahousse L, Verhamme KM, Stricker BH, *et al*. Cardiac effects of current treatments of chronic obstructive pulmonary disease. *Lancet Respir Med* 2016;**4**:149–64.

91. Au DH, Udris EM, Curtis JR, *et al*. Association between chronic heart failure and inhaled beta-2-adrenoceptor agonists. *Am Heart J* 2004;**148**:915–20.

92. Gershon A, Croxford R, Calzavara A, *et al*. Cardiovascular safety of inhaled long-acting bronchodilators in individuals with chronic obstructive pulmonary disease. *JAMA Intern Med* 2013;**173**:1175–85.

93. Bermingham M, O'Callaghan E, Dawkins I, *et al*. Are beta2-agonists responsible for increased mortality in heart failure? *Eur J Heart Fail* 2011;**13**:885–91.

94. Suissa S, Dellaniello S, Ernst P. Long-acting bronchodilator initiation in COPD and the risk of adverse cardio-pulmonary events: a population-based comparative safety study. *Chest* Published Online First: 20 August 2016.

95. Wise RA, Anzueto A, Cotton D, *et al*. Tiotropium Respimat inhaler and the risk of death in COPD. *N Engl J Med* 2013;**369**:1491–501.

96. Tashkin DP, Leimer I, Metzdorf N, *et al*. Cardiac safety of tiotropium in patients with cardiac events: a retrospective analysis of the UPLIFT® trial. *Respir Res* 2015;**16**:65.

97. Vestbo J, Anderson JA, Brook RD, *et al*. Fluticasone furoate and vilanterol and survival in chronic obstructive pulmonary disease with heightened cardiovascular risk (SUMMIT): a double-blind randomised controlled trial. *Lancet Lond Engl* 2016;**387**:1817–26.

98. Rotmensch HH, Liron M, Tupilski M, *et al*. Possible association of pneumonitis with amiodarone therapy. *Am Heart J* 1980;**100**:412–13.

99. Sunderji R, Kanji Z, Gin K. Pulmonary effects of low dose amiodarone: a review of the risks and recommendations for surveillance. *Can J Cardiol* 2000;**16**:1435–40.

100. Effect of prophylactic amiodarone on mortality after acute myocardial infarction and in congestive heart failure: meta-analysis of individual data from 6500 patients in randomised trials. Amiodarone Trials Meta-Analysis Investigators. *Lancet Lond Engl* 1997;**350**:1417–24.

101. Goldschlager N, Epstein AE, Naccarelli GV, *et al*. A practical guide for clinicians who treat patients with amiodarone: 2007. *Heart Rhythm* 2007;**4**:1250–9.

102. Al-Shammari B, Khalifa M, Bakheet SA, *et al*. A mechanistic study on the amiodarone-induced pulmonary toxicity. *Oxid Med Cell Longev* 2016;**2016**:6265853.

103. Epstein AE, Olshansky B, Naccarelli GV, *et al*. Practical management guide for clinicians who treat patients with amiodarone. *Am J Med* 2016;**129**:468–75.

104. Vogelmeier CF, Criner GJ, Martinez FJ, Anzueto A, Barnes PJ, Bourbeau J, et al. Global Strategy for the Diagnosis, Management, and Prevention of Chronic Obstructive Lung Disease 2017 Report: GOLD Executive Summary. *Eur Respir J*. 2017 Jan 30;

105. Adler D, Pépin J-L, Dupuis-Lozeron E, Espa-Cervena K, Merlet-Violet R, Muller H, et al. Comorbidities and Subgroups of Patients Surviving Severe Acute Hypercapnic Respiratory Failure in the Intensive Care Unit. *Am J Respir Crit Care Med*. 2017 Jul 15;196(2):200–7.

106. Abroug F, Ouanes-Besbes L, Nciri N, Sellami N, Addad F, Hamda KB, et al. Association of Left-Heart Dysfunction with Severe Exacerbation of Chronic Obstructive Pulmonary Disease. *Am J Respir Crit Care Med*. 2006 Nov 1;174(9):990–6.

107. Boussuges A, Pinet C, Molenat F, Burnet H, Ambrosi P, Badier M, et al. Left atrial and ventricular filling in chronic obstructive pulmonary disease. An echocardiographic and Doppler study. *Am J Respir Crit Care Med*. 2000 Aug;162(2 Pt 1):670–5.

108. Huang Y-S, Feng Y-C, Zhang J, Bai L, Huang W, Li M, et al. Impact of chronic obstructive pulmonary diseases on left ventricular diastolic function in hospitalized elderly patients. *Clin Interv Aging*. 2015;10:81–7.

109. Kwon B-J, Kim D-B, Jang S-W, Yoo K-D, Moon K-W, Shim BJ, et al. Prognosis of heart failure patients with reduced and preserved ejection fraction and coexistent chronic obstructive pulmonary disease. *Eur J Heart Fail*. 2010 Dec;12(12):1339–44.

110. López-Sánchez M, Muñoz-Esquerre M, Huertas D, Gonzalez-Costello J, Ribas J, Manresa F, et al. High Prevalence of Left Ventricle Diastolic Dysfunction in Severe COPD Associated with A Low Exercise Capacity: A Cross-Sectional Study. *PLoS ONE* [Internet]. 2013 Jun 27 [cited 2017 Aug 31];8(6). Available from: http://www.ncbi.nlm.nih.gov/pmc/articles/PMC3694927/

111. Marcun R, Stankovic I, Vidakovic R, Farkas J, Kadivec S, Putnikovic B, et al. Prognostic implications of heart failure with preserved ejection fraction in patients with an exacerbation of chronic obstructive pulmonary disease. *Intern Emerg Med*. 2016 Jun;11(4):519–27.

112. Rutten FH, Cramer M-JM, Grobbee DE, Sachs APE, Kirkels JH, Lammers J-WJ, et al. Unrecognized heart failure in elderly patients with stable chronic obstructive pulmonary disease. *Eur Heart J*. 2005 Sep;26(18):1887–94.

35

Pulmonary hypertension

J. Simon R. Gibbs

Introduction

Pulmonary hypertension is at once a cause of heart failure as well as being caused by heart failure in some patients. It is becoming recognized as an increasing global health problem affecting 1% of the global population, rising to 10% in those aged >65 years.[1] As many as 30 million people worldwide aged >65 years might be affected by pulmonary hypertension due to left heart disease. Pulmonary hypertension worsens symptoms and increases mortality independently of its causative underlying disease. This chapter explores the haemodynamic and clinical classifications of pulmonary hypertension, its investigation, diagnosis, and treatment.

Haemodynamic definitions in pulmonary hypertension

Pulmonary hypertension is defined as a mean pulmonary artery pressure ≥25 mmHg at rest. Pulmonary hypertension is subdivided into pre-capillary and post-capillary pulmonary hypertension depending on the left heart filling pressures.

Pre-capillary pulmonary hypertension is associated with a pulmonary artery wedge pressure (PAWP) or left ventricular end-diastolic pressure ≤15 mmHg. In post-capillary pulmonary hypertension, PAWP is >15 mmHg.

Post-capillary pulmonary hypertension may be further subdivided into isolated post-capillary pulmonary hypertension (IPCPH) where there is no significant increase in vascular resistance in the pulmonary circulation and the driver of pulmonary hypertension is the elevated left heart filling pressures; and combined post-capillary and pre-capillary pulmonary hypertension (CPCPH) which is associated with increased pulmonary vascular resistance (PVR) in addition to the increased left heart filling pressures.[2] These subdivisions of post-capillary pulmonary hypertension were devised to identify patients with raised PVR who may be suitable for clinical trials and are of uncertain clinical value.

Clinical classification of pulmonary hypertension

For the purposes of clinical management, a classification is used which groups together diseases with similar pathophysiology, clinical presentation, and response to treatment. This classification contains five groups:[3] pulmonary arterial hypertension; pulmonary hypertension due to left heart disease; pulmonary hypertension due to lung diseases and/or hypoxia; chronic thromboembolic pulmonary hypertension and other pulmonary artery obstructions; and pulmonary hypertension with unclear and/or multifactorial mechanisms (see Box 35.1). The classification is in evolution as understanding of disease mechanisms and treatments improves.

Pulmonary arterial hypertension

Pulmonary arterial hypertension (PAH) is a rare form of pulmonary hypertension with an incidence of 1.1–7.6 per million adults per year and a prevalence of 6.6–26.0 per million.[4-6] Registries report that 58–81% of patients with PAH are female, although this female predominance is not seen in the elderly or consistently in other types of pulmonary hypertension.[7,8] There is a ratio of two females per male in heritable PAH.[9] Contemporary survival is 72–93% at one year[10-12] and 55–77% at three years[4,5,13,14] with females having better survival than males.[15]

The diagnosis requires pre-capillary haemodynamics (i.e. normal left ventricular filling pressure) plus a raised PVR >3 Wood units.[3] Other causes of pulmonary hypertension must be excluded. Some aetiologies of PAH may cause pulmonary hypertension by different mechanisms despite being grouped under PAH. For example, scleroderma-associated PAH may cause any one or combination of: PAH, pulmonary veno-occlusive disease (PVOD), pulmonary hypertension related to diffuse parenchymal lung disease, or pulmonary hypertension related to left ventricular disease.

PAH is associated with endothelial dysfunction which results in vasoconstriction and dysregulated proliferation of pulmonary artery smooth muscle cells, local inflammation and endothelial cells resistant to apoptosis.[16] These changes increase resistance to blood flow in small pulmonary arteries. Increased PVR causes right ventricular hypertrophy and dilation eventually leading to progressive right ventricular failure and ultimately death. The disease may progress rapidly over weeks to months in some patients whereas in others it may show little progress over years. Disease associated with *BMPR2* mutations occurs in younger patients and may be particularly aggressive.[17]

PVOD/pulmonary capillary haemangiomatosis (PCH) is a rare and rapidly progressive form of PAH with a predilection for

Box 35.1 Comprehensive clinical classification of pulmonary hypertension

1. Pulmonary arterial hypertension
   1.1 Idiopatic
   1.2 Heritable
      1.2.1 *BMPR2* mutation
      1.2.2 Other mutations
   1.3 Drugs and toxins induced
   1.4 Associated with:
      1.4.1 Connective tissue disease
      1.4.2 Human immunodeficiency virus (HIV) infection
      1.4.3 Portal hypertension
      1.4.4 Congenital heart diseases
      1.4.5 Schistosomiasis
      1.4.6 Chronic haemolytic anaemia
   1.5 Associated with significant venous or capillary involvement
      1.5.1 Pulmonary veno-occlusive disease
      1.5.2 Pulmonary capillary haemangiomatosis
   1.6 Persistent pulmonary hypertension of the newborn
2. Pulmonary hypertension due to left heart disease
   2.1 Left ventricular systolic dysfunction
   2.2 Left ventricular diastolic dysfunction
   2.3 Valvular disease
   2.4 Congenital/acquired left heart inflow/outflow tract obstruction and congenital cardiomyopathies
   2.5 Congenital/acquired pulmonary veins stenosis
3. Pulmonary hypertension due to lung disease and/or hypoxia
   3.1 Chronic obstructive pulmonary disease
   3.2 Interstitial lung disease
   3.3 Other pulmonary diseases with mixed restrictive and obstructive pattern
   3.4 Sleep-disordered breathing
   3.5 Alveolar hypoventilation disorders
   3.6 Chronic exposure to high altitude
   3.7 Developmental lung disease
4. Chronic thromboembolic pulmonary hypertension and other pulmonary artery obstructions
   4.1 Chronic thromboembolic pulmonary
   4.2 Other pulmonary artery obstructions
      4.2.1 Angiosarcoma
      4.2.2 Other intravascular tumors
      4.2.3 Arteritis
      4.2.4 Congenital pulmonary arteries stenosis
      4.2.5 Parasites (hydatidosis)
5. Pulmonary hypertension with unclear and/or multifactorial mechanisms
   5.1 Haematological disorders: chronic haemolytic anaemia, myeloproliferative disorders, splenectomy
   5.2 Systemic disorders, sarcoidosis, pulmonary histiocytosis, lymphangioleiomyomatosis
   5.3 Metabolic disorders: glycogen storage disease, Gaucher disease, thyroid disorders
   5.4 Others: pulmonary tumoral thrombothic microangiopathy, fibrosing mediastinitis, chronic renal failure (with/without dialysis). Segmental pulmonary hypertension

Reproduced from Galie N, Humbert M, Vachiery JL, *et al.* 2015 ESC/ERS Guidelines for the diagnosis and treatment of pulmonary hypertension: The Joint Task Force for the Diagnosis and Treatment of Pulmonary Hypertension of the European Society of Cardiology (ESC) and the European Respiratory Society (ERS): Endorsed by: Association for European Paediatric and Congenital Cardiology (AEPC), International Society for Heart and Lung Transplantation (ISHLT). *European Heart Journal* 2016;**37**:67–119 with permission from Oxford University Press.

pulmonary veins. In its familial form it is associated with a rare autosomal recessive mutation of the *EIF2AK4* gene.[18] Family members who develop the disease must have the mutation on both copies of their gene and thus only a single generation in a family is affected.

Pulmonary hypertension due to left heart disease

Left heart disease is a common cause of pulmonary hypertension particularly in the elderly. The presence of left ventricular dysfunction, aortic and/or mitral valve disease, hypertension, diabetes mellitus, ischaemic heart disease, atrial fibrillation and raised body mass index suggest this cause. The pathophysiology of pulmonary hypertension due to left heart disease is illustrated in **Figure 35.1**. Left ventricular disease requires an elevation of filling pressure to maintain cardiac output. This results in enlargement of the left atrium due to raised pressure whose effect on the pulmonary circulation may be exacerbated by increased stiffness of the left atrium. Functional mitral regurgitation also increases left atrial pressure and typically this worsens on exercise.[19] Pulmonary artery pressure must increase to compensate for the raised left atrial pressure and gives rise to pulmonary vascular remodelling.

Pulmonary hypertension due to lung disease

Lung disease and/or hypoxia is another common cause of pulmonary hypertension associated with pre-capillary haemodynamics and poor survival.[20] Typically, the lung diseases responsible are chronic obstructive pulmonary disease (COPD), idiopathic pulmonary fibrosis (IPF), and combined pulmonary fibrosis and emphysema (CPFE).[21] The pathophysiology is associated with loss of lung units, hypoxic pulmonary vasoconstriction, pulmonary vascular remodelling, and hyperinflation. Haemodynamics are divided into lung disease causing pulmonary hypertension (mean pulmonary artery pressure ≥ 25 mmHg) or severe pulmonary hypertension (mean pulmonary artery pressure >35 mmHg or mean pulmonary artery pressure ≥ 25 mmHg in the presence of a low cardiac output (<2.5 L/min/m^2) not explained by other causes.[21] Severe pulmonary hypertension in the setting of isolated lung disease is uncommon and additional left heart disease or chronic thromboembolic disease should be considered.

Chronic thromboembolic pulmonary hypertension

Chronic thromboembolic pulmonary hypertension (CTEPH) is a rare form of pulmonary hypertension with an incidence of 0.9–4.0 cases per million population per annum.[1,22] Around 75% of patients present with a history of pulmonary embolism.[22] The risk of a patient with pulmonary embolism going on to develop CTEPH appears to be very low despite cohort studies suggesting that it occurs in 1.0–8.8% of all cases of pulmonary embolism;[23–25] these numbers are likely to be an exaggeration. If CTEPH develops after pulmonary embolism, it does so within two years of the initial event.[26]

The mechanism of persistent thrombosis may be related to disordered angiogenesis and results in thrombotic material becoming incorporated within the pulmonary artery wall as fibrous material.[27,28] The disease manifests as proximal obstructions in the pulmonary arteries as well as a distal small vessel disease which includes PAH-like lesions of muscularized arterioles.[28] Note that some patients with previous pulmonary embolism complain of persistent

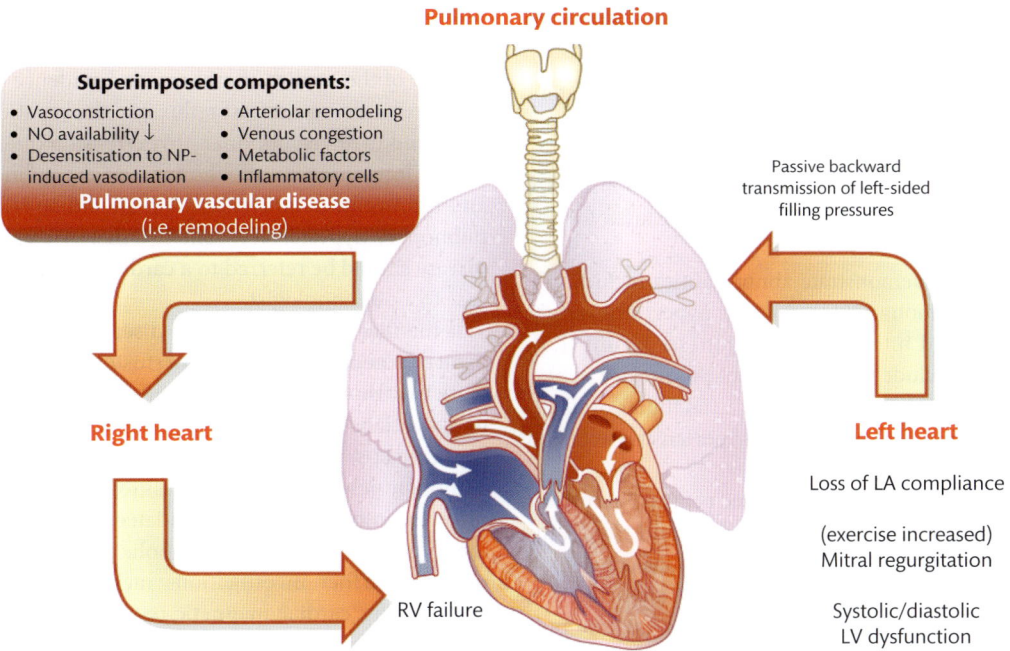

Figure 35.1 Cardiopulmonary interaction and pathobiology of pulmonary hypertension (PH) in left ventricular heart failure.
Reproduced from Rosenkranz S, Gibbs JS, Wachter R, De Marco T, Vonk-Noordegraaf A and Vachiery JL. Left ventricular heart failure and pulmonary hypertension. *European Heart Journal* 2016;**37**:942–54, with permission from Oxford University Press.

breathlessness which may be related to ventilation perfusion mismatch as a result of pulmonary arterial obstructions even in the absence of pulmonary hypertension.

Pulmonary hypertension with unclear and/or multifactorial mechanisms

The group of diseases causing pulmonary hypertension with unclear and/or multifactorial mechanisms are a diverse collection of conditions, some of which are rare. Each should be assessed individually at a specialist pulmonary hypertension centre.

Clinical presentation

Pulmonary hypertension presents with non-specific symptoms and their progression is usually related to deteriorating right ventricular function. The main symptoms of breathlessness, fatigue, syncope, and angina occur initially on exertion and only in late disease at rest. Some patients develop symptoms of heart failure before a diagnosis is made and complain of abdominal distension and swollen ankles. Symptom severity is classified according to World Health Organization (WHO) functional class (**Box 35.2**). Occasionally patients present with symptoms related to activation of the Bezold–Jarisch reflex, including exercise-induced nausea and vomiting. Some patients also complain of dry cough.

Patients may also present with complications of pulmonary hypertension such as haemoptysis related to rupture of hypertrophied bronchial arteries. Pulmonary artery expansion may give rise to hoarseness from left recurrent laryngeal nerve compression, wheeze caused by large airway compression, and angina pectoris caused by left main-stem coronary artery compression.

Physical examination may reveal signs of right ventricular hypertrophy with accentuation of the pulmonary second sound, a right ventricular third sound, tricuspid regurgitation and pulmonary regurgitation. In severe pulmonary hypertension the jugular venous pressure may be elevated and there may be hepatomegaly, ascites, peripheral oedema and signs of low cardiac output with cool peripheries. Adventitial sounds in the chest are usually absent. The examination may also reveal signs of systemic diseases underlying pulmonary hypertension itself.

Box 35.2 World Health Organization functional class

- Class I: Patients with pulmonary hypertension but without resulting limitation of physical activity. Ordinary physical activity does not cause undue dyspnoea or fatigue, chest pain or near syncope.
- Class II: Patients with pulmonary hypertension resulting in slight limitation of physical activity. They are comfortable at rest. Ordinary physical activity causes undue dyspnoea or fatigue, chest pain or near syncope.
- Class III: Patients with pulmonary hypertension resulting in marked limitation of physical activity. They are comfortable at rest. Less than ordinary activity causes undue dyspnoea or fatigue, chest pain or near syncope.
- Class IV: Patients with pulmonary hypertension with inability to carry out any physical activity without symptoms. These patients' manifest signs of right heart failure. Dyspnoea and/or fatigue may even be present at rest. Discomfort is increased by any physical activity.

Reproduced from Galie N, Humbert M, Vachiery JL, *et al.* 2015 ESC/ERS Guidelines for the diagnosis and treatment of pulmonary hypertension: The Joint Task Force for the Diagnosis and Treatment of Pulmonary Hypertension of the European Society of Cardiology (ESC) and the European Respiratory Society (ERS): Endorsed by: Association for European Paediatric and Congenital Cardiology (AEPC), International Society for Heart and Lung Transplantation (ISHLT). *European Heart Journal* 2016;**37**:67–119 with permission from Oxford University Press.

Investigation and diagnosis

The investigation of a patient with suspected pulmonary hypertension should begin with an ECG, chest radiograph, pulmonary function tests, routine blood tests, and an echocardiogram. These simple investigations may confirm that further investigation of pulmonary hypertension is necessary or may reveal alternative causes for the patient symptoms.

Although the ECG may demonstrate abnormalities including P pulmonale, right axis deviation, right ventricular hypertrophy, right bundle branch block, and QT interval prolongation (see Figure 31.5), a normal ECG does not exclude the diagnosis of pulmonary hypertension. Supraventricular arrhythmias such as atrial flutter or fibrillation may be observed in severe pulmonary hypertension and lead to decompensation of heart failure.

The plain chest radiograph may show enlarged central pulmonary arteries as well as enlargement of the right atrium and right ventricle. It may also reveal evidence of pulmonary venous congestion caused by left heart disease as well as parenchymal abnormalities in lung disease. A normal chest radiograph does not exclude pulmonary hypertension, and minor but significant pulmonary artery enlargement may go unreported.

Pulmonary function tests are used to identify patients with parenchymal lung disease or airways disease. Mild to moderate reduction of lung volumes is seen in PAH.[29,30] Lung diffusing capacity may be normal or mildly reduced in PAH. Marked reduction of TLCO (<45% of predicted transfer capacity for carbon monoxide) is usually associated with PVOD, PAH associated with scleroderma and/or parenchymal lung disease.[30] Low diffusing capacity is associated with a poor prognosis. Patients with COPD demonstrate evidence of airflow obstruction and increased residual volumes with a low diffusing capacity. CPFE may pseudo-normalize spirometry, although computed tomography (CT) will reveal the diagnosis.[31,32] This emphasizes the importance of combining imaging with pulmonary function tests to assess lung disease.

Transthoracic echocardiography is used to estimate an echocardiographic probability of pulmonary hypertension in patients in whom it is suspected. The echocardiography algorithm recommended in European guidelines calculates probability based initially on peak tricuspid regurgitation velocity (TRV) as low, intermediate, or high risk.[3] Additional echocardiographic information is required to determine risk when the peak TRV is ≤3.4 m/s. These additional measurements concerning the right ventricle, pulmonary artery, and inferior vena cava and right atrium were chosen because they can be reliably made in most patients. Taking into account co-morbid diseases associated with pulmonary hypertension, patients who are at intermediate or high risk should undergo further investigation for pulmonary hypertension whereas in those at low risk an alternative diagnosis should be sought (**Figure 35.2**). At this stage, patients who are at high risk and who have a family history of PAH, or rapidly progressing symptoms and/or syncope, may be considered for direct fast-track referral to a specialist pulmonary hypertension centre.

The next step in investigating pulmonary hypertension is to determine whether it is caused by left heart disease and/or lung disease. This will normally require CT of the chest as well as arterial blood gases. Whereas high-resolution CT of the chest is recommended, CT pulmonary angiography captures the lung windows as well as providing evidence for pulmonary thromboembolism/CTEPH, sinus venosus defect and anomalies of pulmonary venous drainage, the size of the cardiac chambers, and evidence of raised right atrial pressure based on contrast reflux into the hepatic veins. Patients who are found to have pulmonary hypertension due to left heart disease and/or lung disease and who have severe pulmonary hypertension and right ventricular dysfunction should be referred to a specialist pulmonary hypertension centre. Otherwise patients with left heart disease should be referred to a cardiologist and those with lung disease to a pulmonologist.

If the diagnosis of left heart disease or lung disease is not confirmed, a nuclear ventilation perfusion scan should be undertaken to detect thromboembolism and the patient should be referred to a specialist pulmonary hypertension centre. The nuclear scan is the most sensitive technique at present for detecting CTEPH.[33] Although newer imaging modalities will likely supersede this, no other techniques have been validated. If the appearances of the scan are consistent with thromboembolic disease then the patient should undergo further investigations including two of CT pulmonary angiography, cardiac magnetic resonance pulmonary angiography, and selective pulmonary angiography (see **Figure 35.3**). These investigations are best carried out in a specialist pulmonary hypertension centre to provide imaging of a standard sufficient to make a treatment decision about surgery for CTEPH.

Patients with a negative ventilation perfusion scan require further evaluation for PAH or pulmonary hypertension with unclear and/or multifactorial mechanisms to determine the aetiology including serology to test for rare causes of PAH causes as well as liver ultrasound to look for evidence of portal hypertension. Further investigation for possible causes of pulmonary hypertension may be necessary.

Cardiac catheterization comes at the end of the list of investigations since it can be used to answer questions raised by other investigations. Haemodynamic testing requires accurate pressure measurements with particular attention to PAWP since errors in this measurement may result in an incorrect haemodynamic diagnosis.[34,35] Where doubt exists about a PAWP measurement, left ventricular end-diastolic pressure should be measured directly. The zero calibration of fluid-filled catheter pressure transducers should be at a point half the height of the chest when the patient is lying on the catheterization table.[36] Pressures should be measured at end expiration during free breathing as well as during held expiration. The recordings should be reviewed to verify that the measurements are valid. An example of pressure traces found in pulmonary hypertension is shown in **Figure 35.4**. Cardiac output measurement is also prone to errors and should be measured either by direct Fick (using measured oxygen consumption) or thermodilution (not useful if a right-to-left shunt is present).[37] The use of fluid loading and exercise testing during haemodynamic catheterization is used by many laboratories—for example, to differentiate pre- and post-capillary haemodynamics in some patients—but is not validated. How the results of these interventions should be used for clinical diagnosis is uncertain.

Diagnosis and diagnostic controversies

The final step in diagnosis is to review of the results of comprehensive investigation at a multidisciplinary team meeting to determine the final diagnosis according to the clinical classification. Where

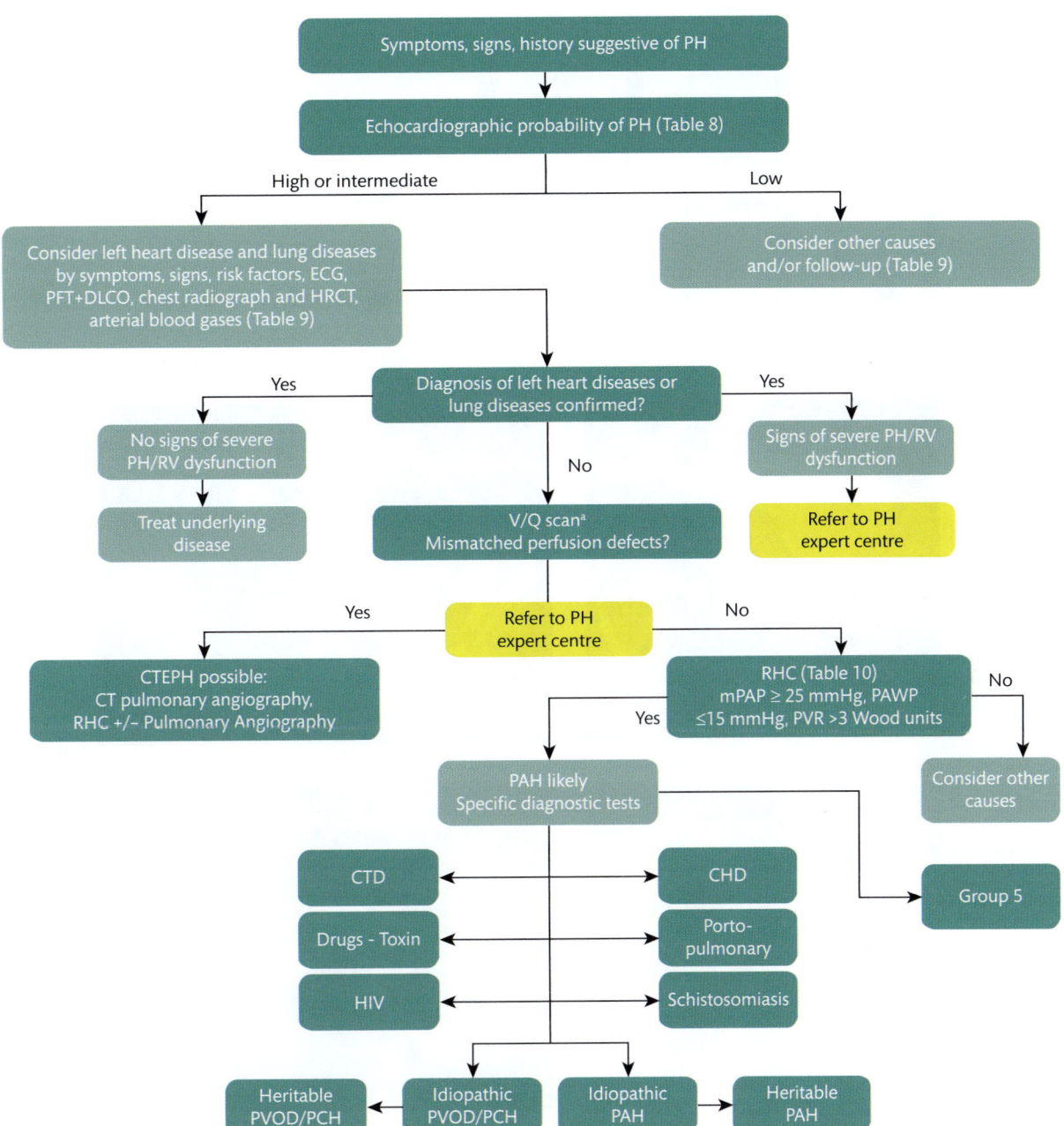

CHD = congenital heart diseases; CT = computed tomography; CTD = connective tissue disease; CTEPH = chronic thromboembolic pulmonary hypertension; DLCO = carbon monoxide diffusing capacity; ECG = electrocardiogram; HIV = Human immunodeficiency virus; HR-CT = high resolution CT; mPAP = mean pulmonary arterial pressure; PA = pulmonary angiography; PAH = pulmonary arterial hypertension; PAWP = pulmonary artery wedge pressure; PFT = pulmonary function tests; PH = pulmonary hypertension; PVOD/PCH = pulmonary veno-occlusive disease or pulmonary capillary hemangiomathosis; PVR = pulmonary vascular resistance; RHC = right heart catheterisation; RV = right ventricular; V/Q = ventilation/perfusion.
a CT pulmonary angiography alone may miss diagnosis of chronic thromboembolic pulmonary hypertension.

Figure 35.2 Diagnostic algorithm for pulmonary hypertension (2015).

Reproduced from Galie N, Humbert M, Vachiery JL, *et al.* 2015 ESC/ERS Guidelines for the diagnosis and treatment of pulmonary hypertension: The Joint Task Force for the Diagnosis and Treatment of Pulmonary Hypertension of the European Society of Cardiology (ESC) and the European Respiratory Society (ERS): Endorsed by: Association for European Paediatric and Congenital Cardiology (AEPC), International Society for Heart and Lung Transplantation (ISHLT). *European Heart Journal* 2016;**37**:67–119 with permission from Oxford University Press.

doubt exists, the most likely diagnosis can be tested with a therapeutic trial.

With increasing age and multiple co-morbidities, patients may have several causes of pulmonary hypertension. In patients with multiple cardiovascular risk factors and pre-capillary haemodynamics, the differential diagnosis between pulmonary hypertension due to left heart disease, especially heart failure with normal ejection fraction (HFnEF), and idiopathic PAH may require consideration. This clinical challenge arises when cardiac imaging does not detect left ventricular dysfunction or valvular heart disease. In the presence of

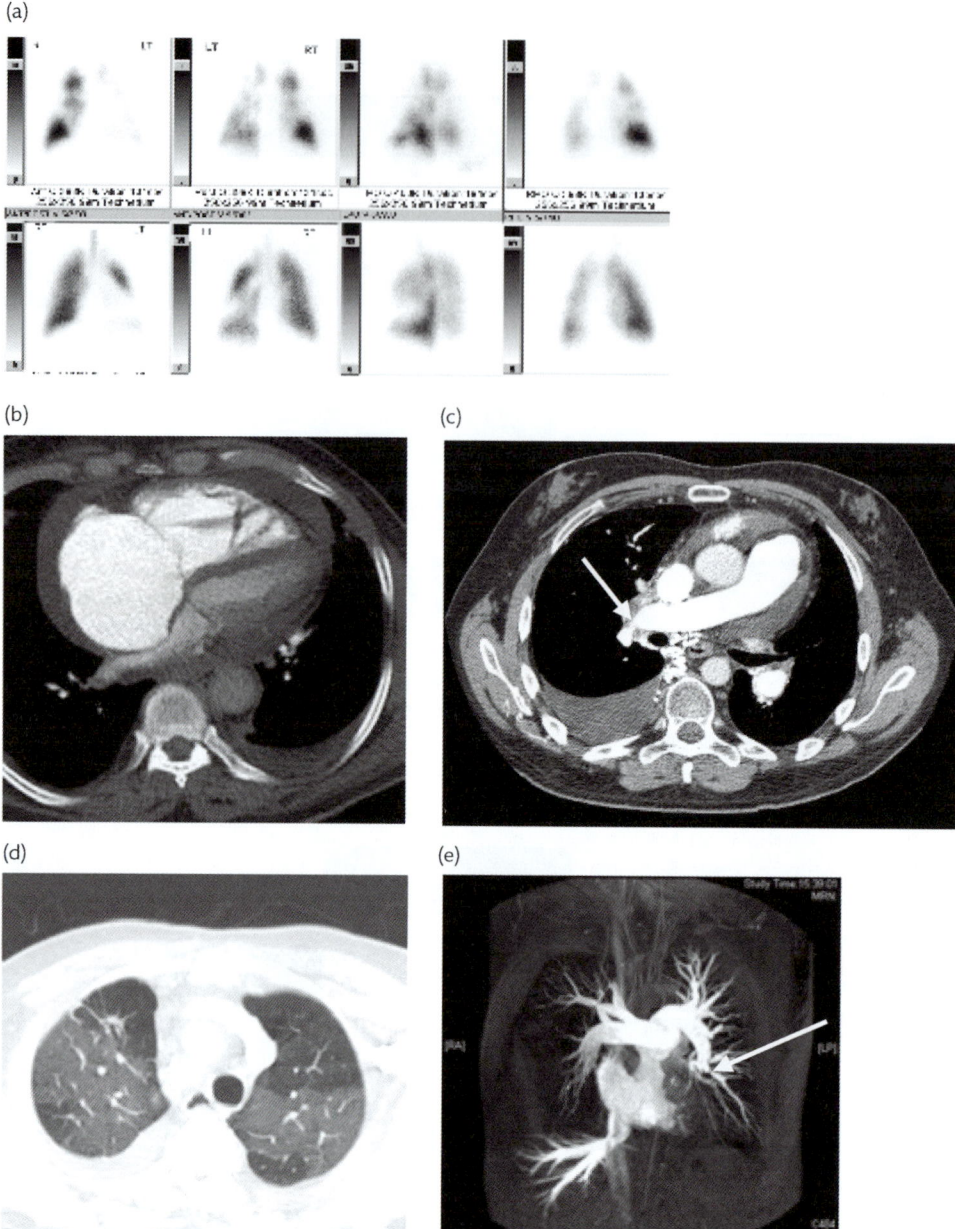

Figure 35.3 Typical imaging findings in chronic thromboembolic pulmonary hypertension (CTEPH). Nuclear ventilation perfusion scan (a) showing perfusion images (*top row*) and matching ventilation images (*bottom row*). Ventilated areas of lung show patchy perfusion mismatch. Computed tomography pulmonary angiogram shows an enlarged right atrium and dilated, hypertrophied right ventricle (b); a web causing stenosis of the right pulmonary artery (arrow) (c); mosaic perfusion of lung parenchyma (d) showing dark underperfused lung and denser normally perfused lung; and magnetic resonance angiography (e) showing a left pulmonary artery web (arrow) as well as contrast reflux into the hepatic veins indication raised right atrial pressure.

cardiovascular risk factors and particularly left atrial dilation in a patient sinus rhythm, a diagnosis of pulmonary hypertension related to heart failure is most likely. Reliance on invasive haemodynamics alone to detect post-capillary pulmonary hypertension in patients with cardiovascular risk factors should be treated cautiously since these measurements are affected by several confounding factors, including normalization of left ventricular filling pressure with diuretics.[38] Of note, current guidelines recommend optimization of a patient's fluid balance before cardiac catheterization.

While it has been suggested that patients with several cardiovascular risk factors and pre-capillary haemodynamics should be classified as having 'atypical' PAH, unless there is a clear-cut definition, this diagnosis will not lead to evidence-based treatment. A continuous spectrum of the clinical phenotypes between idiopathic PAH and pulmonary hypertension due to heart failure with preserved ejection fraction (HFpEF) has been observed,[39] although current evidence suggests that PAH and pulmonary hypertension due to HNpEF are distinct diseases.

PVOD/PCH typically presents with rapid onset of progressive breathlessness, marked hypoxaemia, finger clubbing, and pleural effusions.[40] It is a differential diagnosis of pulmonary hypertension presenting with pulmonary oedema (itself usually caused by left

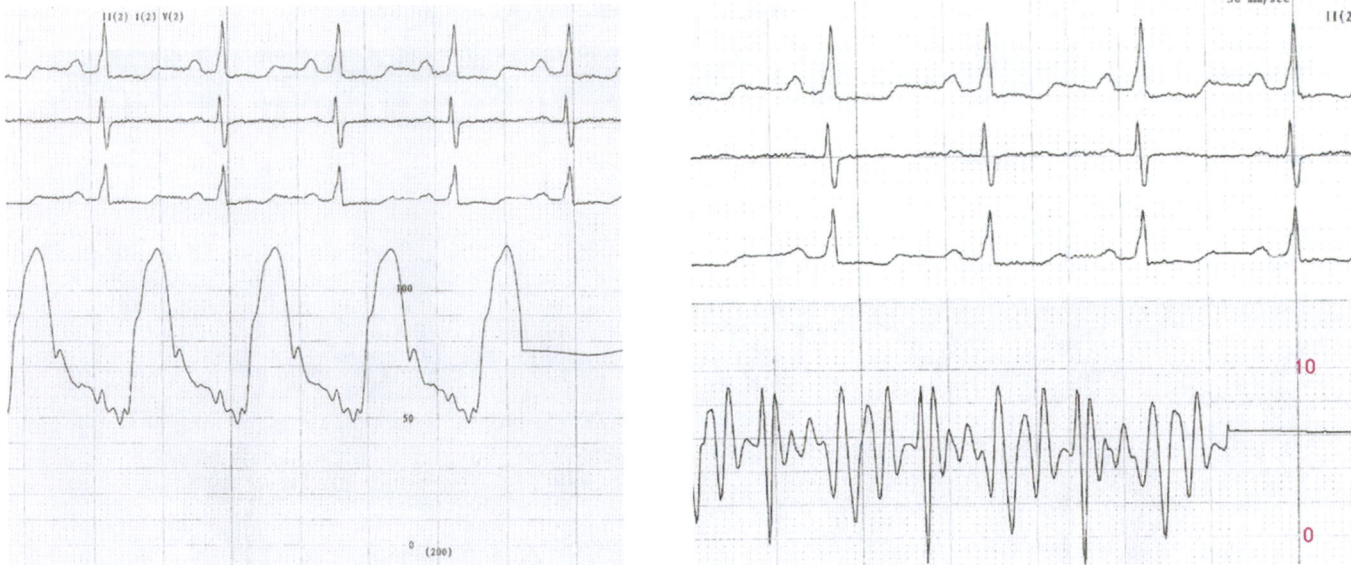

Figure 35.4 Invasive haemodynamics in pulmonary hypertension. Cardiac catheterization in a patient with pulmonary artery hypertension (PAH). The pulmonary artery pressure is high (*left*) whilst the pulmonary capillary wedge pressure (*right*) is normal.

heart disease) and thus requires exclusion of raised left ventricular filling pressure. Pulmonary function tests reveal low pulmonary diffusing capacity (TLCO <45% of predicted). The CT findings of pleural effusions, mediastinal lymphadenopathy, interlobular septal thickening, and parenchymal ground glass appearances are consistent with pulmonary oedema. If the PAWP is normal at the time of imaging and left heart function is normal on cardiac imaging, then the CT findings suggest PVOD/PCH (which remains a clinical diagnosis in most patients). Diagnostic certainty could be reached by lung biopsy but the high mortality of lung biopsy in pulmonary hypertension prohibits its use. Additional diagnostic information may be obtained by bronchoalveolar lavage in selected patients.

Treatment of pulmonary hypertension

Evidence from randomized controlled trials with drugs for pulmonary hypertension shows that patients with PAH gain benefit (and one of these treatments gives benefit in CTEPH), whereas patients with pulmonary hypertension due to left heart disease and pulmonary hypertension due to lung disease do not benefit and may even deteriorate on treatment directed at pulmonary hypertension.

Pulmonary arterial hypertension

For patients with a new diagnosis of PAH the first step towards treatment is to undertake a comprehensive prognostic evaluation and risk assessment (Table 35.1). This involves assessment of symptoms of breathlessness and syncope, the rate of progression of those symptoms, and clinical signs of right heart failure. Exercise capacity is assessed with a 6 min walk test and a cardiopulmonary exercise test (except in syncopal patients). B-type natriuretic peptide levels (NT-proBNP or BNP plasma levels) are included in the assessment. Cardiac imaging is used to determine right atrial area and whether a pericardial effusion is present; and haemodynamics are measured invasively including right atrial pressure, cardiac index, and mixed venous oxygen saturation. Based on this risk assessment, patients

are stratified as low risk, intermediate risk, or high risk. The aim of treatment is to obtain a low-risk risk profile.[41]

General treatment measures apply to all patients with PAH. These include: avoiding becoming pregnant since pulmonary hypertension carries a high maternal mortality; immunization against influenza and pneumococcal pneumonia; providing psychological and social support; supervised exercise training in physically deconditioned patients on stable medical therapy; in-flight administration of oxygen in patients in WHO functional classes III and IV and those with a PaO_2 consistently <8 kPa (60 mmHg); and the use of regional or epidural anaesthesia in patients requiring general surgery. Patients should be discouraged from excessive physical activity that leads to distressing symptoms.

Supportive drug therapy includes diuretics for decompensated right heart failure, and long-term oxygen therapy in patients whose PaO_2 is consistently <8 kPa (based on data from patients with COPD). The patients with idiopathic or heritable PAH and PAH associated with anorexigens may be considered for oral anticoagulation. Correction of anaemia and/or iron deficiency may be considered. Pulmonary haemodynamics may worsen in the presence of certain cardiovascular drugs including angiotensin converting enzyme inhibitors, angiotensin II receptor antagonists, β-blockers, and ivabradine.

At diagnosis all patients with idiopathic or heritable PAH and PAH associated with anorexigens should undergo acute vasoreactivity testing in the cardiac catheterization laboratory with nitric oxide or, if this is unavailable, with intravenous adenosine or epoprostenol (Figure 35.5). Patients with a positive vasoreactivity study, defined as a 10 mmHg fall in mean pulmonary artery pressure to a level <40 mmHg while maintaining or increasing cardiac output, should be treated with calcium channel blockers.[42,43] Nifedipine, diltiazem, or amlodipine are started at a low dose and progressively uptitrated to doses of 120 to 240 mg per day for nifedipine, 240 to 720 mg for diltiazem, and up to 20 mg for amlodipine. Uptitration may be limited by systemic hypotension or side-effects such as ankle swelling. The aim of treatment is to achieve WHO functional class I or II with near

Table 35.1 Risk assessment for pulmonary artery hypertension according to European guidelines 2015

Determinants of prognosis[a] (estimated 1-year mortality)	Low risk (<5%)	Intermediate risk (5–10%)	High risk (>10%)
Clinical signs of right heart failure	Absent	Absent	Present
Progression of symptoms	No	Slow	Rapid
Syncope	No	Occasional syncope[b]	Repeated syncope[c]
WHO functional class	I, II	III	IV
6MWD	>440 m	165–440 m	<165 m
Cardiopulmonary exercise testing	Peak VO$_2$ >15 mL/min/kg (>65% predicted) VE/VCO$_2$ slope <36	Peak VO$_2$ 11–15 mL/min/kg (35–65% predicted) VE/VCO$_2$ slope 36–44.9	Peak VO$_2$ <11 mL/min/kg (<35% predicted) VE/VCO$_2$ ≥45
NT-proBNP plasma levels	BNP <50 ng/L NT-proBNP <300 ng/mL	BNP 50–300 ng/L NT-proBNP 300–1400 ng/L	BNP >300 ng/L NT-proBNP >1400 ng/L
Imaging (echocardiography, CMR imaging)	RA area <18 cm² No pericardial effusion	RA area 18–26 cm² No or minimal, pericardial effusion	RA area >26 cm² Pericardial effusion
Haemodynamics	RAP <8 mmHg CI ≥2.5 L/min/m² SvO$_2$ >65%	RAP 8–14 mmHg CI 2.0–2.4 L/min/m² SvO$_2$ 60–65%	RAP >14 mmHg CI <2.0 L/min/m² SvO$_2$ <60%

[a] Most of the proposed variables and cut-off values are based on expert opinion. They may provide information and may be used to guide therapeutic decisions. but application to individual patients must be done carefully. One must also note that most of these variables have been validated mostly for IPAH and the cut-off levels used above may not necessarily apply to other forms of PAH. Furthermore, the use of approved therapies and their influence on the variables should be considered in the evaluation of the risk.

[b] Occasional syncope during brisk or heavy exercise, or occasional orthostatic syncope in an otherwise stable patient.

[c] Repeated episodes of syncope. Even with little or regular physical activity.

6MWD, 6 min walking distance; BNP, brain natriuretic peptide; CI, cardiac index; CMR, cardiac magnetic resonance; NT-proBNP, N-terminal pro-brain natriuretic peptide; RA, right atrium; RAP, right atrial pressure; SvO$_2$, mixed venous oxygen saturation; VE/VCO$_2$, ventilator equivalents for carbon dioxide; VO$_2$, oxygen consumption; WHO, World Health Organization.

Reproduced from Galie N, Humbert M, Vachiery JL, et al. 2015 ESC/ERS Guidelines for the diagnosis and treatment of pulmonary hypertension: The Joint Task Force for the Diagnosis and Treatment of Pulmonary Hypertension of the European Society of Cardiology (ESC) and the European Respiratory Society (ERS): Endorsed by: Association for European Paediatric and Congenital Cardiology (AEPC), International Society for Heart and Lung Transplantation (ISHLT). *European Heart Journal* 2016;**37**:67–119 with permission from Oxford University Press.

normalization of pulmonary haemodynamics. Vigilant long-term monitoring of these patients is important since they may suddenly fail to respond to calcium channel blockers despite a satisfactory initial response. In such circumstances they should be transitioned to other pulmonary hypertension drug therapies. Patients with a negative vasoreactivity study or those in whom the study was omitted should not be treated with calcium channel blockers since they may cause harm. Patients with other causes of PAH including connective tissue disease, HIV, portal hypertension, and PVOD should not undergo a vasoreactivity study since it does not predict a beneficial long-term response to calcium channel blockers.[44]

Patients with PAH should be offered drug therapy affecting one or more of three biochemical pathways shown in **Figure 35.6**.

Prostacyclin analogues

The first group of drugs to undergo a randomized controlled trial were the prostacyclin analogues which stimulate prostacyclin receptors. Prostacyclin is produced by endothelial cells and acts as a powerful vasodilator and inhibitor of platelet aggregation.[45] The parenteral prostacyclin analogues include epoprostenol, iloprost, and treprostinil.

- Epoprostenol has been shown to be beneficial in idiopathic PAH and PAH associated with scleroderma in three un-blinded randomized trials. It improves haemodynamics, symptoms, and exercise capacity and is the only drug shown to improve survival in a randomized controlled trial.[46–48] The drug is delivered via a permanent tunnelled intravenous

catheter with an infusion that runs continuously. Epoprostenol has a half-life of up to 5 min and acute withdrawal of a chronic infusion may result in rebound pulmonary hypertension with serious consequences. The main risk of a permanent intravenous catheter is septicaemia. Problems may also occur with catheter obstruction or fracture, infusion pump malfunction and a variety of problems with intravenous line connectors. This treatment should only be administered in patients who are capable and willing to manage such an intravenous infusion system. Some patients resist the use of intravenous prostacyclin analogues over oral agents, preferring to keep an intravenous infusion as a last resort. This may not, however, always be the best or safest treatment approach. Some epoprostenol preparations are unstable at room temperature for more than eight hours, but temperature-stable preparations are now available.

- Iloprost is a stable prostacyclin analogue which can be administered by inhalation of an aerosol or by intravenous infusion. Inhaled iloprost has been shown to improve haemodynamics and exercise capacity in a randomized controlled trial (RCT).[49] A further RCT of patients pre-treated with bosentan almost improved exercise capacity ($P < 0.051$).[50] Inhaled iloprost needs to be taken six to nine times a day. The frequency of inhalations, which take a few minutes, makes it inconvenient for some patients. Intravenous iloprost administered as a continuous infusion has been shown to be beneficial in a small series of patients.[51]

- Treprostinil is a stable prostacyclin analogue which can be administered by continuous subcutaneous infusion where it improves exercise capacity, haemodynamics, and symptoms, as well as by

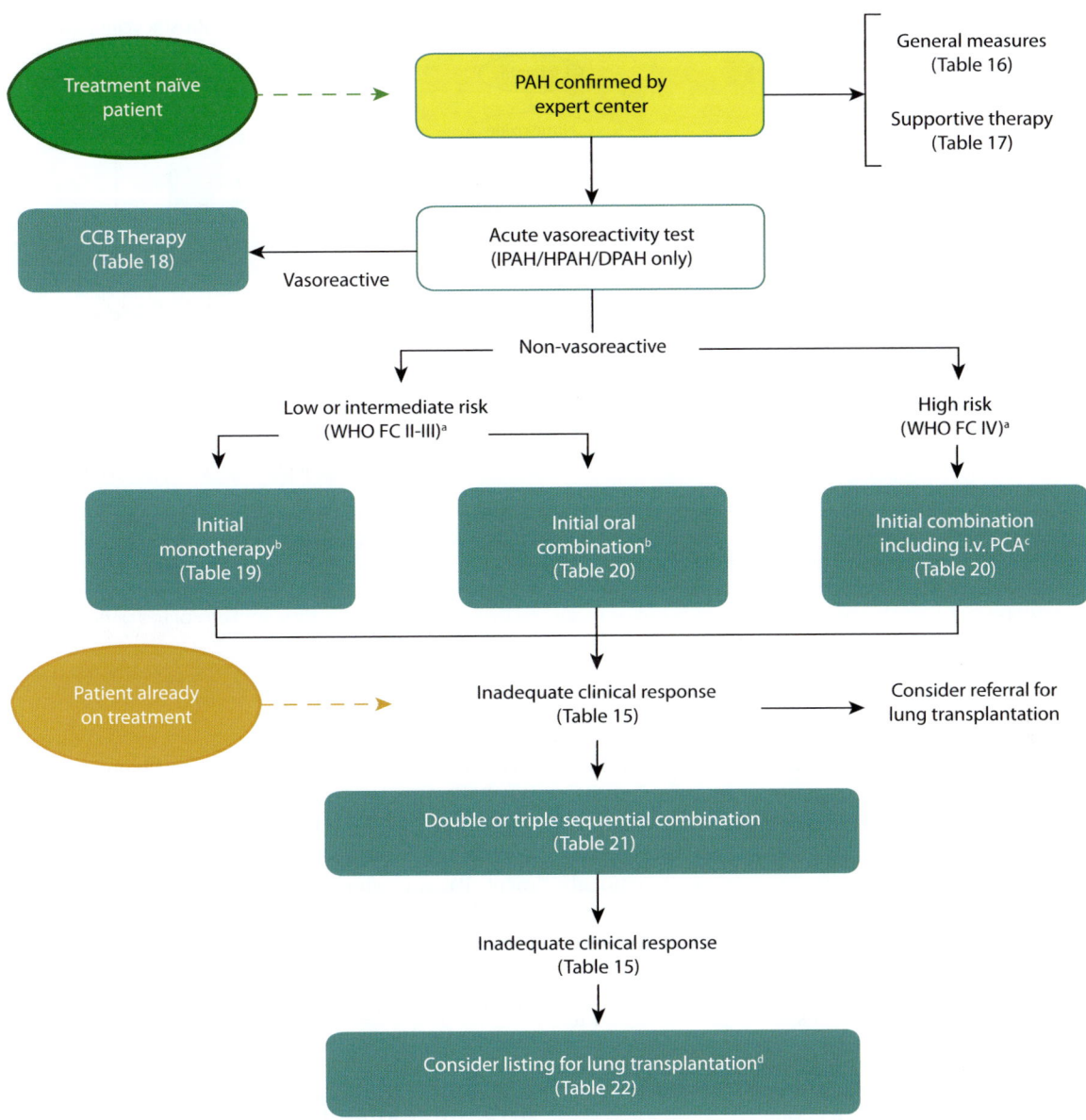

CCB = calcium channel blockers; DPAH = drug-induced PAH; HPAH = heritable PAH; IPAH = Idiopathic PAH; i.v. = intravenous; PAH = pulmonary arterial hypertension; PCA = prostacyclin analogues; WHO-FC = World Health Organization functional class.
[a]Some WHO-FC III patients may be considered high risk (See Table 13).
[b]Initial combination with ambrisentan plus tadalafil has proven to be superior to initial monotherapy with ambrisentan or tadalafil in delaying clinical failure.
[c]Intravenous epoprostenol should be prioritised as it has reduced the 3 months rate for mortality in high risk PAH patients also as monotherapy.
[d]Consider also balloon atrial septostomy.

Figure 35.5 Evidence-based treatment algorithm for pulmonary arterial hypertension (PAH) only (2015).

Reproduced from Galie N, Humbert M, Vachiery JL, *et al.* 2015 ESC/ERS Guidelines for the diagnosis and treatment of pulmonary hypertension: The Joint Task Force for the Diagnosis and Treatment of Pulmonary Hypertension of the European Society of Cardiology (ESC) and the European Respiratory Society (ERS): Endorsed by: Association for European Paediatric and Congenital Cardiology (AEPC), International Society for Heart and Lung Transplantation (ISHLT). *European Heart Journal* 2016;**37**:67–119 with permission from Oxford University Press.

intravenous infusion or inhalation. It has a longer half-life than epoprostenol and has been shown to be effective in RCTs of the subcutaneous,[52] inhaled,[53] and oral[54] preparations, although not all oral trials have been positive.[55,56] A major side-effect of subcutaneous infusion is local pain caused by stimulation of prostacyclin pain receptors.

All prostacyclin analogues may cause side-effects which include flushing, headache, jaw pain, generalized aching, nausea, vomiting, and diarrhoea.

Selexipag is an oral selective prostacyclin receptor (IP) agonist. Selexipag reduced composite morbidity and mortality in a randomized controlled trial.[57] This effect was demonstrated in treatment-naive patients as well as those on oral monotherapy or dual combination therapy. Selexipag is not a replacement for intravenous epoprostenol in high-risk patients.

Nitric oxide pathway

Drugs targeting the nitric oxide pathway are phosphodiesterase 5 (PDE5) inhibitors and guanylate cyclase stimulators. The PDE5

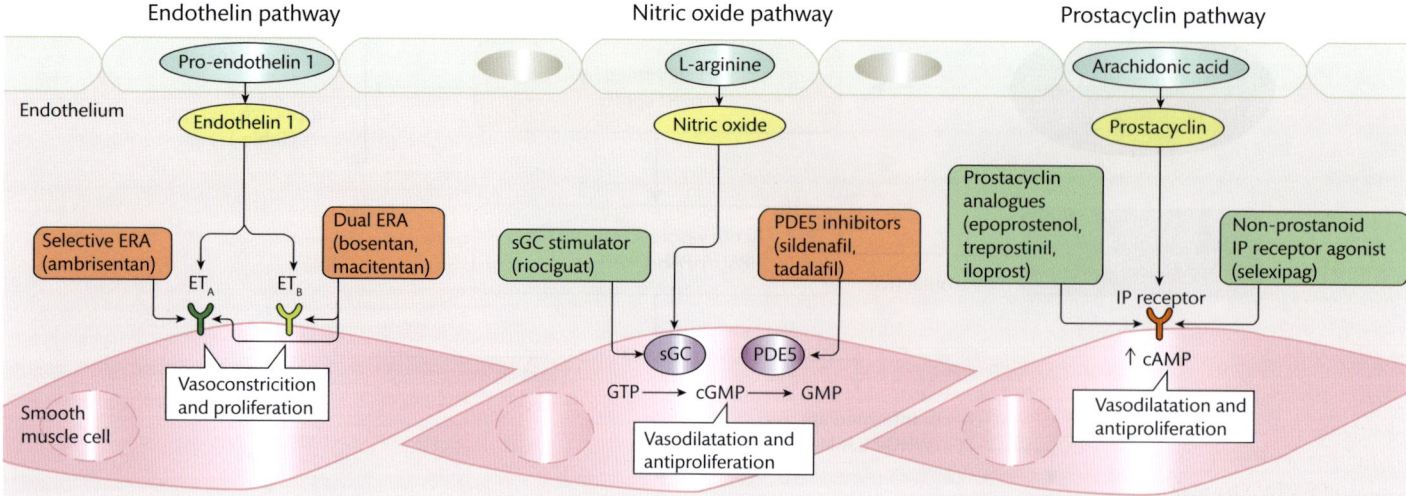

Figure 35.6 Pulmonary hypertension drugs approved for the treatment of PAH98 The endothelin 1, nitric oxide, and prostacyclin signalling pathways are crucial therapeutic targets for pulmonary arterial hypertension (PAH). This disease is characterized by upregulation of vasoconstricting endothelin 1 and decreased production of vasodilatory nitric oxide and prostacyclin. The endothelin 1 pathway can be blocked by either selective or non-selective endothelin 1 receptor antagonists (ERAs); the nitric oxide pathway can be enhanced by inhibition of phosphodiesterase 5 (PDE5) or stimulation of soluble guanylate cyclase (sGC); and the prostacyclin pathway can be enhanced by administration of prostanoid analogues or non-prostanoid IP receptor agonists. ETA, endothelin A; ETB, endothelin B.
Reproduced from Lau EMT, Giannoulatou E, Celermajer DS and Humbert M. Epidemiology and treatment of pulmonary arterial hypertension. *Nature Reviews Cardiology* 2017;**14**:603–614 with permission from Springer.

inhibitors, sildenafil, tadalafil and vardenafil, have demonstrated improvement in exercise capacity, symptoms (not vardenafil), haemodynamics and time to clinical worsening (not sildenafil) in randomized controlled trials.[58–62] Riociguat, a guanylate cyclase stimulator, improved exercise capacity, haemodynamics, functional class and time to clinical worsening in a RCT.[63] PDE5 inhibitors and riociguat should not be combined because of the risk of systemic hypotension.[64]

Endothelin receptor antagonists

Endothelin receptor antagonists block the effects of endothelin system activation in PAH. Endothelin-1 is a vasoconstrictor and mitogen and binds to endothelin A and B receptors.[65] Three drugs are available. Ambrisentan binds to type A receptors whereas bosentan and macitentan bind to type A and B receptors. The first two drugs have been shown to be effective at improving symptoms, exercise capacity, haemodynamics and time to clinical worsening.[66–70] Macitentan reduced the composite endpoint of morbidity and mortality and also increased exercise capacity.[71] Liver function tests are required monthly for ambrisentan and bosentan in Europe. Macitentan requires liver function tests less frequently.

Treatment strategy

Patients presenting with PAH who are at high risk should be offered treatment with intravenous prostacyclin analogues in addition to an oral therapy.[3] Patients who are at intermediate or low risk may be offered either monotherapy or dual oral combination therapy although initial dual therapy is preferred based on the results of the AMBITION trial.[72] Initial triple combination therapy is being tested in a RCT.

Patients require lifelong follow-up at three- to six-monthly intervals. In addition to clinical assessment they require an electrocardiogram, an exercise test and blood tests including (NT-pro)BNP. An echocardiogram, cardiac catheterization and blood gas analysis may be considered less frequently. The data from these assessments is used to review the risk assessment which informs treatment. Patients who remain at intermediate or high risk should be considered for escalation of treatment and where appropriate lung transplantation.

Pulmonary hypertension drug therapies may cause pulmonary oedema in patients with PVOD/PCH and have a poor outcome. The primary treatment in these patients should be lung transplantation.[40]

Treatment of pulmonary hypertension due to left heart disease

Treatment of the underlying myocardial or valvular heart disease should be the main aim of treatment. Risk factors for cardiovascular disease should be managed. Treatment of co-morbid diseases such as COPD, pulmonary thromboembolism and sleep apnoea should also be undertaken.

Evidence from RCTs does not support the treatment of left heart disease with drug directed therapies against pulmonary hypertension. In 1958 Paul Wood observed in patients with mitral stenosis that 'a sufficiently high (pulmonary vascular) resistance protects the pulmonary capillaries and venous radicals from developing dangerously high pressure'.[73] He also observed that patients with pulmonary vascular resistance below 5 Wood units were prone to develop pulmonary oedema whereas those with higher resistance did not.

Based on these observations, one might predict that pulmonary hypertension drug therapies would not demonstrate a beneficial effect in left heart disease patients. This notion has been confirmed

by demonstrating that nitric oxide raises PAWP[74] and may lead to pulmonary oedema in stable severe heart failure.[75] Studying patients with raised pulmonary vascular resistance undergoing mitral valve surgery demonstrated that the pulmonary artery pressure fell rapidly over 2 to 5 days post operatively, suggesting that the underlying primary pathology in the pulmonary circulation was vasoconstriction, albeit with medial hypertrophy of the pulmonary arteries.[76]

In patients with HFnEF a randomized controlled trial of epoprostenol showed a strong trend towards reduced survival while improving haemodynamics and not improving exercise performance or quality of life.[77] A trial of bosentan in severe chronic heart failure demonstrated no effect of bosentan on survival, time to hospitalization for worsening heart failure or discontinuation of study drug compared to placebo.[78] An important criticism of these trials is that patients who entered the studies were not required to have pulmonary hypertension.

Multicentre RCTs of pulmonary hypertension drugs in HFnEF have shown similarly negative results. In three studies, patients did not have pulmonary hypertension. One study of riociguat investigated patients with isolated post-capillary pulmonary hypertension (IPCPH).[79] An RCT of sildenafil showed no change in mean pulmonary artery pressure at 12 weeks but once again these patients had IPCPH.[80] In SOCRATES-PRESERVED, vericiguat did not alter $\log_{10}$ NT-proBNP and left atrial volume at 12 weeks compared to placebo.[81] Pulmonary hypertension was once again not an entry requirement of the trial. The results of the MELODY trial with macitentan in patients with CPCPH are awaited. If any group of patients is likely to respond to pulmonary hypertension drug therapies, it is those with raised pulmonary vascular resistance (CPCPH) rather than those with IPCPH.

These data are in contrast to a single-centre randomized trial investigating the effects of sildenafil on right ventricular performance and haemodynamics in 44 highly selected patients with CPCPH.[82] At six months sildenafil significantly improved mean pulmonary artery pressure and right ventricular function while it increased tricuspid annular systolic excursion and ejection rate and reduced right atrial pressure. These results require further confirmation in an RCT before sildenafil can be recommended as a therapy for treating pulmonary hypertension in heart failure.

Treatment of pulmonary hypertension due to lung disease and/or hypoxaemia

Guidelines recommend the use of long-term oxygen therapy in patients with chronic hypoxaemia although benefit has only been demonstrated in patients with COPD. Oxygen therapy does not normalize haemodynamics or reverse pulmonary vascular remodelling and therefore pulmonary hypertension drug therapy has been considered as a treatment option in such patients.

Nitric oxide worsens gas exchange in patients with COPD.[83] A meta-analysis of pulmonary hypertension drug therapy in COPD shows no significant effect on 6 min walk test distance.[84] Similar results were shown in diffuse parenchymal lung disease.[84] Clinical trials have shown no significant improvement in symptom burden or exercise capacity. Whereas haemodynamics in COPD tend to improve with pulmonary hypertension drugs, in diffuse parenchymal

lung disease, the effect on haemodynamics is inconsistent.[84] Only registry data suggest that PDE5 inhibitors may improve symptoms and functional class.[85] A randomized trial of treatment of IPF with ambrisentan demonstrated more disease progression and respiratory hospitalization in the group receiving ambrisentan and the authors concluded that ambrisentan should not be used to treat patients with IPF.[86] In 2017, a randomized trial of riociguat in idiopathic interstitial pneumonia was discontinued because of safety concerns.[87]

Treatment of chronic thromboembolic pulmonary hypertension

All patients with CTEPH should receive lifelong anticoagulation. At the time of diagnosis patients should be assessed for pulmonary endarterectomy by a CTEPH multidisciplinary team, since, in specialized surgical centres, this operation has an excellent outcome.[88,89] Patients who are technically not operable should be offered pulmonary hypertension drug therapy with riociguat. Riociguat is the only drug approved for patients with inoperable CTEPH and for patients with persistent symptomatic pulmonary hypertension following pulmonary endarterectomy.[90] Macitentan was also effective in a phase 2 trial.[91] Balloon pulmonary angioplasty may be considered in addition to medical therapy or pulmonary endarterectomy where there is persistent symptomatic pulmonary hypertension.[92,93] Currently this technique is not an alternative to surgery and its role in the future will depend on experience being obtained. Severely symptomatic patients who have exhausted these therapies may be considered for lung transplantation.

Treatment of pulmonary hypertension with unclear and/or multifactorial mechanisms

Despite attempting RCTs in sickle-cell disease, no positive results have been obtained. In a trial using sildenafil there was an excess incidence of patients being hospitalized for pain in the sildenafil-treated group.[94] Another trial with bosentan failed to recruit enough patients and had to be discontinued.[95]

A small randomized trial of bosentan in sarcoidosis was negative.[96] Other diseases in this group are rare and have not been subject to RCTs.

Conclusions

Pulmonary hypertension due to left heart disease and pulmonary hypertension due to lung disease are important health problems worldwide. Whereas drug therapies have been developed for PAH—and anticoagulation, surgery, drug therapy, and balloon pulmonary angioplasty for CTEPH—the treatment of pulmonary hypertension due to left heart disease and pulmonary hypertension due to lung disease is that of the underlying condition. PAH remains a condition with high mortality; current treatments slow down but do not halt progression to right ventricular failure. Treatment strategies with existing drugs have shown benefit with initial combination and

sequential combination therapy. Treatments to support the right ventricle to treat and prevent its failure are in early-stage development and are yet to be tested. Lung transplantation remains a treatment of last resort in eligible patients.

REFERENCES

1. Hoeper MM, Humbert M, Souza R, *et al*. A global view of pulmonary hypertension. *Lancet Resp Med* 2016;**4**:306–22.
2. Vachiery JL, Adir Y, Barbera JA, *et al*. Pulmonary hypertension due to left heart diseases. *J Am Coll Cardiol* 2013;**62**:D100–8.
3. Galie N, Humbert M, Vachiery JL, *et al*. 2015 ESC/ERS Guidelines for the diagnosis and treatment of pulmonary hypertension: The Joint Task Force for the Diagnosis and Treatment of Pulmonary Hypertension of the European Society of Cardiology (ESC) and the European Respiratory Society (ERS): Endorsed by: Association for European Paediatric and Congenital Cardiology (AEPC), International Society for Heart and Lung Transplantation (ISHLT). *Eur Heart J* 2016;**37**:67–119.
4. Escribano-Subias P, Blanco I, Lopez-Meseguer M, *et al*.; REHAP investigators. Survival in pulmonary hypertension in Spain: insights from the Spanish registry. *Eur Resp J* 2012;**40**:596–603.
5. Humbert M, Sitbon O, Chaouat A, *et al*. Pulmonary arterial hypertension in France: results from a national registry. *Am J Resp Crit Care Med* 2006;**173**:1023–30.
6. Peacock AJ, Murphy NF, McMurray JJ, Caballero L, Stewart S. An epidemiological study of pulmonary arterial hypertension. *Eur Resp J* 2007;**30**:104–9.
7. Kawut SM, Horn EM, Berekashvili KK, *et al*. New predictors of outcome in idiopathic pulmonary arterial hypertension. *Am J Cardiol* 2005;**95**:199–203.
8. Korsholm K, Andersen A, Kirkfeldt RE, *et al*. Survival in an incident cohort of patients with pulmonary arterial hypertension in Denmark. *Pulmon Circ* 2015;**5**:364–9.
9. Girerd B, Montani D, Eyries M, *et al*. Absence of influence of gender and BMPR2 mutation type on clinical phenotypes of pulmonary arterial hypertension. *Resp Res* 2010;**11**:73.
10. Alves JL, Jr, Gavilanes F, Jardim C, *et al*. Pulmonary arterial hypertension in the southern hemisphere: results from a registry of incident Brazilian cases. *Chest* 2015;**147**:495–501.
11. Idrees M, Alnajashi K, Abdulhameed J, *et al*. and Registry Taskforce SAPH. Saudi experience in the management of pulmonary arterial hypertension; the outcome of PAH therapy with the exclusion of chronic parenteral prostacyclin. *Ann Thoracic Med* 2015;**10**:204–11.
12. Ling Y, Johnson MK, Kiely DG, *et al*. Changing demographics, epidemiology, and survival of incident pulmonary arterial hypertension: results from the pulmonary hypertension registry of the United Kingdom and Ireland. *Am J Resp Crit Care Med* 2012;**186**:790–6.
13. Barst RJ, Gibbs JS, Ghofrani HA, *et al*. Updated evidence-based treatment algorithm in pulmonary arterial hypertension. *J Am Coll Cardiol* 2009;**54**:S78–84.
14. Humbert M, Sitbon O, Yaici A, *et al*. and French Pulmonary Arterial Hypertension Network. Survival in incident and prevalent cohorts of patients with pulmonary arterial hypertension. *Eur Resp J* 2010;**36**:549–55.
15. Ventetuolo CE, Praestgaard A, Palevsky HI, *et al*. Sex and haemodynamics in pulmonary arterial hypertension. *Eur Resp J* 2014;**43**:523–30.
16. Tuder RM, Archer SL, Dorfmuller P, *et al*. Relevant issues in the pathology and pathobiology of pulmonary hypertension. *J Am Coll Cardiol* 2013;**62**:D4–12.
17. Evans JD, Girerd B, Montani D, *et al*. BMPR2 mutations and survival in pulmonary arterial hypertension: an individual participant data meta-analysis. *Lancet Resp Med* 2016;**4**:129–37.
18. Eyries M, Montani D, Girerd B, *et al*. EIF2AK4 mutations cause pulmonary veno-occlusive disease, a recessive form of pulmonary hypertension. *Nature Genet* 2014;**46**:65–9.
19. Tumminello G, Lancellotti P, Lempereur M, D'Orio V, Pierard LA. Determinants of pulmonary artery hypertension at rest and during exercise in patients with heart failure. *Eur Heart J* 2007;**28**:569–74.
20. Harari S, Elia D, Humbert M. Pulmonary hypertension in parenchymal lung diseases: any future for new therapies? *Chest* 2018;**153**:217–23.
21. Seeger W, Adir Y, Barbera JA, *et al*. Pulmonary hypertension in chronic lung diseases. *J Am Coll Cardiol* 2013;**62**:D109–16.
22. Pepke-Zaba J, Delcroix M, Lang I, *et al*. Chronic thromboembolic pulmonary hypertension (CTEPH): results from an international prospective registry. *Circulation* 2011;**124**:1973–81.
23. Dentali F, Donadini M, Gianni M, *et al*. Incidence of chronic pulmonary hypertension in patients with previous pulmonary embolism. *Thromb Res* 2009;**124**:256–8.
24. Pengo V, Lensing AW, Prins MH, *et al*. and Thromboembolic Pulmonary Hypertension Study Group. Incidence of chronic thromboembolic pulmonary hypertension after pulmonary embolism. *N Engl J Med* 2004;**350**:2257–64.
25. Becattini C, Agnelli G, Pesavento R, *et al*. Incidence of chronic thromboembolic pulmonary hypertension after a first episode of pulmonary embolism. *Chest* 2006;**130**:172–5.
26. Klok FA, Zondag W, van Kralingen KW, *et al*. Patient outcomes after acute pulmonary embolism. A pooled survival analysis of different adverse events. *Am J Resp Crit Care Med* 2010;**181**:501–6.
27. Quarck R, Delcroix M. Is inflammation a potential therapeutic target in chronic thromboembolic pulmonary hypertension? *Eur Resp J* 2014;**44**:842–5.
28. Simonneau G, Torbicki A, Dorfmuller P, Kim N. The pathophysiology of chronic thromboembolic pulmonary hypertension. *Eur Resp Rev* 2017;**26**:160112.
29. Sun XG, Hansen JE, Oudiz RJ, Wasserman K. Pulmonary function in primary pulmonary hypertension. *J Am Coll Cardiol* 2003;**41**:1028–35.
30. Trip P, Nossent EJ, de Man FS, *et al*. Severely reduced diffusion capacity in idiopathic pulmonary arterial hypertension: patient characteristics and treatment responses. *Eur Resp J* 2013;**42**:1575–85.
31. Cottin V, Nunes H, Brillet PY, *et al*. and Groupe d'Etude et de Recherche sur les Maladies Orphelines Pulmonaires. Combined pulmonary fibrosis and emphysema: a distinct underrecognised entity. *Eur Resp J* 2005;**26**:586–93.
32. Jankowich MD, Rounds SIS. Combined pulmonary fibrosis and emphysema syndrome: a review. *Chest* 2012;**141**:222–231.
33. Tunariu N, Gibbs SJ, Win Z, *et al*. Ventilation–perfusion scintigraphy is more sensitive than multidetector CTPA in detecting chronic thromboembolic pulmonary disease as a treatable cause of pulmonary hypertension. *J Nucl Med* 2007;**48**:680–4.
34. LeVarge BL, Pomerantsev E, Channick RN. Reliance on end-expiratory wedge pressure leads to misclassification of pulmonary hypertension. *Eur Resp J* 2014;**44**:425–34.

35. Ryan JJ, Rich JD, Thiruvoipati T, *et al.* Current practice for determining pulmonary capillary wedge pressure predisposes to serious errors in the classification of patients with pulmonary hypertension. *Am Heart J* 2012;**163**:589–94.

36. Kovacs G, Avian A, Pienn M, Naeije R, Olschewski H. Reading pulmonary vascular pressure tracings. How to handle the problems of zero leveling and respiratory swings. *Am J Resp Crit Care Med* 2014;**190**:252–7.

37. Hoeper MM, Maier R, Tongers J, *et al.* Determination of cardiac output by the Fick method, thermodilution, and acetylene rebreathing in pulmonary hypertension. *Am J Resp Crit Care Med* 1999;**160**:535–41.

38. Dumitrescu D, Gerhardt F, Viethen T, Erdmann E, Rosenkranz S. [70-year-old woman with cardiac hypertrophy and severe pulmonary hypertension: pre- or postcapillary?] *Deut medizin Wochenschr* 2011;**136**:2594–8.

39. Opitz CF, Hoeper MM, Gibbs JS, *et al.* Pre-capillary, combined, and post-capillary pulmonary hypertension: a pathophysiological continuum. *J Am Coll Cardiol* 2016;**68**:368–78.

40. Montani D, Girerd B, Jais X, *et al.* Clinical phenotypes and outcomes of heritable and sporadic pulmonary veno-occlusive disease: a population-based study. *Lancet Resp Med* 2017;**5**:125–134.

41. Hoeper MM, Kramer T, Pan Z, *et al.* Mortality in pulmonary arterial hypertension: prediction by the 2015 European pulmonary hypertension guidelines risk stratification model. *Eur Resp J* 2017;**50**:1700740.

42. Rich S, Brundage BH. High dose calcium channel-blocking therapy for primary pulmonary hypertension: evidence for long-term reduction in pulmonary arterial pressure and regression of right ventricular hypertrophy. *Circulation* 1987;**76**:135–41.

43. Sitbon O, Humbert M, Jais X, *et al.* Long-term response to calcium channel blockers in idiopathic pulmonary arterial hypertension. *Circulation* 2005;**111**:3105–11.

44. Montani D, Savale L, Natali D, *et al.* Long-term response to calcium-channel blockers in non-idiopathic pulmonary arterial hypertension. *Eur Heart J* 2010;**31**:1898–907.

45. Moncada S, Higgs EA, Vane JR. Human arterial and venous tissues generate prostacyclin (prostaglandin x), a potent inhibitor of platelet aggregation. *Lancet* 1977;**1**:18–20.

46. Rubin LJ, Mendoza J, Hood M, *et al.* Treatment of primary pulmonary hypertension with continuous intravenous prostacyclin (epoprostenol). Results of a randomized trial. *Ann Intern Med* 1990;**112**:485–91.

47. Barst RJ, Rubin LJ, Long WA, *et al.* and Primary Pulmonary Hypertension Study Group. A comparison of continuous intravenous epoprostenol (prostacyclin) with conventional therapy for primary pulmonary hypertension. *N Engl J Med* 1996;**334**:296–301.

48. Badesch DB, Tapson VF, McGoon MD, *et al.* Continuous intravenous epoprostenol for pulmonary hypertension due to the scleroderma spectrum of disease. A randomized, controlled trial. *Ann Intern Med* 2000;**132**:425–34.

49. Olschewski H, Simonneau G, Galie N, *et al.* and Aerosolized Iloprost Randomized Study Group. Inhaled iloprost for severe pulmonary hypertension. *N Engl J Med* 2002;**347**:322–9.

50. McLaughlin VV, Oudiz RJ, Frost A, *et al.* Randomized study of adding inhaled iloprost to existing bosentan in pulmonary arterial hypertension. *Am J Resp Crit Care Med* 2006;**174**:1257–63.

51. Higenbottam T, Butt AY, McMahon A, Westerbeck R, Sharples L. Long-term intravenous prostaglandin (epoprostenol or iloprost) for treatment of severe pulmonary hypertension. *Heart* 1998;**80**:151–5.

52. Simonneau G, Barst RJ, Galie N, *et al.* and Treprostinil Study Group. Continuous subcutaneous infusion of treprostinil, a prostacyclin analogue, in patients with pulmonary arterial hypertension: a double-blind, randomized, placebo-controlled trial. *Am J Resp Crit Care Med* 2002;**165**:800–4.

53. McLaughlin VV, Benza RL, Rubin LJ, *et al.* Addition of inhaled treprostinil to oral therapy for pulmonary arterial hypertension: a randomized controlled clinical trial. *J Am Coll Cardiol* 2010;**55**:1915–22.

54. Jing ZC, Parikh K, Pulido T, *et al.* Efficacy and safety of oral treprostinil monotherapy for the treatment of pulmonary arterial hypertension: a randomized, controlled trial. *Circulation* 2013;**127**:624–33.

55. Tapson VF, Torres F, Kermeen F, *et al.* Oral treprostinil for the treatment of pulmonary arterial hypertension in patients on background endothelin receptor antagonist and/or phosphodiesterase type 5 inhibitor therapy (the FREEDOM-C study): a randomized controlled trial. *Chest* 2012;**142**:1383–90.

56. Tapson VF, Jing ZC, Xu KF, *et al.*; FREEDOM-C2 Study Team. Oral treprostinil for the treatment of pulmonary arterial hypertension in patients receiving background endothelin receptor antagonist and phosphodiesterase type 5 inhibitor therapy (the FREEDOM-C2 study): a randomized controlled trial. *Chest* 2013;**144**:952–8.

57. Sitbon O, Channick R, Chin KM, *et al.*; GRIPHON Investigators. Selexipag for the treatment of pulmonary arterial hypertension. *N Engl J Med* 2015;**373**:2522–33.

58. Galie N, Brundage BH, Ghofrani HA, *et al.* Pulmonary Arterial Hypertension and Response to Tadalafil Study Group. Tadalafil therapy for pulmonary arterial hypertension. *Circulation* 2009;**119**:2894–903.

59. Galie N, Ghofrani HA, Torbicki A, *et al.* and Sildenafil Use in Pulmonary Arterial Hypertension Study Group. Sildenafil citrate therapy for pulmonary arterial hypertension. *N Engl J Med* 2005;**353**:2148–57.

60. Jing ZC, Yu ZX, Shen JY, *et al.*, Efficacy and Safety of Vardenafil in the Treatment of Pulmonary Arterial Hypertension Study Group. Vardenafil in pulmonary arterial hypertension: a randomized, double-blind, placebo-controlled study. *Am J Resp Crit Care Med* 2011;**183**:1723–9.

61. Sastry BK, Narasimhan C, Reddy NK. Raju BS. Clinical efficacy of sildenafil in primary pulmonary hypertension: a randomized, placebo-controlled, double-blind, crossover study. *J Am Coll Cardiol* 2004;**43**:1149–53.

62. Singh TP, Rohit M, Grover A, Malhotra S. Vijayvergiya R. A randomized, placebo-controlled, double-blind, crossover study to evaluate the efficacy of oral sildenafil therapy in severe pulmonary artery hypertension. *Am Heart J* 2006;**151**:851 e1–5.

63. Ghofrani HA, Galie N, Grimminger F, *et al.*; PATENT-1 Study Group. Riociguat for the treatment of pulmonary arterial hypertension. *N Engl J Med* 2013;**369**:330–40.

64. Galie N, Muller K, Scalise AV, Grunig E. PATENT PLUS: a blinded, randomised and extension study of riociguat plus sildenafil in pulmonary arterial hypertension. *Eur Resp J* 2015;**45**:1314–22.

65. Giaid A, Yanagisawa M, Langleben D, *et al.* Expression of endothelin-1 in the lungs of patients with pulmonary hypertension. *N Engl J Med* 1993;**328**:1732–9.

66. Channick RN, Simonneau G, Sitbon O, *et al.* Effects of the dual endothelin-receptor antagonist bosentan in patients with

pulmonary hypertension: a randomised placebo-controlled study. *Lancet* 2001;**358**:1119–23.

67. Galie N, Beghetti M, Gatzoulis MA, *et al.* and Bosentan Randomized Trial of Endothelin Antagonist Therapy I. Bosentan therapy in patients with Eisenmenger syndrome: a multicenter, double-blind, randomized, placebo-controlled study. *Circulation* 2006;**114**:48–54.

68. Galie N, Olschewski H, Oudiz RJ, *et al.* and Ambrisentan in Pulmonary Arterial Hypertension RD-BP-CMESG. Ambrisentan for the treatment of pulmonary arterial hypertension: results of the ambrisentan in pulmonary arterial hypertension, randomized, double-blind, placebo-controlled, multicenter, efficacy (ARIES) study 1 and 2. *Circulation* 2008;**117**:3010–19.

69. Galie N, Rubin L, Hoeper M, *et al.* Treatment of patients with mildly symptomatic pulmonary arterial hypertension with bosentan (EARLY study): a double-blind, randomised controlled trial. *Lancet* 2008;**371**:2093–100.

70. Rubin LJ, Badesch DB, Barst RJ, *et al.* Bosentan therapy for pulmonary arterial hypertension. *N Engl J Med* 2002;**346**:896–903.

71. Pulido T, Adzerikho I, Channick RN, *et al.*; SERAPHIN Investigators. Macitentan and morbidity and mortality in pulmonary arterial hypertension. *N Engl J Med* 2013;**369**:809–18.

72. Galie N, Barbera JA, Frost AE, *et al.*; AMBITION Investigators. Initial use of ambrisentan plus tadalafil in pulmonary arterial hypertension. *N Engl J Med* 2015;**373**:834–44.

73. Wood P, Besterman EM, Towers MK, McIlroy MB. The effect of acetylcholine on pulmonary vascular resistance and left atrial pressure in mitral stenosis. *Br Heart J* 1957;**19**:279–86.

74. Loh E, Stamler JS, Hare JM, Loscalzo J, Colucci WS. Cardiovascular effects of inhaled nitric oxide in patients with left ventricular dysfunction. *Circulation* 1994;**90**:2780–5.

75. Bocchi EA, Bacal F, Auler Junior JO, *et al.* Inhaled nitric oxide leading to pulmonary edema in stable severe heart failure. *Am J Cardiol* 1994;**74**:70–2.

76. Dalen JE, Matloff JM, Evans GL, *et al.* Early reduction of pulmonary vascular resistance after mitral-valve replacement. *N Engl J Med* 1967;**277**:387–94.

77. Califf RM, Adams KF, McKenna WJ, *et al.* A randomized controlled trial of epoprostenol therapy for severe congestive heart failure: The Flolan International Randomized Survival Trial (FIRST). *Am Heart J* 1997;**134**:44–54.

78. Packer M, McMurray J, Massie BM, *et al.* Clinical effects of endothelin receptor antagonism with bosentan in patients with severe chronic heart failure: results of a pilot study. *J Cardiac Fail* 2005;**11**:12–20.

79. Bonderman D, Pretsch I, Steringer-Mascherbauer R, *et al.* Acute hemodynamic effects of riociguat in patients with pulmonary hypertension associated with diastolic heart failure (DILATE-1): a randomized, double-blind, placebo-controlled, single-dose study. *Chest* 2014;**146**:1274–85.

80. Hoendermis ES, Liu LC, Hummel YM, *et al.* Effects of sildenafil on invasive haemodynamics and exercise capacity in heart failure patients with preserved ejection fraction and pulmonary hypertension: a randomized controlled trial. *Eur Heart J* 2015;**36**:2565–73.

81. Pieske B, Maggioni AP, Lam CSP, *et al.* Vericiguat in patients with worsening chronic heart failure and preserved ejection fraction: results of the SOluble guanylate Cyclase stimulatoR in heArT failurE patientS with PRESERVED EF (SOCRATES-PRESERVED) study. *Eur Heart J* 2017;**38**:1119–27.

82. Guazzi M, Vicenzi M, Arena R, Guazzi MD. Pulmonary hypertension in heart failure with preserved ejection fraction: a

target of phosphodiesterase-5 inhibition in a 1-year study. *Circulation* 2011;**124**:164–74.

83. Barbera JA. Nitric oxide in chronic obstructive pulmonary disease. *Monaldi Arch Chest Dis* 1996;**51**:528–32.

84. Prins KW, Duval S, Markowitz J, Pritzker M, Thenappan T. Chronic use of PAH-specific therapy in World Health Organization Group III Pulmonary Hypertension: a systematic review and meta-analysis. *Pulmon Circ* 2017;**7**:145–55.

85. Hoeper MM, Behr J, Held M, *et al.* Pulmonary hypertension in patients with chronic fibrosing idiopathic interstitial pneumonias. *PloS One* 2015;**10**:e0141911.

86. Raghu G, Behr J, Brown KK, *et al.*; ARTEMIS-IPF Investigators. Treatment of idiopathic pulmonary fibrosis with ambrisentan: a parallel, randomized trial. *Ann Intern Med* 2013;**158**:641–9.

87. Nathan SD, Behr J, Collard HR, *et al.* Riociguat for idiopathic interstitial pneumonia-associated pulmonary hypertension (RISE-IIP): a randomised, placebo-controlled phase 2b study. *Lancet Respir Med* 2019;**7**:780–790.

88. Jenkins DP, Madani M, Mayer E, *et al.* Surgical treatment of chronic thromboembolic pulmonary hypertension. *Eur Resp J* 2013;**41**:735–42.

89. Madani MM, Auger WR, Pretorius V, *et al.* Pulmonary endarterectomy: recent changes in a single institution's experience of more than 2,700 patients. *Ann Thoracic Surg* 2012;**94**:97–103; discussion 103.

90. Ghofrani HA, D'Armini AM, Grimminger F, *et al.*; CHEST-1 Study Group. Riociguat for the treatment of chronic thromboembolic pulmonary hypertension. *N Engl J Med* 2013;**369**:319–29.

91. Ghofrani HA, Simonneau G, D'Armini AM, *et al.*; MERIT study investigators. Macitentan for the treatment of inoperable chronic thromboembolic pulmonary hypertension (MERIT-1): results from the multicentre, phase 2, randomised, double-blind, placebo-controlled study. *Lancet Resp Med* 2017;**5**:785–94.

92. Sugimura K, Fukumoto Y, Satoh K, *et al.* Percutaneous transluminal pulmonary angioplasty markedly improves pulmonary hemodynamics and long-term prognosis in patients with chronic thromboembolic pulmonary hypertension. *Circ J* 2012;**76**:485–8.

93. Andreassen AK, Ragnarsson A, Gude E, Geiran O, Andersen R. Balloon pulmonary angioplasty in patients with inoperable chronic thromboembolic pulmonary hypertension. *Heart* 2013;**99**:1415–20.

94. Machado RF, Barst RJ, Yovetich NA, *et al.*; walk-PHaSST Investigators and Patients. Hospitalization for pain in patients with sickle cell disease treated with sildenafil for elevated TRV and low exercise capacity. *Blood* 2011;**118**:855–64.

95. Barst RJ, Mubarak KK, Machado RF, *et al.*; ASSET study group. Exercise capacity and haemodynamics in patients with sickle cell disease with pulmonary hypertension treated with bosentan: results of the ASSET studies. *Br J Haematol* 2010;**149**:426–35.

96. Baughman RP, Culver DA, Cordova FC, *et al.* Bosentan for sarcoidosis-associated pulmonary hypertension: a double-blind placebo controlled randomized trial. *Chest* 2014;**145**:810–17.

97. Rosenkranz S, Gibbs JS, Wachter R, *et al.* Left ventricular heart failure and pulmonary hypertension. *Eur Heart J* 2016;**37**:942–54.

98. Lau EMT, Giannoulatou E, Celermajer DS, Humbert M. Epidemiology and treatment of pulmonary arterial hypertension. *Nature Rev Cardiol* 2017;**14**:603–14.

RECOMMENDED READING

Galie N, Humbert M, Vachiery JL, *et al.* 2015 ESC/ERS Guidelines for the diagnosis and treatment of pulmonary hypertension: The Joint Task Force for the Diagnosis and Treatment of Pulmonary Hypertension of the European Society of Cardiology (ESC) and the European Respiratory Society (ERS): Endorsed by: Association for European Paediatric and Congenital Cardiology (AEPC), International Society for Heart and Lung Transplantation (ISHLT). *Eur Heart J* 2016;**37**:67–119.

Hoeper MM, Humbert M, Souza R, *et al.* A global view of pulmonary hypertension. *Lancet Resp Med* 2016;**4**:306–22.

Hoeper MM, Lam CSP, Vachiery JL, *et al.* Pulmonary hypertension in heart failure with preserved ejection fraction: a plea for proper phenotyping and further research. *Eur Heart J* 2017;**38**: 2869–73.

Rosenkranz S, Gibbs JS, Wachter R, *et al.* Left ventricular heart failure and pulmonary hypertension. *Eur Heart J* 2016;**37**: 942–54.

36

Diabetes mellitus

Andrew Jamieson

Introduction

Heart failure and diabetes mellitus (DM) are both increasing in prevalence worldwide, and HF is a serious and increasingly common co-morbidity in the patient with DM. The patient with heart failure and DM may present particular problems in relation to a number of management areas, and as a consequence, it is increasingly important that practitioners dealing with patients with heart failure have some knowledge of the interplay between DM and heart failure, and the potential pitfalls encountered when treating the diabetic patient with heart failure, and vice versa.

Epidemiology

The initial observations from the Framingham Heart Study population demonstrated that heart failure was twice as common in men with DM, and five times as common in women with DM aged 45–74 years as compared to their age-matched controls, and the risk of heart failure was independent of age, the presence of hypertension, obesity, coronary artery disease (CAD), or dyslipidaemia.[1] Furthermore, in patients with DM aged ≤65 years, the prevalence of heart failure was even higher compared with the control subjects (men with DM: four-fold increase; women with DM: eight-fold increase). The increased risk of developing heart failure conferred by DM in women was confirmed in the HERS study population where DM was the strongest predictor of heart failure, more so than the presence of CAD.[2]

The presence of DM itself is an independent predictor of developing heart failure following myocardial infarction,[3] and if developed predicts a poorer outcome than in non-diabetic patients, greater even than the presence of CAD.[4,5] Furthermore, patients hospitalized with heart failure have a poorer outcome if they have DM, with a blood glucose level of >10 mmol/L being associated with a poor outcome.[6,7]

Epidemiology of heart failure in patients with diabetes mellitus

Prevalence of heart failure in patients with DM

Population-based studies have estimated that 0.3–0.5% of the population have both DM and heart failure,[8,9] whilst the prevalence of heart failure in patients with DM is 12–22%, the prevalence increasing with age (Table 36.1).[8,10]

Prevalence of DM in patients with heart failure

The prevalence of DM in patients with heart failure varies significantly dependent upon the population studied. The background prevalence of DM is 4–7% in northern hemisphere populations,[8,11] but varies from 6% to 44% in patients with varying degrees of severity of heart failure (Table 36.2). Studies of treatment of heart failure due to left ventricular systolic dysfunction (LVSD) have consistently demonstrated that 20–30% of patients with heart failure

Table 36.1 Prevalence and incidence of heart failure and diabetes mellitus in related circumstances

Study type	Prevalence			Incidence	
	General population	HF in DM	DM in HF	HF in DM	DM in HF
Population-based studies[a]	DM: 4–15% (population and age dependent) HF: 1–4% (age dependent)[8,9,11]	12% 22% aged >64 years[10]	6–44%[18,19]	HR 1.74–8 (age dependent) OR 2.0–2.8[1,8,10]	28.8% with DM vs 18.3% without DM (3 years)[26]
Clinical trials	N/A	N/A	11–41%[12–16]	2.3–11.9 per 1000 person-years (HbA1c related)[20] 13.3% in placebo group of MICROHOPE (4.2 years)[23]	5.9–7.4% (3 years) 13–20% (7.7 years, NYHA class dependent)[27–29]

HF, heart failure; DM, diabetes mellitus; HR, hazard ratio; OR, odds ratio; N/A, not applicable; HbA1c, glycated haemoglobin; NYHA, New York Heart Association.

[a] Includes epidemiological, registry and population based studies with endpoints including hospitalization.

Table 36.2 Prevalence of diabetes mellitus in populations with and without LVSD based on a measure of LVEF

	Study type	Mean age, years (range)	LVEF measure	Prevalence of LVSD (%)	Symptomatic/ asymptomatic (%)	Prevalence of DM with LVSD (%)	Prevalence of DM without LVSD (%)
Glasgow[30]	Epidemiological	50 (25–74)	<30% <35%	2.9 7.7	77% asymptomatic	12.4	2.5
ECHOES, England[9]	Epidemiological: primary care	61 (>45)	<40%	1.8	1.0/0.8	30	3.8
Olmstead, USA[31]	Epidemiological	63 (>45)	≤50% ≤40%	6.5 1.8	N/A	17 15	6.8
Copenhagen[32]	Prospective: hospital	69 (N/A)	<45%	All included	All included were symptomatic	25.5	N/A

LVEF, left ventricular ejection fraction; LVSD, left ventricular systolic dysfunction; DM, diabetes mellitus; N/A, not applicable.

have DM[12–16] with a similar prevalence observed in patients with heart failure and preserved LV function (CHARM-Preserved population).[17]

By contrast, hospitalization-based studies have demonstrated consistently higher prevalence of DM in patients with heart failure ranging from 34% to 44%.[18,19] Whilst it would appear that intervention studies underestimate the true prevalence of DM in patients with heart failure, it is still abundantly clear that the prevalence of DM in patients with heart failure is significantly higher than the background prevalence of DM in the non-heart-failure-affected population.

Incidence of heart failure in DM

The Framingham study identified DM as an important independent risk factor for developing heart failure.[1] This has been confirmed by a number of population-based studies in the USA and Europe which all confirm with some consistency an age-adjusted odds ratio for developing heart failure of around 2 compared with non-diabetic subjects.[1,8,10] The annual incidence of heart failure in patients with DM has been assessed in five studies.[20–24] The UKPDS reported heart failure incidence rates of 2.3–11.9 per 1000 patient-years over a 10-year follow-up period. The DIABHYCAR study estimated the annual incidence rate of heart failure requiring hospitalization in subjects with DM at 1% (10 per 1000 patient-years). A large diabetic population (48 000 subjects with a mean age of 58 years) was studied and demonstrated an incidence rate of 4.5–9.2 per 1000 patient-years. This study only recorded those who were hospitalized and heart failure was the principal diagnosis, thus excluding less severe cases and underestimating the true incidence of heart failure. The MICRO-HOPE substudy placebo group of patients with DM had an incidence of heart failure of 13.3% over 4.5 years.

A retrospective cohort study of >16 000 patients with and without type 2 DM followed for 6 years confirmed that patients with DM were much more likely to develop heart failure than those without (incidence rate 30.9 vs 12.4 cases per 1000 person-years, giving a rate ratio of 2.5), and that the rate of developing heart failure was greatest in younger age groups (aged 45–54 years with DM vs no DM, odds ratio: 8.6; aged 75–84 years, odds ratio: 1.2). In addition to the effect of age, the authors concluded that poor glycaemic control and obesity were also important factors affecting the development of heart failure in patients with type 2 DM.

Thus, the incidence of heart failure in DM is significantly greater than the non-diabetic population, and whilst the size of the diabetic population increases, the potential burden of heart failure

co-morbidity is increasing too, perhaps at a rate greater than expected based on the rise in diabetes cases.[25]

Incidence of DM in heart failure

In one population-based study in elderly Italians, the odds ratio for developing DM in patients with heart failure was 1.6 versus patients without heart failure, with the absolute incidence of DM in the heart failure group 28% over 3 years.[26] Within the context of clinical trials, the incidence of DM in patients with heart failure ranged from 5.9% to 7.4% over 3 years,[27,28] whilst the BIPS demonstrated an incidence of DM in patients without heart failure of 13% over a mean of 7.7 years versus 15% in patients with New York Heart Association (NYHA) class II and 20% in patients with NYHA class III heart failure.[29] Clearly DM is an independent risk factor for developing heart failure, but it is also clear that heart failure is an independent risk factor for developing DM. However, the mechanism behind this increased risk is unclear.

Rising prevalence of diabetes mellitus

The worldwide prevalence of DM is alarmingly high, with current estimates suggesting that there are >200 million people with diabetes worldwide with the total number projected to be 300 million by 2025,[33] and that in developed countries >25% of people aged ≥65 years will have diabetes. Patients with diabetes have an excess burden of vascular complications, both macrovascular, i.e. coronary artery disease, cerebrovascular disease, peripheral arterial disease and heart failure, and microvascular, i.e. diabetic retinopathy, nephropathy and neuropathy, and three out of four deaths in patients with DM are attributed to cardiovascular causes.[20] In addition to hyperglycaemia, the diabetic patient has an increased prevalence of other key cardiovascular risk factors, namely hypertension, obesity, dyslipidaemia and chronic kidney disease (CKD), and it is likely that the interaction of hyperglycaemia with a whole range of cardiovascular risk factors, conventional or otherwise, leads to the development of structural and functional changes in the vasculature and myocardium which contribute to the excess prevalence of heart failure in patients with DM.

The rise in the prevalence of obesity together with the reclassification of the diagnostic criteria for DM has led to an increased awareness of diabetes leading to the implementation of screening of individuals at risk for developing DM, e.g. those with obesity or positive family history of DM. Similarly, improved patient access to diagnostic testing, the application of evidence-based cardiovascular

prevention strategies for patients with DM, improved detection and treatment of renal disease, increasing use of percutaneous coronary intervention, coronary artery bypass graft surgery, and peripheral vascular intervention have all contributed to the increase in size of the patient population with DM, and in particular those surviving with heart failure or the substrates to develop heart failure.

Diagnosis and aetiology of diabetes mellitus

Diagnosis of diabetes mellitus

In 1997 the diagnostic criteria and aetiological classification of DM were updated.[34] The critical changes made were: the lowering of the level of fasting blood glucose required to diagnose DM to ≥7 mmol/L; to propose the routine use of fasting blood glucose rather than the standard 75 g oral glucose tolerance test; and the introduction of a new category of abnormal glucose regulation—'impaired fasting glucose' (Table 36.3).

Most recently, the use of a single measure of HbA1c (the glycosylated fraction of haemoglobin typically used to monitor glycaemic control in DM patients) to diagnose DM (random HbA1c ≥6.5%) has been advocated, although this is still a matter of hot debate.[35,36]

Aetiology of diabetes mellitus

Type 1 DM accounts for 5–10% of cases of DM and is characterized by an absolute deficiency of insulin, most commonly in the context of associated cellular autoimmunity directed towards the pancreatic beta cells. Between 80% and 90% of those affected have evidence of autoimmunity against pancreatic beta cells, e.g. the presence of anti-islet cell antibodies, or anti-GAD$_{65}$ antibodies. As a consequence,

Table 36.3 Diagnostic criteria and classification of aetiology of diabetes mellitus

Diagnostic criteria for diabetes mellitus	Classification of diabetes mellitus
Fasting blood glucose ≥7 mmol/L	Type 1 diabetes mellitus Autoimmunity: islet cell antibodies present in the majority of individuals, e.g anti-GAD65 antibodies
2 h post 75 g OGTT Blood glucose ≥11.1 mmol/L	Type 2 diabetes mellitus Insulin resistance and centripetal obesity
Random blood glucose ≥11.1 mmol/L[a]	Others: Pancreatic disease, e.g. cystic fibrosis, acute or chronic pancreatitis, pancreatectomy. Endocrine disease, e.g. acromegaly, thyrotoxicosis, Cushing's syndrome, primary hyperaldosteronism, hereditary haemochromatosis.
Impaired fasting flood glucose FBG ≥6 and <7 mmol/L	

OGTT, oral glucose tolerance test.

[a] In the presence of symptoms compatible with diabetes mellitus, e.g. polydipsia, polyuria. A further fasting sample is required 4–6 weeks later if there are no symptoms present to confirm the diagnosis.

Source data from The Expert Committee on the Diagnosis and Classification of Diabetes Mellitus. Report of the Expert Committee on the Diagnosis and Classification of Diabetes Mellitus. *Diabetes Care* 1997;**20**:1183–1197.

individuals with type 1 DM require insulin therapy lifelong from diagnosis and are prone to developing ketoacidosis. Individuals with type 1 DM are at high risk of developing the classic manifestations of DM such as diabetic retinopathy and nephropathy in young adulthood, and have a reduced life expectancy principally due to cardiovascular deaths.

Type 2 DM is characterized by the presence of peripheral tissue insulin resistance and elevated insulin concentrations and is typically found in individuals who are centrally obese. As time progresses, the continuum from normal glucose tolerance to the development of DM in susceptible individuals with insulin resistance is associated with a gradual rise in fasting and meal-stimulated insulin concentrations associated with rising levels of fasting and postprandial blood glucose. The precise mechanism of insulin resistance is still unclear, although peripheral tissue resistance (principally adipose tissue and skeletal muscle) to the transmembrane and intracellular effects of insulin associated with fasting and postprandial hyperinsulinaemia, the presence of centripetal obesity, and abnormal regulation of hepatic glucose production and fatty acid metabolism are contributory features. At some point, the progressive rise in insulin concentration will plateau for a variable period of time, and subsequently begin to fall, leading to an eventual state of relative or absolute insulin deficiency. This fall in insulin production is related to the presence of impaired beta cell function, which is virtually always present when type 2 DM is diagnosed. The rate of decline in beta cell function in cases of type 2 DM varies between individuals but clearly contributes to the progressive hyperglycaemia seen in type 2 DM, the progressive failure of glycaemic response to agents such as sulfonylurea drugs (SUs), and the increasing requirement for exogenous insulin to maintain levels of glycaemic control as the duration of type 2 DM continues.

Based on the key aetiological observations regarding the development of type 2 DM, interventions to control blood glucose levels in patients with type 2 DM are directed at reducing insulin resistance, directly stimulating remaining beta cell insulin release, and modifying meal-related insulin release. Insulin therapy in type 2 DM is usually initiated when one, or a combination, of these approaches has been tried and deemed to have failed by the treating clinician.

Risk factors for developing heart failure in diabetic patients

The two most common risk factors for the development of heart failure are the presence of CAD and arterial hypertension. Both of these are more prevalent in patients with DM than non-diabetic subjects, and clearly this impacts upon the increased prevalence and incidence of heart failure in diabetic patients.

In addition to these two major risk factors, a number of features associated with DM have been identified as independent risk factors for developing heart failure: poor glycaemic control, increasing body mass index (BMI), increasing age, the use of insulin,[24] the presence of any measurable renal insult from microalbuminuria to end-stage renal failure,[10,24] and duration of DM. For instance, a 1% reduction in HbA1c in UKPDS reduced the risk of heart failure by 16%,[20] whereas a 2.5 unit increase in BMI increased the risk of heart failure by 12%.[24]

Diabetic cardiomyopathy

Although most registry-based studies and intervention trials for the treatment of chronic heart failure suggest that the principal cause of LVSD in patients with DM is ischaemic in origin, a sizeable proportion appear to arise from the entity referred to as 'diabetic cardiomyopathy', i.e. heart failure occurring in a patient with DM in the absence of CAD or hypertension.[37]

The existence of a specific diabetic cardiomyopathy has long been debated, and attempts made to characterize specific pathological and diagnostic features. The initial description was based on a small number of individuals noted to have a clinical diagnosis of heart failure but with no evidence of prior CAD or hypertension.[38] Using this simple clinical approach suggested that diabetic cardiomyopathy was a rare entity. However, further investigation has revealed a raft of abnormalities in the diabetic heart which suggests not only that diabetic cardiomyopathy is a real entity, but also that it is extremely prevalent in patients with DM. The full extent of these abnormalities are out with the scope of this review, but key features are summarized in Table 36.4.[37,39]

The initial feature of diabetic cardiomyopathy appears to be the development of features of LVSD. Early studies using conventional two-dimensional transthoracic echocardiography are likely to have failed to appreciate the presence of the subtle abnormalities consistent with diastolic dysfunction and thus to have underestimated the true prevalence of diabetic cardiomyopathy. The assessment of transmitral flow, use of Valsalva manoeuvre, pulmonary venous blood flow, and the use of tissue Doppler assessment of longitudinal function greatly increase the ability to detect LVSD in patients with symptoms or signs of heart failure.[39] Thus, in those patients with no echocardiographic features of LVSD, but clinical features of heart failure, and with evidence of LVSD, a diagnosis of diastolic heart failure can be made, and this early feature correlates closely with HbA1c in diabetic patients.[40] Whilst it is suggested (perhaps erroneously) that diastolic heart failure may account for 50% of all heart failure cases,[31] studies of patients with both type 1 and type 2 DM have suggested that diastolic dysfunction is as common in asymptomatic patients without overt CAD.[41–43]

Once present, diastolic dysfunction has a prognosis similar to systolic dysfunction and the combination of either left ventricular hypertrophy, CAD, or both has a profound deleterious effect on the diabetic heart.[3–7] Thus, in addition to optimizing glycaemic control, rigorous attention to blood pressure and cardiovascular risk modification is essential in the patient with DM.

Treating hyperglycaemia in diabetes mellitus

Whilst fasting and postprandial hyperglycaemia are the key diagnostic features of DM—and this is clearly responsible for the development of the microvascular complications of DM, and is an important factor in the genesis of the excess burden of cardiovascular complications seen in patients with DM—the management of the patient with DM should not be simply glucocentric.

The management of cardiovascular risk, with the purpose of reducing end-organ damage—specifically heart failure—is complex and requires meticulous attention to the control of blood pressure, aggressive modification of dyslipidaemia, appropriate use of antiplatelet therapy, and constant attention to lifestyle modification (Table 36.5).

Crucially, the UKPDS demonstrated the benefit of treating hypertension in diabetics by revealing a reduction in both microvascular and macrovascular complications, and notably a reduction in new cases of heart failure of 44%.[44] However, this benefit did not persist after relaxation of blood pressure control, suggesting that aggressive blood pressure control should be instituted when first detected and maintained lifelong.[45,46]

Treating hyperglycaemia to reduce the vascular complications of DM seems intuitively straightforward. However, the first study attempting to address this question, the controversial UGDP,[47]

Table 36.4 Clinical, pathological, and molecular features of diabetic cardiomyopathy

Clinical features	Pathological features
• Absence of arterial hypertension • Absence of coronary artery disease • Symptoms and/or signs of heart failure	• Myocardial fibrosis • Cardiomyocyte hypertrophy • Increased myocardial fat
Echocardiographic features	**Molecular mechanisms**
• Left ventricular diastolic dysfunction evidenced by: reduced early and increased late diastolic transmitral flow (reversed E:A ratio) restrictive LV filling pattern • Tissue Doppler measurements at mitral valve annulus to quantify longitudinal myocardial lengthening/shortening • Left atrial volume index >40 mL/min²	• Conventional coronary risk factors • Hyperglycaemia • Reactive oxygen species • Nitric oxide • Poly-(ADP-ribose) polymerase • Protein kinase C • Altered intracellular calcium homeostasis • Dysfunctional RAAS • Hypoxia-inducible factor-1 • VEGF
Cardiac magnetic resonance imaging	
• Greater morphological and functional parameter assessment • Comparable measures of LV filling to echocardiography • Allows other assessments, e.g. myocardial fat measurement	

LV, left ventricle; RAAS, renin–angiotensin–aldosterone system; VEGF, vascular endothelial growth factor.

Table 36.5 'Four corners' approach to modifying risk of cardiovascular disease in patients with diabetes mellitus

Hypertension	Hyperglycaemia
• Aggressive treatment of hypertension to minimize risk of development of LVH and subsequent LVSD. • Target based blood pressure: ≤130/75 mmHg. • Lower blood pressure target in presence of end-organ damage, e.g. microalbuminuria: ≤120/70 mmHg. • Promote use of RAS blockade: ACEi/ARB/MRA. • Do not avoid use of β-blocker therapy due to presence of DM or fear of hypoglycaemic unawareness. Use evidence-based therapies, e.g. carvedilol, bisoprolol. • Patients with DM are at increased risk of hyperkalaemia during treatment with MRA/ACEi/ARB therapy, and monitoring of eGFR and serum K⁺ is recommended.	• Optimal long-term control of hyperglycaemia. • A target HbA1c between 6.0% and 7.5% is likely to minimize the microvascular and macrovascular adverse effects of hyperglycaemia. • Complex combinations of oral agents, GLP-1 analogues and insulin may be required to reach this target. • Complex regimens to lower HbA1c are associated with greater risks of significant hypoglycaemia, weight gain and possibly cardiovascular adverse effects. • Patients with established heart failure should not receive TZD therapy except in isolated supervised circumstances. • Metformin is safe in stable CHF but monitoring of renal function and temporary cessation during intercurrent illness is required.
Hyperlipidaemia	**Anti-platelet therapy/smoking cessation**
• Patients with known vascular disease should receive lipid-lowering therapy with an HMG–CoA reductase inhibitor in line with local/national guidance, e.g. NICE, JBS2. • Diabetes is recognized as a 'CHD-equivalent' in some national guidelines, and lowering of total and LDL-cholesterol with an HMG–CoA reductase inhibitor is recommended even in the absence of clinical vascular disease. • Addition of other therapies, including fibrates, should be considered. • Patients with early diabetic cardiomyopathy may benefit from treatment with HMG–CoA reductase inhibitor therapy more than those with advanced heart failure.	• Antiplatelet therapy with aspirin or clopidogrel should be used when there is evidence of existing vascular disease, i.e. in line with guidance on secondary prevention of CHD. Use of Aspirin in patients with DM but without clinically apparent vascular disease is not routinely recommended due to concerns regarding risk-benefits of this approach, i.e. risk of bleeding vs. reduction in vascular events. • There are no data to support the use of aspirin in the absence of vascular disease in patients with diabetes. • Smoking cessation will limit the risk of further vascular events, including progressive retinopathy in diabetic patients.

LVH, left ventricular hypertrophy; LVSD, left ventricular systolic dysfunction; Hb1Ac, glycated haemoglobin; RAS, renal artery stenosis; ACEi, angiotensin converting enzyme inhibitor; ARB, angiotensin receptor blocker; MRA, mineralocorticoid receptor antagonist; GLP-1, glucagon-like peptide 1; DM, diabetes mellitus; TZD, thiazolidinediones; eGFR, estimated glomerular filtration rate; NICE, National Institute for Health and Care Excellence; JBS2, Joint British Societies' guidelines; CHD, coronary heart disease; LDL, low-density lipoprotein.

suggested that pharmacological measures to lower blood glucose levels in patients with type 2 DM with the SU drug tolbutamide actually resulted in an excess of cardiovascular deaths. This study has been the centre of much controversy and more recently a number of well-conducted, informative studies have assessed the benefit, if any, of blood glucose lowering via pharmacological intervention in patients with type 1 and type 2 DM.

Principal among these studies has been the UKPDS.[48] This UK-based study assessed the value of 'tight' glycaemic control, i.e. treatment based on achieving near-normal fasting or postprandial blood glucose levels, versus 'conventional' glycaemic control, i.e. treatment based on symptom control. Within the UKPDS, tight control required the introduction of escalating doses of oral hypoglycaemic agents, insulin, or both.

Overall, the application of the tight control approach resulted in an absolute reduction in HbA1c (the standard measure of long-term glycaemic control) of ~1% compared to the conventional treatment group.[48] This difference in glycaemic control was translated into a number of clear benefits in terms of vascular risk modification (Table 36.4). Whilst there was no clear significant benefit of tight glycaemic control on the overall risk of myocardial infarction, treatment with metformin in obese patients with type 2 DM did result in a significant reduction in the risk of myocardial infarction, and overall it was demonstrated that the risk of developing heart failure increased by 8% for every 1% absolute rise in HbA1c in keeping with the intuitive notion of good glycaemic control reducing the risk of heart failure.[20]

Prolonged follow-up of the UKPDS demonstrated that even though the tight control group and the conventional control group gravitated towards each other in terms of long-term HbA1c measures after study completion, a legacy effect was demonstrable in the tight control group beyond the period of strict tight control.[49]

Perhaps of even greater interest was that after cessation of tight control, although measures of diabetes control deteriorated, there was the emergence at 10 years of clear benefits in terms of a reduction in myocardial infarction of 15% ($P = 0.01$) in the SU-treated group, and a reduction in myocardial infarction of 33% ($P < 0.005$) and death from any cause of 27% ($P = 0.002$) in those overweight patients treated with metformin.[49]

The cornerstone of the management of all patients with DM is, and always has been, lifestyle modification aimed at maximizing daily activity, stopping tobacco exposure, attaining as near an ideal weight and BMI as practicable, and encouraging healthy eating habits to minimize salt, saturated fat, refined carbohydrate, and excess calorie intake.[50] However, in the case of type 1 DM and the vast majority of cases of type 2 DM, adjunctive therapy with either oral agents, insulin, or both is necessary, not just to relieve the symptoms of hyperglycaemia, but to achieve as near-normal blood glucose control as possible with the hope of minimizing DM-related complications including heart failure.

Oral hypoglycaemic agents

Until the mid 1990s, the only oral agents available for treating hyperglycaemia in DM were old drugs, or their mildly altered derivatives. Since the late 1990s, however, two new classes of agents have become widely available for treating hyperglycaemia in DM, with other novel agents in development (Table 36.6).

Metformin

Metformin is a biguanide drug which has been available for treating type 2 DM for more than 40 years. Its precise mode of action is unclear, but it does reduce hepatic gluconeogenesis and peripheral

Table 36.6 Drug classes used to lower blood glucose in patients with diabetes mellitus

Class of agent	Example	Typical use	Side-effects
Biguanide	Metformin	First line after lifestyle modification. Combined with all other classes.	Gastrointestinal upset Vitamin B_{12} deficiency (rare) Lactic acidosis (rare, associated with intercurrent hypoxia-associated illness)
Sulfonylurea	Glipizide Gliclazide Glimepiride	Second line in addition to metformin or if metformin contraindicated	Hypoglycaemia Weight gain Relatively rapid loss of efficacy
Thiazolidinedione (glitazone)	Pioglitazone Rosiglitazone	Second line in addition to metformin or if metformin contraindicated (rarely used now)	Fluid retention, heart failure, osteoporosis
α-Glucosidase inhibitor	Acarbose	Second line in addition to metformin or if metformin contraindicated (little used in the UK)	Gastrointestinal upset, especially flatulence
Meglitinide	Repaglinide Nateglinide		Hypoglycaemia
DPP-IV inhibitor	Sitagliptin Vildagliptin Alogliptin Linagliptin Saxagliptin	Second line in addition to metformin or if metformin contraindicated. May be used with SU.	Minor. Saxagliptin may increase heart failure risk.
SGLT-2 inhibitors	Dapagliflozin Empgliflozin Canagliflozin	Second line in addition to metformin or if metformin contraindicated. Likely to become first-line in those who have heart failure. May be used with SU.	Genital infections (candida), possibly lower limb amputation (canagliflozin), increased risk of Diabetic ketoacidosis (all).
Incretin mimetics	Exenatide Liraglutide Dulaglutide Semaglutide (subcutaneous or oral)	Second line to metformin or first line if known atherosclerotic vascular disease. Can be used with insulin and in renal impairment (semaglutide).	Nausea, gastrointestinal upset Acute pancreatitis (exenatide).
Insulin	Rapid-acting Long-acting Human/analogue/porcine	All cases of type 1 DM. Type 2 DM after metformin monotherapy has failed or after trials of multiple oral agents.	Hypoglycaemia Weight gain

DPP-IV, dipeptidyl peptidase-4; SU, sulfonylurea; SGLT-2, sodium-glucose linked co-transporter 2; DM, diabetes mellitus.

insulin resistance, leading to a reduction in both fasting and post-prandial hyperglycaemia.

Metformin is widely used for the treatment of type 2 DM world-wide, with most national guidelines suggesting it as the first-line oral agent for type 2 DM once lifestyle modification has been implemented, and no longer sufficient to maintain the set glycaemic target.[51] Metformin is often used in combination with other oral agents, insulin, and other injectable agents in type 2 DM, and is often used in patients with type 1 DM when there is clinical evidence of insulin resistance.

Metformin's popularity stems from its positive association with reducing cardiovascular events in obese patients with type 2 DM in the UKPDS.[52] Within the UKPDS, metformin treatment was associated with a reduction of myocardial infarction which was sustained at 10 years of follow-up.[49]

The major limitation to treatment with metformin is its propensity to cause gastrointestinal upset, particularly nausea and diarrhoea, which necessitates discontinuation of the drug in up to 20% of cases. Much less common is the potential for megaloblastic anaemia due to interference with vitamin B_{12} absorption. Metformin is renally excreted, and can accumulate in the presence of renal impairment. Current guidance in the UK suggests that withdrawal of metformin be considered when serum creatinine reaches 150 μmol/L, or when estimated glomerular filtration rate (eGFR) falls to <30 mL/min.[53]

Of greater concern, although much less common, is the association between metformin and lactic acidosis. This association, although well documented, is rare and spontaneous isolated cases of metformin-induced lactic acidosis are extremely infrequent (<1 case per 100 000 treated patients).[54,55]

In clinical practice, it is wise to withdraw metformin in patients with heart failure who experience intercurrent illness that might be associated with tissue hypoxia, e.g. acute decompensated heart failure, myocardial infarction, or pneumonia. Similarly, patients with heart failure treated with metformin should have regular monitoring of renal function to ensure that metformin is withdrawn in the event of a rapid decline in renal function, or in the context of a slow decline to a level where concern about accumulation outweighs potential benefits on glycaemic control and cardiovascular event reduction.

Sulfonylurea drugs

Initial experience with SU drugs was tempered by the UGDP experience.[47] Subsequent investigations using newer agents with different properties have established the class as a popular choice for treating hyperglycaemia in patients who are no longer satisfactorily controlled on metformin alone.

The use of SUs has been controversial since the UGDP. Some observational and retrospective studies suggest that SUs are associated with increased cardiovascular mortality.[56,57] However, neither the

UKPDS nor ADVANCE study demonstrated any adverse cardiovascular mortality effects associated with their use.[49,58] Their rapid onset of action and low cost is particularly attractive when treating symptomatic patients, but on the downside, use of SUs to achieve tight glycaemic control is associated with weight gain and significant potential for symptomatic hypoglycaemia.[58,59] Furthermore, SUs appear to exhibit a rather more rapid decline in efficacy over time than either metformin or thiazolidinediones,[60] making their use as first-line agents less attractive.

Thiazolidinediones

Thiazolidinediones (TZDs, glitazones) are modulators of the peroxisome proliferator-activated receptor-γ and increase insulin sensitivity of skeletal muscle, adipose tissue, and liver to insulin.[61] TZDs have a similar magnitude and duration of effect on glycaemic control to metformin as single therapy,[60] with lower risks of hypoglycaemia than SUs. However, TZDs have two adverse effects which have limited their use in the treatment of patients with DM, and especially those with or at risk of developing heart failure, namely weight gain and fluid retention.

Weight gain with TZDs is similar to or greater than that seen with SUs, although it is often associated with some modest benefits on lipid profiles.[60] Fluid retention is mediated via the kidney, and peripheral oedema and heart failure are both increased in users of TZDs.[62] Although it appears that TZDs do not directly affect left ventricular function,[62] there is no question that they do cause heart failure, even in the presence of normal left ventricular function.[63,64]

Perhaps the greatest controversy surrounding TZDs is the suggestion that they may increase the risk of myocardial infarction or death. Initial evidence suggested that pioglitazone may have a modest beneficial effect on cardiovascular outcomes in patients with type 2 DM (secondary end-point of myocardial infarction, stroke, and premature death: 16%, $P = 0.027$;[65] the primary end-point was not affected). However, a controversial meta-analysis of data pertaining to rosiglitazone suggested that it was associated with a 43% increased risk of myocardial infarction (OR: 1.43; $P = 0.03$).[66] This result was followed by a raft of publications which have confirmed that both TZDs result in increased rates of peripheral oedema, heart failure, and hospitalization due to heart failure.[54,63] A retrospective cohort study of adverse cardiovascular events associated with TZD use demonstrated no difference in the incidence of acute myocardial infarction related to use of pioglitazone versus rosiglitazone, but did demonstrate a reduction in risk of both death (adjusted hazard ratio: 0.86; 95% CI: 0.75–0.98) and heart failure (0.77; 0.69–0.87) for users of pioglitazone versus rosiglitazone. This translated into numbers needed to harm of 120 for heart failure and 293 for death, for users of rosiglitazone rather than pioglitazone.[63] However, it should be borne in mind that the absolute event rates quoted (risk of myocardial infarction plus heart failure plus death, pioglitazone 5.3% vs rosiglitazone 6.9% over 6 years) equate to a 10-year CVD risk that barely reaches 10%.

TZDs are available for use in the treatment of type 2 DM worldwide, either in combination with oral agents, or with insulin in selected cases. They are not recommended for use in patients with known heart failure, and should be used with caution in patients at risk of developing heart failure.[64]

Dipeptidyl peptidase-4 inhibitors (DPP-IV)

Insulin secretion after meals is enhanced by the release of endogenous incretin peptides from the small intestinal wall. The secretion of these incretins, e.g. glucagon like peptide 1 (GLP-1), are reduced in type 2 DM and contribute to the development of hyperglycaemia.

One means of maximizing the effect of endogenous incretins is to increase their biological half-life by inhibiting their natural catabolism by the enzyme dipeptidyl peptidase-4 (DPP-IV). Oral agents that perform this function are available as once-daily treatments, and are generally well tolerated with limited risk of hypoglycaemia or weight gain when used as a single agent or in combination with metformin. Co-administration with SUs or insulin does not enhance the weight gain or hypoglycaemia risk above that of the co-administered drug.

One concern that arose during the clinical studies of the different DPP-IV agents was the potential for increased cases of clinical heart failure or hospital admissions due to worsening heart failure.

Three agents have been studied in patients with type 2 DM with increased risk of cardiovascular events, or following acute coronary syndromes.[67,68,69] One of these trials (SAVOR-TIMI 53) studied Saxagliptin in patients with type 2 DM at increased risk of cardiovascular events. Although there was no observed change in mortality or non-fatal myocardial infarction or stroke, there was an increased rate of admission to hospital with worsening heart failure (3.5% vs 2.8%; HR: 1.27; 95% CI: 1.07–1.51; $P = 0.007$).[69] This risk was highest in patients with a prior diagnosis of heart failure, reduced eGFR and elevated N-terminal B-type pronatriuetic peptide. Of interest, the risk of hospitalization subsided to that of the placebo arm after around 10 months of use. Other agents have not demonstrated a significant increase in hospitalization due to heart failure.[67,68]

Glucagon-like peptide-1 receptor agonists

Rather than slow down catabolism of endogenous incretins, exogenous administration of glucagon-like peptide-1 (GLP-1) receptor agonists or analogues of it have been used to treat hyperglycaemia in type 2 DM, and as an adjunct to the treatment of type 1 DM or obesity.

Their use in the treatment of heart failure is ongoing in clinical trials but an early analysis of the use of liraglutide in patients following an episode of acute heart failure did not reveal any positive effect.[70]

In patients with type 2 DM at risk of cardiovascular events, the addition of liraglutide to standard therapy was studied in the LEADER trial.[71] In patients receiving liraglutide there was a lower rate of death from cardiovascular causes and there was a non-significant reduction in the cases of hospitalization for heart failure. The study of another GLP-1 analogue, semaglutide,[72] in patients with type 2 DM suggested that there was also benefit in reduction of combined cardiovascular end-points, but did not show a significant reduction in hospitalization due to heart failure. Further investigation of oral semaglutide in patients with diabetes mellitus and the presence of cardiovascular risk factors or established cardiovascular disease suggested that oral semaglutide reduced MACE events but did not impact on heart failure admissions.[73]

Sodium-glucose-linked co-transporter 2 inhibitors

Inhibition of glucose reabsorption at the proximal convoluted tubule by sodium-glucose-linked co-transporter 2 (SGLT-2) inhibitors is an effective way of reducing blood glucose in patients with type 2 DM. It is associated with persistent glycosuria (a loss of around 300 calories per day), with the principal side-effect of an increase in genital and urinary tract infections. The EMPA-REG Outcome study examined the use of empagliflozin in patients with type 2 DM at high risk of cardiovascular events, and this saw a 14% relative risk reduction in the primary end-point of cardiovascular death, non-fatal myocardial infarction, and stroke ($P = 0.04$).[73] In a further analysis, there was a 34% relative reduction in cardiovascular deaths and hospitalizations due to heart failure in those treated with empagliflozin (2.7% vs 4.1%; HR: 0.66; 95% CI: 0.55–0.79; $P < 0.001$).[74] As such, there are several ongoing clinical trials of SGLT-2 inhibitors in patients with heart failure.

The DAPA-HF trial investigated the use of dapagliflozin in patients with heart failure with NYHA class II–IV, an ejection fraction ≤40% and eGFR>30mL/min. Treatment with dapagliflozin reduced the primary endpoint of worsening heart failure, or cardiovascular death by 26% compared to placebo (HR: 0.74; 95% CI: 0.65–0.85; $P < 0.0001$). Furthermore, there were significant reductions in all-cause and cardiovascular mortality, and heart failure hospitalisation, and an improvement in quality of life. This effect was seen in those with or without diabetes mellitus.[76] A similar effect was seen in the EMPEROR-REDUCED study with empagliflozin where the primary endpoint of CV death or hospitalisation for heart failure was reduced by 25%.[77] These drugs are well tolerated, with no excess of renal impairment (and indeed appear renal-protective,[78] volume depletion, or hypoglycaemia. Indeed, the only adverse more common with SGLT2-inhibitors than placebo is genital fungal infection, and patients should be counselled accordingly. As such, the SGLT2-inhibitors dapagliflozin and empagliflozin have become cornerstone agents in the management of HFrEF. There are two ongoing studies in HFpEF (DELIVER and EMPEROR-PRESERVED) which are due to report shortly.

Insulin

Insulin is the longest-serving therapeutic option for the treatment of DM. Multiple formulations exist, and numerous means of administration of insulin are used in an attempt to mimic physiological insulin profiles and restore normal blood glucose profiles in patients with DM.

The use of insulin in the treatment of patients with type 2 DM is increasingly common, principally due to the increasing use of glycaemic targets promoted by national and international expert committees.[67] Patients with heart failure exhibit increased resistance to insulin, mediated via a variety of different mechanisms including excess catecholamine production. As a consequence, insulin doses required to achieve adequate glycaemic control are substantially higher than in patients with type 1 DM, or in those without heart failure.

The use of insulin is an independent predictor for the development of heart failure and increased mortality in patients with DM.[24,68,69,70] One retrospective cohort study of patients with DM without heart failure showed that those commenced on insulin had a higher rate of hospitalization due to heart failure than those commenced on SUs (HR: 1.56; $P = 0.05$).[70]

Within the UKPDS insulin treatment did not not increase the incidence of heart failure or mortality,[48] whereas insulin-treated patients in the CHARM study had a greater risk of mortality than non-insulin treated patients.[71] A further retrospective analysis of patients with advanced heart failure suggested that insulin treatment was an independent predictor of mortality (HR: 4.30; 95% CI: 1.69–10.94).[69]

At present, there are no prospective evaluations of insulin therapy in patients with DM—with or without heart failure—to advise on the precise role of insulin treatment.

Heart failure treatment in patients with diabetes mellitus

The majority of the benefit of treatments for heart failure in patients with DM are inferred from subgroups of the major intervention trials for the treatment of heart failure (Table 36.7). There are no specific data in relation to the effect of digoxin in patients with heart failure and DM. In A-HeFT, DM did not affect the benefit of hydralazine plus isosorbide dinitrate.[103] Thiazide diuretics have the potential to increase fasting blood glucose levels, although their effect on reducing blood pressure, preventing heart failure, and on reducing strokes far outweighs any minor effect on glycaemic control.[94]

Angiotensin converting enzyme inhibitors and angiotensin receptor blockers

ACE inhibitors are widely used to treat hypertension, micro-albuminuria, and proteinuria in patients with DM.[101] Their benefits in the treatment of heart failure are well established, although in patients with DM the benefits are less apparent (Table 36.7).[104]

β-Blockers

β-Blockers are effective treatments for heart failure. In patients with heart failure and DM the benefits of β-blocker therapy are similar to those seen in non-diabetic subjects in reducing mortality and hospitalization due to heart failure (Table 36.7).[104] One concern regarding the application of β-blocker therapy in patients with DM is the potential for this class of drugs to alter insulin sensitivity and alter hypoglycaemia awareness.

Hypoglycaemia results in a pronounced activation of the sympathetic nervous system, cortisol, and glucagon release. These responses aim to increase hepatic glucose output, and to increase blood supply to the brain and other glucose-sensitive tissues. The UKPDS assessed the rates of hypoglycaemia in patients with hypertension and DM and discerned no difference in the rate of hypoglycaemia in patients treated with atenolol or captopril,[44] whereas one study of elderly diabetic patients suggested that insulin-treated patients were more likely to experience severe hypoglycaemia than those treated with SUs.[105]

In general, there are few or no data to suggest that β-blockers used to treat heart failure in patients with DM specifically affect hypoglycaemic awareness, recovery from symptomatic hypoglycaemia,

Table 36.7 Treatment of diabetic patients with or without heart failure: results of selected intervention studies

Study name	Total study population	Diabetes	No diabetes	Mortality risk ratio (95% confidence interval)		
				Diabetes	No diabetes	Diabetes vs no diabetes
β-Blockers						
MERIT-HF[12]	3991	985	3006	0.81 (0.57–1.15)	0.62 (0.48–0.79)	
CIBIS-II[84]	2647	312	2335	0.81 (0.52–1.27)	0.66 (0.54–0.81)	
COPERNICUS[85]	2287	586	1701	0.68 (0.47–1.00)	0.67 (0.52–0.85)	
Pooled data		1883	7042	0.77 (0.61–0.96)	0.65 (0.57–0.74)	1.19 (0.91–1.55)
ACEi: heart failure						
CONSENSUS[14]	253	56	197	1.06 (0.65–1.74)	0.64 (0.46–0.88)2231	
SAVE[86]	2231	492	1739	0.89 (0.68–1.16)	0.82 (0.68–0.99)	
SMILE[87]	1556	303	1253	0.44 (0.22–0.87)	0.79 (0.5–1.15)	
SOLVD−prevention[88]	4228	647	3581	0.75 (0.55–1.02)	0.97 (0.83–1.15)	
SOLVD−treatment[88]	2569	663	1906	1.01 (0.85–1.21)	0.84 (0.74–0.95)	
TRACE[5]	1749	237	1512	0.73(0.57–0.94)	0.85 (0.74–0.97)	
Pooled data		2398	10188	0.84 (0.70–1.00)	0.85 (0.78–0.92)	1.00 (0.80–1.25)
DM without HF	Placebo rate of HF	ACEi-treated rate of HF				
HOPE[89]	11–15%	9%				
EUROPA[90]	No difference with respect to DM status					
Aldosterone antagonists						
RALES[91]	No difference shown or outcomes not stratified with respect to with diabetes					
EPHESUS[92]						
ARBs						
Val-HeFT[93]	Valsartan therapy did not prevent the primary endpoint in patients with HF and DM					
CHARM overall[94,95]	Trend to lesser effect of candesartan on preventing HF in patients with DM					
CHARM preserved[17]	Non-significant trend in reduction in HF in patients with DM					
I-PRESERVED[96]	No effect of irbesartan on reducing onset of HF, and no benefit with respect to DM diagnosis					
Others (not specifically targeting patient with DM or HF)						
IDNT[97]	Irbesartan more effective than amlodipine in preventing new HF in patients with DM					
VALUE[98]	Valsartan more effective than amlodipine in preventing new HF in patients with DM					
RENAAL[99]	Losartan reduces HF incidence in patients with DM and preserved LV function by 32%					
LIFE[100]	Losartan reduced the risk of developing HF in patients with DM more than atenolol; RR: 0.41.					
Renin inhibitors						
ATMOSPHERE[102]	Aliskiren addition to enalpril of no benefit and higher rates of hypotension, hyperkalaemia and worsening serum creatinine					

ACEi, angiotensin converting enzyme inhibitors; ARBs, angiotensin receptor blockers; DM, diabetes mellitus; HF, heart failure.

or adversely alter lipid metabolism to the detriment of patients.[105] Furthermore, the benefits of treatment with β-blockers in terms of reduction in critical endpoints far outweighs any potential effects on other measures.

Practice points

Table 36.8 lists a number of key practice points that are worth paying attention to in day to day practice when dealing with the patient with heart failure and DM.

Summary

Diabetes mellitus and heart failure are increasingly common conditions, and they therefore frequently coexist. Diabetes complicates the management, and imparts a greater risk of morbidity and mortality on the patient with heart failure. Optimizing cardiovascular risk factors is essential for limiting adverse outcomes for both conditions, and patients with diabetes mellitus are, at present, still less likely to receive optimal care whether due to fear of application of some evidence-based strategies, or the inability to tolerate a number of therapeutic agents. Glycaemic control is an important factor in

Table 36.8 Practice points for daily management of patients with heart failure and diabetes mellitus

Practice point	Risks	Action
Hyperkalaemia	• Long standing DM • Type 4 renal tubular acidosis • ACEi/ARB/MRA use • NSAID use	• Monitor serum potassium regularly and during intercurrent illness • Withdraw or modify doses of offending drugs
Hypoglycaemia	• Sulfonylurea use • Insulin use • Injection site lipohypertrophy • Unexpected exercise/missed meals • Worsening renal function	• Measure renal function • Examine injection sites • Modify dose/timing of SU or insulin • Correct any reversible causes of renal impairment
Renal impairment	• DM duration • Hypertension • Cigarette smoking • ACEi/ARB/renin inhibitors • Peripheral vascular disease • Dehydration/ excessive diuretic use • NSAID use	• Correct any intercurrent precipitant • Withhold metformin and ACEi/ARB/renin inhibitors until condition improved • Consider withdrawal or dose modification of metformin and ACEi/ARB/MRA
Heart failure	• TZDs • Saxagliptin • Insulin initiation • Pre-existing hypertension, atrial fibrillation, LBBB on ECG	• Modify treatment to exclude TZD or saxagliptin if indicated • Avoid commencement of TZD if possible • Consider alteration of loop diuretic dose • Monitor for signs of worsening heart failure if initiating TZD, saxagliptin or insulin

DM, diabetes mellitus; ACEi, angiotensin converting enzyme inhibitor; ARB, angiotensin receptor blocker; NSAID, non-steroidal anit-inflammatory drug; SU, 7 sulfonylurea drug; MRA, mineralocorticoid receptor antagonist; TZD, thiazolidinediones; LBBB, left bundle branch block; ECG, electrocardiogram.

the management of the patient with diabetes mellitus and heart failure; when optimized, patient-specific approaches are most likely to minimize adverse events while maximizing the opportunity for reducing long-term complications. The role of the newest agents has become clearer, with heart failure guidelines likely to endorse SGLT2 inhibitors as first line agents for the patient with heart failure and DM. However, it is clear that these agents have effects beyond DM, as they have been found to improve morbidity and mortality even in those HF patients who do not have DM.

REFERENCES

1. Kannel WB, Hjortland M, Castelli WP. Role of diabetes in congestive heart failure: the Framinhgam study. *Am J Cardiol* 1974;**34**:29–34.
2. Bibbins-Domingo K, Lin F, Vittinghoff E. Predictors of heart failure among women with coronary disease. *Circulation* 2004;**110**:1424–30.
3. Carrabba N, Valenti R, Parodi G, Santoro GM, Antoniucci D. Left ventricular remodelling and heart failure in diabetic patients treated with primary angioplasty for acute myocardial infarction. *Circulation* 2004;**110**:1974–9.
4. Mukamal, KJ, Nesto RW, Cohen MC, *et al.* mpact of diabetes on long-term survival after acute myocardial infarction: comparability of risk with prior myocardial infarction. *Diabetes Care* 2001;**24**:1422–7.
5. Melchior T, Kober L, Madsen CR, *et al.* Accelerating impact of diabetes mellitus on mortality in the years following an acute myocardial infarction: TRACE Study Group Trandolapril Cardiac Evaluation. *Eur Heart J* 1999;**20**:973–8.
6. Newton JD, Squire IB. Glucose and haemoglobin in the assessment of prognosis after first hospitalisation for heart failure. *Heart* 2006;**92**:1441–6.

7. Berry C, Brett M, Stevenson K, McMurray JJV, Norrie J. Nature and prognostic importance of abnormal glucose tolerance and diabetes in acute heart failure. *Heart* 2008;**94**:296–304.
8. Thrainsdottir IS, Aspelund T, Thorgeirsson G, *et al.* The association between glucose abnormalities and heart failure in the population-based Reykjavik study. *Diabetes Care* 2005;**28**:612–16.
9. Davies M, Hobbs F, Davis R, *et al.* Prevalence of left-ventricular systolic dysfunction and heart failure in the Echocardiographic Heart of England Screening study: a population based study. *Lancet* 2001;**358**:439–44.
10. Bertoni AG, Hundley WG, Massing MW, *et al.* Heart failure prevalence, incidence, and mortality in the elderly with diabetes. *Diabetes Care* 2004;**27**:699–703.
11. Harris MI, Flegal KM, Cowie CC, *et al.* Prevalence of diabetes, impaired fasting glucose, and impaired glucose tolerance in U.S. Adults. The Third National Health and Nutrition Examination Survey 1988–1994. *Diabetes Care* 1998;**21**:518–24.
12. MERIT-HF Investigators. Effect of metoprolol CR/XL in chronic heart failure. Metoprolol CR/XL Randomised Intervention Trial in Congestive Heart Failure (MERIT-HF). *Lancet* 1999;**353**:2001–2007.
13. Poole-Wilson PA, Swedberg K, Cleland JG, *et al.* Comparison of carvedilol and metoprolol on outcomes in patients with chronic heart failure in the Carvedilol or Metoprolol European Trial (COMET): randomised controlled trial. *Lancet* 2003;**362**:7–13.
14. CONSENSUS Trial Study Group. Effects of enalapril on mortality in severe congestive heart failure. Results of the Cooperative North Scandinavian Enalapril Survival Study (CONSENSUS). *N Engl J Med* 1987;**316**:1429–35.
15. Cohn JN, Tognoni G. A randomised trial of the angiotensin-receptor blocker valsartan in chronic heart failure. *N Engl J Med* 2001;**345**:1667–75.
16. Pitt B, Poole-Wilson PA, Segal R, *et al.* Effect of losartan compared with captopril on mortality in patients with

symptomatic heart failure: randomised trial—the Losartan Heart Failure Survival Study Elite II. *Lancet* 2000;**355**:1582–7.

17. Yusuf S, Pfeffer MA, Swedberg K, *et al.* Effects of candesartan in patients with chronic heart failure and preserved left ventricular ejection fraction: the CHARM-preserved Trial. *Lancet* 2003;**362**:777–781.

18. Adams KF Jr, Fonarow GC, Emerman CL, *et al.*; ADHERE Scientific Advisory Committee and Investigators. Characteristics and outcomes of patients hospitalised for heart failure in the United States: rationale, design, and preliminary observations from the first 100,000 cases in the Acute Decompensated Heart Failure National Registry (ADHERE). *Am Heart J* 2005;**149**:209–16.

19. Greenberg BH, Abraham WT, Albert NM, *et al.* Influence of diabetes on characteristics and outcomes in patients hospitalised with heart failure: a report from the Organized Program to Initiate Lifesaving Treatment in Hospitalized Patients with Heart Failure (OPTIMIZE-HF). *Am J Heart* 2007 **154**:27.e1–277.e8.

20. Stratton IM, Adler AI, Neil HAW, *et al.* Association of glycaemia with macrovascular and microvascular complications of type 2 diabetes (UKPDS 35): prospective observational study. *Br Med J* 2000;**321**:405–12.

21. Vaur I, Gueret P, Lievre M, Chabaud S, Passa P. Development of congestive heart failure in type 2 diabetic patients with microalbuminuria or proteinuria: observations from the DIABHYCAR (Type 2 DIABetes, Hypertension, Cardiovascular, Events and Ramipril) study. *Diabetes Care* 2003;**26**:855–60.

22. Iribarren C, Karter AJ, Go AS, *et al.* Glycemic control and heart failure among adult patients with diabetes. *Circulation* 2001;**103**:2668–73.

23. Heart Outcome Prevention Evaluation (HOPE) Study Investigators. Effects of ramipril on cardiovascular and microvascular outcomes in people with diabetes mellitus: results of the HOPE study and MICRO-HOPE substudy. *Lancet* 2000;**355**:253–9.

24. Nichols GA, Gullion CM, Koro CE, Ephross SE, Brown JB. The incidence of congestive heart failure in type 2 diabetes. *Diabetes Care* 2004;**27**:1879–84.

25. Kamalesh M, Nair G. Increasing prevalence of diabetes among patients with congestive heart failure. *Int J Cardiol* 2005;**104**:77–80.

26. Amato L, Paolisso G, Cacciatore F, *et al.* Congestive heart failure predicts the development of non-insulin-dependent diabetes mellitus in the elderly. The Osservatorio Geriatrico Regione Campania Group. *Diabetes Metab* 1997;**23**:213–18.

27. Yusuf S, Ostergren JB, Gerstein HC, *et al.* Effects of candesartan on the development of a new diagnosis of diabetes mellitus in patients with heart failure. *Circulation* 2005;**112**:48–53.

28. Vermes E, Ducharme A, Bourassa MG, *et al.* Enalapril reduces the incidence of diabetes in patients with chronic heart failure: insight from the studies of left ventricular dysfunction (SOLVD). *Circulation* 2003;**107**:1291–6.

29. Tenenbaum A, Motro M, Fisman EZ, *et al.* Functional class in patients with heart failure is associated with the development of diabetes. *Am J Med* 2003;**114**:271–5.

30. McDonagh TA, Morrison CE, Lawrence A, *et al.* Symptomatic and asymptomatic left-ventricular systolic dysfunction in an urban population. *Lancet* 1997;**350**:829–33.

31. Redfield MM, Jacobsen SJ, Burnett JC Jr, *et al.* Burden of systolic and diastolic ventricular dysfunction in the community: appreciating the scope of the heart failure epidemic. *JAMA* 2003;**289**:194–202.

32. Kistorp C, Galatius S, Gustafsson F, *et al.* Prevalence and characteristics of diabetic patients in a chronic heart failure population. *Int J Cardiol* 2005;**100**:281–7.

33. King H, Aubert RE, Herman WH. Global burden of diabetes, 1995–2025: prevalence, numerical estimates, and projections. *Diabetes Care* 1998;**21**:1414–31.

34. Expert Committee on the Diagnosis and Classification of Diabetes Mellitus. Report of the Expert Committee on the Diagnosis and Classification of Diabetes Mellitus. *Diabetes Care* 1997;**20**:1183–97.

35. International Expert Committee. International expert committee report on the role of the A1c assay in the diagnosis of diabetes. *Diabetes Care* 2009;**32**:1327–34.

36. Kilpatrick ES, Bloomgarden ZT, Zimmet PZ. Is haemoglobin A1c a step forward for diagnosing diabetes? *Br Med J* 2009;**339**:b4432.

37. Boudina S, Abel ED. Diabetic cardiomyopathy revisited. *Circulation* 2007;**115**:3213–23.

38. Rubler S, Dlugash J, Yuceoglu YZ, *et al.* New type of cardiomyopathy associated with diabetic glomerulosclerosis. *Am J Cardiol* 1972;**30**:595–602.

39. Khhavandi K, Khavandi A, Asghar O, *et al.* Dilated cardiomyopathy—a distinct disease? *Best Pract Res Clin Endocrinol Metab* 2009;**23**:347–60.

40. Shishehbor MH, Hoogwerf BJ, Schoeenhagen P, *et al.* Relation of hemoglobin A1c to left ventricular relaxation in patients with type 1 diabetes mellitus and without overt heart disease. *Am J Cardiol* 2003;**91**:1514–17, A9.

41. Poirer P, Bogaty P, Garneau C, Marois L, Dumesnil JG. Diastolic dysfunction in normotensive men with well-controlled type 2 diabetes: importance of maneuvers in echocardiographic screening for preclinical diabetic cardiomyopathy. *Diabetes Care* 2001;**24**:5–10.

42. Shivalkar B, Dhondt D, Goovaerts I, *et al.* Flow mediated dilatation and cardiac function in type 1 diabetes mellitus. *Am J Cardiol* 2006;**97**:77–82.

43. Di Bonito P, Moio N, Cavuto L, *et al.* Early detection of diabetic cardiomyopathy: usefulness of tissue Doppler imaging. *Diabet Med* 2005;**22**:1720–5.

44. UKPDS Group. Tight blood pressure control and risk of macrovascular and microvascular complications in type 2 diabetes. *Br Med J* 1998;**317**:703–13.

45. Holman RR, Paul SK, Bethel MA, Neil HAW, Matthews DR. Long-term follow-up after tight control of blood pressure in type 2 diabetes. *N Engl J Med* 2008;**359**:1565–76.

46. Group AC, Patel A, MacMahon S, *et al.* Intensive blood glucose control and vascular outcomes in patients with type 2 diabetes. *N Engl J Med* 2008;**358**:2560–72.

47. Meinert CL, Knatterud GL, Prout TE, *et al.* A study of the effects of hypoglycemic agents on vascular complications in patients with adult-onset diabetes. *Diabetes* 1970;**19**:789–830.

48. UKPDS Group. UKPDS 33: intensive blood-glucose control with sulphonylureas or insulin compared with conventional treatment and risk of complications in patients with type 2 diabetes. *Lancet* 1998;**352**:837–51.

49. Holman RR, Paul SK, Bethel MA, Matthews DR, Neil HAW. 10-year follow-up of intensive glucose control in type 2 diabetes. *N Engl J Med* 2008;**359**:1577–89.

50. SIGN Guideline Committee. SIGN 55—Management of Diabetes. Scottish Intercollegiate Guideline Network, ISBN 1899893 82 2. 2001.

51. Nathan DM, Buse JB, Davidson MB, *et al.* Medical management of hyperglycaemia in type 2 diabetes: a consensus algorithm for the initiation and adjustment of therapy. *Diabetes Care* 2009;**32**:193–203.

52. UKPDS study group. Effect of intensive blood-glucose control with metformin on complications in overweight patients with type 2 diabetes (UKPDS 34). *Lancet* 1998;**352**:854–65.

53. Shaw JS, Wilmot RL, Kilpatrick ES. Establishing pragmatic estimated GFR thresholds to guide metformin prescribing. *Diabetic Med* 2007;**24**:1160–3.

54. Bolen S, Feldman L, Vassy J, *et al.* Systematic review: comparative effectiveness and safety of oral medications for type 2 diabetes mellitus. *Ann Intern Med* 2007;**147**:386–99.

55. Salpeter S, Greyber E, Pasternak G, *et al.* Risk of fatal and nonfatal lactic acidosis with metformin use in type 2 diabetes mellitus. *Cochrane Database Syst Rev* 2006;(1):CD002967.

56. Evans J, Ogston S, Emslie-Smith A, Morris A. Risk of mortality and adverse cardiovascular outcomes in type 2 diabetes: a comparison of patients treated with sulphonylureas and metformin. *Diabetologia* 2006;**49**:930–6.

57. Tzoulaki I, Molokhia M, Curcin V, *et al.* Risk of cardiovascular disease and all cause mortality among patients with type 2 diabetes prescribed oral antidiabetes drugs: retrospective cohort study using UK general practice research database. *Br Med J* 2009;**339**:b4731.

58. ADVANCE Collaborative Group. Intensive blood glucose lowering in type 2 diabetes. *N Engl J Med* 2008;**358**:2560–72.

59. Action to Control Cardiovascular Risk in Diabetes Study Group. Effects of intensive glucose lowering in type 2 diabetes. *N Engl J Med* 2008;**358**:2545–59.

60. Kahn SE, Haffner SM, Heise MA, *et al.* Glycemic durability of rosiglitazone, metformin, or glyburide monotherapy. *N Engl J Med* 2006;**355**:2427–43.

61. Yki-Jarvinen H. Drug therapy: thiazolidinediones. *N Engl J Med* 2004;**351**:1106–10.

62. Dargie HJ, Hildebrandt PR, Riegger GAJ, *et al.* A randomised, placebo-controlled trial assessing the effects of rosiglitazone on echocardiographic function and cardiac status in type-2 diabetic patients with NYHA functional class I/II heart failure. *J Am Coll Cardiol* 2007;**49**:1696–1704.

63. Juurlink DN, Gomes T, Lipscombe LL, *et al.* Adverse cardiovascular events during treatment with pioglitazone and rosiglitazone: population based cohort study. *Br Med J* 2009;**339**:2942–8.

64. Jamieson A, Abousleiman Y. Thiazolidinedione-associated congestive heart failure and pulmonary edema. *Mayo Clin Proc* 2004;**79**:571–7.

65. Dormandy J, Charbonnel B, Eckland D, *et al.* Secondary prevention of macrovascular events in patients with type 2 diabetes in the PROactive Study (PROspective pioglitAzone Clinical Trial In macroVascular Events): a randomised controlled trial. *Lancet* 2005;**366**:1279–89.

66. Nissen SE, Wolski K. Effect of rosiglitazone on the risk of myocardial infarction and death from cardiovascular causes. *N Engl J Med* 2007;**356**:2457–71.

67. McGuire DK, Van de Werf F, Armstrong PW, *et al.*; Trial Evaluating Cardiovascular Outcomes With Sitagliptin (TECOS) Study Group. Association between sitagliptin use and heart failure hospitalization and related outcomes in type 2 diabetes mellitus: secondary analysis of a randomized clinical trial. *JAMA Cardiol* 2016;**1**:126–35.

68. White WB, Cannon CP, Heller SR, *et al.*; EXAMINE Investigators. Alogliptin after acute coronary syndrome in patients with type 2 diabetes. *N Engl J Med* 2013;**369**:1327–35.

69. Scirica BM, Bhatt DL, Braunwald E, *et al.*; SAVOR-TIMI 53 Steering Committee and Investigators. Saxagliptin and cardiovascular outcomes in patients with type 2 diabetes mellitus. *N Engl J Med* 2013;**369**:1317–26.

70. Margulies, KB, Hernandez AF, Redfield MM, *et al.*, for the NHLBI Heart Failure Clinical Research Network. Effects of liraglutide on clinical stability among patients with advanced heart failure and reduced ejection fraction: a randomized clinical trial. *JAMA* 2016;**316**:500–8.

71. Marso SP, Daniels GH, Brown-Frandsen K, *et al.*; LEADER Steering Committee; LEADER Trial Investigators. Liraglutide and cardiovascular outcomes in type 2 diabetes. *N Engl J Med* 2016;**375**:311–22.

72. Marso S, Holst AG, Vilsbøll T. Semaglutide and cardiovascular outcomes in patients with type 2 diabetes. *N Engl J Med* 2017;**376**:891–2.

73. Husain M, Birkenfeld AL, Donsmark M, *et al.* Oral semaglutide and cardiovascular outcomes in patients with type 2 diabetes. *N Engl J Med* 2019;**381**:841–51.

74. Zinman B, Wanner C, Lachin JM, *et al.*, for the EMPA-REG OUTCOME Investigators. Empagliflozin, cardiovascular outcomes, and mortality in type 2 diabetes. *N Engl J Med* 2015;**373**:2117–28.

75. Fitchett D, Zinman B, Wanner C, *et al.*; EMPA-REG OUTCOME® trial investigators. Heart failure outcomes with empagliflozin in patients with type 2 diabetes at high cardiovascular risk: results of the EMPA-REG OUTCOME® trial. *Eur Heart J* 2016;**37**:1526–34.

76. McMurray JJV, Solomon SD, Inzucchi L, *et al.* Dapagliflozin in patients with heart failure and reduced ejection fraction. *N Engl J Med* 2019;**381**:1995–2008.

77. Rådholm K, Figtree G, Perkovic V, *et al.* Canagliflozin and heart failure in type 2 diabetes mellitus. *Circulation* 2018;**138**(5):458–68.

78. Heerspink HJ, Stefánsson BV, Correa-Rotter R, *et al.* Dapagliflozin in patients with chronic kidney disease. *N Engl J Med* 2020;**383**:1436–46.

79. Neal B, Perkovic V, Mahaffey KW, *et al.*, for the CANVAS Program Collaborative Group. Canagliflozin and cardiovascular and renal events in type 2 diabetes. *N Engl J Med* 2017;**377**:644–57.

80. Summary of Revisions for the 2016 Clinical Practice Recommendations. *Diabetes Care* 2016;**39** Suppl 1:S1–S2.

81. Domanski M, Krause-Steinrauf H, Deedwania P, *et al.* The effect of diabetes on outcomes of patients with advanced heart failure in the BEST trial. *J Am Coll Cardiol* 2003 **42**:914–22.

82. Smooke S, Horwich TB, Fonarow GC. Insulin-treated diabetes is associated with a marked increase in mortality in patients with advanced heart failure. *Am Heart J* 2005 **149**:168–74.

83. Karter AJ, Ahmed AT, Liu J, Moffet HH, Parker MM. Pioglitazone initiation and subsequent hospitalisation for congestive heart failure. *Diabet Med* 2005;**22**:986–93.

84. Pocock SJ, Wang D, Pfeffer MA, *et al.* Predictors of mortality and morbidity in patients with chronic heart failure. *Eur Heart J* 2005 **27**:65–75.

85. Erdmann E, Lechat P, Verkenne P, Wiemann H. Results from post-hoc analyses of the CIBIS II trial: effect of bisoprolol in high-risk patient groups with chronic heart failure. *Eur J Heart Fail* 2001;**3**:469–79.

86. Packer M, Fowler MB, Roecker EB, *et al.* Effect of carvedilol on the morbidity of patients with severe chronic heart failure. *Circulation* 2002;**106**:2194–9.

87. Moye LA, Pfeffer MA, Wun CC, *et al.* Uniformity of captopril benefit in the SAVE Study: subgroupanalysis. Survival and

Ventricular Enlargement Study. *Eur Heart J* 1994;**15**(Suppl B):2e8; discussion 26e30.

88. Gustafsson I, Torp-Pedersen C, Køber L, Gustafsson F, Per Hildebrandt P, on behalf of the Trace Study Group. Effect of the angiotensin-converting enzyme inhibitor trandolapril on mortality and morbidity in diabetic patients with left ventricular dysfunction after acute myocardial infarction. *J Am Coll Cardiol* 1999;**34**:83–9.

89. Shindler DM, Kostis JB, Yusuf S, *et al.* Diabetes mellitus, a predictor of morbidity and mortality in the Studies of Left Ventricular Dysfunction (SOLVD) Trials and Registry. *Am J Cardiol* 1996;**77**:1017e20.

90. Arnold JM, Yusuf S, Young J, *et al.* Prevention of heart failure in patients in the Heart Outcomes Prevention Evaluation (HOPE) Study. *Circulation* 2003;**107**:1284e90.

91. Fox KM. Efficacy of perindopril in reduction of cardiovascular events among patients with stable coronary artery disease: randomised, double blind, placebo-controlled, multicentre trial (the EUROPA study). *Lancet* 2003;**362**:782e8.

92. Pitt B, Zannad F, Remme WJ, *et al.* The effect of spironolactone on morbidity and mortality in patients with severe heart failure. Randomized Aldactone Evaluation Study Investigators. *N Engl J Med* 1999;**341**:709e17.

93. Pitt B, Remme W, Zannad F, *et al.* Eplerenone, a selective aldosterone blocker, in patients with left ventricular dysfunction after myocardial infarction. *N Engl J Med* 2003;**348**:1309–21.

94. Conn JN, Tognoni G. A randomized trial of the angiotensin-receptor blocker valsartan in chronic heart failure. *N Engl J Med* 2001;**345**:1667–75.

95. Pfeffer MA, Swedberg K, Granger CB, *et al.* Effects of candesartan on mortality and morbidity in patients with chronic heart failure: the CHARM-Overall programme. *Lancet* 2003;**362**:759–66.

96. Yusuf S, Ostergren JB, Gerstein HC, *et al.* Effects of candesartan on the development of a new diagnosis of diabetes mellitus in patients with heart failure. *Circulation* 2005;**112**:48–53.

97. Massie BM, Carson PE, McMurray JJV, *et al.* Irbesartan in patients with heart failure and preserved ejection fraction. *N Engl J Med* 2008;**359**:2456–67.

98. Parving HH, Lehnert H, Brochner-Mortensen J, *et al.* The effect of irbesartan on the development of diabetic nephropathy in patients with type 2 diabetes. *N Engl J Med* 2001;**345**:870–8.

99. Julius S, Kjeldsen SE, Weber M, *et al.* Outcomes in hypertensive patients at high cardiovascular risk treated with regimens based on valsartan or amlodipine: the VALUE randomised trial. *Lancet* 2004;**363**:2022–31.

100. Brenner BM, Cooper ME, de Zeeuw D, *et al.* Effects of losartan on renal and cardiovascular outcomes in patients with type 2 diabetes and nephropathy. *N Engl J Med* 2001;**345**:861–9.

101. Lindholm LH, Ibsen H, Borch-Johnsen K, *et al.* Risk of new-onset diabetes in the Losartan Intervention For Endpoint reduction in hypertension study. *J Hypertens* 2002;**20**:1879–86.

102. McMurray JJV, Krum H, Abraham WT, *et al.*; ATMOSPHERE Committees Investigators. Aliskiren, enalapril, or aliskiren and enalapril in heart failure. *N Engl J Med* 2016;**374**:1521–32.

103. Taylor AL, Ziesche S, Yancy C, *et al.* Combination of isosorbide dinitrate and hydralazine in blacks with heart failure. *N Engl J Med* 2004;**351**:2049–57.

104. Shekelle PG, Rich MW, Morton C, *et al.* Efficacy of angiotensin-converting enzyme inhibitors and beta blockers in the management of left ventricular systolic dysfunction according to race, gender, and diabetic status: a meta-analysis. *J Am Coll Cardiol* 2003;**41**:1529–38.

105. Shorr RI, Ray WA, Daugherty JR, Griffin MR. Antihypertensives and the risk of serious hypoglycaemia in older persons using insulin or sulphonylureas. *JAMA* 1997;**278**:40–3.

37

Valvular heart disease

Hannah Z. R. McConkey and Bernard Prendergast

Introduction

As the population ages, the clinical importance and burden of valvular heart disease (VHD) increases and is highly relevant to everyday cardiac care. Where symptomatology is subjective and confounded by co-morbidities, the clinician is faced with the challenge of evaluating a conundrum of complex physiological parameters (see Table 37.1)[1] whilst also balancing the potential risks and benefits of intervention by means of surgical valve replacement or percutaneous intervention. Meanwhile, there are currently no medical or pharmacological therapies to halt progression of VHD or reverse valve destruction, which in developed nations is increasingly caused by degenerative pathology rather than rheumatic heart disease.

The emergence of transcatheter aortic valve implantation (TAVI) and percutaneous edge-to-edge repair for mainstream treatment of aortic stenosis (AS) and mitral regurgitation (MR), respectively, has paved the way for further innovative percutaneous options in this field. At the time of writing, there are 35 products either approved or in design for the percutaneous treatment of MR alone—an exciting, emergent area which has attracted significant financial investment.

The EuroHeart Failure Survey,[2] involving >11 000 patients with suspected or confirmed heart failure, revealed that moderate or severe VHD contributed to the development of heart failure in 29% of patients (the most common cause being secondary MR). A US population-based study of nearly 12 000 participants identified moderate VHD in 2.5% of the overall adult population and a marked increase of prevalence with age (11.7% in those aged >75 years).[3] These findings were confirmed in a prospective UK population-based study,[4] which also demonstrated that the population with VHD is destined to double in the next three decades as a function of the ageing population.

The most recent AHA/ACC[5] and ESC guidelines[6] place a strong emphasis on the assessment of left ventricular (LV) function in the management of VHD, especially in asymptomatic subjects (see Table 37.2). Accurate assessment of VHD when there is LV dysfunction and coexisting heart failure is challenging since transvalvular

Table 37.1 The complex interplay of multiple valve pathology

The presence of:	Impacts the diagnosis of:			
	Aortic stenosis	Aortic regurgitation	Mitral stenosis	Mitral regurgitation
AS	N/A	Unreliable PHT	Unreliable PHT due to impaired ventricular relaxation. LFLG MS can occur.	High mitral regurgitant volume. Increased area of MR jet. Mitral ROA less affected than volume.
AR	Increased LVOT V_{max} in AR may affect AS gradient if using Simplified Bernoulli formula. Continuity equation is applicable. Peak V_{max} reflects the severity of both AS and AR.	N/A	AR jet can be mistaken for MS jet. Continuity equation unreliable. Unreliable PHT due to overestimation of the MVA.	Doppler volumetric method invalid
MS	LFLG AS common	MS can blunt pulse pressure increase in AR	N/A	Not affected
MR	LFLG AS common MR jet can be mistaken for AS jet on CW spectral Doppler	Doppler volumetric method inapplicable. Unreliable PHT	Continuity equation unreliable due to underestimation of MVA due to increased antegrade mitral flow. Unreliable PHT	N/A

AS, aortic stenosis; N/A, not applicable; PHT, pressure half-time; LFLG, low flow-low gradient; MS, mitral stenosis; MR, mitral regurgitation; ROA, regurgitant orifice area; LVOT, left ventricular outflow tract; V_{max}, maximum velocity; AR, aortic regurgitation; MVA, mitral valve area; CW, continuous wave.

Table 37.2 The role of left ventricular function in valvular heart disease management

	Status	ESC 2017	ACC/AHA 2014/2017
AS	Asymptomatic, LVEF <50%	I, C	I, B
	Severe LFLG, LV dysfunction, flow reserve present	I, C	IIa, B
	Severe LFLG, LV dysfunction, no flow reserve	IIa, C	
Primary MR	Asymptomatic, LV dysfunction, LVESd ≥40-45mm	I, B	I, B
	Symptomatic, LVEF >30%	I, B	I, B
	Symptomatic, LVEF <30%	IIa/b, C	IIb, C
AR	Asymptomatic, LVEF <50%	I, B	I, B
	Asymptomatic, LVEF >50%, LVESd >50mm / LVESd >25mm/m^2	IIa, B	IIa, B

ACC, American College of Cardiology; AHA, American Heart Association; ESC, European Society of Cardiology; LFLG, Low flow low gradient; LVEF, left ventricular ejection fraction; LVESd, left ventricular end systolic diameter.

pressures are heavily flow dependent. For example, in paradoxical low flow–low gradient AS, indexed stroke volume is impaired although LV ejection fraction (LVEF) is 'normal', with resulting disproportionately low pressure gradients across the aortic valve and underdiagnosis of severe AS.

Acute valve pathology is poorly tolerated, leading to rapid onset pulmonary oedema and circulatory collapse. Initial treatment should focus on urgent echocardiography, delineation of the aetiology of decompensation, instigation of circulatory support, and organization of intervention. Intervention should not be delayed since mortality is at least 75% within the first 24 h. Intra-aortic balloon counterpulsation accompanied by vasodilator therapy and inotropic support may provide temporary stability in patients with cardiogenic shock secondary to acute mitral regurgitation prior to early surgery.

This chapter focuses predominantly on chronic VHD and incorporates discussion of cardiac physiology, clinical features, quantification using echocardiography, and clinical management for individual valve lesions.

Mitral valve disease

Mitral regurgitation

Mitral valve anatomy is intricate and there are numerous ways in which function may be impacted. Primary MR relates to disease of the valve leaflets (myxomatous degeneration, infective endocarditis) and predominantly causes eccentric jets which can be challenging to quantify. In contrast, secondary MR arises as a consequence of disease affecting the left ventricular myocardium, most commonly in the context of ischaemic heart disease.[7] So-called 'ischaemic MR' results from disruption of the subvalve apparatus (the chordae or papillary muscles) secondary to regional wall motion abnormalities which disrupt the normal tethering of the valve leaflets, or papillary muscle dysfunction or rupture following acute myocardial infarction (the latter leading to acute, torrential MR). Similarly, the mitral annulus is subject to stretch in ischaemic heart disease, dilated cardiomyopathy, and volume-overloaded states, resulting in central, functional MR (see Figure 37.1). The mitral valve is obliquely located in the heart and immediately adjacent to the aortic valve—both

are prone to late regurgitation following chest radiotherapy which causes fibrotic thickening, valvular retraction, and calcification.

Although mild MR may be found in up to 19% of the population, the most common cause of moderate–severe MR is myxomatous degeneration, with a prevalence of ~2% (5:1 male preponderance, even age distribution). Myxomatous infiltration and fibroelastic deficiency result in chordal stretching and valve prolapse, principally affecting the posterior leaflet.

Transoesophageal echocardiography plays a key role in defining the mechanism of MR and can help predict the likelihood of successful mitral valve repair with implications for the mode and timing of surgery. It is also highly sensitive in the detection of thrombus, vegetations, and abscesses, which may not be apparent on transthoracic imaging.

Cardiac physiology in MR

During ventricular contraction, blood is ejected from the LV both into the aorta and through the regurgitant mitral valve into the left atrium (LA), thereby increasing LA pressure. Chronic MR causes compensatory LV dilatation and eccentric hypertrophy due to increased preload and afterload, increased total stroke volume, and left atrial dilatation (with higher likelihood of atrial fibrillation (AF)). As a consequence of the bidirectional ejection of blood into the aorta and LA, LV ejection fraction is falsely elevated (and should be supranormal in this state). Functional recovery is possible if mitral valve intervention is undertaken at an early stage. However, if permitted to progress, MR results in irreversible structural and functional deterioration and surgical outcomes are poor.

Clinical examination

The LV apical impulse is usually brisk and hyperdynamic due to volume overload and may be laterally displaced as a result of LV dilatation. Carotid upstroke is sharp in compensated MR, but volume is diminished in the presence of advanced heart failure. The systolic murmur can vary depending on the mechanism of mitral regurgitation and its severity—it is a holosystolic murmur, best heard at the apex in the left lateral decubitus position and radiating to the axilla in severe degenerative MR. S1 is often soft and a split S2 is common, with late systolic murmurs typical of mitral valve prolapse or papillary muscle dysfunction.

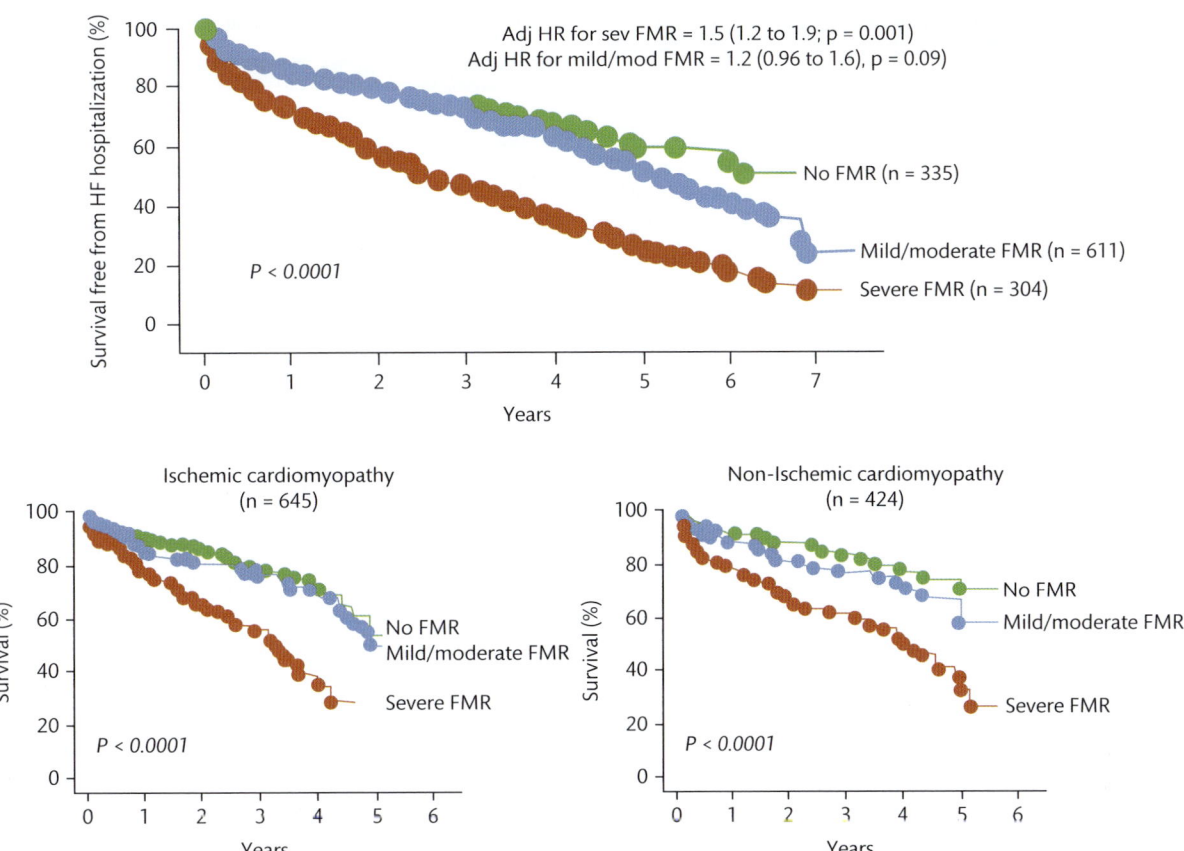

Figure 37.1 Functional MR (FMR) prognosis in ischaemic and non-ischaemic cardiomyopathy

Reproduced from Asgar, A. W., Mack, M. J. & Stone, G. W. Secondary mitral regurgitation in heart failure. *Journal of the American College of Cardiology* 65, 1231–1248 (2015) with permission from Elsevier.

Management: surgery

Primary MR should be treated with valve repair if possible, in all patients with symptoms, and in asymptomatic patients with LV systolic dysfunction or dilatation, new onset AF, pulmonary hypertension, or a high likelihood of repair and low surgical risk.

Secondary MR is a disease of the LV causing annular dilatation or disruption of the subvalvular apparatus (with normal valve leaflets) and is strongly associated with poor prognosis in patients with heart failure. The objective of any treatment is therefore to improve symptomatic heart failure, reduce hospital admissions, and demonstrate a mortality benefit. First-line treatment is with guideline-directed medical therapy for LV dysfunction, i.e. angiotensin converting enzyme inhibitors or angiotensin-receptor neprilysin inhibitors, β-blockers, and mineralocorticoid receptor antagonists. Cardiac resynchronization should be considered in appropriate subsets if symptoms persist despite medical treatment.

Surgery should only be considered in secondary MR if symptoms are unresponsive to medical and cardiac device therapy. When indicated, valve repair using an undersized, rigid ring annuloplasty is preferred to replacement although long-term survival advantage has yet to be convincingly demonstrated. In particular, valve repair for severe secondary MR has the advantage of lower operative risk than valve replacement but higher likelihood of significant postoperative MR[8] and heart-failure-related adverse events.[9,10] Moreover, in moderate ischaemic MR, there is no demonstrable advantage in adding

mitral valve repair to coronary artery bypass grafting at the time of cardiac surgery.[11] When valve replacement is performed, a mechanical prosthesis is recommended if there are no contraindications to long-term anticoagulation or if the patient is aged <65–70 years with reasonable life expectancy.

Management: novel transcatheter therapies

- Edge-to-edge repair
- Chordal repair
- Enhanced coaptation
- Direct annuloplasty
- Indirect annuloplasty
- Hybrid surgical
- Ventricular remodelling
- Mitral valve replacement

The COAPT and MITRA-FR trials have investigated the role of transcatheter edge-to-edge repair in patients with secondary MR as an addition to optimized guideline-directed medical therapy (including cardiac resynchronization when appropriate). Although the trials demonstrated differing outcomes, the overall consensus is that edge-to-edge repair offers symptomatic and prognostic benefits when undertaken by experienced operators in carefully selected patients with refractory symptoms despite optimal medical therapy.

Mitral stenosis

The declining incidence of mitral stenosis (MS) parallels that of acute rheumatic fever, which induces an exaggerated immune response to group A β-haemolytic streptococcal infection and an associated pancarditis. Proteins produced by streptococci display molecular mimicry triggering an immune response, particularly to M-proteins and human cardiac antigens such as myosin and valvular endothelium. T-cells infiltrate the valve, activated by the binding of antistreptococcal carbohydrates, with release of tumour necrosis factor and interleukins. The resulting multiple inflammatory foci (Aschoff bodies, perivascular mononuclear infiltrate) become progressively thickened and calcified over subsequent decades, with commissural fusion leading to a small effective orifice area and high pressure gradient across the valve during ventricular diastole. Occasionally, mitral annular calcification (MAC) results in severe MS—a degree of MAC is found in 8.5–10% of the population aged >50 years but rarely has significant haemodynamic impact.

Cardiac physiology in mitral stenosis

Mitral stenosis manifests as gradual obstruction to left ventricular inflow and decreased preload. Progressive valve stenosis curtails the free flow of blood from the LA to the LV, eventually causing LA dilatation and impaired LV filling with reduced stroke volume and cardiac output. As stenosis severity progresses, pulmonary congestion and reduced cardiac output manifest as congestive cardiac failure despite preserved LV ejection fraction. Back pressure and congestion through the lung capillary bed and into the right ventricle (RV) cause pressure overload, pulmonary hypertension, and right heart failure.

Symptoms can include dyspnoea, chest pain due to pulmonary hypertension, and haemoptysis secondary to alveolar, capillary, or bronchial vein rupture. Progressive LA dilatation can compress surrounding structures: the left recurrent laryngeal nerve causing hoarseness; the oesophagus causing dysphagia; and the left main bronchus causing left lung collapse. The onset of AF can precipitate decompensation and increases the risk of systemic embolism.

Clinical examination

A malar flush may be evident and patients are often in AF. MS is associated with a sharp, brief, 'tapping' thrust of the non-displaced apex beat during systole (which is in fact a palpable S1 as high LA pressure causes abrupt mitral valve closure). S1 is loud followed by an opening snap and rumbling mid-diastolic murmur, heard best in the left lateral decubitus position during expiration. The murmur becomes longer in duration (and the opening snap closer to S2) as the stenosis becomes more severe.

Management

All attempts should be made to maintain sinus rhythm or optimize rate control in AF where restoration of sinus rhythm is not possible. β-Blockers prolong LV diastolic filling and are of particular value. Anticoagulation with warfarin is recommended in patients with AF, LA thrombus, or a previous embolic event (note

Table 37.3 Quantification of valve severity (mitral regurgitation)

Mitral regurgitation	Mild	Moderate	Severe
Jet area/LA size (%)	<20%		>40%
PISA radius (cm) (Nyquist 40 cm/s)	<0.4		>1.0
Vena contracta (cm)	<0.3		≥0.7
Regurgitant volume (mL/beat)	≤30	31–59	≥60
Regurgitant fraction (%)	<30	31–49	≥50
Regurgitant orifice area (cm²)	<0.2	0.21–0.39	≥0.4

LA, left atrium; PISA, proximal isovelocity surface area.

that non-vitamin K antagonist oral anticoagulants (NOACs) are not currently approved in valvular AF). Diuretic and nitrate therapy provide symptomatic relief in the setting of pulmonary congestion.

Intervention should only be performed in symptomatic patients with a mitral valve area (MVA) ≤1.5 cm². It can also be considered in asymptomatic patients who are at high risk of thromboembolism and/or haemodynamic decompensation (systolic pulmonary pressure >50 mmHg at rest, need for major non-cardiac surgery, desire for pregnancy), have no unfavourable clinical characteristics (advanced age, history of prior commissurotomy, New York Heart Association functional class IV, permanent AF, severe pulmonary hypertension) and favourable anatomy for percutaneous mitral commissurotomy.[8] Anatomical distribution of calcification, degree of commissural fusion, and extent of MR are the key characteristics that determine best treatment (see Tables 37.3 and 37.4). Percutaneous mitral commissurotomy may also be considered in symptomatic patients with unfavourable anatomy (Wilkins score >8 (see Table 37.5),[12] Cormier group 3 (see Table 37.6),[13] very small mitral valve area, severe tricuspid regurgitation) and no unfavourable clinical characteristics.

Percutaneous mitral commissurotomy (see Figure 37.2), achieves a good result in over 80% of cases with improved MVA >1.5 cm² and at most mild MR. Procedural risks include mortality (0.5–4%), haemopericardium (0.5–10%), embolism (0.5–5%), and severe MR (2–10%). Contraindications include LA thrombus, significant MR, severe or bicommissural calcification, absence of commissural fusion, and severe aortic valve disease or the need for coronary artery bypass grafting.

Open surgical mitral commissurotomy is rarely performed and reserved for patients with adverse anatomical characteristics unsuitable for percutaneous techniques. The alternative is conventional mitral valve replacement—valve repair techniques are challenging in mitral stenosis and have limited efficacy.

Table 37.4 Quantification of valve severity (mitral stenosis)

Mitral stenosis	Normal	Mild	Moderate	Severe
Pressure half-time (ms)	40–70	71–139	140–219	≥220
Mean pressure fall (mmHg)		<5	5–10	>10
Valve area (cm²)	4-6	1.6–2.0	1.0–1.5	<1.0

Table 37.5 Wilkins score[12]

Grade	Mobility	Subvalvular thickening	Thickening	Calcification
1	Highly mobile valve with only leaflet tips restricted	Minimal thickening just below the mitral leaflets	Leaflets near normal thickness (4–5 mm)	Single area of increased echo brightness
2	Leaflet mid and base portions have normal mobility	Thickening of chordal structures extending to one-third of chordal length	Mid-leaflets normal, considerable thickening of margins (5–8 mm)	Scattered areas of brightness confined to leaflet margins
3	Valve continues to move forward in diastole, mainly from the base	Thickening extending to distal third of chords	Thickening extending through the entire leaflet (5–8 mm)	Brightness extending into the mid-portion of the leaflets
4	No or minimal forward movement of the leaflets in diastole	Extensive thickening and shortening of all chordal structures extending to the papillary muscles	Considerable thickening of all leaflet tissue (>8–10 mm)	Extensive brightness throughout much of the leaflet tissue

Source data from Wilkins, G. T., Weyman, A. E., Abascal, V. M., Block, P. C. & Palacios, I. F. Percutaneous balloon dilatation of the mitral valve: an analysis of echocardiographic variables related to outcome and the mechanism of dilatation. British Heart Journal **60**, 299–308 (1988).

Table 37.6 Cormier score[13]

Echocardiographic group	Mitral valve anatomy
Group 1	Pliable non-calcified anterior mitral leaflet and mild subvalvular disease (i.e. thin chordae ≥10 mm long)
Group 2	Pliable non-calcified anterior mitral leaflet and severe subvalvular disease (i.e. thickened chordae <10 mm long)
Group 3	Calcification of mitral valve of any extent (fluoroscopy) whatever the state of subvalvular apparatus

Source data from Ormier, B. et al. [Evaluation by two-dimensional and doppler echocardiography of the results of percutaneous mitral valvuloplasty]. *Arch Mal Coeur Vaiss* **82**, 185–191 (1989).

Aortic valve disease

Aortic stenosis

Severe symptomatic aortic stenosis (AS) has a bleak prognosis and is the third most prevalent form of cardiovascular disease in western countries after hypertension and coronary artery disease. Moreover, the clinical importance and burden of AS are set to increase as the population ages. AS usually results from degenerative calcification of a trileaflet valve, thickening and calcification of a congenital bicuspid valve or, less frequently, rheumatic heart disease. Progressive thickening of the aortic valve over years leads to breathlessness (raised diastolic filling pressures), angina (impaired coronary flow reserve), decompensated heart failure (left ventricular dysfunction), and exertional syncope (low cardiac output due to fixed LV outflow tract obstruction). Once symptomatic, life-expectancy is shorter than most cancers, and decompensation is often swift and accelerated with the onset of AF.

Cardiac physiology in AS

AS is characterized by progressive valve narrowing, frequently accompanied by changes in myocardial deformation properties and subclinical LV dysfunction (see Table 37.7). At a certain point in the natural history, adaptive, compensatory LV hypertrophy that increases contractile force and reduces systolic wall stress becomes maladaptive, resulting in cardiac decompensation. Myocardial hypertrophy is detrimental to overall survival and correlates with myocardial fibrosis, impaired longitudinal shortening, and worsening diastolic function.[14] Myocardial fibrosis is a crucial determinant of cardiac dysfunction and prognosis, and has long been associated with AS, even in the absence of significant epicardial coronary artery disease. Replacement fibrosis may be the result of myocyte apoptosis owing to extensive hypertrophy and eventually accounts for progression to heart failure.

Clinical examination

Clinical examination findings depend on disease severity. Patients with severe AS exhibit a heaving apex beat, a loud ejection systolic murmur (best heard in the aortic area during expiration and

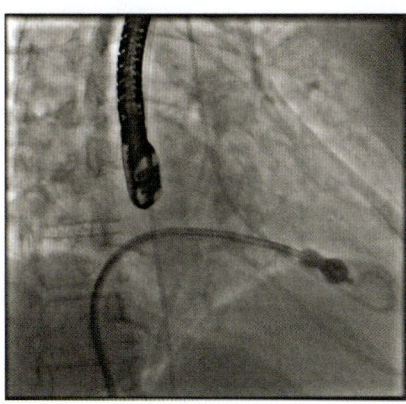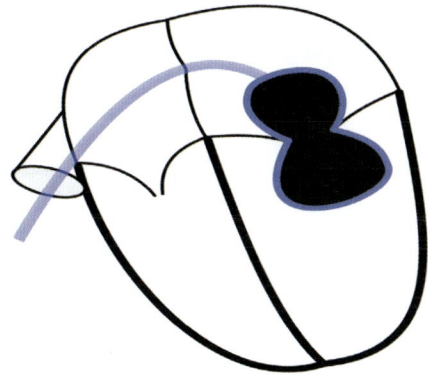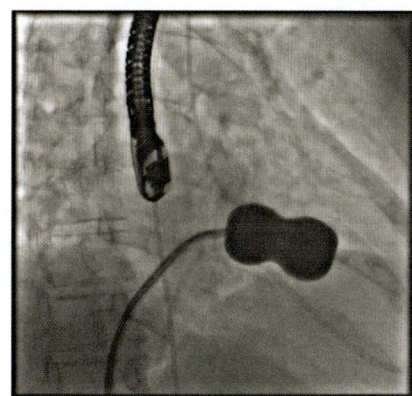

Figure 37.2 Percutaneous mitral commissurotomy demonstrating trans-septal puncture and balloon inflation across the mitral valve.
Image courtesy of Professor Simon Redwood.

Table 37.7 Quantification of valve severity (aortic stenosis)

Aortic stenosis	Normal	Mild	Moderate	Severe
Peak velocity (m/s)	–	<2.9	3.0–3.9	>4.0
Mean pressure fall (mmHg)	–	<25	25–40	>40
Valve area (cm²)	>2.0	1.5–2.0	1.0–1.4	<1.0
Velocity ratio (m/s)	–	≥0.5	0.25–0.5	≤0.25

radiating to the carotid arteries) and an often inaudible S2. Pulses are slow-rising and there is a narrow pulse pressure. S4 may be audible in severe AS, and signs of decompensation may be evident. In end-stage disease, the murmur may become quieter due to a lower stroke volume from a 'burnt out' LV.

Classification

There are distinct and poorly understood pathological and physiological differences among patients with AS and aortic valve area (AVA) <1 cm². Flow and stroke volume may both be reduced or normal in patients with preserved and reduced LV ejection fraction. Whilst there is a clear consensus that symptomatic AS with AVA <1 cm², peak velocity (V_{max}) >4 m/s and mean pressure gradient (MPG) >40 mmHg (normal flow, high gradient, AS) warrant intervention, diagnostic ambiguity exists in patients with small AVA and low pressure gradients (despite preserved LV ejection fraction) where lower stroke volumes contribute significantly to discrepancies. A large proportion of AS patients have discordant parameters, and where stroke volume is low, it is important to rule out a myocardial cause (pseudo-stenosis) (see **Figure 37.3**).

Medical therapy

Whereas there is no effective medical treatment, symptomatic patients can be palliated with cautious diuretics (which relieve preload but may cause hypovolaemia and syncope) and β-blockade (which reduces myocardial oxygen demand). Attempts should be made to restore sinus rhythm since AF can lead to rapid decompensation in the setting of a stiff ventricle. Agents that reduce afterload (e.g. GTN) should be avoided and angiotensin converting enzyme (ACE) inhibitors have been traditionally contraindicated. However, the RIAS study demonstrated a modest but progressive reduction in LV mass associated with ramipril in patients with asymptomatic moderate–severe AS, coupled with improved myocardial physiology and slower progression of valve stenosis.[15] ACE inhibitors may therefore be beneficial in moderate and severe AS. Despite promising retrospective studies suggesting that statin therapy may slow the progression of AS, prospective large trials (SEAS and SALTIRE) found no change with aggressive lipid-lowering therapy.[16,17]

Balloon valvuloplasty

Balloon aortic valvuloplasty was first developed in 1985 but fell into disrepute due to high rates of restenosis. However, the procedure has seen a resurgence in the last few years, allowing a bridge to definitive treatment with TAVI in unstable patients, and a means of temporary relief of AS in high risk symptomatic patients who are scheduled for elective non-cardiac surgery (2014 ESC/ESA Guidelines on non-cardiac surgery, Class IIa, Level C)[18]. Current indications are: cardiogenic shock; severely impaired LV systolic function or presentation in pulmonary oedema; symptomatic ambiguity where

there is significant pulmonary disease (to allow assessment of symptomatic improvement); palliation for those with a life expectancy <1 year.

Transcatheter aortic valve implantation

There have been over 30000 TAVIs performed in the UK since a national service began in 2007 (>750 000 worldwide) with an average patient age of 81 years (mean logistic EUROscore: 20). A plethora of devices are now available (see **Figure 37.4**) and **Figure 37.5** demonstrates a schematically how a TAVI is performed. Less than 2% of patients suffer a stroke, and emergency cardiac surgery for haemorrhage, coronary obstruction, annular rupture, or device embolization is rare. In-hospital mortality is now 1.3% (from British Cardiovascular Intervention Society audit data).

Treatment of aortic stenosis with left ventricle impairment

The PARTNER A trial compared the outcomes of high risk patients with AS and LV ejection fraction <50% undergoing TAVI and surgical AVR and found equivalent rates of mortality and LV functional recovery.[19] Similarly, the PARTNER II study demonstrated no difference in outcomes of intermediate risk patients with EF <55% undergoing TAVI or surgical AVR (HR: 0.84; 0.56–1.25; $P = 0.27$);[20] more recent trials in low risk patients demonstrate equivalent outcomes to surgery at two-year follow-up.[21,22] Patients with no flow reserve undergoing valve intervention have a higher operative mortality[23] although survival is still superior with intervention than with conservative management. Although paravalvular regurgitation following TAVI is related to medium- and long-term mortality, this issue has been largely overcome with contemporary device designs.

Aortic regurgitation

Chronic aortic regurgitation (AR) is caused by either gradual disruption of the normal valve leaflets (congenital bicuspid, unicuspid or quadricuspid valve, rheumatic fever, collagen vascular disease, infective endocarditis, atherosclerotic degeneration) or aortic root enlargement (uncontrolled hypertension, Marfan syndrome, ankylosing spondylitis). Once symptoms develop, untreated severe AR carries a mortality risk of 10–20% per year—similar to outcomes in asymptomatic patients with LV dilatation.

Cardiac physiology

Both preload (as a result of volume overload) and afterload (as a result of increased end-diastolic volume and wall stress) are elevated in AR. LV remodelling causes eccentric hypertrophy to maintain normal wall stress but rising LV end-diastolic pressure (LVEDP) and reduction of the aortic–LV gradient shorten the murmur to early diastole once haemodynamic decompensation develops. Tachycardia is well tolerated due to a shortened diastolic interval.

Clinical examination

Aortic regurgitation is characterized by volume overload and the LV apex is usually heaving and laterally displaced. There is a wide pulse pressure with brisk upstroke and a collapsing ('water-hammer') pulse due to increased stroke volume, accompanied by a decrescendo, blowing, early diastolic murmur, heard best on expiration while the patient leans forward. A loud S2 is consistent with a dilated

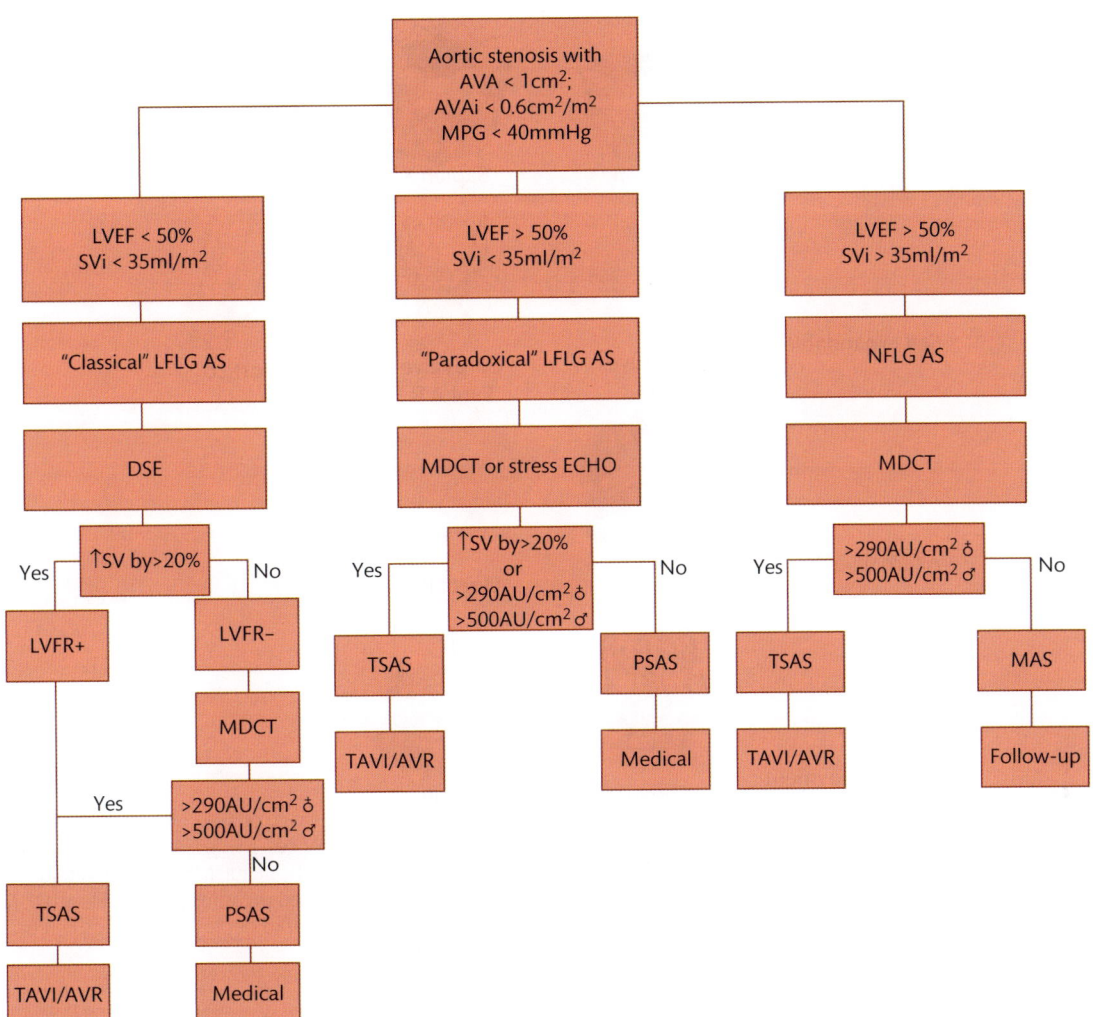

Figure 37.3 Diagnostic flow chart for patients with low gradient AS. SVi: indexed stroke volume, DSE: Dobutamine stress echocardiogram, LVFR: left ventricular flow reserve, MDCT: multidetector computed tomography, TSAS: true-severe aortic stenosis, AU: Agaston units, PSAS: pseudo-severe aortic stenosis, NFLG: normal flow low gradient, MAS: moderate aortic stenosis.

aortic root whereas a soft S2 is common with abnormally thickened or retracted leaflets. Several eponymous syndromes are associated with aortic regurgitation: Corrigan sign (visible carotid pulsation), de Musset sign (head nodding with each heart beat), Traube sign (pistol shot sounds heard over the femoral artery), Müller sign (visible pulsation of the uvula), Quincke sign (capillary pulsations in the nailbed), and Durozier sign (systolic murmur audible 2 cm proximal to the stethoscope and diastolic murmur 2 cm distal when the femoral arteries are compressed). The Austin–Flint murmur, a late diastolic murmur similar to that in MS, is caused by restricted mitral valve opening as a consequence of raised LVEDP and the jet of AR.

Management

All symptomatic patients should be offered cardiac surgery along with those who are asymptomatic but have progressive LV dilatation (LV end-diastolic diameter >70 mm, LV end-systolic diameter >50 mm) or declining LV function (ejection fraction ≤50%). Optimal blood pressure control is key in asymptomatic patients and vasodilator therapy can be useful in symptomatic patients awaiting surgery. β-Blockers have no

proven role and may exacerbate AR as a result of prolonged diastole. Paradoxically, β-blockade may slow aortic root dilatation and reduce the risk of aortic complications in patients with Marfan syndrome.

Right-sided valvular heart disease

Indications for intervention

The adult population rarely present with primary right-sided VHD and epidemiological data are scarce. Pulmonary hypertension associated with left-sided VHD may cause regurgitation of either or both right heart valves. Tricuspid stenosis may be associated with rheumatic mitral and aortic valve disease, and is occasionally seen as a feature of carcinoid syndrome or secondary to pacing lead fibrosis. Surgery is indicated in patients with symptomatic severe tricuspid stenosis, or severe tricuspid regurgitation at the time of planned left-sided valve surgery. A number of approaches to the percutaneous treatment of tricuspid valve disease are currently under investigation.

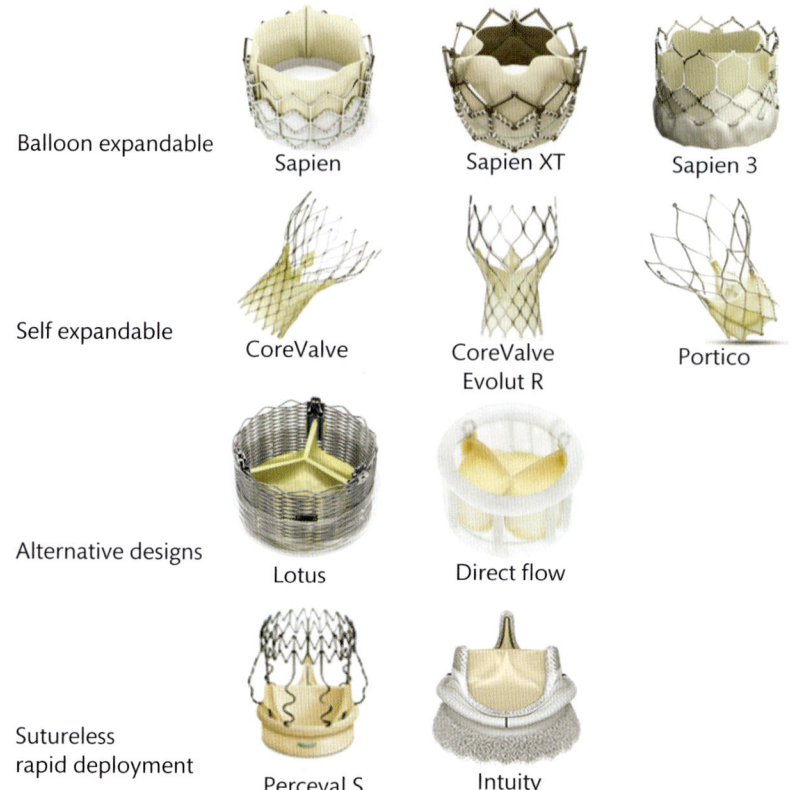

Balloon expandable
Sapien   Sapien XT   Sapien 3

Self expandable
CoreValve   CoreValve Evolut R   Portico

Alternative designs
Lotus   Direct flow

Sutureless rapid deployment
Perceval S   Intuity

Figure 37.4 Transcatheter prosthetic heart valves. Balloon expandable valves (all by Edwards Lifesciences, Irvine CA). Self-expandable valves: CoreValve and CoreValve Evolut R (Medtronic, Minneapolis, MN, USA), Portico (St Jude Medical, St Paul, MN, USA). Alternative Designs: Lotus (Boston Scientific, Natick, MA, USA) which is a pre-loaded, repositionable and retrievable stent-mounted prosthesis, Direct Flow (DF Medical, Santa Rosa, CA, USA) which is a non-metallic, repositionable and retrievable conformable valve. Sutureless, rapid deployment valves Perceval S (Sorin, Saluggia, Italy) and Intuity (Edwards Lifesciences, Irvine, CA, USA).
Reproduced from Weiss, D. *et al.* Available transcatheter aortic valve replacement technology. *Curr Atheroscler Rep* 17, 488 (2015).

Peripheral oedema is the principal symptom of right heart disease and may be accompanied by ascites, abdominal discomfort, anorexia, and dyspnoea. Tricuspid regurgitation is characterized by a quiet pansystolic murmur and a right ventricular heave with peripheral oedema, pulsatile hepatomegaly, and ascites.

Conclusion

Early diagnosis, definition of pathophysiological mechanisms, and prompt intervention are vital in the optimal management of the patient with VHD and heart failure. Acute haemodynamic decompensation is very poorly tolerated with high mortality in the first 24–48 h,

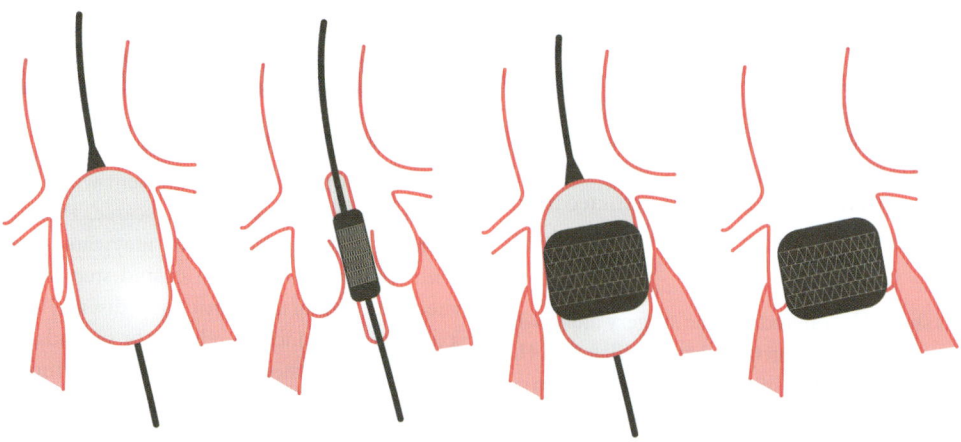

Figure 37.5 TAVI using a balloon-expandable valve.

Table 37.8 Quantification of valve severity (aortic regurgitation)

Aortic regurgitation	Mild	Moderate	Severe
Vena contracta width (cm)	<0.3		>0.6
Jet width/LVOT diameter (%)	<25		≥65
Regurgitant volume (mL/beat)	<30	31–59	≥60
Regurgitant fraction (%)	<30	31–49	≥50
Regurgitant orifice area (cm²)	<0.1	0.11–0.29	≥0.3
End-diastolic velocity (upper DAo)			>20 cm/s
Pressure half-time (ms)	>500		<200

LVOT, left ventricular outflow tract; DAo, descending aorta.

Table 37.9 Valve quantification (right sided valves)

Tricuspid stenosis	Normal	Mild	Moderate	Severe
Mean pressure fall (mmHg)				≥5
Inflow VTI (cm)				>60
Valve area (cm²)	>7			<1.0
Tricuspid regurgitation	**Mild**	**Moderate**		**Severe**
Jet area (cm²)	<5	5–10		>10
Vena contracta width (cm)		<0.7		>0.7
PISA radius (cm)	<0.5	0.6–0.9		>0.9
CW jet density/contour	Soft/parabolic	Dense/variable		Dense/triangular
RA/RV/IVC size	Normal	Normal/dilated		Dilated
Hepatic vein flow	S > D	Systolic blunting		D > S
Pulmonary stenosis	Mild	Moderate		Severe
Peak velocity (m/s)	<3	3–4		≥4
Pulmonary regurgitation	**Mild**	**Moderate**		**Severe**
Jet size (CFM) (cm)	Narrow, <1	Intermediate		Wide, large
Regurgitant fraction (%)	<40	40–60		>60
CW jet density/deceleration rate	Soft/slow	Dense/variable		Dense/steep
RVOT VTI/LVOT VTI	↑	↑↑		↑↑↑

VTI, velocity time integral; PISA, proximal isovelocity surface area; CW, continuous wave; RA, right atrium; RV, right ventricle; IVC, inferior vena cava; S, systolic waveform; D, diastolic waveform; CFM, colour flow mapping; RVOT, right ventricular outflow tract; LVOT, left ventricular outflow tract.

whereas chronic progressive VHD is associated with compensatory mechanisms that allow careful assessment and planning of surgical or percutaneous intervention. Multidisciplinary heart teams encompassing expertise in VHD and heart failure, cardiac imaging, intervention, and surgery are pivotal in discerning the best treatment option for individual patients in this rapidly evolving field.

REFERENCES

1. Unger P, Rosenhek R, Dedobbeleer C, Berrebi A, Lancellotti, P. Management of multiple valve disease. *Heart* 2011;**97**:272–7.
2. Cleland JGF, Swedberg K, Follath F, *et al.* The EuroHeart Failure survey programme—a survey on the quality of care among patients with heart failure in Europe. Part 1: patient characteristics and diagnosis. *Eur Heart J* 2003;**24**:442–63.
3. Nkomo VT, Gardin JM, Skelton TN, *et al.* Burden of valvular heart diseases: a population-based study. *Lancet* 2006;**368**:1005–11.
4. d'Arcy JL, Coffey S, Loudon MA, *et al.* Large-scale community echocardiographic screening reveals a major burden of undiagnosed valvular heart disease in older people: the OxVALVE Population Cohort Study. *Eur Heart J* 2016;**37**:3515–22.
5. Nishimura RA, Otto CM, Bonow RO, *et al.* 2017 AHA/ACC Focused Update of the 2014 AHA/ACC Guideline for the Management of Patients With Valvular Heart Disease: A Report of the American College of Cardiology/American Heart Association Task Force on Clinical Practice Guidelines. *Circulation* 2017;**135**(25):e1159–95.
6. Baumgartner H, Falk V, Bax JJ, *et al.* 2017 ESC/EACTS Guidelines for the management of valvular heart disease. *Eur Heart J* 2017;**38**(36):2739–91.
7. Asgar AW, Mack MJ, Stone GW. Secondary mitral regurgitation in heart failure. *J Am Coll Cardiol* 2015;**65**:1231–48.
8. Vahanian A, Alfieri O, Andreotti F, *et al.* Guidelines on the management of valvular heart disease (version 2012): the Joint Task Force on the Management of Valvular Heart Disease of the European Society of Cardiology (ESC) and the European Association for Cardio-Thoracic Surgery (EACTS). *Eur J Cardio-thoracic Surg* 2012;**42**:S1–44.
9. Smith PK, Puskas JD, Ascheim DD, *et al.* Surgical treatment of moderate ischemic mitral regurgitation. *N Engl J Med* 2014;**371**:2178–88.
10. Salmasi MY, Acharya M, Humayun N, *et al.* Is valve repair preferable to valve replacement in ischaemic mitral regurgitation? A systematic review and meta-analysis. *Eur J Cardiothor Surg* 2016;**50**:17–28.
11. Goldstein D, Moskowitz AJ, Gelijns AC, *et al.* Two-year outcomes of surgical treatment of severe ischemic mitral regurgitation. *N Engl J Med* 2016;**374**:344–53.
12. Wilkins GT, Weyman AE, Abascal VM, Block PC, Palacios IF. Percutaneous balloon dilatation of the mitral valve: an analysis of echocardiographic variables related to outcome and the mechanism of dilatation. *Br Heart J* 1988;**60**:299–308.
13. Cormier B, Vahanian A, Michel PL, *et al.* [Evaluation by two-dimensional and doppler echocardiography of the results of percutaneous mitral valvuloplasty.] *Arch Mal Coeur Vaiss* 1989;**82**:185–91.
14. Shah ASV Chin CWL, Vassiliou V, *et al.* Left ventricular hypertrophy with strain and aortic stenosis. *Circulation* 2014;**130**:1607–16.
15. Bull S, Loudon M, Francis JM, *et al.* A prospective, double-blind, randomized controlled trial of the angiotensin-converting enzyme inhibitor Ramipril In Aortic Stenosis (RIAS trial). *Eur Heart J Cardiovasc Imaging* 2015;**16**:834–41.
16. Cowell SJ, Newby DE, Prescott RJ, *et al.* A randomized trial of intensive lipid-lowering therapy in calcific aortic stenosis. *N Engl J Med* 2005;**352**:2389–97.

17. Rossebø AB, Pedersen TR, Boman K, *et al.* Intensive lipid lowering with simvastatin and ezetimibe in aortic stenosis. *N Engl J Med* 2008;**359**:1343–56.

18. 2014 ESC/ESA Guidelines on non-cardiac surgery: cardiovascular assessment and management. *Eur Heart J* 2014;**35**:2383–2431.

19. Elmariah S, Palacios IF, McAndrew T, *et al.* Outcomes of transcatheter and surgical aortic valve replacement in high-risk patients with aortic stenosis and left ventricular dysfunction: results from the Placement of Aortic Transcatheter Valves (PARTNER) trial (cohort A). *Circulation. Cardiovasc Intervent* 2013;**6**:604–14.

20. Leon MB, Smith CR, Mack MJ, *et al.* Transcatheter or surgical aortic-valve replacement in intermediate-risk patients. *N Engl J Med* 2016;**374**:1609–20.

21. Mack MJ, Leon MB, Thourani VH, *et al.* Transcatheter aortic-valve replacement with a balloon-expandable valve in low-risk patients. *N Engl J Med* 2019;**380**:1695–1705.

22. Popma JJ, Deeb GM, Yakubov SJ, *et al.* Transcatheter aortic-valve replacement with a self-expanding valve in low-risk patients. *N Engl J Med* 2019;**380**:1706–15.

23. Monin JL. Low-gradient aortic stenosis: operative risk stratification and predictors for long-term outcome: a multicenter study using dobutamine stress hemodynamics. *Circulation* 2003;**108**:319–24.

RECOMMENDED READING

2014 ESC/ESA Guidelines on non-cardiac surgery: cardiovascular assessment and management. *European Heart Journal* 2014;**35**:2383–2431.

Carabello BA. Introduction to aortic stenosis. *Circ Res* 2013;**113**:179–85.

Chambers JB, Myerson SG, Rajani R, *et al.* Multimodality imaging in heart valve disease. *Open Heart* 2016;**3**:e000330.

Unger P, Clavel M-A, Lindman BR, Mathieu P, Pibarot P. Pathophysiology and management of multivalvular disease. *Nat Rev Cardiol* 2016;**13**:429–40.

38

Sleep-disordered breathing

Anita K. Simonds

Introduction and definitions

Respiration during sleep in patients with heart failure is likely to be unstable for several reasons. During wakefulness, ventilation is under the control of cortical and chemical influences, but during sleep, chemical control driven by the partial pressure of carbon dioxide (Pco_2) predominates and relatively small decreases in Pco_2 can destabilize breathing, leading to central sleep apnoea. Muscle tone also falls quickly with the onset of sleep, particularly affecting upper airway muscles, predisposing the individual to obstructive sleep apnoea. Furthermore in sleep there is an increase in parasympathetic activity and reduction in sympathetic autonomic tone, resulting in a fall in minute ventilation and in cardiac output.[1]

Irregular breathing during sleep in heart failure has been observed for centuries, with Cheyne–Stokes respiration (CSR) being the classic example.[2,3] A rapid increase of knowledge in sleep medicine over the last few decades has identified a range of sleep-disordered breathing conditions, all of which have relevance to the cardiac patient. Sleep-disordered breathing (SDB) is a generic term used to cover the respiratory disturbances during sleep that include obstructive sleep apnoea (OSA), central sleep apnoea (CSA), CSR/periodic breathing, and obstructive and central hypoventilation. In adults, an apnoea is defined by 10 s of cessation in airflow; obstructive apnoeas are accompanied by respiratory effort; and in central events, effort is absent (Figure 38.1). Hypopnoeas are partial events and are variously defined: most definitions include a reduction of >30% in respiratory airflow or thoracoabdominal excursion together with arterial desaturation of 2–4%, or >50% reduction in airflow without desaturation.

The syndrome of OSA is defined by the presence of >15 obstructive apnoeas and hypopnoeas per hour; or >5 obstructive apnoeas and hypopnoeas per hour associated with symptoms such as daytime sleepiness and fatigue, nocturnal choking, or unrefreshing sleep. The apnoea–hypopnoea index (AHI) is the total number of these events per hour of sleep. Severe SDB is considered to be present if there are >30 apnoeas and hypopnoeas per hour. The respiratory disturbance index (RDI) is used to express the total number of respiratory events per hour of study time and therefore may differ from the AHI as any episodes of wakefulness during the monitoring period will be included in the RDI. New metrics such as hypoxic burden and arousal intensity are now being evaluated to see if they are able to quantify the pathophysiological consequences of OSA and response to treatment more effectively than AHI or RDI.[4]

Effects of sleep in heart failure

The prevalence of SDB has been examined in a variety of studies (Table 38.1).[5-13] The results vary according to whether data are derived from community screening or referrals to a sleep laboratory,

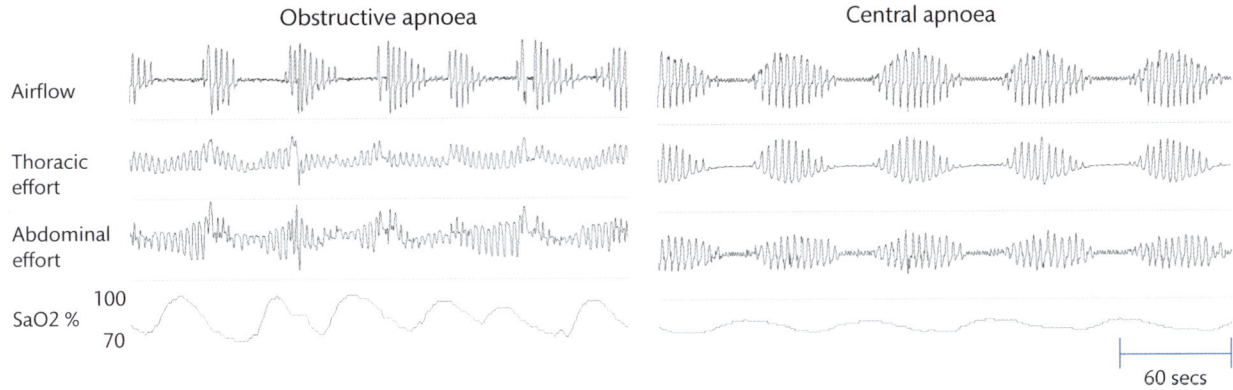

Figure 38.1 Classification of obstructive and central sleep apnoea.

Table 38.1 Prevalence of sleep-disordered breathing in heart failure

Study	No. of patients	NYHA class	Male (%)	LVEF (%)	SDB severity (AHI)	OSA (%)	CSA (%)
Lanfranchi et al.[5]	47	I	89	27 (6)	>15/h	11	55
Ferrier et al.[6]	53	I–II	77	34 (9)	>10/h	15	53
Javaheri et al.[7]	100	II	100	25 (7)	>15/h	37	12
Oldenburg et al.[8]	700	>II	80	28 (7)	>15/h	19	33
Schulz et al.[9]	203	II, III	75	28	>10/h	43	28
Vazir et al.[10]	55	II	100	31 (10)	>15/h	15	38
MacDonald et al.[11]	108	>II	85	20	>15/h	30	31
Bitter et al.[12]	244	II–IV	64	>55	>15/h	24	23
Yumino et al.[13]	218	II–IV	77	<45	>15/h	26	21

NYHA, New York Heart Association; LVEF, left ventricular ejection fraction; SDB, sleep-disordered breathing; AHI, apnoea–hypopnoea index; OSA, obstructive sleep apnoea; CSA, central sleep apnoea.

as subjects in the latter group are likely to have symptoms. Most recent findings in optimally medically treated heart failure patients, however, suggest that SDB is present in around 50% of patients with chronic heart failure. For example, Bitter et al.[12] found an AHI >15 in 47% of patients with heart failure and normal left ventricular ejection fraction (LVEF) and Yumino et al.[13] have noted that the prevalence of OSA and CSA has not changed despite increased use of beta blockers and spironolactone therapy. These results compare to a prevalence of obstructive apnoea syndrome in 4% of males and 2% of females in the general population.[14] Previously it was assumed that SDB, especially CSR, was solely a marker or epiphenomenon of end-stage heart failure, but it is becoming clearer that SDB is found in patients with mild heart failure[10] and is likely to contribute to functional cardiac decline through a range of mechanisms including hypoxaemia, increased sympathetic drive and oxidative stress.[15] Treatment to control SDB is therefore an important potential management tool.

Diagnosis of sleep-disordered breathing

Establishing the diagnosis of SDB almost always involves a sleep study to determine whether respiratory disturbances are present and to determine their nature, frequency, and pathophysiological consequences. It is often asserted that detailed polysomnography (assessment of ECG, electro-oculogram, and chin electromyogram to establish sleep stage and arousals, chest and abdominal effort sensors, airflow detection, oximetry, periodic limb, and snoring monitoring) is the reference standard technique. However, the diagnosis can usually be secured by monitoring of respiratory variables such as pulse oximetry, airflow, respiratory effort, snoring, and position. Oximetry alone may establish the diagnosis in severe OSA and can be used to screen heart failure patients for SDB but cannot differentiate between obstructive and central sleep apnoeas.[16] Further trials are in progress to establish the most effective method to screen patients including use of the simple 'ApneaLink' device (ResMed Co., Abingdon, UK) which detects airflow,[17] and heart rate variation analysis from 24 h ECG monitoring. Clearly screening becomes more relevant if therapy is available. This is the case in OSA, but the management of CSA in heart failure remains controversial (see 'Central sleep apnoea').

In many patients, a mixture of obstructive and central apnoeas and hypopnoeas is present. OSA is diagnosed if >50% of the events are obstructive and CSA diagnosed when >50% of the events are central.

Night-to-night variation in sleep-disordered breathing

In one study examining stable heart failure patients over four consecutive nights in the home, Vazir et al.[18] showed that there was minimal change in the AHI, but around 40% of patients demonstrated a shift in the type of events either from OSA to CSA or vice versa. Remarkably, there is also within-night variation in some patients. Tkacova et al.[19] carried out polysomnography in 12 stable patients with mean LVEF of 28.4% (±3.2%) NYHA class II or III, mean age 62.5 years. During the night, circulation time and periodic breathing cycle length increased, while transcutaneous PCO_2 level fell. The changes were accompanied by a reduction in obstructive events as the night progressed and an increase in central events. As discussed below, the increase in cycle length is likely to reflect worsening heart failure overnight, which in turn leads to a shift from OSA to CSA.

Obstructive sleep apnoea

Mechanisms

Obstructive apnoea occurs when the pharynx collapses during sleep, usually at nasopharyngeal, oropharyngeal, and/or hypopharyngeal levels. The obstruction is observed as pharyngeal dilator muscle tone is reduced with the onset of sleep. In addition, the supine posture favours airway collapse, and any obesity causing thickening of the neck adds to anatomical narrowing. In the recumbent position, fluid shift from the legs may increase pharyngeal oedema. Muscle tone is at its nadir in rapid eye movement sleep. Anatomical narrowing of the upper airway will exacerbate airway compromise and individuals with low respiratory arousal threshold and hypersensitive respiratory drive (known as high loop gain) also comprise pathophysiological phenotypes which are prone to OSA.[20] Systematic studies have now confirmed a clear association between displacement of peripheral oedema in the supine position, an increased distension of neck veins/pharyngeal oedema, and AHI.[21]

As a result of airway collapse, arterial oxygen saturation falls and the patient makes increasing respiratory efforts to overcome the obstruction. The pulmonary stretch receptors are stimulated, which causes disinhibition of central sympathetic outflow, thereby increasing heart rate. Arousal to a lighter stage of sleep terminates the apnoea but the associated cortical activity also causes a burst of sympathetic activity and loss of vagal tone. The post-apnoeic period is thus characterized by a surge in sympathetic outflow and a brisk increase in blood pressure and heart rate. Once arousal has opened the airway, deeper sleep ensues, the pharynx collapses, and the cycle begins again. Elevated sympathetic nerve activity (already present in heart failure) is augmented and is associated with increased mortality: sympathetic activation can be reduced by overnight continuous positive airways pressure (CPAP) therapy.[22]

Sleep apnoea may directly affect cardiac output. During the respiratory effort against the occluded airway there is a reduction in intrathoracic pressure. In turn, there is a consequent increase in left ventricular transmural pressure and therefore the afterload against which the left ventricle has to eject blood. Venous return is augmented, producing right ventricular distension which may shift the interventricular septum to the left, so reducing left ventricular filling.[15]

OSA may also have proinflammatory, oxidative stress and endothelial effects. Patients with OSA have higher plasma C-reactive protein levels than controls[23] and increased reactive oxygen species in neutrophils and monocytes.[8] In OSA patients with ischaemic heart disease, raised levels of soluble circulating adhesion molecules and increased expression of the adhesion molecules CD15 and CD11c have been reported. Patients with OSA treated with CPAP support appear to have downregulation of the expression of CD15 and CD11c in monocytes.[24] Such changes suggest that OSA might be associated with the development of atherosclerosis, but as yet there is no clear evidence that it does. Hypoxaemia increases production of angiogenic promoters such as vascular endothelial growth factor (VEGF). In patients with OSA, VEGF level is proportional to the number of apnoeas and degree of nocturnal hypoxaemia,[25] but again, no direct link has been demonstrated between OSA and angiogenesis. In mice, intermittent hypoxaemia combined with a high-cholesterol diet causes lipid peroxidation and provokes aortic atherosclerosis, suggesting that effect of OSA and hypercholesterolaemia may be additive.[26] A randomized trial has shown that CPAP in OSA reduces carotid intima-media thickness, suggesting a causal relationship which is potentially reversible.[27]

Pathophysiological consequences

The pathophysiological consequences of sleep apnoea are outlined in Figure 38.2. In general, they can be divided into the effects of hypoxaemia, the impact of arousals including sympathetic hyperactivity and sleep fragmentation, and the effects on haemodynamics.[28] In practice, the pathophysiological changes have combined consequences which are likely to converge to exacerbate the progression of cardiac failure and increase mortality.

A prospective epidemiological study has shown that OSA is an independent risk factor for the development of systemic hypertension, and nocturnal blood pressure in patients with hypertension who also have OSA is higher than those without SDB.[29] In patients with heart failure, elevated daytime blood pressure is increased in proportion to the AHI (in other words, daytime blood pressure is increased in relation to the severity of OSA). In a related effect, OSA diminishes or prevents the usual fall in heart rate and blood pressure

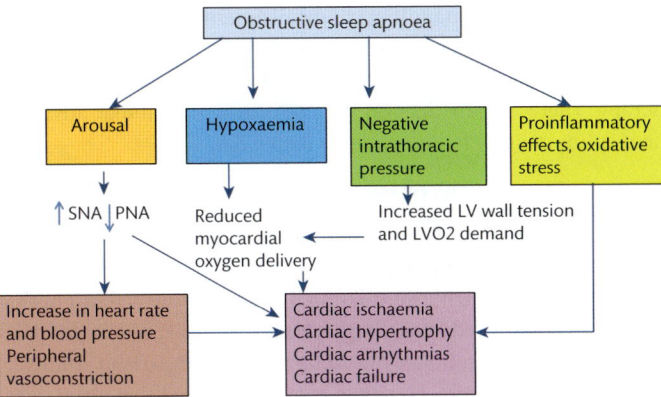

Figure 38.2 Pathophysiological consequences of obstructive sleep apnoea. LV, left ventricle; SNA, sympathetic nervous system activity; PNA, parasympathetic nervous system activity.

that occurs during sleep, and heightened sympathetic tone may predispose individuals to arrhythmia.

Each deep inspiratory effort to open the occluded airway during an apnoea can be associated with very marked swings in intrathoracic pressure. Negative intrathoracic pressures of >60 cmH₂O have been recorded. These frequent pressure swings are associated with an increase in afterload and large falls in stroke volume can be seen as a consequence. The repetitive falls in stroke volume occur on a background of arterial hypoxaemia. The repetitive stimuli every night could play a role in myocyte and contractile dysfunction, setting up a progressive cycle of cardiac decline.

The presence of OSA has an impact on survival in patients with heart failure. Kasai et al.[30] studied 88 patients with heart failure (NYHA II or III, LVEF 36%) and moderate–severe OSA to establish outcome in those who either were untreated, received CPAP therapy, or who were provided with CPAP but did not comply. During an average follow-up period of 25 months, 44.3% of patients died or were hospitalized. On multivariate analysis, the risk of death and hospitalization was increased in the untreated group (hazard ratio (HR): 2.03; 95% confidence interval (CI): 1.07–3.68; P = 0.030) and in the poorly compliant CPAP group (4.02; 1.33–12.3; P = 0.014). However, this was a non-randomized observational study. The results are supported by other work, although Roebuck et al.[31] showed no impact of CPAP on survival in heart failure patients with OSA. Compliance with CPAP was not documented in the latter study, however, so it is possible that patients in the treatment group did not receive effective CPAP.

It should be noted that a randomised trial of CPAP for primary prevention of cardiovascular events[32] and several trials of CPAP for secondary prevention of cardiovascular events in patients with OSA[33,34,35] have produced no reduction in coronary heart disease, death or stoke. Sleepy patients and those with marked hypoxaemia were excluded from these trials, so it is not clear whether these subgroups might benefit. Duration of nightly CPAP use tended to be low, and this is often the case in non sleepy patients.

Management of obstructive sleep apnoea in heart failure

Strategies include optimization of therapy for heart failure, weight loss, positional modification during sleep, positive pressure

ventilatory devices, mandibular advancement splints, and oxygen therapy. While optimization of cardiac function and achieving ideal body weight are sensible, the burden of evidence concerns CPAP therapy. There are few data on the use of the mandibular advancement splint in heart failure patients with OSA.

Impact of treatment of heart failure

Interventions to improve cardiac function are likely to prove beneficial by decreasing both upper airway oedema and pulmonary oedema, thereby stabilizing ventilation. It was previously thought that β-blockers could predispose individuals with heart failure to OSA, but this has not been borne out in treatment comparison studies.[36] A preliminary report by Garrigue et al.[37] suggested that atrial overdrive pacing at a rate of 15 beats/min faster than mean nocturnal heart rate reduced AHI in a group of patients with both OSA and CSA. Whereas an impact on CSA is plausible via an improvement in cardiac output leading to a decrease in heart–lung circulation time and left ventricular filling pressure, the effect on obstructive events is more difficult to explain. Subsequent work has not, however, confirmed the finding and thus the role of atrial overdrive pacing has not been convincingly demonstrated.

Of more relevance is cardiac resynchronization therapy (CRT). Again, it might be expected to be more effective in heart failure patients with CSA, and Stanchina et al.[38] have examined the impact of CRT in heart failure patients with OSA. They found that mean ejection fraction increased from 22% (±1.7) to 33.6% (±2.0) and AHI fell from 40.9 (±6.4) to 29.5 (±5.9) with CRT. As AHI still remained abnormal, it is not surprisingly that there was no improvement in sleep architecture or sleep-related symptoms.

Since upper airway anatomy and body habitus contributes to OSA, cardiac transplantation might be expected not to reduce this component of SDB compared to potential beneficial effects on CSA. This seems indeed to be the case, and some transplant patients may develop OSA.

Positive airway pressure therapy

In an early uncontrolled study of the effects of CPAP on patients with dilated cardiomyopathy and OSA, CPAP therapy for a month increased LVEF from 37% to 49% and breathlessness was reduced.[39] The improvements were lost when CPAP was withdrawn. In a randomized study of 24 patients with mean LVEF <45% and AHI >20, CPAP lowered daytime heart rate and systolic blood pressure and increased LVEF by 9% over 30 days compared to no change in a matched control group who did not receive CPAP.[40] In a further randomized study in congestive heart failure (CHF) patients with OSA, CPAP improved LVEF more modestly (5%) and peak exercise capacity did not change. There was a reduction in daytime sleepiness.[41] More recent outcome data suggest that there is a decrease in mortality in heart failure patients with OSA treated with CPAP compared to those who did not receive CPAP.[29] It is important to stress, however, that the patients were not randomized, so the two treatment groups may represent different populations. As outlined above, it would now be problematic ethically to have a control group of patients with proven symptomatic OSA randomized to no CPAP therapy.

The impact of CPAP on rehospitalization rates in heart failure patients with sleep-disordered breathing has recently been assessed. Sharma et al.[42] carried out sleep studies in patients admitted with CHF. Those with sleep-disordered breathing on CPAP had reduced admission rate, and those highly compliant with CPAP therapy had fewest readmissions over the 6 months post discharge compared to 6 months pre-admission, and a greater reduction in clinical events.

Central sleep apnoea

Mechanisms

CSA and CSR represent forms of periodic breathing. All patients with CSR have central apnoeas, but not all individuals with CSA have the waxing and waning hyperpnoea and hypopnoea pattern of CSR (see **Figure 38.1**, *right*). In contrast to OSA, CSA/CSR arises as a consequence of heart failure itself. Pulmonary congestion and hypoxaemia stimulate receptors within the lung that cause hyperventilation which in turn lead to low arterial CO_2 levels. Lung congestion may be increased on lying flat at night as venous return from the limbs increases. If P_{CO_2} falls below the threshold required to stimulate breathing, a central apnoea occurs and continues until P_{CO_2} rises above the apnoeic threshold. Termination of the apnoea may be accompanied by arousal which stimulates breathing and drives down CO_2 again, leading to a self-perpetuating oscillation between apnoea and hyperpnoea. Prolonged circulation time delays information on arterial blood gas tensions from the lungs reaching the central chemoreceptors in particular, and thereby adds to periodicity such that the length of the ventilatory phase is inversely proportional to cardiac output.[43]

Pathophysiological consequences

Like OSA, CSA is associated with cyclical hypoxaemia, arousal from sleep and sympathetic activation. Passive airway collapse may occur at the end of a central event. Risk factors for the development of CSA/CSR are male sex (perhaps because of higher baseline chemosensitivity in males), age, and the presence of atrial fibrillation. It used to be thought that CSA/CSR was a paraphenomenon and simply represented the presence of severe heart failure. This is unlikely to be the case as prevalence studies have shown a high prevalence of CSA in patients with mild heart failure.[10,12] Importantly, patients with heart failure and CSA/CSR have a worse prognosis than those without this form of SDB.[44]

Controversy surrounds the question of the pathophysiological risk/benefits gained from CSR. Despite being associated with end-stage disease, periodic hyperventilation may augment cardiac output and increase end-expiratory lung volume, thereby improving oxygenation and creating a respiratory alkalosis which may offset the detrimental effects of acidosis. It is for that reason that abolishment of CSA, for example, by positive pressure techniques, may or may not be beneficial.

Treatment

Impact of treatment for heart failure on central sleep apnoea

Therapies that improve cardiac function should also decrease CSA/CSR. Use of angiotensin converting enzyme (ACE) inhibitor therapy

and diuretic therapy to reduce left ventricular filling pressure can produce a decrease in AHI. Vazir et al.[45] showed that a left ventricular assist device reduced CSA/CSR. Similarly, effective cardiac resynchronization therapy can reduce the frequency of CSA.[46] Therefore steps to optimize cardiac function should always be taken first.

Other therapies

A short-term trial of aminophylline produced a reduction in CSA but did not change left or right ventricular function or quality of life.[47] Oxygen therapy at night corrects apnoea-related hypoxaemia and decreases nocturnal noradrenaline level while increasing exercise capacity.[48] However, over a month there was no impact on cardiac function or quality of life.[37] Long term trials of nocturnal oxygen therapy are in progress. Acetazolamide may reduce apnoeas in the short term but long-term effects have not been examined. In addition, oxygen therapy in heart failure can reduce cardiac output and be associated with a rise in pulmonary capillary pressure,[49] so cannot currently be recommended in normoxic heart failure patients.[50,51]

From a theoretical viewpoint, increasing P_{CO_2} by either inhaling CO_2 or rebreathing dead space might be expected to stabilize periodic breathing by raising P_{CO_2} above the apnoeic threshold. Simple inhalation of CO_2 does not seem effective: whereas it may reduce apnoeas, cortical arousals are increased.[52] Similarly, breathing dead space has been shown to reduce central apnoeas but the benefit was offset by an increased work of breathing.[53] Notwithstanding concerns on the safety of asking patients to breathe CO_2 overnight, Mebrate et al.[54] have shown in an experimental model that targeted short-burst CO_2 in a small portion of the ventilatory cycle may stabilize ventilation, but this remains a highly exploratory approach.

Positive pressure therapy

Following the success of CPAP therapy in the management of OSA in heart failure patients, CPAP use has been extended to patients with CSA. However, the mechanisms of OSA and CSA are clearly different and there is no equivalent respiratory end-point (opening the airway) to titrate therapy against. Furthermore, CPAP therapy can mildly reduce P_{CO_2} which might destabilize breathing further. Despite these physiological considerations, initial short-term uncontrolled trials suggested benefit from CPAP in treating CSA in terms of control of SDB and a reduction in ventricular ectopics. In a randomized study of 20 patients with heart failure and CSA, those who complied with CPAP therapy had a significant reduction in the combined rate of mortality/transplantation over 5 years.[55] However, the improved outcome disappeared when outcome was analysed on an intention-to-treat basis.

As a consequence of this work, the Canadian Positive Airway Pressure Trial for patients with congestive cardiac failure and CSA (CANPAP)[56] recruited 258 patients randomized to receive CPAP or usual therapy. In the patients treated with CPAP, mean nocturnal arterial oxygen saturation increased and there was a small improvement in LVEF. There was an early excess of deaths in the CPAP-treated group, but after 2 years the primary end-point of combined mortality and transplantation was identical in CPAP and control groups. Recruitment and event rate were slowed by advances in medical and device therapy as the trial progressed, leaving it underpowered, and so the trial was terminated prematurely.[44] A post-hoc analysis suggested that there might be improved survival in patients

in whom apnoeas/hypopnoeas and CSR was suppressed.[57] This might indicate that therapies better able to suppress SDB may be more effective.

Adaptive servoventilation (ASV) is a form of ventilation that has been designed to smooth out periodic breathing in CSA/CSR by providing ventilatory support during apnoeic periods and reducing the support as spontaneous ventilation begins again (see **Figure 38.3**). Over a relatively short period, breathing is captured and periodicity removed. As a result, arterial P_{CO_2} is stabilized, in turn stabilizing breathing further. Positive pressure is provided in expiration to maintain upper airway patency and control any mixed or obstructive respiratory events.

Small studies show that ASV leads to good control of AHI: in a one-night cross-over study, ASV was more effective at controlling AHI, reducing arousals, and normalizing sleep quality than oxygen therapy, CPAP, or bilevel non-invasive ventilation.[58] In addition, ASV appeared to be better tolerated by patients than CPAP and so more likely to be effective long term.[48] In a 'real world' study, heart failure patients with CSA/CSR who accepted ASV had a significant improvement in LVEF compared to those who did not receive ASV for six months.[59] Conversely, Pepperell et al.[59] showed improvement in sleep-related symptoms and nocturnal sympathetic measures but no change in ejection fraction. A further randomized Japanese trial[60] and meta-analysis[61] showed favourable results. This set the scene for a large multicentre trial (SERVE-HF).

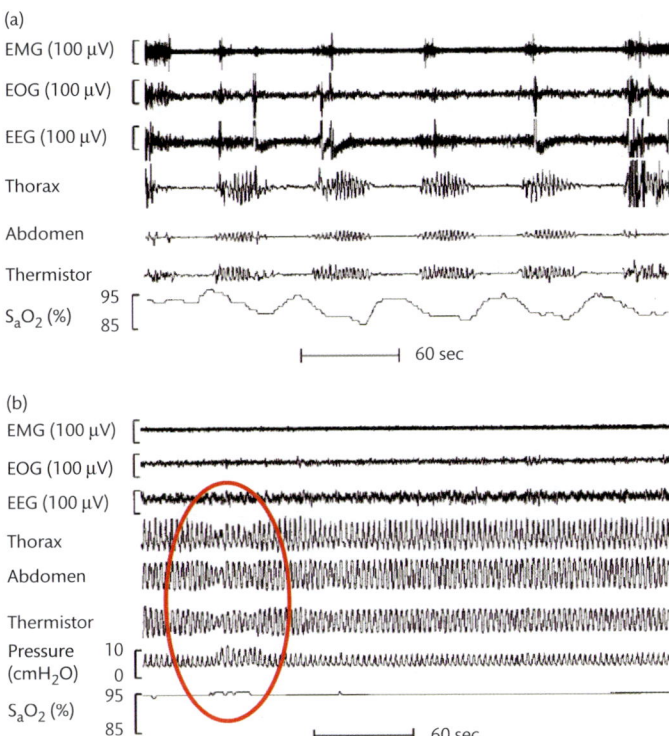

Figure 38.3 Effect of assisted servo-ventilation on sleep apnoea. (a) Untreated, the patient shows regular periods of apnoea with no thoracic or abdominal muscular effort. (b) On treatment. An impending apnoea (characterized by decline in thoracic and abdominal effort, outlined in red) is detected and treated.

Reproduced from Teschler H, Dohring J, Wang YM, Berthon Jones M. Adaptive pressure support servo-ventilation: a novel treatment for Cheyne-Stokes respiration in heart failure and central sleep apnea. Am J Resp Crit Care Med 2001;164:614–619.

The SERVE-HF trial was designed to examine the effects of ASV in heart failure patients with reduced systolic ejection fraction and predominant CSA/CSR using long-term, hard clinical end-points of cardiac and all-cause mortality, and hospital admissions. Contrary to expectations raised by smaller trials, SERVE-HF showed no difference in the primary end-point of hospitalization rate for worsening heart failure, or in time to death, life-saving cardiac intervention (e.g. implantation of LV assist device), or resuscitation after sudden cardiac arrest in the ASV group compared to controls.[62] All-cause mortality and cardiovascular mortality were actually increased in the ASV group (HR for death from any cause: 1.28; 95% CI: 1.06–1.55; $P = 0.01$; HR for cardiovascular death: 1.34; 95% CI: 1.09–1.65; $P = 0.0006$) (Figure 38.4). This was despite ASV reducing AHI successfully and improving mean arterial oxygen saturation overnight. Further analysis has shown that risk of death was higher in those with a greater proportion of CSR and that the signal for cardiovascular death was stronger in those with very low LV ejection fraction.

A substudy of the trial in which echocardiographic and cardiac magnetic resonance imaging (CMR) end-points were studied at baseline and after 12 months showed no significant differences for changes in left ventricular dimensions, wall thickness, diastolic function or right ventricular dimensions and ejection fraction (echocardiography), or in any of the CMR variables assessed. In addition, plasma N-terminal proB-type natriuretic peptide concentration decreased from baseline in both groups; levels at 12 months were similar in the two groups and there were no significant differences between treatment groups in changes in cardiac, renal, and systemic inflammation biomarkers.

This lack of an effect of ASV on cardiac function and evidence of increased sudden death suggest an arhythmogenic aetiology—possibly due to autonomic or metabolic effects induced by ASV. It is possible that ASV removes some possible protective function of CSA/CSR; another possibility is that CSR during the day was left untreated by ASV, and might, indeed, have worsened as a consequence of ASV treatment. These mechanisms are being investigated further. The Advent-HF trial[63] is currently recruiting non-somnolent heart failure patients with OSA and CSA, so should help clarify whether this risk affects all systolic heart failure patients with SDB. The ASV device used in the Advent-HF trial delivers lower end-expiratory and minimum pressure support than were used in SERVE-HF, which might offer an advantage if overventilation and metabolic alkalosis is a causative factor in the deaths associated with SERVE-HF.

These findings mean that pending further trials ASV should *not* be used in patients with systolic heart failure (LVEF ≤45%). Patients already on ASV fulfilling these criteria should have the ASV withdrawn. ASV can be considered in patients with OSA or OSA/CSA and heart failure with normal ejection fraction or in patients with complex sleep apnoea and no evidence of heart failure, as there is no evidence of harm in these groups: there is, however, no strong evidence base in support of such treatment.

Heart failure in neuromuscular disease

It should not be forgotten that some forms of inherited neuromuscular disease have associated cardiac muscle involvement. Cardiomyopathy is almost inevitable in Duchenne muscular dystrophy, and cardiac involvement is seen in Becker and Emery–Dreifuss muscular dystrophies, myotonic dystrophy, some forms of limb girdle muscular dystrophy (LGMD 1B, LGMD 1D, LGMD2C-2 sarcoglycanopathies), and some other myopathies such as acid maltase deficiency. Many of these patients also have respiratory muscle weakness resulting in ventilatory failure.

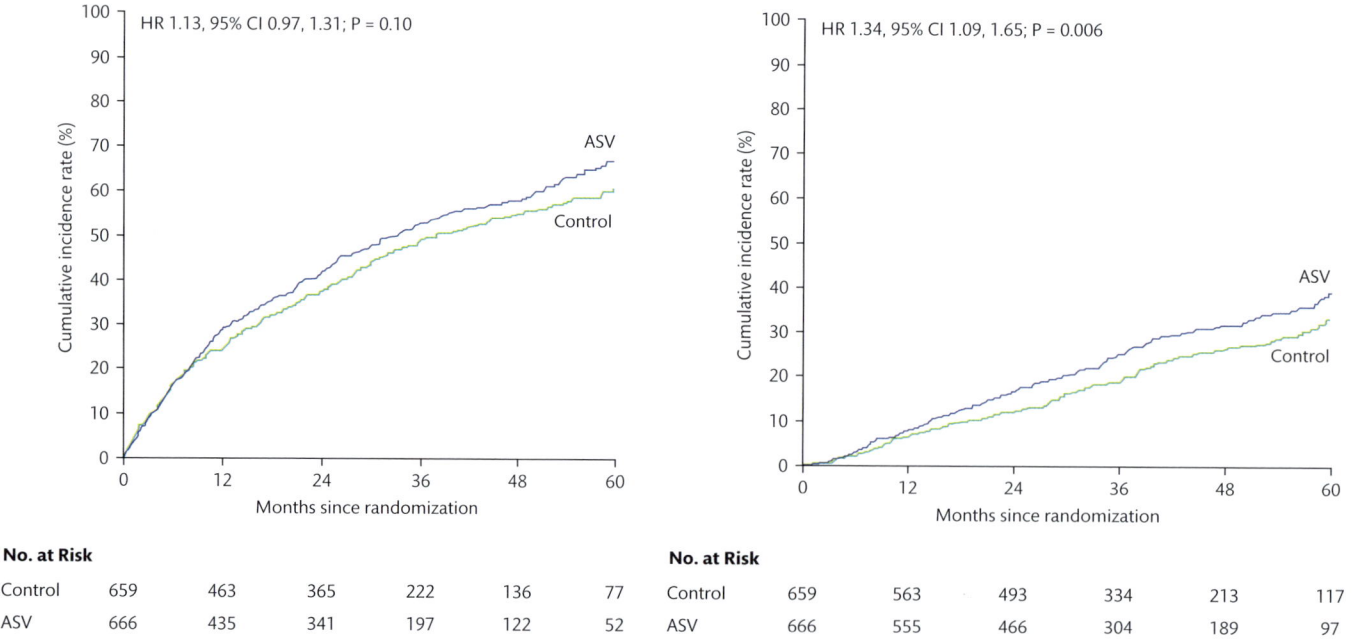

Figure 38.4 Results of the SERVE-HF trial. Adaptive servoventilation had no effect on the primary end-point (a), but was associated with a statistically significant increase in the risk of cardiovascular death.
Source data from Cowie MR, Woehrle H, Wegscheider K, Angermann C, d'Ortho M-P, Erdmann E et al. Adaptive servo-ventilation for central sleep apnea in systolic heart Failure. *N Engl J Med* 2015;**373**:1095–1105.

In some groups, the introduction of non-invasive ventilation to control nocturnal hypoventilation has increased survival and reduced respiratory complications so that the cardiomyopathy becomes a key prognostic determinant. A combination of non-invasive ventilation and optimal cardiac failure therapy means that many patients with Duchenne muscular dystrophy are now living into their 30s and beyond. Anticipation of problems with serial monitoring by yearly ECG and echocardiogram is part of the standard of care in these conditions as the previous nihilistic approach to care is now unjustified.[64]

Duboc[65] has carried out a randomized controlled trial of perindopril in Duchenne patients aged between 9.5 and 13 years (LVEF >55%) for 3 years, after which both perindopril and placebo limbs received open-label perindopril 2–4 mg/day as tolerated for a further 2 years. LVEF was similar in both groups after 3 years, but after 5 years a single patient in the phase I perindopril group had an LVEF <45%, whereas eight patients had LVEF <45% in the phase I placebo group ($P = 0.02$). Currently, a trial of combined prophylactic ACE inhibitor and β-blocker is in progress in children with Duchenne muscular dystrophy.

Clinical features and implications

It is important to realize that the symptoms of OSA and CSA may differ. While OSA patients are classically sleepy during the daytime as quantified by Epworth sleepiness score (ESS),[66] patients with CSA (and some heart failure patients with OSA) do not routinely complain of sleepiness. The ESS is usually within the normal range (<10). Snoring, choking episodes and struggling to breathe are noted by partners of patients with OSA but not those with CSA. Patients with CSA may, however, complain of poor quality, fragmented sleep together with tiredness or fatigue. In addition, despite the lack of subjective sleepiness, objective measures of vigilance are reduced, and daytime activity, as measured by actigraphy watches, is reduced in heart failure patients with all forms of SDB compared to those with no SDB.[67] Current guidelines suggest that sleep-disordered breathing should be considered in patients with difficult-to-control or drug-resistant hypertension and refractory malignant dysrrythmias, especially if they occur during sleep.[68,69] It is important to note that awareness of sleep-disordered breathing, although increasing, remains low. In a US study of Medicare recipients, only 2% of newly diagnosed heart failure patients were tested for sleep apnoea over a 2-year period. Nevertheless, those who underwent sleep studies, who were diagnosed and who were treated for sleep apnoea had better survival than those who were not.[70]

Practicalities of assessment in the clinic and therapy

The lack of typical symptoms raises the question of how to identify heart failure patients with SDB in the clinic. A story of snoring, witnessed apnoea, and daytime sleepiness should be specifically asked for as the symptoms may be present in some, particularly those with higher body mass index (BMI). Clinicians should also be aware that sleep can be disturbed by restless legs, nocturia, paroxysmal

Box 38.1 The Stop-Bang questionnaire

1 Do you snore loudly?
2 Do you often feel tired, fatigued or sleepy during the daytime?
3 Has anyone *observed* you stop breathing while you sleep?
4 Do you have or are you being treated for high blood *pressure*?
5 *Body mass index ≥35 kg/m²*
6 *Age >50 years?*
7 *Neck circumference >40 cm?*
8 *Gender—male?*

High risk of obstructive sleep apnoea (OSA): answering 'yes' to ≥3 items; low risk of OSA: answering 'yes' to <3 items

nocturnal dyspnoea, anxiety, and depression. Daytime sleepiness can be assessed by the ESS: in addition, the STOP-Bang questionnaire has a sensitivity of >80% when identifying patients with moderate–severe OSA (Box 38.1). SDB occurs in up to three-quarters of CHF patients with chronic atrial fibrillation (AF),[56] so there should be a low threshold for asking about symptoms and carrying out a sleep study in this group. As the presence of SDB cannot be easily predicted in others, a variety of screening mechanisms is being investigated. Screening is, of course, only justified where effective treatment is available for the condition detected. At present, there is good evidence in favour of treating OSA in patients with CHF, but in light of the negative results from the SERVE-HF trial,[62] the optimal management of CSA/CSR is less clear. ASV should be avoided in patients with CSA and systolic heart failure with LVEF <45%. Screening methods that can be used in the home include oximetry, analysis of heart rate variation, and apnoea detection, but more detailed techniques are required to differentiate OSA from CSA.

CPAP treatment is best started by experienced teams, and a good link between cardiology departments and sleep departments is highly recommended. In patients with labile heart failure and poor cardiac output, initiating CPAP is more safely done with the patient in hospital with haemodynamic monitoring. In CHF patients with OSA, outpatient set-up is usually effective as long as there is careful explanation of the anticipated benefit, the importance of fitting of mask interface, and support in the home.[71] Autoset variable pressure devices can be used to determine the correct pressure setting overnight, but for long-term use, fixed-level standard CPAP machines are usually sufficient. Continued input from the CPAP team to maintain compliance and adherence is helpful. Patients with heart failure often have other comorbidities. In those with additional severe chronic obstructive pulmonary disease or obesity resulting in nocturnal hypoventilation, obstructive hypopnoeas or even obesity–hypoventilation syndrome and daytime hypercapnia, non-invasive ventilation is likely to be preferable to autoset devices.

REFERENCES

1. Naughton MT. Respiratory sleep disorders in patients with congestive cardiac failure. *J Thorac Dis* 2015;7:1298–1310.
2. Cheyne J. A case of apoplexy in which the fleshy part of the heart was converted into fat. *Dublin Hosp Rep* 1818;2:216–23.
3. Stokes W. Fatty degeneration of the heart. In: *The diseases of the heart and aorta*, pp. 320–327. Dublin, 1854.

4. Malhotra A, Ayappa I, Ayas N, *et al.* Metrics of sleep apnea severity: beyond the apnea-hypopnea index. *Sleep J* 2020;**44**:1–16.

5. Lanfranchi PA, Somers VK, Braghiroli A, *et al.* Central sleep apnea in left ventricular dysfunction: prevalence and implications for arrhythmic risk. *Circulation* 2003;**107**:727–32.

6. Ferrier K, Campbell A, Yee B, *et al.* Sleep-disordered breathing occurs frequently in stable outpatients with congestive heart failure. *Chest* 2005;**128**:2116–22.

7. Javaheri S, Parker TJ, Liming JD, *et al.* Sleep apnea in 81 ambulatory male patients with stable heart failure: types and their prevalences, consequences and presentations. *Circulation* 1998;**97**:2154–9.

8. Oldenburg O, Lamp B, Teschler H, Horstkotte D, Topfer V. Sleep-disordered breathing in patients with symptomatic heart failure: a contemporary study of prevalence in and characteristics of 700 patients. *Eur J Heart Fail* 2007;**9**:251–7.

9. Schulz R, Blau A, Borgel J, *et al.* Sleep apnoea in heart failure—results of a German survey. *Eur Respir J* 2007;**29**:1201–5.

10. Vazir A, Hastings PC, Dayer M, *et al.* A high prevalence of sleep disordered breathing in men with mild symptomatic chronic heart failure due to left ventricular systolic dysfunction. *Eur J Heart Fail* 2007;**9**:243–50.

11. MacDonald M, Fang J, Pittman SD, White DP, Malhotra A. The current prevalence of sleep disordered breathing in congestive heart failure patients treated with beta blockers. *J Clin Sleep Med* 2008;**4**:38–42.

12. Bitter T, Faber L, Hering D, *et al.* Sleep disordered breathing in heart failure with normal left ventricular ejection fraction. *Eur J Heart Fail* 2009;**11**:602–8.

13. Yumino D, Wang H, Floras JS, *et al.* Prevalence and physiological predictors of sleep apnea in patients with heart failure and systolic dysfunction. *J Card Fail* 2009;**15**:279–85.

14. Young T, Palta M, Dempsey J, *et al.* The occurrence of sleep-disordered breathing among middle-aged adults. *N Engl J Med* 1993;**328**:1230–5.

15. Kasai T, Bradley TD. Obstructive sleep apnea and heart failure. *J Am Coll Cardiol* 2011;**57**:119–27.

16. Ward NR, Cowie MC, Rosen SD, *et al.* Utility of overnight pulse oximetry and heart rate variability analysis to screen for sleep-disordered breathing in chronic heart failure. *Thorax* 2012;**67**:1000–5.

17. Clark AL, Crabbe S, Aziz A, Reddy P, Greenstone M. Use of a screening tool for detection of sleep-disordered breathing. *J Laryngol Otol* 2009;**123**:746–9.

18. Vazir A, Hastings PC, Papaioannou I, *et al.* Variation in severity and type of sleep-disordered breathing throughhout 4 nights in patients with heart failure. *Respir Med* 2008;**102**:831–9.

19. Tkacova R, Niroumand M, Lorenzi-Filho L, Douglas TD. Overnight shift from obstructive to central apneas in patients with heart failure. *Circulation* 2001;**103**:238.

20. Bonsignore MR, Suarez Giron MC, Marrone O, *et al.* Personalised medicine in sleep respiratory disorders: focus on obstructive sleep apnoea diagnosis and treatment. *Eur Resp Rev* 2017;26.

21. Yumino D, Redolfi S, Ruttanaumpawan P, *et al.* Nocturnal rostral fluid shift: a unifying concept for the pathogenesis of obstructive and central sleep apnea in heart failure. *Circulation* 2010;**121**:1598–1605.

22. Usui K, Bradley TD, Spaak J, *et al.* Inhibition of awake sympathetic nerve activity of heart failure patients with obstructive sleep apnea by nocturnal continuous positive airway pressure. *J Am Coll Cardiol* 2005;**45**:2008–11.

23. Shamsuzzaman AS, Winnicki M, Lanfranchi P, *et al.* Elevated C-reactive protein in patients with obstructive sleep apnea. *Circulation* 2002;**105**:2462–4.

24. Dyugovskaya L, Lavie P, Lavie L, *et al.* Increased adhesion molecule expression and production of reactive oxygen species in leucocytes of sleep apnea patients. *Am J Respir Crit Care Med* 2002;**165**:934–9.

25. Schulz R, Hummel C, Heinemann S, *et al.* Serum levels of vascular endothelial growth factor are elevated in patients with obstructive sleep apnea and severe nighttime hypoxia. *Am J Respir Crit Care Med* 2002;**165**:67–70.

26. Savransky V, Nanayakkara A, Li J, *et al.* Chronic intermittent hypoxia induces atherosclerosis. *Am J Resp Crit Care Med* 2007;**175**:1290–7.

27. Drager LF, Bortolotto LA, Figueiredo AC, Krieger EM, Lorenzi GF. Effects of continuous positive airway pressure on early signs of atherosclerosis in obstructive sleep apnea. *Am J Resp Crit Care Med* 2007;**176**:706–12.

28. Somers VK, White DP, Amin R, *et al.* Sleep apnea and cardiovascular disease. AHA/ACCF Scientific Statement. *Circulation* 2008;**118**:1080–1111.

29. Peppard PE, Young T, Palta M, Skatrud J. Prospective study of the association between sleep-disordered breathing and hypertension. *N Engl J Med* 2000;**342**:1378–84.

30. Kasai T, Narui K, Dohi T, *et al.* Prognosis of patients with heart failure and obstructive sleep apnea treated with continuous positive airway pressure. *Chest* 2008;**133**(690):696.

31. Roebuck T, Solin P, Kaye DM, *et al.* Increased long-term mortality in heart failure due to sleep apnoea is not yet proven. *Eur Respir J* 2004;**23**(735):740.

32. Barbe F, Duran-Cantolla J, Sanchez-De-La-Toree M, *et al.* Effect of continous positive airway pressure on incidence of hypertension and cardiovascular events in nonsleepy patients with obstructive sleep apnea. *JAMA* 2012;**307**:2161–68.

33. Pekker Y, Glantz H, Eulenburg C, et al. Effect of positive airway pressure on cardiovascular outcomes in coronary artery disease patients with non-sleepy apnea. The RICCADSA randomised controlled trial. *Am J Resp Crit Care Med* 2016;**194**:613–620.

34. McEvoy RD, Antic NA, Heweley E, et al. CPAP for prevention of cardiovascular events in obstructive sleep apnea. *N Engl J Med* 2016;**375**:919–931.

35. Sanches-de-la-Torre M, Sanchez-de-la Torre A, Bertran S, *et al.* Effect of obstructive sleep apnoea and its treatment with continuous posiitve airway pressure on the presence of cardiovascular events in patients with acute coronary syndrome (ISAAC study): a randomised controlled trial. *Lancet Respir Med* 2020;**8**:359–367.

36. Kraiczi H, Hedner J, Peker Y, Grote L. Comparison of atenolol, amlodipine, enalapril, hydrochlorthiazide and losartan for antihypertensive treatment of patients with obstructive sleep apnea. *Am J Respir Crit Care Med* 2000;**161**:1423–8.

37. Garrigue S, Bordier O, Jais P, *et al.* Benefit of atrial pacing in sleep apnea syndrome. *N Engl J Med* 2002;**346**:404–12.

38. Stanchina ML, Ellison K, Malhotra A, *et al.* The impact of cardiac resynchronisation therapy on obstructive sleep apnea in heart failure. *Chest* 20097;**132**:433–9.

39. Malone S, Liu PP, Holloway R, *et al.* Obstructive sleep apnoea in patients with dilated cardiomyopathy: effects of continuous positive airway pressure. *Lancet* 1991;**338**:1480–4.

40. Kaneko Y, Floras JS, Usui K, *et al.* Cardiovascular effects of continuous positive airway pressure in patinents with heart failure and obstructive sleep apnoea. *N Engl J Med* 2003;**348**:1233–41.

41. Mansfield DR, Gollogly NC, Kaye DM, *et al.* Controlled trial of continuous positive airway pressure in obstructive sleep apnoea and heart failure. *Am J Respir Crit Care Med* 2004;**169**:361–6.

42. Sharma S, Mather P, Gupta A, *et al.* Effect of early intervention with positive pressure therapy for sleep disordered breathing on six month readmission rates in hospitalized patients with heart failure. *Am J Cardiol* 2016;**117**:940–5.

43. Bradley TD, Floras JS. Sleep apnea and heart failure. Part II. Central sleep apnea. *Circulation* 2003;**107**:1822–6.

44. Lanfranchi PA, Braghiroli A, Bosimini E, *et al.* Prognostic value of nocturnal Cheyne–Stokes respiration in chronic heart failure. *Circulation* 1999;**99**:1435–40.

45. Vazir A, Hastings PC, Morrell MJ, *et al.* Resolution of central sleep apnoea following implantation of a left ventricular assist device. *Int J Cardiol* 2010;**138**:317–19.

46. Oldenburg O, Faber L, Vogt J, *et al.* Influence of cardiac resynchronisation therapy on different types of sleep disordered breathing. *Eur J Heart Fail* 2007;**9**:820–6.

47. Javaheri S, Parker TJ, Wexler L, *et al.* Effect of theophylline on sleep-disordered breathing in heart failure. *N Engl J Med* 1996;**335**:562–7.

48. Andreas S, Clemens C, Sandholzer H, *et al.* Improvement in exercise capacity with treatment of Cheyne–Stokes respiration in patients with congestive cardiac failure. *J Am Coll Cardiol* 1996;**27**:1486–90.

49. Mak S, Azevedo ER, Liu PP, *et al.* Effect of hyperoxia on left ventricular function and filling pressures in patients with and without congestive heart failure. *Chest* 2001;**120**:467–473.

50. Clark AL, Johnson MJ, Squire I. Does home oxygen benefit people with chronic heart failure? *Br Med J* 2011;**342**:d234.

51. Clark AL, Johnson M, Fairhurst C, *et al.* Does home oxygen therapy (HOT) in addition to standard care reduce disease severity and improve symptoms in people with chronic heart failure? A randomised trial of home oxygen therapy for patients with chronic heart failure. *Health Technol Assess* 2015;**19**:1–120.

52. Szollosi I, Jones M, Morrell M. Effect of CO_2 inhalation on central sleep apnoea and arousals from sleep. *Respiration* 2004;**71**:493–8.

53. Szollosi I, O'Driscoll DM, Dayer MJ, *et al.* Adaptive servo-ventilation and deadspace: effects on central sleep apnoea. *J Sleep Res* 2006;**15**:199–205.

54. Mebrate Y, Willson K, Manisty CH, *et al.* Dynamic CO_2 therapy in periodic breathing: a modelling study to determine optimal timing and dosage regimes. *J Appl Physiol* 2009;**107**:696–706.

55. Sin DD, Logan AG, Fitzgerald FS, *et al.* Effects of continuous positive airway pressure on cardiovascular outcomes in heart failure patients with and without Cheyne–Stokes respiration. *Circulation* 2000;**102**:61–6.

56. Bradley TD, Logan AG, Kimoff J, *et al.* Continuous positive airway pressure for central sleep apnea and heart failure. *N Engl J Med* 2005;**353**:2025–33.

57. Artzt M, Floras JS, Logan AG, *et al.* Suppression of central sleep apnea by continuous positive pressure airway pressure and transplant-free survival in heart failure. A post hoc analysis of the Canadian Continuous Positive Airway Pressure for patients with central sleep apnea and heart failure trial (CANPAP). *Circulation* 2007;**115**:3173–80.

58. Teschler H, Dohring J, Wang YM, Berthon-Jones M. Adaptive pressure support servo-ventilation: a novel treatment for Cheyne–Stokes respiration in heart failure and central sleep apnea. *Am J Resp Crit Care Med* 2001;**164**:614–19.

59. Pepperell JC, Maskell NA, Jones DR, *et al.* A randomise controlled trial of adaptive ventilation for Cheyne–Stokes breathing in heart failure. *Am J Resp Crit Care Med* 2003;**168**:1109–14.

60. Momomura S, Seino Y, Kihara Y, *et al.* Adaptive servo-ventilation therapy for patients with chronic heart failure in confirmatory, multicenter, randomized, controlled study. *Circulation* 2015;**579**:981–90.

61. Nakamura S, Asai K, Kubota Y, *et al.* Impact of sleep disordered breathing and efficacy of positive airway pressure on mortality in patients with chronic heart failure and sleep disordered breathing: a meta-analysis. *Clin Res Cardiol* 2015;**104**:208–16.

62. Cowie MR, Woehrle H, Wegscheider K, *et al.* Adaptive servo-ventilation for central sleep apnea in systolic heart Failure. *N Engl J Med* 2015;**373**:1095–105.

63. Bradley TD, Floras JS. Adaptive servo-ventilation and treatment of central sleep apnea in heart failure. Let's not throw the baby out with the bathwater. *Am J Resp Crit Care Med* 2015;**193**:357–9.

64. Bushby K, Muntoni F, Bourke JP. 107th International Workshop: the management of cardiac involvement in muscular dystrophy and myotonic dystrophy. *Neuromusc Disord* 2003;**13**:166–72.

65. Duboc D, Meaune C, Lerebours G, *et al.* Effect of perindopril on the onset and progression of left ventricular dysfunction in Duchenne muscular dystrophy. *J Am Coll Cardiol* 2005;**45**:855–7.

66. Johns MW. Daytime sleepiness, snoring, and obstructive sleep apnea. The Epworth Sleepiness Scale. *Chest* 1993;**103**:30–6.

67. Hastings PC, Vazir A, O'Driscoll DM, Morrell MJ, Simonds AK. Symptom burden of sleep-disordered breathing in mild-to-moderate congestive heart failure patients. *Eur Respir J* 2006;**27**:748–55.

68. McKelvie RS, Moe GW, Cheung A, *et al.* The 2011 Canadian Cardiovascular Society Heart Failure management guideline update: focus on sleep apnea, renal dysfunction, mechanical circulatory support and palliative care. *Can J Cardiol* 2011;**27**:319–38.

69. Ponikowski P, Voors AA, Anker SD, *et al.* 2016 ESC Guidelines for the diagnosis and treatment of acute and chronic heart failure. Task Force for the diagnosis and treatment of acute and chronic heart failure of the European Society of Cardiology. *Eur Heart J* 2016;**37**:2129–200.

70. Javaheri S, Caref EB, Chen E, Tong KB, Abraham WT. Sleep apnea testing and outcomes in a large cohort of Medicare beneficiaries with newly diagnosed heart failure. *Am J Respir Crit Care Med* 2011;**183**:539–46.

71. Simonds AK. Positive airway pressure treatment. In: Simonds AK, de Backer W (eds), *ERS Handbook, Respiratory sleep medicine*, 1st ed., pp. 157–163. European Respiratory Society, Sheffield, 2012.

39

Arthritis

Sam Rodgers and Niki L. Walker

Introduction

Heart failure and arthritis are both common in adults, and both increase in incidence and prevalence with age. The term arthritis covers a wide spectrum of disease (**Box 39.1**). Broadly, the diseases involve the cartilage, bone, tensile structures (ligaments, tendons and muscles), or synovial tissue. Pathological processes can impact on any of these structures. The most common arthritis is osteoarthritis resulting from cartilage fragmentation and loss, usually with wear and age. The major target for autoimmune and inflammatory arthritides is the synovium.

The main focus of this chapter is the interaction of heart failure with the inflammatory arthritides. Systemic inflammation in the patient with arthritis is linked to heart failure by:

- myocardial disease, resulting in:
  - ventricular systolic dysfunction, e.g. myocarditis
  - ventricular diastolic dysfunction, e.g. amyloidosis;
- pericardial disease, e.g. pericarditis with effusion;
- coronary artery disease, both acute inflammatory arteritis and traditional atheromatous disease;
- conduction disease, usually bradyarrhythmias related to myocardial fibrosis;
- valvular disease, this may occur with the seronegative spondyloarthropathies such as ankylosing spondylitis, or with endocarditic lesions including the non-bacterial Libman–Sacks endocarditis.

Box 39.1 Categories of arthritis

- Monoarthritis
- Osteoarthritis
- Septic arthritis
- Crystal arthritis (gout and calcium pyrophosphate dihydrate)
- Trauma with haemarthrosis
- Polyarthritis
- Rheumatoid arthritis
- Psoriatic arthritis
- Ankylosing spondylitis
- Reactive arthritis (bacterial or viral)
- Osteoarthritis
- Connective tissue disease (e.g. systemic lupus erythematosus)
- Systemic disease (including malignancy, endocarditis, sarcoidosis, sickle cell disease, familial Mediterranean fever)

The presentation of arthritis may offer a clue to the cause of heart failure. For example, pseudogout caused by calcium pyrophosphate dihydrate crystals may be precipitated by hypothyroidism, which might in turn explain new-onset heart failure or decompensation of chronic heart failure.

Heart failure and arthritis may coexist. When both are present, the pharmacotherapy of either condition may impact on the other, to a beneficial or detrimental effect. For example, gout may be triggered by diuretic use in the management of heart failure.

Epidemiology of heart failure and rheumatoid arthritis

Most of the evidence relating to arthritis and heart failure is from the extensive study of rheumatoid arthritis (RA). The recurring theme is that the clinical presentation and outcome of heart failure is different in patients with RA compared to heart failure in the general population.

RA is one of the most common chronic rheumatic diseases, affecting 1% of the population. Premature death, predominantly from cardiovascular disease, is associated with an 8–15-year reduction in lifespan compared to age-matched controls.[1] In a recent UK case–control study, patients with RA were at increased risk of incident cardiovascular disease including acute myocardial infarction, sudden cardiac death (and resuscitated cardiac arrest), and particularly of heart failure with an adjusted incidence ratio (after adjustment for cardiovascular risk factors) of 1.61 (95% confidence interval (CI): 1.43–1.83) compared to a matched population without RA (**Figure 39.1**).[2]

The extent of cardiac involvement in arthritis has been a source of ongoing interest for decades. In 1943, Bayles described postmortem findings in the heart of patients with RA.[3] Excess cardiovascular mortality in patients with RA was reported as early as 1975.[4]

To quantify the frequency of heart failure among patients with RA, Wolfe *et al.*[5] asked 13 171 participants in the National Data Bank for Rheumatic Diseases: 'During the last 6 months were you diagnosed or treated for heart failure?' Those with a positive reply were then interviewed by the research team to confirm validity. The frequency of heart failure increases with age and is always greater in men than in women (**Figure 39.2**).

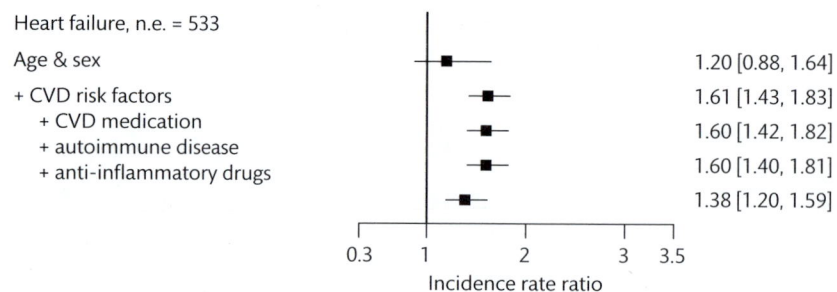

Heart failure, n.e. = 533

Age & sex   1.20 [0.88, 1.64]

+ CVD risk factors   1.61 [1.43, 1.83]
  + CVD medication   1.60 [1.42, 1.82]
  + autoimmune disease   1.60 [1.40, 1.81]
  + anti-inflammatory drugs   1.38 [1.20, 1.59]

0.3   1   2   3   3.5
Incidence rate ratio

Figure 39.1 The adjusted incidence ratio of heart failure after adjustment for cardiovascular disease risk (CVD) factors compared to a matched population without rheumatoid arthritis was 1.61 (95% CI: 1.43–1.83). CVD risk factors included index of multiple deprivation, smoking status, systolic blood pressure, body mass index, and diabetes mellitus.
Reproduced from Pujades-Rodriguez M, Duyx B, Thomas SL, Stogiannis D, Rahman A, Smeeth L, et al. Rheumatoid arthritis and incidence of twelve initial presentations of cardiovascular disease: A population record-linkage cohort study in England. *PLoS One* 2016;**11**(3).

In a population-based inception cohort of 603 individuals with RA and 603 patients without RA living in Rochester, Minnesota, mortality rates were 39.0 and 29.2 per 1000 person-years, respectively (**Figure 39.3**). At 30 years follow-up, there was a higher incidence of heart failure in patients with RA (37.1% vs 27.7% in non-RA; *P* < 0.001).[6]

A community-based cohort study of patients with heart failure compared 103 patients with RA to 852 without.[7] The patients with RA were more likely to be female, and were less likely to be obese, or to have hypertension or ischaemic heart disease. Their symptoms and signs at presentation were often more subtle and consequently they were less likely to have an echocardiogram. Patients with RA were more likely to have heart failure with preserved systolic function (**Figure 39.4**) but had higher mortality at one year (**Figure 39.5**). These findings illustrate the difficulties in the assessment and management (and study) of patients with RA.

Epidemiology of heart failure and psoriatic arthritis

Psoriasis is a systemic inflammatory condition that affects 1–3% of the population and manifests primarily as a skin disorder. However, of those affected, 6–11% have psoriatic arthropathy. There is a 31% higher risk of heart failure among patients with psoriatic arthropathy than among the general population (odds ratio (OR): 1.31; 95% CI: 1.11–1.55), and a 68% increased risk of myocardial infarction (1.68; 1.31–2.15).[8]

However, diabetes, hypertension, hyperlipidaemia, smoking, and obesity are more common than usual in patients with mild psoriasis and even more common in those with severe psoriasis, complicating the interpretation of the data.[9] Gelfand *et al.* found that the relative risk of myocardial infarction associated with psoriasis is greatest in young patients with severe psoriasis, falls with age, but is higher than normal even after controlling for traditional cardiovascular risk factors (**Figure 39.6**).[10] In a study from the USA, the 10-year risk of coronary disease was 28% greater among patients with psoriasis than in the general population.[11] However, a very large Dutch cohort found that psoriasis was not a clinically relevant independent

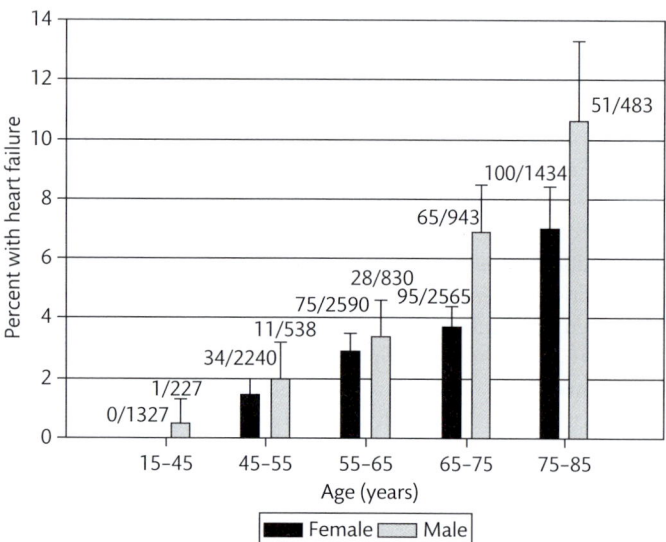

Figure 39.2 Frequency of heart failure in 13 171 rheumatoid arthritis patients stratified by age and sex. Rates increase with age (*P* < 0.001) and are always greater in men than in women (*P* < 0.001).
Reproduced from Wolfe F, Michaud K. Heart failure in rheumatoid arthritis: rates, predictors, and the effect of anti-tumor necrosis factor therapy. *American Journal of Medicine* 2004. p. 305–11 with permission from Elsevier.

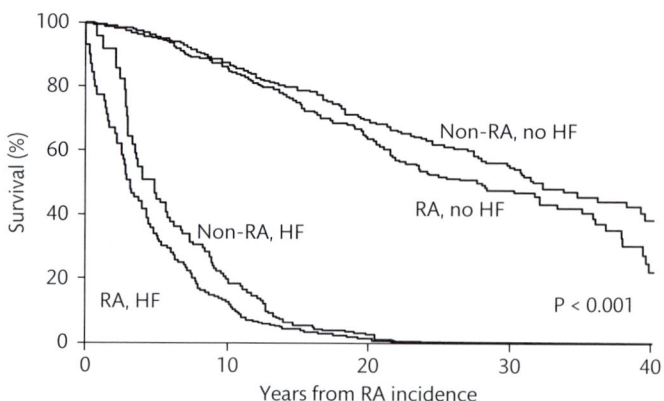

Figure 39.3 The impact of rheumatoid arthritis (RA) on survival, and the cumulative impact of heart failure (HF) with RA on survival.
Reproduced from Nicola PJ, Crowson CS, Maradit-Kremers H, Ballman KV, Roger VL, Jacobsen SJ, et al. Contribution of congestive heart failure and ischemic heart disease to excess mortality in rheumatoid arthritis. *Arthritis Rheum* 2006;**54**(1):60–7 with permission from John Wiley and Sons.

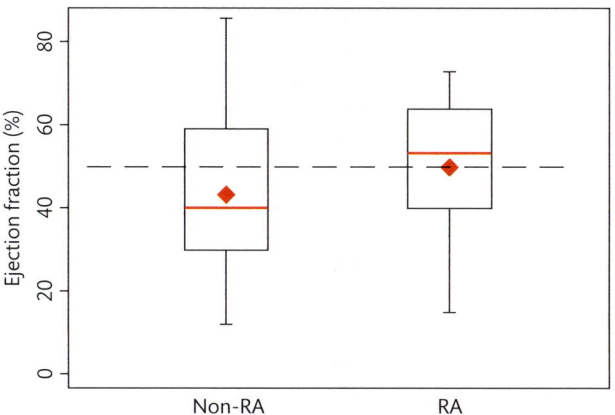

Figure 39.4 Patients with rheumatoid arthritis (RA) and heart failure are more likely to have preserved systolic function (left ventricular ejection fraction >50%) than patients without RA.

Reproduced from Davis JM, Roger VL, Crowson CS, Kremers HM, Therneau TM, Gabriel SE. The presentation and outcome of heart failure in patients with rheumatoid arthritis differs from that in the general population. *Arthritis Rheum* 2008;**58**(9):2603–11 with permission from John Wiley and Sons.

risk factor for ischaemic heart disease hospitalization.[12] It remains to be seen whether aggressive control of the traditional risk factors and of systemic inflammation will have any impact on the evolution of coronary artery disease in patients with psoriasis and more specifically psoriatic arthropathy.

Arthritis, atherosclerosis, and inflammation

Classic risk factors alone do not explain excess vascular disease in RA. In one report[13] there was a 3.96-fold higher incidence of

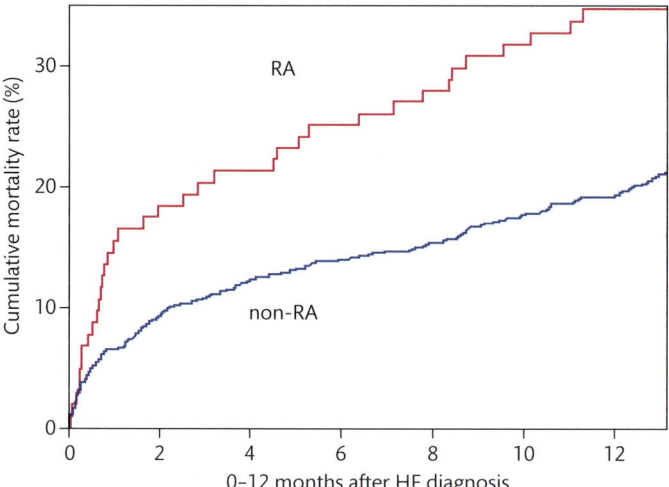

Figure 39.5 Mortality rate following a diagnosis of heart failure (HF) is higher among patients with rheumatoid arthritis (RA). There is early separation of the curves with 30-day mortality of 15.5% in the RA group compared with 6.6% in the non-RA group. The curves continue to separate for at least the first year, and Figure 39.3 suggests that the divergence may persist out to approximately 10 years.

Reproduced from Davis JM, Roger VL, Crowson CS, Kremers HM, Therneau TM, Gabriel SE. The presentation and outcome of heart failure in patients with rheumatoid arthritis differs from that in the general population. *Arthritis Rheum* 2008;**58**(9):2603–11 with permission from John Wiley and Sons.

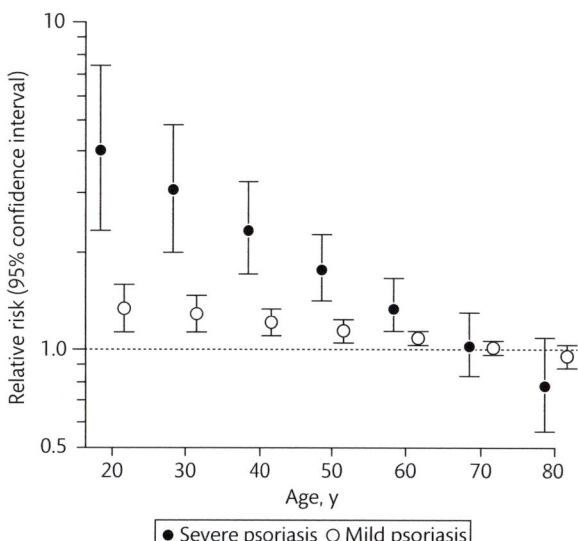

● Severe psoriasis ○ Mild psoriasis

Figure 39.6 Adjusted relative risk of myocardial infarction in patients with psoriasis based on age and risk shown on a logarithmic scale. The data are divided between those with mild or severe psoriasis.

Source data from Gelfand JM, Neimann AL, Shin DB, Wang X, Margolis DJ, Troxel AB. Risk of myocardial infarction in patients with psoriasis. *J Am Med Assoc* [Internet] 2006;**296**(14):1735–41.

cardiovascular events among patients with RA compared to controls which was only minimally reduced to 3.17 after correction for conventional risk factors.

The role of autoimmune processes is well described in several arthritic conditions including RA and systemic lupus erythematosus (SLE). There is increasing evidence that active autoimmune arthritis is associated with heart disease including heart failure.

Parallels can be drawn between coronary heart disease, with inflammatory molecules and immune cells in the cap region of unstable atheromatous plaques, and the inflammatory process in synovitis. Cytokines (particularly tumour necrosis factor-α (TNFα), interleukin-1β (IL-1β), and IL-6) can be identified in both heart failure and the inflammatory arthritides. TNFα is implicated in the pathogenesis of heart failure and cardiac cachexia.[14] In a follow-up study of the SOLVD (Studies Of Left Ventricular Dysfunction) population, concentrations of TNFα were significantly higher in patients with heart failure compared with normal controls.[15] Furthermore, in a study of patients with advanced heart failure, higher concentrations of cytokines were associated with a worse prognosis (**Figure 39.7**).[16]

TNFα alongside other cytokines (IL-1β, IL-6)—which are produced in abundance from the inflamed synovium of individuals with RA—appear to have independent pathophysiological importance in the development of clinical heart failure and this effect worsens with time. The process is mechanistically complex and not yet fully understood.[17]

Dyslipidaemia is common among patients with RA, but can be difficult to interpret due to a complex association between serum lipid concentrations and systemic inflammation. For instance, one population-based study[18] examined the risk of cardiovascular disease and heart failure among 651 adults with RA associated with inflammatory markers (erythrocyte sedimentation rate (ESR) and C-reactive protein) and serum lipid profile. In contrast to the

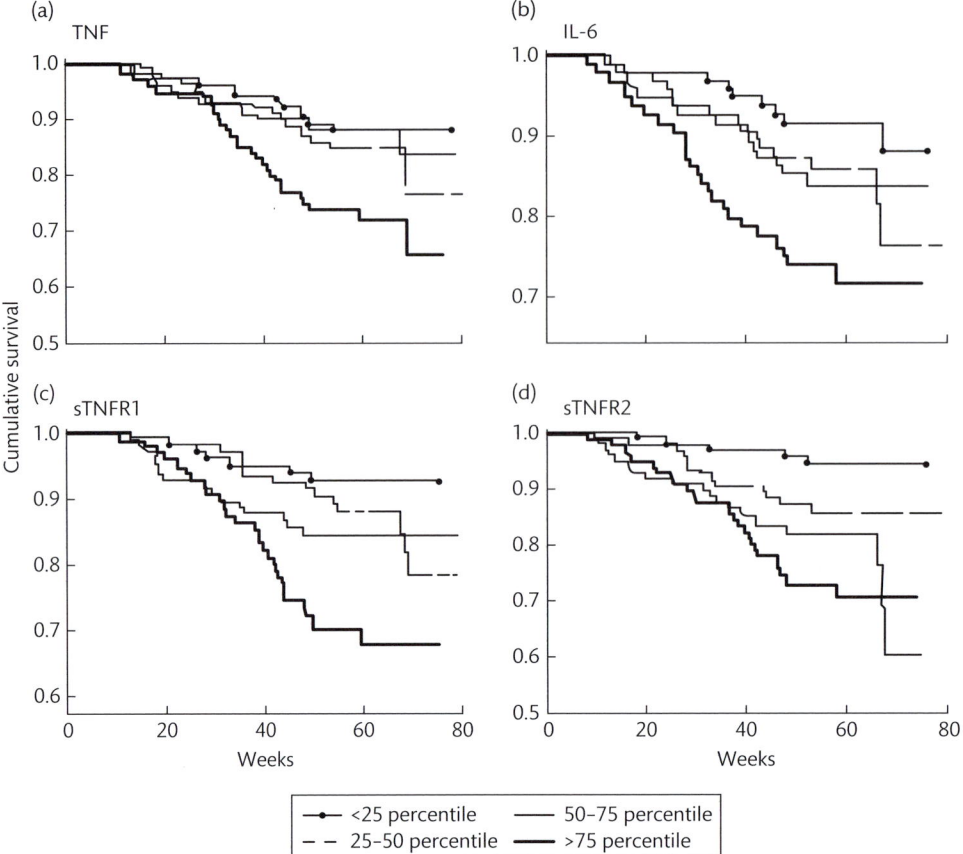

Figure 39.7 Circulating levels of TNFα, IL-6, soluble TNF receptor 1 (sTNFR1), and sTNFR2 in relation to patient survival during follow-up. Circulating levels of cytokines and cytokine receptors were arbitrarily divided into quartiles.

Reproduced from Deswal a, Petersen NJ, Feldman a M, Young JB, White BG, Mann DL. Cytokines and cytokine receptors in advanced heart failure: an analysis of the cytokine database from the Vesnarinone trial (VEST). *Circulation* 2001;103(16):2055–9 with permission from Wolters Kluwer.

commonly accepted paradigm, the highest risk of cardiovascular disease and heart failure was seen in patients with a low total cholesterol (TCh) and high high-density lipoprotein (HDL). For the development of heart failure, hazard ratio (HR) (95% confidence interval (CI)) for high serum concentrations of TCh and HDL, respectively, were 0.92 (0.85–0.99) and 1.35 (1.09–1.68). However, increasing inflammatory markers, particularly ESR, were strongly predictive of cardiovascular disease and mortality.

Figure 39.8 illustrates the complex relationship between serum lipid levels and risk of cardiovascular disease. The risk is greatest with a total cholesterol <4 mmol/L, at which level, inflammatory indices are high. Estimating the cardiovascular risk of patients with RA is more difficult than in the general population[19] and the paradoxical association with serum lipids may contribute to this. Traditional tools such as the Framingham risk score have been shown to underestimate risk among these patients,[20] and clinically this manifests as under-treatment of risk factors.[21]

The pleiotropic effects of statins are thought to include anti-inflammatory, anti-fibrotic, and antioxidant effects;[22] prevention of left ventricular hypertrophy;[23] reduction of endothelial dysfunction;[24,25] inhibition of neurohormonal activation; and prevention of cardiac arrhythmias.[26] The Trial of Atorvastatin in Rheumatoid Arthritis (TARA) study showed that atorvastatin improved lipid profile and reduced RA disease activity score, suggesting a clinically important anti-inflammatory effect.[27]

Sattar *et al.* hypothesized that it is the severity and chronicity of the systemic inflammation that is particularly damaging.[28] Even when the arthritis is clinically quiescent, cytokine production remains high and continues to promote vascular risk (**Figure 39.9**).

The consequence of the inflammatory process on cardiac structure and function has been investigated with cardiac magnetic resonance imaging in patients with no clinically evident heart disease.[29]

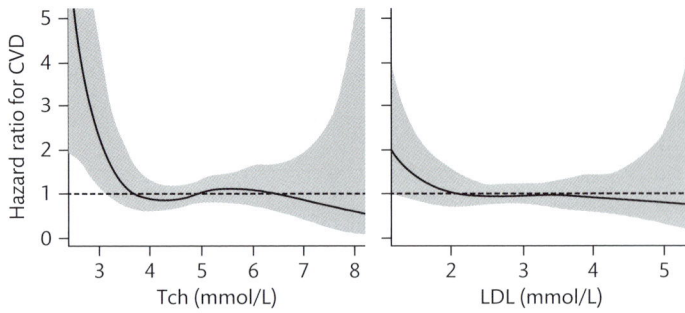

Figure 39.8 Hazard ratios for cardiovascular disease (CVD) in rheumatoid arthritis according to total cholesterol (TCh) and low-density lipid (LDL) concentrations. Shaded area represents 95% confidence intervals.

Source data from Myasoedova E, Crowson CS, Kremers HM, Roger VL, Fitz-Gibbon PD, Therneau TM, *et al*. Lipid paradox in rheumatoid arthritis: the impact of serum lipid measures and systemic inflammation on the risk of cardiovascular disease. *Ann Rheum Dis* 2011;70(3):482–7.

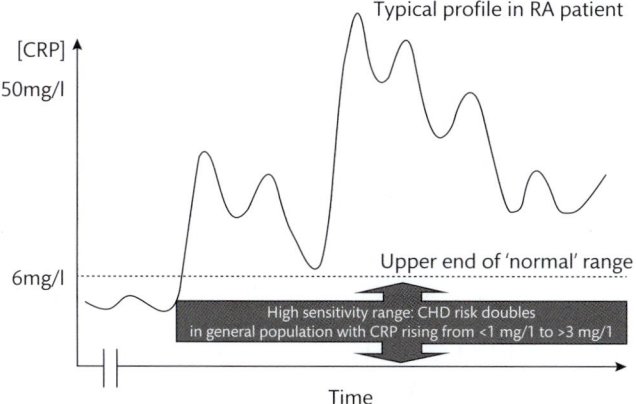

Figure 39.9 Graphic illustrating the high levels of systemic inflammation, as measured with serum C- reactive protein (CRP), found in rheumatoid arthritis (RA) and the recurrent and relapsing nature of the disease. Note that even when the disease activity subsides the CRP levels do not fall.

Reproduced from Sattar N, McCarey DW, Capell H, McInnes IB. Explaining how "high-grade" systemic inflammation accelerates vascular risk in rheumatoid arthritis. *Circulation* 2003;108(24):2957–63 with permission from Wolters Kluwer.

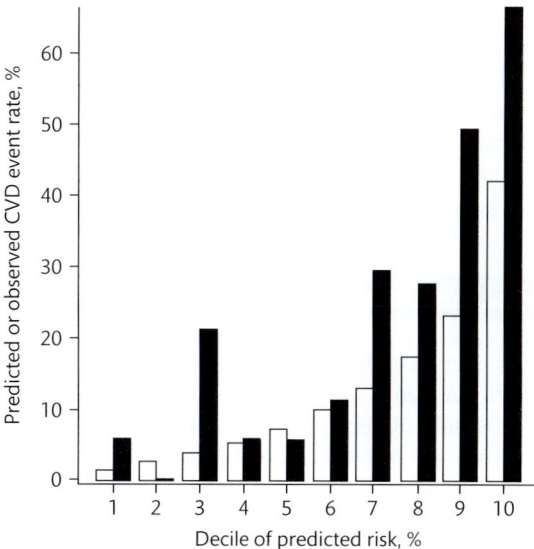

Figure 39.10 Comparison of observed (solid bars) and predicted (open bars) 10-year risk for cardiovascular disease. Groupings are as per decile of predicted risk as calculated by the Framingham risk score. Observed risk was obtained using Kaplan-Meier method.

Reproduced from Crowson CS, Matteson EL, Roger VL, Therneau TM, Gabriel SE. Usefulness of risk scores to estimate the risk of cardiovascular disease in patients with rheumatoid arthritis. *Am J Cardiol* 2012;110(3):420–4 with permission from Elsevier.

Patients with RA have a markedly lower left ventricular (LV) mass than those without (mean LV mass 119 g in RA vs 145 g in non-RA, $P < 0.001$). They have a slightly lower ejection fraction (65% vs 68%, $P = 0.003$) and stroke volume (80 vs 86 mL, $P = 0.019$) than normal. Worsening disease severity (as measured by higher titres of antibodies to cyclic citrullinated peptide) and the use of biologic agents were associated with worse cardiac function.

Heart failure and arthritis: mechanisms

Ischaemic cardiomyopathy

In patients with RA, the risk of coronary artery disease is high in both men and women (approximately two-fold higher than among the normal population[30]) and increases with the severity of RA, disease duration and evidence of extra-articular disease.[31] Additionally, there is evidence that cardiovascular risk is underestimated in RA. Crowson *et al.* examined 525 RA patients prospectively and found that cardiovascular events were two-fold more common in men and 65% more common in women than predicted by Framingham risk score (**Figure 39.10**).[20] A recent meta-analysis of 24 observational studies, with 111 758 patients, found that the risk of coronary artery disease-related mortality was 59% higher in patients with RA than in the general population.[32] Patients with RA tend to be undertreated compared to non-RA patients. As an example, one study examined 400 patients with RA and only 7% of those at high risk by the Framingham score were receiving lipid-lowering therapy.[21] More aggressive primary and secondary prevention of cardiovascular disease is required.

Patients with RA seem to present differently with their coronary disease compared with the wider population. They are twice as likely to experience unrecognized myocardial infarctions and sudden death, and less likely to report angina or to undergo coronary artery bypass grafting.[33] The lower frequency of presentation with acute myocardial ischaemia limits the therapeutic options available. It may be that persistent silent ischaemia causes a reduction in systolic function. Interestingly, the increased risk of coronary artery disease precedes the diagnosis of RA, and the risk cannot be explained by a higher prevalence of traditional CHD risk factors. Whether the risk is related to subclinical inflammation is not clear.

The differential diagnosis of chest pain in patients with systemic inflammatory athritides includes:

- ischaemic heart disease;
- costochondral or sternoclavicular joint pain;
- pericarditis—acute pericarditis causes chest pain with ECG changes, and may be associated with a friction rub. Echocardiography may demonstrate a pericardial effusion; but it should be noted that incidental small effusions are not uncommon in RA or SLE;
- coronary arteritis—this is an uncommon manifestation of longstanding, severe RA, often as part of a more general rheumatoid vasculitis. It may present as acute myocardial infarction in children or adolescents with SLE;
- aortitis with aortic dissection;
- pulmonary hypertension secondary to arthritis-related interstitial lung disease—it is thought that the pain, which is exertional, is caused by right ventricular ischaemia.

Inflammatory cardiomyopathy

Myocarditis is an uncommon presentation of inflammatory arthritis. In patients with SLE, asymptomatic myocarditis affects between 8% and 25% of patients,[34,35] and is more common in African-American patients. Myocarditis should be considered if there is a persistent tachycardia with non-specific ST- and T-wave abnormalities. Echocardiography may show systolic or diastolic dysfunction, although the diagnosis of myocarditis is difficult to confirm using echo alone. CMR is the reference standard method of confirming the presence of myocardial inflammatory changes, as well as accurately assessing ventricular performance.[36]

Occasionally, an endomyocardial biopsy is required. Histology demonstrates mononuclear cell infiltration of the myocardium. In established cases with a more prolonged myocarditic process, the inflammation may lead to fibrosis, which may be present clinically as dilated cardiomyopathy. In addition to heart failure, myocarditis can cause conduction abnormalities usually consequent to fibrosis. These may present as bradycardia or tachyarrhythmias.

Diastolic dysfunction

There is a higher prevalence of impaired left ventricular relaxation in patients with RA than in healthy age- and sex-matched controls (66% vs 43%).[37] Diastolic dysfunction may predate clinically apparent heart failure. In a study of patients with SLE without clinically evident cardiovascular disease, there was no significant abnormality in systolic function, but there was evidence of diastolic dysfunction.[38] The greater the disease duration, the greater the likelihood of diastolic dysfunction.

Amyloidosis

Reactive, or secondary (AA) amyloidosis refers to predominantly extracellular tissue deposition of fibrils composed of fragments of serum amyloid A protein, an acute phase reactant. Significant deposition of AA amyloid in the heart is uncommon and is rarely the cause of death. In poorly controlled chronic inflammatory arthritis—mainly seropositive rheumatoid arthritis and ankylosing spondylitis—cardiac AA amyloidosis can occur.

Cardiac involvement may be suspected by low-voltage complexes in the limb leads or a pseudo-infarct pattern on electrocardiography. Left ventricular wall thickening with evidence of diastolic dysfunction is the earliest echocardiographic abnormality. Right ventricular diastolic dysfunction can also occur. If AA amyloidosis is clinically suspected and suggested on non-invasive tests then it can be diagnosed by rectal, subcutaneous abdominal fat, skin, or, if necessary, cardiac biopsies.

Among patients with AA amyloidosis due to RA, up to 40% have cardiac involvement,[39] but cardiac failure attributable to AA amyloidosis is rare: in only one out of 374 patients with AA amyloidosis (60% of whom had chronic inflammatory arthritis) was heart failure caused by the amyloid. Only two out of 224 patients undergoing echocardiography had findings consistent with cardiac infiltration.[40]

Pharmacology-related heart failure

Many of the agents used to treat arthritis can adversely affect heart failure, and in some cases may be the cause of heart failure.

Non-steroidal anti-inflammatory drugs

These are at the frontline of disease control. Non-steroidal anti-inflammatory drugs (NSAIDs) have both analgesic and anti-inflammatory properties, but do not alter the disease progression. NSAIDs have several potential adverse cardiovascular effects including interference with the antiplatelet action of aspirin, an increase in cardiovascular events including myocardial infarction, and exacerbation of established heart failure.

The attenuation of the antiplatelet effect of aspirin is well described with both ibuprofen and naproxen.[41,42] The presumed mechanism is competitive binding at the cyclooxygenase (COX)-1 receptor. The impact of this interaction is the potential increase in thrombotic coronary events, with consequent heart failure, although there is no proven clinical relevance.

Studies have not demonstrated an association between NSAID use and an increase in incident heart failure.[43] However, in established heart failure, NSAID use is associated with relapse of heart failure symptoms and increased mortality. One possible mechanism is an increase in afterload resulting from NSAID-induced systemic vasoconstriction. The effect is exacerbated by hyponatraemia. In a large observational study from Denmark[44] the adjusted risk of rehospitalization for heart failure was significantly increased in patients on diclofenac or ibuprofen (adjusted HR: 1.35 and 1.16, respectively). There was a dose-dependent increase in risk of death, which was highest with diclofenac (adjusted HR: 2.08). Higher doses of ibuprofen (>1200 mg/day) and naproxen (>500 mg/day), but not lower doses, were also associated with an increased risk of death (adjusted HR: 1.31 and 1.22, respectively).

COX-2-selective inhibitors

In an attempt to overcome the gastrointestinal adverse effects of non-selective NSAIDS, COX-2-selective inhibitors were developed. Unfortunately, because of significant cardiovascular toxicity many of the agents have been withdrawn. COX-2-selective inhibitors increase ischaemic coronary events, presumably because COX-2-selective inhibitors reduce prostacyclin production by vascular endothelium without inhibiting production of the prothrombotic platelet thromboxane A_2.

In a cohort study to assess the impact of COX-2-selective inhibitors on the incidence of heart failure, crude rates of hospitalization for heart failure per 100 patient-years of exposure were 0.9 for the controls, 2.4 for the patients treated with rofecoxib, and 1.3 for the patients treated with celecoxib. Adjusting for potential confounding risk factors, the risk of hospitalization with heart failure compared to controls was significantly higher in patients treated with rofecoxib but not celecoxib.[45]

The PRECISION (Prospective Randomized Evaluation of Celecoxib Integrated Safety versus Ibuprofen or Naproxen) trial has recently reported.[45] At moderate doses, celecoxib was non-inferior to ibuprofen or naproxen in terms of cardiovascular adverse events including hospitalization for congestive heart failure, and had significantly lower rates of gastrointestinal upset than either comparator.

In summary, the current evidence suggests that both selective and non-selective NSAIDs should be used with caution in patients with established heart failure. If new heart failure develops, the drug's potential cardiovascular adverse effects (including myocardial infarction) should be considered as a potential mechanism.

Glucocorticoids

Glucocorticoids are frequently used to achieve inflammatory control in an acute flare of arthritis. Glucocorticoids are associated with higher rates of heart failure, myocardial infarction, stroke, and all-cause mortality in a dose-dependent manner.[46] The risk of heart failure increases with the daily dose of glucocorticoids, with a relative risk of 3.72 at doses ≥7.5 mg/day of prednisolone. Ongoing steroid use is associated with a higher risk than intermittent courses.

Antimalarial drugs

Chloroquine and hydroxychloroquine are disease-modifying agents used in the management of several of the arthritides, including RA and SLE. They have a beneficial effect on the lipid profile in SLE. Side-effects include: generalized myopathy, retinopathy, neuropathy, and rarely a cardiomyopathy. Toxicity may also cause conduction abnormalities. Antimalarial cardiomyopathy presents as a restrictive cardiomyopathy, with or without conduction abnormalities such as atrioventricular or bundle branch block. In most cases of chloroquine and hydroxychloroquine cardiomyopathies, non-cardiac toxicities are also present.[47] The diagnosis is confirmed by biopsy. The characteristic pathological appearance by light microscopy of large myocardiocytes containing intracytoplasmic vacuoles can be confirmed by electron microscopic evidence of curvilinear bodies.[48] Prompt withdrawal of the causative agent results in partial or complete resolution in most cases, but progression to death or transplantation despite discontinuation of therapy has been reported.[49]

TNFα inhibitors

TNFα is a key agent in systemic inflammation, stimulating the release of other inflammatory cytokines (including IL-1β, IL-6, IL-8); causing upregulation of endothelial adhesion molecules and chemokines; and inducing the migration of leucocytes to targeted organs. The failing heart produces TNFα, but the normal heart does not. Clinical trials of TNFα blockers in advanced heart failure have been disappointing.[30,51]

There is ongoing debate as to whether anti-TNFα therapy—which is being used increasingly in the treatment of systemic inflammatory diseases including arthritis—affects the risk of heart failure.[5] At present there is no compelling evidence that TNFα blockers worsen heart failure. TNFα antagonist therapies in rheumatoid arthritis may ameliorate the deleterious cardiac effects of circulating TNFα. Blocking TNFα in patients with RA but with no evidence of heart failure decreases N-terminal pro-B-type brain natriuretic peptide (NT-proBNP) levels by around 18%, suggesting at worst that there is no treatment-induced deterioration in cardiac function, and a potential cardiovascular risk benefit.[52] Despite this, the current recommendation is to avoid use of anti-TNFα agents in patients with heart failure, especially in those with New York Heart Association (NYHA) classes III or IV.[17]

TNFα blockers offer a significant advance in the management of inflammatory arthritis and so it is important that they should be available to as many patients as appropriate. In patients with NYHA class I or II, TNFα blockers may be considered, but a baseline echo should be performed and careful clinical and echocardiographic follow-up should be employed. High doses of the agents should be avoided. If clinical heart failure symptoms develop or deteriorate then the TNFα blocker should be discontinued.

Arthritis resulting from heart failure

Gout

Gout is the clinical syndrome that results from the deposition of urate crystals in the joints. Gouty arthritis occurs when granulocytes phagocytose the crystals and then secrete inflammatory mediators that produce an intense inflammatory reaction, resulting in an exceedingly painful acute arthritis. Joint destruction can eventually result. The inflammatory process becomes self-perpetuating with increased lactic acid production reducing the synovial fluid pH, which favours further deposition of urate crystals.[53]

The key laboratory finding is hyperuricaemia, although serum urate concentrations may be normal in patients with acute gout. Urate levels vary with age and sex, and also blood pressure, renal function, diet, and alcohol intake. However, the incidence of gouty arthritis among men with urate levels >540 μmol/L (9.0 mg/dL) is <5% per year.[54]

Patients with chronic heart failure frequently develop gout. Multiple factors contribute to hyperuricaemia in patients with heart failure, including hypertension and hyperlipidaemia, which may be key in the aetiology of the heart failure; chronic renal failure, which may be consequent upon the pharmacotherapy of heart failure; and diuretics therapy. Although all diuretics can cause hyperuricaemia, loop diuretics are the most likely culprits, then thiazides. Mineralocorticoid receptor antagonists are least likely to raise uric acid concentrations.[55,56] Diuretic-induced hyperuricaemia can be minimized by the concurrent prescription of angiotensin converting enzyme inhibitors or an angiotensin II receptor blocker.[57,58] This has been postulated to be mediated by inhibition of the proximal sodium and urate reabsorption induced by angiotensin II.

Interestingly, there is a negative correlation between serum urate concentrations and maximal oxygen uptake and a positive correlation with increasing NYHA functional class in patients with heart failure.[59] Increasing urate level also correlates strongly with increasing levels of markers of inflammation in patients with chronic heart failure, such as TNFα and its soluble receptors.[60]

The management of acute gout in patients with heart failure can be challenging. Usually, acute gout is managed with NSAIDs, but NSAIDs may be detrimental in heart failure by causing sodium and water retention, hyperkalaemia, and renal failure. Therefore, a modified approach has been described using a combination of NSAIDs and colchicine, which allows the early withdrawal of the NSAID (**Figure 39.11**). Naproxen is probably the NSAID of choice, at as low a dose as possible.

Colchicine was established as a therapy for acute gout almost 250 years ago. If given soon after the onset of symptoms, it almost invariably achieves resolution of symptoms. Colchicine is an antimitotic agent which decreases the functional activity of locally infiltrating granulocytes and inhibits the release of proinflammatory mediators.[61] However, the serum urate levels are unchanged. The side-effects of diarrhoea and vomiting may limit tolerability, but are less likely when doses of ≤1.8 mg in total during 24 h are given; a regimen which has high efficacy if initiated at the very onset (within hours) of a flare.[62]

Glucocorticoids can be used in acute gout both as anti-inflammatory agents and to reduce the serum urate concentration. Oral glucocorticoids are problematic in heart failure because of the mineralocorticoid effect of fluid retention, but local joint aspiration and then injection with glucocorticoid targets the site of inflammation and reduces the systemic dose needed, as well as relieving the tense, hot, swollen joint by removing some of the synovial fluid. This is a particularly useful adjuvant in patients who are struggling with painful acute gout despite NSAID and colchicine. In particularly resistant disease or where choice of therapy is severely limited by co-morbidity or tolerance, IL-1-inhibiting agents, such as anakinra, may be tried.

In the longer term, the serum urate level should be addressed. Patient education about diet modification, reducing the amount of meat,

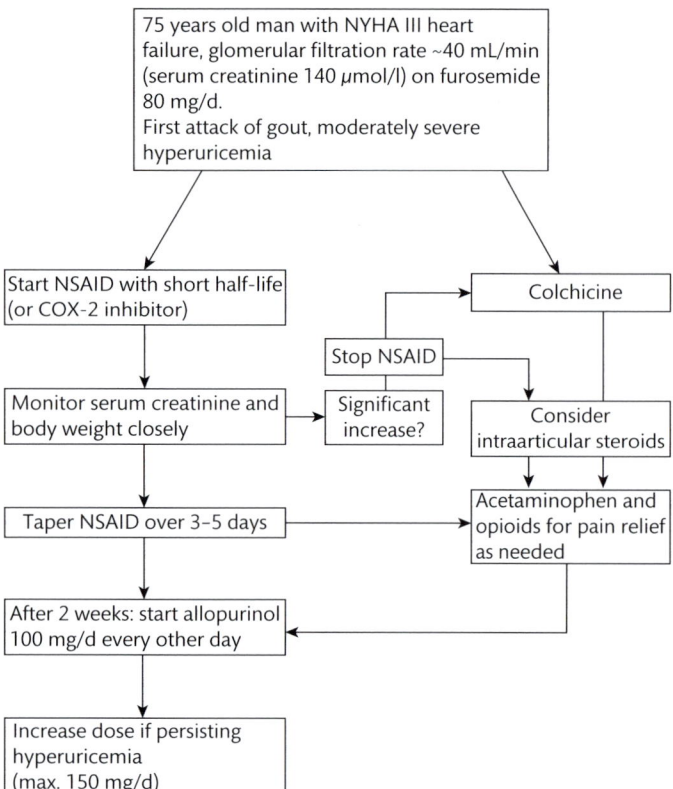

Figure 39.11 Suggested management of acute gout in a typical patient with heart failure.

Reproduced from Spieker LE, Ruschitzka FT, Lüscher TF, Noll G. The management of hyperuricemia and gout in patients with heart failure. *Eur J Heart Fail* 2002 Aug 10 [cited 2017 Feb 15];4(4):403–10 with permission from John Wiley and Sons.

pulses, and alcohol, is important but usually fails to achieve adequate urate reduction. Therefore, pharmacological prophylaxis should be considered, starting cautiously two weeks after the acute episode. The dose should be uptitrated over the following weeks to reduce the likelihood of a further acute attack. In recurrent attacks in a patient already established on urate-lowering therapy, this should be continued.

There are two classes of drug available in the management of hyperuricaemia: uricosuric agents (e.g. probenicid) and xanthine oxidase inhibitors (allopurinol). Allopurinol inhibits xanthine oxidase, thus stopping the synthesis of uric acid, and is most widely used. The dose of allopurinol should be reduced if renal failure coexists or develops. An additional potential benefit of allopurinol is its effect in reducing oxidative stress by inhibiting xanthine oxidase in the vascular endothelium, thereby preventing the formation of superoxide free radicals. In patients with heart failure, allopurinol reduces markers of oxidative stress and improves endothelium-dependent vasodilatation.[63] There are also studies demonstrating that allopurinol improves left ventricular efficiency[64] and reverses ventricular remodelling.[65] However, there are no trial data to suggest that xanthine oxidase inhibitors improve prognosis in patients with cardiovascular disease.[66]

Pseudogout

Pseudogout is an acute synovitis precipitated by calcium pyrophosphate dihydrate (CPPD) crystal deposition in joints. Clinically such an episode resembles gout caused by urate crystal deposition. The diagnosis of pseudogout is made by aspiration of the affected joint, and demonstration of positively birefringent CPPD crystals by polarized light microscopy.

The management of an acute episode of pseudogout is similar to that of gout, with NSAID and colchicine being the first-line agents and then local glucocorticoid if required. Long-term prophylaxis is different from that for gout. Patients suffering recurrent attacks of pseudogout can be successfully treated using colchicine 0.6 mg twice daily as oral prophylaxis.[67]

Pseudogout may reveal the underlying cause of heart failure. The majority of cases of CPPD crystal deposition are idiopathic, and it is more common in the elderly (mean age at symptomatic presentation is 72 years). However, some metabolic and endocrine conditions such as haemochromatosis and hypothyroidism may cause crystal deposition at a younger age;[68] and may, of course, be the cause of heart failure.

Clinical syndromes

In the assessment of patients with heart failure and arthritis there are several possible presentations:

Established heart failure with new presentation of arthritis

The onset of arthritis in patients with heart failure may be the evolution of an incidental arthritis, a complication of the aetiology of the heart failure, or may be related to the pharmacotherapy of heart failure.

Established arthritis with asymptomatic left ventricular systolic dysfunction or without symptoms of heart failure

At present, there is no evidence to support screening of asymptomatic patients with arthritis for cardiac dysfunction. However, there is a role for risk assessment with the established risk models. The EULAR recommendations recently made the following statement: 'Annual cardiovascular risk assessment using national guidelines is recommended for all patients with RA and should be considered for all patients with ankylosing spondylitis and psoriatic arthropathy. Any cardiovascular risk factors identified should be managed according to local guidelines. If no local guidelines are available, cardiovascular risk management should be carried out according to the SCORE function. In addition to appropriate cardiovascular risk management, aggressive suppression of the inflammatory process is recommended to further lower the cardiovascular risk.'[69]

Established arthritis with new-onset heart failure

New-onset heart failure may be the first manifestation of incidental heart disease, may be a consequence of the arthritis, or may be the result of pharmacotherapy. The cause of the heart failure may be myocardial, pericardial, valvular, rhythm-related, or due to coronary artery disease.

Investigations should be the same as for any other patient with new-onset heart failure. The differentiation between constrictive pericarditis and restrictive cardiomyopathy may be a problem, and advanced imaging together with cardiac catheterization may be needed. Endomyocardial biopsy can provide tissue to identify potentially treatable causes such as antimalarial-induced cardiomyopathy.

Summary

The interactions between heart failure and arthritis are complex. With an ageing population, it is becoming more common for patients to be limited by both conditions. Teasing apart the cause and effect of the disease processes and the impact of the various therapies can be challenging. The trend towards earlier disease recognition and more aggressive management of both heart failure and arthritis may mean that their negative impact will be attenuated. In both conditions, maintaining the patient's physical activity and independence brings significant physical and psychological benefits.

REFERENCES

1. Wolfe F, Freundlich B, Straus WL. Increase in cardiovascular and cerebrovascular disease prevalence in rheumatoid arthritis. *J Rheumatol* 2003;**30**(1):36–40.
2. Pujades-Rodriguez M, Duyx B, Thomas SL, *et al.* Rheumatoid arthritis and incidence of twelve initial presentations of cardiovascular disease: a population record-linkage cohort study in England. *PLoS One* 2016;**11**(3):e0151245. doi:10.1371/journal. pone.0151245. PMID: 26978266; PMCID: PMC4792375.
3. Bayles TB. Rheumatic heart disease in autopsied cases of rheumatoid arthritis: (abstract). *Ann Intern Med* 1943;**19**(1):113–14.
4. Isomäki HA, Mutru O, Koota K. Death rate and causes of death in patients with rheumatoid arthritis. *Scand J Rheumatol* 1975;**4**(4):205–8.
5. Wolfe F, Michaud K. Heart failure in rheumatoid arthritis: rates, predictors, and the effect of anti-tumor necrosis factor therapy. *Am J Med* 2004;**116**(5):305–11.
6. Nicola PJ, Crowson CS, Maradit-Kremers H, *et al.* Contribution of congestive heart failure and ischemic heart disease to excess mortality in rheumatoid arthritis. *Arthritis Rheum* 2006;**54**(1):60–7.
7. Davis JM, Roger VL, Crowson CS, *et al.* The presentation and outcome of heart failure in patients with rheumatoid arthritis differs from that in the general population. *Arthritis Rheum* 2008;**58**(9):2603–11.
8. Polachek A, Touma Z, Anderson M, Eder L. Risk of cardiovascular morbidity in patients with psoriatic arthritis: a meta-analysis of observational studies. *Arthritis Care Res (Hoboken)* 2016;**69**(1):67–74.
9. Neimann AL, Shin DB, Wang X, *et al.* Prevalence of cardiovascular risk factors in patients with psoriasis. *J Am Acad Dermatol* 2006;**55**(5):829–35.
10. Gelfand JM, Neimann AL, Shin DB, *et al.* Risk of myocardial infarction in patients with psoriasis. *J Am Med Assoc* 2006;**296**(14):1735–41.
11. Kimball AB, Guerin A, Latremouille-Viau D, *et al.* Coronary heart disease and stroke risk in patients with psoriasis: retrospective analysis. *Am J Med* 2010;**123**(4):350–7.
12. Wakkee M, Herings RM, Nijsten T. Psoriasis may not be an independent risk factor for acute ischemic heart disease hospitalizations: results of a large population-based Dutch cohort. *J Invest Dermatol* 2010;**130**(4):962–7.
13. del Rincon ID, Williams K, Stern MP, Freeman GL, Escalante A. High incidence of cardiovascular events in a rheumatoid arthritis cohort not explained by traditional cardiac risk factors. *Arthritis Rheum* 2001;**44**(12):2737–45.
14. Feldman AM, Combes A, Wagner D, *et al.* The role of tumor necrosis factor in the pathophysiology of heart failure. *J Am Coll Cardiol* 2000;**35**(3):537–44.
15. Torre-Amione G, Kapadia S, Benedict C, *et al.* Proinflammatory cytokine levels in patients with depressed left ventricular ejection fraction: a report from the Studies of Left Ventricular Dysfunction (SOLVD). *J Am Coll Cardiol* 1996;**27**(5):1201–6.
16. Deswal A, Petersen NJ, Feldman AM, *et al.* Cytokines and cytokine receptors in advanced heart failure: an analysis of the cytokine database from the Vesnarinone trial (VEST). *Circulation* 2001;**103**(16):2055–9.
17. Danila MI, Patkar NM, Curtis JR, Saag KG, Teng GG. Biologics and heart failure in rheumatoid arthritis: are we any wiser? *Curr Opin Rheumatol* 2008;**20**(3):327–33.
18. Myasoedova E, Crowson CS, Kremers HM, *et al.* Lipid paradox in rheumatoid arthritis: the impact of serum lipid measures and systemic inflammation on the risk of cardiovascular disease. *Ann Rheum Dis* 2011;**70**(3):482–7.
19. Mackey RH, Kuller LH, Moreland LW. Cardiovascular disease risk in patients with rheumatic diseases. *Clin Geriatric Med* 2017;**33**(1):105–17.
20. Crowson CS, Matteson EL, Roger VL, Therneau TM, Gabriel SE. Usefulness of risk scores to estimate the risk of cardiovascular disease in patients with rheumatoid arthritis. *Am J Cardiol* 2012;**110**(3):420–4.
21. Huizinga T, Nigrovic P, Ruderman E, Schulze-Koops H. Statin use in rheumatoid arthritis in relation to actual cardiovascular risk: evidence for substantial undertreatment of lipid-associated cardiovascular risk? Commentary. *Int J Adv Rheumatol* 2010;**8**(3):124.
22. Mathur N, Ramasubbu K, Mann DL. Spectrum of pleiotropic effects of statins in heart failure. *Heart Fail Clin* 2008;**4**(2):153–61.
23. Jain MK, Ridker PM. Anti-inflammatory effects of statins: clinical evidence and basic mechanisms. *Nat Rev Drug Discov* 2005;**4**(12):977–87.
24. Laufs U, La Fata V, Plutzky J, Liao JK. Upregulation of endothelial nitric oxide synthase by HMG CoA reductase inhibitors. *Circulation* 1998;**97**(12):1129–35.
25. Dilaveris P, Giannopoulos G, Riga M, Synetos A, Stefanadis C. Beneficial effects of statins on endothelial dysfunction and vascular stiffness. *Curr Vasc Pharmacol* 2007;**5**(3):227–37.
26. Levantesi G, Scarano M, Marfisi R, *et al.* Meta-analysis of effect of statin treatment on risk of sudden death. *Am J Cardiol* 2007;**100**(11):1644–50.
27. McCarey DW, McInnes IB, Madhok R, *et al.* Trial of Atorvastatin in Rheumatoid Arthritis (TARA): double-blind, randomised placebo-controlled trial. *Lancet* 2004;**363**(9426):2015–21.
28. Sattar N, McCarey DW, Capell H, McInnes IB. Explaining how "high-grade" systemic inflammation accelerates vascular risk in rheumatoid arthritis. *Circulation* 2003;**108**(24):2957–63.
29. Giles JT, Malayeri AA, Fernandes V, *et al.* Left ventricular structure and function in patients with rheumatoid arthritis, as assessed by cardiac magnetic resonance imaging. *Arthritis Rheum* 2010;**62**(4):940–51.
30. Sattar N, McInnes IB. Vascular comorbidity in rheumatoid arthritis: potential mechanisms and solutions. *Curr Opin Rheumatol* 2005;**17**(3):286–92.
31. Van Doornum S, McColl G, Wicks IP. Accelerated atherosclerosis: an extraarticular feature of rheumatoid arthritis? *Arthritis Rheum* 2002;**46**(4):862–73.

32. Aviña-Zubieta JA, Choi HK, Sadatsafavi M, *et al.* Risk of cardiovascular mortality in patients with rheumatoid arthritis: a meta-analysis of observational studies. *Arthritis Rheum* 2008;**59**(12):1690–7.

33. Maradit-Kremers H, Crowson CS, Nicola PJ, *et al.* Increased unrecognized coronary heart disease and sudden deaths in rheumatoid arthritis: a population-based cohort study. *Arthritis Rheum* 2005;**52**(2):402–11.

34. Mandell BF. Cardiovascular involvement in systemic lupus erythematosus. *Semin Arthritis Rheum* 1987;**17**(2):126–41.

35. Apte M, McGwin GJ, Vilá LM, *et al.* Associated factors and impact of myocarditis in patients with SLE from LUMINA, a multiethnic US cohort. *Rheumatology* 2008;**47**(3):362–7.

36. Mavrogeni S, Dimitroulas T, Sfikakis PP, Kitas GD. Heart involvement in rheumatoid arthritis: multimodality imaging and the emerging role of cardiac magnetic resonance. *Semin Arthritis Rheum* 2013;**43**(3):314–24.

37. Di Franco M, Paradiso M, Mammarella A, *et al.* Diastolic function abnormalities in rheumatoid arthritis. Evaluation by echo Doppler transmitral flow and pulmonary venous flow: relation with duration of disease. *Ann Rheum Dis* 2000;**59**(3):227–9.

38. Wislowska M, Dereń D, Kochmański M, Sypuła S, Rozbicka J. Systolic and diastolic heart function in SLE patients. *Rheumatol Int* 2009;**29**(12):1469–76.

39. Okuda Y, Takasugi K, Oyama T, Onuma M, Oyama H. [Amyloidosis in rheumatoid arthritis—clinical study of 124 histologically proven cases.] *Ryumachi* 1994;**34**(6):939–46.

40. Gallimore JR, Sabin CA, Gillmore JD, *et al.* Natural history and outcome in systemic AA amyloidosis. *N Engl J Med* 2007;**356**(23):2361–71.

41. Catella-Lawson F, Reilly MP, Kapoor SC, *et al.* Cyclooxygenase inhibitors and the antiplatelet effects of aspirin. *N Engl J Med* 2001;**345**(25):1809–17.

42. Capone ML, Sciulli MG, Tacconelli S, *et al.* Pharmacodynamic interaction of naproxen with low-dose aspirin in healthy subjects. *J Am Coll Cardiol* 2005;**45**(8):1295–301.

43. Feenstra J, Heerdink ER, Grobbee DE, Stricker BHC. Association of nonsteroidal anti-inflammatory drugs with first occurrence of heart failure and with relapsing heart failure: the Rotterdam Study. *Arch Intern Med* 2002;**162**(3):265–70.

44. Gislason GH, Rasmussen JN, Abildstrom SZ, *et al.* Increased mortality and cardiovascular morbidity associated with use of nonsteroidal anti-inflammatory drugs in chronic heart failure. *Arch Intern Med* 2009;**169**(2):141–9.

45. Nissen SE, Yeomans ND, Solomon DH, *et al.* Cardiovascular safety of celecoxib, naproxen, or ibuprofen for arthritis. *N Engl J Med* 2016;**375**(26):2519–29.

46. Wei L, MacDonald TM, Walker BR. Taking glucocorticoids by prescription is associated with subsequent cardiovascular disease. *Ann Intern Med* 2004;**141**(10):764–70.

47. Costedoat-Chalumeau N, Hulot JS, Amoura Z, *et al.* Cardiomyopathy related to antimalarial therapy with illustrative case report. *Cardiology* 2007;**107**(2):73–80.

48. Roos JM, Aubry M-C, Edwards WD. Chloroquine cardiotoxicity: clinicopathologic features in three patients and comparison with three patients with Fabry disease. *Cardiovasc Pathol* 2002;**11**(5):277–83.

49. Joyce E, Fabre A, Mahon N. Hydroxychloroquine cardiotoxicity presenting as a rapidly evolving biventricular cardiomyopathy: key diagnostic features and literature review. *Eur Hear J Acute Cardiovasc Care* 2013;**2**(1):77–83.

50. Mann DL, McMurray JJV, Packer M, *et al.* Targeted anticytokine therapy in patients with chronic heart failure. *Circulation* 2004;**109**:1594–602.

51. Chung ES, Packer M, Lo KH, Fasanmade AA. Randomized, double-blind, placebo-controlled, pilot trial of infliximab, a chimeric monoclonal antibody to tumor necrosis factor-α, in patients with moderate-to-severe heart failure: results of the anti-TNF Therapy Against Congestive Heart Failure (ATTACH) trial. *Circulation* 2003;**107**(25):3133–40.

52. Peters MJL, Welsh P, McInnes IB, *et al.* Tumour necrosis factor α blockade reduces circulating N-terminal pro-brain natriuretic peptide levels in patients with active rheumatoid arthritis: results from a prospective cohort study. *Ann Rheum Dis* 2010;**69**(7):1281–5.

53. Spieker LE, Ruschitzka FT, Lüscher TF, Noll G. The management of hyperuricemia and gout in patients with heart failure. *Eur J Heart Fail* 2002;**4**(4):403–10.

54. Lin KC, Lin HY, Chou P. The interaction between uric acid level and other risk factors on the development of gout among asymptomatic hyperuricemic men in a prospective study. *J Rheumatol* 2000;**27**(6):1501–5.

55. Waller PC, Ramsay LE. Predicting acute gout in diuretic-treated hypertensive patients. *J Hum Hypertens* 1989;**3**(6):457–61.

56. Schrijver G, Weinberger MH. Hydrochlorothiazide and spironolactone in hypertension. *Clin Pharmacol Ther* 1979;**25**(1):33–42.

57. Weinberger MH. Influence of an angiotensin converting-enzyme inhibitor on diuretic-induced metabolic effects in hypertension. *Hypertension* 1983;**5**(5 Pt 2):III132–8.

58. Shahinfar S, Simpson RL, Carides AD, *et al.* Safety of losartan in hypertensive patients with thiazide-induced hyperuricemia. *Kidney Int* 1999;**56**(5):1879–85.

59. Leyva F, Anker S, Swan JW, *et al.* Serum uric acid as an index of impaired oxidative metabolism in chronic heart failure. *Eur Hear J* 1997;**18**(5):858–65.

60. Leyva F, Anker SD, Godsland IF, *et al.* Uric acid in chronic heart failure: a marker of chronic inflammation. *Eur Hear J* 1998;**19**:1814–22.

61. Spilberg I, Mandell B, Mehta J, Simchowitz L, Rosenberg D. Mechanism of action of colchicine in acute urate crystal-induced arthritis. *J Clin Invest* 1979;**64**(3):775–80.

62. Terkeltaub RA, Furst DE, Bennett K, *et al.* High versus low dosing of oral colchicine for early acute gout flare: twenty-four-hour outcome of the first multicenter, randomized, double-blind, placebo-controlled, parallel-group, dose-comparison colchicine study. *Arthritis Rheum* 2010;**62**(4):1060–8.

63. Farquharson CAJ, Butler R, Hill A, Belch JJF, Struthers AD. Allopurinol improves endothelial dysfunction in chronic heart failure. *Circulation* 2002;**106**(2):221–6.

64. Cappola TP, Kass DA, Nelson GS, *et al.* Allopurinol improves myocardial efficiency in patients with idiopathic dilated cardiomyopathy. *Circulation* 2001;**104**(20):2407–11.

65. Minhas KM, Saraiva RM, Schuleri KH, *et al.* Xanthine oxidoreductase inhibition causes reverse remodeling in rats with dilated cardiomyopathy. *Circ Res* 2006;**98**(2):271–9.

66. Zhang J, Dierckx R, Mohee K, Clark AL, Cleland JG. Xanthine oxidase inhibition for the treatment of cardiovascular disease: an

updated systematic review and meta-analysis. *ESC Heart Fail* 2017;**4**:40–5.

67. Alvarellos A, Spilberg I. Colchicine prophylaxis in pseudogout. *J Rheumatol* 1986;**13**(4):804–5.

68. Jones AC, Chuck AJ, Arie EA, Green DJ, Doherty M. Diseases associated with calcium pyrophosphate deposition disease. *Semin Arthritis Rheum* 1992;**22**(3):188–202.

69. Peters MJL, Symmons DPM, McCarey D, *et al.* EULAR evidence-based recommendations for cardiovascular risk management in patients with rheumatoid arthritis and other forms of inflammatory arthritis. *Ann Rheum Dis* 2010;**69**(2):325–31.

40

Arrhythmias

Ashley M. Nisbet and Derek T. Connelly

Introduction

Both atrial and ventricular arrhythmias are common in patients with heart failure and cardiomyopathy, regardless of underlying aetiology. Arrhythmias contribute significantly to symptoms, morbidity including periodic decompensations, and to mortality in the form of ventricular arrhythmias causing sudden cardiac death. The diagnosis and management of arrhythmias is an important element in the clinical management of patients with heart failure.

Atrial fibrillation in heart failure

Epidemiology

Atrial fibrillation (AF) and heart failure are common and often coexist. They have been called the 'two new epidemics of cardiovascular disease'[1] and the burden of each is growing as the population ages, with the incidence of both doubling for each successive decade of age. AF is estimated to occur in 15–30% of patients with heart failure throughout the course of the disease. The prevalence of AF increases with New York Heart Association (NYHA) class (**Figure 40.1**). In NYHA classes I–III, the reported prevalence

is 4–15%.[2–4] In NYHA classes III–IV, the reported prevalence is 25–50%.[5–7] AF and heart failure often coexist in part because the disease processes that predispose to heart failure also predispose to AF.[8] These include hypertension, coronary artery disease, valvular heart disease, and diabetes mellitus. Furthermore, there is a propensity for AF in patients with echocardiographic abnormalities such as left atrial enlargement, left ventricular (LV) hypertrophy and dilatation, and reduced left ventricular ejection fraction (LVEF), as are frequently found in patients with heart failure.[9]

Haemodynamic consequences

Atrial fibrillation is associated with adverse haemodynamic consequences, which may exacerbate heart failure.[10] There may be an associated decrease in cardiac output with the onset of AF in heart failure and this is likely to be multifactorial. A reduction in cardiac output may result from loss of atrioventricular synchrony, which impairs diastolic filling of the left ventricle and reduced stroke volume, as well as increasing mean atrial diastolic pressure, further contributing to atrial enlargement and perpetuating the substrate for the arrhythmia. The irregular ventricular rate and rapid ventricular response in AF also contribute to the adverse haemodynamics by decreasing cardiac output, increasing right atrial pressure, and elevating pulmonary artery capillary wedge pressure irrespective of heart rate. This impairs volume homeostasis and thus exacerbates fluid retention, which ultimately further elevates filling pressures. Furthermore, the presence of mitral regurgitation results in left atrial volume and pressure overload, resulting in dilatation, providing the substrate for the development of AF, which then perpetuates the problem by further increasing LA pressures.

Electrophysiological consequences

There is evidence of cellular electrophysiological remodelling in heart failure that predisposes to AF. Volume and pressure overload in the atria results in stretch induced reductions in atrial myocyte refractory periods, reduced conduction velocity and increased triggered activity.[11] This increases automaticity and heterogeneity of depolarization and repolarization within the atria resulting in an environment able to initiate and sustain spontaneous re-entrant atrial arrhythmias. In heart failure, there is evidence of reduction in atrial myocyte L-type calcium current, and this can both contribute to AF and occur as a result of AF.[12] Neurohormonal alterations in heart

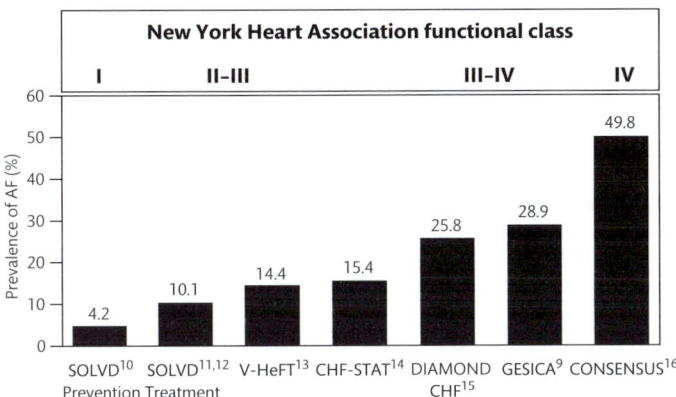

Figure 40.1 Prevalence of atrial fibrillation (AF) with NYHA class.
Reproduced from Maisel WH, Stevenson LW. Atrial fibrillation in heart failure: epidemiology, pathophysiology, and rationale for therapy. *Am J Cardiol* 2003;**91**(6A):2D–8D.

failure, such as activation of the renin–angiotensin–aldosterone system, result in extracellular matrix fibrosis.[13] Atrial fibrosis results in further areas of slow conduction, again predisposing to AF. Furthermore, alterations in connexin expression and activity have been observed in rapid pacing models of AF.[14] The resultant changes in atrial conducting properties contribute to the maintenance of the arrhythmia.

Effect on mortality and prognosis

The presence of AF is associated with an increased mortality regardless of age or gender, with 50–90% increased risk of death observed in the Framingham Heart Study.[15,16] The co-existence of AF and heart failure is associated with an increased risk of mortality and heart failure progression. In a retrospective review of the SOLVD trials, the increase in observed all-cause mortality occurred in the presence of both symptomatic and asymptomatic left ventricular systolic dysfunction (LVSD).[2] This was due to an increased risk of pump-failure death. Furthermore, AF resulted in an increased risk of the composite end-point of death from any cause or hospitalization for worsening heart failure. This confirmed the findings of earlier studies of the negative prognostic effect of AF in heart failure. However, there has been some debate over the years about this issue, with some studies suggesting that the coincidence of AF in heart failure may be neutral[3] or indeed beneficial.[17] The reasons for the apparent beneficial effect of AF in heart failure are not clear, although it may be a spurious effect due to underestimation of the LVEF while in AF with a rapid ventricular response, leading to an improvement of greater magnitude compared with the absence of AF. Alternatively, if the LVSD is a consequence of the tachycardia (sometimes known as a tachycardiomyopathy), effective treatment of the arrhythmia would result in an improvement in LVEF and a better outcome.

In the V-HeFT trials, baseline AF was not related to overall mortality or sudden death.[3] The disparities in the findings of these studies were addressed by Wang et al.[15] using the Framingham Heart Study population. This study aimed to address the temporal relationship of AF and heart failure and their joint effect on mortality. In this study, 1470 developed AF or heart failure or both. In this study, male patients with heart failure who developed AF had a 60% higher mortality than those who remained in sinus rhythm; for women with heart failure, the development of AF was associated with mortality rates more than doubling.

Some clinical trials of medications and devices have published the outcomes in patients with AF versus patients in sinus rhythm, and the results are not always consistent. In the CIBIS-2 study,[18] 2018 patients were randomly allocated to the β-blocker bisoprolol or placebo; 16% of these patients had AF. The mortality rate in the placebo groups was the same in both patients with AF and sinus rhythm, but whereas bisoprolol improved survival in the sinus rhythm group, there was no evidence of benefit in the subgroup of patients with AF. In the COMET trial,[19] 3029 patients with heart failure were randomized to carvedilol or metoprolol; of these, 600 (20%) had AF. The patients with AF had a 29% increased risk of mortality compared to those in sinus rhythm; however, in multivariate analysis, AF was no longer a predictor of mortality. In the CHARM programme, 18% of patients had AF, and the presence of AF predicted a higher risk of cardiovascular morbidity and mortality regardless of baseline ejection fraction.[20] Conversely, in the SCD-HeFT trial[21] of implantable cardioverter–defibrillator (ICD) therapy and amiodarone versus placebo in patients with heart failure and LVSD, after adjusting for differences in baseline variables, there was no difference in mortality between patients with sinus rhythm and AF.

Thus, the effect of AF on mortality (and the magnitude of the effect) has remained unclear, with somewhat conflicting findings across several studies. The mechanisms by which AF might be associated with an increase in mortality are multifactorial. Patients with AF tend to be older, and might be more likely to have other features such as mitral regurgitation (which in itself might mask the severity of LV dysfunction). The presence of AF in heart failure may simply be a marker of the severity of the left ventricular dysfunction. The presence of paroxysmal AF may reflect underlying sinus node disease, and this population may be predisposed to an increased risk of fatal bradyarrhythmias. Furthermore, the increase in mortality in heart failure with AF may reflect an increase in fatal thromboembolic events.

Further light has been shed on the interplay between AF and heart failure in an analysis of outcomes in two contemporary randomized clinical trials in patients with heart failure and reduced ejection fraction (PARADIGM-HF and ATMOSPHERE). Mogensen et al.[22] documented the outcomes in patients with pre-existing chronic AF, paroxysmal AF, and new-onset AF. Of 15 415 patients in these two trials, 5481 (35.6%) had a history of AF at randomization; of these, 1465 (30%) were paroxysmal. A further 369 patients developed AF during the course of the trials. Compared with the patients in sinus rhythm, the patients with permanent AF had similar survival and similar rates of heart failure hospitalization and stroke. Patients with paroxysmal AF had a 20–35% higher risk of heart failure hospitalization and stroke but similar mortality. However, those who developed new-onset AF during the course of the trials had the worst outcomes, with risks of mortality, heart failure hospitalization, and stroke more than twice as high as the other groups.

Aims of treatment of atrial fibrillation in heart failure

The adverse haemodynamic and prognostic effects of AF in heart failure underpin the rationale for treatment. The reduction in cardiac output and exercise capacity in individuals with heart failure and AF would suggest that restoration of sinus rhythm should be the target of treatment, but there is currently little evidence in favour of this strategy. The AF-CHF study showed no mortality benefit from a rhythm control versus a rate control strategy in heart failure patients.[23] Overall the aim of treatment of AF in heart failure is to improve symptoms and quality of life, to improve prognosis if possible, and to reduce the risk of thromboembolic complications. This may be via either the restoration and maintenance of sinus rhythm, or control of ventricular rate, and anticoagulation.

Rhythm control

The maintenance of sinus rhythm may be achieved by means of direct current cardioversion and/or the use of antiarrhythmic drugs. The rationale for this 'rhythm-control' approach includes the possibility of fewer symptoms, better exercise tolerance, a lower risk of stroke, eventual discontinuation of long-term anticoagulant therapy, better quality of life, and better survival, if sinus rhythm can be maintained. However, the AF-CHF study has failed to demonstrate any survival benefit from adopting a rhythm control strategy in AF in the context of heart failure. Furthermore, AF is often poorly responsive

to antiarrhythmic drugs, which may also have serious adverse effects. Class I antiarrhythmic drugs are proarrhythmic and therefore contraindicated in the presence of heart failure. If a rhythm control strategy is adopted, the first-line antiarrhythmic drug is amiodarone, with sotalol or dofetilide suitable alternatives. However, in both AF-CHF[23] and AFFIRM,[24] a rhythm control strategy resulted in more frequent hospitalizations, whether for recurrence of AF, repeat cardioversions, or bradyarrhythmias.

A further strategy for restoration of sinus rhythm is catheter ablation of AF via pulmonary vein isolation, with or without more extensive left atrial ablation. The commonest techniques involve either the delivery of multiple radiofrequency lesions around the pulmonary veins, or the use of a balloon catheter irrigated with liquid nitrogen to perform cryo-ablation around these veins. These techniques are used extensively in patients with symptomatic AF and structurally normal hearts (or with mild structural disease).[25–27] Several recent small studies have examined the efficacy of catheter ablation in restoring and maintaining sinus rhythm in patients with heart failure due to LVSD. Two recent meta-analyses of these studies[28,29] concluded that ablation is superior to rate control in improving LVEF, quality of life, and functional capacity in patients with heart failure and AF. A larger trial, the CASTLE-AF study[30] has recently been completed. In this trial, 363 patients with AF and heart failure due to LVSD were randomized to ablation versus medical therapy and followed for up to five years. This trial showed that the patients randomized to an ablation strategy experienced a significant 38% reduction in the combined primary end-point of mortality and hospitalization for worsening heart failure: 51 patients in the ablation group met this end-point, versus 82 patients in the medical therapy group. All-cause mortality was also significantly lower (by 47%) in the patients treated by ablation—there were 24 deaths in patients treated by ablation, versus 46 deaths in the medial therapy limb, corresponding to a 47% risk reduction in all-cause mortality. Subgroup analyses suggest that the patients most likely to gain from the ablation procedure are those with LVEF >25%, those with NYHA class II heart failure symptoms, and possibly younger patients (age <65 years). There has been some criticism of the validity of this trial,[31] and further trials are ongoing or planned to determine whether the results are generalizable or not.

Rate control

A strategy of controlling the ventricular rate in AF via the use of atrioventricular (AV) nodal blocking drugs may be desirable in heart failure. Drugs used to control the ventricular rate may be less toxic than antiarrhythmic agents used to restore or maintain sinus rhythm, although in heart failure some commonly used agents may be contraindicated. Calcium channel blockers should be avoided in the context of heart failure as a result of their negative inotropic effects, which may result in hospital admissions for worsening heart failure. Traditionally, first-line therapy for rate control in AF in the context of LVSD has been β-blockade (if no evidence of decompensation), with one of the β-blockers licensed for use in heart failure (bisoprolol, slow-release metoprolol, or carvedilol) plus or minus digoxin if required. There is evidence that carvedilol is beneficial in patients with heart failure and AF. The COMET trial randomized patients with heart failure to carvedilol or metoprolol, and 600 out of the 3029 patient in the trial had AF. Although patients with AF had a higher mortality rate than those in sinus rhythm, the AF patients treated with carvedilol had a 16% lower mortality than those treated with metoprolol.[19] The evidence for bisoprolol is less clear. The CIBIS-2 trial recruited 2018 patients with heart failure and randomized them to bisoprolol or placebo, of whom 321 had AF. In the AF subgroup of the CIBIS-2 trial there was no difference in mortality between those treated with bisoprolol or placebo.[18]

The target heart rate for rate control in patients with heart failure and AF remains unknown. Traditionally, physicians have uptitrated rate control medications, aiming to achieve a resting heart rate of <80/min. This approach was challenged by the RACE-2 trial[32] which demonstrated in 614 patients with AF that 'lenient' rate control (aiming for a resting heart rate <110/min) was just as effective and easier to achieve than 'strict' rate control (resting heart rate <80/min). However, only 10% of the patients in this trial had a history of heart failure and LVSD, and a similar trial in a heart failure population would be a useful addition to the evidence base.

The role for digoxin remains unclear. Although digoxin is often added to β-blockade in order to achieve rate control, a systematic review and meta-analysis of the literature on digoxin[33] has shown that the use of this drug is associated with a 29% increase in mortality when used in patients with AF and a 14% increase in mortality when used in patients with heart failure. Whether this represents an adverse effect of the drug or implies that digoxin might be used in patients with more resistant symptoms or with co-morbidities that preclude full β-blocker use remains unclear.

An alternative to drug therapy for ventricular rate control is ablation of the AV node and permanent pacemaker implantation.[34] This strategy may be appropriate if drug therapy is ineffective or poorly tolerated. Short-term studies have shown that biventricular pacing appears to result in superior haemodynamic effects when compared to right ventricular pacing.[35] A meta-analysis of studies comparing biventricular versus right ventricular pacing for patients with heart failure and AF undergoing AV nodal ablation[36] showed that biventricular pacing was not associated with significantly improved survival when compared with right ventricular-only pacing, but biventricular pacing was associated with an improvement in symptoms and ejection fraction. Furthermore, a systematic review and meta-analysis by Gasparini et al.[37] showed that, in patients with heart failure and AF undergoing cardiac resynchronization therapy (CRT) device implantation, AV nodal ablation appeared to be associated with better survival than treatment with rate-limiting drugs. Based on studies such as these, the most recent guidelines from the European Society of Cardiology[38] state that CRT should be considered for certain patients with heart failure and AF (with LVEF ≤35% and QRS duration >130 ms, in NYHA classes III–IVd despite optimal medical therapy) in order to improve symptoms and reduce morbidity and mortality, 'provided a strategy to ensure biventricular capture is in place'.

Anticoagulation

Patients with AF are at increased risk of thromboembolic events. This risk is further increased in the presence of LVSD—the risk of stroke is 2.5-fold greater in a patient with moderate–severe LVSD.[16] The use of vitamin K antagonists, primarily warfarin, has been recommended in AF (target international normalized ratio (INR) range: 2.0–3.0), whether persistent or paroxysmal, in heart failure to reduce the risk of thromboembolic complications.

It is highly effective in the reduction of ischaemic stroke in patients with AF, reducing the risk of stroke by 64% in comparison to placebo and by 37% when compared with antiplatelet therapy.[39] Warfarin does have a number of limitations, however. There is a very narrow therapeutic window, and, if INR >3.0, there is significantly increased risk of intracranial bleeding. It has a slow onset of action, there is significant genetic variation in the response, and there are multiple food and drug interactions with warfarin.

In recent years several new oral anticoagulants (often referred to as DOACs: the direct acting oral anticoagulants; or NOACs: the non-vitamin K-dependent oral anticoagulants) have been approved for use in 'non-valvular' AF. At the present time, four drugs have been licensed for this indication in patients with non-valvular AF and one or more risk factors for stroke. The first drug to be licensed, dabigatran, acts as a direct thrombin (factor II) inhibitor, and the other three drugs (rivaroxaban, apixaban, and edoxaban) act by inhibiting factor Xa. Each of these drugs has been compared to warfarin in large randomized clinical trials in patients with AF and one or more risk factors for stroke. A meta-analysis of these trials[40] has confirmed the efficacy of these drugs, showing that they reduce the risk of stroke by 19% and reduce all-cause mortality by 10% compared to warfarin. The risk of intracranial bleeding is substantially lower with these new drugs compared to warfarin, although some of these drugs can be associated with a higher risk of gastrointestinal bleeding.

Each of the trials of NOACs versus warfarin included a significant proportion of patients with heart failure (between 30% and 62% of patients) and the benefits of the NOACs have been confirmed in patients with heart failure and AF. The most recent European Society of Cardiology guidelines on AF[41] now recommend use of NOACs in preference to warfarin, except in patients with either a mechanical prosthetic valve or moderate–severe mitral stenosis, where the NOACs are contraindicated and warfarin is the anticoagulant of choice.

Atrial flutter

Atrial flutter is a common supraventricular tachyarrhythmia encountered in heart failure patients. It is a macro-re-entrant arrhythmia, in either the right (typical atrial flutter) or left (atypical atrial flutter) atrium. It is typically initiated by a premature impulse within the atrium, and propagated as a result of differences in the conduction properties and refractory periods of the atrial tissue. The atrial rate in atrial flutter is typically between 240 and 350 beats/min.

In typical atrial flutter, the macro-re-entrant circuit is confined to the right atrium. The wavefront can occur in either a clockwise or counterclockwise direction around the right atrium. The activation wavefront emerges from a zone of slow conduction between the tricuspid valve annulus and the os of the coronary sinus and then, in the case of counterclockwise flutter, ascends the inter-atrial septum, spreads to the posterior right atrium and then downwards and laterally between the tricuspid valve and crista terminalis. The wavefront then crosses via an isthmus between the inferior vena cava and the tricuspid valve annulus. This isthmus is the target for radiofrequency ablation, to create a line of functional conduction block in the circuit, terminating and preventing recurrence of the tachycardia.

Treatment of atrial flutter

The treatment goals in atrial flutter are essentially the same as those in the management of AF, namely, either rate or rhythm control and anticoagulation. In atrial flutter, the re-entrant nature of the arrhythmia makes it more readily amenable to catheter ablation and this is an effective treatment, including in the heart failure population. Radiofrequency ablation for atrial flutter has a high long-term success rate (~90%), and patients with heart failure and atrial flutter should be prioritized for this treatment, particularly if they have recurrent atrial flutter despite antiarrhythmic drug therapy. Although there are few randomized trials comparing flutter ablation with medical therapy, it is generally accepted that cavotricuspid isthmus ablation is a safe and appropriate first-line treatment for atrial flutter.[42,43] The most recent guidelines from the European Heart Rhythm Society state that 'In patients with depressed LV systolic function, ablation (for atrial flutter) may be considered to revert dysfunction due to tachycardiomyopathy, and prevent recurrences'.[44]

Atypical or left atrial flutter is much less common. It may occur as a complication of radiofrequency ablation in the left atrium for AF. It can be difficult to control with antiarrhythmic drugs. Radiofrequency ablation of the left atrial circuit is feasible, but tends to be technically more difficult than ablation for right atrial flutter, with a lower success rate.

Tachycardiomyopathy

Tachycardiomyopathy is a rare but potentially curable cause of heart failure, in particular dilated cardiomyopathy. Arrhythmias are frequently a consequence of cardiomyopathy of heart failure and can therefore be easily overlooked as the potential cause. Incessant AF, ectopic atrial tachycardia, atrial flutter, AV re-entrant tachycardia, AV nodal re-entrant tachycardia, atrial flutter, and ventricular tachycardia (VT) have all been shown to cause tachycardiomyopathy. In cases of tachycardiomyopathy, the eventual recognition and treatment of the tachyarrhythmia can lead to complete resolution of the cardiomyopathy.[45-47] This diagnosis should be considered in patients with heart failure and persistent tachycardia, particularly when the tachycardia persists despite β-blocker therapy. Careful and expert analysis of the ECG is required, since some atrial tachycardias may be very difficult to distinguish from sinus tachycardia (**Figure 40.2**).

Ventricular arrhythmias

Prevalence and effect on mortality

Despite recent advances in the treatment of chronic heart failure, mortality remains high, and sudden arrhythmic death is accepted to be the cause in ~40% of cases. In studies of the cause of sudden unexpected death in heart failure, where Holter recordings were available, ventricular tachyarrhythmias are responsible in ~80% of cases.[48] Several studies in patients with heart failure have demonstrated a high prevalence of ventricular arrhythmias, including complex ventricular premature beats, non-sustained VT (NSVT) and sustained VT, and these appear to be independent predictors of mortality.[49] In the GESICA study,[6] ventricular couplets were found in 59% of the population and in >90% of the patients with NSVT. Couplets and/or NSVT were detected in 62.7% of the study population, with a 50.8% mortality rate. The remaining 37.3% without

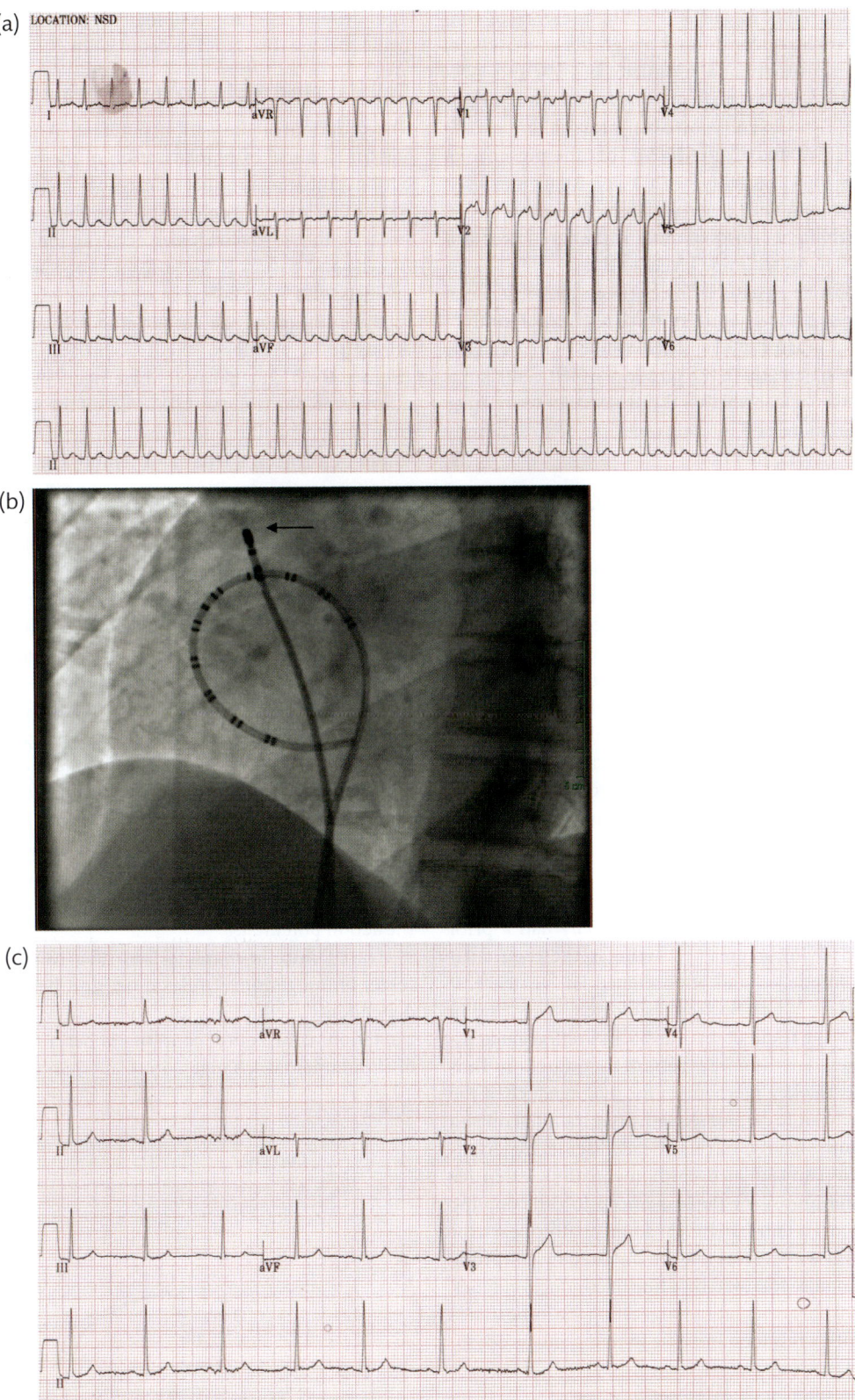

Figure 40.2 (a) Twelve-lead ECG of incessant atrial tachycardia in a 16-year-old boy who presented with severe heart failure resistant to medical therapy. (b) Catheter position (arrowed) at which this arrhythmia was successfully ablated (~2 cm from the sino-atrial node). (c) Twelve-lead ECG in sinus rhythm after successful ablation of atrial tachycardia. Thereafter his rhythm remained normal, his symptoms resolved, and his left ventricular function soon returned to normal.

couplets had a lower mortality rate of 26.3%. The presence of ventricular premature complexes constituted a significant marker of sudden death, with a sensitivity and specificity of 89% and 42%, respectively. Furthermore, the negative predictive value was 95.5%. The incidence of NSVT has been reported in heart failure as 28–80%. The GESICA-GEMA study[50] concluded that the presence of NSVT correlates with total mortality, with a persistent increased risk of 1.63 after adjustment with other variables. However, NSVT was also associated with higher doses of diuretic therapy, lower systolic blood pressure, higher creatinine levels, and faster heart rates, all of which tend to indicate an association between the presence of NSVT and worsening of clinical status. In the UK-HEART study,[51] the presence of NSVT was associated with a two-fold increase in the risk of sudden death, particularly in the presence of left ventricular dilatation. Therefore it is unclear whether the presence of ventricular arrhythmias confers an increased mortality risk *per se* or is simply indicative of worse LV systolic function.

Mechanisms and pathogenesis of ventricular arrhythmias in heart failure

Multiple factors are responsible for the initiation and maintenance of ventricular arrhythmias in heart failure. The mechanisms differ with aetiology, although re-entry, the mechanism thought to be responsible for most ventricular arrhythmias, is common to both ischaemic and non-ischaemic aetiologies. Furthermore, cardiac failure is characterized by ventricular hypertrophy, manifest as an increase in LV mass, cellular hypertrophy, alterations in cellular ionic currents, and changes in the histological features of the ventricular interstitium. Also, the presence of coronary artery disease increases the risk of further myocardial ischaemia, which is proarrhythmic.

Re-entry

In ischaemic cardiomyopathy, patients have typically had a prior myocardial infarction, having an area of scarring in the ventricular myocardium, and a remodelled and often dilated left ventricle. It is often possible to induce VT at electrophysiological study, and in hearts that are failing as the result of myocardial infarction a macro-re-entrant circuit may exist in the border zone of the infarction. Thus scar-related re-entry is the key mechanism for maintenance of the arrhythmia. In non-ischaemic cardiomyopathy (e.g. familial dilated or hypertrophic cardiomyopathy, valvular heart disease, hypertension, post-viral or idiopathic dilated cardiomyopathy), extensive myocardial damage and fibrosis or the loss of cell-to-cell coupling provide the substrates for re-entry. In the cardiomyopathic heart, for example, new re-entrant wave fronts may be initiated by epicardial breakthrough of the impulse followed by a line of conduction block parallel to the epicardial fibre orientation, suggesting the importance of increased fibrosis with a resultant increase in tissue anisotropy.

Automaticity and triggered activity

Abnormal automaticity may arise in hypertrophied and failing hearts in the setting of a reduction in resting membrane potential or acceleration of phase 4 diastolic depolarization such that the threshold for activation of the Na current is reached rapidly. Triggered activity, arising from either early afterdepolarizations or delayed afterdepolarizations, also contribute to ventricular arrhythmias in patients with both ischaemic and non-ischaemic cardiomyopathy.

The cellular electrophysiological mechanisms underlying these principles are discussed in detail below.

Cellular electrophysiology in heart failure

The duration of the action potential is primarily responsible for the time-course of repolarization of the heart. Prolongation of the action potential produces delays in cardiac repolarization, manifest as QT interval prolongation on the surface ECG, which can be proarrhythmic. Prolongation of the action potential is characteristic of cells and tissues isolated from ventricles of animals and human subjects with heart failure independent of the mechanism. A change in the duration of the action potential occurs as a result of alterations in the profiles of the depolarizing and repolarizing currents (**Figure 40.3**). Furthermore, heterogeneity of action potential duration across the transmural surface of the ventricular wall may be an important contributor to arrhythmogenesis.[52] Experimental models finding enhanced spatial and temporal dispersion of monophasic action potential duration, refractoriness, and electrocardiographic QT intervals in humans and animals with heart failure are consistent with an exaggerated dispersion of action potential duration that may predispose to ventricular arrhythmias.[53,54]

Repolarization in the mammalian heart is achieved primarily by the activity of potassium-selective ionic currents. Functional downregulation of K currents is a recurring theme in hypertrophied and failing ventricular myocardium; reduction in the current density of the transient outward K current (I_{to}) is arguably the most consistent ionic current change. Downregulation of I_{to}, without a significant change in the voltage dependence or kinetics of the current, has also been observed in cells isolated from terminally failing human hearts. I_{to} is a transient current and therefore downregulation itself may not produce large effects on the action potential duration. However, it does profoundly influence phase 1 and the level of the plateau, thereby affecting all of the currents that are active later in the action potential.

Heart failure is characterized by a reduction in the developed force, prolongation of relaxation, and blunting of the frequency-dependent facilitation of contraction. The abnormalities in excitation–contraction coupling in heart failure are a consequence of fundamental changes in Ca^{2+} handling within ventricular

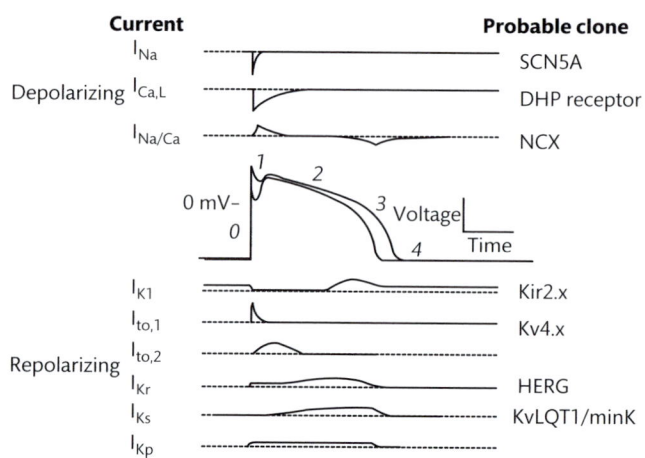

Figure 40.3 Ionic currents contributing to the ventricular action potential.

myocytes.[55–57] The L-type Ca current is the primary source of Ca^{2+} entry, triggering release of Ca^{2+} from the sarcoplasmic reticulum and initiating actin–myosin crossbridge cycling. Studies of L-type Ca current in cells isolated from failing human hearts exhibit either no change, or a decrease in current density or dihydropyridine binding sites. Ventricular myocytes isolated from failing hearts exhibit attenuated augmentation of the L-type Ca current by β-adrenergic stimulation and depression of rate-dependent potentiation compared to cells isolated from control hearts. Depression of the L-type Ca current results in slowing of the decay of the whole-cell current, a change that could alter excitation–contraction coupling and would tend to prolong the action potential duration, the latter of which would be proarrhythmic. The amplitude of the intracellular Ca^{2+} transient and its rate of decay are reduced in intact muscles and cells isolated from failing ventricles compared with normal controls. The changes in the Ca^{2+} transient are the result of defective function of the sarcoplasmic reticulum (SR), but the precise molecular mechanism(s) of this defect is controversial. The SR Ca^{2+}–ATPase (SERCA2a) and the Na^+–Ca^{2+} exchanger (NCX) are primary mediators of Ca^{2+} removal from the cytoplasm. SERCA2a is inhibited by unphosphorylated phospholamban (PLB) by direct protein–protein interaction; when PLB is phosphorylated, SERCA2a inhibition is relieved. Ca^{2+} entry into the cell through the L-type Ca channel stimulates release of Ca^{2+} from the SR by the ryanodine receptor (RyR) in a process known as Ca^{2+}-induced Ca^{2+} release. The level of ventricular RyR mRNA decreases in some studies of terminal human heart failure. The NCX importantly contributes to control of intracellular $[Ca^{2+}]$, extruding cytoplasmic Ca^{2+} by electrogenically exchanging it for extracellular Na^+. Most studies from hypertrophied and failing hearts have demonstrated an increase in both NCX mRNA and protein, suggesting that enhanced NCX function compensates for defective SR removal of Ca^{2+} from the cytoplasm in the failing heart. The characteristic slow decay of the Ca^{2+} transient and increased diastolic $[Ca^{2+}]$ can predispose to oscillatory release of Ca^{2+} from the SR and delayed afterdepolarization-mediated triggered arrhythmias. The slow decay of the Ca^{2+} transient will influence ion flux through the NCX and may also predispose to late phase 3 early afterdepolarization-mediated triggered arrhythmias.

The Na^+–K^+ ATPase (Na, K pump) transports K^+ into the cell and Na^+ out with a stoichiometry of 2:3, therefore generating an outward repolarizing current. The expression and function of the Na^+–K^+ ATPase are reduced in failing compared with control hearts which may have arrhythmogenic consequences. This reduction in the outward repolarizing current would tend to prolong action potential duration. Furthermore reduced function of the Na^+–K^+ ATPase would lead to an increase in intracellular $[Na^+]$ and enhanced reversed mode NCX, increasing depolarizing current.

The hyperpolarization-activated 'funny' or pacemaker current (I_f) in the heart is a non-selective cation current that was originally described in automatic tissues such as the sino-atrial node. More recently I_f has been demonstrated in ventricular cells from animal and human hearts, activating at very negative voltages outside the physiological range. Although I_f is found in higher density in ventricular myocytes from failing human hearts, the difference from controls did not reach statistical significance. It is therefore unclear whether this current has a role to play in abnormal automaticity and the induction of ventricular arrhythmias in heart failure.

Conduction delay and re-entry

Alterations in anisotropic conduction may contribute to the production of arrhythmias in hypertrophic and failing hearts. Alterations in intracellular $[Ca^{2+}]$ and redistribution of gap junctions affect intercellular conduction. Microfibrosis separates myocytes and myocyte bundles, altering anisotropic conduction leading to spatial non-uniformities of electrical activation. Diminished intercellular coupling slows conduction, which predisposes to re-entry. Slowed ventricular conduction is manifest on the surface ECG as QRS prolongation, which is an independent risk factor for sudden cardiac death.[58,59] Furthermore, QRS duration is a major criterion for risk stratification and identification of patients suitable for advanced therapies for heart failure, namely CRT (biventricular pacemakers) and ICDs.[60,61]

Neurohormonal modulation and the pathogenesis of arrhythmias

In the presence of impaired cardiac function, the body attempts to maintain circulatory homeostasis through a complex series of

Table 40.1 Cellular electrophysiological changes linked to arrhythmia mechanisms in heart failure

Arrhythmogenic mechanism	Molecular changes in hypertrophy/HF	
Abnormal automaticity		
Reduced resting membrane potential	Enhanced phase 4 diastolic depolarization	$\uparrow I_{Ca-T}$, I_{K1}, $\uparrow I_f$
	Reduced maximum diastolic potential	
Triggered activity		
EAD-mediated	APD	$\downarrow$ K currents, $\uparrow$ NCX,
	($\uparrow$ APD and altered profile)	Altered I_{Ca-L} density and kinetics,
Late EAD-mediated and DAD-mediated	Increased $[Ca^{2+}]_i$	Slowed Ca^{2+} transient, $\uparrow$ NCX
Re-entry		
Reactivation	Prolonged APD	
Slowed conduction and block	Anisotropic conduction	Microfibrosis in the interstitium

HF = heart failure; I_{Ca}-T = T-type calcium current; I_{K1} = inward-rectifying potassium current; I_f = hyperpolarization-activated ('funny') pacemaker current; EAD = early after depolarization; APD = action potential duration; NCX - Na+-Ca++ exchanger; ICaL = L-type Calcium current; DAD = delayed afterdepolarization; $[Ca^{2+}]_i$ = intracellular calcium concentration.

neurohormonal changes. These changes in neurohormonal signalling have prominent effects on the electrophysiology of the failing heart.

The β_1, β_2, and α_1 adrenergic receptors mediate the effects of increased circulating epinephrine and norepinephrine released from cardiac nerve terminals in the heart. These receptor subtypes are coupled to different signalling systems. The β_1 and β_2 receptors are coupled by stimulatory G proteins to adenylyl cyclase; activation results in increased cellular levels of cAMP. The α_1 receptor is coupled by a G protein to phospholipase C (PLC) which hydrolyses inositol phospholipids increasing cellular inositol 1,4,5-trisphosphate and diacylglycerol. Angiotensin II (AT1) receptors are also coupled to PLC. Activation of the AT1 receptor or the α-adrenergic pathway initiates a kinase cascade, triggering cell growth and altering the level of intracellular Ca^{2+}. This increases the cellular Ca load, and the possible adverse consequences of increased Ca^{2+} load include activation of phospholipases, proteases, and endonucleases culminating in cell necrosis or apoptosis and progression of heart failure.

The β and α signalling pathways significantly affect the function of a number of ion channels and transporters. The net effect of β-adrenergic stimulation is to shorten the ventricular action potential duration due to an increase in the current density and a hyperpolarizing shift of the activation of I_K, despite β_1 receptor stimulation of depolarizing current through the L-type Ca channel. α_1-Adrenergic receptor stimulation inhibits several K currents in the mammalian heart, including I_{to}, I_{K1}, and I_K in rat ventricle with the net effect of prolonging action potential duration.

Mechanical load is an important modulator of excitability in the heart. The effect of altered haemodynamic load may be exaggerated in the failing compared with the normal ventricle. In doxorubicin-induced heart failure in the rabbit, increased load produced exaggerated shortening of the action potential duration and enhanced arrhythmia susceptibility in failing compared to control hearts.[62] The effect of load is not likely to be distributed uniformly across the ventricular wall or throughout the myocardium, and thus has the potential to increase dispersion in action potential duration with arrhythmogenic consequences.

Myocardial ischaemia in the pathogenesis of arrhythmias in heart failure

Myocardial ischaemia is proarrhythmic and has a role in increasing the risk of sudden death in heart failure. Ischaemia results in QT interval prolongation and polymorphic VT, which may degenerate into ventricular fibrillation. The presence of electrolyte abnormalities, sympathetic stimulation, and ventricular hypertrophy all increase the risk of arrhythmias in myocardial ischaemia and are often coexistent in heart failure. The potential for myocardial ischaemia precipitating ventricular tachyarrhythmia is well recognized in patients with ischaemic cardiomyopathy; however, there is a significant incidence of undiagnosed coronary artery disease in 'non-ischaemic' cardiomyopathy, with one study reporting a 40% incidence of 'acute' coronary lesions in individuals with a sudden cardiac death but no previous documented history of ischaemic heart disease.[63] This emphasizes the importance of optimal anti-ischaemic therapies in individuals with ischaemic and perhaps also non-ischaemic cardiomyopathies.

Electrolyte abnormalities

Electrolyte abnormalities, notably hypo- or hyperkalaemia or hypomagnesaemia, are associated with an increased risk of ventricular tachyarrhythmias. Hypokalaemia or hypomagnesaemia may occur as a result of diuretic therapy and predispose to QT interval prolongation. The presence of hypomagnesaemia impairs the repletion of potassium stores and appears to be implicated in ventricular tachyarrhythmias. Conversely, hyperkalaemia may predispose to bradyarrhythmias or sinusoidal VT, and may occur as a result of impaired renal function or secondary to drug therapy (e.g. angiotensin converting enzyme (ACE) inhibitors, angiotensin receptor blockers, aldosterone antagonists, or potassium supplements).

Types of ventricular arrhythmias

Ventricular premature beats

Ventricular premature beats (VPBs) are single ventricular impulses caused by re-entry within the ventricle or abnormal automaticity of ventricular cells. VPBs, also called premature ventricular contractions or complexes (PVCs), may occur erratically or at predictable intervals (e.g. every third (trigeminy) or second (bigeminy) beat). VPBs may increase with stimulants (e.g. anxiety, stress, alcohol, caffeine, sympathomimetic drugs), hypoxia, or electrolyte abnormalities. VPBs may be asymptomatic or cause palpitations or may be experienced as missed or skipped beats; the VPB itself is not sensed but rather the following augmented sinus beat. When VPBs are very frequent, particularly when they represent every second heart beat, mild haemodynamic symptoms are possible because the sinus rate has been effectively halved. Diagnosis is by ECG showing a wide QRS complex without a preceding P wave, typically followed by a fully compensatory pause.

There are several different patterns of premature ventricular contractions. In bigeminy, one VPB occurs after every normal beat, in an alternating pattern. In trigeminy, one VPB occurs after every two normal beats. In quadrigeminy, one VPB occurs after every three normal beats of the heart. Unifocal premature ventricular contractions occur where the depolarizations are triggered from a single site in the ventricles, resulting in a single QRS morphology of VPBs. Multifocal premature ventricular contractions arise from more than one site in the ventricles, resulting in VPBs with more than one QRS morphology. If three or more VPBs occur in a row it is defined as VT. Ventricular premature beats are of variable prognostic importance, and may be associated with an increased risk of sustained ventricular tachyarrhythmias and sudden cardiac death in selected patients. One report evaluated intracardiac electrograms in patients with an ICD. Among those with a reduced LVEF, monomorphic VT was most often initiated by multiple VPBs, which had morphology different from the VT.[64] There is no evidence, however, that suppression of VPBs improves mortality in the presence of heart failure, and in fact the use of class I antiarrhythmics may be proarrhythmic in this patient group, resulting in increased mortality.

For patients with very frequent ventricular premature beats of a single morphology, some investigators have attempted to eliminate the ventricular premature beats by radiofrequency ablation. Several small studies have reported some success at this technique, often with demonstration of an improvement in LV size and ejection fraction post ablation. A meta-analysis of 15 studies in a total of 712 patients has been published; 336 of the patients had reduced LVEF prior to ablation.[65] The mean 'burden' of ventricular premature beats was 24%, the long-term success rate for ablation ranged from 66% to

90%, and the mean increase in LVEF post ablation was 7.7%. For patients who had LVSD at baseline, the overall mean increase in LVEF post ablation was 12.4%.

Ventricular tachycardia

Three or more beats in a row on an ECG that originate from the ventricle at a rate of >100 beats/min constitute a ventricular tachycardia (VT). If the fast rhythm self-terminates within 30 s, it is defined as non-sustained ventricular tachycardia (NSVT). Ventricular tachycardia lasting >30 s or requiring cardioversion (either pharmacological, electrical, or by overdrive pacing) for haemodynamic compromise within that time is defined as sustained VT. Occasionally an atrial impulse arrives when the AV node and the His–Purkinje system are not refractory and AV conduction can occur. This results in a capture beat in which ventricular conduction occurs over the normal pathways, resulting in a normal-appearing (narrow) QRS complex. A capture beat occurs at a shorter RR interval than the RR interval of the VT. AV conduction also may occur simultaneously with depolarization of the ventricular focus. In this instance, the ventricle will be depolarized in part over the normal pathway and in part from the ventricular focus. The resulting QRS complex will be intermediate in morphology between a normal QRS and a QRS of ventricular origin. In this instance, the RR interval will not change. This is called a fusion beat. Ventricular tachycardia may be monomorphic (all QRSs with the same shape) or polymorphic (varying QRS shapes during the tachycardia).

Several algorithms have been derived to assist in the ECG diagnosis of VT, including the distinction between VT and SVT with bundle branch block.[66] The Brugada algorithm[67] is widely used and is summarized in **Figure 40.4**. Such algorithms are guidelines and should be used with caution in certain circumstances such as in the context of acute myocardial infarction, complex congenital

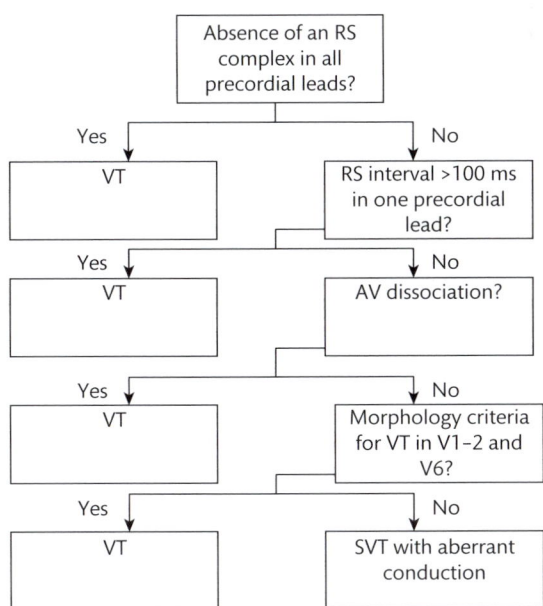

Figure 40.4 Algorithm for analysis of 12-lead ECG of wide QRS complex tachycardia.

Source data from Brugada P, Brugada J, Mont L, Smeets J, Andries EW. A new approach to the differential diagnosis of a regular tachycardia with a wide QRS complex. *Circulation* 1991;**83**(5):1649–59.

heart disease, electrolyte abnormalities, and in patients already on antiarrhythmic drugs, especially Class 1C agents.

The prognostic significance of NSVT in heart failure is uncertain. The GESICA-GEMA study showed that in patients with CHF, NSVT is an independent marker for increased overall mortality rate and sudden death. The absence of NSVT and ventricular premature beats in a 24 h Holter indicated a low probability of sudden death. However, on the contrary, the CHF-STAT study reported that NSVT is frequently seen in patients with heart failure and may be associated with worsened survival by univariate analysis. However, after adjusting other variables, especially for LVEF, NSVT was not an *independent* predictor of all-cause mortality or sudden death. These results have serious implications in that suppression of these arrhythmias may not improve survival.

Torsades de pointes

Torsades de pointes or polymorphic VT is a form of VT in which the QRS morphology appears to be constantly changing. As its name suggests, its electrical activity appears to be twisted into a helix or turning about a fixed point. This form of VT may occur due to drug toxicity or an idiosyncratic reaction to type IA antiarrhythmic agents such as quinidine, procainamide, or disopyramide, or other agents that prolong the QT interval. Myocardial ischaemia, hypokalaemia, hypomagnesaemia and bradycardias can also initiate torsades de pointes. This arrhythmia is usually precipitated by prolongation of the QT interval.

Treatment of ventricular arrhythmias in heart failure

Treatment of modulating factors

The initiation and maintenance of ventricular arrhythmias in heart failure occur via several mechanisms as outlined above, and implicit in this are the electrophysiological changes in the failing ventricle in response to changes in myocardial load and stretch. Contemporary heart failure treatment includes the use of ACE inhibitors which have been shown to confer a survival benefit in heart failure.[7,68] Furthermore, the V-HeFT-II study showed a significant reduction in sudden death (39% RRR) in patients treated with enalapril compared to a hydralazine and isosorbide dinitrate combination.[69] Of note, this effect was most marked in patients with less severe heart failure symptoms and may be explained in part by the effect of the drug to prevent the development of myocardial stretch and fibrosis known to be implicated in the genesis of ventricular arrhythmias. This antiarrhythmic effect is evident from the Holter recordings of the patients receiving enalapril, who had fewer complex ventricular arrhythmias compared to the hydralazine and nitrate-treated group. Furthermore, ACE inhibitors have some β-blocking properties and stabilize electrolyte concentrations (including their potassium sparing effect) in heart failure patients, further protecting from ventricular arrhythmias.

Aldosterone is another neurohumoral agent responsible for some of the deleterious haemodynamic effects of heart failure. Via its potent mineralocorticoid effects, it promotes imbalance of sodium, potassium, magnesium, and water retention, as well as promoting myocardial fibrosis, further adding to the substrate for arrhythmias.

Spironolactone is an aldosterone antagonist which has been shown to reduce all-cause mortality in heart failure.[70] Furthermore, there was a significant reduction in sudden cardiac death in the spironolactone-treated group, suggesting an effect on the frequency of ventricular arrhythmias. A further study has demonstrated that spironolactone reduces the frequency of VPBs and NSVT in Holter monitoring and monitored treadmill testing of heart failure patients compared to standard medical therapy alone.[71] Further evidence for the antiarrhythmic effect of aldosterone antagonism comes from the EPHESUS trial of eplerenone for patients with LV dysfunction post myocardial infarction, which reported a significant reduction in sudden cardiac death at 30 days compared to placebo.[72]

Antiarrhythmic drug treatment for ventricular arrhythmias in heart failure

Drug treatment of ventricular arrhythmias in heart failure presents a difficult challenge. With increasing degrees of LV dysfunction, the efficacy of antiarrhythmic drugs decreases. Furthermore, with increasing degrees of heart failure, antiarrhythmic drugs demonstrate a greater negative inotropic effect, more frequent proarrhythmic effects, and more frequent bradyarrhythmias. The use of class I antiarrhythmic agents is contraindicated in the presence of LVSD post myocardial infarction.[73] Amiodarone, an iodine-containing benzofuran originally classified as a class III antiarrhythmic agent with minor class II effects, and later recognized to have class I and class IV effects, is widely used for the prevention of sustained VT and fibrillation. If patients with heart failure require antiarrhythmic drug therapy for ventricular arrhythmias, amiodarone is the drug of choice as there is evidence of a reduction in arrhythmic death.[74-76] Interestingly, the SCD-HEFT trial failed to show any reduction in mortality with amiodarone treatment compared to placebo in NYHA class II heart failure and was associated with decreased survival in NYHA class III.[77] There is no evidence for the prophylactic use of amiodarone in patients with depressed left ventricular systolic function in the absence of an arrhythmic indication for the drug.[76] Dronedarone is a novel antiarrhythmic drug which is a non-iodinated benzofuran derivative related to amiodarone. Clinical trials of the effectiveness of this drug for the management of AF show promising results. Its use in heart failure was investigated in the ANDROMEDA study.[78] This trial was terminated early because of an observed excess of deaths in the dronedarone treatment group, largely due to worsening heart failure, with an increased risk of death in the presence of severely reduced LVEF. It is therefore contraindicated in heart failure.

Device therapy

There have been several studies of ICD therapy for the primary or secondary prevention of sudden cardiac death (SCD). SCD occurs in approximately 50 000–70 000 people annually in the UK and represents the largest proportion of the deaths attributable to coronary heart disease. Approximately 85–90% of SCD is due to the first recognized arrhythmic event; the remaining 10–15% is due to recurrent events. The survival rates for out-of-hospital sudden cardiac episodes are <5% in most industrialized countries, including the UK. People who survive a first episode of a life-threatening ventricular arrhythmia are at high risk of further episodes. Prevention of SCD is either primary, defined as prevention of a first life-threatening arrhythmic event, or secondary, which refers to the prevention of

an additional life-threatening event in survivors of sustained VT or ventricular fibrillation (VF) or patients with recurrent unstable rhythms. Apart from a history of previous VT or VF, risk factors for SCD include a prior myocardial infarction, coronary artery disease, heart failure, LVEF <35%, prolonged QRS duration, and certain familial cardiac conditions (including long QT syndrome, Brugada syndrome, hypertrophic cardiomyopathy, and arrhythmogenic right ventricular cardiomyopathy). The incidence of SCD increases with age.

The use of the ICD in secondary prevention has been extensively investigated. Three trials involving a total of 1850 survivors of cardiac arrest (AVID[79]; CASH[80]; and CIDS[81]) have since been the subject of three different meta-analyses. These meta-analyses reported that, compared with amiodarone or another antiarrhythmic drug, treatment with ICDs resulted in a 50% reduction in the risk of cardiac death (95% confidence interval (CI) average: 35–65, with small differences between meta-analyses) and a 25–28% risk reduction in all-cause mortality (95% CI average: 10–40%, with small differences between meta-analyses).

There is evidence of mortality benefit conferred by the implantation of a primary prevention ICD in heart failure with reduced LVEF. MADIT II reported a significant reduction in mortality (31% relative reduction in risk of death at 20 months) in patients with LVEF <30% post myocardial infarction with ICD therapy compared to conventional medical therapy alone.[82] SCD-HEFT was a primary prevention trial of amiodarone versus ICD therapy, finding that ICD therapy led to a 23% relative reduction in mortality after 5 years in patients with heart failure (NYHA classes II–III and LVEF <35%).[77] Furthermore, in patients with advanced heart failure and a prolonged QRS interval, CRT (with or without an ICD[60,61]) significantly reduces mortality. The role of the ICD in the primary and secondary prevention of sudden arrhythmic death is discussed in Chapter 58.

Role of electrophysiological studies and radiofrequency ablation for ventricular arrhythmias

In the heart failure patient, VT encountered in clinical practice is often related to re-entry around a scar, most often a consequence of myocardial infarction. Monomorphic VT can be studied in the electrophysiology laboratory by conventional methods, and may be amenable to radiofrequency ablation. The purpose of mapping in VT is to identify an area of slow conduction (usually the exit point of the re-entrant circuit)—this isthmus is the target for ablation. Electrophysiologic testing is of much less value in patients with NSVT, polymorphic VT or primary VF.

Conventional mapping of VT requires the arrhythmia to be both electrically and haemodynamically stable. This can be a limitation of VT mapping and ablation in heart failure patients, who often decompensate as a consequence of the ventricular arrhythmia. In order to limit the time spent in tachycardia, a number of strategies may be used to approximate the location of the re-entrant circuit. The 12-lead ECG during tachycardia can provide the initial clues to the location via the QRS morphology and axis.[83] Thereafter, mapping in sinus rhythm can be used to identify areas of low-amplitude, fractionated potentials in the peri-infarct zone. Pace-mapping identifies the region of the exit site of the circuit. Thereafter, following induction of VT, activation mapping confirms the exit site and zone of slow conduction, i.e. the target region for ablation.

One of the main limitations of this conventional approach to VT ablation is that the VT might be non-inducible in the electrophysiology laboratory (or several VT morphologies might be inducible and the operator may not be able to determine which is the 'clinical VT'). If the patient has an ICD, the only record of the VT might be the stored electrograms from the device, not a 12-lead electrocardiogram defining the tachycardia. As a consequence, recent strategies for VT ablation have concentrated more on modification of the substrate for VT, either by delivering lesions around areas of scar tissue in the ventricular endocardium (and occasionally the epicardium) or by targeting sites of abnormal electrical signals in the heart, usually low-amplitude signals recorded during electrical diastole which signify areas of slow conduction that might be a substrate for re-entry (Figure 40.5). Invariably these cases are performed with the use of electroanatomical or non-fluoroscopic mapping systems, allowing the operator to build up a three-dimensional reconstruction of the chamber of interest (usually the left ventricle) and to identify areas of dense scar tissue, areas of surviving myocardium within the scare or adjacent to the scar, and areas of slow conduction. The operator can then perform extensive ablation at appropriate sites in sinus rhythm, and the mapping system allows recording and registration of the sites of the ablation lesions.

Polymorphic VT is usually not a target for the ablationist, but there are rare cases of patients with recurrent polymorphic VT and VF in whom each episode of the arrhythmia is triggered by an ectopic beat of a fixed morphology. Many of these ectopic beats arise either from the right ventricular outflow tract or from the Purkinje fibres of the left ventricle, and several case series have documented that ablation of the ectopic focus can occasionally be useful in controlling the arrhythmia. These can of course be hazardous procedures to perform, since the patient might actually be having multiple episodes of life-threatening unstable ventricular arrhythmias during the ablation procedure (Figure 40.6).

The role of ablation for VT occurring in the context of structural heart disease or heart failure has not been established and ICD therapy is currently recommended as first-line therapy to most such patients.[84-86] The decision as to whether and when to offer catheter ablation to patients with VT and structural heart disease varies between hospitals and even between individual clinicians. Most would agree, however, that VT ablation should be considered in patients

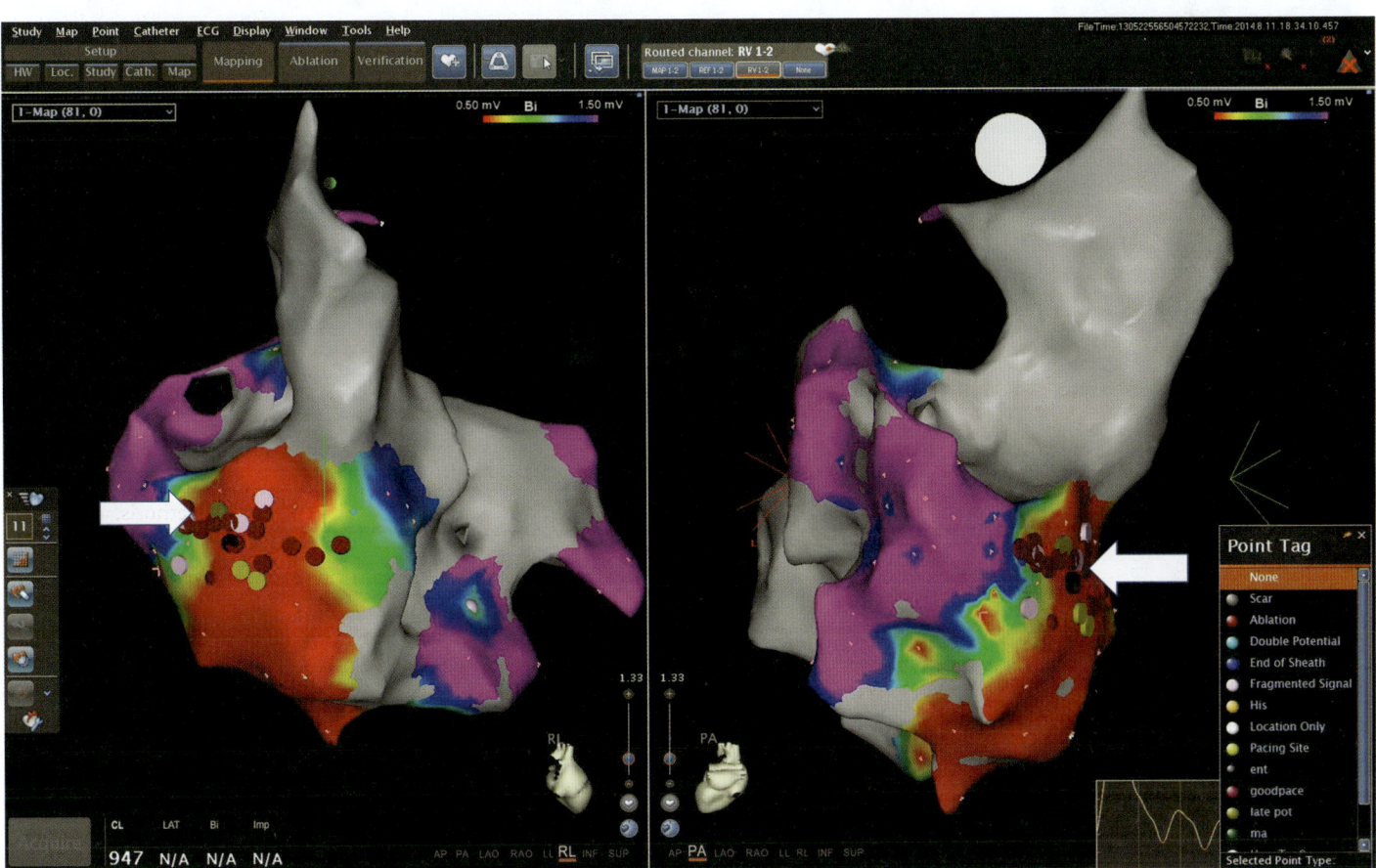

Figure 40.5 Electroanatomic map using the CARTO system (Biosense Webster, Diamond Bar, CA, USA) of left ventricle in a patient who presented with multiple implantable cardioverter–defibrillator shocks for sustained monomorphic ventricular tachycardia (VT) in the context of prior infero-posterior myocardial infarction and left ventricular dysfunction. The red areas represent areas of low voltage due to dense endocardial scar. The VT was demonstrated to be due to re-entry around the infero-posterior infarct scar, and was utilizing a critical isthmus between the infarct and the mitral annulus. Radiofrequency ablation lesions (dark red dots, arrowed) were delivered between the mitral annulus and the infarct scar, resulting in termination of the VT and rendering the VT non-inducible.

Courtesy of Dr G. A. Wright.

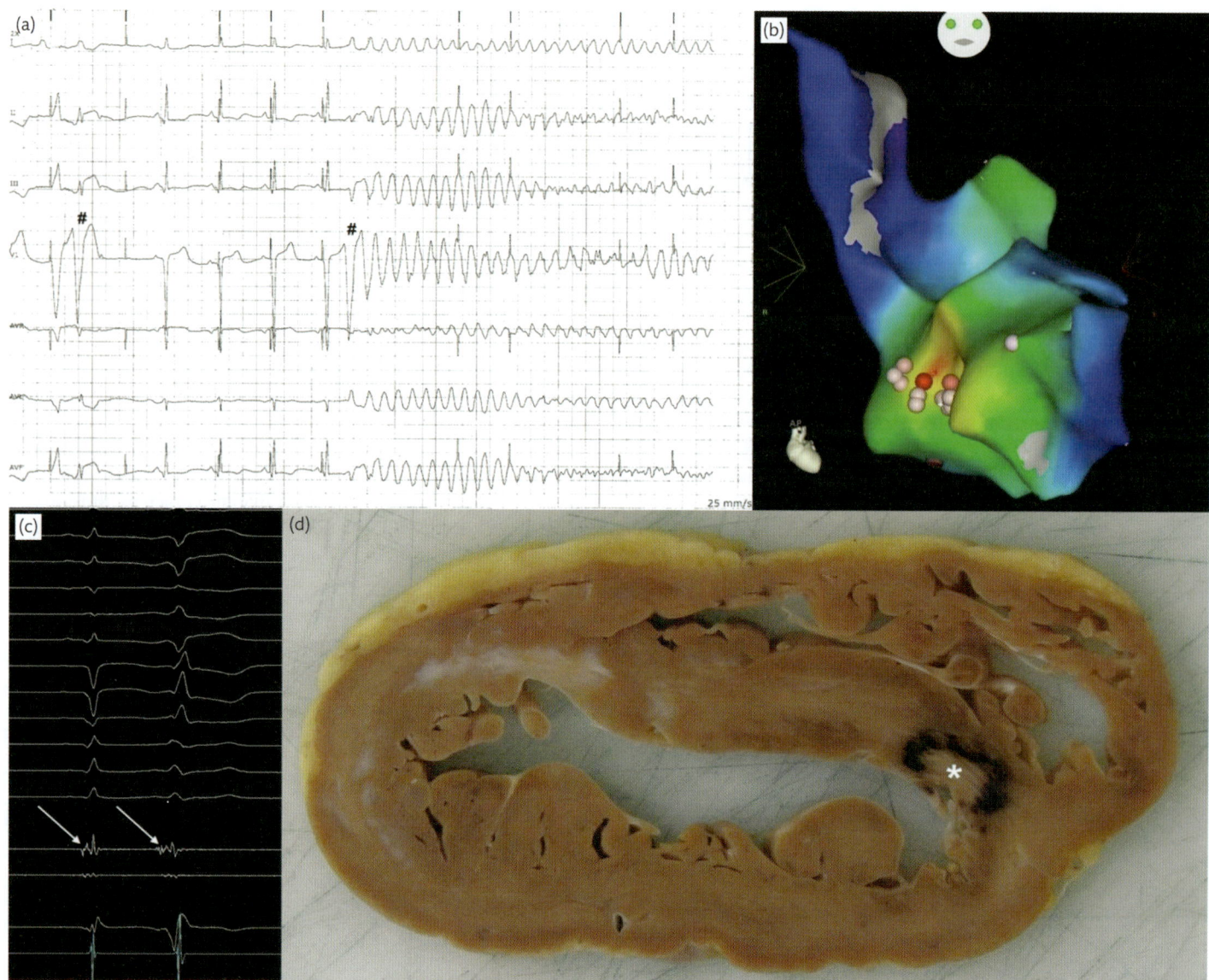

Figure 40.6 (a) ECG from a patient experiencing multiple episodes of polymorphic ventricular tachycardia (VT) and ventricular fibrillation (VF) post anterior myocardial infarction. All the episodes of VT/ VF were initiated by ectopic beats originating from the Purkinje fibres of the left ventricle. (b) Electroanatomic map of LV in this patient documenting the site of ablation of the ectopic focus initiating the VT/ VF. (c) The patient subsequently underwent orthotopic heart transplant. The explanted heart was examined and the ablation lesion is clearly identified, on the septal aspect of the endocardial surface of the LV.

Courtesy of Dr G. A. Wright and Dr A. McPhaden.

with ICDs *in situ* who experience multiple shocks despite appropriate antiarrhythmic drug therapy, particularly if there is a single morphology of haemodynamically well-tolerated VT (or more than one morphology, but likely to be utilizing a single diastolic circuit[85] and no major contraindications to the procedure. Furthermore, VT ablation may need to be considered on an urgent or emergency basis in cases of incessant VT resistant to medical therapy.

Recent studies have investigated whether VT ablation should be more widely used in patients with ICDs *in situ*, in order to reduce the frequency of subsequent ICD shocks. The SMASH-VT Trial[84] randomized 128 patients with prior myocardial infarction and at least one previous episode of a sustained ventricular arrhythmia to medical therapy or ablation. Patients randomized to VT ablation therapy

had a 15% rate of appropriate ICD discharges over a two-year period, whereas those treated medically received ICD discharges in 33% of cases ($P = 0.022$). There were six deaths in the ablation group and 11 deaths in the medically treated group. However, the study was not powered to detect differences in mortality. A similar study in Europe, the V-TACH study,[86] randomized 107 patients with prior myocardial infarction and haemodynamically stable VT either to medical therapy or to ablation. There were fewer recurrences of VT in the ablated group, the mean tome to recurrence of VT was prolonged by a year, and the mean number of ICD shocks was significantly lower in the patients who underwent ablation (0.6 vs 3.4 shocks per year).

A recent Canadian study, the VANISH trial,[87] has addressed the issue of the role of ablation therapy versus escalation of medical

therapy in patients who have had recurrent VT and are already being treated with antiarrhythmic drugs. The trial recruited 259 patients who were already on treatment with either sotalol or amiodarone; patients who had recurrent ventricular arrhythmias on sotalol were randomly allocated either to VT ablation or to amiodarone therapy; patients already on amiodarone were randomized either to VT ablation or to further intensification of drug therapy (either a higher dose of amiodarone or the addition of mexiletine). The study demonstrated that, for those patients who did not have prior amiodarone therapy, treatment with amiodarone was as effective as VT ablation. For those patients already taking amiodarone (and who had recurrent ventricular arrhythmias while taking amiodarone), VT ablation was more likely to be successful than intensification of drug therapy. However, there was no evidence of a mortality difference between the two strategies.

Several small published studies have examined the effectiveness of ablation and other therapies for 'VT storm', defined as either incessant VT (lasting >12 h) or three or more episodes of VT within 24 h. A systematic review and meta-analysis of these studies has concluded that ablation for ventricular arrhythmia storm ablation has high-acute success rates, with a low rate of recurrent storms. Heart failure is the dominant cause of death in the long term, and failure of the acute procedure carries a high mortality.[88]

The main contraindications to VT ablation are problems with either vascular access or access to the left ventricle (e.g. bilateral femoral arterial stenoses, severe aortic stenosis, contraindications to trans-septal puncture), and other potential hazards such as LV thrombus.

Bradycardia in heart failure

Disorders of sinus node function and AV nodal conduction are common, especially in the elderly population, and many patients with heart failure will be prone to these conditions. Furthermore, sinus node dysfunction and AV nodal conduction disorders can both be exacerbated by β-blockers, which are a mainstay of treatment of heart failure due to LVSD. In addition, heart failure itself is often associated with PR interval prolongation and bundle branch block.[89,58,59] In many cases where there is symptomatic bradycardia (even bradycardia induced or exacerbated by drugs, when it is necessary to continue that drug therapy[90] or life-threatening conduction disturbances), the standard treatment is implantation of a permanent pacemaker. Heart failure is an important co-morbidity in many patients undergoing pacemaker implantation, although in only a small minority of cases is it the primary reason for pacemaker implantation in the UK.[91]

Careful individual decision-making is required in selecting the optimum pacing mode[38] in patients with heart failure. In patients with sinus node dysfunction but intact AV conduction, atrial pacing alone (AAI mode) was previously considered. However, the DANPACE trial[92] demonstrated that there is a significant risk of subsequent AV block in these patients, with a need for upgrade of the pacemaker to allow ventricular pacing, and accordingly AAI pacing is now very seldom performed. Modern dual-chamber pacemakers with algorithms to limit unnecessary ventricular pacing are likely to be more appropriate than AAI pacemakers in this population.[93]

Patients with heart failure and AV block (actual or threatened) will require ventricular pacing. There is no strong evidence from clinical trials that dual-chamber pacing (DDD or DDDR) is superior to single-chamber ventricular pacing (VVI or VVIR), even in the heart failure population.[94] Clinical trials of pacing modes in patients without heart failure have been inconclusive; the MOST study in patients with sinus node disease showed better 'heart failure scores' in patients randomized to dual-chamber pacing than to single-chamber ventricular pacing,[95] but the UK-PACE study in elderly patients with AV block showed a trend towards less heart failure during follow-up in patients randomized to fixed-rate ventricular pacing (VVI mode) than in those randomized to rate-adaptive ventricular pacing (VVIR mode) or dual-chamber pacing (DDD mode).[96] A meta-analysis of these and other mode-selection studies showed no significant reduction in heart failure mortality with atrial-based pacing than with ventricular pacing (hazard ratio: 0.89; 95% confidence interval: 0.77–1.03; $P = 0.15$).[94]

There is, however, ample evidence from several studies that right ventricular pacing *per se* is deleterious in patients with left ventricular dysfunction[97] (and may be deleterious even in the normal heart.[98,99] Atrio-biventricular pacing ('CRT') is therefore often considered in patients with heart failure and severe left ventricular dysfunction who are likely to require long-term ventricular pacing. It is worth emphasizing that all the major clinical trials of CRT[60,61,100] deliberately excluded patients with either significant sinus node disease or AV conduction disease (in order that the trials would not be biased by showing a benefit for pacing alone in these patients).

A strategy of implantation of biventricular pacemakers in patients with heart failure and AV block was investigated in the BLOCK-HF trial.[101] The trial recruited patients with an LVEF of <50%, NYHA classes I–III heart failure, and AV block. Patients had a CRT-pacemaker implanted and after implantation the devices were randomly programmed to either biventricular pacing or apical RV pacing.

The biventricular-paced group showed a significant 26% reduction in the primary composite end-point of all-cause mortality, heart failure-related urgent care, or a >15% increase in LV end-systolic volume index over about three years. The benefit was driven almost entirely by the end-point's two clinical components, which together fell by 27%.

Conclusions

The treatment of cardiac arrhythmias in patients with heart failure is a complex and difficult field, where close collaboration is often needed among different medical disciplines. Treatment can do more harm than good: several antiarrhythmic drugs, both old and new, are known to be potentially hazardous in the patient with severe heart failure, because of pro-arrhythmia, negative inotropism, or other factors. Even drugs that are known to be beneficial, such as certain β-blockers, must be used initially in low dosages and titrated gradually in order to avoid clinical deterioration in patients with heart failure.

When treating arrhythmias in these patients, physicians are reminded to consider carefully the significance of the arrhythmia and the aims of treatment. Specifically, one should ask whether the

intended treatment is aimed at improving symptoms or improving prognosis. If it is the former, one should be certain that the arrhythmia is the cause of the symptoms and not merely an epiphenomenon. If it is the latter, one should have good evidence that the treatment has been proven to improve the patient's prognosis. If neither of these criteria is fulfilled, then treatment may not be required. Finally, if the arrhythmia itself does require treatment, one should always consider the different modalities of treatment (drugs, ablation, devices) in order to ensure the optimum outcome for the patient.

REFERENCES

1. Braunwald E. Shattuck lecture—cardiovascular medicine at the turn of the millennium: triumphs, concerns, and opportunities. *N Engl J Med* 1997;**337**(19):1360–9.
2. Dries DL, Exner DV, Gersh BJ, *et al.* Atrial fibrillation is associated with an increased risk for mortality and heart failure progression in patients with asymptomatic and symptomatic left ventricular systolic dysfunction: a retrospective analysis of the SOLVD trials. Studies of Left Ventricular Dysfunction. *J Am Coll Cardiol* 1998;**32**(3):695–703.
3. Carson PE, Johnson GR, Dunkman WB, *et al.* The influence of atrial fibrillation on prognosis in mild to moderate heart failure. The V-HeFT Studies. The V-HeFT VA Cooperative Studies Group. *Circulation* 1993;**87**(6 Suppl):VI102–110.
4. Deedwania PC, Singh BN, Ellenbogen K, *et al.* Spontaneous conversion and maintenance of sinus rhythm by amiodarone in patients with heart failure and atrial fibrillation: observations from the veterans affairs congestive heart failure survival trial of antiarrhythmic therapy (CHF-STAT). The Department of Veterans Affairs CHF-STAT Investigators. *Circulation* 1998;**98**(23):2574–9.
5. Torp-Pedersen C, Moller M, Bloch-Thomsen PE, *et al.* Dofetilide in patients with congestive heart failure and left ventricular dysfunction. Danish Investigations of Arrhythmia and Mortality on Dofetilide Study Group. *N Engl J Med* 1999;**341**(12):857–65.
6. Doval HC, Nul DR, Grancelli HO, *et al.* Randomised trial of low-dose amiodarone in severe congestive heart failure. Grupo de Estudio de la Sobrevida en la Insuficiencia Cardiaca en Argentina (GESICA). *Lancet* 1994;**344**(8921):493–8.
7. CONSENSUS Trial Study Group. Effects of enalapril on mortality in severe congestive heart failure. Results of the Cooperative North Scandinavian Enalapril Survival Study (CONSENSUS). *N Engl J Med* 1987;**316**(23):1429–35.
8. Benjamin EJ, Wolf PA, D'Agostino RB, *et al.* Impact of atrial fibrillation on the risk of death: the Framingham Heart Study. *Circulation* 1998;**98**(10):946–52.
9. Vaziri SM, Larson MG, Benjamin EJ, Levy D. Echocardiographic predictors of nonrheumatic atrial fibrillation. The Framingham Heart Study. *Circulation* 1994;**89**(2):724–30.
10. Maisel WH, Stevenson LW. Atrial fibrillation in heart failure: epidemiology, pathophysiology, and rationale for therapy. *Am J Cardiol* 2003;**91**(6A):2D–8D.
11. Solti F, Vecsey T, Kekesi V, Juhasz-Nagy A. The effect of atrial dilatation on the genesis of atrial arrhythmias. *Cardiovasc Res* 1989;**23**(10):882–6.
12. Nattel S. Ionic determinants of atrial fibrillation and Ca2+ channel abnormalities: cause, consequence, or innocent bystander? *Circ Res* 1999;**85**(5):473–6.
13. Li D, Shinagawa K, Pang L, *et al.* Effects of angiotensin-converting enzyme inhibition on the development of the atrial fibrillation substrate in dogs with ventricular tachypacing-induced congestive heart failure. *Circulation* 2001;**104**(21):2608–14.
14. Li D, Fareh S, Leung TK, Nattel S. Promotion of atrial fibrillation by heart failure in dogs: atrial remodeling of a different sort. *Circulation* 1999;**100**(1):87–95.
15. Wang TJ, Larson MG, Levy D, *et al.* Temporal relations of atrial fibrillation and congestive heart failure and their joint influence on mortality: the Framingham Heart Study. *Circulation* 2003;**107**(23):2920–25.
16. Wang TJ, Massaro JM, Levy D, *et al.* A risk score for predicting stroke or death in individuals with new-onset atrial fibrillation in the community: the Framingham Heart Study. *JAMA* 2003;**290**(8):1049–56.
17. Takarada A, Kurogane H, Hayashi T, *et al.* Prognostic significance of atrial fibrillation in dilated cardiomyopathy. *Jpn Heart J* 1993;**34**(6):749–58.
18. Lechat P, Hulot JS, Escolano S, *et al.* Bisoprolol in AF in HF Heart rate and cardiac rhythm relationships with bisoprolol benefit in chronic heart failure in CIBIS II Trial. *Circulation* 2001;**103**(10):1428–33.
19. Swedberg K, Olsson LG, Charlesworth A, *et al.* Prognostic relevance of atrial fibrillation in patients with chronic heart failure on long-term treatment with beta-blockers: results from COMET. *Eur Heart J* 2005;**26**(13):1303–8.
20. Olsson LG, Swedberg K, Ducharme A, *et al.*; CHARM Investigators. Atrial fibrillation and risk of clinical events in chronic heart failure with and without left ventricular systolic dysfunction: results from the Candesartan in Heart failure-Assessment of Reduction in Mortality and morbidity (CHARM) program. *J Am Coll Cardiol* 2006;**47**(10):1997–2004.
21. Singh SN, Poole J, Anderson J, *et al.*; SCD-HeFT Investigators. Role of amiodarone or implantable cardioverter/defibrillator in patients with atrial fibrillation and heart failure. *Am Heart J* 2006;**152**(5):974.e7–11.
22. Mogensen UM, Jhund PS, Abraham WT, *et al.* Type of atrial fibrillation and outcomes in patients with heart failure and reduced ejection fraction. *J Am Coll Cardiol* 2017;**70**: 2490–500.
23. Roy D, Talajic M, Nattel S, *et al.* Rhythm control versus rate control for atrial fibrillation and heart failure. *N Engl J Med* 2008;**358**(25):2667–77.
24. Wyse DG, Waldo AL, DiMarco JP, *et al.* A comparison of rate control and rhythm control in patients with atrial fibrillation. *N Engl J Med* 2002;**347**(23):1825–33.
25. Hsu LF, Jais P, Sanders P, *et al.* Catheter ablation for atrial fibrillation in congestive heart failure. *N Engl J Med* 2004;**351**(23):2373–83.
26. Chen MS, Marrouche NF, Khaykin Y, *et al.* Pulmonary vein isolation for the treatment of atrial fibrillation in patients with impaired systolic function. *J Am Coll Cardiol* 2004;**43**(6):1004–9.
27. Khan MN, Jais P, Cummings J, *et al.* Pulmonary-vein isolation for atrial fibrillation in patients with heart failure. *N Engl J Med* 2008;**359**:1778–85.
28. Al Halabi S, Qintar M, Hussein A, *et al.* Catheter ablation for atrial fibrillation in heart failure patients: a meta-analysis of randomized controlled trials. *J Am Coll Cardiol Clin Electrophysiol* 2015;**1**:200–9.
29. Anselmino M, Matta M, D'Ascenzo F, *et al.* Catheter ablation of atrial fibrillation in patients with left ventricular systolic dysfunction: a systematic review and meta-analysis. *Circ Arrhythm Electrophysiol* 2014;**7**:1011–18.

30. Marrouche NF, Brachmann J, Andresen D, *et al*. Catheter ablation for atrial fibrillation with heart failure. *N Engl J Med* 2018;**378**:417–27.

31. Packer M, Kowey PR. Building castles in the sky. *Circulation* 2018;**138**:751–3.

32. van Gelder IC, Groenveld HF, Crijns HJGM, *et al*. Lenient versus strict rate control in patients with atrial fibrillation. *N Engl J Med* 2010;**362**;1363–73.

33. Vamos M, Erath JW, Hohnloser SH. Digoxin-associated mortality: a systematic review and meta-analysis of the literature. *Eur Heart J* 2015;**36**:1831–8.

34. Brignole M, Menozzi C, Gianfranchi L, *et al*. Assessment of atrioventricular junction ablation and VVIR pacemaker versus pharmacological treatment in patients with heart failure and chronic atrial fibrillation: a randomized, controlled study. *Circulation* 1998;**98**(10):953–60.

35. Hay I, Melenovsky V, Fetics BJ, *et al*. Short-term effects of right-left heart sequential cardiac resynchronization in patients with heart failure, chronic atrial fibrillation, and atrioventricular nodal block. *Circulation* 2004;**110**(22):3404–10.

36. Chatterjee NA, Upadhyay GA, Ellenbogen KA, Hayes DL, Singh JP. Atrioventricular nodal ablation in atrial fibrillation: a meta-analysis of biventricular vs. right ventricular pacing mode. *Eur J Heart Fail* 2012;**14**:661–7.

37. Gasparini M, Leclercq C, Lunati M, *et al*. Cardiac resynchronization therapy in patients with atrial fibrillation. The CERTIFY Study (Cardiac Resynchronization Therapy in Atrial Fibrillation Patients Multinational Registry) *JACC Heart Fail* 2013;**1**:500–7.

38. Ponikowski P, Voors AA, Anker SD, *et al*. 2016 ESC Guidelines for the diagnosis and treatment of acute and chronic heart failure. *Eur Heart J* 2016;**37**:2129–200.

39. Hart RG, Pearce LA, Aguilar MI. Meta-analysis: antithrombotic therapy to prevent stroke in patients who have nonvalvular atrial fibrillation. *Ann Intern Med* 2007;**146**:857–67.

40. Ruff CT, Giugliano RP, Braunwald E, *et al*. Comparison of the efficacy and safety of new oral anticoagulants with warfarin in patients with atrial fibrillation: a meta-analysis of randomised trials. *Lancet* 2014;**383**(9921):955–62.

41. Kirchhof P, Benussi S, Kotecha D, *et al*. 2016 ESC guidelines for the management of atrial fibrillation developed in collaboration with EACTS. *Eur Heart J* 2016;**37**:2893–962.

42. Perez FJ, Schubert CM, Parvez B, *et al*. Long-term outcomes after catheter ablation of cavo-tricuspid isthmus dependent atrial flutter: a meta-analysis. *Circ Arrhythm Electrophysiol* 2009;**2**:393–401.

43. Rodgers M, McKenna C, Palmer S, *et al*. Curative catheter ablation in atrial fibrillation and typical atrial flutter: systematic review and economic evaluation. *Health Technol Assess* 2008;**12**(34):iii–iv, xi–xiii, 1–198.

44. Katritsis DG, Boriani G, Cosio FG, *et al*. European Heart Rhythm Association Consensus Document on the Management of Supraventricular Arrhythmias: Endorsed by Heart Rhythm Society (HRS), Asia-Pacific Heart Rhythm Society (APHRS), and Sociedad Latinoamericana de Estimulación Cardiaca y Electrofisiologia (SOLAECE). *Europace* 2017;**19**:465–511.

45. Noë P, Van Driel, V, Wittkampf F, Sreeram N. Rapid recovery of cardiac function after catheter ablation of persistent junctional reciprocating tachycardia in children. *Pacing Clin Electrophysiol* 2002;**25**(2):191–4.

46. Aguinaga L, Primo J, Anguera I, *et al*. Long-term follow-up in patients with the permanent form of junctional reciprocating tachycardia treated with radiofrequency ablation. *Pacing Clin Electrophysiol* 1998;**21**(11 Pt 1):2073–8.

47. Walker NL, Cobbe SM, Birnie DH. Tachycardiomyopathy: a diagnosis not to be missed. *Heart* 2004;**90**(2):e7.

48. Nikolic G, Bishop RL, Singh JB. Sudden death recorded during Holter monitoring. *Circulation* 1982;**66**(1):218–25.

49. de Sousa MR, Morillo CA, Rabelo FT, Nogueira Filho AM, Ribeiro AL. Non-sustained ventricular tachycardia as a predictor of sudden cardiac death in patients with left ventricular dysfunction: a meta-analysis. *Eur J Heart Fail* 2008;**10**(10):1007–14.

50. Doval HC, Nul DR, Grancelli HO, *et al*. Nonsustained ventricular tachycardia in severe heart failure. Independent marker of increased mortality due to sudden death. GESICA-GEMA Investigators. *Circulation* 1996;**94**(12):3198–203.

51. Kearney MT, Fox KA, Lee AJ, *et al*. Predicting sudden death in patients with mild to moderate chronic heart failure. *Heart* 2004;**90**(10):1137–43.

52. Akar FG, Rosenbaum DS. Transmural electrophysiological heterogeneities underlying arrhythmogenesis in heart failure. *Circ Res* 2003;**93**(7):638–45.

53. Sicouri S, Antzelevitch C. A subpopulation of cells with unique electrophysiological properties in the deep subepicardium of the canine ventricle. The M cell. *Circ Res* 1991;**68**(6):1729–41.

54. Akar FG, Yan GX, Antzelevitch C, Rosenbaum DS. Unique topographical distribution of M cells underlies reentrant mechanism of torsade de pointes in the long-QT syndrome. *Circulation* 2002;**105**(10):1247–53.

55. Tomaselli GF, Marban E. Electrophysiological remodeling in hypertrophy and heart failure. *Cardiovasc Res* 1999;**42**(2):270–83.

56. McIntosh MA, Cobbe SM, Smith GL. Heterogeneous changes in action potential and intracellular Ca2+ in left ventricular myocyte sub-types from rabbits with heart failure. *Cardiovasc Res* 2000;**45**(2):397–409.

57. Pogwizd SM, Schlotthauer K, Li L, Yuan W, Bers DM. Arrhythmogenesis and contractile dysfunction in heart failure: roles of sodium–calcium exchange, inward rectifier potassium current, and residual beta-adrenergic responsiveness. *Circ Res* 2001;**88**(11):1159–67.

58. Shamim W. Intraventricular conduction delay: a prognostic marker in chronic heart failre. *Int J Cardiol* 1999;**70**:171–8.

59. Shamim W, Yousufuddin M, Cicoria M, *et al*. Incremental changes in QRS duration in serial ECGs over time identify high risk elderly patients with heart failure. *Heart* 2002;**88**(1):47–51.

60. Cleland JGF, Daubert JC, Erdmann E, *et al*. The effect of cardiac resynchronization on morbidity and mortality in heart failure. *N Engl J Med* 2005;**352**;1539–49.

61. Bristow MR, Saxon LA, Boehmer J, *et al*. Cardiac-resynchronization therapy with or without an implantable defibrillator in advanced chronic heart failure. *N Engl J Med* 2004;**350**(21):2140–50.

62. Pye MP, Cobbe SM. Arrhythmogenesis in experimental models of heart failure: the role of increased load. *Cardiovasc Res* 1996;**32**(2):248–57.

63. Uretsky BF, Thygesen K, Armstrong PW, *et al*. Acute coronary findings at autopsy in heart failure patients with sudden death: results from the Assessment of Treatment With Lisinopril and Survival (ATLAS) Trial. *Circulation* 2000;**102**(6):611–16.

64. Saeed M, Link MS, Mahapatra S, *et al*. Analysis of intracardiac electrograms showing monomorphic ventricular tachycardia in patients with implantable cardioverter-defibrillators. *Am J Cardiol* 2000;**85**(5):580–7.

65. Zang M, Zhang T, Mao J, Zhou S, He B. Beneficial effects of catheter ablation of frequent premature ventricular complexes on left ventricular function. *Heart* 2014;**100**:787–93.

66. Wellens HJ. Ventricular tachycardia: diagnosis of broad QRS complex tachycardia. *Heart* 2001;**86**(5):579–85.

67. Brugada P, Brugada J, Mont L, Smeets J, Andries EW. A new approach to the differential diagnosis of a regular tachycardia with a wide QRS complex. *Circulation* 1991;**83**(5):1649–59.

68. Campbell RW. ACE inhibitors and arrhythmias. *Heart* 1996;**76**(3 Suppl 3):79–82.

69. Cohn JN, Johnson G, Ziesche S, et al. A comparison of enalapril with hydralazine-isosorbide dinitrate in the treatment of chronic congestive heart failure. *N Engl J Med* 1991;**325**(5):303–10.

70. Pitt B, Zannad F, Remme WJ, et al. The effect of spironolactone on morbidity and mortality in patients with severe heart failure. Randomized Aldactone Evaluation Study Investigators. *N Engl J Med* 1999;**341**(10):709–17.

71. Ramires FJ, Mansur A, Coelho O, et al. Effect of spironolactone on ventricular arrhythmias in congestive heart failure secondary to idiopathic dilated or to ischemic cardiomyopathy. *Am J Cardiol* 2000;**85**(10):1207–11.

72. Pitt B, Remme W, Zannad F, et al. Eplerenone, a selective aldosterone blocker, in patients with left ventricular dysfunction after myocardial infarction. *N Engl J Med* 2003;**348**(14):1309–21.

73. Greene HL, Roden DM, Katz RJ, et al. The Cardiac Arrhythmia Suppression Trial: first CAST ... then CAST-II. *J Am Coll Cardiol* 1992;**19**(5):894–8.

74. Cairns JA, Connolly SJ, Roberts R, Gent M. Randomised trial of outcome after myocardial infarction in patients with frequent or repetitive ventricular premature depolarisations: CAMIAT. Canadian Amiodarone Myocardial Infarction Arrhythmia Trial Investigators. *Lancet* 1997;**349**(9053):675–82.

75. Julian DG, Camm AJ, Frangin G, et al. Randomised trial of effect of amiodarone on mortality in patients with left-ventricular dysfunction after recent myocardial infarction: EMIAT. European Myocardial Infarct Amiodarone Trial Investigators. *Lancet* 1997;**349**(9053):667–74.

76. Amiodarone Trials Meta-Analysis Investigators. Effect of prophylactic amiodarone on mortality after acute myocardial infarction and in congestive heart failure: meta-analysis of individual data from 6500 patients in randomised trials. *Lancet* 1997;**350**(9089):1417–24.

77. Bardy GH, Lee KL, Mark DB, et al. Amiodarone or an implantable cardioverter-defibrillator for congestive heart failure. *N Engl J Med* 2005;**352**(3):225–37.

78. Kober L, Torp-Pedersen C, McMurray JJV, et al. Increased mortality after dronedarone therapy for severe heart failure. *N Engl J Med* 2008;**358**(25):2678–87.

79. Antiarrhythmics versus Implantable Defibrillators (AVID) Investigators. A comparison of antiarrhythmic-drug therapy with implantable defibrillators in patients resuscitated from near-fatal ventricular arrhythmias. *N Engl J Med* 1997;**337**(22):1576–84.

80. Kuck KH, Cappato R, Siebels J, Ruppel R. Randomized comparison of antiarrhythmic drug therapy with implantable defibrillators in patients resuscitated from cardiac arrest: the Cardiac Arrest Study Hamburg (CASH). *Circulation* 2000;**102**(7):748–54.

81. Connolly SJ, Gent M, Roberts RS, et al. Canadian implantable defibrillator study (CIDS): a randomized trial of the implantable cardioverter defibrillator against amiodarone. *Circulation* 2000;**101**(11):1297–302.

82. Moss AJ, Zareba W, Hall WJ, et al. Prophylactic implantation of a defibrillator in patients with myocardial infarction and reduced ejection fraction. *N Engl J Med* 2002;**346**(12):877–83.

83. Segal OR, Chow AW, Wong T, et al. A novel algorithm for determining endocardial VT exit site from 12-lead surface ECG characteristics in human, infarct-related ventricular tachycardia. *J Cardiovasc Electrophysiol* 2007;**18**(2):161–8.

84. Reddy VY, Reynolds MR, Neuzil P, et al. Prophylactic catheter ablation for the prevention of defibrillator therapy. *N Engl J Med* 2007;**357**(26):2657–65.

85. Estes NA, III. Ablation after ICD implantation—bridging the gap between promise and practice. *N Engl J Med* 2007;**357**(26):2717–9.

86. Kuck KH, Schaumann A, Eckardt L, et al. Catheter ablation of stable ventricular tachycardia before defibrillator implantation in patients with coronary heart disease (VTACH): a multicentre randomised controlled trial. *Lancet* 2010;**375**(9708):31–40.

87. Sapp JL, Wells GA, Parkash R, et al. Ventricular tachycardia ablation versus escalation of antiarrhythmic drugs. *N Engl J Med* 2016;**375**(2):111–21.

88. Nayyar S, Ganesan AN, Brooks AG, et al. Venturing into ventricular arrhythmia storm: a systematic review and meta-analysis. *Eur Heart J* 2013;**34**(8):560–71.

89. Schoeller R, Andresen D, Buttner P, et al. First or second degree atrioventricular block as a risk factor in idiopathic dilated cardiomyopathy. *Am J Cardiol* 1993;**71**(8):720–6.

90. Kusumoto FM, Schoenfeld MH, Barrett C, et al. 2018 ACC/AHA/HRS Guideline on the Evaluation and Management of Patients With Bradycardia and Cardiac Conduction Delay: A Report of the American College of Cardiology/American Heart Association Task Force on Clinical Practice Guidelines and the Heart Rhythm Society. *Circulation* 2019;**140**(8):e382–e482.

91. National Audit of Cardiac Rhythm Management Devices 2020: https://www.nicor.org.uk/wp-content/uploads/2020/12/National-Audit-of-Cardiac-Rhythm-Management-NACRM-FINAL.pdf.

92. Nielsen JC1, Thomsen PE, Højberg S, et al.; DANPACE Investigators. A comparison of single-lead atrial pacing with dual-chamber pacing in sick sinus syndrome. *Eur Heart J* 2011;**32**(6):686–96.

93. Sweeney MO, Shea JB, Fox V, et al. Randomized pilot study of a new atrial-based minimal ventricular pacing mode in dual-chamber implantable cardioverter-defibrillators. *Heart Rhythm* 2004;**1**:160–7.

94. Healey JS, Toff WD, Lamas GA, et al. Cardiovascular outcomes with atrial-based pacing compared with ventricular pacing: meta-analysis of randomized trials, using individual patient data. *Circulation* 2006;**114**:11–17.

95. Lamas GA, Lee KL, Sweeney MO, et al. Ventricular pacing or dual-chamber pacing for sinus-node dysfunction *N Engl J Med* 2002;**346**:1854–62.

96. Toff WD, Camm AJ, Skehan JD. Single-chamber versus dual-chamber pacing for high-grade atrioventricular block. *N Engl J Med* 2005;**353**:145–55.

97. Wilkoff BL, Cook JR, Epstein AE. Dual-chamber pacing or ventricular backup pacing in patients with an implantable defibrillator: the Dual Chamber and VVI Implantable Defibrillator (DAVID) Trial. *JAMA* 2002;**288**:3115–23.

98. Lindsay BD. Deleterious effects of right ventricular pacing. *N Engl J Med* 2009;**361**:2183–85.

99. Yu CM, Chan JYS, Zhang Q, *et al.* Biventricular pacing in patients with bradycardia and normal ejection fraction. *N Engl J Med* 2009;**361**:2123–34.

100. Bradley DJ, Bradley EA, Baughman KL, *et al.* Cardiac resynchronization and death from progressive heart failure: a meta-analysis of randomized controlled trials. *JAMA* 2003;**289**:730–9.

101. Curtis AB, Worley SJ, Adamson PB, *et al.*; Biventricular versus Right Ventricular Pacing in Heart Failure Patients with Atrioventricular Block (BLOCK HF) Trial Investigators. Biventricular pacing for atrioventricular block and systolic dysfunction. *N Engl J Med* 2013;**368**: 1585–93.

41

Pregnancy

Lorna Swan and Niki L. Walker

Introduction

Heart failure is one of the commonest cardiac complications associated with pregnancy. It is the 'common final pathway' of many pre-existing and de-novo cardiac lesions that have either presented or decompensated during pregnancy. Its aetiology varies across the world (**Figure 41.1**), but, no matter the cause, pregnancy may pose a significant challenge when the circulation is 'vulnerable'.

With improvements in paediatric and adult cardiac care there are now large populations of young women who have either stable or 'recovered' left ventricular dysfunction. Many of these patients are well controlled on medical therapy, and are leading lives that are difficult to differentiate from the normal population. The desire to have a family is part of that normality. However, these women do not have a normal outcome during pregnancy and access to detailed pre-conception counselling is essential for all such women of child-bearing age.[1] This chapter will outline the key importance of pre-conception counselling in those with known disease and the need for specialist acute care pathways for those with a new diagnosis.

Physiology of normal pregnancy

Pregnancy is a normal physiological process rather than a disease. However, it is a challenge even to normal hearts. There is a significant increase in cardiac output, retention of sodium and water leading to blood volume expansion, and a reduction in systemic vascular resistance (**Figure 41.2**). The contributors to the fall in vascular resistance and related fall in blood pressure are complex and include hormonal factors and changes in prostacyclin, nitric oxide, and decreased responsiveness to factors including angiotensin II and norepinephrine.[2,3] Pregnancy is also a pro-arrhythmic and pro-thrombotic state.

All of these adaptive changes are in order to optimize the conditions to facilitate foetal growth and development. These changes in maternal physiology begin early after conception, peak during the second trimester, then remain relatively constant until delivery.

At the time of labour and delivery there are further changes in maternal physiology which can be compounded by anxiety, pain

and bleeding. Anaesthesia or analgesia may also have a detrimental physiological impact. Cardiac output increases during labour by almost 25%. This is compounded by an increase in pre-load as each contraction returns blood to the systemic circulation from the uterine sinusoids. Active pushing in the second stage of labour achieves a 50% increase in cardiac output in women with normal hearts, and this increases further with the auto-transfusion that occurs immediately after delivery and uterine contraction.[4]

During active labour, blood pressure increases by 10–25% with each uterine contraction, depending on duration of contraction, pain, anxiety, and position of the mother. In addition, bearing down and pushing create effects of repeated Valsalva manoeuvres. All of these changes can potentially be a challenge to the patient with impaired cardiac reserve. Pre-pregnancy baseline levels of cardiac output and systemic vascular resistance are gradually achieved after at least 12 weeks postpartum.[5]

Epidemiology of heart failure in pregnancy

The incidence of overt heart failure during pregnancy is unknown. Furthermore, there may be many additional women with silent and transient ventricular dysfunction, particularly at the time of delivery or in the setting of pre-eclampsia. The data we do have relate to short-term mortality and severe morbidity. In the latest UK Confidential Enquiry into Maternal Death[6] myocardial disease was the leading cause of maternal cardiac death. The numbers of deaths were small but the more sizable issue is that of severe maternal morbidity. This was highlighted in a national registry from the Netherlands.[7] This registry covers all of the country's 98 maternity units serving a population of 17 million people. In this study, cardiomyopathy was the commonest cause of cardiovascular events significant enough to trigger emergency admission to a high dependency unit in hospital. For every one death due to heart failure there were in excess of 10 women with severe morbidity.

In women of child-bearing age seeking pre-conception counselling, the most common causes of ventricular dysfunction in a western country are idiopathic and familial dilated cardiomyopathy (DCM), previous myocarditis, previous chemotherapeutic agent exposure, prior peripartum cardiomyopathy, and a large group of

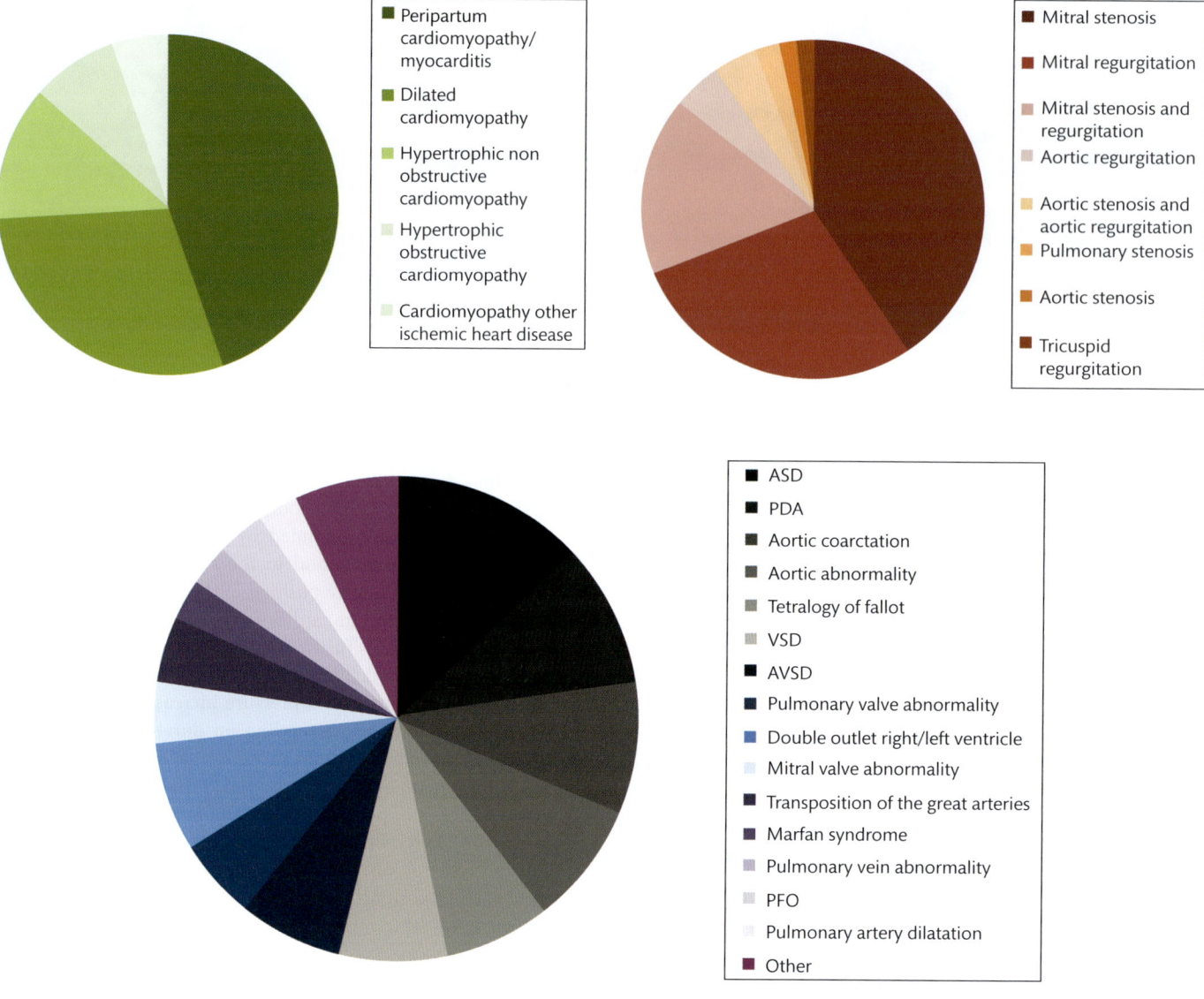

Green–Cardiomyopathy (n = 36). Red–Valve disease (n = 64) and other shades–congenital heart disease (n–71)

Figure 41.1 Causes of heart failure during pregnancy. ASD, atrial septal defect; PDA, patent ductus arteriosus; VSD, ventricular septal defect; AVSD, atrioventricular septal defect; PFO, patent foramen ovale.

Source data from Ruys TP, Roos-Hesselink JW, Hall R, Subirana-Domènech MT, Grando-Ting J, Estensen M, *et al*. Heart failure in pregnant women with cardiac disease: data from the ROPAC. *Heart* 2014;**100**(3):231–8.

diverse congenital heart disease lesions. In other parts of the world valvular heart disease (especially rheumatic mitral stenosis) predominates. Treatment for all types of myocardial dysfunction during pregnancy is improving with a case fatality rate of 10%.[7]

Pre-conception counselling

All women of child-bearing age with known myocardial disease should be offered pre-conception counselling, and it should be remembered that with assisted fertility techniques 'child bearing age' may extend well beyond age 40 years. This counselling should be performed by a specialist team with expertise in maternal cardiac

disease and, at a minimum, should include a high-risk specialist obstetrician and a cardiologist with expertise in pregnancy. Pre-pregnancy counselling needs to comprehensively address multiple issues (**Box 41.1**) pertaining to the mother and the foetus. The most important of these is the risk of precipitating heart failure.

Stratifying risk

There are several useful scoring systems to determine pregnancy risk for women with pre-existing cardiac disease. The original system was the CARPREG score, which awards points for various pre-pregnancy risk factors—this included a history of a prior cardiac event (such as heart failure), and a pre-pregnancy reduction in systemic ventricular dysfunction of <40%. A New York Heart

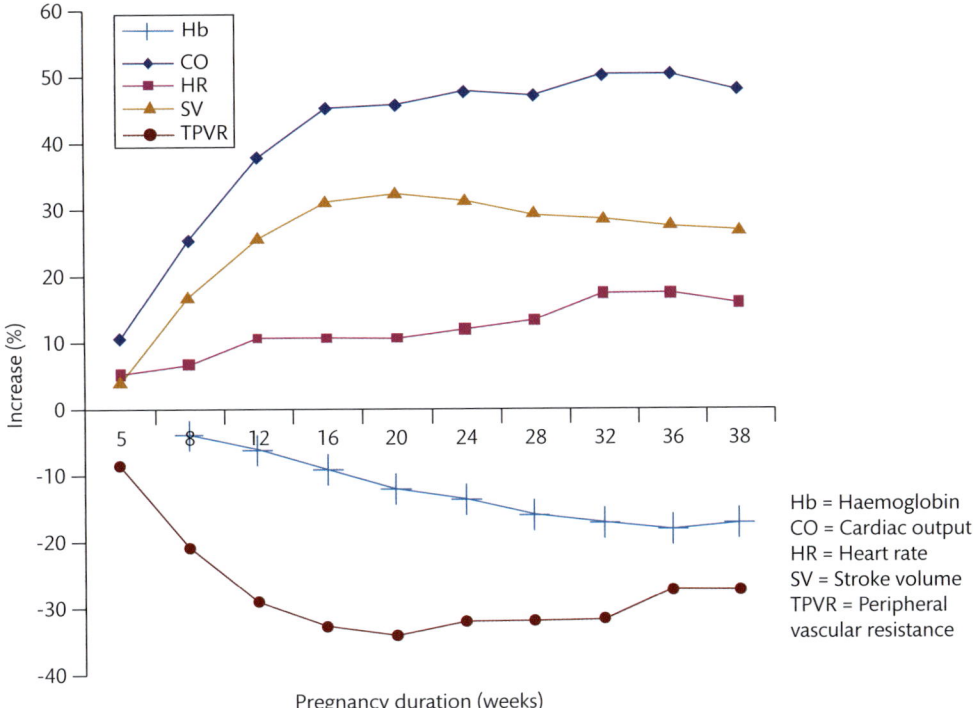

Figure 41.2 Haemodynamic changes of pregnancy.
Reproduced from Emmanuel Y *et al. Best Practice & Research Clinical Obstetrics and Gynaecology* 2015. **29**; 597e.

Association (NYHA) class >II is also a risk factor.[8] A similar scoring system was then described by the ZAHARA investigators although this identified the additional risk factors of the use of cardiac medication pre-pregnancy, and the presence of regurgitant atrioventricular valves.[9] More recently it has been suggested that the most useful scoring system is the modified World Health Organization (mWHO) classification. This allocates patients to a risk group dependent on their underlying cardiac condition (rather than on prior events).[10] In the mWHO classification, patients with moderate ventricular dysfunction would be in risk class III. This group is said to have a 'significantly increased risk of maternal mortality or severe morbidity' and should be cared for in a 'specialist multidisciplinary cardiac obstetric unit'. Those with an ejection fraction of <30% would be in mWHO class IV, where pregnancy should be considered to be contraindicated. Most recently, these risk groups have been applied to various populations of pregnant patients with cardiac disease (ROPAC registry). This demonstrated that women in mWHO Class III had a maternal mortality of 1.5% and a risk of heart failure of 19%. Overall the risk of hospitalization due to cardiac issues was 36%.[11]

Other risk factors to consider

Although a useful overview, the current pregnancy scoring systems are not comprehensive enough to be the only source of information given to a woman planning a high-risk pregnancy. There are multiple other considerations. One important determinant of outcome is the aetiology of ventricular dysfunction, and the expected natural history of the underlying pathology. For example, those with a known progressive disorder such as neuromuscular-related cardiomyopathy[12] are likely to have a poorer pregnancy outcome than patients with a less aggressive cause of ventricular dysfunction.

Ejection fraction is the traditional measure used to assess ventricular function in pregnancy studies. More recently other parameters have been investigation. One of the most promising is stress-echo-determined contractile reserve. In women with recovered peripartum cardiomyopathy (Chapter 12) and a normalized ejection fraction, contractile reserve has given additional information regarding the risk of heart failure in a subsequent pregnancy.

Box 41.1 Pre-conception check list

Maternal factors

- What are the CARPREG, ZAHARA, and modified WHO scores?
- What is the current functional class? Cardiac symptoms?
- Are there arrhythmia issues? Pacing or device issues?
- Risk of ventricular dysfunction?
- Risk of bleeding or thrombosis?
- Are the pulmonary artery pressures normal?
- Risk of ischaemia?
- Risk of dissection?
- Increased risk of hypertension?
- What drugs need to be changed?
- Are there lifestyle issues?
- Any obstetric or non-cardiac issues?
- What is the long-term prognosis?

Fetal factors

- Risk due to low maternal cardiac output?
- Risk of maternal cyanosis?
- Risk due to maternal medication?
- Risk of prematurity or growth restriction?
- Genetic or foetal recurrence risk?

Although the ejection fraction was the same in the two groups, those with a good contractile reserve were much less likely to have a relapse of heart failure than those with a blunted reserve, 23% of whom relapsed.[13] Whether this tool is equally useful in other forms of 'cured' cardiomyopathy patients planning pregnancy is unclear.

Newer risk stratification tools

In more recent studies, pre-pregnancy exercise stress testing has been used as a part of a comprehensive baseline assessment. These studies have not specifically looked at cardiomyopathy patients but at a heterogeneous group of women with cardiac disease. Peak heart rate and peak oxygen uptake are both higher in patients who go on to have a pregnancy without a maternal cardiac event.[14] In a separate study a good chronotropic response was shown to be associated with a better foetal outcome.[15]

Biomarkers are another area of interest. B-type natriuretic peptide (BNP) and N-terminal (NT)-proBNP stay relatively stable throughout a normal pregnancy. In women with heart disease, BNP is significantly elevated in those who have maternal cardiac events.[16] BNP has also been used to predict outcome when measured at 20 weeks.[17] In these studies, NT-proBNP >100 pg/mL is often associated with a maternal cardiac event during pregnancy. Further studies will be needed to assess the utility of a pre-pregnancy BNP level in predicting adverse events. Many units use a serial measurement of BNP to monitor a woman's progress during pregnancy.

Pre-conception medication

One area of difficulty is whether women should be assessed (pre-conception) on or off their full heart failure therapy. Several heart failure medications must be discontinued in pregnancy (such as angiotensin converting enzyme (ACE) inhibitors or spironolactone) due to their associated teratogenicity. Discontinuing these drugs may have a negative impact on cardiac performance. Several authors would suggest that these medications are discontinued and the woman assessed off therapy. Others suggest continuing therapy until conception if a woman is adamant she wishes to proceed with a pregnancy irrespective of her results off treatment. Although several medications need to be discontinued during pregnancy, others should be continued and may need to be increased. This includes β-blockers (see below regarding treatment).

Discussing long-term maternal outcome

The long-term prognosis of a patient with ventricular dysfunction must be part of the pre-conception discussion. There are few data to quantify how a pregnancy, or several pregnancies, impact on long-term outcome but it is believed that pregnancy is likely to have a chronic, adverse effect on systemic ventricular function.[18] Clinicians working in this field all have salutatory anecdotal cases of women who have successfully negotiated pregnancy only to spiral into severe heart failure in the subsequent couple of years. A further consideration is the impact of pregnancy on maternal antibody production, as maternal sensitization reduces the possibility of a successful transplant in the years to come.[19]

Foetal outcomes

When women seek pre-pregnancy advice, their questions rarely focus only on short-term maternal outcomes. Many of their questions surround foetal outcome and whether they will be fit enough

to look after their child in the years to come. These conversations should be handled very openly with the cardiologist, obstetrician, and neonatal team, talking through the potential likely scenarios. One particularly emotive scenario is to discuss with the woman the therapeutic options and foetal issues surrounding severe heart failure decompensation at 24–27 weeks. From epidemiology studies, it is clear that there are two peaks of heart failure during pregnancy. The first occurs at 23–30 weeks and the second post peri-delivery.[20] Pre-conception counselling should include a detailed discussion of the issues of extreme prematurity and foetal outcome if a woman was to require urgent delivery at these earlier gestations due to decompensated heart failure. Even with significant improvements in neonatal care, a baby born at 25 weeks is still at high risk of death or severe morbidity/disability.

Comprehensive pre-conception counselling includes a focus on foetal outcomes. Registry data have shown that women with heart failure have an additional risk of premature delivery, foetal growth restriction, and low birth weight. There are various possible causes for growth restriction including reduced cardiac output and the use of maternal β-blockers. In patients with a known familial cardiomyopathy the risk of recurrent disease in the foetus needs to be considered. The use of comprehensive family genotyping will help quantify this risk. Given the variability in the expression of many of these conditions, prenatal diagnosis (with maternal chorionic villus sampling) and preimplantation genetic diagnosis are only offered in some units and are variably taken up by families.

Antenatal care

There is no single specific template for antenatal care for these women. The precise antenatal care plan will be dependent on the individual risk of patients and their additional needs (Table 41.1). In the first trimester, the keys to care are ensuring that the patient is fully aware of the implications of pregnancy (and offering termination of pregnancy if appropriate), ensuring the woman has access to the expert high-risk cardiac obstetric team, and establishing the correct treatment regimen. Baseline imaging and bloodwork are required and any diagnostic uncertainties need to be clarified where possible. From an obstetric perspective, a dating scan will be required. In women with significant risk of decompensation, serial imaging should be arranged—this is usually transthoracic echo and may need to be performed up to every 4–6 weeks. Cardiac magnetic resonance imaging has a role if there is any diagnostic uncertainty, although the use of gadolinium is contraindicated.[21]

When following patients with echo antenatally, care should be taken to perform a comprehensive study. Focus on the left ventricular ejection fraction alone is inadequate, especially in patients with conditions such as hypertrophic cardiomyopathy.

Antenatal treatment

Care during pregnancy will be guided by maternal symptoms, echo parameters, exercise tolerance and BNP concentrations. The presence of new arrhythmia may also herald decompensation. Furosemide, β-blockers, nitrates, and hydralazine can all be used in pregnancy. Hospitalization with bed-rest may also be of value. Foetal growth and uterine Doppler will also be informative. Early maternal delivery is indicated when there is severe maternal or foetal

Table 41.1 Cardiac drugs in pregnancy

Drug	Class	Previous FDA category[a]	Potential adverse effects
Furosemide	Diuretic	C	Oligohydramnion
Bisoprolol	β-Blocker	C	Foetal growth restriction, bradycardia and hypoglycaemia
Digoxin	Cardiac glycoside	C	Serum levels are unreliable
Hydralazine	Vasodilator	C	Maternal lupus-like syndrome. Foetal arrhythmias
Isosorbide dinitrate	Nitrates	B	Bradycardia
Spironolactone	Aldosterone antagonist	D	Antiandrogen effects; foetal cleft palate (first trimester)
Eplerenone	Aldosterone antagonist	B	Limited data regarding risk
Candesartan	Angiotensin II receptor blocker	D	Renal issues, growth restriction, ossification disorders, foetal death
Enalapril	ACE inhibitor	D	Renal issues, growth restriction, ossification disorders, foetal death

FDA, US Food and Drug Administration; ACE, angiotensin converting enzyme.

[a] FDA categories have now been replaced with a narrative description of risks.

Previous FDA categories: (A) Well-controlled studies have failed to demonstrate foetal risk. (B) Animal studies have failed to demonstrate foetal risk and there are no adequate and well-controlled human studies. (C) Animal studies have shown an adverse effect on the foetus but potential benefits may warrant use of the drug in pregnant women despite potential risks. (D) There is positive evidence of human foetal risk but potential benefits may warrant use despite potential risks. **X** Studies have demonstrated that foetal abnormalities and the risks involved in use of the drug in pregnant women clearly outweigh potential benefits.

compromise not responding to medical therapy. All of these treatment decisions should be made by the multidisciplinary team and the routine obstetric antenatal treatments should not be forgotten (e.g. maternal vaccination against influenza).

New diagnosis of heart failure in pregnancy

Women with no previous cardiac history may present at any stage of pregnancy with a new diagnosis of heart failure. The most common presenting symptom is breathlessness, but fatigue, reduced exercise capacity, and peripheral oedema may also be reported. However, these are all common features in a normal pregnancy.

Differentiating normal pregnancy from pathological breathlessness is based on clinical history, examination, and focused investigations. Because the symptoms of heart failure may overlap with the symptoms of a normal pregnancy, clinicians involved in the care of pregnant women require an index of suspicion before attributing symptoms as normal. For example, orthopnoea is not a normal feature of pregnancy, nor is paroxysmal nocturnal dyspnoea. If a pregnant woman develops new or worsening symptoms suggestive of heart failure, the attending clinician should:

- take a detailed **history**;
- **examine** the patient for evidence of lung crepitations, arrhythmia, peripheral oedema, murmurs;
- check a dipstick **urinalysis** for proteinuria;
- arrange **blood tests** including full blood count, renal function, thyroid function, BNP; and consider troponin assay if there has been a history of chest pain;
- review the **electrocardiogram** for arrhythmia, ST–T changes, bundle branch block or features of ventricular hypertrophy, and establish continuous ECG monitoring as there is a risk of arrhythmias;
- assess ventricular function (both systolic and diastolic) and valvar function with **transthoracic echocardiography**;
- perform a **chest X-ray** if there is clinical doubt. Although one strives to minimize radiation exposure in pregnancy, if there is diagnostic uncertainty it is imperative to perform the required imaging.

The differential diagnosis of new-onset breathlessness in pregnancy includes pulmonary thromboembolism, asthma, pneumonia, and pre-eclampsia. Pre-eclampsia may be recognized by the presence of hypertension with proteinuria. However, it should be recognized that pre-eclampsia and heart failure can coexist. Breathlessness may be the manifestation of acidosis, e.g. in diabetic ketoacidosis.

Once the diagnosis of heart failure has been made, management should be initiated and an aetiology sought. There are three pregnancy-related causes of heart failure (pre-eclampsia, peripartum cardiomyopathy, and amniotic fluid embolism) in addition to the full spectrum of non-pregnancy causes of heart failure that may present in pregnancy. Anthony and Sliwa[22] suggest a classification for non-pregnancy-related aetiologies of heart failure:

- increased vascular resistance;
- diseases of the aortic root;
- heart disease—ventricular dysfunction, obstruction, congenital abnormalities (of the heart or the proximal vessels).

Increased vascular resistance

Pre-eclampsia

Pre-eclampsia is diagnosed when a previously normotensive woman has new-onset hypertension and either proteinuria or end-organ dysfunction after 20 weeks of gestation. It is thought that pre-eclampsia affects 2–8% of pregnancies, with ~0.5% of pregnancies developing severe pre-eclampsia.[23]

The diagnostic criteria for pre-eclampsia are a systemic blood pressure ≥140 mmHg or diastolic blood pressure ≥90 mmHg *and* proteinuria ≥0.3 g/24 h, or protein:creatinine ratio ≥30 mg/mmol, *or* signs of end-organ dysfunction. Signs of end-organ dysfunction include a platelet count <100 000/μL, a serum creatinine doubling or >97 μmol/L (1.1 mg/dL), and elevated serum transaminases of greater than twice upper limit of normal.[24]

Pre-eclampsia can cause pulmonary oedema because the increase in systemic vascular resistance associated with pre-eclampsia results

in increased filling pressures in the left atrium and left ventricle. Occasionally left ventricular systolic dysfunction can be seen on echo with severe pre-eclampsia.

Hypertensive cardiomyopathy secondary to long-standing systemic hypertension may cause diastolic dysfunction that may manifest in pregnancy. Chronic hypertension may predispose the woman to pre-eclampsia, foetal growth restriction, pre-term birth, and placental abruption.[25]

Pulmonary hypertension

Pulmonary hypertension is an mWHO class IV condition when assessing women with heart disease considering pregnancy. In other words, there is a high risk of maternal mortality and morbidity. Therefore, women with pulmonary hypertension should be advised against pregnancy and referred for pre-pregnancy counselling to a clinician with experience in cardiac obstetrics. There should also be careful counselling about contraceptive options if advocating against pregnancy.

Unfortunately, pulmonary hypertension may first manifest in pregnancy. Exertional breathlessness is the most common symptom. Exercise-related syncope is another presentation that should raise concern of the possibility of pulmonary hypertension. The major concern with pulmonary hypertension in pregnancy is the potential for the development of acute right heart failure. This risk persists for at least two weeks postpartum, and women diagnosed with pulmonary hypertension associated with pregnancy should remain in hospital for at least two weeks after delivery.

Aortic root disease and heart failure

Aortic disease may present in pregnancy with heart failure symptoms because of acute aortic dissection or aortic valve regurgitation secondary to aortopathies such as Marfan syndrome. Inflammatory aortopathy, for example Takayasu's arteritis, may cause hypertensive cardiomyopathy or aortic valve dysfunction due to the aortopathy. With the ageing obstetric population there may be an increase in atherosclerotic aortopathy that may cause aortic valve dysfunction or be associated with hypertensive cardiomyopathy.

De-novo heart disease: ventricular dysfunction

Left ventricular systolic dysfunction may arise *de novo* during pregnancy. By definition, these women will not have had access to any pre-conception counselling and may present at any gestation.

Peripartum cardiomyopathy

Peripartum cardiomyopathy, the most concerning of these, is discussed in Chapter 12.

Amniotic fluid embolism syndrome

Amniotic fluid embolism syndrome presents with cardiorespiratory collapse, coagulopathy, and frequently with coma or seizures. Large amounts of amniotic fluid with foetal material enter the maternal circulation and prompt an acute inflammatory and anaphylactoid reaction, with pulmonary hypertension causing acute right ventricular failure, then left ventricular failure with pulmonary oedema. It is rare but important to consider as the need

for prompt and aggressive support is essential to allow a chance for survival.[26]

Ischaemic cardiomyopathy

Ischaemic cardiomyopathy may be acute or chronic. The acute presentation is usually of chest pain with ECG change and consequent left ventricular systolic dysfunction. Acute coronary syndromes presenting in pregnancy remain infrequent, affecting approximately one in 10 000 pregnancies. The aetiology may be atherosclerotic, coronary artery dissection, or, infrequently, related to the anomalous course of a coronary artery.

With an ageing obstetric population, more women are contemplating or pursuing pregnancy who have previously had an acute coronary syndrome. A proportion of these women have an established ischaemic cardiomyopathy, and these patients should have access to specialist pre-conception counselling.[11]

Other cardiomyopathies

A wide range of alternative causes of cardiomyopathy may present for the first time with heart failure in pregnancy. These include:

- **inherited cardiomyopathies**, such as hypertrophic cardiomyopathy, dilated cardiomyopathy, arrhythmogenic right ventricular cardiomyopathy;
- **toxin-related cardiomyopathies**, such as alcohol, illicit drug use with amphetamines, chemotherapy, radiotherapy;
- **acute myocarditis**, such as viral-mediated or autoimmune;
- **tachycardiomyopathy** or cardiomyopathy related to profound bradyarrhythmias.

De-novo heart failure secondary to valve dysfunction

Valvular heart disease may present with heart failure during pregnancy because the haemodynamic challenge of pregnancy unmasks the severity of the lesion. In general, regurgitant lesions are reasonably well-tolerated in pregnancy. The most common cause of valvular heart disease in young women is rheumatic heart disease. Other causes include congenital heart disease, including bicuspid aortic valves.

Mitral stenosis and aortic stenosis may present with breathlessness as the first manifestation of heart failure in pregnancy. The haemodynamic lesion may be further exacerbated by pregnancy-related anaemia or the development of arrhythmias.

Women with established valvular heart disease may have had previous surgical intervention. However, this does not prevent acute heart failure in pregnancy. Valves may re-stenose following valvotomy, bioprosthetic valve replacements may fail acutely in pregnancy, and mechanical valve replacements may thrombose in pregnancy and cause acute heart failure. Therefore, these women should be counselled pre-pregnancy about the potential risks and the need for follow-up during pregnancy.

De-novo heart failure: congenital lesions

Most women with congenital heart disease will be known to their cardiac specialist and will tolerate pregnancy well. These women will have access to pre-conception counselling and should be in optimal health prior to pregnancy. However, the women at greatest risk are those who are undiagnosed (e.g. a woman with an undiagnosed

coarctation of the aorta), or those lost to follow-up who may be unaware of the potential risk or not optimized structurally from a cardiac perspective prior to a planned pregnancy.[27]

Acute heart failure management

The initial assessment of an acutely breathless pregnant or peripartum woman is discussed in 'Foetal outcomes'. Having established a diagnosis of heart failure, a management plan is defined to progress care. The exact management will depend on the stage of pregnancy. If the woman is pregnant but <24 weeks gestation the management is different from that of a postpartum woman.

The available data on maternal deaths, for example the Confidential Enquiry into Maternal Deaths in the UK (CMACE is now superseded by the MBRRACE-UK,[28] i.e. 'Mothers and Babies: Reducing Risk through Audits and Confidential Enquiries across the UK') highlights the importance of *early* recognition of the severity of illness and involvement of key team members including senior obstetrics (both obstetrician and midwife), senior cardiologist, senior intensivists and anaesthetists. A senior neonatologist should be involved in the discussions if the woman is pregnant with a viable foetus. Together this multidisciplinary team must agree the location for care (depends on local service provision considering the needs of the mother first); the timing of delivery if pregnant (rather than postpartum); consider the options to optimize foetal outcome; and deliver strategies to treat acute heart failure.

Location of care

The correct location of care for the woman will depend on local facility configuration and the current needs of the woman. In some centres, the labour ward is a high-dependency setting with input from obstetrics, physicians, and intensivists, whereas in other units the labour ward is the domain of obstetrics alone.

Timing of delivery

The timing of delivery in acute heart failure is difficult. Involvement of the full multidisciplinary team is essential. The key concern is maternal well-being. However, this needs to acknowledge the gestation of the foetus and the mother's wishes. Foetal scans to determine progression of growth can be instructive: if there is evidence of a trend that growth is falling off the previous growth centile, then this may trigger delivery as foetal and maternal well-being are compromised.

In general, urgent delivery of haemodynamically unstable women with acute heart failure is considered advisable. Escalation to inotropes or mechanical circulatory support should trigger plans for an elective caesarean section assuming that the woman re-stabilizes on treatment.

If it is anticipated that the foetus will be delivered before 37 weeks of gestation, then the mother is usually given intramuscular steroids to enhance foetal lung maturity.[29] The administration of bolus steroids in women with decompensated heart failure needs to be supervised with the recognition of the potential for decompensation including the need for increased diuretic doses.

Strategies to treat heart failure

The goals of heart failure treatment are to manage symptoms, optimize haemodynamics and oxygenation, initiate disease-modifying therapies, and to identify and treat precipitants.

Management of symptoms

The mainstays of symptom control are rest and diuretics. The benefit of bed rest should not be underestimated. Thromboprophylaxis should be initiated with bedrest, given the prothrombotic effects of pregnancy and acute heart failure. Most women will be naive to diuretics, therefore initial bolus intravenous doses should be small, for example 20–40 mg furosemide intravenously (or equivalent) and then titrated as response demands. Vasodilatation with intravenous nitrates may be of benefit, particularly in acute hypertension associated with hypertensive cardiomyopathy. Cautious initiation of β-blockers (preferably carvedilol or bisoprolol for their proven benefit in left ventricular systolic dysfunction) may also improve symptoms, but only once the patient is euvolaemic. Introduction of pharmacology to a pregnant woman requires careful counselling to explain the balance of benefit to the mother and potential risks to the foetus. This includes considering whether additional monitoring will be required, e.g. foetal growth scans for women receiving β-blockers.[1]

ACE inhibitors, angiotensin receptor blockers (ARBs), and aldosterone antagonists are teratogenic and should not be used during pregnancy. In some circumstances, spironolactone is considered if the foetus is known to be female, as spironolactone may cause feminization of a male foetus. The woman requires careful counselling in advance of initiating spironolactone (Table 41.2).

Table 41.2 Typical antenatal care for patient with left ventricular systolic dysfunction

Gestation	Care
<10 weeks	• Re-discussing risk and maternal choice to continue with pregnancy. • Stopping teratogenic drugs (ACEi/warfarin) as early as possible. • Optimizing medical therapy.
10–12 weeks	• Booking visit with routine antenatal care. • Introduce women to the high-risk cardiac obstetric team. • Dating scan. • Baseline echo, bloods, BNP. • Consider thrombotic risk. • Review approx. every 4 weeks.
13–26 weeks	• Routine anomaly scan. • Foetal echo (if indicated). • Serial maternal echocardiography and BNP every 4–6 weeks. • Consider CVS if indicated (known cardiomyopathy mutation). • Medication review. • Caution at 24–26 weeks. • Review approx. every 2–4 weeks.
26–40 weeks	• Ongoing routine antenatal care. • Serial maternal echocardiography and BNP every 4–6 weeks. • Delivery planning meeting (before 30th week). • Serial foetal growth scans in last trimester. • Review approx. every 1–2 weeks.
Postnatal	• Inpatient optimization of medication. • Review thrombosis risk. • Careful post-delivery maternal surveillance. • Further imaging if indicated. • Advice regarding breastfeeding. • Advice regarding contraception.

ACEi, angiotensin converting enzyme inhibitor; BNP, B-type natriuretic peptide; CVS, chorionic villus sampling.

The treatment algorithm for acute heart failure proposed by the 2016 European Society of Cardiology heart failure guidelines (Figure 41.3) is appropriate for pregnant women also. The category of 'wet and cold' is particularly concerning, and the potential need for escalation of therapy recognized early.

Optimization of haemodynamics and oxygenation

Current evidence suggests that oxygen should not be used routinely in non-hypoxic patients. However, if the woman is hypoxic then high-flow oxygen should be initiated. Non-invasive positive pressure ventilation may be considered.

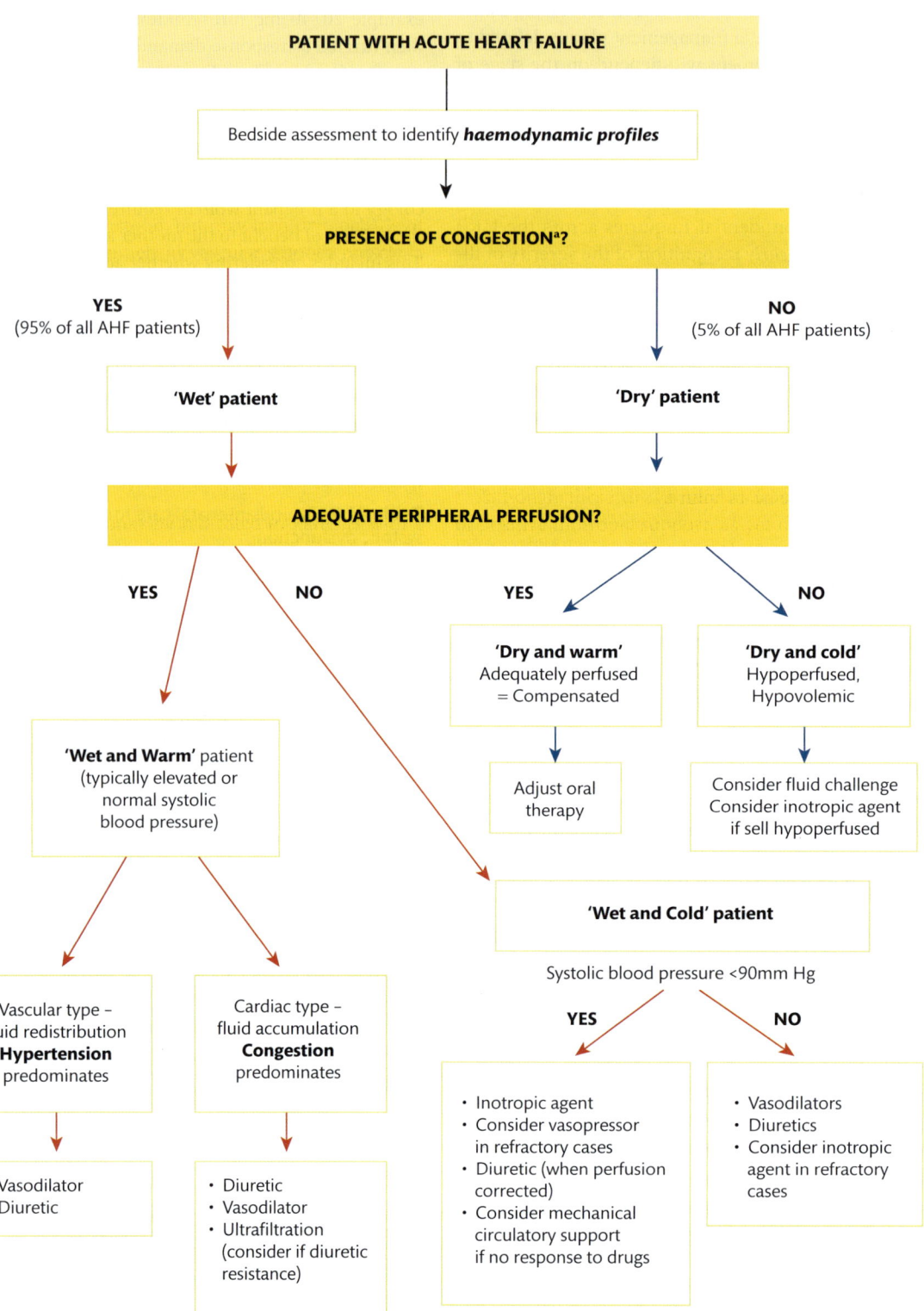

Figure 41.3 Acute heart failure.
Reproduced from Ponikowski P, Voors AA, Anker SD, *et al.* 2016 ESC Guidelines for the diagnosis and treatment of acute and chronic heart failure: The Task Force for the diagnosis and treatment of acute and chronic heart failure of the European Society of Cardiology (ESC). Developed with the special contribution of the Heart Failure Association (HFA) of the ESC. *European Journal of Heart Failure* 2016; **18**(8): 891–975 with permission from Oxford University Press.

Escalation to vasopressors is a significant step and should trigger discussion with the multidisciplinary team, to review the location of care and timing of delivery. Vasopressors should mandate that the woman is cared for in a high-dependency area with continuous ECG monitoring. Indications for vasopressor therapy include clinical features of hypoperfusion and systolic blood pressure <90 mmHg.[30]

The type of vasopressor depends on the clinical setting and familiarity with available agents. Dopamine is a reasonable initial therapy that can be titrated to response.

If there is ongoing haemodynamic instability, then urgent review by the multidisciplinary team is required. The need for emergent delivery needs to be considered. An additional plan to support the mother is required and is likely to need mechanical support of the circulation. Initial efforts may be attempted with an intra-aortic balloon pump, but escalation to extracorporeal membrane oxygenation or ventricular assist devices (plus cardiac transplantation) may be required and need to be planned for.[31] Any instrumentation of the femoral arteries, for example, with an intra-aortic balloon pump, has the potential to trigger urgent delivery, and so obstetric and neonatal support should be sought.

Initiation of disease-modifying therapies

The options for disease-modifying therapy in women with ongoing pregnancy are limited. As already stated, ACE inhibitors, ARBs and mineralocorticoid receptor antagonists are contraindicated in pregnancy. Therefore, β-blockers are the main therapy with proven benefit. There was previous concern about foetal growth restriction with β-blockers; however, with contemporary agents at evidence-based doses the risk is acceptable, though foetal growth monitoring is advised.[1]

After delivery, all the evidence-based therapies can be initiated. Breastfeeding is considered safe with all current recommended therapies, although carvedilol may be the preferred β-blocker as it has the lowest excretion in breast milk.[1]

Identify and treat potential precipitants

Once the woman has stabilized, the focus needs to turn to consider why the acute deterioration has occurred. Common causes include anaemia, infection, and thyroid dysfunction. Arteriovenous malformations can become apparent in pregnancy and cause a high-output cardiac failure.

Arrhythmias may also be the precipitant cause of the acute heart failure. The management of the arrhythmia will depend on the woman's haemodynamic status: if they are unstable then early electrical cardioversion may be required. Early involvement of the multidisciplinary team is essential.

Delivery

As discussed in the previous section, early consideration of the correct location for delivery is essential. What is the woman potentially going to require as a 'bail-out' strategy? Where can that be provided? It is not advisable to transfer a woman in labour; therefore, if a woman needs to be transferred for ongoing care this arrangement should be facilitated early.

An extensive team needs to be available for delivery: this is a group with multiple skills who together can direct a care plan towards an optimal outcome. If the woman has stabilized with medical therapy then a vaginal delivery can be considered. Effective analgesia (regional) to allow an instrumented assisted delivery, if required, should be discussed.[32] If a woman is haemodynamically unstable or has ongoing pulmonary oedema that precludes lying flat for delivery, then a general anaesthetic to facilitate a caesarean section for delivery is appropriate.[33] This approach also allows prompt escalation of therapy, e.g. to mechanical circulatory support, if required.

The management of the third stage of labour has previously included discussion of restricting pharmacotherapy such as oxytocin infusions. However, recent evidence has suggested that there is greater harm from withholding appropriate use of oxytocin because of the destabilizing effects of a major postpartum haemorrhage.[34] Most centres now withhold the bolus dose but utilize the infusion of oxytocin, perhaps for longer than in non-cardiac patients. Prior to discharge post delivery there must be discussion and provision of adequate contraception.

Contraception

Contraceptive advice is an integral part of any pregnancy discussion. In women with significant ventricular impairment and a risk of thrombosis, oestrogens should be avoided. There are, however, several other highly effective alternatives. These include oral progesterone-based tablets (such as Cerezette), subcutaneous implants (Implanon or Nexplanon), or a Mirena Coil.[35] Surgical sterilization is an alternative, especially if utilizing some of the newer percutaneous tubal plugs.

Patients with ventricular dysfunction can also use emergency contraception, if required. This can include the use of a copper coil (effective up to five days after unprotected sex), or agents such as levonorgestrel (Levonelle), which is effective up to 72 h but which interacts with warfarin and bosentan.

Advice about contraceptive choices for women with heart disease can be found from the Faculty of Reproductive and Sexual Healthcare of the Royal College of Obstetricians and Gynaecologists.[36]

Conclusion

Myocardial disease is a leading cause of maternal cardiac death. This usually has an acquired, rather than congenital, aetiology and may appear for the first time during pregnancy. In women of child-bearing age with known pre-existing ventricular dysfunction, a pre-pregnancy assessment should be routinely offered. This should be performed by a multidisciplinary team, and the discussion should focus on maternal and foetal outcomes, including the difficult issue of maternal longevity. There are several risk scores to assist in the estimation of risk associated with pregnancy. These are, however, insufficiently detailed to be the sole tool utilized in counselling the patient. Only in individualizing care with all the available data and highlighting the areas where there is uncertainty will women be in a position to make informed decisions regarding their desires to have a family.

REFERENCES

1. European Society of Gynecology; Association for European Paediatric Cardiology; German Society for Gender Medicine, Regitz-Zagrosek V, Blomstrom Lundqvist C, Borghi C, et al.; ESC Committee for Practice Guidelines. ESC Guidelines on the management of cardiovascular diseases during pregnancy: the Task Force on the Management of Cardiovascular Diseases during Pregnancy of the European Society of Cardiology (ESC). Eur Heart J 2011;32(24):3147–97.

2. Robson SC, Hunter S, Boys RJ, Dunlop W. Serial study of factors influencing changes in cardiac output during human pregnancy. *Am J Physiol* 1989;**256**(4 Pt 2):H1060–5.

3. Sanghavi M, Rutherford JD. Cardiovascular physiology of pregnancy. *Circulation* 2014;**130**:1003–8.

4. Ouzoinian JG, Elkayam U. Physiologic changes during normal pregnancy and delivery. *Cardiol Clin* 2012;**30**(3):317–29.

5. Capeless EL, Clapp JF. When do cardiovascular parameters return to their preconception values? *Am J Obstet Gynecol* 1991;**165**:883.

6. McClure JH, Cooper GM, Clutton-Brock TH, Centre for Maternal and Child Enquiries. Saving mothers' lives: reviewing maternal death to make motherhood safer 2006–8. *Br J Obstet Gynaecol* 2011;**118**(Suppl 1);1–203.

7. Huisman CM, Zwart JJ, Roos-Hesselink JW, Duvekot JJ, van Roosmalen J. Incidence and predictors of maternal cardiovascular mortality and severe morbidity in the Netherlands: a prospective cohort study. *PLoS One* 2013;**8**:e56494.

8. Siu SC, Sermer M, Colman JM, et al. Prospective multicenter study of pregnancy outcomes in women with heart disease. *Circulation* 2001;**104**:515–21.

9. Drenthen W, Boersma E, Balci A, et al. Predictors of pregnancy complications in women with congenital heart disease. *Eur Heart J* 2010;**31**:2124–32.

10. Thorne S, MacGregor A, Nelson-Piercy C. Risks of contraception and pregnancy in heart disease. *Heart* 2006;**92**:1520–5.

11. Roos-Hesselink JW, Ruys TP, Stein JI, et al. Outcome of pregnancy in patients with structural or ischaemic heart disease: results of a registry of the European Society of Cardiology. *Eur Heart J* 2013;**34**:657–65.

12. Wilkinson JD, Landy DC, Colan SD, et al. The pediatric cardiomyopathy registry and heart failure: key results from the first 15 years. *Heart Fail Clin* 2010;**6**:401–13.

13. Fett JD, Fristoe KL, Welsh SN. Risk of heart failure relapse in subsequent pregnancy among peripartum cardiomyopathy mothers. *Int J Gynaecol Obstet* 2010;**109**:34–6.

14. Ohuchi H, Tanabe Y, Kamiya C, et al. Cardiopulmonary variables during exercise predict pregnancy outcome in women with congenital heart disease. *Circ J* 2013;**77**:470–6.

15. Lui GK, Silversides CK, Khairy P, et al. Heart rate response during exercise and pregnancy outcome in women with congenital heart disease. *Circulation* 2011;**123**:242–8.

16. Tanous D, Siu SC, Mason J, et al. B-type natriuretic peptide in pregnant women with heart disease. *J Am Coll Cardiol* 2010;**56**:1247–53.

17. Kampman MA, Balci A, van Veldhuisen DJ, et al. N-terminal pro-B-type natriuretic peptide predicts cardiovascular complications in pregnant women with congenital heart disease. *Eur Heart J* 2014;**35**:708–15.

18. Metz TD, Jackson GM, Yetman AT. Pregnancy outcomes in women who have undergone an atrial switch repair for congenital d-transposition of the great arteries. *Am J Obstet Gynecol* 2011;**205**:273.

19. Hyun J, Park KD, Yoo Y, et al. Effects of different sensitisation events on HLA alloimmunization in solid organ transplantation patients. *Transplant Proc* 2012;**44**(1):222–5.

20. Ruys TP, Roos-Hesselink JW, Hall R, et al. Heart failure in pregnant women with cardiac disease: data from the ROPAC. *Heart* 2014;**100**(3):231–8.

21. Ray JG, Vermeulen MJ, Bharatha A, Montanera WJ, Park AL. Association between MRI exposure during pregnancy and foetal and childhood outcomes. *JAMA* 2016;**316**(9):952–61.

22. Anthony J, Sliwa K. Decompensated heart failure in pregnancy. *Cardiac Fail Rev* 2015;**1**(2):20–6.

23. National Institute for Health and Care Excellence. Hypertension in pregnancy. 2010 NICE clinical guideline 107. https://www.nice.org.uk/guidance/cg107

24. Phipps E, Prasanna D, Brima W, Jim B. Preeclampsia: updates in pathogenesis, definitions and guidelines. *Clin J Am Soc Nephrol* 2016;**11**(6):1102–13.

25. Seely EW, Ecker J. Chronic hypertension in pregnancy. *N Engl J Med* 2011;**365**:439–46.

26. Balinger KJ, Chu Lam MT, Hon HH, Stawicki SP, Anasti JN. Amniotic fluid embolism: despite progress, challenges remain. *Curr Opin Obstet Gynecol* 2015;**27**(6):398–405.

27. Greutmann M, Pieper PG. Pregnancy in women with congenital heart disease. *Eur Heart J* 2015;**36**(37):2491–9.

28. Knight M, Nair M, Tuffnell D, et al. (eds) on behalf of MBRRACE-UK. Saving Lives, Improving Mothers' Care—Surveillance of maternal deaths in the UK 2012–14 and lessons learned to inform maternity care from the UK and Ireland Confidential Enquiries into Maternal Deaths and Morbidity 2009–14. National Perinatal Epidemiology Unit, University of Oxford, Oxford, 2016.

29. Ogunyemi D. Risk factors for acute pulmonary edema in preterm delivery. *Eur J Obstet Gynecol Reprod Biol* 2007:**133**(2):143–7.

30. Bauersachs J, Arrigo M, Hilfiker-Kleiner D, et al. Current management of patients with severe acute peripartum cardiomyopathy: practical guidance from the Heart Failure association of the European Society of Cardiology Study Group on peripartum cardiomyopathy. *Eur J Heart Fail* 2016;**18**(9):1096–105.

31. Shin JJ, Hamad E, Murthy S, Pina IL. Heart failure in women. *Clin Cardiol* 2012;**35**(3):172–77.

32. Ashikhmina E, Farber MK, Mizuguchi KA. Parturients with hypertrophic cardiomyopathy: case series and review of pregnancy and anesthetic management of labor and delivery. *Int J Obstet Anesth* 2015;**24**(4):344–55.

33. Ituk US, Habib AS, Polin CM, Allen TK. Anesthetic management and outcomes of parturients with dilated cardiomyopathy in an academic centre. *Can J Anaesth* 2015;**62**(3):278–88.

34. Cauldwell M, Von Klemperer K, Uebing A, et al. Why is postpartum haemorrhage more common in women with congenital heart disease? *Int J Cardiol* 2016;**218**:285–90.

35. Roos-Hesselink JW, Cornette J, Sliwa K, et al. Contraception and cardiovascular disease. *Eur Heart J* 2015;**36**(27);1728–34.

36. Faculty of Sexual and Reproductive Healthcare of the Royal College of Obstetrics and Gynaecology. FSRH clinical guideline: contraceptive choices for women with cardiac disease (June 2014). https://www.fsrh.org/standards-and-guidance/documents/ceu-guidance-contraceptive-choices-for-women-with-cardiac/

42

Anxiety and depression

Anna Maddison and John Sharp

Mental health and heart failure

The relationship between psychological and cardiological well-being has become embedded within societies, cultures, and language over centuries. Emotional well-being continues to be conveyed via its assumed impact on cardiological function. Sadness is expressed as 'heartache', perhaps experienced by a spurned lover left 'broken-hearted'. People who show their emotions openly 'wear their heart on their sleeve', while those lacking empathy and compassion are 'hard-hearted' or even 'heartless'. Those encountering challenges might describe a 'sinking heart', whereas others might 'take heart' in response to positive encouragement.

An ever-increasing body of evidence is emerging to demonstrate that the association between emotional and cardiac health is not restricted to excerpts from the prose of poetic scribes. Mental health and cardiac health regularly coexist and their bidirectional interaction influences the genesis, maintenance, and exacerbation of heart failure. The onset of heart failure may be directly related to maladaptive behaviour, including substance abuse/misuse and disordered eating or an iatrogenic consequence of the use of antipsychotic medication in the management of severe and enduring mental health problems. Conversely, heart failure may lead to the development of a range of psychological problems, including cognitive impairment, body image, self-esteem, somatization, and sexual dysfunction. This chapter begins by presenting an overview of the most commonly occurring and frequently studied psychological problems—anxiety and depression—and how these present within heart failure populations. The chapter then examines epidemiological studies that report the prevalence of such problems and have investigated the association between depression, anxiety and heart failure. Finally, evidence from clinical trials is presented to inform the appropriate management of heart failure with depression and anxiety.

Characterizing anxiety in heart failure

Anxiety is a broad term alluding to a feeling of unease, worry, or fear. Anxiety is common and normal, and may be congruous with circumstances and context. For example, being fearful when faced with real-world threats may be appropriate and protective. Similarly, worrying when one encounters a problem or challenge can aid its solution. However, when the experience of anxiety becomes frequent and disruptive, or its occurrence intense and distressing, or when individuals struggle to control the extent to which they worry, the problem may be considered pathological.

Anxiety manifests through a combination of cognitive, behavioural, physical and emotional symptoms. The manner in which these symptoms present often aligns with recognizable patterns characteristic of a range of well-established, discrete anxiety disorders which have shared symptom burden. For example, the experience of acute anxiety, or panic attacks, is common to most, but not all, anxiety disorders. The presence of specific stressors generates a physiological response and a variety of somatic symptoms ranging from muscular tension and increased heart rate to dizziness and feelings of breathlessness depending on the severity of acute anxiety. Additionally, anxiety disorders are usually characterized by maladaptive, often distorted, cognitions whereby individuals overestimate the extent of danger or threat linked to specific situations or bodily sensation. This distorted threat appraisal elicits avoidant behaviours in an attempt to prevent the onset of anxiety. The short-term success of this coping strategy reinforces the value of avoidance as a means of managing anxiety with the long-term detrimental consequence of individuals becoming increasingly reliant on this technique, generalizing its use to any situation provoking anxiety.

Brief descriptions of the anxiety disorders common to heart failure populations are provided below.

Panic disorder

Panic disorder is classified as recurrent attacks of severe acute anxiety, more commonly known as 'panic attacks'. Dominant symptoms include palpitations, chest pain, dizziness, choking sensations, and a feeling of unreality. There is also often a secondary fear of dying, going mad, or losing control.[1] **Figure 42.1** illustrates how cognitions, emotions, behaviour, and physiology combine to elicit and perpetuate panic attacks, and portrays how panic disorder might present in an individual with heart failure.[2]

People with heart failure are often legitimately, and always understandably, concerned about their general physical well-being and, specifically, the functioning of their heart. This leads to a tendency

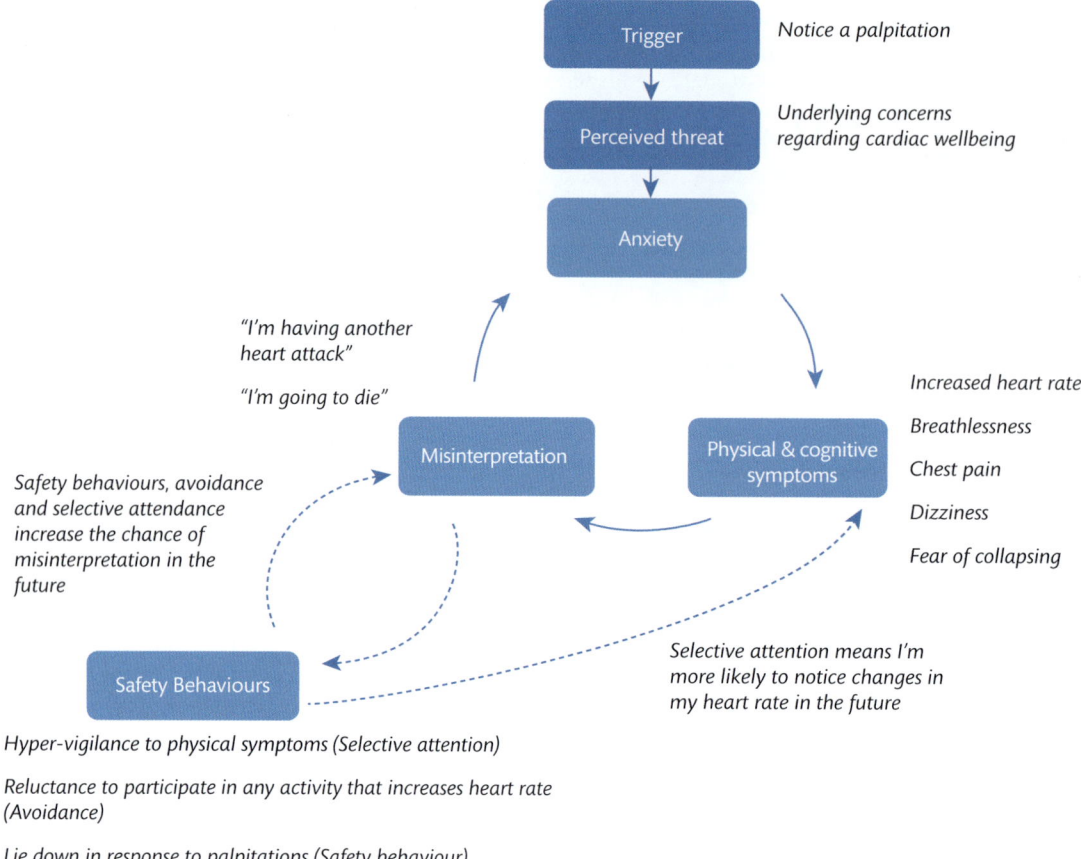

Figure 42.1 The panic cycle.
Source data from Clark DM. A cognitive approach to panic. *Behav Res Ther* 1986;**24**(4):461–470.

to closely monitor for the presence of physical symptoms. Such hypervigilance and attentional bias increases an individual's sensitivity to detect normal physiological symptoms and amplify the symptom experience. Underlying fears and beliefs regarding safety and physical well-being are activated, generating the intrusion of anxious predictions anticipating the potential for imminent catastrophic cardiac events. The prospect of such an event is obviously anxiety-provoking. As previously described, anxiety is manifest by an array of physiological symptoms including accelerated heart rate or palpitations, feelings of breathlessness, and tight chest. Unfortunately, such symptoms can easily be misinterpreted as indicative of an acute cardiac event and, as such, reinforce initial fears and exacerbate the severity of the acute anxiety.

Agoraphobia

The experience of panic attacks is unpleasant and distressing. Unsurprisingly, those who experience panic attacks will often go to great lengths to minimize their likelihood. Consequently, people often avoid situations that they believe increase the chances of panic occurring or places in which they feel unsafe. When people are fearful of having a cardiac event they are often reluctant to leave the perceived safety of their home or to travel any significant distance alone through fear of what might happen to them.

Agoraphobia is characterized by fear and avoidance of at least two of the following situations: crowds; public places; travelling

alone; travelling away from home. When faced with these situations symptoms of anxiety, often escalating to panic attacks, will arise.[1] Agoraphobia is commonly diagnosed with or without the presence of co-morbid panic disorder.

Specific phobias

Acute anxiety may occur as a response to any perceived threat. For reasons that are not always obvious, people may develop fears of a seemingly endless list of often otherwise innocuous stimuli. Specific phobias are characterized as the fear or avoidance of a distinct object or situation, and symptoms of anxiety are restricted to the feared situation. Certain specific phobias can have huge implications for an individual's heart failure care. For example, common specific phobias such as fear of hospitals (nosocomophobia), fear of injection or medical needles (trypanophobia), fear of enclosed spaces (claustrophobia), and fear of surgery (tomophobia) would be exceptionally distressing for individual patients and highly disruptive to the delivery of care.

Post-traumatic stress disorder

When people are exposed to stressful or traumatic events, significant psychological stress may ensue. Post-traumatic stress disorder (PTSD) involves persistent reliving of the event through intrusive flashbacks, vivid memories, and recurring dreams. The individual may experience distress in circumstances resembling or associated

with the event and will avoid such circumstances. Psychological disturbance is manifest through either the inability to recall, partially or completely, important aspects of the event; or through heightened psychological arousal, evident through any two of the following: difficulty sleeping; irritability or outbursts of anger; difficulty concentrating; hyper-vigilance; exaggerated startle response.[1] People with heart failure can endure numerous traumatic—sometimes life-threatening—events, and PTSD is often experienced following implantable cardioverter–defibrillator shocks, myocardial infarction, cardiac arrest, or intensive care unit admission.

Generalized anxiety disorder

Generalized anxiety disorder (GAD) is an anxiety disorder characterized by symptoms that are both persistent and generalized, i.e. not restricted to, or strongly related to, a specific environmental stressor. Individuals worry excessively about a variety of issues to a level that disrupts the ability to perform everyday tasks. The extent of worrying is so distressing that individuals often describe 'worrying about how much they worry'. Such 'meta-worry' conveys the difficulty people with GAD experience in controlling their tendency to worry. The criterion symptoms of GAD include over-arousal features such as: persistent restlessness; muscle tension; sleep disturbance; irritability; difficulty concentrating; fatigue; and meta-worry. Heart failure has wide impact upon the individual, their family, and relationships, and social and vocational functioning. Consequently, worries regarding health, family, and finances are prominent and frequent. For many people with heart failure, such worries become all-consuming, difficult to control, and distressing to endure.

Characterizing depression in heart failure

Depression is an over-used term. It has been adopted within the common lexicon to convey any alterations in affective state including the type of transient feelings of flat mood experienced regularly by everyone. Clinically, it pertains to persistent, severe, recurring episodes of low mood and anhedonia. Depression is the 'common cold' of psychiatry which manifests through a variety of cognitive, behavioural, somatic, and emotional symptoms. The two main classification systems, ICD-10[1] and DSM-5,[3] present broadly similar diagnostic criteria to indicate the presence of a major depressive episode (see Box 42.1).

The severity of depression experienced is determined by the number of symptoms present but must also be associated with clinically significant distress or impairment in social, occupational, or other important areas of life.[3] Episodes of depression are emotionally distressing and may have a profound and ruinous impact on individuals' physical well-being, quality of life, and behaviour, including ability to function socially and vocationally. At its most extreme, depression may lead to suicidal ideation and greatly increases the risk of deliberate self-harm including suicide.

There are numerous competing explanatory models for depression. The dominant psychological theory asserts that negative thinking has a central role in an individual's depressed mood state. Beck's cognitive model[4] recognizes that the manner in which individuals cognitively interpret a situation determines how they respond emotionally, behaviourally, and physically. People predisposed to depression have a tendency to perceive or interpret circumstances negatively. Persistent engagement with negative thoughts

---

Box 42.1 Diagnostic criteria for depression (ICD-10 classification)[1]

Depressive episode

A. *Main symptoms*

Depressed mood to a degree that is definitely abnormal for the individual, present for most of the day and almost every day, largely uninfluenced by circumstances

Loss of interest or pleasure in activities that are normally pleasurable

Decreased energy or increased fatiguability

B. *Additional symptoms*

Loss of confidence and self-esteem

Unreasonable feelings of self-reproach or excessive and inappropriate guilt

Recurrent thoughts of death or suicide, or any suicidal behaviour

Complaints or evidence of diminished ability to think or concentrate, such as indecisiveness or vacillation

Change in psychomotor activity, with agitation or retardation (either subjective or objective)

Sleep disturbance of any type

Change in appetite (decrease or increase) with corresponding weight change)

C. *Somatic syndrome symptoms*

Marked loss of interest or pleasure in activities that are normally pleasurable

Lack of emotional reactions to events or activities that normally produce an emotional response

Waking in the morning ≥2 h before the usual time

Depression worse in the morning

Objective evidence of marked psychomotor retardation or agitation (remarked on or reported by other people)

Marked loss of appetite

Weight loss (≥5% of body weight in the past month)

Marked loss of libido

Further essential requirements

- Symptoms present for at least two weeks
- No hypomanic or manic symptoms
- Not attributable to psychoactive substance use or to any organic mental disorder

Level of severity

Mild:

- 4 symptoms in total
- ≥2 symptoms from main category

Moderate:

- 6 symptoms in total
- ≥2 symptoms from main category

Severe:

- ≥8 symptoms in total
- All 3 main symptoms present

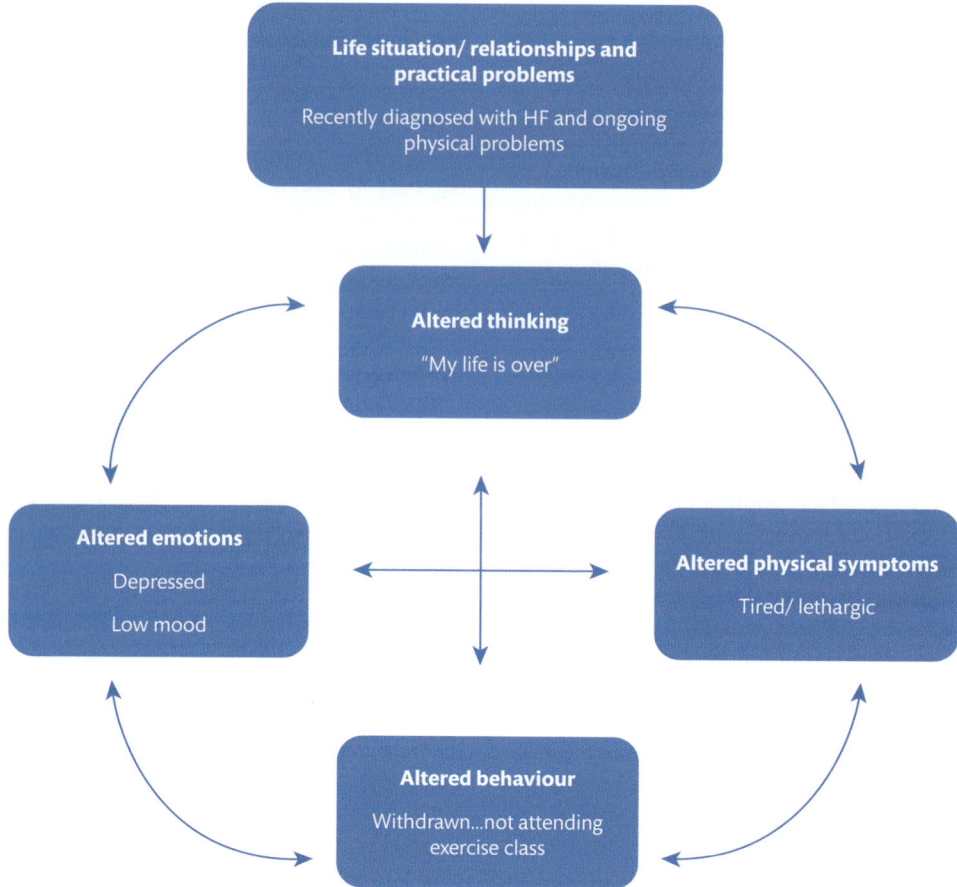

Figure 42.2 A simplified problem-level model of heart failure depression.
Source data from Beck AT. *Depression: Clinical, experimental, and theoretical aspects.* University of Pennsylvania Press; 1967.

and beliefs may cause and/or aggravate depressed mood. The cognitive model predicts that changes in cognitions causally lead to changes in behaviour and emotion, and an abundance of empirical research supports this model.[5]

From diagnosis to final stages, people with heart failure experience multiple losses which can precipitate and perpetuate depression. These include losses of their normal functioning impacting on recreation, relationships, vocation, and income. These in turn can result in the loss of identity, and, in combination with the physical symptoms of heart failure, lead to hopelessness and depression (see Figure 42.2).

Prevalence of anxiety and depression in heart failure

People who have a chronic physical health condition are at increased risk of developing depression and/or anxiety. A rule of thumb states that, as the severity of the physical health condition increases, so too does the prevalence of any co-morbid mental health problem.

Heart failure anxiety

Anxiety is common in the general adult population, with an estimated prevalence rate of 7.3%.[6] The impact of heart failure on individuals' psychological well-being is evident, with heart failure anxiety (HFA) known to be exceptionally prevalent. Estimates for HFA range from 11% to 45%[7] depending on measurement procedures and population sample. A meta-analysis of 73 studies concluded that more than one-quarter (28.8%) of people with a diagnosis of heart failure report clinically significant anxiety, and more than half (55.5%) experience elevated symptoms of anxiety.[8]

Heart failure depression

Within the general adult population, depression has an estimated prevalence of 5%.[9] Heart failure has a substantial impact on individuals' affective state. Heart failure depression (HFD) is well known to be exceptionally prevalent, with estimates ranging from 13%[10] to 77.5%[11] depending on procedures of measurement and features of the population sample. A meta-analysis of 27 studies concluded that one-third (33.6%) of people with a diagnosis of heart failure report clinically significant depressive symptoms and approximately one in five (21.5%) presents with major depression disorder.[12] Further, the prevalence of depression correlated with New York Heart Association (NYHA) functional status with prevalence increasing from 11% in people with NYHA class I (mild) heart failure, 20% in those with class II, 38% in those with class III, and 42% in those with class IV (severe) heart failure.

Impact of co-morbid anxiety and depression

Experiencing an anxiety or affective disorder is unquestionably distressing and often disrupts individuals' ability to function across a range of domains. Treatment for such conditions is justified and warranted for these reasons alone. However, the impact of anxiety and depression is not confined to the experience of the cardinal features of these conditions such as heightened nervousness or excessive worry, lowered affective state or anhedonia. Anxiety and depression are characterized in part by somatic symptoms including disturbed sleep, erratic appetite, fatigue, and experience of pain. The manner in which anxiety and depression affect physical well-being has huge implications for the initial occurrence, maintenance, and exacerbation of heart failure symptoms and outcomes.

Mortality

Among psychological contributors with a demonstrated association with both non-fatal and fatal coronary heart disease events, depression is the best-established independent risk factor for coronary heart disease.[13] Similar associations have been found within heart failure populations. Depression and heart failure have a bidirectional association; the former can long antedate, immediately precede, or be an emotional response to a diagnosis of the latter. Over two decades, prospective studies have revealed depression to be an independent predictor of mortality in heart failure.[14,15] Some studies show that heart failure patients with co-morbid severe depression are four times more likely to die within two years compared with those classified not depressed,[16] whereas others indicate that major depression after heart failure is a significant predictor for subsequent all-cause mortality.[17]

Far fewer studies have considered the effect of anxiety on mortality. Perhaps as a consequence, a meta-analysis found the effect of anxiety on mortality to be inconclusive. However, this systematic review and meta-analysis suggests that depression is an important and independent predictor of all-cause mortality among heart failure patients, whereas anxiety does not appear to have a strong effect.[18]

Morbidity

In addition to increasing the risk of mortality in people with heart failure, multiple studies show that major depression constitutes an independent predictive factor for heart failure patient clinical outcome equal in importance to left ventricular dysfunction, smoking, or history of myocardial infarction. Indeed, depression has been shown to be an independent predictor of future cardiac events in patients with heart failure, regardless of disease severity,[19,20] and both clinical major depressive disorder and subthreshold depressive symptoms associate with greater risk for several adverse outcomes, including hospitalizations, increased health care costs and functional decline.[21]

Healthcare utilization

Depression worsens prognosis and heart failure morbidity and, consequently, leads to greater reliance on healthcare resources. People with co-morbid heart failure and depression have a three-fold increase in hospitalization[22] and medical costs are increased by 25–40%.[23] Whereas a meta-analysis confirmed the trend toward increased health care use, and higher rates of hospitalization and

emergency room visits among depressed patients,[12] a systematic review was unable to determine whether anxiety predicts hospitalizations in heart failure populations due to a lack of research in this area.[24]

Quality of life

Quality of life (QoL) comprises numerous domains frequently influenced by an individual's psychological well-being. Common symptoms of an altered mood state, such as depressed mood, irritability, guilt, hopelessness, low self-esteem, fatigue, sleep disturbance, appetite change, or cognitive impairment, are likely to have a detrimental impact on every aspect of health-related QoL including physical and social functioning and mental health.[25] Indeed, QoL unsurprisingly has a significant positive correlation with level of depression.[26]

Depression and QoL appear to be inextricably linked. For example, people with heart failure reported that financial stressors, overall poor health, past traumatic life experiences, and negative thinking contributed to depressive symptoms.[27] Tautologically, depression has adverse prognostic implications for people with heart failure, including increased risk of somatic symptoms, increased financial burden, and poorer QoL (cf. Newhouse and Jiang[20]). However, specific features inherent in any calculation of health-related QoL, including level of social support and style of coping with heart failure, are important prognostic factors in their own right.[28]

Association of anxiety and depression with heart failure

As outlined, psychological distress, particularly depression, is associated with a poorer QoL, increased use of health care resources, more frequent adverse clinical events and hospitalizations, and twice the risk of mortality for people with heart failure.[29] Although such associations are now well established, the underlying reasons for them remain less well understood.

Indirect mechanisms

The impact of emotional distress on heart failure morbidity and mortality is perhaps most readily understood by the way such conditions alter behaviours known to be linked to positive outcomes. For example, people who suffer from depression often struggle with motivation to complete even basic tasks or make positive health behaviour changes. Individuals who experience anxiety relating to hospitals or medical procedures often avoid situations that provoke their symptoms and therefore deny themselves the opportunity to receive appropriate and necessary care. It is for such reasons that depression and anxiety are associated with a range of behaviours detrimental to heart failure health, including a three-fold increase in the risk of non-adherence to medical treatment regimens,[14,16,19,20,23,26,30–34] poor dietary control,[14,32–34] reduced engagement with exercise,[14,32–34] smoking,[22,33,34] and alcohol use.[20,34]

Depressive symptoms of hopelessness, despair, and impaired social relationships may promote decreased ability to engage in heart failure self-care.[27] A review of psychological determinants of self-care in heart failure concluded that depression, mental well-being, and self-efficacy are each associated with self-care behaviours. Depression was linked with poor physical activity, delay in treatment and overall reported

self-care. Evidence for the effect of anxiety on self-care was inconclusive.[35] However, the same review indicated how depression interferes with individuals' ability to cope. Whereas adaptive coping styles such as active coping, acceptance, and planning are seen in heart failure patients with less depression, more maladaptive methods of coping such as denial and disengagement are displayed in those with higher levels of depression.[36] Such coping styles complicate the management of heart failure, lead to the development of adverse clinical events, and consequently increase the costly tendency to use health care resources including the need for hospital admission.[29]

Direct mechanisms

An abundance of research has investigated biobehavioural mechanisms explaining the effects of depression on cardiovascular morbidity and mortality in people with coronary heart disease.[37] Whereas fewer studies have contemplated direct mechanisms to account for the adverse prognostic effects of depression within heart failure, there have been ample pathophysiological explanations postulated with a number of factors reputed to be implicated in the bidirectional interaction between depression and heart failure. The shared biological processes of heart failure and depression are manifest in the overlapping somatic symptoms presenting across the two conditions. These include difficulties with fatigue, sleep, cognitive

impairment including concentration, and regulating weight. It has been suggested that the biobehavioural processes inherent within heart failure such as activation of inflammatory cascades, dysregulation of neurohormonal axes, and increased arrhythmias, are also likely to be implicated in the genesis, maintenance, and/or exacerbation of depression. These mechanisms have been previously and thoroughly reviewed[21] and both the potential indirect and direct factors that could explain the association between heart failure and depression are illustrated in **Figure 42.3**.

Identifying anxiety and depression in heart failure

The prevalence of both anxiety and depression and the potential impact on morbidity and mortality mandates the systematic and routine consideration of anxiety and depression in all people with heart failure. Emotional well-being is not static and fluctuates according to circumstances. Isolated assessment of psychological well-being is an unreliable means of detecting changes in the level of anxiety or depression and does not permit timely response and access to appropriate intervention. People with heart failure should have their psychological well-being considered at every patient contact. Brief psychometric measures, such as Patient Health Questionnaire 4

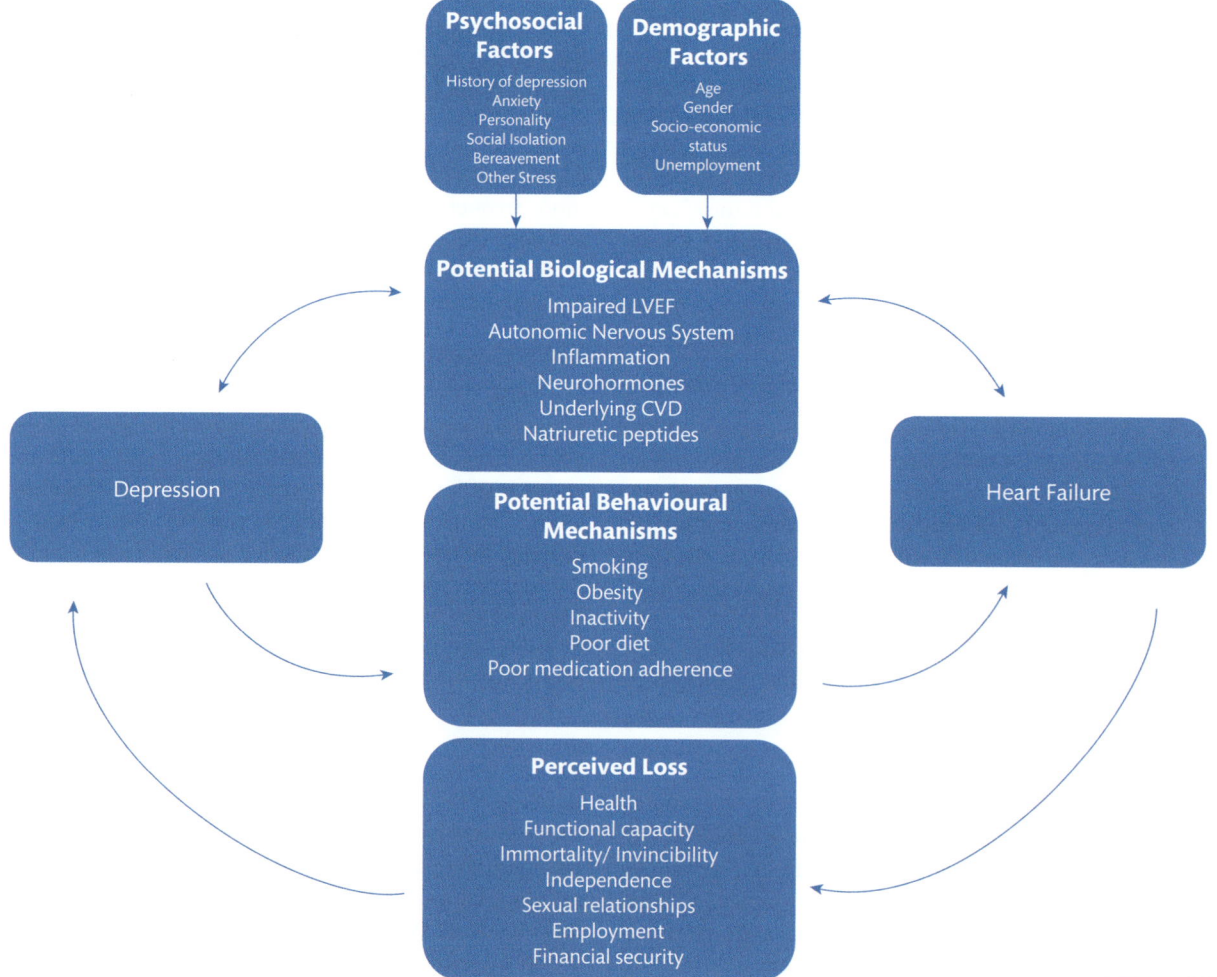

Figure 42.3 Conceptual relationship between depression and heart failure. LVEF, left ventricular ejection fraction; CVD, cardiovascular disease.

(PHQ-4) and Generalized Anxiety Disorder 2 (GAD-2), can rapidly screen for the likely presence of problematic anxiety and depression and can be readily incorporated into existing heart failure case-note documentation.

Screening for depression and anxiety is crucial to identify individuals in need of psychological support. However, evidence demonstrates that screening in isolation does not change clinical practice or improve patient outcomes.[38] A core criterion for the use of screening measures is that they must result in effective treatment, and therefore require being part of a predetermined clinical pathway.

Anxiety

Chest pain and dizziness are two core symptoms exceedingly common in panic attacks; they are also alarming symptoms for a person with heart failure. As many as one in four patients presenting with chest pain at accident and emergency departments have no cardiologic pathology revealed following their inevitable admission.[39] Unfortunately, virtually all such patients presenting with non-cardiac chest pain—likely a consequence of anxiety and panic disorder—fail to have any explanation of possible psychological aetiology, their anxiety recognized, or offered access to appropriate psychological therapy.

Clinical guidelines recommend screening for anxiety using validated tools in the context of a collaborative, stepped care mode. Tools validated for use in the heart failure population include Generalized Anxiety Disorder 7 (GAD-7) and Hospital Anxiety and Depression Scale (HADS). Both forms are self-report measures which take less than five minutes to complete. They should be used in conjunction with clinical judgement to guide decision-making for appropriate intervention.

Depression

Depression in heart failure is under-recognized and under-treated.[23,40] National guidelines recommend screening all patients with heart failure for depression using a validated measure, within the context of a collaborative, stepped care model.[41]

Uncertainty in identifying and diagnosing depression arises in practice due to the overlap of symptoms. Of the nine defining characteristics of depression, many are also symptoms of heart failure. Overlapping symptoms include: fatigue; low energy; change in appetite; change in sleep; reduced concentration; dyspnoea; and reduced physical activity.

Screening tools facilitate recognition of depression, can guide treatment selection, and monitor symptom severity.[33] Screening tools should always be used in conjunction with clinical judgement, taking into account the symptom overlap described above. Validated screening tools for use in the heart failure population include the PHQ-9, HADS, and Beck Depression Inventory, 2nd edition (BDI-II).[41] The PHQ-9 has been used in a considerable amount of cardiac research, has shown acceptable sensitivity and specificity for patients with heart failure, and is recommended by American Heart Association.[33,42]

Management of anxiety and depression in heart failure

There is a significant gap between the demand for psychological therapy services and the available supply. The efficiency of provision

can be increased through the adoption of a collaborative, stepped care model: a model of healthcare delivery where the recommended treatment should be the least restrictive of those currently available, but still likely to provide significant health gain. Such models are self-correcting, allowing for 'stepping up' and 'stepping down' according to patient needs. The main components of a collaborative care model include: a clearly defined clinical care pathway; a person-centred approach taking into account individuals' needs and preferences; integrating case managers to ensure routine screening of depression and anxiety using validated measurement to monitor well-being and track response to treatment; use of a patient registry to allow monitoring of intervention and effective reviews of caseloads by mental health practitioners; stepped care approaches to facilitate simultaneous delivery of multiple interventions and escalation of the intensity of the intervention as required.

Collaborative care models have shown efficacy in the treatment of depression in cardiac settings, with the potential of using nurses as case managers.[43] NICE recommends the use of the stepped care model outlined in Figure 42.4.[44]

Evidence-based interventions

Pharmacological intervention

The multiple overlapping factors in the pathophysiology of HFD suggest a potential role for pharmacotherapy to exploit these hypothesized mechanisms. However, to date there is a lack of evidence regarding drug therapy for HFD. Selective serotonin reuptake inhibitors (SSRIs) are first-line treatments for depression.[45] Randomized clinical trials have demonstrated that sertraline and citalopram are safe for patients with coronary heart disease and effective for moderate, severe, or recurrent depression.[15,33] SSRIs have lower risk of adverse anticholinergic and antihistaminergic side-effects.[15] Tricyclics (e.g. imipramine, amitriptyline, lofepramine) are contraindicated in cardiac populations as they may cause QT interval prolongation, atrioventricular block, bundle branch block, ventricular arrhythmias, hypotension, and disturbances of myocardial contractility.[15,46]

A major clinical trial, SADHART-CHF,[47] hypothesized that the SSRI sertraline would improve both symptoms of depression and cardiovascular status in depressed heart failure patients compared to a matching placebo. All participants also received support provided by staff with previous psychiatric training or experience. There was no significant difference in degree of depression at 12 weeks and the proportion of patients classified as 'worsened', 'improved', or 'unchanged' did not differ significantly between the sertraline and placebo groups. Both conditions demonstrated significant pre- to post-intervention improvements in depression. The authors discussed the possibility that the patient support delivered by psychiatric-trained nursing staff may have been more therapeutically potent than had been intended or foreseen. The apparent benefit of such support—reasoned to have partially confounded any effects of sertraline—hints at the potential benefits of more thorough, deliberate application of 'talking therapies'.

Psychotherapy

Psychological interventions are widely recommended as therapeutic options for the treatment of depression in the general

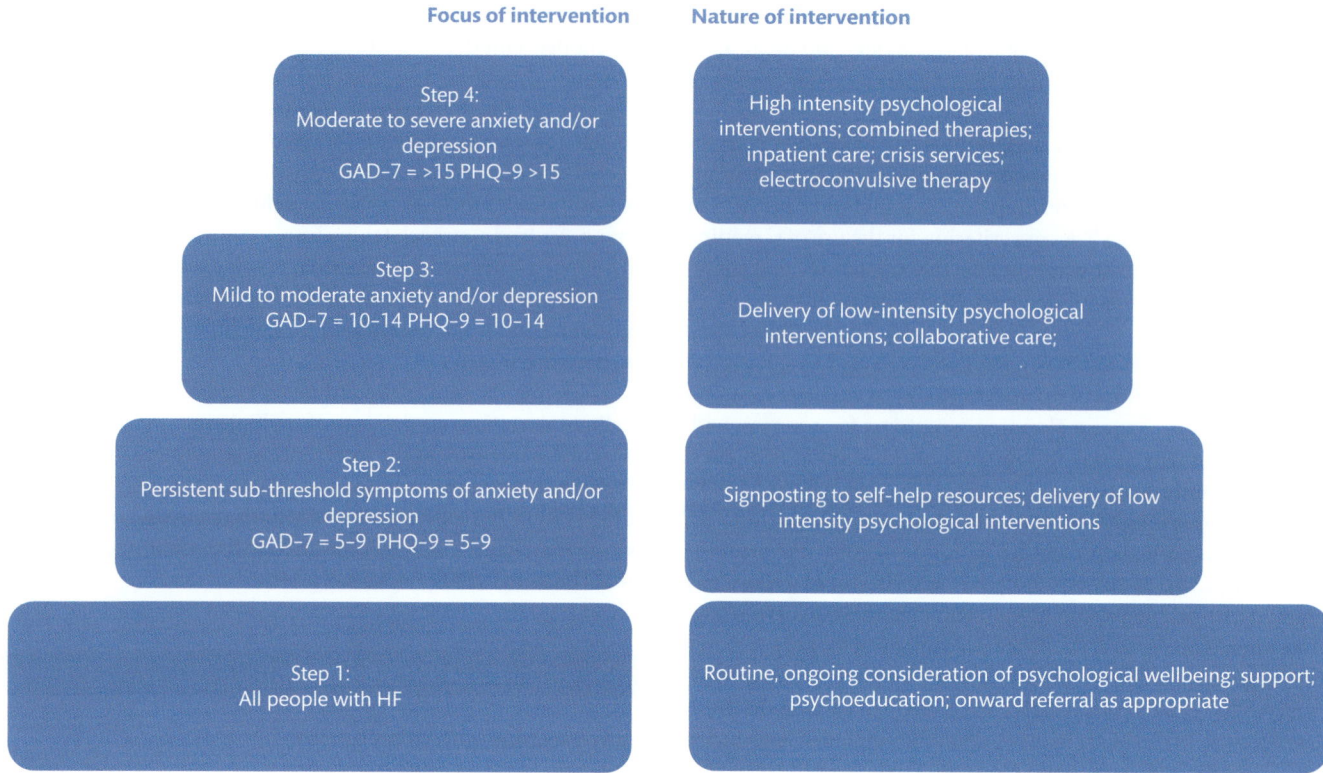

Figure 42.4 Stepped care model for the recognition and treatment of depression in heart failure (HF).

adult population.[48] Whereas there are numerous psychological therapies known to be effective in treating depression within the general population, few trials have explored their efficacy within heart failure populations. The most popular and readily available psychological intervention is cognitive behaviour therapy (CBT). Borne from Beck's cognitive model, CBT aims first to help individuals' identification of selective information processing, leading to engagement with depresso- or anxiogenic cognitions and subsequent behavioural responses that contribute to the genesis, maintenance, and exacerbation of depression and/or anxiety. Intervention involves helping individuals acquire skills to challenge and modify thoughts and beliefs that are distorted or unhelpful and to adjust behaviours that are maladaptive and often self-defeating.

A randomized control trial to determine the efficacy of CBT against usual care demonstrates that CBT targeting both depression and self-care is effective for HFD. There were no significant differences between CBT and usual care for self-care or physical functioning. However, additional benefits of CBT intervention include reduced anxiety and fatigue, improved social functioning, and better health-related QoL.[49] Accordingly, the Scottish Intercollegiate Guidelines Network recommends considering CBT for patients with co-morbid heart failure and depression.[41]

Recently, small-scale randomized controlled trials have similarly hinted at the potential effectiveness of psychotherapy in reducing depression scores, improving subjective measures of heart failure outcomes compared with usual care,[50] and leading to longer cardiac-event free survival compared to a 'usual care' control condition.[51] However, such studies have typically been underpowered and lacked placebo or control conditions.[12] There remains a clear need for larger clinical trials to assist in the understanding of psychological management of HFD.

Conclusion

This chapter has attempted to describe some of the mental health conditions commonly co-occurring with heart failure. In addition to raising awareness of the characteristics and prevalence of depression and anxiety, the objective was to impress the potential impact of such disorders on heart failure morbidity and mortality and to highlight the importance of integrating psychological care within heart failure services. The overriding imperative should be to recognize depression and anxiety as early as possible and intervene appropriately. The underlying indirect (behavioural) and direct (pathophysiological) mechanisms of depression and anxiety were discussed. A brief review of the existing evidence for treatment of co-morbid depression, anxiety, and heart failure was presented as well as appropriate management strategies. Finally, of critical importance is the need for future investigation into psychological therapies for HFD and HFA, to clarify whether treatment of depression and anxiety can improve the poorer prognosis in patients with heart failure.

REFERENCES

1. World Health Organization. *The ICD-10 classification of mental and behavioural disorders: clinical descriptions and diagnostic guidelines*. World Health Organization, Geneva, 1992.

2. Clark DM. A cognitive approach to panic. *Behav Res Ther* 1986;**24**(4):461–70.

3. American Psychiatric Association. *Diagnostic and statistical manual of mental disorders*, 5th edn, 2013.

4. Beck AT. *Depression: clinical, experimental, and theoretical aspects*. University of Pennsylvania Press, 1967.

5. Tang HY, Sayers SL, Weissinger G, Riegel B. The role of depression in medication adherence among heart failure patients. *Clin Nurs Res* 2014;**23**(3):231–44.

6. Baxter AJ, Scott KM, Vos T, Whiteford HA. Global prevalence of anxiety disorders: a systematic review and meta-regression. *Psychol Med* 2013;**43**(5):897–910.

7. Yohannes AM, Willgoss TG, Baldwin RC, Connolly MJ. Depression and anxiety in chronic heart failure and chronic obstructive pulmonary disease: prevalence, relevance, clinical implications and management principles. *Int J Geriatr Psychiatry* 2010;**25**(12):1209–21.

8. Easton K, Coventry P, Lovell K, Carter L, Deaton C. Prevalence and measurement of anxiety in samples of patients with heart failure. *J Cardiovasc Nurs* 2016;**31**(4):367–79.

9. Ohayon MM, Priest RG, Guilleminault C, Caulet M. The prevalence of depressive disorders in the United Kingdom. *Biol Psychiatry* 1999;**45**(3):300–7.

10. Murberg TA. Long-term effect of social relationships on mortality in patients with congestive heart failure. *Int J Psychiatry Med* 2004;**34**(3):207–17.

11. Vaccarino V, Kasl SV, Abramson J, Krumholz HM. Depressive symptoms and risk of functional decline and death in patients with heart failure. *J Am Coll Cardiol* 2001;**38**(1):199–205.

12. Rutledge T, Reis VA, Linke SE, Greenberg BH, Mills PJ. Depression in heart failure: a meta-analytic review of prevalence, intervention effects, and associations with clinical outcomes. *J Am Coll Cardiol* 2006;**48**(8):1527–37.

13. O'Neil A. The relationship between coronary heart disease (CHD) and major depressive disorder (MDD): key mechanisms and the role of quality of life. *Eur J Psychol* 2013;**9**(1):163–84.

14. Freedland KE, Carney RM, Rich MW. Effect of depression on prognosis in heart failure. *Heart Fail Clin* 2011;**7**(1):11–21.

15. Tousoulis D, Antonopoulos AS, Antoniades C, *et al*. Role of depression in heart failure—choosing the right antidepressive treatment. *Int J Cardiol* 2010;**140**(1):12–18.

16. Konstam V, Moser DK, De Jong MJ. Depression and anxiety in heart failure. *J Card Fail* 2005;**11**(6):455–63.

17. Fan H, Yu W, Zhang Q, *et al*. Depression after heart failure and risk of cardiovascular and all-cause mortality: a meta-analysis. *Prev Med* 2014;**63**:36–42.

18. Sokoreli I, de Vries J, Pauws S, Steyerberg E. Depression and anxiety as predictors of mortality among heart failure patients: systematic review and meta-analysis. *Heart Fail Rev* 2016;**21**(1):49–63.

19. Nair N, Farmer C, Gongora E, Dehmer GJ. Commonality between depression and heart failure. *Am J Cardiol* 2012;**109**(5):768–72.

20. Newhouse A, Jiang W. Heart failure and depression. *Heart Fail Clin* 2014;**10**(2):295–304.

21. Kop WJ, Synowski SJ, Gottlieb SS. Depression in heart failure: biobehavioral mechanisms. *Heart Fail Clin* 2011;**7**(1):23–38.

22. Jiang W, Alexander J, Christopher E, *et al*. Relationship of depression to increased risk of mortality and rehospitalization in patients with congestive heart failure. *Arch Intern Med* 2001;**161**(15):1849–56.

23. Norra C, Skobel EC, Arndt M, Schauerte P. High impact of depression in heart failure: early diagnosis and treatment options. *Int J Cardiol* 2008;**125**(2):220–31.

24. Vongmany J, Hickman LD, Lewis J, Newton PJ, Phillips JL. Anxiety in chronic heart failure and the risk of increased hospitalisations and mortality: a systematic review. *Eur J Cardiovasc Nurs* 2016;**15**(7):478–85.

25. Dekker RL. Cognitive therapy for depression in patients with heart failure: a critical review. *Heart Fail Clin* 2011;**7**(1):127–41.

26. Gnanasekaran G. Epidemiology of depression in heart failure. *Heart Fail Clin* 2011;**7**(1):1–10.

27. Dekker RL. Patient perspectives about depressive symptoms in heart failure: a review of the qualitative literature. *J Cardiovasc Nurs* 2014;**29**(1):E9–15.

28. MacMahon KMA, Lip GYH. Psychological factors in heart failure: a review of the literature. *Arch Intern Med* 2002;**162**(5):509–16.

29. Rustad JK, Stern TA, Hebert KA, Musselman DL. Diagnosis and treatment of depression in patients with congestive heart failure: a review of the literature. *Prim Care Companion CNS Disord* 2013;**15**(4):13r01511.

30. Joynt KE, Whellan DJ, O'Connor CM. Why is depression bad for the failing heart? A review of the mechanistic relationship between depression and heart failure. *J Card Fail* 2004;**10**(3):258–71.

31. Lane DA, Chong AY, Lip GY. Psychological interventions for depression in heart failure. *Cochrane Database Syst Rev* 2005;(1):CD003329.

32. Lea P. The effects of depression in heart failure. *Dimens Crit Care Nurs* 2009;**28**(4):164–68.

33. Lichtman JH, Bigger JT, Jr, Blumenthal JA, *et al*. Depression and coronary heart disease: recommendations for screening, referral, and treatment: a science advisory from the American Heart Association Prevention Committee of the Council on Cardiovascular Nursing, Council on Clinical Cardiology, Council on Epidemiology and Prevention, and Interdisciplinary Council on Quality of Care and Outcomes Research: endorsed by the American Psychiatric Association. *Circulation* 2008;**118**(17):1768–75.

34. Moudgil R, Haddad H. Depression in heart failure. *Curr Opin Cardiol* 2013;**28**(2):249–58.

35. Kessing D, Denollet J, Widdershoven J, Kupper N. Psychological determinants of heart failure self-care: systematic review and meta-analysis. *Psychosom Med* 2016;**78**(4):412–31.

36. Allman E, Berry D, Nasir L. Depression and coping in heart failure patients: a review of the literature. *J Cardiovasc Nurs* 2009;**24**(2):106–17.

37. Skala JA, Freedland KE, Carney RM. Coronary heart disease and depression: a review of recent mechanistic research. *Can J Psychiat* 2006;**51**(12):738.

38. Gilbody S, Sheldon T, House A. Screening and case-finding instruments for depression: a meta-analysis. *Can Med Assoc J* 2008;**178**(8):997–1003.

39. Potokar JP, Nutt DJ. Chest pain: panic attack or heart attack? *Int J Clin Pract* 2000;**54**(2):110–14.
40. Guck TP, Elsasser GN, Kavan MG, Eugene J, Eugene J. Depression and congestive heart failure. *Congest Heart Fail* 2003;**9**(3):163–69.
41. Scottish Intercollegiate Guidelines Network. *Management of chronic heart failure.* 2016.
42. Yeager KR, Binkley PF, Saveanu RV, *et al.* Screening and identification of depression among patients with coronary heart disease and congestive heart failure. *Heart Fail Clin* 2011;**7**(1):69–74.
43. Huffman JC, Mastromauro CA, Sowden G, *et al.* Impact of a depression care management program for hospitalized cardiac patients. *Circ Cardiovasc Qual Outcomes* 2011;**4**(2):198–205.
44. National Institute for Health and Care Excellence (NICE). *Depression in adults with a chronic physical health problem: recognition and management.* Clinical Guideline 91. 2009. https://www.nice.org.uk/guidance/cg91
45. Shapiro PA. Treatment of depression in patients with congestive heart failure. *Heart Fail Rev* 2009;**14**(1):7–12.
46. Dimos AK, Stougiannos PN, Kakkavas AT, Trikas AG. Depression and heart failure. *Hellenic J Cardiol* 2009;**50**(3):410–17.
47. Jiang W, O'Connor C, Silva SG, *et al.* Safety and efficacy of sertraline for depression in patients with CHF (SADHART-CHF): a randomized, double-blind, placebo-controlled trial of sertraline for major depression with congestive heart failure. *Am Heart J* 2008;**156**(3):437–44.
48. Middleton H, Shaw I, Hull S, Feder G. NICE Guidelines for the management of depression … are clear for severe depression, but uncertain for mild or moderate depression. *Br Med J* 2005;**330**:267–8.
49. Freedland KE, Carney RM, Rich MW, Steinmeyer BC, Rubin EH. Cognitive behavior therapy for depression and self-care in heart failure patients: a randomized clinical trial. *JAMA Intern Med* 2015;**175**(11):1773–82.
50. Gary RA, Dunbar SB, Higgins MK, Musselman DL, Smith AL. Combined exercise and cognitive behavioral therapy improves outcomes in patients with heart failure. *J Psychosom Res* 2010;**69**(2):119–31.
51. Dekker RL, Moser DK, Peden AR, Lennie TA. Cognitive therapy improves three-month outcomes in hospitalized patients with heart failure. *J Card Fail* 2012;**18**(1):10–20.

RECOMMENDED READING

Freedland KE, Carney RM, Rich MW, Steinmeyer BC, Rubin EH. Cognitive behavior therapy for depression and self-care in heart failure patients: a randomized clinical trial. *JAMA Intern Med* 2015;**175**(11):1773–82.

National Health Sevice (NHS) Education for Scotland. *Emotion matters.* NHS Education for Scotland developed training for all health and social staff, aiming to develop skills in addressing emotional issues with people who are living with a long term condition. http://www.knowledge.scot.nhs.uk/home/learning-and-cpd/learning-spaces/emotion-matters.aspx

National Institute for Health and Care Excellence (NICE). *Depression in adults with a chronic physical health problem: treatment and management.* Clinical Guideline 91. 2009. https://www.nice.org.uk/guidance/cg91

Naylor C, Parsonage M, McDaid D, *et al.* Long-term conditions and mental health. The cost of co-morbidities. The King's Fund and Centre for Mental Health, London, 2012.

Rutledge T, Reis VA, Linke SE, Greenberg BH, Mills PJ. Depression in heart failure: a meta-analytic review of prevalence, intervention effects, and associations with clinical outcomes. *J Am Coll Cardiol* 2006;**48**(8):1527–37.

43

Cognitive impairment

John Baxter and Lesley Young

Introduction

Cognitive impairment is common in older patients, most frequently due to delirium or dementia. Both commonly coexist with heart failure as all are diseases of ageing.[1]

Dementia is a chronic progressive neurological disorder characterized by impairment of memory and at least one other cognitive domain, such as executive functioning. Delirium is a clinical syndrome characterized by altered attention, arousal and disturbances in cognition to varying degrees, usually in the context of an identifiable precipitant.

Dementia and heart failure

Aetiology and epidemiology

Dementia is an umbrella term for a group of neurodegenerative disorders, all of which result in progressive cognitive decline. The most common forms are Alzheimer disease (62%), vascular dementia (17%), mixed Alzheimer and vascular (10%), Lewy body dementia (4%) and fronto-temporal dementia (2%), Parkinson-related dementia (2%) and other rarer types (3%). Dementia is a disease of ageing, with prevalence increasing with age, with ~3% of 65–75-year-olds being affected, increasing to around 40% of those aged >95 years.[2] In patients with heart failure, vascular dementia is the most common aetiology, accounting for 36% in one Swedish study, which found Alzheimer disease in only 16%.[3]

Pathophysiology

Two theories account for the occurrence of dementia in heart failure patients. First, they are both manifestations of a common pathology, such as atherosclerosis. Second, that dementia is a direct consequence of heart failure. Both cerebral hypoperfusion and microemboli are common pathophysiological mechanisms.[4,5]

Clinical features

Common features of all types of dementia include the development of cognitive or behavioural symptoms of sufficient degree to interfere with normal everyday activities, social functioning, or work activities, constituting a decline from the person's baseline not due solely to a coexistent delirium.

As well as impairment of memory and the ability to retain new information, the ICD-10 definition of dementia syndrome also includes declines in other cognitive abilities such as judgement, thinking, planning and organizing, processing of information, a decline in emotional control with reduced motivation, exemplified by issues such as emotional lability, irritability, and apathy, or coarsening of social behaviour. Patients with dementia may also exhibit deficits in higher cortical function such as aphasia, agnosia, and apraxia. The features should have been present for at least six months in order to be confident in a diagnosis of dementia.

Diagnosis

Recognizing the presence of dementia in patients is important. Patients will be more vulnerable to developing delirium in the presence of intercurrent illness, and measures should be taken to prevent delirium where possible, for example avoiding 'deliriogenic' drugs such as opiates, benzodiazepines[6] and those with anticholinergic effects (see Box 43.1). Recognition of dementia should also prompt an assessment of capacity when making important clinical decisions such as those concerning resuscitation, anticoagulation, and use of implantable cardioverter–defibrillator devices.

When assessing cognition in the clinical setting, the use of brief cognitive screening tools will help identify the presence of dementia. The most widely used tool is the Mini Mental State Examination (MMSE).[7] A more recently developed tool is the Montreal Cognitive Assessment (MoCA),[8] which is freely available online (https://www.mocatest.org) and has 100% sensitivity and 87% specificity for dementia with a cut-off of 25/30. Both the MMSE and MoCA take about 10 min to administer. Briefer screening tools (generally <5 min) include Abbreviated Mental Test Score (AMTS),[9] which is scored out of 10, and at a cut-off of 6/10 (sensitivity 81%, specificity 84%) and the six-item Cognitive Impairment Test (6-CIT; sensitivity 90%, specificity 100%).[10]

Management

The main pharmacological intervention for the management of dementia is the use of acetylcholinesterase inhibitors in Alzheimer

Box 43.1 Drugs with anticholinergic effects

High			
Amitriptyline	Nortriptyline	Meperidine	Dipyridamole
Amoxapine	Olanzapine	Methotrimeprazine	Disopyramide
Atropine	Orphenadrine	Molindone	Fentanyl
Benztropine	Oxybutynin	Nefopam	Furosemide
Brompheniramine	Paroxetine	Oxcarbazepine	Fluvoxamine
Carbinoxamine	Perphenazine	Pimozide	Haloperidol
Chlorpheniramine	Promethazine	**Low**	Hydralazine
Chlorpromazine	Propantheline	Alimemazine	Hydrocortisone
Clemastine	Propiverine	Alverine	Iloperidone
Clomipramine	Quetiapine	Alprazolam	Isosorbide
Clozapine	Scopolamine	Aripiprazole	Levocetirizine
Darifenacin	Solifenacin	Asenapine	Loperamide
Desipramine	Thioridazine	Atenolol	Loratadine
Dicyclomine	Tolterodine	Bupropion	Metoprolol
Dimenhydrinate	Trifluoperazine	Captopril	Morphine
Diphenhydramine	Trihexyphenidyl	Cetirizine	Nifedipine
Doxepin	Trimipramine	Chlorthalidone	Paliperidone
Doxylamine	Trospium	Cimetidine	Prednisone
Fesoterodine	**Medium**	Clidinium	Quinidine
Flavoxate	Amantadine	Clorazepate	Ranitidine
Hydroxyzine	Belladonna	Codeine	Risperidone
Hyoscyamine	Carbamazepine	Colchicine	Theophylline
Imipramine	Cyclobenzaprine	Desloratadine	Trazodone
Meclizine	Cyproheptadine	Diazepam	Triamterene
Methocarbamol	Loxapine	Digoxin	Venlafaxine
			Warfarin

Source data from Anticholinergic Cognitive Burden Scale 2012 Update Developed by the Aging Brain Program of the Indiana University Center for Aging Research. https://www.agingbraincare.org

and Lewy body type dementias. Whereas these drugs do not alter the disease progression in dementia, they can be useful in alleviating symptoms and thereby promoting independence. They are generally well tolerated with no absolute contraindications listed and the main side-effects are nausea, vomiting, and diarrhoea. Due to the co-mechanism of action there is a recognized risk of cardiovascular adverse effects, notably sick sinus syndrome and cardiac conduction defects. However, these are rare, with an estimated frequency of bradyarrhythmias, myocardial infarction, and angina of between 1 in 100 and 1 in 10 000, and of more serious sino-atrial block and atrioventricular block of between 1 in 1000 and 1 in 100 000. ECG is not required prior to commencing such treatment as an abnormal ECG has low predictive value in determining risk of subsequent cardiovascular adverse events.[11] Coexistent cardiovascular disease is regarded as a caution to treatment rather than as a contraindication. For patients who develop syncope or symptomatic bradycardia on this class of drug, ECG should be carried out and the drug withheld pending further review of the cause.

Prognosis and clinical outcomes

Prognosis and clinical outcomes are worse in heart failure patients who also have dementia. Hospitalized patients with heart failure and cognitive impairment have a significantly higher mortality than heart failure patients with normal cognition,[12] and they are at higher risk of complications such as delirium, falls, and functional impairment.

Community-dwelling heart failure patients with dementia have a better prognosis, more in line with the general heart failure population. In a Swedish study, community-dwelling heart failure patients with dementia had a one-year survival of 76%.[3]

Delirium and heart failure

Aetiology and epidemiology

Delirium is a clinical syndrome of altered attention, arousal, and cognition resulting from an underlying organic cause. Delirium has been described since ancient times, being recognized as a condition occurring in conjunction with illness, especially sepsis and being associated with a poor prognosis. There are several definitions of delirium (see Table 43.1), the most widely used being those defined by the American Psychiatric Association in the *Diagnostic and statistical manual* and that developed by the World Health Organization. However, all definitions include the following key features:

1. a change in the patient's usual cognitive function;
2. impairment of attention;
3. altered arousal;
4. onset over a short period of time, usually hours to days with a fluctuating picture.

Delirium is common in hospitalized patients, with studies showing a point prevalence in acute general hospitals of ~20%,[13] of whom around half had coexisting dementia. Delirium is an independent predictor of poor outcomes, with the presence of delirium conferring a two-fold increased risk of mortality compared to non-delirious patients.[14] It is also associated with increased length of stay,

Table 43.1 Definitions of delirium

DSM-5 (APA, 2013)	DSM-4 (APA, 2000)	ICD-10 (WHO, 1992)
A. A disturbance in attention (that is reduced ability to direct, focus, sustain and shift attention) and awareness (reduced orientation to the environment).	A. Disturbance of consciousness (that is reduced clarity of awareness of the environment) with reduced ability to focus, sustain or shift attention.	A. Clouding of consciousness (i.e. reduced clarity of awareness of the environment with reduced ability to focus, sustain or shift attention).
B. The disturbance develops over a short period of time (usually hours to a few days), which represents a change from baseline attention and awareness, and tends to fluctuate in severity during the course of a day.	C. The disturbance develops over a short period of time usually hours to days) and tends to fluctuate during the course of the day.	E. Rapid onset and fluctuations of symptoms over the course of the day.
C. An additional disturbance in cognition (e.g. memory deficit, disorientation, language, visuospatial ability or perception).	B. A change in cognition or the development of new perceptual disturbance that is not better accounted for by a pre-existing, established or evolving dementia.	B. Disturbance of cognition, manifest by both: (1) impairment of immediate recall and recent memory with relatively intact remote memory; (2) disorientation in time, place or person. C. At least one of the following psychomotor disturbances: (1) rapid unpredictable shifts from hypo-activity to hyperactivity; (2) increased reaction time; (3) increased or decreased flow of speech; (4) enhanced startle reaction. D. Disturbance of the sleep-wake cycle, manifest by at least one of the following: (1) insomnia which in severe cases, may involve total sleep loss with or without day time drowsiness or reversal of sleep wake cycle; (2) nocturnal worsening of symptoms; (3) disturbing dreams or nightmares which may continue as hallucinations or illusions after awakening.
D. The disturbance in criteria A and C are not better explained by a pre-existing, established or evolving neurocognitive disorder and do not occur in the context of a severely reduced level of arousal such as a coma.		
E. There is evidence form the history, physical examination or laboratory findings that the disturbance is a direct consequence of another medical condition, substance intoxication or withdrawal or exposure to a toxin, or is due to multiple aetiologies.	D. There is evidence from the history, physical examination or laboratory findings that the disturbance is caused by the direct physiological consequences of a general medical condition.	F. Objective evidence from history, physical and neurological examination or laboratory tests of an underlying cerebral or systemic disease (other than psychoactive substance relayed) that can be presumed to be responsible for the clinical manifestations in A–D.
		Emotional disturbances such as depression, anxiety, fear, irritability, euphoria, apathy or wondering perplexity, disturbances in perception (illusions or hallucinations, often visual) and transient delusions are typical, but not specific indications for the diagnosis.

DSM, Diagnostic and statistical manual of mental disorders; APA, American Psychiatric Association; ICD, International classification of diseases; WHO, World Health Organization.

increased risk of institutionalization,[14,15] and with a greater risk of other inpatient complications such as falls, continence problems, and pressure sores.[16]

Whereas a proportion of patients will present to medical attention with delirium already present ('prevalent delirium'), others will develop the condition during the course of their illness ('incident delirium'). There is good evidence that up to 40% of these cases are preventable.[17,18] Identifying both patients at risk of delirium, as well as those who already have delirium, is therefore important in order to implement delirium prevention.[19]

Risk factors for developing delirium include:

- increased age;
- dementia;
- sensory deficits such visual and hearing loss;
- severe illness;
- dehydration;
- immobility.

There is an association between the underlying vulnerability of a person and the severity of the precipitant required to cause delirium: a person with a very low vulnerability to developing delirium would require a significant precipitant to develop a delirium, whereas a person with a high vulnerability requires only a small precipitant to develop delirium.[20]

Any illness can precipitate a delirium in a vulnerable patient and the cause is frequently multifactorial. However, the more common causes of delirium include:

- infections;
- biochemical disturbances, including hypo- and hypernatraemia, hypercalcaemia, hypoglycaemia;

Box 43.2 Check list for capacity assessment

Your patient has capacity until proved otherwise.

Capacity is time and decision specific.

Does your patient have a disorder of the mind or brain?

Can your patient:

1. Understand
2. Retain
3. Weigh up
4. Communicate their decision.

Document your capacity assessment.

- acute kidney injury;
- drugs, particularly those with anticholinergic effects (see Box 43.2);
- pain;
- organ failure, including renal failure, haptic failure, and cardiac failure;
- surgery.

Diagnosis

Clinicians are poor at identifying the presence of delirium.[21] Failure to recognize delirium is associated with worse outcomes,[22] probably because this results in a delay in identifying and treating the precipitating cause. Figure 43.2 shows an initial approach to the assessment of a confused patient.

There are many tools available to screen for and evaluate delirium; however, some are more appropriate for specialist use and research. Any screening tool should address the key areas of attention, acuity of onset, and arousal. This means that more traditional cognitive screening tools used to screen for dementia such as the AMTS are less useful for identifying the delirium. More recently published tools[23] include:

- 4AT (the 4 As Test; see Figure 43.1);[24]
- SQiD (Single Question in Delirium): 'Do you think [name of the patient] has been more confused lately?';[25]
- Short CAM (Confusion Assessment Method).[26]

Although CAM performs well when used by trained staff, its sensitivity and specificity fall when used by non-experts.[27] The 4AT (https://ww.the4AT.com) is a free-to-use tool, specifically designed for use by non-specialists as a brief screen to identify the possible presence of delirium. It has been widely used and validated.[24] In clinical practice, a patient who has altered arousal that is drowsy or agitated, and who has impaired attention, is highly likely to have delirium.

Management

The treatment of delirium is the treatment of the underlying cause (see Table 43.2). There is no proven treatment of delirium as such. Any electrolyte or other biochemical disturbance should be corrected. A full medication review should be undertaken. Many drugs have anticholinergic effects (see Box 43.2) and the effects of these are cumulative. Drugs which may be contributing should be discontinued wherever possible. Careful monitoring of fluid balance and bowel function is also important, as constipation frequently contributes to the development of delirium. Where possible, invasive monitoring such as the use of urinary catheters should be avoided. Patients should be mobilized as soon as possible. Communication with the patient and those close to them is important, as delirium is a frightening experience for both, and explaining the condition and its likely progress can help to alleviate distress. Ensuring that sensory aids such as hearing aids and spectacles are available can also be beneficial. For some patients, the presence of family members can be a reassuring and settling factor, and this should be considered.[19,28]

Role of drugs

There is no evidence for routine use of antipsychotic medication in the prevention or treatment of delirium.[29,30] Although they may have a role in alleviating symptoms from distressing hallucinations or delusions occurring in delirium, drugs should be considered second line to multicomponent non-pharmacological interventions.[19] If antipsychotics are considered, there is little evidence to support the use of newer agents over older agents such as haloperidol and the recommendation from NICE suggests haloperidol or olanzapine, in low doses and for the shortest possible time.[28] Although there is a theoretical risk of prolonged QTc with antipsychotic medications, this is rarely seen in the low doses indicated in the management of delirium,[31] and when used in this manner for delirium there does not appear to be an increased risk of cardiovascular adverse events.[32]

Benzodiazepines are not recommended as first-line agents in the management of delirium, unless antipsychotics are contraindicated (as in Parkinson disease or dementia with Lewy bodies), because of their association with causing or worsening delirium.[6]

Prognosis and clinical outcomes

Whereas most cases of delirium do resolve when the underlying cause has been treated, the delirium often takes much longer to resolve than the precipitant and may take many weeks or occasionally months to fully resolve. However, in a significant minority, the delirium does not resolve. Associated factors include hypoactive delirium, pre-existing dementia, and a more prolonged episode of delirium.[33] Delirium can also result in a worsening of, and accelerated decline in, pre-existing dementia, such that even if the delirium appears to have resolved, the person may have worse cognitive function after an episode of delirium.[34] Delirium is an independent predictor of death, new institutionalization, and increased length of hospital stay.[14]

When considering interventions or treatments that carry a risk of developing delirium, such as surgery, it is important to advise patients and carers of the risk of delirium and that it does carry an increased mortality and risk of permanent cognitive decline.[35]

4AT

Assessment test
for delirium &
cognitive impairment

Patient name:

Date of birth:

Patient number:

(label)

Date: Time:

Tester:

CIRCLE

[1] ALERTNESS
This includes patients who may be markedly drowsy (eg. difficult to rouse and/or obviously sleepy during assessment) or agitated/hyperactive. Observe the patient. If asleep, attempt to wake with speech or gentle touch on shoulder. Ask the patient to state their name and address to assist rating.

Normal (fully alert, but not agitated, throughout assessment)	0
Mild sleepiness for <10 seconds after waking, then normal	0
Clearly abnormal	4

[2] AMT4
Age, date of birth, place (name of the hospital or building), current year.

No mistakes	0
1 mistake	1
2 or more mistakes/untestable	2

[3] ATTENTION
Ask the patient: "Please tell me the months of the year in backwards order, starting at December."
To assist initial understanding one prompt of "what is the month before December?" is permitted.

Months of the year backwards		
	Achieves 7 months or more correctly	0
	Starts but scores <7 months / refuses to start	1
	Untestable (cannot start because unwell, drowsy, inattentive)	2

[4] ACUTE CHANGE OR FLUCTUATING COURSE
Evidence of significant change or fluctuation in: alertness, cognition, other mental function (eg. paranoia, hallucinations) arising over the last 2 weeks and still evident in last 24hrs

No	0
Yes	4

4 or above: possible delirium +/- cognitive impairment
1-3: possible cognitive impairment
0: delirium or severe cognitive impairment unlikely (but delirium still possible if [4] information incomplete)

4AT SCORE ☐

GUIDANCE NOTES   Version 1.2. Information and download: **www.the4AT.com**
The 4AT is a screening instrument designed for rapid initial assessment of delirium and cognitive impairment. A score of 4 or more suggests delirium but is not diagnostic: more detailed assessment of mental status may be required to reach a diagnosis. A score of 1-3 suggests cognitive impairment and more detailed cognitive testing and informant history-taking are required. A score of 0 does not definitively exclude delirium or cognitive impairment: more detailed testing may be required depending on the clinical context. Items 1-3 are rated solely on observation of the patient at the time of assessment. Item 4 requires information from one or more source(s), eg. your own knowledge of the patient, other staff who know the patient (eg. ward nurses), GP letter, case notes, carers. The tester should take account of communication difficulties (hearing impairment, dysphasia, lack of common language) when carrying out the test and interpreting the score.
Alertness: Altered level of alertness is very likely to be delirium in general hospital settings. If the patient shows significant altered alertness during the bedside assessment, score 4 for this item. **AMT4** (Abbreviated Mental Test - 4): This score can be extracted from items in the AMT10 if the latter is done immediately before. **Acute Change or Fluctuating Course:** Fluctuation can occur without delirium in some cases of dementia, but marked fluctuation usually indicates delirium. To help elicit any hallucinations and/or paranoid thoughts ask the patient questions such as, "Are you concerned about anything going on here?"; "Do you feel frightened by anything or anyone?"; "Have you been seeing or hearing anything unusual?"

© 2011-2014 MacLullich, Ryan, Cash

Figure 43.1 The 4AT score.
Reproduced by kind permission of Prof Alisdair MacLullich. See www.the4AT.com for free downloads, updates and further information.

Medico-legal issues

In all patients with cognitive problems, it is important to consider the person's understanding of their diagnosis and their capacity to consent to the care and treatment proposed. In England and Wales, capacity is defined by the Mental Capacity Act (2005) and is assessed using a two-stage functional test.

1. Is there an impairment of, or disturbance in, the functioning of the person's mind or brain?

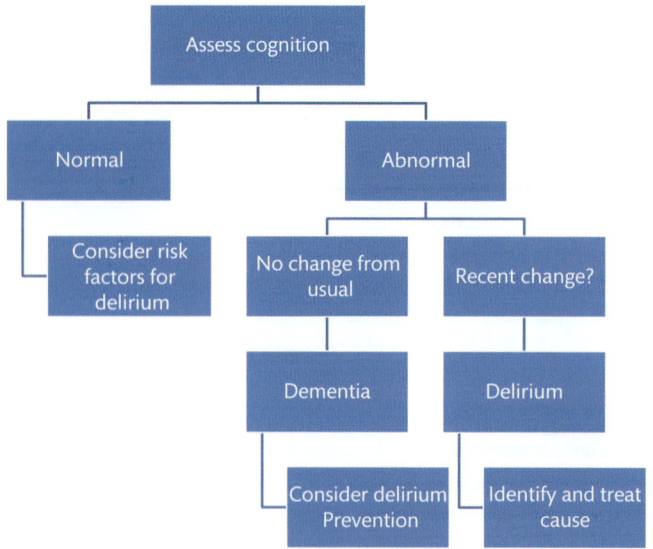

Figure 43.2 Clinical approach to cognition assessment.

2. Is this impairment or disturbance identified in part 1 of sufficient degree such that it impacts on the person's ability to:
   • understand,
   • retain,
   • weigh up,

or

   • communicate information relevant to the decision on question.

Thus, capacity is seen to be specific to the decision in question, i.e. a person may quite possibly have capacity to make one decision, but not another more complicated decision. Capacity is also time specific, in that it may vary over a period of time and must therefore be assessed at the time appropriate to the decision being made. If a person lacks capacity to make a decision for themselves, the Act empowers health care professionals to act on their behalf, as long as the principles of the Act are followed. The principles of the Mental Capacity Act are:

1. A person must be assumed to have capacity unless it is established otherwise. The onus is on the clinician to show that a

Table 43.2 PINCHME: Check list for managing a heart failure patient with delirium

Address five key issues:	
*PA*IN	Ensure your patient is monitored for pain and has adequate regular and PRN (*pro re nata*) analgesia.
	Be cautious in the use of analgesic agents that may exacerbate confusion, especially opiates.
*IN*FECTION	Be rigorous in identifying possible sources of infection.
*CH*F	Review chronic heart failure clinical status and change treatment accordingly.
*M*EDICATION	Review all prescribed drugs and rationalise
*E*NVIRONMENT	Ensure the ward environment is appropriate for delirious patients.

person does not have capacity, rather than the person requiring to prove they do have capacity.

2. A person must be supported in their decision-making. This means that all practical steps must be taken to help a person make a decision, such as providing written information, providing sensory aids, using sign language or translators.

3. A person with capacity has a right to make unwise decisions. Thus, making what could be considered an unwise decision does not mean that a person lacks capacity, even in situations where the consequence of that decision may result in a person's death.

4. Any acts undertaken or decisions made on behalf of a person who lacks capacity must be in done or made in that person's best interests.

5. Any act or decision made on behalf of a person who lacks capacity must be the least restrictive option.

The 2005 MCA introduced the concept of Lasting Power of Attorney (LPA). A person with capacity can appoint an attorney to act on their behalf. Ordinary power of attorney becomes invalid if a person loses capacity, whereas LPA does not. LPA can be appointed for:

• Property and finances—this can be activated while a person still has capacity if they
• Health and welfare—this only comes into effect when the person lacks capacity to make the relevant decisions. The LPA can then make decisions on behalf of the person relating to all aspects of health and personal welfare; this includes decisions about accepting or refusing medical treatment and place of residence.

Health care professionals must consult with any LPA of health and welfare when considering treatment for patients who lack capacity to make these decisions themselves.

When making decisions on behalf of a person who lacks capacity, it is necessary to document the evidence around the capacity assessment and to undertake a best interests assessment. This should include consultation with the patient, if they are able to participate in such a discussion—as, even if they lack capacity, they may be able to express some wishes or views, while not being the ultimate decision-maker. Any LPA for health and welfare must be consulted, and, in the absence of an LPA, discussion with any carers or family who may be able to inform decision-making with respect to the patient's views, wishes, and beliefs must also be consulted, along with other members of the multidisciplinary team. If the patient has no friends or family who can support decision-making, an Independent Mental Capacity Advocate (IMCA) should be appointed to act as an advocate on the patient's behalf, when decisions regarding serious medical treatment need to be made. This includes decisions such as Do Not Attempt Resuscitation. In order to reach a best interests decision, all options for treatment should be explored along with the potential risks and benefits for each option for the individual. As with a person with capacity, an LPA may refuse treatment on a patient's behalf, but cannot demand a treatment that is not deemed to be clinically appropriate or ethical by the clinical team.

The outcome of this decision-making process should be documented. In urgent or emergency situations, access to supporting

information may be more difficult with limited time for consultation; however, any decisions must still be in the person's best interests, and, wherever practicable, discussion should take place with interested parties such as next of kin.

A recent case was taken to the High Court in England with respect to a 'Do not attempt cardiopulmonary resuscitation' (CPR) decision in a patient who lacked capacity.[36] The hospital trust was deemed to be at fault and the patient's human rights were deemed to have been violated because the attending clinical team did not discuss the proposed DNACPR decision with the patient's next of kin prior to placing a DNACPR notice in the patient's notes, despite it having been practicable to do so.[37]

In Scotland, similar principles are set out in the Adults with Incapacity (Scotland) Act (2000), whereby clinicians performing care must follow the general principles of benefit, minimum intervention, considering the individual's wishes and feelings, consultation with appropriate others, and encouraging the exercise of residual capacity. Part 5 of the Act allows a clinician authority to treat an adult with incapacity following the issue of a certificate of incapacity;[38] however, in the case of treatment required for immediate preservation of life or prevention of serious deterioration in a clinical condition, common law permits intervention with the requirement of completing the steps laid out in Part 5 of the Act.

Management of heart failure patients with cognitive impairment

It is very important that heart failure services recognize those patients with cognitive impairment as early as possible. This is because cognitive impairment requires diagnostic work-up and appropriate treatments. Also, the presence of cognitive impairment may require a change in management strategy to ensure that patients receive optimal heart failure treatment, and that adherence to therapy maximized.

There are several scenarios that a health care professional working in a heart failure team may come across:

- the development of cognitive impairment in a patient with known heart failure;
- the development of possible heart failure in a patient with established dementia;
- the co-presentation of cognitive impairment and heart failure.

Establishing the diagnosis of cognitive impairment

Routine cognitive testing for heart failure patients should be considered for selected outpatients and all inpatients aged >65 years (Figure 43.2). It is important that health care professionals have the appropriate skills in undertaking screening assessments. Informal assessments of cognition by a cardiologist are insufficiently sensitive to detect cognitive impairment during routine consultation.[39] Currently routine screening is not recommended by UK or European heart failure guidelines.

Patients who are found to have cognitive impairment should be assessed by appropriate services. For outpatients, referral to a specialized memory clinic offering multidisciplinary assessments, perhaps in the patient's own home, should be considered. Hospitalized heart failure patients with delirium or dementia may require assessments by delirium and dementia teams often involving specialist nurse review supported by a geriatrician or old-age psychiatrist.

Approaches to management

Health care professionals considering therapeutic strategies for heart failure patients should not exclude treatments simply because a patient has cognitive impairment. However, there are additional requirements in determining the optimum heart failure therapy and most appropriate chronic disease management.

There are four steps a health care professional should take when managing heart failure in a patient who has cognitive impairment:

1. Assessment of the patient's ability to participate in treatment decisions (see Box 43.2). Health care professionals need to have the appropriate skill set to assess a patient's capacity to participate in treatment decisions. It is important to remember that capacity assessments are decision and time specific. Hence some patients may have the capacity to agree to medical treatment such as β-blockers or angiotensin converting enzyme inhibitors but may lack capacity to participate in decision-making regarding complex device therapies and other interventional treatments.

2. Ensuring compliance with local legislation. Heart failure health care professionals must ensure they are following legal requirements when managing heart failure patients who lack capacity to participate in accepting indicated treatments. In the UK this would involve compliance with the Mental Capacity Act. Treatments should comply with an advance decision to refuse treatment. Should the patient have granted a lasting power of attorney then the nominated individual must be consulted. Best interest decisions need to be made with the help of relatives, carers and advance health care plans. A referral to an Independent Mental Capacity Advocate should be completed in an unbefriended patient. All decision-making needs to be clearly documented and communicated. Team-based decision-making is the most effective and accountable (see Box 43.3).

3. Altering management strategies to help compliance with treatment. It is important that heart failure services be flexible enough to alter drug regimens, disease surveillance programmes, rehabilitation services, and other service provision to accommodate patients who have cognitive impairment. For example, in patients who are unable to adhere to complex drug regimens,

---

Box 43.3 Check list for decision-making in a patient who lacks capacity to participate in the decision in question:

1 Document your patients capacity;
   i. Date and time your assessment
   ii. If they lack capacity for the decision in question, proceed as follows:
2 Do they have an advanced decision to refuse treatment (ADRT)?
3 Has your patient granted legal power of attorney for medical matters?
4 Best interest decisions should be communicated with relatives or carers, or with independent mental capacity advocates in unbefriended patients.

consideration should be given to alter drug frequencies to match visits from carers who can facilitate compliance. Also methods of disease monitoring may need to be changed, as well as content and delivery of rehabilitation programmes.

4. Heart failure specialists need to be alert to the cardiovascular risks of treatments for cognitive impairment that their patient may be taking. Cognitive-enhancing medication such as acetylcholinesterase inhibitors may cause bradycardia, sick sinus syndrome, and other arrhythmias.

REFERENCES

1. Cannon JA, McMurray JJV, Quinn TJ. Hearts and minds: association, causation and implication of cognitive impairment in heart failure. *Alzheimer's Res Ther* 2015;7:22.
2. Alzheimer's Society. Dementia UK update 2014.
3. Cermakova P, Lund LH, Fereshtehnejad S-M, *et al*. Heart failure and dementia: survival in relation to types of heart failure and different dementia disorders. *Eur J Heart Fail* 2015;17(6):612–19.
4. Ogren JA, Fonarow GC, Woo MA. Cerebral impairment in heart failure. *Curr Heart fail Rep* 2014;11(3);321–9.
5. Kalaria, R. N. (2012). Cerebrovascular disease and mechanisms of cognitive impairment; evidence from clinicopathological studies in humans. *Stroke* 2012;43(9):2526–34.
6. Clegg A, Young John B. Which medications to avoid in people at risk of delirium: a systematic review. *Age Ageing* 2011;40(1):23–9.
7. Folstein MF, Folstein SE, McHugh PR. 'Mini-mental state': a practical method for grading cognitive state of patients for the clinician. *J Psychiat Res* 1975;12(3):189–98.
8. Pendlebury ST, Klaus SP, Mather M, de Brito M, Wharton RM. Routine cognitive screening in older patients admitted to acute medicine: abbreviated mental test score (AMTS) and subjective memory complaint versus Montreal Cognitive Assessment and IQCODE. *Age Ageing* 2015:44(6):1000–5.
9. Qureshi KN, Hodkinson M. Evaluation of a ten question mental test in the institutionalized elderly. *Age Ageing* 1974;3(3):152–7.
10. Sheehan B. Assessment scales in dementia. *Ther Adv Neurol Disord* 2012;5(6):349–58.
11. Rowland JP, Rigby J, Harper AC, Rowland R. Cardiovascular monitoring with acetylcholinesterase inhibitors: a clinical protocol. *Adv Psychiat Treat* 2007:13(3):178–84.
12. Zuccalà G, Pedone C, Cesari M, *et al*. The effects of cognitive impairment on mortality in hospitalised heart failure patients. *Am J Med* 2003;115(2):97–103.
13. Ryan DJ, O'Regan NA, O'Caoimh R, *et al*. Delirium in an adult acute hospital population: predictors, prevalence and detection. *BMJ Open* 2013;3(1):e001772.
14. Siddiqi N, House AO, Holmes JD. Occurrence and outcomes of delirium in medical in-patients: a systematic literature review. *Age Ageing* 2006;35(4):350–64.
15. Mangusan R. Outcomes associated with postoperative delirium after cardiac surgery. *Am J Crit Care* 2015;24(2):156–163.
16. O'Keeffe S, Lavan J. The prognostic significance of delirium in older hospital patients. *J Am Geriat Soc* 1997;45(2):174–8.

17. Inouye SK, Bogardus ST, Charpentier PA, *et al*. A multicomponent intervention to prevent delirium in hospitalized older patients. *N Engl J Med* 1999:340:669–76.
18. Hshieh TT, Yue J, Puelle M, *et al*. Effectiveness of multicomponent nonpharmacological delirium interventions: a meta-analysis. *JAMA Intern Med* 2015;175(4):512–20.
19. Scottish Intercollegiate Guidelines Network (SIGN) 157. *Risk reduction and management of delirium—a national clinical guideline*. March 2019.
20. Inouye SK, Charpentier PA. Precipitating factors for delirium in hospitalized elderly persons. Predictive model and interrelationship with baseline vulnerability. *JAMA* 1996;275(11):852–7.
21. Yanamadala M, Wieland D, Heflin MT. Educational interventions to improve recognition of delirium. *J Am Geriat Soc* 2013;61(11):1983–93.
22. Kakuma R, Du Fort GG, Aresnault L, *et al*. Delirium in older emergency department patients discharged home: effect on survival. *J Am Geriat Soc* 2003;51(4):443–50.
23. De J, Wand APF. Delirium screening tools: a systematic review of delirium screening tools in hospitalized patients. *Gerontologist* 2015;55(6):1079–99.
24. Bellelli G, Morandi A, Davis DHJ, *et al*. Validation of the 4AT, a new instrument for rapid delirium screening: a study in 234 hospitalised older people. *Age Ageing* 2014;43(4):496–502.
25. Sands MB. Single question in delirium (SQiD): testing its efficacy against psychiatrist interview, the Confusion Assessment Method and the Memorial Delirium Assessment Scale. *Palliat Med* 2010;24(6):561–5.
26. Inouye SK, van Dyck CH, Alessi CA, *et al*. Clarifying confusion: the confusion assessment method. A new method for detection of delirium. *Ann Intern Med* 1990;113:941–958
27. Smulter N, Lingehall HC, Gustafson Y, Olofsson B, Engstrom KG. Validation of the Confusion Assessment Method in detecting postoperative delirium in cardiac surgery patients. *Am J Crit Care* 2015;24(6):480–487
28. National Institute for Health and Care Excellence. *Delirium: prevention, diagnosis and management*. Clinical Guideline 103.
29. Inouye SK, Westendrop RGJ, Saczynski JS. Delirium in elderly people. Lancet 2014:383(9920):911–922
30. Neufeld KJ, Yue J, Robinson TN, Inouye SK, Needham D. Antipsychotic medication for prevention and treatment of delirium in hospitalized adults: a systematic review and meta-analysis. *J Am Geriat Soc* 2016:64(4)705–14.
31. Page VJ, Ely EW, Gates S, *et al*. Effects of intravenous haloperidol on the duration of delirium and coma in critically ill patients (Hope-ICU): a randomised, double blind, placebo controlled trial. *Lancet Resp Med* 2013;1(7):515–23.
32. Al-Qadheeb NS, Skrobik Y, Schumaker G, *et al*. Preventing ICU subsyndromal delirium conversion to delirium with low dose IV haloperidol: a double-blind, placebo-controlled pilot study. *Crit Care Med* 2016;44(3):583–91.
33. Bellelli G, Morandi A, Bruni A, *et al*. Duration of post-operative delirium is an independent predictor of 6 month mortality in older adults after hip fracture. *J Am Geriat Soc* 2014;62(7):1335–40.
34. Pandharipande PP, Girard TD, Jackson JC, *et al*., for the BRAIN-ICU Study Investigators. Long-term cognitive impairment after critical illness. *N Engl J Med* 2013;369:1306–16.

35. Saczynski JS, Marcantonio ER, Quach L, *et al.* Cognitive trajectories after postoperative delirium. *N Engl J Med* 2012;**367**:30–9.

36. England and Wales High Court 2015. Winspear v City Hospitals Sunderland NHS foundation Trust EWHC 3250 (QB), 2015 MHLO 104.

37. British Medical Association, Resuscitation Council (UK), Royal College of Nursing. *Decisions relating to cardiopulmonary resuscitation* (3rd edition, 1st revision), 2016.

38. Adults with Incapacity (Scotland) Act 2000: code of practice (third edition) for practitioners authorised to carry out medical treatment or research under part 5 of the Act 2010.

39. Hanon O, Vidal J-S, de Groote P, *et al.* Prevalence of memory disorders in ambulatory patients aged over 70 years with chronic heart failure. *Am J Cardiol* 2014;**113**:1205–10.

SECTION 10
Treatment of acute heart failure

44

Inotropes, pressors, and vasodilators

Susanna Price and Shahana Uddin

Introduction

The management of chronic heart failure (CHF) has changed—from focusing on inotropy to a predominantly neurohormonal and disease-modifying approach to therapeutic intervention. By contrast, in acute heart failure (AHF) and cardiogenic shock the critical inability of the myocardium to maintain a cardiac output sufficient to meet the demands of the peripheral circulation needs urgent intervention to restore adequate perfusion.[1] Thus, acute interventions to support cardiovascular haemodynamics are pivotal, and the use of inotropes, pressors, and vasodilators to support the cardiovascular system remains widespread.[2–4] This is despite continued concerns about the lack of evidence of benefit, and the potential of these agents to increase organ damage and mortality in some patient populations.[4–6] Current recommendations are that in AHF/cardiogenic shock inotropes should be used only in selected patients, with appropriate monitoring, and reduced/withdrawn as soon as adequate organ perfusion is restored, and/or the patient receives mechanical circulatory support.[7] This chapter reviews the pharmacology of positive inotropic drugs, the principles underlying the choice of vasoactive drugs in AHF, and potential future developments in the field.

General mechanisms of action

Inotropes are a diverse collection of pluripotent molecules, with differing pharmacological properties. Of their key shared activities, only one relates to positive inotropy, with the remainder differentially affecting bacterial metabolism and translocation, modification in inflammatory markers and reactive oxygen species, immune-modulatory effects, alteration in coagulation, and with variable effects on the micro- and macro-circulation. In the systemic inflammatory status that defines cardiogenic shock, these additional affects may be key to determining the patient response.

Mechanisms of inotropic effects

Classically, direct inotropic effects are mediated via release of calcium ions from the myocyte sarcoplasmic reticulum and other subsarcolemmal sites, and subsequent interaction between calcium and contractile proteins. The release of calcium is effected via cyclic AMP (cAMP)-dependent or -independent mechanisms (**Figure 44.1**). cAMP increases phosphokinase A (PKA) activity which promotes opening of the cell membrane L-type calcium channels, in turn promoting intracellular calcium entry, and then increasing calcium release via the ryanodine receptor in the sarcoplasmic reticulum. PKA also phosphorylates phospholamban and calmodulin, promoting uptake of calcium into the sarcoplasmic reticulum, and may potentially additionally promote sarcoplasmic reticulum calcium release independently via a voltage-sensitive release mechanism. There are numerous cell membrane receptors on the human myocardium, many of which are linked to G proteins (Gs, Gi, Gq). The different G proteins have a number of specific effects, including the modulation of cAMP formation (Gs, Gi), and production of diacylglycerol and inositol triphosphate (Gq), with resultant changes in intracellular calcium ion concentration.

Current research is now focusing on novel inotropic mechanisms such as increasing the sensitivity of the contractile process,[8] or gene therapies and metabolic energy modulators.[9]

cAMP-dependent mechanisms

The β_1- and β_2-adrenergic receptors found on the surface of cardiomyocytes (**Figure 44.1**; **Table 44.1**) mediate cardiac responses to endogenous and exogenous catecholamines via coupling to the Gs proteins, resulting in production of cAMP.[10] Stimulation of β_1-receptors (but not β_2-receptors) results in PKA-mediated phosphorylation of phospholamban and cardiac contractile proteins[11] and promotes cardiomyocyte apoptosis.[12,13] In heart failure, there is a redistribution in the proportions of β_1- and β_2-receptors on the cardiomyocyte surface, modulating the responses of the myocyte to adrenergic stimulation.[14] The redistribution, together with the relative desensitization of β-receptor pathways found in heart failure, and downregulation of receptor numbers with prolonged administration of β-agonists, may additionally alter the clinical effects of inotropic agents, although the precise implications are not yet fully understood. β-Receptor agonists include the catecholamines (adrenaline, noradrenaline, dopamine, dobutamine, isoprenaline, and dopexamine) which contain a benzene ring with different ethylamine side-chains. They all activate different adrenoreceptors to varying degrees depending on the dosage used (**Table 44.1**).

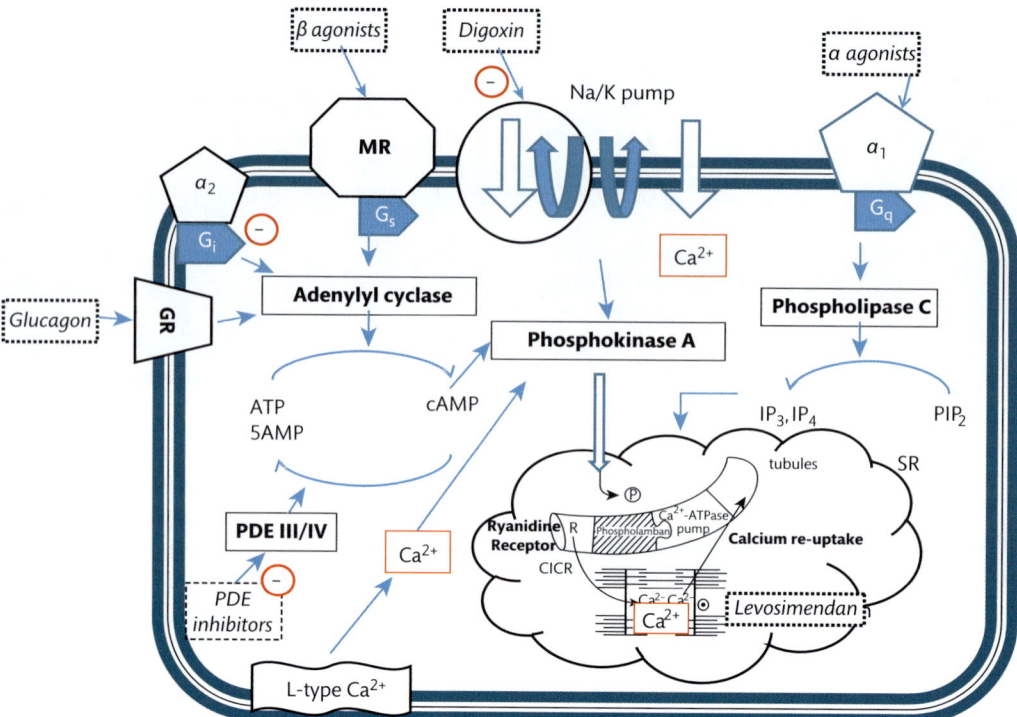

Figure 44.1 Schematic representation of mechanism of action of inotropes on cardiac myocytes. Stimulation/inhibition of cell receptors alters enzyme (in black boxes) activity which in turn alters the availability of substrates to facilitate calcium entry into the sarcoplasmic reticulum and subsequent force of myocardial contraction. Agents affecting receptor or pump activity are shown in dotted boxes. α_1, α_1-adrenoreceptor; α_2, α_1-adrenoreceptor; Gx, various G proteins (s, i, q); MR, various myocyte receptors (including β-adrenoreceptors 5HT receptors, VIP, somatostatin, M2 muscarinic); GR, glucagon receptor; Na/K pump, sodium potassium exchange pump; – within red circle, inhibits; Ca^{2+}, calcium; PDE, phosphodiesterase; SR, sarcoplasmic reticulum.

Phosphodiesterase (PDE) is a ubiquitous enzyme that catalyses the hydrolysis of both cAMP and cGMP. A number of drugs inhibit the different subtypes of the enzyme with varying degrees of specificity (Table 44.2): however, those most relevant to positive inotropic effects relate to PDE III or IV (the biguanides amrinone and milrinone, and the imidazolone derivative enoximone).

cAMP-independent mechanisms

A number of drugs increase intracellular calcium levels via cAMP-independent mechanisms, or exert their positive inotropic effect by increasing sensitivity to calcium. Inhibition of the ATPase-dependent Na^+/K^+ pump leads to a gradual increase in intracellular sodium. This in turn leads to a reduction in the exchange of intracellular calcium with extracellular sodium, thus increasing calcium stores in the sarcoplasmic reticulum (Figure 44.1). The only currently used inotrope with such an action is the cardiac glycoside digoxin.[15] α_1-Receptor agonists (phenylephrine, methoxamine) act on myocardial α_1 receptors resulting in an increase in contractility via Gq protein-mediated increases in inositol phosphatase 3 and calcium release from the sarcoplasmic reticulum, additionally acting to sensitize the contractile proteins (Figure 44.1). Finally, the myofilament calcium sensitizers (pimobendan, levosimendan) augment calcium binding to the calcium-specific regulatory site of cardiac troponin C, stabilizing calcium-induced conformational changes and thus inducing positive inotropy with no related change in intracellular calcium (Figure 44.1).

Mechanisms of vascular dilatation and constriction

The vascular endothelium is highly complex, with synthetic and metabolic capabilities. It reacts to a variety of substances to produce vasodilatation or constriction (Figure 44.2). The drugs used in the management of heart failure may have simultaneous dilator and constrictor effects depending upon the pathological process and the vascular bed studied, and differential effects on the arterial/venous and pulmonary/systemic circulations depending upon the distribution of receptors and the downstream signalling pathways. Several mechanisms have been implicated in the action of drugs used to modify vascular reactivity in heart failure, including cAMP-dependent, cGMP-dependent, and hyperpolarization-mediated dilatation/constriction. These mechanisms depend upon changes in intracellular calcium concentrations and/or myosin light chain phosphorylation, with an increase in intracellular calcium resulting in myosin light chain phosphorylation and thus sustained constriction.[8]

β₂-Adrenergic receptors mediate their dilatory effects on vascular tone by coupling to the Gs proteins, resulting in an increase in adenylyl cyclase activity, and an increase in cAMP. The resultant PKA-mediated phosphorylation of myosin light chain kinase reduces the phosphorylation of myosin light chains themselves. α_1-Receptor agonists and vasopressin (via vascular V_1 receptors) mediate their effects by coupling with the G proteins. An increase

Table 44.1 Pharmacology of differing inotropes, vasodilators, and vasopressors

Agent	Site of action/receptor/enzymes	Dosage/bolus	Onset/infusion	Duration	Metabolism	Elimination	t1/2	Clearance	Side-effects/cautions
Vasodilators									
Nitroglycerine	NO donor (indirect via thiol). Catalyses cGMP. Venous > arterial	Nil	10–20 µg/min. Titrate up to 200 µg/min	Minutes	Short	Hepatic nitrate reductase and thiols	3 min	Liver	Hypotension, headache
Nitroprusside	NO donor (direct). Catalyses cGMP. Arterial = venous	Nil	0.3 µg/kg/min and increase up to 5 µg/kg/min	Minutes	Short	See text	Thiocyanate 2–7 days	Urine	Toxicity. Metabolic acidosis $\uparrow$ ScVO$_2$
Nesiritide	Particulate GC	2 µg/kg	0.015–0.03 µg/kg/min	10 min	Short	See text	18 min	Urine. Endopeptidase	Hypotension
Inotropes									
Dobutamine	β_1,β_2	Nil	2–20 µg/kg/min	5 min	Short	COMT	2 min	Urine	Include: tachycardia, arrhythmia, hypotension, hypertension, myocardial ischaemia
Dopamine	DA$_1$ DA$_2$ β_1,β_2	Nil	3–5 µg/kg/min (>5 µg/kg/min; additional alpha effects)	5 min	10 min	MAO/COMT. Liver, kidney, blood	3 min	Urine	As dobutamine plus: vasoconstriction, bradycardia
Milrinone	PDE III/IV	25–75 mg/kg over 10–20 min	0.375–0.75 µg/kg/min	30 min	Medium	12% hepatic	1–2.5 h	Urine	As dobutamine
Enoximone	PDE III/IV	0.25–0.75 mg/kg	5–20 µg/kg/min	30 min	Medium	Hepatic	4.5 h	Urine	As dobutamine
Isoprenaline	β_1,β_2		0.5–10 µg/min	Minutes	Short	COMT	2 h	Urine	As dobutamine
Levosimendan	Myofilaments. Contractile proteins in SR	12 µg/kg over 10 min (usually avoided due to hypotension)	0.1 µg/kg/min. 0.05–0.2 µg/kg/min	12 min (bolus) 4 h (infusion)	Long	Hepatic. Small bowel	80 h	Urine. Faeces	Tachycardia. Arrhythmia. Hypotension.
Vasopressors									
Noradrenaline	β_1,α_1	Nil	0.02–1 µg/kg/min	Minutes	Short	Uptake 1-MAO. Circulation MAO/COMT	2 min	Urine	Hypertension. Bradycardia. Arrhythmia. Vasoconstriction. Decreased CO.
Metaraminol	$\alpha_1 > \beta$	1–5 mg	5 µg/kg/min	Seconds	Short	Hepatic. Unknown	Unknown	Urine. Tissue uptake	As noradrenaline
Phenylephrine	α_1 Partial	50–100 µg	40–180 µg/min	Seconds	10 min	Hepatic. MAO. GIT	2–3 h	Urine	As noradrenaline
Methoxamine	α_1	1 mg	0.1–0.3 mg/min	Seconds	Minutes	Hepatic	Unknown	Unknown ?urine	As noradrenaline
Adrenaline	Cardiac β_1 Peripheral $\alpha_2\beta_2$	Nil. Except in cardiac arrest	0.05–0.5 µg/kg/min	Minutes	Short	MAO/COMT. Liver, kidney, blood	2 min	Urine	As dobutamine and noradrenaline plus: lactic acidosis

α, alpha-adrenoceptor; β, beta-adrenoceptor; CO, cardiac output; COMT, catechol-O-methyl transferase; DA, dopamine receptor; GC, guanylate cyclase; GIT, gastrointestinal tract; MAO, monoamine oxidase; NO, nitric oxide; PDE, phosphodiesterase; ScVO$_2$, mixed central venous oxygen saturations; SR, sarcoplasmic reticulum.

Table 44.2 Differing phosphodiesterase isoforms, target enzyme system, tissues expressing receptors, and inhibitor drugs

Isoenzyme	Target	Tissues	Inhibitors
I	Calmodulin cGMP > cAMP	Heart, brain, kidney, liver, skeletal muscle, smooth muscle	Vinpocetine Phenothiazines
II	cGMP, cAMP	Adrenal cortex, brain, corpus cavernosum, heart, liver, kidney, airway smooth muscle, platelets	ENHA
III	cAMP > cGMP	Heart, corpus cavernosum, platelets, smooth muscle, liver, kidney, inflammatory cells (T and B lymphocytes, basophils, mast cells, monocytes, macrophages)	Amrinone Cilostamide Cilostazol Imadazodan Milrinone Motapizone Olprinone Pimobendam Piroximone
IV	cAMP	Kidney, lung, heart, skeletal muscle, smooth muscle (vascular, visceral, airway), platelets, inflammatory cells (T and B lymphocytes, basophils, mast cells, monocytes, macrophages, endothelial cells, eosinophils, neutrophils)	Enoximone Rolipram
III and IV	cAMP, CGMP	As above	Benafentrine Piclmilast Tibenelast Tolafentrine Zardavarine
VII	cAMP	Skeletal muscle, heart, kidney, airways, T and B lymphocytes, monocytes, eosinophils	Dipyridamole
Non-specific	cAMP, adenosine		Caffeine Papaverine Theophylline

cGMP, cyclic guanosine monophosphate; cAMP, cyclic adenosine monophosphate; EHNA erythro-9-(2-hydroxy-3-nonyl) adenine.

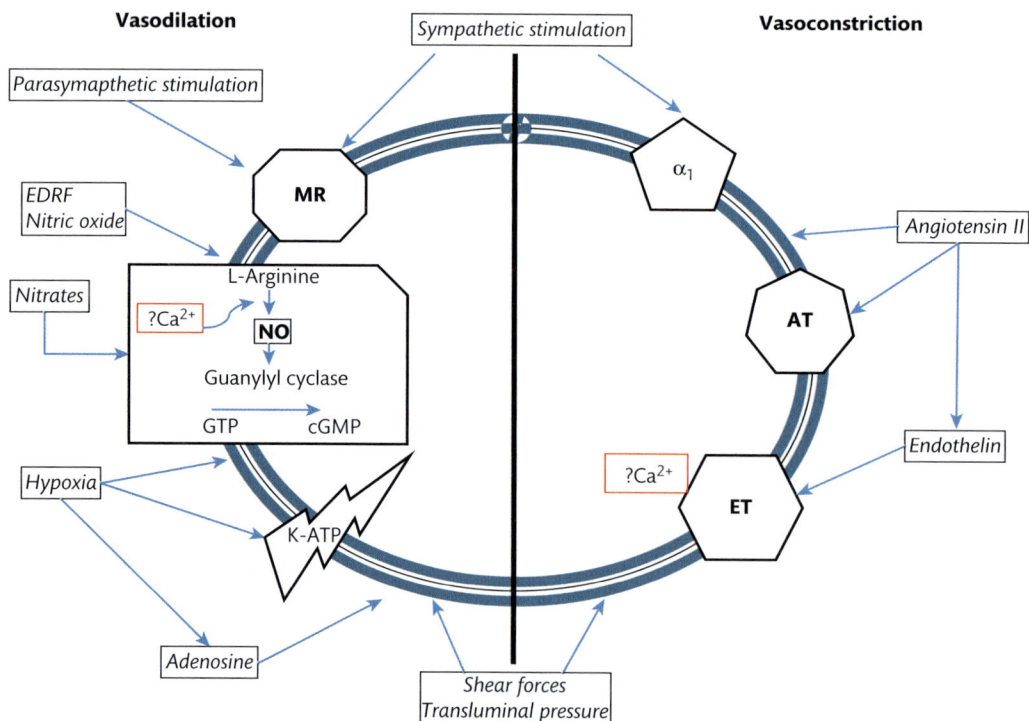

Figure 44.2 Schematic representation of action of agents on vascular smooth muscle. Vasomotor tone results from a balance between vasodilating and vasoconstricting factors which are secreted from and/or act upon vascular endothelial cells. α₁, α₁-adrenoreceptor; MR, various myocyte receptors (including β-adrenoreceptors, 5HT receptors, VIP, somatostatin, M2 muscarinic); K-ATP, potassium ATPase channels; – within red circle, inhibits; Ca²⁺, calcium; AT, angiotensin receptors; ET, endothelin receptors.

in smooth muscle contractility results from Gq and Gi protein-mediated increase in inositol phosphatase 3, and calcium release from the sarcoplasmic reticulum. Nitric oxide donors (inducible NO, nitrates, and nitroprusside) reduce vascular tone via an increase in intracellular cGMP and protein kinase G activity, resulting in the dephosphorylation of myosin light chains. Neseritide acts by binding to the particulate guanylyl cyclase receptor of vascular smooth muscle and endothelial cells, leading to increased intracellular cGMP and thus smooth muscle cell relaxation. Of note, the differential effects on the venous and arterial circulation reflect the relative concentration of guanylyl cyclase in the different vascular beds.

Inotropic agents

Inotropic agents are those which act predominantly by increasing cardiac contractility, although many have combined vasodilator or constrictor effects, depending upon the dosage used (Table 44.1). Numerous studies have failed to show reduced mortality with their use in AHF, with some showing actual harm.[5,6] Routine administration of the drugs in AHF is thus not recommended, especially where there is ongoing myocardial ischaemia or until other reversible cause, such as hypovolaemia, has been corrected. However, on occasion their transient use may be life-saving for individual, selected patients, and studies are underway to evaluate their use during cardiac arrest. Current guidelines recommend that their use be considered in patients with a low cardiac output state, in the presence of signs of hypoperfusion or congestion, the 'wet and cold' patient, despite the use of diuretics and/or dilators.[1,16-18] Additional recommendations are that inotropic drugs should be administered as early as possible and reduced or stopped as soon as adequate organ perfusion is restored. Such guidance demands a rapid diagnosis of inadequate cardiac output and of the presence of potentially reversible cause for deterioration.[1] Treatment algorithms based on the systolic blood pressure and estimated left-sided filling pressures are shown in Figure 44.3.

Dobutamine

A structural analogue of isoprenaline, dobutamine acts as an agonist at β_1 and β_2 receptors. It thus acts as an inotrope, increasing cardiac output while also decreasing vascular resistance. Dobutamine can exacerbate tachycardia and tachyarrhythmias, and in the presence of hypovolaemia may result in profound hypotension. Dosage should be titrated up to 15 µg/kg/min according to clinical effect. When used in patients receiving concomitant β-blocker therapy, the dose may need to be increased to 20 µg/kg/min. Therapy should be weaned gradually while simultaneously optimizing oral therapy.[1]

Dopamine

A naturally occurring precursor of noradrenaline, at low doses (0.5–3 µg/kg/min) dopamine has its predominant activity on the dopaminergic DA_1 and DA_2 receptors. At higher doses (3–10 µg/kg/min), its β_1 effects predominate, with some β_2-mediated peripheral

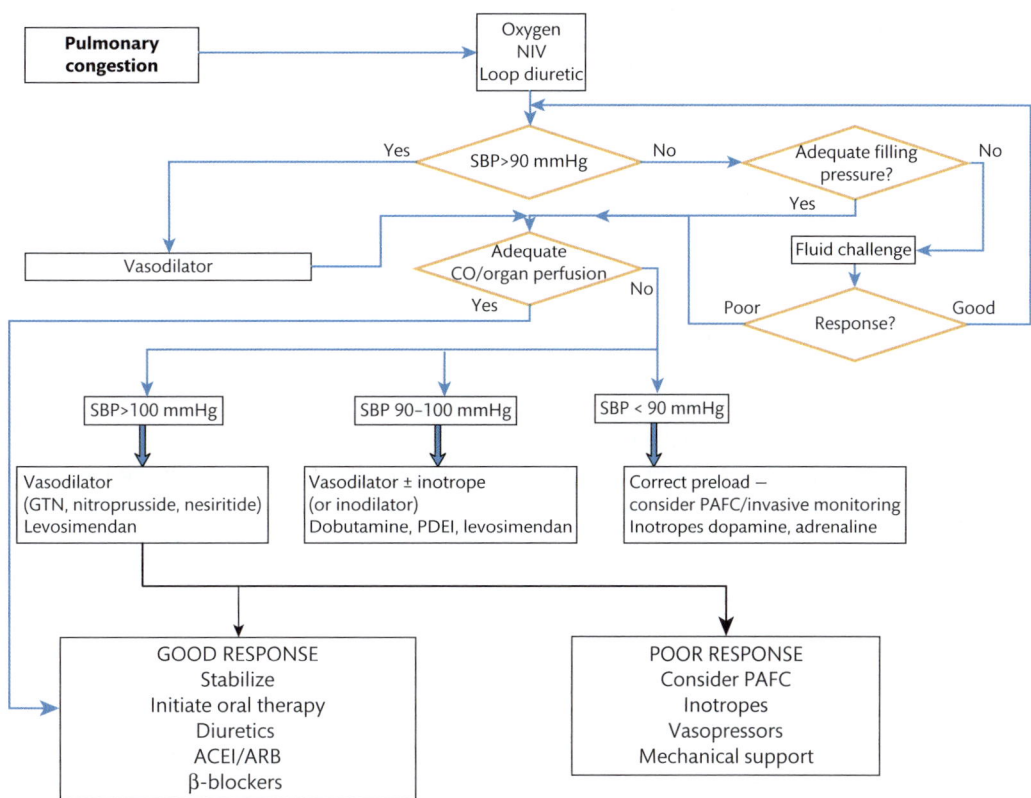

Figure 44.3 Flowchart to aid selection of inotropic or vasodilator therapy depending on clinical status (systolic blood pressure, left atrial filling pressure, end organ perfusion) in pulmonary oedema due to acute heart failure or acute exacerbation of chronic heart failure. NIV, non-invasive ventilation; SBP, systolic blood pressure; CO, cardiac output; PAFC, pulmonary artery flotation catheter; GTN, glyceryl trinitrate; PDEI, phosphodiesterase inhibitor; ACEI, angiotensin converting enzyme inhibitor; ARB, angiotensin receptor blocker.

vasodilatation, thus maintaining mean arterial pressure, venous capacitance, and preload. Higher doses of dopamine should be used with caution as they are associated with an increasing risk of tachycardia, tachyarrhythmias, and α stimulation, resulting in increased systemic vascular resistance.[1]

Milrinone and enoximone

Milrinone and enoximone are predominantly phosphodiesterase III inhibitors (PDEIs), acting as inodilators: that is, their use results in an increase in cardiac output and stroke volume with a concomitant reduction in pulmonary artery pressure, pulmonary capillary wedge pressure (PCWP), and systemic/pulmonary vascular resistance. As their site of action is downstream from the β receptors, they may be used in patients treated with concomitant use of β-blocker therapy. Milrinone and other PDEIs should be used with caution in patients with coronary artery disease, as there may be an increase in medium-term mortality.[5,19] Although milrinone has similar haemodynamic effects to dobutamine, there are some important differences. Milrinone has more significant vasodilatory effects, and appears to cause less tachycardia and increase in myocardial oxygen demand. Further, milrinone is renally cleared and has a longer half-life. It should, therefore, be used with caution in renal impairment. In certain circumstances a loading dose may be used, although this is rarely done in practice because of the potential for provoking profound haemodynamic instability.[1]

Levosimendan

Levosimendan is a calcium sensitizer that exerts its inotropic effect by binding to troponin C in cardiomyocytes. It additionally causes significant vasodilatation through its action on ATP-sensitive potassium channels and has mild PDE inhibitory action at higher doses. Its haemodynamic effects are to increase cardiac output and stroke volume, and to reduce PCWP and systemic/pulmonary vascular resistance. Because of metabolism to active metabolites, its haemodynamic effects persist for several days after discontinuation of treatment. Levosimendan should be used with caution in those with a relatively low systemic vascular resistance. As with milrinone, the drug may be loaded (although in the presence of haemodynamic instability the bolus should be omitted), and is effective even in the presence of β-blockade.[20,21]

Adrenaline

An endogenous catecholamine formed by the methylation of noradrenaline, adrenaline acts on cardiac β₁ and peripheral α₁ receptors, resulting in inotropic and vasoconstrictor effects. Adrenaline additionally acts as a constrictor of venous beds, causing an increase in preload; however, peripheral β₂-receptor activation results in vasodilator activity. The net effect of adrenaline on systemic vascular resistance is thus less predictable than with noradrenaline. Adrenaline is also dromotropic (speeds conduction in the atrioventricular node), and bathmotropic (makes myocytes more electrically excitable). The potential adverse effects of adrenaline are thus (a) to increase myocardial work and oxygen consumption significantly, (b) to have proarrhythmogenic effects, and (c) to induce/exacerbate myocardial ischaemia. Further, stimulation of the Embden–Meyerhof pathway resulting in pyruvate production increases lactic acid, especially in the presence of an impaired citric acid cycle. Although adrenaline is not recommended for the routine

treatment of AHF in current guidelines, it is frequently used at low doses in patients with severe refractory haemodynamic instability as a potentially life-saving measure, and as part of current advanced life-support guidelines in the management of pre-hospital cardiac arrest, where, although it results in a higher rate of survival, there is no benefit in terms of favourable neurological outcome.[22,23]

Isoprenaline

Isoprenaline is a synthetic derivative of dopamine, with potent β₁ and β₂ effects. Its chronotropic effects predominate and it is therefore infrequently used as an inotrope, being more frequently used to provide a temporary increase in heart rate pending institution of definitive pacing, or while awaiting resolution of the bradycardia. One exception is in the presence of significant pulmonary hypertension, where isoprenaline acts both as an inotrope and as a pulmonary vasodilator.[24]

Vasodilator agents

Vasodilators are recommended early in the treatment of AHF in the absence of hypotension (systolic blood pressure <90 mmHg) or severe obstructive valvular disease.[25] However, there is a high incidence of side-effects (Table 44.1). The effects of vasodilators are to reduce both right- and left-sided filling pressures and systemic vascular resistance, resulting in improved haemodynamics and symptoms. Coronary artery flow is usually not compromised unless either a steal phenomenon occurs, or the left ventricular end-diastolic pressure remains high despite a fall in diastolic blood pressure. Dosage and administration of the principal vasodilators used in AHF are shown in Table 44.1.

Organic nitrates

These are prodrugs that undergo complex biotransformation, predominantly in smooth muscle,[26] to form nitric oxide (NO) or S-nitrosothiol, which, via cGMP, results in venous and arterial vasodilatation. Clearance is by extraction, blood hydrolysis, or glutathione–nitrate reductase in the liver. Nitrates are administered as detailed in Table 44.1 and should be titrated up to maximum tolerated dosage. Potential haemodynamic effects include: reduction in right- and left-sided filling pressures; a fall in systemic and pulmonary vascular resistance; and a fall in systolic blood pressure. Therapy is usually associated with little or no change in heart rate, but results in an increase in cardiac output due to reduction in afterload, reversal in ischaemia, and reduction in severity of any mitral regurgitation. Other effects are shown in Table 44.3. The limitations of nitrates include the development of resistance, with a marked attenuation of initial effects within hours of starting therapy in up to 50% of patients.[25,27,28]

Nitroprusside

Sodium nitroprusside is a potent vasodilator and is generally considered the standard against which other vasodilators are assessed. Comprising the sodium (or potassium) salt of a complex molecule containing a ferrous iron atom bound to five cyanide molecules and nitric acid, nitroprusside mediates its effects by decomposition to produce nitrosothiol on contact with red blood cells. This in turn generates cGMP in the vascular smooth muscle, resulting in

Table 44.3 Effects of agents on physiological variables

Agent	CI	SV	HR	PCWP	MPAP	PVR	SBP	SVR	CSBF	MOC
Dopamine	↑	↑	↑↑	↔	↔	↔	↑↓	↓	↑	↑
Isoprenaline	↑	↑/↔	↑↑	↓	↓	↓	↓	↓↓	↓	↑
Noradrenaline	↑	↑	↓	↑	↑	↑↑	↑↑	↑↑	↑	↑
Adrenaline	↑	↑	↑	↑↓	↑	↑↓	↑↑	↑↓	↑	↑↑
Milrinone	↑	↑	↑	↓↓	↓↓	↓↓	↓	↓↓	↔	↑
Enoximone	↑	↑	↑	↓↓	↓↓	↓↓	↓	↓↓	↔	↑
Dobutamine	↑	↑	↑↑	↓	↓	↓	↓/↑	↓	↑	↑↑
Levosimendan	↑	↑	↑	↓	↓↓	↓↓	↓↓	↓	↑	↔
Nitroprusside	↑	↑	↑	↓	↓	↓	↓	↓	↑↓	↓
Neseritide	↑	↑	↔	↓	↓	↓	↓↓	↓	↑	↓
Phenylephrine	↑↓	↑	↓	↑	↑	↑	↑	↑	↓	↓
Metaraminol	↑↓	↑↓	↓	↓	↑	↑	↑	↑	↑	↑

CI, cardiac index; CSBF, coronary sinus blood flow; HR, heart rate; MOC, myocardial oxygen consumption; MPAP, mean pulmonary artery pressure; PCWP, pulmonary capillary wedge pressure; PVR, pulmonary vascular resistance; SBP, systolic blood pressure; SV, stroke volume; SVR, systemic vascular resistance; ↑, increase; ↔, equivocal; ↓, decrease.

NO-mediated vasodilatation. Clearance is via hepatic metabolism to thiocyanate, which is then renally excreted with a half-life of 3–4 days. The administration and dosage of nitroprusside is shown in Table 44.1. The haemodynamic effects of nitroprusside are to reduce systemic and pulmonary vascular venous tone, increase vascular compliance, and reduce afterload and any atrioventricular valvular regurgitation, with the net effect of increasing cardiac output. The main limitation of the drug relates to the toxicity of its metabolites (cyanide and thiocyanate), the presence of which are related to the dose and duration of therapy. Where toxicity is suspected (lactic acidosis, confusion, fits) thiocyanate toxicity should be suspected, and treated using haemofiltration.

Nesiritide

This recombinant DNA preparation of human ventricular brain natriuretic peptide has an elimination half-life of 18 min.[21,25] Clearance is via binding to cell surface receptors, uptake and intracellular proteolysis, proteolytic cleavage via neutral endopeptidases within renal tubular and vascular cells, and renal filtration. The administration and dosage of nesiritide is shown in Table 44.1. The haemodynamic effects are to reduce venous tone, increase vascular compliance, and reduce systemic and pulmonary vascular resistance, with an increase in cardiac output. Other effects of nesiritide are shown in Table 44.3. The main limitations of its usage are hypotension and availability.

Although nesiritide has been widely used in the USA, it has not been licensed for use by the European regulatory authorities, partly because some preliminary studies suggest that it may worsen outcome.[29,30] Recent meta-analysis suggests that although there is symptomatic relief, its use is not associated with increased survival and may cause hypotension. However, there is no associated reduction in urine output nor need for additional dialysis. It remains useful where available for certain patients who remain symptomatic despite therapy.

Vasopressin antagonists

The vasoconstrictor effects of arginine vasopressin have led to development of antagonists proposed for the use in AHF. A dual

$V_{1a/2}$ vasopressin receptor antagonist (Conivaptan) reduces PCWP and right atrial pressure, with no significant change in blood pressure, heart rate, cardiac output, and pulmonary/systemic vascular resistance.[31] The use of vasopressin antagonists is not currently recommended routinely in the treatment of AHF.

Vasopressor agents

Vasopressor agents are not generally recommended in the management of AHF, but the use of vasodilator/inodilators drugs and/or the concomitant presence of sepsis in the critically ill patient with AHF may demand their use. Care must always be exercised to avoid an excessive increase in systemic vascular resistance resulting in a critical deterioration in cardiac output. Further, regional vasoconstriction in key vascular beds may result in life-threatening hypoperfusion which must be rapidly recognized.[24]

Noradrenaline

Noradrenaline is a potent β_1 and α_1 agonist, causing peripheral vasoconstriction especially in the pulmonary and splanchnic beds. The α-mediated increase in systemic vascular resistance opposes its β-mediated inotropic effects, manifesting clinically with an increase in mean arterial pressure and a minor increase in heart rate, but little change in cardiac output. The effects of noradrenaline are dose-related; in low doses the β effects are apparent, whereas in higher doses vasoconstrictive α effects predominate. The dose of noradrenaline should therefore be titrated to achieve a mean arterial pressure consistent with adequate end-organ perfusion, as excessive doses result in tissue ischaemia, progressive metabolic acidosis, and excessive systemic vascular resistance, resulting in a fall in cardiac output. Current subgroup analysis suggests that noradrenaline use may be associated with lower mortality and side-effects when compared to dopamine in the treatment of shock.[24,32]

Metaraminol/phenylephrine

These α agonists cause a rise in systolic and diastolic pressures, a marked increase in systemic and pulmonary vascular resistance, and

a concomitant decrease in cardiac output. Because of the profound constrictor effects and the fall in cardiac output associated with their administration, the only use of these drugs in AHF is in the emergency and short-term support of blood pressure in the peri-arrest situation or in cardiogenic shock, while definitive life-saving treatment is initiated. The advantage over other agents is that they are safe to use peripherally until central venous access is established.[24]

Vasopressin

Arginine vasopressin is released from the posterior pituitary in response to increased serum osmolality or reduced plasma volume. Vasopressin becomes a constrictor in shock states, where its actions are to produce constriction in some vascular beds, and dilatation in others (renal, pulmonary, mesenteric, and vascular). The precise mechanisms are not well understood, but may include blockade of activated ATP-sensitive K^+ channels in vascular smooth muscle, a decrease in the NO second messenger cGMP, and stimulation of endothelin-1 synthesis. As with other constrictors, the use of vasopressin in AHF is generally limited to the short-term support of the circulation of the critically ill patient in whom there is profound and life-threatening vasodilatation, resistant to other agents.[24]

Choice of vasoactive agent

Intravenous vasoactive agents may be indicated in patients with a low cardiac output state determined either clinically and/or by cardiac output monitoring. Their use should also be considered in the presence of significant pulmonary or peripheral congestion despite the appropriate use of diuretics and/or vasodilators. Algorithms to guide the institution of therapy and the potential choice of inotropic drug have been published,[1,7] but the choice and dose of inotropic drug must be tailored to the individual patient's circumstances

(Figure 44.3, Table 44.3). When considering the choice of vasoactive agent, several important principles apply. First, the heart should be considered as two pumps in series, with the effects of reducing and increasing the filling pressures of each considered independently. This is particularly relevant when a wide discrepancy exists between the stroke work equations of the right and left hearts. Second, the underlying pathophysiology of AHF must be considered and the precipitant or cause reversed where possible. Where ischaemia is present, positive inotropic agents which increase myocardial oxygen consumption should be avoided if the haemodynamics allow, and mechanical support may be more beneficial. Finally, repeated re-evaluation of global and regional perfusion is required in order to optimize organ perfusion.

Future directions

There are marked limitations in the management of AHF using the currently established vasoactive agents due to their many adverse effects.[18] Alternative pharmacological agents with potential for short-term use are being developed and are at varying stages of investigation.[9] These have physiologically plausible cellular targets or mechanisms of action as listed (Table 44.4), but have failed to produce long-term benefit in the clinical trials performed to date.

Although these drugs may in future offer alternative methods of positive inotropic support, as yet they are unproven, and all are limited to short-term use in order to support the failing circulation while any reversible cause is treated and either the heart recovers, or mechanical circulatory support/cardiac transplantation is undertaken. Their adverse side-effect profile, and requirement for close patient monitoring, demand that therapy be reduced as soon as the haemodynamic status of the patient allows, while instituting more standard oral therapy. Although some of the newer agents in

Table 44.4 Non-standard agents/previously considered agents in acute heart failure (AHF)

Drug	Mechanism of proposed action	Clinical trial	Results	Comments
Ularatide	Synthetic natriuretic peptides: urodilantin	TRUE AHF[33]	Symptomatic improvement in 48 h, but no long-term benefit (34 months). Associated with ongoing myocardial damage as measured by troponin rise.	Similar pathway to neseritide
Serelaxin[34-36]	Recombinant human relaxin 2	RELAX AHF2	Did not meet primary end-points in reduction of CVS mortality at 180 days. Nor reduced worsening HF when added to standard medical therapy through day 5.	Vasodilatory and end organ protective effects
AAV1/SERCA2a (adeno-associated virus 1/sarco/endoplasmic reticulum Ca^{2+}-ATPase)	Gene therapy to improve SERCA 2a deficiency	CUPID 2[37]	AAV1/SERCA2a did not improve time to recurrent events compared with placebo	Single intracoronary infusion of 1×10^{13} DNase-resistant particles of AAV1/SERCA2a or placebo.
Omecamtiv	Cardiac myosin activators: increase myocardial contractility by improving the crossbridge cycle and thus efficiency of the contractile apparatus	ATOMIC HF[38]	Did not meet primary end point of improvement in dyspnoea in most groups except possibly in high dose group	Increased myocardial function in healthy volunteers, well tolerated in HF and increased in systolic ejection time
Istaroxime	Dual action • non-glycoside Na/K/ATPase inhibitor • stimulates SERCA 2a activity			Inotropy and lusitropy. No increase in myocardial oxygen demand. Increase SBP, decrease HR and PCWP and increase CO

SBP, systolic blood pressure; HR, heart rate, PCWP, pulmonary capillary wedge pressure; CO, cardiac output.

development seem promising, modern demands for a high level of evidence showing outcome benefit will undoubtedly be a significant hurdle in their widespread usage.[34,35,37,38]

REFERENCES

1. Ponikowski P, Voors AA, Anker SD, *et al.* 2016 ESC Guidelines for the diagnosis and treatment of acute and chronic heart failure: The Task Force for the diagnosis and treatment of acute and chronic heart failure of the European Society of Cardiology (ESC) Developed with the special contribution of the Heart Failure Association (HFA) of the ESC. *Eur Heart J* 2016;**37**(27):2129–200.

2. Adams KF, Jr, Fonarow GC, Emerman CL, *et al.* Characteristics and outcomes of patients hospitalized for heart failure in the United States: rationale, design, and preliminary observations from the first 100,000 cases in the Acute Decompensated Heart Failure National Registry (ADHERE). *Am Heart J* 2005;**149**(2):209–16.

3. Abraham WT, Adams KF, Fonarow GC, *et al.* In-hospital mortality in patients with acute decompensated heart failure requiring intravenous vasoactive medications: an analysis from the Acute Decompensated Heart Failure National Registry (ADHERE). *J Am Coll Cardiol* 2005;**46**(1):57–64.

4. Harjola VP, Lassus J, Sionis A, *et al.* Clinical picture and risk prediction of short-term mortality in cardiogenic shock. *Eur J Heart Fail* 2015;**17**(5):501–9.

5. Felker GM, Benza RL, Chandler AB, *et al.* Heart failure etiology and response to milrinone in decompensated heart failure: results from the OPTIME-CHF study. *J Am Coll Cardiol* 2003;**41**(6):997–1003.

6. Gheorghiade M, Gattis WA, Klein L. OPTIME in CHF trial: rethinking the use of inotropes in the management of worsening chronic heart failure resulting in hospitalization. *Eur J Heart Fail* 2003;**5**(1):9–12.

7. Dickstein K, Vardas PE, Auricchio A, *et al.* 2010 Focused Update of ESC Guidelines on device therapy in heart failure: an update of the 2008 ESC Guidelines for the diagnosis and treatment of acute and chronic heart failure and the 2007 ESC Guidelines for cardiac and resynchronization therapy. Developed with the special contribution of the Heart Failure Association and the European Heart Rhythm Association. *Europace* 2010;**12**(11):1526–36.

8. Evers AS, Maze M (eds). *Anesthetic pharmacology: physiologic principles and clinical practice: a companion to Miller's Anesthesia*. Churchill Livingstone, Philadelphia, 2004.

9. von Lueder TG, Krum H. New medical therapies for heart failure. *Nat Rev Cardiol* 2015;**12**(12):730–40.

10. Xiang Y, Kobilka BK. Myocyte adrenoceptor signaling pathways. *Science* 2003;**300**(5625):1530–2.

11. Xiao RP. Beta-adrenergic signaling in the heart: dual coupling of the beta2-adrenergic receptor to G(s) and G(i) proteins. *Sci STKE* 2001;**2001**(104):re15.

12. Communal C, Singh K, Sawyer DB, Colucci WS. Opposing effects of beta(1)- and beta(2)-adrenergic receptors on cardiac myocyte apoptosis: role of a pertussis toxin-sensitive G protein. *Circulation* 1999;**100**(22):2210–2.

13. Zhu WZ, Zheng M, Koch WJ, *et al.* Dual modulation of cell survival and cell death by beta(2)-adrenergic signaling in adult mouse cardiac myocytes. *Proc Natl Acad Sci USA* 2001;**98**(4):1607–12.

14. Nikolaev VO, Moshkov A, Lyon AR, *et al.* Beta2-adrenergic receptor redistribution in heart failure changes cAMP compartmentation. *Science* 2010;**327**(5973):1653–7.

15. Gheorghiade M, Pang PS. Acute heart failure syndromes. *J Am Coll Cardiol* 2009;**53**(7):557–73.

16. Yancy CW, Jessup M, Bozkurt B, *et al.* 2017 ACC/AHA/HFSA Focused Update of the 2013 ACCF/AHA Guideline for the Management of Heart Failure: A Report of the American College of Cardiology/American Heart Association Task Force on Clinical Practice Guidelines and the Heart Failure Society of America. *Circulation* 2017;**136**(6):e137–1e61.

17. Teerlink JR, Metra M, Zaca V, *et al.* Agents with inotropic properties for the management of acute heart failure syndromes. Traditional agents and beyond. *Heart Fail Rev* 2009;**14**(4):243–53.

18. Hasenfuss G, Teerlink JR. Cardiac inotropes: current agents and future directions. *Eur Heart J* 2011;**32**(15):1838–45.

19. Metra M, Nodari S, D'Aloia A, *et al.* Beta-blocker therapy influences the hemodynamic response to inotropic agents in patients with heart failure: a randomized comparison of dobutamine and enoximone before and after chronic treatment with metoprolol or carvedilol. *J Am Coll Cardiol* 2002;**40**(7):1248–58.

20. Nieminen MS, Fruhwald S, Heunks LM, *et al.* Levosimendan: current data, clinical use and future development. *Heart Lung Vessel* 2013;**5**(4):227–45.

21. Delaney A, Bradford C, McCaffrey J, Bagshaw SM, Lee R. Levosimendan for the treatment of acute severe heart failure: a meta-analysis of randomised controlled trials. *Int J Cardiol* 2010;**138**(3):281–9.

22. Nolan JP, Deakin CD, Soar J, *et al.* European Resuscitation Council guidelines for resuscitation 2005. Section 4. Adult advanced life support. *Resuscitation* 2005;**67**(Suppl 1):S39–86.

23. Perkins GD, Chen J, Deakin CD, *et al.* A randomised trial of epinephrine in out-of-hospital cardiac arrest. *N Engl J Med* 2018;**379**(8):711–21.

24. Overgaard CB, Dzavik V. Inotropes and vasopressors: review of physiology and clinical use in cardiovascular disease. *Circulation* 2008;**118**(10):1047–56.

25. Elkayam U, Janmohamed M, Habib M, Hatamizadeh P. Vasodilators in the management of acute heart failure. *Crit Care Med* 2008;**36**(1 Suppl):S95–105.

26. Khot UN, Novaro GM, Popovic ZB, *et al.* Nitroprusside in critically ill patients with left ventricular dysfunction and aortic stenosis. *N Engl J Med* 2003;**348**(18):1756–63.

27. Elkayam U, Roth A, Kumar A, *et al.* Hemodynamic and volumetric effects of venodilation with nitroglycerin in chronic mitral regurgitation. *Am J Cardiol* 1987;**60**(13):1106–11.

28. Dupuis J, Lalonde G, Lemieux R, Rouleau JL. Tolerance to intravenous nitroglycerin in patients with congestive heart failure: role of increased intravascular volume, neurohumoral activation and lack of prevention with N-acetylcysteine. *J Am Coll Cardiol* 1990;**16**(4):923–31.

29. Sackner-Bernstein JD, Skopicki HA, Aaronson KD. Risk of worsening renal function with nesiritide in patients with acutely decompensated heart failure. *Circulation* 2005;**111**(12):1487–91.

30. Sackner-Bernstein JD, Kowalski M, Fox M, Aaronson K. Short-term risk of death after treatment with nesiritide for decompensated heart failure: a pooled analysis of randomized controlled trials. *JAMA* 2005;**293**(15):1900–5.

31. Udelson JE, Smith WB, Hendrix GH, *et al.* Acute hemodynamic effects of conivaptan, a dual V(1A) and V(2) vasopressin receptor

antagonist, in patients with advanced heart failure. *Circulation* 2001;**104**(20):2417–23.

32. De Backer D, Biston P, Devriendt J, *et al.* Comparison of dopamine and norepinephrine in the treatment of shock. *N Engl J Med* 2010;**362**(9):779–89.

33. Packer M, O'Connor C, McMurray JJV, *et al.* Effect of ularitide on cardiovascular mortality in acute heart failure. *N Engl J Med* 2017;**376**(20):1956–64.

34. Tietjens J, Teerlink JR. Serelaxin and acute heart failure. *Heart* 2016;**102**(2):95–9.

35. Teerlink JR, Voors AA, Ponikowski P, *et al.* Serelaxin in addition to standard therapy in acute heart failure: rationale and design of the RELAX-AHF-2 study. *Eur J Heart Fail* 2017;**19**(6):800–9.

36. Teerlink JR, Cotter G, Davison BA, *et al.* Serelaxin, recombinant human relaxin-2, for treatment of acute heart failure (RELAX-AHF): a randomised, placebo-controlled trial. *Lancet* 2013;**381**(9860):29–39.

37. Greenberg B, Butler J, Felker GM, *et al.* Calcium upregulation by percutaneous administration of gene therapy in patients with cardiac disease (CUPID 2): a randomised, multinational, double-blind, placebo-controlled, phase 2b trial. *Lancet* 2016;**387**(10024):1178–86.

38. Teerlink JR, Felker GM, McMurray JJV, *et al.* Acute treatment with omecamtiv mecarbil to increase contractility in acute heart failure: the ATOMIC-AHF Study. *J Am Coll Cardiol* 2016;**67**(12):1444–55.

45

Vasodilators

Susan Piper and Theresa A. McDonagh

Introduction

Vasodilatory compounds have long been used in the treatment of heart failure. Whereas they have mostly been used in the setting of acutely decompensated heart failure, there is evidence to support the use of oral preparations in certain subgroups with chronic heart failure (CHF).

This chapter explores the current evidence and guidelines for the use of vasodilators in clinical practice, both in the acute and chronic setting; and it examines the potential for novel vasodilatory compounds and possible future directions.

Vasodilators in clinical practice

Nitrates

There are two basic types of nitrodilator: those that release nitric oxide (NO) spontaneously (e.g. sodium nitroprusside) and the organic nitrates, that require an enzymatic process to form NO (e.g. isosorbide dinitrate (ISDN), isosorbide mononitrate (ISMN), and nitroglycerine).

Mechanisms of action

Nitric oxide activates smooth-muscle soluble guanylate cyclase (sGC) to form cyclic guanosine monophosphate (cGMP). Increased intracellular cGMP inhibits calcium entry into the cell, thereby decreasing intracellular calcium (Ca^{2+}) concentration and causing smooth muscle relaxation.[1] NO also activates potassium (K^+) channels, leading to hyperpolarization and relaxation. Finally, acting through cGMP, NO can stimulate a cGMP-dependent protein kinase that activates myosin light-chain phosphatase, leading to relaxation and dilation (**Figure 45.1**).

At low doses, organic nitrates induce only venous dilatation, but as the dose increases they cause the arteries, including the coronary arteries, to dilate.[2] They therefore cause balanced vasodilatation of both sides of the circulation, thereby reducing elevated left ventricular (LV) filling pressures and systemic vascular resistance (SVR) without impairing tissue perfusion. Therapy is usually associated with little or no change in heart rate, but results in an increase in cardiac output due to reduction in afterload, reversal in ischaemia, and reduction in severity of any mitral regurgitation.

Unlike the organic nitrates, sodium nitroprusside causes direct relaxation of vascular smooth muscle, resulting in reduction of arteriolar resistance and venous tone to an equivalent extent. This makes nitroprusside particularly useful in settings where acute afterload reduction is required, including hypertensive crises, acute aortic and mitral regurgitation and acute ventricular septal rupture.[3] With its rapid onset and reversibility of action, it has a distinct advantage in acutely unwell patients but it has highly variable individual responses.

Nesiritide

Nesiritide is recombinant B-type natriuretic peptide (BNP) and has venous, arterial, and coronary vasodilatory properties.

Mechanism of action

Nesiritide has natriuretic properties and acts to increase cGMP levels via membrane-bound particulate guanylyl cyclase (pGC) (**Figure 45.1**). Its effects result in both venous and arterial vasodilatation with a subsequent reduction in both preload and afterload. This generates an increase in cardiac output without direct inotropic effects.[4]

Hydralazine

Hydralazine is a potent vasodilator that has been in clinical use for nearly six decades.

Mechanism of action

The mechanism of action of hydralazine remains poorly understood. The scarce functional studies undertaken in human blood vessels indicate a dominant arterial effect but do not provide definitive mechanistic insights.[5]

The evidence currently available suggests that the vasoactive properties of hydralazine may occur via a variety of mechanisms[6-8] including:

- smooth muscle hyperpolarization, most likely through the opening of K^+ channels;[6]
- inhibition of inositol 1,4,5-trisphosphate (IP$_3$)-induced release of calcium from the smooth muscle sarcoplasmic reticulum,

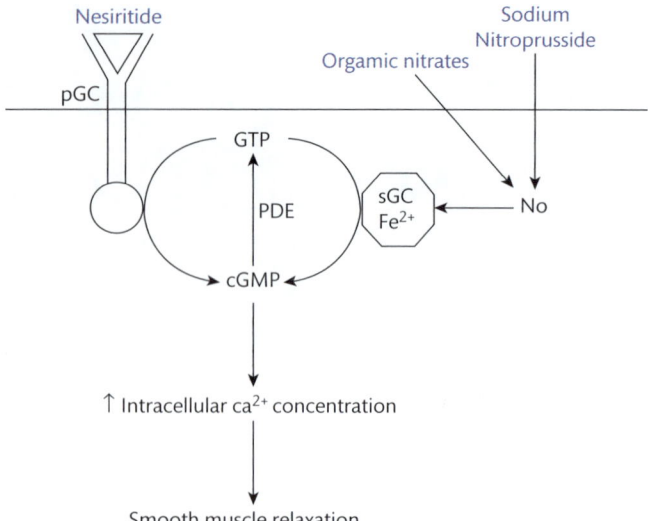

Figure 45.1 Mechanism of action of nitrates and nesiritide.

resulting in the activation of myosin light-chain kinase and muscle relaxation;

- stimulating the formation of NO by the vascular endothelium, leading to cGMP-mediated vasodilation.

In addition to its vasodilatory properties, hydralazine potentially has mild inotropic effects, which are thought to reflect activation of the sympathetic nervous system.[9,10] Moreover, hydralazine has been shown to prolong the effects of ISDN in both experimental and clinical models.[11,12] Such findings potentially explain, at least in part, why the combination of hydralazine and ISDN has shown beneficial effects in heart failure when no such benefit has been demonstrated for either agent in isolation.

Vasodilators for acute heart failure

Hospitalization for acute heart failure (AHF) remains a major clinical challenge, with a high (and increasing) incidence, substantial morbidity and mortality, and few improvements in therapy over recent decades.

Given that several haemodynamic studies have demonstrated that acute pulmonary oedema may result from a rapidly deteriorating cycle of events in which patients with reduced baseline systolic and diastolic reserve are faced with an acute increase in LV filling pressures and high SVR,[13–17] it is unsurprising that vasodilatation should, conceptually, confer significant improvement for such patients.

The use of these agents, however, is still based on limited evidence primarily from small, single-centre studies. Thus, there remains an apparent uncoupling of symptom improvement from outcomes, suggesting that current management strategies do not affect the pathophysiologic processes relating to outcome.[18]

Despite this, current pharmacotherapy for AHF without cardiogenic shock continues to consist primarily of diuretics, supplemented by oxygen, opiates, and vasodilators in selected subsets.

Epidemiology of vasodilator use in acute heart failure

Despite the compelling rationale for vasodilator therapy,[19] the use of nitrates in AHF is less standardized than that of diuretics. In a review of UK practice, Crane[20] demonstrated that <70% of patients presenting with acute pulmonary oedema received nitrates, compared with >80% receiving diuretics.[21] Moreover, data from the EuroHeart Failure Survey showed that the use of nitrates varied from 6% to 70% in different European regions,[22] with the ADHERE registry documenting similar findings in the USA.[23] The discrepancy is, at least in part, due to the lack of controlled data concerning the use of nitrates in AHF[1] and cannot be attributed to differences in blood pressure (BP) alone. Certainly, data from the ADHERE registry indicate that not only is a history of hypertension common in patients hospitalized with pulmonary oedema, but that at presentation most patients in this group are frankly hypertensive. By contrast, only 3% of patients had a first-recorded BP <90 mmHg. Patients who were admitted for pulmonary oedema were more often significantly hypertensive and had preserved systolic function instead of being hypotensive and having reduced systolic function. The ADHERE registry thus demonstrated significant differences between the typical patient hospitalized for acute pulmonary oedema and patients enrolled in randomized clinical trials.

Organic nitrates

Despite their long-history of use, no single study has been sufficiently powered to evaluate the safety of nitrate use carefully. Moreover, whereas haemodynamic effects have been shown in a few small studies,[13,16,24–27] there are no robust trials to show that they relieve symptoms or improve clinical outcomes.

In one of the most quoted papers pertaining to the benefits of nitrate therapy, Cotter et al.[13] demonstrated that the combination of high-dose ISDN given as repeated intravenous boluses after low-dose intravenous furosemide was more effective than high-dose furosemide with low-dose ISDN in reducing the need for mechanical ventilation in 110 patients with severe pulmonary oedema (**Figure 45.2**).

Moreover, Sharon et al.[16] demonstrated that, in a small cohort of only 40 patients presenting with acute pulmonary oedema, the use of high-dose ISDN was safer and more effective than combined treatment with bilevel positive airway pressure and conventional AHF therapy.

In 2002, the Vasodilation in the Management of Acute Congestive Heart Failure (VMAC) trial reported on the use of the recombinant BNP, nesiritide, compared with intravenous nitrates and placebo for the treatment of decompensated heart failure.[27] As part of their analysis, the reporters compared intravenous nitrates with placebo for the first 3 h of admission in 285 patients. Although a significant improvement in pulmonary capillary wedge pressure (PCWP) was observed in the nitroglycerine group at 2 h compared with placebo, this effect was not sustained; overall, apart from the expected significant differences observed in BP, there were no sustained haemodynamic differences between the groups and no differences in global clinical status or dyspnoea, both of which were measured using a non-validated symptom scale.

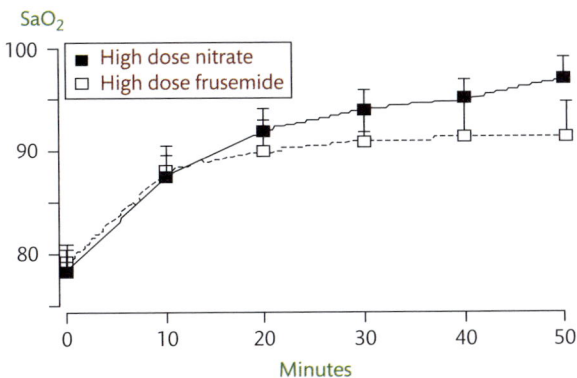

Figure 45.2 Combination of high-dose isosorbide dinitrate given as repeated intravenous boluses after low-dose intravenous furosemide was more effective than high-dose furosemide with low-dose isosorbide dinitrate in reducing the need for mechanical ventilation.

Source data from Cotter G, Metzkor E, Kaluski E, Faigenberg Z, Miller R, Simovitz A, et al. Randomised trial of high-dose isosorbide dinitrate plus low-dose furosemide versus high-dose frusemide plus low-dose isosorbide dinitrate in severe pulmonary oedema. *Lancet.* 1998;**351**(9100):389–93.

More recently, Breidthardt *et al.*[24] showed that, in a study of 128 patients, the use of high-dose transdermal and sublingual ISDN, in addition to standard AHF care, induced a faster and greater decrease in serum BNP compared to standard therapy alone. This did not, however, translate to a significant reduction in intensive care (ICU) admission, 90-day mortality, or rehospitalization rates.

Overall, trials of nitrates in AHF have been small and insufficiently powered to enable firm conclusions to be drawn. In a recent Cochrane review of nitrates for AHF syndromes, Wakai *et al.*[28] attempted to pool such results but found only six trials eligible for inclusion.[13,25–27,29,30] Of these, the study by Cotter *et al.*[13] was excluded for including nitrates in both arms of the trial. A further study by Elkayam *et al.*[26] was excluded due to being a subgroup analysis of VMAC,[27] which was already included in the review.

Of the remaining four trials, both patient populations and study design were heterogeneous, making direct comparisons difficult. Two studies included only patients with AHF following acute myocardial infarction (AMI), one study excluded patients with overt AMI, and one study included participants both with and without acute coronary syndromes. There were a total of 634 patients with AHF across the included studies, with two types of nitrates (ISDN and nitroglycerin) studied. Trials compared nitrates with furosemide and morphine, furosemide alone, hydralazine, prenalterol, intravenous nesiritide, and placebo. Seventy-four per cent of all the patients included in the studies were male. Overall analysis of the four included studies found no evidence to support a difference in symptom relief between intravenous nitrate vasodilator therapy and alternative interventions in patients with AHF. It was recognized, however, that the data were limited and of relatively low methodological quality, two of the four included studies having been performed >25 years ago.[25,30]

Sodium nitroprusside

As with the organic nitrates, data demonstrating the efficacy of sodium nitroprusside are limited, with only small studies demonstrating

haemodynamic benefits that show no robust translation into improvements in either short- or long-term outcomes.

In one of the earliest studies evaluating the haemodynamic effects of sodium nitroprusside in 50 patients with acute myocardial infarction complicated by LV failure, sodium nitroprusside was associated with a greater decrease in PCWP and SVR at 1 h compared with furosemide.[31] Moreover, in the same study, a significant increase in cardiac index at 1 h was also demonstrated. Except for PCWP, these differences were maintained at 48 h, but there was no significant difference in all-cause mortality at 48 h or at 12 months.

Using a larger cohort of 812 men, a subsequent multi-centred, randomized placebo-controlled trial sought to examine the haemodynamic effects on mortality in patients with LV failure and raised LV filling pressure after acute myocardial infarction.[32] There was no significant difference in all-cause mortality at 48 h, 21 days, or 13 weeks, between either the two main treatment groups or pre-specified subgroups (including age, systolic BP, and LV filling pressure). More interestingly, infusion within 9 h of infarction was associated with a significant increase in mortality at 13 weeks, whereas infusion initiated after 9 h was associated with decreased mortality, suggesting that those with persistent pump failure might receive sustained benefit from short-term sodium nitroprusside therapy.

More recently, in a small retrospective case study of 78 patients admitted with AHF treated with sodium nitroprusside (compared with 97 patients who were not) to a mean arterial pressure (MAP) of 65–70 mmHg, there was no significant difference between the two groups in the need for heart transplant or readmission. However, those treated with sodium nitroprusside had a significantly lower all-cause mortality (29% vs 44%; *P* = 0.005).[33] Moreover, sodium nitroprusside remained an independent predictor of survival on multivariate analysis. It is important to note that, at baseline, those who received sodium nitroprusside had significantly higher central venous pressure, PCWP, and MAP as well as significantly lower cardiac index than those who did not, once again highlighting the importance of patient selection when considering the use of vasodilators and the design of trials to test their efficacy.

Nesiritide

After several small trials demonstrating positive haemodynamic effects in the AHF population,[34–36] the VMAC study was designed to address issues of safety and acute effects compared with intravenous nitrates.[27] In total, 489 patients were enrolled, with 204 randomized to nesiritide, 143 to intravenous nitroglycerine, and 142 to placebo for the first 3 h. This was subsequently followed by nesiritide or nitroglycerine added to standard therapy for 24 h. Compared with nitrates, nesiritide showed significantly greater reductions in PCWP up to 36 h after treatment initiation, with a statistically significant improvement in dyspnoea at 3 h post infusion in patients treated with nesiritide over those treated with nitroglycerine or placebo—leading to US Food and Drug Administration (FDA) approval of nesiritide for use in the USA.

Following its approval, however, two meta-analyses raised doubt about the purported mortality benefits and suggested detrimental renal effects.[37,38] Hence, the Acute Study of Clinical Effectiveness of Nesiritide in Decompensated Heart Failure (ASCEND-HF) trial was designed to address these questions.[39] In this large, multi-centre,

randomized, placebo-controlled trial of 7141 patients with AHF, nesiritide, added to standard AHF care, was compared with standard therapy alone. There was no clinical benefit with nesiritide over standard heart failure therapy. There was no significant difference in symptomatic hypotension, but the duration of hypotension was significantly greater in the nesiritide group. There was no difference in renal function between the two groups.

ROSE-AHF was a multicentre, double-blind, placebo-controlled trial designed to test the hypothesis that the addition of low-dose nesiritide or low-dose dopamine to diuretic therapy may enhance decongestion and preserve renal function in patients presenting with AHF associated with renal dysfunction.[40] Compared with placebo, neither low-dose dopamine nor nesiritide demonstrated any benefit in terms of decongestion, renal function, or clinical outcomes.

Despite these findings, nesiritide continues to have approval by the FDA for early relief of dyspnoea in patients with AHF. It is, however, not licensed in several other countries, including the UK, and is unlikely to be so.

Current recommendations for intravenous vasodilator use in AHF

Conflicting results from relatively small studies have led to differing recommendations on the use of intravenous vasodilators in the setting of AHF (Table 45.1).

With similar clinical effects and side-effect profiles (Table 45.2), however, all guidelines recommend that symptoms and BP should be monitored frequently during administration.

2013 ACCF/AHA guideline for the management of heart failure

Vasodilation using intravenous nitroglycerine, nitroprusside, or nesiritide as an adjuvant to diuretic therapy for relief of dyspnoea in patients admitted with AHF receives a class IIb recommendation (*may* be considered) with level of evidence A. Although no specific haemodynamic cut-offs are suggested, this recommendation mandates that symptomatic hypotension is absent before such therapies are considered. Moreover, the American College of Cardiology

Foundation/American Heart Association (ACCF/AHA) guidelines suggest that nitroprusside is potentially of value in severely congested patients with hypertension or severe mitral valve regurgitation complicating LV dysfunction.

2016 ESC guidelines for the diagnosis and treatment of acute and chronic heart failure

The European Society of Cardiology (ESC) gives the use of intravenous vasodilators for symptomatic relief in AHF a class IIa recommendation (*should* be considered) with level of evidence B. These guidelines specify that systolic BP should be >90 mmHg and that patients should not have symptomatic hypotension; they also give separate recommendations for those with hypertensive AHF, where intravenous vasodilators should be considered as initial therapy.

2014 NICE guidelines for diagnosing and managing acute heart failure in adults

In contrast to both the ESC and AHA/ACCF guidelines, the UK National Institute for Health and Care Excellence (NICE) guidelines provide limited advice regarding the use of vasodilators, simply recommending that nitrates and sodium nitroprusside should not be routinely offered to patients with AHF. This is supplemented with the recommendation that if intravenous nitrates are used in specific circumstances—such as for people with concomitant myocardial ischaemia, severe hypertension or regurgitant aortic or mitral valve disease—BP should be monitored closely in a setting where more detailed observation or intervention can be provided, including support for a single failing organ system.[41]

Limitations of intravenous vasodilator use

Hypotension and end-organ perfusion

The use of vasodilators is characterized by several properties that limit their use, most prominently hypotension and subsequent end-organ hypoperfusion. In patients with AHF in whom cardiac reserve is reduced, inappropriate vasodilatation may induce a steep reduction in BP, resulting in haemodynamic instability, ischaemia, renal failure, and potentially overt shock—all of which are related to

Table 45.1 Summary of guidelines for vasodilators in acute heart failure

Professional/governmental body	Guidance	Class	Level
American College of Cardiology Foundation/American Heart Association	If symptomatic hypotension is absent, intravenous nitroglycerin, nitroprusside, or nesiritide may be considered an adjuvant to diuretic therapy for relief of dyspnoea in patients admitted with acutely decompensated heart failure.	IIb	A
European Society of Cardiology	IV vasodilators should be considered for symptomatic relief in AHF with SBP >90 mmHg (and without symptomatic hypotension). Symptoms and blood pressure should be monitored frequently during administration of IV vasodilators.	IIa	B
	In patients with hypertensive AHF, IV vasodilators should be considered as initial therapy to improve symptoms and reduce congestion.	IIa	B
National Institute for Health and Care Excellence	Do not routinely administer nitrates to people with AHF.		
	If intravenous nitrates are used in specific circumstances, such as for people with concomitant myocardial ischaemia, severe hypertension or regurgitant aortic or mitral valve disease, monitor blood pressure closely in a setting where at least level 2 care can be provided.		
	Do not administer sodium nitroprusside to people with AHF.		

AHF, acute heart failure; IV, intravenous; SBP, systolic blood pressure.

Table 45.2 Comparison between clinical effects of intravenous vasodilators in the treatment of acute heart failure

Variables	Nitroprusside	Nitroglycerine	Nesiritide
Clinical studies in heart failure	–	+	+++
Haemodynamic effect	+++	+++	+++
Tolerance	–	++	–
Need for dose titration	+++	+++	–
Effect on coronary blood flow	↓	↑↑	↑
Myocardial ischaemia	↑	↓	NA
Effect on urine output	NA	NA	+/–
Effect on neurohormones	↑	↑	↓
Vascular resitance	+	+	+
Evidence of symptomatic improvement	–	–	–

↓, decreased; ↑, increased; NA, not available; +/–, diverse results in different studies.

increased mortality in patients with AHF. No data exist on optimum vasodilator doses in AHF. Thus, most studies base uptitration on clinical judgement and pre-defined blood pressure targets. Because nesiritide has a longer effective half-life than the organic nitrates or nitroprusside, adverse effects such as hypotension may persist longer.

Over and above its hypotensive potential, nitroprusside use is further complicated both by its light-sensitive nature and by concerns of coronary steal in patients with active ischaemia. As such, it not only requires shielding during administration, but its use in patients with overt or suspected ischaemia is not recommended.

Patient selection and need for monitoring

Due to their potential for profound hypotension, the use of vasodilators is only recommended in patients with adequate BP and in a setting where careful monitoring can be provided. Data from both the ADHERE[42] and OPTIMIZE-HF[43] registries indicate that a substantial proportion of patients with AHF have normal or elevated BP at the time of presentation and that higher BP is associated with lower six-month mortality.[44] The use of vasodilators, however, has not been well studied in this subset of patients. The requirement for careful monitoring ultimately impacts on hospital resources, including the need for appropriate equipment and trained staff/ staffing levels to deal with such patients.

Pseudotolerance and tolerance

Further limitation on the use of the organic nitrates is the phenomenon of tachyphylaxis, with subsequent attenuation of the beneficial haemodynamic effects. This early tolerance (pseudotolerance) is purported to be due to counter-regulatory neurohormonal responses (increased noradrenaline, vasopressin, and renin activity) with resultant sodium and water retention and plasma volume expansion.

With continuing nitrate therapy, there are changes in endothelial and smooth muscle function, resulting in true tolerance. A number of lines of evidence show that therapy with most organic nitrates in clinically used doses impairs responsiveness to stimuli for the release of endothelium-derived NO.[45] Several mechanisms underlying this phenomenon have been described. Most involve the formation of superoxide either via the uncoupling of endothelial NO synthase or via the activation of NADPH oxidase by angiotensin II. These superoxides lead to the inactivation of the vasodilatory effects of NO and subsequent vasoconstriction. Moreover, superoxide directly inhibits smooth muscle guanylate cyclase, leading to a reduction in cGMP levels.

Several studies have assessed the haemodynamic tolerance to nitrates in patients with CHF. In one such study of intravenous nitroglycerine, Packer et al.[46] demonstrated that, after 48 h, those receiving a continuous infusion showed marked attenuation of response to near-baseline levels compared with those receiving two intermittent 12 h infusions. More recently, in a report of the VMAC heart failure trial, nitroglycerine doses had to be increased from a mean of 40–160 μg/min to maintain a reduction in wedge pressure at 12 h, and, even then, the effect was attenuated at 24 h.[26]

Due to the role of angiotensin II in the formation of nitrate tolerance, several studies have investigated the use of angiotensin converting enzyme inhibitor (ACEi) in its prevention. The majority of these have demonstrated that concomitant use of ACEi results in continued haemodynamic response to nitroglycerine therapy despite increased plasma renin activity.[47–49] Moreover, improvements in exercise tolerance, LV function,[47] and endothelial function[50] have been reported in patients receiving ACEi in combination with nitrates. Such results imply that early initiation or maintenance of ACEi therapy in patients with AHF could have beneficial effects on response to nitrate therapy.

Toxicity

Prolonged use of sodium nitroprusside is limited by its potential toxic accumulation of cyanide or thiocyanide, resulting in confusion, hyper-reflexia, and convulsions.

Future directions

Given the limited data and relative contraindications and complications of nitrate therapy, combined with a need for new therapies for

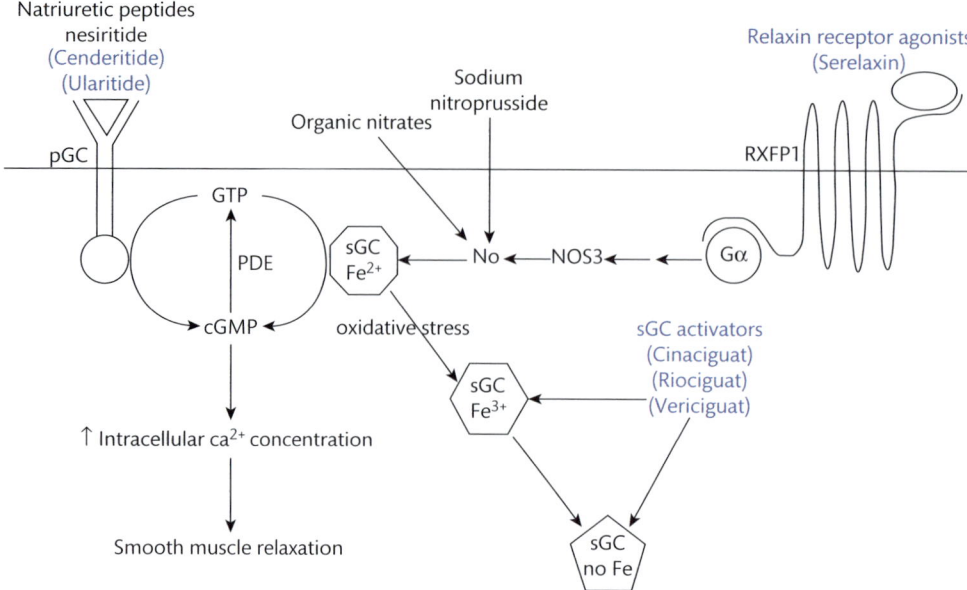

Figure 45.3 Mechanism of action of novel vasodilators.

AHF, several novel agents (**Figure 45.3**) have been investigated, with disappointing results so far.

Relaxin receptor agonists

Relaxin-2 is a naturally occurring peptide that modulates cardiovascular responses to pregnancy. Its actions lead to systemic and renal vasodilation and increased arterial compliance. Unlike the nitrates, it appears to have some inotropic effect and does not appear to reduce venous tone.[51] Furthermore, there is evidence to suggest a renoprotective role, with improvement in renal function observed in several clinical trials.[52,53]

In a study of recombinant human relaxin-2 (serelaxin) in stable patients with CHF, small but potentially important haemodynamic and neurohormonal effects were observed, with increases in cardiac output and decreases in SVR, PCWP, and N-terminal pro B-type natriuretic peptide (NT-proBNP).[54] The RELAXin in Acute Heart Failure (RELAX-AHF) trial,[55] was subsequently designed to evaluate the effects of serelaxin, added to standard therapy, on dyspnoea relief and other clinical efficacy outcomes. There was an improvement in patient-reported dyspnoea (visual analogue scale score) from enrolment to day 5 compared with placebo, but no effect on the patient-reported dyspnoea (Likert scale) at 6, 12, and 24 h. Treatment with serelaxin did not reduce readmissions, nor did it increase survival up to 60 days after hospital discharge. It did, however, apparently reduce cardiovascular and all-cause mortality by 37% at 180 days in a secondary analysis (**Figures 45.4** and **45.5**).

The RELAX-AHF 2 trial was designed to confirm whether the reduction in mortality was reproducible and to assess the effects of serelaxin on worsening heart failure up to day 5. Unfortunately, whereas the results of the trial confirm drug safety, it failed to reach any of its primary end-points, showing no benefit in either cardiovascular mortality or worsening heart failure with serelaxin therapy. It is unlikely that further trials examining the use of serelaxin will be forthcoming.[56]

Soluble guanylate cyclase activators

Unlike the nitrates, sGC activators are capable of activating sGC in a NO independent manner and in nitrate tolerant conditions.[57]

Cinaciguat

Cinaciguat is an intravenous sGC activator developed for the treatment of AHF. Preclinical characterization demonstrated that cinaciguat administration results in vasodilation with preserved glomerular filtration. Moreover, both antihypertrophic and antifibrotic effects were observed.[58,59] Initial studies in a small number of patients with AHF demonstrated significantly reduced PCWP together with a significant increase in cardiac output.[60] Results of the COMPOSE series of phase IIb studies, however, were terminated early due to an excess of hypotension in the cinaciguat arms and subsequent slow enrolment. It is unlikely that further studies will be performed on intravenous cinaciguat in AHF.[59]

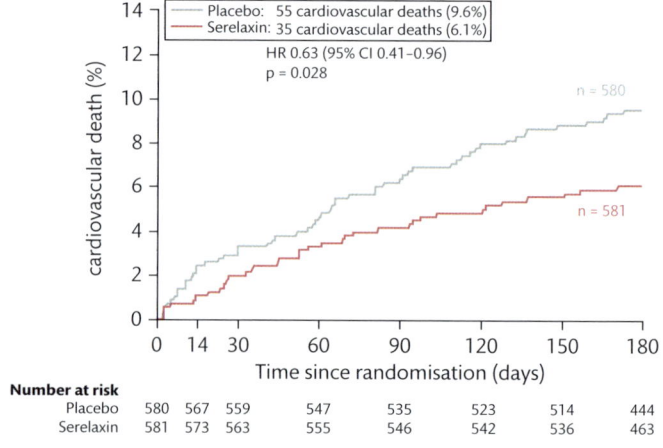

Figure 45.4 Study of recombinant human relaxin-2 (serelaxin) in stable patients with chronic heart failure.

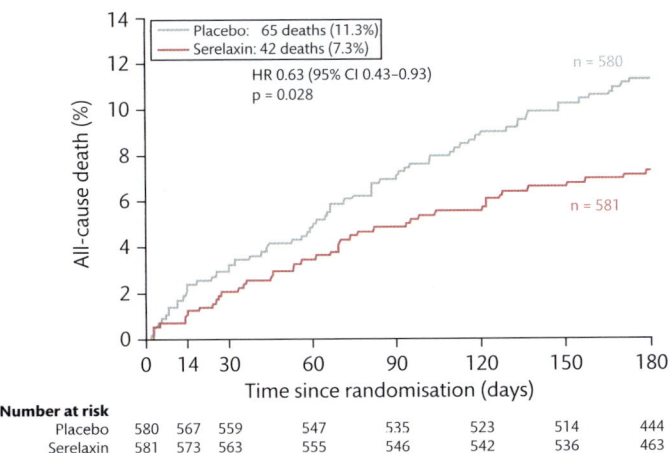

Figure 45.5 Study of recombinant human relaxin-2 (serelaxin) in stable patients with chronic heart failure.

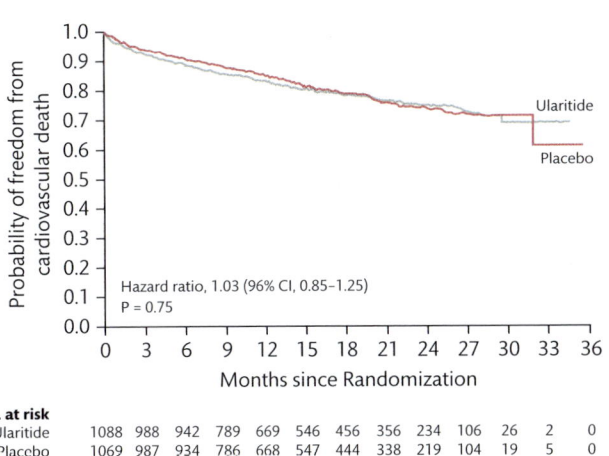

Figure 45.6 TRUE-AHF: a placebo-controlled randomized trial.

Vericiguat

Vericiguat is a novel oral sGC activator that stabilizes nitric oxide binding, thereby sensitizing sGC to endogenous nitric oxide.[1] The SOCRATES-REDUCED trial was a phase 2b study designed to evaluate the tolerability and effect of vericiguat, compared with placebo, on natriuretic peptide concentrations in patients with worsening heart failure and reduced LV ejection fraction.[2] Although no statistical difference in natriuretic peptide concentrations was observed, the drug was well tolerated.

The phase 3 'Vericiguat Global Study in Subjects with Heart Failure with Reduced Ejection Fraction' (VICTORIA) trial aimed to further evaluate the efficacy and safety of vericiguat in patients with a reduced ejection fraction and CHF with recent decompensation.[3] The results of this multinational trial of >5000 patients demonstrated that, compared with placebo, treatment with vericiguat resulted in a significant reduction in the composite primary end-point of cardiovascular death and first hospitalization. As with the SOCRATES-REDUCED trail, the drug was well tolerated, with 89% of participants achieving target dose. There was, however, no significant difference in the secondary outcomes of cardiovascular or all-cause mortality. Overall, these results are promising, with vericiguat as a potential novel treatment for patients with heart failure and high risk of hospitalization.

Natriuretic peptides

Ularitide

Ularitide is a synthetic analogue of urodilatin, a member of the family of A-type natriuretic peptides. Early studies reported favourable haemodynamic effects and possible enhanced natriuresis and diuresis.[61,62] TRUE-AHF was a placebo-controlled randomized trial designed to evaluate the efficacy of intravenous ularitide on clinical status and cardiovascular mortality in patients with acutely decompensated heart failure. Whereas intravenous ularitide was associated with favourable physiological effects, including a significant reduction in NT-proBNP and in-hospital heart failure events in the first 48 h, these did not translate into improvements in the primary end-point or reduced cardiovascular mortality (Figure 45.6).[63]

Cenderitide

Cenderitide is a chimeric natriuretic peptide designed to take advantage of the vasorelaxive properties of C-type natriuretic peptide and the positive renal effects of dendroaspis natriuretic peptide. It induces natriuresis and diuresis together with suppression of plasma aldosterone. Ongoing clinical trials are needed to validate the potential of cenderitide as an effective treatment option for AHF.

Summary

Despite haemodynamic data suggesting that vasodilator therapy should be beneficial in AHF, there is no robust evidence from carefully controlled prospective studies relating to outcomes or to symptom benefit in this patient population. Furthermore, there is no evidence to guide the physician on dose titration and BP targets. Trials to date have been small, underpowered, and have arguably targeted different populations than those identified in large registries. With the current and anticipated future burden of AHF presentations on healthcare services, more is required to establish the role of intravenous vasodilators in patients with acute pulmonary oedema. The development of novel therapies could help to address the current limitations of nitrates in AHF management, but results so far have been disappointing. Large, prospective, well-designed studies are urgently required.

Vasodilators for chronic heart failure

Isosorbide dinitrate and hydralazine

The Vasodilators in Heart Failure Trial (V-HeFT-I) study was the first placebo-controlled clinical trial to study the effect of vasodilator therapy on survival in patients with CHF. A total of 642 men with mild-to-moderate heart failure were randomized to placebo, the α-adrenoceptor antagonist prazosin, or to the combination of hydralazine and ISDN added to standard therapy. V-HeFT-I was undertaken at a time when the benefits of ACEi, β-blockers, and mineralocorticoid receptor antagonists (MRAs) were yet to be discovered and standard therapy consisted solely of a diuretic and digoxin. Two years after randomization, survival in the hydralazine–ISDN group was significantly enhanced compared to the placebo

group ($P = 0.028$). Hydralazine–ISDN also increased exercise capacity and LV ejection fraction compared to the placebo group. Such benefits were demonstrated over and above the BP-lowering effects of the hydralazine–ISDN combination.

The second V-HeFT-II study was performed after the results of CONSENSUS had shown significant mortality benefits of ACEi in patients with CHF and reduced ejection fraction. It sought to compare the efficacy of hydralazine–ISDN with that of enalapril. A total of 804 men with NYHA II–III functional status were randomized to hydralazine–ISDN or enalapril in addition to standard therapy with a diuretic and digoxin. Two years after randomization, a clear early difference was observed with a 27% relative risk reduction in mortality in the enalapril arm (18%) compared with 25% in the hydralazine–ISDN group.

Retrospective analyses of both V-HeFT-I and V-HeFT-II suggested that, compared with Caucasians, African-Americans derived benefit from the hydralazine–ISDN combination.[64,65] In 2004, the African-American Heart Failure (A-HeFT) trial was undertaken to evaluate further the observed benefits of hydralazine and ISDN in the African-American population. A total of 1050 NYHA class III and IV patients were randomized to receive a fixed-dose combination of hydralazine–ISDN or placebo three times daily.[65] By this time, the clinical benefits of ACEi, β-blockers, and MRAs were established and patients in A-HeFT were treated accordingly. The trial was discontinued prematurely at a median follow-up of 10 months following a significant reduction in all-cause mortality in the hydralazine–ISDN treatment group. A composite end-point was used, combining mortality, quality of life (as measured with the Minnesota Living with Heart Failure Questionnaire), and time to first hospitalization; each component was statistically significant in favour of the combination therapy.

Current recommendations for vasodilator use in chronic heart failure

As with the use of intravenous vasodilators, current recommendations for the use of the combination of hydralazine and ISDN are presented with differing levels across the American and European guidelines (Table 45.3).

2013 ACCF/AHA guidelines for the management of heart failure

The combination of hydralazine and ISDN carries two distinct recommendations in the ACCF/AHA guidelines for CHF.[66] The strongest recommendation, class I level of evidence A, is given for their use to reduce morbidity and mortality in patients self-described as African-American with NYHA class III–IV heart failure who are receiving optimal therapy with ACEi and β-blockers.

A class IIa, level of evidence B recommendation is suggested for the combination to reduce morbidity or mortality in patients who cannot be administered ACEi or ARB because of drug intolerance, hypotension, or renal insufficiency.

2016 ESC guidelines for the diagnosis and treatment of acute and chronic heart failure

Although current European guidelines also suggest two recommendations for the use of hydralazine and ISDN in CHF, unlike the ACCF/AHA they suggest the same class and level of evidence for both. These guidelines recommend that the main indication for hydralazine–ISDN is as a *substitute* in patients with intolerance to an ACEi or ARB (class IIb, level of evidence B) but that it should also be considered as an *additional* treatment in African-Americans

Table 45.3 Summary of guidelines for vasodilators in chronic heart failure

Professional/governmental body	Guidance	Class	Level
American College of Cardiology Foundation/American Heart Association	The combination of hydralazine and isosorbide dinitrate is recommended to reduce morbidity and mortality for patients self-described as African-Americans with NYHA class III–IV HFrEF receiving optimal therapy with ACEi and β-blockers, unless contraindicated	I IIa	A B
	A combination of hydralazine and isosorbide dinitrate can be useful to reduce morbidity or mortality in patients with current or prior symptomatic HFrEF who cannot be given an ACEi or ARB because of drug intolerance, hypotension, or renal insufficiency, unless contraindicated		
European Society of Cardiology	Hydralazine and isosorbide dinitrate should be considered in self-identified black patients with LVEF ≤35% or with an LVEF <45% combined with a dilated LV in NYHA class III–IV despite treatment with an ACEI, a β-blocker, and an MRA to reduce the risk of heart failure hospitalization and death.	IIa IIb	B B
	Hydralazine and isosorbide dinitrate may be considered in symptomatic patients with HFrEF who can tolerate neither an ACEi nor an ARB (or they are contra-indicated) to reduce the risk of death.		
National Institute for Health and Care Excellence	Seek specialist advice and consider adding hydralazine in combination with nitrate (especially if the patient is of African or Caribbean origin and has moderate to severe heart failure (NYHA class III–IV)) if a patient remains symptomatic despite optimal therapy with an ACEi and a β-blocker		
Scottish Intercollegiate Guidelines Network	Patients who are intolerant of an ACEi and an angiotensin II receptor blocker due to renal dysfunction or hyperkalaemia should be considered for treatment with a combination of hydralazine and isosorbide dinitrate.		1+ 1++
	African-American patients with heart failure with reduced ejection fraction, NYHA class III or IV, should be given hydralazine and isosorbide dinitrate in addition to standard therapy.		

ACEi, angiotensin converting enzyme inhibitor; HFrEF, heart failure with reduced ejection fraction; LVEF, left ventricular ejection fraction; MRA, mineralocorticoid receptor antagonist; NYHA, New York Heart Association.

who remain symptomatic on other proven therapies (class IIb, level of evidence B).[67]

2010 NICE guideline on diagnosis and management in primary and secondary care for chronic heart failure

Providing perhaps the simplest guidance on the prescription of hydralazine and ISDN for CHF, NICE recommends that physicians seek specialist advice to consider their use in patients who are either intolerant of ACEi and ARBs or who remain symptomatic despite optimal therapy with an ACEi and a β-blocker, especially if the patient is of African or Caribbean origin and has moderate-to-severe heart failure (NYHA class III–IV).[68]

2016 SIGN management of chronic heart failure

The Scottish Intercollegiate Guidelines Network (SIGN) guidelines[69] suggest that the combination *should be given* in addition to standard therapy to African-American patients with heart failure with reduced ejection fraction (HFrEF), NYHA class III or IV. By contrast, the same guidelines suggest that it *should be considered* in patients who are intolerant of an ACEi or ARB due to renal dysfunction or hyperkalaemia.

Limitations of hydralazine use

Sympathetic activation

Acting via the baroreceptor reflex, hydralazine causes sympathetic activation, leading to a rise in heart rate and cardiac output. Hence, caution is recommended in patients with coronary artery disease due to the possibility of myocardial ischaemia.

Systemic lupus erythematosus

Hydralazine metabolism occurs via acetylation, a process that occurs at different rates in different individuals. A rare adverse effect of higher doses of hydralazine, especially in patients who are slow acetylators, is a systemic lupus erythematosus-like syndrome. Although the exact mechanism by which hydralazine induces this syndrome is unclear, studies have demonstrated that it is likely to be associated with the formation of antihistone antibodies to H1 and the H3–H4 complex and a decrease in T-cell DNA methylation, leading to autoantibody formation.[70]

Clinical disease in the form of arthralgia, myalgia, malaise, serositis, and/or rash is thought to occur in 5–10% of patients treated with hydralazine. Although there is no specific test to confirm the diagnosis, the presence of antihistone antibodies in combination with a history of hydralazine use for more than one month makes the diagnosis highly likely. In most cases, symptoms resolve spontaneously upon withdrawal of the drug but full recovery may take several weeks/months.

Future directions

Soluble guanylate cyclase activators

Riociguat and vericiguat are oral sGC stimulators (Table 45.2) in development for the treatment of pulmonary hypertension and CHF.

The phase IIb exploratory randomized controlled trial, LEft ventricular systolic dysfunction associated with Pulmonary Hypertension riociguat Trial (LEPHT), examined the effects of riociguat in addition to standard heart failure therapy in patients with pulmonary hypertension secondary to LV systolic dysfunction. Riociguat was well tolerated and improved cardiac index, pulmonary vascular resistance, SVR, and quality of life, with no significant change in systemic BP or mean pulmonary arterial pressure.[71] Riociguat has been further evaluated in the treatment of pulmonary hypertension, but, due to its short half-life, studies in CHF have focused on the use of vericiguat, a longer-acting compound with a once-daily dosing regimen.[72]

Vericiguat has been evaluated in several preclinical and phase I studies, together with two phase IIb trials. The SOluble guanylate Cyclase stimulatoR in heArT failurE patientS (SOCRATES) trials examined the tolerability, optimal dosing and effects of vericiguat in both reduced ejection fraction (SOCRATES-REDUCED)[73] and preserved ejection fraction (SOCRATES-PRESERVED)[74] patient groups.

In the SOCRATES-REDUCED trial, vericiguat in doses up to 10 mg daily were well tolerated with a clinically significant reduction in NT-proBNP levels in the 10 mg target dose arm.[73] The subsequent, VerICiguaT Global Study in Subjects With Heart Failure With Reduced Ejection Fraction (VICTORIA) trial aims to evaluate the clinical efficacy of vericiguat on a background of heart failure standard therapy for subjects with HFrEF.[75]

The SOCRATES-PRESERVED trial was unable to demonstrate any clinically significant reduction in NT-proBNP or left atrial volumes. Compared with placebo, however, those patients in the 10 mg target-dose arm reported significant improvements in health status, as assessed by the Kansas City Cardiomyopathy Questionnaire (KCCQ) and the generic health-related quality-of-life measure EQ-5D. Further studies examining the benefit of vericiguat in the HFpEF population have been proposed.[74]

Summary

Compared to placebo, the combination of hydralazine and ISDN reduces mortality in patients with CHF, particularly in those of African-American descent. However, compared with ACEi the combination is inferior and there is no evidence to support the use of either drug alone in CHF.[76]

Few studies have assessed their efficacy in the era of contemporary heart-failure pharmacological and device therapies. Although questions remain as to the timing of initiation and the extent of benefit in those not of African-American or similar descent, the use of hydralazine and nitrates remains an important treatment option for those intolerant of the renin–angiotensin system antagonists.

The addition of novel oral sGC activators to standard heart failure therapy in patients with LV systolic dysfunction has produced promising results in phase IIb trials. Further randomized placebo-controlled phase III trials are planned to evaluate the potential benefits of vericiguat on heart failure hospitalization and cardiovascular mortality.

Conclusion

Although there remains a compelling physiological basis for the use of vasodilators, lack of robust evidence has led to differing opinions

about their use both in AHF and CHF. Much of the difference is due to the difficulties in performing clinical trials, particularly in the acute setting where time-limited interventions and the diverse presentation of patients makes the logistics of studies challenging. However, vasodilators remain an important weapon in the arsenal of therapies for the heart failure specialist in the treatment of selected patients. Careful trial design to target those most likely to benefit and the willingness of clinical trialists to perform such studies are required to understand the potential role (if any) of vasodilators in clinical practice.

REFERENCES

1. Vizzardi E, Bonadei I, Rovetta R, *et al.* When should we use nitrates in congestive heart failure? *Cardiovasc Ther* 2013;**31**(1):27–31.
2. Hollenberg SM. Vasodilators in acute heart failure. *Heart Fail Rev* 2007;**12**(2):143–7.
3. Metra M, Teerlink JR, Voors AA, *et al.* Vasodilators in the treatment of acute heart failure: what we know, what we don't. *Heart Fail Rev* 2009;**14**(4):299–307.
4. Mills RM, LeJemtel TH, Horton DP, *et al.* Sustained hemodynamic effects of an infusion of nesiritide (human b-type natriuretic peptide) in heart failure: a randomized, double-blind, placebo-controlled clinical trial. Natrecor Study Group. *J Am Coll Cardiol* 1999;**34**(1):155–62.
5. Lipe S, Moulds RF. In vitro differences between human arteries and veins in their responses to hydralazine. *J Pharmacol Exp Ther* 1981;**217**(1):204–8.
6. Bang L, Nielsen-Kudsk JE, Gruhn N, *et al.* Hydralazine-induced vasodilation involves opening of high conductance Ca²⁺-activated K⁺ channels. *Eur J Pharmacol* 1998;**361**(1):43–9.
7. Ellershaw DC, Gurney AM. Mechanisms of hydralazine induced vasodilation in rabbit aorta and pulmonary artery. *Br J Pharmacol* 2001;**134**(3):621–31.
8. Hermsmeyer K, Trapani A, Abel PW, Worcel M. Effect of hydralazine on tension and membrane potential in the rat caudal artery. *J Pharmacol Exp Ther* 1983;**227**(2):322–6.
9. Leier CV, Desch CE, Magorien RD, *et al.* Positive inotropic effects of hydralazine in human subjects: comparison with prazosin in the setting of congestive heart failure. *Am J Cardiol* 1980;**46**(6):1039–44.
10. Rouleau JL, Chatterjee K, Benge W, Parmley WW, Hiramatsu B. Alterations in left ventricular function and coronary hemodynamics with captopril, hydralazine and prazosin in chronic ischemic heart failure: a comparative study. *Circulation* 1982;**65**(4):671–8.
11. Bauer JA, Fung HL. Concurrent hydralazine administration prevents nitroglycerin-induced hemodynamic tolerance in experimental heart failure. *Circulation* 1991;**84**(1):35–9.
12. Gogia H, Mehra A, Parikh S, *et al.* Prevention of tolerance to hemodynamic effects of nitrates with concomitant use of hydralazine in patients with chronic heart failure. *J Am Coll Cardiol* 1995;**26**(7):1575–80.
13. Cotter G, Metzkor E, Kaluski E, *et al.* Randomised trial of high-dose isosorbide dinitrate plus low-dose furosemide versus high-dose furosemide plus low-dose isosorbide dinitrate in severe pulmonary oedema. *Lancet* 1998;**351**(9100):389–93.
14. Cotter G, Moshkovitz Y, Milovanov O, *et al.* Acute heart failure: a novel approach to its pathogenesis and treatment. *Eur J Heart Fail* 2002;**4**(3):227–34.
15. Cotter G, Moshkovitz Y, Kaluski E, *et al.* The role of cardiac power and systemic vascular resistance in the pathophysiology and diagnosis of patients with acute congestive heart failure. *Eur J Heart Fail* 2003;**5**(4):443–51.
16. Sharon A, Shpirer I, Kaluski E, *et al.* High-dose intravenous isosorbide-dinitrate is safer and better than Bi-PAP ventilation combined with conventional treatment for severe pulmonary edema. *J Am Coll Cardiol* 2000;**36**(3):832–7.
17. Stevenson LW. Tailored therapy to hemodynamic goals for advanced heart failure. *Eur J Heart Fail* 1999;**1**(3):251–7.
18. Leto L, Aspromonte N, Feola M. Efficacy and safety of loop diuretic therapy in acute decompensated heart failure: a clinical review. *Heart Fail Rev* 2014;**19**(2):237–46.
19. Northridge D. Frusemide or nitrates for acute heart failure? *Lancet* 1996;**347**(9002):667–8.
20. Crane SD. Epidemiology, treatment and outcome of acidotic, acute, cardiogenic pulmonary oedema presenting to an emergency department. *Eur J Emerg Med* 2002;**9**(4):320–4.
21. De Luca L, Fonarow GC, Adams KF, Jr, *et al.* Acute heart failure syndromes: clinical scenarios and pathophysiologic targets for therapy. *Heart Fail Rev* 2007;**12**(2):97–104.
22. Komajda M, Follath F, Swedberg K, *et al.* The EuroHeart Failure Survey programme—a survey on the quality of care among patients with heart failure in Europe. Part 2: treatment. *Eur Heart J* 2003;**24**(5):464–74.
23. Fonarow GC, Corday E. Overview of acutely decompensated congestive heart failure (ADHF): a report from the ADHERE registry. *Heart Fail Rev* 2004;**9**(3):179–85.
24. Breidthardt T, Noveanu M, Potocki M, *et al.* Impact of a high-dose nitrate strategy on cardiac stress in acute heart failure: a pilot study. *J Intern Med* 2010;**267**(3):322–30.
25. Nelson GI, Silke B, Ahuja RC, Hussain M, Taylor SH. Haemodynamic advantages of isosorbide dinitrate over frusemide in acute heart-failure following myocardial infarction. *Lancet* 1983;**1**(8327):730–3.
26. Elkayam U, Akhter MW, Singh H, Khan S, Usman A. Comparison of effects on left ventricular filling pressure of intravenous nesiritide and high-dose nitroglycerin in patients with decompensated heart failure. *Am J Cardiol* 2004;**93**(2):237–40.
27. VMAC Investigators (Vasodilatation in the Management of Acute CHF). Intravenous nesiritide vs nitroglycerin for treatment of decompensated congestive heart failure: a randomized controlled trial. *JAMA* 2002;**287**(12):1531–40.
28. Wakai A, McCabe A, Kidney R, *et al.* Nitrates for acute heart failure syndromes. *Cochrane Database Syst Rev* 2013;(8):Cd005151.
29. Beltrame JF, Zeitz CJ, Unger SA, *et al.* Nitrate therapy is an alternative to furosemide/morphine therapy in the management of acute cardiogenic pulmonary edema. *J Card Fail* 1998;**4**(4):271–9.
30. Verma SP, Silke B, Hussain M, *et al.* First-line treatment of left ventricular failure complicating acute myocardial infarction: a randomised evaluation of immediate effects of diuretic, venodilator, arteriodilator, and positive inotropic drugs on left ventricular function. *J Cardiovasc Pharmacol* 1987;**10**(1):38–46.
31. Hockings BE, Cope GD, Clarke GM, Taylor RR. Randomized controlled trial of vasodilator therapy after myocardial infarction. *Am J Cardiol* 1981;**48**(2):345–52.
32. Cohn JN, Franciosa JA, Francis GS, *et al.* Effect of short-term infusion of sodium nitroprusside on mortality rate in acute myocardial infarction complicated by left ventricular

failure: results of a Veterans Administration cooperative study. *N Engl J Med* 1982;**306**(19):1129–35.

33. Mullens W, Abrahams Z, Francis GS, *et al*. Sodium nitroprusside for advanced low-output heart failure. *J Am Coll Cardiol* 2008;**52**(3):200–7.

34. Hobbs RE, Miller LW, Bott-Silverman C, *et al*. Hemodynamic effects of a single intravenous injection of synthetic human brain natriuretic peptide in patients with heart failure secondary to ischemic or idiopathic dilated cardiomyopathy. *Am J Cardiol* 1996;**78**(8):896–901.

35. Marcus LS, Hart D, Packer M, *et al*. Hemodynamic and renal excretory effects of human brain natriuretic peptide infusion in patients with congestive heart failure. A double-blind, placebo-controlled, randomized crossover trial. *Circulation* 1996;**94**(12):3184–9.

36. Abraham WT, Lowes BD, Ferguson DA, *et al*. Systemic hemodynamic, neurohormonal, and renal effects of a steady-state infusion of human brain natriuretic peptide in patients with hemodynamically decompensated heart failure. *J Card Fail* 1998;**4**(1):37–44.

37. Sackner-Bernstein JD, Skopicki HA, Aaronson KD. Risk of worsening renal function with nesiritide in patients with acutely decompensated heart failure. *Circulation* 2005;**111**(12):1487–91.

38. Sackner-Bernstein JD, Kowalski M, Fox M, Aaronson K. Short-term risk of death after treatment with nesiritide for decompensated heart failure: a pooled analysis of randomized controlled trials. *JAMA* 2005;**293**(15):1900–5.

39. O'Connor CM, Starling RC, Hernandez AF, *et al*. Effect of nesiritide in patients with acute decompensated heart failure. *N Engl J Med* 2011;**365**(1):32–43.

40. Chen HH, Anstrom KJ, Givertz MM, *et al*. Low-dose dopamine or low-dose nesiritide in acute heart failure with renal dysfunction: the ROSE acute heart failure randomized trial. *JAMA* 2013;**310**(23):2533–43.

41. National Institute for Health and Care Excellence. *Acute heart failure: diagnosis and management*. NICE; 2014.

42. Adams KF, Jr, Fonarow GC, Emerman CL, *et al*. Characteristics and outcomes of patients hospitalized for heart failure in the United States: rationale, design, and preliminary observations from the first 100,000 cases in the Acute Decompensated Heart Failure National Registry (ADHERE). *Am Heart J* 2005;**149**(2):209–16.

43. Gheorghiade M, Abraham WT, Albert NM, *et al*. Systolic blood pressure at admission, clinical characteristics, and outcomes in patients hospitalized with acute heart failure. *JAMA* 2006;**296**(18):2217–26.

44. Milo-Cotter O, Adams KF, O'Connor CM, *et al*. Acute heart failure associated with high admission blood pressure—a distinct vascular disorder? *Eur J Heart Fail* 2007;**9**(2):178–83.

45. Munzel T, Daiber A, Gori T. Nitrate therapy: new aspects concerning molecular action and tolerance. *Circulation* 2011;**123**(19):2132–44.

46. Packer M, Lee WH, Kessler PD, *et al*. Prevention and reversal of nitrate tolerance in patients with congestive heart failure. *N Engl J Med* 1987;**317**(13):799–804.

47. Elkayam U, Johnson JV, Shotan A, *et al*. Double-blind, placebo-controlled study to evaluate the effect of organic nitrates in patients with chronic heart failure treated with angiotensin-converting enzyme inhibition. *Circulation* 1999;**99**(20):2652–7.

48. Mehra A, Ostrzega E, Shotan A, Johnson JV, Elkayam U. Persistent hemodynamic improvement with short-term nitrate

therapy in patients with chronic congestive heart failure already treated with captopril. *Am J Cardiol* 1992;**70**(15):1310–14.

49. Pizzulli L, Hagendorff A, Zirbes M, *et al*. Influence of captopril on nitroglycerin-mediated vasodilation and development of nitrate tolerance in arterial and venous circulation. *Am Heart J* 1996;**131**(2):342–9.

50. Watanabe H, Kakihana M, Ohtsuka S, Sugishita Y. Preventive effects of angiotensin-converting enzyme inhibitors on nitrate tolerance during continuous transdermal application of nitroglycerin in patients with chronic heart failure. *Jap Circ J* 1998;**62**(5):353–8.

51. Debrah DO, Conrad KP, Jeyabalan A, Danielson LA, Shroff SG. Relaxin increases cardiac output and reduces systemic arterial load in. *Hypertension* 2005;**46**(4):745–50.

52. Smith MC, Danielson LA, Conrad KP, Davison JM. Influence of recombinant human relaxin on renal hemodynamics in healthy volunteers. *J Am Soc Nephrol* 2006;**17**(11):3192–7.

53. Teichman SL, Unemori E, Dschietzig T, *et al*. Relaxin, a pleiotropic vasodilator for the treatment of heart failure. *Heart Fail Rev* 2009;**14**(4):321–9.

54. Dschietzig T, Teichman S, Unemori E, *et al*. Intravenous recombinant human relaxin in compensated heart failure: a safety, tolerability, and pharmacodynamic trial. *J Card Fail* 2009;**15**(3):182–90.

55. Teerlink JR, Cotter G, Davison BA, *et al*. Serelaxin, recombinant human relaxin-2, for treatment of acute heart failure (RELAX-AHF): a randomised, placebo-controlled trial. *Lancet* 2013;**381**(9860):29–39.

56. Metra M, Teerlink JR, Cotter G, *et al*.; RELAX-AHF-2 Committees Investigators. Effects of Serelaxin in Patients with Acute Heart Failure. *N Engl J Med* 2019;**381**:716–26.

57. Zamani P, Greenberg BH. Novel vasodilators in heart failure. *Curr Heart Fail Rep* 2013;**10**(1):1–11.

58. Boerrigter G, Costello-Boerrigter LC, Cataliotti A, *et al*. Targeting heme-oxidized soluble guanylate cyclase in experimental heart failure. *Hypertension* 2007;**49**(5):1128–33.

59. Gheorghiade M, Greene SJ, Filippatos G, *et al*. Cinaciguat, a soluble guanylate cyclase activator: results from the randomized, controlled, phase IIb COMPOSE programme in acute heart failure syndromes. *Eur J Heart Fail* 2012;**14**(9):1056–66.

60. Lapp H, Mitrovic V, Franz N, *et al*. Cinaciguat (BAY 58-2667) improves cardiopulmonary hemodynamics in patients with acute decompensated heart failure. *Circulation* 2009;**119**(21):2781–8.

61. Mitrovic V, Seferovic PM, Simeunovic D, *et al*. Haemodynamic and clinical effects of ularitide in decompensated heart failure. *Eur Heart J* 2006;**27**(23):2823–32.

62. Luss H, Mitrovic V, Seferovic PM, *et al*. Renal effects of ularitide in patients with decompensated heart failure. *Am Heart J* 2008;**155**(6):1012.e1–8.

63. Packer M, O'Connor C, McMurray JJV, *et al*. Effect of ularitide on cardiovascular mortality in acute heart failure. *N Engl J Med* 2017;**376**(20):1956–64.

64. Carson P, Ziesche S, Johnson G, Cohn JN. Racial differences in response to therapy for heart failure: analysis of the vasodilator–heart failure trials. Vasodilator–Heart Failure Trial Study Group. *J Card Fail* 1999;**5**(3):178–87.

65. Taylor AL, Ziesche S, Yancy C, *et al*. Combination of isosorbide dinitrate and hydralazine in blacks with heart failure. *N Engl J Med* 2004;**351**(20):2049–57.

66. Yancy CW, Jessup M, Bozkurt B, *et al*. 2013 ACCF/AHA guideline for the management of heart failure: a report of the American College of Cardiology Foundation/American Heart

Association Task Force on practice guidelines. *Circulation* 2013;**128**(16):e240–327.

67. Ponikowski P, Voors AA, Anker SD, *et al.* 2016 ESC Guidelines for the diagnosis and treatment of acute and chronic heart failure: The Task Force for the diagnosis and treatment of acute and chronic heart failure of the European Society of Cardiology (ESC). Developed with the special contribution of the Heart Failure Association (HFA) of the ESC. *Eur J Heart Fail* 2016;**18**(8):891–975.

68. National Institute for Health and Care Excellence. *Chronic heart failure*. Clinical Guideline 108. NICE, 2010.

69. Scottish Intercollegiate Guidelines Network. *Management of chronic heart failure*. SIGN, 2016.

70. Yung RL, Johnson KJ, Richardson BC. New concepts in the pathogenesis of drug-induced lupus. *Lab Invest* 1995;**73**(6):746–59.

71. Bonderman D, Ghio S, Felix SB, *et al.* Riociguat for patients with pulmonary hypertension caused by systolic left ventricular dysfunction: a phase IIb double-blind, randomized, placebo-controlled, dose-ranging hemodynamic study. *Circulation* 2013;**128**(5):502–11.

72. Follmann M, Ackerstaff J, Redlich G, *et al.* Discovery of the soluble guanylate cyclase stimulator vericiguat (BAY 1021189) for the treatment of chronic heart failure. *J Med Chem* 2017;**60**(12):5146–61.

73. Gheorghiade M, Greene SJ, Butler J, *et al.* Effect of vericiguat, a soluble guanylate cyclase stimulator, on natriuretic peptide levels in patients with worsening chronic heart failure and reduced ejection fraction: the SOCRATES-REDUCED randomized trial. *JAMA* 2015;**314**(21):2251–62.

74. Pieske B, Maggioni AP, Lam CSP, *et al.* Vericiguat in patients with worsening chronic heart failure and preserved ejection fraction: results of the SOluble guanylate Cyclase stimulatoR in heArT failurE patientS with PRESERVED EF (SOCRATES-PRESERVED) study. *Eur Heart J* 2017;**38**(15):1119–27.

75. Merck Sharp & Dohme Corp. A study of vericiguat in participants with heart failure with reduced ejection fraction (HFrEF) (MK-1242-001) (VICTORIA) 2016. https://clinicaltrials.gov/ct2/show/NCT02861534.

76. Farag M, Mabote T, Shoaib A, *et al.* Hydralazine and nitrates alone or combined for the management of chronic heart failure: a systematic review. *Int J Cardiol* 2015;**196**:61–9.

46

Ventilatory support

Christopher Armstrong and Alasdair Gray

Background

Acute heart failure (AHF) is common, accounting for around 5% of all hospital admissions in Europe and consuming ~2% of all health spending in many developed countries.[1] It is the leading cause of hospitalization of patients aged ≥65 years in the UK[2] and results in about one million hospital admissions per year in the USA.[3] Around 12% of all patients are likely to die during hospital admission and up to 56% of patients aged >75 years will die within the year after hospitalization.[4]

Many patients present in pulmonary oedema, with the classical signs and symptoms of acute breathlessness and pulmonary crackles, often with associated orthopnoea, paroxysmal nocturnal dyspnoea, and ankle oedema.[5] Given the exceptionally poor prognosis, optimal management early in their admission is essential.

For many of those presenting with respiratory distress, oxygenation and ventilatory support will be required immediately on arrival to hospital. Various forms of respiratory support may be needed depending on individual patient characteristics, from simple oxygen delivery devices to non-invasive ventilation (continuous positive airway pressure (CPAP) and bilevel positive airway pressure (BiPAP)) or even, occasionally, endotracheal intubation and mechanical ventilation. Positive pressure ventilation has effects on both the respiratory system[6,7] and the cardiovascular system.[8] Its potential benefit has been recognized for many years,[9] and its use is now widespread and advocated in professional guidelines.[2,5,9]

Pathophysiology of oxygenation and ventilatory failure in heart failure

Oxygenation and ventilation are impaired by a number of factors in the setting of congestive heart failure (CHF), be it acute or chronic, systolic or diastolic, and regardless of aetiology. In health, Starling forces ensure that only a small amount of fluid moves from the intravascular space into the pulmonary interstitium. This fluid then flows into the interlobular septae, the peribronchovascular space, and finally the hilum where it is drained by the lymphatic system.[10] CHF causes a rise in left ventricular end-diastolic pressure and subsequently left atrial pressure, which in turn causes a rise in pulmonary capillary pressure. Initially, this is compensated for by recruitment and distension of pulmonary capillaries.[11,12] As the intravascular hydrostatic pressure continues to rise, Starling forces between the vascular colloid and hydrostatic pressures and those of the interstitium are altered sufficiently that increased fluid begins to cross the capillary membrane into the interstitial space. Once the pulmonary capillary pressure reaches ~25 mmHg, the flow of fluid from the intravascular to interstitial space overwhelms the lymphatic system's capacity and fluid begins to accumulate, causing pulmonary oedema.[13] As this progresses, oxygenation and ventilation become impaired through multiple mechanisms.

Oxygenation and ventilation depend on the ability of gases to diffuse across the alveolar membrane, through the basement membrane, interstitium, and across the capillary wall to enter the bloodstream in the case of oxygen, and *vice versa* for carbon dioxide. In pulmonary oedema, fluid collects in the interstitial space, so increasing the distance gas must travel between the alveolus and blood. Fluid then collects in the alveolus itself, so increasing the distance between air and the alveolar membrane. In addition, increasing alveolar fluid causes an increase in surface tension and subsequent alveolar collapse,[14] so reducing the volume of ventilated lung and increasing right-to-left pulmonary shunting of deoxygenated blood. These changes result in both hypoxaemia and hypercapnoea.

Congested lungs are also considerably less compliant,[15-17] requiring a marked increase in the work of breathing[6] and generating significant negative intrapleural pressure. This negative pressure aggravates pulmonary oedema and impairs cardiac function by increasing afterload.[18,19] The associated increased work of breathing causes eventual exhaustion of the respiratory muscles,[20,21] a deterioration in the effort of breathing, and a consequential reduction in oxygenation and ventilation. Moreover, chronic heart failure is associated with cachexia and wasting of the respiratory muscles,[22] so reducing the ability of the chest wall to compensate. Increasing lung fluid volume also causes an element of reversible air flow obstruction, which is postulated to be caused by a combination of C-fibre stretch-receptor-mediated bronchoconstriction, bronchial vessel dilatation, and possibly peribronchial compression due to fluid accumulation.[23]

Raised pulmonary capillary pressures also result in changes to the pulmonary microvasculature and to the parenchyma itself.[24,25] In

acute decompensation these microvascular changes involve hydrostatic damage to the capillary walls and an increase in fluid and protein shift into the interstitium, which can be reversed. In chronic heart failure, however, this accumulation of fluid causes an increase in extracellular collagen proliferation and remodelling of the lung parenchyma, which decreases the diffusion capacity[26] and the compliance of the lung.[27] These changes are not reversible with acute medical interventions and persist even after heart transplant, so represent a gradual decline in underlying baseline function of the lung.

This combination of factors, especially in the setting of acute or chronic heart failure, leads to decompensation with symptoms of acute breathlessness and respiratory distress, requiring oxygenation or ventilatory assistance.

Types of oxygenation and ventilatory support

In patients who are critically ill, high-flow oxygen should be administered immediately as part of the resuscitation process.[28] It is important to recognize that in patients with CHF who are not hypoxic or critically ill, oxygen therapy may be detrimental in patients with left ventricular systolic dysfunction, causing a decrease in cardiac output and a trend towards increase in systemic vascular resistance.[29] Some patients who present with acute heart failure may be dyspnoeic due to pathophysiological responses that are not related to hypoxia.[30] Therefore, supplemental oxygen or ventilatory support should only be given to those who require it.

Oxygen can be delivered in a variety of ways, providing fixed or variable fractions of inspired oxygen (FiO_2) depending on delivery mode and patient variables.[31] The most basic of these is nasal cannulae. Simple nasal cannulae can deliver fixed flow rates between 1 and 5 L/min. The FiO_2 delivered to patients therefore depends on their respiratory rate and tidal volume, and relies on them breathing through their nose. High-flow nasal prongs (HFNPs) can generate flows up to 60 L/min and have been shown to provide positive end-expiratory pressure of up to 8.7 cmH$_2$O,[32,33] although this is reliant on patients keeping their mouth closed. HFNPs can be configured to deliver humidified gas flows and variable FiO_2 and can be used in hypoxaemic non-hypercapnic respiratory failure.[34] They may also be better tolerated than traditional face mask delivery systems.[35]

Face masks can either provide a fixed FiO_2, in the case of a venturi device, or a variable FiO_2, depending on oxygen flow rate and patient factors (e.g. respiratory rate and tidal volume), in the case of a Hudson mask. Venturi masks can be selected to provide a set FiO_2 between 24% and 60% regardless of oxygen flow rate, but patients breathing faster than 30 breaths per minute should have flows increased 50% above the recommended rate where possible to ensure that FiO_2 is maintained.[28] Higher concentrations of oxygen can be achieved with variable flow masks such as a high-concentration reservoir mask (non-rebreathing mask). These can deliver an FiO_2 of 60–90% with flow rates of 10–15 L/min; however, the FiO_2 is variable depending on the seal of the mask and the minute volume of the patient. There is also the risk of impairing breathing with oxygen flows <5 L/min, so these should generally be restricted to seriously ill patients with a significant oxygen requirement.

Non-invasive ventilation (NIV) can be considered to encompass continuous positive airway pressure (CPAP) and bilevel positive airway pressure (BiPAP).

CPAP provides a steady level of positive airway pressure throughout the respiratory cycle, regardless of patient respiratory phase or effort. It can be delivered in a number of ways, from simple portable devices to complex critical care unit ventilators. Basic flow-dependent CPAP valves, which generate positive airway pressure proportional to oxygen flow rate delivered from standard cylinders or wall outlets, are probably the simplest of these and have been shown to work well in emergency settings.[36] More complex ventilator-based systems are commonly used in hospital and can have both the airway pressure and FiO_2 adjusted according to patient response.

BiPAP provides an increased level of positive airway pressure during inspiration (IPAP), triggered by the patient's own initiation of a breath, while continuing to provide expiratory positive airway pressure (EPAP) during exhalation. As with CPAP, the pressure settings for each phase and FiO_2 can be adjusted to the requirements of the patient. BiPAP, however, requires more complex equipment than CPAP and increased provider training.[37] NIV can be delivered through a variety of patient interfaces, from nasal masks to oronasal masks, full-face masks and helmet devices. There is no strong evidence that any specific interface is superior to any other, but nasal masks are less well tolerated due to mouth leak and helmet devices are noisy and may result in increased patient–ventilator dysynchrony in BiPAP mode due to the increased dead space within the helmet.[38] Oro-nasal and full-face masks may, however, cause pressure lesions on the face, particularly on the bridge of the nose in the case of oro-nasal masks, and therefore must be managed carefully and prolonged application avoided. Most guidelines suggest an oro-nasal mask or full-face mask initially, although any interface can be used depending on patient preference and tolerance.[9,39]

Endotracheal intubation and mechanical ventilation is the option of last resort but ensures a secured airway and ability to ventilate the patient. It requires highly trained staff to perform and comes with significant risks to the patient.[40] However, it should not be delayed in the critically ill patient who has failed to respond to medical therapy in combination with oxygenation or NIV, e.g. those with worsening hypoxaemia, hypercapnoea, or acidosis.[2] These patients require urgent intervention and should be managed in the critical care unit.

Mechanisms of action of ventilation

The application of positive airway pressure has been shown to improve both cardiovascular and respiratory dynamics in patients with pulmonary oedema.[41] It does this by altering not only the mechanics of the lung, but also the cardiovascular physiology, having an effect on each system individually and altering the complex interplay between the two (**Box 46.1**).

Positive airway pressure has been shown to improve lung mechanics in pulmonary oedema in a number of ways.[6,7] It improves lung compliance and reduces lung and airway resistance while also reducing the amount of energy used by the respiratory muscles, so reducing the work and metabolic demand of breathing. Tidal volumes are increased, indicating recruitment of previously collapsed alveoli, and respiratory rate is reduced along with minute ventilation volumes, indicating an improvement in respiratory efficiency. Total extravascular lung water is reduced, and there is an increase in lymphatic drainage from the lungs.[42] There is also a reduction in

Respiratory system
- Improves lung compliance
- Reduces lung and airway resistance
- Reduces work of breathing
- Increases tidal volumes
- Improves functional residual capacity
- Reduces respiratory rate
- Increases lung lymphatic drainage

Cardiovascular system
- Reduces excess right ventricular preload
- Reduces pulmonary vascular resistance
- Reduces left heart preload
- Reduces transmural pressure
- Reduces left heart after load
- Reduces pulmonary shunting

pulmonary shunting and in the arteriolar–arterial oxygen gradient.[43] BiPAP has also been shown to decrease the work of breathing further when compared to CPAP by unloading the respiratory muscles to a greater extent.[41] In addition, mechanical ventilation of the lungs has been shown to reduce sympathetic tone, so reducing the sympathetic overload associated with acute heart failure.[44]

Heart failure is associated with excessive preload and afterload, including elevated transmural pressure—the difference in pressure across the cardiac wall between the chambers of the heart and the pleural cavity. These elevations in volume and pressure shift the heart right on the Frank–Starling curve to such an extent that function is impaired.

Right heart preload is determined by right atrial pressure, which in turn is significantly dependent on systemic venous return. Positive airway pressure increases intrathoracic pressure (ITP) and so alters the pressure gradient from the systemic circulation back to the heart and causes a decrease in venous return.[45] In health this can cause underfilled individuals to become hypotensive due to decreased preload. In heart failure, however, it returns the heart to a more efficient point on the Frank–Starling curve, so improving function. Right heart afterload is determined largely by pulmonary vascular resistance (PVR). This is affected by a number of factors, including the level of inflation of the lung and pulmonary vasoconstriction caused by hypoxia. PVR is distributed in a U-shaped curve, increased in both the collapsed lung and hyperinflated lung.[46] It is postulated that this is due to the balance of flow in the lung between intra-alveolar and extra-alveolar vessels.[47] Below normal functional residual capacity (FRC), as may be the case in collapsed lung in pulmonary oedema, compression of extra-alveolar vessels causes increased resistance. Increasing lung volume distends these vessels, so reducing PVR, and it has been shown that restoring lung to near its original functional residual capacity optimizes PVR. This has correlated with ~10 cmH$_2$O in abnormal lungs in dogs.[48] Recruiting alveoli also reduces hypoxia, thereby reducing hypoxic pulmonary vasoconstriction and pulmonary shunting.[49]

As the right and left heart are in series, any reduction in systemic venous return, and therefore right heart output, will cause a decrease in left ventricular preload by reducing the amount of blood flowing from the right ventricle to the left. The predominant effect of the rise in intrathoracic pressure caused by positive airway pressure in the setting of impaired left ventricular function, however, is through a reduction in afterload.[50] Left ventricular afterload is affected by the transmural pressure, that is the difference between the pressure within the left ventricle itself and the pressure outside the heart (within the thorax), and the systemic mean arterial pressure—the pressure against which the left ventricle has to push. In spontaneous breathing, inspiration causes negative intrathoracic pressure. During systole, the left ventricle has to contract against this distending negative pressure, so increasing afterload by adding to left ventricle wall stress and therefore work.[8,51] In pulmonary oedema, these swings in negative pressure are significantly greater due to the increased effort of inflating oedematous lungs, so transmural pressure and therefore afterload is markedly increased. Non-invasive ventilation decreases transmural pressure by increasing ITP, so exerting a contracting rather than distending force on the left ventricle, and thus reducing the effort of systole.[52] NIV also reduces afterload by increasing the pressure gradient between the thorax and the peripheral circulation, so reducing the vascular resistance that the left ventricle must overcome during systole.[53] The combination of these various factors has been shown to increase cardiac output in the failing heart.[8]

Research evidence of clinical benefit

The potential benefits of positive airway pressure were first identified over eighty years ago.[54] Multiple recent trials have investigated both CPAP and BiPAP compared to standard oxygen therapy and each other, which has led to the widespread uptake of this therapeutic intervention.

The benefit of CPAP has been demonstrated in multiple small trials (30–100 patients) since the 1980s.[36,43,55–58] These studies showed that, when compared to standard therapy with oxygen through a face mask, oxygen combined with CPAP increases tidal volumes and the arterial partial pressure of oxygen (PaO_2) while decreasing the alveolar–arterial oxygen tension gradient, respiratory rate, and arterial partial pressure of carbon dioxide ($PaCO_2$). The cardiovascular effects of CPAP included a decrease in systolic blood pressure, heart rate, rate–pressure product (a measure of oxygen demand and therefore work of the heart), and intrapulmonary shunting while increasing the stroke volume index. CPAP patients also had a lower rate of treatment failure requiring intubation and mechanical ventilation. They did not, however, show any significant difference in hospital length of stay or overall mortality between the two groups.

Some trials have also investigated the use of BiPAP when compared to standard oxygen therapy.[59–64] These also demonstrated a benefit with BiPAP with increasing oxygen saturations (SpO_2), PaO_2 and arterial pH with decreasing respiratory rate and $PaCO_2$. They also showed a decrease in intubation rate and a significant shortening of symptom resolution time (defined as maintained oxygen saturations >96% and respiratory rate <30).[60] One early trial suggested an increase in acute myocardial infarction (MI) with BiPAP;[62] however, this was likely due to a larger number of patients with chest pain in the BiPAP group[65] and has not been seen in subsequent larger studies.[63,66] There was, however, no difference in mortality rates or in length of hospital stay when compared to standard oxygen therapy.

With both modes of positive pressure ventilation showing clinical benefit, multiple studies have been performed to compare BiPAP to CPAP, and to standard oxygen therapy.[41,66–74] Small early trials[41,67,68] (recruiting six to 27 patients) appeared to suggest some benefit of BiPAP over CPAP, with greater reduction of dyspnoea, heart rate, blood pressure, pH, and $PaCO_2$,[67] with a reduction in rate of intubation shown in one trial.[68] BiPAP was shown to off-load the respiratory muscles to a greater extent in one small trial[41] (six patients) but there was no difference in the decrease in transmural pressure and none of these trials demonstrated a reduction in mortality or length of stay. Subsequent larger trials[69–73] (36–109 patients) showed that both BiPAP and CPAP improved physiological parameters when compared to standard oxygen therapy but without significant difference between the two modes of NIV. Two studies[69,70] also further investigated changes in the incidence of MI and demonstrated no increase in the BiPAP group compared to controls.

Systematic reviews[75,76] and meta-analyses[77–79] including these studies and others confirmed that both BiPAP and CPAP reduced need to intubate and mortality when compared to standard therapy but that there was no significant difference between the two, including in the incidence of MI. In 2008, Gray et al.[66] recruited 1069 patients (similar in number to all patients recruited to previous studies combined) to a multicentre, prospective randomized trial comparing BiPAP to CPAP and standard oxygen therapy. This showed improvement in physiological parameters as in previous studies but did not demonstrate any significant difference in need to intubate, incidence of MI, or in 7- or 30-day mortality in those assigned to BiPAP or CPAP compared to standard therapy. However, the intubation rate was very low in this study (eight patients in total), and, being a pragmatic study, patients were allowed to cross over from one arm to the other, with 43 and 13 patients from the oxygen arm changing to CPAP and BiPAP respectively who may have been intubated in other studies.

Subsequent more recent systematic reviews[80,81] and meta-analyses,[82–85] some including >3000 patients, have all shown no difference in need for intubation, incidence of MI or mortality between CPAP and BiPAP. They have continued to demonstrate a reduction in intubation rates and mortality for either mode of NIV when compared to standard therapy, even after inclusion of the 3CPO trial in these analyses.[81]

Clinical application

The successful application of NIV relies on a number of factors: appropriate patient selection, appropriate staff expertise and appropriate clinical surroundings. Several guidelines provide advice on the selection of patients most likely to benefit from NIV,[5,86–88] and guidance on the indications and contraindications of NIV use (**Box 46.2**).[5,88] NIV should be used in clinical settings where there are appropriate staffing levels and expertise, usually the emergency department, dedicated respiratory unit, or the critical care unit, with nursing ratios of 2:1 recommended, at least in the first 24 h.[89]

Some small studies have been conducted into applying CPAP and BiPAP in the prehospital environment for acute pulmonary oedema and undifferentiated acute respiratory failure. Three systematic reviews[90–92] of these prehospital trials have shown that prehospital

---

Box 46.2 Indications and contraindications of non-invasive ventilation

Indications

Bedside observations
- Increased dyspnoea: moderate to severe
- Tachypnoea (>25 bpm)
- Signs of increased work of breathing, accessory muscle use, and abdominal paradox

Gas exchange
- Acute or acute on chronic ventilatory failure: $PaCO_2$ >6.0 kPa, pH <7.35
- Hypoxaemia: oxygen saturations <90%, PaO_2/FiO_2 ratio <200

Contraindications

Absolute
- Cardiac arrest
- Upper airway obstruction
- Severe facial or upper airway trauma or burns
- Undrained pnuemothorax
- Unable to fit mask

Relative
- Medically unstable: hypotensive shock
- Uncontrolled cardiac ischaemia or arrhythmia
- Uncontrolled copious upper gastrointestinal bleeding
- Agitated, unco-operative
- Unable to protect airway
- Swallowing impairment
- Excessive secretions not managed by secretion clearance techniques
- Multiple (i.e. two or more) organ failure
- Recent upper airway or upper gastrointestinal surgery

CPAP may reduce intubation rates and subsequent in-hospital mortality but that it does not reduce critical care length of stay. The benefit of BiPAP and the cost-effectiveness of prehospital NIV remain uncertain.

The successful application of NIV relies upon building trust with the patient and taking adequate time to familiarize them with the mask and the sensation of NIV. Thorough explanation of the process coupled with applying the mask by hand, before securing the straps to the patient's face, will increase patient tolerance. To aid this process, initial settings should be kept low. Typically, CPAP is started at ~5 cmH$_2$O and increased to ~10 cmH$_2$O as tolerated. BiPAP is usually initiated with EPAP of ~5 cmH$_2$O and IPAP of ~10 cmH$_2$O, and subsequently increased to a maximum EPAP of 10 cmH$_2$O and IPAP of 20–25 cmH$_2$O to achieve adequate oxygenation and ventilation,[93] with tidal volumes of ~6–8 mL/kg. The opening pressure of the gastro-oesophageal sphincter is ~25 cmH$_2$O, therefore increasing the inspiratory pressure beyond this may lead to significant gastric insufflation and resulting respiratory impairment and must be avoided.[38]

Once on NIV, patients should be reassessed frequently (at least hourly initially) for improvement. Some patients with pulmonary oedema may improve rapidly and might only need a short time (1–3 h) on NIV.[66] Others may require 24–48 h. There is little formal evidence to guide weaning although one study has suggested that protocol-guided weaning can shorten NIV duration and intensive care unit length of stay.[94] In general, resolution of respiratory

distress, normalization of respiratory rate, and oxygen saturations and correction of any respiratory acidosis should prompt a gradual reduction in the FiO_2 and positive airway pressure with close attention paid for any signs of deterioration. Trial without NIV can be performed (for instance to allow face/oral hygiene or drinking/eating), and, if well tolerated, then NIV can be discontinued. Equally, patients should be observed closely for signs of failure of NIV therapy, such as worsening respiratory distress or respiratory failure on blood gas analysis, and prompt intubation and invasive mechanical ventilation should be considered.

NIV should be used in conjunction with medical therapy to correct the underlying cause of pulmonary oedema. Often this will involve intravenous nitrate therapy if initially hypertensive and diuretics in patients with signs of fluid overload.[5] Simultaneous investigation and treatment of precipitating factors such as myocardial ischaemia, arrhythmias, uncontrolled hypertension, infection, mechanical failure (such as valve prolapse or septal/wall rupture) or pulmonary embolism should also be instigated. Occasionally patients will require haemodynamic support in the form of inotropes or vasopressors, and local and international guidelines should be followed in this instance with urgent referral to coronary or critical care (**Figure 46.1**).[5]

Once patients have recovered from their acute illness, they should be referred to specialist heart failure multidisciplinary teams for ongoing management, both in hospital and in the community.

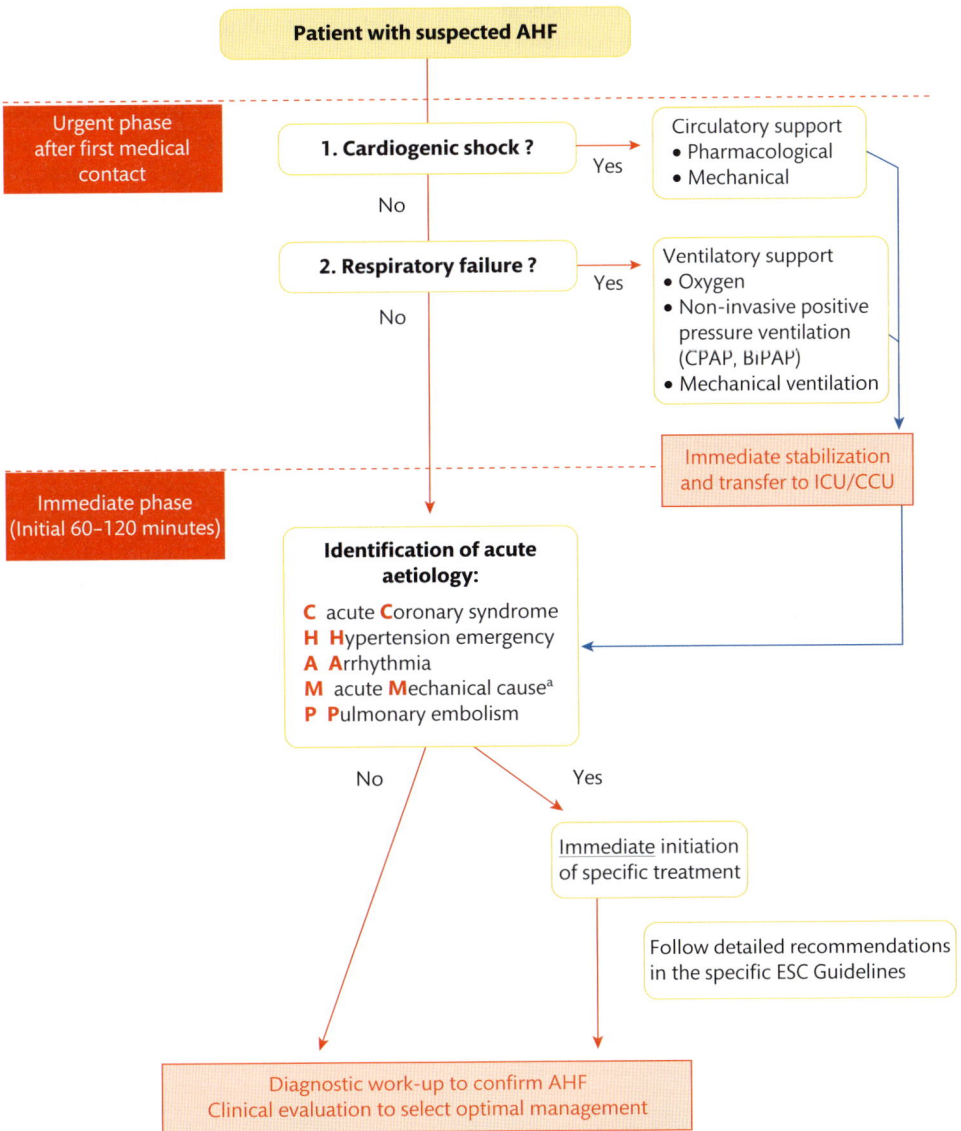

Figure 46.1 Patient with suspected acute heart failure. AHF, acute heart failure; CPAP, continuous positive airway pressure; BiPAP, biphasic positive airway pressure; ICU, intensive care unit; CCU, critical care unit; ESC, European Society of Cardiology.

Reproduced from Ponikowski P, Voors AA, Anker SD, et al. 2016 ESC Guidelines for the diagnosis and treatment of acute and chronic heart failure: The Task Force for the diagnosis and treatment of acute and chronic heart failure of the European Society of Cardiology (ESC). Developed with the special contribution of the Heart Failure Association (HFA) of the ESC. *European Journal of Heart Failure* 2016; **18**(8): 891–975 with permission from Oxford University Press.

Conclusion

Acute heart failure is common, with respiratory distress secondary to pulmonary oedema often being the cause of presentation to hospital. Many patients will require supplemental oxygen and positive pressure ventilation as part of their early and ongoing management.

Positive airway pressure has beneficial effects on both the cardiovascular and respiratory systems: it reduces right heart preload and therefore left heart preload, and reduces afterload by increasing flow away from the left heart and decreasing left ventricular transmural pressures, thereby improving the function of the failing heart. It has been shown to increase lung compliance and tidal volumes, increase alveolar recruitment, improve alveolar–arterial oxygen gradients, and decrease respiratory rate, work of breathing, and intrapulmonary shunting. BiPAP may also confer further benefit on hypercapnic patients by unloading the work of the respiratory muscles.

NIV has been shown to reduce symptoms of respiratory distress, often the most pressing issue for patients. It can be used safely in both prehospital, emergency department, and critical care settings; however, its efficacy in reducing long-term outcomes remains uncertain, with the largest multicentre trial showing no significant difference in mortality or intubation rates despite evidence from smaller trials and meta-analyses suggesting this. Nevertheless, it is now a central part of the management of acute pulmonary oedema in the setting of heart failure. It should be instigated by experienced staff in appropriate clinical settings, with good patient selection imperative to ensure therapeutic success.

REFERENCES

1. Braunschweig F, Cowie MR, Auricchio A. What are the costs of heart failure? *Europace* 2011;**13**(Suppl 2):ii13–ii17.
2. Dworzynski K, Roberts E, Ludman A, Mant J. Diagnosing and managing acute heart failure in adults: summary of NICE guidance. *BMJ* 2014;**349**:g5695.
3. Mozaffarian D, Benjamin EJ, Go AS, *et al.* Heart disease and stroke statistics—2016 update. *Circulation* 2016;**133**(4):e38–e360.
4. Cleland JG, McDonagh T, Rigby AS, *et al.* The national heart failure audit for England and Wales 2008–2009. *Heart* 2011;**97**(11):876–86.
5. Ponikowski P, Voors AA, Anker SD, *et al.* 2016 ESC Guidelines for the diagnosis and treatment of acute and chronic heart failure. *Eur Heart J* 2016;**37**(27):2129–200.
6. Katz JA, Marks JD. Inspiratory work with and without continuous positive airway pressure in patients with acute respiratory failure. *Anesthesiology* 1985;**63**(6):598–607.
7. Lenique F, Habis M, Lofaso F, *et al.* Ventilatory and hemodynamic effects of continuous positive airway pressure in left heart failure. *Am J Respir Crit Care Med* 1997;**155**(2):500–5.
8. Pinsky MR, Summer WR, Wise RA, Permutt S, Bromberger-Barnea B. Augmentation of cardiac function by elevation of intrathoracic pressure. *J Appl Physiol Respir Environ Exerc Physiol* 1983;**54**(4):950–5.
9. Keenan SP, Sinuff T, Burns KEA, *et al.* Clinical practice guidelines for the use of noninvasive positive-pressure ventilation and noninvasive continuous positive airway pressure in the acute care setting. *Can Med Assoc J* 2011;**183**(3):E195–E214.
10. Staub NC. The pathophysiology of pulmonary edema. *Hum Pathol* 1970;**1**(3):419–32.
11. West JB, Dollery CT, Naimark A. Distribution of blood flow in isolated lung; relation to vascular and alveolar pressures. *J Appl Physiol* 1964;**19**:713–24.
12. Glazier JB, Hughes JM, Maloney JE, West JB. Measurements of capillary dimensions and blood volume in rapidly frozen lungs. *J Appl Physiol* 1969;**26**(1):65–76.
13. Gehlbach BK, Geppert E. The pulmonary manifestations of left heart failure. *Chest* 2004;**125**(2):669–82.
14. Allison RC. Initial treatment of pulmonary edema: a physiological approach. *Am J Med Sci* 1991;**302**(6):385–91.
15. Noble WH, Kay JC, Obdrzalek J. Lung mechanics in hypervolemic pulmonary edema. *J Appl Physiol* 1975;**38**(4):681–7.
16. Sharp JT, Griffith GT, Bunnell IL, Greene DG. Ventilatory mechanics in pulmonary edema in man. *J Clin Invest* 1958;**37**(1):111–17.
17. Cosby RS, Stowell EC, Hartwig WR, Mayo M. Pulmonary function in left ventricular failure, including cardiac asthma. *Circulation* 1957;**15**(4):492–501.
18. Buda AJ, Pinsky MR, Ingels NB, Jr, *et al.* Effect of intrathoracic pressure on left ventricular performance. *N Engl J Med* 1979;**301**(9):453–9.
19. Hausknecht MJ, Brin KP, Weisfeldt ML, Permutt S, Yin FC. Effects of left ventricular loading by negative intrathoracic pressure in dogs. *Circ Res* 1988;**62**(3):620–31.
20. Field S, Kelly SM, Macklem PT. The oxygen cost of breathing in patients with cardiorespiratory disease. *Am Rev Respir Dis* 1982;**126**(1):9–13.
21. Aubier M, Trippenbach T, Roussos C. Respiratory muscle fatigue during cardiogenic shock. *J Appl Physiol* 1981;**51**(2):499–508.
22. von Haehling S, Anker SD. Prevalence, incidence and clinical impact of cachexia: facts and numbers-update 2014. *J Cachexia Sarcopenia Muscle* 2014;**5**(4):261–3.
23. Puri S, Dutka DP, Baker BL, Hughes JM, Cleland JG. Acute saline infusion reduces alveolar–capillary membrane conductance and increases airflow obstruction in patients with left ventricular dysfunction. *Circulation* 1999;**99**(9):1190–6.
24. Guazzi M. Alveolar gas diffusion abnormalities in heart failure. *J Card Fail* 2008;**14**(8):695–702.
25. West JB, Mathieu-Costello O. Vulnerability of pulmonary capillaries in heart disease. *Circulation* 1995;**92**(3):622–31.
26. Olson LJ, Snyder EM, Beck KC, Johnson BD. Reduced rate of alveolar–capillary recruitment and fall of pulmonary diffusing capacity during exercise in patients with heart failure. *J Card Fail* 2006;**12**(4):299–306.
27. Mettauer B, Lampert E, Charloux A, *et al.* Lung membrane diffusing capacity, heart failure, and heart transplantation. *Am J Cardiol* 1999;**83**(1):62–7.
28. O'Driscoll BR, Howard LS, Davison AG. BTS guideline for emergency oxygen use in adult patients. *Thorax* 2008;**63**(Suppl 6):vi1–vi68.
29. Park JH, Balmain S, Berry C, Morton JJ, McMurray JJV. Potentially detrimental cardiovascular effects of oxygen in patients with chronic left ventricular systolic dysfunction. *Heart* 2010;**96**(7):533–8.
30. Vaisanen IT, Rasanen J. Continuous positive airway pressure and supplemental oxygen in the treatment of cardiogenic pulmonary edema. *Chest* 1987;**92**(3):481–5.
31. Bateman NT, Leach RM. Acute oxygen therapy. *BMJ* 1998;**317**(7161):798–801.

32. Groves N, Tobin A. High flow nasal oxygen generates positive airway pressure in adult volunteers. *Aust Crit Care* 2007;**20**(4):126–31.

33. Lee JH, Rehder KJ, Williford L, Cheifetz IM, Turner DA. Use of high flow nasal cannula in critically ill infants, children, and adults: a critical review of the literature. *Intensive Care Med* 2013;**39**(2):247–57.

34. Frat JP, Thille AW, Mercat A, *et al*. High-flow oxygen through nasal cannula in acute hypoxemic respiratory failure. *N Engl J Med* 2015;**372**(23):2185–96.

35. Ward JJ. High-flow oxygen administration by nasal cannula for adult and perinatal patients. *Respir Care* 2013;**58**(1):98–122.

36. Moritz F, Benichou J, Vanheste M, *et al*. Boussignac continuous positive airway pressure device in the emergency care of acute cardiogenic pulmonary oedema: a randomized pilot study. *Eur J Emerg Med* 2003;**10**(3):204–8.

37. British Thoracic Society Standards of Care Committee. Non-invasive ventilation in acute respiratory failure. *Thorax* 2002;**57**(3):192–11.

38. Carron M, Freo U, BaHammam AS, *et al*. Complications of non-invasive ventilation techniques: a comprehensive qualitative review of randomized trials. *Br J Anaesth* 2013;**110**(6):896–914.

39. Agarwal R, Gupta D. What is the role of noninvasive ventilation in diastolic heart failure? *Intensive Care Med* 2005;**31**(10):1451; author reply 1452.

40. Loh KS, Irish JC. Traumatic complications of intubation and other airway management procedures. *Anesthesiol Clin North Amer* 2002;**20**(4):953–69.

41. Chadda K, Annane D, Hart N, *et al*. Cardiac and respiratory effects of continuous positive airway pressure and noninvasive ventilation in acute cardiac pulmonary edema. *Crit Care Med* 2002;**30**(11):2457–61.

42. Fernandez Mondejar E, Vazquez Mata G, *et al*. Ventilation with positive end-expiratory pressure reduces extravascular lung water and increases lymphatic flow in hydrostatic pulmonary edema. *Crit Care Med* 1996;**24**(9):1562–7.

43. Lin M, Chiang HT. The efficacy of early continuous positive airway pressure therapy in patients with acute cardiogenic pulmonary edema. *J Formos Med Assoc* 1991;**90**(8):736–43.

44. Kaye DM, Mansfield D, Aggarwal A, Naughton MT, Esler MD. Acute effects of continuous positive airway pressure on cardiac sympathetic tone in congestive heart failure. *Circulation* 2001;**103**(19):2336–8.

45. Pinsky MR. Determinants of pulmonary arterial flow variation during respiration. *J Appl Physiol Respir Environ Exerc Physiol* 1984;**56**(5):1237–45.

46. Whittenberger JL, McGregor M, Berglund E, Borst HG. Influence of state of inflation of the lung on pulmonary vascular resistance. *J Appl Physiol* 1960;**15**:878–82.

47. Luecke T, Pelosi P. Clinical review: Positive end-expiratory pressure and cardiac output. *Crit Care* 2005;**9**(6):607–21.

48. Canada E, Benumof JL, Tousdale FR. Pulmonary vascular resistance correlates in intact normal and abnormal canine lungs. *Crit Care Med* 1982;**10**(11):719–23.

49. Marshall BE, Marshall C, Frasch F, Hanson CW. Role of hypoxic pulmonary vasoconstriction in pulmonary gas exchange and blood flow distribution. 1. Physiologic concepts. *Intensive Care Med* 1994;**20**(4):291–7.

50. Fessler HE, Brower RG, Wise RA, Permutt S. Effects of systolic and diastolic positive pleural pressure pulses with altered cardiac contractility. *J Appl Physiol* 1992;**73**(2):498–505.

51. Scharf SM, Brown R, Tow DE, Parisi AF. Cardiac effects of increased lung volume and decreased pleural pressure in man. *J Appl Physiol* 1979;**47**(2):257–62.

52. Naughton MT, Rahman MA, Hara K, Floras JS, Bradley TD. Effect of continuous positive airway pressure on intrathoracic and left ventricular transmural pressures in patients with congestive heart failure. *Circulation* 1995;**91**(6):1725–31.

53. Klinger JR. Hemodynamics and positive end-expiratory pressure in critically ill patients. *Crit Care Clin* 1996;**12**(4):841–64.

54. Poulton EP. Originally published as Volume 2, Issue 5904 Left-sided heart failure with pulmonary oedema. *Lancet* 1936;**228**(5904):981–3.

55. Rasanen J, Heikkila J, Downs J, *et al*. Continuous positive airway pressure by face mask in acute cardiogenic pulmonary edema. *Am J Cardiol* 1985;**55**(4):296–300.

56. Bersten AD, Holt AW, Vedig AE, Skowronski GA, Baggoley CJ. Treatment of severe cardiogenic pulmonary edema with continuous positive airway pressure delivered by face mask. *N Engl J Med* 1991;**325**(26):1825–30.

57. Lin M, Yang YF, Chiang HT, *et al*. Reappraisal of continuous positive airway pressure therapy in acute cardiogenic pulmonary edema. Short-term results and long-term follow-up. *Chest* 1995;**107**(5):1379–86.

58. Kelly CA, Newby DE, McDonagh TA, *et al*. Randomised controlled trial of continuous positive airway pressure and standard oxygen therapy in acute pulmonary oedema; effects on plasma brain natriuretic peptide concentrations. *Eur Heart J* 2002;**23**(17):1379–86.

59. Rusterholtz T, Kempf J, Berton C, *et al*. Noninvasive pressure support ventilation (NIPSV) with face mask in patients with acute cardiogenic pulmonary edema (ACPE). *Intensive Care Med* 1999;**25**(1):21–8.

60. Masip J, Betbese AJ, Paez J, *et al*. Non-invasive pressure support ventilation versus conventional oxygen therapy in acute cardiogenic pulmonary oedema: a randomised trial. *Lancet* 2000;**356**(9248):2126–32.

61. Levitt MA. A prospective, randomized trial of BiPAP in severe acute congestive heart failure. *J Emerg Med* 2001;**21**(4):363–9.

62. Sharon A, Shpirer I, Kaluski E, *et al*. High-dose intravenous isosorbide-dinitrate is safer and better than Bi-PAP ventilation combined with conventional treatment for severe pulmonary edema. *J Am Coll Cardiol* 2000;**36**(3):832–7.

63. Nava S, Carbone G, DiBattista N, *et al*. Noninvasive ventilation in cardiogenic pulmonary edema: a multicenter randomized trial. *Am J Respir Crit Care Med* 2003;**168**(12):1432–7.

64. Valipour A, Cozzarini W, Burghuber OC. Non-invasive pressure support ventilation in patients with respiratory failure due to severe acute cardiogenic pulmonary edema. *Respiration* 2004;**71**(2):144–51.

65. Masip J. Non-invasive ventilation. *Heart Fail Rev* 2007;**12**(2):119–24.

66. Gray A, Goodacre S, Newby DE, *et al*. Noninvasive ventilation in acute cardiogenic pulmonary edema. *N Engl J Med* 2008;**359**(2):142–51.

67. Mehta S, Jay GD, Woolard RH, *et al*. Randomized, prospective trial of bilevel versus continuous positive airway pressure in acute pulmonary edema. *Crit Care Med* 1997;**25**(4):620–8.

68. Park M, Lorenzi-Filho G, Feltrim MI, *et al*. Oxygen therapy, continuous positive airway pressure, or noninvasive bilevel positive pressure ventilation in the treatment of acute cardiogenic pulmonary edema. *Arq Bras Cardiol* 2001;**76**(3):221–30.

69. Park M, Sangean MC, Volpe Mde S, *et al.* Randomized, prospective trial of oxygen, continuous positive airway pressure, and bilevel positive airway pressure by face mask in acute cardiogenic pulmonary edema. *Crit Care Med* 2004;**32**(12):2407–15.

70. Bellone A, Monari A, Cortellaro F, *et al.* Myocardial infarction rate in acute pulmonary edema: noninvasive pressure support ventilation versus continuous positive airway pressure. *Crit Care Med* 2004;**32**(9):1860–5.

71. Crane SD, Elliott MW, Gilligan P, Richards K, Gray AJ. Randomised controlled comparison of continuous positive airways pressure, bilevel non-invasive ventilation, and standard treatment in emergency department patients with acute cardiogenic pulmonary oedema. *Emerg Med J* 2004;**21**(2):155–61.

72. Bellone A, Vettorello M, Monari A, Cortellaro F, Coen D. Noninvasive pressure support ventilation vs. continuous positive airway pressure in acute hypercapnic pulmonary edema. *Intensive Care Med* 2005;**31**(6):807–11.

73. Moritz F, Brousse B, Gellee B, *et al.* Continuous positive airway pressure versus bilevel noninvasive ventilation in acute cardiogenic pulmonary edema: a randomized multicenter trial. *Ann Emerg Med* 2007;**50**(6):666–75, 675.e1.

74. Liesching T, Nelson DL, Cormier KL, *et al.* Randomized trial of bilevel versus continuous positive airway pressure for acute pulmonary edema. *J Emerg Med* 2014;**46**(1):130–40.

75. Pang D, Keenan SP, Cook DJ, Sibbald WJ. The effect of positive pressure airway support on mortality and the need for intubation in cardiogenic pulmonary edema: a systematic review. *Chest* 1998;**114**(4):1185–92.

76. Vital FM, Saconato H, Ladeira MT, *et al.* Non-invasive positive pressure ventilation (CPAP or bilevel NPPV) for cardiogenic pulmonary edema. *Cochrane Database Syst Rev* 2008;(3):CD005351.

77. Ho KM, Wong K. A comparison of continuous and bi-level positive airway pressure non-invasive ventilation in patients with acute cardiogenic pulmonary oedema: a meta-analysis. *Crit Care* 2006;**10**(2):R49.

78. Winck JC, Azevedo LF, Costa-Pereira A, Antonelli M, Wyatt JC. Efficacy and safety of non-invasive ventilation in the treatment of acute cardiogenic pulmonary edema—a systematic review and meta-analysis. *Crit Care* 2006;**10**(2):R69.

79. Peter JV, Moran JL, Phillips-Hughes J, Graham P, Bersten AD. Effect of non-invasive positive pressure ventilation (NIPPV) on mortality in patients with acute cardiogenic pulmonary oedema: a meta-analysis. *Lancet* 2006;**367**(9517):1155–63.

80. Mehta S, Al-Hashim AH, Keenan SP. Noninvasive ventilation in patients with acute cardiogenic pulmonary edema. *Respir Care* 2009;**54**(2):186–95; discussion 195–7.

81. Vital FM, Ladeira MT, Atallah AN. Non-invasive positive pressure ventilation (CPAP or bilevel NPPV) for cardiogenic pulmonary oedema. *Cochrane Database Syst Rev* 2013;(5):CD005351.

82. Agarwal R, Aggarwal AN, Gupta D. Is noninvasive pressure support ventilation as effective and safe as continuous positive airway pressure in cardiogenic pulmonary oedema? *Singapore Med J* 2009;**50**(6):595–603.

83. Mariani J, Macchia A, Belziti C, *et al.* Noninvasive ventilation in acute cardiogenic pulmonary edema: a meta-analysis of randomized controlled trials. *J Card Fail* 2011;**17**(10):850–9.

84. Li H, Hu C, Xia J, *et al.* A comparison of bilevel and continuous positive airway pressure noninvasive ventilation in acute cardiogenic pulmonary edema. *Am J Emerg Med* 2013;**31**(9):1322–7.

85. Weng CL, Zhao YT, Liu QH, *et al.* Meta-analysis: Noninvasive ventilation in acute cardiogenic pulmonary edema. *Ann Intern Med* 2010;**152**(9):590–600.

86. Mas A, Masip J. Noninvasive ventilation in acute respiratory failure. *Int J Chron Obstruct Pulmon Dis* 2014;**9**:837–52.

87. Barreiro TJ, Gemmel DJ. Noninvasive ventilation. *Crit Care Clin* 2007;**23**(2):201–22, ix.

88. McNeill G, Glossop A. Clinical applications of non-invasive ventilation in critical care. *Contin Educn Anaesth Critical Care Pain* 2012;**12**:33–7.

89. Davidson AC, Banham S, Elliott M, *et al.* BTS/ICS guideline for the ventilatory management of acute hypercapnic respiratory failure in adults. *Thorax* 2016;**71**(Suppl 2):ii1–ii35.

90. Bakke SA, Botker MT, Riddervold IS, Kirkegaard H, Christensen EF. Continuous positive airway pressure and noninvasive ventilation in prehospital treatment of patients with acute respiratory failure: a systematic review of controlled studies. *Scand J Trauma, Resusc Emerg Med* 2014;**22**(1):1–13.

91. Mal S, McLeod S, Iansavichene A, Dukelow A, Lewell M. Effect of out-of-hospital noninvasive positive-pressure support ventilation in adult patients with severe respiratory distress: a systematic review and meta-analysis. *Ann Emerg Med* 2014;**63**(5):600–607. e1.

92. Goodacre S, Stevens JW, Pandor A, *et al.* Prehospital noninvasive ventilation for acute respiratory failure: systematic review, network meta-analysis, and individual patient data meta-analysis. *Acad Emerg Med* 2014;**21**(9):960–70.

93. Masip J. Non-invasive ventilation. *Heart Fail Rev* 2007;**12**(2):119–24.

94. Duan J, Tang X, Huang S, Jia J, Guo S. Protocol-directed versus physician-directed weaning from noninvasive ventilation: the impact in chronic obstructive pulmonary disease patients. *J Trauma Acute Care Surg* 2012;**72**(5):1271–5.

47

Therapeutic control of fluid balance in chronic heart failure

Andrew L. Clark, Alison P. Coletta, and John G. F. Cleland

Introduction

A cardinal clinical feature of heart failure is water retention by the kidneys, leading to increases in atrial and, consequently, pulmonary and systemic venous pressures, which may be termed 'haemodynamic congestion'. This may lead to extravasation of water into tissues, resulting in peripheral or pulmonary oedema, or 'clinical congestion'. Of note, oedema is mostly composed of water, with just a small amount of salt. The term 'congestive heart failure' fell out of favour about 30 years ago because diuretics are rather effective at treating the clinical signs of congestion, at least at rest,[1,2] and there was (at the time) no simple, non-invasive means of assessing 'haemodynamic' congestion. The advent of natriuretic peptide testing (a marker of atrial wall stress), and echocardiographic assessment of atrial volumes and venous distension show that 'haemodynamic congestion' is common,[3] even in patients with few symptoms or signs of heart failure. Congestion is associated with a poor prognosis and is an important potential therapeutic target.

The introduction of diuretics, particularly loop diuretics, revolutionized the management of fluid retention. Previously, tourniquets, venesection, and nitrates had been used to reduce preload in the acute setting.[4] Southey's tubes,[5] introduced by direct skin incision, were used to drain chronic peripheral oedema. William Withering (active 1767–1799) noted that digitalis caused a diuresis, particularly in patients with a rapid irregular pulse, long before the electrocardiogram was available to make a diagnosis of atrial fibrillation. William Stokes (active 1825–1870) advocated the diuretic properties of mercury,[6] and mercurial diuretics were introduced in 1919 after the diuretic effect of organo-mercurial agents (used to treat syphilis) was noted.[6,7]

Sulfonamide-based diuretics were introduced in the 1950s and '60s: first, thiazides[8] and carbonic anhydrase inhibitors, and subsequently loop diuretics such as frusemide (furosemide).[9,10] The steroid-based mineralocorticoid antagonist (MRA), spironolactone, was also introduced in the 1950s. More recently, sodium–glucose co-transporter-2 (SGLT-2) inhibitors have been introduced, which have several properties including natriuresis (leading to weight loss and plasma volume contraction).

Physiologically, the body responds to the development of heart failure in a similar fashion to dehydration, salt deprivation, or moderate blood loss. There is activation of the renin–angiotensin–aldosterone (RAAS), antidiuretic hormone, and sympathetic nervous systems, which have evolved to conserve water, salt, and circulating volume. In heart failure, reversing water and salt retention with diuretics leads to further activation of these neuroendocrine systems (Figure 47.1),[11–14] which might accelerate the progression of heart failure by causing cellular damage and fibrosis in the myocardium, blood vessels, kidneys and possibly other organs. The concept of neurohormonal activation led to a series of landmark trials of a range of neuroendocrine antagonists that improved outcome and supported experimental observations in animal and cell models.

Observational studies show that patients who do not require treatment with loop diuretics have a much better prognosis than those who do, and that higher doses of loop diuretics are strongly associated with a worse prognosis.[15] Such findings have led to recommendations that the dose and use of diuretics for heart failure should be minimized. However, more careful analyses of the data suggest that the use and dose of loop diuretics is merely a surrogate marker for the severity of congestion and that it is the congestion that is lethal. This argues that a sufficient dose of diuretic to control congestion effectively should be used.[3]

Diuretics

Diuretics are the most prescribed treatment for heart failure.[16] The EuroHeart Failure Survey reported that almost 90% of patients with heart failure were prescribed loop diuretic agents.[17] Although most trials investigating new agents for the treatment of heart failure were conducted in the setting of a high background use of loop diuretics, there is relatively little clinical trial evidence to guide the use of diuretics in heart failure. Clinical experience and small-scale studies have shown that diuretics improve the symptoms and signs, but there are no large-scale clinical trials investigating effects on hospitalizations and mortality. Patients who are not congested might not

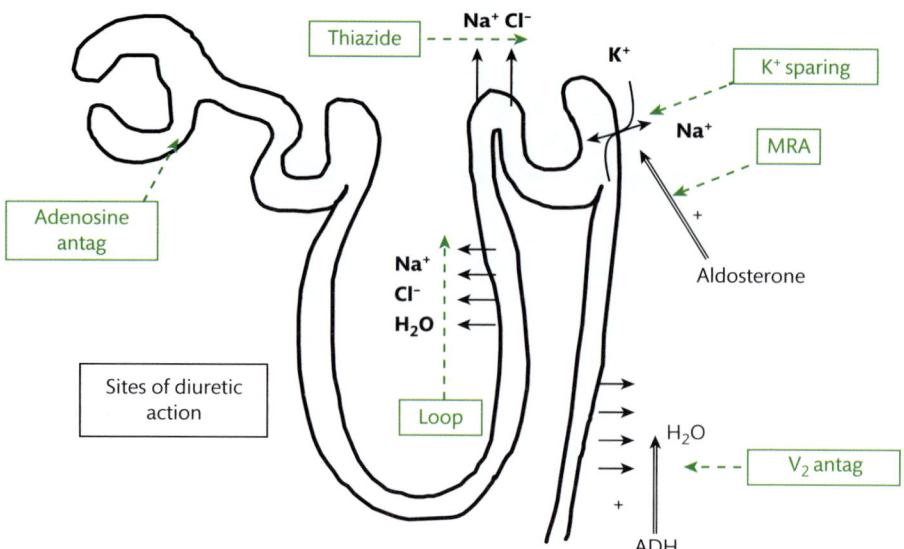

Figure 47.1 Sites of action of different diuretics in the renal tubule. MRA = mineralocorticoid antagonist.

benefit from diuretics; patients *with* congestion might not manage long without them. Stopping diuretics in patients with persisting symptoms or signs of congestion is likely to result in rapid worsening of congestion, necessitating their reintroduction. If an ethics committee were to agree that diuretics could be withdrawn from patients with evidence of congestion, the trial might not need to be very large or last very long.

Treatment with agents such as angiotensin converting enzyme (ACE) inhibitors, β-blockers, MRA, sacubitril–valsartan, and SGLT-2 inhibitors may control congestion in some patients and render treatment with diuretics unnecessary.[18] Indeed, subgroups of patients who were not treated with diuretics were enrolled in the landmark trials. Such patients had a good prognosis and may not have obtained much benefit from the new treatment being investigated. On the other hand, patients on higher doses of loop diuretic have a poor outcome, but that appears to be because they have more severe congestion.[15]

Guidelines suggest that diuretics are essential for the treatment of symptoms of heart failure in patients with water overload but that, when water overload is absent, their dose should be reduced and possibly discontinued.[19] Observational studies conducted in the era before widespread use of echocardiography or natriuretic peptides suggested that many patients could discontinue treatment with diuretics. However, many of these patients lacked objective evidence of heart failure. Randomized trials of withdrawing loop diuretics in patients with symptomatic heart failure were quickly curtailed due to high rates of worsening heart failure.[20]

For stable patients, with well-documented heart failure and few symptoms but elevated plasma concentrations of natriuretic peptides, randomization to withdrawal of medication (including diuretics) for 48 h was associated with an increase in symptoms and a near doubling in plasma natriuretic peptides.[21] By contrast, a randomized trial (188 patients followed for 90 days) from Brazil suggested that it was safe to withdraw lower-doses of loop diuretics (for example, furosemide 40 mg/day) from patients with prior evidence of heart failure with reduced left ventricular ejection fraction (HFrEF) receiving guideline-recommended

treatment who had become asymptomatic.[22] Further trials are to be encouraged.[18]

Mechanism of action

Heart failure is a cardiorenal syndrome. Patients who do not retain water and salt will not develop chronic heart failure. It is possible to develop acute heart failure without water and salt retention due (for instance) to flail mitral valve or a sustained tachyarrhythmia. This will often be accompanied by anuria and shock, and the patient will retain water and salt only if they survive long enough. Oedema is mostly composed of water, with just a small amount of salt. Most patients will have at least mild hyponatraemia, indicating greater retention of water compared to sodium.

Worsening peripheral and pulmonary oedema due to water and salt retention is a common cause of hospitalization for patients with heart failure.[23] Fluid retention may be due to progressive cardiac or renal dysfunction, excessive dietary intake of salt or water, noncompliance with diuretics, or reduced diuretic absorption.

The success of diuretic therapy depends on the ability of the diuretic agent to reduce water and salt reabsorption in the kidney. In the normal kidney, >99% of filtered sodium is reabsorbed; 60–70% in the proximal tubule, 20–25% in the loop of Henle, 5–10% in the distal tubule and 3% in the collecting duct.[24] In heart failure, a reduction in net arteriovenous renal perfusion pressure, activation of the RAAS, antidiuretic hormone and sympathetic stimulation all conspire to increase renal absorption of water and salt. Water retention then causes oedema. In addition to the haemodynamic effects of heart failure on renal function, many patients have intrinsic renal damage, often due to the same problems that caused heart failure (i.e. hypertension, diabetes, and atherosclerosis).[25,26] Renal dysfunction itself also causes water and salt retention and impairs the response to diuretics.[27]

There are four classes of diuretic commonly used in the treatment of heart failure: loop diuretics (furosemide, bumetanide, torasemide, and ethacrynic acid), thiazide diuretics (including hydrochlorthiazide, bendroflumethiazide, and the thiazide-like metolazone), directly acting potassium-sparing diuretics (amiloride

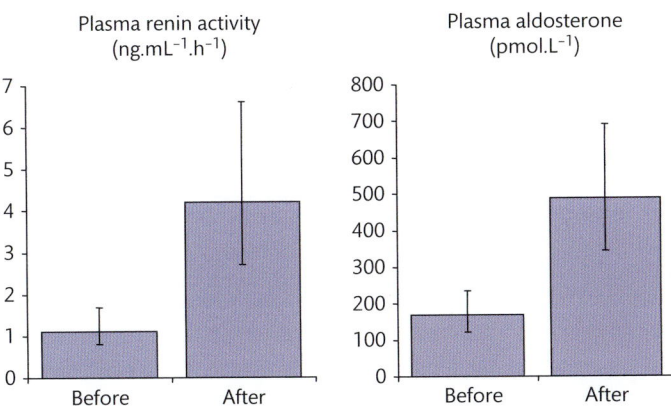

Figure 47.2 The effect of diuretic therapy on neurohormonal activation in resting patients with chronic heart failure. Even more striking effects were seen after exertion.

Source data from Ikram H, Chan W, Espiner EA, Nicholls MG. Haemodynamic and hormone responses to acute and chronic frusemide therapy in congestive heart failure. *Clin Sci* 1980;**59**:443–449.

and triamterene) and mineralocorticoid receptor antagonists (spironolactone, canrenoate, and eplerenone). Each of these has a different site of action in the renal tubule (**Figure 47.2**). Other agents, including vasopressin antagonists (tolvaptan, conivaptan), adenosine antagonists (theophylline), and carbonic anhydrase inhibitors (acetazolamide) are rarely used but this may change as further research evidence becomes available. SGLT-2 inhibitors may also act as diuretic agents, either by effects on renal metabolism or as osmotic diuretics by causing glucosuria. New diuretics are also being developed, such as renal outer-medullary potassium (ROMK) channel inhibitors.[28]

Loop diuretics

Loop diuretics are also called fast-acting, high ceiling, or high-potency diuretics and are the most widely used diuretics for heart failure. The principal site of action of loop diuretics is on the luminal aspect of the thick ascending limb of the loop of Henle, where they inhibit the sodium, potassium and chloride co-transporter. Since ~20–30% of filtered sodium is reabsorbed at the ascending loop of Henle, these are potent diuretics. Existing loop diuretics work from the luminal surface and rely on adequate renal function to deliver them to their site of action. ROMK channel inhibitors may exert effects similar to those of loop diuretics with less potassium-wasting and without the need for glomerular filtration because they act on the interstitial side of the thick ascending limb of the loop of Henle and cortical collecting duct.

Loop diuretics have a rapid onset of action: diuresis occurs within minutes following intravenous administration and within 30 min following oral administration.[29] However, loop diuretics have a short half-life; their duration of action is brief but intense and followed by rebound water and salt retention as the patient's pathophysiology tries to restore balance to the pre-diuretic state. For patients with more severe congestion, loop diuretics may need to be administered more than once a day or be administered by continuous infusion to attenuate rebound sodium reabsorption.

Furosemide is the most widely used loop diuretic but bumetanide and torasemide may have advantages. The oral bioavailability of furosemide is extremely variable, with values between 12% and 112% reported.[30] Furosemide is highly protein-bound (>95%) and must be secreted in the proximal tubule to reach its site of action. Absorption can be delayed by food.[31] Non-steroidal anti-inflammatory drugs may cause salt and water retention and blunt the response to loop diuretics.[32] Compared to furosemide, torasemide and bumetanide have a much higher and more predictable oral bioavailability. Torasemide has a slightly longer half-life (3–4 h) than other loop diuretics, which may delay and/or reduce rebound. Unlike furosemide, which undergoes renal elimination, torasemide and bumetanide undergo substantial hepatic elimination and therefore should not accumulate in patients with poor renal function.[33]

Loop diuretics are generally well tolerated by patients with congestion but do have many adverse effects, including activation of the RAAS and sympathetic nervous system, hypokalaemia, hyponatraemia, renal dysfunction (although they can also improve renal function during treatment of severe congestion), hyperuricaemia, and gout. Violent diuresis may cause bladder retention. High-dose intravenous furosemide may cause deafness, particularly if it is administered rapidly.

Thiazide and thiazide-like diuretics

Thiazide diuretics act on the distal convoluted tubule, where they inhibit sodium and chloride reabsorption. Only 10–15% of filtered sodium is reabsorbed at this site and therefore thiazides have a smaller peak effect than loop diuretics but a much longer duration of action (12–24 h), so rebound sodium retention is less. Accordingly, 24 h sodium excretion may be similar for hydrochlorothiazide 100 mg day and furosemide 40 mg but nocturia may be more common with loop diuretics.[34,35]

Thiazide diuretics are less effective when renal function is impaired. When creatinine clearance is <50 mL/min, the response to thiazides may be poor and a loop diuretic is the treatment of choice.[33] Metolazone is thought to have an additional effect on the proximal tubule, which may enhance its diuretic potency. Unlike other thiazides, metolazone is effective in patients with moderate renal impairment.[36]

Both loop and thiazide diuretics increase the delivery of sodium to the distal convoluted tubule, which causes an increase in sodium reabsorption in exchange for potassium and hence an increase in potassium excretion. Both hypokalaemia and hyponatraemia are more common with thiazide than with loop diuretics.[37,38]

Randomized trials of loop and/or thiazide diuretic agents

Patients are likely to be aware of the potent effects of loop diuretics, rendering blinding of any trial comparing these agents to placebo or a low-potency diuretic futile. Nonetheless, some trials do profess to be double-blind.

Placebo-controlled studies

The available randomized, placebo-controlled studies evaluating diuretic therapy in heart failure are summarized in Table 47.1. Few patients were enrolled, but the results suggest that diuretics improve the symptoms of heart failure as expected.[39–44] A meta-analysis has suggested that conventional diuretics can reduce the risk of worsening heart failure or death compared with placebo.[45]

Table 47.1 Randomized, placebo controlled diuretic studies in heart failure

First author (year)	No. of patients/HF severity	Treatment	Duration	Outcome compared with placebo
Kourouklis (1976)[39]	10	Bumetanide Frusemide Placebo	14 days XO	Both diuretics increased diuresis, and had similar effects on electrolytes.
Sherman (1986)[40]	38 NYHA II–III	Piretanide Placebo	28 days DB/PG	Improved NYHA class (P < 0.05 compared to baseline), no increase in 24 h K excretion
Haerer (1990)[41]	60 NYHA II–III	Piretanide Placebo	21 days SB	44 patients reported subjective improvement, decreased systolic and diastolic diameters on echo, decreased heart volume on CXR. Serum K unchanged.
Kleber (1990)[42]	247 mild HF	Hydrochlorothiazide Ibopamine HCZ plus IB Placebo	8 weeks DB/PG	Weight loss with all active treatments (P < 0). Hypokalaemia greater with HCZ
Patterson (1994)[43]	66 NYHA II–III	Torasemide 5 mg Torasemide 10 mg Torasemide 20 mg Placebo	7 days DB/R/PG	Weight loss with 10 and 20 mg doses
Stewart (1965)[44]	3	Furosemide Bendrofluazide Ethacrynic acid	2 days treatment XO for 32 days	Diuresis

DB, double blind; SB, single blind; PG, parallel group; XO, crossover.
NYHA, New York Heart Association classification; HF, heart failure; HCZ, hydrochlorthiazide; IB, ibopamine; CXR, chest X-ray; K, potassium.

Diuretic withdrawal

Guidelines suggest that diuretics might be withdrawn once symptoms and signs of congestion have resolved. Trials of diuretic withdrawal are shown in Table 47.2.[20–22,46–53] Unfortunately, the diagnosis of heart failure was often not robust in these patients. A large (if variable) proportion of patients was able to stop their diuretics (or perhaps use them only 'as needed'). One of the largest trials (202 elderly patients in primary care) suggested that about half

Table 47.2 Studies of withdrawal of diuretic therapy in heart failure

First author (year)	N	Treatment	Duration	Outcome
Taggart (1983)[46]	42	Diuretic W/D in patients on moderate doses, with no HT, active HF, renal or hepatic oedema	12 weeks	71% completed the study. 29% deteriorated clinically or radiologically. 1 patient died
Richardson (1987)[20]	14	All patients on diuretic at baseline, then W/D DB, rand, to captopril or furosemide plus amiloride, then XO	16 weeks	10 patients remained stable on captopril alone, 4 patients developed pulmonary oedema or breathlessness and required diuretic therapy
Magnani (1988)[47]	94	Diuretic W/D if used and patients randomized to captopril or placebo	1 year	After 1 year, 25% of patients required diuretic in captopril group vs 36% in placebo group
Walma (1993)[48]	15	Diuretic W/D	Pilot study 6 months	Reinstatement of diuretic therapy required in 9 patients
Grinstead (1994)[49]	41	Diuretic W/D and substituted with either lisinopril or placebo	12 weeks	71% of patients required re-initiation of diuretic therapy. There was no difference between lisinopril and placebo
Walma (1997)[50]	202	Patients on long-term diuretics rand DB to diuretic W/D or continuation	6 months	50 patients in the W/D group required diuretic compared with 13 patients in the continuation group
van Kraaij (2000)[51]	32	Patients rand DB to continuation of furosemide therapy or placebo (diuretic W/D)	Pilot study 3 months	W/D successful in 90% of patients
Braunschweig (2002)[52]	4	Haemodynamic study of diuretic W/D	Pilot study 2 weeks	Deterioration in ventricular pressure parameters with signs and symptoms of worsening HF following diuretic W/D
Galve (2005)[53]	26	Diuretic W/D in stable HF patients	3 months	17 patients were able to tolerate W/D with improvements in renal function and glucose metabolism, but ANP increased
Dovancescu (2017)[21]	20	Short-term omission of all heart failure medications, including loop diuretics in stable HF patients. Cross-over trial	48 hours	Six of 20 patients deteriorated by one NYHA class. Left atrial volume increased and NT-proBNP doubled with omission of therapy.
Rohde (2019)[22]	188	Diuretic withdrawal (predominantly 40mg/day of furosemide) in stable patients with HFrEF	90 days	No difference in symptoms or clinical events (5 in each group had a HF hospitalization or died)

W/D, withdrawal; rand, randomized; DB, double blind; ANP, atrial natriuretic peptide.

could successfully stop taking diuretic.[50] Patients with a normal left ventricular ejection fraction were more likely to tolerate diuretic withdrawal, perhaps because the diagnosis was wrong.[51]

In a recent double-blinded trial from Brazil,[22] 188 patients with heart failure, which was both well documented and symptomatically well controlled, were randomized to withdraw or continue treatment with furosemide for 90 days. There was no difference between the groups in self-reported worsening breathlessness, nor in the proportion of patients given extra diuretic therapy. There was no effect on admissions or deaths (although the number of events was very small). Curiously, no difference in the effects on N-terminal pro B-type natriuretic peptide (NT-proBNP) were observed. Perhaps the hot climate in Brazil provides an alternative route to dispose of water and salt, or perhaps adherence to the assigned diuretic strategy was poor.

By contrast, another (smaller) study showed that withdrawing loop diuretics in patients with similarly stable heart failure caused worsening symptoms within 48 h and a doubling of NT-proBNP and increase in left atrial volume.[21]

Thiazide vs loop

Trials comparing thiazide with loop diuretics were small (<100 patients: see Table 47.3).[34,35,44,54–65] The results suggest that both classes had similar efficacy in managing heart failure, although with a trend favouring loop diuretics.[44,61,63] The risk of hypokalaemia was greater with thiazides,[35,44,58,59] but the effects on glucose tolerance and diabetes were similar.[60,66]

Thiazide diuretics are often preferred by patients as they cause less rapid diuresis and less frequent micturition than loop diuretics, which might improve compliance.[62]

Table 47.3 Randomized studies of loop versus thiazide diuretics in heart failure

First author (year)	No. of patients	Diuretics used	Design and duration	Outcome
Stewart (1965)[44]	11	Frusemide Ethacrynic acid Bendrofluazide Mersalyl		Frusemide had greater natriuretic effect than bendrofluazide. More K loss on bendrofluazide
Peltola (1970)[54]	8	Frusemide HCZ	XO Single dose	Both treatments produced similar diuresis. Na and aldosterone excretion greater with HCZ
Levy (1977)[55]	32 NYHA II–III	HCZ + spironolactone Frusemide	DB 16 weeks	Both treatments produced similar control of HF symptoms. Increased plasma renin activity and aldosterone excretion with HCZ
Coodley (1979)[56]	30	Diapamide Frusemide	O/XO 4 days	Urine output greater with frusemide (P-value not stated)
Levy (1979)[57]	32 NYHA II–III	HCZ + spironolactone HCZ + triamterene Frusemide	Open 16 weeks	No clinical benefit of combinations over frusemide. Changes in BUN, plasma renin and aldosterone excretion were greater with HCZ
Gillies (1980)[58]	?	Piretanide Chlorothiazide	3 days	Similar diuresis and weight loss. Greater K loss with thiazide
Gabriel (1981)[59]	18	Bendrofluazide Bumetanide Frusemide	XO 9 months	Patients remained stable with no significant changes in body weight. Bendroflumethiazide had greater effect on plasma K
Pothuizen (1982)[34]	23 NYHA II–III	Frusemide SR HCZ	R / DB 6 weeks	Both treatments produced similar improvement in functional class, less nocturia with frusemide, small reduction in K in both groups
Vermeulen (1982)[35]	38 NYHA I–III	Frusemide HCZ	DB/R 6 weeks	Similar improvement in functional class. More hypokalaemia with HCZ
Pehrsson (1985)[60]	86 NYHA II–III	Frusemide SR Bendroflumethiazide	R/DB 12 weeks	Similar clinical response with both treatments
Gonska (1985)[61]	30 NYHA II–III	Piretanide HCZ + triamterene	O/R 14 days	More patients fully recompensated, and LVEDD and LVESD less on piretanide. Piretanide caused small fall in serum K
Funke-Küpper (1986)[62]	37 NYHA II–III	HCZ + triamterene Frusemide + triamterene	R/XO 16 weeks	Equivalence on maintenance of body weight and symptoms, but patient preference for HCZ due to less acute diuresis
Crawford (1988)[63]	47 General practice	Frusemide + amiloride Cyclopenthiazide + KCl	Open 3 months	Frusemide superior on patient symptom assessment
Heseltine (1988)[64]	70 NYHA II	Frusemide Thiazide	Obs	Postural hypotension and hypokalaemia with thiazide
Allman (1990)[65]	71 mild HF	Frusemide + amiloride Cyclopenthiazide + K⁺	O/R 12 weeks	Similar improvement in oedema, crepitations, orthopnoea, and self-assessed dyspnoea of effort

HCZ, hydrochlorothiazide; DB, double blind; R, randomized; O, open; XO, crossover, Obs, observational study; HF, heart failure; SR, slow release.

Loop vs loop

Non-randomized comparisons between different loop diuretics are shown in Table 47.4.[67,68,70-74] Only studies with >100 participants are shown. These suggest that torasemide might reduce hospital days compared with furosemide,[67] and TORIC, an observational study in 2303 patients with chronic congestive heart failure, suggested that there might be a mortality benefit for torasemide compared with furosemide.[68] A more recent analysis of treatment in >6000 patients suggested that the choice of loop diuretic had little association with outcome.[69]

Randomized studies comparing one loop diuretic with another in heart failure are listed in Table 47.4.[67,68,70-74] The results are generally inconclusive. However, a meta-analysis of comparative trials suggests that, compared to furosemide, treatment with torasemide was associated with better symptom control and trends to fewer hospitalizations and lower mortality.[75] A large-scale trial comparing furosemide and torasemide is ongoing (TRANSFORM-HF; NCT03296813) to determine whether pharmacological differences between agents is associated with clinically different results. For now, switching from furosemide to torasemide and bumetanide should be considered as an alternative to increasing the dose of furosemide for worsening congestion.

Loop vs ACE inhibitor

Studies of patients with heart failure who remained symptomatic despite standard doses of diuretics suggested that higher doses of diuretics or the introduction of ACE inhibitors had similar effects on symptoms and exercise capacity,[76,77] but others have found that increasing diuretic dose gives a better symptomatic response.[78] However, as ACE inhibitors have been shown to improve prognosis, the question addressed by these trials is now somewhat redundant. Withdrawing loop diuretics in symptomatic patients receiving an ACE inhibitor is associated with worsening congestion.[20]

Potassium-sparing diuretics (other than mineralocorticoid receptor antagonists)

Potassium-sparing diuretics inhibit sodium/potassium exchange in the distal convoluted tubule, which is hypertrophied in heart failure due to the use of loop and thiazide diuretics. Potassium-sparing diuretics increase sodium and reduce potassium excretion and cause a mild diuresis. Potassium-sparing diuretics are usually used in combination with loop or thiazide diuretics to reduce potassium loss.[79,80] Potassium-sparing diuretics are more effective than potassium supplements in maintaining serum potassium and magnesium and total body potassium.[81] Avoiding hypokalaemia may account for their association with a better prognosis in observational studies.[82] Their use has largely been superseded by MRAs, although there is no evidence that they are less effective.

Mineralocorticoid receptor antagonists

The mineralocorticoid receptor antagonists spironolactone, canrenone and eplerenone have potassium-sparing, natriuretic, and diuretic effects and each is associated with lower morbidity and mortality in patients with chronic heart failure. Whether the main mechanism of benefit is diuresis and better control of congestion, potassium retention and the avoidance of hypokalaemia or blocking the pro-fibrotic effects of aldosterone is uncertain.[83] MRAs are considered in greater detail elsewhere (Chapter 52). On current evidence, they should be prescribed in preference to the other potassium-sparing diuretics.

Maintaining serum potassium ~4.5 mmol/L is associated with better outcomes in patients with heart failure. Potassium-sparing diuretics and MRAs may cause hyperkalaemia, particularly for patients on other guideline-recommended therapies for heart failure and with impaired renal function. Patients should be counselled about dietary potassium and avoid agents such as trimethoprim or NSAIDs that may cause hyperkalaemia. Serum potassium >5.5 mmol/L requires

Table 47.4 Studies comparing one loop diuretic with another in heart failure (only those with *N* > 100 are shown)

First author (year)	No. of patients	Diuretics used	Design and duration	Outcomes
Non-randomized studies				
Spannheimer (1998)[67]	400	Torasemide Frusemide	Observational pharmaco-economic study, 1 year	80% reduction in hospital days on torasemide
Cosin (TORIC) (2002)[68]	1377	Torasemide Frusemide or other diuretics	Open, non-randomized, post marketing, 1 year	Morbidity/mortality benefit for torasemide
Randomized studies				
Stauch (1990)[70]	104	Torasemide 5 or 10 mg Frusemide 40 mg	4 weeks db/mc/rand	All treatments were effective in reducing body weight and improving NYHA class and cardiac symptoms
Noe (PEACH) (1999)[71]	240	Torasemide Frusemide	6 months rand/open/mc	Similar efficacy and treatment costs
Stroupe (2000)[72]	193	Torasemide Frusemide	1 year rand/open	Fewer hospital admissions with torasemide
Murray (2001)[73]	234	Torasemide Frusemide	1 year rand/open	Fewer cardiovascular readmissions and less fatigue with torasemide
Müller (2003)[74]	237	Torasemide Frusemide	9 months open/rand	Trend to greater clinical improvement and QoL benefit with torasemide

xo, crossover; db, double blind; pg, parallel group; rand, randomized; KCl(sr), slow-release potassium chloride; mc, multicentre; QoL, quality of life.

action. The dose of potassium-retaining agents may be reduced. For patients who are congested, increasing the dose of conventional diuretic agents will increase potassium excretion.

Recently, patiromer[84] and sodium zirconium cyclosilicate,[85] agents that bind potassium in the gut, have been shown to control hyperkalaemia. Whether their long-term use will improve outcome by allowing more patients to attain higher doses of MRAs and other treatments for heart failure is yet to be shown. However, for patients with resistant hypertension or peripheral oedema resistent to other interventions, and in whom there is good reason not to discontinue an MRA, the addition of a potassium-binding agent should be considered.

Carbonic anhydrase inhibitors

The proximal convoluted tubule is rich in carbonic anhydrase. Inhibition of intracellular carbonic anhydrase reduces production of intracellular H^+ ions, thus reducing sodium reabsorption via the Na^+/H^+ co-transporters on the apical membrane. Inhibition of luminal carbonic anhydrase reduces production of water and carbon dioxide, thus increasing urinary bicarbonate.

The carbonic anhydrase inhibitor acetazolamide increases bicarbonate, sodium and water excretion. Unlike other diuretics, which are associated with a metabolic alkalosis, acetazolamide may cause an acidosis (or reverse an alkalosis caused by other agents). Acetazolamide also causes an increase in serum chloride concentration.[86] As there is a strong association between hypochloraemia and adverse outcomes, both in acute[87] and chronic[88] heart failure, this is of some interest. Case reports suggest that acetazolamide might be useful in patients with resistant fluid retention, as an add-on to standard therapy.[89]

The ADVOR trial aims to enrol >500 patients with heart failure hospitalized with fluid retention. Patients will be randomized to acetazolamide or placebo in addition to standard therapy for 3 days.[90] The primary end-point is decongestion on day 4.

Sodium–glucose co-transporter-2 inhibitors

The SGLT-2 reabsorbs filtered glucose from the urinary space in the proximal convoluted tubule. Inhibition of SGLT-2 thus prevents glucose reabsorption, increasing the concentration of glucose in the renal tubules. SGLT-2 inhibitors (sometimes known as gliflozins) are osmotic diuretics. They may have additional effects on the sodium–hydrogen exchanger in the kidney that also promote diuresis.

Gliflozins were originally developed as treatments for diabetes. In the EMPA-REG OUTCOMES trial of patients with type II diabetes,[91] there was a modest reduction in heart failure-related events in the patients treated with empagliflozin relative to placebo. In CANVAS,[92] patients randomized to canagliflozin had a lower risk of mortality, heart attack or stroke, and a lower risk of hospitalization for heart failure. The benefits seemed to be greater in those with pre-existing heart failure.[93] Dapagliflozin, in DECLARE-TIMI 58, had a similar effect. Indeed, the trial would most likely have been neutral had it not been for the striking benefit in patients with HeFREF.[18,94]

The effect of SGLT2 inhibitors on heart failure end-points was unexpected, but led to clinical trials specifically in patients with heart failure, regardless of the presence of diabetes. In DAPA-HF, 4744 patients with symptomatic heart failure and an average LV ejection fraction of ~30% were randomized to dapagliflozin or placebo. Only 42% of patients had pre-existing diabetes. There was a reduction in the primary end-point of worsening heart failure and cardiovascular death from 21.2% in the placebo group to 16.3% in the actively treated group—a hazard ratio of 0.74.[95] The beneficial effect was seen in patients with and those without diabetes at baseline.[96]

Whether the benefits of SGLT-2 inhibitors are due to anything other than their diuretic effect is not yet clear. Congestion is common in patients with heart failure, even when they are apparently clinically euvolaemic,[3] and strongly associated with an adverse outcome.[97] Dapagliflozin markedly reduces LV filling pressures as assessed by pulmonary artery pressure monitoring.[98] However, many other effects of SGLT-2 inhibition have been proposed as beneficial actions, including reducing inflammation and oxidative stress, improving myocardial metabolism (well reviewed by Lopaschuk and Verma[99]) and increasing production of erythropoietin.[18] However, whatever the exact mechanism of action, there are increasing calls for dapagliflozin to become part of the standard management of patients with heart failure.[100]

Diuretic resistance

As chronic heart failure progresses, patients often require higher doses of diuretic to achieve a given therapeutic effect, and commonly reach a state of diuretic resistance when the diuretic response is either diminished or lost before congestion is controlled. A number of mechanisms potentially contribute to diuretic resistance:

- Renal haemodynamics (potentially reversible)
  - Increased renal venous pressure and reduced arterial perfusion pressure reduce the net perfusion pressure across the glomerulus, which will cause glomerular filtration rate (GFR) to decline and trigger water and salt retention.
  - A fall in renal blood flow with consequent afferent arteriolar vasoconstriction will cause GFR to decline.
  - Efferent arteriolar vasodilatation due to ACE inhibitors and angiotensin receptor blockers (ARBs) will also reduce glomerular filtration fraction.
- Chronic kidney disease (potentially irreversible)
  - The hypertension, diabetes and atherosclerosis which lead to heart failure may also damage the kidney.
  - GFR declines with age.
- Furosemide is highly protein-bound and must be secreted by the organic acid transporter in the proximal tubule to reach its site of action. Low GFR may be associated with proximal tubular dysfunction.
- Renal adaptation. Chronic diuretic therapy increases delivery of sodium to the distal convoluted tubule (DCT), which hypertrophies in consequence.[101,102] The hypertrophied DCT is able to retain more sodium (and hence water).
- Rebound: with bolus diuretic dosing, sometimes there is no diuretic at the site of action.
- Decreased absorption of oral diuretic agents. Worsening congestion of the splanchnic circulation may reduce absorption, especially of furosemide.[103,104]
- Drug interactions may interfere with the renal response to diuretic:
  - non-steroidal anti-inflammatory drugs, including aspirin;[105]

- thiazolidinediones/glitazones, endothelin antagonists, dihydro-pyridine calcium antagonists, steroids;
- any agent that reduces GFR including ACE inhibitors and ARBs.

Approaches to managing diuretic resistance include: discontinuing medications that may be exacerbating the problem; giving higher doses and/or more frequent oral dosing of loop diuretics; 'sequential nephron blockade'; and changing the route of diuretic administration from oral to parenteral.

Route of administration

Parenteral administration of diuretic overcomes the problems of variation in oral bioavailability of furosemide (and bumetanide).[106–111] Continuous dosing reduces the risk of ototoxicity associated with large boluses of furosemide.[106] Bumetanide infusions may be associated with a higher rate of side-effects than bolus therapy.[112] There is little evidence to favour continuous infusion of torasemide.[113] Its high oral bioavailability reduces the difference between oral and intravenous torasemide.

In the DOSE trial, patients admitted with fluid retention were randomized in a 2 × 2 factorial trial to: (i) low- or high-dose furosemide (total daily intravenous dose either equal to or 2.5 times the previous daily oral dose), given (ii) either as a bolus or continuous infusion. Improvement in symptoms was similar for each strategy but tended to favour higher doses, which were associated with a greater diuresis and greater weight loss but some transient worsening in renal function.[114]

Subcutaneous rather than intravenous furosemide may be used to try to avoid hospital admission in, for example, patients reaching end of life.[115] Existing formulations of furosemide may cause irritation at the infusion site but a new formulation of furosemide with neutral pH is now being tested in clinical trials.

Sequential nephron blockade (combination therapy)

That combination diuretic therapy might overcome diuretic resistance has been known for a long time; indeed in some of the first trials of loop diuretics they were given on a background of thiazide diuretics (**Figure 47.3**).[44] Enhanced sodium reabsorption due to hypertrophy of DCT after prolonged use of loop diuretics can be blocked with the addition of a thiazide, causing a profound diuresis. Many small observational studies[112,117] and two randomized trials[118,119] have investigated the synergistic effects of combining loop diuretics with thiazide diuretics in heart failure (**Figure 47.4**). Most studies have used metolazone, which may have additional effects on the proximal tubule, possibly making it more potent than other thiazides. However, Channer et al.[119] showed that metolazone and bendroflumethiazide were similarly effective in inducing diuresis in patients with resistant oedema when added to intravenous furosemide. The effects of chlorothiazide and metolazone also appear similar.[120]

Mineralocorticoid receptors are intracellular and the actions of MRAs are mediated by altering nuclear gene transcription. It may thus require several days for the onset of their effects, which may explain the failure of short-term trials of MRAs to improve outcomes.[121,122] Longer-term administration, however, improves the efficacy of loop diuretics.[44] Importantly, MRAs cause retention of much more potassium than can be accommodated in the extracellular space. Potassium must be transferred to the intracellular space

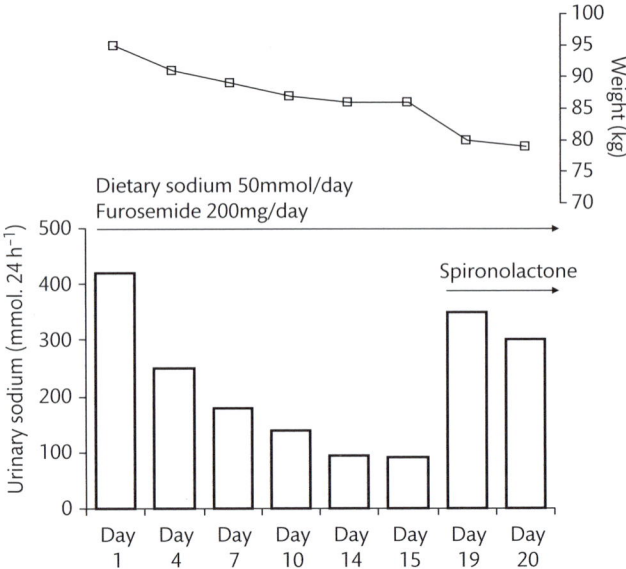

Figure 47.3 Effect of adding spironolactone to furosemide on daily urinary sodium levels.

Source data from Stewart JH, Edwards KDG. Clinical comparison of frusemide with bendrofluazide, mersalyl and ethacrynic acid. Br Med J 1965;**2**:1277–1281.

and consequently intracellular water must increase if intracellular potassium concentration is not to change. Accordingly, weight change may underestimate the loss of extracellular water/oedema after administration of an MRA.

Non-MRA potassium-sparing diuretics, which act on the collecting duct, do not substantially enhance the effects of loop diuretic agents on water excretion but help reduce potassium losses (with some increase in sodium excretion). Whether additional blockade of the proximal renal tubule with acetazolamide further enhances diuresis is uncertain.

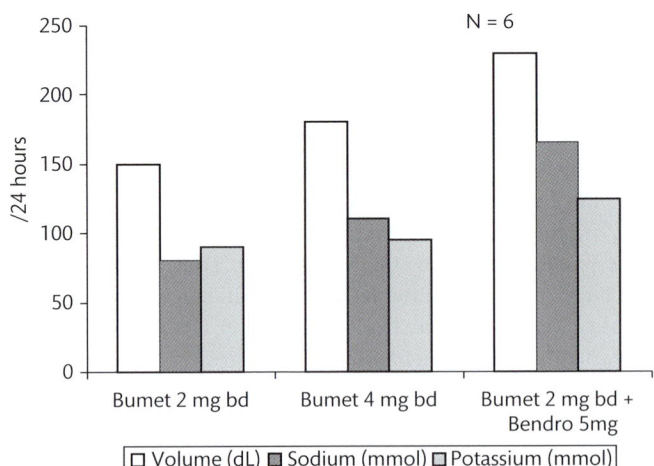

Figure 47.4 Effect of adding a thiazide to a low-dose loop diuretic compared with increasing the dose of loop diuretic, on urine volume and sodium and potassium excretion, measured in six patients over 24 h.

Source data from Dormans TPJ, Gerlag PGG. Combination of high-dose furosemide and hydrochlorothiazide in the treatment of refractory congestive heart failure. Eur Heart J 1996;**17**:1867–1874.

Sequential nephron blockade is effective in patients with diuretic resistance, even when the patient has significant renal impairment.[117] However, combination therapy should be monitored closely as unpredictably large diuretic effects may occur, leading to electrolyte disturbances, hypotension, dehydration, and renal dysfunction. It may take several days before the effect of combination therapy reaches a maximum.

Increase sodium intake

Perhaps counterintuitively, administering salt might be beneficial.[123,124] Urinary excretion of sodium in response to diuretics depends on sodium intake. Severe dietary limitation of sodium will reduce natriuresis, which may inhibit aquaresis (for patients with oedema it is the excess of water that is the real problem). Administration of hypertonic saline may improve diuretic responsiveness, including water excretion. Anecdotally, relaxing dietary sodium restriction may have similar effects.

An alternative is to replace a proportion of the urinary losses of salt and water with intravenous normal saline to avoid excessive reductions in plasma volume,[125] an approach that has been associated with a better-sustained diuresis and a lower risk of renal dysfunction.

Other therapies

There is some evidence that corticosteroids might reduce diuretic resistance,[126,127] perhaps via upregulating responses to natriuretic hormones.[128] There are also concerns that steroids, unchecked by MRA, may cause sodium and water retention.

Aquaretics

Antidiuretic hormone (ADH), also known as arginine vasopressin (AVP), is raised in many patients with chronic heart failure.[129,130] The primary physiological role of AVP is to modulate body water content to maintain plasma osmolality. AVP is released from the posterior pituitary in response to a fall in osmolality, a fall in blood pressure, pain, or opiates. Its effects are mediated through two main receptor subtypes: V1 and V2. V1 receptors are predominantly vascular and mediate vasoconstriction. V2 receptors are found in the collecting ducts of nephrons. Stimulation of V2 receptors causes translocation of pre-formed aquaporin from the interior of collecting duct cells to their surface, allowing water to leave the urine along an osmotic gradient back into the circulation. There are many aquaporins; aquaporin-2 is the one involved in renal osmoregulation.

Tolvaptan, a selective V2 antagonist, is licensed in many countries for treating secondary hyponatraemia (due to inappropriate ADH secretion) rather than heart failure. Tolvaptan causes an aquaresis (i.e. it increases water but not salt excretion) leading to weight loss in patients with chronic heart failure.[131,132]

In EVEREST, 4133 patients admitted with heart failure were randomized to receive tolvaptan or placebo in addition to standard therapy.[133,134] Tolvaptan initially caused an aquaresis, improved breathlessness, and reduced requirements for conventional diuretics, but had no longer-term benefit and did not reduce rehospitalization or mortality. Thirst was a common side-effect. Three smaller trials, each with about 200 patients, confirmed that tolvaptan enhanced furosemide-induced aquaresis but did not lead to strikingly greater improvement in symptoms or renal function (TACTICS-HF[135];

SECRET of CHF[136]; AQUAMARINE[137]). Trials of patients with acute heart failure are dogged by the problem that intravenous furosemide is very effective at inducing diuresis and rapidly improving symptoms for most patients. There might still be a role for tolvaptan in some situations, such as fluid overload with severe hyponatraemia.

Blocking the V2 receptor causes plasma concentrations of AVP to rise, which stimulates thirst but may also activate V1 receptors that may cause vasoconstriction and increase platelet adhesion. A nonselective antagonist might have performed differently.

Hyponatraemia

Low serum sodium is common in end-stage heart failure and is associated with a very bleak outlook. It develops because there is a nonosmotic stimulus to ADH production which causes water retention and dilutional hyponatraemia, although there may be an overall excess in total body sodium.[130,138]

Standard advice for the management of chronic heart failure in many international guidelines[139] is to limit salt intake. However, several studies suggest that the reverse approach might be helpful. In patients with chronic heart failure, a normal salt diet has been associated with better outcomes.[140] The fact that a meta-analysis of the available information on salt restriction was subsequently withdrawn due to concerns about the data contributing to the analysis[141] simply emphasizes the need for data from properly conducted trials rather than reliance on advice from experts.

In patients admitted to hospital with congestion, hyponatraemia is often treated with strict limitation of sodium and fluid intake. There is very little evidence indeed to support such practice. The evidence that does exist suggests that restriction is not associated with better outcomes, but simply makes the patients more thirsty.[142] The opposite approach might, indeed, be more fruitful. Hypertonic saline infusions coupled with continuing diuretic treatment may increase serum sodium concentration and cause net water excretion (the main constituent of oedema) and reduce plasma biomarkers of congestion.[127,143]

It is important to realize that the background dosing of furosemide in these studies was high (0.5–1 g, twice daily), and it might be that the hypertonic saline is simply counteracting the adverse consequences of such high diuretic dosage. However, on an anecdotal basis, hypertonic saline infusions appear to be helpful (**Figure 47.5**).

There might be a specific role for AVP antagonists in the management of hyponatraemia,[133,144] not only for increasing serum sodium concentrations but also for improving hyponatraemia-associated mental dysfunction. Whether the effects of AVP antagonists on serum sodium persist in the longer term is not known. Further trials will be needed to establish their role in managing fluid balance.

Adjunctive therapies

Adenosine antagonists

Within individual nephrons, the distal tubule lies very close to the vascular pole of the glomerulus. At this point, metabolically active cells in the distal tubule, the macula densa, act as detectors of the nephron's GFR. When the sodium load in the distal tubule is

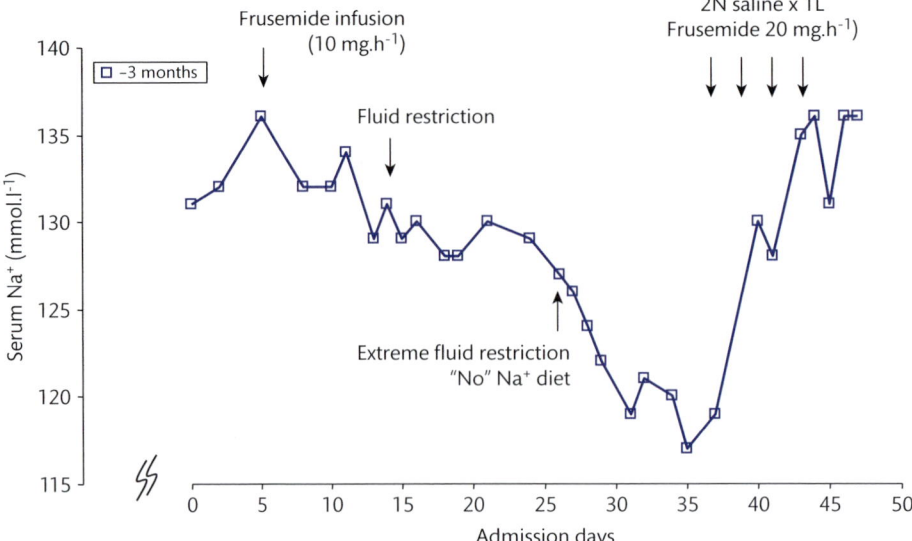

Figure 47.5 Effects of using hypertonic saline in hyponatraemia. The patient had gross fluid retention and rapidly developed symptomatic hyponatraemia when managed with sodium and fluid restriction. The hyponatraemia resolved with hypertonic saline infusion and continued intravenous furosemide. 2 N saline is twice normal saline, i.e. 1.8% saline.

increased, due to diet or diuretics, the macula densa 'interprets' the rise as being due to a high GFR and induces constriction of the afferent glomerular arteriole. This homeostatic mechanism is known as tubulo-glomerular feedback. The precise mediators of tubulo-glomerular feedback are not known, but involve adenosine. Adenosine released by the macula densa causes afferent arteriolar constriction through binding to A_1 receptors in the mesangium.

Adenosine antagonists might improve renal function by increasing GFR and enhancing diuretic efficacy. Gottlieb and colleagues showed that a single dose of the adenosine antagonist, BG9719, increased both urine output and GFR.[145] By contrast, furosemide produced an increase in urine output but decreased GFR. When BG9719 and furosemide were administered together, there was a further increase in urine volume with no reduction in GFR, suggesting that the adenosine antagonist may protect against the adverse effects of loop diuretics.

Another adenosine antagonist, rolofylline, also enhanced the response to loop diuretics and appeared to protect renal function in patients with decompensated heart failure.[146,147] However, a large clinical trial of patients hospitalized with worsening heart failure (PROTECT) showed no benefit on renal function, morbidity, or mortality.[148]

'Renal dose' dopamine

Low-dose dopamine might have a beneficial effect on renal function and enhance a diuresis, particularly in patients with resistant oedema or worsening renal function. In the DAD-HF trial,[149] 60 patients were randomized to high-dose furosemide versus low-dose furosemide plus low-dose dopamine. Each strategy was similarly effective in inducing diuresis, with the patients receiving dopamine less likely to have a decline in renal function. ROSE AHF investigated the effects of two interventions (nesiritide and dopamine) for patients with heart failure and renal dysfunction.[150] Neither treatment improved diuresis or renal function.

There is thus no compelling evidence to support the use of renal dose dopamine but it appears safe from the small amount of data available. It might be used, but more in desperation and hope than in expectation.

Ultrafiltration

Whereas the physical removal of oedema fluid can be achieved by venesection or Southey's tubes, another approach is to use ultrafiltration. In *dialysis*, blood is run against another fluid, dialysate, separated by a semi-permeable membrane. Solutes pass along a concentration gradient, and the fluid compartment of blood is removed by *ultrafiltration*, that is, by the hydrostatic pressure of the blood relative to the dialysate.

For treating patients with heart failure and fluid retention, only the ultrafiltration is needed: fluid is removed from blood by pressure gradient alone. As fluid passes across the membrane, some solutes (including sodium, potassium, and some larger molecules) are 'dragged' along simultaneously. In practice, blood is removed, usually via a large-bore tube, pumped through a filter where the filtrate is removed, and 'concentrated' blood is returned to the patient (**Figure 47.6**). The flow rate can be adjusted to remove fluid at the required rate: depending upon the equipment, large volumes (≥ 1 L/h) can be removed rapidly.

A potential advantage of ultrafiltration is that the filtrate has the same sodium concentration as plasma: for each litre of fluid removed by ultrafiltration, a much higher quantity of sodium is removed than via a litre of urine.[151]

Filtration and peritoneal dialysis for heart failure predates the availability of loop diuretics.[152–154] Recent advances in ultrafiltration technology have been driven by the availability of veno-venous systems which avoid more invasive alternatives. Effective ultrafiltration (e.g. removal of ~5 L of fluid in 24 h) can reduce atrial pressures

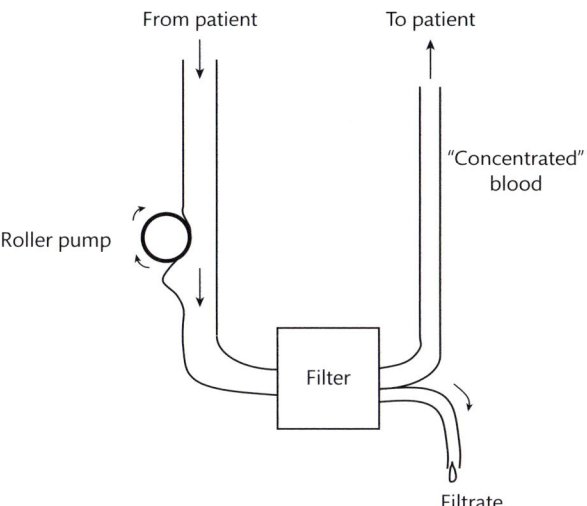

Figure 47.6 Basic ultrafiltration circuit.

rapidly and might increase cardiac output.[155] Even more rapid removal of fluid (>3 L in 8 h) appears safe and effective.[156]

Ultrafiltration can be an effective initial strategy for patients with gross water overload,[157] reducing diuretic resistance,[158] correcting hyponatraemia[157] and reducing length of stay. Intermittent outpatient use may reduce the need for readmission[159] (see Figure 47.7). Ultrafiltration may also have beneficial neurohormonal effects, including reduction of BNP,[158] interleukins and tumour necrosis factor.[160]

In the UNLOAD trial of ultrafiltration, 200 patients admitted to hospital with fluid overload due to heart failure were randomized to receive ultrafiltration or standard intravenous diuretic therapy.[161] Weight and fluid loss was slightly greater in the ultrafiltration group. Although it was not a primary endpoint in the study, heart-failure-related hospitalization at 90 days was reduced.

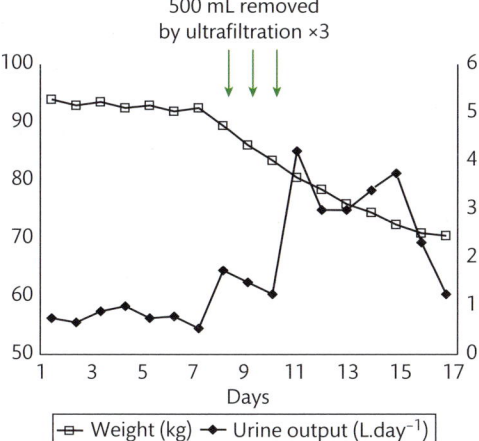

Figure 47.7 Effect of ultrafiltration in restoring urine flow. The patient was a 57-year-old female with underlying ischaemic heart disease (ejection fraction 18%) and intractable fluid retention. Three episodes of ultrafiltration to remove 500 mL of fluid on each occasion were sufficient to restore urine flow. Before filtration, the patient had been receiving 20 mg/h furosemide, bendroflumethiazide, spironolactone, and digoxin for 1 week and dopamine and dobutamine for 72 h.

In CARESS-HF, 188 patients with congestion and worsening renal function (defined as an increase in the serum creatinine level of ≥0.3 mg/dL) were randomized to standard pharmacological therapy or ultrafiltration. Weight loss was similar for each group,[162] but there were more adverse events with ultrafiltration, including worsening renal function, bleeding, and catheter complications. There was no improvement in longer-term outcomes.

The AVOID-HF trial[163] randomized patients with severe water retention to ultrafiltration or standard care but was terminated early by the sponsor because of slow recruitment (and against the advice of the trial steering committee) when only 224 of the 800 planned patients had been enrolled. The primary end-point of heart failure events at 90 days favoured ultrafiltration, but was not significant. The number of patients experiencing a *serious* adverse event of special interest was similar for each group.

The role of ultrafiltration in the standard management of heart failure is not yet clear. There is no definitive evidence that it is better than standard diuretic management, and some evidence that it might worsen renal function. Ultrafiltration clearly helps individual patients who are refractory to treatment. Well-designed trials may yet show advantages for ultrafiltration, if only in those who are truly refractory to diuretic therapy.

Practical tips to managing fluid balance

Day-to-day management

Congestion is central to the concept, pathophysiology, and diagnosis of heart failure and, currently, the most effective treatments for congestion are diuretics. For many patients, the diagnosis of heart failure is first made after admission to hospital with severe symptoms and signs of congestion. These patients require treatment with a loop diuretic, usually furosemide at a dose of 40–80 mg per day, although it could be argued that bumetanide (1–2 mg) or torasemide (20–40 mg) would be a better choice. If the left ventricular ejection fraction is low, or the patient has hypertension, many would start one or more RAAS inhibitors at the same time.

For patients with heart failure and reduced ejection fraction who are in sinus rhythm, heart rate control with β-blockers and/or ivabradine should be instituted when overt signs of congestion have been controlled. For patients presenting with milder symptoms in primary care, thiazide diuretics are a reasonable alternative, provided that GFR is not markedly reduced. Many patients are not even aware of the 'gentle' diuresis that thiazides produce, but metabolic disturbances, such as hypokalaemia and hyponatraemia, as well as nocturia, may be more problematic than with loop diuretics. Combination with MRA or other potassium-sparing diuretics should be considered.

Once the patient has reached clinical euvolaemia—in other words, when breathlessness and peripheral oedema have improved and, for the expert, when jugular venous pressure has normalized—the diuretic may simply be continued without further consideration. Some doctors involve the patient in actively managing their fluid balance, teaching them that 1 kg is equal to 1 L of water and then to weigh themselves regularly (preferably with the same scales at the same time of day), preferably in kilograms. The patient should understand

that diuretics have a different purpose from the rest of their medication: whereas β-blockers, RAAS inhibitors, and SGLT-2 inhibitors are prescribed mainly to stop things getting worse, diuretics are prescribed for the day-to-day relief of symptoms due to fluid retention. This allows patients to modify their diuretic dose.

In general, a target 'dry' weight should be set and the patient should try to deviate from it as little as possible. If weight goes up due to increased salt intake, then either the patient should follow a low-salt diet until weight is corrected or should take an extra dose of diuretic (or do both). If weight is below target, a patient should withhold diuretic until it rises. Some patients will need to take a diuretic every few days and others may be able to stop them for longer periods. Even for patients with severe heart failure, missing a dose of diuretic may be perfectly reasonable before a long journey.

Education about a target weight should include what to do if visiting a hot country (reduce diuretic dose as there will be increased fluid loss due to sweating) or how to manage an episode of diarrhoea. Target weight may need to be revised from time to time, depending on whether the patient is losing or gaining fat or lean-body mass. 'Dry' weight may be estimated clinically by measuring biomarkers of congestion, such as natriuretic peptides, or by imaging the heart and great veins either by ultrasound or other technologies.[3,164]

Patients on long-term diuretic therapy should have their electrolytes and renal function assessed on a regular basis. Many patients with heart failure will have GFR <60 mL/min. Renal dysfunction is not an indication to reduce therapy unless the deterioration in GFR is large or rapid.

If congestion is not well controlled despite standard doses of loop diuretics, then higher doses may be used (e.g. 250–1000 mg of furosemide) or one or more additional classes of diuretic agent may be added, usually an MRA and/or a thiazide, such as bendroflumethiazide (bendrofluazide) 2.5 mg once daily. The safety of sequential nephron blockade compared to high-dose loop diuretic for severely congested patients is uncertain. Checks on electrolytes and renal function should be done at least monthly. Patients taking diuretics more than once per day should be warned to take their second dose ≥4 h before they intend to go to bed to avoid interrupting sleep.

Anasarca

Many patients with chronic heart failure need admission to hospital due to increasing water retention that, when severe, may cause abdominal wall oedema, ascites and pleural effusions: a condition known as *anasarca* (Greek ανα-, throughout; σαρχ, σαρκ-, flesh). It requires active management to avoid prolonged hospital stays.

The patient should be confined to bed with the legs raised.[165] Appropriate antithrombotic prophylaxis is important as patients with anasarca are at high risk of deep vein thrombosis and pulmonary embolism. Intravenous diuretics should generally be used. An infusion prevents rebound water and salt retention. Less well tried alternatives are to use oral torasemide, which is much better absorbed, or sequential nephron blockade with oral agents (such as bumetanide, MRA, metolazone, and even acetazolamide).

Strict monitoring of fluid balance is vital: unless fluid balance is known, it is very difficult to track progress. Fluid intake and urine output must be measured accurately and charted, together with daily weights. The daily weight should be measured at the same time of day with the same scales and with the patient wearing similar clothing.

Urea and electrolytes should be measured daily with careful replacement of potassium as necessary. There is no evidence to support severe fluid restriction,[166,167] although making sure the patient does not drink more than 2 L per day seems sensible. There is no role for salt restriction; indeed there is evidence to support allowing more dietary salt or even giving it intravenously, especially for hyponatraemic patients.

Which (if any) medication should be stopped if a patient is admitted with anasarca remains controversial. Unnecessary medication should certainly be stopped, as should agents likely to worsen renal function, especially non-steroidal anti-inflammatory agents (including aspirin). Standard advice is to stop β-blockers when patients are admitted, but there is some provisional evidence that those patients who continue with β-blockers once they are admitted have a better outcome.[168]

The aim is to reduce weight by 2 kg each day (2 L of fluid loss) until dry weight is achieved. Assessment by an experienced clinician may be adequate to determine fluid status,[3,164] but cardiac imaging or devices for measuring right atrial pressure will improve precision, especially for the less experienced.[3,164] Careful daily assessment is vital. If targets are not met, then treatment should be modified. If the patient is not losing weight, then increasing loop diuretic therapy (to, for example, infusion of 20 mg per hour of furosemide)—and, if not done already, adding a thiazide and spironolactone—are next steps. If this is insufficient, then consider ultrafiltration.

As the patient is reaching dry weight, ACE inhibitor and β-blocker should be started. As a rule of thumb, patients will need to be discharged on more diuretic than they were taking before admission: educating patients on diuretic management is key to avoiding early readmissions.

Worsening renal function during treatment for acute heart failure is associated with worse outcomes.[170] Many doctors think that they should stop diuretic treatment if renal function worsens. However, there are two important findings from the randomized trials relevant to this issue:

- the CARESS trial of ultrafiltration used high-dose loop diuretics in those randomized to pharmacological therapy—with infusion of furosemide at up to 30 mg per hour *and* metolazone 5 mg twice daily.[171] Despite such a dosing scheme (and despite worsening renal function being an inclusion criterion), renal function improved with diuretic therapy (**Figure 47.8**).
- in the DOSE study, worsening renal function was not associated with a worse outcome; and, perhaps paradoxically, improved renal function during the first 72 h of treatment made the composite endpoint of death, re-hospitalization or emergency room visit within 60 days *more* likely.[172]

Thus, although renal function should be monitored, the primary aim of treatment should be the management of oedema and congestion and not excessive concern about renal function.

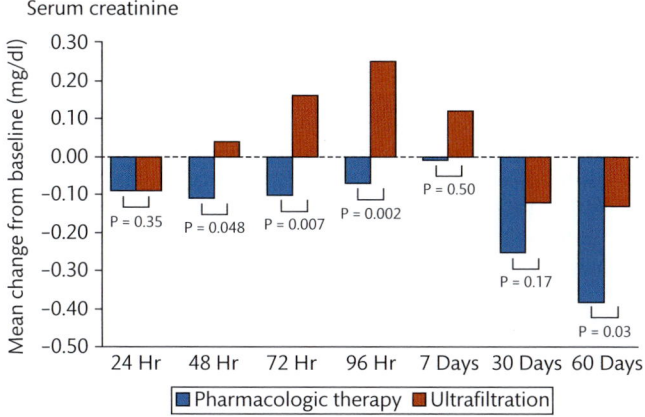

Figure 47.8 Results from the CARRESS-HF trial of ultrafiltration. Note that intensive diuretic therapy caused an improvement in renal function even in a group of patients entered into the trial because of deteriorating renal function at baseline. 1 mg/dL is 88.4 µmol/L.

Source data from Bart BA, Goldsmith SR, Lee KL, Givertz MM, O'Connor CM, Bull DA, Redfield MM, Deswal A, Rouleau JL, LeWinter MM, Ofili EO, Stevenson LW, Semigran MJ, Felker GM, Chen HH, Hernandez AF, Anstrom KJ, McNulty SE, Velazquez EJ, Ibarra JC, Mascette AM, Braunwald E; Heart Failure Clinical Research Network. Ultrafiltration in decompensated heart failure with cardiorenal syndrome. *N Engl J Med* 2012;**367**:2296–304.

Conclusions

Most doctors, when asked which treatment they would choose not to do without for managing congestive heart failure, reply loop diuretics; those who say otherwise have probably not managed many patients. Currently, diuretics are the most important family of treatments for patients with heart failure and one of the most under-researched. Diuretic management resides firmly in the era of opinion-based medicine, perhaps because it is nigh on impossible to manage the congestion without them. Now that tools for measuring congestion have improved and are widely available for clinical practice, we should investigate how to use diuretics more effectively. In this case, 'practice (for more than 60 years) has not made perfect'. There is much to learn.

REFERENCES

1. Task Force on Heart Failure of the European Society of Cardiology. Guidelines for the diagnosis of heart failure. *Eur Heart J* 1995;**16**:741–51.
2. Cleland JG, Habib F. Assessment and diagnosis of heart failure. *J Intern Med* 1996;**239**:317–25.
3. Pellicori P, Shah P, Cuthbert J, *et al.* Prevalence, pattern and clinical relevance of ultrasound indices of congestion in outpatients with heart failure. *Eur J Heart Fail* 2019;**21**:904–16.
4. Krishnakumar N, Harikrishnan S, Tharakan JM. Self-blood letting in congestive cardiac failure. *Int J Cardiol* 2007;**114**:135–6.
5. Southey R. Chronic parenchymatous nephritis of right kidney. Left kidney small and atrophied. Old scrofulous pyelitis. *Trans Clin Soc Lond* 1877;**10**:152–6.
6. Ventura HO, Mehra MR, Young JB. Treatment of heart failure according to William Stokes: the enchanted mercury. *J Card Fail* 2001;7:277–82.
7. Vogl A. The discovery of the organc mercurial diuretics. *Am Heart J* 1950;**39**:881–3.
8. Novello FC, Sprague JM. Benzothiadiazine dioxides as novel diuretics. *J Am Chem Soc* 1957;**79**:2028–29.
9. Robson AO, Kerr DN, Ashcroft R, Teasdale G. The diuretic response to frusemide. *Lancet* 1964;**2**:1085–8.
10. Verel D, Stentiford NH, Rahman F, Saynor R. A clinical trial of frusemide. *Lancet* 1964;**2**:1088–9.
11. Francis GS, Siegel RM, Goldsmith SR, *et al.* Acute vasoconstrictor response to intravenous furosemide in patients with chronic congestive heart failure. *Ann Int Med* 1985;**103**:1–6.
12. Ikram H, Chan W, Espiner EA, Nicholls MG. Haemodynamic and hormone responses to acute and chronic frusemide therapy in congestive heart failure. *Clin Sci* 1980;**59**:443–9.
13. Bayliss J, Norell M, Canepa-Anson R, Sutton G, Poole-Wilson P. Untreated heart failure clinical and neuroendocrine effects of introducing diuretics. *Br Heart J* 1987:**57**:17–22.
14. Anand IS, Florea VG. Diuretics in chronic heart failure- benefits and hazards. *Eur Heart J* 2001;**3**(Suppl):G8–18.
15. Pellicori P, Kallvikbacka-Bennett A, Urbinati A, *et al.* Cardiac dysfunction, congestion and loop diuretics: their relationship to prognosis in heart failure. *Cardiovasc Drugs Ther* 2016;**30**:599–609.
16. Young JB, Weiner DH, Yusuf S, *et al.* Patterns of medication use in patients with heart failure: a report from the Registry of studies of left ventricular dysfunction (SOLVD) *South Med J* 1995;**88**:514–23.
17. Komajda M, Follath F, Swedberg K, *et al.*; Study Group on Diagnosis of the Working Group on Heart Failure of the European Society of Cardiology. The EuroHeart Failure Survey programme--a survey on the quality of care among patients with heart failure in Europe. Part 2: treatment. *Eur Heart J* 2003;**24**:464–74.
18. Cleland JGF, Lyon AR, McDonagh T, McMurray JJV. The year in cardiology: heart failure: The year in cardiology 2019. *Eur Heart J* 2020;**41**:1232–48.
19. van Veldhuisen DJ, van Gilst WH. The pharmacological management of heart failure: too many treatments? *Eur J Heart Fail* 2003;**5**:5–8.
20. Richardson A, Bayliss J, Scriven AJ, *et al.* Double-blind comparison of captopril alone against frusemide plus amiloride in mild heart failure. *Lancet* 1987;**2**:709–11.
21. Dovancescu S, Pellicori P, Mabote T, *et al.* The effects of short-term omission of daily medication on the pathophysiology of heart failure. *Eur J Heart Fail* 2017;**19**:643–9.
22. Rohde LE, Rover MM, Figueiredo Neto JA, *et al.* Short-term diuretic withdrawal in stable outpatients with mild heart failure and no fluid retention receiving optimal therapy: a double-blind, multicentre, randomized trial. *Eur Heart J* 2019;**40**:3605–12.
23. Bennett SJ, Huster GA, Baker SL, *et al.* Characterisation of the precipitants of hospitalisation for heart failure decompensation. *Am J Crit Care* 1998;**7**:168–74.
24. Dormans TPJ, Gerlag PGG, Russel FGM, Smits P. Combination diuretic therapy in severe congestive heart failure. *Drugs* 1998;**2**:165–72.
25. Bourantas CV, Loh HP, Lukaschuk EI, *et al.* Renal artery stenosis: an innocent bystander or an independent predictor of worse outcome in patients with chronic heart failure? A magnetic resonance imaging study. *Eur J Heart Fail* 2012;**14**:764–72.
26. de Silva R, Nikitin NP, Witte KKA, *et al.* Incidence of renal dysfunction over 6 months in patients with chronic heart failure

due to left ventricular systolic dysfunction: contributing factors and relationship to prognosis. *Eur Heart J* 2006:**27**:569–81.

27. Maxwell AP, Ong HY, Nicholls DP. Influence of progressive renal dysfunction in chronic heart failure. *Eur J Heart Fail* 2002;**4**:125–30.

28. Aretz CD, Vadukoot AK, Hopkins CR. Discovery of small molecule renal outer medullary potassium (romk) channel inhibitors: a brief history of medicinal chemistry approaches to develop novel diuretic therapeutics. *J Med Chem* 2019;**62**:8682–94.

29. Brater DC. Pharmacology of diuretics. *Am J Med Sci* 2000;**319**:38–50.

30. Murray MD, Haag KM, Black PK, Hall SD, Brater DC. Variable furosemide absorption and poor predictability of response in elderly patients. *Pharmacother* 1997;**17**:98–106.

31. McCrindle JL, Li Kam Wa TC, Barron W, Prescott LF. Effect of food on the absorption of frusemide and bumetanide in man. *Br J Clin Pharmacol* 1996;**42**:743–6.

32. Kramer BK, Schweda F, Reigger GAJ. Diuretic treatment and diuretic resistance in heart failure. *Am J Med* 1999;**106**:90–6.

33. Brater DC. Drug therapy: diuretic therapy. *N Eng J Med* 1998;**339**:387–97.

34. Pothuizen LM, Chada DR. Treatment of congestive cardiac failure in elderly patients: randomised study of hydrochlorothiazide and slow release furosemide. *Curr Ther Res* 1982;**32**:513–19.

35. Vermeulen A, Chada DR. Slow-release furosemide and hydrochlorothiazide in congestive cardiac failure: a controlled trial. *J Clin Pharmacol* 1982;**22**:513–19.

36. Dargie HJ, Allison MEM, Kennedy AC, Gray MHJ. High dose metolazone in chronic renal failure. *Br Med J* 1972;**4**:196.

37. Robertson JIS. Diuretics, potassium depletion and the risk of arrhythmias. *Eur Heart J* 1984;**5**(Suppl A):25–8.

38. Spital A. Diuretic induced hyponatremia. *Am J Nephrol* 1999;**19**:447–52.

39. Kourouklis CC, Christensen O, Augoustakis D. Bumetanide in congestive heart failure. *Curr Med Res Opin* 1976;**4**:422–31.

40. Sherman LG, Liang CS, Baumgardner S, *et al.* Piretanide a potent diuretic with potassium sparing properties, for the treatment of congestive heart failure. *Clin Pharmacol Ther* 1986;**40**:587–94.

41. Haerer W, Bauer U, Sultan N, *et al.* Acute and chronic effects of a diuretic monotherapy with piretanide in congestive heart failure. A placebo controlled trial. *Cardiovasc Drug Ther* 1990;**4**:515–22.

42. Kleber FX, Thyroff-Freisinger U. Treatment of mild chronic congestive heart failure with ibopamine, hydrochlorthiazide, ibopamine plus hydrochlorthiazide or placebo. *Cardiology* 1990;**77**:67–74.

43. Patterson JH, Kirkwood FA, Applefield MM, Corder CN, Masse BR for the Torasemide Investigators group. Oral torasemide in patients with chronic congestive heart failure: effects on body weight, edema and electrolyte excretion. *Pharmacotherapy* 1994;**14**:514–21.

44. Stewart JH, Edwards KDG. Clinical comparison of frusemide with bendrofluazide, mersalyl and ethacrynic acid. *Br Med J* 1965;**2**:1277–81.

45. Faris R, Flather M, Purcell H, *et al.* Current evidence supporting the role of diuretics in heart failure; a meta analysis of randomised controlled trials. *Int J Cardiol* 2002;**82**:149–58.

46. Taggart AJ, McDevitt DG. Diuretic withdrawal a need for caution. *Curr Med Res Opin* 1983;**8**:501–8.

47. Magnani B. Converting enzyme inhibition and heart failure. *Am J Med* 1988;**84**:87–91.

48. Walma EP, Hoes AW, Prins A, Boukes FS, van der Does E. Withdrawing long-term diuretic therapy in the elderly: a study in general practice in The Netherlands. *Fam Med* 1993;**25**:661–4.

49. Grinstead WC, Francis MJ, Marks GF, *et al.* Discontinuation of chronic diuretic therapy in stable congestive heart failure secondary to coronary artery disease or to idiopathic dilated cardiomyopathy. *Am J Cardiol* 1994;**73**:881–6.

50. Walma EP, Hoes AW, van Dooren C, Prins A, van der Does E. Withdrawal of long term diuretic medication in elderly patients: a double-blind randomised trial. *Br Med J* 1997;**315**:464–8.

51. Van Kraaij DJW, Jansen RWMM, Bouwels LHR, Gribnau FWJ, Hoefnagels WHL. Furosemide withdrawal in elderly patients with preserved left ventricular systolic function. *Am J Cardiol* 2000;**85**:1461–6.

52. Braunschweig F, Linde C, Eriksson MJ, Hofman-Bang C, Ryden L. Continuous haemodynamic monitoring during withdrawal of diuretics in patients with congestive heart failure. *Eur Heart J* 2002;**23**:59–69.

53. Galve E, Mallol A, Catalan R, *et al.* Clinical and neurohormonal consequences of diuretic withdrawal in patients with chronic stabilised heart failure and systolic dysfunction. *Eur J Heart Fail* 2005;**7**:892–8.

54. Peltola P, Lahovaara S, Paasonen MK Effect of furosemide and hydrochlorothiazide on plasma renin activity in man. *Ann Med Exp Fenn* 1970;**48**:122–4.

55. Levy B. The efficacy and safety of furosemide and a combination of spironalactone and hydrochlorothiazide in congestive heart failure. *J Clin Pharmacol* 1977;**17**:420–30.

56. Coodley EL, Nandi PS, Chiotellis P. Evaluation of a new diuretic diapamide in congestive heart failure. *J Clin Pharmacol* 1979;**19**:127–36.

57. Levy B. Fixed-dose combination diuretics in congestive heart failure: an evaluation. *J Clin Pharmacol* 1979;**19**:743–6.

58. Gillies A, Morgan T, Myers J. Comparison of piretanide and chlorothiazide in the treatment of cardiac failure. *Med J Aust* 1980;**1**:170–2.

59. Gabriel R, Baylor P. Comparison of the chronic effects of bendrofluazide, bumetanide and frusemide on plasma biochemical variables. *Postgrad Med J* 1981;**57**:71–4.

60. Pehrsson SK. Multicentre comparison between slow release furosemide and bendroflumethiazide in congestive heart failure. *Eur J Clin Pharmacol* 1985;**28**:235–9.

61. Gonska BD, Kreuzer H. Diuretic monotherapy in heart failure. Comparison of piretanide and hydrochlorothiazide–triamterene. *Dtsch Med Ewochenschr* 1985;**110**:1812–16.

62. Funke Küpper AJ, Fintelman H, Huige MC, *et al.* Cross-over comparison of the fixed combination of hydrochlorothiazide and triamterene and the free combination of furosemide and triamterene in the maintenance treatment of congestive heart failure. *Eur J Clin Pharmacol* 1986;**30**:341–3.

63. Crawford RJ, Allman S, Gibson W, Kitchen S, Richards HH. A comparative study of frusemide–amiloride and cyclopenthiazide–potassium chloride in the treatment of congestive cardiac failure in general practice. *Int J Med Res* 1988;**16**:143–9.

64. Heseltine D, Bramble MG. Loop diuretics cause less postural hypotension than thiazide diuretics in the frail elderly. *Curr Med Res Opin* 1988;**11**:232–5.

65. Allman S, Norris RJ. An open parallel group study comparing frusemide/amiloride diuretic and a diuretic containing cyclopenthiazide with sustained release potassium in the

treatment of congestive cardiac failure—a multicentre general practice study. *Int J Med Res* 1990;**18**:17B–23B.

66. Suter PM, Vetter W. Metabolic effects of antihypertensive drugs. *J Hypertens* 1995;**13**:S11–17.

67. Spannheimer A, Goertz A, Dreckmann-Behrendt B. Comparison of therapies with torasemide or furosemide in patients with congestive heart failure from a pharmacoeconomic viewpoint. *Int J Clin Pract* 1998;**52**:467–71.

68. Cosin J, Diez J, on behalf of the TORIC investigators. Torasemide in chronic heart failure: results of the TORIC study. *Eur J Heart Fail* 2002;**4**:507–13.

69. Täger T, Fröhlich H, Grundtvig M, *et al.* Comparative effectiveness of loop diuretics on mortality in the treatment of patients with chronic heart failure—a multicenter propensity score matched analysis. *Int J Cardiol* 2019;**289**:83–90.

70. Stauch M, Stiehl L. Controlled double blind clinical trial on the efficacy and tolerance of torasemide in comparison with furosemide in patients with congestive heart failure a multicentre study. *Prog Pharmacol Clin Pharmacol* 1990;**8**:121–6.

71. Noe LL, Vreeland MG, Pezzella SM, Trotter JP. A pharmacoeconomic assessment of torsemide and furosemide in the treatment of patients with congestive heart failure. *Clin Ther* 1999;**21**:854–66.

72. Stroupe KT, Forthofer MM, Brater DC, Murray MD. Healthcare costs of patients with heart failure treated with torasemide or furosemide. *Pharmacoecon* 2000;**17**:429–40.

73. Murray MD, Deer MM, Ferguson JA, *et al.* Open label randomised trial of torasemide compared with furosemide therapy for patients with heart failure. *Am J Med* 2001;**111**:513–19.

74. Müller K, Gamba G, Jaquet F, Hess B. Torasemide vs furosemide in primary care patients with chronic heart failure NYHA II to IV—efficacy and quality of life. *Eur J Heart Fail* 2003;**5**:793–801.

75. Abraham B, Megaly M, Sous M, *et al.* Meta-analysis comparing torsemide versus furosemide in patients with heart failure. *Am J Cardiol* 2020;**125**:92–9.

76. Boccanelli A, Zachara E, Liberatore SM, Carboni GP, Prati PL. Addition of captopril versus increasing diuretics in moderate but deteriorating heart failure: a double-blind comparative trial. *Postgrad Med J* 1986;**62**:184–7.

77. Lewis SJ, Roberts CJC. Double-blind comparison of high-dose bumetanide and half-dose bumetanide together with captopril in heart failure. *Curr Ther Res* 1991;**50**(Suppl A):3–13.

78. Cowley AJ, Stainer K, Wynne RD, Rowley JM, Hampton JR. Symptomatic assessment of patients with heart failure; double-blind comparison of increasing doses of diuretics and captopril in moderate heart failure. *Lancet* 1986;**2**:770–2.

79. Ghosh AK, Mankikar G, Strouthidis T, *et al.* A single-blind, comparative study of hydrochlorothiazide/amiloride (Moduret 25) and hydrochlorothiazide/triamterene (Dyazide) in elderly patients with congestive heart failure. *Curr Med Res Opin* 1987;**10**:573–9.

80. Townsend HA, Waddy AL, Eason CT, Richards HH. Frusemide/amiloride combination in heart failure: an open mulit-centre study in general practice. *Curr Med Res Opin* 1984;**9**:132–40.

81. Kohvakka A. Maintenance of potassium balance during long-term diuretic therapy in chronic heart failure patients with thiazide induced hypokalemia. *Int J Clin Pharmacol Ther Toxicol* 1988;**26**:273–7.

82. Domanski M, Norman J, Pitt B, *et al.* Diuretic use, progressive heart failure, and death in patients in the Studies Of Left Ventricular Dysfunction (SOLVD). *J Am Coll Cardiol* 2003;**42**:705–8.

83. Pellicori P, Ferreira JP, Mariottoni B, *et al.* Effects of spironolactone on serum markers of fibrosis in people at high risk of developing heart failure: rationale, design and baseline characteristics of a proof-of-concept, randomised, precision-medicine, prevention trial. The Heart OMics in AGing (HOMAGE) trial. *Eur J Heart Fail* 2020;**22**:1711–23.

84. Pitt B, Anker SD, Bushinsky DA, *et al.*; PEARL-HF Investigators. Evaluation of the efficacy and safety of RLY5016, a polymeric potassium binder, in a double-blind, placebo-controlled study in patients with chronic heart failure (the PEARL-HF) trial. *Eur Heart J* 2011;**32**:820–8.

85. Kosiborod M, Rasmussen HS, Lavin P, *et al.* Effect of sodium zirconium cyclosilicate on potassium lowering for 28 days among outpatients with hyperkalemia: the HARMONIZE randomized clinical trial. *JAMA* 2014;**312**:2223–33.

86. Kataoka H. Acetazolamide as a potent chloride-regaining diuretic: short- and long-term effects, and its pharmacologic role under the 'chloride theory' for heart failure pathophysiology. *Heart Vessels* 2019;**34**:1952–60.

87. Grodin JL, Simon J, Hachamovitch R, *et al.* Prognostic role of serum chloride levels in acute decompensated heart failure. *J Am Coll Cardiol* 2015;**66**:659–66.

88. Cuthbert JJ, Pellicori P, Rigby A, *et al.* Low serum chloride in patients with chronic heart failure: clinical associations and prognostic significance. *Eur J Heart Fail* 2018;**20**:1426–35.

89. Imiela T, Budaj A. Acetazolamide as add-on diuretic therapy in exacerbations of chronic heart failure: a pilot study. *Clin Drug Invest* 2017;**37**:1175–81.

90. Acetazolamide in Decompensated Heart Failure With Volume OveRload (ADVOR). https://clinicaltrials.gov/ct2/show/NCT03505788

91. Zinman B, Wanner C, Lachin JM, *et al.* Empagliflozin, cardiovascular outcomes, and mortality in type 2 diabetes. *N Engl J Med* 2015;**373**:2117–28.

92. Neal B, Perkovic V, Mahaffey KW, *et al.*; CANVAS Program Collaborative Group. Canagliflozin and cardiovascular and renal events in Type 2 diabetes. *N Engl J Med* 2017;**377**:644–57.

93. Rådholm K, Figtree G, Perkovic V, *et al.* Canagliflozin and heart failure in type 2 diabetes mellitus: results from the CANVAS Program. *Circulation* 2018;**138**:458–68.

94. Kato ET, Silverman MG, Mosenzon O, *et al.* Effect of dapagliflozin on heart failure and mortality in type 2 diabetes mellitus. *Circulation* 2019;**139**:2528–36.

95. McMurray JJV, Solomon SD, Inzucchi SE, *et al.*; DAPA-HF Trial Committees and Investigators. Dapagliflozin in patients with heart failure and reduced ejection fraction. *N Engl J Med* 2019;**381**:1995–2008.

96. Petrie MC, Verma S, Docherty KF, *et al.* Effect of dapagliflozin on worsening heart failure and cardiovascular death in patients with heart failure with and without diabetes. *JAMA* 2020;**323**:1353–68.

97. Shoaib A, Mamas MA, Ahmad QS, *et al.* Characteristics and outcome of acute heart failure patients according to the severity of peripheral oedema. *Int J Cardiol* 2019;**285**:40–6.

98. Mullens W, Martens P, Forouzan O, *et al.* Effects of dapagliflozin on congestion assessed by remote pulmonary artery pressure monitoring. *ESC Heart Fail* 2020;**7**:2071–3.

99. Lopaschuk GD, Verma S. Mechanisms of cardiovascular benefits of sodium glucose co-transporter 2 (SGLT2) inhibitors: a state-of-the-art review. *JACC: Basic Transl Sci* 2020;**5**:632–44.

100. US Food and Drug Administration. FDA approves new treatment for a type of heart failure. Press release, May 2020. https://www.fda.gov/news-events/press-announcements/fda-approves-new-treatment-type-heart-failure

101. Kaissling B, Stanton BA. Adaptation of distal tubule and collecting duct to increased sodium delivery: I. Ultrastructure. *Am J Physiol* 1988;**255**:F1256–75.

102. Stanton BA, Kaissling B. Adaptation of distal tubule and collecting duct to increased Na delivery II. Na and K transport. *Am J Physiol* 1988;**255**:1269–75.

103. Brater DC, Day B, Burdette A, Anderson S. Bumetanide and furosemide in heart failure. *Kidney Int* 1984;**26**:183–9.

104. Vasko MR, Cartwright DB, Knochel JP. Furosemide absorption altered in decompensated congestive heart failure. *Ann Intern Med* 1985;**102**:314–18.

105. Bartoli E, Arras S, Faedda R, *et al*. Blunting of furosemide diuresis by aspirin in man. *J Clin Pharmacol* 1980;**20**:452–8.

106. Van Meyel JJ, Smits P, Dormans T, *et al*. Continuous infusion of furosemide in the treatment of patients with congestive heart failure and diuretic resistance. *J Intern Med* 1994;**235**:329–34.

107. Dormans TPJ, Meyel JJM, Gerlag PGG, *et al*. Diuretic efficacy of high dose furosemide in severe heart failure: bolus versus continuous infusion. *J Am Coll Cardiol* 1996;**28**:376–82.

108. Lahav M, Regev A, Ra'anani P, Theodor E. Intermittent administration of furosemide vs continuous infusion preceded by a loading dose for congestive heart failure. *Chest* 1992;**102**:725–31.

109. Pivac N, Rumboldt Z, Sardelic S, *et al*. Diuretic effects of furosemide infusion versus bolus injection in congestive heart failure. *Int J Clin Pharmacol Res* 1998;**18**:121–8.

110. Paterna S, Di Pasquale P, Parrinello G, *et al*. Effects of high dose furosemide and small volume hypertonic saline solution infusion in comparison with a high dose of furosemide as a bolus, in refractory congestive heart failure. *Eur J Heart Fail* 2000;**2**:305–13.

111. Rudy DW, Voelker JR, Greene PK, Esparza FA, Brater DC. Loop diuretics for renal insufficiency: a continuous infusion is more efficacious than bolus therapy. *Ann Intern Med* 1991;**115**:360–66.

112. Howard PA, Dunn MI. Severe musculoskeletal symptoms during continuous infusion of bumetanide. *Chest* 1997;**111**:359–64.

113. Kramer WG, Smith WB, Ferguson J, *et al*. Pharmacodynamics of torsemide administered as an intravenous injection and as a continuous infusion to patients with congestive heart failure. *J Clin Pharmacol* 1996;**36**:265–70.

114. Felker GM, Lee KL, Bull DA, *et al*. Diuretic strategies in patients with acute decompensated heart failure. *N Engl J Med* 2011;**364**:797–805.

115. Zacharias H, Raw J, Nunn A, Parsons S, Johnson M. Is there a role for subcutaneous furosemide in the community and hospice management of end-stage heart failure? *Palliat Med* 2011;**25**:658–63.

116. Kiyingi A, Field MJ, Pawsey CC, *et al*. Metolazone in treatment of severe refractory congestive cardiac failure. *Lancet* 1990;**335**:29–31.

117. Dormans TPJ, Gerlag PGG. Combination of high-dose furosemide and hydrochlorothiazide in the treatment of refractory congestive heart failure. *Eur Heart J* 1996;**17**:1867–74.

118. Sigured B, Olesen KH, Wennevold A. The supra-additive natriuretic effect of addition of bendroflumethiazide and bumetanide in congestive heart failure. *Am Heart J* 1975;**89**:163–70.

119. Channer KS, McLean KA, Lawson-Matthew P, Richardson M. Combination diuretic treatment in severe heart failure: a randomised controlled trial. *Br Heart J* 1994;**71**:146–50.

120. Shulenberger CE, Jiang A, Devabhakthuni S, *et al*. Efficacy and safety of intravenous chlorothiazide versus oral metolazone in patients with acute decompensated heart failure and loop diuretic resistance. *Pharmacotherapy* 2016;**36**:852–60.

121. Butler J, Anstrom KJ, Felker GM, *et al*.; National Heart Lung and Blood Institute Heart Failure Clinical Research Network. Efficacy and safety of spironolactone in acute heart failure: the ATHENA-HF randomized clinical trial. *JAMA Cardiol* 2017;**2**:950–8.

122. de Denus S, Leclair G, Dubé MP, *et al*. Spironolactone metabolite concentrations in decompensated heart failure: insights from the ATHENA-HF trial. *Eur J Heart Fail* 2020;**22**:1451–61.

123. Licata G, Di Pasquale P, Parrinello G, *et al*. Effects of high-dose furosemide and small-volume hypertonic saline solution infusion in comparison with a high dose of furosemide as bolus in refractory congestive heart failure: long-term effects. *Am Heart J* 2003;**145**:459–66.

124. Paterna S, Di Pasquale P, Parrinello G, *et al*. Changes in brain natriuretic peptide levels and bioelectrical impedance measurements after treatment with high-dose furosemide and hypertonic saline solution versus high-dose furosemide alone in refractory congestive heart failure: a double-blind study. *J Am Coll Cardiol* 2005;**45**:1997–2003.

125. Biegus J, Zymlinski R, Siwolowski P, *et al*. Controlled decongestion by Reprieve therapy in acute heart failure: results of the TARGET-1 and TARGET-2 studies. *Eur J Heart Fail* 2019;**21**:1079–87.

126. Liu C, Liu G, Zhou C, *et al*. Potent diuretic effects of prednisone in heart failure patients with refractory diuretic resistance. *Can J Cardiol* 2007;**23**:865–8.

127. Zhang H, Liu C, Ji Z, *et al*. Prednisone adding to usual care treatment for refractory decompensated congestive heart failure. *Int Heart J* 2008;**49**:587–95.

128. Lanier-Smith KL, Currie MG. Effect of glucocorticoids on the binding of atrial natriuretic peptide to endothelial cells. *Eur J Pharmacol* 1990;**178**:105–9.

129. Szatalowicz VL, Arnold PE, Chaimovitz C, *et al*. Radioimmunoassay of plasma arginine vasopressin in hyponatremic patients with congestive heart failure. *N Engl J Med* 1981;**305**:263–6.

130. Francis GS, Benedict C, Johnstone DE, *et al*. Comparison of neuroendocrine activation in patients with left ventricular dysfunction with and without congestive heart failure: a substudy of the Studies of Left Ventricular Dysfunction (SOLVD). *Circulation* 1990;**82**:1724–9.

131. Gheoghiade M, Niazi I, Ouyang J, *et al*. Vasopressin V2-receptor blockade with tolvaptan in patients with chronic heart failure. *Circulation* 2003;**107**:2690–6.

132. Gheorghiade M, Gattis WA, O'Conner C, *et al*. Effects of tolvaptan vasopressin antagonist, in patients hospitalized with worsening heart failure. *JAMA* 2004;**291**:1963–71.

133. Konstam MA, Gheorghiade M, Burnett JC Jr, *et al*.; Efficacy of Vasopressin Antagonism in Heart Failure Outcome Study With Tolvaptan (EVEREST) Investigators. Effects of oral tolvaptan in patients hospitalized for worsening heart failure: the EVEREST Outcome Trial. *JAMA* 2007;**297**:1319–31.

134. Gheorghiade M, Konstam MA, Burnett JC Jr, *et al.*; Efficacy of Vasopressin Antagonism in Heart Failure Outcome Study With Tolvaptan (EVEREST) Investigators. Short-term clinical effects of tolvaptan, an oral vasopressin antagonist, in patients hospitalized for heart failure: the EVEREST Clinical Status Trials. *JAMA* 2007;**297**:1332–43.

135. Felker GM, Mentz RJ, Cole R, *et al.* Efficacy and safety of tolvaptan in patients hospitalized with acute heart failure. *J Am Coll Cardiol* 2017;**69**:1399–406.

136. Konstam MA, Kiernan M, Chandler A, *et al.*; SECRET of CHF Investigators, Coordinators, and Committee Members. Short-term effects of tolvaptan in patients with acute heart failure and volume overload. *J Am Coll Cardiol* 2017;**69**:1409–19.

137. Matsue Y, Suzuki M, Torii S, *et al.* Clinical effectiveness of tolvaptan in patients with acute heart failure and renal dysfunction. *J Card Fail* 2016;**22**:423–32.

138. Robertson GL. Regulation of arginine vasopressin in the syndrome of inappropriate antidiuresis. *Am J Med* 2006;**119**(Suppl 1):S36–S42.

139. Gupta D, Georgiopoulou VV, Kalogeropoulos AP, *et al.* Dietary sodium intake in heart failure. *Circulation* 2012;**126**:479–85.

140. Paterna S, Gaspare P, Fasullo S, Sarullo FM, Di Pasquale P. Normal-sodium diet compared with low-sodium diet in compensated congestive heart failure: is sodium an old enemy or a new friend? *Clin Sci* 2008;**114**:221–30.

141. Jun M, Neal B. Low dietary sodium in heart failure: a need for scientific rigour. *Heart* 2014;**100**:21.

142. Aliti GB, Rabelo ER, Clausell N, *et al.* Aggressive fluid and sodium restriction in acute decompensated heart failure: a randomized clinical trial. *JAMA Intern Med* 2013;**173**:1058–64.

143. Paterna S, Di Pasquale P, Parrinello G, *et al.* Changes in brain natriuretic peptide levels and bioelectrical impedance measurements after treatment with high-dose furosemide and hypertonic saline solution versus high-dose furosemide alone in refractory congestive heart failure: a double-blind study. *J Am Coll Cardiol* 2005;**45**:1997–2003.

144. Schrier RW, Gross P, Gheorghiade M, *et al.*, for the SALT Investigators. Tolvaptan, a selective oral vasopressin V2-receptor antagonist, for hyponatremia. *N Eng J Med* 2006;**355**:2099–112.

145. Gottlieb SS, Brater C, Thomas I, *et al.* BG9719 (CVT-124) an adenosine receptor antagonist protects against the decline in renal function observed with diuretic therapy. *Circulation* 2002;**105**:1348–53.

146. Givertz MM, Massie BM, Fields TK, Pearson LL, Dittrich HC; CKI-201 and CKI-202 Investigators. The effects of KW-3902, an adenosine A1-receptor antagonist, on diuresis and renal function in patients with acute decompensated heart failure and renal impairment or diuretic resistance. *J Am Coll Cardiol* 2007;**50**:1551–60.

147. Cotter G, Dittrich HC, Weatherley BD, *et al.*; Protect Steering Committee, Investigators, and Coordinators. The PROTECT pilot study: a randomized, placebo-controlled, dose-finding study of the adenosine A1 receptor antagonist rolofylline in patients with acute heart failure and renal impairment. *J Card Fail* 2008;**14**:631–40.

148. Massie BM, O'Connor CM, Metra M, *et al.*; PROTECT Investigators and Committees. Rolofylline, an adenosine A1-receptor antagonist, in acute heart failure. *N Engl J Med* 2010;**363**:1419–28.

149. Giamouzis G, Butler J, Starling RC, *et al.* Impact of dopamine infusion on renal function in hospitalized heart failure patients: results of the Dopamine in Acute Decompensated Heart Failure (DAD-HF) Trial. *J Card Fail* 2010;**16**:922–30.

150. Chen HH, Anstrom KJ, Givertz MM, *et al.*; NHLBI Heart Failure Clinical Research Network. Low-dose dopamine or low-dose nesiritide in acute heart failure with renal dysfunction: the ROSE acute heart failure randomized trial. *JAMA* 2013;**310**:2533–43.

151. Ali SS, Olinger CC, Sobotka PA, *et al.* Loop diuretics can cause clinical natriuretic failure: a prescription for volume expansion. *Congest Heart Fail* 2009;**15**:1–4.

152. Kolff WJ, Leonards JR. Reduction of otherwise intractable edema by dialysis or filtration. *Cleveland Clin Q* 1954;**21**:61–71.

153. Mailloux LU, Swartz CD, Onesti G, *et al.* Peritoneal dailysis for refractory congestive heart failure. *J Am Med Assoc* 1967;**199**:873–78.

154. Cairns KB, Porter GA, Kloster FE, Bristow JD, Griswold HE. Clinical and hemodynamic results of peritoneal dialysis for severe cardiac failure. *Am Heart J* 1968;**76**:227–34.

155. Marenzi G, Lauri G, Grazi M, *et al.* Circulatory response to fluid overload removal by extracorporeal ultrafiltration in refractory congestive heart failure. *J Am Coll Cardiol* 2001;**38**:963–8.

156. Bart BA, Boyle A, Bank AJ, *et al.* Ultrafiltration versus usual care for hospitalized patients with heart failure: the Relief for Acutely Fluid-Overloaded Patients With Decompensated Congestive Heart Failure (RAPID-CHF) trial. *J Am Coll Cardiol* 2005;**46**:2043–6.

157. Costanzo MR, Saltzberg M, O'Sullivan J, Sobotka P. Early ultrafiltration in patients with decompensated heart failure and diuretic resistance. *J Am Coll Cardiol* 2005;**46**:2047–51.

158. Libetta C, Sepe V, Zucchi M, *et al.* Intermittent haemodiafiltration in refractory congestive heart failure: BNP and balance of inflammatory cytokines. *Nephrol Dial Transplant* 2007;**22**:2013–19.

159. Sheppard R, Panyon J, Pohwani AL, *et al.* Intermittent outpatient ultrafiltration for the treatment of severe refractory congestive heart failure. *J Card Fail* 2004;**10**:380–3.

160. Bellomo R, Tipping P, Boyce N. Continuous veno-venous hemofiltration with dialysis removes cytokines from the circulation of septic patients. *Crit Care Med* 1993;**21**:522–6.

161. Costanzo MR, Guglin ME, Saltzberg MT, *et al.*; UNLOAD Trial Investigators. Ultrafiltration versus intravenous diuretics for patients hospitalized for acute decompensated heart failure. *J Am Coll Cardiol* 2007;**49**:675–83 (Erratum in: *J Am Coll Cardiol* 2007;**49**:1136).

162. Bart BA, Goldsmith SR, Lee KL, *et al.*; Heart Failure Clinical Research Network. Ultrafiltration in decompensated heart failure with cardiorenal syndrome. *N Engl J Med* 2012;**367**:2296–304.

163. Costanzo MR, Negoianu D, Jaski BE, *et al.* Aquapheresis versus intravenous diuretics and hospitalizations for heart failure. *JACC Heart Fail* 2016;**4**:95–105.

164. Pellicori P, Clark AL, Kallvikbacka-Bennett A, *et al.* Non-invasive measurement of right atrial pressure by near-infrared spectroscopy: preliminary experience. A report from the SICA-HF study. *Eur J Heart Fail* 2017;**19**:883–92.

165. Flapan AD, Davies E, Waugh C, *et al.* The influence of posture on the response to loop diuretics in patients with chronic cardiac failure is reduced by angiotensin converting enzyme inhibition. *Eur J Clin Pharmacol* 1992;**42**:581–5.

166. Travers B, O'Loughlin C, Murphy NF, *et al.* Fluid restriction in the management of decompensated heart failure: no impact on time to clinical stability. *J Card Fail* 2007;**13**:128–32.

167. Holst M, Strömberg A, Lindholm M, Willenheimer R. Liberal versus restricted fluid prescription in stabilised patients with chronic heart failure: result of a randomised cross-over study of the effects on health-related quality of life, physical capacity, thirst and morbidity. *Scand Cardiovasc J* 2008;**42**:316–22.

168. Jondeau G, Neuder Y, Eicher JC, *et al.*; B-CONVINCED Investigators. B-CONVINCED: Beta-blocker CONtinuation Vs. INterruption in patients with Congestive heart failure hospitalizED for a decompensation episode. *Eur Heart J* 2009;**30**:2186–92.

169. Anand IS, Veall N, Kalra GS, *et al.* Treatment of heart failure with diuretics: body compartments, renal function and plasma hormones. *Eur Heart J* 1989;**10**:445–50.

170. Damman K, Valente MAE, Voors AA, *et al.* Renal impairment, worsening renal function, and outcome in patients with heart failure: an updated meta-analysis. *Eur Heart J* 2014;**35**:455–69.

171. Bart BA, Goldsmith SR, Lee KL, *et al.* Cardiorenal rescue study in acute decompensated heart failure: rationale and design of CARRESS-HF, for the Heart Failure Clinical Research Network. *J Card Fail* 2012;**18**:176–82.

172. Brisco MA, Zile MR, Hanberg JS, *et al.* Relevance of changes in serum creatinine during a heart failure trial of decongestive strategies: insights from the DOSE Trial. *J Card Fail* 2016;**22**:753–60.

48

Angiotensin converting enzyme inhibitors and vasodilators

Iain Squire and Andrew L. Clark

Introduction

Until the latter part of the twentieth century, the pharmacological management of chronic heart failure (CHF) was limited to correction of fluid and electrolyte disturbances (diuretics) and augmentation of myocardial contractility (cardiac glycosides). However, during 1980s and 1990s, evidence mounted for the central role to the pathophysiology of CHF of activation of the renin–angiotensin–aldosterone system (RAAS) and adrenergic nervous system.[1] Over those years and into the early part of the twenty-first century century, large randomized, controlled trials provided physicians with enormous amounts of evidence for the benefits to patients with heart failure of angiotensin converting enzyme (ACE) inhibitors, angiotensin receptor antagonists, mineralocorticoid receptor antagonists, and β-receptor blockers, in addition to our old friends diuretics and digoxin.

The degree of activation of the RAAS (**Figure 48.1**) correlates inversely with prognosis in CHF; the agents with which we have become familiar in our management of patients with heart failure inhibit activity of the RAAS, directly (in the case of ACE inhibitors and angiotensin receptor blockers (ARBs)) or indirectly (in the case of β-blockers), emphasizing the crucial role of this system in the heart failure syndrome. Among the agents with proven efficacy in the management of heart failure, of all the classes of agent available to us, ACE inhibitors have the most extensive evidence base. Further, in head-to head comparisons with ARBs, ACE inhibitors have invariably been shown to provide superior clinical benefit.[2–4]

Only very recently have we seen evidence that the clinical benefits of ACE inhibitors can be surpassed, with treatment with the angiotensin receptor–neprilysin inhibitor (ARNI) sacubitril valsartan.[5] The latter agent, and the details of the trial comparing it to enalapril, are discussed in Chapter 49. At the time of writing, it seems likely that ACE inhibitors will retain an important place in the management of a large proportion of patients with CHF. However, with the advent of a new development in the pharmacological management of heart failure, it is appropriate that this chapter reviews the development and pharmacology of ACE inhibitors and their physiological actions. It will also discuss the side-effect profile of ACE inhibitors and the place of vasodilators that do not block the RAAS as potential alternatives to ACE inhibition. It is also timely for us to remind ourselves of the huge clinical impact of ACE inhibitors in the treatment of heart failure.

ACE inhibitors

Development

ACE inhibitors are the result of one of the first successful attempts to design a drug based upon its target. ACE inhibitors for oral administration were *designed* for the purpose of inhibiting ACE, based upon the ACE-inhibiting action of peptides in the venom of *Bothrops jararaca*, the South American pit viper (**Figure 48.2**), and on similarities between ACE and the pancreatic digestive enzyme carboxypeptidase A. The known zinc dependence of ACE led Ondetti and Cushman to incorporate a sulfhydryl molecule in their original dipeptide ACE inhibitor, captopril.[6] Subsequent ACE inhibitor molecules were developed to bind to sites on the ACE molecule other than the zinc moiety, with varying aims of increasing duration of action or potency, or to increase absorption. Of currently

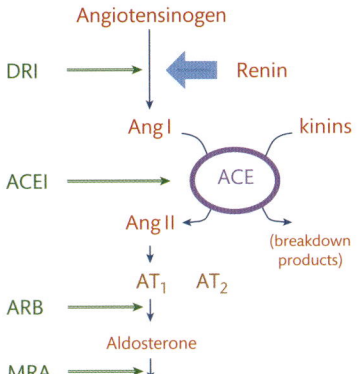

Figure 48.1 The degree of activation of the renin–angiotensin–aldosterone system. DRI, direct angiotensin inhibitor; Ang, angiotensin; ACEI, angiotensin converting enzyme inhibitor; AT$_1$, angiotensin II type 1 receptor; ARB, angiotensin receptor blocker; MRA, mineralocorticoid receptor antagonist.

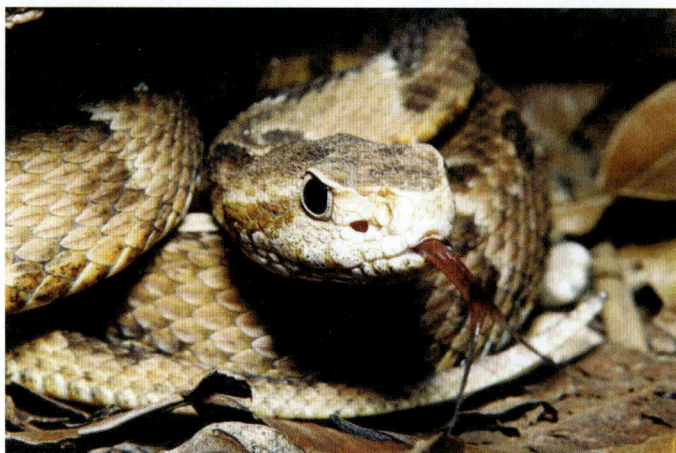

Figure 48.2 *Bothrops jararaca*, the South American pit viper.

available ACE inhibitors, only captopril binds via a sulfhydryl ligand, fosinopril via a phosphinyl group, and the remainder via a carboxyl ligand. The structural differences are associated with pharmacokinetic and pharmacodynamic differences, the clinical significance of which is unclear in the management of patients with heart failure.

Physiology

The RAAS is a ubiquitous endocrine system, and ACE is found in the circulation as well as in many tissues. ACE has a number of potential substrates, the most relevant to the use of ACE inhibitors in heart failure being angiotensin I and bradykinin.

Claims have been made for individual ACE inhibitors having properties of high affinity for, and inhibition of, tissue ACE. In reality, ACE inhibitors block tissue ACE and plasma ACE with the same rank-order of potency. Again, the clinical relevance of differences among ACE inhibitors in this context is unclear. In heart failure, ACE inhibition leads to reduced plasma angiotensin II and aldosterone levels, with subsequently lower systemic blood pressure via reduction in peripheral vascular resistance. In contrast to other vasodilator drugs, the fall in systemic vascular resistance is not accompanied by reflex tachycardia, possibly due to interaction between angiotensin II and the sympathetic nervous system. As a consequence of reduced circulating aldosterone, plasma potassium concentrations increase. Left-sided cardiac pressures fall rapidly after ACE inhibition, as does pulmonary artery pressure, and cardiac index increases. These changes are beneficial in the setting of heart failure and, importantly, are maintained with chronic dosing and in exercise. Cardiac work and myocardial oxygen demand are reduced, and left ventricular ejection fraction (LVEF) tends to increase, at least with chronic treatment.

The magnitude of the blood pressure response to ACE inhibition is often a concern to clinicians caring for patients with heart failure. Indeed, in the early years of ACE inhibitor use, it was common practice for patients to be admitted to hospital for initiation of therapy. This seldom, if ever, happens now, although a fall in blood pressure remains one of the most common issues limiting the use of ACE inhibitors in practice. Prediction of the magnitude of blood pressure response, and assessment of its clinical relevance in an individual patient, is challenging, and we will return to this clinical issue later in the chapter.

In clinical practice, ACE inhibitor therapy is well tolerated in the vast majority of patients. Measured changes in systemic blood pressure are seldom associated with clinically meaningful symptoms, although they do occur in a minority of patients. Whereas accumulation of bradykinin appears to contribute to the fall in blood pressure after ACE inhibition in normal individuals,[8] it is not known whether the accumulation occurs in people with heart failure. It may be argued that bradykinin accumulation to be desirable, given the consistent equivalence or superiority of ACE inhibitors over angiotensin receptor blockers in clinical studies to date. Importantly, the acute haemodynamic response to ACE inhibition is a poor predictor of clinical benefit,[9] a point which should always be remembered by practitioners.

ACE inhibitors in clinical practice

In 1979, captopril, the first orally administered ACE inhibitor, was demonstrated to lower left ventricular filling pressure and systemic vascular resistance in heart failure.[10] Sustained beneficial haemodynamic effects were demonstrated soon afterwards.[11]

The earliest evidence of survival benefit from vasodilator therapy in heart failure came from a number of small studies in the mid 1980s with prazosin, isosorbide dinitrate or hydralazine,[12] followed by the demonstration of the superiority of the combination of isosorbide dinitrate with hydralazine compared to prazosin.[13] The first evidence for the potential benefit of ACE inhibitors came from a trend to increased survival with captopril in the Captopril Multicenter Research trial.[14] Since then, ACE inhibitors have become one of the most extensively investigated classes of drug in any branch of medicine, certainly in heart failure, with tens of thousands of patients enrolled in clinical trials, and many millions treated in clinical practice.

Clinical trials of ACE inhibitors in chronic heart failure

The first randomized, controlled trial to show a clear benefit from ACE inhibition in CHF was the CONSENSUS study.[15] In what would be considered by modern standards a very small trial, 127 patients were randomized to receive enalapril at a dose of 2.5–40 mg once daily, and 126 received matching placebo. The patient group chosen for this trial was at high risk, being a population of patients with advanced heart failure and New York Heart Association (NYHA) class IV symptoms, their background treatment including an average of ~200 mg per day of oral furosemide. The magnitude of the benefit seen with ACE inhibition is startling; over an average follow-up of six months, crude mortality of 44% in the placebo group was reduced to 26% in those treated with enalapril, a relative risk reduction of 40%, which was ascribed entirely to reduction in death from progressive heart failure (Figure 48.3). The survival benefits of enalapril were evident irrespective of whether the patients' background treatment included other vasodilators, which were prescribed in around half of the participants.

Few trials in any area of medicine, before or since, have demonstrated such a large survival benefit from a pharmacological intervention in a chronic disease. Case-fatality in the placebo group was indeed representative of that seen in such patients at the time. An important point is that a consistent finding in trials of ACE inhibition in heart failure is that those patients with the most severe disease have the greatest relative benefit from intervention. It is also relevant to note that by 10 years following the end of the CONSENSUS trial, almost all the participating patients had died[16] (Figure 48.4); in the

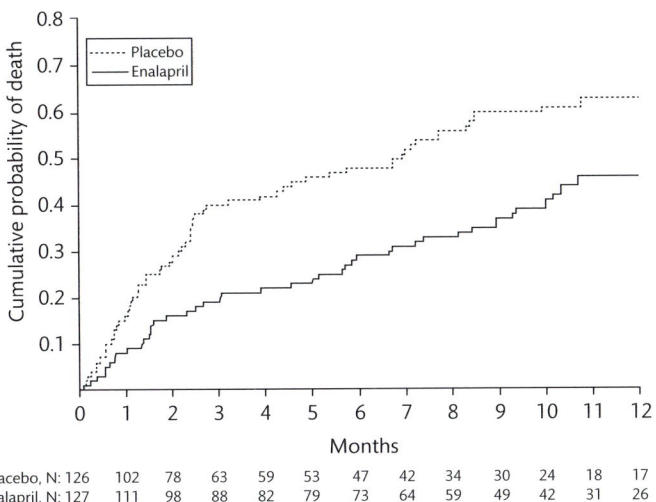

Figure 48.3 Survival in the CONSENSUS trial. 127 patients received enalapril (interrupted line) and 126 received matching placebo (solid line). The primary endpoint was mortality at 6 months.

management of heart failure, even the best treatment does not save, but only extends, life.

The second landmark trial which demonstrated the benefit of enalapril in patients with chronic, symptomatic heart failure was the SOLVD (Studies of Left Ventricular Dysfunction) treatment trial.[17] SOLVD randomized 2569 patients with less symptomatic heart failure, mostly NYHA II–III, to receive enalapril 2.5–10 mg ($n = 1285$), or placebo ($n = 1284$), twice daily. The summary statistics for the results of these two trials are shown in Table 48.1. The absolute and relative risk reductions seen in these trials, and the numbers of patients needed to treat to achieve one event saved, are clear and consistent, and these results are the basis for our use of ACE inhibitors in CHF. The observations are also supported by a meta-analysis of smaller randomized trials, which also reported improved survival, reduced hospitalization, and improvement in quality of life and exercise capacity.[18]

ACE inhibitors in asymptomatic heart failure

Between them, CONSENSUS (NYHA IV) and SOLVD treatment (NYHA II–III) addressed the efficacy of patients with symptomatic heart failure and reduced LVEF. As the aim of treatment with ACE

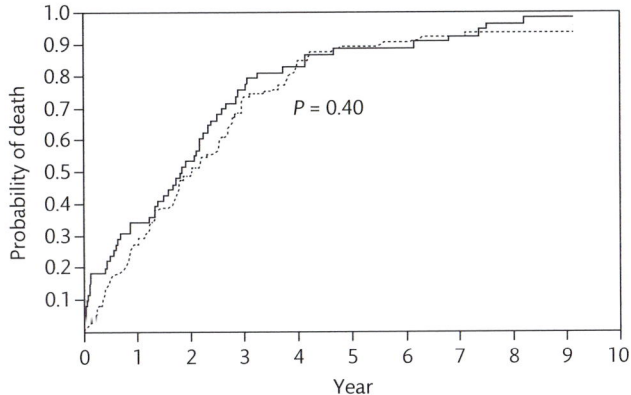

Figure 48.4 CONSENSUS 10 year follow up. Survival following the end of the study (during which time all patients were offered enalapril) is shown.

inhibition is to interfere with pathophysiological processes, rather than to improve symptoms, the SOLVD prevention trial examined the effect of enalapril in patients with asymptomatic left ventricular systolic dysfunction, in the same doses as used in the treatment trial.[19] As shown in Table 48.1, the effects on mortality were of lesser magnitude than in the other trials, but there was a statistically significant benefit in the composite of death or heart failure hospitalization. Thus, there is evidence for the use of ACE inhibitors in chronic left ventricular systolic dysfunction (LVEF ≤40%) irrespective of symptom severity.

Why might the benefit in asymptomatic patients be so much less than in those with symptoms, in the context of similar LVEF? There is of course a myriad of potential explanations, but the observation demonstrates the limitations of assessing the severity of heart failure using LVEF as a dichotomized variable. In the current era, we have much more sensitive tools by which we may make an assessment of heart failure severity, especially plasma biomarkers such as natriuretic peptides. However, in contemporary practice, assessment of LVEF, most commonly by echocardiography, remains central to the assessment and management of the individual patient with heart failure. We should also bear in mind that a number of recent clinical trials in heart failure have required as an eligibility criterion that the patient had to have elevated natriuretic peptide levels as well as, rather than instead of, reduced LVEF.

We might pause here to consider that many of the ACE inhibitors with a licensed indication for the treatment of CHF have never been exposed to investigation in a randomized controlled trial; enalapril has by far and away the most extensive evidence base in CHF, a fact recognized by the US Food and Drug Administration when it mandated that enalapril, at a target dose of 20 mg daily, should be the comparator for sacubitril/valsartan in the recent PARADIGM HF trial.[5]

Clinical trials of ACE inhibitors after acute myocardial infarction

For patients with CHF, starting treatment with an ACE inhibitor is *secondary* prevention therapy introduced at very variable timepoints in the natural history of an individual's disease progression. As the single largest contributing cause of CHF is coronary artery disease, starting ACE inhibitors in patients with acute myocardial infarction (AMI) in the coronary care unit represents an opportunity to start treatment early in the course of the disease. Following the results of CONSENSUS and SOLVD, it was logical that the impact of ACE inhibition should be investigated in patients early following AMI.

The randomized, placebo-controlled clinical trials of ACE inhibition following AMI have varied in terms of eligibility criteria, timing of initiation of therapy in relation to the index event, and duration of follow-up. Overall, the trials can be divided into: (i) those which initiated ACE inhibition in the acute phase of AMI, recruited patients irrespective of evidence of heart failure or LV systolic dysfunction, and continued therapy for a relatively short period of time; and (ii) those which initiated therapy more remote from the index MI, recruited patients with evidence of impaired LV function, and continued therapy over a longer period.

Early ACE inhibition

Four major trials have investigated the effects of ACE inhibition initiated 0–36 h after the onset of symptoms of MI, together

Table 48.1 Summary statistics from CONSENSUS and SOLVD (Treatment) trials

Trial	Number	Deaths			NNT	Additional findings
		No. (%)	RRR	ARR		
CONSENSUS NYHA IV LVEF ≤40%	Enalapril, n = 127	33 (26%)	40%ᵃ (P = 0.002)	18%	7 (over average of 6 months)	Reduced NYHA class; reduced heart size
	Placebo, n = 126	55 (44%)				
SOLVD-T NYHA II–III LVEF ≤35%	Enalapril, n = 1285	452 (35.2%)	16% (P = 0.0036)	4.5%	22 (over average of 41 months)	26% reduction HF hospitalization
	Placebo, n = 1284	510 (39.7%)				
SOLVD-P NYHA I LVEF ≤35%	Enalapril, n = 2111	313 (14.8%)	8% (P = 0.30)	1%	N/A	20% RRR in risk of death or HF hospitalization
	Placebo, n = 2117	334 (15.8%)				

ARR, absolute risk reduction; HF, heart failure; LVEF, left ventricular ejection fraction; NNT, number needed to treat to delay one death; NYHA, New York Heart Association; RRR, relative risk reduction.
ᵃ Six-month mortality RRR. One-year RRR was 31%.

including nearly 100 000 patients.[20–23] These trials—CONSENSUS-II, GISSI-3, ISIS-4 and CCS-1—enrolled patients within 24 h[18–20] or 36 h[21] of onset of symptoms of MI, and investigated captopril,[22,23] lisinopril[21] or enalapril[20] administered over 28 days,[22,23] 42 days,[21] or 6 months.[20]

Reassuringly, in a meta-analysis there was no evidence of heterogeneity among the results of the four trials (**Figure 48.5**).[24] Over the first 30 days of follow-up, mortality was 7.1% in patients allocated to ACE inhibitor, and 7.6% in patients allocated to comparator treatment—a 7% relative risk reduction (P = 0.004) corresponding to approximately five fewer deaths per 1000 patients treated for 30 days. Remarkably, 80% of these deaths were avoided in the first seven days of treatment, corresponding to four fewer deaths per 1000 treated patients. The incidence of non-fatal heart failure was also reduced over the first 30 days.[24]

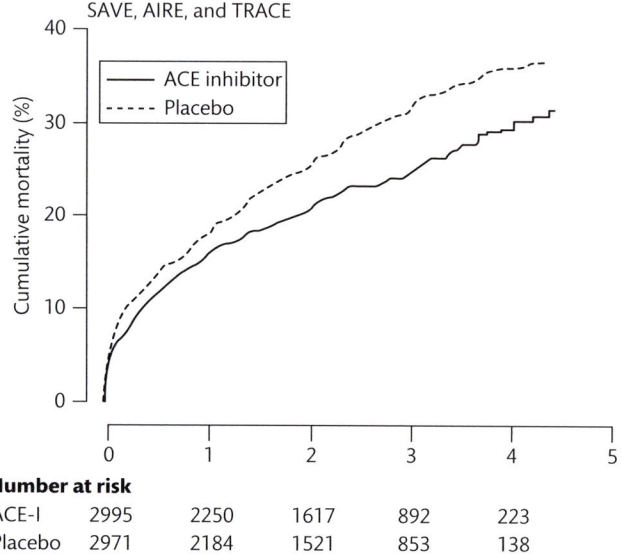

Number at risk

	0	1	2	3	4
ACE-I	2995	2250	1617	892	223
Placebo	2971	2184	1521	853	138

Figure 48.5 Combined Kaplan–Meier mortality curve for the SAVE, AIRE, and TRACE trials of angiotensin converting enzyme inhibition (ACEi) in patients with heart failure or echocardiographic left ventricular systolic dysfunction following acute myocardial infarction.

Reproduced from Flather MD, Yusuf S, Køber L, et al. Long-term ACE-inhibitor therapy in patients with heart failure or left-ventricular dysfunction: a systematic overview of data from individual patients. *Lancet* 2000;**355**:1575–81.

The CONSENSUS-II study[20] is unique among outcome studies of ACE inhibition in heart failure in that treatment was initiated with intravenous enalaprilat, followed by oral enalapril. It is also the only randomized, controlled trial of ACE inhibition in which the point estimate of the magnitude of effect was indicative of harm. The implications are discussed below.

Across the four trials, the absolute and proportional benefits of ACE inhibition were similar in men and women, and across age groups. It is important to note that absolute benefits were greater in patients at higher risk of adverse outcome; thus, patients with high heart rate, high Killip class at entry, with anterior MI or with prior MI or diabetes had greater absolute benefit.

Later ACE inhibition

Several randomized, controlled trials have studied the efficacy of initiation of ACE inhibition after acute MI but commenced beyond the very early phase. The trials are characterized by restriction of eligibility to patients with clinical or echocardiographic evidence of left ventricular dysfunction, and observed the effects of therapy over at least a year.

The three largest such trials were SAVE,[25] AIRE,[26] and TRACE,[27] which respectively studied captopril, ramipril, and trandolapril, each started at least three days after the acute event. As with the trials of early ACE inhibition, meta-analysis shows no evidence of heterogeneity among the results, with significant overall benefit.[28] Across the three trials, median duration of treatment was 31 months, during which case-fatality in patients receiving ACE inhibitor was 23.4% compared to 29.1% for placebo, an absolute reduction of 5.7% and an odds ratio for mortality of 0.74 (95% confidence interval: 0.66–0.83). This equates to 60 fewer deaths per 1000 patients treated for 30 months. Survival benefit was evident within a few weeks of initiation of treatment. ACE inhibition was also associated with reduced risk of hospitalization with heart failure, and of reinfarction.

Adverse events in post-myocardial infarction ACE inhibitor trials

The potential benefits of ACE inhibition after MI are clear; treatment is associated with statistically significant, and clinically meaningful, benefits. The benefits were not achieved without unwanted effects. In the short term, early treatment trials,[20–23] persistent hypotension occurred in 17.6% and 9.3% of ACE inhibitor and control patients

respectively, an excess of 84 per 1000 patients treated. Although there were more cases of cardiogenic shock and renal dysfunction in ACE inhibitor-treated patients compared with placebo (4.6 and 6.2 per 1000 respectively), absolute event rates were very small.

In the trials in which an ACE inhibitor was started later and continued for longer,[25-27] hypotension (14.7% in ACE inhibitor-treated patients compared with 8.7% in placebo-treated patients; odds ratio: 1.86; $P < 0.0001$) and renal dysfunction (5.2% ACE inhibitor compared with 3.6% placebo; odds ratio: 1.49; $P < 0.0001$) were more common with active therapy, but again the absolute rates were low.

ACE inhibition after acute myocardial infarction: which patients?

The studies of early (<36 h) initiation show a relatively small overall benefit using an all-inclusive, unselective approach to treatment; the benefit is seen within the first 7 days, and is of greater absolute magnitude in patients with higher baseline risk. The benefits are countered, to some degree, by a greater likelihood of important adverse events within the same time-frame, including cardiogenic shock.[24] The adverse events were particularly evident in the CONSENSUS II trial, which addressed the hypothesis that very early ACE inhibition with intravenous enalaprilat would be of clinical benefit. That CONSENSUS II refuted the hypothesis serves as a caution against the introduction of powerful pharmacological therapy in the very early period after AMI.[20]

The studies of later introduction of ACE inhibition, recruiting patients with evidence of left ventricular impairment followed for longer periods, showed greater absolute benefit as the studies included only higher-risk patients. Benefit was again evident from an early time after initiation of treatment.

Overall, the data support the prescription of ACE inhibitor from around day 3 after MI, in patients with evidence of left ventricular dysfunction. In patients without evidence of significant left ventricular systolic impairment, additional criteria suggesting that there is likely to be benefit from treatment should be considered: previous or concomitant conditions (e.g. diabetes or previous MI, hypertension), the site (anterior), or extent of MI (high cardiac enzymes or troponin) should encourage the use of ACE inhibitor.

In Europe, current guidelines[29] recommend prescription of ACE inhibitor for patients with LVEF <40%. Other (UK national) guideline documents recommend that ACE inhibition should be *considered* for all patients with heart failure due to left ventricular systolic dysfunction.[30] In reality, in many countries ACE inhibition is prescribed to the majority of patients after MI, or with a diagnosis of heart failure, irrespective of left ventricular function. This is pragmatic, and for the vast majority of patients, safe, but caution should be exercised; after AMI, very early treatment should be avoided, and

care should be taken in patients with impaired renal function and in haemodynamically compromised individuals. In the future, more sophisticated methods may allow identification of patients likely to benefit from therapy, such as the circulating concentration of one or more biomarker.

The patients at highest risk have the most to gain from treatment. However, such patients are often the most challenging to treat with ACE inhibition, and indeed with other pharmacological therapies; they may present with extensive infarction or severe heart failure, low blood pressure, and renal impairment. It is in the management of these individuals that the physician best demonstrates his or her clinical expertise. In practice we try to take a clinically pragmatic approach; our starting point is to consider that if the patient has sufficient blood pressure to maintain cerebral (i.e. no, or minimal, symptoms of hypotension) and renal (maintenance of appropriate renal function) perfusion, then the patient has adequate blood pressure. This at least mitigates against the (often knee-jerk) response to low brachial blood pressure which leads to withdrawal of disease-modifying therapy; always consider what we are denying the patient.

An alternative to ACE inhibitor in chronic heart failure? Comparative studies

A number of studies compared the clinical efficacy of ACE inhibitors to alternative pharmacological therapy. Indeed, one of the earliest trials to investigate the clinical effects of ACE inhibitors in heart failure was a comparison of enalapril against the combination of hydralazine and isosorbide dinitrate, the second Veterans Administration Heart Failure Trial, VHeFT II.[31]

More recent studies have investigated the comparative benefits of ACE inhibitors and angiotensin receptor antagonists, the class of agent which has become the alternative renin–angiotensin–aldosterone inhibitor. The first such trial, ELITE (Evaluation of Losartan in The Elderly), suggested that losartan in a target dose of 50 mg once daily was associated with >40% improved survival compared to captopril.[32] Unsurprisingly, the result stimulated enormous interest in the angiotensin receptor antagonists, and led to a number of large, properly powered studies. ELITE was a safety and tolerability study in only ~700 patients, and the subsequent definitive outcome trial, ELITE II, showed no superiority of losartan over captopril.[33]

ACE inhibitors have also stood up to the test of comparison with angiotensin receptor blockers after MI. Losartan has once again been compared with captopril, in the OPTIMAAL (Optimal Trial In Myocardial Infarction with the angiotensin II antagonist Losartan) trial.[34] The results of this trial, summarized in Table 48.2, confirmed the (statistically non-significant) superiority of the ACE inhibitor captopril, at a mean achieved dose of 45 mg three times daily,

Table 48.2 Summary of clinical end-points for treatment with losartan or with captopril in the OPTIMAAL trial[32]

Clinical end-point	Losartan	Captopril	RR losartan vs captopril	P-value
All-cause mortality	499 (18.2%)	447 (16.4%)	1.13 (0.99–1.28)	0.069
Myocardial reinfarction	384 (14.0%)	379 (13.9%)	1.03 (0.89–1.18)	0.722
Cardiovascular mortality	420 (15.3%)	363 (13.3%)	1.17 (1.01–1.34)	0.032
First all-cause hospitalization	1806 (65.8%)	1774 (64.9%)	1.03 (0.97–1.10)	0.362
First HF hospitalization	306 (11.2%)	265 (9.7%)	1.16 (0.98–1.37)	0.072

HF, heart failure; RR, relative risk.

compared to losartan at a mean dose of 44 mg once daily. A later post-MI trial, VALIANT, studied the comparative survival benefits of captopril, valsartan, or the combination of the two agents. VALIANT demonstrated very similar survival benefit for captopril compared to valsartan, with no evidence of added benefit, and greater side-effects, from the combination of the two.[35]

Overall, the evidence is compelling for the use of ACE inhibitors in patients with left ventricular systolic dysfunction in patients with heart failure or following AMI. No alternative single agent has been shown to be superior to ACE inhibitors in improving both mortality and morbidity.

Side-effect profile

The ACE inhibitors are generally very well tolerated and have a side-effect profile predictable from their pharmacology; they lower glomerular perfusion in the kidney, and blood pressure, and potentially stimulate accumulation of bradykinin. The resulting potential effects are: symptomatic hypotension, renal impairment, and cough. It is important to remember that each of these symptoms is experienced frequently in patients with heart failure irrespective of ACE inhibitor therapy.

Renal impairment is a common accompaniment to heart failure, and there is a small absolute risk of significant worsening following initiation of ACE inhibitor therapy. In the SAVE, TRACE, and SOLVD studies, renal impairment was recorded in 5.2% of patients treated with ACE inhibitor compared to 3.6% of patients receiving placebo.[26] In clinical practice, patients at risk of developing renal dysfunction are not easy to identify, but renovascular disease is more prevalent among patients with peripheral vascular disease. Thus, the finding of reduced or absent peripheral (foot) pulses indicates a patient at risk of renovascular disease. It is important to remember that a degree of deterioration in renal function should not come as a surprise after introduction or uptitration of ACE inhibitor therapy. This is far from universal, and a small change in urea and creatinine or estimated glomerular filtration rate should not lead to withdrawal of ACE therapy. An analysis of randomized trials looking at the effects of RAAS inhibitors in patients with heart failure found that worsening renal function was more common in patients randomized to receive RAAS. However, the worsening renal function in patients with heart failure and reduced ejection fraction was not associated with a worse outcome compared with worsening renal function on placebo. Conversely, in patients with heart failure and normal ejection fraction, worsening renal function on RAAS was strongly associated with worse outcomes.[36] The implication is that worsening renal function should not lead to an ACE inhibitor being stopped in patients with heart failure with reduced ejection fraction, but stopping should be strongly considered in patients with heart failure with normal ejection fraction. Changes in renal function should always be considered in the context of the patient's quality of life and prognosis, and in the context of the potential consequences of denial of disease-modifying ACE inhibitor treatment.

Cough is common in patients with heart failure, and is often incorrectly assumed to be secondary to the ACE inhibitor. However, there is a small increase in the incidence of cough in patients treated with ACE inhibitors, thought to be due to bradykinin accumulation in the airways. There is no proven effective therapy for ACE-inhibitor induced cough and this unwanted effect frequently leads to treatment withdrawal. The reasons for withdrawal of therapy,

and the possible consequences for prognosis, should be discussed with the patient. The clinical response to withdrawal of treatment should always be monitored and reintroduction considered where the cough persists in the absence of ACE inhibitor. When patients are informed of the mortality benefit to be gained from the ACE inhibitor, they are often prepared to tolerate their cough. Angio-oedema occurs as a side-effect in less than 1% of patients treated with ACE inhibitors. Given its potentially life-threatening nature, the clinical suspicion of angio-oedema should lead to complete avoidance of ACE inhibition thereafter.

A lowering of blood pressure is an expected consequence of ACE inhibitor therapy, and this alone should not raise concerns of health care professionals caring for those with heart failure. By contrast, hypotension leading to symptoms is of more concern and may limit therapy. Whereas this is often described as 'first-dose hypotension', and considered by many to occur only at the initiation of treatment, the blood pressure response after an individual dose of an ACE inhibitor is the same after many months of treatment as it was after the very first dose.[37,38]

The variation in the blood pressure response to the very first dose of ACE inhibitor can be gauged from Figure 48.6, which shows the individual mean arterial pressure responses to the first dose of oral enalapril 2.5 mg in 24 patients with heart failure.[39] The maximum mean fall in mean arterial pressure was 15 mmHg, ranging from zero to >40 mmHg; importantly the time to the maximum fall varied enormously, from 2 to 8 h.

Although several physiological variables have been reported to be associated with the magnitude of the blood pressure response to ACE inhibition, it is in reality very difficult to predict in an individual patient with heart failure. Murray et al. attempted to identify clinical variables predicting the magnitude of the blood pressure fall in response to initiation of ACE inhibition in 144 patients with heart failure. Age, sex, NYHA class, diuretic dose, sodium, potassium, creatinine concentration, serum ACE activity, and plasma renin concentration were not predictive of the fall in blood pressure.[39] At best, the combination of plasma renin activity, creatinine, age, the ACE inhibitor, and baseline blood pressure explained <25% of the blood pressure response. In these patients with heart failure, higher

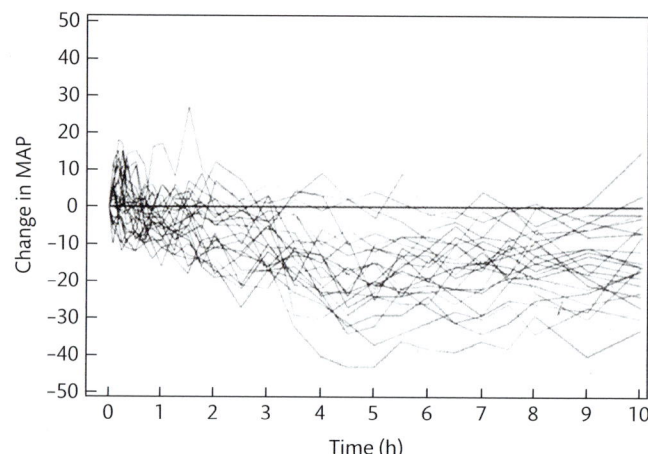

Figure 48.6 Individual change in mean arterial blood pressure (MAP) in 24 patients with heart failure following the first oral dose of enalapril 2.5 mg.

baseline blood pressure was associated with a greater fall in response to ACE inhibition.

Finally, a small fall in haemoglobin may be observed during ACE inhibitor treatment, possibly as a consequence of the role of angiotensin II in the formation of erythroid precursors. The magnitude of fall in haematocrit is seldom >5%, and the overall risk of a clinically significant change is very small and is associated with higher creatinine and with concurrent weight loss,[40] both of which are more common in advanced heart failure.

Initiation and titration

It is clear from the above that adverse events in response to initiation of ACE inhibition, although rare, are unpredictable and potentially important. On this background, all national[30] and international[29] guidelines for the management of heart failure recommend initiation of therapy at a low dose of the individual agent, and careful monitoring of the response of both blood pressure and renal function. This is simple, sound advice.

Summary

The ACE inhibitors are among the most investigated groups of drugs in cardiovascular medicine. Thirty years after the first inkling that ACE inhibitors may have a place in the management of heart failure, they remain a central component of the physician's armamentarium. As a class, ACE inhibitors have transformed not only the management of patients with heart failure, but also our understanding of this complex syndrome. The recent development of the ARNI class of neurohormonal antagonists may alter the relative place of ACE inhibitors in practice. However, ACE inhibitors are likely to remain central to the management of a large proportion of patients with heart failure for the foreseeable future. The magnitude of benefit is large and ACE inhibitors are well tolerated by the vast majority of patients. In such patients with left ventricular systolic dysfunction, all efforts should be made to initiate, and maintain at appropriate doses, treatment with ACE inhibitors.

Aliskiren

It is now possible to interfere with most aspects of the RAAS. Aliskiren is a direct renin inhibitor: it binds to the active site of renin, thereby preventing access to angiotensinogen. Direct renin inhibition thus reduces production of both angiotensin I and II, and should not be compromised by 'ACE escape', the phenomenon by which angiotensin II is generated via non-ACE pathways from angiotensin I. Aliskiren is certainly an effective antihypertensive agent[41] and has been trialled in a number of clinical settings.

In ALTITUDE, 8561 patients with type 2 diabetes and renal impairment were randomized to receive aliskiren or placebo in addition to ACE inhibitor (or ARB).[42] This was an at-risk group without heart failure. Although there was no statistically significant difference between the two groups in the primary end-point (a composite of cardiovascular and renal endpoints) the trial was stopped early as there appeared to be a slight excess of adverse events in the aliskiren group.

In ASTRONAUT, 1639 patients hospitalized with heart failure were randomized to aliskiren or placebo with the aim of seeing whether aliskiren could reduce death or readmission rate.[43]

Aliskiren had no such effect: and, again, adverse events were more common with aliskiren. Repeated statistical testing of the data suggested that there might be a particularly bad outcome associated with aliskiren in people with diabetes, although the most likely explanation is surely chance due to multiple testing.

In ATMOSPHERE, >7000 patients were randomized to receive enalapril, aliskiren, or both.[44] Patients had heart failure with reduced ejection fraction (mean LVEF: 28%). There was no difference among the three groups in the primary end-point of death from cardiovascular causes or first hospitalization for heart failure, with patients in the combination limb having a greater risk of hypotension, decline in renal function and hyperkalaemia.

The conduct of ATMOSPHERE was controversial[45] as the regulators (but not the committee structures of the trial) required aliskiren to be stopped in patients with diabetes as a consequence of the effects seen in ALTITUDE and ASTRONAUT. It is doubtful whether the trial outcome was affected, but it certainly removed a high-risk tranche of patients. Nevertheless, it is difficult to see a role for aliskiren in the management of patients with heart failure in future.

Hydralazine and nitrates

Hydralazine is a direct-acting vasodilator, acting predominantly on the arterial side of the circulation. Nitrates are vasodilators with marked effects on the venous circulation. Used together, the combination therapy potentially offers balanced vasodilation, reducing both preload and afterload for the failing heart.

In the earliest large-scale mortality study for patients with CHF, 652 patients were randomized to receive therapy with the combination of hydralazine and isosorbide dinitrate, prazosin (an α-blocker), or placebo.[13] The study, known as VHeFT 1, showed a small benefit from the hydralazine and isosorbide dinitrate combination over the other limbs of the study.

The next step was VHeFT 2, in which 804 men with CHF were randomized to either the hydralazine and isosorbide dinitrate combination or enalapril.[46] Two-year mortality was significantly lower in patients randomized to enalapril than hydralazine/isosorbide dinitrate, although a striking finding was that combination therapy led to a greater improvement in exercise capacity than did enalapril.

Interest in the hydralazine/nitrate combination largely waned with the results of VHeFT 2. Hydralazine is a difficult drug to use, particularly as some subjects metabolize it slowly (slow acetylators) and are at risk of developing a lupus-like syndrome with its use. Both hydralazine and nitrates are otherwise metabolized rapidly and have to be given frequently to have an effect.

However, reviews of the VHeFT programme suggested that Black patients may have more to gain from hydralazine/nitrate therapy than White patients.[47] The AHeFT (African-American Heart Failure Trial) was thus constructed.[48] More than 1000 African-American patients were randomized to receive isosorbide dinitrate plus hydralazine or placebo in addition to standard therapy for heart failure. All the patients had dilated left ventricles, and nearly 80% were taking either an ACE inhibitor or angiotensin receptor antagonist at baseline. There was a significant improvement in outcome in patients treated with isosorbide dinitrate plus hydralazine.

A meta-analysis of the available data (including 2626 patients) suggests that combination treatment with isosorbide dinitrate plus hydralazine reduces mortality compared with placebo, but is less effective than ACE inhibitors.[49] There is no evidence to support the use of either nitrate or hydralazine as single agents.

The practical consequences are not clear-cut. The results lend support to the common practice of using hydralazine/isosorbide dinitrate in patients with CHF, who, for some reason, cannot tolerate ACE inhibitor or angiotensin receptor blocker. However, there is no clear-cut evidence that such an approach is appropriate in White patients. Equally, it is not clear whether all people with heart failure who identify themselves as Black should be offered hydralazine/isosorbide dinitrate.

Other vasodilators

An important finding from VHeFT 2 was that hydralazine/isosorbide dinitrate had a greater effect on exercise capacity than enalapril, although a lesser effect on mortality.[2] The finding emphasizes the importance of the neurohormonal hypothesis for heart failure—ACE inhibitors are not mediating their benefit primarily through vasodilation. Drugs with more pure vasodilating activity, such as flosequinan, do improve exercise capacity quite strikingly,[50] but are associated with a worse outcome.[51]

Amlodipine, a dihydropyridine calcium antagonist, has been extensively tested in heart failure. The PRAISE trial[52] suggested that amlodipine might be beneficial for patients with heart failure due to causes other than ischaemic heart disease. PRAISE-2 studied 1652 patients with severe heart failure and a normal coronary angiogram randomized to amlodipine or placebo.[53] There was no difference in outcome between the two groups. It is possible that the difference between PRAISE and PRAISE-2 is explained by a beneficial effect of amlodipine in patients with heart failure due to *occult* coronary heart disease: such patients in PRAISE would have been analysed together with patients with dilated cardiomyopathy as there was no requirement for coronary angiography in PRAISE, only PRAISE-2.

The general conclusion from the PRAISE study programme is that there is no routine role for calcium antagonists in patients with CHF, but that if a patient has angina or blood pressure difficult to control with standard heart failure medication, then amlodipine is a safe additional therapy.

REFERENCES

1. Nicholls GG, Riegger AJG. Renin in cardiac failure. In: Robertson JIS, Nicholls MG (eds), *The renin angiotensin system*, pp. 76.1–76.21. Gower Medical Publishing, London, 1993.
2. Pitt B, Poole-Wilson PA, Segal R, *et al.* Effects of losartan compared with captopril on mortality in patients with symptomatic heart failure: the Losartan Heart Failure Survival Study ELITE II. *Lancet* 2000;**355**:1582–7.
3. Dickstein K, Kjekshus J, and the OPTIMAAL Steering Committee. Effects of losartan and captopril on mortality and morbidity in high-risk patients after acute myocardial infarction: the OPTIMAAL randomised trial. *Lancet* 2002;**360**:752–60.
4. Pfeffer MA, McMurray JJ, Velazquez EJ, *et al.* Valsartan, captopril or both in myocardial infarction complicated by heart failure, left ventricular dysfunction, or both. *N Engl J Med* 2003;**349**:1893–906.
5. McMurray JJ, Packer M, Desai AS, *et al.*; PARADIGM-HF Investigators and Committees. Angiotensin–neprilysin inhibition versus enalapril in heart failure. *N Engl J Med* 2014;**371**:993–1004.
6. Cushman DW, Ondetti MA. Personal and historical perspectives: history of the design of captopril and related inhibitors of angiotensin converting enzyme. *Hypertension* 1991;**17**:589–92.
7. Johnston CI. Angiotensin converting enzyme inhibitors. In Robertson JIS, Nicholls MG (eds), *The renin angiotensin system*, pp 87.1–87.15. Gower Medical Publishing, London, 1993.
8. Squire IB, O'Kane KPJ, Anderson N, Reid JL. Bradykinin B2 receptor antagonism attenuates the blood pressure response to acute ACE inhibition in normal man. *Hypertension* 2000;**36**:132–6.
9. Packer M, Medina N, Yushak M, Meller J. Haemodynamic patterns of response during long-term captopril therapy for severe chronic heart failure. *Circulation* 1983;**68**:803–12.
10. Turini GA, Gribic M, Brunner HR, Waeber B, Gavras H. Improvement of chronic congestive heart failure by oral captopril. *Lancet* 1979;**I**:1213–15.
11. Dzau VJ, Colucci WS, Williams GH, *et al.* Sustained effectiveness of converting enzyme inhibition in patients with severe congestive heart failure. *N Engl J Med* 1980;**302**:1373–9.
12. Furberg CD, Yusuf S. Effect of vasodilators on survival in chronic congestive heart failure. *Am J Cardiol* 1985;**55**:1110–13.
13. Cohn J, Archibald DG, Ziesche S, *et al.* Effect of vasodilator therapy on mortality in chronic congestive heart failure. *N Engl J Med* 1986;**314**:1547–55.
14. Captopril Multicenter Research Group. A placebo controlled trial of captopril in refractory chronic congestive heart failure. *J Am Coll Cardiol* 1983;**2**:755–63.
15. CONSENSUS Trial Study Group. Effects of enalapril on mortality in severe congestive heart failure. Results of the cooperative North Scandinavian Enalapril Survival Study (CONSENSUS). *N Engl J Med* 1987;**316**:1429–5.
16. Swedberg K, Kjekshus J, Snappin S, for the CONSENSUS Investigators. Long term survival in severe heart failure patients treated with enalapril. 10 year follow up of CONSENSUS I. *Eur Heart J* 1999;**20**:136–9.
17. SOLVD Investigators. Effects of enalapril on survival in patients with reduced left ventricular ejection fractions and congestive heart failure. *N Engl J Med* 1991;**325**:293–302.
18. McAlister FA, Stewart S, Ferrua S, McMurray JJ. Multidisciplinary strategies for the management of heart failure patients at high risk of admission: a systematic review of randomised trials. *J Am Coll Cardiol* 2004;**44**:810–19.
19. SOLVD Investigators. Effect of enalapril on mortality and the development of heart failure in asymptomatic patients with reduced left ventricular ejection fractions. *N Engl J Med* 1992;**327**:685–91.
20. Swedberg K, Held P, Kjekshus J, *et al.*, on behalf of the CONSENSUS II Study Group. Effects of the early administration of enalapril on mortality in patients with acute myocardial infarction: results of the Cooperative New Scandinavian Enalapril Survival Study II (CONSENSUS II). *N Engl J Med* 1992;**327**:678–84.
21. Gruppo Italiano per lo Studio della Sopravvivenza nell'Infarto Miocardico. ISSI-3: effects of lisinopril and transdermal glyceryl trinitrate singly and together on 6-week mortality and

ventricular function after acute myocardial infarction. *Lancet* 1994;**343**:1115–22.

22. ISIS-4 Collaborative Group. ISIS-4: a randomised factorial trial assessing early oral captopril, oral mononitrate, and intravenous magnesium sulphate in 58050 patients with suspected acute myocardial infarction. *Lancet* 1995;**345**:669–85.

23. Chinese Cardiac Study Collaborative Group. Oral captopril versus placebo among 13,634 patients with suspected acute myocardial infarction: interim report from the Chinese Cardiac Study (CCS-1). *Lancet* 1995;**345**:686–7.

24. ACE Inhibitor Myocardial Infarction Collaborative Group. Indications for ACE inhibitors in the early treatment of acute myocardial infarction; systematic overview of individual data from 100 000 patients in randomized trials. *Circulation* 1998;**97**:2202–12.

25. Pfeffer MA, Braunwald E, Moyé L, et al. Effect of captopril on mortality and morbidity in patients with left ventricular dysfunction after myocardial infarction: results of the survival and ventricular enlargement trial. *N Engl J Med* 1992;**327**:669–77.

26. Acute Infarction Ramipril Efficacy (AIRE) Study Investigators. Effect of ramipril on mortality and morbidity of survivors of acute myocardial infarction with clinical evidence of heart failure. *Lancet* 1993;**342**:821–28.

27. Kober L, Torp-Pedersen C, Carlsen JE, et al. A clinical trial of the angiotensin-converting-enzyme inhibitor trandolapril in patients with left ventricular dysfunction after myocardial infarction. *N Engl J Med* 1995;**333**:1670–76.

28. Flather MD, Yusuf S, Køber L, et al. Long-term ACE-inhibitor therapy in patients with heart failure or left-ventricular dysfunction: a systematic overview of data from individual patients *Lancet* 2000;**355**:1575–81.

29. Task Force for the diagnosis and treatment of acute and chronic heart failure of the European Society of Cardiology. 2016 ESC Guidelines for the diagnosis and treatment of acute and chronic heart failure 2016. *Eur Heart J* 2016;**37**:2129–200.

30. National Institute for Health and Clinical Excellence. *Chronic heart failure in adults*. 2010. https://nice.org.uk/guidance/cg108

31. Cohn JN, Johnson G, Ziesche S, et al. A comparison of enalapril with hydralazine–isosorbide dinitrate in the treatment of chronic congestive heart failure. *N Engl J Med* 1991;**325**:303–10.

32. Pitt B, Segal R, Martinez FA, et al. Randomised trial of losartan versus captopril in patients over 65 with heart failure. *Lancet* 1997;**349**:747–52.

33. Pitt B, Poole-Wilson PA, Segal R, et al. Effect of losartan compared with captopril on mortality in patients with symptomatic heart failure: randomised trial—the Losartan Heart Failure Survival Study ELITE II. *Lancet* 2000;**355**:1582–87.

34. Dickstein K, Kjekshus J, and the OPTIMAAL Steering Committee. Effects of losartan and captopril on mortality and morbidity in high-risk patients after acute myocardial infarction: the OPTIMAAL randomised trial. *Lancet* 2002;**360**:752–60.

35. Pfeffer MA, McMurray JJV, Velazquez EJ, et al. Valsartan, captopril or both in myocardial infarction complicated by heart failure, left ventricular dysfunction, or both. *N Engl J Med* 2003;**349**:1893–906.

36. Beldhuis IE, Streng KW, Ter Maaten JM, et al. Renin–angiotensin system inhibition, worsening renal function, and outcome in heart failure patients with reduced and preserved ejection fraction: a meta-analysis of published study data. *Circ Heart Fail* 2017;**10**(2). pii: e003588.

37. McLay JS, McMurray J, Bridges A, Struthers AD. Practical issues when initiating captopril therapy in chronic heart failure. *Eur Heart J* 1992;**13**:1521–7.

38. Packer M, Lee WH, Yushak M, Medina N. Comparison of captopril and enalapril in patients with severe chronic heart failure. *N Engl J Med* 1986;**315**:847–53.

39. Murray L, Squire IB, Reid JL, Lees KR. Determinants of the blood pressure response to the first dose of ACE inhibitor in mild to moderate congestive heart failure. *Br J Clin Pharmacol* 1998;**45**:559–66.

40. Ishani A, Weinhandl E, Zhao Z, et al. Angiotensin converting enzyme inhibitor as a risk factor for the development of anaemia, and the impact of incident anaemia on mortality in patients with left ventricular dysfunction. *J Am Coll Cardiol* 2005;**45**:391–9.

41. Gradman AH, Schmieder RE, Lins RL, et al. Aliskiren, a novel orally effective renin inhibitor, provides dose-dependent antihypertensive efficacy and placebo-like tolerability in hypertensive patients. *Circulation* 2005;**111**:1012–18.

42. Parving HH, Brenner BM, McMurray JJ, et al.; ALTITUDE Investigators. Cardiorenal end points in a trial of aliskiren for type 2 diabetes. *N Engl J Med* 2012;**367**:2204–13.

43. Gheorghiade M, Bohm M, Greene SJ, et al. Effect of aliskiren on postdischarge mortality and heart failure readmissions among patients hospitalized for heart failure: the ASTRONAUT randomized trial. *JAMA* 2013;**309**:1125–35.

44. McMurray JJ, Krum H, Abraham WT, et al.; ATMOSPHERE Committees Investigators. Aliskiren, enalapril, or aliskiren and enalapril in heart failure. *N Engl J Med* 2016;**374**:1521–32.

45. Swedberg K, Borer JS, Pitt B, Pocock S, Rouleau J. Challenges to data monitoring committees when regulatory authorities intervene. *N Engl J Med* 2016;**374**:1580–4.

46. Cohn JN, Johnson G, Ziesche S, et al. A comparison of enalapril with hydralazine–isosorbide dinitrate in the treatment of chronic congestive heart failure. *N Engl J Med* 1991;**325**:303–10.

47. Carson P, Ziesche S, Johnson G, Cohn JN. Racial differences in response to therapy for heart failure: analysis of the vasodilator heart failure trials. *J Card Fail* 1999;**5**:178–187.

48. Taylor AL, Ziesche S, Yancy C, et al.; African-American Heart Failure Trial Investigators. Combination of isosorbide dinitrate and hydralazine in blacks with heart failure. *N Engl J Med* 2004;**351**:2049–57.

49. Farag M, Mabote T, Shoaib A, et al. Hydralazine and nitrates alone or combined for the management of chronic heart failure: a systematic review. *Int J Cardiol* 2015;**196**:61–9.

50. Cowley AJ, Wynne RD, Stainer K, et al. Flosequinan in heart failure: acute haemodynamic and longer term symptomatic effects. *Br Med J* 1988;**297**:169–73.

51. Packer M, Rouleau J, Swedberg K, et al. Effect of flosequinan on survival in chronic heart failure: preliminary results of the PROFILE study. *Circulation* 1993;**88**(Suppl 1):301.

52. Packer M, O'Connor CM, Ghali JK, et al. Effect of amlodipine on morbidity and mortality in severe chronic heart failure. Prospective Randomized Amlodipine Survival Evaluation Study Group. *N Engl J Med* 1996;**335**:1107–14.

53. Thackray S, Witte K, Clark AL, Cleland JG. Clinical trials update: OPTIME-CHF, PRAISE-2, ALL-HAT. *Eur J Heart Fail* 2000;**2**:209–12.

49

Angiotensin receptor blockers and angiotensin receptor–neprilysin inhibitors

John McMurray

Angiotensin receptor blockers

Angiotensin receptor blockers (ARBs) or angiotensin II receptor antagonists were introduced as a potentially superior alternative to an angiotensin converting enzyme (ACE) inhibitor and, later, as a possible addition to an ACE inhibitor.[1]

Unlike ACE inhibitors which block the generation of angiotensin II from angiotensin I, ARBs antagonize the action of angiotensin II at the angiotensin II type 1 receptor. This receptor mediates the known actions of angiotensin II considered harmful in heart failure, e.g. vasoconstriction and sodium retention.[1]

Theoretically, ARBs should be more effective than ACE inhibitors at blocking the actions of angiotensin II, as angiotensin II can be generated by enzymes other than ACE, such as chymase.[1] Renin–angiotensin system (RAS) 'escape' has been described in patients treated chronically with an ACE inhibitor, possibly because of the existence of alternative enzymatic pathways or simply through substrate (angiotensin I) accumulation. ARBs should also be better tolerated than ACE inhibitors because of a lower risk of cough and angioedema related to bradykinin. ACE, also known as kininase II, is one of the enzymes responsible for the breakdown of bradykinin.[1] However, bradykinin is also a powerful vasodilator, inhibits pathological growth, and has fibrinolytic actions. The potentially incomplete blockade of the RAS by ACE inhibitors, but possibly beneficial action of enhancing bradykinin, provided the rationale for combining an ACE inhibitor and ARB.[1] That ARBs were developed after ACE inhibitors had become evidence-based 'standard of care' in heart failure with reduced ejection fraction (HFrEF) made clinical evaluation of ARBs in these patients challenging. Essentially, three approaches could be considered: (1) a head-to-head comparison with an ACE inhibitor; (2) a placebo-controlled comparison in patients intolerant of an ACE inhibitor; and (3) addition of an ARB to an ACE inhibitor (compared with an ACE inhibitor alone).[2–8] These strategies were tested in ELITE-2 (approach 1), the CHARM Programme (approaches 2 and 3), and

Val-HeFT (approach 3) in patients with HFrEF (Tables 49.1–49.3). Parallel trials in patients with heart failure, left ventricular systolic dysfunction, or both, after myocardial infarction also examined these strategies: OPTIMAAL (approach 1), and VALIANT (approaches 1 and 3).[9,10] Later trials examined similar strategies in patients with other types of cardiovascular disease and chronic kidney disease (Tables 49.1–49.3).[11,12]

In patients with heart failure with preserved ejection fraction (HFpEF) no 'standard of care' exists and, therefore, ARBs were compared with placebo in unselected patients in CHARM-Preserved (one of the three trials in the CHARM Programme) and in I-Preserve.[8,13]

Table 49.1 Trials comparing renin–angiotensin receptor inhibitor monotherapies

Trial	Control	New therapy	Superiority?	Non-inferiority?
HFrEF				
ELITE-2	Captopril 50 mg tid	Losartan 50 mg qd	No	No
ATMOSPHERE	Enalapril 10 mg bid	Aliskiren 300 mg qd	No	No
PARADIGM-HF	Enalapril 10 mg bid	Sacubitril/valsartan 97/103 mg bid	Yes	-
Myocardial infarction				
OPTIMAAL	Captopril 50 mg tid	Losartan 50 mg qd	No	No
VALIANT	Captopril 50 mg tid	Valsartan 160 mg bid	No	Yes
Other				
ONTARGET	Ramipril 10 mg qd	Telmisartan 80 mg qd	No	Yes

Table 49.2 Trials adding a second renin–angiotensin receptor inhibitor to a first

Trial	Mandated evidence-based dose of ACE inhibitor/ARB?	Add-on treatment	Superiority?
HFrEF			
Val-HeFT	No	Valsartan 160 mg bid	Yes
CHARM-Added	No	Candesartan 32 mg qd	Yes
ASTRONAUT	No	Aliskiren 300 mg qd	No
ATMOSPHERE	Yes (enalapril 10 mg bid)	Aliskiren 300 mg qd	No
Myocardial infarction			
VALIANT	Yes (captopril 50 mg tid)	Valsartan 80 mg bid	No
Other			
ON-TARGET	Yes (ramipril 10 mg qd)	Telmisartan 80 mg qd	No
ALTITUDE	No	Aliskiren 300 mg qd	No
VA-NEPHRON-D	Yes (losartan 100 mg qd)	Lisinopril (40 mg qd)	No

ELITE-2

Following favourable findings in a pilot trial, ELITE-2 was designed to compare the effect of losartan 50 mg once daily with captopril 50 mg thrice daily on death from any cause. After a median follow-up of 1.52 years, 280 out of 1578 losartan patients died, compared with 250 out of 1574 patients (hazard ratio (HR): 1.13; 95% confidence interval (CI): 0.95–1.35; P = 0.16). There were 270 versus 293 hospitalizations for heart failure, respectively (HR: 0.92; 95% CI: 0.78–1.08; P = 0.32). Losartan was neither superior nor non-inferior to captopril. The acute myocardial infarction trial comparing the same

Table 49.3 Mean dose of enalapril used in pivotal trials.

Trial	No. in enalapril group	Target dose (mg)	Mean daily dose (mg)
CONSENSUS (1987)[a]	127	20 bid	18.4
SOLVD-T (1991)[b]	1284	10 bid	16.6
SOLVD-P (1992)	2111	10 bid	16.7
V-HeFT II (1991)	403	10 bid	15.0
OVERTURE (2002)	2884	10 bid	17.7
CARMEN (2004)	190 enalapril only 191 enalapril plus carvedilol	10 bid 10 bid	16.8 14.9
CIBIS-3 (2005)	190 enalapril first 191 bisoprolol first	10 bid 10 bid	17.2 15.8
PARADIGM-HF (2014)	4212	10 bid	18.9
ATMOSPHERE (2016)	2336 enalapril only 2340 enalapril plus aliskiren	5–10 bid 5–10 bid	18.6 19.1

[a] 22% reached target dose.
[b] Active run-in; 49% reached target dose.

treatments (OPTIMAAL) reached similar conclusions. Subsequent positive trials in hypertension and chronic kidney disease (CKD) with a higher dose of losartan (100 mg once daily) raised the possibility that 50 mg once daily was a suboptimal dose. A second trial in HFrEF (HEAAL)[14] was designed to compare the effect of 150 mg of losartan once daily with 50 mg daily on a primary composite outcome of death from any cause of heart failure hospitalization. After a median follow-up of 4.7 years, 828 out of 1921 patients in the 150 mg group experienced a primary end-point, compared with 889 of 1913 in the 50 mg group (HR: 0.90; 95% CI: 0.82–0.99; P = 0.027). The number of deaths in each group was 635 and 665, respectively (HR: 0.94; 95% CI: 0.84–1.04; P = 0.24); the number of patients hospitalized with heart failure was 450 and 503, respectively (HR: 0.87; 95% CI: 0.76–0.98; P = 0.025).

Although not definitive, collectively these findings suggest that, dosed adequately, ARBs probably have similar benefits to those of an ACE inhibitor. This conclusion is supported by the findings of CHARM-Alternative.

CHARM-Alternative

The second approach to evaluating the potential value of ARBs in HFrEF was to compare this new treatment with an ACE inhibitor. In CHARM-Alternative, 2028 such individuals were randomized to candesartan 32 mg once daily or placebo, and followed for a median of 2.8 years. Among the 1013 patients assigned to candesartan, 334 experienced the primary end-point of death from cardiovascular causes or heart failure hospitalization. In the placebo group, 406 out of 1015 patients experienced this outcome (HR: 0.77; 95% CI: 0.67–0.89; P = 0.0004). The number of deaths was 265 and 296, respectively (HR: 0.87; 95% CI: 0.74–1.03; P = 0.11) and the number of heart failure hospitalizations was 207 compared with 286, respectively (HR: 0.68; 95% CI: 0.57–0.81; P < 0.0001). As expected, and as seen with ACE inhibitors, there was an excess of hypotension, renal dysfunction and hyperkalaemia in the candesartan group (although no increase in cough).

Val-HeFT and CHARM-Added

Two trials evaluated the approach of adding an ARB to an ACE inhibitor. In Val-HeFT, valsartan 160 mg twice daily was used and candesartan 32 mg once daily was tested in CHARM-Added. Crucially, as it turns out in retrospect, neither trial mandated use of a full, evidence-based, dose of background ACE inhibitor (although the acute infarction trial VALIANT and later trials in patients with other cardiovascular disease and CKD did). In Val-HeFT, 495 out of 2511 valsartan-treated patients died from any cause compared with 484 out of 2499 patients in the placebo group (relative risk (RR): 1.02; 95% CI: 0.88–1.18; P = 0.80) after a mean follow-up of 23 months. The number experiencing a co-primary composite outcome (death, hospitalization for heart failure, cardiac arrest with resuscitation or worsening heart failure treated with intravenous therapy) was 723 and 801, respectively (RR: 0.87; 95% CI: 0.77–0.97; P = 0.009). The number of individuals hospitalized with worsening heart failure was 349 and 463, respectively (HR: 0.725; 95% CI: 0.63–0.83; P = 0.0001).

In CHARM-Added, the primary end-point was a composite of death from cardiovascular causes or hospitalization for heart failure and the median follow-up was 41 months. Of the 1276 patients assigned to candesartan, 483 experienced the primary

outcome, compared with 538 patients in the placebo group (HR: 0.85; 95% CI: 0.75–0.96; *P* = 0.011). The number of deaths from any cause was 377 versus 412, respectively (HR: 0.89; 95% CI: 0.77–1.02; *P* = 0.086). The number of patients hospitalized with heart failure was 309 compared with 356, respectively (HR: 0.83; 95% CI: 0.71–0.96; *P* = 0.014).

Subgroup analysis of Val-HeFT suggested no incremental benefit of adding valsartan to full-dose ACE inhibition whereas the opposite was found in CHARM-Added. In the add-on arm of VALIANT, which had a different design, mandating full-dose background captopril treatment, valsartan did not reduce risk further and the same was found in other combination therapy trials in different disease areas. In retrospect, CHARM-Added seems the outlier with a more recent trial in HFrEF, using a direct renin inhibitor (aliskiren) showing no incremental benefit of combination treatment when aliskiren was added to full-dose enalapril. Interestingly, in that trial (ATMOSPHERE)[15] there were more adverse effects, i.e. there does seem to be an efficacy ceiling for RAS blockade in HFrEF above which there is no additional benefit and only harm. In summary, adequate dosing of RAS blockers is important to maximize benefit (as suggested by both the ATLAS[16] and HEAAL trials). An ARB probably has the same benefit as an ACE inhibitor. There is no value in adding an ARB to a full dose of ACE inhibitor.

CHARM-Preserved and I-Preserve

Two trials compared an ARB with placebo in patients with HFpEF. In CHARM-Preserved, the primary end-point was the composite of cardiovascular death or heart failure hospitalization and the median follow-up was 36.6 months. Of the 1514 patients assigned to candesartan 32 mg once daily, 333 experienced the primary end-point, compared with 366 in the placebo group (HR: 0.89; 95% CI: 0.77–1.03; *P* = 0.118). The number of deaths from any cause was 244 and 237, respectively (HR: 1.02; 95% CI: 0.85–1.22; *P* = 0.84). The number of hospitalizations for heart failure was 241 and 276, respectively (HR: 0.85; 95% CI: 0.72–1.01; *P* = 0.072). Secondary and post-hoc exploratory analyses suggested that candesartan did reduce the risk of heart failure hospitalization.[17]

In I-PRESERVE, 4128 patients were assigned to irbesartan 300 mg once daily or placebo and followed for a mean of 49.5 months for the primary composite outcome of death from any cause or cardiovascular hospitalization (heart failure, myocardial infarction, unstable angina, arrhythmia, or stroke). Of the 2067 patients assigned to irbesartan, 742 experienced the primary outcome compared with 763 in the placebo group (HR: 0.95; 95% CI: 0.86–1.05; *P* = 0.35). The number of deaths from any cause was 445 and 436, respectively (HR: 1.00; 95% CI: 0.88–1.14; *P* = 0.98). The number of patients hospitalized with heart failure was 325 and 336, respectively (HR: 0.95; 95% CI: 0.81–1.10; *P* = 0.50). Irbesartan had no clear benefit on any outcome in this trial.

It is unclear whether these trials really differ in outcome. CHARM-Preserved included patients with an ejection fraction >40% whereas I-Preserve had a higher entry cut-off at ≥45%. Candesartan 32 mg once daily probably gives more intense inhibition of the RAS than irbesartan 300 mg.[18] Recent retrospective analysis of the CHARM trials, in conjunction with similar analyses of other trials, have suggested that ARBs (and additional drugs modulating neurohumoral activity) may be of benefit in patients with heart failure and mildly reduced ejection fraction (HFmrEF).[19,20]

Neprilysin inhibition

In 1981, de Bold and colleagues demonstrated that atrial extracts stimulated urinary sodium and water excretion.[21] This led to the subsequent identification and characterization of the natriuretic peptides, which constitute an endogenous neurohumoral system with diuretic, natriuretic, vasodilating, and growth-inhibiting properties (including inhibition of pathological growth such as hypertrophy and fibrosis). There has long been interest in harnessing the potential benefits of natriuretic peptides in heart failure.[22] Conceptually, this represents a complementary approach to inhibition of the harmful anti-natriuretic, vasoconstrictor, and pathological growth-promoting systems (such as the renin–angiotensin–aldosterone and sympathetic nervous systems), a strategy that has been very successful and which underpins the current pharmacological approach to treating HFrEF.[22] The key question was how to augment natriuretic peptides?

Neprilysin is a membrane-bound endopeptidase found in many tissues, particularly in the kidney.[23] Neprilysin hydrolyses A-type, B-type, and C-type natriuretic peptide (and possibly urodilatin).[24] The enzyme is known by several other names including enkephalinase, neutral endopeptidase 24.11 (NEP), vasopeptidase, and atriopeptidase. Degradation by neprilysin is one of the two major means of elimination of natriuretic peptides, the other being through a clearance receptor (the natriuretic peptide clearance receptor: NPRC or NPR3). Inhibition of neprilysin, therefore, enhances endogenous natriuretic peptide levels.

Although neprilysin inhibitors were originally designed to augment natriuretic peptides, it is now recognized that several other vasoactive substances are metabolized by this enzyme.[25–30] The most obvious of these is bradykinin which can be considered a 'double-edged sword' in heart failure, as described in relation to ACE inhibitors, ARBs and omapatrilat. Other postulated substrates for neprilysin include adrenomedullin, substance P and calcitonin gene-related peptide (other powerful vasodilators), vasoactive intestinal polypeptide, and enkephalins (**Figure 49.1**).[31,32–35] Of recent interest is apelin, an endogenous peptide made in the myocardium which has positive inotropic actions and which seems to be reduced in advanced heart failure.[36] Also of note is glucagon-like peptide-1

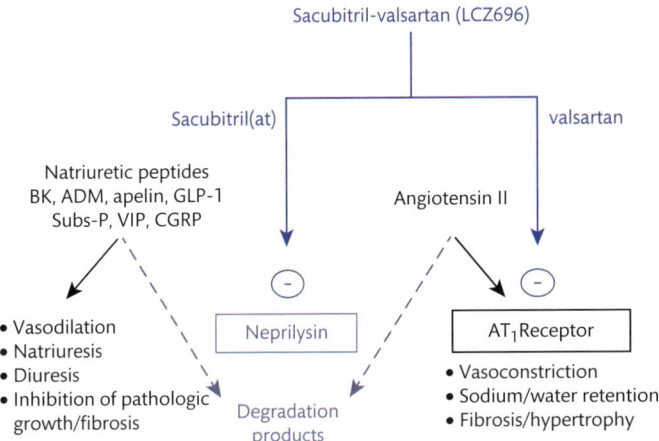

Figure 49.1 Mechanism of action of LCZ696 (sacubitril/valsartan). ADM, adrenomedullin; AT$_1$, angiotensin II type 1; BK, bradykinin; CGRP, calcitonin gene-related peptide; GLP-1, glucagon-like peptide-1; Subs-P, substance P; VIP, vasoactive intestinal (poly)peptide.

(GLP-1) which lowers blood glucose and is a therapeutic target in diabetes.[37] Neprilysin is one of several mechanisms clearing amyloid-β peptides from the central nervous system.[38] As accumulation of these peptides in the brain is implicated in the development of Alzheimer's disease, there has been concern about the potential neurotoxicity of neprilysin inhibitors, a question addressed later in this section.

Neprilysin inhibitors

Two seminal reports in 1989 demonstrated that acute inhibition of neprilysin with oral racecadotril (formerly known as acetorphan) and intravenous candoxatrilat (UK 69579) increased circulating atrial natriuretic peptide levels and urinary sodium excretion in humans.[25,27] Candoxatrilat also reduced right atrial pressure and pulmonary capillary wedge pressure in patients with heart failure (and blood pressure in patients with hypertension).[25] Subsequently, ecadotril (formerly known as sinorphan), the (S)-isomer of acetorphan, was shown to have similar acute haemodynamic effects to candoxatril.[28] Disappointingly, chronic dosing with candoxatril (the orally active pro-drug of candoxatrilat) did not produce a sustained reduction in blood pressure, leading to termination of the development of this agent which was primarily being developed as an antihypertensive.[28] Subsequently it was shown that neprilysin also breaks down angiotensin II[29-31] and that, by increasing levels of this peptide, neprilysin inhibition may cause vasoconstriction, offsetting the vasodilator actions of augmented natriuretic peptides (and other vasodilators).

ACE–neprilysin inhibition

One potential solution to this problem was combined inhibition of ACE and neprilysin, and a series of compounds of this type were developed, the lead example of which was omapatrilat.[39-42] Omapatrilat was shown to have sustained, favourable, haemodynamic, and neurohumoral actions but used in a single daily dose of 40 mg once daily was not superior to enalapril 10 mg twice daily in a head-to-head comparison in patients with chronic HFrEF in the Omapatrilat Versus Enalapril Randomized Trial of Utility in Reducing Events trial (OVERTURE).[40-42] However, although omapatrilat reduced the main secondary outcome of death from any cause of cardiovascular hospitalization by 9% (nominal $P = 0.024$)[42] and in a post-hoc analysis using investigator reported (rather than end-point committee-adjudicated) heart failure hospitalization, the primary composite outcome was also reduced by 11% (nominal $P = 0.012$). These findings and concerns about the dosing strategy (once daily administration of a large dose of omapatrilat causing excessive initial hypotension and not providing sustained ACE or neprilysin inhibition over 24 h) left open the possibility that a strategy of combined neprilysin and renin–angiotensin inhibition might still be useful in HFrEF. However, omapatrilat caused angioedema that was quite common and sometimes life-threatening, leading to termination of the clinical development of this agent (and related compounds in the class).[43] Although both ACE and neprilysin metabolize bradykinin, it had not been expected that inhibition of both enzymes would lead to sufficient bradykinin accumulation to cause the angioedema problem observed. As it turned out, omapatrilat also inhibited aminopeptidase P, a third key enzyme involved in bradykinin metabolism.[44]

Angiotensin receptor neprilysin inhibition

The development of the angiotensin receptor–neprilysin inhibitor (ARNI) sacubitril/valsartan (formerly known as LCZ696) allowed another test of the hypothesis explored in the OVERTURE.[45-47]

However, because sacubitril/valsartan blocked the angiotensin II type 1 receptor rather than ACE, and because sacubitrilat (LBQ657), the active metabolite of sacubitril (AHU377), did not inhibit aminopeptidase P, the risk of angioedema was considered to be less than with omapatrilat (**Figure 49.1**).[45-47] LCZ696 was also developed to be prescribed twice daily ensuring sustained neprilysin and RAS inhibition over the 24 h period.[45-48] The dose of target dose of sacubitril/valsartan used, 97/103 mg twice daily (LCZ696 200 mg twice daily) delivers plasma levels of valsartan equivalent to 160 mg twice daily (i.e. the evidence-based dose) also results in near-complete inhibition of neprilysin.[45-47]

PARADIGM-HF

The Prospective comparison of ARNI with ACEI to Determine Impact on Global Mortality and morbidity in Heart Failure trial (PARADIGM-HF) tested whether sacubitril/valsartan 200 mg (97/103 mg) twice daily was superior to enalapril 10 mg twice daily in reducing the primary end-point which was a composite of cardiovascular death or heart failure hospitalization over a median follow-up of 27 months.[48-50] All patients completed a run-in period of 6–8 weeks during which patients had to tolerate enalapril 10 mg twice daily and then sacubitril/valsartan 200 mg twice daily before randomization. The average dose of enalapril taken in the ACE inhibitor group was greater than in either Cooperative North Scandinavian Enalapril Survival Study (CONSENSUS) or the Studies of Left Ventricular Dysfunction (SOLVD) (**Table 49.3**).

PARADIGM-HF was terminated early, on the recommendation of the Data Monitoring Committee, due to a sustained and highly significant reduction in the risk of the primary end-point and in cardiovascular mortality in the sacubitril/valsartan group compared with the enalapril group. At the end of the trial, there was a 20% relative risk reduction in the primary end-point and each of its components, as well as a 16% reduction in all-cause mortality (**Figure 49.2**). The two major modes of cardiovascular death, sudden death, and death from worsening heart failure were equally and significantly reduced.[51] Both first hospitalizations for heart failure and total (including repeat) hospitalizations were also reduced by 21% and 23% respectively (**Figure 49.2**).[52] PARADIGM-HF showed that, for every 1000 patients switched from enalapril to sacubitril/valsartan, over a median of 27 months there were 47 fewer patients with a primary end-point (cardiovascular death or heart failure hospitalization), 33 fewer cardiovascular deaths, 28 fewer first hospital admissions for heart failure (53 fewer hospitalizations for heart failure overall, including repeat episodes) and 32 fewer deaths from any cause. There was no convincing or consistent heterogeneity in treatment benefit in any of the pre-specified subgroups.[50] Subsequent analyses of PARADIGM-HF have confirmed that the relative reductions in morbidity and mortality and differential rates of adverse events were similar across all age categories and across the spectrum of baseline risk.[53,54]

There was no statistically significant difference in the occurrence of angioedema between treatment groups, although numerically more cases were observed in the sacubitril/valsartan group, compared with the enalapril group (19 patients in the sacubitril/valsartan group and 10 cases in the enalapril group; $P = 0.13$).[50] Hypotension was significantly more common with sacubitril/valsartan than with enalapril (14% vs 9% in the in the sacubitril/valsartan and enalapril groups respectively; $P < 0.001$), although this rarely led to study-drug discontinuation (0.9% and 0.7% in the sacubitril/valsartan and

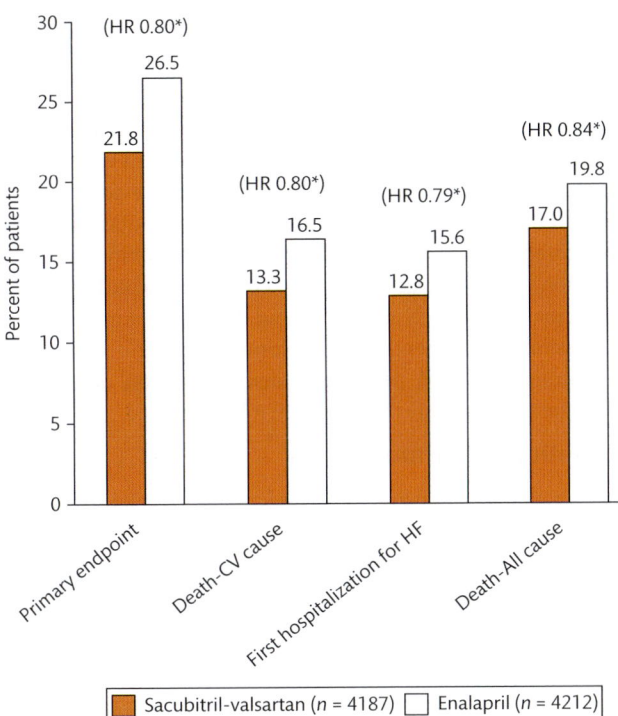

Figure 49.2 Summary of the clinical benefits of sacubitril valsartan (formerly known as LCZ696) over enalapril in PARADIGM-HF. CV, cardiovascular; HFH, heart failure; HR, hazard ratio.

enalapril groups, respectively; $P = 0.38$) (**Figure 49.3**). Conversely, renal dysfunction, hyperkalaemia, and cough were less common with sacubitril/valsartan than with enalapril. Dementia and cognition-related adverse effects were not increased by sacubitril/valsartan in PARADIGM-HF.[55] Many additional analyses from

PARADIGM-HF have been published and a useful summary has been published recently.[56]

Regulatory approval and statistical robustness of results

Regulatory approval of a new drug requires demonstration of effectiveness and safety in either two trials with two-sided $P < 0.05$ or a single, large, internally consistent, multicentre study with $P < 0.00125$.[31] PARADIGM-HF met these criteria. It was large (8399 patients randomized), highly statistically significant ($P = 0.0000004$), internally consistent (lack of subgroup interaction), multicentre (sites were located in 47 countries), and there were large effects on morbidity and mortality (as described above). Even if the argument that it would be unethical to repeat PARADIGM-HF was ignored, to achieve such a statistically significant result for the primary end-point would require four or five trials each with $P < 0.05$ to have the same strength of evidence as provided by a single trial with $P = 0.0000004$.[57]

Which patients with HFrEF should be prescribed sacubitril/valsartan?

The most substantial data on the use of sacubitril/valsartan are in ambulatory patients as these were the only individuals enrolled in PARADIGM-HF. Therefore, that trial provides the best guide to the use of this treatment. The key inclusion and exclusion criteria for PARADIGM-HF were: NYHA functional class II–IV and a reduced ejection fraction (≤40%), receiving a β-blocker and mineralocorticoid receptor antagonist (MRA) as recommended by guidelines, with a systolic blood pressure of ≥100 mmHg and estimated glomerular filtration rate (eGFR) ≥30 mL/min/1.73 m^2 and potassium ≤5.2 mmol/L. The US Food and Drug Administration (FDA) and European Medicines Agency (EMA) product labelling reflects these critieria. The trial had additional enrolment criteria: patients had to have BNP ≥150 pg/mL (NT-proBNP ≥600 pg/mL) or, if hospitalized with heart failure, BNP ≥100 pg/mL (NT-proBNP ≥400 pg/

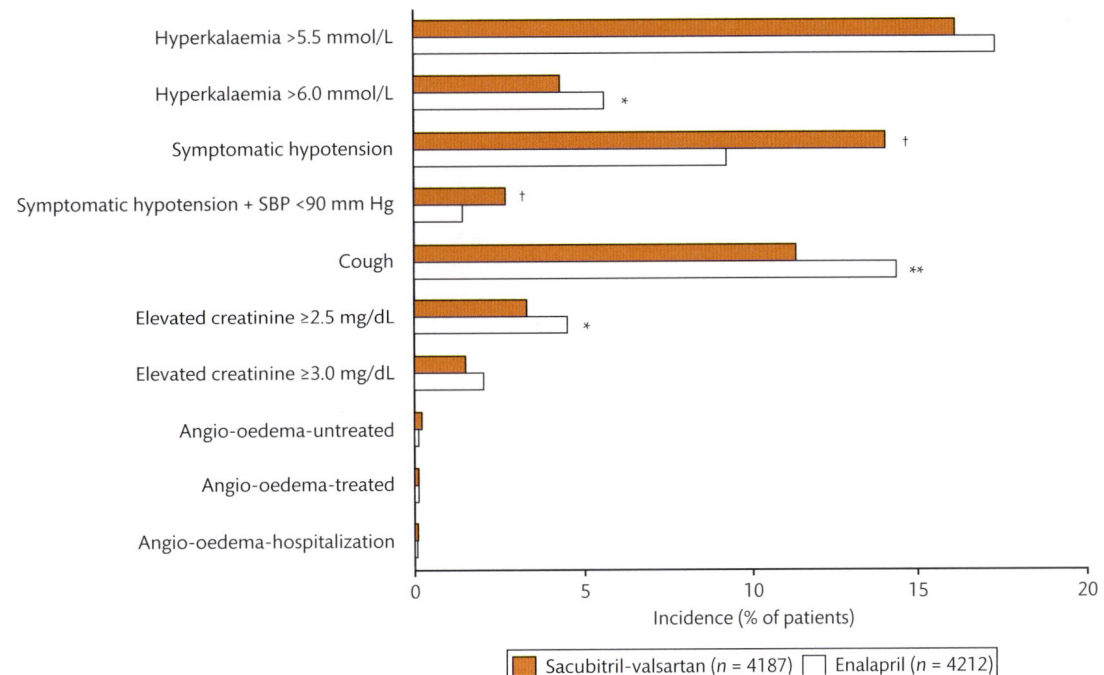

Figure 49.3 Summary of the adverse events after randomization in PARADIGM-HF: comparison of sacubitril/valsartan (formerly known as LCZ696) with enalapril. SBP, systolic blood pressure.

mL) although these are not part of the FDA or EMA labelling, presumably because most patients with HFrEF exceed these thresholds. Moreover, there was no interaction between baseline natriuretic peptide concentration and the effect of treatment and there is no biological basis for assuming that sacubitril/valsartan would lose its effectiveness below these thresholds.[58] The Comparison of Sacubitril–Valsartan versus Enalapril on Effect on NT-proBNP in Patients Stabilized from an Acute Heart Failure Episode (PIONEER-HF) was a second trial comparing sacubitril/valsartan to enalapril. It was conducted among 881 patients with HFrEF hospitalized for worsening heart failure. Although relatively small and short-term (double-blind randomized treatment given for 8 weeks), PIONEER-HF demonstrated the feasibility and safety of initiating treatment with sacubitril/valsartan in hospital. PIONEER-HF was also important because around a third of patients enrolled had new onset heart failure and about half were not treated with an ACE inhibitor or ARB.[59]

When should sacubitril/valsartan be prescribed?

Patients in PARADIGM-HF were treated with an ACE inhibitor or ARB before enrolment and there is a lack of evidence about the effects of sacubitril/valsartan in ACE inhibitor (or ARB)-naive patients. The European Society of Cardiology (ESC) guidelines recommend that patients should be treated with an ACE inhibitor (or ARB) for at least one month before considering switching to sacubitril/valsartan, in keeping with the conduct of PARADIGM-HF.[60] However, the FDA labelling permits initiation of sacubitril/valsartan in ACE inhibitor/ARB-naive patients. Other guidance is consistent with this more liberal approach.[61]

The other significant inconsistency between guidelines reflects the sequencing of treatments. Not only do the ESC guidelines recommend prior treatment with an ACE inhibitor (or ARB) before switching to sacubitril/valsartan, but they also advise addition of MRA to background ACE inhibitor/ARB (and β-blocker) therapy before considering switching to sacubitril/valsartan. This is not required in the US guidelines. The demonstration that hyperkalaemia is more common with the combination of MRA and ACE inhibitor/ARB than with the combination of MRA and sacubitril/valsartan may argue against the recommended ESC sequencing.[62]

How should sacubitril/valsartan be prescribed?

Sacubitril/valsartan should not be given in conjunction with another ARB or renin inhibitor (because of the risk of renal impairment and hyperkalaemia), or an ACE inhibitor (risk of renal impairment, hyperkalaemia, and angioedema). Due to the potential risk of angioedema when used concurrently with an ACE inhibitor, sacubitril/valsartan must not be started for at least 36 h after discontinuing an ACE inhibitor.[58,60] The starting dose of sacubitril/valsartan is usually 100 mg (49/51 mg) twice daily. This can be reduced in potentially vulnerable groups to 50 mg (24/26 mg) twice daily, e.g. those with a low systolic blood pressure (<10 mmHg), renal impairment (eGFR <60 mL/min/1.73 m^2) or a higher potassium (≥5 mmol/L) and those not already taking the equivalent of enalapril 10 mg daily. The dose should be doubled every 2–4 weeks as tolerated by the patient to the target dose of 200 mg (97/103 mg) twice daily.[63]

Patients should also be prescribed other evidence-based drugs (β-blocker, SGLT2 inhibitor, MRA, ivabradine, and digoxin) and devices (cardiac resynchronization therapy, implantable cardioverter–defibrillator), as appropriate.

Adverse effects and cautions

Patients should be monitored for symptoms of hypotension, and non-disease-modifying vasodilator drugs (e.g. calcium channel blockers, nitrates, α-adrenoceptor antagonists) discontinued if hypotension is a problem. Diuretic dose may be reduced if the patient is euvolaemic, although patients must be carefully followed-up for evidence of fluid retention if this action is taken. Renal function and potassium should be monitored as with the use of any other RAAS blocker. If renal dysfunction or hyperkalaemia occurs, consider discontinuing other non-essential drugs such as non-steroidal anti-inflammatory drugs and potassium supplements. The development of angioedema should lead to immediate and permanent discontinuation of sacubitril/valsartan and appropriate therapy until it has resolved.

Natriuretic peptide monitoring

Because sacubitril/valsartan increases levels of circulating BNP, this peptide is not reliable for monitoring patients whereas NT-proBNP, which is not a substrate for neprilysin, is still useful.[58]

Heart failure with mildly reduced and preserved ejection fraction

The Prospective comparison of ARni with Arb Global Outcomes in heart failure with preserved ejectioN fraction (PARAGON-HF; NCT01920711).[64]

PARAGON-HF and HFmrEF/HFpEF

The Prospective comparison of ARni with Arb Global Outcomes in heart failure with preserved ejectioN fraction (PARAGON- HF; NCT01920711) compared sacubitril/valsartan with valsartan in 4822 patients with an ejection fraction of ≥45%.[65] Sacubitril/valsartan led to a modest reduction in the primary composite outcome of total heart failure hospitalizations and cardiovascular deaths which was of borderline statistical significance (rate ratio, 0.87; 95% CI, 0.75 to 1.01; P = 0.06). In a prespecified subgroup analysis, there was a significant interaction between baseline ejection fraction and the effect of sacubitril/valsartan, with more benefit in patients with an ejection fraction at or below the median value of 57%. This finding has led to an expanded approval for the use of sacubitril/valsartan in patients with HFmrEF, as well as HFrEF, in some countries.[66]

REFERENCES

1. McMurray JJ, Pfeffer MA, Swedberg K, Dzau VJ. Which inhibitor of the renin–angiotensin system should be used in chronic heart failure and acute myocardial infarction? *Circulation* 2004;**110**:3281–8.
2. Cohn JN, Tognoni G; Valsartan Heart Failure Trial Investigators. A randomized trial of the angiotensin-receptor blocker valsartan in chronic heart failure. *N Engl J Med* 2001;**345**:1667–75.
3. Maggioni AP, Anand I, Gottlieb SO, et al.; Val-HeFT Investigators (Valsartan Heart Failure Trial). Effects of valsartan on morbidity and mortality in patients with heart failure not receiving angiotensin-converting enzyme inhibitors. *J Am Coll Cardiol* 2002;**40**:1414–21.
4. Pitt B, Poole-Wilson PA, Segal R, et al. Effect of losartan compared with captopril on mortality in patients with symptomatic heart failure: randomised trial—the Losartan Heart Failure Survival Study ELITE II. *Lancet* 2000;**355**:1582–7.
5. Pfeffer MA, Swedberg K, Granger CB, et al.; CHARM Investigators and Committees. Effects of candesartan on mortality and morbidity in patients with chronic heart failure: the CHARM-Overall programme. Lancet 2003;**362**:759–66.

6. McMurray JJ, Ostergren J, Swedberg K, *et al.*; CHARM Investigators and Committees. Effects of candesartan in patients with chronic heart failure and reduced left-ventricular systolic function taking angiotensin-converting-enzyme inhibitors: the CHARM-Added trial. *Lancet* 2003;**362**:767–71.

7. Granger CB, McMurray JJ, Yusuf S, *et al.*; CHARM Investigators and Committees. Effects of candesartan in patients with chronic heart failure and reduced left-ventricular systolic function intolerant to angiotensin-converting-enzyme inhibitors: the CHARM-Alternative trial. *Lancet* 2003;**362**:772–6.

8. Yusuf S, Pfeffer MA, Swedberg K, *et al.*; CHARM Investigators and Committees. Effects of candesartan in patients with chronic heart failure and preserved left-ventricular ejection fraction: the CHARM-Preserved Trial. *Lancet* 2003;**362**:777–81.

9. Dickstein K, Kjekshus J; OPTIMAAL Steering Committee of the OPTIMAAL Study Group. Effects of losartan and captopril on mortality and morbidity in high-risk patients after acute myocardial infarction: the OPTIMAAL randomised trial. Optimal Trial in Myocardial Infarction with Angiotensin II Antagonist Losartan. *Lancet* 2002;**360**:752–60.

10. Pfeffer MA, McMurray JJ, Velazquez EJ, *et al.*; Valsartan in Acute Myocardial Infarction Trial Investigators. Valsartan, captopril, or both in myocardial infarction complicated by heart failure, left ventricular dysfunction, or both. *N Engl J Med* 2003;**349**:1893–906.

11. ONTARGET Investigators, Yusuf S, Teo KK, Pogue J, *et al.* Telmisartan, ramipril, or both in patients at high risk for vascular events. *N Engl J Med* 2008;**358**:1547–59.

12. Fried LF, Emanuele N, Zhang JH, *et al.*; VA NEPHRON-D Investigators. Combined angiotensin inhibition for the treatment of diabetic nephropathy. *N Engl J Med* 2013;**369**:1892–903.

13. Massie BM, Carson PE, McMurray JJ, *et al.*; I-PRESERVE Investigators. Irbesartan in patients with heart failure and preserved ejection fraction. *N Engl J Med* 2008;**359**:2456–67.

14. Konstam MA, Neaton JD, Dickstein K, *et al.*; HEAAL Investigators. Effects of high-dose versus low-dose losartan on clinical outcomes in patients with heart failure (HEAAL study): a randomised, double-blind trial. *Lancet* 2009;**374**:1840–8.

15. McMurray JJ, Krum H, Abraham WT, *et al.*; ATMOSPHERE Committees Investigators. Aliskiren, enalapril, or aliskiren and enalapril in heart failure. *N Engl J Med* 2016;**374**:1521–32.

16. Packer M, Poole-Wilson PA, Armstrong PW, *et al.* Comparative effects of low and high doses of the angiotensin-converting enzyme inhibitor, lisinopril, on morbidity and mortality in chronic heart failure. ATLAS Study Group. *Circulation* 1999;**100**:2312–18.

17. Rogers JK, Pocock SJ, McMurray JJ, *et al.* Analysing recurrent hospitalizations in heart failure: a review of statistical methodology, with application to CHARM-Preserved. *Eur J Heart Fail* 2014;**16**:33–40.

18. Belz GG, Butzer R, Kober S, Mutschler E. Pharmacodynamic studies on the angiotensin II type 1 antagonists irbesartan and candesartan based on angiotensin II dose response in humans. *J Cardiovasc Pharmacol* 2002;**39**:561–8.

19. Lund LH, Claggett B, Liu J, *et al.* Heart failure with mid-range ejection fraction in CHARM: characteristics, outcomes and effect of candesartan across the entire ejection fraction spectrum. *Eur J Heart Fail* 2018;**20**:1230–39.

20. Dewan P, Jackson A, Lam CSP, et al. Interactions between left ventricular ejection fraction, sex and effect of neurohumoral modulators in heart failure. *Eur J Heart Fail.* 2020;**22**:898–901.

21. deBold AI, Borenstein HB, Veress AT, Sonnenberg H. A rapid and potent natriuretic response to intravenous injection of atrial myocardial extract in rats. *Life Sci* 1981;**28**:89–94.

22. McMurray J, Struthers AD. Significance of atrial natriuretic factor in chronic heart failure. *Br J Hosp Med* 1988;**40**:55–7.

23. Kerr MA, Kenny AJ. The purification and specificity of a neutral endopeptidase from rabbit kidney brush border. *Biochem J* 1974;**137**:477–88.

24. Vanneste Y, Michel A, Dimaline R, Najdovski T, Deschodt-Lanckman M. Hydrolysis of alpha-human atrial natriuretic peptide in vitro by human kidney membranes and purified endopeptidase-24.11. Evidence for a novel cleavage site. *Biochem J* 1988;**254**:531–7.

25. Northridge DB, Jardine AG, Alabaster CT, *et al.* Effects of UK 69 578: a novel atriopeptidase inhibitor. *Lancet* 1989;**2**:591–3.

26. Cha YM, Dzeja PP, Redfield MM, Shen WK, Terzic A. Bioenergetic protection of failing atrial and ventricular myocardium by vasopeptidase inhibitor omapatrilat. *Am J Physiol Heart Circ Physiol* 2006;**290**:H1686–92.

27. Gros C, Souque A, Schwartz JC, *et al.* Protection of atrial natriuretic factor against degradation: diuretic and natriuretic responses after in vivo inhibition of enkephalinase (EC 3.4.24.11) by acetorphan. *Proc Natl Acad Sci USA* 1989;**86**:7580–4.

28. Kahn JC, Patey M, Dubois-Rande JL, *et al.* Effect of sinorphan on plasma atrial natriuretic factor in congestive heart failure. *Lancet* 1990;**335**:118–9.

29. Richards AM, Wittert GA, Espiner EA, *et al.* Effect of inhibition of endopeptidase 24.11 on responses to angiotensin II in human volunteers. *Circ Res* 1992;**71**:1501–7.

30. Ferro CJ, Spratt JC, Haynes WG, Webb DJ. Inhibition of neutral endopeptidase causes vasoconstriction of human resistance vessels in vivo. *Circulation* 1998;**97**:2323–30.

31. Dalzell JR, Seed A, Berry C, *et al.* Effects of neutral endopeptidase (neprilysin) inhibition on the response to other vasoactive peptides in small human resistance arteries: studies with thiorphan and omapatrilat. *Cardiovasc Ther* 2014;**32**:13–18.

32. Wilkinson IB, McEniery CM, Bongaerts KH, *et al.* Adrenomedullin (ADM) in the human forearm vascular bed: effect of neutral endopeptidase inhibition and comparison with proadrenomedullin NH2-terminal 20 peptide (PAMP). *Br J Clin Pharmacol* 2001;**52**:159–64.

33. Matsas R, Rattray M, Kenny AJ, Turner AJ. The metabolism of neuropeptides. Endopeptidase-24.11 in human synaptic membrane preparations hydrolyses substance P. *Biochem J* 1985;**228**:487–92.

34. Katayama M, Nadel JA, Bunnett NW, *et al.* Catabolism of calcitonin gene-related peptide and substance P by neutral endopeptidase. *Peptides* 1991;**12**:563–7.

35. McDowell G, Coutie W, Shaw C, *et al.* The effect of the neutral endopeptidase inhibitor drug, candoxatril, on circulating levels of two of the most potent vasoactive peptides. *Br J Clin Pharmacol* 1997;**43**:329–32.

36. McKinnie SM, Fischer C, Tran KM, *et al.* The metalloprotease neprilysin degrades and inactivates apelin peptides. *Chembiochemistry* 2016;**17**:1495–8.

37. Plamboeck A, Holst JJ, Carr RD, Deacon CF. Neutral endopeptidase 24.11 and dipeptidyl peptidase IV are both mediators of the degradation of glucagon-like peptide 1 in the anaesthetised pig. *Diabetologia* 2005;**48**:1882–90.

38. Baranello RJ, Bharani KL, Padmaraju V, *et al.* Amyloid-beta protein clearance and degradation (ABCD) pathways and their role in Alzheimer's disease. *Curr Alzheimer Res* 2015;**12**:32–46.

39. Trippodo NC, Robl JA, Asaad MM, *et al.* Cardiovascular effects of the novel dual inhibitor of neutral endopeptidase and angiotensin-converting enzyme BMS 182657 in experimental hypertension and heart failure. *J Pharmacol Exp Ther* 1995;**275**:745–52.

40. McClean DR, Ikram H, Garlick AH, *et al.* The clinical, cardiac, renal, arterial and neurohormonal effects of omapatrilat, a vasopeptidase inhibitor, in patients with chronic heart failure. *J Am Coll Cardiol* 2000;**36**:479–86.

41. Rouleau JL, Pfeffer MA, Stewart DJ, *et al.* Comparison of vasopeptidase inhibitor, omapatrilat, and lisinopril on exercise tolerance and morbidity in patients with heart failure: IMPRESS randomised trial. *Lancet* 2000;**356**:615–20.

42. Packer M, Califf RM, Konstam MA, *et al.* Comparison of omapatrilat and enalapril in patients with chronic heart failure: the Omapatrilat Versus Enalapril Randomized Trial of Utility in Reducing Events (OVERTURE). *Circulation* 2002;**106**:920–6.

43. Kostis JB, Packer M, Black HR, *et al.* Omapatrilat and enalapril in patients with hypertension: the Omapatrilat Cardiovascular Treatment vs. Enalapril (OCTAVE) trial. *Am J Hypertens* 2004;**17**:103–11.

44. Fryer RM, Segreti J, Banfor PN, *et al.* Effect of bradykinin metabolism inhibitors on evoked hypotension in rats: rank efficacy of enzymes associated with bradykinin-mediated angioedema. *Br J Pharmacol* 2008;**153**:947–55.

45. Gu J, Noe A, Chandra P, *et al.* Pharmacokinetics and pharmacodynamics of LCZ696, a novel dual-acting angiotensin receptor-neprilysin inhibitor (ARNi). *J Clin Pharmacol* 2010;**50**:401–14.

46. Hegde LG, Yu C, Renner T, *et al.* Concomitant angiotensin AT1 receptor antagonism and neprilysin inhibition produces omapatrilat-like antihypertensive effects without promoting tracheal plasma extravasation in the rat. *J Cardiovasc Pharmacol* 2011;**57**:495–504.

47. Ruilope LM, Dukat A, Böhm M, *et al.* Blood-pressure reduction with LCZ696, a novel dual-acting inhibitor of the angiotensin II receptor and neprilysin: a randomised, double-blind, placebo-controlled, active comparator study. *Lancet* 2010;**375**:1255–66.

48. McMurray JJ, Packer M, Desai AS, *et al.*; PARADIGM-HF Committees and Investigators. Dual angiotensin receptor and neprilysin inhibition as an alternative to angiotensin-converting enzyme inhibition in patients with chronic systolic heart failure: rationale for and design of the Prospective comparison of ARNI with ACEI to Determine Impact on Global Mortality and morbidity in Heart Failure trial (PARADIGM-HF). *Eur J Heart Fail* 2013;**15**:1062–73.

49. McMurray JJ, Packer M, Desai AS, *et al.*; PARADIGM-HF Committees Investigators. Baseline characteristics and treatment of patients in Prospective comparison of ARNI with ACEI to Determine Impact on Global Mortality and morbidity in Heart Failure trial (PARADIGM-HF). *Eur J Heart Fail* 2014;**16**:817–25.

50. McMurray JJ, Packer M, Desai AS, *et al.*; PARADIGM-HF Investigators and Committees. Angiotensin–neprilysin inhibition versus enalapril in heart failure. *N Engl J Med* 2014;**371**:993–1004.

51. Desai AS, McMurray JJ, Packer M, *et al.* Effect of the angiotensin-receptor–neprilysin inhibitor LCZ696 compared with enalapril on mode of death in heart failure patients. *Eur Heart J* 2015;**36**:1990–7.

52. Packer M, McMurray JJ, Desai AS, *et al.*; PARADIGM-HF Investigators and Coordinators. Angiotensin receptor neprilysin inhibition compared with enalapril on the risk of clinical progression in surviving patients with heart failure. *Circulation* 2015;**131**:54–61.

53. Jhund PS, Fu M, Bayram E, *et al.*; PARADIGM-HF Investigators and Committees. Efficacy and safety of LCZ696 (sacubitril-valsartan) according to age: insights from PARADIGM-HF. *Eur Heart J* 2015;**36**:2576–84.

54. Simpson J, Jhund PS, Silva Cardoso J, *et al.*; PARADIGM-HF Investigators and Committees. Comparing LCZ696 with enalapril according to baseline risk using the MAGGIC and EMPHASIS-HF risk scores: an analysis of mortality and morbidity in PARADIGM-HF. *J Am Coll Cardiol* 2015;**66**:2059–71.

55. Cannon JA, Shen L, Jhund PS, *et al.*; PARADIGM-HF Investigators and Committees. Dementia-related adverse events in PARADIGM-HF and other trials in heart failure with reduced ejection fraction. *Eur J Heart Fail* 2017;**19**:129–37.

56. Docherty KF, Vaduganathan M, Solomon SD, McMurray JJV. Sacubitril/Valsartan: Neprilysin Inhibition 5 Years After PARADIGM-HF. *JACC Heart Fail* 2020 Oct;**8**(10):800–10.

57. Jhund PS, McMurray JJ. The neprilysin pathway in heart failure: a review and guide on the use of sacubitril/valsartan. *Heart* 2016;**102**:1342–7.

58. Zile MR, Claggett BL, Prescott MF, *et al.* Prognostic implications of changes in N-terminal pro-B-type natriuretic peptide in patients with heart failure. *J Am Coll Cardiol* 2016;**68**:2425–2436.

59. Velazquez EJ, Morrow DA, DeVore AD, et al. PIONEER-HF Investigators. Angiotensin-neprilysin inhibition in acute decompensated heart failure. *N Engl J Med* 2019;**380**:539–48.

60. Ponikowski P, Voors AA, Anker SD, *et al.*; Authors/Task Force Members;Document Reviewers. 2016 ESC Guidelines for the diagnosis and treatment of acute and chronic heart failure: The Task Force for the diagnosis and treatment of acute and chronic heart failure of the European Society of Cardiology (ESC). Developed with the special contribution of the Heart Failure Association (HFA) of the ESC. *Eur J Heart Fail* 2016;**18**:891–975.

61. Writing Committee, Maddox TM, Januzzi JL Jr, *et al.* Update to the 2017 ACC Expert Consensus Decision Pathway for Optimization of Heart Failure Treatment: Answers to 10 Pivotal Issues About Heart Failure With Reduced Ejection Fraction: A Report of the American College of Cardiology Solution Set Oversight Committee. *J Am Coll Cardiol.* 2021 Feb 16;**77**(6):772–810. doi: 10.1016/j.jacc.2020.11.022. Epub 2021 Jan 11. PMID: 33446410.

62. McDonald M, Virani S, Chan M, et al. CCS/CHFS Heart Failure Guidelines Update: Defining a New Pharmacologic Standard of Care for Heart Failure With Reduced Ejection Fraction. *Can J Cardiol.* 2021 Apr;**37**(4):531–46. doi: 10.1016/j.cjca.2021.01.017. PMID: 33827756.

63. Desai AS, Vardeny O, Claggett B, *et al.* Reduced risk of hyperkalemia during treatment of heart failure with mineralocorticoid receptor antagonists by use of sacubitril/valsartan compared with enalapril: a secondary analysis of the PARADIGM-HF Trial. *JAMA Cardiol* 2017;**2**:79–85.

64. Senni M, McMurray JJ, Wachter R, *et al.* Initiating sacubitril/valsartan (LCZ696) in heart failure: results of TITRATION, a double-blind, randomized comparison of two uptitration regimens. *Eur J Heart Fail* 2016;**18**:1193–202.

65. Solomon SD, McMurray JJV, Anand IS, et al. PARAGON-HF Investigators and committees. Angiotensin-Neprilysin inhibition in heart failure with preserved ejection fraction. *N Engl J Med.* 2019 Oct 24;**381**(17):1609–20. doi: 10.1056/NEJMoa1908655. Epub 2019 Sep 1. PMID: 31475794.

66. Solomon SD, McMurray JJV. Making the case for an expanded indication for Sacubitril/Valsartan in heart failure. *J Card Fail.* 2021 Jun;**27**(6):693–95. doi: 10.1016/j.cardfail.2021.04.008. Epub 2021 Apr 16. PMID: 33872760.

β-Adrenoreceptor antagonists

Simon A. S. Beggs, Roy S. Gardner, and Theresa A. McDonagh

Background

Sir James Black's quest for a substance that would block the potentially harmful effects of adrenaline on the ischaemic heart led to his invention of the β-adrenoreceptor (AR) antagonists pronethalol and propranalol between 1959 and 1962.[1] The ubiquitous nature of adrenaline ensured that these β-AR antagonists, commonly referred to in clinical practice as β-blockers, found a role in multiple aspects of cardiovascular therapeutics.[2] Sir James could not have predicted the colossal impact his discovery of β-blockers subsequently would have in improving the lives and preventing the deaths of countless patients over the subsequent 50 years. Regarded by basic scientists as the father of analytical pharmacology, he was also a committed exponent of what we now regard as translational medical research. Sir James's achievement in discovering β-blockers followed by histamine type 2 antagonists (H$_2$ blockers), the first effective treatment for peptic ulcer, was recognized by the award of the Nobel Prize in 1986.

Black's original hypothesis was that patients with stable angina pectoris might benefit by reducing the work of the heart, rather than increasing the blood flow. So the first clinical study with the initial β-blocker pronethalol was carried out in angina pectoris by Pritchard.[3] In a careful dose–response study he showed that there was clinical improvement in 16 out of 17 patients. Pritchard noted that during the dose–response period there was also a fall in blood pressure. This serendipitous observation was confirmed in a subsequent study with propranolol, showing a significant decrease in blood pressure in 17 out of 18 patients. Further clinical studies showed that propranolol had anti-arrhythmic properties, and much later that it reduced mortality in patients with myocardial infarction (MI).[4] Most recently β-blockers have conclusively been shown to be of great benefit in heart failure, clearly demonstrating the extensive role of sympathetic nervous activity in cardiovascular disease.[5,6] The pharmacological properties of β-blockers that have been used in heart failure studies are summarized in Table 50.1.

Using β-blockers in heart failure seems counterintuitive given that the increased sympathetic activity that occurs in patients with heart failure is required to support the failing heart. Early studies of propranolol in experimental heart failure in calves[7,8] fuelled a natural concern at inhibiting the very system on which the heart appeared to depend for support. Based on such clinical considerations, there was a universally agreed view that the use of the non-selective β-blockers available at that time was contraindicated in heart failure.[9]

Despite these experimental findings and clinical anecdotage, the early published studies of β-blockade in patients with heart failure

Table 50.1 Pharmacological properties of β-blockers evaluated in chronic heart failure trials

Component	In-vitro K_D[33]		β$_1$/ β$_2$ ratio	MSP	Partial agonism	$t_{1/2}$ (h)	Dose (mg)	Vasodilation
β$_1$-Selective								
Atenolol	β$_1$: −6.66	β$_2$: −5.99	4.7	No	No		50–100	No
Bisoprolol	−7.83	−6.70	13.5	No	No	10–12	10–20	No
Nebivolol	0.88	48	55	–	No	10.3–31.9	5–10	Yes
Xamoterol	–	–	40	No	Yes (43% of isoprenaline)	13	200 bd	No
Non-selective								
Bucindolol	–	–	?	No	Yes	3.6–9.0	50–200	Yes weak AR$_1$
Carvedilol	−8.75	−9.40	4.5 (β$_2$)	Yes	No	2–4	15–50	Yes (AR$_1$)[a]
β$_2$-Selective								
ICI 118551	−6.52	−9.26	549.5	Yes	No	3	25–50	No

AR, adrenoreceptor; bd, twice daily.
[a] α-AR blockade.

in the UK and Sweden did point tantalizingly to potential benefit in selected patients, but it was not until the 1970s that the somewhat counterintuitive notion of using β-blockers to treat patients with heart failure began to be taken seriously. The initial clinical studies of the effects of β-blockade in heart failure were performed both by Gibson et al. at the National Heart Institute, London[9] and by Waagstein and colleagues in Gothenburg.[10,11] Both groups studied the β_1 cardioselective blocker practolol (ICI50172), and the Swedish investigators also used alprenolol, which has partial agonist activity, in patients with idiopathic dilated cardiomyopathy. The initial studies from both groups involved the parenteral administration of practolol to patients in severe heart failure with supraventricular tachycardia. The marked reduction in heart rate was accompanied by significant clinical improvement without side-effects. A subsequent long-term study with the β_1-selective blocker metoprolol in patients with dilated cardiomyopathy showed that after 3 years of treatment, the survival in the β-blocker-treated group was 52%, compared to only 10% for matched controls.[12]

The idea that β-blockers might be of value in heart failure was consistent with the developing 'neuroendocrine hypothesis' of heart failure. This was prompted when the CONSENSUS study showed a huge 60% reduction in mortality by the angiotensin converting enzyme (ACE) inhibitor enalapril.[13] Subsequently it was suggested that several neurohormonal systems, principally the renin–angiotensin–aldosterone system (RAAS) and the sympathetic nervous system, could be responsible for the apparently inexorable deterioration of cardiac function and high mortality in heart failure.

Thereafter, inhibition of this neuroendocrine response by ACE inhibitors,[13,14] selective inhibition of angiotensin II receptors by angiotensin receptor blockers (ARBs)[15] and angiotensin receptor–neprilysin inhibitors (ARNIs),[16] and of aldosterone receptors,[17] together with β-blockers has become the standard evidence-based

approach to the medical treatment of heart failure. This combination of treatments markedly improves survival by reducing both sudden cardiac death and death due to worsening heart failure. It also leads to improved ventricular function due to amelioration of ventricular remodelling consequent upon myocardial cell loss from MI or other heart muscle disorders.

The evidence

There can be few medicines whose efficacy in heart failure has been so clearly demonstrated as β-blockers insofar as the two major outcomes of survival and need for hospital admission are concerned. Following the early pioneering and hypothesis-generating studies of the potential value of β-blockers in MI and heart failure—performed in the UK and Sweden with practolol, alprenolol, and metoprolol—there are now data from >15 000 patients from randomized placebo-controlled trials that, collectively, demonstrate impressive statistically and clinically important reductions in death and unscheduled admissions to hospital for worsening heart failure. A summary of the major trials can be found in Table 50.2.

Survival

Interest in the use of β-blockers in chronic heart failure rapidly increased when the results of the US Carvedilol Heart Failure Trial Programme on survival in >1000 patients with NYHA class II–IV heart failure were disclosed in 1996.[18] This was a series of double-blind randomized controlled trials (RCTs) in heart failure that individually investigated dose, haemodynamics, exercise capacity, and symptoms while collectively assessing the impact of β-blockade on mortality. The reduction in mortality reported in this programme greatly strengthened the hypothesis that β-blockers could indeed

Table 50.2 Major β-blocker trials

	CIBIS II	BEST	MERIT-HF	MDC	SENIORS	GAXST	XAMOTEROL in Severe Heart Failure Study Group
Patients (n)	2647	2708	3991	383	2128	433	352
β-Blocker	Bisoprolol	Bucindolol	Metoprolol CR/XL	Metoprolol	Nebivolol	Xamoterol	Xamoterol
NYHA class	III–IV	III–IV	II–IV	I–IV	II–IV	II–III	III–IV
LVEF	≤35%	≤35%	≤40%	<40%	33%	N/A	N/A
Mean follow-up (months)	14	24	12	12	21	3	13 weeks
Mean dose achieved (mg/day)	7.5	152	159	100–150	1.25–10	200 mg bd	200 mg tid
Primary end-point	All-cause mortality	All-cause mortality	All-cause mortality	Exercise LV function	All-cause mortality Hospitalization	Effort tolerance improved 37%	9.2% died vs 3.7% placebo
Results	All-cause mortality reduced 34%	All-cause mortality reduced 10%	All-cause mortality reduced 34%	EF increased Exercise increased	All-cause mortality reduced	Reduced oedema/ pulmonary congestion	Trial suspended
P-value	<0.001	0.13	0.0062	0.0001 0.046	0.039	N/A	N/A

BEST, β-Blocker Evaluation of Survival Trial; CIBIS II, Cardiac Insufficiency Bisoprolol Study II; CR/XL, controlled release/extended release; EF, ejection fraction; GASXT, German and Austrian Xamoterol Trial; LV, left ventricular; MDC, Metoprolol in Dilated Cardiomyopathy; MERIT-HF, Metoprolol CR/XL Randomized Intervention Trial in Congestive Heart Failure; N/A, not applicable.

improve survival, and to a similar extent as had been demonstrated in the definitive ACE inhibitor studies in heart failure of the previous decade. It also lent even greater credence to the neuroendocrine hypothesis of heart failure promulgated in the wake of the early ACE inhibitor studies—that activation of a number of neural and endocrine systems, notably the RAAS and sympathetic nervous system, was not simply a reflection of the presence and severity of heart failure, but also directly contributed to poor outcomes in patients with heart failure through deleterious effects on the myocardium, blood vessels, and kidney.

The carvedilol heart failure programme was an ambitious enterprise of great significance to the development of a comprehensive evidence base for the use of β-blockers together with ACE inhibitors in patients with heart failure due to left ventricular systolic dysfunction (LVSD). Nevertheless, the survival benefit was based on a relatively small number of deaths, 31 (7.8%) on placebo versus 22 (3.2%) on carvedilol, representing absolute and relative reductions in mortality of 4.6% and 65% respectively. The overall mortality was relatively low and it was clear that the results of further ongoing and new studies in larger and more diverse patient groups were required to establish as securely as with ACE inhibitors a strong evidence base for the safety and efficacy of β-blockers to improve clinical status and outcome in heart failure.

In 1998 the results of the CIBIS II trial of bisoprolol (β1 selective) in >2000 patients—essentially the first large single RCT of β-blockade in heart failure—showed a survival advantage for patients randomized to bisoprolol. The risk reduction for all-cause mortality in the treatment group was 34% in a trial where the mortality rate in the placebo group was 17.3%, the highest studied thus far in a large clinical trial.[19] The trial patients included patients in NYHA classes III–IV. CIBIS II also drew attention to the remarkable relative reduction of 44% in the sudden death rate, and the important reductions not only in hospital admission for worsening heart failure but also on all-cause hospital admissions. Notably, CIBIS II was stopped early after an interim analysis revealed the remarkable survival advantage in the bisoprolol arm.

Later that year the MERIT-HF trial of metoprolol succinate, in an even larger study of almost 4000 patients, essentially completed the evidence base for the impressive improvement in outcome in terms of survival and admission to hospital afforded by chronic treatment with β-blockers.[20] It also confirmed the marked reduction in sudden cardiac death demonstrated by the preceding trials. Thus in the short space of three years the cumulative evidence for the efficacy of β-blockers raised the profile of β-blockers as having at least as salutary an additional beneficial effect on morbidity and mortality as ACE inhibitors when given in conjunction with them.

Remodelling

Unfavourable changes to the geometry, structure, and function of the left (or right) ventricles accompany several disease processes affecting the myocardium, among which MI is the most typical and frequent cause. Myocyte loss or dysfunction can set in train a series of cellular processes including myocyte hypertrophy and renewal, as well as interstitial fibrosis and dilatation of the left ventricle, causing the chamber to become more spherical than elliptical. This results in increased wall tension, reduced contractility, impaired filling, and ultimately the clinical syndrome of heart failure.[21]

In 1997 the Australia and New Zealand (ANZ) trial in 415 patients convincingly demonstrated that carvedilol improved left ventricular systolic function, although exercise capacity did not change.[22] The ANZ trial also contributed to the evidence that clinical outcomes improved on β-blockers. Subsequently the CAPRICORN trial of carvedilol showed that similar benefits may occur with β-blockers in conjunction with ACE inhibitors in patients with post-MI left ventricular dysfunction or heart failure.[23,24] The totality of data from these and other mechanistic trials indicate that β-blockers have a clinically important beneficial effect on remodelling in heart failure.

Arrhythmia

It is said that it was the sudden, unexpected death of the young James Black's father following a very stressful day at work that caused him to consider the possibility that high levels of adrenaline from excess sympathetic nervous activity could have been responsible and that blocking these effects of adrenaline on the heart might prevent such tragedies. Perspicacious in the extreme, perhaps, but there is no doubt that a major feature of β-blocker therapy is the reduction in sudden death observed both after MI and in heart failure. Given the pro-arrhythmic effects of catecholamines, the major anti-arrhythmic effects of β-blockers is scarcely surprising. The precise mechanism by which β-blockers achieve this effect is unclear, but substantial reductions in serious ventricular arrhythmias including ventricular tachycardia and ventricular fibrillation were noted during ambulatory ECG monitoring in CAPRICORN.[23–25]

Of considerable importance also is the suppression of supraventricular arrhythmias, especially atrial fibrillation (AF) and atrial flutter, which, in patients with heart failure often precipitate acute heart failure and decompensation in patients with known chronic heart failure.

The downside of the anti-arrhythmic properties of β-blockers is bradycardia, which may limit the maximum tolerated dose in individual patients and lead to various degrees of heart block, most commonly first degree but occasionally second degree and complete heart block. In the latter it is usually in the context of pre-existing conduction disturbance and in such cases permanent pacing may be required.

Specific patient subgroups

Severe heart failure

Despite the impressive results of the US Carvedilol programme and the CIBIS II and MERIT-HF trials, many questions still remained to be answered about β-blocking therapy, including its safety and efficacy in very severe heart failure. For, although patients with NYHA classes III and IV were included in the preceding trials, they were relatively few in number and had to have been clinically stable for some time before entry to these trials. This question has best been addressed in the COPERNICUS trial of carvedilol in >2000 patients with NYHA class III or IV heart failure in which there was a total of >500 deaths, the largest yet recorded in a heart failure trial. Carvedilol reduced all-cause mortality.[26] Overall, significant survival benefit was also derived by patients in a pre-specified subgroup at even higher risk due to, among other criteria, recent decompensation or a severely depressed ejection fraction of ≤14%. Carvedilol

reduced all-cause mortality by 39% in this subgroup, and decreased the combined risk of all-cause mortality or hospitalizations by 29%. Notably, among patients in this subgroup who received placebo, the annualized mortality rate was 24%. COPERNICUS indicated that, far from being hazardous, it is in the highest-risk groups of patients that β-blockers can exert their greatest effects. It must be stressed, however, that these benefits of β-blockers were obtained in the context of a standard of patient care as near optimal as possible.

Heart failure after myocardial infarction

The powerful effects of β-blockers on survival in patients with cardiovascular disease was first demonstrated in the β-blocker trials in MI of the previous decade. The first of these trials, and still the most impressive in terms of outcome benefits, was the Norwegian multicentre trial of timolol, published in 1980. This was followed by several other trials with metoprolol, propranolol, practolol, oxprenolol, sotalol, and alprenolol in which the results on survival and recurrent MI, though more variable, were directionally similar to those of the timolol trial. Subsequent meta-analyses confirmed the powerful beneficial effects of β-blockers in the post-MI patient on survival and recurrent MI.[4] Patients with heart failure were included in some of these studies but generally they were excluded because of safety concerns. Consequently it soon became apparent that, in clinical practice, the prescription rate of β-blockers in patients whose MI was complicated by heart failure remained low. This was the reason for carrying out a specific trial in post-MI patients with significant left ventricular dysfunction and/or heart failure, the CAPRICORN trial with carvedilol, in ~2000 patients.[23] The impact on survival reflected in a relative risk reduction of 23% (absolute reduction 3%) was identical to that calculated in meta-analyses of the previous MI trials, and the effects on sudden death and recurrent MI were also statistically and clinically highly significant. The CAPRICORN trial therefore completed the spectrum of post-MI trials by indicating that patients with heart failure or severe left ventricular dysfunction post-MI should definitely and specifically be considered for β-blocker therapy. An important practical contribution was the experience gained in initiating β-blocker treatment safely in patients with acute heart failure, guided by specific clinical indicators which could be applied for the safe use of β-blockers in patients with heart failure however caused.

Heart failure with preserved ejection fraction

Over many years the main experimental and clinical focus of interest in heart failure encompassing particularly the neuroendocrine hypothesis for the development and progression of heart failure has been on LVSD, or heart failure with reduced ejection fraction (HFrEF). It is now recognized that a significant proportion of patients who present with the heart failure syndrome have heart failure with preserved ejection fraction (HFpEF).

These patients more often are older, with a history of hypertension and evidence of left ventricular hypertrophy.[27] Contemporary estimations indicate that they are possibly as numerous as those with HFrEF. Most of the 'landmark' clinical trials of β-blockers in heart failure have been in patients with HFrEF, whereas such data in patients with HFpEF are few. Theoretically the risk/benefit ratio should be favourable in HFpEF, with less myocardial depression and improved ventricular filling from a slower heart rate.

The two largest RCTs to evaluate the efficacy of β-blockers in reducing adverse outcomes in HFpEF are SENIORS and J-DHF. In the SENIORS trial, the effects of nebivolol, a β1-selective β-blocker with a nitric-oxide-based vasodilator activity, was studied in a large group of patients aged ≥70 years. A secure clinical diagnosis of heart failure was required but no specific value of ejection fraction mandated: thus, HFpEF patients were included in SENIORS, but were not the sole focus of the trial.[28] The composite 1-year end-point of all-cause mortality or cardiovascular hospitalizations was significantly reduced by nebivolol regardless of ejection fraction. Nebivolol is licensed for the treatment of heart failure in some countries but it has not been approved in the USA. The efficacy of treatment with β-blockers in a Japanese population with HFpEF was subsequently examined in the J-DHF trial, wherein 245 patients with LVEF >40% were randomized to placebo or carvedilol.[29] After a median follow-up of 3.2 years, there was no significant difference in the rates of cardiovascular death and unplanned hospitalization for heart failure (the composite primary end-point), although there were just 29 and 34 events in the treatment group and placebo group, respectively. The median carvedilol dose achieved in J-DHF was only 7.5 mg/day (compared to 37 mg/day in COPERNICUS, for example), and the authors hypothesized that reduced therapeutic efficacy at lower doses contributed to the neutral outcome of the trial. Having intended to recruit 800 patients, the trial also fell very significantly short of this target, reducing its statistical power. Every one of the eight primary and secondary end-points in J-DHF showed a non-significant trend to a benefit of carvedilol therapy. The consistency of this finding is striking, and it is intriguing to speculate what a well-powered trial would have revealed.

Several observational cohort studies—both retrospective and prospective—have examined the association between β-blocker therapy and clinical outcomes in large HFpEF populations. Although meta-analyses of these non-randomized studies suggest that β-blockers are associated with lower all-cause mortality, this association was not maintained in simultaneous meta-analyses of the two RCTs discussed above.[30,31]

The efficacy of β-blockers in HFpEF thus remains an unresolved issue. Nevertheless, β-blockers are frequently indicated in patients with HFpEF due to concomitant—predominantly cardiovascular—co-morbidity, and thus their use in this population is common.

Obstructive airways disease

It is always a significant clinical disappointment when contra-indications prevent the use of life-enhancing and life-saving medicines. Since β2-adrenergic receptor blockade encourages bronchoconstriction, asthma and chronic obstructive pulmonary disease (COPD) were formerly considered contraindications to β-blockers. However, a series of small RCTs examining the safety profile of β-blockers in patients with heart failure and concomitant moderate-to-severe COPD appear to have confirmed the tolerability of cardioselective agents.[32-35] Of interest, in an open-label, triple crossover trial, forced expiratory volume in 1 min was greatest with bisoprolol (2.0 L) and lowest with carvedilol (1.85 L), appearing to support an association between cardioselectivity and lung function.[34] β-Blockers may thus be considered safe in all but severe COPD. Asthma remains a relative contraindication to β-blocker therapy, and should only be used under specialist supervision, with

consideration of the risks for and against their use.[36,37] In both COPD and asthma, β_1-selective agents are preferred.

Differentiating between COPD and asthma is not always straightforward, and in the presence of diagnostic doubt it is advisable to seek a formal opinion from a respiratory specialist as to the correct underlying diagnosis. Ultimately the decision lies with the physician who, aware of the balance of risks of exacerbating bronchoconstriction and of withholding a most effective treatment for heart failure and preventing sudden cardiac death, can give an informed opinion.

Gender

Men and women do not always respond equally to medicines, but as far as β-blockers are concerned a meta-analysis involving the major trials (USCTP, CIBIS II, MERIT-HF, and COPERNICUS) confirms equal benefit in terms of major outcomes.[38]

Atrial fibrillation

The reported prevalence of AF in contemporary HFrEF series varies from 13% to 27%, increasing with the severity of heart failure, and occurring in up to half of those patients who are most symptomatic.[39,40] The concomitant presence of AF confers higher rates of both mortality and hospital admission in patients with HFrEF.[41] The seminal RCTs that evaluated β-blockers in heart failure did include patients with AF, although there is increasing doubt that the prognostic benefits of β-blockers do indeed apply in these patients. A 2014 meta-analysis utilizing individual patient-level data from ten major RCTs randomizing 18 254 patients with heart failure to either a β-blocker or placebo determined that β-blocker therapy effected a reduction in all-cause mortality (the primary outcome) in those patients with sinus rhythm on their baseline ECG, but not in those with AF.[42] The P-value for interaction between the sinus rhythm and AF groups was significant (P = 0.002). This lack of efficacy in patients with AF was consistent across demographic features and comorbidities, and held true for secondary outcomes such as first heart-failure-related hospital admission and a range of composite clinical outcomes. A previous meta-analysis utilizing trial-level data from a smaller number of RCTs broadly supports these findings.[43] These meta-analyses are retrospective and not wholly supported by observational data,[44] and it would be desirable to clarify this issue with a high-quality RCT of β-blocker therapy in patients with HFrEF and concomitant AF. However, it is now unlikely that such a study will be conducted, both because β-blockers are so firmly entrenched in accepted practice, and because they are now off-patent.

Why β-blockers should be less efficacious in the HFrEF subpopulation with AF remains unclear, although multiple theories have been advanced.[42,45] Of interest in this regard, slower ventricular rates are associated with better survival for patients in sinus rhythm but this association is either attenuated or non-existent in patients with AF.[44,46] In any case, when considered alongside other heart failure therapies where there are differences in the evidence of efficacy for patients in AF and sinus rhythm—such as cardiac resynchronization therapy and ivabradine—these concerns regarding the benefits of β-blockers add to the impression of 'AF–HFrEF' patients as a qualitatively distinct population, rather than being merely patients with HFrEF and a concomitant, 'bystander' comorbidity. It is important

therefore to highlight that no evidence of harm from β-blockers was detected among AF patients in the aforementioned meta-analyses. On this basis, and because the analyses were retrospective, the most recent European Society of Cardiology guidelines on the management of heart failure did not make separate recommendation regarding β-blockers in HFrEF according to cardiac rhythm.[36]

Elderly patients

As with female or Black patients, or those with significant comorbidity such as severe renal impairment, patients of advanced age were markedly under-represented in the major β-blocker trials that cemented the current evidence base. The mean age of patients in the US Carvedilol trials, CIBIS II, MERIT-HF, CAPRICORN and COPERNICUS, for example, was 58, 61, 64, 63, and 63 respectively. By contrast, patients admitted to hospital with heart failure in the UK have a mean age of 78 years.[47] Whilst it is hardly surprising that younger patients are more suited to the potentially onerous requirements of clinical trial participation, the changes in pharmacokinetics and pharmacodynamics that accompany advancing age mean that extrapolations about drug effects (and side-effects) to an older population are hazardous. The SENIORS trial was specifically designed to address this issue, thus examining the effects of nebivolol in heart failure patients aged ≥70 years. The choice of study drug was a considered one: it was theorized that, in an elderly heart failure population, the vasodilating properties of nebivolol might confer superior tolerability vis-à-vis other β-blockers. Treatment discontinuation rates (for reasons other than death) were high, but were similar between the nebivolol and placebo groups (27% and 25% respectively), and >80% of the nebivolol arm achieved ≥50% of the target dose.

Treatment with nebivolol reduced the composite risk of all-cause mortality or cardiovascular hospital admission (the primary endpoint) by 15%, and this effect remained consistent across multiple subgroups, including age. Especially since half of the trial population were in fact aged ≥75 years, this implies that nebivolol is efficacious in patients who are very substantially older than in the other major β-blocker trials. In a retrospective analysis, the investigators examined the subgroup of SENIORS patients who were most similar to those in previous β-blocker trials (namely, those aged 70–74 years and with LVEF ≤35%). In this cohort, the risk reduction for the primary end-point was greater (27%), and the reduction in all-cause mortality (38%) was similar to that found in other trials. This implies that elderly patients with higher LVEF derive less benefit from β-blocker therapy. Nevertheless, SENIORS demonstrated that nebivolol is both efficacious and tolerable in elderly patients with heart failure.

This conclusion is supported by a meta-analysis of all-cause mortality data from the US Carvedilol trials, BEST, CIBIS II, COPERNICUS, and MERIT-HF, which demonstrated no significant reduction in the treatment effect of β-blockers in 'elderly' patients as compared to 'non-elderly'.[48] A more recent, large patient-level meta-analysis of patients with HFrEF in sinus rhythm reinforced the case for β-blockers in elderly patients, despite noting that the treatment effect was attenuated in older patients.[49] In summary, there is good evidence for a prognostic benefit of β-blockers in elderly patients and, whereas genuine contraindications and patient preference may override this principle, those of a more mature

vintage should not be denied optimal therapy merely because 'they are too old'.

Pharmacological differences among β-blockers

Selective and non-selective β-blockers

The human heart contains both β_1 and β_2 ARs in a ratio of approximately 4:1. It is commonly believed that the harmful effects of increased sympathetic activity are mediated by the β_1 receptor through G-protein-coupled stimulation of cyclic AMP (cAMP) leading to activation of a number of downstream signalling pathways associated with ventricular and vascular remodelling.

Nevertheless, there has been prolonged debate as to the relative merits clinically of β_1 'selective' and 'non-selective' β_1 and β_2 AR antagonists in cardiovascular disease generally. Insofar as heart failure is concerned, this issue seemed to be resolved when the β_1-selective β-blockers bisoprolol and metoprolol, and the non-selective β-blocker carvedilol, were all shown to reduce all-cause death substantially and to the similar extent of about one-third in, respectively, the CIBIS II, MERIT-HF, and COPERNICUS trials. But interest in potential differences, initiated by the remarkable two-thirds reduction in mortality in the US carvedilol trials, was heightened by the results of the COMET trial, in which the non-selective β-blocker carvedilol was associated with a statistically and clinically significant lower mortality than the β_1-selective β-blocker metoprolol.[50] Although carvedilol has other potentially valuable ancillary properties, including β_1 AR blockade, there are no supportive outcome data from large clinical trials in heart failure for benefit of α_1 blockade[51] or antioxidant activity.

The question of β-blocker dose was addressed in COMET, in which the study design aimed to effect comparable reductions in heart rate between the two groups, since the molecular effects in the myocardium are similar when equipotent doses of carvedilol and metoprolol, in terms of inhibition of exercise-induced tachycardia, are compared.[52]

The resting heart-rate reduction of 13.3 beats/min in COMET with carvedilol 50 mg/day (mean dose at the onset of maintenance phase 42mg/day) was very similar to that achieved with the same dose in the US carvedilol studies on which the COMET dose was based. The heart-rate reduction with the dose of 100 mg/day metoprolol tartrate (mean dose at the onset of maintenance phase 85mg/day), however, was only 11.7 beats/min compared with 15 beats/min achieved with 100 mg/day to 150 mg/day in the Metoprolol in Dilated Cardiomyopathy trial (MDC) on which the dose of metoprolol in COMET was based.[53] Moreover, the major study of metoprolol in heart failure that addressed outcome was the MERIT-HF study, in which the preparation of metoprolol used was metoprolol succinate, a controlled/extended release formulation (metoprolol CR/XL), at a target dose of 200 mg/day. The mean dose actually taken and the mean reduction in heart rate achieved were 159 mg (equivalent to 106 mg of metoprolol tartrate) and 14 beats/min, similar to that found in the MDC trial. Thus the greater benefit in outcomes with carvedilol over metoprolol in the COMET trial might suggest that equivalent blockade of cardiac β_1 receptors may not have been achieved in the metoprolol arm.

Experimental data on β-blocker pharmacology (**Figure 50.1**) challenge the conventional wisdom regarding the primacy of the β_1 receptor in health and disease and heart failure in particular. First, receptor-binding studies using cultured human cells have questioned the validity of previous clinical classifications of β-blockers as 'selective' or 'non-selective'.[54] For example, carvedilol in human tissue is a more potent blocker of β_2 than of β_1 receptors, while the β_2 effects of drugs formerly classified as 'selective' β_1 antagonists such as bisoprolol and metoprolol could be clinically more significant than previously appreciated.[54] Secondly, in health, the β_1 ARs are located on the cell crests, ensuring their wide distribution over the entire cell surface (**Figure 50.2**).[55] This facilitates, following their stimulation, wide diffusion of the Gs-protein-coupled production of the second messenger cAMP throughout the cytoplasm where it increases the strength and frequency of myocyte contraction. The effects of cAMP following stimulation of the β_2 ARs, residing in the base of the T

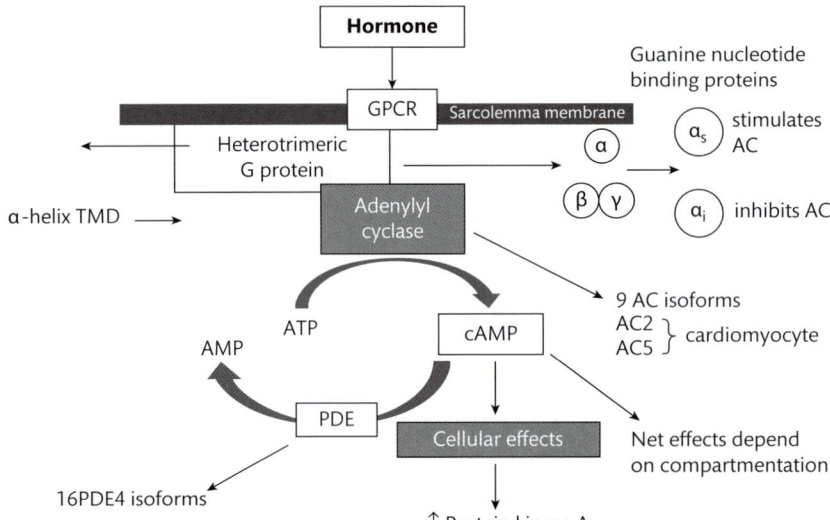

Figure 50.1 Different β_1/β_2 coupling mechanisms to downstream effectors. Note that β_2 adrenoceptors, when phosphorylated, can activate the Gi proteins which in turn activate various kinases to initiate apoptotic, fibrotic, and inflammatory processes. The original model pathway in shown in green; subsequent discoveries of cAMP modulation are in red.

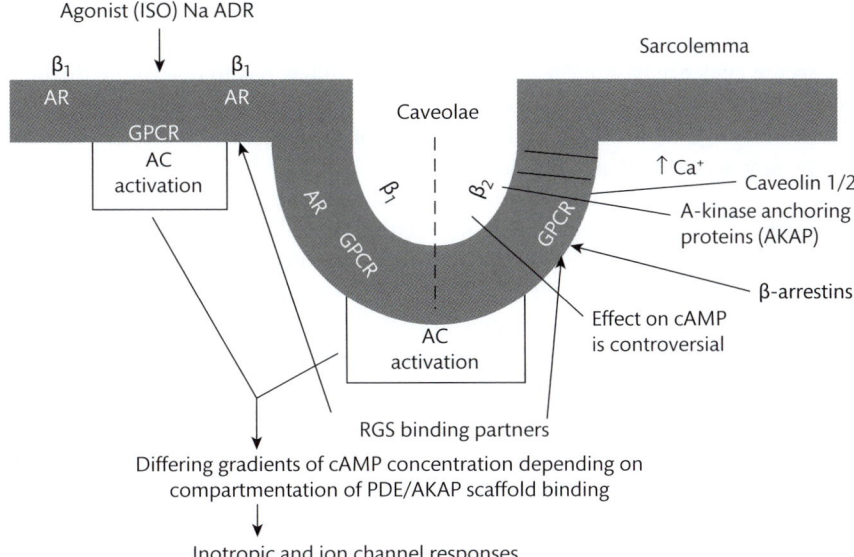

Figure 50.2 The differing downstream effects of activation of protein kinase A by cAMP. Note the complex effects of phosphorylation of different cardiomyocyte cytosolic mediators and its role in β₂ adrenoceptor downregulation.

tubules of the cell membrane, are more localized. Studies show, however, that this compartmentalization of β-AR function is disrupted, leading to relocation of β_2 ARs to the cell surface where their subsequent stimulation causes a pattern of cAMP release similar to that of β_1 receptor stimulation. Thirdly, β_1 but not β_2 receptors are downregulated in heart failure,[56,57] thereby changing the effective ratio of functioning β_1 and β_2 activity from 4:1 to 3:2.

It has also been hypothesized that carvedilol may have a protective effect by stimulating the β-arrestin signalling pathway in the presence of chronic catecholamine stimulation, leading to inhibition of mycocyte apoptosis, as is the case in heart failure. By contrast, G-protein-dependent signalling may be cardiotoxic under these same conditions.[58] Thus there remains a place for further investigation of the relative roles of β_1 and β_2 receptor function in heart failure.

Intrinsic sympathomimesis (partial agonism)

Several β-adrenoceptor antagonists have partial agonist activity, which it was hoped might protect against β-blocker-induced myocardial depression while also ameliorating or preventing some common side-effects including excessive bradycardia due to either β_1 or β_2 antagonism, cold hands, and bronchoconstriction due to β_2 antagonism. Partial agonism has never been shown conclusively to have beneficial effects, however, and in terms of outcome no improvement has been seen in post-MI trials.

The role of partial agonism in heart failure was investigated through the clinical development programme of the β_1 selective partial agonist xamoterol (Corwin).[59,60] It was hypothesized that xamoterol would be useful in protecting the heart from the adverse effects of increased sympathetic stimulation during daytime activities while providing support for the heart through expression of partial agonism during periods of low sympathetic traffic during rest. Ambulatory ECG monitoring showed a clear reduction of the heart rate during the day and a substantial increase nocturnally, in keeping with its significant degree of β_1 agonism. The clinical trials that led to the licensing of xamoterol for mild-to-moderate heart

failure demonstrated clear evidence of benefit by improving quality of life and increasing exercise capacity.[59] Unfortunately the large trial set up to investigate its efficacy and safety in severe heart failure was stopped by the data-monitoring committee because of excess mortality in the xamoterol arm.[60] There was no pattern to the mode of death, and no plausible explanation for the adverse outcome could be discerned from all the data collected. Despite the ambulatory monitoring studies no definite association between the heart rate findings and mortality could be determined. It remains tantalizing to speculate that had xamoterol been introduced at a very small dose and titrated slowly to the target dose, in keeping with modern β-blocking therapy in heart failure, the outcome of that trial might have been very different.

The only other β-blocker with partial agonism to be studied in a large RCT in heart failure is bucindolol. Unlike all the other landmark trials of β-blockers, the BEST trial of bucindolol failed to show a convincing increase in survival,[61,62] suggesting the possibility of detrimental effects in Black Americans but benefit in White subjects. It cannot be concluded that partial β-receptor partial agonism was culpable, but it has been suggested that genetic polymorphisms among the subjects could have influenced the result. Bucindolol is known to be strongly sympatholytic and in BEST, as in the MOXCON study of moxonidine in heart failure, sympatholysis was associated with poor survival. Polymorphism of two genes concerned with β_1 AR function, the glycine moiety of the β-arginine/glycine 389 and the preadrenergic junctional α_2c-Del 3222–3225 AR, were linked to sympatholysis and poorer survival.[63,64]

Practical aspects of β-blocker use

Who should receive β-blockers?

β-Blockers are a class 1 (A) recommendation in the major guidelines on heart failure treatment because of the overwhelming evidence of benefit, especially in patients with LVSD (HFrEF).[36,65] The

evidence for benefit in patients with HFpEF is much less complete at present, due not to adverse results but to a relative dearth of trials similar to those on which the secure evidence base for β-blockers in HFrEF has been built. The data in SENIORS, the only large trial to address this issue, is consistent with the trials in HFrEF and their meta-analyses. In SENIORS, a pragmatic, more modern, approach was taken in comparison to some older trials by including patients with 'heart failure' as determined by a clinical diagnosis made in a specialist setting. The results revealed no heterogeneity of effect between those with impaired or significantly unimpaired left ventricular systolic function. Since the overarching view of the progression of heart failure and its pharmacological treatment is based on antagonizing the putative deleterious effects of neuroendocrine systems, especially the RAAS and the sympathetic nervous system,[66] it is not unreasonable to believe that inhibitors of these systems should be beneficial in heart failure *per se*, both HFrEF and HFpEF, to an extent depending on the degree of activation of these systems. There are also other reasons for prescribing β-blockers due to the protean nature of their indications, including hypertension and angina pectoris, conditions that are present in many patients either as a comorbidity or as a cause of their heart failure. The anti-arrhythmic effects of β-blockers are particularly relevant in heart failure for preventing or gaining rate control of AF and for preventing sudden cardiac death from serious ventricular arrhythmia. In the specific case of HFpEF there may also be pathophysiological justification for β-blockade including the promotion of better filling by reducing the heart rate.[67] For all these reasons β-blockers should be considered in all patients with heart failure in the absence of a specific-disease-related or other standard contraindication.

Research and especially clinical trials of medications has traditionally been dominated by studies in LVSD, although more recently complemented by studies of a variety of medications in patients with preserved ejection fractions. Very little is known about the effects of the major 'heart failure' medications including β-blockers in patients with other forms of specific heart disease such as valvular heart diseases and specific heart muscle disorders, apart from their indication for rate control in AF. In those circumstances clinical judgement is required to identify those patients with characteristics that might suggest benefit from β-blockers.

Which β-blocker should be prescribed and at what dose?

In both Europe and the USA, bisoprolol, carvedilol, and metoprolol are approved by the relevant regulatory bodies for the treatment of heart failure due to LVSD because of the strong evidence for benefit for all three medicines. In the UK, but not in the USA, nebivolol is also licensed for the treatment of heart failure in patients aged ≥70 years. Currently it has not been approved for heart failure by either the European Medicines Agency or the US Food and Drug Administration. No other β-blocker has been licensed in the heart failure indication because of the absence of large trials confirming safety and efficacy. In these circumstances it is recommended that, where possible, licensed medicines should be prescribed at a dose and in a manner that was tested in the relevant clinical trials.

Pharmacoepidemiological data[68,69] provide a perspective on outcomes of different classes of β-blockers from managed care databases such as, for example, the DECIDE programme and the North Carolina Medicaid/Medicare patients. The objective of these studies was to determine the outcomes of patients taking either β-blockers approved by the FDA—namely carvedilol, metoprolol succinate, and bisoprolol fumarate, which are considered to have evidence-based treatment for heart failure—or atenolol. In DECIDE, there was no difference between atenolol and carvedilol in either mortality or rehospitalization rates, whereas there appeared to be an increased risk using short-acting metoprolol tartrate.[68] The Medicare/Medicaid study showed that there was no difference between outcomes in either approved or unapproved β-blockers, and both showed a substantial benefit compared with no β-blocker treatment.[69]

Pharmacoepidemiology data are available for atenolol—one of the most widely prescribed β-blockers in the world—for many other indications, which suggests that long-term outcomes were similar in patients on licensed β-blockers and atenolol. This is by no means equivalent to data on safety and efficacy but it does give some comfort to patients and clinicians practising in economically challenged countries throughout the world.

At what stage of heart failure should β-blockers be prescribed?

Data from the large heart failure trials were obtained in patients with NYHA class II–IV heart failure who were clinically stable at the time of initiation of treatment. The earlier trials recruited largely ambulant outpatients of milder severity and greater stability, whereas studies such as CAPRICORN[23] and COPERNICUS[26] included inpatients recovering from an acute MI or recent decompensation of chronic heart failure respectively. These trials demonstrated the safety of inpatient prescribing in an environment where the availability of specialist expertise in heart failure and adherence to a clear protocol for initiation and uptitration allowed the safe introduction and continuation of β-blockade.

Subsequently the additional benefit obtained from initiating treatment during an acute admission has been confirmed in clinical practice.[70] A different but still important question is whether β-blockers should be used in patients with asymptomatic LVSD, which differs technically from NYHA functional class I heart failure in that these patients have never had symptomatic heart failure at any point. A proportion of the patients with post-MI LVSD in CAPRICORN were asymptomatic, and on this basis international guidelines recommend β-blockers in patients with asymptomatic LVSD and a history of MI 'in order to prevent or delay the onset of heart failure or prolong life'.[36] β-Blocker therapy was also shown to reverse left ventricular (LV) remodelling in patients with asymptomatic LVSD in the smaller REVERT trial, which randomized 149 such patients to metoprolol succinate or placebo.[71] In almost half of this group, LVSD was of non-ischaemic aetiology. The success of metoprolol in attenuating LV remodelling in REVERT suggests a pathologic basis for the benefit of β-blockers in asymptomatic, non-ischaemic LVSD, and therefore a mechanistic justification for their use in this population. However, although LV remodelling is frequently regarded as a surrogate for important clinical outcomes, REVERT was insufficiently powered to determine whether metoprolol therapy affected rates of mortality or hospitalization. Therefore, there is thought to be insufficient evidence currently to

recommend β-blockers for asymptomatic LVSD in the absence of a previous MI.[36]

How should β-blockers be used?

A detailed exposition of initiation, titration, and chronic dosing is beyond the scope of this chapter but it is crucially important that patients are clinically stable at the time of initiation even though this may be only a few days after an episode of decompensation or of an acute MI. Acute blockade of β-adrenergic receptors in patients who are already 'decompensated' carries the potential to cause disastrous haemodynamic upset due to a reduction in cardiac output and increase in filling pressures. Recognition of 'stability' is a matter of clinical judgement but cardinal signs include absence of fluid retention (euvolaemia) and of other signs of circulatory failure such as hypotension (systolic blood pressure ≥90 mmHg), peripheral hypoperfusion, and oliguria. These criteria are a matter for local implementation guidelines, ideally in the context of a multidisciplinary heart failure programme within which the safe and effective use of β-blockers is best achieved (Chapter 62).

The clinical trials all have had detailed initial dose titration schedules and a final target dose and these are a practical guide to management. As a rule of thumb, the mantra 'start low, go slow' is sound advice.

What is the optimum prescription rate for β-blockers in heart failure?

Adherence to medication and doses achieved in clinical trials are often much higher than in 'real life' clinical practice for several very good reasons related to the selection criteria of the former circumstance and the clinical status and frailty of unselected patients in the latter. Nevertheless, in clinical practice it is possible to achieve target doses in a high percentage of patients depending on the skill, patience and time available to the health professionals concerned. In this light, it is greatly satisfying to witness the consistent improvement in prescription rates achieved in UK clinical practice. Nationally, the proportion of patients prescribed a β-blocker following a hospital admission for heart failure has risen remarkably, from 31% to 38% (varying according to gender) in 2005–2006,[72] to 87% in 2015–2016.[47] Similarly, the latest clinical audit data from the ESC Heart Failure Long-Term Registry indicate a pan-European β-blocker prescription rate of 92.7% among patients with chronic heart failure.[73] In parallel, β-blocker prescription rates achieved in large randomized heart failure trials have risen steadily (see Table 50.3), yet it is important to note that the 'prescription gap' between the spheres of clinical practice and clinical trials has closed substantially in recent years.

It remains the case, however, that titration of medical therapy in heart failure is complex for many reasons, and should be conducted

Table 50.3 β-Blocker use in selected heart failure trials by year

	USCTP	COPERNICUS	CAPRICORN	CARMEN[a]	COMET[b]	MOCHA	PRECISE	REVERT
Patients (n)	1094	2289	1959	479	3029		278	366
NYHA class	II–IV	NA	NA	I–III	II–IV	II–III	II–III	II
LVEF	≤35%	<25%	Post-MI ≤40%	≤39%	26%	23%	22%	23%
Mean follow-up (months)	6.5	10.4	15	18	58	6	6	12
Mean dose achieved (mg/day)	45	37	20	CAR: 47.9[c] CAR: 48.7[d]	CAR: 41.8 MET: 85.0	6.25 12.5 bd 25.0	6.25 bd upwards	6.25 bd
Primary end-point	Safety	All-cause mortality	All-cause mortality or all-cause mortality or CV hospitalization combined	LV remodelling	All-cause mortality	Exercise tolerance Quality of life	Improved EF	CHF progression^
Results	All-cause mortality reduced 65%[e]	All-cause mortality reduced 35%	All-cause mortality reduced 23%	LVESVI reduced in combination with enalapril	17% relative risk reduction in favour of carvedilol	All-cause mortality reduced 73%	Morbidity and mortality reduced	Mortality Hospitalization EF^^ all reduced
P-value	0.0001	0.00013	0.031	<0.002	0.0017	0.001 Hospitalization rate 0.01	0.001/0.029	^0.008 ^^0.03

CAPRICORN, Carvedilol Postinfarct Survival Controlled Evaluation; CAR, carvedilol; CARMEN, Carvedilol Ace Inhibitor Remodelling Mild Heart Failure Evaluation; CHF, chronic heart failure; COMET, Carvedilol or Metoprolol European Trial; COPERNICUS, Carvedilol Prospective Randomized Cumulative Survival; CV, cardiovascular; EF, ejection fraction; LVEF, left ventricular ejection fraction; LVESVI, left ventricular end-systolic volume index; MET, metoprolol; MI, myocardial infarction; MOCHA, Multi-Center Oral Carvedilol Heart Failure Assessment; NYHA, New York Heart Association class; PRECISE, Prospective Randomized Trial of the Optimal Evaluation of Cardiac Symptoms and Revascularization; REVERT, REversal of VEntricular Remodeling with Toprol-XL; RRR, relative risk reduction; USCTP, US Carvedilol Heart Failure Study Programme.

[a] Compared with enalapril alone or in combination with enalapril.
[b] Carvedilol vs metoprolol.
[c] Dose of carvedilol achieved as monotherapy.
[d] Dose of carvedilol achieved as part of combination therapy with enalapril.
[e] End-point.

in a multidisciplinary setting such as in the clinical trials within which the data on safety and efficacy were obtained.

When should β-blockers be withdrawn or reduced?

'Withdrawal' effects due to excess sympathetic stimulation have been noted after abrupt cessation of β-blockers in circumstances other than heart failure. In hypertension this has led to loss of control of blood pressure and in angina pectoris to acute exacerbations.[90] There has therefore been concern over the possible consequences of sudden withdrawal of β-blockers in patients with heart failure, especially in the situation of acute decompensation. In order to avoid this potential hazard many have simply reduced the dose to that of initiation with uptitration when stabilization has occurred. No detriment has been reported by continuing with the maintenance dose, both from registry data and B-CONVINCED, a randomized trial designed to address this specific issue.[91,92] In B-CONVINCED, continuation of β-blocker therapy during an acute decompensation was also associated with a higher rate of β-blocker therapy at three months, with a clear benefit of this inferred.[92] Nevertheless, no hard-and-fast rule need apply and there will be clinical situations in which acute, partial, or no withdrawal will be appropriate according to the individual circumstances.

Reduction or withdrawal of β-blockers may be necessary in very advanced heart failure associated with hypotension and deteriorating renal function as part of a general review of the overall medicines prescription since all 'evidence-based medicines' for heart failure can lower the blood pressure to an extent that renal function is compromised. This is often temporary, but in the state of terminal care it is reasonable to continue only those medicines that will contribute positively to the palliative care of the patient.

Finally, when typical side-effects occur, it should be recalled that patients randomized to placebo in β-blocker trials report side-effects at comparable rates to those receiving the study drug. Indeed, non-specific adverse effects such as fatigue may in fact be more common in placebo groups.[93] Moreover, where β-blocker therapy is associated with a higher incidence of adverse effects—as it is with hypotension, dizziness, and bradycardia—the increases in risk remain small in absolute terms.[93] Supporting this, a pooled analysis of nine major β-blocker trials determined study drug withdrawal to be greater across the placebo groups than β-blocker groups.[93]

Conclusions

The use of β-blockers in heart failure has been both a revelation and a revolution. Sir James Black, the inventor of by far the most successful class of medicines for cardiovascular disease, died in 2010 at the age of 85. Modest to the end about his immense contribution to cardiovascular science and medicine, his quests for new mechanisms and medicines had never ceased. Without prejudice to his many colleagues with whom he was still working, it may be said that the β-blocker odyssey of discovery has not ended.

REFERENCES

1. Fitzgerald D. The importance of chance and the prepared mind in the discovery of beta blockers. *Dialog Cardiovasc Med* 2000;**5**:172–5.

2. Cruickshank JM, Pritchard BNC. *β-Blockers in clinical practice*. Churchill Livingstone, London, 1994.

3. Pritchard BNC, Dickinson CJ, Alleyne GAO, et al. Effect of pronethalol in angina pectoris. *Br Med J* 1963;ii:1226–7.

4. Yusuf S, Peto R, Lewis J, Collins R, Sleight I. Beta blockade during and after myocardial infarction: an overview of the randomized trials. *Prog Cardiovasc Dis* 1985;**27**:335–71.

5. McMurray J. Major β blocker mortality trials in chronic heart failure: a critical review. *Heart* 1999;**82**(Suppl IV):IV14–22.

6. Chidsey CA, Vogel JHK. Adrenergic mechanisms in heart failure. In Kattus AA, Ross G, Hall VE (eds), *Cardiovascular β-adrenergic responses: UCLA Forum in Medical Sciences 13*, pp. 81–92. University of California Press, Berkeley, 1970.

7. Chidsey CA, Braunwald E. Sympathetic activity and neurotransmitter depletion in congestive heart failure. *Pharmacol Rev* 1966;**18**:685–700.

8. Epstein SE, Braunwald E. Circulatory effects and clinical applications of β-adrenergic receptor inhibition. In Kattus AA, Ross G, Hall VE (eds), *Cardiovascular β-adrenergic responses: UCLA Forum in Medical Sciences 13*, pp. 139–49. University of California Press, Berkeley, 1970.

9. Gibson DG, Balcon R, Souten E. Clinical use of ICI 50172 as an anti-dysrhythmic agent in heart failure. *Br Med J* 1968;**3**:161–3.

10. Waagstein F, Hjalmaison A, Vernauskas E, Wallentin I. Effects of chronic β-adrenergic receptor blockade in congestive cardiomyopathy. *Br Heart J* 1975;**37**:1022–36.

11. Swedberg K, Hjalmarson A, Waagstein F, Wallentin I. Beneficial effects of long-term β-blockade in congestive cardiomopathy. *Br Heart J* 1980;**44**:117–33.

12. Swedberg K, Hjalmarson A, Waagstein F, Wallentin I. Prolongation of survival in congestive cardiomyopathy by beta-receptor blockade. *Lancet* 1979;**1**(8131):1374–6.

13. CONSENSUS Trial Study Group. Effects of enalapril on mortality in severe congestive heart failure. Results of the Cooperative North Scandinavian Enalapril Survival Study (CONSENSUS). *N Engl J Med* 1987;**316**:1429–35.

14. SOLVD Investigators. Effect of enalapril on survival in patients with reduced left ventricular ejection fractions and congestive heart failure. *N Engl J Med* 1991;**325**:293–302.

15. Granger CB, McMurray JJ, Yusuf S, et al. Effects of candesartan in patients with chronic heart failure and reduced left-ventricular systolic function intolerant to angiotensin-converting-enzyme inhibitors: the CHARM-Alternative trial. *Lancet* 2003;**362**:772–6.

16. McMurray JJ, Packer M, Desai AS, et al. Angiotensin–neprilysin inhibition versus enalapril in heart failure. *N Engl J Med* 2014;**371**:993–1004.

17. Pitt B, Zannad F, Remme WJ, et al. The effect of spironolactone on morbidity and mortality in patients with severe heart failure. Randomized Aldactone Evaluation Study Investigators. *N Engl J Med* 1999;**341**:709–17.

18. Packer M, Bristow MR, Cohn JN, et al. The effects of carvedilol on morbidity and mortality in chronic heart failure. *N Engl J Med* 1996;**334**:1249–55.

19. CIBIS II investigators and committees. The Cardiac Insufficiency Bisoprolol Study: a randomized trial. *Lancet* 1999;**353**:9–13.

20. MERIT HF Study Group. Effect of metoprolol CR/XL in chronic heart failure: CR/XL Randomised Intervention Trial in Congestive Heart Failure (MERIT HF). *Lancet* 1999;**353**:2001–7.

21. Mann DL. Basic mechanisms of left ventricular remodeling: the contribution of wall stress. *J Card Fail* 2004;**10**(6 Suppl):S202–6.

22. Australia/New Zealand Heart Failure Research Collaborative Group. Randomised, placebo-controlled trial of carvedilol in

patients with congestive heart failure due to ischaemic heart disease. *Lancet* 1997;**349**:375–80.

23. Dargie HJ. Effect of carvedilol on outcome after myocardial infarction in patients with left-ventricular dysfunction: the CAPRICORN randomised trial. *Lancet* 2001;**357**(9266):1385–90.

24. Doughty RN, Whalley GA, Walsh HA, et al. Effects of carvedilol on left ventricular remodeling after acute myocardial infarction: the CAPRICORN Echo Substudy. *Circulation* 2004;**109**(2):201–6.

25. McMurray J, Køber L, Robertson M, et al. Antiarrhythmic effect of carvedilol after acute myocardial infarction. Results of the Carvedilol Post-Infarct Survival Control in Left Ventricular Dysfunction (CAPRICORN) Trial. *J Am Coll Cardiol* 2005;**45**:525–30.

26. Packer M, Coats AJ, Fowler MB, et al. Effect of carvedilol on survival in severe chronic heart failure. *N Engl J Med* 2001;**344**:1651–8.

27. Zile M. Heart failure with preserved ejection fraction: is this diastolic heart failure? *J Am Coll Cardiol* 2003;**41**:1519–22.

28. Flather MD, Shibata MC, Coats AJ, et al. Randomized trial to determine the effect of nebivolol on mortality and cardiovascular hospital admission in elderly patients with heart failure. (SENIORS). *Eur Heart J* 2005;**26**:215–25.

29. Yamamoto K, Origasa H, Hori M on behalf of the J-DHF investigators. Effects of carvedilol on heart failure with preserved ejection fraction: the Japanese Diastolic Heart Failure Study (J-DHF). *Eur J Heart Fail* 2013;**15**:110–18.

30. Bavishi C, Chatterjee S, Ather S, et al. Beta-blockers in heart failure with preserved ejection fraction: a meta-analysis. *Heart Fail Rev* 2015;**20**:193–201.

31. Fukuta H, Goto T, Wakami K, et al. The effect of beta-blockers on mortality in heart failure with preserved ejection fraction: a meta-analysis of observational cohort and randomized controlled studies. *Int J Card* 2017;**228**:4–10.

32. Hawkins NM, Macdonald MR, Petrie MC, et al. Bisoprolol in patients with heart failure and moderate to severe chronic obstructive pulmonary disease: a randomized controlled trial. *Eur J Heart Fail* 2009;**11**:684–90.

33. Lainscak M, Podbregar M, Kovacic D, et al. Differences between bisoprolol and carvedilol in patients with chronic heart failure and chronic obstructive pulmonary disease: a randomized trial. *Resp Med* 2011;**105**(Suppl 1):S44–S49.

34. Jabbour A, Macdonald PS, Keogh AM, et al. Differences between beta-blockers in patients with chronic heart failure and chronic obstructive pulmonary disease: a randomized crossover trial. *J Am Coll Cardiol* 2010;**55**:1780–7.

35. Andrus MR, Holloway KP, Clark DB. Use of beta-blockers in patients with COPD. *Ann Pharmacother* 2004;**38**(1):142–5.

36. Ponikowski P, Voors AA, Anker SD, et al. 2016 ESC Guidelines for the diagnosis and treatment of acute and chronic heart failure: The Task Force for the diagnosis and treatment of acute and chronic heart failure of the European Society of Cardiology (ESC). Developed with the special contribution of the Heart Failure Association (HFA) of the ESC. *Eur J Heart Fail* 2016;**18**(8):891–975.

37. Global Initiative for Asthma. Global strategy for asthma management and prevention 2016. Available via http://ginasthma.org/2016-gina-report-global-strategy-for-asthma-management-and-prevention/

38. Fonarow GC. A review of evidence-based beta-blockers in special populations with heart failure. *Rev Cardiovasc Med* 2008;**9**(2):84–95.

39. Maisel WH, Stevenson LW. Atrial fibrillation in heart failure: epidemiology, pathophysiology, and rationale for therapy. *Am J Cardiol* 2003;**91**(6A):2D–8D.

40. McMurray JJV, van Veldhuisen DJ. β Blockers, atrial fibrillation, and heart failure. *Lancet* 2014–15;**384**(9961):2181–3.

41. Wang TJ, Larson MG, Levy D, et al. Temporal relations of atrial fibrillation and congestive heart failure and their joint influence on mortality: the Framingham Heart Study. *Circulation* 2003;**107**:2920–25.

42. Kotecha D, Holmes J, Krum H, et al. Efficacy of β blockers in patients with heart failure plus atrial fibrillation: an individual-patient-data meta-analysis. *Lancet* 2014;**384**:2235–43.

43. Rienstra M, Damman K, Mulder BA, et al. Beta-blockers and outcome in heart failure and atrial fibrillation: a meta-analysis. *JACC: Heart Failure* 2013;**1**:21–8.

44. Li SJ, Sartipy U, Lund LH, et al. Prognostic significance of resting heart rate and use of β-blockers in atrial fibrillation and sinus rhythm in patients with heart failure and reduced ejection fraction findings from the Swedish Heart Failure Registry. *Circ Heart Fail* 2015;**8**:871–9.

45. Bristow MR, Aleong RG. Treatment of the heart failure patient with atrial fibrillation: a major unmet need. *JACC: Heart Fail* 2013;**1**(1):29–30.

46. Cullington D, Goode K, Zhang J, et al. Is heart rate important for patients with heart failure in atrial fibrillation? *JACC Heart Fail* 2014;**2**(3):213–20.

47. National Institute for Cardiovascular Outcomes Research (NICOR). *National Heart Failure Audit April 2015—March 2016*. https://www.ucl.ac.uk/nicor/audits/heartfailure/reports

48. Dulin BR, Haas SJ, Abraham WT, et al. Do elderly systolic heart failure patients benefit from beta blockers to the same extent as the non-elderly? Meta-analysis of >12,000 patients in large-scale clinical trials. *Am J Cardiol* 2005;**95**(7):896–8.

49. Kotecha D, Manzano L, Krum H, et al. Effect of age and sex on efficacy and tolerability of β blockers in patients with heart failure with reduced ejection fraction: individual patient data meta-analysis. *BMJ* 2016;**353**:i1855.

50. Poole-Wilson P, Swedberg K, Cleland JG, et al. Comparison of carvedilol and metoprolol on clinical outcomes in patients with chronic heart failure in the Carvedilol Or Metoprolol European Trial (COMET): randomised controlled trial. *Lancet* 2003;**362**:7–13.

51. Cohn JN, Archibald DG, Ziesche S, et al. Effect of vasodilator therapy on mortality in chronic congestive heart failure. *N Engl J Med* 1986;**314**:1547–52.

52. Dargie HJ. Beta blockers in heart failure. *Lancet* 2003;**362**(9377):2–3.

53. Waagstein F, Bristow MR, Swedberg K, et al. Beneficial effects of metoprolol in idiopathic dilated cardiomyopathy. Metoprolol in Dilated Cardiomyopathy (MDC) Trial Study Group. *Lancet* 1993;**342**(8885):1441–6.

54. Baker JG. The selectivity of β-adrenoceptor antagonists at the human β_1, β_2, and β_3 adrenoceptors. *Br J Pharmacol* 2005;**144**:317–22.

55. Nikolaev VO, Moshkov A, Lyon AR, et al. Beta2-adrenergic receptor redistribution in heart failure changes cAMP compartmentation. *Science* 2010;**327**:1653–7.

56. Bristow MR, Ginsburg R, Umans V, et al. Beta 1- and beta 2-adrenergic-receptor subpopulations in nonfailing and failing human ventricular myocardium: coupling of both receptor subtypes to muscle contraction and selective beta 1-receptor down-regulation in heart failure. *Circ Res* 1986;**59**:297–309.

57. Brodde O-E. β_1- and β_2-Adrenoceptors in the human heart: properties, function and alterations in chronic heart failure. *Pharmacol Rev* 1991;**43**:203–41.

58. Wisler JW, DeWire SM, Whalen EJ, et al. A unique mechanism of β-blocker action: carvedilol stimulates β-arrestin signaling. *Proc Natl Acad Sci USA* 2007;**104**:16659–62.

59. Marlow HF. Review of clinical experience with xamoterol. Effects on exercise capacity and symptoms in heart failure. *Circulation* 1990;**81**(2 Suppl):III93–8.

60. Xamoterol in Severe Heart Failure Study Group. Xamoterol in severe heart failure. *Lancet* 1990;**336**(8706):1–6.

61. BEST Investigators. A trial of the β-adrenergic blocker bucindolol in patients with advanced chronic heart failure. *N Engl J Med* 2001;**344**:1659–67.

62. Domanski MJ, Krause-Steinrauf H, Massie BM, et al. A comparative analysis of the results from 4 trials of beta-blocker therapy for heart failure: BEST, CIBIS-II, MERIT-HF, and COPERNICUS. *J Card Fail* 2003;**9**(5):354–63.

63. Cohn JN, Pfeffer MA, Rouleau J, et al. Adverse mortality effect of central sympathetic inhibition with sustained-release moxonidine in patients with heart failure (MOXCON). *Eur J Heart Fail* 2003;**5**(5):659–67.

64. Bristow MR, Murphy GA, Krause-Steinrauf H, et al. An alpha2C-adrenergic receptor polymorphism alters the norepinephrine-lowering effects and therapeutic response of the beta-blocker bucindolol in chronic heart failure. *Circ Heart Fail* 2010;**3**(1):21–8.

65. Yancy CB, Jessup M, Bozkurt B, et al. 2013 ACCF/AHA Guideline for the Management of Heart Failure. A Report of the American College of Cardiology Foundation/American Heart Association Task Force on Practice Guidelines. *Circulation* 2013;**128**:e240–e327.

66. Mann DL. Basic mechanisms of disease progression in the failing heart: the role of excessive adrenergic drive. *Prog Cardiovasc Dis* 1998;**41**(1 Suppl 1):1–8.

67. Zile MR. Diastolic heart failure. Diagnosis, prognosis, treatment. *Minerva Cardioangiol* 2003;**51**(2):131–42.

68. Go AS, Yang J, Gurwitz JH, et al. Comparative effectiveness of different beta-adrenergic antagonists on mortality among adults with heart failure in clinical practice. *Arch Intern Med* 2008;**168**(22):2415–21.

69. Kramer JM, Curtis LH, Dupree CS, et al. Comparative effectiveness of beta-blockers in elderly patients with heart failure. *Arch Intern Med* 2008;**168**(22):2422–8; discussion 8–32.

70. Martinez-Selles M, Datino T, Alhama M. Rapid carvedilol up-titration in hospitalized patients with left ventricular systolic dysfunction—data from the Carvedilol in Hospital: Up-titration Limits after Acute Patients Admission registry. *J Cardiovasc Med (Hagerstown)* 2010;**11**(5):352–8.

71. Colucci WS, Kolias TJ, Adams KF, et al. Metoprolol reverses left ventricular remodeling in patients with asymptomatic systolic dysfunction: the REversal of VEntricular Remodeling with Toprol-XL (REVERT) trial. *Circulation* 2007;**116**:49e56.

72. Nicol ED, Fittall B, Roughton M, et al. NHS heart failure survey: a survey of acute heart failure admissions in England, Wales and Northern Ireland. *Heart* 2008;**94**(2):172–7.

73. Maggioni AP, Anker SD, Dahlstrom U, et al. Are hospitalized or ambulatory patients with heart failure treated in accordance with European Society of Cardiology guidelines? Evidence from 12,440 patients of the ESC Heart Failure Long-Term Registry. *Eur J Heart Fail* 2013;**15**(10):1173–84.

74. SOLVD Investigators. Effect of enalapril on mortality and the development of heart failure in asymptomatic patients with reduced left ventricular ejection fractions. *N Engl J Med* 1992;**327**(10):685–91.

75. Digitalis Investigation Group. The effect of digoxin on mortality and morbidity in patients with heart failure. *N Engl J Med* 1997;**336**(8):525–33.

76. Pitt B, Zannad F, Remme WJ, et al. The effect of spironolactone on morbidity and mortality in patients with severe heart failure. *N Engl J Med* 1999;**341**(10):709–17.

77. Cohn JN, Tognoni G. A randomized trial of the angiotensin-receptor blocker valsartan in chronic heart failure. *N Engl J Med* 2001;**345**(23):1667–75.

78. Bardy GH, Lee KL, Mark DB, et al. Amiodarone or an implantable cardioverter–defibrillator for congestive heart failure. *N Engl J Med* 2005;**352**:225–37.

79. Pfeffer MA, Swedberg K, Granger CB, et al. Effects of candesartan on mortality and morbidity in patients with chronic heart failure: the CHARM-Overall programme. *Lancet* 2003;**362**:759–66.

80. Pitt B, Remme W, Zannad F, et al. Eplerenone, a selective aldosterone blocker, in patients with left ventricular dysfunction after myocardial infarction. *N Engl J Med* 2003;**348**:1309–21.

81. Bristow MR, Saxon LA, Boehmer J, et al. Cardiac-resynchronization therapy with or without an implantable defibrillator in advanced chronic heart failure. *N Engl J Med* 2004;**350**(21):2140–50.

82. Konstam MA, Neaton JD, Dickstein K. Effects of high-dose versus low-dose losartan on clinical outcomes in patients with heart failure (HEAAL study): a randomised, double-blind trial. *Lancet* 2009;**374**:1840–48.

83. Cleland JGF, Daubert JC, Erdmann E, et al. The effect of cardiac resynchronization on morbidity and mortality in heart failure. *N Engl J Med* 2005;**352**(15):1539–49.

84. GISSI-HF investigators. Effect of rosuvastatin in patients with chronic heart failure (the GISSI-HF trial): a randomised, double-blind, placebo-controlled trial. *Lancet* 2008;**372**:1231–39.

85. Kjekshus J, Apetrei E, Barrios V, et al. Rosuvastatin in older patients with systolic heart failure. *N Engl J Med* 2007;**357**:2248–61.

86. Tang ASL, Wells GA, Talajic M, et al. Cardiac-resynchronization therapy for mild-to-moderate heart failure. *N Engl J Med* 2010;**363**:2385–95.

87. Swedberg K, Komajda M, Böhm M, et al. Ivabradine and outcomes in chronic heart failure (SHIFT): a randomised placebo-controlled study. *Lancet* 2010;**376**:875–85.

88. Zannad F, McMurray JJV, Krum H, et al. Eplerenone in patients with systolic heart failure and mild symptoms. *N Engl J Med* 2011;**364**:11–21.

89. Køber L, Thune JJ, Nielsen JC, et al. Defibrillator implantation in patients with nonischemic systolic heart failure. *N Engl J Med* 2016;**375**(13):1221–30.

90. Teichert M, de Smet PA, Hofman A, Witteman JC, Stricker BH. Discontinuation of beta-blockers and the risk of myocardial infarction in the elderly. *Drug Saf* 2007;**30**(6):541–9.

91. Fonarow GC, Abraham WT, Albert NM, et al. Influence of beta-blocker continuation or withdrawal on outcomes in patients hospitalized with heart failure: findings from the OPTIMIZE-HF program. *J Am Coll Cardiol* 2008;**52**(3):190–9.

92. Jondeau G, Neuder Y, Eicher JC, et al. B-CONVINCED: Beta-blocker CONtinuation Vs. INterruption in patients with Congestive heart failure hospitalizED for a decompensation episode. *Eur Heart J* 2009;**30**:2186–92.

93. Ko DT, Hebert PR, Coffey CS, et al. Adverse effects of β-blocker therapy for patients with heart failure. a quantitative overview of randomized trials. *Arch Intern Med* 2004;**164**(13):1389–94.

51

Sodium–glucose co-transporter-2 inhibitors

Matthew M. Y. Lee, Kieran F. Docherty, and Pardeep S. Jhund

Introduction

The sodium–glucose co-transporter 2 inhibitors (SGLT2i) were initially developed as glucose-lowering drugs for the treatment of type 2 diabetes mellitus (T2DM).[1] Through inhibition of the SGLT2 co-transporter (located in the first segment of the proximal convoluted tubule of the kidney), they cause excretion of glucose in the urine, thus reducing blood sugar.[1] In patients with T2DM, this urinary glucose excretion reduces glycated haemoglobin A1c (HbA1c) by around 0.5–1% with the degree of glycosuria being dependent on circulating glucose levels and kidney function. Glycosuria decreases with lower kidney function and with lower circulating glucose, therefore the risk of hypoglycaemia is low. As required by regulatory agencies these drugs were tested in large, randomized controlled trials to ensure that no excess of cardiovascular (CV) events were observed with this new therapy for T2DM.

Clinical trial evidence for SGLT2i in patients with T2DM

Patients with T2DM are at higher risk of death, heart failure, and ischaemic events (myocardial infarction and stroke).[2] After observing that the thiazolidinediones were associated with a higher risk of myocardial infarction,[3] both the US Food and Drug Administration and the European Medicines Agency mandated that new drugs for the treatment of diabetes demonstrate CV safety in large prospective CV outcome trials. These trials were designed to demonstrate that there was no excess of adverse CV outcomes with these drugs. The first of these trials with SGLT2i was the Empagliflozin Cardiovascular Outcome Event Trial in Type 2 Diabetes Mellitus Patients (EMPA-REG OUTCOME) and as well as showing safety with empagliflozin they also reported a significant reduction in the primary end-point of major adverse cardiac events (a composite of non-fatal myocardial infarction, non-fatal stroke or CV death) with a relative risk reduction of 14%.[4] An even larger relative risk reduction (35%) in the risk of hospitalization for heart failure (HHF) was reported, stimulating interest in these drugs as potential treatments for heart failure.[4,5] The results of EMPA-REG OUTCOME were replicated with other SGLT2i (dapagliflozin, canagliflozin, ertugliflozin) in similar trials in T2DM.[6–9] A meta-analysis of these SGLT2i trials including 46,969 unique patients demonstrated that SGLT2i reduced the risk of major adverse cardiac events (hazard ratio (HR): 0.90; 95% confidence interval (CI): 0.85–0.95), CV death/HHF (HR: 0.78; 95% CI: 0.73–0.84), and kidney outcomes (HR: 0.62; 95% CI: 0.56–0.70).[10] The reduction in risk of HHF was highly consistent across the trials (HR: 0.68; CI: 0.61–0.76) and achieving nominal statistical significance in each of the trials.[10] Collectively, these showed the role of SGLT2i in the prevention of heart failure in T2DM patients with a baseline prevalence of heart failure of ~10%, and with similar effects in those with versus without heart failure.[5,11,12] Finally, and importantly for patients with heart failure, the Canagliflozin and Renal Events in Diabetes with Established Nephropathy Clinical Evaluation (CREDENCE) trial examined a primary cardiorenal composite end-point in patients with T2DM and albuminuric chronic kidney disease. In this trial, canagliflozin reduced the primary cardio-renal composite end-point of end-stage kidney disease (dialysis, transplantation, or a sustained estimated glomerular filtration rate (eGFR) of <15 mL/min/1.73 m^2), a doubling of serum creatinine level, or death from renal or CV causes, by 30%, confirming the renal benefits seen in the secondary analyses of trials in patients with T2DM.[8] In light of this evidence, SLGT2i have been adopted into treatment guidelines for T2DM.[13,14]

Beyond glucose-lowering

Importantly, the benefits of SGLT2i were independent of glucose-lowering effects,[15] and a plethora of potential explanatory mechanisms that confer CV and renal protection suggested that these drugs may be useful in patients with heart failure. As noted above, there was a large and consistent relative risk reduction for HHF. However, these trials were not initially designed to examine heart failure patients in detail, and whether the patients had heart failure with reduced ejection (HFrEF) or heart failure with preserved ejection fraction (HFpEF) was unclear. Some of the proposed mechanisms

of action of SGLT2i in T2DM, such as haemodynamic alterations or renal benefits, were thought potentially to have led to the observed reduction in HHF.

Whereas it was clear that these drugs were beneficial to those with T2DM, it was less clear whether the benefits would extend to those with heart failure, or to those without T2DM. Since many patients with heart failure have T2DM or dysglycaemia, the possibility that a glucose-lowering drug may improve outcomes in those with dysglycaemia and heart failure was an attractive proposition. Similarly, the putative mechanisms of action would also be beneficial in those without T2DM and therefore randomized trials were designed to test these drugs in heart failure.

Clinical trial evidence for SGLT2i in patients with HFrEF

Two large, prospective randomized controlled trials of SGLT2i in HFrEF have now been completed. The first of these trials to report was the Dapagliflozin and Prevention of Adverse-Outcomes in Heart Failure (DAPA-HF) trial which compared the SGLT2i dapagliflozin at a dose of 10 mg once daily with placebo in 4744 patients with chronic HFrEF.[16-18] Patients were eligible for inclusion if they had a left ventricular ejection fraction (LVEF) ≤40%, were in New York Heart Association (NYHA) functional classifications II–IV, had elevated levels of natriuretic peptides, eGFR ≥30 mL/min/1.73m², and were optimally treated with guideline-recommended pharmacological and device therapy for HFrEF for at least one month prior to screening.[16] Exclusion criteria included a history of type 1 diabetes mellitus and symptomatic hypotension or systolic blood pressure <95 mmHg. Importantly, both patients with and without T2DM were included in DAPA-HF and 55% of patients did not have T2DM at baseline. The majority of patients randomized were in NYHA functional class II (68%), mean age was 66 years, 56% had an ischaemic aetiology of HFrEF, mean LVEF was 31% and median N-terminal prohormone of B-type natriuretic peptide (NT-proBNP) level was 1437 pg/mL. Patients were well treated with background HFrEF therapy with 83% taking an angiotensin converting enzyme inhibitor or angiotensin receptor blocker, 96% a β-blocker, 11% an angiotensin receptor–neprilysin inhibitor (sacubitril–valsartan), 71% a mineralocorticoid receptor antagonist (MRA), 26% had an implantable cardioverter–defibrillator (ICD) (including cardiac resynchronization therapy (CRT) defibrillator), and 7% had a CRT device.

The primary outcome of DAPA-HF was a composite of time to first worsening heart failure event (defined as HHF or an urgent visit requiring use of intravenous therapy for heart failure) or CV death. Dapagliflozin, compared with placebo, reduced the risk of the primary composite outcome by 26% (HR: 0.74; 95% CI: 0.65–0.85) with a number needed to treat to prevent one primary composite outcome event of 21 over a median follow-up of 18 months.[18] The benefit of dapagliflozin in reducing the risk of the primary outcome was apparent early in the trial, with sustained statistical evidence of benefit from 28 days following randomization.[19] The risk of both individual components of the primary outcome, worsening heart failure event or CV death, was significantly reduced with dapagliflozin by 30% (95% CI: 17–41) and 18% (95% CI: 2–31), respectively. Similarly, the risk of death from any cause was reduced by 17% (95% CI: 3–29). Furthermore, a composite outcome of total

(first and recurrent) HHF and CV death occurred less frequently with dapagliflozin compared with placebo (rate ratio: 0.75; 95% CI: 0.65–0.88). The prespecified secondary outcome of worsening renal function (a composite of a reduction ≥50% in eGFR sustained for ≥28 days, end-stage renal disease (eGFR <15 mL/min/1.73 m² or dialysis treatment with both sustained for ≥28 days), or kidney transplantation, or death from renal causes) occurred less frequently with dapagliflozin than placebo but this difference did not reach statistical significance. The benefits of dapagliflozin on clinical outcomes were accompanied by substantial beneficial effects on patient's self-reported symptom burden, degree of functional limitation and quality of life, as measured by the Kansas City Cardiomyopathy Questionnaire (KCCQ); compared with placebo, patients randomized to dapagliflozin were less likely to report a clinically meaningful (≥5-point) deterioration in KCCQ Total Symptom Score, and more likely to report clinically meaningful improvements in this patient-reported outcome measure.[18,20] The safety profile of dapagliflozin was favourable, with no significant increase compared with placebo in the occurrence of the adverse events of volume depletion, renal adverse events, amputation, fracture, hypoglycaemia and diabetic ketoacidosis.[18]

Following on from the positive results of DAPA-HF, the Empagliflozin Outcome Trial in Patients with Chronic Heart Failure and a Reduced Ejection Fraction (EMPEROR-Reduced) reported on the safety and efficacy of empagliflozin at a dose of 10 mg once daily, compared with placebo.[21,22] As in DAPA-HF, patients were eligible for inclusion in EMPEROR-Reduced irrespective of diabetes status. There were some key differences in the design of EMPEROR-Reduced compared to DAPA-HF; patients were eligible for inclusion with a greater degree of renal dysfunction (eGFR ≥20 mL/min/1.73 m²), and higher levels of NT-proBNP were required for patients with a higher LVEF (up to a maximum of 40%) than in DAPA-HF.[21] This was with the aim of recruiting a higher-risk population than that in DAPA-HF and, accordingly, the 3730 patients in EMPEROR-Reduced had a higher baseline median NT-proBNP, lower mean eGFR and LVEF than those in DAPA-HF. Another notable difference between the two trials was the greater proportion of patients taking sacubitril–valsartan in EMPEROR-Reduced than in DAPA-HF (19% vs 11%).[22]

Empagliflozin, compared with placebo, reduced the risk of the primary composite outcome of time to first HHF or CV death by 25% (HR: 0.75; 95% CI: 0.65–0.86).[22] The number needed to treat over a median follow-up of 16 months was 19. The risk of time to first HHF and the total number of HHF was significantly reduced by 31% (95% CI: 19–41) and 30% (95% CI: 15–42), respectively. No significant difference between the treatment groups was observed in the risk of death from CV causes or death from any cause. The benefits of empagliflozin in improving symptoms, functional limitations and quality of life were similar to those seen with dapagliflozin in DAPA-HF.[22,23] As well as reducing the risk of a composite renal outcome of worsening renal function events, empagliflozin significantly reduced the rate of decline in eGFR over time compared with placebo, a finding which was also seen with dapagliflozin in a post-hoc analysis of DAPA-HF.[22,24,25] As with dapagliflozin, empagliflozin was well tolerated; however, uncomplicated genital infections did occur more frequently with empagliflozin compared with placebo (this adverse event was not routinely recorded in DAPA-HF).[22] There were no diabetic ketoacidosis adverse events in EMPEROR-Reduced.

In addition to the primary results of DAPA-HF and EMPEROR-Reduced, a series of prespecified and post-hoc secondary analyses from both trials have provided further insight into the additive benefits of SGLT2i in the management of HFrEF.

One of the key questions prior to the results of DAPA-HF and EMPEROR-Reduced was whether the effect of SGLT2i in patients with HFrEF was modified by the presence or absence of diabetes. Both trials reported a consistent effect of the addition of an SGLT2i on outcomes irrespective of diabetes status at baseline.[26,27] Moreover, the benefits were consistent when examined across the range of HbA1c at baseline in both trials, confirming that the benefits of this class of drug in HFrEF are independent of diabetes status.[26,27]

Another important question was whether the effect of SGLT2i varied by the use or not of sacubitril–valsartan? The mechanism of action of SGLT2i is physiologically distinct from that of sacubitril–valsartan, therefore it is perhaps of no surprise that the benefits of both dapagliflozin and empagliflozin have been shown to be additive and independent to those offered not only by sacubitril–valsartan but also by other guideline-recommended pharmacological and device therapies including MRA, ICD, CRT and the percentage of target renin–angiotensin system blocker and β-blocker dose taken.[28–31] Initiation of an MRA during follow-up in EMPEROR-Reduced was less frequent with empagliflozin than placebo, and, in those on an MRA at baseline, both the risk of discontinuation of MRA and severe hyperkalaemia were reduced with empagliflozin.[32]

Further to the benefits on the clinical outcomes detailed above in DAPA-HF, dapagliflozin reduced the incidence of the augmentation of oral heart failure therapy in the outpatient setting in response to worsening signs and symptoms of heart failure, the occurrence of which has been shown to be associated with a worse prognosis than that of those who do not experience this event.[33] In EMPEROR-Reduced, empagliflozin significantly reduced the risk of the total number of HHF requiring intensive care and those requiring a vasopressor or positive inotropic drug or mechanical or surgical intervention.[34] Additionally, a greater proportion of patients reported an improvement, and fewer reported a worsening in NYHA functional class with empagliflozin as compared with placebo, an effect that was evident from as early as 28 days following randomization.[34]

In both trials, the benefits of the addition of an SGLT2i to background HFrEF therapy were consistent across a range of prespecified subgroups including age, sex, LVEF, baseline body mass index, aetiology of heart failure, and baseline plasma levels of NT-proBNP.[18,22] In DAPA-HF, approximately one-quarter of patients were aged ≥75 years with consistent evidence of benefit of dapagliflozin in this age group and no suggestion of an increased risk of adverse events related to treatment versus placebo as compared to younger patients.[35] The duration of history of heart failure did not modify the efficacy of dapagliflozin in DAPA-HF, and in both trials, in those who had been previously hospitalized for worsening heart failure, there was no suggestion of an interaction between treatment effect and the proximity of the previous hospitalization to randomization.[19,36] The effect of the addition of an SGLT2i on systolic blood pressure was minimal in both trials, with a between-treatment difference in the change from baseline to two weeks of −2.5 mmHg in DAPA-HF.[37] Furthermore, the benefit and safety of dapagliflozin was consistent across the range of systolic blood pressure in patients in DAPA-HF. Further consistency of the effect and safety of the addition of an SGLT2i to HFrEF therapy has been reported across

the range of renal function as measured by eGFR at baseline.[24,25] Both trials, consistent with the evidence from trials in patients with diabetes and/or chronic kidney disease, observed a temporary reduction in eGFR shortly following initiation of an SGLT2i which was seen to subsequently resolve. This is thought to be secondary to changes in intraglomerular haemodynamics and, as noted above, both dapagliflozin and empagliflozin attenuated the decline in eGFR during follow-up compared with placebo.

Both DAPA-HF and EMPEROR-Reduced provide convincing evidence of the benefit of the addition of an SGLT2i to guideline-recommended medical and device therapy in improving outcomes and symptoms in a broad range of patients with HFrEF (Figure 51.1). Taken together, the data from these two trials yield a pooled estimate in a trial-level data meta-analysis of 26% (95% CI: 18–32%) reduction in the risk of HHF or CV death, 31% reduction (95% CI: 22–38%) in the risk of HHF, 14% reduction (95% CI: 2–24%) in the risk of CV death, and 13% reduction (95% CI: 2–23%) in the risk of all-cause mortality.[38] Furthermore, and importantly, when combined there was a convincing reduction in kidney outcomes (38% relative risk reduction (95% CI: 10–57%)). Combination treatment with an SGLT2i, sacubitril–valsartan, an MRA, and a β-blocker has been estimated to provide on average an additional 6.3 years of overall survival and 8.3 years free from CV death or first HHF, when compared to treatment with a RAS-blocker and a β-blocker alone.[39]

Both DAPA-HF and EMPEROR-Reduced examined the addition of an SGLT2i to background HFrEF therapy in outpatients with HFrEF. The Effect of Sotagliflozin on Cardiovascular Events in Patients with Type 2 Diabetes Post Worsening Heart Failure (SOLOIST-WHF) trial examined the safety and efficacy of commencing the combined SGLT1/SGLT2 inhibitor sotagliflozin in patients with T2DM stabilized from an episode of worsening heart failure requiring intravenous diuretic therapy.[40] Sotagliflozin, which was commenced while patients were hospitalized or shortly after discharge, was well tolerated and, compared with placebo, reduced the risk of the primary composite outcome of the total number of HHF, urgent heart failure visits, and CV death by 33% (HR: 0.67; 95% CI: 0.52–0.85). SOLOIST-WHF included patients with heart failure across the spectrum of LVEF, thus supplying for the first time data regarding the effect of SGLT2i in patients with HFpEF. In a prespecified subgroup analysis, the benefits of sotagliflozin were consistent in those with LVEF <50% or ≥50%; however, this finding requires confirmation in larger, adequately powered, randomized controlled trials. Two ongoing dedicated HFpEF trials will provide definitive evidence for the potential role of SGLT2i in improving morbidity and mortality in HFpEF (the Dapagliflozin Evaluation to Improve the LIVEs of Patients With PReserved Ejection Fraction Heart Failure trial (DELIVER; ClinicalTrials.gov identifier NCT03619213) and the EMPagliflozin outcomE tRial in Patients With chrOnic heaRt Failure With Preserved Ejection Fraction (EMPEROR-Preserved; NCT03057951)).[41]

Potential mechanisms of action of SGLT2i

There is substantial interest in elucidating mechanisms of actions of SGLT2i in broad populations beyond T2DM in light of the findings described above.[42] SGLT2i are likely to exhibit a broad range of beneficial effects, beyond their modest effects on lowering glucose (HbA1c reduction of 0.5 to 1.0%), body weight (reduction of ~2 kg)

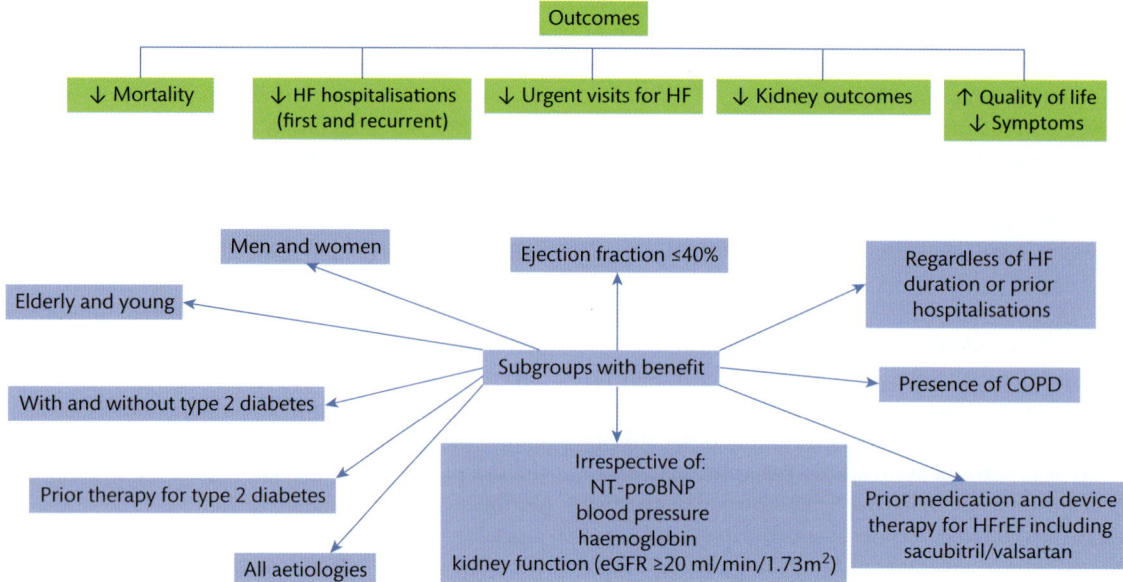

Figure 51.1 Benefits of sodium–glucose co-transporter 2 inhibitor (SGLT2i) in heart failure with reduced ejection fraction (HFrEF).
COPD, chronic obstructive pulmonary disease; eGFR, estimated glomerular filtration rate; HF, heart failure; NT-proBNP, N-terminal prohormone of B-type natriuretic peptide.

and blood pressure (reduction in systolic and diastolic readings of ~4 and ~2 mmHg respectively) (**Figure 51.2**).[43] Notably, the efficacy of SGLT2i in reducing the risk of worsening heart failure or CV death was consistent in those with and without diabetes.[26,27] Furthermore, the rapidity of efficacy (within weeks) seen with SGLT2i suggests mechanisms which cannot be explained wholly by structural changes either in the heart or the degree of atherosclerosis.

The most common prevailing mechanistic explanations and hypotheses include:

- prevention of adverse cardiac remodelling
- diuresis and natriuresis
- reduced preload and afterload

- reduced plasma volume
- blood pressure reduction
- improved vascular function
- reduced pulmonary pressures
- glucose-lowering
- glycosuria
- weight loss
- reduced body mass
- inhibition of sympathetic nervous system
- reduced intraglomerular pressure
- reduced albuminuria
- stimulation of erythropoietin production

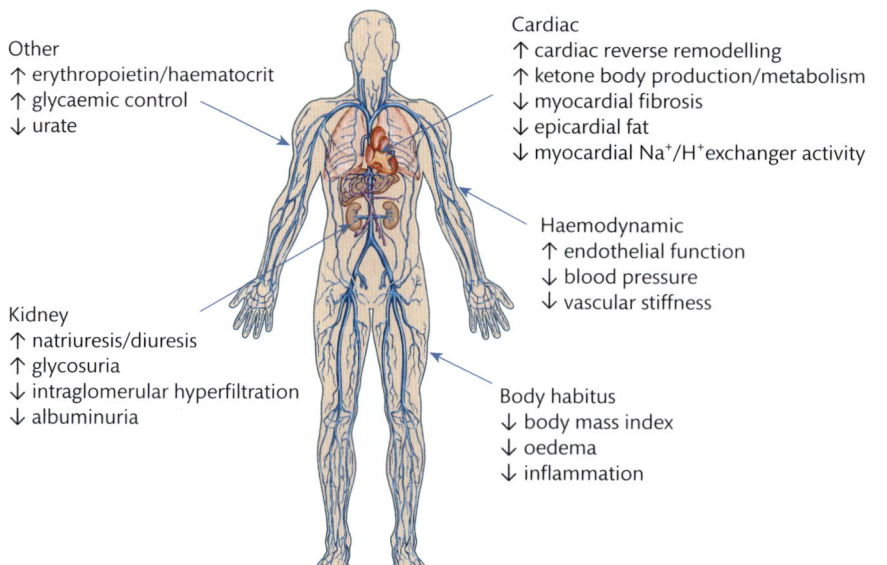

Figure 51.2 Potential mechanisms of action of sodium–glucose co-transporter 2 inhibitor (SGLT2i).

- improved myocardial efficiency and energetics
- decreased epicardial fat mass
- reduced inflammation
- reduced oxidative stress
- increased circulating provascular progenitor cells
- inhibition of Na^+/H^+ exchanger (NHE)
- reduction in hyperuricaemia
- increased autophagy
- lysosomal degradation
- prevention of ischaemia/reperfusion injury,

each of which are discussed in turn. Most studies have so far examined patients with T2DM with few specifically examining patients with heart failure.

Adverse left ventricular (LV) remodelling with progressive LV dilatation is pathognomonic of HFrEF, and several pharmacological therapies with prognostic benefit in HFrEF have also been shown to reverse adverse remodelling.[44] In patients with HFrEF, randomized placebo-controlled trials have found that, compared to placebo, empagliflozin reduced LV end-diastolic and end-systolic volumes indexed to body surface area (BSA), measured on cardiovascular magnetic resonance (CMR) and transthoracic echocardiography.[45–47] Two studies reported that empagliflozin was associated with reduction in LV mass indexed to BSA.[46,47] It has been reported that empagliflozin reduced extracellular volume on CMR, a marker of extracellular myocardial remodelling, and may account for these findings.[48]

The 'diuretic hypothesis' is quoted as a potential mechanism of benefit of heart failure and for the early reduction in outcomes observed. SGLT2i induce diuresis and prevent sodium and water retention, thereby potentially reducing peripheral and pulmonary congestion. In patients with acute decompensated heart failure, a trial of 80 patients reported that empagliflozin had an early effect on diuresis and reduction in whole body water content.[49] However, two analyses in patients with HFrEF suggest that 'diuresis' is not a dominant mechanism. In DAPA-HF, dapagliflozin efficacy and safety were consistent across subgroups of patients according to diuretic use and diuretic dose did not change in most patients during follow-up, with mean diuretic dose not differing between the dapagliflozin and placebo groups after randomization.[50] In EMPEROR-Reduced, the benefits of empagliflozin were not more marked in patients with recent volume overload, suggesting that diuresis did not play a dominant role in mediating the clinical benefits of SGLT2i in HFrEF.[51] Furthermore, volume-related adverse events were not more common with SGLT2i in trials of patients with HFrEF, again suggesting that volume depletion is not a major mechanism of action in the longer term.[18,22] The finding that the natriuresis induced by SGLT2i is attenuated over time through compensatory mechanisms would refute the 'diuretic hypothesis' as being the only mechanism that explains the results of the trials of SGLT2i.

Resorption of glucose and sodium in the proximal convoluted tubule is coupled, therefore SGLT2i results in a mild negative sodium–water balance.[1] SGLT2i cause an acute natriuretic effect which returns to baseline over several weeks. In patients with heart failure, treatment for 14 days with empagliflozin resulted in a significant natriuresis, particularly when combined with loop diuretics, resulting in an improvement in blood volume.[52] In patients with HFrEF and T2DM, empagliflozin, when used in combination with

loop diuretic, caused a significant increase in 24 h urine volume, but without an increase in urinary sodium at 6 weeks.[53]

Potentially beneficial haemodynamic changes have been observed with SGLT2i. In patients with T2DM, SGLT2i reduce systolic blood pressure by ~4 mmHg and diastolic blood pressure by ~2 mmHg,[54] and have favourable effects on markers of arterial stiffness and vascular resistance.[55] A meta-analysis did not find sufficient evidence for blood pressure reduction *per se* to explain the CV benefits seen with SGLT2i.[56] In patients with HFrEF randomized to dapagliflozin, the magnitude of blood pressure lowering was smaller at lower starting blood pressure (only around 1 or 2 mmHg at lower systolic blood pressures), again suggesting that, for many patients, blood pressure lowering alone does not explain the reduction in CV events.[37] Some studies have suggested that SGLT2i can produce rapid reductions in pulmonary artery pressures independent of loop diuretic management,[57] and reduce pulmonary capillary wedge pressure.[58]

A notable effect of the caloric loss induced by SGLT2i (SGLT2i cause a urinary loss of ~70 g of glucose per day equating to ~1300 kcal/day)[59] is that there is a body weight loss of ~2 kg in patients receiving these drugs.[54] In patients with T2DM, SGLT2i reduce adipose tissue mass (both visceral and subcutaneous),[60] with preservation of muscle mass,[61] and transient (rather than permanent) loss of extracellular fluid.[62]

Despite reducing plasma volume, SGLT2i do not increase heart rate,[54] as might be seen with other diuretics due to reflex-mediated sympathetic activation.[63] This may suggest cardiac sympathetic inhibition and/or increased parasympathetic tone.[64] SGLT2i increases distal renal sodium delivery, with the resultant tubuloglomerular feedback causing glomerular afferent arteriolar vasoconstriction, thereby reducing hyperfiltration and a fall in renal plasma and reduction in GFR.[43] SGLT2i cause an initial fall in eGFR within 4–5 weeks, followed by progressive recovery over time.[65,66] Another proposed mechanism that relies on the complex interplay between the heart and the kidney is that SGLT2i increase erythropoietin production after 1 month of treatment, which is accompanied by an increase in haematocrit, reduced ferritin, and red blood cell haemoglobin concentration.[67] Whether changes in haemoglobin levels in heart failure seen with SGLT2i are due to haemoconcentration or erythropoiesis remains unknown.

Chronic SGLT2i shifts substrate utilization from carbohydrate to lipid.[68] SGLT2i increase circulating ketone levels; β-hydroxybutyrate is freely taken up by the heart and oxidized in preference to fatty acids, thereby potentially improving myocardial efficiency.[69] An experimental model of diabetic mice showed that empagliflozin enhances the cardiac energy pool by increasing cardiac energy production from glucose and fatty acid oxidation, but not ketone oxidation.[70] In patients with diabetes, SGLT2i reduce epicardial adipose tissue volume/thickness.[71] In patients undergoing heart surgery, adipose samples were obtained and treated with dapagliflozin and/or insulin—dapagliflozin increased glucose uptake, reduced the secretion of proinflammatory chemokines and improved the differentiation of epicardial adipose tissue cells.[72]

SGLT2i have been proposed to reduce cardiac oxidative stress and inflammation and induce a state of fasting mimicry.[73] In patients with diabetes, SGLT2i attenuate the inflammatory profile.[74] In patients with T2DM and CAD, SGLT2i reduced proinflammatory M1 cells while increasing the number of M2 polarized, anti-inflammatory cells, and cells which are involved in vessel repair.[75]

Other proposed mechanisms of action of SGLT2i include effects on NHE-1 in the heart and NHE-3 in the kidney (thereby reducing cardiomyocyte calcium,[76] and improving cardiomyocyte excitation–contraction coupling and mitochondrial antioxidant capacity).[76] SGLT2i increase renal urate elimination,[77] decreasing plasma uric acid,[78] although it is unclear if urate is a biomarker and/or mediator of disease in heart failure. SGLT2i may restore normal diurnal metabolism, promote autophagy and lysosomal degradation, thereby improving mitochondrial morphology and function, and there is some data to suggest that they may protect against myocardial ischaemia/reperfusion injury.[79]

Summary

The SGLT2i clearly improve morbidity, mortality, and patient-reported quality of life in patients with HFrEF and are a core element of the treatment of HFrEF. They are well tolerated and provide additional benefit to the drugs and devices that are currently used to treat HFrEF. Although the potential mechanism by which they exert these effects is unclear they do appear to induce a degree of cardiac remodelling. Whether these drugs are similarly beneficial in HFpEF remains to be determined.

REFERENCES

1. Zelniker TA, Braunwald E. Mechanisms of cardiorenal effects of sodium–glucose cotransporter 2 inhibitors: JACC state-of-the-art review. *J Am Coll Cardiol* 2020;**75**:422–34.
2. Cavender MA, Steg PG, Smith SCJ, et al. Impact of diabetes mellitus on hospitalization for heart failure, cardiovascular events, and death: outcomes at 4 years from the Reduction of Atherothrombosis for Continued Health (REACH) Registry. *Circulation* 2015;**132**:923–31.
3. Nissen SE, Wolski K. Effect of rosiglitazone on the risk of myocardial infarction and death from cardiovascular causes. *N Engl J Med* 2007;**356**:2457–71.
4. Zinman B, Wanner C, Lachin JM, et al. Empagliflozin, cardiovascular outcomes, and mortality in type 2 diabetes. *N Engl J Med* 2015;**373**:2117–28.
5. Fitchett D, Zinman B, Wanner C, et al. Heart failure outcomes with empagliflozin in patients with type 2 diabetes at high cardiovascular risk: results of the EMPA-REG OUTCOME® trial. *Eur Heart J* 2016;**37**:1526–34.
6. Neal B, Perkovic V, Mahaffey KW, et al. Canagliflozin and cardiovascular and renal events in type 2 diabetes. *N Engl J Med* 2017;**377**:644–57.
7. Wiviott SD, Raz I, Bonaca MP, et al. Dapagliflozin and cardiovascular outcomes in type 2 diabetes. *N Engl J Med* 2019;**380**:347–57.
8. Perkovic V, Jardine MJ, Neal B, et al. Canagliflozin and renal outcomes in type 2 diabetes and nephropathy. *N Engl J Med* 2019;**380**:2295–306.
9. Cannon CP, Pratley R, Dagogo-Jack S, et al. Cardiovascular outcomes with ertugliflozin in type 2 diabetes. *N Engl J Med* 2020;**383**:1425–35.
10. McGuire DK, Shih WJ, Cosentino F, et al. Association of SGLT2 inhibitors with cardiovascular and kidney outcomes in patients with type 2 diabetes: a meta-analysis. *JAMA Cardiol* 2021;**6**:148–58.
11. Rådholm K, Figtree G, Perkovic V, et al. Canagliflozin and heart failure in type 2 diabetes mellitus: results from the CANVAS Program. *Circulation* 2018;**138**:458–68.
12. Kato ET, Silverman MG, Mosenzon O, et al. Effect of dapagliflozin on heart failure and mortality in type 2 diabetes mellitus. *Circulation* 2019;**139**:2528–36.
13. Cosentino F, Grant PJ, Aboyans V, et al. 2019 ESC Guidelines on diabetes, pre-diabetes, and cardiovascular diseases developed in collaboration with the EASD. *Eur Heart J* 2020;**41**:255–323.
14. American Diabetes Association. 9. Pharmacologic approaches to glycemic treatment: standards of medical care in diabetes—2020. *Diabetes Care* 2020;**43**:S98 LP-S110.
15. Inzucchi SE, Kosiborod M, Fitchett D, et al. Improvement in cardiovascular outcomes with empagliflozin is independent of glycemic control. *Circulation* 2018;**138**:1904–7.
16. McMurray JJV, DeMets DL, Inzucchi SE, et al. A trial to evaluate the effect of the sodium–glucose co-transporter 2 inhibitor dapagliflozin on morbidity and mortality in patients with heart failure and reduced left ventricular ejection fraction (DAPA-HF). *Eur J Heart Fail* 2019;**381**:665–75.
17. McMurray JJV, DeMets DL, Inzucchi SE, et al. The Dapagliflozin and Prevention of Adverse-outcomes in Heart Failure (DAPA-HF) trial: baseline characteristics. *Eur J Heart Fail* 2019;**21**:1402–11.
18. McMurray JJV, Solomon SD, Inzucchi SE, et al. Dapagliflozin in patients with heart failure and reduced ejection fraction. *N Engl J Med* 2019;**381**:1995–2008.
19. Berg DD, Jhund PS, Docherty KF, et al. Time to clinical benefit of dapagliflozin and significance of prior heart failure hospitalization in patients with heart failure with reduced ejection fraction. *JAMA Cardiol* 2021 Feb 17;e207585. doi: 10.1001/jamacardio.2020.7585. Online ahead of print.
20. Kosiborod MN, Jhund PS, Docherty KF, et al. Effects of dapagliflozin on symptoms, function, and quality of life in patients with heart failure and reduced ejection fraction. *Circulation* 2020;**141**:90–9.
21. Packer M, Butler J, Filippatos GS, et al. Evaluation of the effect of sodium–glucose co-transporter 2 inhibition with empagliflozin on morbidity and mortality of patients with chronic heart failure and a reduced ejection fraction: rationale for and design of the EMPEROR-Reduced trial. *Eur J Heart Fail* 2019;**21**:1270–8.
22. Packer M, Anker SD, Butler J, et al. Cardiovascular and renal outcomes with empagliflozin in heart failure. *N Engl J Med* 2020;**383**:1413–24.
23. Butler J, Anker SD, Filippatos G, et al. Empagliflozin and health-related quality of life outcomes in patients with heart failure with reduced ejection fraction: the EMPEROR-Reduced trial. *Eur Heart J* 2021;**42**:1203–12.
24. Zannad F, Ferreira JP, Pocock SJ, et al. Cardiac and kidney benefits of empagliflozin in heart failure across the spectrum of kidney function: insights from EMPEROR-Reduced. *Circulation* 2021;**143**:310–21.
25. Jhund PS, Solomon SD, Docherty KF, et al. Efficacy of dapagliflozin on renal function and outcomes in patients with heart failure with reduced ejection fraction: results of DAPA-HF. *Circulation* 2021;**143**:298–309.
26. Petrie MC, Verma S, Docherty KF, et al. Effect of dapagliflozin on worsening heart failure and cardiovascular death in patients with heart failure with and without diabetes. *JAMA* 2020;**323**:1353–68.

27. Anker SD, Butler J, Filippatos G, *et al.* Effect of empagliflozin on cardiovascular and renal outcomes in patients with heart failure by baseline diabetes status: results from the EMPEROR-Reduced trial. *Circulation* 2021;**143**:337–49.

28. Docherty KF, Jhund PS, Inzucchi SE, *et al.* Effects of dapagliflozin in DAPA-HF according to background heart failure therapy. *Eur Heart J* 2020;**41**:2379–92.

29. Solomon SD, Jhund PS, Claggett BL, *et al.* Effect of dapagliflozin in patients with HFrEF treated with sacubitril/valsartan: the DAPA-HF trial. *JACC Hear Fail* 2020;**8**:811–18.

30. Packer M, Anker SD, Butler J, *et al.* Influence of neprilysin inhibition on the efficacy and safety of empagliflozin in patients with chronic heart failure and a reduced ejection fraction: the EMPEROR-Reduced trial. *Eur Heart J* 2021;**42**:671–80.

31. Shen L, Kristensen SL, Bengtsson O, *et al.* Dapagliflozin in HFrEF patients treated with mineralocorticoid receptor antagonists: an analysis of DAPA-HF. *JACC Heart Fail* 2021;**9**:254–64.

32. Ferreira JP, Zannad F, Pocock SJ, *et al.* Interplay of mineralocorticoid receptor antagonists and empagliflozin in heart failure: EMPEROR-Reduced. *J Am Coll Cardiol* 2021;**77**:1397–407.

33. Docherty KF, Jhund PS, Anand I, *et al.* Effect of dapagliflozin on outpatient worsening of patients with heart failure and reduced ejection fraction. *Circulation* 2020;**142**:1623–32.

34. Packer M, Anker SD, Butler J, *et al.* Effect of empagliflozin on the clinical stability of patients with heart failure and a reduced ejection fraction. *Circulation* 2021;**143**:326–36.

35. Martinez FA, Serenelli M, Nicolau JC, *et al.* Efficacy and safety of dapagliflozin in heart failure with reduced ejection fraction according to age: insights from DAPA-HF. *Circulation* 2020;**141**:100–11.

36. Yeoh SE, Dewan P, Jhund PS, *et al.* Patient characteristics, clinical outcomes, and effect of dapagliflozin in relation to duration of heart failure: is it ever too late to start a new therapy? *Circ Heart Fail* 2020;**13**:e007879.

37. Serenelli M, Böhm M, Inzucchi SE, *et al.* Effect of dapagliflozin according to baseline systolic blood pressure in the Dapagliflozin and Prevention of Adverse Outcomes in Heart Failure trial (DAPA-HF). *Eur Heart J* 2020;**41**:3402–18.

38. Zannad F, Ferreira JP, Pocock SJ, *et al.* SGLT2 inhibitors in patients with heart failure with reduced ejection fraction: a meta-analysis of the EMPEROR-Reduced and DAPA-HF trials. *Lancet* 2020;**396**:819–29.

39. Vaduganathan M, Claggett BL, Jhund PS, *et al.* Estimating lifetime benefits of comprehensive disease-modifying pharmacological therapies in patients with heart failure with reduced ejection fraction: a comparative analysis of three randomised controlled trials. *Lancet* 2020;**396**:121–8.

40. Bhatt DL, Szarek M, Steg PG, *et al.* Sotagliflozin in patients with diabetes and recent worsening heart failure. *N Engl J Med* 2021;**384**:117–28.

41. Anker SD, Butler J, Filippatos GS, *et al.* Evaluation of the effects of sodium–glucose co-transporter 2 inhibition with empagliflozin on morbidity and mortality in patients with chronic heart failure and a preserved ejection fraction: rationale for and design of the EMPEROR-Preserved Trial. *Eur J Heart Fail* 2019;**21**:1279–87.

42. Lee MMY, Petrie MC, McMurray JJV, Sattar N. How Do SGLT2 (sodium-glucose cotransporter 2) inhibitors and GLP-1 (glucagon-like peptide-1) receptor agonists reduce cardiovascular outcomes?: completed and ongoing mechanistic trials. *Arterioscler Thromb Vasc Biol* 2020;**40**:506–22.

43. Cowie MR, Fisher M. SGLT2 inhibitors: mechanisms of cardiovascular benefit beyond glycaemic control. *Nat Rev Cardiol* 2020;**17**:761–72.

44. Konstam MA, Kramer DG, Patel AR, Maron MS, Udelson JE. Left ventricular remodeling in heart failure: current concepts in clinical significance and assessment. *JACC Cardiovasc Imaging* 2011;**4**:98–108.

45. Lee MMY, Brooksbank KJM, Wetherall K, *et al.* Effect of empagliflozin on left ventricular volumes in patients with type 2 diabetes, or prediabetes, and heart failure with reduced ejection fraction (SUGAR-DM-HF). *Circulation* 2021;**143**:516–25.

46. Santos-Gallego CG, Vargas-Delgado AP, Requena JA, *et al.* Randomized trial of empagliflozin in non-diabetic patients with heart failure and reduced ejection fraction. *J Am Coll Cardiol* 2021;**77**:243–55.

47. Omar M, Jensen J, Ali M, *et al.* Associations of empagliflozin with left ventricular volumes, mass, and function in patients with heart failure and reduced ejection fraction: a substudy of the Empire HF randomized clinical trial. *JAMA Cardiol* 2021:e206827.

48. Mason T, Coelho-Filho OR, Verma S, *et al.* Empagliflozin reduces myocardial extracellular volume in patients with type 2 diabetes and coronary artery disease. *JACC Cardiovasc Imaging* 2021 Jan 4;**S1936-878X**(20)30939-6. doi: 10.1016/j.jcmg.2020.10.017. Online ahead of print.

49. Damman K, Beusekamp JC, Boorsma EM, *et al.* Randomized, double-blind, placebo-controlled, multicentre pilot study on the effects of empagliflozin on clinical outcomes in patients with acute decompensated heart failure (EMPA-RESPONSE-AHF). *Eur J Heart Fail* 2020;**22**:713–22.

50. Jackson AM, Dewan P, Anand IS, *et al.* Dapagliflozin and diuretic use in patients with heart failure and reduced ejection fraction in DAPA-HF. *Circulation* 2020;**142**:1040–54.

51. Packer M, Anker SD, Butler J, *et al.* Empagliflozin in patients with heart failure, reduced ejection fraction, and volume overload: EMPEROR-Reduced trial. *J Am Coll Cardiol* 2021;**77**:1381–92.

52. Griffin M, Rao VS, Ivey-Miranda J, *et al.* Empagliflozin in heart failure: diuretic and cardiorenal effects. *Circulation* 2020;**142**:1028–39.

53. Mordi NA, Mordi IR, Singh JS, McCrimmon RJ, Struthers AD, Lang CC. Renal and cardiovascular effects of SGLT2 inhibition in combination with loop diuretics in patients with type 2 diabetes and chronic heart failure: the RECEDE-CHF Trial. *Circulation* 2020;**142**:1713–24.

54. Storgaard H, Gluud LL, Bennett C, *et al.* Benefits and harms of sodium-glucose co-transporter 2 inhibitors in patients with type 2 diabetes: a systematic review and meta-analysis. *PLoS One* 2016;**11**:e0166125.

55. Striepe K, Jumar A, Ott C, *et al.* Effects of the selective sodium–glucose cotransporter 2 inhibitor empagliflozin on vascular function and central hemodynamics in patients with type 2 diabetes mellitus. *Circulation* 2017;**136**:1167–9.

56. Benham JL, Booth JE, Sigal RJ, Daskalopoulou SS, Leung AA, Rabi DM. Systematic review and meta-analysis: SGLT2 inhibitors, blood pressure and cardiovascular outcomes. *Int J Cardiol Hear Vasc* 2021;**33**:100725.

57. Nassif ME, Qintar M, Windsor SL, *et al.* Empagliflozin effects on pulmonary artery pressure in patients with heart failure: results from EMpagliflozin Evaluation By MeasuRing ImpAct on HemodynamiCs in PatiEnts with Heart Failure (EMBRACE-HF) trial. *Circulation* 2021 Feb 8. doi: 10.1161/CIRCULATIONAHA.120.052503. Online ahead of print.

58. Omar M, Jensen J, Frederiksen PH, *et al.* Effect of empagliflozin on hemodynamics in patients with heart failure and reduced ejection fraction. *J Am Coll Cardiol* 2020;**76**:2740–51.

59. Rajeev SP, Cuthbertson DJ, Wilding JPH. Energy balance and metabolic changes with sodium-glucose co-transporter 2 inhibition. *Diabetes Obes Metab* 2016;**18**:125–34.

60. Bolinder J, Ljunggren Ö, Kullberg J, *et al.* Effects of dapagliflozin on body weight, total fat mass, and regional adipose tissue distribution in patients with type 2 diabetes mellitus with inadequate glycemic control on metformin. *J Clin Endocrinol Metab* 2012;**97**:1020–31.

61. Inoue H, Morino K, Ugi S, *et al.* Ipragliflozin, a sodium-glucose cotransporter 2 inhibitor, reduces bodyweight and fat mass, but not muscle mass, in Japanese type 2 diabetes patients treated with insulin: a randomized clinical trial. *J Diabetes Investig* 2019;**10**:1012–21.

62. Schork A, Saynisch J, Vosseler A, *et al.* Effect of SGLT2 inhibitors on body composition, fluid status and renin–angiotensin–aldosterone system in type 2 diabetes: a prospective study using bioimpedance spectroscopy. *Cardiovasc Diabetol* 2019;**18**:46.

63. Jordan J, Tank J, Heusser K, *et al.* The effect of empagliflozin on muscle sympathetic nerve activity in patients with type II diabetes mellitus. *J Am Soc Hypertens* 2017;**11**:604–12.

64. Scheen AJ. Effect of SGLT2 inhibitors on the sympathetic nervous system and blood pressure. *Curr Cardiol Rep* 2019;**21**:70.

65. Cefalu WT, Leiter LA, Yoon K-H, *et al.* Efficacy and safety of canagliflozin versus glimepiride in patients with type 2 diabetes inadequately controlled with metformin (CANTATA-SU): 52 week results from a randomised, double-blind, phase 3 non-inferiority trial. *Lancet* 2013;**382**:941–50.

66. Barnett AH, Mithal A, Manassie J, *et al.* Efficacy and safety of empagliflozin added to existing antidiabetes treatment in patients with type 2 diabetes and chronic kidney disease: a randomised, double-blind, placebo-controlled trial. *Lancet Diabetes Endocrinol* 2014;**2**:369–84.

67. Mazer CD, Hare GMT, Connelly PW, *et al.* Effect of empagliflozin on erythropoietin levels, iron stores, and red blood cell morphology in patients with type 2 diabetes mellitus and coronary artery disease. *Circulation* 2020;**141**:704–7.

68. Ferrannini E, Muscelli E, Frascerra S, *et al.* Metabolic response to sodium–glucose cotransporter 2 inhibition in type 2 diabetic patients. *J Clin Invest* 2014;**124**:499–508.

69. Mudaliar S, Alloju S, Henry RR. Can a shift in fuel energetics explain the beneficial cardiorenal outcomes in the EMPA-REG OUTCOME study? A unifying hypothesis. *Diabetes Care* 2016;**39**:1115–22.

70. Verma S, Rawat S, Ho KL, *et al.* Empagliflozin increases cardiac energy production in diabetes: novel translational insights into the heart failure benefits of SGLT2 inhibitors. *JACC Basic to Transl Sci* 2018;**3**:575–87.

71. Fukuda T, Bouchi R, Terashima M, *et al.* Ipragliflozin reduces epicardial fat accumulation in non-obese type 2 diabetic patients with visceral obesity: a pilot study. *Diabetes Ther* 2017;**8**:851–61.

72. Díaz-Rodríguez E, Agra RM, Fernández ÁL, *et al.* Effects of dapagliflozin on human epicardial adipose tissue: modulation of insulin resistance, inflammatory chemokine production, and differentiation ability. *Cardiovasc Res* 2018;**114**:336–46.

73. Packer M. Cardioprotective effects of sirtuin-1 and its downstream effectors: potential role in mediating the heart failure benefits of SGLT2 (sodium–glucose cotransporter 2) inhibitors. *Circ Heart Fail* 2020;**13**:e007197.

74. Heerspink HJL, Perco P, Mulder S, *et al.* Canagliflozin reduces inflammation and fibrosis biomarkers: a potential mechanism of action for beneficial effects of SGLT2 inhibitors in diabetic kidney disease. *Diabetologia* 2019;**62**:1154–66.

75. Hess DA, Terenzi DC, Trac JZ, *et al.* SGLT2 Inhibition with empagliflozin increases circulating provascular progenitor cells in people with type 2 diabetes mellitus. *Cell Metab* 2019;**30**:609–13.

76. Clancy CE, Chen-Izu Y, Bers DM, *et al.* Deranged sodium to sudden death. *J Physiol* 2015;**593**:1331–45.

77. Chino Y, Samukawa Y, Sakai S, *et al.* SGLT2 inhibitor lowers serum uric acid through alteration of uric acid transport activity in renal tubule by increased glycosuria. *Biopharm Drug Dispos* 2014;**35**:391–404.

78. Zhao Y, Xu L, Tian D, *et al.* Effects of sodium–glucose co-transporter 2 (SGLT2) inhibitors on serum uric acid level: a meta-analysis of randomized controlled trials. *Diabetes Obes Metab* 2018;**20**:458–62.

79. Lim VG, Bell RM, Arjun S, Kolatsi-Joannou M, Long DA, Yellon DM. SGLT2 inhibitor, canagliflozin, attenuates myocardial infarction in the diabetic and nondiabetic heart. *JACC Basic Transl Sci* 2019;**4**:15–26.

52

Mineralocorticoid receptor antagonists

S. Rekhraj, Ben. R. Szwejkowski, and Allan D. Struthers

Background

There are numerous neurohormonal mechanisms involved in the pathophysiology of heart failure, including the renin–angiotensin–aldosterone system (RAAS), the sympathetic nervous system, and arginine vasopressin (AVP). With regards to the RAAS, plasma aldosterone levels are 20-fold higher in heart failure than in normal subjects. In normal subjects with normal sodium intake, plasma aldosterone levels are 5–15 ng/dL (139–416 pmol/L) compared to plasma levels up to 300 ng/dL (8322 pmol/L) in heart failure patients.[1] Aldosterone has been known for a long time to be a predictor of poor prognosis in chronic heart failure (CHF) patients, as shown in the hormonal data from the CONSENSUS and SAVE study.[2,3]

Angiotensin converting enzyme inhibitors (ACEi) were studied in the 1980s as a treatment for CHF. After favourable responses in small studies, numerous large-scale multicentre studies showed that ACEi reduced cardiovascular events and mortality in patients with CHF due to left ventricular systolic dysfunction (LVSD), which is now called heart failure with reduced ejection fraction (HFrEF).

The main pharmacological effect thought to mediate the benefits of ACEi was blocking the pharmacological effects of angiotensin II (AII). However, since AII causes aldosterone release, there was an unwritten assumption that the lowering of aldosterone might contribute to the benefits of ACEi. In those early days, it was thought that the only real effect of aldosterone was to retain sodium (and water) and to excrete potassium (K+). Therefore, it was assumed that one of the many benefits of ACEi was to reduce the antidiuretic effects of aldosterone. This was the case in part because spironolactone had been known for a long time to be an excellent diuretic in hepatic ascites. The fact that spironolactone was usually used at very high dose in cirrhosis and in the absence of ACEi could have alerted us that the above diuretic effect might not be that relevant to ACEi-treated CHF patients.

However, events moved on and what then surprised most people and became clear was that, whereas ACEi undoubtedly delivered major clinical benefits in CHF, they did so without maintaining aldosterone suppression in the long term.[4] Although initially surprising, a consideration of basic physiology should have alerted us that ACEi were unlikely to maintain aldosterone suppression. This is because AII is not the only secretagogue for aldosterone and that another major secretagogue is potassium (K+) (**Figure 52.1**). Therefore, when an ACEi reduces AII, this will decrease aldosterone release, but when the ACEi concurrently increases K+, this will tend to increase aldosterone release. These two effects might cancel each other out in the medium to long term.

Indeed, in populations in general, there is usually a U-shaped relationship between K+ and aldosterone levels. At low levels of K+, aldosterone will be high and cause the low K+ (due to primary hyperaldosteronism), whereas at high levels of K+, aldosterone levels will also be high, but in this latter instance it will be K+ that is causing the high levels of aldosterone rather than the other way around.

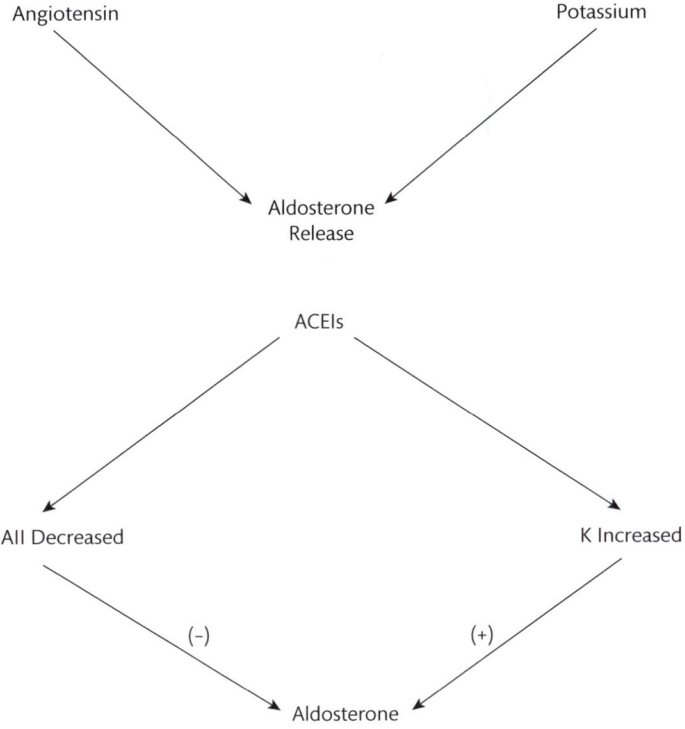

Figure 52.1 Angiotensin converting enzyme inhibitors and aldosterone release.

Although the above explains why ACEi only marginally reduce aldosterone in the long term it was still thought in the early 1980s that the only real biological effect of aldosterone was as an antidiuretic substance acting on Na$^+$/K$^+$ in the renal tubules. Although diuresis is clearly important in CHF, it turned out that this view grossly underappreciated the biological effects of aldosterone in CHF. Indeed, such extra renal effects of aldosterone only became appreciated in the 1990s.

It was the experimental work of Karl Weber that first pointed out the wider biological effects of aldosterone—especially on the heart. In a series of elegant studies, Brilla et al. (1993) were able to show that aldosterone promotes myocardial fibrosis in rats.[5] It did appear that the animals needed to be salt replete for aldosterone to promote myocardial fibrosis. Whereas in most clinical situations, salt repletion would be associated with low levels of aldosterone, this is not the case in CHF where salt/fluid retention uniquely coexists with unsuppressed levels of aldosterone.

Three events then occurred together in the early 1990s to advance this issue. First, in a commentary article in 1993, Zannad floated the idea that such adverse effects of aldosterone (on myocardial and vascular fibrosis) might pertain in ACEi-treated patients and that adding spironolactone to an ACEi should be explored as a possible new therapeutic option.[6] When this article was published, two other groups were already exploring this idea.

Second, beginning in 1992, Barr et al. began to explore the effects of adding spironolactone (target dose of 50 mg) to an ACEi in patients with CHF due to LVSD.[7] The focus of this study was on different myocardial effects of aldosterone, i.e. on cardiac sympathetic activity and on ventricular arrhythmias. Previous animal studies had shown that aldosterone reduced norepinephrine uptake and disposal in the myocardium in vivo. This group was also the first ever to demonstrate in humans that adding spironolactone to ACEi produced beneficial cardiac effects.[7] In this study, spironolactone clearly reduced ventricular arrhythmias and reduced cardiac sympathetic activity (as assessed by cardiac nuclear MIBG scans).[7] Furthermore, somewhat surprisingly, spironolactone was well tolerated in terms of its effect on plasma potassium and creatinine. These effects on sympathetic activity and on arrhythmias may help explain the later somewhat surprising finding from RALES and EMPHASIS-HF that aldosterone blockade was very effective at reducing sudden cardiac deaths (as opposed to deaths from progressive heart failure). This early study was later used also as a way of showing that spironolactone reduced myocardial fibrosis in man.[8] This paper showed that spironolactone consistently reduced plasma levels of procollagen type III amino-terminal peptide (PIIINP), which is a recognized biomarker for myocardial collagen. Later Zannad et al. showed the importance of this effect from the RALES study where it appeared that the mortality-reducing effect of spironolactone closely tracked with high levels of PIIINP being reduced by spironolactone.[9]

Third, the other group exploring the feasibility of spironolactone in CHF in the early 1990s was the company GD Searle (the makers of spironolactone). Their main rationale was that spironolactone might be an effective add-on diuretic in CHF since CHF is a disease characterized by fluid retention. This was also relevant to GD Searle at the time as they had developed a new selective aldosterone antagonist (also known as a mineralocorticoid receptor antagonist (MRA)), now called eplerenone, which had the huge advantage of being a cleaner drug without the anti-androgen effect of spironolactone (and therefore without causing the troublesome gynaecomastia seen in men taking spironolactone, a non-selective mineralocorticoid antagonist (MRA)). GD Searle enlisted Bert Pitt to explore the potential of spironolactone in this regard. Pitt has commented that GD Searle initially approached other CHF investigators in the USA with this idea but at least one felt that in the era of ACEi, there would be little benefit in blocking aldosterone as well. The latter was a common view at the time.

Pitt initially explored this idea by doing a dose-ranging study with spironolactone in ACEi-treated CHF patients.[10] This was an entirely sensible initial approach as dose was crucial here, as the concept could easily have been 'throttled at birth' if definitive studies were undertaken at the wrong dose and problems with hyperkalaemia and renal dysfunction were marked. What this dose-ranging study found was that, at very low doses, spironolactone reduced levels of N-terminal pro B-type natriuretic peptide (NT-proBNP). Indeed, higher doses produced little extra reduction in NT-proBNP. By contrast, problems with hyperkalaemia and renal dysfunction showed a clear dose–response relationship. From this dose-ranging study, it was decided that the dose of 25–50 mg spironolactone per day was appropriate for the RALES study. This view was boosted at the time by the results of Barr et al. who had already shown that this same dose had other beneficial cardiac effects in man, as described above.[7]

Much experimental work was done to explore whether aldosterone blockade might have a therapeutic role outside of CHF. Rocha and Funder did a series of animal studies that suggested that aldosterone blockade had anti-inflammatory effects and improved vascular and renal function.[11] Farquharson and Struthers, and MacDonald et al. were able to show that in human CHF, spironolactone clearly improved endothelial dysfunction, but this group was unable to find a similar effect on endothelial dysfunction in non-CHF patients such as normotensive diabetics, hypertensive diabetics, or angina patients.[12–16] Similarly, Godfrey et al. found no effect of spironolactone on the inflammatory biomarker, C-reactive protein.[17]

Mineralocorticoid receptor antagonists

There are currently two mineralocorticoid receptor antagonists available in clinical practice: spironolactone and eplerenone. Spironolactone is a non-selective competitive mineralocorticoid receptor antagonist which is extensively metabolized by the liver into its active metabolites. Spironolactone and its metabolites are >90% bound to plasma protein. The metabolites are excreted primarily in the urine and secondarily in bile. It is structurally similar to progesterone, which explains its anti-androgen side-effects such as breast pain, gynaecomastia, and impotence in males, and menstrual irregularities in premenstrual females.[18]

Eplerenone is a selective antagonist of the mineralocorticoid receptor which has been derived from spironolactone. The substitution of the 17α-thoacetyl group in spironolactone with a carbomethoxy group increases its selectivity for the aldosterone receptor over other steroid receptors. This results in lower endocrine side-effects (1%) compared to spironolactone (10%).[19,20] Approximately 50% of eplerenone is bound to plasma proteins and it is primarily metabolized by CYP4503A4.[21]

Aldosterone antagonists (MRAs) in HFrEF

Spironolactone (RALES)

The Randomized Aldactone Evaluation Study (RALES study) (n = 1663) (Table 52.1) began recruiting in 1996 and was terminated early when the overwhelmingly positive results appeared, leading to a major landmark publication in 1999.[19] This randomized, double-blind, placebo-controlled study assessed the use of spironolactone in severe heart failure patients (New York Heart Association (NYHA) class III or IV, mean left ventricular ejection fraction (LVEF) 25%) on medical treatment including ACEi, loop diuretic, and in most cases digoxin. Patients were excluded if baseline bloods indicated a serum creatinine >220 µmol/L or potassium >5 mmol/L. Patients were commenced on 25 mg spironolactone once daily, which was uptitrated to 50 mg after two months if there was no evidence of hyperkalaemia. Spironolactone therapy was associated with a 30% reduction in total mortality, 36% reduction in heart failure mortality, and 29% reduction in sudden cardiac death. These patients also had a 35% reduced risk of heart failure admissions and 41% had an improvement in NYHA class (compared to 33% in placebo group). Although these are very impressive results, it should be noted that in this study only a small number of patients were on β-blocker therapy (11% in spironolactone group compared to 10% in placebo group) compared to our current heart failure population. Nevertheless, this small subgroup on β-blockers appeared to benefit equally from spironolactone.[10] Gynaecomastia or breast pain was reported in 10% of men in the spironolactone group compared to 1% in placebo group (P < 0.001). Only after publication of this landmark study was the scientific community really convinced about endogenous aldosterone promoting mortality in CHF, and so began to use spironolactone.

However, as often happens in real clinical practice, clinicians did not exert enough caution in using the drug, and reports appeared of high levels of hyperkalaemia appearing after RALES was published.[22] Scrutiny revealed that in routine practice, spironolactone was often used in the wrong patients at the wrong (too high) dose and that careful monitoring was not undertaken. Wei et al. subsequently showed that when the drug was used at the correct dose in the correct patients and where appropriate monitoring was undertaken, the incidence of hyperkalaemia was reassuringly low and as low as it had been in the RALES trial where the only patient to die of hyperkalaemia was in the placebo group.[23]

Eplerenone (EPHESUS and EMPHASIS-HF)

Although RALES was very positive, it was felt that confirmatory evidence was required. This was especially the case since eplerenone, a new selective mineralocorticoid receptor antagonist with little anti-androgen activity, came on the scene. This led to the Eplerenone Post-acute Myocardial Infarction Heart failure Efficacy and Survival Study (EPHESUS) study (Table 52.1), a randomized multicentre double-blinded, placebo-controlled study that assessed the use of eplerenone in 6632 patients who were 3–14 days post-myocardial infarction (MI) with LVSD in the presence of either coincidental diabetes or symptoms of heart failure. The patients were recruited over a period of two years (1999 until 2001) and were already on maximal therapy, which included drugs such as β-blockers, ACEi, angiotensin receptor blockers (ARBs) and diuretics and coronary revascularization. By comparison with RALES, EPHESUS recruited more patients (6632 vs 1663) with a higher LVEF (33% vs 25.6%) and a higher usage of β-blockers (75% vs 11%). Although the results were not quite as impressive as RALES, there was a significant reduction in all-cause mortality (15%), cardiovascular mortality (17%), and a 15% relative risk reduction in heart failure hospitalization.[20] A retrospective sub-analysis of diabetic patients in the EPHESUS study noted that eplerenone therapy in diabetics was associated with a greater absolute risk reduction of all-cause and cardiovascular mortality or cardiovascular hospitalization compared to non-diabetics.[24]

Therefore, strong positive results were seen in patients with severe CHF (RALES study) and in post-MI patients with LVSD (EPHESUS). The normal procedure in developing new treatments in CHF is to study them first in severe CHF and then to do similar studies in milder versions of CHF. This was certainly the case with ACEi, which first were studied in the CONSENSUS study and then in milder patients in the SOLVD studies. Therefore, the next study to be undertaken was the Eplerenone in Mild Patients Hospitalization and Survival Study in Heart failure (EMPHASIS-HF) (Table 52.1). This multicentre RCT (n = 2737) assessed the use of eplerenone in patients with mild symptoms of heart failure (NYHA class II), severe LVSD (LVEF ≤30%, or if LVEF was 30–35% the QRS duration had to be >130 ms on ECG) and already on an ACEi or ARB (or both), and a β-blocker at maximum tolerated dose. Patients had to have had either a cardiovascular hospitalization in the previous six months or an elevated plasma natriuretic peptide concentration. Patients with an acute MI, significant heart failure symptoms (NYHA class III–IV), on potassium sparing diuretics, serum potassium >5 mmol/L

Table 52.1 Randomized controlled trials of aldosterone antagonists (mineralocorticoid receptor antagonists) in heart failure with reduced rejection fraction

Trial (drug vs placebo)	No. of patients	NYHA class (%)	Mean LVEF (%)	Mean follow-up (years)	Mortality reduction (%)	Withdrawal due to intolerance (% versus placebo)
RALES (spironolactone)	1663	0.5 II 70.5 III 29 IV	25	1.9	30	8 versus 5
EPHESUS (eplerenone)	6632	Post-MI	33	1.3	15	4 versus 3
EMPHASIS-HF (eplerenone)	2737	II	26	1.75	24	14 versus 16

NYHA, New York Heart Association; LVEF, left ventricular ejection fraction

Source data from Gardner, R., McDonagh, T., and Walker, N., *Oxford Specialist Handbook Heart Failure* 2e, Oxford University Press, Oxford, 2014.

and significant renal impairment (estimated glomerular filtration rate <30 mL/min) were excluded. This study was stopped prematurely at 21 months due to evidence of benefit with eplerenone, including significant reductions in the primary outcome (composite of heart failure hospitalization or cardiovascular mortality) (37%), all-cause mortality (24%), all cause hospitalization (23%), and heart failure hospitalization (42%). Eplerenone was associated with a non-significant increase in incidence of serious hyperkalaemia (serum potassium ≥6 meq/L), hospitalization for hyperkalaemia, or worsening renal failure.[25]

Mineralocorticoid antagonists (MRA) in HFpEF

Not all clinical CHF patients have LVSD. There is a large and well-recognized group of heart failure patients with LVEF ≥50%, now called HFpEF (heart failure with preserved ejection fraction). Several therapies (ACEi and ARBs) have been investigated in HFpEF patients but sadly none of them has produced significant benefit.

Studies assessing the use of mineralocorticoid antagonists have also been performed in the HFpEF patient group. The Aldosterone Receptor Blockade in Diastolic Heart Failure study (Aldo-DHF) of 422 patients with NYHA class II or III, preserved LVEF (>50%), and evidence of diastolic dysfunction found that 25 mg spironolactone for 12 months resulted in a significant improvement in diastolic function (E/e′; 95% CI: −2 to −0.9; $P < 0.0001$) and BNP levels, but did not improve heart failure symptoms, quality of life, or maximum exercise capacity compared to placebo.[26]

The Treatment Of Preserved Cardiac function heart failure with an Aldosterone anTagonist (TOPCAT) study was a large ($n = 3445$), National Institutes of Health-sponsored study to see whether spironolactone (15 to 45 mg daily) was of benefit in symptomatic heart failure patients with LVEF ≥45%. At a mean follow-up of 3.3 years, spironolactone did not significantly reduce the primary composite outcome of death from cardiovascular causes, aborted cardiac arrest, or heart failure hospitalization compared to placebo (spironolactone 18.6%, placebo 20.4%; $P = 0.14$). Spironolactone only significantly reduced heart failure hospitalizations compared to the placebo group (12% vs 14.2%; $P = 0.04$).[27] There was a significant increase in hyperkalaemia (18.7% vs 9.1% in placebo) and serum creatinine levels with spironolactone, highlighting the importance of monitoring patients taking spironolactone with blood tests. Post-hoc analysis highlighted substantial regional variation with patients from the Americas (51% of patients) benefiting from taking spironolactone but not patients from Russia/Georgia (49% patients) (**Figure 52.2**). This study raised questions regarding the regional variation in HFpEF diagnosis and regional discrepancy in the reported and actual use of spironolactone by measuring canrenone concentration (an active metabolite of spironolactone), which may explain the regional discrepancy.[28] Further subgroup analysis has also found that patients from Americas with LVEF at the lower end of the spectrum were more likely to benefit from taking spironolactone compared to those with higher LVEF.[29] There are currently two ongoing trials assessing spironolactone in patients with HFpEF, including SPIRRIT-HFpEF and SPIRRIT.

The 2017 American College of Cardiology/American Heart Association (ACC/AHA) heart failure guidelines have given MRAs a class 2b indication for HFpEF patients with elevated natriuretic

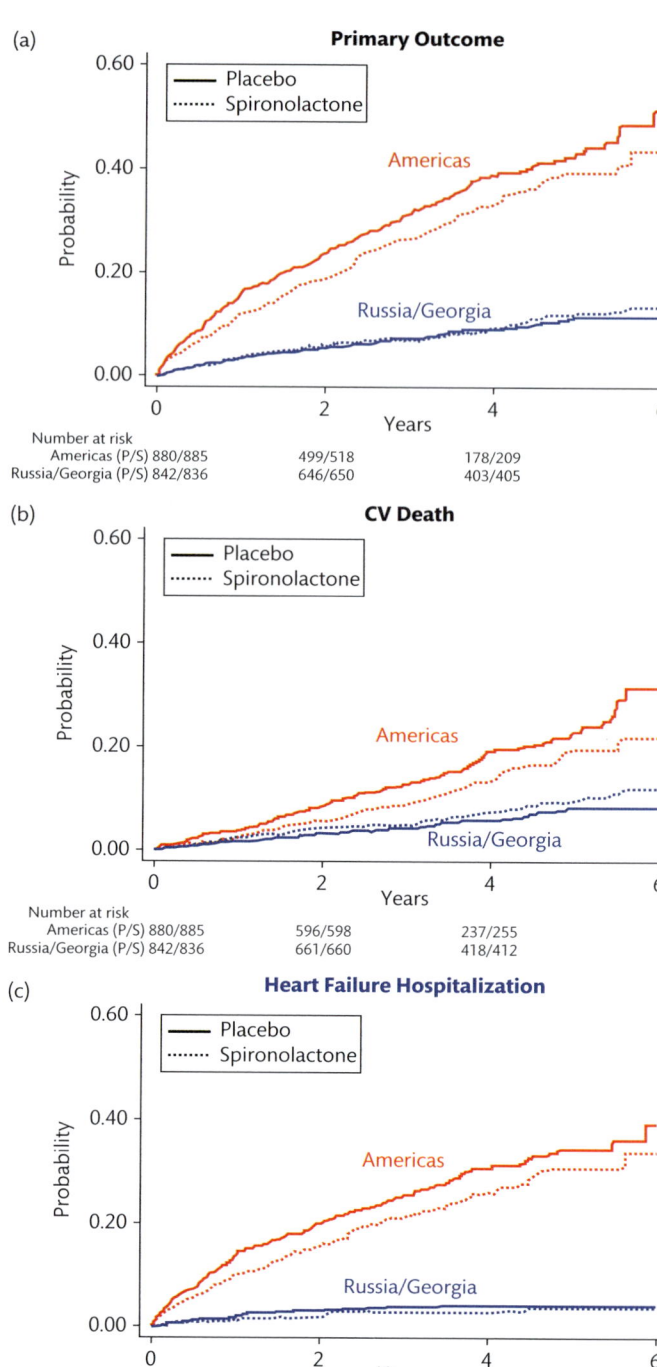

Figure 52.2 Kaplan–Meier plots of primary outcome (death from cardiovascular causes, aborted cardiac arrest or heart failure hospitalization) and two major components. (a) Time to primary outcome; (b) time to cardiovascular (CV) death; (c) time to first confirmed hospitalization for heart failure.

Reproduced from Pfeffer MA, Claggett B, Assmann SF, Boineau R, Anand IS, Clausell N, et al. Regional variation in patients and outcomes in the Treatment of Preserved Cardiac Function Heart Failure With an Aldosterone Antagonist (TOPCAT) trial. *Circulation*. 2015 Jan 6;**131**(1):34–42.

peptides or those who have been hospitalized for heart failure in the last 12 months based on the subgroup analysis of TOPCAT.[30] However, this is not so in the last European Society of Cardiology heart failure guidelines 2016.[31]

Elderly heart failure patients

Similar to other heart failure medication, MRAs are under-used in the treatment of elderly patients with heart failure. A recent meta-analysis of RALES, EMPHASIS-HF, and TOPCAT found that MRAs had a beneficial effect on reducing morbidity and mortality in elderly patients (aged ≥75 years) with heart failure which was more marked in the patients with HFREF but was also seen in the HFPEF group. However, worsening of renal function occurred more frequently in the older group compared to the younger patients.[32] It is therefore important to monitor renal function closely, especially when using MRAs in this group of patients.

Summary

Overall, the results for aldosterone blockade in CHF due to LVSD (HFrEF) have been very impressive, with three large, undoubtedly positive results. These are the RALES study, the EPHESUS study, and the EMPHASIS-HF study. Importantly there are no neutral or negative studies for aldosterone blockade in HFrEF. In both the ACC/AHA and ESC guidelines, MRAs have a class 1 indication for use in patients with chronic severe HFREF and in patients with HFREF early post MI who either have heart failure symptoms or diabetes. The advent of sacubitril–valsartan from the PARADIGM-HF trial should not influence the position of MRAs as third-line drugs in the treatment of HFrEF. However, efforts should be made ultimately to establish patients on both agents.

The position of MRAs for HFpEF is currently unclear, especially due to the results of the TOPCAT study. There are ongoing trials to help address this question. A related issue is that the PATHWAY-2 study has shown that spironolactone is a particularly effective antihypertensive in patients with resistant hypertension.[33] Since HFpEF and hypertension commonly coexist (and sometimes the latter in its resistant form), many HFpEF patients may end up receiving an MRA because they have coincidental (resistant) hypertension rather than because they have HFpEF *per se*.

REFERENCES

1. Weber KT. Aldosterone in congestive heart failure. *N Engl J Med* 2001;**345**(23):1689–97.
2. Swedberg K, Eneroth P, Kjekshus J, Wilhelmsen L. Hormones regulating cardiovascular function in patients with severe congestive heart failure and their relation to mortality. CONSENSUS Trial Study Group. *Circulation* 1990;**82**(5):1730–6.
3. Vantrimpont P, Rouleau JL, Ciampi A, *et al*. Two-year time course and significance of neurohumoral activation in the Survival and Ventricular Enlargement (SAVE) Study. *Eur Heart J* 1998;**19**(10):1552–63.
4. MacFadyen RJ, Lee AF, Morton JJ, Pringle SD, Struthers AD. How often are angiotensin II and aldosterone concentrations raised during chronic ACE inhibitor treatment in cardiac failure? *Heart* 1999;**82**(1):57–61.
5. Brilla CG, Matsubara LS, Weber KT. Anti-aldosterone treatment and the prevention of myocardial fibrosis in primary and secondary hyperaldosteronism. *J Mol Cell Cardiol* 1993;**25**(5):563–75.
6. Zannad F. Angiotensin converting enzyme inhibitor and spironolactone combination therapy. New objectives in congestive heart failure treatment. *Am J Cardiol* 1993;**71**(3):34A–9A.
7. Barr CS, Lang CC, Hanson J, *et al*. Effects of adding spironolactone to an angiotensin-converting enzyme inhibitor in chronic congestive heart failure secondary to coronary artery disease. *Am J Cardiol* 1995;**76**(17):1259–65.
8. MacFadyen RJ, Barr CS, Struthers AD. Aldosterone blockade reduces vascular collagen turnover, improves heart rate variability and reduces early morning rise in heart rate in heart failure patients. *Cardiovasc Res* 1997;**35**(1):30–4.
9. Zannad F, Alla F, Dousset B, Perez A, Pitt B. Limitation of excessive extracellular matrix turnover may contribute to survival benefit of spironolactone therapy in patients with congestive heart failure: insights from the randomized aldactone evaluation study (RALES). Rales Investigators. *Circulation* 2000;**102**(22):2700–6.
10. Anonymous. Effectiveness of spironolactone added to an angiotensin-converting enzyme inhibitor and a loop diuretic for severe chronic congestive heart failure (the Randomized Aldactone Evaluation Study [RALES]). *Am J Cardiol* 1996;**78**(8):902–7.
11. Rocha R, Funder JW. The pathophysiology of aldosterone in the cardiovascular system. *Ann NY Acad Sci* 2002;**970**:89–100.
12. Farquharson CA, Struthers AD. Spironolactone increases nitric oxide bioactivity, improves endothelial vasodilator dysfunction, and suppresses vascular angiotensin I/angiotensin II conversion in patients with chronic heart failure. *Circulation* 2000;**101**(6):594–7.
13. Macdonald JE, Kennedy N, Struthers AD. Effects of spironolactone on endothelial function, vascular angiotensin converting enzyme activity, and other prognostic markers in patients with mild heart failure already taking optimal treatment. *Heart* 2004;**90**(7):765–70.
14. Davies JI, Band M, Morris A, Struthers AD. Spironolactone impairs endothelial function and heart rate variability in patients with type 2 diabetes. *Diabetologia* 2004;**47**(10):1687–94.
15. Swaminathan K, Davies J, George J, *et al*. Spironolactone for poorly controlled hypertension in type 2 diabetes: conflicting effects on blood pressure, endothelial function, glycaemic control and hormonal profiles. *Diabetologia* 2008;**51**(5):762–8.
16. Shah NC, Pringle SD, Donnan PT, Struthers AD. Spironolactone has antiarrhythmic activity in ischaemic cardiac patients without cardiac failure. *J Hypertens* 2007;**25**(11):2345–51.
17. Godfrey V, Farquharson CA, Macdonald JE, Yee KM, Struthers AD. Effect of spironolactone on C-reactive protein levels in patients with heart disease. *Int J Cardiol* 2007;**117**(2):282–4.
18. Sica DA. Pharmacokinetics and pharmacodynamics of mineralocorticoid blocking agents and their effects on potassium homeostasis. *Heart Fail Rev* 2005;**10**(1):23–9.
19. Pitt B, Zannad F, Remme WJ, *et al*. The effect of spironolactone on morbidity and mortality in patients with severe heart failure. Randomized Aldactone Evaluation Study Investigators. *N Engl J Med* 1999;**341**(10):709–17.
20. Pitt B, Remme W, Zannad F, *et al*. Eplerenone, a selective aldosterone blocker, in patients with left ventricular dysfunction after myocardial infarction. *N Engl J Med* 2003;**348**(14):1309–21.
21. Brown NJ. Eplerenone: cardiovascular protection. *Circulation* 2003;**107**(19):2512–18.
22. Juurlink DN, Mamdani MM, Lee DS, *et al*. Rates of hyperkalemia after publication of the Randomized Aldactone Evaluation Study. *N Engl J Med* 2004;**351**(6):543–51.

23. Wei L, Struthers AD, Fahey T, Watson AD, Macdonald TM. Spironolactone use and renal toxicity: population based longitudinal analysis. *BMJ* 2010;**340**:c1768.

24. O'Keefe JH, Abuissa H, Pitt B. Eplerenone improves prognosis in postmyocardial infarction diabetic patients with heart failure: results from EPHESUS. *Diabetes Obes Metab* 2008;**10**(6):492–7.

25. Zannad F, McMurray JJ, Krum H, *et al.* Eplerenone in patients with systolic heart failure and mild symptoms. *N Engl J Med* 2011;**364**(1):11–21.

26. Edelmann F, Wachter R, Schmidt AG, *et al.* Effect of spironolactone on diastolic function and exercise capacity in patients with heart failure with preserved ejection fraction: the Aldo-DHF randomized controlled trial. *JAMA* 2013;**309**(8):781–91.

27. Pitt B, Pfeffer MA, Assmann SF, *et al.* Spironolactone for heart failure with preserved ejection fraction. *N Engl J Med* 2014;**370**(15):1383–92.

28. de Denus S, O'Meara E, Desai AS, *et al.* Spironolactone metabolites in TOPCAT—new insights into regional variation. *N Engl J Med* 2017;**376**(17):1690–2.

29. Solomon SD, Claggett B, Lewis EF, *et al.* Influence of ejection fraction on outcomes and efficacy of spironolactone in patients with heart failure with preserved ejection fraction. *Eur Heart J* 2016;**37**(5):455–62.

30. Yancy CW, Jessup M, Bozkurt B, *et al.* 2017 ACC/AHA/HFSA Focused Update of the 2013 ACCF/AHA Guideline for the Management of Heart Failure: A Report of the American College of Cardiology/American Heart Association Task Force on Clinical Practice Guidelines and the Heart Failure Society of America. *J Am Coll Cardiol* 2017;**70**(6):776–803.

31. Ponikowski P, Voors AA, Anker SD, *et al.* 2016 ESC Guidelines for the diagnosis and treatment of acute and chronic heart failure: The Task Force for the diagnosis and treatment of acute and chronic heart failure of the European Society of Cardiology (ESC) developed with the special contribution of the Heart Failure Association (HFA) of the ESC. *Eur Heart J* 2016;**37**(27):2129–200.

32. Ferreira JP, Rossello X, Eschalier R, *et al.* MRAs in elderly HF patients: individual patient-data meta-analysis of RALES, EMPAHSIS-HF, and TOPCAT. *JACC Heart Fail* 2019;**7**(12):1012–21.

33. Williams B, MacDonald TM, Morant S, *et al.* Spironolactone versus placebo, bisoprolol, and doxazosin to determine the optimal treatment for drug-resistant hypertension (PATHWAY-2): a randomised, double-blind, crossover trial. *Lancet* 2015;**386**(10008):2059–68.

53

Digoxin

Joseph J. Cuthbert and Andrew L. Clark

History

Digitalis has been used in medical practice for thousands of years. Ancient Indian Ayurvedic texts refer to using the roots of yellow oleander (which contain the cardiac glycosides thevetin A and B),[1] and there is evidence that the Romans used digitalis for medical purposes.[2]

The first detailed account of the clinical effects of digoxin was by William Withering (**Figure 53.1a**) in his 1785 publication *An account of the foxglove and some of its medical uses: with practical remarks on dropsy and other diseases*.[3] In a case-series of 163 patients, Withering reported his experiences and those of others in using the leaves of *Digitalis purpurea* to treat, among other things, breathlessness, dropsy (peripheral oedema) and hydrothorax (pleural effusion) while noting side-effects such as nausea, vomiting, and bradycardia. The active ingredients of digitalis include the most widely used today, namely digoxin. Due to the difficulty and expense of chemical synthesis, digoxin is still a semi-synthetic derivative of the leaves of *Digitalis lanata* (**Figure 53.1b**).[4]

Digoxin remained the only treatment for heart failure until the introduction of intravenous mercurial diuretics in the 1950s and, in 1958, oral chlorothiazide.[5] In the control arm of the CONSENSUS trial, 94% of patients were taking digoxin.[6] The use of digoxin as a treatment for patients with heart failure has declined ever since (**Table 53.1**), with the emergence of medications with proven prognostic benefit (angiotensin converting enzyme inhibitors (ACEi), β-blockers, and mineralocorticoid receptor antagonists (MRA)).

Digoxin is used for ventricular rate control in patients with atrial fibrillation (AF), a common co-morbidity in patients with heart failure. A patient with heart failure who is taking digoxin is likely to be taking it for rate control rather than for heart failure itself.

However, there are few robust clinical trials of digoxin in patients with heart failure on which clinical practice can be based. The most rigorous investigation into the clinical effects of digoxin was the DIG study, published in 1997. It found that digoxin had no impact on mortality in patients with heart failure who were also treated with ACEi and diuretic, but that it did reduce the risk of hospitalization compared to placebo.[7] The scarcity of data from randomized controlled trials means that information on the safety and efficacy of digoxin in patients with heart failure and/or AF is largely derived from observational data, the different interpretations of which have caused much controversy and debate.

Despite the decline in its use, digoxin is still cautiously recommended by the European Society of Cardiology (ESC) in its guidelines both for heart failure and for AF. In the heart failure guidelines, digoxin is recommended for the treatment of heart failure in patients in sinus rhythm who are symptomatic despite 'triple therapy' (ACEi, β-blocker, and MRA) or for ventricular rate control in patients with heart failure and AF when other options have been exhausted.[8] The guidelines carry the significant caveat that digoxin's effects have not been tested in randomized controlled trials in the modern age of triple therapy for heart failure.

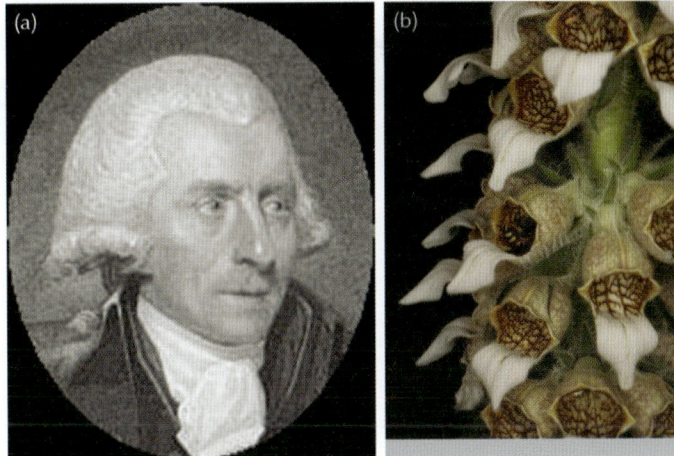

Figure 53.1 (a) William Withering (1741–1799). (b) *Digitalis lanata*. (a, b) Wellcome Images.

Table 53.1 Change in use of digoxin (and other cardiac glycosides) with time seen through the lens of the characteristics of patients recruited to some landmark clinic trials

	CONSENSUS[a]	SOLVD[b]	CIBIS[c]	CARE-HF[d]	EMPHASIS-HF[e]	PARADIGM[f]
Year	1987	1991	1999	2005	2011	2014
Intervention	Enalapril	Enalapril	Bisoprolol	CRT	Eplerenone	Sacubitril–valsartan
Digoxin	94%	68%	51%	45%	27%	31%
β-Blocker	2%	7%	0%	74%	87%	93%
AF	47%	7.9%	20%	0%	30%	37%

Data are shown for the placebo/control therapy groups. Year is year of publication of the main paper from the study; β-Blocker is the percentage of patients taking a β-adrenoceptor antagonist; AF is the percentage of patients in atrial fibrillation at baseline.
[a] *N Engl J Med* 1987;**316**:1429–35.
[b] *N Engl J Med* 1991;**325**:293–302.
[c] *Lancet* 1999;**353**:9–13.
[d] *N Engl J Med* 2005;**352**:1539–49.
[e] *N Engl J Med* 2011;**364**:11–21.
[f] *N Engl J Med* 2014;**371**:993–1004.

Cardiac glycosides

Digoxin is only one of many cardiac glycosides (also known as cardiotonic steroids) that have been studied to varying degrees over the years (Table 53.2).[9–21] Two of the more commonly used medications, digoxin and digitoxin, are derived from *Digitalis* plant species. Ouabain, another cardiac glycoside predominantly used in research, is derived from *Acokanthera schimperi* and *Strophanthus gratus* plants, both native to Eastern Africa where it is used as arrow poison. Marinobufagenin is another naturally occurring cardiac glycoside so-called as it derived from the giant toad species *Bufo marinus*. All have a similar mechanism of action with subtle differences (Table 53.2).

Some of these pharmacological compounds are also secreted endogenously. Molecules chemically indistinguishable from digoxin[22] and ouabain[23] have been identified in human urine and plasma respectively. The latter has been more extensively studied: possibly excreted from the adrenal glands[24] or hypothalamus,[25] it may have a role in the pathogenesis of hypertension.[26] Marinobufagenin has

also been identified in human plasma after periods of hypoventilation in normal subjects.[27] Plasma marinobufagenin is significantly higher in patients with primary hyperaldosteronism than patients with essential hypertension.[28]

The primary *pharmacological* mechanism of action of cardiac glycosides is inhibition of the sodium–potassium–adenosine triphosphatase (Na^+-K^+-ATPase) enzyme. Interestingly, at very low (physiological) concentrations, endogenous cardiac glycosides, such as digitalis-like factor and endogenous ouabain, *stimulate* the Na^+-K^+-ATPase pump.[29] The exact role of endogenous cardiac glycosides is not fully understood but may include important roles in sodium homeostasis[30] and cellular signalling pathways via changes in calcium ion concentrations.[31]

Mechanism of action

Digoxin has three effects that have theoretical benefit in clinical practice: a positive inotropic effect, a negative chronotropic effect, and an inhibitory effect on renin release (Figure 53.2).

Table 53.2 Pharmacological differences between digoxin, ouabain, and digitoxin

Drug	Derivation	Pharmacological differences from digoxin	Clinical use
Digoxin	*Digitalis lanata* *Digitalis purpurea*	*Comparator*	*See text*
Digitoxin	*D. lanata* *D. purpurea*	Less profound reduction in heart rate compared to digoxin.[9] More lipophilic[2] and has a longer half-life[10] than digoxin and ouabain. More predictably absorbed than digoxin,[11] and metabolism not affected by renal function.[12] Greater positive inotropic effect than ouabain or digoxin.[13]	Digitoxin has fallen behind digoxin use in clinical practice due to concerns surrounding toxicity with the longer half-life. There are no modern trials of digitoxin.
Ouabain	*Acokanthera schimperi* *Strophanthus gratus*	Faster onset of action compared to digoxin.[14] More hydrophilic than digoxin and digitoxin.[15] Binds to the apical aspect of Na^+-K^+-ATPase pump only (digoxin penetrates the cell membrane).[2] Increases cellular metabolic activity in animal studies via activation of intracellular signalling pathways.[16,17] Digoxin is not known to have a similar effect.	Research only, recent studies include: • investigating the protective effect of ouabain against reperfusion injury in rabbit myocytes;[18] • investigating the potential of ouabain (and other cardiac glycosides) for the treatment of some cancers such as lymphoma;[19,20] • investigating the effect of ouabain on reducing C-reactive protein synthesis.[21]

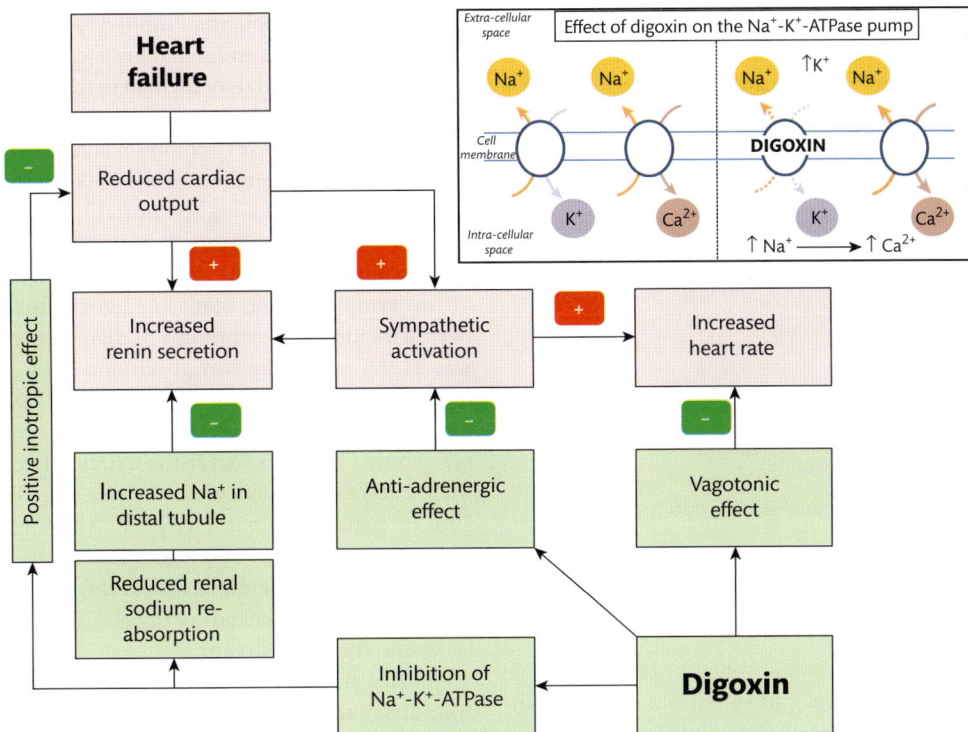

Figure 53.2 Theoretical beneficial effects of digoxin in patients with heart failure.

Positive inotropic effect

Digoxin inhibits the Na^+-K^+-ATPase enzyme on the plasma membranes of cardiac myocytes. Na^+-K^+-ATPase is a pump, removing sodium ions from the myocyte in exchange for potassium ions in order to maintain the resting potential. Inhibition of Na^+-K^+-ATPase thus increases intracellular sodium concentration. This, in turn, increases the activity of the sodium–calcium exchanger that removes sodium ions in exchange for calcium ions; the end result is a subsequent rise in intracellular calcium which is thought to mediate positive inotropy.

Myocardial contraction is stimulated by binding of myosin to actin which causes shortening of the sarcomere. In diastole, myosin binding sites on actin are covered by tropomyosin. In systole, calcium ions bind to troponin C, causing a conformational change that removes tropomyosin from the myosin binding sites, allowing actin and myosin to bind, causing contraction. The force of myocardial contraction is a function of intracellular calcium concentration.[32] Inhibition of the Na^+-K^+-ATPase pump increases intracellular calcium levels, thus shifting the Frank–Starling curve upwards and to the left: for a given preload, the contractile strength of the myocardium is increased in the presence of digoxin (**Figure 53.3**).

Negative chronotropic effect

Digoxin reduces resting heart rate, but has little effect on exercise-induced tachycardia in patients with AF. Any chronotropic effect is thus unlikely to be due to a direct effect on atrioventricular nodal conduction.[33] The mechanisms by which digoxin, and other cardiac

glycosides, slow heart rate are likely to stem from vagotonic and anti-adrenergic effects. The evidence to support both mechanisms comes from disparate studies in animals, normal subjects and patients with heart failure.

Vagotonic effect

- Infusion of digoxin causes bradycardia and hypotension in cats, but the effect is much diminished after a reduction of blood flow to the carotid sinus or vagotomy.[34]
- In cats, infusion of ouabain increases the excitability of the branch of the vagus nerve supplying the sinus node as well as the magnitude of the action potential.[35]
- In patients with heart failure, digoxin increases variables associated with enhanced parasympathetic activity, such as increased heart rate variability.

Inhibition of the sympathetic nervous system

- In patients with sinus bradycardia, digoxin slows the sinus rate even when given with atropine.[36]
- In animal studies, digitalis causes sinus bradycardia after vagotomy or cardiac sympathectomy, but not both.[37]
- In patients with chronic heart failure, digoxin reduces plasma noradrenaline concentrations[24] and reduces efferent sympathetic nerve activity.[38]

Inhibition of renin release

William Withering describes several cases of increased urinary frequency after treatment with digitalis, leading him to believe that

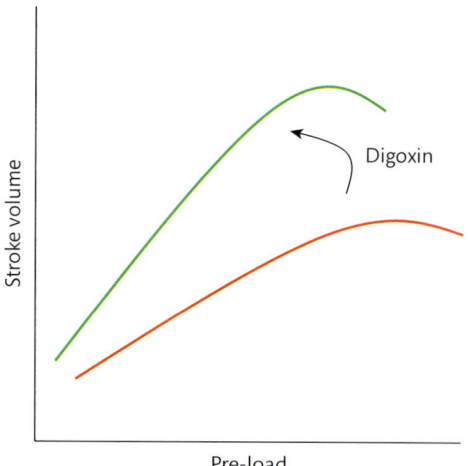

Figure 53.3 Effect of digoxin on the Frank–Starling curve.

the drug may have diuretic action.[3] More modern research suggests that this may be through inhibition of the renin–angiotensin–aldosterone system.

- Intravenous digoxin causes a rapid and significant reduction in serum renin levels in normal subjects,[39] patients with hypertension,[40] and patients with heart failure.[41]
- Inhibition of renal Na^+-K^+-ATPase by ouabain reduces tubular sodium reabsorption, promoting natriuresis and suppressing renin secretion.[42]
- Renin secretion is governed, in part, by sympathetic activation: digoxin-induced sympathetic inhibition may in turn contribute to reduced renin secretion.

Pharmacokinetics

Digoxin is absorbed in the small intestine: 67% is absorbed from tablets and up to 100% from encapsulated elixir preparations.[43] Clinical effects can be seen within 30 min if digoxin is given intravenously and after 2 h if given orally. Peak effect is seen after 4 and 6 h for intravenous and oral administration respectively.

Digoxin metabolism occurs in the liver, independent of the cytochrome P450 system, but ~80% of the drug will be excreted, unchanged, in the urine. The half-life of digoxin is dependent on renal function: for subjects with normal renal function, the half-life is ~40 h but can be as long as 5 days in patients with moderate-to-severe renal impairment. Similarly, time to steady-state serum levels varies with renal function: without loading doses, patients with normal renal function will achieve steady state within 7 days, but in patients with renal impairment, it may take up to 20 days for serum levels to reach a steady state.[44] Digoxin is highly tissue-bound and has a large volume of distribution, making dialysis ineffective for treating toxicity.[32]

Digoxin toxicity

In early clinical practice, it was usual to increase digoxin dose until adverse effects were seen.[45] As a consequence, digoxin toxicity was common (~25% of patients admitted to hospital who were taking digoxin had symptoms and signs consistent with toxicity).[46] Before the large-scale clinical trials of digoxin in the mid-1990s, the therapeutic window was considered to lie between serum levels of 0.8 and 2.0 ng/mL, with toxicity very common at levels above the upper limit.[35] However, post-hoc analysis of the DIG study found a higher rate of digoxin toxicity and a higher mortality rate in patients with serum digoxin levels >1.2 ng/mL.[47] The current recommended therapeutic window is 0.6–1.2 ng/mL.

The symptoms and signs of digoxin toxicity are diverse. The overall incidence of symptoms of 'digoxin toxicity' in the DIG study was 11.9% in the digoxin group and 7.9% in the placebo group, highlighting the non-specific nature of many adverse effects of digoxin. They are usually grouped into cardiac and extracardiac symptoms (Table 53.3). Of the extracardiac features, gastrointestinal side-effects, particularly nausea, are common, affecting 30–70% of patients with toxicity.[48,49] Although the risk of adverse cardiac consequences of digoxin toxicity are exacerbated by hypokalaemia, *hyper*kalaemia is a worrying sign of severe toxicity: as a result of systemic blockade of the Na^+-K^+-ATPase pump, potassium leaks into the bloodstream.

Cardiac side-effects include bradyarrhythmias due to reduced sino-atrial and atrioventricular node conduction and, paradoxically, tachyarrhythmia.[50,51] Inhibition of the Na^+-K^+-ATPase pump causes accumulation of intracellular calcium. Intracellular calcium ions are usually sequestered by the endoplasmic reticulum during diastole. At toxic digoxin levels, the sarcoplasmic reticulum becomes saturated with calcium ions and there is spontaneous release of calcium into the intracellular space during diastole. This, combined with ongoing calcium uptake by the sodium–calcium exchanger, causes high intracellular calcium concentrations resulting in small depolarizations termed 'delayed afterdepolarizations' (DAD) (Figure 53.4).[52,53] Discrete DADs can combine, reach threshold, and trigger rapid repetitive electrical impulses.[54]

ECG changes associated with digoxin therapy

Changes in intracellular ion concentrations due to treatment with digoxin can cause electrical changes that are detectable on ECG. However, ECG changes can be seen at therapeutic serum levels when patients have no symptoms of toxicity. Thus, the ECG changes are classed as either digitalis 'effect' or digitalis toxicity.[55]

Table 53.3 Symptoms and signs of digoxin toxicity

Extracardiac	Cardiac
• Fatigue	Premature ventricular complexes
• Nausea	
• Vomiting	Bradycardia
• Anorexia	• Atrioventricular block
• Diarrhoea	• Sino-atrial block
• Hyperkalaemia	• Asystole
• Blurred vision	
• Yellow–green discoloration to vision	Tachycardia
• Headache	• Accelerated junctional rhythm
• Weakness	• Supraventricular tachycardia
	• Sustained ventricular tachycardia
	Ventricular fibrillation

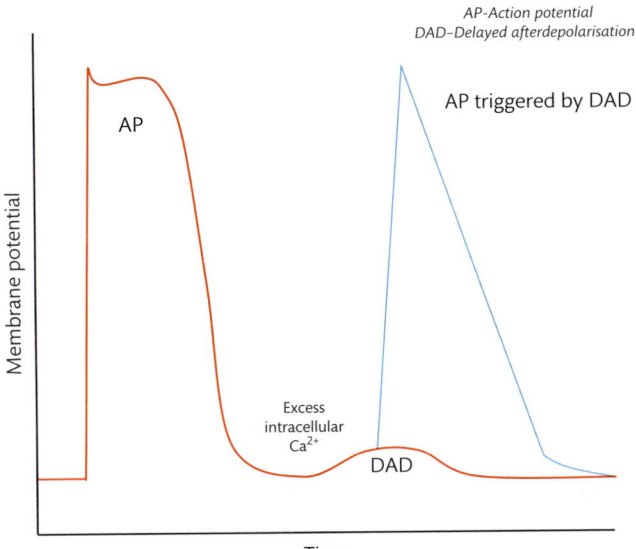

AP–Action potential
DAD–Delayed afterdepolarisation

Figure 53.4 Delayed afterdepolarization.

ECG changes associated with digitalis effect:

- reduced T-wave amplitude
- shortening of the QT interval
- 'reverse-tick' ST depression
- ventricular bigeminy.

ECG changes associated with toxicity:

- Frank T-wave inversion
- arrhythmia
- changes consistent with hyperkalaemia:
  - peaked T waves ('tall, tented T waves')
  - broad, small or absent P waves
  - broadened QRS
  - sine-wave pattern: T waves fused with a broad QRS
  - idioventricular rhythm.

Treatment of digoxin toxicity

Since 1990, the overall incidence of digoxin toxicity has declined with the rate of digoxin prescriptions;[56] however, the incidence per treated patient may have remained the same.[57] Digoxin-specific antibody fragments can be used to treat digoxin toxicity. They bind to digoxin molecules, forming an inactive compound that is excreted in the urine. Given intravenously, a clinical response can be seen after 20 min with peak effect seen after 90 min. Dose is determined by serum levels or amount ingested (if known), or by the patient's body weight and haemodynamic (in)stability.[58]

There are no evidence-based guidelines describing which patients should receive digoxin-specific antibodies and therefore treatment varies.[59] There is a consensus that treatment should be given to patients with suspected digoxin toxicity in the following circumstances:[60,61]

- cardiac arrest or life threatening arrhythmia
- serum potassium ≥5.0 mmol/L.

Treatment with digoxin-specific antibodies is expensive (~£1,000 per vial),[62] and other indications for treatment will depend on local protocols based on a cost-benefit analysis, but may include:

- acute ingestion of >10 mg in adults
- evidence of end-organ damage
- severe gastrointestinal symptoms
- serum levels >12 ng/mL
- significant clinical features of digoxin toxicity (e.g. symptomatic bradycardia) with serum levels >1.6 ng/mL.

Clinical trials of digoxin

The alarming symptoms and incidence of digoxin toxicity led to trials of digoxin withdrawal in patients with heart failure in the mid-twentieth century. Initial non-randomized studies found that stopping digoxin may be safe in the majority of patients with heart failure in sinus rhythm,[63] but was associated with increased risk of worsening symptoms and tachycardia in patients with heart failure and AF.[64]

These findings stimulated placebo-controlled crossover trials of digoxin withdrawal vs continuation in the 1970s and 1980s (Table 53.4).[65–70] These studies were small and the results were variable, making it difficult to draw meaningful conclusions. The two largest digoxin withdrawal trials were published in 1993 (the RADIANCE and PROVED studies).

The RADIANCE trial (N = 178, average age 60 years, 75% New York Heart Association (NYHA) class II, average left ventricular ejection fraction (LVEF) 26% in the digoxin arm, all of whom were in sinus rhythm and taking ACEi, diuretic and digoxin) was a prospective, multicentre, randomized, controlled trial of digoxin withdrawal vs continuation of therapy.[71] The primary end-points were rate of study withdrawal due to worsening heart failure symptoms, time to study withdrawal, and changes in exercise capacity measured by maximal treadmill exercise time and 6 min walk test distance (6MWT). After 12 weeks, therapeutic intervention to treat worsening heart failure symptoms was required for 23 patients in the placebo group and four in the digoxin group (P < 0.001). Digoxin withdrawal was associated with a relative risk of 5.9 of worsening heart failure symptoms compared to continuing treatment; the risk increased over time. Digoxin withdrawal was associated with a lower maximal exercise time and 6MWT distance compared to continuing treatment.

In the PROVED trial, 88 patients (average age 64 years, 92% NYHA class II, average LVEF 27%, all in sinus rhythm) were randomized to either withdrawal or continuation of digoxin treatment; the primary end-points were the same as the RADIANCE study.[72] After 12 weeks, patients in whom digoxin had been stopped had lower maximal exercise time, higher rate of 'treatment failure' (defined as needing therapeutic intervention to treat worsening heart failure) and shorter time to treatment failure than patients who had continued digoxin.

However, the numerous digoxin withdrawal studies can give no data on the benefits (or risks) of *initiating* digoxin treatment. Indeed, the conclusion that digoxin is advantageous because withdrawal appears to trigger a clinical deterioration is flawed for two reasons:

Table 53.4 Table of digoxin withdrawal studies prior to PROVED and RADIANCE (1970–1990)

Study	N	Trial design	Findings
Dobbs *et al.* (1977)[52]	46	6 weeks, randomized, double-blind, placebo-controlled crossover.	• 35% of patients on placebo had worsening signs or symptoms of heart failure: 50% of whom improved on restarting digoxin.
Fleg *et al.* (1982)[53]	30	3 months, randomized, double-blind, placebo-controlled crossover.	• Small increase in left ventricular end-diastolic diameter. • No cases of worsening heart failure. • No change in exercise capacity.
Lee *et al.* (1982)[54]	25	9 weeks, randomized, double-blind, placebo-controlled crossover.	• After the switch from placebo to digoxin, 56% patients improved and 44% patients were clinically unchanged based on a clinico-radiographic scoring system.
Taggart *et al.* (1983)[55]	22	3 months, randomized, double-blind, placebo-controlled crossover.	• 64% of patients remained stable. • 23% patients deteriorated on while on placebo compared to 14% on digoxin (not significant).
Guyatt *et al.* (1988)[56]	20	7 weeks, randomized, double-blind, placebo-controlled crossover.	• 35% patients deteriorated while taking placebo, none while taking digoxin. • Small but significant improvements in breathlessness and exercise capacity with digoxin treatment.
Pugh *et al.* (1989)[57]	44	Two separate periods of 8 weeks, randomized, double-blind, placebo-controlled crossover.	• 64% of patients remained stable • 25% of patients deteriorated while on placebo compared to 11% on digoxin. • Significant increase in the number of clinical deteriorations in the placebo treatment periods compared to the digoxin treatment periods (N = 13 vs N = 5, P = 0.02).

- such studies only include the patients who can tolerate digoxin and have survived long-term digoxin therapy without notable ill-effects—the absence of patients who have either died or become too unwell to participate in the trials due to adverse effects of the drug inevitably biases the findings.

- it may be that digoxin is beneficial *enough* to conceal any harm that it is causing; thus treatment withdrawal 'unmasks' the adverse effects of the drug and the patient deteriorates as a result.[73]

Randomized controlled trials involving digoxin as a treatment for heart failure

In the 'Comparison of oral milrinone, digoxin, and their combination in the treatment of patients with chronic heart failure' study (average age 60 years, 34% NYHA II, average LVEF 26% in the digoxin group) Di Bianco *et al.* randomized 230 patients to either digoxin, milrinone, both, or placebo for 12 weeks. Patients treated with digoxin were able to exercise for longer (aged >65 years, P = 0.026) and had lower rate of treatment for worsening heart failure (15% vs 47%, P < 0.001) compared to those in the placebo group. However, there was no difference in mortality rate.[74]

In the Captopril–Digoxin study (average age 57 years, 82% NYHA II, average LVEF 25%), 300 patients were randomized to captopril, digoxin, or placebo for 6 months. Digoxin had no effect on exercise time or NYHA class compared to placebo after 6 months of treatment (whereas captopril significantly improved both end-points).[75]

In the German–Austrian Xamoterol study (median age 62 years, 63% NYHA II), 433 patients were randomized to xamoterol, placebo, or digoxin in a 2:1:1 ratio. Again, digoxin had no effect on exercise duration or work done compared to placebo.[76]

The DIG trial

The definitive trial of digoxin efficacy in patients with heart failure was published in 1997. In the Digitalis Investigation Group (DIG) study, 6800 patients (average age 63 years, 54% NYHA II, average LVEF 28%, *all in sinus rhythm*) were randomized to receive either digoxin (median dose 250 µg/day) or placebo.[7] The primary outcome

was all-cause mortality, and secondary outcomes included hospitalization for worsening heart failure and death from terminal heart failure or other cardiovascular causes. After an average follow-up of 37 months, digoxin had no impact on survival (**Figure 53.5**) but was associated with a lower rate of heart failure hospitalization (26.8% vs 34.7%; P < 0.001).

Multiple post-hoc analyses have been performed on the data from DIG in an attempt to define the role that digoxin might play in contemporary heart failure management. For example, there was a lower rate of the combined end-point of death or hospitalization due to worsening heart failure in the digoxin arm compared to placebo.[7] However, whereas hospitalization due to worsening heart failure was significantly reduced with digoxin, the reduction in *death* due to worsening heart failure was not statistically significant (P = 0.06) and the combination of the two outcomes was not a specified end-point of the study.

One more recent report suggested that low serum digoxin concentrations (0.5–0.9 ng/mL) are associated with lower one-year

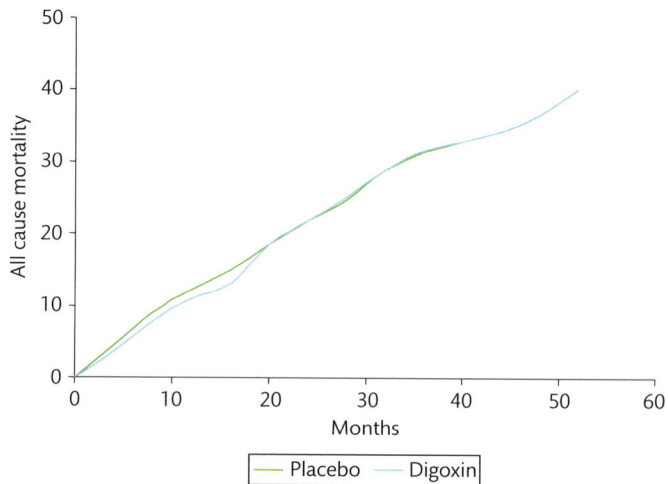

Figure 53.5 Primary outcome from DIG trial.

all-cause mortality, cardiovascular mortality, and heart failure mortality compared to placebo in patients with heart failure who are concurrently treated with ACEi and diuretics.[77] This was usually achieved with doses of ≤125 µg/day. Higher concentrations are associated with greater mortality.[78] However, the conclusions of all post-hoc analyses must be overridden by the fact that DIG was neutral as regards mortality.

Digoxin for heart failure with a normal ejection fraction

The DIG study had an ancillary trial which recruited 988 patients with LVEF >45% to the same trial protocol. The primary end-point was a combination of death from worsening heart failure or hospitalization with heart failure. Although the risk of adverse outcome was numerically lower with digoxin compared to placebo, the association was not statistically significant. Digoxin is yet another drug that may be beneficial in patients with reduced ejection fraction, but has no prognostic benefit in patients with a normal ejection fraction.

The digoxin controversy

Disagreement about which patients should be treated with digoxin and for what clinical purpose began ~100 years ago and persists to this day. In his 1913 textbook, *Diseases of the heart*, Sir James Mackenzie recommended digoxin only for patients with heart failure *and* atrial fibrillation.[79] His contemporary, the American physician Thomas Christian, advocated its use in patients with heart failure regardless of cardiac rhythm.[80] It is still unclear which patients should be taking digoxin: the strength of the recommendation for treatment with digoxin in current ESC guidelines for both heart failure and AF is level B only, and, in the UK, the National Institute for Health and Care Excellence recommends digoxin only as a second-line treatment for rate control in AF.[8,81,82]

In the DIG study, there was a trend towards an increased risk of *cardiovascular* death in the digoxin group compared to placebo, including a significantly increased risk of death from arrhythmia, coronary artery disease, bradyarrhythmia, low-output states, or cardiac surgery ($P = 0.04$).[7] The risk of hospitalization for cardiovascular causes other than worsening heart failure, arrhythmia, ischaemic heart disease, or stroke was also greater in the digoxin group compared to placebo (risk ratio: 1.20). It is possible that any benefit on heart failure from treatment with digoxin is negated by other adverse cardiovascular effects, thus giving an overall neutral effect.

The problem with observational reports

There are numerous observational reports suggesting that digoxin may be associated with an increased risk of mortality: a recent meta-analysis of propensity-matched data from observational reports of patients with heart failure and/or AF found a risk ratio for all-cause mortality of 1.18 ($P < 0.001$) with digoxin compared to placebo.[83] However, there was a proportional relationship between the strength of the association between digoxin and increased risk of mortality on the one hand, and the risk of observational bias in the study on the other. Analysis of all randomized controlled data ($N = 8406$, largely DIG study patients) found no association between digoxin and mortality (relative risk: 0.99; $P = 0.75$).[61]

Perhaps the most compelling argument against the use of observational reports to inform practice regarding the use of digoxin in patients with heart failure comes from a post-hoc analysis of the DIG trial which was published in 2019. *Pre-trial* treatment with digoxin was associated with a worse outcome after adjustment for prognostic variables regardless of whether patients were subsequently randomized to placebo or digoxin *during* the trial (hazard ratio: 1.22, $P < 0.001$ for mortality; 1.47, $P < 0.001$ for heart failure hospitalization).[84] Despite there being no significant differences between patients randomized to placebo or digoxin at baseline, the patients who were pre-treated with digoxin had more severe symptoms and signs of heart failure than those who were not pre-treated. Indeed, the prescription bias for pre-trial digoxin use was so great that not only did it persist despite multivariable adjustment for baseline characteristics, the direction of treatment effect with randomized data (reduced risk of heart failure hospitalization with digoxin) was the *opposite* of that suggested by the observational data in the same population (increased risk of hospitalization with digoxin).

Observational data can mislead clinical practice—consider the true effect of flecainide in patients with ventricular ectopy following a myocardial infarction (MI).[85] Similarly with digoxin, misleading observational data may have led to under-use of a medication that is potentially beneficial.[86]

DIG was conducted in an era before the widespread use of β-blockers, ivabradine, MRA, cardiac resynchronization therapy, and implantable cardioverter–defibrillators in patients with heart failure. The role of digoxin in modern medical therapy for heart failure is thus unclear, particularly for patients in sinus rhythm. Ivabradine can also slow ventricular rate and may confer prognostic benefit:[87] however, it is perhaps worth noting that in a post-hoc analysis of the data from DIG, there was a similar risk reduction in the primary end-point used in SHIFT, namely cardiovascular death or hospitalization for heart failure.[88] In the absence of more recent randomized data, the results from DIG are the best available evidence on which we should base the clinical use of digoxin.

Clinical use

Digoxin is recommended for ventricular rate control in patients with heart failure and AF or atrial flutter, and for patients in sinus rhythm with symptomatic heart failure due to a reduced ejection fraction despite triple therapy (ACEi, β-blocker, and MRA) in order to reduce the risk of hospital admission.[8,89,90]

Treatment with digoxin requires careful monitoring of serum levels and patient response to treatment. Rapid digitalization is only required in patients with a fast ventricular rate that is causing, or contributing to, clinical deterioration. For patients with normal renal function, the daily dose is 125–250 µg. In the elderly or patients with renal dysfunction, a lower dose of 62.5–125 µg should be used. In patients with heart failure, AF, and a rapid ventricular rate, digoxin dose is dependent on clinical response. The optimal dose is less clear for patients with heart failure in sinus rhythm, as long as serum levels do not exceed the recommended upper limit (1.2 ng/mL).

Despite digoxin having a defined therapeutic window, there is no evidence to support regular monitoring of digoxin levels as it does not affect outcomes. Digoxin levels should only be tested regularly if digoxin toxicity is suspected or has happened in the past.[80] Hypokalaemia[91] and, possibly, hypomagnesaemia[92] increase

myocardial sensitivity to digoxin and toxic effects may be seen even when digoxin levels are within the 'therapeutic' range. Patients with heart failure require regular monitoring of renal function and serum electrolytes to detect and treat abnormalities associated with treatment,[87] such as hypokalaemia: this is all the more important in patients with heart failure who are taking digoxin.

Contraindications

There are numerous contraindications and cautions with digoxin therapy.

- Obstructive cardiomyopathy (including hypertrophic obstructive cardiomyopathy and hypertropic sub-aortic stenosis): the positive inotropic effect can worsen left ventricular outflow obstruction.
- Wolff–Parkinson–White with AF: digoxin can accelerate anterograde conduction down the bypass-tract, causing ventricular tachycardia or fibrillation.
- Digoxin may be harmful in the acute phase following MI due to the vasoconstrictive effect of increased intracellular calcium on vascular smooth muscle, causing coronary vasoconstriction, and may increase infarct size.[93]
- Second- or third-degree heart block and sick sinus syndrome can all be worsened by digoxin. It is especially unsafe in patients in whom the conduction abnormality is unstable such as following MI or myocarditis.
- The risk of digoxin toxicity increases with age and decreasing renal function. The safety of digoxin therapy for elderly patients and/or those with renal impairment should be very carefully considered.
- Care should be taken with the combination of digoxin and other drugs that inhibit atrioventricular nodal conduction, or drugs that may increase serum digoxin levels such as amiodarone, and erythromycin and tetracycline antibiotics.

Summary

Despite being the subject of scientific scrutiny for more than 200 years, what role digoxin should play in modern medical management of heart failure remains uncertain.

Observational data suggest that starting digoxin therapy may be harmful, but these are highly susceptible to bias. Digoxin withdrawal trial data suggest that withdrawing digoxin therapy may be harmful in patients with heart failure, but cannot be relied upon to determine whether or not digoxin confers any clinical benefit. The only randomized controlled data on digoxin in patients with heart failure suggests that, whereas it does not reduce the risk of mortality, it does not increase the overall risk of death either. The same data tell us that digoxin does reduce the risk of hospital admissions with heart failure; an event that is associated with high healthcare costs, and high patient morbidity and mortality.

It is possible that the cardiovascular benefits of digoxin (increased vagal tone, sympathetic nervous inhibition and inhibition of renin secretion) are now provided by other medications that have more robust evidence to support their use, such as β-blockers, MRA, ivabradine and, more recently, angiotensin receptor–neprilysin inhibitors. However, digoxin is the only available medication

for ventricular rate control in AF that does not also reduce blood pressure—a useful effect in patients with heart failure, who tend to be taking at least two medications that can cause hypotension. For this reason, it is likely to be around for many years to come.

REFERENCES

1. Sharma J. Cardiovascular system and its diseases in the ancient Indian literature. *Indian J Dis* 1986;**9**:32.
2. Yusuf S. Clinical experience in protecting the failing heart. *Clin Cardiol* 1993;**16**:1127–29.
3. Withering W. *An account of the foxglove and some of its medical uses: with practical remarks on dropsy and other diseases.* G. G. J. & J. Robinson, London, 1785.
4. Hollman A. Drugs for atrial fibrillation. Digoxin comes from *Digitalis lanata. BMJ* 1996;**312**(7035):912.
5. Silverman ME. A view from the millennium: the practice of cardiology circa 1950 and thereafter. *J Am Coll Cardiol* 1999;**33**(5):1141–51.
6. Consensus Trial Study Group. Effects of enalapril on mortality in severe congestive heart failure. *N Engl J Med* 1987;**316**:1429–35.
7. Digitalis Investigation Group. The effect of digoxin on mortality and morbidity in patients with heart failure. *N Engl J Med* 1997;**336**:525–33.
8. Ponikowski P, Voors AA, Anker SD, *et al.* 2016 ESC Guidelines for the diagnosis and treatment of acute and chronic heart failure. *Eur J Heart Fail* 2016;**18**:891–975.
9. Aravanis C, Luisada A. Clinical comparison of six digitalis preparations by the parenteral route. *Am J Cardiol* 1958;**74**:706–16.
10. Belz GG, Breithaupt-Grögler K, Osowski U. Treatment of congestive heart failure—current status of use of digitoxin. *Eur J Clin Invest* 2001;**31 Suppl 2**:10–17.
11. Wagner JG. Appraisal of digoxin bioavailability and pharmacokinetics in relation to cardiac therapy. *Am Heart J* 1974;**88**:133–8.
12. Kirch W, Ohnhaus EE, Dylewicz P, Pabst J, Storstein L. Bioavailability and elimination of digitoxin in patients with hepatorenal insufficiency. *Am Heart J* 1986;**111**:325–9.
13. Runge TM, Stephens JC, Holden P, *et al.* Pharmacodynamic distinctions between ouabain, digoxin and digitoxin. *Arch Int Pharmacodyn Ther* 1975;**214**(1):31–45.
14. Fuerstenwerth H. On the differences between ouabain and digitalis glycosides. *Am J Ther* 2014;**21**(1):35–42.
15. Joubert PH. Are all cardiac glycosides pharmacodynamically similar? *Eur J Clin Pharmacol* 1990;**39**(4):317–20.
16. Tian J, Xie ZJ. The Na-K-ATPase and calcium-signalling microdomains. *Physiology (Bethesda)* 2008;**23**:205–11.
17. Li J, Zelenin S, Aperia A, *et al.* Low doses of ouabain protect from serum deprivation-triggered apoptosis and stimulate kidney cell proliferation via activation of NFkappaB. *J Am Soc Nephrol* 2006;**17**:1848–57.
18. Morgan EE, Li Z, Stebal C, *et al.* Preconditioning by sub-inotropic doses of ouabain in the Langendorff-perfused rabbit heart. *J Cardiovasc Pharmacol* 2010;**55**:234–9.
19. Meng L, Wen Y, Zhou M, *et al.* Ouabain induces apoptosis and autophagy in Burkitt's lymphoma Raji cells. *Biomed Pharmacother* 2016;**84**:1841–8.
20. Newman RA, Yang P, Pawlus AD, Block KI. Cardiac glycosides as novel cancer therapeutic agents. *Mol Interv* 2008;**8**(1):36–49.
21. Kolkhof P, Geerts A, Schäfer S, *et al.* Cardiac glycosides potently inhibit C-reactive protein synthesis in human hepatocytes. *Biochem Biophys Res Commun* 2010;**394**:233–9.

22. Goto A, Ishiguro T, Yamada K, *et al.* Isolation of a urinary digitalis-like factor indistinguishable from digoxin. *Biochem Biophys Res Commun* 1990;**173**(3):1093–101.

23. Hamlyn JM, Blaustein MP, Bova S, *et al.* Identification and characterization of a ouabain-like compound from human plasma. *Proc Natl Acad Sci USA* 1991;**88**(14):6259–63.

24. El-Masri MA, Clark BJ, Qazzaz HM, Valdes Jr R. Human adrenal cells in culture produce both ouabain-like and dihydroouabain-like factors. *Clin Chem* 2002;**48**:1720–30.

25. Murrell JR, Randall JD, Rosoff J, *et al.* Endogenous ouabain: upregulation of steroidogenic genes in hypertensive hypothalamus but not adrenal. *Circulation* 2005;**112**:1301–8.

26. Hamlym JM, Manunta P. Endogenous ouabain: a link between sodium intake and hypertension. *Curr Hypertens Rep* 2011;**13**:14–20.

27. Bagrov AY, Fedorova OV, Austin-Lane JL, Dmitrieva RI, Anderson DE. Endogenous marinobufagenin-like immunoreactive factor and Na+, K+ ATPase inhibition during voluntary hypoventilation. *Hypertension* 1995;**26**(5):781–8.

28. Tomaschitz A, Piecha G, Ritz E *et al.* Marinobufagenin in essential hypertension and primary aldosteronism: a cardiotonic steroid with clinical and diagnostic implications. *Clin Exp Hypertens* 2015;**37**(2):108–15.

29. Gao J, Wymore RS, Wang Y, *et al.* Isoform-specific stimulation of cardiac Na/K pumps by nanomolar concentrations of glycosides. *J Gen Physiol* 2002;**119**:297–312.

30. Jaitovich A, Bertorello AM. Salt, Na+/K+-ATPase and hypertension. *Life Sci* 2010;**86**:73–8.

31. Aizman O, Uhlen P, Lal M, Brismar H, Aperia A. Ouabain, a steroid hormone that signals with slow calcium oscillations. *Proc Natl Acad Sci USA* 2001;**98**(23):13420–4.

32. Bers DM. Calcium fluxes involved in control of cardiac myocyte contraction. *Circ Res* 2000;**87**:275–281.

33. Beasley R, Smith DA, McHaffie DJ. Exercise heart rates at different serum digoxin concentrations in patients with atrial fibrillation. *BMJ* 1985;**290**:9–11.

34. Chai CY, Wang HH, Hoffman BF, Wang SC. Mechanisms of bradycardia induced by digitalis substances. *Am J Physiol* 1967;**212**(1):26–34.

35. Ten Eick RE, Hoffman BF. The effect of digitalis on the excitability of autonomic nerves. *J Pharmacol Exp Ther* 1969;**169**(1):95–108.

36. Reiffel JA, Bigger JT, Cramer M. Effects of digoxin on sinus nodal function before and after vagal blockade in patients with sinus nodal dysfunction. *Am J Cardiol* 1979;**43**:983–9.

37. Ten Eick RE, Hoffman BF. Chronotropic effect of cardiac glycosides in cats, dogs and rabbits. *Circ Res* 1969;**25**:365–77.

38. Ferguson DW, Berg WJ, Sanders JS, *et al.* Sympathoinhibitory responses to digitalis glycosides in heart failure patients. Direct evidence from sympathetic neural recordings. *Circulation* 1989;**80**(1):65–77.

39. Antonello A, Cargnielli G, Ferrari M, Melacini P, Montanaro D. Effect of digoxin on plasma renin activity in man. *Lancet* 1976;**II**:850.

40. Montanaro D, Antonello A, Baggio B, *et al.* Effect of digoxin on plasma renin activity in hypertensive patients. *Int J Clin Pharmacol Ther Toxicol* 1980;**18**:322–3.

41. Covit AB, Schaer GL, Sealey JE, Laragh JH, Cody RJ. Suppression of the renin–angiotensin system by intravenous digoxin in chronic congestive heart failure. *Am J Med* 1983;**75**(3):445–7.

42. Torretti J, Hendler E, Weinstein E, Longnecker RE, Epstein FH. Functional significance of Na-K-ATPase in the kidney: effects of ouabain inhibition. *Am J Physiol* 1972;**222**(6):1398–405.

43. Aronson JK. Clinical pharmacokinetics of digoxin 1980. *Clin. Pharmacokinet* 1980;**5**:137.

44. GlaxoSmith-Kline. Product information: Lanoxin, digoxin 2006. GSK, Greenville, NC, 2006.

45. Bauman JL, Didomenico RJ, Galanter WL. Mechanisms, manifestations, and management of digoxin toxicity in the modern era. *Am J Cardiovasc Drugs* 2006;**6**(2):77–86.

46. Beller GA, Smith TW, Abelmann WH, *et al.* Digitalis intoxication: a prospective clinical study with serum level correlations. *N Engl J Med* 1971;**284**:989–97.

47. Rathore SS, Curtis JP, Wang Y, *et al.* Association of serum digoxin concentration and outcomes in patients with heart failure. *JAMA* 2003;**289**:871–8.

48. Mahdyoon H, Battilana G, Rosman H, *et al.* The evolving pattern of digoxin intoxication: observations at a large urban hospital from 1980 to 1988. *Am Heart J* 1990;**120**:1189–94.

49. Williamson KM, Thrasher KA, Fulton KB, *et al.* Digoxin toxicity: an evaluation in current clinical practice. *Arch Intern Med* 1998;**158**:2444–9.

50. Abad-Santos F, Carcas AJ, Ibanez C, *et al.* Digoxin level and clinical manifestations as determinants in the diagnosis of digoxin toxicity. *Ther Drug Monit* 2000;**22**:163–8.

51. Antman EM, Wenger TL, Butler Jr VP, *et al.* Treatment of 150 cases of life-threatening digitalis intoxication with digoxin-specific Fab antibody fragments: final report of a multicenter study. *Circulation* 1990;**81**:1744–52.

52. Hauptman PJ, Kelly RA. Digitalis. *Circulation* 1999;**99**:1265–70.

53. Xie JT, Cunningham PM, January CT. Digoxin-induced delay afterdepolarisations: biphasis effects of digoxin on action potential duration and the Q-T interval in cardiac Purkinje fibers. *Methods Find Exp Clin Pharmacol* 1995;**17**:113–20.

54. Rocchetti M, Besana A, Mostacciuolo G, *et al.* Diverse toxicity associated with cardiac Na+/K+ pump inhibition: evaluation of electrophysiological mechanisms. *J Pharmacol Exp Ther* 2003;**305**:765–71.

55. Wetherell H. Digoxin and the heart. *Br J Cardiol* 2015;**22**:96–7.

56. Haynes K, Heitjan D, Kanetsky P, Hennessy S. Declining public health burden of digoxin toxicity from 1991 to 2004. *Clin Pharmacol Ther* 2008;**84**(1):90–4.

57. Schmiedl S, Rottenkolber M, Szymanski J, Hasford J, Thuermann PA. Declining public health burden of digoxin toxicity: decreased use or safer prescribing? *Clin Pharmacol Ther* 2009;**85**(2):143–4.

58. Nelson L, Goldfrank LR. *Goldfrank's Toxicologic emergencies*, 9th edn. McGraw-Hill Medical, New York, 2011.

59. Kirrane BM, Olmedo RE, Nelson LS, *et al.* Inconsistent approach to the treatment of chronic digoxin toxicity in the United States. *Hum Exp Toxicol* 2009;**28**(5):285–92.

60. Pincus M. Management of digoxin toxicity. *Aust Prescr* 2016;**39**(1):18–20.

61. Kanji S, MacLean RD. Cardiac glycoside toxicity: more than 200 years and counting. *Crit Care Clin* 2012;**28**(4):527–35.

62. Gandhi AJ, Vlasses PH, Morton DJ, Bauman JL. Economic impact of digoxin toxicity. *Pharmacoeconomics* 1997;**12**(2 Pt 1):175–81.

63. Dall JL. Maintenance digoxin in elderly patients. *Br Med J* 1970;**2**(5711):705–6.

64. Rogen AS. Maintenance treatment with Digitalis. *Br Med J* 1943;**1**(4300):694–5.

65. Dobbs, SM, Kenyon WI, Dobbs RJ. Maintenance digoxin after an episode of heart failure: placebo-controlled trial in outpatients. *BMJ* 1977;**1**:749–52.

66. Fleg JL, Gottlieb SH, Lakatta EG. Is digoxin really important in treatment of compensated heart failure? A placebo-controlled crossover study in patients with sinus rhythm. *Am J Med* 1982;**73**(2):244–50.

67. Lee DC, Johnson RA, Bingham JB, *et al*. Heart failure in outpatients: a randomized trial of digoxin versus placebo. *N Engl J Med* 1982;**306**(12):699–705.

68. Taggart AJ, Johnston GD, McDevitt DG. Digoxin withdrawal after cardiac failure in patients with sinus rhythm. *J Cardiovasc Pharmacol* 1983;**5**(2):229–34.

69. Guyatt GH, Sullivan MJ, Fallen EL, *et al*. A controlled trial of digoxin in congestive heart failure. *Am J Cardiol* 1988;**61**(4):371–5.

70. Pugh SE, White NJ, Aronson JK, Grahame-Smith DG, Bloomfield JG. Clinical, haemodynamic, and pharmacological effects of withdrawal and reintroduction of digoxin in patients with heart failure in sinus rhythm after long term treatment. *Br Heart J* 1989;**61**(6):529–39.

71. Packer M, Gheorghiade M, Young JB, *et al*. Withdrawal of digoxin from patients with chronic heart failure treated with angiotensin-converting-enzyme inhibitors. RADIANCE Study. *N Engl J Med* 1993;**329**(1):1–7.

72. Uretsky BF, Young JB, Shahidi FE, *et al*. Randomized study assessing the effect of digoxin withdrawal in patients with mild to moderate chronic congestive heart failure: results of the PROVED trial. PROVED Investigative Group. *J Am Coll Cardiol* 1993;**22**(4):955–62.

73. Poole-Wilson PA. Digoxin withdrawal in patients with heart failure. *J Am Coll Cardiol* 1994;**24**(2):578–9.

74. DiBianco R, Shabetai R, Kostuk W, *et al*. A comparison of oral milrinone, digoxin, and their combination in the treatment of patients with chronic heart failure. *N Engl J Med* 1989;**320**(11):677–83.

75. Captopril–Digoxin Multicenter Research Group. Comparative effects of therapy with captopril and digoxin in patients with mild to moderate heart failure. *JAMA* 1988;**259**(4):539–44.

76. German and Austrian Xamoterol Study Group. Double-blind placebo-controlled comparison of digoxin and xamoterol in chronic heart failure. *Lancet* 1988;**1**(8584):489–93.

77. Ahmed A, Rich MW, Love TE, *et al*. Digoxin and reduction in mortality and hospitalization in heart failure: a comprehensive post hoc analysis of the DIG trial. *Eur Heart J* 2006;**27**:178–86.

78. Rathore SS, Curtis JP, Wang Y, Bristow MR, Krumholz HM. Association of serum digoxin concentration and outcomes in patients with heart failure. *JAMA* 2003;**289**:871–8.

79. Mackenzie J. *Diseases of the heart*, 3rd edn. Oxford University Press, London, 1913.

80. Christian H. Digitalis effects in chronic cardiac cases with regular rhythm in contrast to auricular fibrillation. *Med Clin North Am* 1922;**5**:1173–90.

81. National Institute for Health and Clinical Excellence. *CG180. Atrial fibrillation: management*. NICE, London, 2014. https://www.nice.org.uk/guidance/cg180

82. Kirchhof P, Benussi S, Kotecha D, *et al*. 2016 ESC Guidelines for the management of atrial fibrillation developed in collaboration with EACTS. *Europace* 2016;**18**(11):1609–78.

83. Ziff OJ, Lane DA, Samra M, *et al*. Safety and efficacy of digoxin: systematic review and meta-analysis of observational and controlled trial data. *BMJ* 2015;**351**:h4451.

84. Aguirre Dávila L, Weber K, Bavendiek U, *et al*. Digoxin-mortality: randomized vs. observational comparison in the DIG trial. *Eur Heart J* 2019;**40**(40):3336–41.

85. Echt DS, Liebson PR, Mitchell LB, *et al*. Mortality and morbidity in patients receiving encainide, flecainide, or placebo. The Cardiac Arrhythmia Suppression Trial. *N Engl J Med* 1991;**324**(12):781–8.

86. Cole GD, Francis DP. Trials are best, ignore the rest: safety and efficacy of digoxin. *BMJ* 2015;**351**:h4662.

87. Swedberg K, Komajda M, Böhm M, *et al*.; SHIFT Investigators. Ivabradine and outcomes in chronic heart failure (SHIFT): a randomised placebo-controlled study. *Lancet* 2010;**376**(9744):875–85.

88. Castagno D, Petrie MC, Claggett B, McMurray J. Should we SHIFT our thinking about digoxin? Observations on ivabradine and heart rate reduction in heart failure. *Eur Heart J* 2012;**33**:1137–41.

89. National Institute for Health and Clinical Excellence. *CG108. Chronic heart failure in adults: management*. NICE, London, 2010. https://www.nice.org.uk/Guidance/CG108

90. Yancy CW, Jessup M, Bozkurt B, *et al*. 2013 ACCF/AHA Guideline for the management of heart failure. A Report of the American College of Cardiology Foundation/American Heart Association Task Force on Practice Guidelines. *Circulation* 2013;**128**:e240–e327.

91. Marcus FI, Nimmo L, Kapadia GG, Goldsmith C. The effect of acute hypokalemia on the myocardial concentration and body distribution of tritiated digoxin in the dog. *J Pharmacol Exp Ther* 1971;**178**:271–81.

92. Raja Rao MP, Panduranga P, Sulaiman K, Al-Jufaili M. Digoxin toxicity with normal digoxin and serum potassium levels: beware of magnesium, the hidden malefactor. *J Emerg Med* 2013;**45**(2):e31–4.

93. Indolfi C, Piscione F, Russolillo E, *et al*. Digoxin-induced vasoconstriction of normal and atherosclerotic epicardial coronary arteries. *Am J Cardiol* 1991;**68**(13):1274–8.

54

Ivabradine

Martin R. Cowie

What is ivabradine and how does it work?

The cells of the sinoatrial (SA) node generate a cyclical change in their resting membrane potential that drives them towards the threshold that triggers an action potential. The spontaneous depolarization current is a combined Na^+/K^+ inward current, termed the I_{funny} current $(I_{(f)})$. It is voltage-regulated and activated by hyperpolarization at around –40/–45 mV, at which point Na^+ and K^+ enter the SA cell, stopping the repolarization and facilitating the depolarization process. The $I_{(f)}$ current channel closes briefly at the very beginning of the action potential, but when the cell hyperpolarizes again the channel is activated and the cycle continues (**Figure 54.1a**).[1]

Ivabradine binds to the hyperpolarization-activated cyclic nucleotide (HCN4) channel, which regulates the $I_{(f)}$ current. It diffuses across the cellular membrane and binds intracellularly to the HCN4 channel when it is in its open state.[2] By blocking the channel and stopping the $I_{(f)}$ current, the depolarization of the SA node cells is prolonged, resulting in a lowering of the heart rate (**Figure 54.1b**). At a higher heart rate the drug is more effective as more $I_{(f)}$ channels are open.[3]

Comparing ivabradine to a β-blocker

β-Blockers work by blocking the β-adrenoreceptor and thus lowering the sympathetic activation of the heart and thereby reducing heart rate. This is done, in part at least, by lowering cAMP levels intracellularly—with the negative chronotropic effect mediated by a decline in activation of the $I_{(f)}$ current. However, the lower cAMP levels also have a negative inotropic (and lusitropic) effect. Unlike β-blockers, ivabradine is a specific heart-rate-lowering agent—working directly through the $I_{(f)}$ current—without any change in intracellular cAMP.

Pharmacokinetics of ivabradine

Ivabradine is water-soluble, with fast intestinal absorption and high first pass metabolism giving it a bioavailability of 40%. It is primarily metabolized by the cytochrome p450 system (CYP3A4) in the liver and intestinal wall to an active N-desmethylated derivative. Its plasma concentration peaks in 1 h under fasting conditions. Food intake delays this peak by 1 h and increases plasma exposure by 20–30%. It has a half-life of 11 h, with an average plasma concentration at steady state after a dosage of 5 mg twice daily of 10 ng/mL. Ivabradine is 70% plasma protein bound with a steady-state volume of distribution of 100 L. The drug is eliminated via both faeces and urine, but renal clearance only contributes to ~20% of ivabradine elimination, so the impact of renal impairment (down to a creatinine clearance of 15 mL/min) on its pharmacokinetics is minimal. There are limited data in moderate or severe hepatic impairment, but mild hepatic impairment (Child Pugh score ≤7) can increase the plasma concentration by up to 20%.[4]

Although metabolized by CYP3A4, ivabradine has low affinity for induction or inhibition of this complex, and thus does not modify CYP3A4 substrate metabolism. However, the concomitant use of *potent* CYP3A4 inhibitors such as azole antifungals (ketoconazole, itraconazole), macrolide antibiotics (clarithromycin, erythromycin), or HIV protease inhibitors, is contraindicated, as they may increase plasma exposure 7–8-fold. *Moderate* CYP3A4 inhibitors such as diltiazem or verapamil result in a 2–3-fold increase in ivabradine exposure and an additional heart rate reduction of 5 beats/min and are considered contraindicated. Grapefruit juice increases ivabradine exposure 2-fold and should be avoided. CYP3A4 inducers (e.g. rifampicin, barbiturates, phenytoin, *Hypericum perforatum* (St John's Wort)) may decrease ivabradine exposure and activity. If these drugs cannot be avoided, dose increase for ivabradine may be required.[5]

Clinical trials with ivabradine

HFrEF: the SHIFT trial

The key outcome study with ivabradine is in patients with heart failure with reduced left ventricular ejection fraction (HFrEF): the Systolic heart failure treatment with the If-inhibitor ivabradine trial (SHIFT).[6] The trial evaluated the effect of heart rate reduction by ivabradine (in addition to guideline-based treatment) on cardiovascular outcomes, symptoms and quality of life, in patients with

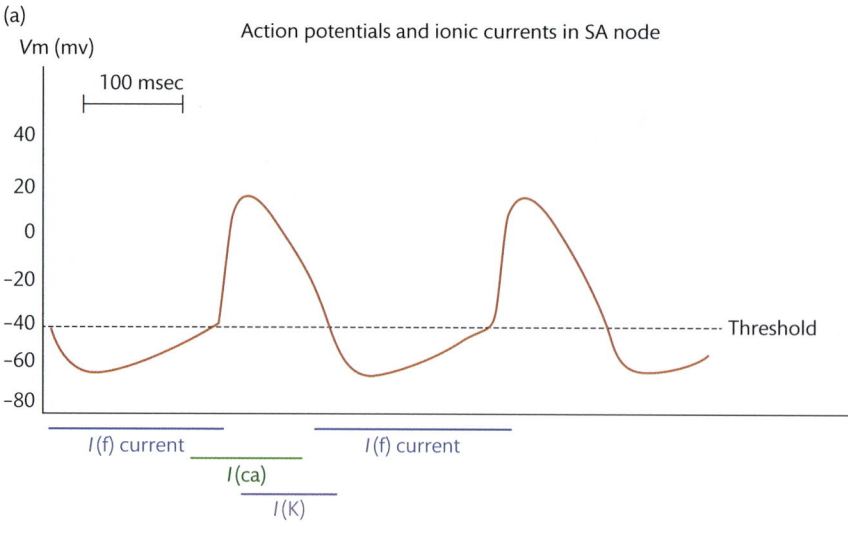

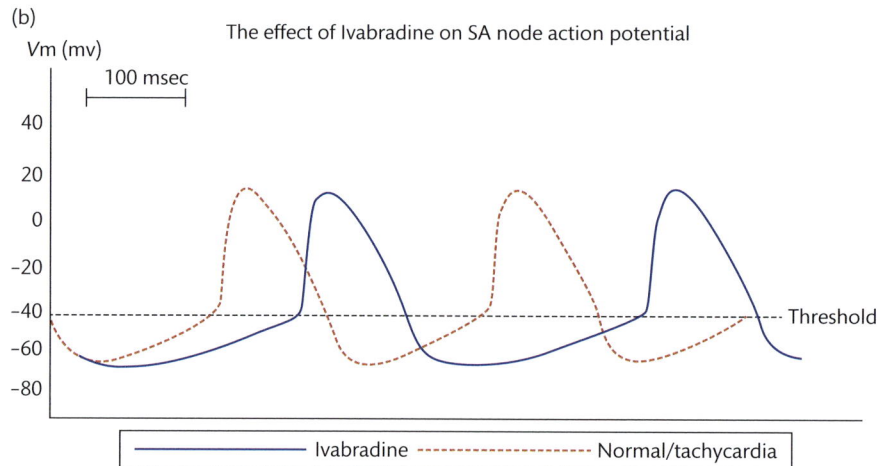

Figure 54.1 (a) The If current is open during the slow depolarization phase. Once the threshold is reached the ICa current opens and the action potential fires. Repolarization then begins with the opening of the IK current, and the cycle begins again. (b) The lowering of heart rate as seen in ivabradine treatment with prolongation of the depolarization phase.

Reproduced from Thorup L, Simonson U, Grimm D, Hedegaard ER. Ivabradine: current and future treatment of heart failure. *Basic Clin Pharmacol Toxicol* 2017. Doi 10.1111/bcpt.12784 with permission from John Wiley and Sons.

HFrEF, sinus rhythm, and a baseline heart rate ≥70 bpm. In this placebo-controlled, double-blind study, ivabradine significantly reduced heart rate by an average of 11 bpm at 28 days, 9 bpm at 1 year, and 8 bpm at the end of the study.[7] Ivabradine was associated with a lower incidence of the primary end-point (a composite of cardiovascular (CV) death or admission to hospital for worsening heart failure) compared to placebo. The result was primarily driven by a reduction in hospital admission for worsening heart failure. In those patients with a resting heart rate ≥75 bpm at baseline (64% of all patients), ivabradine significantly reduced all primary and secondary end-points including all-cause mortality and CV mortality (**Figure 54.2**):[8] this is the population for which the European and UK medicines regulators have awarded a licence.

Interestingly, after 1 month of treatment in the SHIFT study, patients with the lowest achieved heart rate (≤60 beats/min) achieved the lowest subsequent event rates at follow-up, suggesting that although 70 or 75 bpm might be the threshold for introducing ivabradine in patients with HFrEF, the 'target' heart rate might be 60 bpm.[9]

Quality-of-life impact

In the SHIFT Study, a subgroup of 1944 had their heart failure-related quality of life assessed. The incidence of clinical events (CV mortality or hospital admission for heart failure) was associated with the quality-of-life score (Kansas City Cardiomyopathy Questionnaire (KCCQ)): the worse the quality of life the higher the risk of events during follow-up.[10] Overall, there was a modest but statistically significant change in KCCQ scores at 12 months, with a strong relationship in both placebo and ivabradine-treated groups between the reduction in heart rate from baseline to 12 months and the improvement in quality of life. For those who achieved >10 beats/min reduction, the average improvement in the overall summary score was ≥5 points (generally considered the minimally important difference in KCCQ).

Ventricular remodelling

Ivabradine, in humans and at the doses currently recommended, only affects heart rate, and has no direct effect on the ventricular

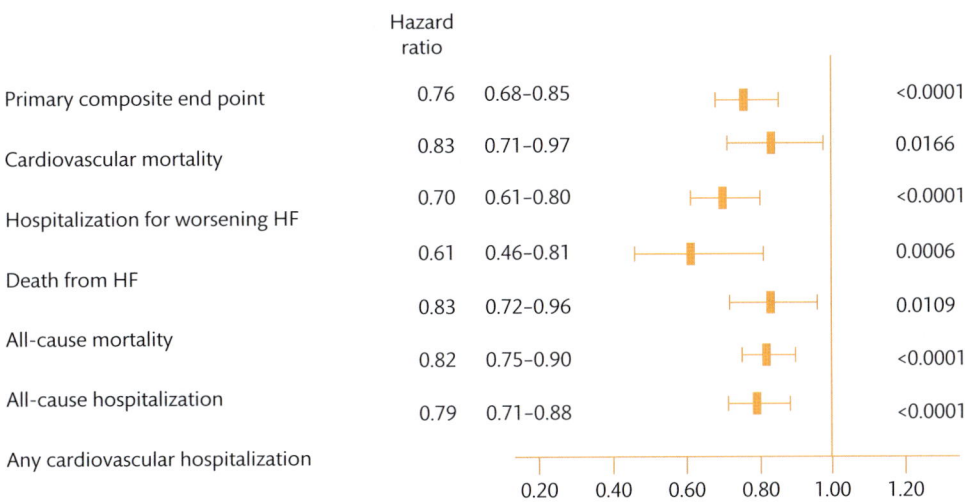

	Hazard ratio			
Primary composite end point	0.76	0.68–0.85		<0.0001
Cardiovascular mortality	0.83	0.71–0.97		0.0166
Hospitalization for worsening HF	0.70	0.61–0.80		<0.0001
Death from HF	0.61	0.46–0.81		0.0006
All-cause mortality	0.83	0.72–0.96		0.0109
All-cause hospitalization	0.82	0.75–0.90		<0.0001
Any cardiovascular hospitalization	0.79	0.71–0.88		<0.0001

Figure 54.2 Effect of ivabradine on outcomes in patients with HR ≥75 beats/min in the SHIFT Trial.
Reproduced from Bohm M, Borer J, Ford I et al. Heart rate at baseline influences the effect of ivabradine on cardiovascular outcomes in chronic heart failure: analysis from the SHIFT Study. *Clin Res Cardiol* 2013; 102: 11–22.

myocardium or conducting system.[11] It is, therefore, interesting to see the effect of greater heart rate lowering on ventricular remodelling in patients with HFrEF. In the echo sub-study of the SHIFT study (411 patients) treatment with ivabradine was associated with an overall reduction in LV end-systolic volume index compared to placebo of –6 mL/m² (95% CI: –9 to –3; $P < 0.001$) at 8 months.[12] The effect was seen irrespective of whether the patient was on a β-blocker or not, the aetiology of the heart failure, or the baseline left ventricular ejection fraction (LVEF). If one uses the left ventricular end-systolic volume (LVESVI) criteria often used to identify those who have responded to cardiac resynchronization therapy (a reduction in LVESVI ≥15%), 38% fulfilled this criterion with ivabradine compared to 25% for those on placebo ($P = 0.005$).[12] The degree of heart rate reduction during follow-up was associated with the increase in LVEF.

Animal models suggest that the reduction in heart rate with ivabradine is associated with reverse remodelling (both structurally and electrophysiologically), reduced sarcoplasmic reticulum calcium overload, reduced local renin–angiotensin–aldosterone stimulation, and reduced sympathetic drive.[13–18]

Sub-populations with co-morbidity

Age does not modify the effect of additional heart rate lowering with ivabradine on outcome,[19] nor does the presence of renal dysfunction,[20] chronic obstructive airways disease,[21] or diabetes mellitus,[22] although these subpopulations are at overall higher absolute risk.

More severe chronic heart failure

Lower systolic blood pressure is associated with greater risk of in-hospital and post-discharge mortality, as well as CV hospitalization (primarily for worsening heart failure).[23] In the SHIFT trial, evidence for benefit from greater heart rate lowering was seen across the blood pressure range in the trial,[24] and overall there was no impact of the use of ivabradine on systolic blood pressure. This has encouraged physicians to use the drug in patients with low blood pressure, where the addition or uptitration of other disease-modifying therapies may be difficult. Similarly, pre-specified analysis of patients with 'severe' heart failure (ejection fraction ≤20% and/or NYHA class IV: a total

of 712 patients) from the SHIFT trial has shown that benefit was also seen in this high-risk group.[25]

Duration of heart failure

Recently, an analysis has been presented that shows that although patients with a longer duration of heart failure have a higher risk of CV mortality and heart failure hospitalization, the beneficial effect of heart rate lowering is similar across the whole population.[26] This suggests that even in those who have had heart failure for some years (and who have been chronically exposed to other drug therapies) there is benefit from additional heart rate lowering.

Acute heart failure

In the SHIFT trial, patients had chronic heart failure and were recruited at least four weeks after a heart failure admission.[27] The drug's licence lists cardiogenic shock, severe hypotension (blood pressure <90/50 mmHg), unstable or acute heart failure, and acute myocardial infarction as specific contraindications to its use. However, since many patients do not see a cardiologist in the UK after discharge from hospital with heart failure, or have to wait many weeks,[28] or have had heart failure for years and are already on multiple disease-modifying medications (and patients with the lowest ejection fraction and the most severe symptoms also gained benefit from the additional heart rate lowering with ivabradine[25]), there has been the suggestion that ivabradine should be introduced during the inpatient phase, particularly as it is clear that heart rate at discharge is strongly predictive of subsequent mortality and rehospitalization risk.[29]

A small trial in one Spanish hospital randomized 71 patients within 24 h of admission with heart failure to either β-blocker introduction and uptitration, or the same regimen combined with ivabradine.[30] Heart rate at discharge, 1 month and 4 months after discharge, was significantly lower in those randomized to the combined approach (4 months: heart rate 60.6 ± 7.5 vs 67.8 ± 8 bpm, $P = 0.004$), and this was associated with lower plasma B-type natriuretic peptide (BNP) concentrations (259 ± 78 vs 554 ± 192 pg/mL; $P = 0.02$) and better LVEF (44.8 ± 14.4% vs 38.1 ± 6.1% $P = 0.039$). There was no difference in mortality or rehospitalization rates in this

small study. The authors also reported no difference in the incidence of adverse effects between the two groups.

A multicentre randomized (open-label) study of pre-discharge initiation of ivabradine—PRIME-HF (Pre-discharge initiation of ivabradine in the management of heart failure) was terminated early due to funding issues. At six months, 40% of patients randomised to pre-discharge initiation were taking ivabradine, compared with only 12% of those randomised to usual care (p = 0.002), with a greater reduction in heart rate (–10 beats/min versus 0.7 beats/min, p = 0.01). Patient-reported outcomes, β-blockade and safety events were similar in both arms of the trial.[31]

Heart failure with preserved ejection fraction

There has been one proof-of-principle study of ivabradine in patients with heart failure with preserved ejection fraction (HFpEF): Effect of ivabradine versus placebo on cardiac function, exercise tolerance, and neuroendocrine activation in patients with chronic heart failure with preserved ejection fraction (EDIFY).[32] EDIFY failed to show any change in three co-primary end-points of plasma N-terminal (NT)-proBNP concentration, echo-Doppler E/e' ratio, or distance on the 6 min walk test in a randomized double-blind, placebo-controlled trial in 179 patients over 8 months with NYHA class II or III HFpEF with ejection fraction ≥45% and NTproBNP concentration at baseline of ≥220 pg/mL (BNP ≥80 pg/mL). The lack of effect was seen despite a placebo-corrected reduction in heart rate of 8 bpm at 8 months, with a target dose of ivabradine 7.5 mg bd. The study was not powered for clinical end-points, and there is no plan currently to perform a large phase III outcome study.

Current recommendations for ivabradine in the treatment of HFrEF

In the UK (and EU) ivabradine is indicated in 'chronic heart failure (NYHA class II to IV) with systolic dysfunction, in patients in sinus rhythm, and whose heart rate is ≥75 bpm, in combination with standard therapy including β-blocker therapy or when β-blocker therapy is contraindicated or not tolerated'.

In England, The National Institute for Health and Care Excellence (NICE) recommends ivabradine as an option for treating stable chronic HFrEF (NYHA class II–IV; LVEF ≤35%) who are in sinus rhythm and with a heart rate ≥75 bpm, in combination with 'standard' therapy including β-blocker, angiotensin converting enzyme (ACE) inhibitors and aldosterone antagonists, or when β-blocker therapy is contraindicated or not tolerated. Additionally, NICE recommends that ivabradine should only be initiated after a stabilization period of 4 weeks on optimized 'standard' therapy with ACE inhibitors, β-blocker, and mineralocorticoid receptor antagonists (MRAs), and that it should be initiated by a heart failure specialist with access to a multidisciplinary heart failure team. Dose titration and monitoring should be carried out by a heart failure specialist, or in primary care by either a GP with a special interest in heart failure or a heart failure nurse specialist.[33] In Scotland, the Scottish Medicines Consortium has used the EU licence wording, but restricted its use for initiation only in patients whose resting heart rate remains ≥75 beats/min despite 'optimal' standard therapy.[34]

The current European Society of Cardiology guideline for heart failure[35] recommends that ivabradine 'should be considered' to reduce the risk of hospitalization and CV death in symptomatic chronic heart failure patients with LVEF ≤35%, in sinus rhythm, and a resting heart rate ≥70 bpm despite treatment with an evidence-based dose of β-blocker (or maximum tolerated dose below that), ACE inhibitor (or angiotensin receptor blocker) and MRA (**Figure 54.3**).

The most recent update to the US guidelines also gives a Level IIa recommendation—'should be considered'—to reduce hospitalization for patients with symptomatic (NYHA class II–III) stable chronic HFrEF (LVEF ≤35%) who are receiving guideline evidenced medicine, including a β-blocker at maximum tolerated dose and who are in sinus rhythm with a heart rate of ≥70 bpm at rest.[36]

Other studies

Ivabradine has also been studied in two other large randomized placebo-controlled trials: BEAUTIFUL[37] and SIGNIFY.[38] In the BEAUTIFUL study of 10 917 patients with LVSD and coronary artery disease (CAD) (no class IV heart failure or instability in past 3 months) and a heart rate ≥60 bpm randomized to either ivabradine (target 7.5 mg bd) or placebo, in addition to usual care, there was no difference in the composite end-point of CV death or hospitalization for acute myocardial infarction or new onset or worsening heart failure over a mean follow-up of 19 months. In a pre-specified sub-group of patients with heart rate ≥70 bpm, there was no difference in the primary end-point, but there was a reduction in the risk of hospitalization for fatal or non-fatal myocardial infarction and coronary revascularization. In the larger SIGNIFY trial, which excluded patients with reduced ejection fraction or heart failure symptoms, but enrolled patients with chronic CAD (often with activity-limiting angina) and a resting heart rate ≥70 bpm, over a median follow-up of 28 months there was no difference in the primary outcome of a composite of cardiovascular death or non-fatal myocardial infarction.[38] For those with activity-limiting angina, ivabradine was associated with an increase in the incidence of the primary composite end-point. Bradycardia (both symptomatic and asymptomatic) was substantially more common in the ivabradine group than with placebo, and was more frequent than in either SHIFT or BEAUTIFUL, presumably related to the higher initiating (7.5 mg bd) and target dose (10 mg bd), and the concomitant use of CYP3A4 inhibitors such as verapamil in a small number of patients. The patient population in SIGNIFY does not overlap with that in SHIFT.

Adverse effects

Adverse effects observed with ivabradine include bradycardia, atrial fibrillation, and visual disturbances.

Overall, in the SHIFT study serious adverse events were reported in a *lower* proportion of patients randomized to ivabradine than to placebo (45% vs 48%; P = 0.025).[6] Overall tolerability similar to placebo was also reported from the BEAUTIFUL Study.[37] There was minimal difference in the number of patients withdrawing from study medication between the two groups (14% ivabradine versus 13% placebo; P = 0.051) and the only statistically significant increase with ivabradine was for symptomatic bradycardia (20 patients (1%) vs 5 (<1%); P = 0.002) and asymptomatic bradycardia (28 patients (1%) vs 5 (<1%); P < 0.0001).

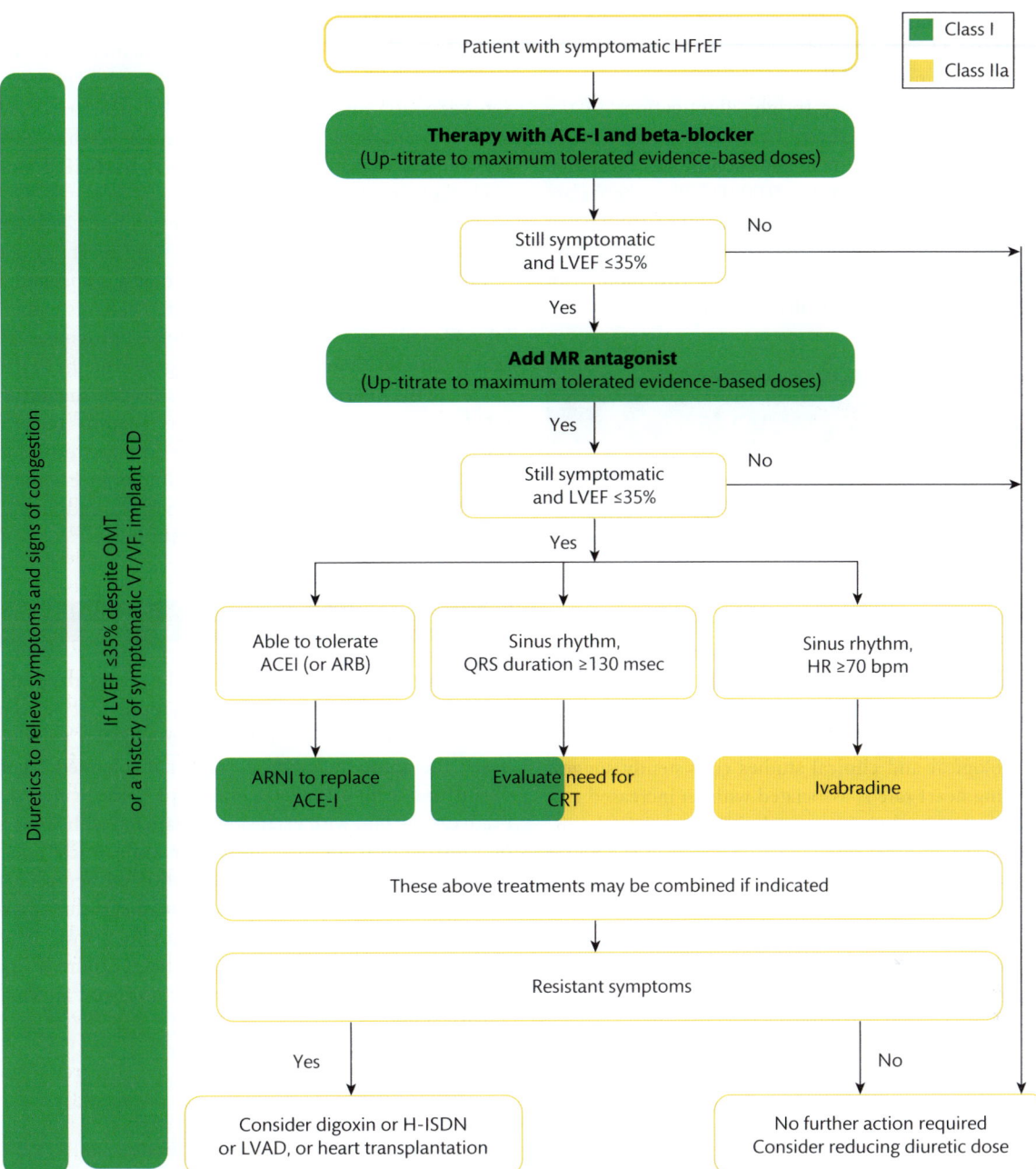

Figure 54.3 European Society of Cardiology 2016 treatment algorithm for patients with symptomatic HFrEF, illustrating the place of ivabradine. Reproduced from Ponikowski P, Voors AA, Anker SD, *et al.* 2016 ESC Guidelines for the diagnosis and treatment of acute and chronic heart failure: The Task Force for the diagnosis and treatment of acute and chronic heart failure of the European Society of Cardiology (ESC). Developed with the special contribution of the Heart Failure Association (HFA) of the ESC. *Eur J Heart Fail* 2016;**18**:891-975.

Of cardiac side-effects in SHIFT, heart failure was less common in the ivabradine group (25% vs 29%; P = 0.0005), but bradycardia was more common (symptomatic 5% vs 1%, asymptomatic 6% vs 1%; both P < 0.0001).

Atrial fibrillation was more common in the ivabradine group in SHIFT (9% vs 8% in placebo group P = 0.012).[6] In a pooled analysis of BEAUTIFUL and SHIFT,[39] AF was reported as an adverse event by investigators in 8% of patients on ivabradine and 7% of patients on placebo (P = 0.054). Whether the AF was brief or persistent was not recorded. In the EU/UK licensed population, the risk of AF as

an adverse event was 4.8% per person-year with ivabradine and 4.2% per person-year (PY) in the placebo arm, an absolute difference of 0.6% per PY. But the serious sequelae of AF—ischaemic stroke and worsening heart failure—were less common in the ivabradine-treated group: 0.6% per PY for ischaemic stroke on ivabradine vs 0.9% PY for placebo, and 14.4% per PY for worsening heart failure for ivabradine versus 17.7% per PY for placebo. So, although there may be a higher incidence of (an episode) of AF, this did not appear to confer a higher risk of more serious sequelae, at least over the duration of the trials.[40] Holter sub-studies in BEAUTIFUL and

SHIFT were also performed and neither reported any statistically significant increase in AF episodes, when comparing the two arms at baseline, 1 month or 8 months.[19,41]

In the SHIFT study, phosphenes (bright illuminations in the periphery of the visual field exacerbated by sudden changes in the ambient level of brightness) were more common in the ivabradine group (3% vs 1% in placebo group; $P < 0.0001$).[6] Phosphenes are due to cross-reactivity with the I_h channel (another subtype of hyperpolarized voltage-gated channels) in retinal tissue.[42] The phenomenon is generally transient, disappearing by two months of therapy, and rarely leads to the need to discontinue treatment.

A higher β-blocker dosage to achieve lower heart rate?

Treatment with β-blocker is central to the therapy of HFrEF, with the benefits likely to be related to reductions in myocardial ischaemia, arrhythmia, and left ventricular wall stress. Additionally, β-blocker may potentially reduce catecholamine-induced myocyte apoptosis. There has been debate about whether it is a 'target' dose of β-blocker that maximizes the effect or whether achieved heart rate is the more important marker of adequate treatment. It is often forgotten that there are marked inter-individual variations in the pharmacodynamics of β-blocker, and the so-called 'target' doses in the heart failure trials were based on doses in angina and hypertension. Epidemiological and clinical studies consistently suggest that a higher resting heart rate is associated with an increased risk of cardiovascular events, and meta-regression of randomized clinical trial data suggest that heart rate reduction achieved is a better marker of likely benefit in heart failure than the dosage of β-blocker (see **Figure 54.4**).[43–45] In a meta-analysis of 23 β-blocker trials, univariable meta-regression revealed no association between dose achieved and mortality benefits, but a strong association between heart rate reduction (18% (95% CI: 6–29%) relative risk reduction per 5 beats/min reduction; $P = 0.006$).[44] This raises the question

of whether β-blocker dose could be increased above trial doses if heart rate reduction is small (at the risk of increasing side-effects), or whether, as in the SHIFT study, a better method of maximizing heart rate reduction might be to add another heart-rate-lowering agent, such as ivabradine. It should be remembered that ~90% of patients randomized to ivabradine or placebo in the SHIFT study were on a β-blocker already.[6]

In a large series of patients referred to one UK heart failure service, the use of a β-blocker and the resting heart rate at clinic review 4 months after referral were independently associated with survival to 3 years, but β-blocker dose was not.[46] Patients with a heart rate of 58–64 beats/min at 4 months had the best prognosis, a 'sweet point' that is remarkably similar to that suggested by the SHIFT study.[7]

Currently, international guidelines do not suggest a target heart rate for patients with HFrEF and sinus rhythm—but advocate introduction and uptitration of β-blocker to target dose for all patients unless there is a contraindication or intolerance—and if the patient is still symptomatic then the addition of ivabradine if the heart rate at rest remains above 70 (or 75) beats/min.

Conclusions

Ivabradine is a specific heart-rate-lowering drug that works in sinus rhythm. The clinical evidence supports its use in patients with chronic HFrEF in sinus rhythm—in addition to other guideline-based therapies, including β-blocker if tolerated. There is no evidence for benefit in patients with HFpEF. The principal side-effect is bradycardia, but, with exclusion of patients with sinus node disease or a resting heart rate <75 beats/min and clinical review of the resulting heart rate reduction on initiation of therapy, ivabradine appears to be a useful addition to the armamentarium for patients with HFrEF. The SHIFT trial suggests that patients will benefit in terms of a reduction in CV mortality and heart failure hospitalization, a greater degree of LV reverse remodelling, and an improvement in quality of life.

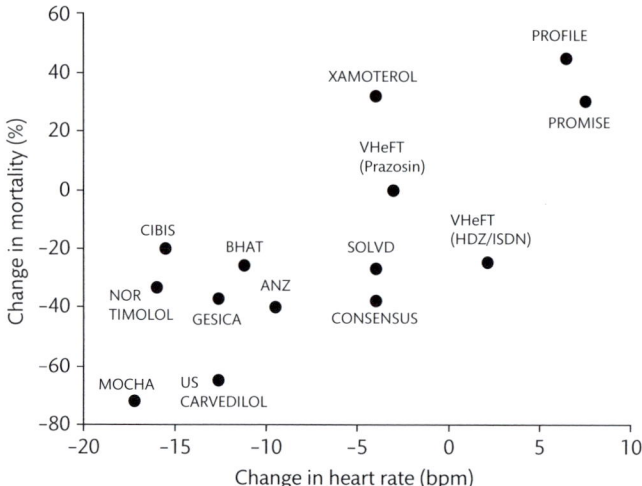

Figure 54.4 The relation between heart rate reduction on the x-axis and reduction in mortality in major randomized trials in patients with chronic heart failure.

Reproduced from Kjekshus J, Gullestad L. Heart rate as a therapeutic target in heart failure. *Eur Heart J* 1999; Suppl H: H64–9 with permission from Oxford University Press.

REFERENCES

1. Thorup L, Simonson U, Grimm D, Hedegaard ER. Ivabradine: current and future treatment of heart failure. *Basic Clin Pharmacol Toxicol* 2017;**121**(2):89–97.
2. Bucchi A, Baruscotti M, DiFrancesco D. Current-dependent block of rabbit sino-atrial node I(f) channels by ivabradine. *J Gen Physiol* 2002;**120**:1–13.
3. DiFrancesco D. If current inhibitors: properties of drug-channel interaction. In Fox K (ed.), *Selective and specific If channel inhibition in cardiology*, pp. 1–13. Science Press Ltd, London, 2004.
4. Rosa GM, Ferrero S, Ghione P, Valbusa A, Brunelli C. An evaluation of the pharmacokinetics and pharmacodynamics of ivabradine for the treatment of heart failure. *Expert Opin Drug Metab Toxicol* 2014;**10**:279–91.
5. http://www.ema.europa.eu/docs/en_GB/document_library/ EPAR_-_Product_Information/human/000597/WC500043590. pdf (last accessed 25 June 2017).
6. Swedberg K, Komajda M, Bohm M, *et al.* Ivabradine and outcomes in chronic heart failure (SHIFT): a randomised placebo-controlled study. *Lancet* 2010;**376**:875–85.

7. Bohm M, Swedberg K, Komajhda M, et al. Heart rate as a risk factor in chronic heart failure (SHIFT): the association between heart rate and outcomes in a randomised placebo-controlled trial. *Lancet* 2010;**376**:886–94.

8. Bohm M, Borer J, Ford I, et al. Heart rate at baseline influences the effect of ivabradine on cardiovascular outcomes in chronic heart failure: analysis from the SHIFT Study. *Clin Res Cardiol* 2013;**102**:11–22.

9. Bohm M, Swedberg K, Komajda M, et al. Heart rate as a risk factor in chronic heart failure (SHIFT): the association between heart rate and outcomes in a randomised placebo-controlled trial. *Lancet* 2010;**376**:886–94.

10. Ekman I, Chassany O, Komajda M, et al. Heart rate reduction with ivabradine and health related quality of life in patients with chronic heart failure: results from the SHIFT study. *Eur Heart J* 2011;**32**:2395–2404.

11. Camm AJ, Lau CP. Electrophysiological effects of a single intravenous administration of ivabraine (S16257) in adult patients with normal baseline electrophysiology. *Drugs R & D* 2003;**4**:83–9

12. Tardif J-C, O'Meara E, Komajda M, et al. Effects of selective heart rate reduction with ivabradine on left ventricular remodelling and function: results from the SHIFT echocardiographic substudy. *Eur Heart J* 2011;**32**:2507–15.

13. Mulder P, Barbier S, Chagraoui A, et al. Long-term heart rate reduction induced by the selective I(f) current inhibitor ivabradine improves left ventricular function and intrinsic myocardial structure in congestive heart failure. *Circulation* 2004;**109**:1674–9.

14. Ceconi C, Comini L, Suffredini S, et al. Heart rate reduction with ivabradine prevents the global phenotype of left ventricular remodeling. *Am J Physiol Heart Circ Physiol* 2010;**300**:H366–H373.

15. Dedkov EI, Zheng W, Christensen LP, et al. Preservation of coronary reserve by ivabradine-induced reduction in heart rate in infarcted rats is associated with decrease in perivascular collagen. *Am J Physiol Heart Circ Physiol* 2007;**293**:H590–H598.

16. Milliez P, Messaoudi S, Nehme J, et al. Beneficial effects of delayed ivabradine treatment on cardiac anatomical and electrical remodelling in rat severe chronic heart failure. *Am J Physiol Heart Circ Physiol* 2009;**296**:H435–H441.

17. Vercauteren M, Favre J, Mulder P, et al. Protection of endothelial function by long-term heart rate reduction induced by ivabradine in a rat model of chronic heart failure. *Eur Heart J* 2007;**28**(Suppl):48. P468.

18. Gupta RC, Wang M, Ilsar I, et al. Heart rate reduction with ivabradine improves sarcoplasmic reticulum calcium cycling in left ventricular myocardium of dogs with moderate heart failure. *J Am Coll Cardiol* 2011;**57**:E323.

19. Tavazzi L, Swedberg K, Komajda M, et al. Efficacy and safety of ivabradine in chronic heart failure across the age spectrum: insights from the SHIFT study. *Eur J Heart Fail* 2013;**15**:1296–303.

20. Voors AA, van Veldhuisen DJ, Robertson M, et al. The effect of heart rate reduction with ivabradine on renal function in patients with chronic heart failure: an analysis from SHIFT. *Eur J Heart Fail* 2014;**16**:426–34.

21. Tavazzi L, Swedberg K, Komajda M, et al. Clinical profiles and outcomes in patients with chronic heart failure and chronic obstructive pulmonary disease: an efficacy and safety analysis of SHIFT study. *Int J Cardiol* 2013,**170**.182–88.

22. Komajda M, Tavazzi L, Francq BG, et al. Efficacy and safety of ivabradine in patients with chronic systolic heart failure and diabetes: an analysis from the SHIFT trial. *Eur J Heart Fail* 2015;**17**:1294–301.

23. Ambrosy AP, Vaduganathan M, Mentz RJ, et al. Clinical profile and prognostic value of low systolic blood pressure in patients hospitalized for heart failure with reduced ejection fraction: insights from the efficacy of vasopressin antagonism in heart failure outcome study with tolvaptan (EVEREST) trial. *Am Heart J* 2013;**165**:216–25.

24. Komajda M, Bohm M, Borer JS, et al. Efficacy and safety of ivabradine in patients with chronic systolic heart failure according to blood pressure level in SHIFT. *Eur J Heart Fail* 2014;**16**:810–16.

25. Borer JS, Bohm M, Ford I, et al. efficacy and safety of ivabradine in patients with severe chronic systolic heart failure (from the SHIFT Study). *Am J Cardiol* 2014;**113**:497–503.

26. Bohm M, Komajda M, Borer JS, et al. Duration of chronic heart failure affects outcomes with preserved effects of heart rate reduction with ivabradine: findings from SHIFT. *Eur J Heart Fail* 2017;**19**(Suppl S1): 225.

27. Swedberg K, Komajda M, Bohm M, et al. Rationale and design of a randomized, double-blind, placebo-controlled outcome trial of ivabradine in chronic heart failure: the systolic heart failure treatment with the If inhibitor ivabradine trial (SHIFT). *Eur J Heart Fail* 2010;**12**:75–81.

28. Bottle A, Goudie R, Bell D, Aylin P, Cowie MR. use of hospital services by age and comorbidity after an index heart failure admission in England: an observational study. *BMJ Open* 2016;**6**:e010669.

29. Habal MV, Liu PP, Austin PC, et al. Association of heart rate at hospital discharge with mortality and hospitalizations in patients with heart failure. *Circ Heart Fail* 2014;**7**:12–20.

30. Hidalgo FJ, Anguita M, Castillo JC, et al. Effect of early treatment with ivabradine combined with beta-blockers versus beta-blockers alone in patients hospitalised with heart failure and reduced left ventricular ejection fraction (ETHIC-AHF): a randomised study. *Int J Cardiol* 2016;**217**:7–11.

31. Mentz RJ, De Vore AD, Tasissa G, et al. Predischarge initiation of ivabradine in the management of heart failure: results of the PRIME-HF Trial. *Am Heart J* 2020;**223**:98–105.

32. Komajda M, Isnard R, Cohen-Solal A, et al. Effect of ivabradine in patients with heart failure with preserved ejection fraction: the EDIFY randomized placebo-controlled trial. *Eur J Heart Fail* 2017;**19**(11):1495–1503.

33. National Institute for Health and Care Excellence. Ivabradine for treating chronic heart failure. Technology appraisal guidance No. 267 (28 November 2012). https://www.nice.org.uk/guidance/ta267/resources/ivabradine-for-treating-chronic-heart-failure-pdf-82600557030853

34. Scottish Medicines Consortium. SMC No. 805/12, issued 7 September 2012. https://www.scottishmedicines.org.uk/files/advice/ivabradine_Procoralan.pdf

35. Ponikowski P, Voors AA, Anker SD, et al. 2016 ESC Guidelines for the diagnosis and treatment of acute and chronic heart failure: The Task Force for the diagnosis and treatment of acute and chronic heart failure of the European Society of Cardiology (ESC). Developed with the special contribution of the Heart Failure Association (HFA) of the ESC. *Eur J Heart Fail* 2016;**18**:891–975.

36. Writing Committee Members; ACC/AHA Task Force Members. 2016 ACC/AHA/HFSA focused update on new pharmacological therapy for heart failure: an update of the 2013 ACCF/AHA Guideline for the management of heart failure: a report of the American College of Cardiology/American Heart Association Task Force on Clinical Practice Guidelines and the Heart Failure Society of America. *J Cardiac Fail* 2016;**22**:659–69.

37. Fox K, Ford I, Steg PG, Tendera M, Ferrari R; BEAUTIFUL Investigators. Ivabradine for patients with stable coronary artery disease and left-ventricular systolic dysfunction (BEAUTIFUL): a randomised, double-blind, placebo-controlled trial. *Lancet* 2008;**372**:807–16.

38. Fox K, Ford I, Steg PG, *et al.* (SIGNIFY Investigators) Ivabradine in stable coronary artery disease without clinical heart failure. *N Engl J Med* 2014;**371**:1091–9.

39. Fox K, Komajda M, Ford I, *et al.* effect of ivabradine in patients with left ventricular systolic dysfunction: a pooled analysis of individual patient data from the BEAUTIFUl and SHIFT trials. *Eur Heart J* 2013;**34**:2263–70.

40. Cowie MR. Ivabradine and atrial fibrillation: what should we tell our patients? *Heart* 2014;**100**:1487–8.

41. Tendera M, Talajic M, Robertson M, *et al.* Safety of ivabradine in patients with coronary artery disease and left ventricular systolic dysfunction (from the BEAUTIFUL Holter Substudy). *Am J Cardiol* 2011;**107**:805–11.

42. Cervetto L, Demontis GC, Gargini C. Cellular mechanisms underlying the pharmacological induction of phosphenes. *Br J Pharmacol* 2007;**150**:383–90.

43. Flannery G, Gehrig-Mills R, Billah B, Krum H. Analysis of randomized controlled trials on the effect of magnitude of heart rate reduction on clinical outcomes in patients with systolic chronic heart failure receiving beta-blockers. *Am J Cardiol* 2008;**101**:865–9.

44. McAlister FA, Wiebe N, Ezekowitz JA, Leung AA, Armstrong PW. Meta-analysis: beta-blocker dose, heart rate reduction, and death in patients with heart failure. *Ann Intern Med* 2009;**150**:784–94.

45. Kjekshus J, Gullestad L. Heart rate as a therapeutic target in heart failure. *Eur Heart J* 1999;**Suppl H**:H64–9.

46. Cullington D, Goode KM, Clark AL, Cleland JGF. Heart rate achieved or beta-blocker dose in patients with chronic heart failure: which is the better target? *Eur J Heart Fail* 2012;**14**:737–47.

55

Antithrobotics

John G. F. Cleland

Introduction

Heart failure is a prothrombotic state because it is associated with vascular disease (predominantly atherosclerosis and endothelial dysfunction), activation of haemostatic systems (largely due to endothelial dysfunction) and blood stasis (due to atrial fibrillation, chamber dilation, venous congestion, and bed rest). Despite many reasons to consider giving antithrombotic agents to patients with heart failure, this practice is not well supported by randomized trials.[1-6] Very few trials had a control group that did not receive antithrombotic therapy and trials comparing different antithrombotic agents generally failed to show important differences in morbidity or mortality among them.

Heart failure, Virchow's triad

Virchow recognized three major factors leading to thrombosis: blood stasis, disease of the vessel wall, and changes in the consistency of blood (Figure 55.1).[7] All three are relevant in heart failure. Blood stasis is more likely when there is venous congestion and bed rest is required or when cardiac chambers are dilated and there is atrial fibrillation. Most patients with heart failure will have atherosclerosis, causing turbulent arterial flow; ulcerated plaque is intensely thrombogenic. The endothelium sits between the blood

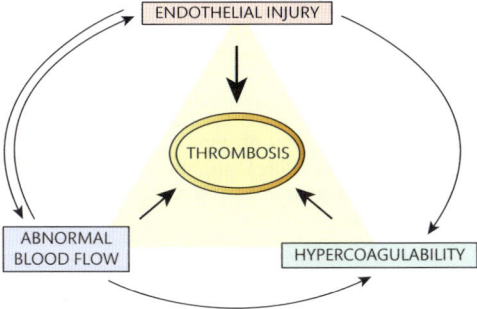

Figure 55.1 Virchow's Triad illustrating the three principle mechanisms promoting the risk of thrombosis. Low blood flow (stasis) may predominate in the venous system and atrial appendage and endothelial injury or disruption may predominate in the arterial circulation.

and the rest of the vascular wall and could be considered to belong to either or both compartments. Heart failure is associated with activation of cytokine–inflammatory pathways, endothelial dysfunction, and reduced production of nitric oxide, a potent vasodilator and inhibitor of platelet aggregation. The inflamed endothelium also secretes endothelin, a potent vascoconstrictor, and haemostatic factors, such as thrombin and von Willebrand factor.[8-13]

Thrombin generation may cause microvascular dysfunction, occlusion, and fibrosis (Figure 55.2),[14,15] which may be important pathophysiological pathways for disease progression and the development of atrial and ventricular arrhythmias.[16-18]

Counter-regulatory systems are also activated that cause vasodilation and/or have antithrombotic effects, including prostaglandin E, prostacyclin, and tissue plasminogen. Pharmacological intervention with aspirin or other non-steroidal anti-inflammatory agents will block prostaglandin and prostacyclin production and may aggravate vascular dysfunction and, paradoxically, the risk of thrombotic vascular occlusion.[19]

Theoretical considerations: atherosclerosis

Plaque rupture leading to thrombotic occlusion of the arterial lumen is conventionally considered the major cause of myocardial infarction and ischaemic stroke.[20] Antithrombotic agents are designed to prevent development and propagation of thrombus and therefore vascular occlusion. However, atherosclerotic plaque provokes the development of a fragile capillary network in the plaque itself, which increases the risk of plaque haemorrhage (Figure 55.3). Plaque growth and rupture may primarily be haemorrhagic events,[21] accounting for the large amount of haemosiderin in plaque. An antithrombotic agent is likely to increase the risk of plaque haemorrhage. Treating the plaque rather than the risk of thrombosis seems the more logical strategy.

Ultimately, it is likely that both thrombosis and haemorrhage contribute to arterial occlusive events; their relative importance will depend on the clinical setting. When plaque has ulcerated, thrombosis will be the dominant risk. When plaque is stable, haemorrhage may be the greater risk. Thus, antithrombotic agents may be useless or worse, due to the risks of dyspepsia, ulcers, and bleeding, for most patients for most of the clinical course of their disease.[22] It is dangerous to base treatment on theory rather than evidence.

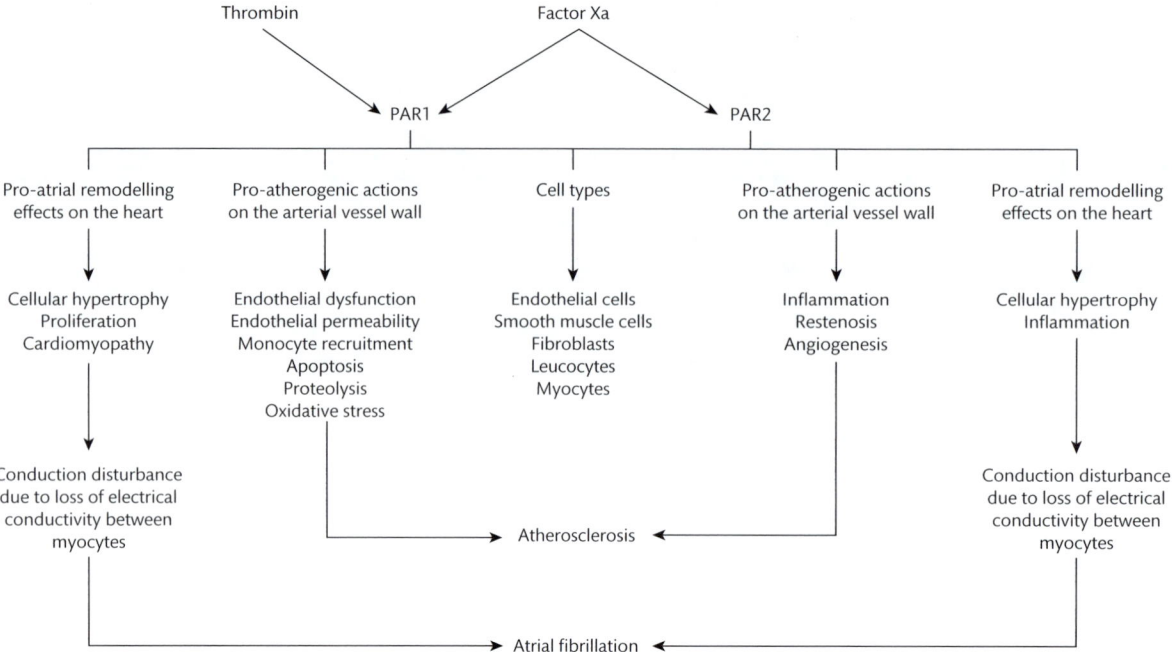

Figure 55.2 Potential effects of thrombin and factor Xa (and their inhibition) on cell hypertrophy and proliferation, inflammation, atherosclerosis, and arrhythmias.

Theoretical considerations: atrial fibrillation

Heart failure and atrial fibrillation might both be expected to increase the risk of stroke, since they are both associated with greater age, atherosclerotic disease, left atrial dilation, and increased blood coagulability. It might be assumed that these risks are additive or worse. However, patients with heart failure also have a shorter life-span and therefore they have less time at risk of getting a stroke.[23-25] Not all strokes in patients with atrial fibrillation are cardio-embolic. Heart failure is associated with lower blood pressure, either because of the disease or its treatment, potentially reducing the risk of ischaemic and haemorrhagic stroke compared to people of a similar age and atherosclerotic burden. Indeed, the risk

of stroke associated with atrial fibrillation may be less than additive (**Tables 55.1** and **55.2**).[41] Again, it is dangerous to assume that theory will translate into practice.

Theoretical considerations: aspirin

Aspirin might reduce the risk of thrombosis by inhibiting thromboxane generation and platelet adhesion but increase the risk of bleeding into atheromatous plaque and the risk of platelet adhesion by inhibiting prostacyclin production (**Figure 55.4**).[42] Increased occult or overt gastrointestinal blood loss may contribute to iron deficiency, which is increasingly recognized as a common and important problem in people with heart disease.[43,44]

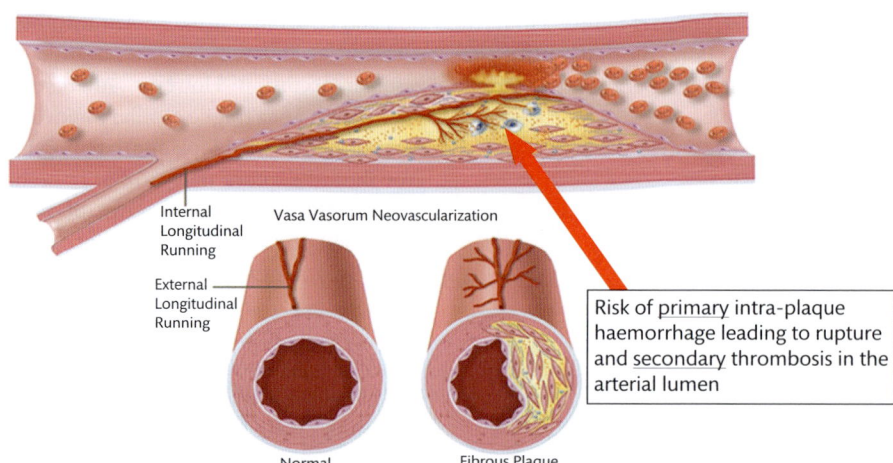

Figure 55.3 Importance of haemorrhage from vasa vasorum to the development of acute arterial vascular events such as myocardial infarction and stroke.

Reproduced from Taruya A, Tanaka A, Nishiguchi T, Matsuo Y, Ozaki Y, Kashiwagi M, Shiono Y, Orii M, Yamano T, Ino Y, Hirata K, Kubo T, Akasaka T. Vasa vasorum restructuring in human atherosclerotic plaque vulnerability: a clinical optical coherence tomography study. *J Am Coll Cardiol* 2015;**65**(23):2469–2477 with permission from Elsevier.

Potential Risks & Benefits of Aspirin

◊ **Potential Benefits (Mediated by Inhibition of Thromboxane Production)**

 • *Reduced Platelet Aggregation, Reducing the Risk of Arterial Thrombosis*

◊ **Potential Risks (Mediated by Inhibition of Prostaglandin E & Prostacyclin Production)**

 • *Increased Risk of Haemorrhage from*

  Δ *Vasa Vasorum into Atheromatous Plaque With Subsequent Risk Of Rupture*

  Δ *Cerebral Vessels (Intracranial Haemorrhage)*

  Δ Gastro-Intestinal Tract

   ◊ *Potentially Massive & Life-Threatening*

   ◊ *Potentially 'Silent' Leading to Iron Deficiency & Anaemia*

 • *Increased Adhesion of Platelets to Vascular Wall*

 • *Altered Renal Haemodynamics Leading to a Reduction in Glomerular Filtration Rate*

 • *Sodium, Chloride & Water Retention*

 • *Reduced Free Water Clearance Leading to Hyponatraemia*

 • *Potassium Retention Leading to Hyperkalaemia*

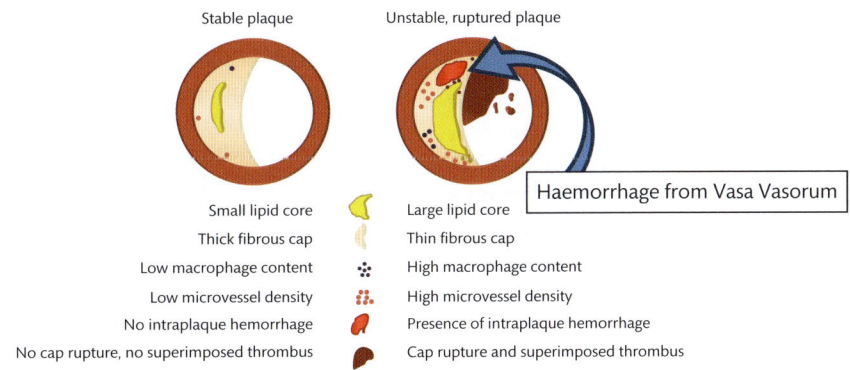

Figure 55.4 Potential risks and benefits of aspirin.

Enhanced vascular-wall production of prostacyclin is a potentially important mechanism of action for angiotensin converting-enzyme inhibitors, which may be blocked by aspirin and account for why angiotensin converting enzyme (ACE) inhibitors appear less effective (or even ineffective) in patients taking aspirin.[45] Aspirin may also detract from the benefits of β-blockers[46] and mineralocorticoid antagonists.[47] Renal prostaglandins may be important in maintaining glomerular filtration and water balance and their inhibition may exacerbate renal dysfunction and hyponatraemia.[23,48] Aspirin, in low doses, may have fewer acute adverse effects but may take a long-term toll.[49,50] Again, evidence is required to determine the importance of theoretical benefits and risks.

Theoretical considerations: other antiplatelet agents

Clopidogrel does not interfere with prostaglandin synthesis, which may benefit vascular and renal function[50] and is less likely to cause duodenal erosions. Theoretically, clopidogrel and prasugrel might be better antiplatelet agents than aspirin for patients with heart failure.[2] Ticagrelor inhibits the cellular uptake of adenosine with the unfortunate side-effect of causing or exacerbating breathlessness in some patients. This may create diagnostic confusion for patients with heart failure.

Theoretical considerations: anticoagulants

Warfarin potentially reduces the risk of venous thrombosis, pulmonary and systemic embolism, in addition to arterial events. This broad spectrum of effects is appealing but warfarin requires monitoring and, in most trials, is associated with a greater risk of major bleeding than aspirin. For patients with advanced heart failure, anticoagulant control may be difficult, due to varying hepatic congestion, complex therapeutic regimens, concomitant therapies (including aspirin and amiodarone) and frequent use of antibiotics, all of which lead to an increased risk either of thrombosis or haemorrhage.

Some of these problems may be overcome by switching to directly acting oral anticoagulants (DOACs) that do not require monitoring and for which control seems less susceptible to changing haemodynamics.[51] Dabigatran is a direct thrombin antagonist and apixaban, edoxaban, and rivaroxaban are factor Xa antagonists which reduce thrombin generation.[9] Animal experimental models suggest that inhibiting thrombin generation may have diverse effects including reductions in vasomotor tone, cellular proliferation, inflammation and fibrosis, including the atrial myocardium and, therefore, the propensity for atrial fibrillation.[15,52] These effects may occur at doses lower than required for conventional anticoagulation [**Figure 55.2**].

What sort of benefits and harms might antithrombotic therapy cause?

The conventional response to this question is that antithrombotic therapy might reduce the risk of arterial events, such as myocardial infarction and stroke, and venous thromboembolism, potentially reducing mortality.[3] However, the commonest clinically overt manifestation of an acute arterial vascular event in patients with heart failure is probably sudden death.[53] Postmortem studies find a high prevalence of acute coronary occlusion not only in patients who died suddenly but also among those who appeared to die of worsening heart failure without a clinically overt vascular event.[54,55] Vascular occlusion may also cause bowel or renal infarction with potentially fatal consequences.

Accordingly, antithrombotic therapy could potentially reduce mortality by reducing sudden death, myocardial infarction, stroke, pulmonary embolism or worsening heart failure. A reduction in stroke alone might be used as a justification for antithrombotic treatment, but for patients with heart failure about 30% of strokes are rapidly fatal and about 50% are associated with little or no chronic disability; fewer than 20% of strokes are associated with persistent moderate or severe disability.[32]

An increased risk of bleeding is the obvious concern. This may be clinically overt and occur into the bowel or other vital organ.[56,57] Aspirin may be of special concern due to its effects on the gastric and duodenal mucosa. Peptic ulcer disease and colonic tumours or angiodysplasia will increase the risk of bleeding. Occult blood loss may suffice to cause or aggravate iron deficiency anaemia.[43] DOACs may be less likely to cause bleeding than warfarin, especially intracranial bleeding (Tables 55.1 and 55.2).[23,40] Proton pump inhibitors might reduce the risk of gastrointestinal bleeding but may increase the risk of iron deficiency, bone fractures, clostridial infection, cardiovascular events, and possibly cancer.[58–60] Prescribing potentially toxic agents (proton pump inhibitors) to reduce the side-effects of antithrombotic agents is irrational unless there is conclusive evidence of benefit.

As noted above, aspirin might also detract from the benefits of many of the agents used to treat heart failure (including diuretics, ACE inhibitors and mineralocorticoid antagonists) and may also adversely affect renal function.

Randomized controlled trials of antithrombotic agents

A brief review of the evidence in patients without heart failure

Sinus rhythm

The contemporary use of antithrombotic agents in heart failure depends on extrapolation from other therapeutic areas and therefore it is appropriate first to examine the evidence for the efficacy of these agents for coronary artery disease and atrial fibrillation.

The mythology surrounding the supposed long-term benefit of aspirin in patients with coronary artery disease is astounding.[5,57,61,62] It is based on just one substantial, positive trial in which aspirin was given for just 28 days after a myocardial infarction and on a meta-analysis comprising large but neutral trials combined with a few, small, outrageously positive trials, strongly suggesting that the meta-analysis is driven merely by publication bias. None of the substantial long-term post-infarction trials used <300 mg/day of aspirin and many used higher doses. Great weight was put on the reduction of clinically overt, non-fatal myocardial infarction. However, coronary occlusion often leads to sudden death and up to half of patients with a myocardial scar indicating myocardial infarction cannot recall a relevant clinical event.[63] Accordingly, non-fatal, clinically overt myocardial infarction may be an unreliable indicator of therapeutic benefit. Randomized controlled trials comparing aspirin to placebo have generally found trends to increases in silent myocardial infarction and sudden death, suggesting that aspirin may conceal rather than prevent coronary events.[5] Aspirin-induced dyspepsia may further cloud the picture when it comes to non-fatal events. In summary, there is remarkably little evidence of benefit with long-term aspirin therapy for patients with coronary artery disease. Recently, two large primary prevention trials suggested little or no benefit with aspirin and a third suggested harm.[64]

The situation is no better with other antiplatelet agents. For instance, in a recent large study, ticagrelor reduced non-fatal events but neither disability nor mortality.[65] The value of preventing events that are not subsequently associated with disability or mortality is questionable. Reducing disability and death, rather than events of uncertain significance, should be the preferred primary outcome for most large cardiovascular trials.

Intriguingly, a study of low-dose rivaroxaban, a factor Xa antagonist, added to antiplatelet therapy after acute myocardial infarction (ATLAS-ACS), suggested a substantial reduction in mortality among patients with a clinical diagnosis of heart failure.[66] Recently, the COMPASS Trial compared the effects of rivaroxaban 5 mg bd alone to aspirin 100 mg/day or a combination of rivaroxaban 2.5 mg bd and aspirin 100 mg/day among 27 395 patients with coronary or peripheral disease, about 22% of whom had clinically overt heart failure. The study was stopped early because the combination was clearly superior to aspirin alone.[67] However, the outcome of those assigned to rivaroxaban was not clearly inferior to those assigned combination therapy.[67] There appeared to be an advantage to rivaroxaban plus aspirin compared to the other two groups for the first 18 months but by 3 years there was little difference between rivaroxaban alone compared to the combination. Moreover, the trial is likely to have underestimated the benefits of rivaroxaban alone because the trial was stopped early due to the benefit in the combination arm. The excess risk of bleeding noted with rivaroxaban 5 mg bd might have been less had 2.5 mg bd been used.

The COMPASS trial still does not provide evidence for the safety or efficacy of aspirin but does show the efficacy of low-dose rivaroxaban, which may be effective in the presence or absence of aspirin. It is unclear whether the effects of rivaroxaban are due to a reduction in thrombosis or a reduction in thrombin-mediated inflammation, fibrosis, and microvascular dysfunction.[14]

Atrial fibrillation

For patients with atrial fibrillation, anticoagulation reduces the risk of disabling stroke by about 2% per year,[68] which translates into a reduction in mortality. There is no reason to expect that patients with heart failure will not benefit similarly (Table 55.2).[69] Interestingly, one large trial showed that patients with atrial fibrillation who receive anticoagulants have a lower risk of stroke if they also have heart failure.[40] This may be either because of the competing risk of death (dead patients don't get strokes) or because patients on 'triple'

Table 55.1 Randomized trials of antithrombotic agents in patients with heart failure in sinus rhythm

Trial	Age (years) Women (%)	CAD	APT	LVEF	Compared	n	Duration (months)	Stroke[a]	MI	CV death	Composite: stroke, MI and CV death	All-cause Mortality	Bleeding
WASH[26]	63 years; 26%	60%	No	≤35%	No ATT / Asp / Warf	99 / 91 / 89	27	N = 2 / N = 2 / N = 0	N = 7 / N = 8 / N = 3	NR	10.6[b] / 11.6[b] / 9.3[b]; HR: ~0.81[b]	9.4 / 13.2 / 11.0; HR: ~0.83[b]	N = 0 / N = 1 / N = 4
HELAS[27]	55 years; 22%; 62 years; 11%	DCM IHD	Yes if CAD	<35%	DCM Pla / Warf / IHD Asp / Warf	44 / 38 / 61 / 54	22	N = 1 / N = C / N = 2 / N = 2	N = 0 / N = 1 / N = 0 / N = 1	NR	NR	7.4 / 2.9 / 8.1 / 11.1	N = 0 / N = 3 / N = 0 / N = 4
WATCH[28]	63 years; 15%	73%	No	≤35%	Asp / Clop / Warf	523 / 524 / 540	21	1.3 / 1.3 / **0.3**; **HR: ~0.24**	1.5 / 1.4 / 2.2; HR: ~1.55	NR	NR	10.3 / 10.5 / 9.7; HR: ~0.95	2.1 / 1.2 / **3.0**; **HR: ~1.44**
WARCEF[25,29]	61 years; 20%	>49%	No	≤35%	Asp / Warf	1163 / 1142	42	1.4 (−0.1[c]) / **0.7 (+0.1[c])**; **HR: 0.52 (0.33–0.82)**	0.9 / 0.8; HR: 0.98 (0.58–1.64)	NR	7.9 / 7.5; HR: 0.93 (0.79–1.10)	6.5 / 6.6; HR: 1.01 (0.85–1.20)	0.9 / **1.8**; **HR: 2.05 (1.36–3.12)**
COMMANDER[30-32]	66 years; 23%	100%	Yes	<40%	Pla / Riv	2515 / 2507	21	1.6 (3.5 TIA) / **1.1 (2.4 TIA)**; **HR: 0.67 (0.47, 0.95)**	2.5 / 2.1; HR: 0.83 (0.63, 1.08)	10.0 / 9.5; HR: 0.95 (0.84, 1.08)	12.7 / 11.5; HR: 0.91 (0.81, 1.02)	11.6 / 11.4; HR: 0.98 (0.87, 1.10)	1.2 / **2.0**; **HR: 1.68 (1.18, 2.39)**
COMPASS-HF[33,34]	66 years; 23%	97%	No	<40%	Asp / Riv / Riv+Asp	240 / 245 / 236	23	1.5 / – / 1.1; HR: 0.74 (0.23, 2.35)	2.2 / −1.3 / –; HR: 0.56 (0.20, 1.55)	4.1 / −3.5 / –; HR: 0.84 (0.43, 1.64)	6.3 / 6.6 / 5.3; HR: 1.07 / HR: 0.82	5.2 / 5.7 / 5.1; HR: 1.13 / HR: 0.96	1.1 / 2.1 / 2.5; HR: 1.96 / HR: 2.30
				>40%	Asp / Riv / Riv+Asp	1418 / 1405 / 1427		0.9 / −0.4 / –; HR: ~ −0.39	1.3 / −1.2 / –; HR: ~ −0.88	1.8 / −1.2 / –; HR: ~ −0.66	3.6 / 2.8 / **2.5**; HR: 0.77 / **HR: 0.68**	2.8 / 2.1 / **1.8**; HR: 0.75 / **HR: 0.63**	1.0 / **1.6** / 1.2; **HR: 1.68** / HR: 1.14
				NK	Asp / Riv / Riv+Asp	321 / 310 / 300		NR	NR	NR	4.9 / 3.0 / **2.6**; HR: 0.64 / **HR: 0.53**	4.5 / 2.9 / 2.2; HR: 0.65 / **HR: 0.49**	0.6 / 0.3 / 1.2; HR: 0.67 / HR: 1.66
ATLAS-ACS with Heart Failure[35]	64 years; 34%	100%	Yes	NK	Pla / Riv 2.5bd	558 / 562	24	0.9 / 0.8; HR: 0.68 (0.25,1.80)	4.5 / 3.2; HR: 0.68 (0.44, 1.04)	4.5 / **2.1**; **HR: 0.45 (0.27, 0.74)**	8.6 / **5.3**; **HR: 0.59 (0.42, 0.81)**	4.7 / **2.1**; **HR: 0.43 (0.26, 0.71)**	N = 2 / N = 3

CAD, coronary artery disease; LVEF, left ventricular ejection fraction; MI, myocardial infarction; CV, cardiovascular; APT, antiplatelet therapy; Asp, aspirin; Warf, warfarin; Riv, rivaroxaban; Apix, apixaban; NR, not reported; NK, not known.
WASH: Warfarin Aspirin Study of Heart Failure; HELAS: Heart failure Long-term Antithrombotic Study; WATCH: Warfarin and Antiplatelet Therapy in Chronic Heart Failure WARCEF: Warfarin versus Aspirin in Reduced Cardiac Ejection Fraction; COMMANDER: A Study to Assess the Effectiveness and Safety of Rivaroxaban in Reducing the Risk of Death, Myocardial Infarction, or Stroke in Participants with Heart Failure and Coronary Artery Disease Following an Episode of Decompensated Heart Failure; COMPASS: Cardiovascular Outcomes for People Using Anticoagulation Strategies; ATLAS-ACS: Anti-Xa Therapy to Lower Cardiovascular Events in Addition to Standard Therapy in Subjects with Acute Coronary Syndrome.

Bold type indicates a statistically significant result (for COMPASS-HF comparisons are with aspirin 100 mg/day).

HR, hazard ratio with 95% confidence interval (95% CI not included for COMPASS-HF to reduce complexity; HR for rivaroxaban versus aspirin appears above HR for combination versus aspirin. ~HR, recalculated approximate HR from summary data.

[a] Intracerebral haemorrhage not included in stroke rates. Composite includes all-cause rather than cardiovascular mortality.

[b] For aspirin compared to warfarin. Composite includes all-cause rather than cardiovascular mortality. Note that the rate of stroke leading to death or moderately severe disability was reduced from about 0.8 to 0.4% per year.

TIA, rate of stroke or transient ischaemic attack.

therapy for heart failure generally have low blood pressure that may reduce the risk of thrombotic and haemorrhagic stroke; not all strokes in patients with atrial fibrillation are embolic.

For patients with heart failure: effects on symptoms, signs, exercise capacity and biochemistry

Antiplatelet agents

There are few studies comparing the effects of aspirin to a control group not receiving any antithrombotic therapy but several have compared aspirin to clopidogrel. For patients with heart failure, clopidogrel does not appear to have any relevant off-target effects; it just inhibits platelet aggregation. Compared to no treatment or to clopidogrel, several small, well-controlled trials suggest that aspirin causes a decline in glomerular filtration rate, sodium retention, a rise in natriuretic peptides, and a decline in exercise capacity.[2,70-75] This may not be a sufficiently large effect to matter for most patients but in patients with advanced heart failure, or with important renal dysfunction, switching from aspirin to clopidogrel or just stopping aspirin should be considered.[50]

Anticoagulants

There is no evidence that warfarin or the new anticoagulant agents have effects on the symptoms, signs, electrolytes, or renal function for patients with heart failure.

Effects on morbidity and mortality in patients with heart failure[76,77]

Five substantial randomized controlled trials of antithrombotic agents for patients with heart failure and reduced left ventricular ejection fraction (LVEF) in sinus rhythm have been published[25-28,78,79] and a substantial subset of the COMPASS trial had heart failure, mainly with preserved LVEF (HFpEF). These trials generally showed a reduction in stroke but, with the exception of patients with HFpEF in COMPASS, did not show a reduction in mortality. Showing that two interventions have similar effects does not prove that either is effective. They might be equally deleterious or ineffective.[1]

Trials comparing warfarin with aspirin or clopidogrel in patients with chronic heart failure and reduced LVEF (HFrEF) in sinus rhythm

WASH was a pilot trial including 279 patients randomized to no antithrombotic treatment, warfarin, or aspirin (Table 55.1). It showed little difference between the three groups over a follow-up of more than two years but hinted at a higher rate of hospitalization for heart failure with aspirin. HELAS was similarly small and inconclusive. WATCH compared warfarin, aspirin, and clopidogrel, showing a reduction in stroke rates from twelve events (~1.3% per year) for each of the antiplatelet agents to just three patients (0.3% per year) with warfarin. Again, patients assigned to aspirin tended to have a higher rate of hospitalization for heart failure. However, there were more major bleeds on warfarin and there was no difference in mortality. WARCEF compared aspirin and warfarin and came to similar conclusions, although no increase in hospitalization for heart failure were observed with aspirin. However, warfarin was associated with lower mortality in patients aged <60 years (from 5.4% to 4.1% per year; HR: 0.65 (0.48–0.89)) but not in those aged ≥60 years (from 7.5% to 9.0% per year; HR: 1.18 (0.94, 1.49)).[29] This difference might reflect less intense anticoagulation and a lower rate of bleeding events among younger patients in WARCEF.[29]

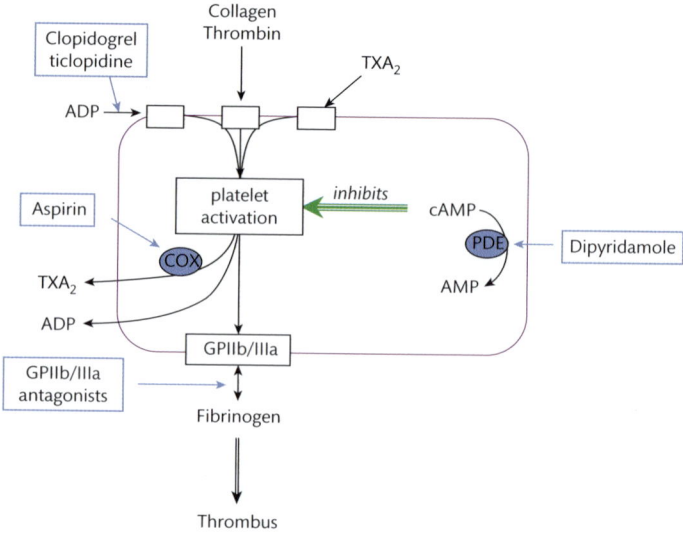

Figure 55.5 The mechanism of action of orally active antiplatelet agents. Once a platelet is activated, it releases ADP and TXA$_2$, thereby recruiting more platelets. The final common pathway of platelet activation is formation of the GPIIb/IIIa complex. cAMP is a powerful inhibitor of platelet activation, the breakdown of which is catalysed by PDE. ADP, adenosine diphosphate; cAMP, cyclic adenosine monophosphate; AMP, adenosine monophosphate; TXA$_2$, thromboxane A$_2$; COX, cyclooxygenase; PDE, phosphodiesterase.

Overall, these trials suggest that, compared to mortality, stroke is a relatively rare event (~1.4% per year) among patients with HFrEF in sinus rhythm receiving no antithrombotic therapy or an antiplatelet agent (Table 55.1; Figure 55.5). The stroke rate is about half the rate (3.3% per year) observed in AVVEROES for patients with heart failure and atrial fibrillation treated with aspirin (Table 55.2). Whether in sinus rhythm or atrial fibrillation, warfarin reduces the risk of stroke by about half.[80] The reduction in the risk of stroke is of a similar magnitude to the increased risk of major bleeding events, which are also distressing and may be fatal (Table 55.1). After a stroke most patients will either die (30%) or make a good recovery (50%); only about 20% will survive with persistent moderate or severe disability; the reduction in non-fatal, disabling stroke by anticoagulation may be closer to 0.1% per year.[32]

Rates of hospitalizations for worsening heart failure were higher for patients assigned to aspirin in WASH and WATCH but not in WARCEF.[26,28,81] Mortality was similar regardless of antithrombotic regimen (aspirin, warfarin, or DOAC) in these trials (Table 55.1). Patients with very low left ventricular ejection fraction (e.g. <15%) and those with gross atrial dilation, who are at greater risk of atrial fibrillation, might be at increased risk of stroke and might warrant anticoagulation, although the evidence is weak.[82]

The COMMANDER-HF trial, comparing rivaroxaban to placebo on a background antiplatelet therapy in patients with HFrEF and CAD

COMMANDER-HF included 5022 patients with HFrEF, CAD in sinus rhythm, who had a recent hospitalization for worsening heart failure.[9] The trial compared rivaroxaban 2.5 mg bd to placebo on top of background antiplatelet therapy (aspirin alone in 58%; dual-antiplatelet therapy in 35%). Rivaroxaban did not improve survival,

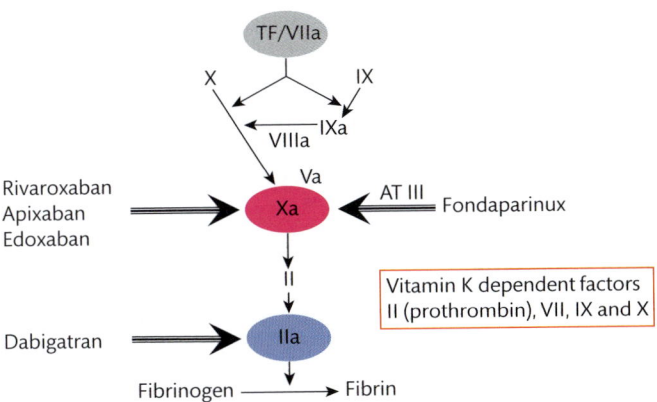

Figure 55.6 Mechanisms of action of anticoagulants. The clotting factors are shown as Roman numerals; AT III, antithrombin III.

Source data from Weitz JI & Bates SM. New anticoagulants. *J Thromb Haemost* 2005;**3**:1843–1853.

although a composite of vascular outcomes (stroke, myocardial infarction and sudden death) was reduced, driven mainly by a reduction in stroke (**Table 55.1**; **Figure 55.6**).[30–33] The reduction in stroke was of similar magnitude to the effect of warfarin observed in the WATCH and WARCEF trials (**Table 55.1**).

The COMMANDER-HF trial suggests that for patients with stable CAD and more advanced heart failure, hospitalizations and deaths due to worsening heart failure are not greatly influenced by antithrombotic therapy and that the driver of disease progression is myocardial dysfunction rather than thrombotic events (**Figure 55.7**). However, patients with less severe heart failure might benefit because they are at low risk of dying from progressive myocardial dysfunction.[33] Patients with an acute coronary syndrome might benefit because they are at greater risk of further vascular events.[83]

Heart failure subsets in the COMPASS trial

COMPASS included 4250 patients with HFpEF, 721 had HFrEF, and LVEF was unknown for 931 patients.[34] As noted above, the overall trial was stopped early for benefit on the primary end-point (a composite of CV death, stroke, or myocardial infarction) with the combination of rivaroxaban and aspirin compared to aspirin alone; rivaroxaban 5 mg bd alone appeared to exert similar benefit.

HFpEF

All-cause mortality was lower for patients with HFpEF assigned to combination therapy (hazard ratio (HR): 0.63; 0.44–0.90) or rivaroxaban alone (HR: 0.75; 0.53–1.06) with an estimated 4% absolute reduction in mortality at two years—rather similar to the effect of sacubitril–valsartan or dapagliflozin (**Figure 55.7**).[33] The risk of the composite outcome of stroke, myocardial infarction, and cardiovascular death was also lower with rivaroxaban. This suggests that coronary events are an important driver of events in HFpEF, although other mechanisms for rivaroxaban's effects discussed earlier cannot be excluded. There was no excess risk of major bleeding with the combination of rivaroxaban 2.5 mg bd and aspirin compared to aspirin alone for patients with HFpEF (HR: 1.14; 0.68–1.91), in contrast to those without heart failure (HR: 1.79; 1.45–2.21). Rivaroxaban 5 mg bd was associated with a somewhat higher risk of bleeding. Whether rivaroxaban 2.5 mg bd alone rather than in combination with aspirin is the safest, effective regimen should be explored. Of note, this is the first randomized trial to show that an intervention can reduce mortality in HFpEF.

HFrEF

The smaller subset of patients with HFrEF had a higher annual mortality (5.2%) compared to those with HFpEF (2.8%) but did not appear to obtain similar benefits, apart, perhaps, from a modest reduction in stroke.

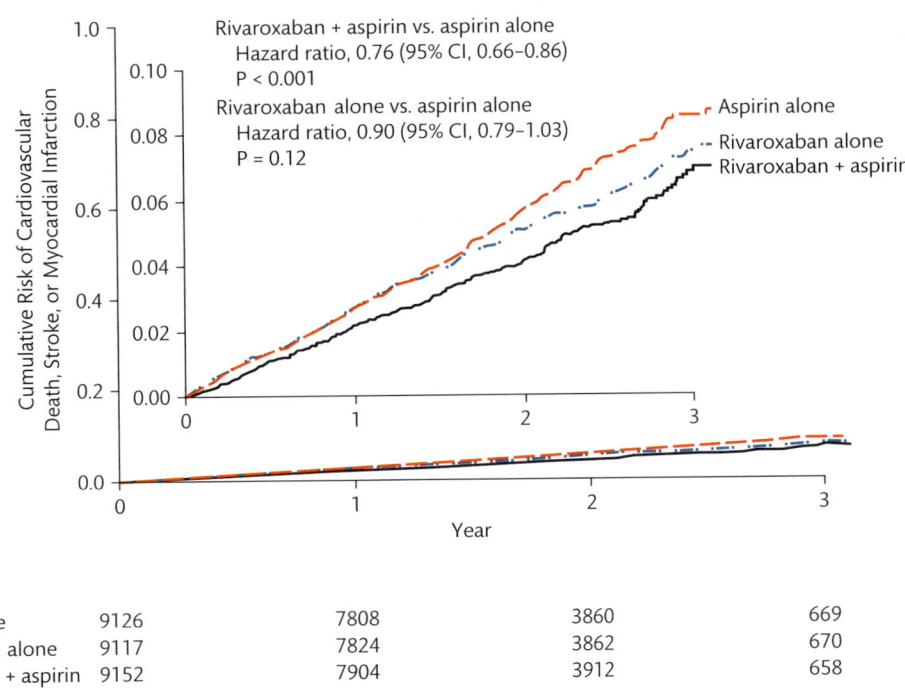

Figure 55.7 Results of the COMPASS trial. Note the similar effects of rivaroxaban alone versus the combination on longer-term outcomes.

Reproduced from Rivaroxaban for the Prevention of Major Cardiovascular Events in Coronary or Peripheral Artery Disease (COMPASS). 2017.

Effects on morbidity and mortality in patients in atrial fibrillation

There are no placebo-controlled trials of anticoagulants specifically in patients with heart failure and atrial fibrillation (Table 55.2). Many patients included in trials of atrial fibrillation comparing anticoagulants to aspirin were reported to have heart failure and it is likely that diagnosis was overlooked in many more. Aspirin is effectively a placebo, or worse, for patients with atrial fibrillation with or without heart failure; it is not known to reduce the risk of stroke or death in this setting. Compared to aspirin, warfarin and DOACs reduce the risk of stroke with a similar relative benefit in patients with or without heart failure, but this may not translate into a reduction in mortality compared to aspirin (Table 55.2). In other words, the effect of anticoagulants compared to aspirin on vascular events in sinus rhythm and atrial fibrillation may be rather similar, although the magnitude of the reduction in stroke may be slightly larger (perhaps 2% per year in atrial fibrillation compared to 1% per year in sinus rhythm).

Once anticoagulated, patients with heart failure may be at no greater, and possibly lower,[40] risk of stroke compared to those without heart failure (Table 55.2; Figure 55.8), either because they have a shorter life-span and therefore reduced exposure to the risk of stroke or because treatment for heart failure reduces blood pressure and therefore ischaemic and haemorrhagic stroke, even if the rate of cardio-embolic stroke is not reduced. Patients with heart failure might also be more adherent to anticoagulant medication. Patients with and without heart failure have similar rates of major bleeds on anticoagulants.

DOACs may be slightly more effective in reducing stroke than warfarin and less likely to cause major bleeds, especially intracranial,[23,84] and this might translate into a slightly lower mortality. In relative terms, these advantages are similar for patients with and without heart failure, although the lower risk of major bleeds may be more pronounced and the effect on mortality less for patients with heart failure.[85] At doses investigated in trials, dabigatran and apixaban may reduce the risk of stroke more than other DOACs and edoxaban 30 mg/day may be associated with the lowest risk of bleeding.[86]

Hospital admissions with (acute) heart failure

Heart failure is a common reason for hospitalization, which may entail a sustained period of bed rest that increases the risk of venous thromboembolism. Clinical trials have identified that, without prophylactic heparin, about 7% of acutely ill medical admissions, a substantial minority of whom had heart failure, will develop a proximal or symptomatic deep vein thrombosis (DVT). The risk of DVT is reduced by anticoagulation, either with heparin or a DOAC (Table 55.3).[87–94] The risk of clinically apparent pulmonary thromboembolism (PTE) is rather low (<0.5%) and may be reduced by about one-third with prophylactic anticoagulation. Anticoagulation doubles the risk of major bleeding, although low-molecular-weight heparin may carry a lower risk than either unfractionated heparin or DOAC (Table 55.3).[87] Many PTEs might be missed and might be fatal, but prophylactic anticoagulation is not associated with a reduction in mortality. Extending anticoagulation for a few weeks after hospitalization may reduce the incidence of DVT but increases the risk of major haemorrhage and does not reduce mortality (Table 55.3).

In patients admitted with an acute coronary syndrome and who have or develop heart failure, treatment with antiplatelet agents and rivaroxaban 2.5 mg bd was associated with a substantial reduction in mortality in the ATLAS-ACS trial.[95]

Being pragmatic

If you are an evidenced-based clinician, then, for patients with HFrEF in sinus rhythm, you should avoid using antithrombotic therapy for patients with chronic heart failure regardless of aetiology or left ventricular phenotype. If the weight of peer-pressure demands use of an antithrombotic agent, then this may be based on theoretical considerations or by focusing on the effect on stroke or by adopting the simplest, low-risk strategy. As noted above, the reduction in the risk of non-fatal, disabling stroke with anticoagulants compared to aspirin may be as little as 0.1% per year and there is no difference in mortality. This argues in favour of aspirin. However, there is no evidence that outcomes with clopidogrel are inferior to aspirin and some evidence that clopidogrel has less unfavourable effects on symptoms and renal function. Clopidogrel is also a better choice based on theoretical mechanisms of action and harm. It has no deleterious effects on vascular or renal function, does not exacerbate congestion, and is less likely to cause gastrointestinal ulceration. It is relatively inexpensive. Accordingly, clopidogrel is the most appropriate antithrombotic for patients with HFrEF in sinus rhythm.

For patients with HFpEF in sinus rhythm who have CAD, the combination of aspirin (75–100 mg/day) plus rivaroxaban 2.5 mg bd is the most effective regimen identified so far.[33,34] It is based on a subgroup analysis, but the overall trial was positive and the benefits were no less and possibly greater among patients with HFpEF. This is also an appropriate therapeutic choice for patients with heart failure and an acute coronary syndrome.

For patients in atrial fibrillation, there are strong arguments in favour of anticoagulation with DOACs despite a dearth of placebo-controlled clinical trials specifically targeting this population. Compared to aspirin, DOACs reduce the risk of stroke by about 2% per year (perhaps 0.4% per year of non-fatal, disabling stroke) and generally appear safer and perhaps slightly more effective in reducing stroke and mortality compared to warfarin.

For acutely ill patients who are thought to need DVT prophylaxis and are not already taking anticoagulants because of atrial fibrillation, subcutaneous low-molecular-weight heparin or DOAC may be considered; patients might prefer the latter. Extending the use of DOACs for 4–6 weeks after discharge appears to have little clinical benefit but may reduce the rate of DVT identified by routine ultrasound investigation, which is not current clinical practice.

There are still roles for warfarin. In urban populations in countries where the cost of anticoagulant monitoring is substantially lower than the cost of DOAC, warfarin may be preferred for the management of atrial fibrillation on the basis of cost, but rural populations may not have ready access to monitoring. Warfarin is still the anticoagulant of choice for patients with a surgically implanted mechanical prosthetic valve.[96,97] The complex antithrombotic regimens for patients with left ventricular assist devices are discussed elsewhere.

Table 55.2 Contemporary randomized trials of antithrombotic agents for atrial fibrillation providing information on heart failure and a meta-analysis of trials comparing antiplatelet therapy with warfarin (separate data for heart failure not available)

Trial	Age (years) Women (%)	CAD	APT	LVEF	Compared	n	Duration (months)	Events per 100 patients per year					
								Stroke[a]	MI[a]	CV death[a]	Composite: stroke, MI and CV death[a]	All-cause mortality[a]	Bleeding[a]
Meta-analysis prior to AVERROES[36]	NR	NR	NA	NR 20–35% had heart failure	APT Warf	4783 4815	23	2.1 **1.4** **HR: 0.68 [0.54, 0.85]**	0.7 0.5 HR: 0.69 [0.47, 1.01]	2.1 2.0 HR: 0.93 [0.75, 1.15]	3.5 2.6 **HR: 0.74 [0.61, 0.90]**	3.2 3.2 HR: 0.99 [0.83, 1.18]	0.6 1.1 HR: 1.9 [1.07, 3.39] – non-CNS
AVERROES[37]	70 years; 41%	NR	No	NR[b]	Asp Apix	2791 2808	13	3.4 (if HF 3.3) **1.5 (if HF 1.3)** **HR: 0.46 (0.33, 0.65)**	0.9 0.8 HR: 0.86 (0.50, 1.48)	3.1 2.7 HR: 0.87 (0.65, 1.17)	6.4 **4.2** **HR: 0.66 (0.53, 0.83)**	4.4 3.5 HR: 0.79 (0.62, 1.02)	1.2 (if HF 1.4) 1.4 (if HF 1.3) HR: 1.13 (0.74, 1.75)
Trials comparing warfarin and direct oral anticoagulants (DOAC) showing rates with and without heart failure[c]													
SPORTIF[38]	71 years 71 years	37% 56%	19% 19%	NR	LVD/Diu – Neither – Either	3774 3555	19	1.5[d] 1.3[d]	0.7 1.4	NR	NR	2.1 5.0	1.8 2.6
ARISTOTLE[39]	71 years; 35% 68 years; 21% 69 years; 42%	29% 43% 48%	30% 34% 32%	60% 35% 46%	No HF LVSD HF-PEF	8728 2736 3207	22	1.3 1.4 1.5	NR	NR	3.5 8.1 5.3	2.4 **7.1** **4.3**	2.5 3.1 2.6
ROCKET[40]	74 years; 40% 72 years; 39%	10% 22%	33% 42%	[e]	No HF HF[e]	5138 9033		2.4 1.9	0.7 1.2	1.8 3.6	3.7 5.1	3.5 5.5	15.4 14.0

CAD, coronary artery disease; LVEF, left ventricular ejection fraction; MI, myocardial infarction. CV, cardiovascular; APT, antiplatelet therapy; Asp, aspirin; Apix, apixaban; NK, not known; NR, not reported; LVD, left ventricular dysfunction; Diu, loop diuretic.

AVERROES, Apixaban Versus Acetylsalicylic Acid Stroke in Atrial Fibrillation Patients Who Have Failed or Are Unsuitable for Vitamin K Antagonist Treatment; SPORTIF, Stroke Prevention by Oral Thrombin Inhibitor in Atrial Fibrillation; ARISTOTLE, Apixaban for Reduction in Stroke and Other Thromboembolic Events in Atrial Fibrillation; ROCKET, Rivaroxaban Oral Direct Factor Xa Inhibition Compared with Vitamin K Antagonism for Prevention of Stroke and Embolism Trial in Atrial Fibrillation.

'nor–CNS': bleeds not involving the central nervous system—single antiplatelet only (risk of bleeding similar for warfarin and dual antiplatelet therapy).

[a] Rates of events expressed per hundred patient-years.

[b] N: ≤35% in 5% of participants; 39% had heart failure. 'if HF', rates for patients with heart failure or LVEF≤35% in the AVERROES trial.

HR, hazard ratio with 95% confidence interval. Bold type indicates a statistically significant result.

[c] Trials comparing warfarin and DOAC suggested similar or lower risk of stroke and mortality with DOAC and a lower risk of major bleeding (especially intracranial) without interactions according to the presence or absence of heart failure.

[d] Stroke or systemic embolic event.

[e] ROCKET: 34% had LVEF ≤40% and 30% in NYHA III/IV; stroke event rate similar for LVEF above or below 40% and for NYHA III/IV versus I/II

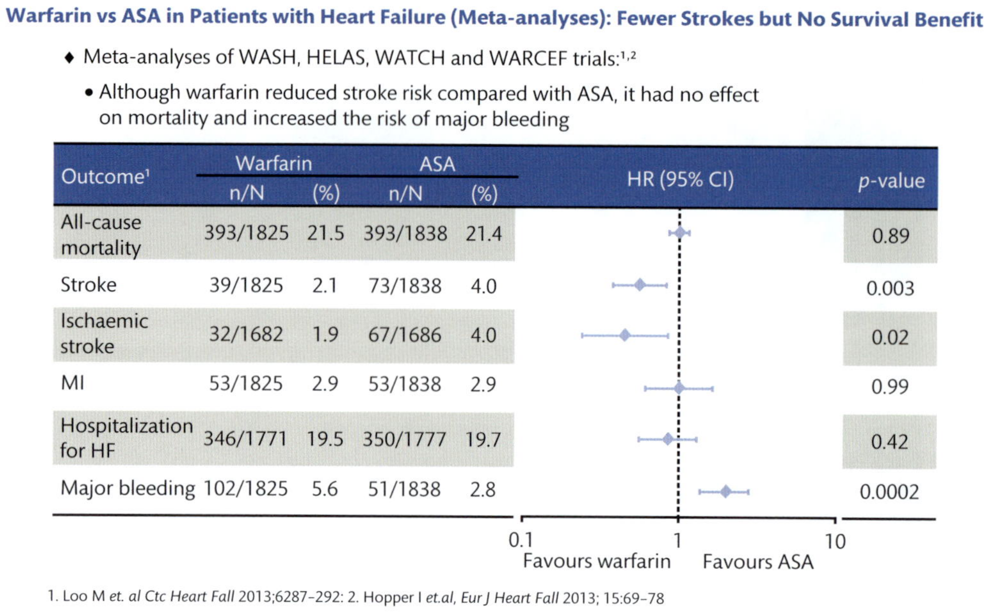

Warfarin vs ASA in Patients with Heart Failure (Meta-analyses): Fewer Strokes but No Survival Benefit

- ◆ Meta-analyses of WASH, HELAS, WATCH and WARCEF trials:[1,2]
  - Although warfarin reduced stroke risk compared with ASA, it had no effect on mortality and increased the risk of major bleeding

Outcome[1]	Warfarin n/N	Warfarin (%)	ASA n/N	ASA (%)	HR (95% CI)	p-value
All-cause mortality	393/1825	21.5	393/1838	21.4		0.89
Stroke	39/1825	2.1	73/1838	4.0		0.003
Ischaemic stroke	32/1682	1.9	67/1686	4.0		0.02
MI	53/1825	2.9	53/1838	2.9		0.99
Hospitalization for HF	346/1771	19.5	350/1777	19.7		0.42
Major bleeding	102/1825	5.6	51/1838	2.8		0.0002

0.1   1   10
Favours warfarin   Favours ASA

1. Loo M et. al Ctc Heart Fall 2013;6287–292: 2. Hopper I et.al, Eur J Heart Fall 2013; 15:69–78

Figure 55.8 Meta-analysis of trials comparing warfarin with aspirin in patients with heart failure.

Table 55.3 Trials of anticoagulants for the prophylaxis of venous thromboembolism for patients hospitalized for an acute medical illness

	Age Women (%) Heart failure (%)	Duration	Intervention	DVT	PTE	Death	Major bleed
Meta-analysis 2014 (individual trials published 1981–2011)[87]	NR NR NR	Inpatient	Placebo Heparin[a]	172 (6.7%) of 2580 **112 (3.8%) of 2931 HR: 0.41 (0.25, 0.67)**	50 (0.4%) of 13 871 33 (0.2%) of 14 100 HR: 0.66 (0.43, 1.02)	732 (5.3%) of 13 775 717 (5.1%) of 14 011 HR: 0.97 (0.87, 1.08)	24 (0.4%) of 6710 44 (0.6%) of 7094 HR: 1.65 (1.01, 2.71)
Meta-analysis 2014 (individual trials published 1995–2010)[87]	NR NR NR	Inpatient	UFH LMWH	193 (6.5%) of 2981 **151 (5.1%) of 2961 HR: 0.77 (0.62, 0.96)**	12 (0.4%) of 2981 10 (0.3%) of 2961 HR: 0.86 (0.39, 1.90)	62(2.2%) of 2807 49 (1.8%) of 2798 HR: 0.79 (0.54, 1.16)	29 (1.0%) of 2981 **12 (0.6%) of 2061 HR: 0.43 (0.22, 0.83)**
		Days	**N =**				
ADOPT 2011[88]	67 years 51% 47%	6–14 30	LMWH: 2284 Apixa: 2211	64 (2.8%) 57 (2.6%) RR: ~0.92[b]	8 (0.2%) 7 (0.2%) RR: ~1.0[b]	133 (4.1%) 131 (4.1%) RR: ~1.0[b]	6 (0.2%) **15 (0.5%) RR: 2.58 (1.02, 7.24)**
MAGELLAN 2013[89]	71 years 46% 32%	6–14 31–39	LMWH: 4051 Riva: 4050	175 (5.7%)[c] **131 (4.4%)c RR: 0.77 (0.62, 0.96)**	44 (1.5%)[d] 29 (0.9%)[d] RR: ~0.6[b]	153 (4.8%) 159 (5.1%) RR: ~1.0[b]	15 (0.4%) **43 (1.1%) RR: 2.9 (1.6, 5.2)**
MARINER 2018[90]	70 years 48% 40%	45 post-discharge	Pla: 6012 Riva: 6007	25 (0.4%)[e] **11 (0.2%)e HR: 0.44 (0.22, 0.89)**	5 confirmed; 41 not[f] 3 confirmed; 40 not[f] HR: ~1.0[b]	89 (1.5%) 71 (1.2%) HR: 0.80 (0.58, 1.09)	9 (0.15%) 17 (0.3%) HR: 1.88 (0.84, 4.23)

PTE, pulmonary thromboembolism, fatal or non-fatal and diagnosed clinically; NR, not reported.

ADOPT, Apixaban Dosing to Optimize Protection from Thrombosis; MAGELLAN, Rivaroxaban for thromboprophylaxis in acutely ill medical patients; MARINER, Medically Ill Patient Assessment of Rivaroxaban versus Placebo in Reducing Post-Discharge Venous Thrombo-Embolism Risk.

Deep venous thrombosis (DVT) could be symptomatic or asymptomatic and detected by a fibrinogen uptake test, ultrasound, venography or plethysmography.

[a] Four trials of unfractionated heparin (UFH) and six of low-molecular weight heparin (LMWH); trials varied in events reported and hence denominator for each outcome differs.

[b] Approximate recalculated.

[c] Patients had routine venous ultrasound leading to high rates of asymptomatic DVT.

[d] Symptomatic PTE or fatal venous thromboembolism.

[e] Symptomatic DVT or non-fatal PTE.

[f] Deaths possibly related to unconfirmed PTE.

REFERENCES

1. Cleland JGF. What do cardiology and homeopathy have in common?: a belief in aspirin? *JACC Heart Fail* 2017;**5**(8):611–14.

2. Cleland JG, Mumtaz S, Cecchini L. Role of antithrombotic agents in heart failure. *Curr Cardiol Rep* 2012;**14**(3):314–25.

3. Cleland JG. Anticoagulant and antiplatelet therapy in heart failure. *Curr Opin Cardiol* 1997;**12**(3):276–87.

4. Cleland JG. Long-term aspirin for coronary artery disease: are we being deceived by a biased presentation of the evidence? *Future Cardiol* 2010;**6**(2):141–6.

5. Cleland JG. Is aspirin useful in primary prevention? *Eur Heart J* 2013;**34**(44):3412–18.

6. Cleland JGF, Cowburn PJ, Falk RH. Should all patients with atrial fibrillation receive warfarin? Evidence from randomised clinical trials. *Eur Heart J* 1996;**17**:674–81.

7. Lip GYH, Gibbs CR. Does heart failure confer a hypercoagulable state? Virchow's triad revisited. *J Am Coll Cardiol* 1999;**33**:1424–6.

8. Sbarouni E, Bradshaw A, Andreotti F, *et al.* Relationship between hemostatic abnormalities and neuroendocrine activity in heart failure. *Am Heart J* 1994;**127**(3):607–12.

9. Zannad F, Greenberg B, Cleland JG, *et al.* Rationale and design of a randomized, double-blind, event-driven, multicentre study comparing the efficacy and safety of oral rivaroxaban with placebo for reducing the risk of death, myocardial infarction or stroke in subjects with heart failure and significant coronary artery disease following an exacerbation of heart failure: the COMMANDER HF trial. *Eur J Heart Fail* 2015;**17**(7):735–42.

10. Loh PH, Goode K, Tin L, *et al.* Prognostic values of laboratory markers for haemostasis, rheology, inflammation and endothelial function in patients with left ventricular systolic dysfunction. *Eur Heart J* 2006;**27**(Suppl):P513.

11. Marcucci R, Gori AM, Giannotti F, *et al.* Markers of hypercoagulability and inflammation predict mortality in patients with heart failure. *J Thromb Haemost* 2006;**4**(5):1017–22.

12. Zorlu A, Yilmaz MB, Yucel H, *et al.* Increased d-dimer levels predict cardiovascular mortality in patients with systolic heart failure. *J Thromb Thrombolysis* 2012;**33**(4):322–8.

13. Kohan DE, Cleland JG, Rubin LJ, Theodorescu D, Barton M. Clinical trials with endothelin receptor antagonists: what went wrong and where can we improve? *Life Sci* 2012;**91**:528–39.

14. Borissoff JI, Spronk HM, Ten CH. The hemostatic system as a modulator of atherosclerosis. *N Engl J Med* 2011;**364**(18):1746–60.

15. Spronk HM, De Jong AM, Crijns HJ, *et al.* Pleiotropic effects of factor Xa and thrombin: what to expect from novel anticoagulants. *Cardiovasc Res* 2014;**101**(3):344–51.

16. Zorlu A, Akkaya E, Altay H, *et al.* The relationship between D-dimer level and the development of atrial fibrillation in patients with systolic heart failure. *J Thromb Thrombolysis* 2012;**33**(4):343–8.

17. Spronk HM, De Jong AM, Verheule S, *et al.* Hypercoagulability causes atrial fibrosis and promotes atrial fibrillation. *Eur Heart J* 2017;**38**(1):38–50.

18. Halliday BP, Gulati A, Ali A, *et al.* Association between midwall late gadolinium enhancement and sudden cardiac death in patients with dilated cardiomyopathy and mild and moderate left ventricular systolic dysfunction. *Circulation* 2017;**135**(22):2106–15.

19. Davie AP, Love MP, McMurray JJV. Even low-dose aspirin inhibits arachidonic acid-induced vasodilation in heart failure. *Clin Pharmacol Ther* 2000;**67**(5):530–7.

20. Taruya A, Tanaka A, Nishiguchi T, *et al.* Vasa vasorum restructuring in human atherosclerotic plaque vulnerability: a clinical optical coherence tomography study. *J Am Coll Cardiol* 2015;**65**(23):2469–77.

21. Kolodgie FD, Gold HK, Burke AP, *et al.* Intraplaque hemorrhage and progression of coronary atheroma. *N Engl J Med* 2003;**349**(24):2316–25.

22. Cleland JG. Chronic aspirin therapy for the prevention of cardiovascular events: a waste of time, or worse? *Nat Clin Pract Cardiovasc Med* 2006;**3**(5):234–5.

23. Ruff CT, Giugliano RP, Braunwald E, *et al.* Comparison of the efficacy and safety of new oral anticoagulants with warfarin in patients with atrial fibrillation: a meta-analysis of randomised trials. *Lancet* 2014;**383**(9921):955–62.

24. Cleland JGF. Anticoagulant and antiplatelet therapy in heart failure. *Curr Opin Cardiol* 1997;**12**:276–87.

25. Homma S, Thompson JL, Pullicino PM, *et al.* Warfarin and aspirin in patients with heart failure and sinus rhythm. *N Engl J Med* 2012;**366**(20):1859–69.

26. Cleland JG, Findlay I, Jafri S, *et al.* The Warfarin/Aspirin Study in Heart failure (WASH): a randomized trial comparing antithrombotic strategies for patients with heart failure. *Am Heart J* 2004;**148**(1):157–64.

27. Cokkinos DV, Haralabopoulos GC, Kostis JB, Toutouzas PK. Efficacy of antithrombotic therapy in chronic heart failure: the HELAS study. *Eur J Heart Fail* 2006;**8**(4):428–32.

28. Massie BM, Collins JF, Ammon SE, *et al.* Randomized trial of warfarin, aspirin, and clopidogrel in patients with chronic heart failure: the Warfarin and Antiplatelet Therapy in Chronic Heart Failure (WATCH) trial. *Circulation* 2009;**119**(12):1616–24.

29. Homma S, Thompson JL, Sanford AR, *et al.* Benefit of warfarin compared with aspirin in patients with heart failure in sinus rhythm: a subgroup analysis of WARCEF, a randomized controlled trial. *Circ Heart Fail* 2013;**6**(5):988–97.

30. Zannad F, Anker SD, Byra WM, *et al.*; COMMANDER HF Investigators. Rivaroxaban in patients with heart failure, sinus rhythm, and coronary disease. *N Engl J Med* 2018;**379**(14):1332–42.

31. Greenberg B, Neaton JD, Anker SD, *et al.* Association of rivaroxaban with thromboembolic events in patients with heart failure, coronary disease, and sinus rhythm: a post hoc analysis of the COMMANDER HF Trial. *JAMA Cardiol* 2019;**4**(6):515–23.

32. Mehra MR, Vaduganathan M, Fu M, *et al.* A comprehensive analysis of the effects of rivaroxaban on stroke or transient ischaemic attack in patients with heart failure, coronary artery disease, and sinus rhythm: the COMMANDER HF trial. *Eur Heart J* 2019;**40**(44):3593–602.

33. Cleland JGF, Lyon AR, McDonagh T, McMurray JJV. The year in cardiology: heart failure. *Eur Heart J* 2020;**41**(12):1232–48.

34. Branch KR, Probstfield JL, Eikelboom JW, *et al.* Rivaroxaban with or without aspirin in patients with heart failure and chronic coronary or peripheral artery disease. *Circulation* 2019;**140**(7):529–37.

35. Korjian S, Braunwald E, Daaboul Y, *et al.* Usefulness of rivaroxaban for secondary prevention of acute coronary syndrome in patients with history of congestive heart failure (from the ATLAS-ACS-2 TIMI-51 Trial). *Am J Cardiol* 2018;**122**(11):1896–901.

36. Aguilar MI, Hart R, Pearce LA. Oral anticoagulants versus antiplatelet therapy for preventing stroke in patients with non-valvular atrial fibrillation and no history of stroke or transient ischemic attacks. *Cochrane Database Syst Rev* 2007;(3):CD006186.

37. Connolly SJ, Eikelboom J, Joyner C, *et al.*; AVERROES Steering Committee and Investigators. Apixaban in patients with atrial fibrillation. *N Engl J Med* 2011;**364**:806–17.

38. Cleland JG, Shelton R, Nikitin N, *et al.* Prevalence of markers of heart failure in patients with atrial fibrillation and the effects of ximelagatran compared to warfarin on the incidence of morbid and fatal events: a report from the SPORTIF III and V trials. *Eur J Heart Fail* 2007;**9**(6–7):730–9.

39. Granger CB, Alexander JH, McMurray JJ, *et al.*; ARISTOTLE Committees and Investigators. Apixaban versus warfarin in patients with atrial fibrillation. *N Engl J Med* 2011;**365**(11):981–92.

40. van DS, Hellkamp AS, Patel MR, *et al.* Efficacy and safety of rivaroxaban in patients with heart failure and nonvalvular atrial fibrillation: insights from ROCKET AF. *Circ Heart Fail* 2013;**6**(4):740–7.

41. Hart RG, Pearce LA, McBride R, Rothbart RM, Asinger RW. Factors associated with ischemic stroke during aspirin therapy in atrial fibrillation: analysis of 2012 participants in the SPAF I–III clinical trials. The Stroke Prevention in Atrial Fibrillation (SPAF) Investigators. *Stroke* 1999;**30**:1223-9.

42. Davie AP, Love MP, McMurray JJ. Even low-dose aspirin inhibits arachidonic acid-induced vasodilation in heart failure. *Clin Pharmacol Ther* 2000;**67**:530–7.

43. Cleland JG, Zhang J, Pellicori P, *et al.* Prevalence and outcomes of anemia and hematinic deficiencies in patients with chronic heart failure. *JAMA Cardiol* 2016;**1**(5):539–47.

44. Anker SD, Kirwan BA, Van Veldhuisen DJ, *et al.* Effects of ferric carboxymaltose on hospitalisations and mortality rates in iron-deficient heart failure patients: an individual patient data meta-analysis. *Eur J Heart Fail* 2018;**20**(1):125–33.

45. Dagenais GR, Pogue J, Fox K, Simoons ML, Yusuf S. Angiotensin-converting-enzyme inhibitors in stable vascular disease without left ventricular systolic dysfunction or heart failure: a combined analysis of three trials. *Lancet* 2006;**368**(9535):581–8.

46. Lindenfeld J, Robertson AD, Lowes BD, Bristow MR, for the MOCHA Investigators. Aspirin impairs reverse myocardial remodeling in patients with heart failure treated with beta-blockers. *J Am Coll Cardiol* 2001;**38**(7):1950–6.

47. Cleland JG. Does aspirin detract from the benefits of mineralocorticoid receptor antagonists in patients with heart failure and a reduced left ventricular ejection fraction? Probably! *Eur J Heart Fail* 2017;**19**(9):1086–8.

48. Dzau VJ, Packer M, Lilly LS, *et al.* Prostaglandins in severe congestive heart failure. Relation to activation of the renin–angiotensin system and hyponatremia. *N Engl J Med* 1984;**310**(6):347–52.

49. Juhlin T, Bjorkman S, Gunnarsson B, *et al.* Acute administration of diclofenac, but possibly not long term low dose aspirin, causes detrimental renal effects in heart failure patients treated with ACE-inhibitors. *Eur J Heart Fail* 2004;**6**(7):909–16.

50. de Silva R, Nikitin NP, Witte KK, *et al.* Effects of applying a standardised management algorithm for moderate to severe renal dysfunction in patients with chronic stable heart failure. *Eur J Heart Fail* 2007;**9**:415–23.

51. Patel MR, Mahaffey KW, Garg J, *et al.* Rivaroxaban versus warfarin in nonvalvular atrial fibrillation. *N Engl J Med* 2011;**365**(10):883–91.

52. Jumeau C, Rupin A, Chieng-Yane P, *et al.* Direct thrombin inhibitors prevent left atrial remodeling associated with heart failure in rats. *JACC Basic Transl Sci* 2016;**1**(5):328–39.

53. Cleland JGF, Massie BM, Packer M. Sudden death in heart failure: vascular or electrical? *Eur J Heart Fail* 1999;**1**:41–5.

54. Uretsky BF, Thygesen K, Armstrong PW, *et al.* Acute coronary findings at autopsy in heart failure patients with sudden death: results from the assessment of treatment with lisinopril and survival (ATLAS) trial. *Circulation* 2000;**102**(6):611–16.

55. Orn S, Cleland JG, Romo M, Kjekshus J, Dickstein K. Recurrent infarction causes the most deaths following myocardial infarction with left ventricular dysfunction. *Am J Med* 2005;**118**(7):752–8.

56. Morant SV, McMahon AD, Cleland JG, Davey PG, MacDonald TM. Cardiovascular prophylaxis with aspirin: costs of supply and management of upper gastrointestinal and renal toxicity. *Br J Clin Pharmacol* 2004;**57**:188–98.

57. Cleland JG. Is aspirin 'the weakest link' in cardiovascular prophylaxis? The surprising lack of evidence supporting the use of aspirin for cardiovascular disease. *Prog Cardiovasc Dis* 2002;**44**:275–92.

58. Abraham NS. Proton pump inhibitors: potential adverse effects. *Curr Opin Gastroenterol* 2012;**28**(6):615–20.

59. Shah NH, LePendu P, Bauer-Mehren A, *et al.* Proton pump inhibitor usage and the risk of myocardial infarction in the general population. *PLoS One* 2015;**10**(6):e0124653.

60. Schoenfeld AJ, Grady D. Adverse effects associated with proton pump inhibitors. *JAMA Intern Med* 2016;**176**(2):172–4.

61. Cleland JG, Parsons S. Aspirin for heart failure: theory- or evidence-based? *Circ Heart Fail* 2014;**7**(2):237–8.

62. Cleland JG. Chronic aspirin is effective—if data are massaged sufficiently. *BMJ* 2002;**324**(7332):295.

63. Schelbert EB, Cao JJ, Sigurdsson S, *et al.* Prevalence and prognosis of unrecognized myocardial infarction determined by cardiac magnetic resonance in older adults. *JAMA* 2012;**308**(9):890–6.

64. Raber I, McCarthy CP, Vaduganathan M, *et al.* The rise and fall of aspirin in the primary prevention of cardiovascular disease. *Lancet* 2019;**393**:2155–67.

65. Bonaca MP, Bhatt DL, Cohen M, *et al.* Long-term use of ticagrelor in patients with prior myocardial infarction. *N Engl J Med* 2015;**372**(19):1791–800.

66. Mega JL, Braunwald E, Wiviott SD, *et al.* Rivaroxaban in patients with a recent acute coronary syndrome. *N Engl J Med* 2012;**366**(1):9–19.

67. Eikelboom JW, Connolly SJ, Bosch J, *et al.* Rivaroxaban with or without aspirin in stable cardiovascular disease. *N Engl J Med* 2017;**377**(14):1319–30.

68. Connolly SJ, Eikelboom J, Joyner C, *et al.*; AVERROES Steering Committee and Investigators. Apixaban in patients with atrial fibrillation. *N Engl J Med* 2011;**364**:806–17.

69. Rivaroxaban for the Prevention of Major Cardiovascular Events in Coronary or Peripheral Artery Disease (COMPASS). 2017.

70. Jug B, Sebestjen M, Sabovic M, Keber I. Clopidogrel is associated with a lesser increase in NT-proBNP when compared to aspirin in patients with ischemic heart failure. *J Card Fail* 2006;**12**(6):446–51.

71. Kindsvater S, Leclerc K, Ward J. Effects of coadministration of aspirin or clopidogrel on exercise testing in patients with heart

failure receiving angiotensin-converting enzyme inhibitors. *Am J Cardiol* 2003;**91**(11):1350–2.

72. Meune C, Mahe I, Cohen-Solal A. Comparative effect of aspirin and clopidogrel on arterial function in CHF. *Int J Cardiol* 2006;**106**(1):61–6.

73. Meune C, Wahbi K, Fulla Y, *et al.* Effects of aspirin and clopidogrel on plasma brain natriuretic peptide in patients with heart failure receiving ACE inhibitors. *Eur J Heart Fail* 2007;**9**(2):197–201.

74. Parsons S, Rigby AS, Gittus C, *et al.* The clopidogrel or aspirin in chronic heart failure (CACHE) study. *Eur J Heart Fail* 2014;**16**:267–8.

75. Serebruany VL, Malinin AI, Jerome SD, *et al.* Effects of clopidogrel and aspirin combination versus aspirin alone on platelet aggregation and major receptor expression in patients with heart failure: the Plavix Use for Treatment of Congestive Heart Failure (PLUTO-CHF) trial. *Am Heart J* 2003;**146**(4):713–20.

76. Hopper I, Skiba M, Krum H. Updated meta-analysis on antithrombotic therapy in patients with heart failure and sinus rhythm. *Eur J Heart Fail* 2013;**15**(1):69–78.

77. Lee M, Saver JL, Hong KS, Wu HC, Ovbiagele B. Risk–benefit profile of warfarin versus aspirin in patients with heart failure and sinus rhythm: a meta-analysis. *Circ Heart Fail* 2013;**6**(2):287–92.

78. Shantsila E, Lip GY. Antiplatelet versus anticoagulation treatment for patients with heart failure in sinus rhythm. *Cochrane Database Syst Rev* 2016;(9):CD003333.

79. Lip GY, Shantsila E. Anticoagulation versus placebo for heart failure in sinus rhythm. *Cochrane Database Syst Rev* 2014;(3):CD003336.

80. Liew AY, Eikelboom JW, Connolly SJ, O'Donnell M, Hart RG. Efficacy and safety of warfarin vs. antiplatelet therapy in patients with systolic heart failure and sinus rhythm: a systematic review and meta-analysis of randomized controlled trials. *Int J Stroke* 2014;**9**(2):199–206.

81. Teerlink JR, Qian M, Bello NA, *et al.* Aspirin does not increase heart failure events in heart failure patients: from the WARCEF Trial. *JACC Heart Fail* 2017;**5**(8):603–10.

82. Di Tullio MR, Qian M, Thompson JL, *et al.* Left ventricular ejection fraction and risk of stroke and cardiac events in heart failure: data from the Warfarin Versus Aspirin in Reduced Ejection Fraction Trial. *Stroke* 2016;**47**(8):2031–7.

83. Gibson CM, Mega JL, Burton P, *et al.* Rationale and design of the Anti-Xa therapy to lower cardiovascular events in addition to standard therapy in subjects with acute coronary syndrome–thrombolysis in myocardial infarction 51 (ATLAS-ACS 2 TIMI 51) trial: a randomized, double-blind, placebo-controlled study to evaluate the efficacy and safety of rivaroxaban in subjects with acute coronary syndrome. *Am Heart J* 2011;**161**:815–21.

84. Savarese G, Giugliano RP, Rosano GM, *et al.* Efficacy and safety of novel oral anticoagulants in patients with atrial fibrillation and heart failure: a meta-analysis. *JACC Heart Fail* 2016;**4**(11):870–80.

85. McMurray JJ, Ezekowitz JA, Lewis BS, *et al.*; ARISTOTLE Committees and Investigators. Left ventricular systolic dysfunction, heart failure, and the risk of stroke and systemic embolism in patients with atrial fibrillation: insights from the ARISTOTLE trial. *Circ Heart Fail* 2013;**6**(3):451–60.

86. Jin H, Zhu K, Wang L, Zhou W, Zhi H. Efficacy and safety of non-vitamin K anticoagulants and warfarin in patients with atrial fibrillation and heart failure: a network meta-analysis. *Thromb Res* 2020;**196**:109–19.

87. Alikhan R, Bedenis R, Cohen AT. Heparin for the prevention of venous thromboembolism in acutely ill medical patients (excluding stroke and myocardial infarction). *Cochrane Database Syst Rev* 2014;(5):CD003747.

88. Goldhaber SZ, Leizorovicz A, Kakkar AK, *et al.*; ADOPT Trial Investigators. Apixaban versus enoxaparin for thromboprophylaxis in medically ill patients. *N Engl J Med* 2011;**365**(23):2167–77.

89. Cohen AT, Spiro TE, Büller HR, *et al.*; MAGELLAN Investigators. Rivaroxaban for thromboprophylaxis in acutely ill medical patients. *N Engl J Med* 2013;**368**(6):513–23.

90. Spyropoulos AC, Ageno W, Albers GW, *et al.*; MARINER Investigators. Rivaroxaban for thromboprophylaxis after hospitalization for medical illness. *N Engl J Med* 2018;**379**(12):1118–27.

91. Dentali F, Douketis JD, Gianni M, Lim W, Crowther MA. Meta-analysis: anticoagulant prophylaxis to prevent symptomatic venous thromboembolism in hospitalized medical patients. *Ann Intern Med* 2007;**146**(4):278–88.

92. Liew AY, Piran S, Eikelboom JW, Douketis JD. Extended-duration versus short-duration pharmacological thromboprophylaxis in acutely ill hospitalized medical patients: a systematic review and meta-analysis of randomized controlled trials. *J Thromb Thrombolysis* 2017;**43**(3):291–301.

93. Cohen AT, Davidson BL, Gallus AS, *et al.* Efficacy and safety of fondaparinux for the prevention of venous thromboembolism in older acute medical patients: randomised placebo controlled trial. *BMJ* 2006;**332**(7537):325–9.

94. Cohen AT, Spiro TE, Buller HR, *et al.* Rivaroxaban for thromboprophylaxis in acutely ill medical patients. *N Engl J Med* 2013;**368**(6):513–23.

95. Korjian S, Braunwald E, Daaboul Y, *et al.* Usefulness of rivaroxaban for secondary prevention of acute coronary syndrome in patients with history of congestive heart failure (from the ATLAS-ACS-2 TIMI-51 Trial). *Am J Cardiol* 2018;**122**:1896–1901.

96. Eikelboom JW, Connolly SJ, Brueckmann M, *et al.*; RE-ALIGN Investigators. Dabigatran versus warfarin in patients with mechanical heart valves. *N Engl J Med* 2013;**369**(13):1206–14.

97. Roost E, Weber A, Alberio L, *et al.* Rivaroxaban in patients with mechanical heart valves: a pilot study. *Thromb Res* 2020;**186**:1–6.

56

Problems with polypharmacy, alternative therapies and medication adherence

Paul Forsyth and Steve McGlynn

Introduction

Heart failure is often the long-term consequence of several different intertwined co-morbidities, both cardiac and non-cardiac, and therefore rarely exists in isolation. Polypharmacy is common in heart failure, both due to the treatment of heart failure itself and also due to the treatment of other underlying co-morbidities.

All medicines have negative aspects to their use, in terms of effects other than that for which they are being taken. These include detrimental physiological effects on morbidity or mortality in patients with heart failure. Therefore, polypharmacy brings with it the challenges, especially in elderly patients, of how to cope with medication that may have harmful effects and how to manage with drug interactions.

In the case of 'conventional' medicines many of these adverse effects are known, although post-marketing surveillance programmes may uncover other effects not seen in the clinical trials used to support the marketing authorization/licensing of the product. However, the adverse effects of some earlier products—which pre-date evidence-based randomized controlled trial methodology—and/or products not exposed to a scientific examination (e.g. alterative therapies) may be unknown.

This chapter reviews the potentially detrimental effects of conventional (prescribed and over-the-counter (OTC)) and alternative medicines. It also discusses the challenges in ensuring optimal medication adherence to the treatments known to improve outcomes in heart failure.

Adverse effects of conventional medicines on heart failure

Conventional medicines used for other cardiac and non-cardiac disease may have adverse cardiovascular effects on patients with heart failure. These include both prescribed medicines and OTC medicines, used to self-medicate minor ailments.

Conventional medicines may have an adverse effect on outcomes via a variety of mechanisms. These include, among others, promotion of fluid retention, negative inotropic effects, positive chronotropic effects, pro-arrhythmic effects, cardiotoxic effects, and drug–drug interactions. Whereas the use of medicines associated with adverse effects should be avoided if possible, clinical need may require the use of such medicines if it is deemed to be in the patient's overall interest. In such cases, the prescriber needs to be aware of the cautions and contraindications for that product when making the decision to use it (see summary in Table 56.1).

Fluid retention

Certain medicines can cause, or exacerbate, fluid retention by either physical (osmotic) or pharmacological effects. The most obvious example of the former is the sodium load associated with some medicines, usually present as an excipient (e.g. high doses of soluble tablets, particularly analgesics), but also as the sodium salt of the medicine (e.g. parenteral antibiotics).[1]

Pharmacological effects include interference with renal physiology (e.g. non-steroidal anti-inflammatory drugs (NSAIDs) inhibit renal prostaglandin synthesis) and aldosterone-like activity (e.g. corticosteroids and mineralocorticoids). Practical examples of common drugs known to worsen fluid retention through pharmacological effects include:

- *Thiazolidinediones (e.g. glitazones)*: treatment is associated with increased rate of heart failure type events and therefore should be avoided in all cases.[2]
- *Minoxidil*: treatment is associated with worse clinical outcomes in patients with heart failure and should also be avoided in all cases.[3]
- *NSAIDs*: treatment is associated with increased risk of decompensated heart failure and is therefore best avoided, in favour of other analgesics.[4] The association with increased risk of myocardial infarction is an additional reason to avoid their use if possible.[5]
- *Corticosteroids (e.g. prednisolone)*: treatment can be detrimental and is associated with increasing levels of fluid overload, especially in patients with more severe symptoms at baseline.[6] Therefore close monitoring of clinical symptoms is needed where the benefit of use outweighs the risk.

Table 56.1 Commonly used drugs contraindicated or cautioned in patients with heart failure

Medication	Main harmful effect	General advice
Cardiac medication		
Anti-arrhythmics (class I and III), excluding amiodarone	• Negatively inotropic effect • Pro-arrhythmic	Do not use
Calcium channel blockers (except amlodipine and felodipine)	• Negatively inotropic effect	Do not use
Minoxidil	• Stimulation of renin–angiotensin–aldosterone system • Sodium and water retention	Do not use
Moxonidine	• Sodium and water retention	Do not use
Non-cardiac medication		
Anthracycline agents/HER2/VEGF	• Cardiotoxic	Close cardiac monitoring should be carried out, including cardiac imaging and electrocardiogram. Multidisciplinary working between cardiology and oncology services is recommended.
Corticosteroids	• Sodium and water retention	Close monitoring of heart failure symptoms needed
Itraconazole	• Negatively inotropic effect	Do not use unless the benefit clearly outweighs the risk
NSAIDs	• Sodium and water retention	Best avoided in favour of other analgesics if possible
Thiazolidinediones (glitazones)	• Fluid retention	Do not use
Tricyclic antidepressants	• Negatively inotropic effect • Pro-arrhythmic	Best avoided in favour of other antidepressants or other neuropathic analgesics if possible

HER2, human epidermal growth factor receptor 2; NSAID, non-steroidal anti-inflammatory; VEGF, vascular endothelial growth factor.

Negative inotropic effects

A number of cardiac medicines, mainly the class I (e.g. flecainide, disopyramide) and class IV (e.g. diltiazem, verapamil) anti-arrhythmics reduce cardiac output by reducing myocardial contractility and are contraindicated in patients with heart failure. Of the class III anti-arrhythmics, dronedarone and sotalol are contraindicated:

- *Non-dihydropyridine calcium-channel blockers (e.g. diltiazem and verapamil)*: have been shown to be unsafe in patients with heart failure[7] and should therefore be avoided in all cases.
- *Class I and III anti-arrhythmic drugs (excluding amiodarone)*: treatment is not recommended for routine use in heart failure because of increased rates of decompensation, arrhythmic events, and death.[8–11]

The commonly used anti-fungal drug itraconazole has also been shown to be negatively inotropic and is best only used where the benefit clearly outweighs the risk.[1,12]

Pro-arrhythmic effects

A number of other medicines, both cardiac and non-cardiac, have potential pro-arrhythmic effects. The most common mechanism for these effects is potassium channel blocking and subsequent prolongation of the QTc interval. Other mechanisms include pharmacodynamic interactions, where the concurrent use of more than one drug that prolongs the QTc interval increases the risk, and pharmacokinetic interactions, where certain drugs that do not prolong the QTc interval themselves cause prolongation of QTc by affecting the metabolism of other drugs that do (see Drug–drug interaction). These effects are well documented due to the risk associated with their use, particularly in patients with congenital or acquired long QTc.[13,14]

In recent years some non-cardiac medicines have been withdrawn from the market due to QTc prolongation. For several others their effects on QTc prolongation mean that they are used with caution, or contraindicated, especially where the QTc interval is already prolonged.

Practical examples of common drugs known to be pro-arrhythmic and generally avoided are:

- *Class I and III anti-arrhythmic drugs (excluding amiodarone)*: see Negative inotropic effects.
- *Tricyclic antidepressants (e.g. amitriptyline)*: treatment is associated with elevated risk of adverse cardiovascular outcomes, including heart failure, and is therefore best avoided, in favour of other antidepressants.[15]

However, several medications prolong QTc interval and extra vigilance is required by healthcare professionals to be alert to the risk of drug-induced QTc prolongation in heart failure patients. Commonly used medicines associated with prolonging QTc are listed in **Box 56.1** and a comprehensive list of medicines that are associated with prolonged QTc is maintained at the CredibleMeds® website.[14]

Cardiotoxic effects

Certain chemotherapy agents can cause or worsen heart failure, mainly through cardiotoxic effects. Older anthracycline type agents, such as doxorubicin, and newer human epidermal growth factor receptor 2 (HER2) blocking agents, such as trastuzumab, and vascular endothelial growth factor (VEGF) inhibitors are known to cause and worsen heart failure.[16] Angiotensin converting enzyme inhibitors, β-blockers, and dexrazoxane may confer some cardioprotection in certain patients, although the evidence is limited.[16,17]

Box 56.1 Common drugs that prolong QTc interval[14]

Antimicrobials
- Azithromycin
- Ciprofloxacin
- Clarithromycin
- Erythromycin
- Fluconazole
- Levofloxacin
- Moxifloxacin.

Cardiac medicines
- Amiodarone
- Disopyramide
- Dronedarone
- Flecainide
- Sotalol
- Ranolazine.

Antiemetics
- Domperidone
- Droperidol
- Ondansetron.

Antipsychotics
- Most antipsychotics have a risk of QT prolongation, and should be used with caution in patients with other risk factors. The following are listed as high risk in the sources described above.
- Chlorpromazine
- Haloperidol
- Pimozide
- Sulpiride.

Antidepressants
- Many antidepressants have been associated with QT prolongation in overdose. For this reason they should be used with caution. The following are listed as high risk at therapeutic doses in the sources described above.
- Citalopram
- Escitalopram.

Others
- Anagrelide
- Hydroxyzine
- Methadone
- Quinine
- Tolterodine
- Lithium
- Some antimalarials
- Some antiretrovirals
- Protein kinase inhibitors and some other oncology drugs—seek specialist advice if unsure.

This list is not exhaustive. Potential drug–drug interactions can be checked at Woosley, RL and Romero, KA, www.Crediblemeds.org, QTdrugs List, Accessed 25th July 2016, AZCERT, Inc. 1822 Innovation Park Dr., Oro Valley, AZ 85755.

A careful cardiovascular work-up, including electrocardiogram and cardiac imaging, should be undertaken prior to the initiation of such cardiotoxic chemotherapy agents and regular cardiovascular evaluation should be routine.[16] Multidisciplinary working between cardiology and oncology services is recommended and clinicians should be vigilant with patients with existing cardiac comorbidities, such as coronary artery disease and hypertension.[16]

Blood pressure effects

Aggressive blood pressure control is known to reduce the risk of developing heart failure[18] and many patients end up taking a variety of blood pressure lowering medications long before they develop heart failure. In established heart failure, however, poor cardiac output often leads to hypotension and this is commonly exacerbated by evidence-based heart failure therapies, which also lower blood pressure. In practical terms, hypotension frequently limits the full therapeutic optimization of heart failure therapies intended to improve mortality and morbidity. In this context, the use of other medicines with hypotensive effects, but without clear mortality or morbidity benefits, should be reviewed and if possible avoided. These include medication used to treat:

- hypertension itself, such as thiazide diuretics (e.g. indapamide) and dihydropyridine calcium channel blockers (e.g. amlodipine). Moxonidine, a centrally acting antihypertensive, is associated with excess mortality and morbidity in one large heart failure trial and should therefore be avoided in all cases.[19] Doxazosin, an α-blocker, is less effective than other hypertensive medications at preventing heart failure but its effects in the established condition are less clear.[20]
- stable angina, including long-acting nitrates, potassium channel openers (e.g. nicorandil), and dihydropyridine calcium channel blockers (e.g. amlodipine).
- benign prostatic hypertrophy, including α-blockers.[1]
- Parkinson disease, such as levodopa and bromocriptine.
- psychiatric disorders, such as antipsychotics and tricyclic antidepressants.[1]
- urinary incontinence, such as antimuscarinics (e.g. oxybutynin).

Positive chronotropic effects

Strict heart rate control in heart failure patients in sinus rhythm is associated with improved outcomes.[21] Consequently, any medicines that increase heart rate may negate some of the benefits of rate control medication.

High doses of inhaled, nebulized, or oral β-agonist bronchodilators, such as salbutamol, used in obstructive airways disease may cause persistent tachycardia. Numerous OTC medicines used to treat the symptoms of the common cold contain indirect-acting sympathomimetics, such as pseudoephedrine. Although these should only be used for short-term treatment, they have the potential to increase heart rate. Case reports exist linking the use of such positive chronotropic agents with heart failure admissions.[22]

Drug–drug interactions

Drug–drug interactions fall within two broad types: pharmacodynamic and pharmacokinetic.

Pharmacodynamic interactions result from two or more medicines having additive or opposing effects. The most common additive effect seen in heart failure patients is hypotension. The majority of heart failure medicines reduce blood pressure, as do some other cardiac and non-cardiac medicines (see Blood pressure effects). Another common additive effect seen in heart failure patients is nephrotoxicity and hyperkalaemia, often caused by dual inhibition of the renin–angiotensin–aldosterone pathway. In the management of heart failure, the beneficial effects of some medicines may be reduced due to the opposing effects of non-cardiovascular medicines

(e.g. β-agonists and β-antagonists, diuretics, and NSAIDS/corticosteroids). However, most of these types of interactions are well understood and consequently this chapter does not discuss them in depth.

Pharmacokinetic interactions involve one or more medicines affecting how the body handles a medicine. This may involve the absorption, distribution, metabolism, or excretion. The resulting change in plasma concentration may affect the pharmacological effect of the medicine. Most of the clinically significant interactions involve inhibition or induction of metabolic hepatic enzyme systems (e.g. cytochrome P450 3A4, CYP3A4)[23] or cellular transport proteins (e.g. P-glycoprotein (P-gp)).[24] There is significant overlap between those medicines that affect enzymes belonging to the P450 system and those that affect P-glycoprotein. Both mechanisms can change plasma drug concentrations and therefore both efficacy and toxicity.[23,24]

As inhibition is due to competition between the two interacting medicines at the site of metabolism or transport, the degree of inhibition is related to the concentration of the interacting medicine at that site. When an inhibiting medicine is commenced, the level of inhibition will rise as the plasma or tissue concentration rises until the steady-state concentration is reached after about four to five half-lives.

A smaller number of interactions involve induction of hepatic enzymes or transport systems, resulting in reduced plasma and tissue concentrations of the affected medicine. Since induction requires upregulation of the system, the rate of reduction of the induced drug plasma or tissue concentrations is usually much slower than when inhibition occurs.

A full discussion of drug–drug interactions is out with the scope of this chapter. Cardiac medicines most likely to be a problem are those with narrow therapeutic indices (e.g. digoxin) or those where the interaction results in a significant change in plasma concentration.

Commonly used evidenced-based heart failure medicines that have clinically significant pharmacokinetic interactions are listed in Table 56.2.[25]

Over-the-counter medicines

Over-the-counter medicines are generally conventional medicines that have been deemed by the medicines regulatory authorities (e.g. European Medicines Agency) to be appropriate for supply to the public without the intervention of a medical or non-medical prescriber.[26]

The adverse effects profile of OTC medicines and the contraindications and cautions to their use are generally well known, at least to health care practitioners. Patients may be less aware of the risks associated with their use, particularly in patients with existing heart disease.

Although many OTC medicines may be available from any retail outlet, some countries have a restricted list of OTC medicines that can only be sold from pharmacies, under the supervision of a pharmacist.

Table 56.2 Common pharmacokinetic drug–drug interactions involving heart failure medicines[25]

Medicine	Examples of interacting medicines	Effect and advice
Bisoprolol	Rifampicin	Slight reduction in half-life. No dose increase usually required.
Carvedilol	Rifampicin, barbiturates	Decreased plasma carvedilol concentrations. Close monitoring needed.
Carvedilol	Cimetidine, ketoconazole, fluoxetine, haloperidol, verapamil,[a] erythromycin	Increased plasma carvedilol concentrations. Close monitoring needed.
Nebivolol	Paroxetine, fluoxetine, thioridazine, quinidine	Possible increased plasma nebivolol concentrations. Close monitoring needed.
Eplerenone	Strong interaction: ketoconazole, itraconazole,[a] ritonavir, nelfinavir, clarithromycin, telithromycin, nefazadone. Moderate interaction: erythromycin, saquinavir, amiodarone, diltiazem,[a] verapamil,[a] fluconazole.	Increased plasma eplerenone concentrations. The concomitant use of eplerenone with strong CYP3A4 inhibitors is contraindicated. In cases of the concomitant use of eplerenone with moderate inhibitors of CYP3A4, eplerenone dosing should not exceed 25 mg daily.
Eplerenone	Rifampicin, carbamazepine, phenytoin, phenobarbital, St John's wort	Reduced plasma eplerenone concentrations. The concomitant use of these medication is not recommended.
Ivabradine	Strong interaction: ketoconazole, itraconazole,[a] clarithromycin, erythromycin, nelfinavir, ritonavir, nefazodone diltiazem,[a] verapamil,[a] grapefruit juice. Moderate interaction: saquinavir, amiodarone, fluconazole.	Increased plasma ivabradine concentrations. The concomitant use of strong and some moderate CYP3A4 inhibitors (e.g. diltiazem and verapamil) is contraindicated. The concomitant use of ivabradine with other moderate CYP3A4 inhibitors may be considered but the starting dose of ivabradine should be reduced (e.g. 2.5 mg twice daily) and close heart rate monitoring is needed.
Ivabradine	Rifampicin, barbiturates, phenytoin, St John's wort	Decreased plasma ivabradine concentrations. The concomitant use of CYP3A4 inducing medicines may require an adjustment of the dose of ivabradine.
Furosemide	Sacubitril/valsartan	Co-administration of sacubitril/valsartan and furosemide reduces serum furosemide exposure and reduces the urinary excretion of sodium. Clinical relevance is unclear. Close monitoring of symptoms is recommended.
Digoxin	Amiodarone, disopyramide,[a] flecainide,[a] propafeneone,[a] quinidine,[a] diltiazem,[a] verapamil,[a] eplerenone, spironolactone, macrolide antibiotics, trimethoprim, itraconazole,[a] quinine, hydroxychloroquine, atorvastatin	Increased plasma digoxin concentrations. Close monitoring needed, especially when starting these medications in patients when digoxin is dosed near the upper limit of therapeutic range at baseline.
Digoxin	Rifampicin, St John's wort	Decreased plasma digoxin concentrations. Close monitoring needed.

[a] Medications best avoided in heart failure patients.

Source data from The electronic Medicines Compendium (eMC), DataPharm Ltd 2016. http://www.medicines.org.uk/emc/.

Table 56.3 UK over-the-counter (OTC) medicines with cardiovascular effects

OTC medication	Indication	Possible effect
Cystitis preparations	Cystitis symptoms	Fluid retention (via sodium content) Hyperkalaemia (via potassium content)
Hyoscine butylbromide	Irritable bowel syndrome	Tachycardia
NSAIDs	Pain/inflammation	Fluid retention Increased cardiovascular events
Soluble analgesics	Pain	Fluid retention (via sodium content)
Sumatriptan	Migraine	Myocardial ischaemia
Sympathomimetic decongestants	Nasal congestion	Tachycardia
Tamsulosin	Urinary retention	Hypotension
Tranexamic acid	Dysmenorrhoea	Prothrombotic

NSAID, non-steroidal anti-inflammatory.

The OTC medicines most likely to have an adverse effect on heart function are those that are associated with fluid retention or increased heart rate, with NSAIDs and sympathomimetic decongestants being the most commonly available (see Fluid retention and Positive chronotropic effects).

Additionally, some OTC products may contain significant quantities of sodium (e.g. soluble analgesics, cystitis relief products).[1] A typical soluble paracetamol or combined paracetamol/codeine tablet in the UK contains as much sodium as 1 g of salt. Another excipient in some cold and flu remedies is caffeine. Although this is claimed to enhance absorption of the analgesic, it will also have central nervous system and cardiovascular stimulant effects.

Certain OTC products may contain substantial quantities of potassium (e.g. other cystitis relief products), which may interact with prognostically important heart failure medicines, such as angiotensin converting enzyme inhibitors, angiotensin receptor blockers, and mineralocorticoid receptor antagonists.

See Table 56.3 for a list of widely used OTC products (available in the UK) with cardiovascular effects.

Complementary and alternative medicines

Complementary and alternative medicines (CAMs) cover a wide range of treatment types and modalities. These include: herbal medicines and traditional Chinese remedies; nutriceuticals; homeopathy; acupuncture; reflexology; osteopathy; chiropractic; aromatherapy; hypnosis; macrobiotic diets; chelation therapy; and faith healing.

This chapter will, however, only consider the use of herbal medicines and traditional Chinese remedies, as the other treatments are unlikely to have clinically significant effects on conventional medications.

The use of conventional medicines in the management of heart failure, and heart disease in general, is largely underpinned by an evidence base that describes how the medicine should be used and the potential benefits, and risks, that patients may experience from their use. Conversely, there is a lack of evidence supporting the use of CAMs that patients may turn to when conventional medicines are perceived to be inadequate. Additionally, CAMs used to treat both heart, and other, disease, may have adverse cardiovascular effects.

A systematic review of this issue found that: 22–68% of cardiovascular patients used biological therapies and 2–46% of patients used herbal remedies. Physicians knew about this use in 8–65% of patients but 35–92% of physicians were unaware. In heart failure, up to 82% of patients who used a CAM took it for cardiovascular health reasons.[27]

Herbal and traditional medicines with cardiovascular effects

It is perhaps unsurprising that botanical products have pharmacological effects since many commonly used conventional medicines have botanical sources (e.g. aspirin from willow, digoxin from foxglove, warfarin from sweet clover, morphine from poppy). Among the concerns regarding the use of such products in patients with cardiovascular disease are lack of safety data, lack of data on interaction with conventional medicines, and variable product quality.[28] In the past there was no regulation of the herbal and traditional Chinese medicine market in Europe. However, they now come under the authority of the same bodies that regulate conventional medicines.

As herbal products are likely to contain pharmacologically active constituents, their possible detrimental effects in patients with heart disease may mirror the detrimental effects possible with conventional medicines, and when used for perceived cardiovascular benefits they may enhance the effects of conventional medicines used in heart disease.[1,29,30] Indeed, many herbal medicines used for a wide variety of conditions may have potentially detrimental effects (see Table 56.4).

Medication adherence

So far this chapter has assumed that patients are actually taking all of the medications that they are prescribed and/or buy. However, this is not always the case. Non-adherence to medication in cardiovascular disease is a significant threat to global health systems, due to the subsequent morbidity which results from it, and the development of interventions to positively impact on this is a priority.[31,32]

There are various terminologies used to describe whether patients take their medication or not, most commonly compliance and adherence. The outdated concept of compliance involves the

Table 56.4 Examples of herbal and traditional Chinese medicines with possible cardiovascular effects

Product	Supposed uses in herbal or traditional Chinese medicine (limited evidence base)	Pharmacology	Issue
Aconite	• Neuralgia • Rheumatism	• Class I anti-arrhythmic effects • Reduced sympathetic activity	• Pro-arrhythmia • Bradycardia
Bitter orange	• Nausea, indigestion, constipation	• Unclear	• Tachycardia • Hypertension
Black cohosh	• Rheumatism • Menopausal symptoms	• Unclear, multiple mechanisms proposed	• Possible oestrogenic effects
Danshen	• Coronary Heart Disease	• Antithrombotic	• Bleeding risk • Digoxin assay interference
Dong quai	• Menopause symptoms	• Unclear	• Bleeding risk
Ephedra	• Colds • Flu • Wheeze • Asthma • Weight management	• Sympathomimetic	• Hypertension • Tachycardia
Garlic	• Cardiovascular disease prevention	• Antithrombotic	• Bleeding risk • Hypotension
Ginkgo	• Dementia • Cognitive impairment • Vascular disease	• Antithrombotic • Cytochrome P450 inhibition	• Bleeding risk • Drug interactions
Ginseng	• 'Immune system stimulant' • Angina/myocardial infarction • Heart failure	• Nitric oxide synthesis • CYP3A4 inhibition • (Digoxin assay interference, Siberian Ginseng)	• Hypotension • Hypertension • Interactions e.g. coumarins • (False high digoxin levels)
Hawthorn	• Digestive problems • Kidney problems • Heart failure • Angina	• Digitalis-like effects • Vasodilator	• Digoxin toxicity • Hypotension
Liquorice root	• Stomach ulcers • Bronchitis • Sore throats (antiviral) • Hepatitis	• Contains glycyrrhizin: Inhibits corticosteroid metabolism	• Fluid retention • Hypertension • Hypokalaemia
Motherwort	• Anxiety • 'Cardiac debility' • Insomnia • Amenorrhoea	• Smooth muscle relaxant/ vasodilator • Antithrombotic	• Hypotension • Bleeding risk
Rauwolfia	• Hypertension	• Catecholamine depletion	• Hypotension
Saw palmetto	• Benign prostatic hyperplasia	• α_1 antagonist • Cyclooxygenase inhibitor	• Hypotension • Bleeding risk
St John's wort	• Depression • Anxiety • Insomnia	• CYP3A4 induction • P-glycoprotein induction	• Numerous • Interactions: • Coumarins • Digoxin • Anti-arrhythmics • Some β-blockers • Calcium channel blockers • Statins • Many others
Yohimbine (Yohimbe)	• Aphrodisiac • Erectile dysfunction	• Monoamine oxidase inhibitors • α_2 antagonist • Increases catecholaminergic stimulation	• Hypotension • Hypertension • Tachycardia

This table does not include supplements (e.g. minerals, co-enzyme q10, etc.).

doctor giving the patient instructions that must be followed; alternatively the notion of adherence acknowledges a partnership in the prescribing process where an agreement is reached between the clinician and the patient. The majority of academic literature now refers to adherence as the preferred term. Perhaps the most widely cited and most comprehensible definition of adherence is from the World Health Organization (WHO); 'the extent to which a person's behaviour—taking medication, following a diet, and/or executing lifestyle changes, corresponds with agreed recommendations from a health care provider'.[32]

The consequences of non-adherence

Pharmacological treatment is the cornerstone of heart failure management, for patients with reduced ejection fraction. In clinical studies from the 1980s, the one-year mortality for patients with heart failure was >50%,[33] but improved pharmacological treatment options have seen this fall to <10% in the modern era.[34,35]

Unsurprisingly, non-adherence to medication in patients with heart failure is well known to be associated with poorer outcomes.[36,37] A sub-analysis of the Candesartan in Heart failure: Assessment of Reduction in Mortality and morbidity (CHARM) trial showed that adherence levels of ≥80% were associated with lower all-cause mortality (hazard ratio: 0.66; 95% confidence interval: 0.58–0.76; $P < 0.0001$).[36]

Interestingly in the CHARM-analysis patients that were adherent with placebo >80% of the time had better outcomes than patients who were non-adherent with candesartan.[36] Interpretation of this finding is not straightforward due to the observational nature of the data (i.e. patients were not randomly assigned to adhere or not, as this would be unethical). It is possible that non-adherent patients in the candesartan arm of the trial were also non-adherent with multiple other prognostically important drugs, such as β-blockers and mineralocorticoid receptor antagonists, raising the importance of clinicians reviewing adherence with first-line agents before adding in second-line therapies. It is equally possible that adherence to drug therapy may be a surrogate indicator of healthier behaviours in general (e.g. better diet, better attendance at healthcare appointments, etc.) which impact on the outcome of interest; the so-called 'healthy adherer' phenomenon.[38] As such, a healthy degree of caution is advised when interpreting direct associations between medication adherence and outcomes in observational studies.

The scale of non-adherence

The quoted scale of medication non-adherence in heart failure varies significantly across the literature from 2% to 90%.[39] This variation results from patient selection bias, the particular method of measuring adherence used and the definition of non-adherence within each individual study.

One population-level cohort study from a Scottish hospital over a 10-year period, using prescription refill records, shows that 35.9% of patients were non-adherent at the <80% level, a commonly accepted clinically relevant threshold.[40]

There is, however, no 'reference standard' measure for medication adherence. Each particular method has strengths and limitations (see Table 56.5). Objective measures, such a pill counts and prescription refill records, are generally regarded as more reliable. When directly compared in the same patient cohort, objective measures of adherence are known to predict outcomes and self-reported measures do not.[41] This is in part due to patients often overestimating their adherence.

Barriers to medication adherence

Many clinicians wrongly attribute sole personal blame for non-adherence to the patient. Medication adherence is influenced by a number of complex interwoven factors. The WHO divided these into five distinct factors:[32]

1. *Patient-related factors*: the motivation levels of a patient and the presence of depression can often impact on likely adherence levels.[42] The ability of a patient to fit medication-taking into their daily routine is also vitally important.[43] Cognitive impairment, which is often undiagnosed, is also a barrier to medication adherence in heart failure.[44]

2. *Condition-related factors*: the symptom burden of a patient has an impact on adherence levels, with asymptomatic patients being more likely to be non-adherent.[39] Those patients with a previous hospitalization are also more likely to adhere.[45] Comorbidity burden is also known to have a detrimental effect on adherence.[46]

3. *Treatment-related factors*: those with perceived side-effects or those with higher levels of poly-pharmacy are less likely to adhere.[39]

Table 56.5 Pros and cons of different methods for measuring medication adherence

Method	Pros	Cons
Patient-reported	• Cheap • Easy to conduct in clinical setting	• Subjective (patients often over-estimate) • Not all patients able to carry it out (e.g. cognitively impaired patients)
Pill counts	• Objective • Gives quantitative data • Easy to conduct in clinical setting	• Time-consuming • Can be altered by patient (e.g. hiding tablets) • Careful interpretation needed when accounting for hospitalizations
Prescribing/dispensing records	• Objective • Cheap • Gives quantitative result • Easy to conduct in clinical setting	• Depending on the healthcare system, prescribing and dispensing can be automated and not patient initiated • Careful interpretation needed when accounting for hospitalizations
Electronic (e.g. MEMS lids on medication bottles)	• Objective • Gives quantitative data	• Expensive • Can be difficult to interpret when patients take more than one dose out of a medication bottle at one time
Blood/urine analysis	• Objective	• Expensive • Blood tests are invasive • Not possible to determine exact adherence level • Metabolism variation between patients

MEMS, Medication Event Monitoring System.

4. *Health care system-related factors*: patients with better relationships with their clinicians and those with higher levels of satisfaction with their care are more likely to adhere.[39] Prescription medication costs also affect adherence levels.[47]

5. *Socio-economic factors*: the level of social support that a patient has can influence medication adherence levels. Examples of this include: married patients having higher adherence that non-married patients and likewise those with carers having higher adherence than those who do not.[39]

Interventions to improve adherence

The existing literature on interventions to improve medication adherence is limited by small patient numbers and significant heterogeneity in adherence measurement methodology and the components of interventions.

A systematic review on interventions to improve medication adherence in heart failure shows that patient education and self-management training alone is not effective.[48] This is undoubtedly due to the complexities of non-adherence. Why would patient education be expected to help those patients with medication non-adherence related to cognitive impairment, depression, social isolation, or poor relationships with their clinicians?

Intensified longitudinal support, particularly involving pharmacists, may be beneficial to some patients.[48] A recent German randomized controlled trial also showed that longitudinal pharmacist intervention can improve both adherence and quality of life in patients with chronic heart failure.[49] However, such interventions need to be tailored to the specific needs of the patient, depending on the particular individual barriers that the patient is experiencing. Concern remains that the positive effects of such an intensive intervention often dissipate when intervention ceases.[48]

Since many of the barriers to medication adherence are frequently social and multi-morbidity related it seems sensible that the potential solutions must include these aspects.[39,50] Unfortunately, such initiatives often have limited impact,[51] and a convincing evidence base for an effective solution with widespread generalizability is still sadly elusive.

Conclusion

Polypharmacy and multi-morbidity are growing epidemics. Heart failure is a syndrome where multi-morbidity (both cardiac and non-cardiac) and polypharmacy (including complementary therapies) are both common. Therefore, clinicians increasingly need to deal with medications for other conditions that may be detrimental to heart failure or may interact with prognostically important evidence-based heart failure therapies. Polypharmacy also brings with it the challenges of maintaining medication adherence with treatments proven to improve patient outcomes.

These complex issues are often difficult to manage, without exact solutions, and are as much an art as a science. However, undoubtedly there is a need for close review, good patient communication, and a team-based multi-disciplinary approach. Further research into these areas is also greatly needed.

REFERENCES

1. Page RL, O'Bryant CL, Cheng D, *et al*. Drugs that may cause or exacerbate heart failure: a scientific statement from the American Heart Association. *Circulation* 2016;**134**(6):e32–69.
2. Komajda M, McMurray JJV, Beck-Nielsen H, *et al*. Heart failure events with rosiglitazone in type 2 diabetes: data from the RECORD clinical trial. *Eur Heart J* 2010;**31**:824–31.
3. Franciosa JA, Jordan RA, Wilen MM, Leddy CL. Minoxidil in patients with chronic left heart failure: contrasting hemodynamic and clinical effects in a controlled trial. *Circulation* 1984;**70**(1):63–8.
4. Scott PA, Kingsley GH, Scott DL. Non-steroidal anti-inflammatory drugs and cardiac failure: meta-analyses of observational studies and randomised controlled trials. *Eur J Heart Fail* 2008;**10**:1102–7.
5. Hippisley-Cox J, Coupland C. Risk of myocardial infarction in patients taking cyclo-oxygenase-2 inhibitors or conventional non-steroidal anti-inflammatory drugs: population based nested case–control analysis. *Br Med J* 2005;**330**(7504):1366–9.
6. Grenne MA, Gordon A, Boltax AJ. Clinical and cardiodynamic effects of adrenocortical steroids in congestive heart failure. *Circulation* 1960;**21**:661–71.
7. Goldstein RE, Boccuzzi SJ, Cruess D, Nattel S. Diltiazem increases late-onset congestive heart failure in postinfarction patients with early reduction in ejection fraction. The Adverse Experience Committee and the Multicenter Diltiazem Postinfarction Research Group. *Circulation* 1991;**83**:52–60.
8. Køber L, Torp-Pedersen C, McMurray JJV, *et al*. Increased mortality after dronedarone therapy for severe heart failure. *N Engl J Med* 2008;**358**:2678–87.
9. Echt DS, Liebson PR, Mitchell LB, *et al*. Mortality and morbidity in patients receiving encainide, flecainide, or placebo. The Cardiac Arrhythmia Suppression Trial. *N Engl J Med* 1991;**324**:781–8.
10. Ravid S, Podrid PJ, Lampert S, Lown B. Congestive heart failure induced by six of the newer antiarrhythmic drugs. *J Am Coll Cardiol* 1989;**14**(5):1326–30.
11. Waldo AL, Camm AJ, DeRuyter H, *et al*. Effect of d-sotalol on mortality in patients with left ventricular dysfunction after recent and remote myocardial infarction. *Lancet* 1996;**348**(9019):7–12.
12. Qu Y, Fang M, Gao B, *et al*. Itraconazole decreases left ventricular contractility in isolated rabbit heart: mechanism of action. *Toxicol Appl Pharmacol* 2013;**268**(2):113–22.
13. Link MG, Yan G-X, Kowey PR. Evaluation of toxicity for heart failure therapeutics: studying effects on QT interval. *Circ Heart Fail* 2010;**3**:547–55.
14. Woosley RL, Romero KA. QTdrugs List, AZCERT, Inc. 1822 Innovation Park Dr., Oro Valley, AZ 85755. www.Crediblemeds.org (accessed 2 August 2020).
15. Hamer M, Batty GD, Seldenrijk A, Kivimaki M. Antidepressant medication use and future risk of cardiovascular disease: The Scottish Health Survey. *Eur Heart J* 2011;**32**(4):437–42.
16. Zamorano JL, Lancellotti P, Rodriguez Muñoz D, *et al*. 2016 ESC Position Paper on cancer treatments and cardiovascular toxicity developed under the auspices of the ESC Committee for Practice Guidelines. *Eur J Heart Fail* 2017;**19**:9–42.
17. van Dalen EC, Caron HN, Dickinson HO, Kremer LCM. Cardioprotective interventions for cancer patients receiving anthracyclines. *Cochrane Database Syst Rev* 2005;(6):CD003917.
18. Wright JT, Williamson JD, Whelton PK, *et al*., SPRINT Research Group. A randomized trial of intensive versus standard blood-pressure control. *N Engl J Med* 2015;**373**:2103–16.

19. Cohn JN, Pfeffer MA, Rouleau J, *et al.*, MOXCON Investigators. Adverse mortality effect of central sympathetic inhibition with sustained-release moxonidine in patients with heart failure (MOXCON). *Eur J Heart Fail* 2003;**5**:659–67.

20. ALLHAT Collaborative Research Group. Major cardiovascular events in hypertensive patients randomized to doxazosin vs chlorthalidone. *JAMA* 2000;**283**:1967–75.

21. Flannery G, Gehrig-Mills R, Billah B, Krum H. Analysis of randomized controlled trials on the effect of magnitude of heart rate reduction on clinical outcomes in patients with systolic chronic heart failure receiving beta-blockers. *Am J Cardiol* 2008;**101**(6):865–9.

22. Mendoza I, Lago R, Cardona R, Morris L. Stress cardiomyopathy induced by common surgical and medical interventions. When patients get more than they asked for. *J Card Fail* 2010;**16**(8 Suppl 1):S110.

23. Cheng JWM, Frishman WH, Aronow WS. Updates on cytochrome P450-mediated cardiovascular drug interactions. *Am J Ther* 2009;**16**:155–63.

24. Wessler JD, Grip LT, Mendell J, Giugliano RP. The P-glycoprotein transport system and cardiovascular drugs. *J Am Coll Cardiol* 2013;**61**:2495–502.

25. Electronic Medicines Compendium (eMC), DataPharm Ltd, 2016. http://www.medicines.org.uk/emc/ (accessed 2 August 2020).

26. Bond C. The over-the-counter pharmaceutical market—policy and practice. https://www.lse.ac.uk/lse-health/assets/documents/eurohealth/issues/eurohealth-v14n3.pdf?from_serp=1 (accessed 2 Aug 2020).

27. Grant SJ, Bin YS, Kiat H, Chang DH-T. The use of complementary and alternative medicine by people with cardiovascular disease: a systematic review. *BMC Public Health* 2012;**12**:299–17.

28. Zhang J, Wider B, Shang H, Li X, Ernst E. Quality of herbal medicines: challenges and solutions. *Complement Ther Med* 2012;**20**:100–6.

29. Tachjian A, Maria V, Jahanjir A. Use of herbal products and potential interactions in patients with cardiovascular disease. *J Am Coll Cardiol* 2010;**55**(6):515–25.

30. Tsai HH, Lin HW, Pickard AS, Tsai HY, Mahady GB. Evaluation of documented drug interactions and contraindications associated with herbs and dietary supplements: a systematic literature review. *Int J Clin Pract* 2012;**66**:1056–78.

31. Kolandaivelu K, Leiden BB, O'Gara PT, Bhatt DL. Non-adherence to cardiovascular medications. *Eur Heart J* 2014;**35**(46):3267–76.

32. Sabaté E, editor. Adherence to long-term therapies: evidence for action. World Health Organization, Geneva, 2003. http://apps.who.int/iris/bitstream/10665/42682/1/9241545992.pdf (accessed 27 July 2016).

33. CONSENSUS Trial Study Group. Effects of enalapril on mortality in severe congestive heart failure. Results of the Cooperative North Scandinavian Enalapril Survival Study (CONSENSUS). *N Engl J Med* 1987;**316**:1429–35.

34. Zannad F, McMurray JJV, Krum H, *et al.* Eplerenone in patients with systolic heart failure and mild symptoms. *N Engl J Med* 2011;**364**:11–21.

35. McMurray JJ, Packer M, Desai AS, *et al.*, PARADIGM-HF Investigators and Committees. Angiotensin–neprilysin inhibition versus enalapril in heart failure. *N Engl J Med* 2014;**371**:993–1004.

36. Granger BB, Swedberg K, Ekman I, *et al.* Adherence to candesartan and placebo and outcomes in chronic heart failure in the CHARM programme: double-blind, randomised, controlled clinical trial. *Lancet* 2005;**366**(9502):2005–11.

37. Fitzgerald AA, Powers JD, Ho PM, *et al.* Impact of medication nonadherence on hospitalizations and mortality in heart failure. *J Card Fail* 2011;**17**(8):664–9.

38. Simpson SH, Eurich DT, Majumdar SR, *et al.* A meta-analysis of the association between adherence to drug therapy and mortality. *Br Med J* 2006;**333**(7557):15–18.

39. Wu J-R, Moser DK, Lennie TA, Burkhart PV. Medication adherence in patients who have heart failure: a review of the literature. *Nurs Clin North Am* 2008;**43**(1):133–53.

40. Yeong LJ, Ogston SA, Hall C, *et al.* Adherence to heart failure therapy and outcome: a population based study. *Heart* 2013;**99**:A12.

41. Wu J-R, Moser DK, Chung ML, Lennie TA. Objectively measured, but not self-reported, medication adherence independently predicts event-free survival in patients with heart failure. *J Card Fail* 2008;**14**(3):203–10.

42. Morgan AL, Masoudi FA, Havranek EP, *et al.* Difficulty taking medications, depression, and health status in heart failure patients. *J Card Fail* 2006;**12**(1):54–60.

43. George J, Shalansky SJ. Predictors of refill non-adherence in patients with heart failure. *Br J Clin Pharmacol* 2007;**63**(4):488–93.

44. Hawkins LA, Kilian S, Firek A, *et al.* Cognitive impairment and medication adherence in outpatients with heart failure. *Heart Lung J Acute Crit Care* 2012;**41**(6):572–82.

45. Monane M, Bohn RL, Gurwitz JH, Glynn RJ, Avorn J. Noncompliance with congestive heart failure therapy in the elderly. *Arch Intern Med* 1994;**154**(4):433–7.

46. Forsyth P, Richardson J, Lowrie R. Patient-reported barriers to medication adherence in heart failure in Scotland. *Int J Pharm Pract* 2019;**27**:443–50.

47. Jackson JE, Doescher MP, Saver BG, Fishman P. Prescription drug coverage, health, and medication acquisition among seniors with one or more chronic conditions. *Med Care* 2004;**42**(11):1056–65.

48. Molloy GJ, O'Carroll RE, Witham MD, McMurdo MET. Interventions to enhance adherence to medications in patients with heart failure a systematic review. *Circ Heart Fail* 2012;**5**(1):126–33.

49. Schulz M, Griese-Mammen N, Anker SD, *et al.* Pharmacy-based interdisciplinary intervention for patients with chronic heart failure: results of the PHARM-CHF randomized controlled trial. *Eur J Heart Fail* 2019;**21**:1012–21.

50. Wamala S, Merlo J, Bostrom G, Hogstedt C, Agren G. Socioeconomic disadvantage and primary non-adherence with medication in Sweden. *Int J Qual Health Care* 2007;**19**(3):134–40.

51. Ruppar TM, Delgado JM, Temple J. Medication adherence interventions for heart failure patients: a meta-analysis. *Eur J Cardiovasc Nurs* 2015;**14**(5):395–404.

FURTHER READING

Page RL, O'Bryant CL, Cheng D, *et al.* Drugs that may cause or exacerbate heart failure: a scientific statement from the American Heart Association. *Circulation* 2016;**134**(6):e32–69.

Tsai HH, Lin HW, Pickard AS, Tsai HY, Mahady GB. Evaluation of documented drug interactions and contraindications associated with herbs and dietary supplements: a systematic literature review. *Int J Clin Pract* 2012;**66**:1056–78.

Wu J-R, Moser DK, Lennie TA, Burkhart PV. Medication adherence in patients who have heart failure: a review of the literature. *Nurs Clin North Am* 2008;**43**(1):133–53.

57

Cardiac rehabilitation and chronic heart failure

Massimo F. Piepoli and Andrew L. Clark

Introduction

All patients with established chronic heart failure (CHF), with or without implantable cardioverter–defibrillator (ICD) and with or without cardiac resynchronization therapy (CRT), require a multifactorial cardiac rehabilitation approach. The role of the multidisciplinary approach will be considered elsewhere (see Chapter XX).

The traditional model of care delivery is thought to contribute to frequent hospitalizations. During these brief episodic encounters, little attention is paid to the numerous barriers to effective CHF treatment and the possible treatment of the common modifiable factors that are the cause of disease progression and thus hospital readmissions. To face these limitations, a CHF multidimensional management programme is necessary to curb the rising cost of management and to improve morbidity and mortality for individual patients.[1]

Cardiac rehabilitation is the ideal comprehensive structured disease intervention since it best addresses the complex interplay of medical, psychological, and behavioural factors facing patients with CHF. It is a coordinated multidimensional intervention designed to stabilize or slow disease progression, alleviate symptoms, improve exercise tolerance, and enhance quality of life, thereby reducing morbidity and mortality.[2] In populations of patients with CHF, such a programme has been shown to improve functional capacity, recovery, emotional well-being, and reduce hospital admission.

Exercise training as a key component in cardiac rehabilitation programme may improve survival and reduce hospitalization in stable heart failure patients. It is recommended for all stable patients with CHF. There is no evidence that it should be limited to any particular heart failure patient subgroup based on aetiology, New York Heart Association (NYHA) class, left ventricular function, or medication (class of recommendation I, level of evidence A).[3]

Despite the virtues of cardiac rehabilitation, only a small percentage of eligible heart failure patients ever get referred, due to barriers such as lack of physician and patient-family awareness of its benefits, and logistical or financial constraints. Patients with CHF are a patient population that challenges cardiac rehabilitation with the need to employ active strategies to disseminate and implement appropriate standards of care.

Core components of cardiac rehabilitation in CHF

Box 57.1 lists the core components of cardiac rehabilitation.

Rest as therapy in CHF

For many years, standard medical advice was that exercise should be avoided for patients with CHF, with standard textbooks bearing such advice as 'Reduced physical activity is critical in the care of patients with heart failure throughout their entire course'.[9] There are some small studies suggesting that rest as a specific intervention may have some modest beneficial effects in terms of reducing heart size,[10-12] but these studies were carried out at a time when modern medical therapy was in its infancy and CHF had an exceptionally high mortality rate. A common problem with long-term rest has been thromboembolic complications and sudden death. Rest as an intervention has not been trialled in the modern therapeutic era.

Safety of exercise training in CHF

Part of the concern about exercise comes from the possibility that it might be dangerous, particularly in patients with underlying ischaemic heart disease. The increased wall stress imposed by exercise might be expected to result in further cardiac enlargement. An influential paper reported on the effects of training in patients who had a moderate-sized anterior myocardial infarct.[13] There appeared to be some echocardiographic evidence of worsening cardiac function despite an improvement in exercise capacity. Further work in animal models[14] suggested that training may worsen left ventricular function.

These observations were alarming: no treatment that worsens left ventricular function is likely to confer long-term benefit. However, the Judgutt study was relatively small, uncontrolled, and used a strenuous training programme. A key study was the EAMI trial in which 95 patients were randomized following an anterior myocardial infarction to a training regime or usual therapy.

Box 57.1 Core components of cardiac rehabilitation in chronic heart failure

1 Clinical assessment and risk stratification

Careful history, physical examination, cardiac imaging and biochemical assays are essential accurately to describe fluid status, and functional capacity. Defining the severity of heart failure is vital before an appropriate rehabilitation programme can be started.[4,5] Note the following:

- **Clinical history**: including screening for cardiovascular risk factors, co-morbidities, and disabilities. Likely concurrent problems such as claudication or cerebrovascular disease should be identified.
- **Symptoms**: what limits the patient on exertion—as well as using the NYHA class for dyspnoea severity, it is vital to know whether other symptoms are limiting the patient.
- **Adherence**: to the medical regime and self-monitoring (weight, blood pressure, symptoms).
- **Physical examination**: general health status with particular care for **haemodynamic and fluid status**: signs of congestion, peripheral and central oedema suggest that further manipulation of diuretic therapy is necessary before an exercise regimen can be prescribed safely. Blood pressure, heart rate and rhythm are also essential. Signs of **cachexia** should be sought: reduced muscle mass, muscle strength and endurance will limit exercise capacity at least initially.
- **ECG**: heart rate, rhythm, QRS width, repolarization abnormalities, arrhythmias (particularly atrial fibrillation).
- **Blood testing**: for routine biochemical assay: serum electrolytes, urea and creatinine should be monitored as part of usual care.
- **Usual physical activity level** is an important consideration. For some patients with a sedentary lifestyle, the idea of an exercise programme may be a startling departure. Domestic, occupational, and recreational needs should be explored; readiness to change behaviour and self-confidence should be assessed, together with describing any barriers to increased physical activity. Encouraging social support in making positive changes may be key for some patients.
- **Exercise capacity**: an assessment of exercise capacity before any exercise training regimen is important. Maximal symptom-limited incremental cardiopulmonary exercise tests with metabolic gas exchange measurements are reference standard tools wisely used in research or in assessing patients for possible advanced therapies such as transplantation. Protocols with small increments (such as 5–10 W/min on a cycle ergometer or modified Bruce or Naughton protocols on a treadmill) are indicated. Other tests such as the 6 or 12 min walk tests are perfectly reasonable in daily practice to assess exercise tolerance and have the merit of perhaps more resembling normal life for the patient.
- **Education**: clear, comprehensible information on the basic purpose of the cardiac rehabilitation programme and the role of each component should be provided to each patient.

The assessment should lead to the formulation of a tailored, patient-specific, treatment plan and document short-term goals within the core components of care that guide intervention strategies.

2 Identification and treatment of causative factors and/or correction of precipitating factors

Coexisting conditions are responsible for 40% of preventable hospital re-admission. Causative factors (including hypertension, coronary artery disease, arrhythmias), and precipitating factors (such as non-compliance to drug, non-steroidal anti-inflammatory and cyclooxygenase-2 inhibitors drug misuse, nasal decongestants, infection, pulmonary emboli, dietary indiscretion, inactivity, hyperthyroidism) must be clearly identified. As the disease progresses and the patient ages, medication and remedies directed at the underlying pathology may be relevant and the need for treatment of coexisting symptoms may outweigh the possible adverse consequences of some therapies for heart failure care.

3 Pharmacological therapy optimization

According to clinical assessment, medical therapy should be oriented to achieve normal jugular venous pressure, resolution of orthopnea and oedema, systolic blood pressure of ≥80 mmHg, stable renal function, and the ability to walk the hospital ward without dizziness or dyspnoea.

Attendance at supervised exercise training session makes it possible to ensure that the patient is taking appropriate medical therapy. Treatment must be tailored according to the individual characteristics with the goal to prescribe according to international guidelines with adequate doses. A careful upward dosage titration is required in the introduction of both ACE inhibitors and β-blockers till the highest tolerated dosages. The uptitration schedule usually extends the convalescent period after the patient has been discharged from the hospital.

The simultaneous presence of competing co-morbidities further complicates pharmacological management. The ever-increasing complexity of polypharmacotherapy is intimidating, meaning that some therapies may not be used, especially by practitioners who lack the time and expertise to pursue the kind of 'micromanagement' required with complex regimens. Although little evidence is available to guide polypharmacotherapy, collaborative disease management programmes (such as those provided in cardiac rehabilitation settings) that include a careful review of medications can be very helpful for patients with CHF and multiple co-morbidities.[6]

Educating patients about their condition and motivating their adherence to a course of therapy are steps towards success. A clear and comprehensible explanation of the basic purpose and action of each drug is required. Patients' understanding and adherence of drug regimen should be periodically refreshed.

4 Physical activity and exercise training programme

As the CHF syndrome starts and develops, the natural tendency for patients is to do whatever seems reasonable to avoid symptoms. Hence the recognition that effort induces undue breathlessness leads to progressive inactivity, contributing to skeletal muscle detraining and general unfitness that contribute to further progression of the heart failure syndrome. A sedentary lifestyle, with little or no physical activity during leisure time or at work, is a risk factor for the development and progress of cardiovascular disease.[7,8]

Although patients with a lower left ventricular ejection fraction at study entry showed ventricular enlargement after six months, there was no difference between the control and training groups.[15] Similar findings have been reported elsewhere,[16] and data from the longer-term ELVD-CHF study suggested that training actually reduced left ventricular volumes and increased left ventricular ejection fraction.[17]

Training might, of course, have some other dangerous effects, such as potentially increasing the risk of ventricular arrhythmias. The majority of early studies in the field used carefully supervised training regimens in carefully selected patients. Incremental exercise testing in patients with CHF is safe,[18,19] and now that large studies of relatively unselected and unsupervised patients have been conducted, the safety of training is now established.[20]

Training in other patient groups

The benefits of exercise training for patients with ischaemic heart disease,[21] and following myocardial infarction,[22,23] have been known for many years. Training can actually improve left ventricular systolic function in 'normal' older men,[24] and rehabilitation is helpful after cardiac events in older people,[25,26] the population most likely to suffer from CHF. Training apparently improves endurance exercise more than peak exercise capacity,[27] the very improvement likely to have the greatest symptomatic benefit for older patients who rarely,

if ever, need to undertake maximal exercise. Given the effects of ageing on muscle strength and bulk, it is not surprising that training might be more generally helpful in older subjects.[28]

The nature of these studies means that they must have included many patients with significant left ventricular impairment, and the lack of cardiac complication in the studies is further evidence that training is safe.

Rationale for training in patients with CHF

Although the pathophysiology of CHF is usually discussed principally in terms of changes to central haemodynamic function, much research over the last 20 years or so has emphasized the fact that CHF is a multisystem disorder with abnormalities affecting many body systems from the central nervous system to bowel wall function to immunological function. The greatest contributor to exercise limitation appears to be changes to skeletal (rather than cardiac) muscle function (see discussions in Chapter 2 and Chapter 33).

A striking feature of the peripheral changes seen is how closely they resemble the effects of detraining in normal subjects. Activation of the renin–angiotensin[29] and sympathetic[30] systems, loss of skeletal muscle bulk and depletion of oxidative enzymes[31,32] are all seen in both conditions (see Table 57.1). Bearing in mind (i) the apparent safety of training regimes (ii) the similarity of CHF to detraining, and (iii) the beneficial effects of training in very similar patient groups, training as a specific intervention for patients with CHF was an inevitable progression.

Early studies

Early uncontrolled work including patients with severe left ventricular dysfunction showed promising results.[33,34] Sullivan *et al.* were among the first to assess training systematically, finding that a training regimen improved exercise capacity by ~20% (as assessed by peak oxygen consumption).[35,36] An important observation was that central haemodynamics at matched workloads was unchanged after training, and the changes responsible were presumably peripheral as reflected in a fall in arterial and venous lactate during exertion.

In a crossover trial, Coats *et al.*[37,38] demonstrated that exercise training improved exercise capacity by a similar proportion and helped improve symptoms. Since these pioneering studies, the beneficial effects of training on peak exercise capacity have been repeatedly confirmed, and, indeed, the effects are greater than (and additive to) the effects of angiotensin converting enzyme (ACE) inhibitors.[39]

Table 57.1 Similarities between the chronic heart failure syndrome and detraining in normal subjects

Variable	Detraining	Heart failure
Heart rate	↑	↑
Exercise capacity	↓	↓
Muscle size	↓	↓
Muscle enzymes	↓	↓
Sympathetic	↑	↑
Renin:angiotensin	↑	↑
Heart rate variability	↓	↓

Benefits of training

Gas exchange and ventilation

Training programmes produce a variety of improvements in heart failure patients, not simply an improvement in peak exercise capacity. There is improvement in endurance exercise capacity and an increase in both anaerobic and ventilatory thresholds.[36,40] In addition, the increased ventilatory response to exercise (as reflected in the increase in the association between ventilation and carbon dioxide production) is improved by training,[41] an effect not seen in normal subjects.[42] In addition, ventilation at matched submaximal workloads is reduced by training.[36,43] Peak exercise ventilation is increased, reflecting the increased overall exercise capacity following training.[44]

Exercise capacity

As well as increasing maximal exercise capacity, training regimes also improve submaximal exercise capacity. This is perhaps a more important observation, as patients rarely encounter peak exertion in daily life. Training induces an increase both in the duration of exercise at a fixed workload,[36] and an increase in the distance covered in a 6 min walk test.[40,45]

Quality of life

Quality-of-life measures are consistently improved by training, which is not something necessarily seen with all treatments that improve prognosis. The effect on quality of life may be more important than effects on abstract measures that do not really reflect day-to-day life. Patients' self-assessment scores during exercise tests are improved,[37,40] and there are improvements in anxiety and depression following training.[46]

The best evidence for the effects of training on quality of life comes from the HF-ACTION study. Using the Kansas City Cardiomyopathy Questionnaire, the investigators found a marked benefit on quality of life persisting through the three years of the study.[47] The effect was the same regardless of the aetiology of the heart failure.

Sympathovagal balance

The abnormal sympathovagal balance of CHF is improved by training, as shown by an increase in heart rate variability and reduction in noradrenaline spillover.[37] There is an improvement in circadian variability of heart rate in some studies,[48] although others have reported that only daytime heart rate variability is increased.[44]

Neurohormonal effects

Training has a beneficial effect on the neurohormonal activation of CHF, causing reductions in angiotensin, aldosterone, and arginine vasopressin.[49] It can also reduce sympathetic activation and natriuretic peptide levels.[50]

Haemodynamic effects

As a consequence of increasing exercise performance, training has been found in many studies to increase maximal cardiac output and heart rate. The effects on submaximal cardiac output are not completely clear: whereas most investigators suggest that, at matched workload, cardiac output is unchanged by training,[35,43] some have reported modest increases.[37] However, it is unlikely that changes to

cardiac output mediate any benefit, as most patients have normal cardiac output responses to submaximal exercise before training.[51,52]

There is some evidence to suggest that training might improve diastolic cardiac function with improved early diastolic filling and increases in peak filling rates at matched heart rates during exercise.[53,54] Other changes include a reduction in both cardiac volume and systemic vascular resistance together with increased endothelium-dependent vasodilation.[55,56] That arm vasodilation is improved after leg training[57] suggests that there are some structural effects of training on the vasculature.[58]

Effects on skeletal muscle

Studies examining skeletal muscle histology have shown that mitochondrial density is increased by training, along with a shift back toward type I muscle fibres and an increase in the ratio of capillaries to myocytes.[59–61] Many of these changes correlate with the improvement in exercise capacity seen, suggesting that the mechanism for improvement lies with changes to skeletal muscle rather than in any haemodynamic changes. Additional effects include a decrease in myocyte phosphocreatine depletion during, and a shortening in the recovery time of phosphocreatine following, exercise.[62] Selective training of ventilatory muscle may also be beneficial.[63]

Other effects in skeletal muscle include an increase in insulin-like growth factor,[64] suggesting that the insulin resistance of heart failure may be partially reversible by training. In addition, training also has a general antioxidant effect in skeletal muscle with an increase in skeletal muscle antioxidant enzymes.[65] A potential link to the improvement in exercise capacity and reduction in ventilatory response induced by training is via the abnormal activation of the ergoreflexes[66] closely associated with the abnormal exercise physiology of patients with CHF: the ergoreflex is reduced by training.[67]

Type and intensity of exercise

Formal studies of training have generally used quite strenuous training stimuli. Different studies have used different techniques ranging from home cycle training to supervised rowing (see **Table 57.2**). Aerobic exercise training for stable patients is the most studied form and is the most highly recommended mode of training.

In the past, isometric exercise was not advised as there appeared to be unfavourable effects and potentially adverse haemodynamic consequences.[71,72] However, a resistive component of a training regime does seem to produce benefits above what is gained from endurance training alone.[73] It may even be possible to achieve some benefits with very localized training,[74] including of respiratory muscle alone.[75]

The strenuous endurance approach is reasonably easy to follow for supervised patients in short-term clinical trials, but is not broadly applicable for most patients with CHF. There is some evidence that rather more gentle regimens can have a beneficial effect. Belardinelli *et al.*[69] found beneficial effects in patients with mild CHF with low-intensity training at only 40% of peak oxygen consumption, a finding confirmed in patients with more severe heart failure who trained at low workloads (<50% of maximal) using supine cycle exercise in a deliberate attempt to minimize ventricular wall stress.[70]

A further consideration is that most patients with CHF are elderly, and many have co-morbidities that will greatly limit their capacity to take part in formal training programmes. One possible alternative approach is that of electrical muscle stimulation. It is possible to induce painless muscle contraction using large electrode plates, and devices can be programmed to deliver stimulation to several large muscle groups in the legs (quadriceps, gluteals, and hamstrings).[76] In normal subjects, such a device can have a training effect,[77] and we have shown that electrical muscle stimulation can have a beneficial training effect in patients with CHF (**Figure 57.1**).[78] Whether programmed electrical muscle stimulation leads to prolonged benefits is not yet known.

Duration of benefit

An important observation is that the improvement in exercise capacity is proportional to compliance with the training regimen.[38] That the benefits are not just short-term gains was confirmed by Kavanagh who demonstrated that the effects lasted for at least a

Table 57.2 Pivotal studies on exercise training in heart failure

Lead author	Type of training	Intensity of training	Frequency	Duration	S/U	↑ peak VO$_2$
Sullivan[35]	Cycle, walking	75%	60 min, 3–5/week	16–24 weeks	S	23%
Coats[37]	Cycle	60–80%	20 min, 5/week	8 weeks	U	18%
Meyer[40]	Cycle, walking (interval[a])	50%	45 min, 11/week	3 weeks	S	20%
Kiilavuori[43]	Walking, cycling	55%	30 min, 3/week	6 months	S: 3 months U: 3 months	12%
Keteyian[44]	Treadmill, cycle, rowing	60–80%	45 min, 3/week	24 weeks	S	16%
Kavanagh[45]	Walking	55%	10–21 km per week	52 weeks	Initially S[b]	17%
Hambrecht[68]	Cycle	near max	40 min daily	6 months	S: 3 weeks U: 6 months[c]	33%
Belardinelli[69]	Cycle	40%	30 min, 3/week	8 weeks	S	17%
Demopoulos[70]	Cycle	<50%	60 min, 4/week	12 weeks	S	22%

S, supervised; U, unsupervised.

[a] Interval training is characterized by repeated short bursts of exercise with recovery periods between.
[b] Initially supervised, but then mainly home based with regular review visits.
[c] Additional twice weekly supervised group sessions.

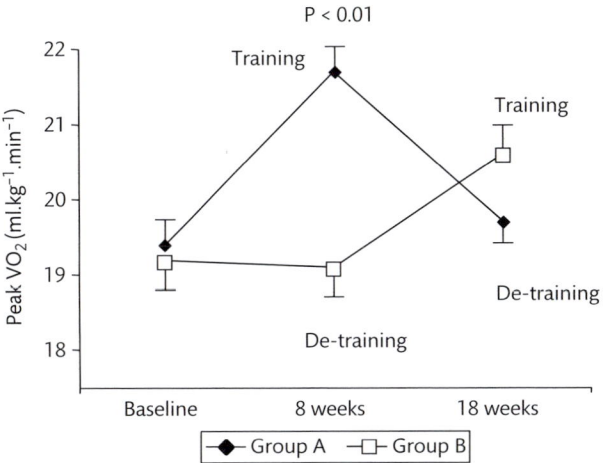

Figure 57.1 The improvement in peak oxygen capacity (VO$_2$) seen after training using programmed muscle stimulation. $P < 0.01$.

Source data from Banerjee P, Caulfield B, Crowe L, Clark AL. Prolonged electrical muscle stimulation exercise improves strength, peak VO$_2$, and exercise capacity in patients with stable chronic heart failure. *J Card Fail* 2009;**15**:319–26.

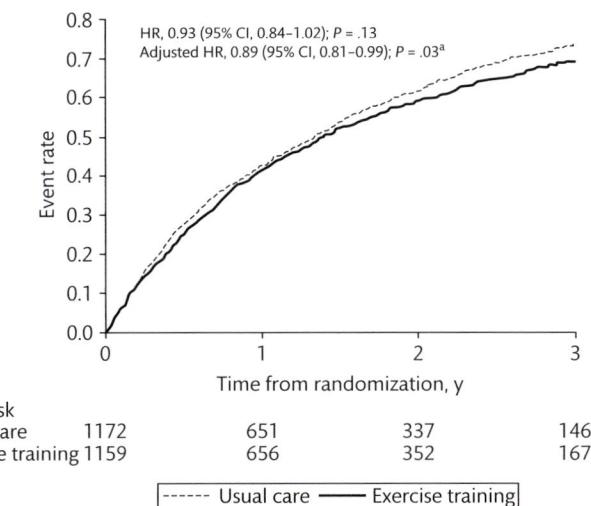

Figure 57.2 The primary end-point, all-cause death and hospitalization, of the HF-ACTION trial. Adjustment was for factors found to be strongly associated with outcome at baseline. HR, hazard ratio; CI, confidence interval.

Source data from O'Connor CM, Whellan DJ, Lee KL, Keteyian SJ, Cooper LS, Ellis SJ, Leifer ES, Kraus WE, Kitzman DW, Blumenthal JA, Rendall DS, Miller NH, Fleg JL, Schulman KA, McKelvie RS, Zannad F, Piña IL; HF-ACTION Investigators. Efficacy and safety of exercise training in patients with chronic heart failure: HF-ACTION randomized controlled trial. *JAMA* 2009;**301**:1439–50.

year, reaching a plateau at around 16 weeks to 6 months.[45] The HF-ACTION study demonstrates that the benefits of training persist for longer—up to 3 years.[47]

Effect on mortality

A key question has been whether the apparently beneficial changes seen in the multitude of relatively small-scale studies translate into improvements in outcome. The ExtraMatch collaborative[79] included 721 patients who had been randomized into trials of exercise training. Follow-up was limited to just over 700 days, but there was a strong suggestion that patients randomized to training were not only less likely to be admitted to hospital, but had a better prognosis.

Mounting a sufficiently large study to answer the question definitively has been very difficult, in part because of the problem of sponsorship, and in part because of the difficulty of running the trial. Blinding the intervention is, of course, impossible, and many patients randomized to usual care are likely to take up exercise once included in any study. There are also likely to be problems with dropouts: compliance with the training regimen is difficult to monitor, and it is easier for individual patients to resile from training than, say, from a drug trial—where the randomization and blinding makes it far less likely that crossovers will be a problem.

The HF-ACTION study[20] randomized 2331 patients to receive a training programme or usual care. The training programme consisted of 36 supervised 30 min sessions three times per week followed by home exercise five times per week at moderate intensity for 40 min. The control group were simply encouraged to take exercise. The primary end-point was all-cause death and hospitalization.

Although the training group had a marked improvement in exercise capacity over the course of the trial, there was no effect on the primary end-point. However, when adjustment was made for other prognostic indicators, there was a modest benefit in favour of training (see **Figure 57.2**). The effect appears to be modest, but should be set in the context that at three years only 30% of patients in the intervention group were adhering to the recommended 120 min per week, and the median exercise duration per week was only around 50 min. The additional benefit of striking improvement in

long-term quality of life[47] means that a structured exercise programme should now be part of the routine management of patients with CHF.

Approach to the patient

Improving adherence to a physical activity and exercise training programme is vital: without compliance, the programme is worthless. A step-by-step approach is helpful (**Figure 57.3**).

Assessment

Assess current physical activity level and determine domestic, occupational, and recreational needs. Evaluate activities relevant to age, sex, and daily life. Assess readiness to change behaviour, self-confidence, barriers to increased physical activity, and social support in making positive changes.

Educational processes and support

- A minimum of 30–60 min per session of moderately intense aerobic activity, preferable daily, or at least three or four per week. Supervised group activity is helpful initially for many patients to restore confidence (many will have been told by well-meaning friends or family to 'take it easy'), and to allow the mutually supportive atmosphere that comes with having many patients facing the same challenges together.

- **Emphasize**: sedentary lifestyle as risk factor, and benefits of physical activity: any increase in activity has a positive health benefit

- **Recommend**: gradual increases in daily lifestyle activities over time, and how to incorporate it into daily routine.

- **Advise**: individualize physical activity according to patient's age, past habits, co-morbidities, preferences, and goals.

- **Reassure**: regarding the safety of the recommended protocol.

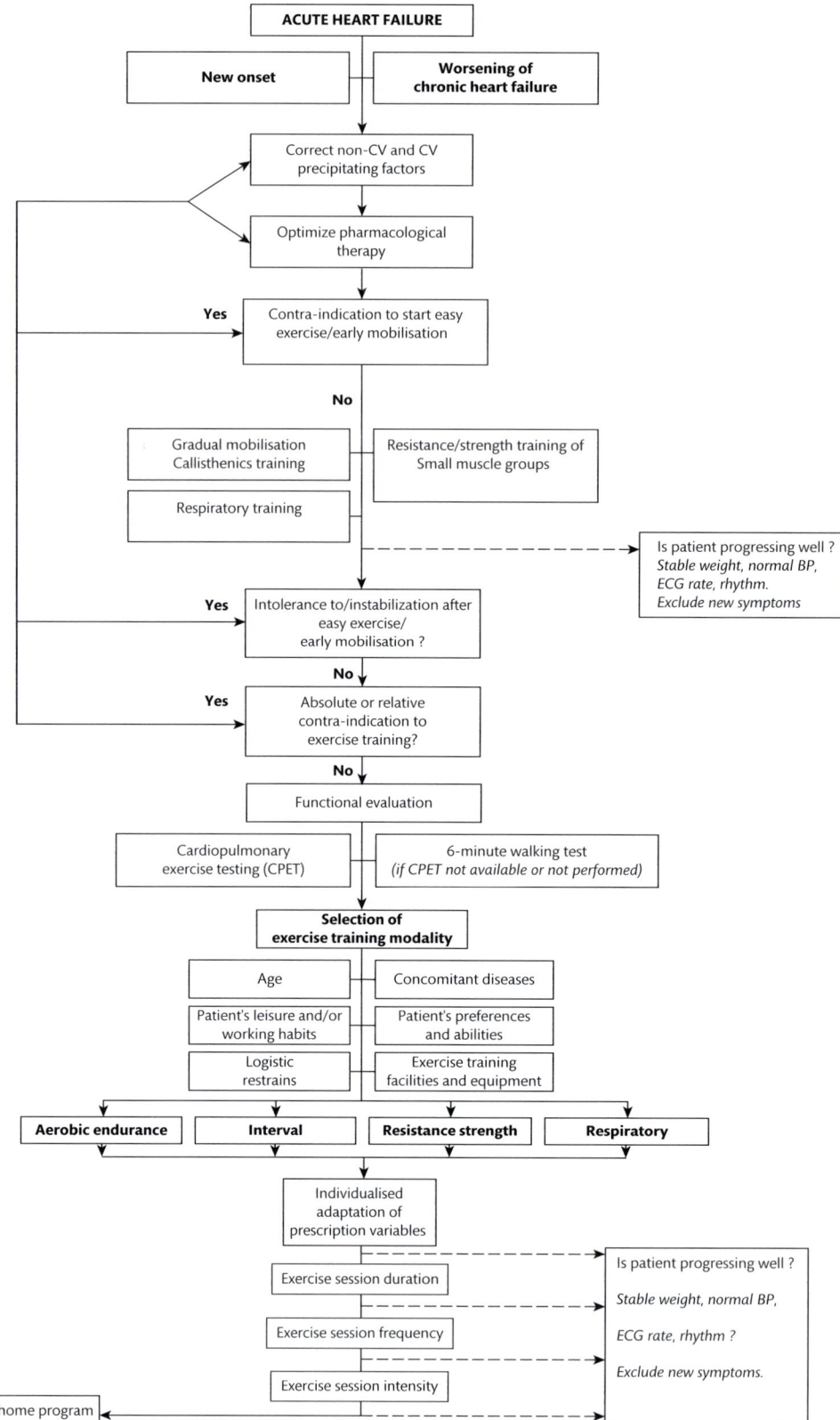

Figure 57.3 Step-by-step approach to implement physical training programme in acute heart failure patients.

Source data from Piepoli MF, Conraads V, Corrà U, Dickstein K, Francis DP, Jaarsma T, McMurray J, Pieske B, Piotrowicz E, Schmid JP, Anker SD, Solal AC, Filippatos GS, Hoes AW, Gielen S, Giannuzzi P, Ponikowski PP. Exercise training in heart failure: from theory to practice. A consensus document of the Heart Failure Association and the European Association for Cardiovascular Prevention and Rehabilitation. *Eur J Heart Fail.* 2011 Apr;**13**(4):347–57.

- **Encourage**: involvement in leisure activities that are enjoyable and in group exercise training programme as patients tend to revert to previous sedentary habits over time.
- **Forewarn**: patients need to be forewarned of the risk of relapses: thus education should underline how benefits may be achieved and the need for its lifelong continuation. If physical activity interruption has occurred, physical, social, and psychological barriers to attendance should be explored, and alternative approaches suggested.[80]
- **Exercise programme**
  - Initial stage: intensity should be kept at a low level (50% of peak exercise capacity), increasing duration from 15 to 30 min, two or three times per week according to perceived symptoms and clinical status for the first 1–2 weeks.
  - Improvement stage: a gradual increase of intensity (60%, 70% to 80% of peak exercise capacity, as tolerated) is the primary aim. Prolongation of exercise sessions is a secondary goal.

The expected outcomes from exercise training programmes are highlighted in Box 57.2.

Specific issues

Exercise training and β-blockers

There is some obvious difficulty in determining heart rate targets in patients taking β-blockers. Patients on β-blockers benefit to the same extent as those not taking them,[81,82] and in HF-ACTION, nearly 95% of patients were taking a β-blocker at baseline. The heart rate at maximum exertion at baseline allows an appropriate target heart rate for training to be determined.

Exercise training and atrial fibrillation

Key here is to make sure that there is adequate control of ventricular rate during exercise. Almost always, a β-blocker will be needed to control heart rate rather than simply digoxin alone. In HF-ACTION, just over one-fifth of the patients had atrial fibrillation at baseline, and there is no reason to exclude patients with atrial fibrillation from a training regime.

Exercise training and patients with ICD or CRT

There appear to be no adverse consequences for patients with ICDs or CRT undergoing a training programme.[83,84] There is a risk of device discharge from a rapidly accelerating heart rate,[84] and, certainly to start with, supervision by qualified staff is important, particularly to monitor the heart rate response to exercise. Training intensity should be determined by the heart rate response and established at a level to increase the heart rate to between 20 and 30 beats below the ICD detection rate.

Left ventricular assist device

The native heart–left ventricular assist device (LVAD) complex responds physiologically to exercise and has a circulatory reserve with the capability to meet the demands of daily activities. Long-term support by an LVAD is now possible and patients can be managed in outpatient clinics. Early initiation of exercise therapy in patients with an LVAD is associated with improvements in exercise capacity. Exercise training also may improve functional status at a later period after LVAD implantation, supporting the use of LVAD as a destination therapy. Scientific data on content, setting, duration, and safety of exercise training in LVAD patients are few. Beneficial results have been reported for various training modalities in different settings, but no standard exercise training programme has been established. A recent snapshot among European centres implanting LVAD reported that the majority (58%) had a functioning exercise training programme for patients with an LVAD. Most of the exercise programmes (84%) include aerobic endurance training, mostly cycling (73%) or walking (62%) at low intensity intervals. Some programmes apply resistance training (47%), respiratory muscle training (55%), or balance training (44%).

Heart failure with preserved ejection fraction

Exercise training reduces diastolic dysfunction in patients with dilated cardiomyopathy. Meta-analyses suggest that aerobic exercise training in heart failure with preserved ejection fraction improves both cardiorespiratory fitness and quality of life, but the data are far less compelling than for patients with heart failure and a reduced ejection fraction.

Counselling and education

The role of the multidisciplinary team in delivering counselling and education is considered elsewhere. In relation to the exercise component, however, some factors are particularly important.

Obesity

Obesity has numerous adverse haemodynamic, cardiac structure, and function effects. On the other hand, obese CHF patients have a better prognosis than underweight patients.[85,86] Obesity should not be seen as a contraindication to exercise training, and training may help weight control.

Cigarette smoking

Cigarette smoking should be strongly discouraged in patients with CHF. In addition to the well-established adverse effects of smoking on CAD, which is the underlying cause of a substantial proportion of patients, smoking has adverse haemodynamic effects in patients with CHF, including increasing heart rate and systemic blood pressure, and mildly increasing pulmonary artery pressure, ventricular filling pressure, and total systemic and pulmonary vascular resistance. Increased peripheral vasoconstriction may contribute to a modest reduction in stroke volume. Finally, the increased susceptibility of patients with CHF to bronchospasm is exacerbated by cigarette smoke.

Box 57.2 Expected outcomes from exercise training programmes for patients with chronic heart failure

- Increased participation in domestic, occupational, and recreational activities.
- Improved psychosocial well-being, prevention of disability, and enhancement of opportunities for independent self-care, improved aerobic fitness.
- Increased cardiorespiratory fitness and enhanced flexibility, muscular endurance, and strength.
- Reduction of symptoms, attenuated physiologic responses to physical challenges, and improved psychosocial well-being.

Psychosocial management

Depression is extremely common in the heart failure population[87] with a wide range of quoted prevalence rates across studies due to the use of different diagnostic instruments and the inclusion of different patient populations. Treatment of depression is an important clinical strategy as it is associated with more frequent hospital admissions, decline in activities of daily living, worse NYHA functional classification and increased medical costs. However, depression frequently goes undiagnosed.

The depressed patient is far less likely to comply with a training regimen, and its recognition at an early stage is important. Patients may be unwilling to disclose emotional distress to their physicians for fear of being stigmatized with the label of mental illness. On the other hand, physicians may not address depression because they have not been adequately trained to recognize both typical and atypical depressive symptoms, because of time constraints in high-volume settings, or because they do not know how to best treat the condition. Recognition and management of depression may be enhanced through the use of multidisciplinary team or disease management programmes.[88,89]

Continuum of care

A good cardiac rehabilitation programme is characterized by a continuum of services that spans inpatient and outpatient rehabilitation.

Inpatients

Inpatient rehabilitation should begin as soon as possible after hospital admission and should be part of routine daily care for every heart failure inpatient. The main elements are appropriate strategies for optimal therapy, education with full participation of patient/caregiver, reassurance and support, mobilization when possible, and group education, according to clinical assessment and risk stratification. Progression of mobilization should be developed according to the patient's clinical condition, functional capacity, age, and co-morbidity under careful medical review and supervision.

Outpatients

As the length of stay for acute heart failure and procedures continues to decrease, patient and family attendance in outpatient cardiac rehabilitation assumes ever greater importance. Structured outpatient cardiac rehabilitation is a crucial issue for the development of a life-long approach to prevention of relapse of heart failure. Attendance should start soon after discharge from the hospital. Outpatient cardiac rehabilitation may be provided in a range of settings, such as heart failure clinics, non-clinic settings (community health centres and general medical practices), or a combination of these. It may also be provided on an individual basis at home, including a combination of home visits, telephone support, telemedicine, and specially developed self-education materials.

The main elements of outpatient cardiac rehabilitation include assessment, review and follow-up, therapy optimization, low- or moderate-intensity physical activity and exercise training, education, discussion, and counselling. The evaluation of ongoing cardiac rehabilitation programme objectives on a regular basis is a key to success.

The challenge of rehabilitation

Although the benefits of exercise rehabilitation, at least for patients with CHF and reduced left ventricular ejection fraction, are clear-cut, many services struggle to deliver rehabilitation to more than a fraction of the potential patients. Partly this is because rehabilitation is not seen to be 'glamorous' for health care professionals, and in many health care systems few doctors train specifically in rehabilitation. Partly, it is because there is very limited commercial drive behind rehabilitation compared with, for example, device or pharmacological therapy; partly, it is because patients themselves may be reluctant to make a long-term commitment to changes in lifestyle that may be very alien. Finally, health care systems themselves are not well-adapted to delivering rehabilitation to the potentially enormous numbers of patients for whom it might be helpful.

Guidelines help to drive change; and regulatory requirements help, too. In the UK, the National Institute for Health and Care Excellence encourages programmes of cardiac rehabilitation as part of their quality standards which will further help drive change.[90]Perhaps the biggest driver for change with the greatest likelihood of increasing access for patients with heart failure may be will be patient demand.

REFERENCES

1. Sagar VA, Davies EJ, Briscoe S, et al. Exercise-based rehabilitation for heart failure: systematic review and meta-analysis. *Open Heart* 2015;**2**(1):e000163.
2. Piepoli MF, Corrà U, Benzer W, et al. Secondary prevention through cardiac rehabilitation—from knowledge to implementation. A Position Paper from the Cardiac Rehabilitation Section of the European Association of Cardiovascular Prevention and Rehabilitation. *Eur J Cardiovasc Prev Rehabil* 2010;**17**(1):1–17.
3. Piepoli MF, Hoes AW, Agewall S, et al. 2016 European Guidelines on cardiovascular disease prevention in clinical practice: The Sixth Joint Task Force of the European Society of Cardiology and Other Societies on Cardiovascular Disease Prevention in Clinical Practice. *Eur J Prev Cardiol* 2016;**23**(11):NP1–NP96.
4. Ponikowski P, Voors AA, Anker SD, et al.; Authors/Task Force Members2016 ESC Guidelines for the diagnosis and treatment of acute and chronic heart failure: The Task Force for the diagnosis and treatment of acute and chronic heart failure of the European Society of Cardiology (ESC). *Eur J Heart Fail* 2016;**37**(27):2129–200.
5. Piepoli MF, Conraads V, Corrà U, et al. Exercise training in heart failure: from theory to practice. A consensus document of the Heart Failure Association and the European Association for Cardiovascular Prevention and Rehabilitation. *Eur J Heart Fail* 2011;**13**(4):347–57.
6. Masoudi FA, Krumholz HM. Polipharmacy and comorbidity in heart failure. *BMJ* 2003;**327**:514–15.
7. Exercise and physical activity in the prevention and treatment of atherosclerotic cardiovascular disease. A statement from the Council on Clinical Cardiology (subcommittee on Exercise, Rehabilitation, and Prevention) and the Council on Nutrition, Physical Activity, and Metabolism (subcommittee on Physical Activity). *Circulation* 2003;**107**:3109–16.
8. Giannuzzi P, Mezzani A, Saner H, et al. Physical activity for primary and secondary prevention. Position paper of the Working Group on Cardiac Rehabilitation and Exercise Physiology of the

European Society of Cardiology. *Eur J Cardiovasc Prev Rehabil* 2003;**10**(5):319–27.

9. Braunwald E. *Heart disease*, 3rd edn. Saunders, Philadelphia, 1988.

10. Burch GE, Walsh JJ, Black WC. Value of prolonged bed rest in management of cardiomegaly. *JAMA* 1963;**183**:81–7.

11. Burch GE, McDonald CD. Prolonged bed rest in the treatment of ischemic cardiomyopathy. *Chest* 1971;**60**:424–30.

12. McDonald CD, Burch GE, Walsh JJ. Prolonged bed rest in the treatment of idiopathic cardiomyopathy. *Am J Med* 1972;**52**:41–50.

13. Jugdutt BI, Michorowski BL, Kappagoda CT. Exercise training after anterior Q wave myocardial infarction: importance of left ventricular function and topography. *J Am Coll Cardiol* 1988;**12**:362–72.

14. Gaudron P, Hu K, Schamberger R, *et al*. Effect of endurance training early or late after coronary artery occlusion on left ventricular remodelling, hemodynamics, and survival in rats with chronic transmural myocardial infarction. *Circulation* 1994;**89**:402–12.

15. Gianuzzi P, Tavazzi L, Temporelli PL, *et al*., for the EAMI study group. Long-term physical training and left ventricular remodelling after anterior myocardial infarction (EAMI) trial. *J Am Coll Cardiol* 1993;**22**:1821–9.

16. Ehansi AA, Miller TR, Miller TA, Ballard EA, Schechtman KB. Comparison of adaptations to a 12-month exercise program and late outcome inpatients with healed myocardial infarction and ejection fraction <45% and >50%. *Am J Cardiol* 1997;**79**:1258–60.

17. Giannuzzi P, Temporelli PL, Corrà U, Tavazzi L; ELVD-CHF Study Group. Antiremodeling effect of long-term exercise training in patients with stable chronic heart failure: results of the Exercise in Left Ventricular Dysfunction and Chronic Heart Failure (ELVD-CHF) Trial. *Circulation* 2003;**108**:554–9.

18. Tristani FE, Hughes CV, Archibald DG, *et al*. Safety of graded symptom-limited exercise testing in patients with congestive heart failure. *Circulation* 1987;**76**(Suppl VI):54–8.

19. Keteyian SJ, Isaac D, Thadani U, *et al*.; HF-ACTION Investigators. Safety of symptom-limited cardiopulmonary exercise testing in patients with chronic heart failure due to severe left ventricular systolic dysfunction. *Am Heart J* 2009;**158**(4 Suppl):S72–7.

20. O'Connor CM, Whellan DJ, Lee KL, *et al*.; HF-ACTION Investigators. Efficacy and safety of exercise training in patients with chronic heart failure: HF-ACTION randomized controlled trial. *JAMA* 2009;**301**:1439–50.

21. Clausen JP. Circulatory adjustments to dynamic exercise and effect of physical training in normal subjects and in patients with coronary artery disease. *Prog Cardiovasc Dis* 1976;**18**:459–95.

22. Oldridge NB, Guyatt GH, Fisher ME, Rimm AA. Cardiac rehabilitation after myocardial infarction: combined experience of randomized clinical trials. *JAMA* 1988;**260**:945–50.

23. O'Connor GT, Buring JE, Yusuf S, *et al*. An overview of randomized trials of rehabilitation with exercise after myocardial infarction. *Circulation* 1989;**80**:234–44.

24. Ehansi AA, Ogawa T, Miller TR, Spina RJ, Jilka SM. Exercise training improves left ventricular systolic function in older men. *Circulation* 1991;**83**:96–103.

25. Lavie CJ, Milani RV. Effects of cardiac rehabilitation and exercise training programs in patients ≥75 years of age. *Am J Cardiol* 1996;**78**:675–7.

26. Levine CJ, Milani RV. Benefits of cardiac rehabilitation and exercise training in elderly women. *Am J Cardiol* 1997;**79**:664–6.

27. Ades PA, Waldmann ML, Poehlman ET, *et al*. Exercise conditioning in older coronary patients: submaximal lactate response and endurance capacity. *Circulation* 1993;**88**:572–5.

28. Fielding RA. Effects of exercise training in the elderly: impact of progressive resistance training on skeletal muscle and whole-body protein metabolism. *Proc Nutr Soc* 1996;**54**:665–75.

29. Hespel P, Lijnen P, Faggard R, *et al*. Effects of physical endurance training on the plasma renin–angiotensin–aldosterone system in normal man. *J Endocr* 1988;**116**:443–9.

30. Cooksey JD, Reilly P, Brown S, Bomze H, Cryer PE. Exercise training and plasma catecholamines in patients with ischemic heart disease. *Am J Cardiol* 1978;**42**:372–6.

31. Holloszy JO. Adaptations of muscular tissue to training. *Prog Cardiovasc Dis* 1976;**18**:445–58.

32. Refenberick DH, Gamble JG, Max SR. Response of mitochondrial enzymes to decreased muscular activity. *Am J Physiol* 1973;**225**:1295–59.

33. Lee AP, Ice R, Blessey R, Sanmarco ME. Long term effects of physical training on coronary patients with impaired LV function. *Circulation* 1978;**60**:1519–26.

34. Conn EH, Williams RS, Wallace AG. Exercise responses before and after physical conditioning in patients with severely depressed left ventricular function. *Am J Cardiol* 1982;**49**:296–300.

35. Sullivan MJ, Higginbotham MB, Cobb FR. Exercise training in patients with severe left ventricular dysfunction: hemodynamic and metabolic effects. *Circulation* 1988;**78**:506–16.

36. Sullivan MJ, Higginbotham MB, Cobb FR. Exercise training in patients with chronic heart failure delays ventilatory anaerobic threshold and improves submaximal exercise performance. *Circulation* 1989;**79**:324–9.

37. Coats AJS, Adamopoulos S, Meyer T, Conway J, Sleight P. Physical training in chronic heart failure. *Lancet* 1990;**335**:63–6.

38. Coats AJS, Adamopoulos S, Radaelli A, *et al*. Controlled trial of physical training in chronic heart failure: exercise performance, hemodynamics, ventilation, and autonomic function. *Circulation* 1992;**85**:2119–31.

39. Meyer TE, Casadei B, Coats AJS, *et al*. Angiotensin-converting enzyme inhibition and physical training in heart failure. *J Intern Med* 1991;**230**:407–13.

40. Meyer K, Schwaibold M, Westbrook S, *et al*. Effect of short-term exercise training and activity restriction on functional capacity in patients with severe chronic congestive heart failure. *Am J Cardiol* 1996;**78**:1017–22.

41. Davey P, Meyer T, Coats A, *et al*. Ventilation in chronic heart failure: effects of physical training. *Br Heart J* 1992;**68**:473–7.

42. Clark AL, Skypala I, Coats AJS. Ventilatory efficiency is unchanged after physical training in health persons despite an increase in exercise tolerance. *J Cardiovasc Risk* 1994;**1**:347–51.

43. Kiilavuori K, Toivonen L, Naveri H, Leinonen H. Reversal of autonomic derangements by physical training in chronic heart failure assessed by heart rate variability. *Eur Heart J* 1995;**16**:490–5.

44. Keteyian SJ, Levine AB, Brawner CA, *et al*. Exercise training in patients with heart failure. *Ann Intern Med* 1996;**124**:1051–7.

45. Kavanagh T, Myers MG, Baigrie RS, *et al*. Quality of life and cardiorespiratory function in chronic heart failure: effects of 12 months' aerobic training. *Heart* 1996;**76**:42–9.

46. Kostis JB, Rosen RC, Cosgrove NM, Shindler DM, Wilson AC. Nonpharmacologic therapy improves functional and emotional status in congestive heart failure. *Chest* 1994;**106**:996–1001.

47. Flynn KE, Piña IL, Whellan DJ, *et al*. Effects of exercise training on health status in patients with chronic heart failure: HF-ACTION randomized controlled trial. *JAMA* 2009;**301**:1439–50.

48. Adamopoulos S, Ponikowski P, Cerqetani E, *et al*. Circadian pattern of heart rate variability in chronic heart failure patients—effects of physical training. *Eur Heart J* 1995;**16**:1380–6.

49. Braith RW, Welsch MA, Feigenbaum MS, Kluess HA, Pepine CJ. Neuroendocrine activation in heart failure is modified by endurance exercise training. *J Am Coll Cardiol* 1999;**34**:1170–5.

50. Passino C, Severino S, Poletti R, *et al*. Aerobic training decreases B-type natriuretic peptide expression and adrenergic activation in patients with heart failure. *J Am Coll Cardiol* 2006;**47**:1835–9.

51. Wilson JR, Mancini DM, Dunkman WB. Exertional fatigue due to skeletal muscle dysfunction in patients with heart failure. *Circulation* 1993;**87**:470–5.

52. Wilson JR, Rayos G, Yeoh TK, Gothard P. Dissociation between peak exercise oxygen consumption and hemodynamic dysfunction in potential heart transplantation candidates. *J Am Coll Cardiol* 1995;**26**:429–35.

53. Belardinelli R, Georgiou D, Cianci G, *et al*. Exercise training improves left ventricular diastolic filling in patients with dilated cardiomyopathy. Clinical and prognostic implications. *Circulation* 1995;**91**:2775–84.

54. Belardinelli R, Georgiou D, Cianci G, Purcaro A. Effects of exercise training on left ventricular filling at rest and during exercise in patients with ischemic cardiomyopathy and severe left ventricular dysfunction. *Am Heart J* 1996;**132**:61–70.

55. Katz SD, Yuen J, Bijou R, LeJemtel TH. Training improves endothelium-dependent vasodilation in resistance vessels of patients with heart failure. *J Appl Physiol* 1997;**82**:1488–92.

56. Hambrecht R, Hilbrich L, Erbs S, *et al*. Correction of endothelial dysfunction in chronic heart failure: additional effects of exercise training and oral L-arginine supplementation. *J Am Coll Cardiol* 2000;**35**:706–13.

57. Linke A, Schoene N, Gielen S, *et al*. Endothelial dysfunction in patients with chronic heart failure: systemic effects of lower-limb exercise training. *J Am Coll Cardiol* 2001;**37**:392–7.

58. Hambrecht R, Gielen S, Linke A, *et al*. Effects of exercise training on left ventricular function and peripheral resistance in patients with chronic heart failure: a randomized trial. *JAMA* 2000;**283**:3095–101.

59. Hambrecht R, Niebauer J, Fiehn E, *et al*. Physical training in patients with stable chronic heart failure: effects on cardiorespiratory fitness and ultrastructural abnormalities of leg muscles. *J Am Coll Cardiol* 1995;**25**:1239–49.

60. Hambrecht R, Fiehn E, Yu J, *et al*. Effects of endurance training on mitochondrial ultrastructure and fiber type distribution in skeletal muscle of patients with stable chronic heart failure. *J Am Coll Cardiol* 1997;**29**:1067–73.

61. Magnusson G, Gordon A, Kaijser L, *et al*. High intensity knee extensor training in patients with chronic heart failure. *Eur Heart J* 1996;**17**:1048–55.

62. Adamopoulos S, Coats AJS, Brunotte F, *et al*. Physical training improves skeletal muscle metabolic abnormalities in patients with chronic heart failure. *J Am Coll Cardiol* 1993;**23**:1101–6.

63. Mancini DM, Henson D, LaManca J, Donchez L, Levine S. Benefit of selective respiratory muscle training on exercise capacity in patients with chronic congestive heart failure. *Circulation* 1995;**91**:320–9.

64. Hambrecht R, Schulze PC, Gielen S, *et al*. Effects of exercise training on insulin-like growth factor-I expression in the skeletal muscle of non-cachectic patients with chronic heart failure. *Eur J Cardiovasc Prev Rehabil* 2005;**12**:401–6.

65. Linke A, Adams V, Schulze PC, *et al*. Antioxidative effects of exercise training in patients with chronic heart failure: increase in radical scavenger enzyme activity in skeletal muscle. *Circulation* 2005;**111**:1763–70.

66. Piepoli M, Clark AL, Coats AJ. Muscle metaboreceptors in hemodynamic, autonomic, and ventilatory responses to exercise in men. *Am J Physiol* 1995;**269**(4 Pt 2):H1428–36.

67. Piepoli M, Clark AL, Volterrani M, *et al*. Contribution of muscle afferents to the hemodynamic, autonomic, and ventilatory responses to exercise in patients with chronic heart failure: effects of physical training. *Circulation* 1996;**93**:940–52.

68. Hambrecht R, Niebauer J, Fiehn E, *et al*. Physical training in patients with stable chronic heart failure: effects on cardiorespiratory fitness and ultrastructural abnormalities of leg muscles. *J Am Coll Cardiol* 1995;**25**:1239–49.

69. Belardinelli R, Georgiou D, Scocco V, Barstow TJ, Purcaro A. Low intensity exercise training in patients with chronic heart failure. *J Am Coll Cardiol* 1995;**26**:975–82.

70. Demopoulos L, Bijou R, Fergus I, *et al*. Exercise training in patients with severe congestive heart failure: enhancing peak aerobic capacity whilst minimizing the increase in ventricular wall stress. *J Am Coll Cardiol* 1997;**29**:597–603.

71. Elkayam U, Roth A, Weber L, *et al*. Isometric exercise in patients with chronic advanced heart failure: hemodynamic and neurohormonal evaluation. *Circulation* 1985;**72**:975–81.

72. Reddy HK, Weber KT, Janicki JS, McElroy PA. Hemodynamic, ventilatory and metabolic effects of light isometric exercise in patients with chronic heart failure. *J Am Coll Cardiol* 1988;**12**:353–8.

73. McKelvie RS, McCartney N, Tomlinson C, Bauer R, MacDougall JD. Comparison of hemodynamic responses to cycling and resistance exercise in congestive heart failure secondary to ischemic cardiomyopathy. *Am J Cardiol* 1995;**76**:977–9.

74. Ohtsubo M, Yonezawa K, Nishijima H, *et al*. Metabolic abnormality of calf skeletal muscle is improved by localised muscle training without changes in blood flow in chronic heart failure. *Heart* 1997;**78**:437–43.

75. Mancini DM, Henson D, LaManca J, Donchez L, Levine S. Benefit of selective respiratory muscle training on exercise capacity in patients with chronic congestive heart failure. *Circulation* 1995;**91**:320–9.

76. Banerjee P, Clark A, Witte K, Crowe L, Caulfield B. Electrical stimulation of unloaded muscles causes cardiovascular exercise by increasing oxygen demand. *Eur J Cardiovasc Prev Rehabil* 2005;**12**:503–8.

77. Banerjee P, Caulfield B, Crowe L, Clark A. Prolonged electrical muscle stimulation exercise improves strength and aerobic capacity in healthy sedentary adults. *J Appl Physiol* 2005;**99**:2307–11.

78. Banerjee P, Caulfield B, Crowe L, Clark AL. Prolonged electrical muscle stimulation exercise improves strength, peak VO_2, and exercise capacity in patients with stable chronic heart failure. *J Card Fail* 2009;**15**:319–26.

79. Piepoli MF, Davos C, Francis DP, Coats AJ; ExTraMATCH Collaborative. Exercise training meta-analysis of trials in patients with chronic heart failure (ExTraMATCH). *BMJ* 2004;**328**:189.

80. Graham I, Atar D, Borch-Johnsen K, *et al*.; Fourth Joint Task Force of the European Society of Cardiology and other societies on cardiovascular disease prevention in clinical practice. *Eur J Cardiovasc Prev Rehab* 2007;**14**(Suppl 2):S1–113.

81. Forissier JF, Vernochet P, Bertrand P, Charbonnier B, Monpère C. Influence of carvedilol on the benefits of physical training in patients with moderate chronic heart failure. *Eur J Heart Fail* 2001;**3**:335–42.

82. Curnier D, Galinier M, Pathak A, *et al.* Rehabilitation of patients with congestive heart failure with or without beta-blockade therapy. *J Card Fail* 2001;**7**:241–8.

83. Fan S, Lyon CE, Savage PD, *et al.* Outcomes and adverse events among patients with implantable cardiac defibrillators in cardiac rehabilitation: a case-controlled study. *J Cardiopulm Rehabil Prev* 2009;**29**:40–3.

84. Vanhees L, Kornaat M, Defoor J, *et al.* Effect of exercise training in patients with an implantable cardioverter defibrillator. *Eur Heart J* 2004;**25**:1120–6.

85. Davos CH, Doehner W, Rauchhaus M, *et al.* Body mass and survival in patients with chronic heart failure without cachexia: the importance of obesity. *J Card Fail* 2003;**9**:29–35.

86. Horwich TB, Fonarow GC, Hamilton MA, *et al.* The relationship between obesity and mortality in patients with advanced heart failure. *J Am Coll Cardiol* 2001;**38**:789–95.

87. Haworth JE, Moniz-Cook E, Clark AL, *et al.* Prevalence and predictors of anxiety and depression in a sample of chronic heart failure patients with left ventricular systolic dysfunction. *Eur J Heart Fail* 2005;**7**:803–8.

88. Sullivan M, Simon G, Spertus J, Russo J. Depression-related costs in heart failure care. *Arch Intern Med* 2002;**162**:1860–66.

89. Rumsfeld JS, Havranek E, Masoudi FA, *et al.* Depressive symptoms are the strongest predictors of short-term declines in health status in patients with heart failure. *J Am Coll Cardiol* 2003;**42**:1811–17.

90. National Institute for Health and Care Excellence. *Chronic heart failure in adults Quality standard (QS9).* June 2011. Last updated: February 2016.

58

Non-pharmacological management

Lynda Blue[†]

Introduction

Managing heart failure not only presents a challenge to patients and their caregivers but it also significantly impacts on health care systems and health care professionals involved in the management of their care. Patient numbers are large and continue to increase, with many patients living with multiple co-morbidities and associated complex needs.

Patients are expected to adapt to multiple pharmacological regimens and lifestyle changes that usually require regular adjustment and adherence. Furthermore, a growing number of patients are being considered for advanced therapies. It is therefore important that patients receive lifestyle and self-management advice that is tailored to their information needs.

National and international guidelines predominantly concentrate on evidence-based pharmacological treatments but also provide best practice guidance recommendations on lifestyle advice and self-care management strategies.

Although there is limited evidence that non-pharmacological strategies in isolation improve mortality, morbidity, or quality of life, it is recommended that adopting a multidisciplinary framework enhances the care management of patients with heart failure.[1]

A blended approach consisting of pharmacological and non-pharmacological strategies enables patients and their caregivers the opportunity to achieve the best quality of life, without offering unrealistic expectations of cure. Health care professionals have a critical role in informing patients and their caregivers to feel knowledgeable and empowered in managing their condition effectively.

Education

Education is an important component of heart failure management programmes. Knowledge is generally defined as a quality, whereby an individual has the ability to understand, reflect, and to reach conclusions that can be used to bring about a change; whereas adherence is the extent to which a person's behaviour concurs with professional health advice. Empowering patients to be knowledgeable about the

implementation of appropriate treatment strategies at an early stage is an important educational outcome.

Barriers to effective learning can be wide-ranging and difficult to overcome and may be associated with functional, psychological, literacy, cognitive, and significant symptom burden limitations.

Heart failure can be difficult to manage. Complex treatment regimens can be confusing for many people, particularly if they live alone and have very little or no social support or require to have frequent adjustment of their medications. Awareness of these barriers must be a requisite of any health care professional who is involved in the management of patients and caregivers living with heart failure. To increase long-term success, individual care planning and management should always be aligned with patient and caregiver goals to encourage shared decision-making and improved health outcomes.

The timing of information-sharing is important as many patients may not always be ready to receive, understand, or absorb information provided by health care professionals. An example is during an inpatient episode when the diagnosis of heart failure has just been given. For many patients it may only be when they go home that they are able to formulate questions about their condition and seek to clarify treatment options.

It is important at hospital discharge and subsequent consultations that patients and/or caregivers are provided with information in a language that they understand. This should be supported with written materials about heart failure, approved heart failure websites, monitoring tools, e.g. weight/symptom monitoring charts and who to contact and what to do in response to symptom deterioration. It is also important that educational resources are available and tailored specifically to meet the needs of patients with impaired hearing or vision, and multicultural issues.

Self-care

The reference standard of patient self-care in heart failure has been defined as 'daily activities that maintain clinical stability'.[2] Self-care is an essential part of heart failure management because patients and their caregivers have to live with the consequences of heart failure and are responsible for the management of their condition in their own environment. Effective self-care not only requires patients to be adherent to prescribed treatment regimens such as medication, diet and exercise, but also to monitor and recognize symptom deterioration, and respond by either adapting behaviours or by seeking appropriate assistance.

To enable self-care to be successful it is important that patients and their caregivers have trust in, and are able to work in partnership with,

†Lynda Blue very sadly died during the production of this book. She was a pioneer of the role of specialist heart failure nurses and made an outstanding contribution to lives of patients with heart failure. Obituary available at https://www.heraldscotland.com/opinion/17353506.obituary-lynda-blue-pioneering-nurse-heart-failure-specialist/

their healthcare professional team. This involves shared decision-making, setting mutually agreed goals for learning, and regular review.

The European Society of Cardiology (2016) identified important topics and self-care skills to include in patient education and the professional behaviours to optimize learning and facilitate shared decision-making (Table 58.1).[1]

A number of psychosocial variables may complicate self-care behaviour in heart failure patients.[3]

Table 58.1 Key topics and self-care skills to include in patient education and the professional behaviour to optimize learning and facilitate shared decision-making

Education topic	Patient skills	Professional behaviours
Definition. Aetiology and trajectory of HF (including prognosis)	• Understand the cause of HF, symptoms, and disease trajectory • Make realistic decisions including decisions about treatment at end-of-life	• Provide oral and written information that takes account of educational grade and health literacy • Recognize HF disease barriers to communication and provide information at regular time intervals • Sensitively communicate information on prognosis at time of diagnosis, during decision-making about treatment options, when there is a change in the clinical condition, and whenever the patient requests
Symptom monitoring and self-care	• Monitor and recognize changes in signs and symptoms • Know how and when to contact a healthcare professional • In line with professional advice. Know when to self-manage diuretic therapy and fluid intake	• Provide individualized information to support self-management such as: • In the case of increasing dyspnoea or oedema or a sudden unexpected weight gain of >2 kg in 3 days. Patients may increase their diuretic dose and/or alert their healthcare team • Use of flexible diuretic regimen • Self-care support aids such as dosette box when appropriate
Pharmacological treatment	• Understand the indication, dosing, and side-effects of drugs • Recognize the common side-effects and know when to notify a healthcare professional • Recognize the benefits of taking medication as prescribed	• Provide written and oral information on dosing, effects, and side-effects (see web tables 7.4–7.8) practical guidance on use of pharmacological agents)
Implanted devices and percutaneous/surgical interventions	• Understand the indications and aims of procedures/implanted devices. • Recognize the common complications and know when to notify a healthcare professional • Recognize the importance and benefits of procedures/implanted devices	• Provide written and oral information on benefits and side-effects • Provide written and oral information on regular control of device functioning, along with documentation of regular check-up
Immunization	• Receive immunization against influenza and pneumococcal disease	• Advise on local guidance and immunization practice
Diet and alcohol	• Avoid excessive fluid intake • Recognize need for altered fluid intake such as: • Increase intake during periods of high heat and humidity. Nausea/vomiting • Fluid restriction of 1.5–2 L/day may be considered in patients with severe HF to relieve symptoms and congestion • Monitor body weight and prevent malnutrition • Eat healthily. Avoid excessive salt intake (>6 g/day) and maintain a healthy body weight. • Abstain from or avoid excessive alcohol intake, especially for alcohol-induced cardiomyopathy	• Individualize information on fluid intake to take into account body weight and periods of high heat and humidity. Adjust advice during periods of acute decompensation and consider altering these restrictions towards end of life • Tailor alcohol advise to aetiology of HF, e.g. abstinence in alcoholic cardiomyopathy • Normal alcohol guidelines apply (2 units per day in men or 1 unit per day in women). 1 unit in 10 mL of pure alcohol (e.g. 1 glass of wine ½ pint of beer. 1 measure of spirit). • For management of obesity (see Section 11.15)
Smoking and recreational substance use	• Stop smoking and taking recreational substances	• Refer to specialist for smoking cessation and drug withdrawal and replacement therapy • Consider referral for cognitive behavioural therapy and psychological support if patient wishes support to stop smoking
Exercise	• Undertake regular exercise sufficiently to provoke mild or moderate breathlessness	• Advise on exercise that recognizes physical and functional limitations, such as frailty, co-morbidities • Referral to exercise programme when appropriate
Travel and leisure	• Prepare travel and leisure activities according to physical capacity • Monitor and adapt fluid intake according to humidity (flights and humid climates) • Be aware of adverse reactions to sun exposure with certain medications (such as amiodarone) • Consider effect of high altitude on oxygenation • Take medicine in cabin luggage in the plane, have a list with you of treatment and the dosage with the generic name	• Refer to local country-specific driving regulations regarding ICD • Provide advice regarding flight security devices in presence of ICD
Sleep and breathing (see co-morbidities Section 11.16)	• Recognize problems with sleeping, their relationship with HF, and how to optimize sleep.	• Provide advice such as timing of diuretics, environment for sleep, device support • In presence of sleep-disordered breathing provide advice on weight reduction/control
Sexual activity (see co-morbidities Section 11.7)	• Be reassured about engaging in sex, provided sexual activity dose not provoke undue symptoms • Recognize problems with sexual activity, their relationship with HF and applied treatment and how to treat erectile dysfunction	• Provide advice on elimination factors predisposing to erectile dysfunction and available pharmacological treatment of erectile dysfunction • Refer to specialist for sexual counselling when necessary

HF, heart failure; ICD, implantable cardioverter–defibrillator.

Reproduced from Ponikowski P, Voors A, Anker SD, *et al.* ESC Guidelines for the diagnosis and treatment of acute and chronic heart failure of the European Society of Cardiology (ESC). Developed with the special contribution of the Heart Failure Association (HFA) of the ESC. *European Heart Journal* 2016;**37**:2129–2200 with permission from Oxford University Press.

Depression and anxiety can impair the patient's ability to perform self-care behaviours as it may impair cognition, energy, and motivation, leading to poorer understanding and clinical outcomes.

Approximately 20% of patients with heart failure are thought to be depressed.[4] Many more might be detected if a more sensitive tool is used to screen for depression on a regular basis. Health professionals should consider using validated assessment tools to help identify anxiety and depression in heart failure patients. This assessment should be within the context of a collaborative, stepped-care model which includes a locally defined clinical care pathway.[5]

Managing anxiety and depression can vary depending on local services and can incorporate non-pharmacological and pharmacological treatment. The evidence for psychological and pharmacological management of patients is, however, limited and requires future research.[5]

Cognitive behavioural therapy (CBT) has been reported to improve depression in patients with long-term conditions. A recent randomized controlled trial exploring the impact of CBT on depression and self-care in patients with heart failure found an improvement in depression compared to usual care after six months of treatment. The CBT intervention was not statistically significant in heart failure care but there were improvements in secondary outcomes of anxiety, fatigue, mental, and heart-failure-related quality of life, social functioning, and hospitalizations.[6] The Scottish Intercollegiate Guidelines Network recommends that cognitive behavioural therapy should be considered for patients with heart failure and clinical depression.[5]

Health literacy has also been linked to a patient's ability to self-manage and low health literacy has been shown to be an independent predictor of mortality.[7] One small before-and-after study of self-care management programmes for low-literacy individuals gives an indication that programmes tailored to literacy levels can lead to improved heart failure knowledge, improved self-weighing, increased accuracy of dose adjustment over time, and improved symptoms.[8] Self-management programmes should be tailored to individual patient requirements, paying particular emphasis to those with low literacy.[5]

To evaluate the effectiveness of interventions aimed at improving self-care behaviours of heart failure patients, a valid, reliable and user-friendly scale—the European Heart Failure Self-care Behaviour scale (EHFScB-9)—was developed and is used in various countries.[9] This scale is considered easy to administer and is practicable for use in everyday clinical practice. It reflects the actions that a heart failure patient undertakes to maintain life, healthy functioning, and well-being. The nine-item scale includes behaviours such as adherence to medication, diet, exercise, as well as self-management of symptoms, daily weighing, and response to fluid retention and when to seek advice when symptoms arise (Table 58.2). The EHFScB-9 was evaluated in 2013 as a reliable measure of heart failure self-care.[10]

Adherence to treatment

Treatment adherence is an essential component of self-care management in chronic heart failure. It has been shown to decrease morbidity, mortality, and improve general well-being.

Table 58.2 European Heart Failure Self-care Behaviour scale

		I completely agree	I don't agree at all
1	I weigh myself every day	1 2 3	4 5
2	If my shortness of breath increases, I contact my doctor or nurse	1 2 3	4 5
3	If my feet/legs become more swollen than usual, I contact my doctor or nurse	1 2 3	4 5
4	If I gain 2 kg in 1 week, I contact my doctor or nurse	1 2 3	4 5
5	I limit the amount of fluids I drink (not more than 1.5–2 litres per day)	1 2 3	4 5
6	If I experience increased fatigue, I contact my doctor or nurse	1 2 3	4 5
7	I eat a low salt diet	1 2 3	4 5
8	I take my medication as prescribed	1 2 3	4 5
9	I exercise regularly	1 2 3	4 5

Reproduced from Jaarsma T, Arestedt KF, Martensson J, Dracup K, Stromberg A. The European Heart Failure Heart Failure Self-care Behaviour scale revised into a nine-item scale (EHFScB-9): a reliable and valid international instrument. *Eur J Heart Fail* 2009;**11**:99–105 with permission from John Wiley and Sons.

Non-adherence to medication is multidimensional and may be intentional or unintentional. It can occur as a consequence of poor knowledge and understanding related to the condition, role of medication, absence of symptoms, diuretic inconvenience, cognitive decline, patient attitudes, or to lack of support related to frequent medication and dose adjustment in line with evidence-based treatment regimens.[11–13]

The World Health Organization reports that non-adherence to long-term therapies is related to health systems, socio-economic factors, condition, therapy, and patient characteristics.[14] Greater adherence is stimulated through various strategies such as a positive patient–professional relationship, education, and interdisciplinary team working. Prompting patients and carers in a timely manner about the importance of adherence to pharmacological and non-pharmacological strategies is essential to prevent adverse health outcomes.[15]

Using an integrated multi-professional educational approach is paramount to encourage greater patient and carer awareness and understanding about their condition and its treatment regimens. The role of the wider professional team, such as the community pharmacists, is unique and can contribute to promoting longer-term adherence aids and strategies. In addition, they can be a channel of communication between patients, their nurse, physician, and/or GP to remove any barriers in relation to seamless adjustment or facilitation of patient prescriptions in the community if any problems arise.[7]

An integrated team approach can also encourage patients to realize that different professionals are consistently sharing the same vital information, advice, and resources that may help the patient to make connections with changes in their condition, symptoms, and the requirement for medication adjustment. Following a comprehensive education and instruction process, it may be possible for many patients to alter their own diuretic regimen in response to a sustained weight gain and deteriorating symptoms.

Symptom monitoring/recognition

Several studies have demonstrated that patients delay seeking advice when their symptoms worsen.[16,17] This delay may be due to patients not being knowledgeable about their condition and not able to recognize the significance should their symptoms deteriorate.

It is important that patients are provided with individualized information and tools to support them to monitor and recognize changes in signs and symptoms and know how and when to contact their health care team/GP. It is also important to explore patients' understanding about their symptoms and to assess and document cognitive and psychological ability to self-manage.

Educating patients to understand the significance of a sudden change in weight—either a gain or loss—is vital to ensure that early clinical deterioration is detected and managed appropriately. By directly linking changes in body weight to clinical deterioration, patients can be empowered to respond accordingly by increasing or decreasing their diuretic dose appropriately; commonly known as a flexible diuretic regimen.

A key component of weight management is to determine, where possible, the patient's ideal 'dry' weight (when a patient who has had signs of fluid retention after diuretic treatment reaches a steady weight at which there are no further signs of fluid overload). Patients should be encouraged to weigh themselves daily at the same time, usually morning in minimal clothes, and record their weight in the chart/diary provided. It is important that patients understand that a sustained weight gain of >2 kg over 3 days may indicate that they are retaining too much fluid and they should be advised to increase their diuretic dose as outlined above and/or alert their healthcare team.

It is also important for patients to be advised that if they have a sustained weight loss of >2 kg over 3 days they may need to reduce or omit their diuretics, and then to contact their healthcare team in case they are volume-depleted due to excessive diuretic usage.

Fatigue management

Fatigue is a prominent and difficult symptom to manage in heart failure and can have a profound effect on patients' quality of life and their ability to perform everyday activities. Fatigue can occur as a direct consequence of cardiac and other clinical factors such as ageing, anaemia, poor sleep quality and psychosocial distress. It can also inhibit a patient's ability to adhere effectively to heart failure self-care behaviours to sustain good health and well-being. It is important that fatigue is acknowledged by the patient, carer, and the professional as a real symptom that originates from their heart failure condition or other multiple co-morbidities. Many patients describe their fatigue as idleness and do not fully understand that it is a real symptom that requires careful assessment and management in the same way that they would assess and manage their other symptoms. Fatigue is different from tiredness and may not always be helped by improved sleep quality. It is paramount that patients are assessed to ensure that their symptom of fatigue is not exacerbated by an underlying reversible cause such as anaemia, depression, sleep deprivation, or dehydration which may be easily treated. Patients should receive optimal tolerated doses of

evidence-based heart failure treatments to ensure that their clinical outcomes can be improved overall. Non-pharmacological management of fatigue in partnership with the wider multi-professional team should also be considered and may include attention to nutritional status; exercise tolerance, realistic goal-setting and the promotion of energy conservation strategies. Adherence to these factors combined with robust assessment and acknowledgement of fatigue will help to ensure that patients' general health and well-being is optimized.

Breathlessness management

Non-pharmacological management strategies for breathlessness should begin with a comprehensive assessment using validated assessment tools. The reference standard New York Heart Association (NYHA) classification tool is used widely in clinical practice (Table 58.3). However, there are several other validated breathlessness assessment tools that can be used.

Enquiry about the severity of the breathlessness, any recent changes and the impact the breathlessness is having on their everyday activities including sleep will alert the professional to any new symptoms associated with nocturnal dyspnoea, increasing orthopnoea or new-onset nocturnal cough. The management of acute breathlessness symptoms may be different from the management of chronic breathlessness. Assessment of chronic breathlessness should determine if the breathlessness is secondary to exertion, anxiety or both, as effective management of exertional and anxiety-induced breathlessness will require different strategies.

Non-pharmacological management of breathlessness should include working in partnership with the wider professional team. The unique contribution of the physiotherapist and occupational therapist should not be underestimated as they can provide invaluable information regarding energy conservation to minimize the risk of breathlessness associated with everyday activities. Additional partnership working may demonstrate the potential benefits of relaxation therapy, alternative treatments, and tailored programmes for individual patients to improve their breathlessness. Correct posture and gentle exercise advice regarding simple breathing techniques to increase the air flow should not be overlooked either. Advising patients to sit near an open window or to use a small electric fan can be of significant benefit to breathless patients. It is thought that the

Table 58.3 New York Heart Association functional classification (NYHA)

Class	Patient symptoms
I	No limitation of physical activity. Ordinary physical activity does not cause undue breathlessness, fatigue, or palpitations.
II	Slight limitation of physical activity. Comfortable at rest, but ordinary physical activity results in fatigue, palpitation, dyspnoea (shortness of breath).
III	Marked limitation of physical activity. Comfortable at rest, but less than ordinary physical activity results in undue breathlessness, fatigue, or palpitations.
IV	Unable to carry on any physical activity without discomfort. Symptoms at rest can be present. If physical activity is undertaken, discomfort is increases.

air flow has a desired effect on the sensory receptors found on the face and/or in the respiratory system in general.[18] The use of relaxation, complementary, and distraction therapy has been shown in small-scale studies to reduce the anxiety that very often precipitates an acute breathlessness event. Many of these therapies are under-utilized in heart failure due to the limited evidence base. However, for many patients who are living with the impact of breathlessness on a day-to-day basis they may be absolutely crucial.

Diet and alcohol

Careful fluid management is a key component of self-care in heart failure and should include individualized information on fluid intake, avoiding excessive fluid intake, and adjusting accordingly in relation to body weight during periods of high heat and humidity. During acute decompensation, health care professionals may consider advising patients to restrict their fluid intake to 1.5–2 L per day to relieve symptoms and congestion.[1]

It is also important to advise patients to monitor their weight to prevent malnutrition and/or obesity by eating healthily, avoid excessive salt intake (<6 g/day) and maintain a healthy body weight.[1]

Patients with heart failure should be advised to refrain from excessive alcohol consumption. Normal alcohol guidelines apply (2 units per day for men or 1 unit per day for women).[1] Long-term excessive alcohol consumption is an important cause of dilated cardiomyopathy.[5] When the aetiology is alcohol-related, patients should be strongly encouraged to stop drinking alcohol. Two prospective studies of patients with severe alcoholic cardiomyopathy found that after six months of total abstinence from alcohol, left ventricular function had significantly improved with an accompanying reduction in the cardiothoracic ratio on chest X-ray.[19,20]

Smoking/recreational substance abuse

Patients with heart failure should be encouraged to stop smoking and taking recreational substances. Professionals should discuss with patients about being referred for specialist advice for smoking cessation and drug withdrawal and replacement therapy. Consider referral for cognitive behavioural therapy and psychological support if patients wish to stop smoking and they are in agreement.[1]

Non-prescription medication

Many people take non-prescription medications such as herbal remedies, alternative medicines and over-the-counter preparations. Over-the-counter preparations may exacerbate heart failure symptoms and must be highlighted to the patient and caregiver. The main drug group of concern is non-steroidal anti-inflammatory drugs (NSAIDs), which can easily be bought over the counter. NSAIDs may lead to fluid retention and worsening renal failure, increasing the risk of hospitalization in patients with heart failure.[21]

A study of the use of non-prescription therapy in persons with heart failure found that 84.3% had used at least one drug that had not been recommended by their physician: 75.8% used over-the-counter drugs, 21.3% had used herbal remedies, and 20.9% had used vitamins and minerals. Importantly the patients were unaware of the possible interaction with heart failure therapies and rarely informed their physician that they were using these therapies.[22]

Sexual activity

Patients should be reassured that the safety of engaging in sexual activity can be sensibly correlated to the severity of their heart failure symptoms and should be considered in the same way as other physical demands. It is therefore reasonable for patients with NYHA I–II classification heart failure to engage in sensible sexual activity without provoking distressing symptoms. However, for patients with NYHA classification III or IV heart failure, sexual activity is not recommended until their heart failure status is stabilized and optimally managed.[23] Optimum evidenced-based treatments and adopting positions that decrease the physical exertion and breathing demand may positively influence sexual activity for heart failure patients.

Approximately 60–87% of heart failure patients experience loss of sexual interest.[23] It is therefore essential that advice, information, and referral to specialist services is appropriately and sensitively considered by health care professionals.[1] Many heart failure patients regard improving their quality of life, which may include sexual activity, as more important than improving survival.[23] Health care professionals should ensure comprehensive assessment of unmet needs to include optimal physical and psychological care management for patients who continue to experience difficulties associated with sexual activity.[1]

Immunization

Influenza infection is a major public health concern across the world as it is associated with high rates of morbidity and mortality each year.[24] Respiratory infections are reported to be a major cause of avoidable heart failure-related deaths and hospitalizations, particularly during winter months.[25]

Although there is general agreement in recommending that heart failure patients with no contraindications should be offered an annual influenza vaccine and one pneumococcal vaccination,[1,5] the degree of clinical effectiveness is controversial and there are few recent studies on this subject available.

An observational study of 59 202 heart failure patients in England during 1990–2013 found that cardiovascular hospitalizations fell by 30% in the year following influenza vaccination, compared with adjacent years with no vaccine, and the rate of respiratory infections fell by 16% during the year following vaccination. The study also looked at influenza uptake by heart failure patients through the 24-year period examined. During that time, the vaccination rose from <10% in 1990 to >60% in 2006 and gradually declined to <50% in 2013. The author attributed the rise in

uptake during the period from 1990 to 2006 in part to incentives that primary care physicians in England began receiving to administer influenza vaccine to their patients.[26]

Travel

Patients with stable compensated heart failure should be reassured about their safety to travel. However, they should be advised to make sure that they have adequate medical cover included in their travel insurance and that the insurance company is fully aware of their diagnosis and any hospitalizations that have occurred in the previous 12 months. General travel information should always include advice about medication and the importance of carrying extra medication doses in their hand luggage in addition to their regular supply. A full list of medications using the generic name will make certain that the exact drug equivalent can be issued overseas if a problem occurs. A brief letter from the GP or physician describing the traveller's medical problem and treatment may be helpful if illness does occur while travelling.

The safest and most suitable mode of travel should always be considered and where possible discussed with either the GP or physician. Most people with stable heart failure can travel as safely as everyone else, but the specific method of travel needs to be considered carefully well in advance.

The National Institute for Health and Care Excellence suggests that air travel is possible for individuals with heart failure depending on their clinical condition at the time of travel.[27] A British Cardiovascular Society working group published guidance on air travel with heart disease. In relation to chronic heart failure, if the patient has been treated in hospital or at home for pulmonary oedema, the restriction is that the person can fly six weeks after treatment, if stabilized and not acutely unwell. With NYHA classifications I and II, there is no restriction to air travel. However, with NYHA classification III, in-flight oxygen may be required. Patients with severe limitation of activity with symptoms at rest, correlating to NYHA classification IV, are advised not to fly without medical assistance and in-flight oxygen.[28]

Patients with heart failure who do wish to travel by air should be advised to check with their GP/physician that they are fit enough to travel. An anticipatory plan should include: letting the airport know in advance if assistance will be required, taking medications in cabin luggage in the plane, having a list of treatments and dosage with the generic name, awareness of time zone changes to ensure timely medication administration, diuretic adjustment, managing the increased risk of dehydration particularly in hot climates, and deep venous thrombosis prophylactic strategies.

The need for oxygen supplementation during the flight should also be considered and discussed as appropriately indicated with the healthcare professional in preparation for travel. It is also important that patients are advised to monitor and adapt their fluid intake according to humidity (flights and humid climates).[1]

If a patient has a cardiac device, they should be advised to take their advice identification/card with them and inform the airport staff that they have a device inserted. Modern cardiac devices are well shielded against interference, although the metal casing may still trigger the security alarm. Airport staff should be alerted by the patient that hand-held metal detectors should be avoided. Patients should also be advised that the Medicines and Healthcare products Regulatory Agency can provide them with further advice and information on the safety aspects of airport systems and cardiac devices.[29]

Travelling by car has many advantages, especially for patients who are prescribed diuretics. Car travel can enable route planning and regular stops, allowing mobilization every two to three hours, which may reduce the development of dependent oedema and deep venous thromboemboli.

Patients with a diagnosis of heart failure can continue to drive a car provided there are no symptoms likely to affect safe driving.

Patients should check driving regulations in their respective countries. In the UK, for example, the Driver and Vehicle Licensing Agency (DVLA) recommendation for drivers who have had a cardiac resynchronization therapy (pacemaker) implanted is that they must notify the DVLA and driving can resume after at least one month following implementation if there are no symptoms likely to affect safe driving and no other disqualifying condition.[30] The DVLA recommendation for drivers who have had an implantable cardioverter defibrillator is outlined in (Box 58.1).[30]

Discussion

Providing effective non-pharmacological advice is an important component of heart failure care. The consequences of failing to address this issue adequately can be both considerable and wide ranging for patients and their caregivers, as well as incurring significant economic costs on the health care system generally.

Heart failure patients need continuous, long-term support in the community and should ideally be seen as soon as possible following hospital discharge. A community-based health care professional can provide advice and support which complements the information given on hospital discharge. Furthermore, a comprehensive assessment of both patients' and caregivers' needs and knowledge base is essential to inform future education and care requirements. Deviating from recommended treatments and self-care behaviours can often lead to exacerbation of symptoms and reduced quality of life, which very often results in increased health utilization and escalation of the associated costs.

Effective self-care management requires professionals to support patients and carers to feel empowered to inform shared decision-making and agreed goals. This should increase their ability to interpret symptoms, willingness to participate and seek help at an early stage.

As heart failure management continues to evolve, the requirement for effective and responsive strategies increases. Key areas for further research and development will include the use of digital technology in supporting health care professionals, patients, and their caregivers to implement self-care behaviours effectively. To address many of the issues discussed in this chapter requires an integrated health care system across invisible care boundaries.

Box 58.1 Implantable cardioverter–defibrillator (ICD)

Group 1: car and lorry drivers

In all cases of ICD for sustained ventricular arrhythmia associated with incapacity, driving must stop for 6 months from the date of ICD implantation and any resumption requires:

- the device being under regular review with interrogation
- no other disqualifying condition.

Group 2: bus and lorry drivers

ICD implantation is a permanent bar to Group 2 licensing. In all cases of ICD implantation (including prophylactic ICD implantation) driving must stop permanently and:

- the DVLA must be notified
- the licence will be refused or revoked permanently.

	Group 1: car and motorcycle	Group 2: bus and lorry
ICD for sustained ventricular arrhythmia associated with incapacity		
Without further sequelae	✗ Must not drive and may need to notify the DVLA. Driving may resume after 6 months from a first implant—except that any of the sequelae 1–4 below require further specific restrictions and may require notification to the DVLA.	✗ Must not drive and must notify the DVLA. Licence will be refused or revoked permanently.
1. With any shock therapy and/or pacing for symptomatic tachycardia	✗ Must not drive and must notify the DVLA. Must not drive for a further 6 months from the time of any shock therapy or pacing for symptomatic tachycardia.	✗ Must not drive and must notify the DVLA. Licence will be refused or revoked permanently.
2. With incapacity following implantation or therapy (whether caused by device or arrhythmia)	✗ Must not drive and may need to notify the DVLA. Must not drive for 2 years after symptoms of incapacity and must notify the DVLA. Exceptions to this 2-year requirement apply as follows, but the minimum initial restriction after implantation still applies (i.e. must not drive for 6 months). 1. If therapy delivery was due to an inappropriate cause such as atrial fibrillation or, for example, programming issues: ▪ driving may resume 1 month after complete control of any cause to the satisfaction of the cardiologist. 2. If therapy delivery was due to sustained ventricular tachycardia or ventricular fibrillation: ▪ driving may resume 6 months after event ▪ provided preventive steps against recurrence have been taken with anti-arrhythmic drugs or ablation procedure, for example, ▪ and provided there is an absence of further symptomatic therapy.	✗ Must not drive and must notify the DVLA. Licence will be refused or revoked permanently.
3. With any revision of electrodes or anti-arrhythmic drug treatment	✗ Must not drive but need not notify the DVLA. Driving may resume 1 month after electrode revision or drug alteration. The minimum initial restriction after implantation still applies (must not drive for 6 months).	✗ Must not drive and must notify the DVLA. Licence will be refused or revoked permanently.
4. With defibrillator box change	✗ Must not drive but need not notify the DVLA. Driving may resume 1 week after box change. The minimum initial restriction after implantation still applies (must not drive for 6 months).	✗ Must not drive and must notify the DVLA. Licence will be refused or revoked permanently.
ICD for sustained ventricular arrhythmia not associated with incapacity		
	✗ Must not drive for 1 month and may need to notify the DVLA. Driving may resume 1 month after implantation and the DVLA need not be notified, provided: ▪ presentation was a 'non-disqualifying' cardiac event, i.e. haemodynamically stable sustained ventricular tachycardia without incapacity ▪ LV ejection fraction is greater than 35% ▪ no fast ventricular tachycardia (VT) induced on electrophysiological study, i.e. RR interval of less than 250 milliseconds ▪ during the post-implantation study, any induced VT could be pace-terminated by the ICD twice, without acceleration. Note: should ICD subsequently deliver anti-tachycardia pacing and/or shock therapy (except during normal clinical testing), the DVLA must be notified and the restrictions must be applied as for sustained ventricular arrhythmia associated with incapacity).	✗ Must not drive and must notify the DVLA. Licence will be refused or revoked permanently.
Prophylactic ICD		
In asymptomatic individuals with a high risk of significant arrhythmia	✗ Must not drive and must notify the DVLA: ▪ driving may resume 1 month after implantation (need not notify the DVLA if remains asymptomatic and no ICD therapy needed) ▪ should the ICD subsequently deliver anti-tachycardia pacing and/or shock therapy (except during normal clinical testing), the DVLA must be notified and the restrictions must be noted as for sustained ventricular arrhythmia associated with incapacity) ▪ need not notify the DVLA if remains asymptomatic and no ICD therapy needed.	Must not drive and must notify the DVLA. Licence will be refused or revoked permanently.

Reproduced from Driver and Vehicle Licensing Agency. Assessing fitness to drive: guide for medical professionals. 11 March 2016. https://www.gov.uk/guidance/cardiovascular-disorders-assessing-fitness-to-drive#implantable-cardioverter-defibrillator-icd

REFERENCES

1. Ponikowski P, Voors A, Anker SD, *et al*. ESC Guidelines for the diagnosis and treatment of acute and chronic heart failure of the European Society of Cardiology (ESC). Developed with the special contribution of the Heart Failure Association (HFA) of the ESC. *Eur Heart J* 2016;**37**:2129–200.
2. McGreal MH, Hogan MJ, Walsh-Irwin C, *et al*. Heart failure self-care interventions to reduce clinical events and symptom burden. *Res Rep Clin Cardiol* 2014;**5**:243–57.
3. Riegel B, Moser DK, Anker SD, *et al*. American Heart Association Council on Cardiovascular Nursing; American Heart Association Council on Cardiovascular Nursing; American Heart Association Council on Clinical Cardiology; American Heart Association Council on Nutrition, Physical Activity, and Metabolism; American Heart Association Interdisciplinary Council on Quality of Care and Outcomes Research. State of the science: promoting self-care in persons with heart failure: a scientific statement from the American Heart Association. *Circulation* 2009;**120**:1141–63.
4. Lainscak M, Blue L, Clark AL, *et al*. Self-care management of heart failure: practical recommendations from the Patient Care Committee of the Heart Failure Association of the ESC. *Eur J Heart Fail* 2011;**13**:115–26.
5. Scottish Intercollegiate Guidelines Network. *Guideline 147: Management of chronic heart failure: a national clinical guideline*. SIGN, Edinburgh, 2016.
6. Freedland KE, Carney RM, RICH MW, *et al*. Cognitive behaviour therapy for depression and self-care in heart failure patients: a randomized clinical trial. *JAMA Intern Med* 2015;**175**(11):1773–82.
7. Lowrie R, Johansson L, Forsyth P, *et al*. Experiences of a community pharmacy service to support adherence and self-management in chronic heart failure. *Int J Clinical Pharm* 2014; **36**:154–62.
8. DeWalt DA, Pignone M, Malone R, *et al*. Development and pilot testing of a disease management program for low literacy patients with heart failure. *Patient Educ Couns* 2004;**55**(1):78–86.
9. Jaarsma T, Arestedt KF, Martensson J, Dracup K, Stromberg A. The European Heart Failure Heart Failure Self-care Behaviour scale revised into a nine-item scale (EHFScB-9): a reliable and valid international instrument. *Eur J Heart Fail* 2009;**11**:99–105.
10. Vellone E, Jaarsma T, Stromberg A, *et al*. The European Heart Failure Self-care Behavioural Scale: new insights into functional, reliability, precision and scoring procedure. *Patient Ed Counsell* 2014;**94**(1):79–102.
11. Fitzgerald AA, Powers JD, Ho PM, *et al*. Impact of medication nonadherence on hospitalizations and mortality in heart failure. *J Card Fail* 2011;**17**(8):664–9.
12. Corotto PS, McCarey MM, Adams S, Khazanie P, Whellan DJ. Heart failure patient adherence: epidemiology, cause, and treatment. *Heart Fail Clin* 2013;**9**(1):49–58.
13. Oosterom-Calo R, van Ballegooijen AJ, Terwee CB, *et al*. Determinants of adherence to heart failure medication: a systematic literature review. *Heart Fail Rev* 2013;**18**(4):409–27.
14. World Health Organization. *Adherence to long term therapies: evidence for action*. Switzerland: WHO; 2003.
15. Wu JR, Moser DK, Lennie TA, *et al*. Factors influencing medication adherence in patients with heart failure. *Heart Lung* 2008;**37**(1):8–16.
16. Patel H, Shafazand M, Scahaufelberger M, Ekman I. Reasons for seeking acute care in chronic heart failure. *Eur J Heart Fail* 2007;**9**:702–8.
17. Clark AM, Freydberg CN, McAlister, *et al*. Patient and informal caregivers' knowledge of heart failure: necessary but insufficient for effective self-care. *Eur J Heart Fail* 2009;**11**:617–21.
18. Booth S, Moffat C, Burkin J, Galbraith S, Bausewein C. Nonpharmacological interventions for breathlessness. *Curr Opin Supp Pall Care* 2011;**5**(2):77–86.
19. Guillo P, Mansourati J, Maheu B, *et al*. Long-term prognosis in patients with alcoholic cardiomyopathy and severe heart failure after total abstinence. *Am J Cardiol* 1997;**79**(9):1276–8.
20. Jacob AJ, McLaren KM, Boon NA. Effects of abstinence on alcoholic heart muscle disease. *Am J Cardiol* 1991;**68**(8):805–7.
21. Garcia RLA, Hernandez-Diaz S. Nonsteroidal inflammatory drugs as a trigger of clinical heart failure. *Epidemiology* 2003;**14**:240–6.
22. Dal Corso E, Bondiani AL, Zanolla L, Vassanelli C. Nurse educational activity on non-prescriptive therapies in patients with chronic heart failure. *Eur J Cardiovasc Nurs* 2007;**6**:314–20.
23. Levine GN, Steinke EE, Bakaeen FG, *et al*. Sexual activity and cardiovascular disease. A scientific statement from the American Heart Association. *Circulation* 2012;**125**:1058–72.
24. Wang CS, Wang ST, Lai CT, Lin LJ, Chou P. Impact of influenza vaccination on major cause specific mortality. *Vaccine* 2007;**25**:1196–203.
25. Stewart S, MacIntyre K, Capewell S, McMurray JJV. Heart failure in a cold climate: seasonal variation in heart failure-related morbidity and mortality. *J Am Coll Cardiol* 2002;**39**:760.
26. Zoler ML. Flu vaccination cut hospitalizations in heart failure patients. *Fam Pract News*, May 2016.
27. National Institute for Health and Care Excellence. *Chronic heart failure in adults: management*. NICE, London, 2010. http://tinyurl.com/z5bmvnp (accessed December 2016).
28. Smith D, Toff W, Joy M, *et al*. Fitness to fly for patients with cardiovascular disease. *Heart* 2010;**96**(1):Suppl 2:ii1–16.
29. British Heart Foundation. *Holidays and travel*. http://tinyurl.com/op39968 (accessed December 2016).
30. Driver and Vehicle Licensing Agency. *Assessing fitness to drive: guide for medical professionals*. 11 March 2016. https://www.gov.uk/guidance/cardiovascular-disorders-assessing-fitness-to-drive#implantable-cardioverter-defibrillator-icd (accessed January 2017).

SECTION 13

Device therapy for heart failure

59

Implantable cardioverter–defibrillators

Jane A. Cannon and Derek T. Connelly

Introduction

The implantable cardioverter–defibrillator (ICD) is established as an effective therapy for ventricular arrhythmias and is now routinely used for both primary and secondary prevention of sudden cardiac death in at-risk populations. Patients with heart failure have an increased propensity to arrhythmic sudden death and large randomized trials have demonstrated a clear mortality benefit following ICD implantation in selected heart failure patients. Despite this, the optimal use of ICDs in patients with heart failure remains a particularly challenging area of clinical practice. This is primarily due to the fact that patients with heart failure are exposed to competing risks, which are both dynamic and difficult to quantify. As the cost and morbidity associated with ICD implantation are not insignificant, careful consideration of the risks and benefits associated with ICD implantation in each individual patient is required. This chapter reviews ICD therapy and considers the rationale for ICD implantation in patients with heart failure.

Sudden cardiac death in heart failure

Heart failure is not only a common condition associated with an extremely high mortality, it is a diverse, complex clinical syndrome in which patients are exposed to competing risks, of sudden arrhythmic death, or death from progressive pump failure.[1,2] Prevention of arrhythmic sudden cardiac death (SCD) constitutes a particular challenge because accurate risk prediction in such a large and heterogeneous population is extremely difficult.[3] Achieving effective prevention of SCD in heart failure is one of the principal challenges facing contemporary cardiovascular medicine.

Incidence and prevalence

Sudden cardiac deaths are, by definition, unexpected and are often unwitnessed, making the classification of the exact cause of death difficult in many cases. Estimates of the prevalence of SCD in heart failure come mainly from observational studies or from clinical trials, in which the definition of SCD is necessarily both arbitrary and pragmatic.[4] The accepted definition is death from a cardiac cause that is sudden and unexpected, in the absence of progressive cardiac deterioration, either within 1 h of cardiac symptoms, in bed during sleep or within 24 h of last being seen alive.[5] Where these tight definitions in end-point classification are used, as much as 50% of total mortality in heart failure is due to SCD.[6,7]

Aetiology

Sudden cardiac death may be caused by a number of different underlying pathologies, including ventricular arrhythmia, acute cardiogenic shock, tamponade, and acute pulmonary embolism. The relative importance of arrhythmic or vascular events as causes of SCD in heart failure is debated.[7] Data regarding the specific aetiology of SCD are difficult to gather, but where they are available, recordings from monitored episodes of SCD show that the cause is ventricular arrhythmia in ~85% of cases.[8–11] To what extent these ventricular arrhythmias are primary or secondary to myocardial ischaemia is more difficult to ascertain. Autopsy data from the Assessment of Treatment with Lisinopril and Survival (ATLAS) trial suggested that myocardial infarction (MI) may be implicated in as many as 40% of sudden deaths in patients with heart failure.[12] However, a review of 157 episodes of ambulatory SCD that occurred during Holter monitoring concluded that the incidence of ST changes prior to ventricular arrhythmias was low.[11] Data from the second Multicenter Automatic Defibrillator Trial (MADIT-II) showed that 51% of deaths in the conventional therapy arm met accepted criteria for SCD, compared with 27% of deaths in the ICD arm,[5] suggesting that around a quarter of all deaths and around half of sudden deaths were due to arrhythmia and amenable to ICD treatment.

Risk stratification for SCD in heart failure

At present, left ventricular ejection fraction (LVEF) is used to risk-stratify patients with heart failure for ICD therapy. Although this method has identified populations in whom significant mortality reductions have been demonstrated, the 7% absolute risk reduction observed with an ICD in the Sudden Cardiac Death in Heart Failure Trial (SCDHeFT) was achieved with only 21% of patients receiving appropriate therapy over five years,[13] suggesting that the use of LVEF alone is suboptimal. A number of non-invasive risk stratification tools have been proposed as having predictive value for arrhythmic events; however, none has the required sensitivity or

specificity to predict SCD accurately.[14,15] The search for improved risk stratification tools continues and the challenge of delivering effective population-wide prevention of SCD through ICD therapy is dependent upon their development.

Pharmacological therapy to prevent arrhythmic SCD in heart failure

Until recently, attempts to prevent SCD have relied upon pharmacological therapy to reverse LV remodelling. Disease-modifying therapy with β-blockers,[16] angiotensin converting enzyme inhibitors (ACEi),[17] angiotensin receptor–neprilysin inhibitors,[18] angiotensin receptor blockers,[2] and aldosterone antagonists[19] reduces the risk of SCD in patients with heart failure and after MI. However, even patients on optimal medical therapy remain at high risk of SCD[2,6] and specific anti-arrhythmic drug therapy has failed to improve survival.[13,20,21]

Competing risks in heart failure

Patients with heart failure are exposed to competing risks. Heart failure carries a risk of sudden death along with a risk of death from progressive pump failure. In addition, many patients with heart failure are elderly and have co-morbidities, which will also influence survival. An interaction is recognized between severity of heart failure symptoms and mode of death, which was exemplified in an analysis of cause-specific mortality by New York Heart Association (NYHA) class at enrolment in the Metoprolol CR/XL Randomised Intervention Trial In Congestive Heart Failure (MERIT-HF) study, which included 3991 patients with NYHA II–IV heart failure and LVEF ≤40%.[6] As shown in **Figure 59.1**, the proportion of sudden deaths reduced with increasing NYHA class (64%, 59%, and 33% respectively), whereas the proportion of deaths due to worsening heart failure increased (24%, 26%, and 56% respectively).

Due to these competing risks in a population with heart failure, any treatment that significantly reduces the risk of SCD will be expected to increase the risk of death from worsening heart failure since more patients will be alive to be exposed to this risk. For this reason, ICD trials have been designed to assess their impact on overall mortality, assuming that a reduction in arrhythmic sudden death will occur, but accepting that conversion to death from worsening heart failure within a short time-scale is not a desirable outcome. The correct targeting of ICD therapy is crucial to ensure that patients not only gain sufficient survival benefit to justify the risks of implantation but also can enjoy improved survival free of debilitating heart failure for a reasonable length of time. This reinforces the need for accurate prognostication in patients with heart failure, such that ICD therapy can be appropriately directed. It also underlines the importance of optimization of medical therapy for heart failure when ICD therapy is being considered, and following implantation.

The implantable–cardioverter defibrillator

The concept of transvenous defibrillation for ventricular arrhythmias was developed by Mirowski and colleagues in the 1970s[22] and the first ICDs were implanted in patients with recurrent refractory ventricular arrhythmias in 1980.[23,24] These early devices incorporated large pulse generators implanted in the abdomen and connected to epicardial sensing and shocking electrodes, tunnelled from the chest. The implant procedure required thoracotomy and was associated with a considerable complication rate. Since then, significant improvements in technology have resulted in systems with smaller pulse generators that can be implanted prepectorally under local anaesthesia, and which employ transvenous lead systems integrated for pacing, tachycardia detection, and administration of therapies. The components of an ICD system are shown in **Figure 59.2**.

Pulse generator

An ICD pulse generator comprises a power source, capacitors for storing electrical charge and the circuits and microprocessors necessary to manage its output. It must combine a pacing capability with

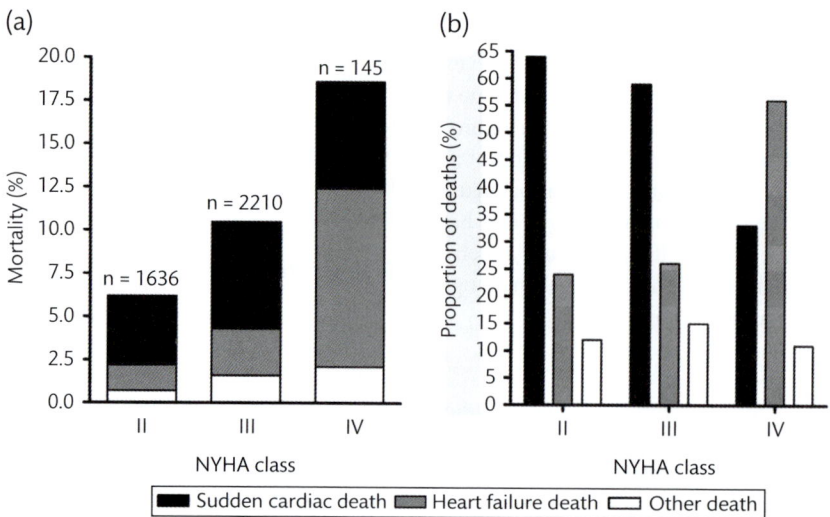

Figure 59.1 (a) Crude mortality rates in the MERIT-HF study according to NYHA class at randomization. The adjudicated cause of death is shown by the colour of the bar. Mean follow-up was one year, mortality data from active and placebo arms are pooled, and the group size is stated in each case. (b) Proportion of total deaths in each NYHA class attributable to sudden cardiac death, heart failure or other causes.

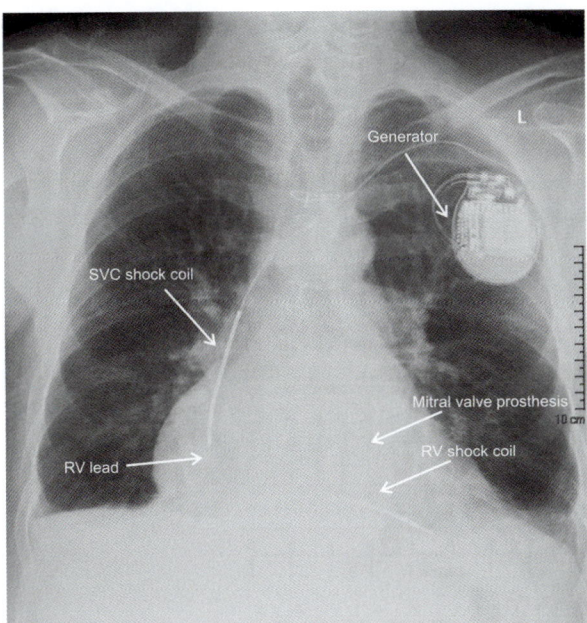

Figure 59.2 Chest radiograph from a patient with a transvenous ICD. The generator, right ventricular (RV), and the shock coils are indicated. SVC, superior vena cava.

the potential to deliver high-energy shocks within seconds of tachycardia detection. This means that specialized anode/cathode configurations are required to allow maintenance of high current and voltage during charging of the high-voltage capacitors for a defibrillation shock. As a consequence, ICD pulse generators are larger than those used in conventional pacemaker systems, and usually have a shorter battery life. The ICD pulse generator also incorporates the circuitry for the monitoring and programming functions necessary for these devices. In most ICD configurations, as described below, the pulse generator or 'can' may also form an active part of the lead system.

Lead systems

ICD lead systems must combine sensing, pacing, and defibrillation functions. In order to achieve this, the right ventricular (RV) endocardial lead contains a series of separately insulated conductors running in parallel. Standard coil conductors are required for pacing and sensing: one attached to the distal tip electrode and a second attached to the proximal ring electrode will supply bipolar sensing and stimulation. Delivery of a defibrillation shock is achieved using a high-voltage cable conductor connected to a shock coil on the external surface of the lead. In single-coil systems the coil is positioned on the distal portion of the lead and therefore sits in the RV apex, and the shock energy is passed between the coil and the pulse generator (an 'active can' configuration). In a two-coil system, there is a second coil positioned more proximally which sits in the superior vena cava (SVC), with defibrillation energy being passed between the RV coil and both the SVC coil and the can. The Jewel Active Can Study randomized ICD recipients to receive ICDs with either active or passive can configuration and found that the active can system was associated with lower defibrillation thresholds and shorter implant times without any adverse events at three months.[25]

Dual-chamber ICD systems incorporate a standard atrial lead in addition to the integrated RV defibrillation lead. The atrial lead can be used for sensing or stimulating in the right atrium and is used when dual-chamber pacing is desirable, or when atrial electrograms will improve tachycardia differentiation. Cardiac resynchronization therapy defibrillator (CRT-D) devices have an additional LV epicardial lead, which is used to provide atrio-biventricular pacing.

Detection algorithms

Rate sensing

The effectiveness of an ICD depends upon its ability to detect the occurrence of those ventricular arrhythmias that require treatment. In a single-chamber system, the determination of ventricular tachyarrhythmia is principally achieved by measuring the rate of the sensed ventricular electrogram. The sensing function of an integrated ICD lead is therefore critical to its function, particularly during ventricular fibrillation (VF). In order to avoid undersensing of small-amplitude potentials during VF, ICDs employ automatic algorithms that adjust their sensitivity over the cardiac cycle. Heart rate intervals, usually referred to as 'detection zones', are set for ventricular tachycardia (VT) and VF. The detection algorithm will stipulate a certain number of consecutive R–R intervals within the detection interval before designating a tachycardia to be VT or VF. Following administration of therapy, a series of usually less stringent redetection rate criteria are applied to ascertain whether it has been successful.

Supraventricular tachycardia discrimination

The major disadvantage with identification of VT or VF by rate-sensing algorithms is that atrial fibrillation (AF) or supraventricular tachycardia (SVT), occurring within the detection zone, may trigger clinically inappropriate therapies (see **Figure 59.3**). Several different algorithms are available to aid the identification of SVT occurring within the VT detection zone, so that therapy can be appropriately withheld. These include analyses of the R–R interval stability, the time-scale of tachycardia onset, and the electrogram morphology. All of these algorithms have potential pitfalls and may result in delayed therapy for VT. As such they are optional and the ICD is always programmed to deliver therapy if a tachycardia designated as SVT persists within the VT detection zone. In dual-chamber systems, atrial electrograms can be used to improve arrhythmia classification, by identifying atrioventricular dissociation.[26] However, in MADIT-II rates of inappropriate therapies were not different between dual-chamber and single-chamber devices.[27] This comparison may be confounded by the fact that stored electrograms from a dual-chamber device give more information regarding the tachycardia and inappropriate therapies may therefore be identified more often than with a single-chamber system. In the Detect Supraventricular Tachycardia Study, the dual-chamber detection group experienced a modest reduction in the proportion of SVTs that were inappropriately detected as VT (30.9% vs 39.5%), but this did not translate into a reduction in inappropriate shocks.[28] Nevertheless, the availability of atrial electrograms can often be invaluable in 'troubleshooting' and in planning subsequent treatment for the patient, including changes in programming, drug therapy, and ablation (see **Figure 59.4**).

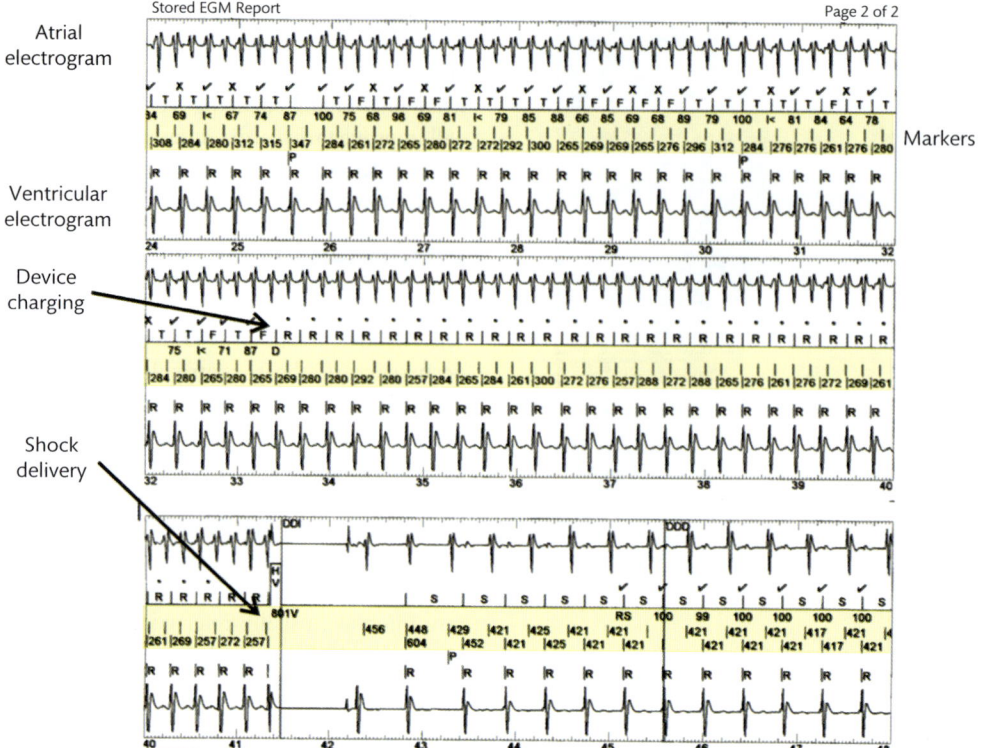

Figure 59.3 Inappropriate ICD therapy. Stored electrograms from a dual-chamber ICD in a patient who experienced multiple inappropriate therapies for atrial fibrillation and flutter. Upper panel shows the atrial electrogram and the ventricular electrograms are shown below; the electrograms are separated by a series of markers, highlighted in yellow, which display the timing of the sensed atrial and ventricular activity along with the corresponding cycle lengths. The electrograms show a ventricular tachyarrhythmia with an atrial rate greater than the ventricular rate. Due to the persistent high ventricular rate, the ICD charges and administers a shock, which restores sinus rhythm. In this case, the presence of an atrial electrogram allows the identification of the higher atrial rate during the tachycardia and clear demonstration of inappropriate shock therapy for rapidly conducted atrial fibrillation. The patient went on to have AF ablation (shown in Figure 58.4).

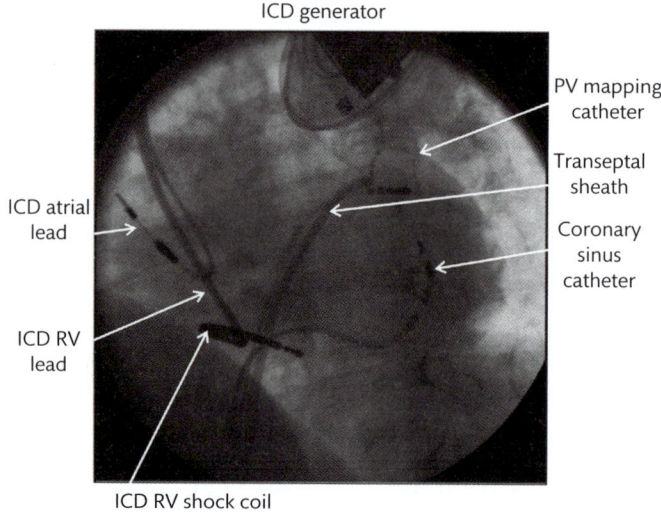

Figure 59.4 Atrial fibrillation ablation in an ICD patient. Fluoroscopy images from a pulmonary vein (PV) isolation procedure from the same patient as in Figure 58.3. The ICD generator, atrial lead and right ventricle (RV) shock coil are all indicated. There is a catheter in the coronary sinus and a transeptal sheath from which the circular ablation catheter has been placed at the ostium of the left superior pulmonary vein.

Programmable therapies

Modern ICD systems incorporate complex programmable pacing and anti-tachyarrhythmia therapies. Optimal ICD programming should always be based on the individual's needs and subject to regular review.

Pacing

All transvenous ICDs have programmable pacing functions, and, depending on the device and lead systems used, pacing capabilities can range from back-up VVI pacing with single-chamber systems, though 'physiologic' (DDDR) pacing with dual-chamber ICDs to atrio-biventricular pacing with cardiac resynchronization therapy defibrillators (CRT-Ds). The rationale for provision of back-up VVI capabilities with all ICDs is to protect from post-shock bradycardia, which may be sufficient to cause haemodynamic compromise in the absence of bradycardia pacing. In dual-chamber systems, the atrial lead can sense atrial electrograms and therefore makes improved SVT discrimination possible and will also allow provision of atrially based pacing as a treatment for atrial arrhythmias or in the event that the patient were to develop conducting system disease. Cardiac resynchronization therapy pacing (CRT-P), which employs atrio-biventricular pacing to correct interventricular dyssynchrony, has

been shown to improve outcome in patients with severe symptomatic heart failure despite optimal medical therapy, who also have LV dysfunction and QRS prolongation,[29] and is combined with a defibrillator function (CRT-D) in these patients when an ICD indication also exists.

Anti-tachycardia pacing

Overdrive or anti-tachycardia pacing (ATP) is an effective therapy for VT,[30] and ICDs can be programmed to administer various types of ATP for tachycardias falling within the VT detection zone. ATP is administered using trains of stimuli, either in a burst (constant cycle length) or a ramp (decremental cycle length) configuration, with the ATP cycle length determined to be a proportion of the tachycardia cycle length (see **Figure 59.5**). Unlike defibrillation shocks, ATP is seldom uncomfortable for the patient and successful ATP should therefore improve device tolerability, having also the potential advantage of minimizing the impact of therapies on battery life. However, there is a risk of tachycardia acceleration during ATP, and prolonged VT during multiple unsuccessful attempts at ATP may lead to haemodynamic compromise. In addition, rapid

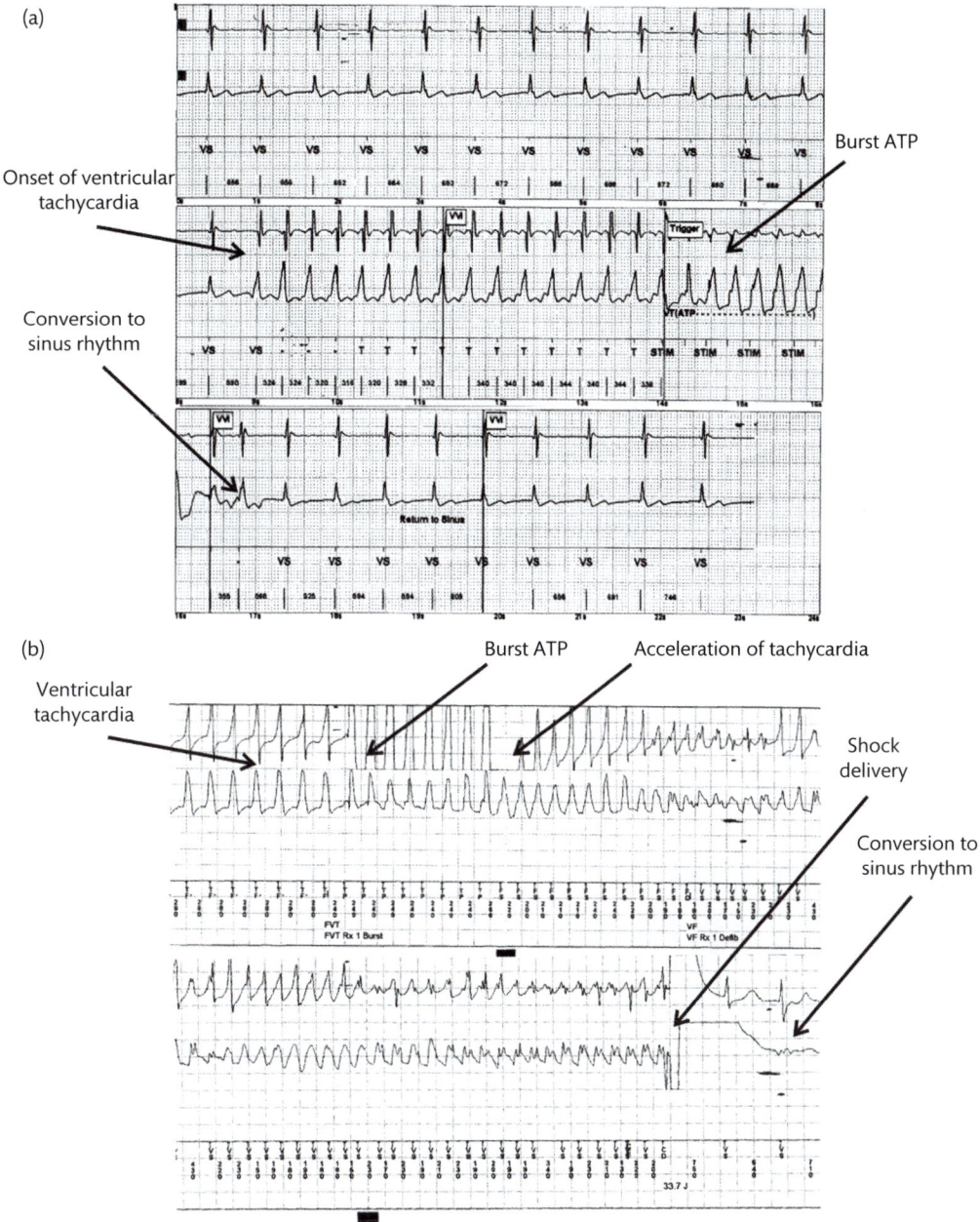

Figure 59.5 Anti-tachycardia pacing for ventricular tachycardia. (a) Stored electrograms from an ICD in a patient who received a successful burst of anti-tachycardia pacing (ATP) for ventricular tachycardia (VT). The upper panel shows sinus rhythm, and the onset of VT is shown in the middle panel. The tachycardia is then sensed by the ICD and a burst of ATP is administered, which results in conversion to sinus rhythm. (b) Stored electrograms from an ICD in a patient who received an unsuccessful burst of ATP for VT. The upper panel shows VT with a burst of ATP which results in acceleration of the tachycardia into the ventricular fibrillation (VF) zone. The tachycardia is re-sensed and the device charges before delivering a shock, which results in conversion to sinus rhythm.

VTs (>200 bpm) are less likely to respond to ATP and more likely to cause haemodynamic compromise, particularly in patients with pre-existing LV dysfunction.[30] In order to optimize ATP delivery, most devices therefore allow programming of two VT detection zones with differential ATP protocols. A slow VT zone can therefore be programmed with less aggressive (and therefore lower risk of acceleration) ATP algorithms and may include more attempts before a shock is eventually delivered. Alternatively, a fast VT zone can be programmed with a lower number of more aggressive ATP protocols before defaulting to defibrillation.

Defibrillation

The mainstay of effective tachycardia treatment by an ICD is the defibrillator capability. In the event of detection of a tachycardia within the VF detection zone or the failure of ATP to terminate a tachycardia, the ICD will deliver a defibrillation shock. Defibrillation shocks are effective in terminating spontaneously occurring VT and VF in the majority of cases.[31] An example of successful VF termination by an ICD is shown in **Figure 59.6**. Effective defibrillation depends on a sufficient voltage (the defibrillation threshold) being delivered to depolarize the bulk of the myocardium. In order to ensure effective defibrillation, the pulse generator must be able to charge the high-voltage capacitor such that the threshold voltage is

consistently surpassed. Historically, assessment of the defibrillation threshold has been a critical component of the ICD implant and programming procedure, though prospective data have failed to show clinical benefit associated with this practice.[32]

ICD therapies as end-points in clinical trials

Appropriate ICD therapies are often used as end-points in studies of ICD recipients. In interpreting such studies it is important to note that appropriate ICD therapies are not a surrogate for sudden cardiac death. An analysis from the DEFINITE trial suggested that patients in the ICD arm experienced appropriate ICD shocks for VF/VT at a rate twice that of the SCD rate in the medical therapy arm, suggesting that around half of the ventricular arrhythmic events treated by an ICD may have been well tolerated or self-terminating and would not have resulted in the patient's death.[33]

Reducing inappropriate therapies

Inappropriate device-delivered therapy is defined as therapy delivered for non-ventricular tachyarrhythmias and occurs in 8–40% of patients with ICDs *in situ*.[34] The Multicentre Automatic Defibrillator Implantation Trial—Reduce Inappropriate Therapy (MADIT-RIT)[35] randomly assigned 1500 patients with a primary prevention indication to receive an ICD with one of three

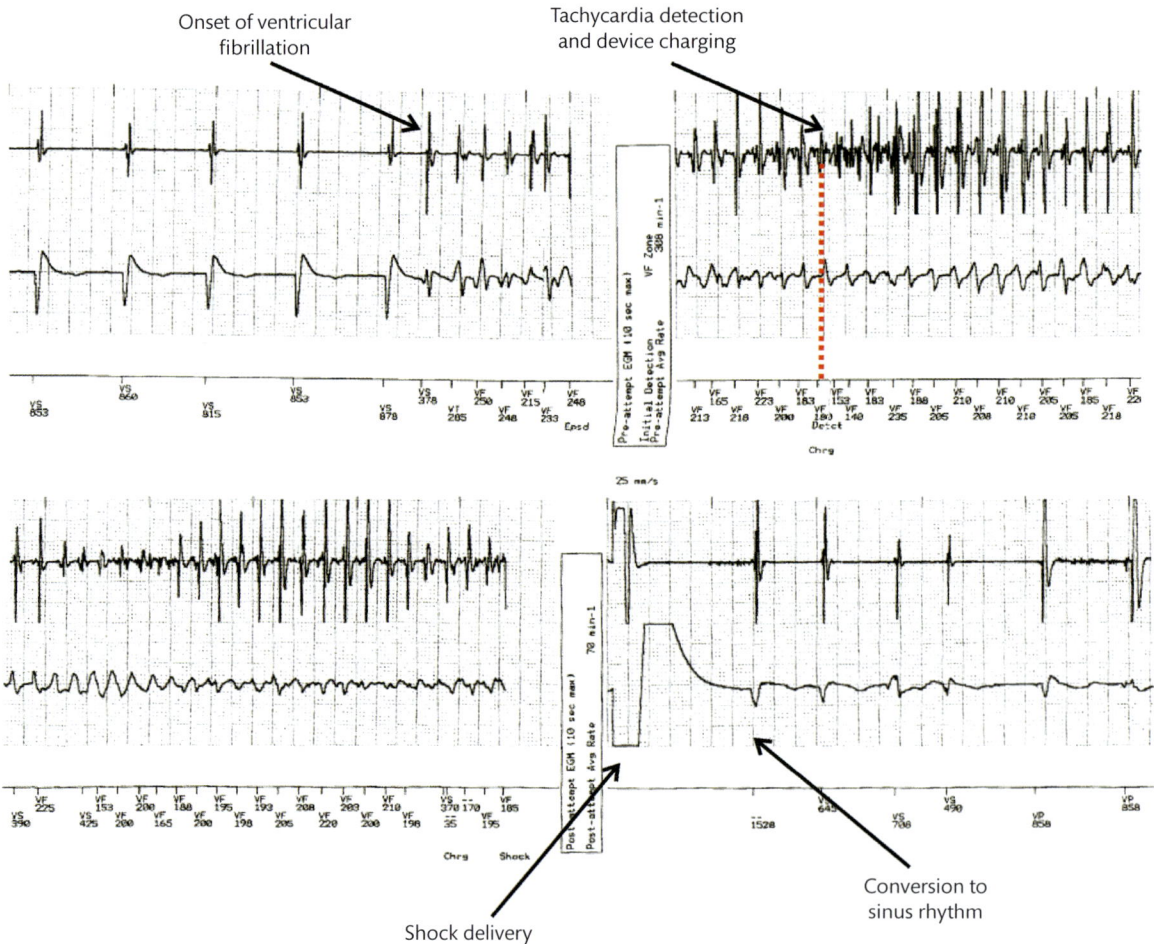

Figure 59.6 Termination of ventricular fibrillation by an ICD shock. Stored electrograms from an ICD in a patient who received a successful shock for ventricular tachycardia (VT). The upper panel shows sinus rhythm, with the onset of VF, which is then sensed by the ICD and a high-energy shock is administered, which results in conversion to sinus rhythm.

programming configurations (conventional therapy, high-rate therapy or delayed therapy). The primary objective was to determine whether programmed high-rate therapy (with a 2.5 s delay before the initiation of therapy at a heart rate of ≥200 beats per minute (bpm)) or delayed therapy (with a 60 s delay at 170 to 199 bpm, a 12 s delay at 200 to 249 bpm, and a 2.5 s delay at ≥250 bpm) was associated with a decrease in the number of patients with a first occurrence of inappropriate anti-tachycardia pacing or shocks as compared with conventional programming (with a 2.5 s delay at 170–199 bpm and a 1.0 s delay at ≥200 bpm). After an average follow-up of 1.4 years, high-rate and delayed therapy were associated with reductions in inappropriate therapy (hazard ratio (HR) with high-rate vs conventional therapy: 0.21; 95% confidence interval (CI): 0.13–0.34; $P < 0.001$; HR with delayed therapy vs conventional therapy: 0.24; 95% CI: 0.24–0.85; $P < 0.001$) and a reduction in all-cause mortality (HR with high-rate vs conventional therapy: 0.45; 95% CI: 0.24–0.85; $P = 0.01$; HR with delayed therapy vs conventional therapy: 0.56; 95% CI: 0.30–1.02; $P = 0.06$).

These results were supported by a recent meta-analysis on the impact of prolonged ICD arrhythmia detection times on outcomes.[36] Four prospective studies, enrolling 4896 patients, were identified. Summary estimates of the relative risk (RR) of death, syncope, and appropriate and inappropriate shocks were calculated using random effect models. In the long detection group there were significant reductions in mortality (RR: 0.77; 95% CI: 0.62–0.96) and inappropriate shocks (0.50; 0.39–0.65), without significant increase in syncope (1.23; 0.84–1.79).

The use of longer detection times and higher arrhythmia detection rates can therefore significantly reduce the burden of inappropriate shock therapy in ICD recipients without significant increase in syncope.

Implantation

The implant procedure is usually performed under conscious sedation with local anaesthesia, although in some complex cases general anaesthesia may be preferable. An operating theatre environment is used and strict surgical aseptic techniques are adhered to. A single incision, ~5 cm in length, is made inferior to the left clavicle, and a pocket is made for the generator, either subcutaneously or deep to the pectoralis major muscle. A lead is introduced to the subclavian or cephalic vein using a Seldinger technique and advanced under fluoroscopy to the apex of the right ventricle. If necessary a right atrial pacing lead may also be implanted. Additionally, if a patient with heart failure requires CRT, an LV epicardial lead is placed via the coronary veins. As for permanent pacing, accurate lead placement, with close attention to achieving optimal threshold, impedance, and stability is crucial. Once the leads are secured in place they are connected to the generator which is buried in the subcutaneous or submuscular pocket, which is then closed in layers using absorbable sutures.

Following publication of the Shockless IMPlant Evaluation (SIMPLE) trial,[37] defibrillation threshold testing is less frequently performed. Although generally well tolerated, this trial showed that routine defibrillation testing at the time of ICD implantation does not improve shock efficacy nor reduce arrhythmic death. In some circumstances defibrillation threshold testing may still be required, for example with implantation of right-sided defibrillators. In instances when it is required, it is performed by inducing ventricular

fibrillation (either by delivering a small shock on the T-wave or a short burst of AC or DC current) and programming the device to terminate the arrhythmia. Conventionally, effective shock energy ≥10 J less than the maximum deliverable by the device is acceptable. An external defibrillator is available should the implanted device fail to terminate the arrhythmia.

Following ICD implantation, patients are usually discharged home the following day provided that a chest X-ray shows satisfactory lead positions and no evidence of pneumothorax and that all device checks are satisfactory.

Complications

ICD implantation has numerous potential complications and it is estimated that as many as one-quarter of those who receive an ICD will experience a complication over a five-year period.[38]

Procedure-related complications

The complications of ICD implantation are similar to those associated with pacemaker implantation, and include haematoma, infection, pneumothorax, and lead displacement. A recent study has estimated that an index complication occurs in ~10% of patients, with mechanical complications being the most common.[39] Implant-related mortality is very rare; published rates of 30-day mortality are ~1% and usually related to the severity of the patient's cardiac disease.[40]

Failure of ICD therapy

It is important to recognize that an ICD is not a cure. Patients are still at risk of a ventricular arrhythmia, which may cause syncope or cardiac arrest. In a retrospective analysis of 320 deaths in 4889 patients enrolled in preclinical trials, 90 out of 317 (28%) classifiable deaths were sudden, and of these sudden deaths a cause was identifiable for 68.[41] Sixteen percent of all deaths in patients with a functioning ICD in place were found to be due to VT/VF, in 17 out of 50 the ICD failed to terminate the arrhythmia, in nine there was incessantly recurrent ventricular arrhythmia, and in 20 immediate post-shock electromechanical dissociation (EMD) was the terminal rhythm. The mechanism of post-shock EMD is unclear, and in some cases factors such as global myocardial ischaemia are likely to be implicated.

Myocardial damage by ICD shocks

Studies in animal models suggest that high-energy defibrillation shocks can cause myocardial damage, although the energies required for damage are significantly higher than those required for effective defibrillation.[42] In MADIT-II, the risk of heart failure was increased following appropriate, but not inappropriate, shocks, suggesting that the effects of the defibrillation shock on the myocardium was not implicated in producing subsequent myocardial dysfunction but rather that the occurrence of a ventricular arrhythmia identified patients at particular risk of developing heart failure.[43] Conversely, all-cause mortality was increased following an inappropriate shock, but not following ATP,[26] suggesting that, under some circumstances, the shock may indeed have adverse consequences. Myocardial damage as indicated by troponin elevation is not infrequently detectable following defibrillation threshold testing at ICD implant,[44] during which the duration of VF is minimized. Patients with severe LV dysfunction are most at risk of developing haemodynamic instability

during routine defibrillation testing at ICD implantation,[45] and in a limited multivariable analysis the only variable that independently predicted post-shock EMD was the presence of NYHA class III/IV heart failure.[40] It is therefore possible that, in some patients with severe LV dysfunction and heart failure, therapeutic defibrillation energy may be sufficient to cause myocardial damage or LV dysfunction, particularly where multiple shocks are administered in close succession.

Inappropriate shocks

In the long term, the most common adverse event associated with ICD therapy is an inappropriate shock from the device. These are commonly due to AF or an SVT occurring within the VT/VF detection zones (see **Figure 59.5**), but may occur due to abnormal sensing as a result of hardware problems such as conductor fracture or insulation break of the ventricular lead. The reason for inappropriate shocks can usually be diagnosed by interrogation of the device. Inappropriate shocks are not only unpleasant for the patient,[46] they limit battery longevity, may cause myocardial damage,[47] and are associated with poor outcomes.[27,48] Patients with heart failure have a high incidence of AF, which occurs in up to 30% of patients with NYHA class II/III heart failure,[49] putting them at particular risk of receiving inappropriate therapies. In MADIT-II, 31% of all shocks administered were judged to be inappropriate and 11.5% of patients in the ICD arm received inappropriate shocks over the two-year period.[27] Of these, 44% were due to atrial fibrillation, 36% by SVT and 20% by abnormal sensing. In the Sudden Cardiac Death in Heart Failure (SCDHeFT) Trial, which implanted single-chamber shock-only devices in patients with symptomatic heart failure, 32% of shocks were inappropriate and 17% of patients in the ICD arm received inappropriate shocks over five years.[48] The PainFree Study showed similar rates of inappropriate shocks, which accounted for 40% of all shocks and occurred in 15% of patients.[45]

In ICD recipients, the occurrence of inappropriate shocks is associated with an increased risk of mortality.[27,48] As the commonest cause of inappropriate shocks is AF with a ventricular rate within the VT/VF detection zone, and since AF is associated with higher mortality in patients with LVSD and heart failure, this association is perhaps expected. However, the possibility of a direct adverse effect of a defibrillation shock remains. The occurrence of anti-tachycardia pacing (either appropriate or inappropriate) is not associated with adverse outcomes, suggesting that the risk associated with defibrillation shocks may relate to the shock rather than to the arrhythmia which triggered it; however, it may equally reflect the fact that ATP is generally reserved for slower, less dangerous arrhythmias.

On an individual basis, inappropriate shocks for SVT can be minimized by judicious programming and appropriate use of β-blockers and other anti-arrhythmic drugs.[50] There is little evidence that dual-chamber detection algorithms have a significant impact on the rate of inappropriate ICD shocks. In MADIT-II, use of the stability algorithm, designed to prevent inappropriate shocks due to AF, was associated with a lower rate of inappropriate shocks.[27]

Psychological problems

Although a minority of patients may develop an adverse psychological reaction to ICD implantation, it is important to be aware that these patients often improve over time as they become accustomed to having the device and that they adapt to their physical limitations.

Although clear associations between the underlying condition, the presence of the ICD, and delivery of therapies and psychological stress are difficult to establish, it is clear that ICD patients do experience a degree of psychological morbidity compared to other patients with cardiovascular disease.[51] Many individual patients tolerate defibrillation shocks very poorly, particularly if they experience multiple shocks (whether appropriate or inappropriate). For this reason, anti-arrhythmic drugs may have a role in reducing the incidence of both ventricular and supraventricular arrhythmias in patients with ICDs.[50]

Lifestyle implications

Inevitably many patients with ICDs face lifestyle restrictions. Although the implant procedure is similar to pacemaker implantation, follow-up of patients with ICDs tends to be more complex, although this may change with the development of systems for remote ICD monitoring.

Quality of life

Patients with heart failure do not simply live longer with an ICD, but live longer with their heart failure symptoms and so are at risk of experiencing a deterioration in those symptoms. ICD therapy in heart failure patients therefore carries a risk of increasing survival but reducing quality of life (QoL). An analysis of health-related QoL from SCDHeFT found that QoL was greater in the ICD arm at 3 and 12 months, but equalled that in the medical therapy arm at 30 months,[52] at least providing reassurance that ICD therapy does not significantly impair QOL in patients with symptomatic heart failure. It is noteworthy that ICD shocks occurring in the month before interview were associated with a reduction in QoL.

Driving

The regulations regarding fitness to drive in patients with ICDs vary between countries, and are subject to periodic review. In the UK, the Driver and Vehicle Licensing Agency publishes its recommendations on its website.[53] Patients who have received an ICD for secondary prevention may be allowed to drive provided that the device has been implanted for at least six months and has not delivered shock therapy or symptomatic ATP for six months, and if previous discharges have not been accompanied by incapacity. Patients must stop driving for one month if the device (lead or generator) is revised, or if any change is made to their anti-arrhythmic treatment. Patients who have a primary prevention ICD implanted need only refrain from driving for one month, unless they subsequently receive shocks from the device. Patients with ICDs are permanently disqualified from driving commercial vehicles. The guidelines in the USA are largely similar, except that primary prevention ICD patients are only restricted from driving until recovery from the procedure (at least one week).[54] The European Heart Rhythm Association guidelines differ in that they recommend that patients need only refrain from driving for three months following a secondary prevention implant or an appropriate therapy.[55]

Sources of electromagnetic interference

Modern pacemakers and ICDs are well protected against external sources of electromagnetic interference. Although devices are being developed that will be safe to use in magnetic resonance imaging (MRI) scanners, at the present time ICD recipients are advised that

they cannot undergo MRI scanning. Cellular telephones (mobile phones) can occasionally interfere with ICDs and pacemakers, but only if the telephone is within 15 cm (6 in.) of the generator. There have been occasional reports of interference to pacemakers and ICDs caused by electronic article surveillance gates, but only if the patient is in the vicinity of the gates for several seconds.[56] Very occasionally patients with these devices work in environments where high-intensity electrical or magnetic fields might interfere with the device, and such scenarios require specialist assessment, which often involves collaboration between the patient's cardiologist, the engineers employed by the device manufacturer, and the occupational health physician at the place of work.

Evidence for ICD implantation in LV dysfunction and heart failure

Secondary prevention

Rationale

ICD implantation in survivors of life-threatening ventricular tachyarrhythmia is referred to as secondary prevention. For the purposes of clinical trial enrolment, life-threatening ventricular arrhythmias are defined as VF or sustained VT, meaning VT that lasts for ≥30 s or requires emergency intervention to terminate the arrhythmia because of cardiac arrest, syncope, haemodynamic compromise, or heart failure. In the absence of an identifiable and reversible precipitant, these patients are at high risk of recurrent ventricular arrhythmia.[57]

Secondary prevention ICD trials

Three large randomized trials have examined the efficacy of ICD implantation in these patients,[58–60] and the recruited populations are summarized in Table 59.1. Of the three, only the Antiarrhythmics Versus Implantable Defibrillator (AVID) trial demonstrated a statistically significant reduction in mortality associated with ICD use.[58] The Canadian Implantable Defibrillator Study (CIDS) was terminated early after results from AVID were reported,[59] and the Cardiac Arrest Study of Hamburg (CASH) trial showed a nonsignificant benefit.[60] However, all three studies reported a similar absolute risk reduction (~6% over 2 years) and meta-analysis showed a 28% relative reduction in mortality in the ICD group compared to amiodarone therapy.[61] In a non-prespecified subgroup analysis of the AVID trial, patients with LVEF ≤35% had more to gain from ICD implantation than those with preserved LVEF in whom there was no significant difference in mortality compared to amiodarone,[62] a finding which was borne out in the meta-analysis.[61] However, the idea that those patients with preserved LVEF following

life-threatening arrhythmias may not benefit from ICD implantation has not been prospectively evaluated, and, as such, is not reflected in the consensus guidelines governing secondary prevention ICD implantation. ICD implantation is recommended for all survivors of life-threatening ventricular arrhythmias, regardless of LVEF,[63] unless a reversible cause is identified (class I, level of evidence A), and remains the only evidence-based therapy for this group of patients. Those ventricular arrhythmias identified to be associated with a reversible cause, such as myocardial ischaemia, infarction, electrolyte disturbance, or a pro-arrhythmic drug effect were excluded from the secondary prevention trials, although data from the AVID registry suggest a poor outcome in these patients.[64] It is common practice not to implant ICDs for VT/VF that occurred during the acute phase of ST segment elevation MI, but whether the same applies to non-ST segment elevation MI is unclear. Perhaps in acknowledgement of this uncertainty, along with the fact that low-grade myocardial ischaemia may be difficult to completely reverse, ischaemia is not listed as a reversible cause in the consensus guidelines.

Primary prevention

Rationale

The majority of victims of SCD do not experience a prior arrhythmic event to identify them as high risk,[15] so a primary prevention ICD strategy is also required. Such a strategy relies on effective means of identifying patients at high risk. The current method of identifying such patients is the presence of a severely impaired LVEF, usually either as a result of prior myocardial infarction or idiopathic dilated cardiomyopathy.

Primary prevention ICD trials

A significant mortality benefit has been demonstrated in large randomized trials of prophylactic ICD therapy in patients with left ventricular systolic dysfunction and a history of either chronic heart failure or MI; the recruited populations are summarized in Table 59.2.

Coronary disease, LVSD and non-sustained/inducible ventricular arrhythmias

The first Multicenter Automatic Defibrillator Implantation Trial (MADIT) recruited patients with prior MI, LVEF ≤35%, spontaneous non-sustained VT and inducible sustained VT at electrophysiological study (EPS) that could not be suppressed acutely using anti-arrhythmic therapy, and randomized them to chronic anti-arrhythmic therapy (mostly amiodarone) or ICD implantation.[65] The Multicenter UnSustained Tachycardia Trial (MUSTT) recruited a similar population and was designed to assess the efficacy

Table 59.1 Summary of populations enrolled in the main secondary prevention ICD trials

Trial	n	Age (years)	LVEF (%)	NYHA class I or II/III or IV	ACEi (%)	β-Blocker (%)
AVID[58]	1016	65	~32	50/10	68	~25
CIDS[59]	659	~63	~33	40/10	NA	~25
CASH[60]	288	~58	~45	83/17	~40	~33[a]

ACEi, angiotensin converting enzyme inhibitor; LVEF, left ventricular ejection fraction; NYHA, New York Heart Association.
[a] Randomized therapy.

Table 59.2 Summary of populations enrolled in the main primary prevention ICD trials

Trial	*n*	Age (years)	LVEF (%)	NYHA class I/II/III/IV (%)	ACEi (%)	β-Blocker (%)	MRA (%)
Coronary disease, LVSD, and non-sustained/inducible ventricular arrhythmias							
MADIT[65]	196	~63	~26	~65% II or III	~57	~21	N/A
MUSTT[66]	704	~67	~30	35/40/25/0	~75	~40	N/A
Coronary disease and LVSD							
MADIT-II[67]	1232	~65	~23	35/35/25/5	70	70	N/A
LVSD early after acute MI							
DINAMIT[68]	674	~62	~28	7/30/15/0	95	87	N/A
Non-ischaemic cardiomyopathy							
DEFINITE[69]	458	~58	~21	22/57/21/0	85	85	N/A
DANISH[70]	1116	~64	~25	0/54/45/1	97	92	58
Symptomatic heart failure and LVSD							
SCDHeFT[13]	2521	~60	~25	0/70/30/0	85	69	20

ACEi, angiotensin converting enzyme inhibitor; LVEF, left ventricular ejection fraction; LVSD, left ventricular systolic dysfunction; MI, myocardial infartion; NYHA, New York Heart Association; N/A, not available.

of EPS-guided pharmacological therapy, but included a provision for patients to receive an ICD in a non-randomized fashion if anti-arrhythmic drugs failed to suppress inducible ventricular arrhythmias.[66] Both of these studies implanted relatively small numbers of ICDs in highly selected patients and demonstrated a sizeable survival advantage with an ICD, the relative reductions in all-cause mortality being 54% and 60%, respectively.

Coronary disease and LVSD

More recently, results from larger studies with less stringent and non-invasive entry criteria have led to the expansion of primary prevention ICD therapy. MADIT-II randomized 1232 patients with ischaemic cardiomyopathy and LVEF of ≤30% to receive an ICD or be treated with conventional therapy alone.[67] No documentation of spontaneous or inducible ventricular arrhythmia was required for enrolment. The patients were well treated, with 70% receiving ACEi and a similar proportion on β-blockers at the last follow-up visit, 57% having previously undergone coronary arterial bypass grafting, and 44% having had a history of percutaneous coronary intervention. The trial was designed to be stopped after a prespecified boundary treatment effect had been observed, which occurred after a mean follow-up of 20 months, with an observed mortality of 14.2% in the ICD group compared to 19.8% in the conventionally treated group. This equates to a relative risk reduction of 31%, less than that achieved in MADIT and MUSTT, but of a similar magnitude to that seen in the secondary prevention trials. The prespecified subgroup analyses did not identify any statistically significant differences in the magnitude of benefit across age (<60 vs 60–69 vs ≥70 years), sex, NYHA class (I vs ≥II), ejection fraction (dichotomized at 25%) and QRS duration (<120 vs 120–150 vs >150 ms), either in terms of reduction in all-cause mortality[67] or of the reduction in sudden cardiac death.[5] There was an observed trend for greater benefit associated with an ICD in patients with a QRS complex width of ≥120 ms.

LVSD early after acute MI

It is important to note that patients with a history of MI within the preceding 3 months were ineligible for recruitment into MADIT-II.

Data from studies of ICD implantation early after MI suggest that the benefit seen in MADIT-II cannot be extrapolated to within 4–6 weeks of acute MI. The Defibrillator in Acute Myocardial Infarction Trial (DINAMIT) demonstrated a trend towards harm with an ICD in patients with LVEF ≤35% and abnormal autonomic function in the early phase (6–40 days) following MI.[68] There was a reduction in the rate of arrhythmic death, which was offset by an increase in non-arrhythmic death in the ICD arm. The reason for the increase in non-arrhythmic death remains unclear, but was recapitulated in the Immediate Risk Stratification Improves Survival (IRIS) trial. The IRIS protocol identified post-MI patients as high risk on the basis of either resting tachycardia in combination with LVEF ≤40% or the presence of non-sustained VT regardless of LVEF,[71] and so included a proportion (~33%) of patients with ischaemic cardiomyopathy and preserved LV function, a group in whom there was no pre-existing evidence for ICD implantation. However, survival benefit was not demonstrated for either high-risk group despite a significant reduction in arrhythmic mortality.[72] It has been suggested that, in this population, the occurrence of ventricular arrhythmia identifies a group at such high risk of overall cardiac mortality that the presence of an ICD will simply convert the mode of death within a relatively short timescale, an effect that is not evident in the trials of chronic ischaemic cardiomyopathy. Whether this is the case, or whether some aspect of ICD implantation actively increases cardiac mortality in the early phase following MI, once again, in a manner that is not observed in chronic ischaemic cardiomyopathy, remains to be established. In either case, published guidelines have taken account of this in recommending that primary prevention ICDs should not be implanted within 4–6 weeks of MI.[63]

Non-ischaemic cardiomyopathy

Until recently, the Defibrillators in Non-Ischemic Cardiomyopathy Treatment Evaluation (DEFINITE) trial was the largest trial to investigate the use of ICDs in patients with non-ischaemic cardiomyopathy. In all, 458 patients with LVEF ≤35%, and either premature ventricular complexes or non-sustained VT on ambulatory

monitoring were randomized to receive optimal medical therapy or optimal medical therapy plus an ICD.[69] The entry criteria only specified a history of heart failure, but the enrolled population had a high prevalence of current symptomatic heart failure (78% NYHA II/III). The trial did not reach statistical significance but demonstrated a trend towards improved survival in the ICD arm over 2 years (7.9 vs 14.1%, $P = 0.08$).

More recently, the DANISH trial was carried out to assess the efficacy of ICDs in patients with non-ischaemic systolic heart failure on mortality.[70] The study enrolled 1116 patients with systolic heart failure not caused by coronary artery disease and randomized them to conventional therapy (contemporary heart failure medication including cardiac resynchronization therapy, where appropriate) or an ICD added to conventional therapy. After a median follow-up period of 5.6 years there was no reduction in the primary endpoint of all-cause mortality for patients randomized to ICD therapy (HR: 0.87; 95% CI: 0.68–1.12; $P = 0.28$). This was despite a significant reduction in sudden cardiac death in the ICD group (HR: 0.50; 95% CI: 0.31–0.82; $P = 0.005$).

Prescription rates of contemporary evidence-based medical therapy were high in DANISH unlike previous ICD trials, with the majority of patients (58%) receiving CRT. The results from this trial suggest that patients with an already relatively low risk of sudden cardiac death because of their non-ischaemic (compared with ischaemic) aetiology, on optimal *contemporary* medical and device treatment have little room for further reduction in sudden cardiac death to reduce cardiovascular death and consequently all-cause mortality.

Of note, however, there was a significant interaction between the effect of ICD treatment and age, with ICD treatment conferring more of a benefit in younger compared with older patients: patients aged <59 years, HR: 0.51 (95% CI: 0.29–0.92); patients aged ≥59 to <68 years, HR: 0.75 (0.48–1.16); patients aged ≥68 years, HR: 1.19 (0.81–1.73). Subgroup analyses can, however, be underpowered to detect true differences in treatment effects or conversely may yield spurious false-positive results from multiple comparisons, and so caution must always be taken in interpretation of subgroup analyses. Overall, however, the findings from this study suggest that in patients with non-ischaemic heart failure, ICD treatment reduces all-cause mortality in younger patients with little co-morbidity.

Heart failure and LVSD

The Sudden Cardiac Death in Heart Failure trial (SCD-HeFT) is the largest ICD trial so far published.[13] In this study, 2521 patients with NYHA class II or III heart failure were randomized to receive optimal medical therapy with placebo, medical therapy plus amiodarone, or medical therapy with implantation of a single-chamber, shock-only ICD. Approximately half of the patients had an ischaemic aetiology, half had non-ischaemic dilated cardiomyopathy, and the majority (70%) were in NYHA class II. After a follow-up period of 5 years the mortality in the medical therapy arm was 36.1% (7.2% per year) and amiodarone had no effect on mortality. The ICD group displayed a 23% reduction in mortality compared to medical therapy ($P = 0.007$), which equated to a 7% absolute risk reduction over 5 years. In subgroup analyses, the benefit from ICD therapy was most pronounced in those with an LVEF of <30% and in the patients

with relatively mild symptoms (NYHA class II vs III). Importantly, a similar magnitude of benefit was seen in patients with ischaemic and non-ischaemic cardiomyopathy. The mortality benefit was attributable to a 60% reduction in sudden death with no observed effect of ICD therapy on heart failure deaths.[73] Indeed, the heart failure status of surviving patients, as assessed by LVEF and NYHA class, improved over the course of the study, possibly reflecting benefit from optimized medical therapy and regular medical contact.[74]

Guidelines for the use of ICD therapy in heart failure

Guidelines from the UK, Europe, and the USA all recommend the use of ICDs for secondary prevention in survivors of life-threatening ventricular arrhythmias in the absence of an identifiable reversible cause, and where survival with a good quality of life of at least one year can reasonably be expected.

For primary prevention indications, however, consensus guidelines vary, as summarized in Table 59.3. The ACC/AHA/HRS joint guidelines (which were updated in 2012) have determined the following class I indications for primary prevention ICD implantation: syncope and inducible VT/VF at EPS; LVEF ≤35% due to prior MI (≥40 days post MI) and NYHA II/III chronic heart failure; LVEF ≤30% due to prior MI (≥40 days post MI) and NYHA I; LVEF ≤35% due to non-ischaemic cardiomyopathy and NYHA II/III; LVEF ≤40% due to prior MI (≥40 days post MI) and non-sustained VT with inducible VT/VF at EPS.[63] The guidelines explicitly state that these criteria assume that the patient is established on optimal medical therapy. Patients who do not have a reasonable expectation of survival with a reasonable functional status for a period of one year are again specifically excluded from ICD implantation, regardless of the indication. Refractory NYHA class IV heart failure, in patients who are not candidates for cardiac transplantation or CRT-D, also negates any indication for ICD implantation. Other exclusions (listed as class III recommendations in the guideline) include incessant VT/VF, significant psychiatric illness, or the identification of completely reversible causes for the occurrence of VT/VF.

The current European Society of Cardiology guidelines[75,76] give a class 1A recommendation for primary prevention ICD implantation in patients with symptomatic heart failure (NYHA class II–III) and LVEF ≤35% of ischaemic aetiology (at least 6 weeks after myocardial infarction) after ≥3 months of optimal medical therapy who are expected to survive for at least 1 year with good functional status. This is reduced to a class IB recommendation if the aetiology of heart failure is non-ischaemic.

In the UK, the National Institute for Health and Care Excellence (NICE)[77] published an ICD guidance which was reviewed in 2014. In these updated guidelines ICDs are recommended for patients with heart failure who have left ventricular systolic dysfunction with an ejection fraction of ≤35% in NYHA functional class I–III with a QRS duration of ≥120 ms. The guidelines also state that ICD implantation should be considered in those patients at high risk of sudden cardiac death who fulfil the above heart failure criterion but who have a QRS duration <120 ms. The Scottish Intercollegiate Guidelines Network (SIGN) also published an update on the use of primary prevention ICDs in patients with heart failure in 2018.[78] These recommendations are identical to those outlined by NICE.

Table 59.3 Guidelines for primary prevention ICD implantation

Condition	ACC/AHA/HRS (2012)[63]	ESC (2015–2016)[75,76]	NICE (2014)[77]	SIGN (2018)[78]
Coronary disease, LVSD and inducible arrhythmias				
LVEF ≤40%	Class I[a]	Class I[a]	NR	NR
LVEF ≤35%	Class I[a]	Class I[a]	Recommended[b]	Prioritize[b]
Coronary disease, LVSD and non-sustained arrhythmias				
LVEF ≤40%	NR	Class I[a]	NR	NR
LVEF ≤35%	Class IIa[a]	Class I[a]	Recommended[b]	Prioritize[b]
Coronary disease and LVSD				
LVEF ≤30%	Class I[a]	Class IIa[a]	NR	Consider[b]
LVEF ≤30% and QRSd ≥120 ms	Class I[a]	Class IIa[a]	Recommended[b]	Prioritize[b]
LVEF ≤35% and NYHA II/III	Class I[a]	Class I[a,c]	NR	Consider[b]
Non-ischaemic cardiomyopathy				
NYHA I	Class IIb	Class IIb	NR	NR
NYHA II/III	Class I	Class I[c]	NR	NR
Syncope	Class IIa	Class IIb	NR	NR
Symptomatic heart failure and LVSD				
NYHA II/III	Class I	Class I[a,c]	NR	NR

LVEF, left ventricular ejection fraction; LVSD, left ventricular systolic dysfunction; MI, myocardial infarction; NYHA, New York Heart Association; NR, not recommended.

[a] At least 40 days post acute myocardial infarction.

[b] At least 4 weeks post acute myocardial infarction.

[c] Chronic Heart Failure Guideline 2008.

Cost-effectiveness of primary prevention ICD therapy in heart failure

The available evidence suggests that improved outcomes can be achieved with primary prevention ICDs in patients with heart failure, and these indications are now included in international consensus guidelines. However, there is a significant cost associated with ICD therapy, and, because the potential primary prevention population is large, ICD therapy may therefore have major implications for finite health budgets.[79] The cost-effectiveness of ICD therapy depends heavily on the healthcare system in which it is assessed and the time-window over which it is considered, particularly as the majority of the cost is associated with the hardware and implant, and the fact that survival benefit takes some time to manifest.[80] Cost-effectiveness analyses were prespecified in SCDHeFT, cost data were collected prospectively, and survival benefit was extrapolated beyond the five year follow-up. The incremental cost per quality-adjusted life-year (QALY) saved was around $41,000,[81] which is congruent with estimates from other primary prevention studies.[82]

Based on average selling prices aggregated across all manufacturers of ICDs sold in the UK to the NHS in the financial year of 2011, the cost of a complete ICD system is estimated at £9,692. This is lower than the estimated cost in previous years. It follows, then, that as the price of ICDs falls and battery longevity improves, the cost per QALY is likely also to improve.

The Markov model, used as the basis for the NICE guidance, estimated the incremental cost-effectiveness ratio (ICER) of primary prevention ICD implantation in the UK as £19,479 per QALY gained. In the broader heart failure population including those with mild-to-moderate heart failure and in patients with non-ischaemic cardiomyopathy, the ICER ranged between £14,231 and £29,756 per QALY gained. This is compared to an estimated ICER of £35,000–45,000 per QALY calculated using the Buxton and Sharples model in 2006.[83]

However, these estimates are dependent on the survival benefit associated with the ICD persisting for around 7–8 years, which in elderly patients with NYHA III heart failure may be unrealistic. Using a limit of $50,000 per life-year saved as a threshold for an acceptable cost-effectiveness profile,[84] this suggests that the cost of primary prevention ICD therapy in heart failure is acceptable in economic terms, provided that the real benefits are similar to those observed in SCDHeFT, and persist beyond five years.

The importance of heart failure in ICD trials

Although SCD-HeFT and DANISH were the only primary prevention ICD trials to mandate symptomatic heart failure at enrolment, patients with low ejection fraction heart failure were also enrolled into the other trials—in DEFINITE and MADIT-II, the prevalence of NYHA II/III heart failure was ~78%[69] and ~60%,[67] respectively (Table 59.2). Moreover, patients with asymptomatic LVSD remain at risk of developing symptomatic heart failure. Although ICDs reduced mortality overall in heart failure patients in SCDHeFT, those patients in the ICD arm who received an appropriate shock had five-fold greater mortality than those who received no shock.[48] Patients receiving inappropriate shocks displayed a doubling of mortality.

The most common cause of death in patients who received an ICD shock was progressive heart failure, accounting for 40% of all deaths in this group. These findings underline the central confounding factor as regards ICD therapy in patients with heart failure—the existence of competing risks dictates that a reduction in sudden death will result in an increase in heart failure death.

Relationship between NYHA class and ICD benefit

The results from randomized trials of ICD therapy have produced conflicting results in terms of the relationship of severity of heart failure symptoms (as determined by NYHA class) and the magnitude of benefit derived from an ICD. In MADIT-II a similar magnitude of benefit was identified for patients with NYHA I symptoms, who constituted around 35% of the population, compared with those with an NYHA class ≥II.[67] In DEFINITE, patients with NYHA class III heart failure may have greater benefit from ICD therapy than those in class II.[69] In a prespecified subgroup analysis of SCDHeFT, the benefit seen with an ICD appeared confined to the 70% of the population who had NYHA class II symptoms.[13] The reasons for these contradictory findings are not immediately apparent, and it is important to note both the limitations of NYHA class in grading heart failure severity and the fact that these studies were not powered to detect differences between subgroups. The numbers of NYHA class IV patients enrolled in ICD trials is sufficiently small that outcomes cannot be extrapolated to this group, and it is likely that in this group the risk of heart failure death is such that any benefit from an ICD would be offset. Therefore patients with NYHA class IV heart failure who are not candidates for CRT or cardiac transplantation should not have ICDs implanted.

Relationship between LVEF and benefit in ICD trials

Data from AVID,[58] CIDS,[59] MADIT,[67] and SCDHeFT[13] all suggest that those patients with the most severely depressed ejection fraction have the most to gain from ICD therapy, despite having a higher overall mortality and a higher absolute risk of death from progressive heart failure. Conversely, data from MADIT-II showed similar benefit across different LVEF <35%.[85] There is, however, evidence to suggest that there may be a lower limit for ICD benefit, with one analysis suggesting that all deaths in patients with prior MI and LVEF <10% were non-arrhythmic.[86]

Emergence of heart failure following ICD implantation

The results of the Dual Chamber and VVI Defibrillator (DAVID) study raised concerns over the use of dual-chamber pacing in patients with ICDs without standard indications for pacing.[87] The study randomized 506 dual-chamber ICD recipients to receive either DDD rate-responsive pacing at 70 bpm or VVI pacing at 40 bpm, and was based on the hypothesis that provision of DDDR pacing in patients with LV dysfunction would suppress atrial arrhythmias, allow optimization of medical therapy and would therefore improve heart failure outcomes. All of the enrolled patients had LV dysfunction (LVEF ≤40%) and half had symptomatic heart failure (NYHA class ≥II). Enrolment was stopped early after the observation that those randomized to DDDR pacing were significantly more likely to experience the composite primary end-point of all-cause mortality or hospitalization for heart failure at one year than those receiving VVI pacing. There was also a trend towards the same result for each of the components of the composite primary

end-point. DDDR programming was associated with a significantly higher level of RV apical pacing, with a mean of 58.9% vs 3.5% in the VVI arm. The subsequent Intrinsic-RV study demonstrated non-inferiority of DDDR pacing vs VVI for the same composite primary end-point when an AV search hysteresis algorithm was used to minimize RV apical pacing during DDDR (10% vs 3% in the VVI arm). Cumulative RV apical pacing >2% was shown to be associated with an increased risk for both subsequent appropriate ICD shocks and for heart failure events.[88] Similar results were seen in the second Multicenter Automatic Defibrillator Implantation Trial (MADIT-II) when cumulative RV apical pacing was dichotomized at 50% (median pacing rates 0.2% vs 95.6%).[89] This may at least in part explain the greater number of heart failure events seen in the ICD arm of MADIT-II in which ~40% of the ICDs implanted were dual-chamber devices.[67] Recipients of dual-chamber ICDs experienced a relatively high proportion of RV apical pacing, compared to little or none in the group who received single-chamber ICDs. The increased risk of first or recurrent heart failure associated with an ICD in MADIT-II was present in those who received single- and dual-chamber devices, but was greater in those with dual-chamber ICDs.[43] It therefore appears that RV apical pacing in ICD recipients may induce ventricular dyssynchrony, worsen LV function, and thereby induce or exacerbate clinical heart failure.

Although the bulk of the evidence for ICD effectiveness comes from trials which implanted single-chamber devices,[13,58–60,65] registry data suggest that a significant proportion of ICDs are dual-chamber devices.[90] Whereas there are theoretical potential benefits to dual-chamber devices in terms of SVT discrimination and provision of physiologic pacing should conducting system disease develop, there are insufficient data to support routine dual-chamber ICD implantation in patients without standard indications for bradycardia pacing, and concerns regarding dual-chamber pacing are especially pertinent in patients with pre-existing heart failure. The evidence certainly supports the use of algorithms to minimize ventricular pacing in ICD recipients, whether single- or dual-chamber devices are used.

In the ICD arm of MADIT-II, the emergence of symptomatic heart failure was more common after appropriate, but not inappropriate, shocks,[43] suggesting that the increased risk of heart failure in defibrillator recipients is in part related to the survival benefit conferred by the device. In addition, the risk of heart failure and non-sudden cardiac death seen with single-chamber ICDs was less than that associated with dual-chamber devices, but was greater than that observed in the conventional therapy arm,[43] suggesting that in a number of patients ICDs convert risk of sudden death to risk of death from worsening heart failure. In MADIT-II, those patients with single-chamber devices continued to experience a mortality benefit from the device after a hospitalization for heart failure, whereas those patients with dual-chamber ICDs saw a reduction in ICD-associated benefit following a heart failure event, and in fact had a similar survival to the conventional therapy group.[43] In the AVID trial, a hospital admission for heart failure was an independent predictor of mortality in patients treated with ICDs following life-threatening ventricular arrhythmias.[91]

Overall, it appears that the presence of heart failure increases the risk of ventricular arrhythmia associated with a given level of left ventricular dysfunction, therefore increasing the potential benefit from ICD therapy while also increasing the likelihood of death from

worsening heart failure. Moreover, although ICDs reduce mortality, patients who experience an ICD shock experience a worse outcome than those who do not, and survival worsens following a shock. In some patients, the occurrence of a ventricular arrhythmia marks the onset of deterioration in their heart failure, which will result in death from progressive heart failure. In other patients, surviving an ICD shock may simply allow them to live longer, during which time they will develop heart failure. In either case, patients with ICDs are at risk of developing or worsening heart failure and accordingly should be targeted for aggressive medical management.

Cardiac resynchronization therapy in combination with an ICD

Rationale

QRS prolongation in heart failure indicates underlying interventricular dyssynchrony and is associated with poor prognosis, in terms of heart failure, sudden death, and overall mortality. Cardiac resynchronization therapy pacing employs atrio-biventricular pacing to reduce interventricular dyssynchrony and produce improvements in LV function and mortality. CRT-P is covered in Chapter 60, but is discussed briefly here as it can be combined with a defibrillator (CRT-D), when an ICD indication also exists. A CRT-D system is shown in **Figure 59.7**.

Evidence for CRT-D in heart failure

The Comparison of Medical Therapy, Pacing and Defibrillators in Chronic Heart Failure (COMPANION) trial enrolled 1520 patients in sinus rhythm with NYHA III/IV heart failure, LVEF ≤35%, and QRS duration ≥120 ms and randomized them to optimal medical therapy alone, medical therapy plus CRT-P or plus CRT-D.[92] The primary end-point—a composite of death or first hospitalization for heart failure—was reduced by both CRT-P and CRT-D, although the secondary end-point—all-cause mortality—was only significantly reduced in the CRT-D arm. The subsequent Cardiac Resynchronisation in Heart Failure (CARE-HF) study demonstrated that addition of an ICD was not required for survival benefit with CRT. CARE-HF randomized similar patients to continue optimal medical therapy or to receive CRT-P in addition.[29] Interventricular dyssynchrony was defined as QRS duration ≥150 ms, or QRS duration 120–149 ms with echocardiographic evidence of mechanical dyssynchrony, although this subset constituted a minority of the enrolled patients. There was a significant improvement in the composite end-point of all-cause mortality or an unplanned hospitalization for a major cardiovascular event. The extended follow-up confirmed a reduction in all-cause mortality, including significant reductions in both sudden death and death from worsening heart failure.[93]

Following the observation of increased heart failure events with an ICD in MADIT-II, the MADIT-CRT Trial was designed to test the hypothesis that the addition of CRT to an ICD would provide additional benefit for high-risk but minimally symptomatic patients.[94] A total of 1820 patients with LVSD (LVEF ≤30%) and QRS prolongation (≥130 ms) who were minimally symptomatic (NYHA I/II heart failure) were randomized to receive CRT-D or an ICD (programmed to VVI or DDI at 40 bpm). The primary end-point, which was a composite of all-cause mortality or a non-fatal heart failure event, was experienced by 17.2% of the CRT-D group and 25.3% of the ICD group over a 4.5-year period, equating to a relative risk reduction of 34% with CRT-D over ICD. This benefit was driven primarily by an 8.9% reduction in non-fatal heart failure events with CRT-D, without any demonstrable survival advantage. The benefit of CRT-D appeared to be concentrated in those patients with QRS duration ≥150 ms (~65% of the recruited population) and was accompanied by 11% absolute improvement in LVEF at one year, as opposed to 3% seen in the ICD arm. These findings are congruent with those seen in trials of CRT-P in minimally symptomatic patients, in which favourable LV reverse remodelling and a reduction in heart failure events have been observed.[95] It is worth noting that the majority of those enrolled (~85%) were in NYHA functional class II, and that a notable proportion (~10%) had a past history of class III symptoms. A pragmatic interpretation might therefore be that CRT-D is likely to reduce heart failure morbidity in ICD candidates with NHYA II heart failure and a very broad QRS complex, particularly those who have a history of more severe heart failure symptomatology.

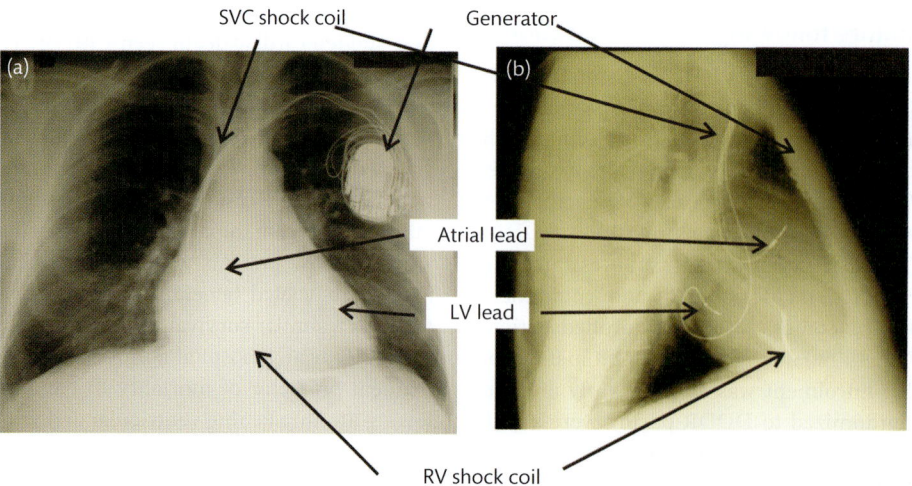

Figure 59.7 A cardiac resynchronization therapy–defibrillator (CRT-D) system PA (a) and lateral (b) chest radiographs in a patient with a CRT-D system. The generator, right ventricular (RV), left ventricular (LV) and atrial leads, along with the shock coils are indicated. SVC, superior vena cava.

Overall, the results from these CRT-D trials once again emphasize the importance of the interplay between heart failure and sudden death in patients with LV dysfunction, and the limitations of NHYA class as a tool to assess the severity of heart failure symptoms. The presence of heart failure indicates a substrate for sudden death which may be modified by medical therapy and CRT, and the occurrence of heart failure is constantly present as a competing risk that cannot be modified by an ICD.

Cost effectiveness of CRT-D in heart failure

Using estimates of cost and benefit based on data from the COMPANION and CARE-HF trials, the incremental cost, from a UK healthcare perspective, of adding an ICD to CRT-P in patients with heart failure has been estimated.[96] The incremental cost of CRT-D over CRT-P was around €48,000 per QALY saved. This may be around the threshold level for an acceptable cost-effectiveness profile, but it does significantly exceed the estimates for CRT-P over optimal medical therapy—around €7,500 per QALY saved.

Palliative care and device deactivation

Heart failure is a chronic condition associated with high mortality and, even with contemporary optimal medical therapy; some recipients will inevitably experience a progression in the severity of their heart failure to refractory end-stage disease. The prognostic benefit of an ICD is likely to change with progression to end-stage heart failure, and with these patients experiencing a heavy symptom burden, effective palliation is clearly extremely important. Given that a key principle of palliative care is withholding treatments that do not improve symptomatology and that may produce unpleasant side-effects, it would seem pertinent that the option of ICD deactivation is discussed.

Device deactivation requires a sensitive discussion with patients, who have likely previously accepted the ICD on the basis that it would be a life-saving intervention. Such discussions are best introduced early as soon as a deterioration in heart failure status is recognized, and for some patients it may be appropriate to raise the possibility of future device deactivation at the time of implantation or generator replacement.[97] Patients may have a preference for device deactivation, and physicians should certainly recognize the need to consider ICD deactivation when: death is imminent, when other therapies are withdrawn, or when a decision not to attempt resuscitation has been taken.[98–100]

Counselling patients with heart failure for an ICD

Patients with heart failure may overestimate the potential benefit associated with ICD therapy compared with that observed in clinical trials, underlining the importance of appropriate counselling, a task made more difficult by the lack of accurate risk stratification algorithms for different modes of death in patients with heart failure.[101] A useful outline for such discussions has been suggested by Stevenson and Desai and is based on the available clinical trial evidence for ICD benefit in patients with heart failure and LV dysfunction.[102] It focuses on a five-year time-period and quantifies the risks and benefits associated with an ICD in terms of expected events affecting 100 patients: seven or eight patients will have their life saved as a result of the ICD; 30 will die anyway, some having

requested that the device be switched off; 10–20 patients will have a shock they did not need; five to 15 will experience some other complication, and the rest will not experience their device at all.[102] This approach quantifies the risks and benefits in a way which is accessible to patients, and makes clear to the physician the importance of individual choice in this decision-making process.

Future developments in ICD therapy for patients with heart failure

Predicting heart failure death

Effective targeting of ICD therapy to patients with heart failure who are most likely to benefit depends on identifying two key subpopulations—those who will die of progressive heart failure or other causes before receiving a life-saving therapy from their device, and those who are at such low risk from an arrhythmia that they are very unlikely to derive meaningful benefit from an ICD. Ideally, then, each potential ICD recipient should undergo two types of assessment which must be combined to give a balanced reflection of whether they would be likely to benefit from ICD implantation.

A number of attempts have been made to develop a risk score to predict mortality in patients undergoing defibrillator implantation for primary prevention of sudden cardiac death. Detailed clinical data of 2717 consecutive patients receiving ICD therapy were collected as part of a large observational study.[103] Using these data, a risk score incorporating Peripheral vascular disease, Age ≥70 years, Creatinine ≥2.0 mg/dL, and left ventricular Ejection fraction ≤20% (PACE) accurately predicted 1-year mortality in the study validation group. Despite ICD therapy, patients with a PACE score of ≥3 had a >4-fold excess 1-year mortality compared to patients with a score of <3 (16.5% vs 3.5%; $P < 0.0001$). Unfortunately it was not possible to determine the risk reduction provided by ICD therapy in this cohort due to the lack of a control group. Nevertheless the investigators concluded that this simple risk score was able to accurately predict 1-year mortality in ICD patients using a cut-off score of ≥3 to denote those at high risk of death.

Other risk models derived from clinical trials have not shown statistically significant survival benefits for patients in the highest 10–20% of predicted risk after ICD implantation. The MADIT II model used a previously developed risk score including five clinical factors (NYHA class >II, age >70 years, blood urea nitrogen >26 mg/dL, QRS duration >0.12 s, and atrial fibrillation) to evaluate 8-year ICD survival benefit within risk score categories among 1191 MADIT II patients.[104] Patients with low (0 risk factors, $n = 345$) and intermediate risk (one or two risk factors, $n = 646$) demonstrated a significantly higher probability of survival at 8-year follow-up when treated by ICD as compared with non-ICD therapy (75% vs 58%, $P < 0.004$; and 47% vs 31%, $P < 0.001$, respectively). Neither the 14% of ICD patients with three or more risk factors nor the 5% of ICD patients in the prespecified very-high-risk group had a statistically significant 8-year survival benefit.

The Seattle Heart Failure Model is another such multivariable model, which uses routine clinical variables to predict mortality risk in patients with heart failure.[105] When applied to the SCDHeFT population to produce quintiles of risk, this model was able to separate groups with greater benefit from ICD therapy (quintile 2

relative risk: 0.48 (0.26–0.89; P = 0.019) vs quintile 5 relative risk 0.98 (0.71–1.82; P = 0.89)).[106] The development of such models to include powerful risk predictors, such as B-type natriuretic peptides, and to predict cause-specific mortality may well lead to improvements in our ability to risk-stratify patients with heart failure and in our ability to select ICD candidates in the future.

Impact of non-cardiac co-morbidities

The effect of non-cardiac co-morbidities must also be taken into account when trying to quantify risk of death that would not be modifiable by an ICD. In an analysis of the impact of non-cardiac co-morbidities on outcome in 2500 ICD recipients over two years in an Ontario registry, co-morbidities such as peripheral vascular disease, pulmonary disease, and renal impairment were significant determinants of mortality following ICD implantation, and risk increased incrementally with increasing numbers of co-morbidities.[107]

Subcutaneous ICDs

Although effective at reducing SCD, transvenous ICD systems are costly and associated with potential hazard, and in reality the eligible population is often elderly with significant co-morbidity, making physicians reluctant to treat. The subcutaneous ICD is a more novel device offering a number of potential advantages to the traditional transvenous ICD system.[108] It is comprised of a subcutaneous defibrillation lead, which runs parallel to the left sternal edge and along the inferior border of the heart to a generator implanted in the axilla (**Figure 59.8**).

In addition to early studies demonstrating the safety and feasibility of the SCD, outcome data have also been published from the Evaluation oF FactORs ImpacTing CLinical Outcome and Cost EffectiveneSS of the S-ICD (EFFORTLESS S-ICD) Registry.[109] This registry was created to provide 'real-world' systematically collected system performance data over a long time-period to look primarily at survival end-points. To date, it has demonstrated that the device

is being successfully implanted in a broad spectrum of patients with 98% first procedure induced VF conversion efficacy. A first shock conversion efficacy was reported at 88% for discrete episodes of spontaneous VT/VF, in line with rates published in transvenous ICD and CRT-D cohorts. The S-ICD procedure has been associated with lower rates of pneumothorax and lead displacement but with a higher rate of procedure-related infection (4%). This is thought to be due to procedural inexperience. The inappropriate shock rates (7%) reported in the EFFORTLESS registry are comparable with the standard transvenous ICD registries and trials ranging from 4% to 18%—with the main cause of inappropriate shocks from the S-ICD system being due to T-wave oversensing.

In summary, data from this registry show that there is appropriate system performance with clinical event rates and inappropriate shock rates comparable with those reported for conventional transvenous ICDs.

Whether the associated cost will be significantly lower than for transvenous systems remains to be seen. These devices are shock-only and do not have the capability to perform ATP or bradycardia pacing outside the post-shock period. However, this is largely the same profile of therapies as that which produced a mortality benefit in heart failure patients enrolled in the SCDHeFT trial. If proved safe and effective, subcutaneous ICD systems may be an option for providing protection from life-threatening arrhythmias in patients with heart failure.

More recently the PRAETORIAN trial randomly allocated 489 patients to either a subcutaneous or transvenous ICD.[110] The primary end-point of device-related complications and/or inappropriate shocks occurred in 48 patients in each group, over a follow-up period of more than four years. There were numerically somewhat more inappropriate shocks with the transvenous ICD, but fewer complications requiring reoperation. The mortality rate and the rate of appropriate ICD shocks did not differ significantly between the two groups.

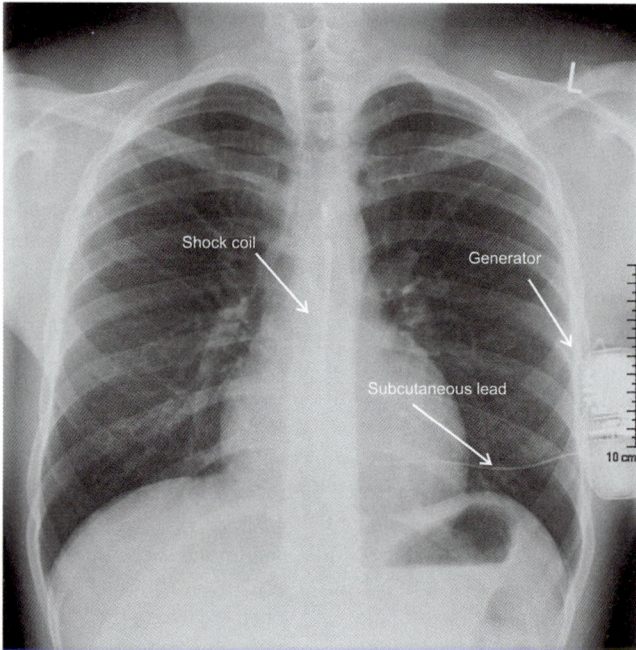

Figure 59.8 A subcutaneous ICD system.

Summary

The prevention of arrhythmic sudden death in patients with heart failure is an important aim, and one which is now achievable through the use of primary prevention ICDs, which provide highly effective treatment for life-threatening ventricular arrhythmias. In selected populations of patients with heart failure and left ventricular dysfunction, randomized trial evidence suggests that the ICD is a well-tolerated, effective, and even cost-effective therapy. However, patients with heart failure are exposed to competing risks and the prevention of sudden death in heart failure leads not only to increased survival but also to consequent increases in non-arrhythmic mortality, hospitalization for heart failure and death from progressive pump failure. This means that patients with heart failure should be carefully selected for ICD implantation, with the individual risk of sudden death and heart failure death being considered as far as possible. Given the difficulties inherent in such individualized risk prediction, it is important to recognize that there is often no correct answer, and each patient must be appropriately counselled and involved in the decision. In order to maximize the benefit afforded by an ICD, all recipients must have optimal medical therapy for heart failure and be managed by a specialist team with expertise in heart failure.

The evidence thus far has suggested that, in patients with left ventricular dysfunction, such a complex interdependence exists between arrhythmic sudden death and heart failure that ICD therapy and optimal management for heart failure should always be considered together. Due to the cumulative effect of evidence-based medication available for the treatment of heart failure, however, the rate of sudden death has declined substantially over time. A recent publication examined data from 40 195 ambulatory patients with heart failure and reduced ejection fraction enrolled into 12 clinical trials spanning the period from 1995 through 2014.[111] A 44% decline in the rate of sudden death was seen over the 19-year period, suggesting that it may become more difficult to show a significant benefit of ICD implantation for primary prevention in patients with heart failure with reduced ejection fraction in this current era.

Acknowledgement

We thank Dr Rachel C. Myles for her contributions towards an earlier version of this chapter.

REFERENCES

1. McMurray JJ, Pfeffer MA. Heart failure. *Lancet* 2005;**365**:1877–89.
2. Pfeffer MA, Swedberg K, Granger CB, *et al*. Effects of candesartan on mortality and morbidity in patients with chronic heart failure: the CHARM-Overall programme. *Lancet* 2003;**362**:759–66.
3. Gehi A, Haas D, Fuster V. Primary prophylaxis with the implantable cardioverter-defibrillator: the need for improved risk stratification. *JAMA* 2005;**294**:958–60.
4. Myerburg RJ, Castellanos A. Emerging paradigms of the epidemiology and demographics of sudden cardiac arrest. *Heart Rhythm* 2006;**3**:235–9.
5. Greenberg H, Case RB, Moss AJ, *et al*. Analysis of mortality events in the Multicenter Automatic Defibrillator Implantation Trial (MADIT-II). *J Am Coll Cardiol* 2004;**43**:1459–65.
6. Anonymous. Effect of metoprolol CR/XL in chronic heart failure: Metoprolol CR/XL Randomised Intervention Trial in Congestive Heart Failure (MERIT-HF). *Lancet* 1999;**353**:2001–7.
7. Cleland JG, Massie BM, Packer M. Sudden death in heart failure: vascular or electrical? *Eur J Heart Fail* 1999;**1**:41–5.
8. Engdahl J, Holmberg M, Karlson BW, *et al*. The epidemiology of out-of-hospital 'sudden' cardiac arrest. *Resuscitation* 2002;**52**:235–45.
9. Luu M, Stevenson WG, Stevenson LW, *et al*. Diverse mechanisms of unexpected cardiac arrest in advanced heart failure. *Circulation* 1989;**80**:1675–80.
10. Leclercq JF, Maisonblanche P, Cauchemez B, Coumel P. Respective role of sympathetic tone and of cardiac pauses in the genesis of 62 cases of ventricular fibrillation recorded during Holter monitoring. *Eur Heart J* 1988;**9**:1276–83.
11. Bayes de Luna A, Coumel P, Leclercq JF. Ambulatory sudden cardiac death: mechanisms of production of fatal arrhythmia on the basis of data from 157 cases. *Am Heart J* 1989;**117**:151–9.
12. Uretsky BF, Thygesen K, Armstrong PW, *et al*. Acute coronary findings at autopsy in heart failure patients with sudden death: results from the assessment of treatment with lisinopril and survival (ATLAS) trial. *Circulation* 2000;**102**:611–16.

13. Bardy GH, Lee KL, Mark DB, *et al*. Amiodarone or an implantable cardioverter-defibrillator for congestive heart failure. *N Engl J Med* 2005;**352**:225–37.
14. Bailey JJ, Berson AS, Handelsman H, Hodges M. Utility of current risk stratification tests for predicting major arrhythmic events after myocardial infarction. *J Am Coll Cardiol* 2001;**38**:1902–11.
15. Huikuri HV, Castellanos A, Myerburg RJ. Sudden death due to cardiac arrhythmias. *N Engl J Med* 2001;**345**:1473–82.
16. Kendall MJ, Lynch KP, Hjalmarson A, Kjekshus J. Beta-blockers and sudden cardiac death. *Ann Intern Med* 1995;**123**:358–67.
17. Domanski MJ, Exner DV, Borkowf CB, *et al*. Effect of angiotensin converting enzyme inhibition on sudden cardiac death in patients following acute myocardial infarction. A meta-analysis of randomized clinical trials. *J Am Coll Cardiol* 1999;**33**:598–604.
18. McMurray JJV, Packer M, Desai AS, Gong J, for the PARADIGM-HF Investigators and Committees. *N Engl J Med* 2014;**371**:993–1004.
19. Pitt B, Zannad F, Remme WJ, *et al*. The effect of spironolactone on morbidity and mortality in patients with severe heart failure. Randomized Aldactone Evaluation Study Investigators. *N Engl J Med* 1999;**341**:709–17.
20. Waldo AL, Camm AJ, deRuyter H, *et al*. Effect of d-sotalol on mortality in patients with left ventricular dysfunction after recent and remote myocardial infarction. The SWORD Investigators. Survival With ORal d-Sotalol. *Lancet* 1996;**348**:7–12.
21. Echt DS, Liebson PR, Mitchell LB, *et al*. Mortality and morbidity in patients receiving encainide, flecainide, or placebo. The Cardiac Arrhythmia Suppression Trial. *N Engl J Med* 1991;**324**:781–8.
22. Mirowski M, Mower MM, Langer A, *et al*. A chronically implanted system for automatic defibrillation in active conscious dogs. Experimental model for treatment of sudden death from ventricular fibrillation. *Circulation* 1978;**58**:90–4.
23. Mirowski M, Reid PR, Mower M, *et al*. Termination of malignant ventricular arrhythmias with an implanted automatic defibrillator in human beings. *N Engl J Med* 1980;**303**:322.
24. Mirowski M, Mower MM, Reid PR. The automatic implantable defibrillator. *American Heart Journal* 1980;**100**:1089–92.
25. Haffajee C, Martin D, Bhandari A, *et al*. A multicenter, randomized trial comparing an active can implantable defibrillator with a passive can system. Jewel Active Can Investigators. *Pacing Clin Electrophysiol* 1997;**20**:215–19.
26. Kouakam C, Kacet S, Hazard JR, *et al*. Performance of a dual-chamber implantable defibrillator algorithm for discrimination of ventricular from supraventricular tachycardia. *Europace* 2004;**6**:32–42.
27. Daubert JP, Zareba W, Cannom DS, *et al*. Inappropriate implantable cardioverter-defibrillator shocks in MADIT II: frequency, mechanisms, predictors, and survival impact. *J Am Coll Cardiol* 2008;**51**:1357–65.
28. Friedman PA, McClelland RL, Bamlet WR, *et al*. Dual-chamber versus single-chamber detection enhancements for implantable defibrillator rhythm diagnosis: the detect supraventricular tachycardia study. *Circulation* 2006;**113**:2871–79.
29. Cleland JG, Daubert JC, Erdmann E, *et al*. The effect of cardiac resynchronization on morbidity and mortality in heart failure. *N Engl J Med* 2005;**352**:1539–49.
30. Wathen MS, Sweeney MO, DeGroot PJ, *et al*. Shock reduction using antitachycardia pacing for spontaneous rapid ventricular tachycardia in patients with coronary artery disease. *Circulation* 2001;**104**:796–801.

31. Gold MR, Higgins S, Klein R, *et al.* Efficacy and temporal stability of reduced safety margins for ventricular defibrillation: primary results from the Low Energy Safety Study (LESS). *Circulation* 2002;**105**:2043–8.

32. Blatt JA, Poole JE, Johnson GW, *et al.* No benefit from defibrillation threshold testing in the SCD-HeFT (Sudden Cardiac Death in Heart Failure Trial). *J Am Coll Cardiol* 2008;**52**:551–6.

33. Ellenbogen KA, Levine JH, Berger RD, *et al.* Are implantable cardioverter defibrillator shocks a surrogate for sudden cardiac death in patients with nonischemic cardiomyopathy? *Circulation* 2006;**113**:776–82.

34. Daubert JP, Zareba W, Cannom DS, *et al.* Inappropriate implantable cardioverter-defibrillator shocks in MADIT II: Frequency, mechanisms, predictors, and survival impact. *J Am Coll Cardiol* 2008;**51**:1357–65

35. Moss AJ, Schuger A, Beck CA, Brown MW, for the MADIT-RIT Trial Investigators. Reduction in inappropriate therapy and mortality through ICD programming. *New Engl J Med* 2012;**367**:2275–83.

36. Scott PA, Silberbauer J, McDonagh TA, Murgatroyd FD. Impact of prolonged implantable cardioverter–defibrillator arrhythmia detection times on outcomes: a meta-analysis. *Heart Rhythm* 2014;**11**:828–35

37. Healey JS, Hohnloser SH, Glikson M, on behalf of the SIMPLE Investigators. Cardioverter defibrillator implantation without indiction of ventricular fibrillation: a single-blind, non-inferiority, randomised controlled trial. *Lancet* 2015;**385**:785–91.

38. Alter P, Waldhans S, Plachta E, *et al.* Complications of implantable cardioverter defibrillator therapy in 440 consecutive patients. *Pacing Clin Electrophysiol* 2005;**28**:926–32.

39. Al Khatib SM, Greiner MA, Peterson ED, *et al.* Patient and implanting physician factors associated with mortality and complications following implantable cardioverter–defibrillator implantation, 2002–2005. *Circ Arrhythm Electrophysiol* 2008;**1**:240–9.

40. Saksena S. Defibrillation thresholds and perioperative mortality associated with endocardial and epicardial defibrillation lead systems. The PCD investigators and participating institutions. *Pacing Clin Electrophysiol* 1993;**16**:202–7.

41. Mitchell LB, Pineda EA, Titus JL, *et al.* Sudden death in patients with implantable cardioverter defibrillators: the importance of post-shock electromechanical dissociation. *J Am Coll Cardiol* 2002;**39**:1323-1328.

42. Wilson CM, Allen JD, Bridges JB, Adgey AA. Death and damage caused by multiple direct current shocks: studies in an animal model. *Eur Heart J* 1988;**9**:1257–65.

43. Goldenberg I, Moss AJ, Hall WJ, *et al.* for the Multicenter Automatic Defibrillator Implantation Trial (MADIT) II Investigators. Causes and consequences of heart failure after prophylactic implantation of a defibrillator in the Multicenter Automatic Defibrillator Implantation Trial II. *Circulation* 2006;**113**:2810–17.

44. Hurst TM, Hinrichs M, Breidenbach C, *et al.* Detection of myocardial injury during transvenous implantation of automatic cardioverter–defibrillators. *J Am Coll Cardiol* 1999;**34**:402–8.

45. Sweeney MO, Wathen MS, Volosin K, *et al.* Appropriate and inappropriate ventricular therapies, quality of life, and mortality among primary and secondary prevention implantable cardioverter defibrillator patients: results from the Pacing Fast VT REduces Shock ThErapies (PainFREE Rx II) Trial. *Circulation* 2005;**111**:2898–905.

46. Ahmad M, Bloomstein L, Roelke M, *et al.* Patients' attitudes toward implanted defibrillator shocks. *Pacing Clin Electrophysiol* 2000;**23**:934–8.

47. Hasdemir C, Shah N, Rao AP, *et al.* Analysis of troponin I levels after spontaneous implantable cardioverter defibrillator shocks. *J Cardiovasc Electrophysiol* 2002;**13**:144–50.

48. Poole JE, Johnson GW, Hellkamp AS, *et al.* Prognostic Importance of Defibrillator Shocks in Patients with Heart Failure. *N Engl J Med* 2008;**359**:1009–17.

49. Maisel WH, Stevenson LW. Atrial fibrillation in heart failure: epidemiology, pathophysiology, and rationale for therapy. *Am J Cardiol* 2003;**91**:2–8.

50. Pacifico A, Hohnloser SH, Williams JH, *et al.* Prevention of implantable-defibrillator shocks by treatment with sotalol. d,l-Sotalol Implantable Cardioverter-Defibrillator Study Group. *N Engl J Med* 1999;**340**:1855–62.

51. Burke JL, Hallas CN, Clark-Carter D, *et al.* The psychosocial impact of the implantable cardioverter defibrillator: a meta-analytic review. *Br J Health Psychol* 2003;**8**:165–78.

52. Mark DB, Anstrom KJ, Sun JL, *et al.* Quality of life with defibrillator therapy or amiodarone in heart failure. *N Engl J Med* 2008;**359**:999–1008.

53. Driver and Vehicle Licensing Agency. Assessing fitness to drive: a guide for medical professionals. https://www.gov.uk/government/publications/assessing-fitness-to-drive-a-guide-for-medical-professionals

54. Epstein AE, Baessler CA, Curtis AB, *et al.* Addendum to "Personal and public safety issues related to arrhythmias that may affect consciousness: implications for regulation and physician recommendations: a medical/ scientific statement from the American Heart Association and the North American Society of Pacing and Electrophysiology". Public safety issues in patients with implantable defibrillators. A scientific statement from the American Heart Association and the Heart Rhythm Society. *Circulation* 2007;**115**:1170–6.

55. Vijgen J, Botto G, Camm J, *et al.* Consensus statement of the European Heart Rhythm Association: updated recommendations for driving by patients with implantable cardioverter defibrillators. *Europace* 2009;**11**:1097–1107.

56. McIvor ME, Reddinger J, Floden E, Sheppard RC. Study of Pacemaker and Implantable Cardioverter Defibrillator Triggering by Electronic Article Surveillance Devices (SPICED TEAS). *Pacing Clin Electrophysiol* 1998;**21**:1847–61.

57. Cobb LA. Resuscitation from out-of-hospital ventricular fibrillation: 4 years follow-up. *Circulation* 1975;**52**:III223–III235.

58. Antiarrhythmics versus Implantable Defibrillators (AVID) Investigators. A comparison of antiarrhythmic-drug therapy with implantable defibrillators in patients resuscitated from near-fatal ventricular arrhythmias. *N Engl J Med* 1997;**337**:1576–83.

59. Connolly SJ, Gent M, Roberts RS, *et al.* Canadian implantable defibrillator study (CIDS): a randomized trial of the implantable cardioverter defibrillator against amiodarone. *Circulation* 2000;**101**:1297–302.

60. Kuck KH, Cappato R, Siebels J, Ruppel R. Randomized comparison of antiarrhythmic drug therapy with implantable defibrillators in patients resuscitated from cardiac arrest: the Cardiac Arrest Study Hamburg (CASH). *Circulation* 2000;**102**:748–54.

61. Connolly SJ, Hallstrom AP, Cappato R, *et al.* Meta-analysis of the implantable cardioverter defibrillator secondary prevention trials. AVID, CASH and CIDS studies. Antiarrhythmics vs Implantable

Defibrillator study. Cardiac Arrest Study Hamburg. Canadian Implantable Defibrillator Study. *Eur Heart J* 2000;**21**:2071–8.

62. Domanski MJ, Epstein A, Hallstrom A, *et al*. Survival of antiarrhythmic or implantable cardioverter defibrillator treated patients with varying degrees of left ventricular dysfunction who survived malignant ventricular arrhythmias. *J Cardiovasc Electrophysiol* 2002;**13**:580–3.

63. ACC/AHA/HRS 2012 Focused Update of the 2008 Guidelines for Device-Based Therapy of Cardiac Rhythm Abnormalities. *Circulation* 2012;**126**:1784–1800.

64. Wyse DG, Friedman PL, Brodsky MA, *et al*. Life-threatening ventricular arrhythmias due to transient or correctable causes: high risk for death in follow-up. *J Am Coll Cardiol* 2001;**38**:1718–24.

65. Moss AJ, Hall WJ, Cannom DS, *et al*. Improved survival with an implanted defibrillator in patients with coronary disease at high risk for ventricular arrhythmia. Multicenter Automatic Defibrillator Implantation Trial Investigators. *N Engl J Med* 1996;**335**:1933–40.

66. Buxton AE, Lee KL, DiCarlo L, *et al*. Electrophysiologic testing to identify patients with coronary artery disease who are at risk for sudden death. Multicenter Unsustained Tachycardia Trial Investigators. *N Engl J Med* 2000;**342**:1937–45.

67. Moss AJ, Zareba W, Hall WJ, *et al*. Prophylactic implantation of a defibrillator in patients with myocardial infarction and reduced ejection fraction. *N Engl J Med* 2002;**346**:877–83.

68. Hohnloser SH, Kuck KH, Dorian P, *et al*. Prophylactic use of an implantable cardioverter–defibrillator after acute myocardial infarction. *N Engl J Med* 2004;**351**:2481–8.

69. Kadish A, Dyer A, Daubert JP, *et al*.; Defibrillators in Non-Ischemic Cardiomyopathy Treatment Evaluation (DEFINITE) Investigators. Prophylactic defibrillator implantation in patients with nonischemic dilated cardiomyopathy. *N Engl J Med* 2004;**350**:2151–8.

70. Kober L, Thune JJ, Nielsen JC, Haarbo J, DANISH Investigators. Defibrillator implantation in patients with nonischemic systolic heart failure. *N Engl J Med* 2016;**375**:1221–30.

71. Steinbeck G, Andresen D, Senges J, *et al*. IRIS Investigators as Joint Study of the German University Hospitals and German Society of Leading Cardiological Hospital Physicians (ALKK). Immediate Risk-Stratification Improves Survival (IRIS): study protocol. *Europace* 2004;**6**:392–9.

72. Steinbeck G, Andresen D, Seidl K, *et al*.; the IRIS Investigators. Defibrillator implantation early after myocardial infarction. *N Engl J Med* 2009;**361**:1427–36.

73. Packer DL, Bernstein R, Wood F, *et al*. Impact of amiodarone versus implantable cardioverter defibrillator therapy on the mode of death in congestive heart failure patients in the SCDHeFT trial. *Heart Rhythm* 2005;**2**:S38–S39.

74. Bardy GH, Lee KL, Boehmer JP, *et al*. The progression of congestive heart failure over the course of the sudden cardiac death in heart failure trial (SCD-HeFT). *Heart Rhythm* 2005;**2**:S39.

75. Priori SG, Blomstrom-Lundqvist C, Mazzanti A, *et al*. 2015 ESC Guidelines for the management of patients with ventricular arrhythmias and the prevention of sudden cardiac death. *Eur Heart J* 2015;**36**:2793–867.

76. Ponikowski P, Voors AA, Anker SD, *et al*. 2016 ESC Guidelines for the diagnosis and treatment of acute and chronic heart failure. *Eur Heart J* 2016;**37**:2129–200.

77. National Institute for Health and Care Excellence. Technology appraisal 314 (2014). Implantable cardioverter defibrillators and cardiac resynchronisation therapy for arrhythmias and heart failure. https://www.nice.org.uk/guidance/ta314

78. Connelly DT, Colquhoun I, Dunn M, *et al*. Cardiac arrhythmias in coronary heart disease. SIGN guideline 152, September 2018. http://www.sign.ac.uk/media/1089/sign152.pdf

79. Hlatky MA, Mark DB. The high cost of implantable defibrillators. *Eur Heart J* 2007;**28**:388–91.

80. Camm J, Klein H, Nisam S. The cost of implantable defibrillators: perceptions and reality. *Eur Heart J* 2007;**28**:392–7.

81. Mark DB, Nelson CL, Anstrom KJ, *et al*. Cost-effectiveness of defibrillator therapy or amiodarone in chronic stable heart failure: results from the Sudden Cardiac Death in Heart Failure Trial (SCD-HeFT). *Circulation* 2006;**114**:135–42.

82. Sanders GD, Hlatky MA, Owens DK. Cost-effectiveness of implantable cardioverter–defibrillators. *N Engl J Med* 2005;**353**:1471–80.

83. Buxton M, Caine N, Chase D, *et al*. A review of the evidence on the effects and costs of implantable cardioverter defibrillator (ICD) therapy in different patient groups, and modelling of cost-effectiveness and cost-utility for these groups in a UK context. *Health Technol Assess* 2006;**10**(27):iii–iv, ix–xi, 1–164.

84. Mark DB, Hlatky MA. Medical economics and the assessment of value in cardiovascular medicine: Part I. *Circulation* 2002;**106**:516–20.

85. Zareba W, Piotrowicz K, McNitt S, Moss AJ. Implantable cardioverter–defibrillator efficacy in patients with heart failure and left ventricular dysfunction (from the MADIT II population). *Am J Cardiol* 2005;**95**:1487–591.

86. Yap YG, Duong T, Bland JM, *et al*. Optimising the dichotomy limit for left ventricular ejection fraction in selecting patients for defibrillator therapy after myocardial infarction. *Heart* 2007;**93**:832–6.

87. Wilkoff BL, Cook JR, Epstein AE, *et al*. Dual Chamber and VVI Implantable Defibrillator Trial Investigators. Dual-chamber pacing or ventricular backup pacing in patients with an implantable defibrillator: the Dual Chamber and VVI Implantable Defibrillator (DAVID) Trial. *JAMA* 2002;**288**:3115–23.

88. Gardiwal A, Yu H, Oswald H, *et al*. Right ventricular pacing is an independent predictor for ventricular tachycardia/ventricular fibrillation occurrence and heart failure events in patients with an implantable cardioverter-defibrillator. *Europace* 2008;**10**:358–63.

89. Steinberg JS, Fischer A, Wang P, *et al*. MADIT II, I. The clinical implications of cumulative right ventricular pacing in the multicenter automatic defibrillator trial II. *J Cardiovasc Electrophysiol* 2005;**16**:359–65.

90. Proclemer A, Ghidina M, Gregori D, *et al*. Impact of the main implantable cardioverter–defibrillator trials in clinical practice: data from the Italian ICD Registry for the years 2005–07. *Europace* 2009;**11**:465–75.

91. Hallstrom AP, Greene HL, Wilkoff BL, *et al*. Relationship between rehospitalization and future death in patients treated for potentially lethal arrhythmia. *J Cardiovasc Electrophysiol* 2001;**12**:990–5.

92. Bristow MR, Saxon LA, Boehmer J, *et al*. Cardiac-resynchronization therapy with or without an implantable defibrillator in advanced chronic heart failure. *N Engl J Med* 2004;**350**:2140–50.

93. Cleland JG, Daubert JC, Erdmann E, *et al*. Longer-term effects of cardiac resynchronization therapy on mortality in heart failure [the CArdiac REsynchronization-Heart Failure (CARE-HF) trial extension phase]. *Eur Heart J* 2006;**27**:1928–32.

94. Moss AJ, Hall WJ, Cannom DS, *et al.* Cardiac-resynchronization therapy for the prevention of heart-failure events. *N Engl J Med* 2009;**361**:1329–38.

95. Linde C, Abraham WT, Gold MR, *et al.* Randomized trial of cardiac resynchronization in mildly symptomatic heart failure patients and in asymptomatic patients with left ventricular dysfunction and previous heart failure symptoms. *J Am Coll Cardiol* 2008;**52**:1834–43.

96. Yao G, Freemantle N, Calvert MJ, *et al.* The long-term cost-effectiveness of cardiac resynchronization therapy with or without an implantable cardioverter-defibrillator. *Eur Heart J* 2007;**28**:42–51.

97. Kramer DB, Buxton MD, Zimetbaum PJ. Time for a change—a new approach to ICD replacement. *N Engl J Med* 2012;**366**:219–93.

98. Pettit SJ, Browne S, Hogg KJ, *et al.* ICDs in end stage heart failure. *BMJ Support Palliat Care* 2012;**2**:94–7.

99. Pettit SJ, Jackson CE, Gardner RS. Deactivation of implantable cardioverter–defibrillators at end of life. *Future Cardiol* 2013;**9**:885–96.

100. Berger JT. The ethics of deactivating implanted cardioverter defibrillators. *Ann Intern Med* 2005;**142**:631–4.

101. Anderson KP. Risk assessment for defibrillator therapy: Il Trittico. *J Am Coll Cardiol* 2007;**50**:1158–60.

102. Stevenson LW, Desai AS. Selecting patients for discussion of the ICD as primary prevention for sudden death in heart failure. *J Card Fail* 2006;**12**:407–12.

103. Kramer DB, Friedman PA, Kallinen LM, *et al.* Development and validation of a risk score to predict early mortality in recipients of implantable cardioverter–defibrillators. *Heart Rhythm* 2012;**9**:42–6.

104. Barsheshet A, Moss AJ, Huang DT, *et al.* Applicability of a risk score for predication of the long-term (8 year) benefit of the implantable cardioverter-defibrillator. *J Am Coll Cardiol* 2012;**59**:2075–9.

105. Levy WC, Mozaffarian D, Linker DT, *et al.* The Seattle Heart Failure Model: prediction of survival in heart failure. *Circulation* 2006;**113**:1424–33.

106. Levy WC, Lee KL, Hellkamp AS, *et al.* Maximising survival benefit with primary prevention ICD therapy in a heart failure population. *Circulation* 2009;**120**:835–42.

107. Lee DS, Tu JV, Austin PC, *et al.* Effect of cardiac and noncardiac conditions on survival after defibrillator implantation. *J Am Coll Cardiol* 2007;**49**:2408–15.

108. Bardy GH, Smith WM, Hood MA, *et al.* An entirely subcutaneous implantable cardioverter–defibrillator. *N Engl J Med* 2010;**363**:36–44.

109. Lambiase PD, Barr C, Theuns DA, *et al.* EFFORTLESS Investigators. *Eur Heart J* 2014;**35**:1657–65.

110. Knops RE, Olde Nordkamp LRA, Delnoy PPHM, *et al.*, for the PRAETORIAN investigators. Subcutaneous or transvenous defibrillator therapy. *N Engl J Med* 2020;**383**:526–36.

111. Shen L, Jhund PS, Petrie MC, *et al.* Declining risk of sudden death in heart failure. *N Engl J Med* 2017;**377**:41–51.

60

Cardiac resynchronization therapy

Paul M. Haydock and Peter J. Cowburn

Introduction

Cardiac resynchronization therapy (CRT), or biventricular pacing (BVP), is now well established as a therapeutic option for selected, symptomatic patients with heart failure due to left ventricular systolic dysfunction and reduced ejection fraction (HFrEF) and a prolonged QRS interval. Numerous well-designed trials, in conjunction with more than a decade of clinical experience, have demonstrated the efficacy of CRT in improving symptoms, reducing hospitalizations, and prolonging survival, when combined with optimal medical therapy in this patient group.[1–6]

CRT improves electromechanical dyssynchrony and maximizes the efficiency of the cardiac contraction sequence, leading to an acute haemodynamic benefit, and, over time, a reduction in left ventricular (LV) volumes and an increase in left ventricular ejection fraction (LVEF). A prolonged QRS width (>130 ms) is a marker of likely benefit, with ~70% of such patients showing symptomatic improvement with CRT.[7] Cardiac resynchronization therapy can be delivered as a pacing system alone (CRT-P) or in addition to an implantable cardioverter–defibrillator (ICD)—CRT-D. Advances in device and lead technologies continue to improve successful delivery of CRT, and modern telecommunication technologies enable remote monitoring of device variables and various surrogate markers of heart failure, potentially offering the ability to predict subclinical deterioration and thus allow for timely therapeutic intervention.

History of pacing in heart failure

In the early 1990s, dual-chamber endocardial pacing with a short atrioventricular (AV) delay (100 ms) was reported to improve LVEF, NYHA class, and exercise duration in studies of small numbers of patients with end-stage dilated cardiomyopathy.[8,9] The benefits occurred predominantly in patients with a long PR interval. The mechanism appeared to be that a reduction in AV delay led to improved diastolic filling and a reduction in diastolic mitral regurgitation.[10] However, these promising results were not confirmed in later studies[11,12] and subsequently the DAVID study[13] demonstrated that chronic right ventricular (RV) pacing was detrimental for patients with left ventricular systolic dysfunction (LVSD). This is presumed to be a result of the uncoordinated contraction, or 'dyssynchrony', created by RV apical pacing.

The haemodynamic effects of temporary pacing with right, left, and simultaneous ventricular activation were described in the 1970s.[14] However, it was only in 1994 that Cazeau and colleagues successfully implanted what would now be recognized as a cardiac resynchronization pacemaker in a patient with NHYA class IV heart failure who had first degree AV block and left bundle branch block (LBBB).[15] All four chambers were paced, using a coronary sinus lead to pace the left atrium and an epicardial lead to pace the LV free wall. The patient made a remarkable recovery and this led to further observational studies of biventricular pacing using transvenous leads to pace the left ventricle via the cardiac veins. Cazeau's work stimulated a large number of research studies looking at the acute haemodynamic effects of atrio-biventricular pacing, which would become known as cardiac resynchronization therapy.

Acute haemodynamic effects of CRT

Leclercq *et al.*[16] studied the acute haemodynamic effects of biventricular pacing (BVP) in patients with end-stage HFrEF and QRS prolongation. Cardiac index (CI) was significantly increased by BVP in comparison with AAI or RV DDD pacing. Pulmonary capillary wedge pressure (PCWP) decreased significantly during BVP compared to AAI pacing. The authors noted that 12/18 patients 'responded' to CRT (which they defined as an increase of ≥10% in CI and a reduction in PCWP of ≥10%), whereas six patients were 'non-responders'.

Kass *et al.*[17] demonstrated that DDD LV free wall pacing raised dP/dt_{max} and pulse pressure compared with normal conduction. Isolated LV pacing increased dP/dt_{max} to a greater extent than BVP. The AV delay for optimal haemodynamics in the study averaged 125 ms, and AV delay had less influence on LV function than did pacing site. Of note, pacing efficacy was not associated with QRS narrowing. Auricchio *et al.*[18] described similar hemodynamic changes with increased pulse pressure and dP/dt_{max} with patient-specific optimal AV delay in individuals with QRS >150 ms. Patients with narrower

QRS, however, showed predominantly deleterious effects on LVSD with ventricular pacing.

It is important to note from these data that the acute haemodynamic changes observed with CRT are associated with a modest lowering of myocardial oxygen consumption. By contrast, inotropic agents, such as dobutamine, increase myocardial oxygen demand while achieving similar haemodynamic changes.[19] Given the adverse outcomes observed with the use of inotropic agents in heart failure,[20] the findings offered great hope for the long-term benefits of CRT.

CRT also results in an acute reduction in the volume of mitral regurgitation. There are several mechanisms for functional mitral regurgitation in patients with heart failure, including mitral valve annular dilation, alterations in LV geometry, and LV dyssynchrony.[21] Functional mitral regurgitation is reduced acutely following CRT due to an increase in LV dP/dt_{max} and an increase in transmitral pressure gradient. There is a consequent improvement in closure of the mitral valve leaflets during LV systole.[22] In patients with markedly prolonged AV interval, there may be presystolic mitral regurgitation, which can be reduced by improved AV timing. Over time, left atrial and LV remodelling may also result in a further reduction in the severity of functional mitral regurgitation.

Dyssynchrony between papillary muscle contractions may also contribute to mitral regurgitation in patients with heart failure and QRS prolongation. Mechanical activation strain mapping has demonstrated a marked reduction in interpapillary muscle time delay with CRT.[23] Where LV dyssynchrony involves the posterior papillary muscle, CRT may lead to an immediate reduction in MR.[24] Figure 60.1 demonstrates an acute rise in arterial blood pressure and a fall in pulmonary artery pressure following onset of CRT. Figure 60.2 demonstrates a sharp reduction in PCWP with onset of CRT in the same patient, with a reduction in the v-wave due to MR.

Outcome studies of CRT

There have now been 16 randomized controlled trials of CRT with a total of ~9500 patients (Table 60.1).[1-5,25-36] The initial studies required surgical placement of the LV lead.[26,27] However, subsequent developments have led to catheter techniques for implanting the LV lead transvenously via the coronary sinus, the method of choice for delivering CRT. Most trials demonstrating the benefits of CRT have compared CRT-D to ICD alone, though a small number have compared CRT-P to back-up pacing. Two large, landmark clinical trials—COMPANION and CARE-HF—compared optimal medical therapy (OMT) alone with OMT plus CRT.

The early studies demonstrated an improvement in symptoms, exercise capacity, and quality of life comparable to, or better than, those obtained in pharmacological studies.[1,2,26,28] The size of the benefit was a 0.5–0.8 point reduction in New York Heart Association (NYHA) class, a 20% increase in 6 min walk distance, and a 10–15% increase in exercise capacity as measured by peak Vo_2. Quality of life (assessed predominantly by the Minnesota Living with Heart Failure Questionnaire) also improved with CRT. These early studies had short follow-up times of 3–6 months and were not powered to assess heart failure morbidity and mortality.

The much larger COMPANION study compared CRT-D and CRT-P with medical therapy over a 12-month period.[4] CRT, with or without a defibrillator, improved hospital-free survival (CRT-P 19% event reduction, CRT-D, 20%) and reduced hospitalization for heart failure (CRT-P 34% reduction, CRT-D 40%) compared with medical therapy alone. The secondary end-point of all-cause mortality was significantly reduced only by CRT-D (36% reduction, $P < 0.003$), but the study was not suitably powered to assess the effect of CRT-P alone, which itself showed a strong trend towards reducing mortality (24% reduction, $P = 0.059$).

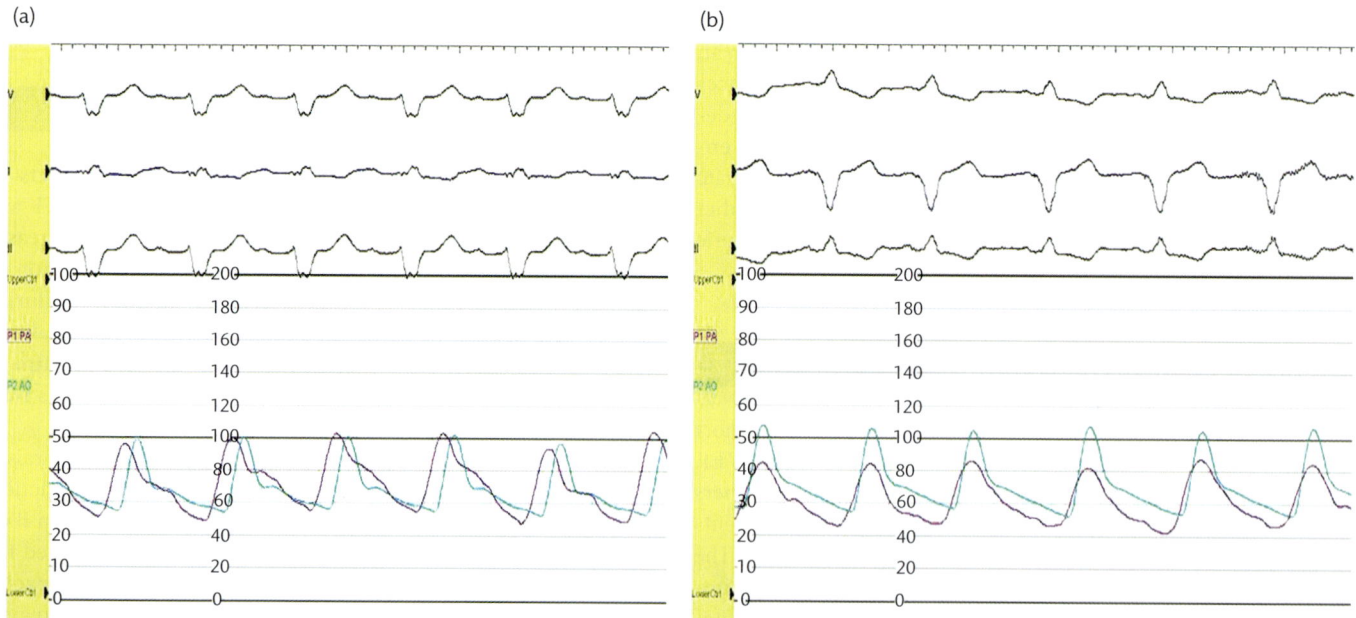

Figure 60.1 (a) A patient with first-degree heart block and left bundle branch block. Simultaneous aortic and pulmonary artery pressures are shown. There is clear interventricular mechanical delay, with the pulmonary arterial trace preceding the aortic trace. (b) The same patient following commencement of cardiac resynchronization therapy. The PR interval has normalized and the QRS morphology has changed. Aortic pressure has increased and pulmonary artery pressure has fallen. Note the marked reduction in interventricular mechanical delay.

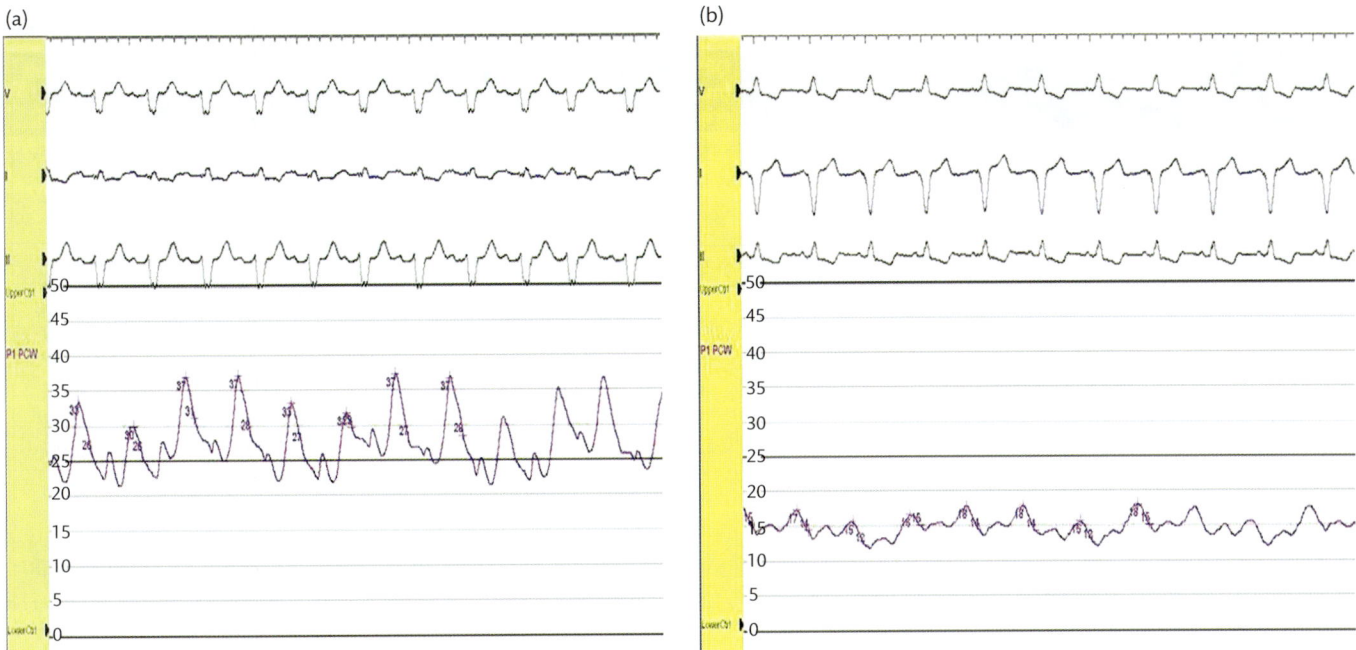

Figure 60.2 (a) A recording of the pulmonary artery capillary wedge pressure (PCWP) in the same patient as shown in Figure 60.1 The mean PCWP is elevated in excess of 25 mmHg with a large V wave secondary to mitral regurgitation. (b) The mean PCWP has fallen to 15 mmHg following commencement of cardiac resynchronization therapy. Note how the V wave is much less marked.

The CARE-HF study[3] was the largest study comparing CRT-P with medical therapy. Both groups were in NYHA class III or IV and were well treated, with 72% on β-blockers, 95% on angiotensin converting enzyme inhibitors or angiotensin receptor blockers, and 57% receiving spironolactone. Patients were followed for a mean of 29.4 months. CRT-P was associated with a 37% reduction in the composite primary end-point of mortality and hospitalization for a major cardiovascular event. All-cause mortality was also reduced by 36% and the risk of unplanned hospitalization for heart failure was reduced by 52% (**Figure 60.3**). There was also a significant reduction in sudden arrhythmic death with CRT alone in the extended follow-up phase,[31] which, taken together with results of the COMPANION study, suggests that there may be only a marginal additional survival benefit of CRT-D compared to CRT-P in patients with advanced heart failure.

The REVERSE,[37] RAFT,[35] and MADIT-CRT[34] trials have investigated the use of CRT in patients with heart failure and less severe symptoms. Each trial confirmed the benefit of CRT in patients with prolonged QRS and LV impairment. Both MADIT-CRT and RAFT compared CRT-D with ICD alone, whereas in REVERSE, all patients were implanted with a CRT-D device and then were programmed CRT on or off. The trials differ in their patient selection criteria and overall length of follow-up, but taken together they provide compelling evidence for the benefits of CRT in mild-to-moderate heart failure in patients with LVEF <40% and prolonged QRS. The principal benefits in the medium term appear to relate to reduction in heart failure hospitalization and beneficial remodelling. In the longer term, mortality benefits are seen in RAFT and in the MADIT-CRT population but the data suggest that QRSd >150 ms is strongly associated with benefit and that the mortality benefits may only be seen in those with LBBB morphology rather than simply a prolonged QRS.[38]

Long-term effects of CRT

Remodelling

Several randomized studies have demonstrated that CRT is associated with a greater reduction in LV internal dimensions and volumes, and an increase in LVEF, when compared with medical therapy alone. Although the majority of such beneficial remodelling occurs between 3 and 9 months after CRT, there is evidence for ongoing remodelling up to 18 months post implant. Less beneficial remodelling is seen in those with ischaemic heart disease (IHD), due to myocardial scar tissue. Patients with no mechanical dyssynchrony or with RV dysfunction at baseline have also been shown to have less beneficial remodelling.[39]

At a molecular level, CRT is associated with reductions in interstitial fibrosis, and reduced levels of the proinflammatory cytokine tumour necrosis factor α, as well as a reduction in cellular apoptosis.[40] Improvement in LV function following CRT is also associated with favourable changes in genes that regulate the contractile apparatus and mediate pathological hypertrophy.[41] However, LV remodelling occurs in only 50–66% of individuals following CRT, and clinical improvement is not confined solely to those patients who exhibit favourable remodelling.[42] There is a suggestion, however, that such remodelling is associated with improvements in overall prognosis: a decrease in left ventricular end-systolic volumes (LVESV) of >10% following CRT was associated with lower mortality in one observational study.[43]

Table 60.1 The randomized CRT trials

RCT	Authors, country, publication date	N	Mean age (years)	NYHA class	QRSd (ms) entry criteria	Mean QRSd (ms)	LVEF (%) entry criteria	Follow-up (months)	Primary end-point	Main result
MUSTIC-SR	Cazeau et al. Europe, 2001	58	63	III	>150	176	<35	3	6MWT	Positive effect of CRT
MUSTIC-AF	Leclerq et al. Europe, 2002	43	63	III	>200	209	<35	3	6MWT	No significant effect
MIRACLE	Abraham et al. USA, 2002	453	64	III, IV	>130	167	<35	6	6MWT, QoL, NYHA Class	Positive effect of CRT
PATH-CHF	Aurrichio et al. Germany, 2002	41	60	III, IV	>130	175	<35	6	6MWT, peak VO$_2$	Positive effect of CRT
PATH-CHF II	Aurrichio et al. Germany, 2003	86	60	II–IV	>120	155	<35	3	6MWT, peak VO$_2$	No difference in primary end-point
MIRACLE-ICD	Young et al. USA, 2003	369	63	III, IV	>130	165	<35	6	6MWT, QoL, NYHA class	Positive effect of CRT
CONTAK-CD	Higgins et al. USA, 2003	445	66	II–IV	>120	160	<35	6	HF progression	No significant effect of CRT
COMPANION	Bristow et al. USA, 2003	1520	67	III, IV	>120	160[a]	<35	12	All cause mortality and hospitalization	37% reduction in primary end-point
MIRACLE-ICD II	Abraham et al. USA 2004	186	60	II	>130	164	<35	6	Peak VO$_2$	No significant effect of CRT
CARE-HF	Cleland et al. Europe 2006	813	67	III, IV	>120	160a	<35	36.4	All cause mortality and hospitalization	55% reduction in primary end-point
HOBIPACE	Kindermann et al. Germany 2006	30	70	NA	NA	174	<35	3	LVEF, LVESV, peak VO$_2$	Positive effect of CRT
REVERSE	Linde et al. Europe/North America 2008	610	62	I, II	>120	154	<40	12	HF clinical composite response	No difference with CRT
MADIT-CRT	Moss et al. Europe/USA 2009	1820	65	I, II	>130	NA	<30	28.8	All cause mortality or non-fatal HF event	44% reduction in primary end-point
RAFT	Tang et al. Europe/ North America/ Australia 2010	1798	66	II, III	>120b	157	<30	40	All cause mortality and hospitalization	25% reduction in primary end-point in CRT group
BLOCK-HF	Curtis et al. North America 2013	691	73	I–III	NA	123	≤50	37	All cause mortality, intravenous diuretic therapy or ≥15% increase in LVESVi	26% reduction in primary end-point in CRT group
EchoCRT	Ruschitzka et al. Europe/North America/Australia 2013	855	58	III, IV	<130	106	≤35	19.4	All cause mortality or first hospitalization for HF	Terminated on grounds of futility. Signal for excess mortality with CRT

6MWT, six-minute walk test; AF, atrial fibrillation; CARE-HF, CArdiac REsynchronization-Heart Failure; COMPANION, Comparison of Medical Therapy Pacing and Defibrillation Therapy in Heart Failure; HF, heart failure; HOPIPACE, Homburg Biventricular Pacing Evaluation; ICD, implantable cardioverter–defibrillator; LVEF, left ventricular ejection fraction; MADIT-CRT, Multicenter Automated Defibrillator Implantation Trial with Cardiac Resynchronization Therapy; MIRACLE, Multicentre InSync Randomized CLinical Evaluation; MUSTIC, MUltisite STimulation In Cardiomyopathies; NA, not available; NYHA, New York Heart Association; PATH-CHF, PAcing THerapies in Congestive Heart Failure; QoL, quality of life; REVERSE, REsynchronization reVErsus Remodeling in Systolic left vEntricular dysfunction; SR, sinus rhythm; RAFT, Resynchronization–Defibrillation for Ambulatory Heart Failure Trial; BLOCK-HF, Biventricular versus Right Ventricular Pacing in Heart Failure Patients with Atrioventricular Block; LVESVi, Left Ventricular End-Systolic Volume index; EchoCRT, Echocardiography Guided Cardiac Resynchronization Therapy.

[a] Median.
[b] Intrinsic QRS duration. Paced QRS duration for entry ≥200 ms.

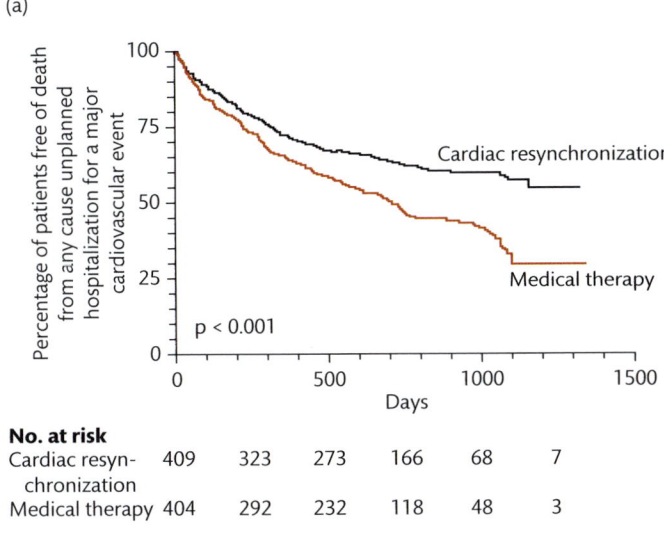

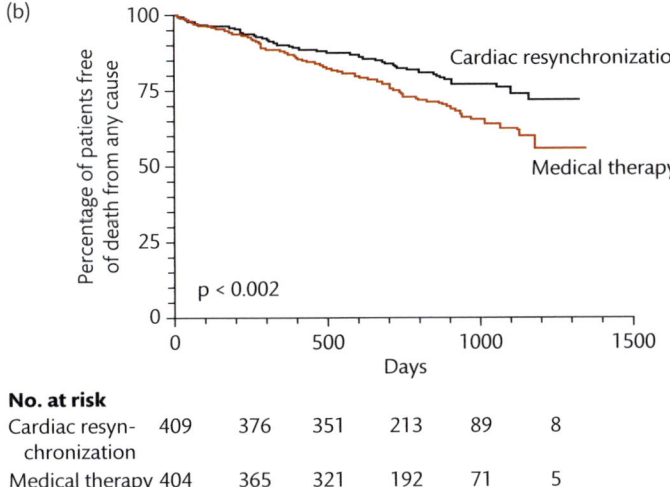

Figure 60.3 CARE-HF study: Kaplan–Meier estimates of time to primary end-point (a) and the principal secondary outcome (b). The primary outcome was death from any cause or unplanned hospitalization for a major cardiovascular event. The principal secondary outcome was death from any cause.

Source date from Saberwal B, Ahsan S. NICE guidelines for use of implantable cardioverter defibrillators. *Br J Hosp Med (Lond)* 2015;**76**:316–17.

Cardiac energy metabolism and perfusion

Functional studies using positron emission tomography have demonstrated that CRT increases stroke volume without increasing metabolic demand.[44] Following CRT, there is a more homogeneous pattern of regional myocardial oxygen and glucose metabolism with an increase in global myocardial perfusion reserve.[45,46] These effects of CRT are maintained for at least 13 months, resulting in a return of regional myocardial perfusion pattern similar to that of patients with mild heart failure and no LBBB.[47]

Cardiac cycle changes

CRT alters cardiac timing so that the proportion of each cardiac cycle spent as isovolumic contraction/relaxation ('wasted time') is reduced. The Tei index ((isovolumic contraction + relaxation time)/ the total ejection time) is increased in patients with heart failure and is reduced with successful CRT.[48,49]

Natriuretic peptides

CRT causes a fall in circulating levels of both atrial natriuretic peptide (ANP) and B-type natriuretic peptide (BNP). CRT results in a greater decrease in BNP than medical therapy alone at 3 months, with further reductions at 18 months, correlating with the improvement in LV function.[50] A high BNP at 1 month following CRT is associated with a worse prognosis, and reduction of BNP at 3 months is a strong predictor of an improvement in exercise capacity, LVEF, and reduction in volume of mitral regurgitation.[51,52] ANP fell with CRT in a sub-group of patients with renal impairment taking part in the MIRACLE study (glomerular filtration rate: 30–60 mL/min/1.73 m^2). In the same group, glomerular filtration rate increased. However, noradrenaline, plasma renin activity, aldosterone, and big endothelin were all unchanged.[53]

Autonomic nervous system

CRT has a sustained sympatho-inibitory effect as measured directly by muscle sympathetic nerve activity.[54] Plasma noradrenaline levels do not change.[53–55] CRT improved heart rate variability (HRV)—a sign of improved autonomic function—in patients with symptomatic heart failure randomized to CRT-ON in the pilot phase of the MIRACLE study.[55] Baroreflex sensitivity also improved by 30% in patients responding to CRT with reduction in LVESV of ≥15% at 6 months. HRV increased by 30% in such responders in the same study.[56] Together, these findings suggest that improvement in autonomic function occurs following CRT and may be part of its beneficial effect.

There is also evidence that central sleep apnoea, which is common in patients with heart failure, may also be improved by CRT (± atrial overdrive pacing).[57] The exact mechanism is unclear, but may involve stabilization of fluctuating parasympathetic tone.

Patient selection

The current selection criteria for CRT are based on the results of the randomized controlled trials described above. The vast majority of patients recruited to trials demonstrating a benefit for CRT had severe LVSD combined with symptoms refractory to maximally tolerated medical therapy, and had a prolonged QRS width. Indeed, there is clear evidence that patients without prolongation of the QRS complex derive no benefit from CRT, and that CRT may be harmful in this group.[5]

Table 60.2 Guidelines for CRT implantation from the Heart Failure Association of the ESC 2016[64]

Recommendations	Class[a]	Level[b]	Ref.[c]
CRT is recommended for symptomatic patients with HF in sinus rhythm with a QRS duration ≥150 ms and LBBB QRS morphology and with LVEF ≤35% despite OMT in order to improve symptoms and reduce morbidity and mortality.	I	A	261–272
CRT should be considered for symptomatic patients with HF in sinus rhythm with a QRS duration ≥150 ms and non-LBBB QRS morphology and with LVEF ≤35% despite OMT in order to improve symptoms and reduce morbidity and mortality.	IIa	B	261–272
CRT is recommended for symptomatic patients with HF in sinus rhythm with a QRS duration of 130–149 ms and LBB QRS morphology and with LVEF ≤35% despite OMT in order to improve symptoms and reduce morbidity and mortality.	I	B	266, 273
CRT is recommended for symptomatic patients with HF in sinus rhythm with a QRS duration of 130–149 ms and LBB QRS morphology and with LVEF ≤35% despite OMT in order to improve symptoms and reduce morbidity and mortality.	IIb	B	266, 273
CRT rather than RV pacing is recommended for patients with HFrEF regardless of NYHA class who have an indication for ventricular pacing and high degree AV black in order to reduce morbidity. This includes patients with AF (see Section 10.1)	I	A	274–277
CRT should be considered for patients with LVEF ≤35% in NYHA class III–IV[d] despite OMT in order to improve symptoms and reduce morbidity and mortality they are in AF and have a QRS duration ≥130 ms provided a strategy to ensure bi-ventricular capture is in place or the patient is expected to return to sinus rhythm.	IIa	B	275, 278–281
Patients with HFrEF who have received a conventional pacemaker or an ICD and subsequently develop worsening HF despite OMT and who have a high proportion of RV pacing may be considered for upgrade to CRT. This does not apply to patients with stable HF.	IIb	B	282
CRT is contra-indicated patients with a QRS duration < 130 MSEC	III	A	266, 283–285

AF, atrial fibrillation; AV, atrioventricular; CRT, cardiac resynchronization therapy; HF, heart failure; HFrEF, heart failure with reduced ejection fraction; ICD, implantable cardioverter defibrillator; LBBB, left bundle branch block; LVEF, left ventricular ejection fraction; NYHA, New York Heart Association; OMT, optimal medical therapy; QRS, Q, R and S waves (combination of three of the graphical deflections); RV, right ventricular.
[a] Class of recommendation.
[b] Level of evidence.
[c] Reference(s) supporting recommendations.
[d] Use judgement for patients with end stage heart failure who might be managed conservatively rather than with treatments to improve symptoms or prognosis.
Reproduced from Ponikowski P, Voors AA, Anker SD, et al. 2016 ESC Guidelines for the diagnosis and treatment of acute and chronic heart failure: The Task Force for the diagnosis and treatment of acute and chronic heart failure of the European Society of Cardiology (ESC). Developed with the special contribution of the Heart Failure Association (HFA) of the ESC. Eur J Heart Fail 2016;**18**:891–975 with permission from Oxford University Press.

National and international guidelines for the appropriate use of CRT in patients with heart failure have been continuously updated in the light of emerging, available evidence. This will undoubtedly continue as novel technologies and algorithms are assessed in the future and experience from large-scale registries informs clinical practice.

Much emphasis has been placed on the importance of reliably identifying those patients who will 'respond' to CRT. This concept is, however, in itself difficult to define and quantify accurately. Clinical trials allow physicians to observe the overall benefit of CRT in a specific cohort in terms of survival advantage or reduced hospitalizations in the cohort as a whole. How this relates to the *individual* patient is more difficult to predict in clinical practice. Defining individual patient response to CRT remains controversial and there is poor concordance in the literature between the definition of 'response,'[58] with

various echocardiographic indices and measures of performance used by different investigators. Many clinicians would place value on the way a patient feels following the procedure, but assessing this robustly in the research arena is virtually impossible.[59]

What is clear is that specific factors should be considered when assessing the patient for potential CRT. Guidelines from ESC/EHRA[60] as well as the Heart Failure Association of the ESC in Europe,[61] ACCF/AHA/HRS in North America,[62] and NICE in the UK[63] will be useful reference documents for clinicians when considering patients for CRT—and they are broadly similar. The most contemporary guidelines are those of the HFA and they principally differ from the others in making a strong recommendation that CRT is contraindicated in patients with QRS duration <130 ms—principally based on the findings of the Echo-CRT study[5] (see **Tables 60.2** and **60.3**).

Table 60.3 UK NICE guidelines for the implantation of CRT 2015[63]

QRS interval	NYHA class			
	I	II	III	IV
<120 ms	ICD if there is a high risk of sudden cardiac death			ICD and CRT not clinically indicated
120–149 ms without LBBB	ICD	ICD	ICD	CRT-P
≥150 ms with or without LBBB	CRT-D	CRT-D	CRT-P or CRT-D	CRT-P

LBBB, left bundle branch block; NYHA, New York Heart Association.
Source data from Saberwal B, Ahsan S. NICE guidelines for use of implantable cardioverter defibrillators. Br J Hosp Med (Lond) 2015;**76**:316–17.

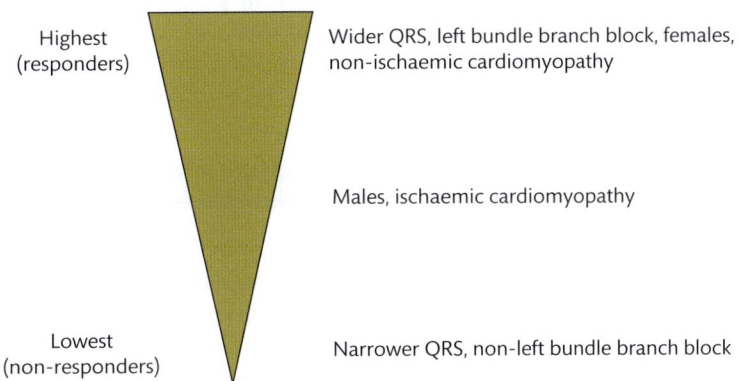

Magnitude of benefit from CRT

Highest (responders) — Wider QRS, left bundle branch block, females, non-ischaemic cardiomyopathy

Males, ischaemic cardiomyopathy

Lowest (non-responders) — Narrower QRS, non-left bundle branch block

Figure 60.4 Factors influencing the decision to implant cardiac resynchronization therapy.

Reproduced from Brignole M, Auricchio A, Baron-Esquivias G, et al. 2013 ESC Guidelines on cardiac pacing and cardiac resynchronization therapy: the Task Force on cardiac pacing and resynchronization therapy of the European Society of Cardiology (ESC). Developed in collaboration with the European Heart Rhythm Association (EHRA). *European Heart Journal* 2013;**34**:2281–329 with permission from Oxford University Press.

Given the various pathophysiological processes countered by CRT, it is likely that the dominant mechanism of benefit will vary between individuals, and that no single factor will accurately predict 'response'. However, on the basis of the available evidence the variables outlined in **Figure 60.4** should be considered.

Ejection fraction

Low ejection fraction was a key inclusion criterion for entry into all of the trials of CRT other than BLOCK-HF, which included patients with any LVEF <50% and an indication for pacing.[36] The majority of trials have specified LVEF <35%, though two of the largest—RAFT and MADIT-CRT—specified LVEF <30%.[34,35] Data for the benefit of CRT in less severe impairment of LV function largely comes from the REVERSE study which recruited patients with LVEF <40%.[37] However, even in this study, mean LVEF was 27%. Post-hoc analysis of the 29% of patients with LVEF >30% suggested that the benefits of CRT in terms of reverse remodelling and clinical outcome were independent of the LVEF.[65]

Despite their inclusion criteria, studies have randomized small numbers of patients with LVEF 35–40%: however, an individual participant data meta-analysis of patients across five randomized controlled trials of CRT suggests that the benefits of CRT are no different in this group.[7]

Subgroup analyses of the available data clearly show that lower LVEF is associated with a favourable outcome in CRT. There is also no evidence that patients with normal LVEF will benefit from CRT, but data from BLOCK-HF support a strategy of considering CRT to reduce morbidity in those with only mild LV impairment where long-term ventricular pacing is mandated.

QRS duration

Prolongation of QRS interval is the most widely used criterion for selection for CRT. A QRS width of ≥120 ms was the entry requirement for the majority of the randomized controlled trials, but the QRS width of the patients actually enrolled in all the studies was considerably higher (see **Table 60.1**); the mean QRS duration in patients receiving CRT was 167 ms in MIRACLE[2] and the median QRS was 150–160 ms in COMPANION, CARE-HF, REVERSE, RAFT, and MADIT-CRT.[3,4,34,35,37]

The RethinQ trial demonstrated no benefit from CRT on improving peak Vo₂ or quality of life in patients with heart failure and QRS width <120 ms[66] and the LESSER-EARTH trial, also investigating those with QRS width <120 ms, was terminated after recruiting only 85 patients due to futility and safety concerns.[67] Recent data have suggested that CRT may be harmful in patients with QRS width <130 ms,[5] and an individual patient data meta-analysis of five key trials of CRT (not including COMPANION and MADIT-CRT) appears to demonstrate a continuous relation between the mortality benefit of CRT and increasingly prolonged QRS.[7] The Echo-CRT trial recruited patients with NYHA II/IV heart failure and LVEF <35% but QRSd <130 ms. It was terminated early on the advice of the data and safety monitoring board after a mean follow-up period of 19.4 months on the basis of futility. At this time, interim analysis demonstrated a 20% increased risk of the combined primary endpoint of death or first hospitalization for heart failure. Although this was statistically non-significant, there was a significantly increased risk of death in the CRT group (hazard ratio: 1.81; 95% confidence interval: 1.11–2.93). When combined with data from the meta-analysis, there is a strong signal of harm with CRT in those with QRS width <130 ms—indeed, the meta-analysis paper suggests that significant benefit may only be seen in CRT when the QRS width is somewhere between 140 and 150 ms (see **Figure 60.5**).

QRS morphology

Guidelines give the strongest recommendations to patients with LBBB. The recommendations are based on sub-group analyses of individual trials, suggesting that those with LBBB show greater benefits with CRT than those without.[68] Data from the MADIT-CRT follow-up study add weight to the recommendations, with only those mildly symptomatic patients with LBBB gaining a long-term mortality

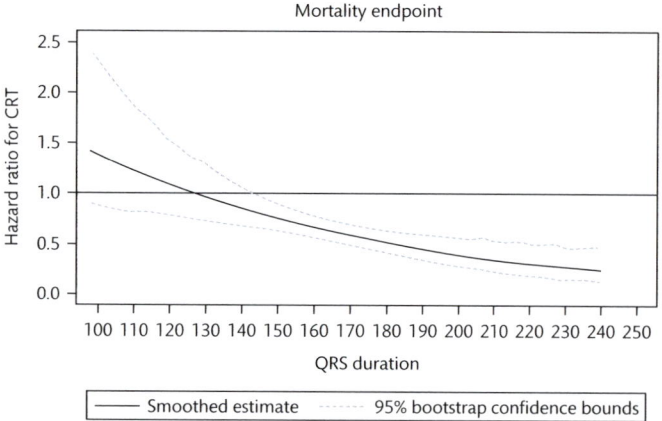

Figure 60.5 The relationship between the effect of cardiac resynchronization therapy on all-cause mortality and QRS duration. Reproduced from Cleland JG, Abraham WT, Linde C et al. An individual patient meta-analysis of five randomized trials assessing the effects of cardiac resynchronization therapy on morbidity and mortality in patients with symptomatic heart failure. European Heart Journal 2013;34:3547–56.

benefit.[38] However, decision-making based on QRS morphology remains controversial and two separate independent patient data meta-analyses have suggested that QRS morphology is largely confounded by QRS width, and that once QRS width is accounted for, there is little evidence that those with LBBB benefit more than those with other prolonged QRS morphologies.[7,69] Certainly, LBBB tends to be broader than RBBB or other non-specific interventricular conduction delay patterns. It should be borne in mind that none of the trials selected patients on the basis of QRS morphology and that they were not powered for sub-group analyses.

Mechanical dyssynchrony

The observation that response to CRT is heterogeneous among individuals with similar patterns of electrical abnormality on the surface ECG stimulated extensive research into methods of assessing mechanical dyssynchrony by various imaging modalities—principally echocardiography. Multiple non-randomized single-centre studies have proposed various methods for assessing dyssynchrony using multiple echocardiographic variables.[70] The definition of response to CRT in such studies was not standardized and the results have been difficult to replicate.

CARE-HF included a dyssynchrony assessment in all patients. Those with QRSd <150 ms were required to fulfil predefined criteria for dyssynchrony in order to be enrolled, but the absolute number of these patients in the trial was small (10% of the total). Results of a pre-defined sub-group analysis did suggest that rates of the primary composite end-point were lower in those receiving CRT with interventricular conduction delay >49 ms (normal <40 ms), but patients without dyssynchrony at baseline still derived benefit from CRT.[71]

In the PROSPECT study, designed to identify the best echocardiographic measure of dyssynchrony for predicting response to CRT, none of the 12 variables studied could reliably predict response to CRT as measured by a clinical composite score and a reduction in

LVESV of >15%.[72] These findings essentially dismissed the ability of echo to predict response to CRT, although many questioned the methodology of the trial, and research in the area continues. Assessment of mechanical dyssynchrony, however, is not included in any current guidelines for selecting patients for CRT.

Severity of heart failure symptoms

In patients with acute, decompensated heart failure there is no randomized trial evidence for the benefit of CRT. Case series have described the effects of CRT on inotrope-dependent patients and we have previously published the outcomes of 10 consecutive hospitalized patients requiring inotropic support for a mean of 11 days prior to CRT. The mean QRS was 205 ms. All patients were weaned from inotropic support after a mean of 2 days and all patients were successfully discharged from hospital. Renal function improved, diuretic requirements were reduced, and hyponatraemia was corrected. Seven patients were alive at 1 year.[73] These promising results have been reproduced by others, but it is clear that some of these patients do very badly and that publication bias is likely to lead to reporting of successful series only.

Early trials recruited patients with severe symptomatic heart failure in NYHA class III/IV. However, due to the recruitment criteria, patients with class IV symptoms were not well represented: 14% in the COMPANION trial and 6% in CARE-HF. Sub-group analysis of the 217 ambulatory, NYHA IV patients in COMPANION has demonstrated longer event-free survival (composite of all cause mortality and hospitalizations) with CRT, with a trend for reduced mortality.[74]

There is now convincing evidence that patients with less severe heart failure—with NYHA class II symptoms—benefit from CRT. Data from REVERSE, MADIT-CRT, and RAFT have all demonstrated significant reductions in time to first hospitalization or heart failure events over medium-term follow-up.[34,37] Mortality benefit for CRT NYHA class II has been demonstrated over the longer term in the follow-on study of MADIT-CRT (7 years) and the RAFT study (mean follow-up 40 months).[35,38]

CRT in atrial fibrillation

There is minimal data from randomized trials to support the use of CRT in patients with atrial fibrillation (AF). The MUSTIC-AF study recruited 59 patients with chronic AF and a slow ventricular rate requiring pacing to compare RV pacing to CRT.[25] Only 37 patients completed the trial per protocol, and there was no significant difference in exercise capacity between the two treatment phases. The PAVE study compared chronic biventricular pacing to RV pacing in 184 patients undergoing ablation of the AV node.[75] This was not a study of patients with heart failure and the mean LVEF was 46%. Six months post ablation, patients receiving CRT had a greater improvement in 6 min walk time (and had a higher LVEF) than those with an RV pacing system. The beneficial effect of CRT appeared to be greater in patients with LVEF ≤45%, or with NYHA class II/III symptoms.

Part of the problem with AF is that any benefit of CRT is likely to be seen only when 100% ventricular pacing is achieved.[76–78]

Patients with AF have no capacity to improve AV dyssynchrony, and poor rate control may mean that 100% pacing is hard to achieve. Algorithms are available that attempt to maximize biventricular pacing in patients with AF: either the base rate of the pacemaker can be programmed to adjust automatically to a rate above the sensed ventricular rate in AF; or 'ventricular sense response' (VSR) pacing can be employed, which attempts to deliver biventricular pacing in response to a sensed ventricular event, with a resulting fusion complex. Although VSR seems reasonable, it may lead to false reassurance that effective biventricular pacing is being delivered when the haemodynamics are not likely to be the same as pure CRT. Meta-analysis of cohort studies has suggested that patients in AF may improve after CRT but with less functional benefit.[79] There are case series suggesting that AV node ablation and CRT improve long-term outcome compared to CRT alone,[80] but others report a similar benefit without need for AV node ablation.[81]

There is a clear need for a suitably powered, randomized outcome trial in patients with AF, but such a trial may never be carried out, particularly because patients in AF are eligible for CRT according to all current guidelines (class IIa indication). Recent large registry data are supportive.[82] If the decision is made to proceed with CRT in a patient in AF, it is important to be aware that some patients spontaneously revert to sinus rhythm following CRT, and some can be successfully cardioverted. It is therefore appropriate to implant an atrial lead in patients with recent-onset AF, or in patients where the duration of AF is unknown. If rate control is not adequately achieved by standard medical therapy (β-blockade and digoxin), then AV node ablation should be considered.

CRT in patients with an indication for pacing

In patients with LVSD and high-degree AV block, CRT improves LV function, quality of life, and exercise capacity compared to RV pacing alone.[32] BLOCK-HF demonstrated significant reduction in a composite primary end-point of death, decompensation requiring intravenous diuretics, or 15% increase in LVESV index in those managed with CRT rather than RV pacing. Most of the events related to changes in LV dimensions over a mean follow-up of 37 months. The study recruited patients with EF <50% and the average EF was around 40%. Comparison of groups receiving ICD (mean LVEF 33%) and standard pacemaker (mean LVEF 43%) showed similar benefits when compared with CRT-D or CRT-P respectively.[36]

CRT may have advantages over RV apical pacing in patients with normal LV function in preventing adverse remodelling and reductions in EF. However, the published evidence had a limited follow-up period and the effects on these indices failed to translate into meaningful clinical differences between groups.[83]

In patients with pre-existing chronic RV pacing who have LVSD and symptomatic heart failure, upgrading to a biventricular device improves acute haemodynamic variables. The improvement is maintained in the medium term and is associated with improvement in symptoms and reduction in admissions for heart failure.[84] During longer-term follow-up, patients with CRT upgrade appear to gain a similar mortality and morbidity benefit and similar LV reverse remodelling to patients with native LBBB treated with CRT.[85]

CRT outcome by age and gender

As with most randomized controlled trials of heart failure, the average age of patients recruited for the CRT trials was relatively young at 64 years (see Table 60.1). In the MIRACLE and MIRACLE ICD trials, 174 out of 839 patients were aged >75 years. CRT led to a similar improvement in NYHA class and LVEF regardless of age.[86] Observational studies suggest that the benefits of CRT also extend to octogenarians, implying that there should be no upper age limit for CRT.[87] The role of a primary prevention ICD is less clear in elderly patients, however, as these patients are more likely to die of other non-cardiac conditions.[88]

Women are less commonly recruited to clinical trials and are less well represented in the CRT trials. Although numbers are smaller, the benefit from CRT appears similar in men and women. Interestingly, there is some evidence that response rates in women are superior to those seen in men;[3,4,34] however, fewer women than men undergo CRT in both the USA and Europe, for reasons which are unclear. Approximately 24–27% of CRT implants are in women and a relatively higher percentage of these patients received CRT-P (as opposed to CRT-D) when compared with men: 30% of CRT-P recipients vs 21% of CRT-D recipients in a contemporary European dataset.[6,89] Although this may represent a sex bias, a meta-analysis reporting on the outcome of 934 women in five ICD trials has suggested that primary prevention ICDs offer no prognostic benefit in women.[90]

Aetiology of heart failure

Patients with both ischaemic and non-ischaemic causes of heart failure benefit from CRT.[2,4,33,34] Patients with non-ischaemic causes of heart failure exhibit greater remodelling after CRT—which might be expected, as fibrotic scar in IHD patients is unlikely to respond to CRT—yet patients with IHD seem to derive equivalent morbidity and mortality benefit from CRT. MR is reduced to a similar degree in patients with IHD and non-ischaemic cardiomyopathy.[7,39,69] Data from the DANISH trial support the use of CRT in heart failure of both ischaemic and non-ischaemic aetiology, but cast doubt on the routine inclusion of an ICD in non-ischaemic patients.[88]

Congenital heart disease and CRT

The role of CRT in patients with congenital heart disease is complicated by the anatomical and physiological heterogeneity of the population and the lack of any randomized trials. The most frequent indication for CRT in case series is as an upgrade in patients with single-site ventricular pacing and heart failure. Venous access can be challenging (sometimes through surgically redirected atria) and coronary sinus anatomy is highly variable. Surgically placed epicardial leads are sometimes required. Evidence from case studies suggests that some patients benefit from CRT, but the risks of the procedure are higher, lead placement may be sub-optimal, and some patients may deteriorate following CRT.[91,92] Careful planning and MDT discussion with adult congenital heart disease specialists is essential when considering CRT in this cohort.

The CRT procedure

The dominant method of CRT implantation is transvenous, using the subclavian, 'axillary' (properly, the extrathoracic subclavian approach), or cephalic veins to access the venous system. Standard endocardial pacing leads are positioned in the right atrial appendage and right ventricle. When implanting a CRT-D system, a single- or dual-coil defibrillator lead is used instead of an RV pacing lead. A variety of pre-shaped guide catheters is available to help intubate the coronary sinus (CS). Contrast is sometimes required to guide cannulation, but its use should be minimized to reduce the risk of nephrotoxicity.[93] After the CS is cannulated, a balloon occlusion venogram is usually obtained (**Figure 60.6**) in at least two projections (antero-posterior and left anterior oblique) to demonstrate the coronary venous anatomy. The anatomy of the CS is variable and most operators aim to place the LV lead in an epicardial venous tributary overlying the lateral border of the left ventricle.

Placement of the LV lead is more technically challenging than standard pacing, often demanding guide wires or inner, pre-shaped, sub-selection catheters to access the target vein. The LV lead is usually delivered over the wire; once it is positioned, the guide catheters are split and removed. The LV lead can be unipolar, bipolar or quadripolar. Unipolar leads are now seldom used, but have historically been employed where the calibre of the preferred target vein is small or the veins are very tortuous. Improved manufacturing processes mean that low-profile bipolar and quadripolar leads are now widely available. Several manufacturers provide pre-shaped leads of varying designs to access veins of differing lengths, calibre, and tortuosity. Most are not actively fixed in the vein, but their pre-formed shape helps to give them stability once delivered to a favourable position. For very large veins, there are leads with active fixation mechanisms. Advances in the design of equipment for LV lead placement have improved the success rate of implantation, but failure rates of up to 5% are reported due to unsuitable venous anatomy, inadequate pacing thresholds, and phrenic nerve stimulation. With bipolar leads, where the electrodes are at the distal portion of the lead,

favourable lead position is often sacrificed for lead stability. The spacing of the four poles along the length of different quadripolar leads removes the trade-off to a certain extent and offers more programming options. Quadripolar leads can increase the chances of successful LV pacing as the number of pacing vectors allows for the selection of the best configuration for the individual patient.[94] Case series data suggest that quadripolar leads may have advantages in preventing hospitalization when compared with bipolar leads.[95]

Surgical placement of epicardial LV leads may still be considered in selected patients, where venous anatomy prohibits LV lead placement by standard methods. Small case series have also demonstrated the feasibility of endocardial LV lead implantation either via atrial septal or ventricular septal puncture. These approaches are at least feasible, but it is a high-risk strategy and effective systemic anticoagulation is vital to prevent stroke and systemic embolization.[96,97]

Complications of CRT

The majority of CRT-related complications pertain to the placement or potential dislodgement of the LV lead. LV lead complications in BLOCK-HF were reported in 6.4% of patients. In a report of >2000 patients taking part in the MIRACLE, MIRACLE ICD, and InSync III studies, the implant attempt succeeded in 91.6% of patients.[98] Dissection or perforation of the CS occurred in 2.2% of patients. A pericardial effusion or tamponade occurred in 0.4% of cases, with one-half requiring pericardiocentesis. Lead revision (predominantly LV lead) was needed in 7.7% of patients during 6-month follow-up. Pocket infection developed in 1%, with two-thirds of patients requiring explanation of the device. Procedure-related mortality was 0.3%. Similar complication rates are reported from the major clinical trials.[99] European registry data suggest an in-hospital mortality of 0.5% in the 'real world' and rates of LV lead-related complication of 4% (2% lead displacement and 2% phrenic nerve stimulation).[6] An analysis of all implants in Denmark over the course of 1 year (209

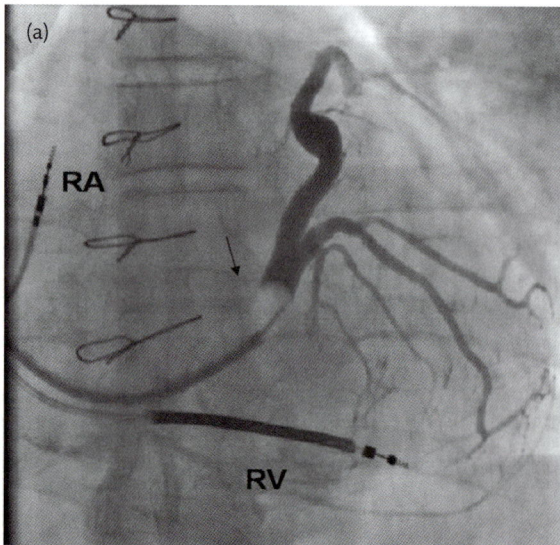
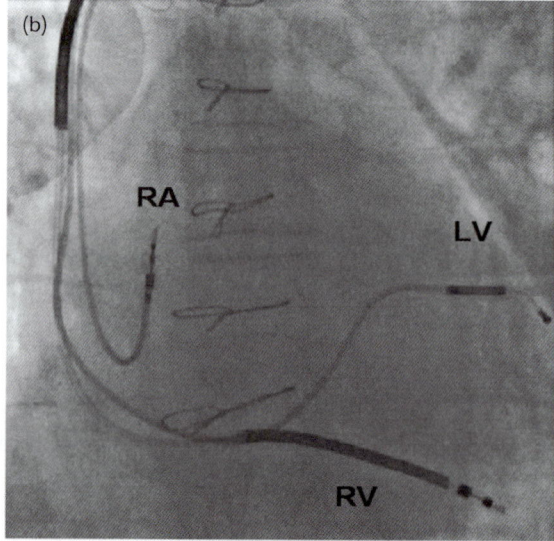

Figure 60.6 (a) AP projection of coronary sinus venogram using balloon occlusion catheter (arrow) demonstrating a lateral vein. (b) Final positions of right atrial (RA) lead, right ventricular (RV) dual-coil defibrillator lead and left ventricular (LV) lead.

CRT-P and 445 CRT-D) showed a 2.9% LV lead-related complication rate in CRT-P but only a 1.8% rate in CRT-D.[100]

Intravenous contrast is required for CS venography and to identify the os of the CS if cannulation is difficult. Contrast nephropathy is a serious complication of the procedure and at-risk patients should be pre-hydrated.[93]

Patients are at risk of the same complications as standard device insertion such as pneumothorax and infection. Analysis of all device implants in Denmark suggests a cumulative rate of any complication following CRT-P of 8% and 16% following CRT-D over a period of 6 months. Periprocedural complication rates in Europe are quoted as 9% for CRT-D and 12% for CRT-P, perhaps reflecting the fact that sicker patients tend to receive CRT-P in many countries in Europe. Re-intervention for lead revision carries a considerably higher risk of complication.[101] Despite these risks, CRT remains a safe and effective procedure. A knowledge of the factors associated with increased risk of complication is essential when consenting patients for CRT. Data suggest that, despite perceptions, younger patients appear to have a greater risk of procedure-related complications, as do those of low body mass index, and women have a higher complication rate than men.[100]

Left ventricular lead placement

The importance of LV lead positioning in achieving a good outcome from CRT[102] cannot be overstated. The positioning of the LV lead is limited by coronary venous anatomy, but there are usually several options in most patients. Haemodynamic studies have shown that placement of the LV lead over the area with the most delayed electrical activation results in the greatest rise in LV dP/dt_{max} and pulse pressure.[103] Areas of slow conduction can be identified using non-contact mapping, and haemodynamic benefit is more marked when the chosen pacing site is outside these areas.[104] In the majority of patients, the area of most delayed contraction occurs at the lateral free wall of the left ventricle, which is targeted using lateral or posterolateral veins. The anterior vein is usually orientated away from the free wall, making it less attractive; however, a lateral branch can be used. The LV lead is typically positioned midway between the base and apex of the heart within the chosen vein.

On the basis of early haemodynamic studies, the lateral or posterolateral veins have been preferentially targeted in the clinical trials. However, these veins are not always the best in an individual patient. Van Campen et al. examined nine different pacing configurations in 48 patients. The site most frequently associated with the greatest increase in cardiac output was the combination of LV pacing from a posterolateral vein with RV apical pacing, but this was true in only 29% of patients.[105] Although anteriorly positioned veins have often been considered sub-optimal, the combination of RV apical pacing with an anterolateral vein produced optimal haemodynamic benefit in 19% of patients in the same study.

Analysis of intracardiac electrograms during LV lead placement allows for the measurement of electrical delay from the onset of the QRS complex on the surface ECG to the time of depolarization in the LV segment in which the lead is placed (QLV). Increasing QLV is associated with greater haemodynamic response (assessed non-invasively using echo to assess changes in dP/dt) and longer electrical delays predict increasing event-free survival (closer relationship in the non-ischaemic population).[106] In a pre-specified sub-study of the SMART-AV trial, longer QLV intervals (>120 ms) were strongly associated with echocardiographically assessed reverse remodelling and improvements in quality of life.[107] Other methods of measuring intracardiac electrical delay have also been proposed. RV–LV interval measurements can be made by means of near-field ECG analysis via the CRT device. The baseline interval is independently associated with a response to CRT with longer RV–LV measurements predicting a better outcome. The best cut-off for predicting response to CRT is an RV–LV interval of 80 ms best (sensitivity 0.63, specificity 0.62), suggesting that the clinical utility is, at best, modest.[108] From the same data, it would also appear that mortality and hospitalization outcomes throughout 2 years of follow-up were worse in those with shorter RV–LV intervals at implant.

The advent of advanced imaging techniques and quadripolar LV leads has increased the possibility of individualizing pacing configuration to improve response to CRT. The use of echocardiographic speckle-tracking to guide LV lead placement at the latest site of LV contraction, and away from scar tissue, has shown promise in two randomized trials.[109,110]

Quadripolar leads allow multiple pacing vectors to be tested in an attempt to activate the LV segment with the highest degree of latency. Response rates increase in case series employing quadripolar leads with the best pacing vector selected by acute haemodynamic response.[111] Quadripolar leads also have the potential to allow for multi-point pacing (MPP) of the LV, which may benefit patients with very pronounced intraventricular dyssynchrony. Again, case series have demonstrated improved response rates with such therapy[112,113] and early data from a non-inferiority study of MPP vs standard biventricular pacing suggest that appropriately optimized MPP could increase response rates to 87%. Larger trials are undoubtedly needed to further assess this promising development.[114]

Right ventricular lead placement

The optimal position of the RV lead for CRT is controversial. Data from a single trial suggest that there is no difference between RV apical and RV high septal pacing sites in clinical outcome and LV reverse remodelling.[115] However, an apparent benefit was observed with RV high septal position if the LV lead was placed in the posterolateral vein. RV apical position appeared superior with anterolateral LV lead placement. It may be that it is important to achieve maximal separation between RV and LV lead tips to achieve optimal resynchronization.[116,117] An example demonstrating the lead separation achieved with RV apical pacing and antero-apical LV pacing is shown in **Figure 60.7**.

Optimization of CRT

In patients who do not have a beneficial response to CRT, guidelines recommend an attempt at post-implant optimization of pacing variables, in an attempt to improve overall haemodynamics and encourage beneficial remodelling. Alterations in pacemaker programming allow changes in timing between atria and ventricles (AV delay) and between right and left ventricle (VV delay). Devices themselves are pre-programmed with 'out-of-the-box'

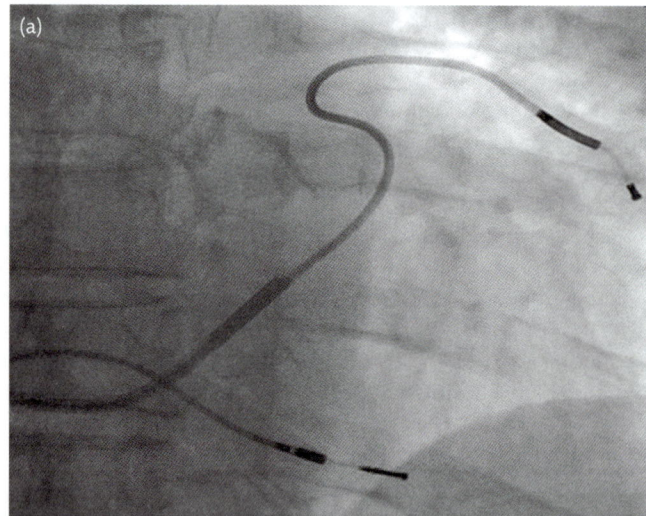

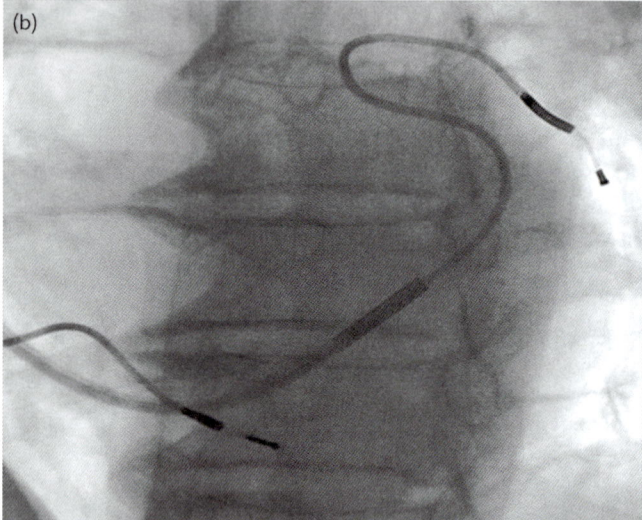

Figure 60.7 Anterolateral LV lead placement with RV apical pacing should no longer be considered a 'sub-optimal' position. (a) RV and LV lead positioning in the AP view; (b) the same leads in LAO view demonstrating excellent lead separation.

settings and the recommendation of the EHRA is for an AV delay of 100–120 ms and no programmed VV delay (simultaneous activation of both ventricles). Short AV delays facilitate biventricular pacing by preventing intrinsic conduction (which potentially causes dyssynchrony), and simultaneous biventricular activation seems the most robust method of eliminating interventricular dyssynchrony. However, the optimal AV delay is variable between individuals, and intraventricular dyssynchrony, most commonly associated with scar in the LV, means that a VV delay of zero may be suboptimal. The ideal VV timing is highly dependent on the pattern of activation within the individual ventricle, and on the final lead positions.

The EHRA propose an approach to optimization based on continuous reassessment of the individual patient's response to CRT—first seeking to optimize AV delay and then addressing VV delay (**Figure 60.8**).

A long AV delay causes late ventricular contraction; diastolic filling time (DFT) is reduced, causing fusion of the E and A waves of the mitral inflow Doppler. The atrial contribution to filling terminates before depolarization of the ventricle, resulting in wasted

diastole and suboptimal preload for ventricular contraction. AV optimization thus has a clear physiological basis with evidence of acute haemodynamic benefit[18] and was used as standard practice in the major CRT trials. The goal of AV optimization is to maximize DFT and to allow complete end-diastolic filling before the onset of LV contraction. AV programming of CRT can eliminate 'diastolic' mitral regurgitation. The most commonly employed method for AV delay optimization is an iterative method using MV pulse-wave Doppler. DFT is measured from the start of the E wave to the end of the A wave. A long AV delay is programmed and reduced in 20 ms steps until the A wave truncates. The interval is then increased in 10 ms increments. The shortest AV delay without A-wave truncation is selected.[118]

AV optimization is not routinely undertaken in all institutions. Most commonly this is due to a lack of appropriately trained staff to undertake what can be a time-consuming procedure. However, there is also a lack of robust, stand-alone evidence of its benefits, and the SMART-AV trial, involving 980 patients, failed to demonstrate any incremental improvement in response to CRT when either echo- or device-based optimization of AV delay was compared with an empirical fixed AV delay of 120 ms.[119] It is also worth noting that optimization is carried out at rest; however, the haemodynamic benefits of CRT may be more marked during exercise, suggesting that optimization should also be carried out at higher heart rates.[120] Most CRT pacemakers can programme a rate-adaptive AV delay to mimic the physiological shortening of AV delay that occurs with exercise, but the clinical value has not been fully evaluated in CRT where an increase in AV delay may actually be of benefit.[121]

VV optimization is intended to restore synchronous ventricular contraction. Sub-optimal LV lead position and regional conduction delays can affect ventricular timing; hence tailored ventricular pacing is potentially valuable. Acute haemodynamic studies have shown a benefit from VV optimization.[18,122] Small studies have also shown that echocardiographically optimized sequential biventricular pacing can improve LV function, dyssynchrony, and LV filling compared to simultaneous pacing.[123]

Again, however, large-scale trial evidence supporting routine VV optimization is lacking. Perhaps we should not be surprised—optimization is, by its nature, individualized to the patient and to the specifics of the final pacing configuration. The heterogeneity of individual cases means that any effect of optimization may be very difficult to determine in a randomly selected cohort of patients entered into a trial. Guidelines recommending an individual approach to CRT optimization based on empirical physiological concepts seem reasonable, particularly given the lack of harm apparent in any study of optimizing AV and VV delay.

In view of the challenges associated with echo-guided optimization, various groups have proposed ECG variables which might predict improved response to CRT, and device companies have developed and tested different algorithms utilizing intracardiac electrograms to facilitate 'auto-optimization'. Despite an apparent lack of relationship between acute haemodynamic benefits of CRT and QRS narrowing in response to pacing, multiple authors have observed that narrowing of the QRS (indexed to the baseline QRS) duration appears to be associated with better response to CRT.[124] Certainly, a large cohort study of patients who deteriorated following CRT found that QRS *widening* indexed to the baseline QRS duration was associated with deterioration in LV function.[125] However, such

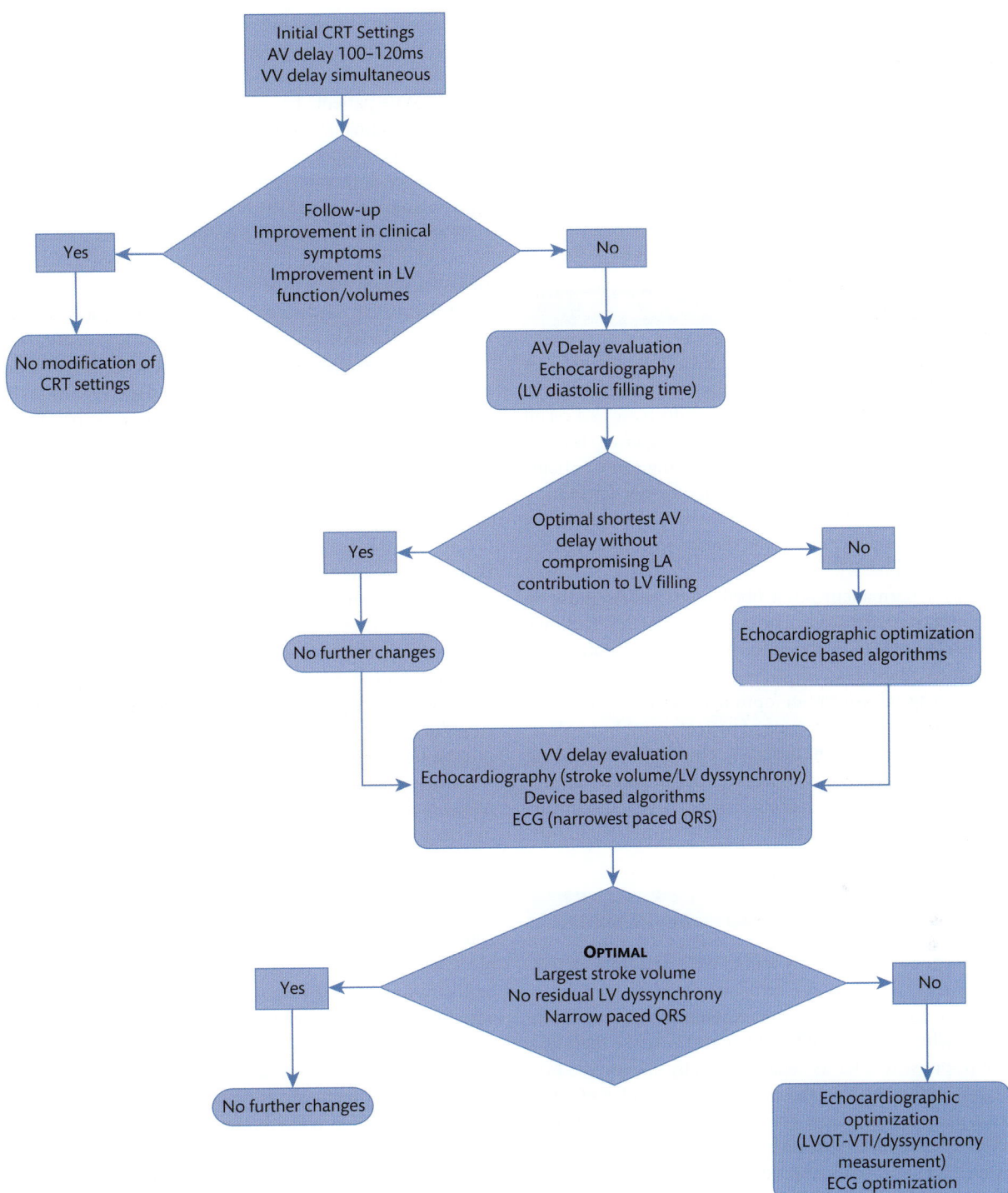

Figure 60.8 Algorithm for cardiac resynchronization therapy optimization, as proposed by the European Heart Rhythm Association.

Source data from Brignole M, Auricchio A, Baron-Esquivias G, *et al.* 2013 ESC Guidelines on cardiac pacing and cardiac resynchronization therapy: the Task Force on cardiac pacing and resynchronization therapy of the European Society of Cardiology (ESC). Developed in collaboration with the European Heart Rhythm Association (EHRA). *European Heart Journal* 2013;**34**:2281–329.

data are taken from small studies. Outcome data are also lacking and there is a lack of concordance in the literature. Indeed, an analysis of the REVERSE study found that the change in QRS duration with pacing was not an independent predictor of outcome.[126]

Studies comparing device-based optimization algorithms with standard of care (FREEDOM[127], CLEAR[128]) or echo-based optimization (Adaptive-CRT[129]) have involved >2000 patients. The studies all used a composite heart failure score as their primary outcome measure, and all demonstrated non-inferiority to the comparator. Evidence for benefits of the therapies over standard care is generally lacking. Some data support the use of Adaptive-CRT, in which an algorithm periodically monitors intrinsic conduction

and delivers preferential LV pacing only when intrinsic RV conduction is normal. The algorithm may improve outcome compared with echo-based optimization of CRT.[130] In the sub-group of patients with normal AV conduction at baseline, there was a lower risk of death or heart failure hospitalization on the Adaptive-CRT arm.[131] Automatically optimized atrioventricular and interventricular delays, based on a peak endocardial acceleration signal system, have also demonstrated greater improvements in patient-reported symptoms compared with standard care.[128]

Optimization of medical therapy

After CRT, patients often have an increase in systolic blood pressure, allowing further uptitration of renin–angiotensin–aldosterone system antagonism. Diuretic requirements may decrease as a result of improved LV performance.[73] Patients are no longer at risk of a β-blocker-induced bradycardia, potentially allowing some patients to be β-blocked for the first time and allowing further uptitration of dose in other patients. Optimization of medical therapy offers the potential to improve patient outcome further, in addition to the benefit achieved through CRT.

In patients with permanent atrial fibrillation, efforts must be made to maximize the percentage of biventricular pacing. This may involve aggressive β-blockade, the use of digoxin, and potentially consideration of AV node ablation.

When considering all aspects of 'optimization' post-CRT, it is clear that a robust system for follow-up of patients must be in place. Ideally this should involve a team including physicians specializing in heart failure with expertise in all aspects of CRT implantation and follow-up, appropriately trained cardiac physiologists and echocardiographers, heart failure specialist nurses, and electrophysiologists.

CRT response

Some patients respond spectacularly well to CRT, and some deteriorate, but the issue of CRT 'response' remains controversial. There is no good definition of a 'responder' or 'non-responder'. Approximately 70% of patients who undergo CRT feel better. However, there is a large placebo response to CRT as demonstrated by improved 6 min walk times and quality of life in the control group of MIRACLE.[28] The fact that a patient's symptoms may not have improved, or their LV volumes have not reduced, is used by many to indicate lack of 'response', but such an approach ignores the fact the patient may have had a mortality benefit, or might (without the device) have deteriorated further. For example, in an observational study of patients with CRT admitted with acute decompensation of their heart failure (who might therefore be thought to be 'non-responders'), when the CRT was switched off, the patients' haemodynamic state deteriorated further.[132]

The reasons for a lack of symptomatic response to CRT are multi-factorial and include poor patient selection, sub-optimal lead placement, device-programming issues, arrhythmias, or failure to optimize medical therapy. Prior knowledge of CS anatomy and identification of areas with non-viable myocardium may help plan LV lead placement. Contrast-enhanced magnetic resonance imaging can identify transmural scar in the posterolateral wall; patients with

such scars do not respond to CRT by clinical and echo criteria.[133] Factors that predicted a poor response to CRT in the CARE-HF trial were an ischaemic aetiology, high BNP, and increasing severity of MR.[134] Male patients have lower response rates, and shorter baseline QRS widths are associated with less favourable response. By contrast, patients with low blood pressure and echocardiographic evidence of interventricular mechanical delay obtained greater benefit from CRT in CARE-HF.[71]

Whereas it is important to identify patients who are most likely to respond to CRT, it is perhaps more important to identify patients in whom CRT may actually be harmful. A sub-analysis of the PROSPECT study defined super-responders as having a reduction in LVESV of ≥30%, responders a reduction of 15–29%, non-responders a reduction of 0–14%, and 'negative responders' an increase in LVESV.[135] Super-responders were more likely to be female, had non-ischaemic heart failure, a wider baseline QRS complex, and more extensive mechanical dyssynchrony at baseline. The percentage of clinical responders and non-responders is shown in **Figure 60.6**: note that 15–20% of patients may actually do worse following CRT.

Can we do more to predict which patients may do badly? In patients with narrower QRS, haemodynamics mostly deteriorate in acute studies, which seems to translate into poorer long-term outcomes in clinical trials.[18] It is clearly impractical to measure dP/dt_{max} invasively on all patients undergoing CRT, but it has been assessed within 24 h of implant non-invasively using echocardiography, and increasing dP/dt_{max} predicts better long-term clinical outcome.[136] Another measure of acute haemodynamic benefit is a prompt rise in systolic blood pressure after the onset of CRT; an increase of >5 mmHg predicts better event-free survival at 2 years.[137] Ideally, we need a method of assessing response at the time of implant so that the operator has the option of testing other lead positions—or alternative pacing vectors, particularly when quadripolar leads are used—if an inadequate or deleterious response is observed. Measuring systolic blood pressure response using an arterial line is one possibility. Alternatives may include assessment of the ECG at the time of implant, with some data suggesting that a positive deflection in lead V1 on the resting ECG in response to biventricular pacing is associated with improved response by echocardiographic variables.[138]

In a study of 75 patients who deteriorated following CRT, a multi-disciplinary team following a protocol-driven assessment recommended further management including additional medical therapy, treating underlying arrhythmias, reprogramming the device, and repositioning the LV lead. The most common problem encountered was sub-optimal AV timing in 47% of patients; however, 12% of patients had an immediate improvement in haemodynamics when CRT was turned off (the majority of these patients had a narrow QRS).[139]

CRT-P versus CRT-D

The debate as to which patient should receive CRT-P or CRT-D is controversial. CRT-D is approximately four times more expensive than CRT-P and thus cost-effectiveness is an issue.[140] In older patients, CRT-D may be less cost-effective than CRT-P.[141] CRT-D should only be considered for patients where there is expectation of survival for more than 1 year with good functional status.

Patients who took part in the clinical trials of CRT and primary prevention ICDs are generally younger than typical patients with heart failure and have predominantly single-organ disease. Older patients with renal impairment and other co-morbidities—particularly with a non-ischaemic aetiology—are less likely to benefit from ICD therapy.[88,142] COMPANION compared CRT-P with CRT-D, though the results are presented as comparisons with medical therapy. CRT-D improved survival compared with medical therapy (36% reduction in mortality), whereas CRT-P reduced mortality by 24%, which was not statistically significant ($P = 0.06$). However, although not formally analysed and reported, there was clearly no statistically significant difference in mortality between CRT-P and CRT-D.[4] In the DANISH trial, ICD implant was compared to standard care in patients who did not have coronary artery disease: 58% of patients in both arms had CRT (322 CRT-D vs 323 CRT-P). The 9% relative risk reduction in all-cause mortality for CRT-D vs CRT-P was not significant.[88]

Patient perspectives are also highly relevant. A CRT-P device is smaller, has no risk of inappropriate shocks, and is at less risk of device advisories, which have been an ongoing problem with ICDs.[143] An ICD may change the mode of death; in an older patient, a peaceful arrhythmic death, rather than dying in discomfort with refractory heart failure, may be a patient's preference. Patients often have unrealistic expectations about the life-saving effects of an ICD, due at least in part to inadequate explanation or oversimplification by medical and nursing staff. Realistic advice for a patient receiving an ICD for primary prevention is that for every 100 patients receiving an ICD, over the next 5 years, ~30 patients would die anyway, 10–20 patients would have a shock they do not need, 5–15 patients would have other complications from the device, and only seven or eight patients would be saved by the ICD.[144] They should also be aware that some patients choose to have their device inactivated to allow a natural death.

Telemonitoring

Advances in telecommunications and device technology allow the remote monitoring of surrogate markers of heart failure severity such as patient activity, heart rate variability, and intrathoracic impedance. Such markers may help predict subclinical heart failure decompensation, allowing medical intervention to prevent hospitalization.[145,146] In order to realize the full potential of telemonitoring, though, device services will need to be reconfigured and more closely integrated with heart failure clinics. Randomized studies continue to evaluate the effectiveness of remote monitoring in this setting but have so far yielded disappointing results, and there are, at present, no data to support the routine use of telemonitoring in clinical practice.[147–149]

Conclusion

CRT offers an important therapeutic option for patients with HFrEF and a prolonged QRS. Successful CRT depends on appropriate patient selection, successful implantation of the device with optimal LV lead positioning, appropriate device programming, and further optimization of medical therapy. A lack of clinical response should lead to careful reassessment, although it must be appreciated that an apparent lack of clinical response does not mean that the patient will not derive benefit from CRT. Further research is still needed to refine the selection criteria for CRT and to help optimize LV lead placement at the time of implantation to maximize patient benefit.

REFERENCES

1. Cazeau S, Leclercq C, Lavergne T, et al. Effects of multisite biventricular pacing in patients with heart failure and intraventricular conduction delay. N Engl J Med 2001;**344**:873–80.
2. Abraham WT, Fisher WG, Smith AL, et al. Cardiac resynchronization in chronic heart failure. N Engl J Med 2002;**346**:1845–53.
3. Cleland JGF, Daubert J-C, Erdmann E, et al. The effect of cardiac resynchronization on morbidity and mortality in heart failure. N Engl J Med 2005;**352**:1539–49.
4. Bristow MR, Saxon LA, Boehmer J, et al. Cardiac-resynchronization therapy with or without an implantable defibrillator in advanced chronic heart failure. N Engl J Med 2004;**350**:2140–50.
5. Ruschitzka F, Abraham WT, Singh JP, et al. Cardiac-resynchronization therapy in heart failure with a narrow QRS complex. N Engl J Med 2013;**369**:1395–405.
6. Dickstein K, Bogale N, Priori S, et al. The European cardiac resynchronization therapy survey. Eur Heart J 2009;**30**:2450–60.
7. Cleland JG, Abraham WT, Linde C, et al. An individual patient meta-analysis of five randomized trials assessing the effects of cardiac resynchronization therapy on morbidity and mortality in patients with symptomatic heart failure. Eur Heart J 2013;**34**:3547–56.
8. Hochleitner M, Hörtnagl H, Ng CK, et al. Usefulness of physiologic dual-chamber pacing in drug-resistant idiopathic dilated cardiomyopathy. Am J Cardiol 1990;**66**:198–202.
9. Brecker SJ, Xiao HB, Sparrow J, et al. Effects of dual-chamber pacing with short atrioventricular delay in dilated cardiomyopathy. Lancet 1992;**340**:1308–12.
10. Nishimura RA, Hayes DL, Holmes DR, et al. Mechanism of hemodynamic improvement by dual-chamber pacing for severe left ventricular dysfunction: an acute Doppler and catheterization hemodynamic study. J Am Coll Cardiol 1995;**25**:281–8.
11. Linde C, Gadler F, Edner M, et al. Results of atrioventricular synchronous pacing with optimized delay in patients with severe congestive heart failure. Am J Cardiol 1995;**75**:919–23.
12. Gold MR, Feliciano Z, Gottlieb SS, et al. Dual-chamber pacing with a short atrioventricular delay in congestive heart failure: a randomized study. J Am Coll Cardiol 1995;**26**:967–73.
13. Wilkoff BL, Cook JR, Epstein AE, et al. Dual-chamber pacing or ventricular backup pacing in patients with an implantable defibrillator: the Dual Chamber and VVI Implantable Defibrillator (DAVID) Trial. JAMA 2002;**288**:3115–23.
14. Gibson DG, Chamberlain DA, Coltart DJ, et al. Effect of changes in ventricular activation on cardiac haemodynamics in man. Comparison of right ventricular, left ventricular, and simultaneous pacing of both ventricles. Br Heart J 1971;**33**:397–400.
15. Cazeau S, Ritter P, Bakdach S, et al. Four chamber pacing in dilated cardiomyopathy. Pacing Clin Electrophysiol 1994;**17**:1974–9.
16. Leclercq C, Cazeau S, Le Breton H, et al. Acute hemodynamic effects of biventricular DDD pacing in patients with end-stage heart failure. J Am Coll Cardiol 1998;**32**:1825–31.

17. Kass DA, Chen CH, Curry C, *et al.* Improved left ventricular mechanics from acute VDD pacing in patients with dilated cardiomyopathy and ventricular conduction delay. *Circulation* 1999;**99**:1567–73.

18. Auricchio A, Stellbrink C, Block M, *et al.* Effect of pacing chamber and atrioventricular delay on acute systolic function of paced patients with congestive heart failure. The Pacing Therapies for Congestive Heart Failure Study Group. The Guidant Congestive Heart Failure Research Group. *Circulation* 1999;**99**:2993–3001.

19. Nelson GS, Berger RD, Fetics BJ, *et al.* Left ventricular or biventricular pacing improves cardiac function at diminished energy cost in patients with dilated cardiomyopathy and left bundle-branch block. *Circulation* 2000;**102**:3053–9.

20. Tavazzi L, Maggioni AP, Lucci D, *et al.* Nationwide survey on acute heart failure in cardiology ward services in Italy. *Eur Heart J* 2006;**27**:1207–15.

21. Agricola E, Oppizzi M, Galderisi M, *et al.* Role of regional mechanical dyssynchrony as a determinant of functional mitral regurgitation in patients with left ventricular systolic dysfunction. *Heart* 2006;**92**:1390–5.

22. Breithardt OA, Sinha AM, Schwammenthal E, *et al.* Acute effects of cardiac resynchronization therapy on functional mitral regurgitation in advanced systolic heart failure. *J Am Coll Cardiol* 2003;**41**:765–70.

23. Kanzaki H, Bazaz R, Schwartzman D, *et al.* A mechanism for immediate reduction in mitral regurgitation after cardiac resynchronization therapy: insights from mechanical activation strain mapping. *J Am Coll Cardiol* 2004;**44**:1619–25.

24. Ypenburg C, Lancellotti P, Tops LF, *et al.* Mechanism of improvement in mitral regurgitation after cardiac resynchronization therapy. *Eur Heart J* 2008;**29**:757–65.

25. Leclercq C, Walker S, Linde C, *et al.* Comparative effects of permanent biventricular and right-univentricular pacing in heart failure patients with chronic atrial fibrillation. *Eur Heart J* 2002;**23**:1780–7.

26. Auricchio A, Stellbrink C, Butter C, *et al.* Clinical efficacy of cardiac resynchronization therapy using left ventricular pacing in heart failure patients stratified by severity of ventricular conduction delay. *J Am Coll Cardiol* 2003;**42**:2109–16.

27. Auricchio A, Stellbrink C, Sack S, *et al.* Long-term clinical effect of hemodynamically optimized cardiac resynchronization therapy in patients with heart failure and ventricular conduction delay. *J Am Coll Cardiol* 2002;**39**:2026–33.

28. Young JB, Abraham WT, Smith AL, *et al.* Combined cardiac resynchronization and implantable cardioversion defibrillation in advanced chronic heart failure: the MIRACLE ICD Trial. *JAMA* 2003;**289**:2685–94.

29. Higgins SL, Hummel JD, Niazi IK, *et al.* Cardiac resynchronization therapy for the treatment of heart failure in patients with intraventricular conduction delay and malignant ventricular tachyarrhythmias. *J Am Coll Cardiol* 2003;**42**:1454–9.

30. Abraham WT, Young JB, Leon AR, *et al.* Effects of cardiac resynchronization on disease progression in patients with left ventricular systolic dysfunction, an indication for an implantable cardioverter–defibrillator, and mildly symptomatic chronic heart failure. *Circulation* 2004;**110**:2864–8.

31. Cleland JGF, Daubert J-C, Erdmann E, *et al.* Longer-term effects of cardiac resynchronization therapy on mortality in heart failure [the CArdiac REsynchronization-Heart Failure (CARE-HF) trial extension phase *Eur Heart J* 2006;**27**:1928–32.

32. Kindermann M, Hennen B, Jung J, *et al.* Biventricular versus conventional right ventricular stimulation for patients with standard pacing indication and left ventricular dysfunction: the Homburg Biventricular Pacing Evaluation (HOBIPACE). *J Am Coll Cardiol* 2006;**47**:1927–37.

33. Linde C, Abraham WT, Gold MR, *et al.* Randomized trial of cardiac resynchronization in mildly symptomatic heart failure patients and in asymptomatic patients with left ventricular dysfunction and previous heart failure symptoms. *J Am Coll Cardiol* 2008;**52**:1834–43.

34. Moss AJ, Hall WJ, Cannom DS, *et al.* Cardiac-resynchronization therapy for the prevention of heart-failure events. *N Engl J Med* 2009;**361**:1329–38.

35. Tang ASL, Wells GA, Talajic M, *et al.* Cardiac-resynchronization therapy for mild-to-moderate heart failure. *N Engl J Med* 2010;**363**:2385–95.

36. Curtis AB, Worley SJ, Adamson PB, *et al.* Biventricular pacing for atrioventricular block and systolic dysfunction. *N Engl J Med* 2013;**368**:1585–93.

37. Daubert C, Gold MR, Abraham WT, *et al.* Prevention of disease progression by cardiac resynchronization therapy in patients with asymptomatic or mildly symptomatic left ventricular dysfunction: insights from the European cohort of the REVERSE (Resynchronization Reverses Remodeling in Systolic Left Ventricular Dysfunction) trial. *J Am Coll Cardiol* 2009;**54**:1837–46.

38. Goldenberg I, Kutyifa V, Klein HU, *et al.* Survival with cardiac-resynchronization therapy in mild heart failure. *N Engl J Med* 2014;**370**:1694–701.

39. Ghio S, Freemantle N, Scelsi L, *et al.* Long-term left ventricular reverse remodelling with cardiac resynchronization therapy: results from the CARE-HF trial. *Eur J Heart Fail* 2009;**11**:480–8.

40. D'Ascia C, Cittadini A, Monti MG, *et al.* Effects of biventricular pacing on interstitial remodelling, tumor necrosis factor-alpha expression, and apoptotic death in failing human myocardium. *Eur Heart J* 2006;**27**:201–6.

41. Vanderheyden M, Mullens W, Delrue L, *et al.* Myocardial gene expression in heart failure patients treated with cardiac resynchronization therapy responders versus nonresponders. *J Am Coll Cardiol* 2008;**51**:129–36.

42. Mangiavacchi M, Gasparini M, Faletra F, *et al.* Clinical predictors of marked improvement in left ventricular performance after cardiac resynchronization therapy in patients with chronic heart failure. *Am Heart J* 2006;**151**:477.e1–477.e6.

43. Yu C-M, Bleeker GB, Fung JW-H, *et al.* Left ventricular reverse remodeling but not clinical improvement predicts long-term survival after cardiac resynchronization therapy. *Circulation* 2005;**112**:1580–6.

44. Ukkonen H, Beanlands RSB, Burwash IG, *et al.* Effect of cardiac resynchronization on myocardial efficiency and regional oxidative metabolism. *Circulation* 2003;**107**:28–31.

45. Nowak B, Sinha AM, Schaefer WM, *et al.* Cardiac resynchronization therapy homogenizes myocardial glucose metabolism and perfusion in dilated cardiomyopathy and left bundle branch block. *J Am Coll Cardiol* 2003;**41**:1523–8.

46. Knaapen P, van Campen LMC, de Cock CC, *et al.* Effects of cardiac resynchronization therapy on myocardial perfusion reserve. *Circulation* 2004;**110**:646–51.

47. Lindner O, Sörensen J, Vogt J, *et al.* Cardiac efficiency and oxygen consumption measured with 11C-acetate PET after long-term cardiac resynchronization therapy. *J Nucl Med* 2006;**47**:378–83.

48. Duncan AM, Lim E, Clague J, et al. Comparison of segmental and global markers of dyssynchrony in predicting clinical response to cardiac resynchronization. *Eur Heart J* 2006;**27**:2426–32.

49. St John Sutton MG, Plappert T, Abraham WT, et al. Effect of cardiac resynchronization therapy on left ventricular size and function in chronic heart failure. *Circulation* 2003;**107**:1985–90.

50. Fruhwald FM, Fahrleitner-Pammer A, Berger R, et al. Early and sustained effects of cardiac resynchronization therapy on N-terminal pro-B-type natriuretic peptide in patients with moderate to severe heart failure and cardiac dyssynchrony. *Eur Heart J* 2007;**28**:1592–7.

51. Pitzalis MV, Iacoviello M, Di Serio F, et al. Prognostic value of brain natriuretic peptide in the management of patients receiving cardiac resynchronization therapy. *Eur J Heart Fail* 2006;**8**:509–14.

52. Kubánek M, Málek I, Bytesník J, et al. Decrease in plasma B-type natriuretic peptide early after initiation of cardiac resynchronization therapy predicts clinical improvement at 12 months. *Eur J Heart Fail* 2006;**8**:832–40.

53. Boerrigter G, Costello-Boerrigter LC, Abraham WT, et al. Cardiac resynchronization therapy improves renal function in human heart failure with reduced glomerular filtration rate. *J Cardiac Fail* 2008;**14**:539–46.

54. Grassi G, Vincenti A, Brambilla R, et al. Sustained sympathoinhibitory effects of cardiac resynchronization therapy in severe heart failure. *Hypertension* 2004;**44**:727–31.

55. Adamson PB, Kleckner KJ, VanHout WL, et al. Cardiac resynchronization therapy improves heart rate variability in patients with symptomatic heart failure. *Circulation* 2003;**108**:266–9.

56. Gademan MGJ, van Bommel RJ, Borleffs CJW, et al. Biventricular pacing-induced acute response in baroreflex sensitivity has predictive value for midterm response to cardiac resynchronization therapy. *Am J Physiol Heart Circ Physiol* 2009;**297**:H233–7.

57. Lamba J, Simpson CS, Redfearn DP, et al. Cardiac resynchronization therapy for the treatment of sleep apnoea: a meta-analysis. *Europace* 2011;**13**:1174–9.

58. Jessup M. Defining success in heart failure: the end-point mess. *Circulation* 2010;**121**:1977–80.

59. Fornwalt BK, Sprague WW, BeDell P, et al. Agreement is poor among current criteria used to define response to cardiac resynchronization therapy. *Circulation* 2010;**121**:1985–91.

60. Brignole M, Auricchio A, Baron-Esquivias G, et al. 2013 ESC Guidelines on cardiac pacing and cardiac resynchronization therapy: the Task Force on cardiac pacing and resynchronization therapy of the European Society of Cardiology (ESC). Developed in collaboration with the European Heart Rhythm Association (EHRA). *Eur Heart J* 2013;**34**:2281–329.

61. Ponikowski P, Voors AA, Anker SD, et al. 2016 ESC Guidelines for the diagnosis and treatment of acute and chronic heart failure: The Task Force for the diagnosis and treatment of acute and chronic heart failure of the European Society of Cardiology (ESC). Developed with the special contribution of the Heart Failure Association (HFA) of the ESC. *Eur Heart J* 2016;**37**:2129–200.

62. Tracy CM, Epstein AE, Darbar D, et al. 2012 ACCF/AHA/HRS focused update of the 2008 guidelines for device-based therapy of cardiac rhythm abnormalities: a report of the American College of Cardiology Foundation/American Heart Association Task Force on Practice Guidelines and the Heart Rhythm Society. [Corrected.] *Circulation* 2012;**126**:1784–800.

63. Saberwal B, Ahsan S. NICE guidelines for use of implantable cardioverter defibrillators. *Br J Hosp Med (Lond)* 2015;**76**:316–17.

64. Ponikowski P, Voors AA, Anker SD, et al. 2016 ESC Guidelines for the diagnosis and treatment of acute and chronic heart failure: The Task Force for the diagnosis and treatment of acute and chronic heart failure of the European Society of Cardiology (ESC). Developed with the special contribution of the Heart Failure Association (HFA) of the ESC. *Eur J Heart Fail* 2016;**18**:891–975.

65. Linde C, Daubert C, Abraham WT, et al. Impact of ejection fraction on the clinical response to cardiac resynchronization therapy in mild heart failure. *Circ Heart Fail* 2013;**6**:1180–9.

66. Beshai JF, Grimm RA, Nagueh SF, et al. Cardiac-resynchronization therapy in heart failure with narrow QRS complexes. *N Engl J Med* 2007;**357**:2461–71.

67. Thibault B, Harel F, Ducharme A, et al. Cardiac resynchronization therapy in patients with heart failure and a QRS complex. *Circulation* 2013;**127**:873–81.

68. Birnie DH, Ha A, Higginson L, et al. Impact of QRS morphology and duration on outcomes after cardiac resynchronization therapy: results from the Resynchronization-Defibrillation for Ambulatory Heart Failure Trial (RAFT). *Circ Heart Fail* 2013;**6**:1190–8.

69. Woods B, Hawkins N, Mealing S, et al. Individual patient data network meta-analysis of mortality effects of implantable cardiac devices. *Heart* 2015;**101**:1800–6.

70. Hawkins NM, Petrie MC, MacDonald MR, et al. Selecting patients for cardiac resynchronization therapy: electrical or mechanical dyssynchrony? *Eur Heart J* 2006;**27**:1270–81.

71. Richardson M, Freemantle N, Calvert MJ, et al. Predictors and treatment response with cardiac resynchronization therapy in patients with heart failure characterized by dyssynchrony: a pre-defined analysis from the CARE-HF trial. *Eur Heart J* 2007;**28**:1827–34.

72. Chung ES, Leon AR, Tavazzi L, et al. Results of the Predictors of Response to CRT (PROSPECT) trial. *Circulation* 2008;**117**:2608–16.

73. Cowburn PJ, Patel H, Jolliffe RE, et al. Cardiac resynchronization therapy: an option for inotrope-supported patients with end-stage heart failure? *Eur J Heart Fail* 2005;**7**:215–7.

74. Lindenfeld J, Feldman AM, Saxon L, et al. Effects of cardiac resynchronization therapy with or without a defibrillator on survival and hospitalizations in patients with New York Heart Association class IV heart failure. *Circulation* 2007;**115**:204–12.

75. Doshi RN, Daoud EG, Fellows C, et al. Left ventricular-based cardiac stimulation post AV nodal ablation evaluation (the PAVE study). *J Cardiovasc Electrophysiol* 2005;**16**:1160–5.

76. Koplan BA, Kaplan AJ, Weiner S, et al. Heart failure decompensation and all-cause mortality in relation to percent biventricular pacing in patients with heart failure: is a goal of 100% biventricular pacing necessary? *J Am Coll Cardiol* 2009;**53**:355–60.

77. Hayes DL, Boehmer JP, Day JD, et al. Cardiac resynchronization therapy and the relationship of percent biventricular pacing to symptoms and survival. *Heart Rhythm* 2011;**8**:1469–75.

78. Cheng A, Landman SR, Stadler RW. Reasons for loss of cardiac resynchronization therapy pacing: insights from 32 844 patients. *Circ Arrhythm Electrophysiol* 2012;**5**:884–8.

79. Upadhyay GA, Choudhry NK, Auricchio A, et al. Cardiac resynchronization in patients with atrial fibrillation: a meta-analysis of prospective cohort studies. *J Am Coll Cardiol* 2008;**52**:1239–46.

80. Gasparini M, Auricchio A, Metra M, *et al.* Long-term survival in patients undergoing cardiac resynchronization therapy: the importance of performing atrio-ventricular junction ablation in patients with permanent atrial fibrillation. *Eur Heart J* 2008;**29**:1644–52.

81. Khadjooi K, Foley PW, Chalil S, *et al.* Long-term effects of cardiac resynchronisation therapy in patients with atrial fibrillation. *Heart* 2008;**94**:879–83.

82. Khazanie P, Greiner MA, Al-Khatib SM, *et al.* Comparative effectiveness of cardiac resynchronization therapy among patients with heart failure and atrial fibrillation: findings from the National Cardiovascular Data Registry's Implantable Cardioverter-Defibrillator Registry. *Circ Heart Fail* 2016;**9**(6):e002324.

83. Yu C-M, Chan JY-S, Zhang Q, *et al.* Biventricular pacing in patients with bradycardia and normal ejection fraction. *N Engl J Med* 2009;**361**:2123–34.

84. Shimano M, Tsuji Y, Yoshida Y, *et al.* Acute and chronic effects of cardiac resynchronization in patients developing heart failure with long-term pacemaker therapy for acquired complete atrioventricular block. *Europace* 2007;**9**:869–74.

85. Foley PWX, Muhyaldeen SA, Chalil S, *et al.* Long-term effects of upgrading from right ventricular pacing to cardiac resynchronization therapy in patients with heart failure. *Europace* 2009;**11**:495–501.

86. Kron J, Aranda JM, Miles WM, *et al.* Benefit of cardiac resynchronization in elderly patients: results from the Multicenter InSync Randomized Clinical Evaluation (MIRACLE) and Multicenter InSync ICD Randomized Clinical Evaluation (MIRACLE-ICD) trials. *J Interv Card Electrophysiol* 2009;**25**:91–6.

87. Foley PWX, Chalil S, Khadjooi K, *et al.* Long-term effects of cardiac resynchronization therapy in octogenarians: a comparative study with a younger population. *Europace* 2008;**10**:1302–7.

88. Køber L, Thune JJ, Nielsen JC, *et al.* Defibrillator implantation in patients with nonischemic systolic heart failure. *N Engl J Med* 2016;**375**:1221–30.

89. Alaeddini J, Wood MA, Amin MS, *et al.* Gender disparity in the use of cardiac resynchronization therapy in the United States. *Pacing Clin Electrophysiol* 2008;**31**:468–72.

90. Ghanbari H, Dalloul G, Hasan R, *et al.* Effectiveness of implantable cardioverter-defibrillators for the primary prevention of sudden cardiac death in women with advanced heart failure: a meta-analysis of randomized controlled trials. *Arch Intern Med* 2009;**169**:1500–6.

91. Janousek J, Tomek V, Chaloupecký VA, *et al.* Cardiac resynchronization therapy: a novel adjunct to the treatment and prevention of systemic right ventricular failure. *J Am Coll Cardiol* 2004;**44**:1927–31.

92. Kiesewetter C, Michael K, Morgan J, *et al.* Left ventricular dysfunction after cardiac resynchronization therapy in congenital heart disease patients with a failing systemic right ventricle. *Pacing Clin Electrophysiol* 2008;**31**:159–62.

93. Cowburn PJ, Patel H, Pipes RR, *et al.* Contrast nephropathy post cardiac resynchronization therapy: an under-recognized complication with important morbidity. *Eur J Heart Fail* 2005;**7**:899–903.

94. Shetty AK, Duckett SG, Bostock J, *et al.* Use of a quadripolar left ventricular lead to achieve successful implantation in patients with previous failed attempts at cardiac resynchronization therapy. *Europace* 2011;**13**:992–6.

95. Forleo GB, Di Biase L, Bharmi R, *et al.* Hospitalization rates and associated cost analysis of cardiac resynchronization therapy with an implantable defibrillator and quadripolar vs. bipolar left ventricular leads: a comparative effectiveness study. *Europace* 2015;**17**:101–7.

96. Morgan JM, Biffi M, Gellér L, *et al.* ALternate Site Cardiac ResYNChronization (ALSYNC): a prospective and multicentre study of left ventricular endocardial pacing for cardiac resynchronization therapy. *Eur Heart J* 2016;**37**:2118–27.

97. Domenichini G, Diab I, Campbell NG, *et al.* A highly effective technique for transseptal endocardial left ventricular lead placement for delivery of cardiac resynchronization therapy. *Heart Rhythm* 2015;**12**:943–9.

98. Leon AR, Abraham WT, Curtis AB, *et al.* Safety of transvenous cardiac resynchronization system implantation in patients with chronic heart failure: combined results of over 2,000 patients from a multicenter study program. *J Am Coll Cardiol* 2005;**46**:2348–56.

99. van Rees JB, de Bie MK, Thijssen J, *et al.* Implantation-related complications of implantable cardioverter–defibrillators and cardiac resynchronization therapy devices: a systematic review of randomized clinical trials. *J Am Coll Cardiol* 2011;**58**:995–1000.

100. Kirkfeldt RE, Johansen JB, Nohr EA, *et al.* Complications after cardiac implantable electronic device implantations: an analysis of a complete, nationwide cohort in Denmark. *Eur Heart J* 2014;**35**:1186–94.

101. Poole JE, Gleva MJ, Mela T, *et al.* Complication rates associated with pacemaker or implantable cardioverter–defibrillator generator replacements and upgrade procedures: results from the REPLACE registry. *Circulation* 2010;**122**:1553–61.

102. Cowburn PJ, Leclercq C. How to improve outcomes with cardiac resynchronisation therapy: importance of lead positioning. *Heart Fail Rev* 2012;**17**:781–9.

103. Butter C, Auricchio A, Stellbrink C, *et al.* Effect of resynchronization therapy stimulation site on the systolic function of heart failure patients. *Circulation* 2001;**104**:3026–9.

104. Lambiase PD, Rinaldi A, Hauck J, *et al.* Non-contact left ventricular endocardial mapping in cardiac resynchronisation therapy. *Heart* 2004;**90**:44–51.

105. van Campen CMC, Visser FC, de Cock CC, *et al.* Comparison of the haemodynamics of different pacing sites in patients undergoing resynchronisation treatment: need for individualisation of lead localisation. *Heart* 2006;**92**:1795–800.

106. Singh JP, Fan D, Heist EK, *et al.* Left ventricular lead electrical delay predicts response to cardiac resynchronization therapy. *Heart Rhythm* 2006;**3**:1285–92.

107. Gold MR, Birgersdotter-Green U, Singh JP, *et al.* The relationship between ventricular electrical delay and left ventricular remodelling with cardiac resynchronization therapy. *Eur Heart J* 2011;**32**:2516–24.

108. D'Onofrio A, Botto G, Mantica M, *et al.* The interventricular conduction time is associated with response to cardiac resynchronization therapy: interventricular electrical delay. *Int J Cardiol* 2013;**168**:5067–8.

109. Khan FZ, Virdee MS, Palmer CR, *et al.* Targeted left ventricular lead placement to guide cardiac resynchronization therapy: the TARGET study: a randomized, controlled trial. *J Am Coll Cardiol* 2012;**59**:1509–18.

110. Saba S, Marek J, Schwartzman D, *et al.* Echocardiography-guided left ventricular lead placement for cardiac resynchronization therapy: results of the Speckle Tracking

Assisted Resynchronization Therapy for Electrode Region trial. *Circ Heart Fail* 2013;**6**:427–34.

111. Asbach S, Hartmann M, Wengenmayer T, *et al.* Vector selection of a quadripolar left ventricular pacing lead affects acute hemodynamic response to cardiac resynchronization therapy: a randomized cross-over trial. *PLoS One* 2013;**8**:e67235.

112. Zanon F, Baracca E, Pastore G, *et al.* Multipoint pacing by a left ventricular quadripolar lead improves the acute hemodynamic response to CRT compared with conventional biventricular pacing at any site. *Heart Rhythm* 2015;**12**:975–81.

113. Forleo GB, Santini L, Giammaria M, *et al.* Multipoint pacing via a quadripolar left-ventricular lead: preliminary results from the Italian registry on multipoint left-ventricular pacing in cardiac resynchronization therapy (IRON-MPP). *Europace* 2017;**19**(7):1170–7.

114. Rinaldi CA, Burri H, Thibault B, *et al.* A review of multisite pacing to achieve cardiac resynchronization therapy. *Europace* 2015;**17**:7–17.

115. Haghjoo M, Bonakdar HR, Jorat MV, *et al.* Effect of right ventricular lead location on response to cardiac resynchronization therapy in patients with end-stage heart failure. *Europace* 2009;**11**:356–63.

116. Buck S, Maass AH, Nieuwland W, *et al.* Impact of interventricular lead distance and the decrease in septal-to-lateral delay on response to cardiac resynchronization therapy. *Europace* 2008;**10**:1313–9.

117. Heist EK, Fan D, Mela T, *et al.* Radiographic left ventricular–right ventricular interlead distance predicts the acute hemodynamic response to cardiac resynchronization therapy. *Am J Cardiol* 2005;**96**:685–90.

118. Stanton T, Hawkins NM, Hogg KJ, *et al.* How should we optimize cardiac resynchronization therapy? *Eur Heart J* 2008;**29**:2458–72.

119. Ellenbogen KA, Gold MR, Meyer TE, *et al.* Primary results from the SmartDelay determined AV optimization: a comparison to other AV delay methods used in cardiac resynchronization therapy (SMART-AV) trial: a randomized trial comparing empirical, echocardiography-guided, and algorithmic atrioventricular delay programming in cardiac resynchronization therapy. *Circulation* 2010;**122**:2660–8.

120. Whinnett ZI, Davies JER, Willson K, *et al.* Haemodynamic effects of changes in atrioventricular and interventricular delay in cardiac resynchronisation therapy show a consistent pattern: analysis of shape, magnitude and relative importance of atrioventricular and interventricular delay. *Heart* 2006;**92**:1628–34.

121. Scharf C, Li P, Muntwyler J, *et al.* Rate-dependent AV delay optimization in cardiac resynchronization therapy. *Pacing Clin Electrophysiol* 2005;**28**:279–84.

122. Kurzidim K, Reinke H, Sperzel J, *et al.* Invasive optimization of cardiac resynchronization therapy: role of sequential biventricular and left ventricular pacing. *Pacing Clin Electrophysiol* 2005;**28**:754–61.

123. Boriani G, Biffi M, Müller CP, *et al.* A prospective randomized evaluation of VV delay optimization in CRT-D recipients: echocardiographic observations from the RHYTHM II ICD study. *Pacing Clin Electrophysiol* 2009;**32** Suppl 1:S120–5.

124. Stabile G, Iuliano A, La Rocca V, *et al.* Geometrical and electrical predictors of cardiac resynchronization therapy response. *Expert Rev Cardiovasc Ther* 2014;**12**:873–84.

125. Rickard J, Jackson G, Spragg DD, *et al.* QRS prolongation induced by cardiac resynchronization therapy correlates

with deterioration in left ventricular function. *Heart Rhythm* 2012;**9**:1674–8.

126. Gold MR, Thébault C, Linde C, *et al.* Effect of QRS duration and morphology on cardiac resynchronization therapy outcomes in mild heart failure: results from the Resynchronization Reverses Remodeling in Systolic Left Ventricular Dysfunction (REVERSE) study. *Circulation* 2012;**126**:822–9.

127. Abraham WT, Gras D, Yu C-M, *et al.* Rationale and design of a randomized clinical trial to assess the safety and efficacy of frequent optimization of cardiac resynchronization therapy: the Frequent Optimization Study Using the QuickOpt Method (FREEDOM) trial. *Am Heart J* 2010;**159**:944–948.e1.

128. Ritter P, Delnoy PPHM, Padeletti L, *et al.* A randomized pilot study of optimization of cardiac resynchronization therapy in sinus rhythm patients using a peak endocardial acceleration sensor vs. standard methods. *Europace* 2012;**14**:1324–33.

129. Martin DO, Lemke B, Birnie D, *et al.* Investigation of a novel algorithm for synchronized left-ventricular pacing and ambulatory optimization of cardiac resynchronization therapy: results of the adaptive CRT trial. *Heart Rhythm* 2012;**9**:1807–14.

130. Singh JP, Abraham WT, Chung ES, *et al.* Clinical response with adaptive CRT algorithm compared with CRT with echocardiography-optimized atrioventricular delay: a retrospective analysis of multicentre trials. *Europace* 2013;**15**:1622–8.

131. Birnie D, Lemke B, Aonuma K, *et al.* Clinical outcomes with synchronized left ventricular pacing: analysis of the adaptive CRT trial. *Heart Rhythm* 2013;**10**:1368–74.

132. Mullens W, Verga T, Grimm RA, *et al.* Persistent hemodynamic benefits of cardiac resynchronization therapy with disease progression in advanced heart failure. *J Am Coll Cardiol* 2009;**53**:600–7.

133. Bleeker GB, Kaandorp TAM, Lamb HJ, *et al.* Effect of posterolateral scar tissue on clinical and echocardiographic improvement after cardiac resynchronization therapy. *Circulation* 2006;**113**:969–76.

134. Cleland JGF, Freemantle N, Daubert JC, *et al.* Long-term effect of cardiac resynchronisation in patients reporting mild symptoms of heart failure: a report from the CARE-HF study. *Heart* 2008;**94**:278–83.

135. van Bommel RJ, Bax JJ, Abraham WT, *et al.* Characteristics of heart failure patients associated with good and poor response to cardiac resynchronization therapy: a PROSPECT (Predictors of Response to CRT) sub-analysis. *EurHeart J* 2009;**30**:2470–7.

136. Tournoux FB, Alabiad C, Fan D, *et al.* Echocardiographic measures of acute haemodynamic response after cardiac resynchronization therapy predict long-term clinical outcome. *Eur Heart J* 2007;**28**:1143–8.

137. Tanaka Y, Tada H, Yamashita E, *et al.* Change in blood pressure just after initiation of cardiac resynchronization therapy predicts long-term clinical outcome in patients with advanced heart failure. *Circ J* 2009;**73**:288–94.

138. Bode WD, Bode MF, Gettes L, *et al.* Prominent R wave in ECG lead V1 predicts improvement of left ventricular ejection fraction after cardiac resynchronization therapy in patients with or without left bundle branch block. *Heart Rhythm* 2015;**12**:2141–7.

139. Mullens W, Grimm RA, Verga T, *et al.* Insights from a cardiac resynchronization optimization clinic as part of a heart failure disease management program. *J Am Coll Cardiol* 2009;**53**:765–73.

140. Yao G, Freemantle N, Calvert MJ, *et al.* The long-term cost-effectiveness of cardiac resynchronization therapy with or without an implantable cardioverter–defibrillator. *Eur Heart J* 2007;**28**:42–51.

141. Mealing S, Woods B, Hawkins N, *et al.* Cost-effectiveness of implantable cardiac devices in patients with systolic heart failure. *Heart* 2016;**102**:1742–9.

142. Goldenberg I, Vyas AK, Hall WJ, *et al.* Risk stratification for primary implantation of a cardioverter–defibrillator in patients with ischemic left ventricular dysfunction. *J Am Coll Cardiol* 2008;**51**:288–96.

143. Maisel WH. Pacemaker and ICD generator reliability: meta-analysis of device registries. *JAMA* 2006;**295**:1929–34.

144. Stevenson LW, Desai AS. Selecting patients for discussion of the ICD as primary prevention for sudden death in heart failure. *J Cardiac Fail* 2006;**12**:407–12.

145. Adamson PB, Smith AL, Abraham WT, *et al.* Continuous autonomic assessment in patients with symptomatic heart failure: prognostic value of heart rate variability measured by an implanted cardiac resynchronization device. *Circulation* 2004;**110**(16):2389–94.

146. Yu C-M, Wang L, Chau E, *et al.* Intrathoracic impedance monitoring in patients with heart failure: correlation with fluid status and feasibility of early warning preceding hospitalization. *Circulation* 2005;**112**:841–8.

147. Morgan JM, Dimitrov BD, Gill J, *et al.* Rationale and study design of the REM-HF study: remote management of heart failure using implanted devices and formalized follow-up procedures. *Eur J Heart Fail* 2014;**16**:1039–45.

148. Boriani G, Da Costa A, Ricci RP, *et al.* The MOnitoring Resynchronization dEvices and CARdiac patiEnts (MORE-CARE) randomized controlled trial: phase 1 results on dynamics of early intervention with remote monitoring. *J Med Internet Res* 2013;**15**:e167.

149. Cowie MR. REM-HF: Remote monitoring: an evaluation of implantable devices for management of heart failure patients. European Society of Cardiology 2016 Congress, Rome, Italy, 28 August 2016; Abstract 1223.

SECTION 14
Surgical therapy for heart failure

61

Heart transplantation

Georgios Karagiannis, Diana Garcia Saez, Margaret M. Burke, André R. Simon, and Nicholas R. Banner

Introduction

Clinical organ transplantation began in the mid-twentieth century, initially with renal transplants. Surgical techniques for heart transplantation began to be developed during the same period, notably by Cass and Brock in the UK, and Lower and Shumway in the USA.[1–3] The drugs then available for prophylaxis against rejection were limited to corticosteroids and azathioprine.[4] The first human heart transplant was performed in 1967;[5] the story of the pioneers in this field has been told elsewhere.[6] The initial results of clinical heart transplantation were disappointing because of relatively ineffective pharmacological immunosuppression, lack of effective monitoring for acute rejection and of therapeutic options for complications including infection and cardiac allograft vasculopathy.[7] The results of organ transplantation improved markedly following the introduction of ciclosporin as an immunosuppressive agent, first for kidney transplantation and subsequently for the heart and other organs.[8,9] Various surgical techniques have been used for transplantation but, in the current era, most surgeons use the bicaval technique, whereby recipient's heart is replaced orthotopically by the transplanted heart using a composite left atrial anastomosis and separate anastomoses for each caval vein.

Heart transplantation was introduced as a treatment for heart failure at a time when the other therapeutic options were very limited (diuretics and digoxin). In subsequent decades considerable progress has been made in the therapy of chronic heart failure based principally on the paradigm of neurohormonal antagonism (angiotensin converting enzyme inhibitors, β-blockers, aldosterone antagonists, angiotensin receptor blockers and, more recently, angiotensin receptor blocker–neprilysin inhibitor combination) coupled with the use of implantable defibrillators to prevent sudden arrhythmic death and, for selected patients, cardiac resynchronization therapy.[10] In the same period, immunosuppression and management after heart transplantation have also improved. Heart transplantation has never been tested against medical therapy in a randomized clinical trial. However, the very low medium-term mortality rates after heart transplantation compared with medical therapy for heart failure, coupled with the results of studies using statistical modelling, indicate that heart transplantation can provide a long-term benefit for many patients with advanced heart failure.[11] Far less progress has been made with the medical management of acute heart failure and many of the therapies used provide marginal or only temporary benefit to such patients. An increasing proportion of heart transplant operations are being performed on an urgent basis in patients with decompensated heart failure who have become dependent on inotropes or short-term circulatory support.[12] In this group, provided that candidates are selected appropriately, heart transplantation is highly efficacious and provides an early survival benefit.[11] However, the scarcity of donor hearts that are suitable for transplantation has prolonged waiting times significantly, making careful selection of transplant candidates essential.[13] Moreover, this development, coupled with advances in technology, has led to an increased use of ventricular assist devices to maintain patients before heart transplantation ('bridge to transplantation'),[14] and now as an alternative therapy for patients who are ineligible for transplantation (destination therapy).[10,15]

Recipient selection

The International Society for Heart and Lung Transplantation (ISHLT) has published guidelines for the care of patients prior to transplantation and case selection.[16,17] For patients with chronic stable heart failure the decision about transplantation should be made after optimizing medical therapy, including the maximum possible use of neurohormonal antagonists and electrical device therapy.[10] The aetiology of the heart failure should be determined and any alternative treatments should be considered. In the setting of advanced heart failure of ischaemic aetiology, high-risk myocardial revascularization is an alternative therapeutic option (when substantial myocardial viability and hibernation are present), although there is no clear evidence that it prolongs survival.[18] Other interventions, including left ventricular reconstruction, surgical or percutaneous ischaemic mitral regurgitation repair, or percutaneous revascularization, can improve heart failure symptoms, but lack proven survival benefit, especially in significantly remodelled ventricles.[18,19] Ambulatory heart failure patients who are on optimal medical therapy can be risk-stratified using the

cardiopulmonary exercise test, natriuretic peptides, as well as scoring systems such as the Heart Failure Survival Score or the Seattle Heart Failure Score.[20–22]

The scarcity of donor hearts has led most countries to introduce methods for prioritizing recipients for transplantation.[23] For example, patients with refractory decompensated heart failure who have become truly inotrope dependent have a dismal prognosis with ongoing medical therapy and should be considered as candidates for urgent transplantation or mechanical circulatory support.[24] In all potential candidates, the presence of co-morbidity, risk factors, and contraindications to transplantation should be determined. Contraindications may be absolute (e.g. an active malignancy that limits the patient's prognosis and would be exacerbated by pharmacological immunosuppression) or relative (e.g. renal or other organ dysfunction).[23] Many of the risk factors for heart transplantation such as renal dysfunction and pulmonary hypertension are complications of the heart failure and directly related to its severity and duration. The dilemma of whether to attempt to transplant such patients has been reduced by the availability of mechanical circulatory support as an alternative strategy to improve patients' health and make them a more suitable heart transplant candidate in the future.[14]

Pulmonary hypertension secondary to left heart failure is an important problem because of the risk of donor right ventricular failure after the transplant procedure. Its prevalence is increasing because of improved survival in chronic heart failure patients with medical therapy. Right heart catheterization should be used to distinguish passive from reactive pulmonary hypertension with a truly increased resistance to blood flow within the pulmonary circulation. In the case of reactive pulmonary hypertension, the traditional approach has been to use pharmacological testing to assess its reversibility;[25] however, the reproducibility and predictive value of such tests is moderate at best. In the most recent era, patients with severe pulmonary hypertension have been rendered more suitable for heart transplantation by bridging them with a mechanical left ventricular assist device (LVAD). Device support provides a long-term reduction in left atrial pressure, usually leading to a favourable remodelling in the pulmonary circulation, and a regression of reactive pulmonary hypertension.

Mechanical circulatory support prior to transplantation

In the current era, ~50% of the patients receiving a heart transplant are on mechanical circulatory support.[26] However, many patients are referred at a very advanced stage of their disease with secondary organ dysfunction, particularly renal failure, chronic congestive hepatopathy, and pulmonary hypertension. Although, in principle, mechanical circulatory support can improve the haemodynamic state of those with refractory decompensated heart failure and so make them suitable for transplantation,[27] this increases the risk of surgery significantly and so referral should be made at an earlier stage whenever possible.[23]

Since heart failure is a progressive condition, the scarcity of hearts suitable for transplantation and the consequent increase in waiting times has led to many patients deteriorating during the waiting period. Although some may be stabilized with intravenous support until a suitable heart becomes available under an urgent allocation scheme, others need mechanical circulatory support (bridge to transplantation). In the acute heart failure setting mechanical circulatory support, in the form of a temporary LVAD, intra-aortic balloon pump, or extracorporeal membrane oxygenation, may be required to stabilize the patient until suitability for heart transplantation is assessed (bridge to decision).[28]

Whereas inotropes may help to produce a short-term improvement in the patient's haemodynamic state and organ function, their efficacy is often limited by the severity of the patient's myocardial dysfunction. In addition the longer-term use of inotropes has been shown to have a detrimental effect on outcome and so, for the patient who is suitable for surgical therapy, their role should be a temporary one before early transplantation, or the implantation of a mechanical circulatory support device.[29]

Historically, the intra-aortic balloon pump has had an important role in maintaining patients prior to transplantation. However, the degree of circulatory support provided is limited and, with increased waiting times, this form of treatment is often impractical. The use of veno-arterial extracorporeal membrane oxygenation (ECMO) in end-stage refractory cardiogenic shock patients may be helpful as salvage treatment, but, as short-term support method, is usually followed by an insertion of a longer-term form of circulatory support.[30] However, the use of ECMO prior to transplantation is related with significantly increased risk.

Mechanical circulatory support with a durable implantable LVAD has now become a standard therapy to stabilize and then maintain patients until transplantation becomes possible.[14] Circulatory support can allow physiological recovery of other organ systems and, with modern implantable devices, the patient can be rehabilitated and achieve an improved functional status prior to transplant. However, the advantages of this strategy should be weighed against the increased complexity of the subsequent transplant surgery. The technology has evolved considerably over the last several decades, with devices progressing from large external pneumatically driven pulsatile pumps to smaller, implantable, electrically driven, continuous flow devices. Currently, the most commonly used devices are the Thoratec HeartMate II (a second-generation device) and the HeartWare LVAD (a third-generation device), but there is an increasing trend towards the use of the third-generation devices (including the Thoratec HeartMate III).[31,32] Because of their small size, continuous-flow devices are easier to implant. Their chief limitation is that they provide univentricular support and that this may be inadequate for patients with decompensated heart failure or very poor right ventricular function. Such patients may require biventricular support.[33] An alternative would be to use a total artificial heart that can provide biventricular support and total cardiac replacement, but there is limited evidence to support this approach and outcomes may be poor.[34]

Surgical planning

Transplantation is a complex process and detailed plans should be made at the time of listing. Patients who have undergone previous cardiac surgery, and especially those who have received a left ventricular assist device, should undergo computed tomography coupled with a review of the previous surgical records to establish the

necessary approach. Some recipients have particular tissue requirements, and a modified operative technique may be needed for those with adult congenital heart disease (ACHD), particularly if there is an abnormal atrial situs.[35] Excellent coordination is required to minimize the organ ischaemia time during transplantation. Patients with ventricular assist devices are sometimes planned to undergo anaesthesia prior to the explant of the donor heart by the retrieval team to allow surgery to commence immediately thereafter; this can increase the time for opening and mobilization of the ventricular assist device and recipient heart while the donor heart is in transit. The risk of this approach is minimal for patients who are already on circulatory support. Use of ex-vivo normothermic preservation (e.g. Organ Care System, TransMedics, Inc.) may sometimes be used to facilitate transplantation of ACHD and LVAD patients.[36]

Donor selection and management

The function of the donor heart may be affected by pre-existing cardiovascular disease in the donor, the effect of brain-stem death, the management that the donor receives in the intensive care unit and the impact of myocardial ischaemia during cold storage. Over the last decades, increased mean donor age and higher prevalence of comorbidities, such as diabetes or hypertension, necessitated methods to improve evaluation of organ quality and organ preservation.[37]

Brain-stem death produces a transient massive increase in sympathetic activity that often leads to severe hypertension (Cushing's reflex) and catecholamine-mediated injury to the myocardium, leading to potentially irreversible myocardial dysfunction. Multiple homeostatic defects also develop.[38] Active management of the donor from the time of the diagnosis of brain-stem death by either an outreach team from the transplant centre or a separately constituted organ procurement organization helps to increase the yield of usable hearts.[39]

Assessment of the donor heart is based on clinical examination, ECG, and echocardiography coupled with haemodynamic studies using a pulmonary artery flotation catheter (PAFC) and, finally, by direct surgical inspection at the time of organ retrieval coupled with direct haemodynamic measurements. Coronary angiography can be useful for the evaluation of coronary artery disease in high-risk donors, but is often not logistically possible in community hospitals.

The ECG can be used to rapidly screen for major abnormalities, such as Q waves, indicating prior myocardial infarction or signs of left ventricular hypertrophy. Repolarization changes are common after brain death and do not preclude organ donation. Transthoracic or transoesophageal echocardiography can be used to screen for structural lesions including valvar heart disease and to assess ventricular function. Ventricular performance is influenced by the loading conditions (systemic vascular resistance is often low after brain-stem death and filling pressures are frequently abnormal). All these factors can be assessed using a PAFC and the results used to direct subsequent therapy. It has been found that left ventricular dysfunction is often reversible after a period of donor resuscitation, so donor hearts should not be declined on the basis of a single echocardiogram showing a low ejection fraction.[40]

Most transplant centres follow the general approach advocated by the Crystal City Conference.[39] However, the evidence for this approach is largely observational and there have been few clinical trials of donor management. This limitation was underscored by a clinical study which found no benefit from hormonal resuscitation as proposed in the Crystal City guidelines.[41] The final assessment and decision about the donor heart suitability for transplantation is made at the time of retrieval by the surgeon. Transoesophageal echocardiography at this stage can provide a final assessment of ventricular function and the presence or absence of any ventricular hypertrophy. The surgeon should also palpate the coronary arteries. In view of the subjective nature of this assessment process, the experience of the retrieving surgeon is of critical importance.

Donor recipient matching

The system for donor organ allocation varies between countries. Organs can either be allocated using a 'patient-oriented' system, where priority is given to patients according to their clinical status within a geographical zone, or a 'centre-oriented' system, where organs are allocated to individual transplant centres who then use them according to priority. The current system in the UK is hybrid: patients can be registered on the national super-urgent and urgent heart allocation scheme provided that they meet specific criteria and that there is centre-based allocation of hearts not required for the urgent scheme. Such national allocation systems are associated with decreased waiting list mortality.[42] Donor–recipient matching requires ABO blood group compatibility, size matching, and a negative virtual or actual HLA cross match in those with clinically important preformed antibodies (high concentration measured with mean fluorescence intensity, in-vitro complement fixation).[43]

Organ retrieval and myocardial protection

The donor operation is usually performed as part of a multi-organ retrieval procedure. At the start of the retrieval, blood flow into the right ventricle is restricted by ligation of the superior caval vein. The inferior caval vein is then opened and the left atrium is vented, to prevent left ventricular distension, either through an incision into the left atrial appendage or into the left atrium between the inferior pulmonary veins. At this point, the ascending aorta is cross-clamped and cold cardioplegia solution is administered via the aortic root to achieve hypothermic diastolic arrest. The heart is then quickly excised with adequate lengths of aorta, pulmonary artery, venae cavae, and the left atrium. Cold storage at 4–8°C is used to transport the heart to the transplant centre. Although most hearts tolerate ischaemia at this temperature for several hours, postoperative cardiac dysfunction and the risk of primary graft failure remain significant problems, especially when hearts from older donors are used.[44]

Alternative methods for protecting the myocardium have been explored. There has been particular interest in the possibility of transporting hearts in a warm perfused beating state.[45] The PROCEED II trial assessed the efficacy and safety of the Organ Care System in human heart transplantation and showed similar short-term outcomes of donor hearts preserved with the system as to those of hearts preserved with standard cold storage, but with a significant reduction in the cold ischaemia time.[36] The potential ability to re-animate and assess hearts from donors after circulatory death before

transplantation also is beginning to increase the pool of donor hearts for transplantation with promising short-term results.[46,47]

Recipient operation (bicaval technique)

A orthotopic heart transplant in a patient with non-ischaemic dilated cardiomyopathy and no previous cardiac surgery is a routine procedure that has historically been used for training of future transplant surgeons. At the other end of the spectrum, transplants in patients who have undergone multiple previous operations, have abnormal anatomy because of ACHD, or who have had a prior LVAD, may be technically challenging. In such cases the donor and recipient surgery needs to be carefully coordinated to allow adequate time for dissection of the recipient heart and haemostasis prior to the arrival of the donor heart, thereby minimizing the organ ischaemia time.

The operation is performed using full cardiopulmonary bypass and most surgeons use a modest degree of hypothermia. Recipient cardiectomy is performed by division of the atria adjacent to the atrioventricular groove and division of the great arteries just distal to the sinotubular junction. This allows the recipient heart to yield homograft valves for other patients. In the bicaval technique, the recipient right atrium is then resected by separating it from the superior and inferior venae cavae (SVC and IVC, respectively) and from the remnant of the recipient left atrium. The left atrium is then trimmed, leaving the posterior wall and surrounding tissue as a bridge between the recipient's four pulmonary veins.[3]

The donor heart is inspected for any damage during the retrieval process and for the presence of a persistent foramen ovale which, if present, should be closed to eliminate the risk of right-to-left shunting postoperatively. The donor left atrium is trimmed to remove the pulmonary venous ostia and the posterior wall that lies between them, creating a defect that can be anastomosed to the corresponding tissue in the recipient (**Figure 61.1a,b**). The left atrial anastomosis is performed first and requires attention because it will be relatively inaccessible at the end of the procedure. The donor and recipient pulmonary arteries are then trimmed to an appropriate length to avoid kinking or torsion as they are anastomosed end to

end. The donor and recipient aortas are then similarly trimmed and anastomosed. At this point, the aortic cross-clamp may be released to re-establish coronary perfusion and minimize the total ischaemia time. The rest of the operation is then performed in a decompressed heart under supportive cardiopulmonary bypass. Suction is used to clear the myocardial venous return to the coronary sinus and right atrium.

The post-ischaemic heart is normally kept on supportive cardiopulmonary bypass for a period of up to an hour, keeping the heart 'empty' to minimize myocardial work but maintaining coronary and systemic organ perfusion. Most hearts spontaneously return to sinus rhythm following release of the aortic cross-clamp and restoration of coronary perfusion. However, some require internal cardioversion from ventricular fibrillation. Transient atrioventricular block is common but usually resolves within the first few hours. Initial sinus node dysfunction is also common but ultimately requires the implantation of a permanent pacemaker in <5% of recipients.

Bleeding may be a concern in patients undergoing redo surgery or transplantation following bridging with an LVAD. Early reversal of anticoagulation and the monitoring of haemostatic function with a thromboelastogram can be of assistance in the management of such patients. Platelet transfusion may be required, especially in those who have been receiving dual antiplatelet drug therapy, but the use of blood products appears associated with a higher risk of right heart failure. Care must be taken to avoid technical complications with the anastomoses; the most likely problems are kinking or torsion at the pulmonary anastomosis which can contribute to postoperative right ventricular dysfunction or stenosis at either the SVC or IVC anastomosis.

The immediate post-bypass period is of critical importance. It is often at this stage that problems related to donor right ventricular failure become apparent. Pulmonary vascular resistance should be managed with inhaled and systemic vasodilator therapy. Inhaled nitric oxide may be used prophylactically in patients with a known elevation of pulmonary vascular resistance and should be initiated early where there is any sign of right ventricular distension or dysfunction. Before separating the patient from cardiopulmonary

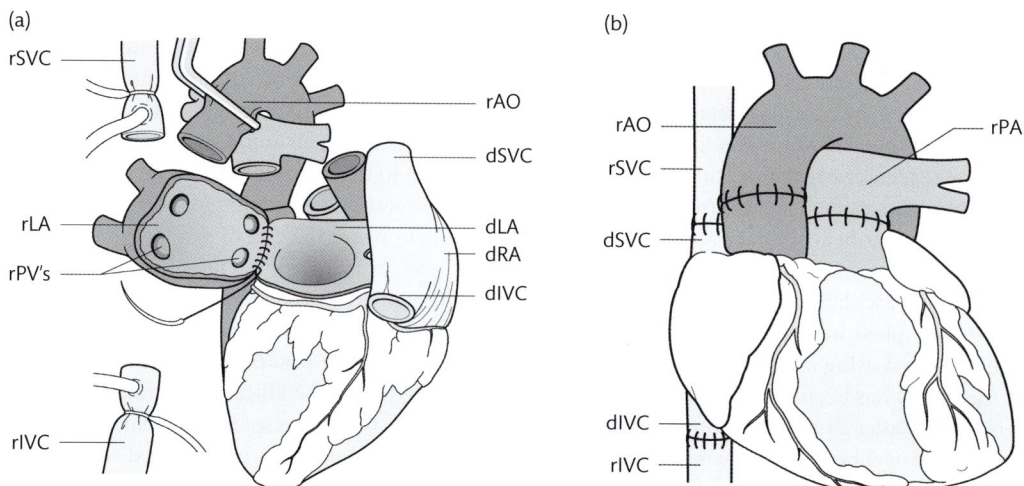

Figure 61.1 (a, b) Orthotopic heart transplantation using the bicaval technique. See text for details. r, recipient; d, donor; AO, aorta; SVC superior vena cava; IVC, inferior vena cava; PA, pulmonary artery; LA, left atrium, RA, right atrium; PVs, pulmonary veins.

bypass, a PAFC should be inserted to allow continuous monitoring of cardiac output and pulmonary artery pressures. Some surgeons also use a left atrial line to allow direct monitoring of left-sided filling pressures.[48] Failure to achieve satisfactory haemodynamics with adequate cardiac output and acceptable filling pressures, without the use of excessive inotropic support, should prompt a complete diagnostic reassessment to exclude technical problems. If necessary, short-term support with temporary ventricular assist devices or central veno-arterial (VA) ECMO should be considered at an early stage to reduce myocardial work and maintain coronary perfusion while also providing adequate systemic perfusion thereby avoiding a slide into multi-system organ failure.[49]

Postoperative care

When the transplanted heart is performing well the patient can be returned to the intensive care unit with only low doses of inotropes being administered. Some centres support the heart rate pharmacologically with an infusion of isoproterenol, whereas others prefer to use atrial pacing. In the early period, the post-ischaemic ventricles often have reduced compliance, producing a limitation in stroke volume. Therefore, the best cardiac output can usually be achieved at relatively fast heart rate, typically 90–110 beats per minute. The overall management plan is similar to that used for patients after coronary bypass surgery although there are the additional concerns of pharmacological immunosuppression and prophylaxis against infection. For the uncomplicated cardiac transplant, extubation is usually possible following the weaning of nitrous oxide on day 1 or 2, inotropes are slowly weaned during the first postoperative week, and mediastinal and pericardial drains are removed once drainage has ceased, typically on the third or fourth postoperative day. Atrial pacing is usually weaned once inotropic support has stopped, with care to ensure that there is an adequate underlying sinus rate.

The complications that may occur in the early postoperative period are summarized in Box 61.1 and their differential diagnosis and management have been reviewed in detail elsewhere.[50] Primary graft dysfunction should be recognized promptly and treated aggressively.[51] The ISHLT has introduced a standardized grading system for primary graft dysfunction and its severity is related postoperative outcome.[51,52] Complex surgical techniques, evolving resistance of nosocomial pathogens, pharmacological immunosuppression and increasing number of patients with circulatory support devices (some with pre-existing chronic infection) necessitate strict preventive measures and management protocols.[53] Fungal infections are becoming a more frequent problem postoperatively with significant prognostic implications and challenging treatment. Finally, the risk of infection by *Mycobacterium chimaera*, which has been recently recognized, can cause life-threatening infections several months after transplantation.[54]

Allograft rejection

Allograft rejection is clinically categorized according to its temporal occurrence (hyper-acute, acute, and chronic) and by the underlying

Box 61.1 Postoperative cardiac and circulatory problems that may occur after orthotopic heart transplantation

- Haemorrhage
  - Surgical
  - Coagulopathic
- Pericardial effusion
  - Potential space after resection of enlarged native heart
  - Inflammatory response after surgery
  - Bleeding into pericardial space
  - Complication of rejection (uncommon)
  - Drug complication (sirolimus)
  - Rarely infection (mediastinitis)
- Cardiac tamponade
- Acute right ventricular failure
  - Recipient pulmonary hypertension
  - Primary graft failure
- Acute biventricular failure
  - Primary graft failure
  - Hyper-acute rejection
  - Accelerated acute rejection
- Technical anastomotic complications
  - Pulmonary artery (stenosis, torsion)
  - Superior caval vein (stenosis)
  - Inferior caval vein (stenosis)
- Systemic inflammatory response
  - Pre-existing infection (e.g. ventricular assist device complication)
  - Prolonged cardiopulmonary bypass
  - As a complication of primary graft failure
  - Pseudosepsis (milrinone accumulation in renal failure)
- Brady- and tachyarrhythmia
  - Sinus node dysfunction
  - Atrioventricular block
  - Atrial arrhythmia, especially atrial flutter
- Acute kidney injury

mechanism (cellular, antibody-mediated, and mixed). In the non-sensitized patient, cellular rejection is the most common form of acute rejection. The immunological response is initiated and driven by the helper T-cell, and most of the immunosuppressive drugs in current use act at various stages in the T-cell activation cascade (Figure 61.2).

Antibody-mediated rejection on the other hand is the result of B-cell proliferation and differentiation and may cause several clinical syndromes. Sensitized patients with pre-formed donor-specific HLA antibody may be subject to hyper-acute rejection, which develops in the first few minutes to hours after the operation and can be aggressive or even catastrophic in nature. It can be avoided by performing a direct or virtual cross-match prior to transplantation, and avoiding donor–recipient pairs where there is donor-specific antibody in the recipient.[43] ABO-incompatible transplantation can also cause hyper-acute rejection in adult patients and should be avoided. Patients with low levels of anti-donor HLA antibody may escape hyper-acute rejection, but then suffer early accelerated acute rejection in the first few days and weeks after the transplant due to an anamnestic antibody response. Some other patients develop de-novo HLA donor-specific antibody months or years after the transplant. Many of these cases remain asymptomatic, although the presence of donor-specific antibodies is a risk factor for late allograft failure.[55] In other cases, however, acute antibody-mediated rejection with allograft dysfunction may occur.

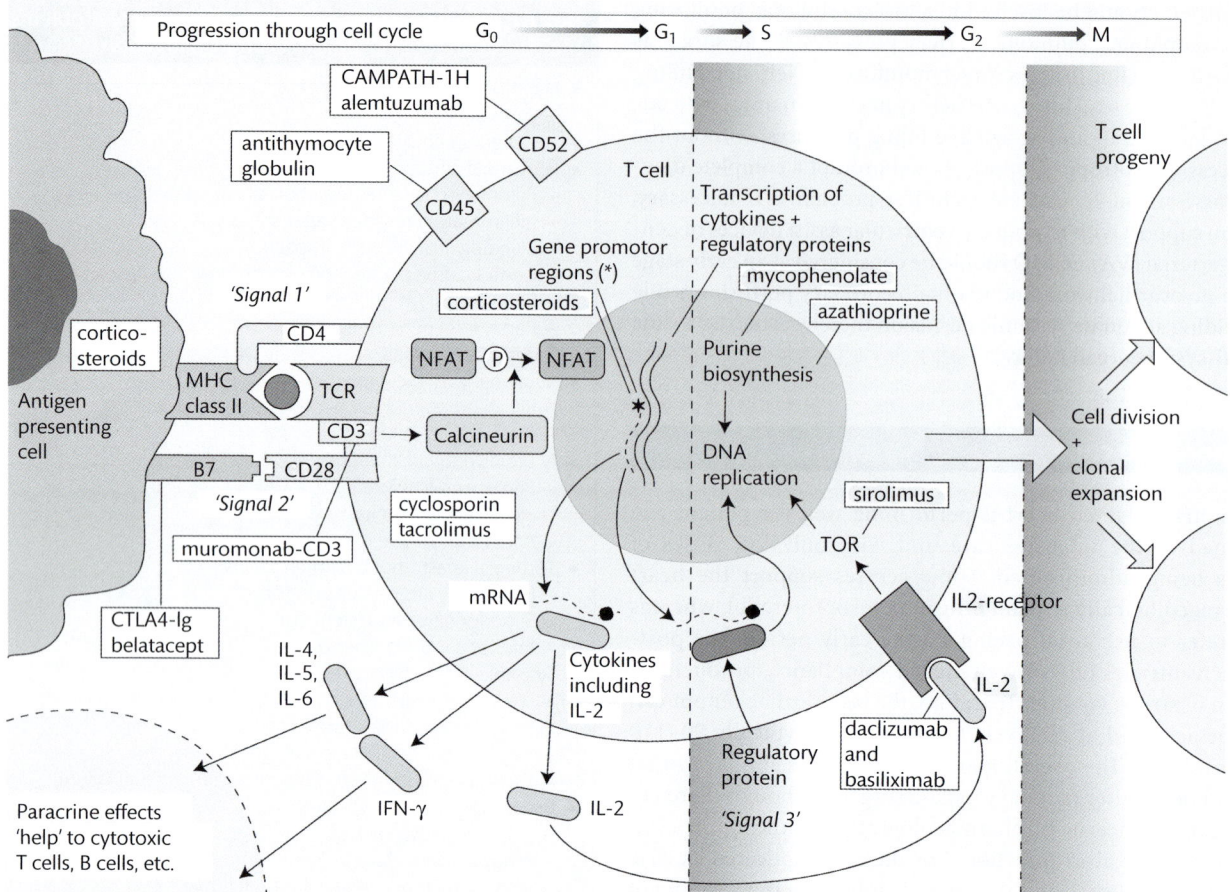

Figure 61.2 Steps in the T-cell activation cascade. Simplified model of the events which occur during the T-cell activation. The early, calcium-dependent, phase of activation begins when the receptor of a CD4-positive helper T-cell (TCR) binds to a complementary MHC class II molecule with an associated peptide in its antigen-presentation grove, 'Signal 1'. Full activation also requires a second signal ('Signal 2') which is caused by binding between complementary adhesion molecules on the surface of the antigen-presenting T-cell. Signal transduction from the TCR occurs via the CD3 complex. Subsequent intracellular signalling involves the inositol triphosphate/diacylglycerol pathway and mobilization of intracellular calcium. This leads to activation of the protein phosphatase calcineurin. Calcineurin dephosphorylates the nuclear factor of activated T-cells (NFAT), allowing its active moiety to translocate to the nucleus and so bind to the promoter regions of various genes encoding cytokines such as interleukin-2 (IL-2), regulatory proteins and the IL-2 receptor. The pattern of cytokine expression depends on the nature of the T-cell (Th1 or Th2) and can lead to either recruitment of cytotoxic CD8-positive T-cells and other effector cells or the provision of help to B-cells for antibody production. The expression of IL-2 leads to autocrine stimulation for the T-cell. Binding of IL-2 to its receptor initiates a second sequence of intracellular signals involving the mammalian target of rapamycin (TOR), which leads to DNA synthesis and replication and which culminates in cell division. The sites of action of various immunosuppressive agents are shown. Polyclonal anti-thymocyte globulin is shown as binding to the common leukocyte antigen (CD45) although, in reality, it contains antibodies which bind to many different T-cell antigens. IL, interleukin; MHC, major histocompatibility complex; NFAT nuclear factor of activated T-cells; TCR, T-cell receptor; TOR; target of rapamycin; IFN, interferon; CTLA4-Ig, the genetically engineered fusion protein between extracellular domain of CTLA4 (CD152) and the Fc portion of human immunoglobulin that acts as a competitive antagonist for CD28; CAMPATH-1H (alemtuzumab), a humanized monoclonal against CD52.

Source data from Banner NR, Lyster H. Pharmacological immunosuppression. In: *Lung Transplantation*. Banner NR, Polak JM, Yacoub M, Eds. Cambridge, Cambridge University Press, 2003.

Chronic allograft dysfunction may develop many years after the transplant and is principally associated with cardiac allograft vasculopathy, although restrictive cardiomyopathy and, less commonly, dilated cardiomyopathy may also occur.

The reference standard method for diagnosing acute cardiac rejection is the endomyocardial biopsy (EMB), which was first introduced by Philip Caves in 1973.[56] Traditionally, biopsies have been performed routinely during the first few years after heart transplantation with the aim of diagnosing rejection at an early stage before cardiac allograft dysfunction has become established.[7] Additional biopsies are performed when there is clinical or other evidence of allograft dysfunction. However, with the current more effective immunosuppression regimens, the yield from routine surveillance biopsies has fallen considerably, diminishing the value of this procedure.[57] Nevertheless, most transplant centres continue to use biopsies in the early phase after transplantation when the risk of rejection is highest and while the immunosuppression is weaned down to the chronic maintenance level. Serious complications of EMB are rare but include cardiac tamponade, coronary septal branch to right ventricular fistulae, tricuspid regurgitation, myocardial infarction and infection, as well as those of vascular access. These risks and the high cost of the procedure have led to a search for alternative, less invasive

diagnostic methods. Tests based on cardiac function, particularly echo-Doppler methods, have lacked sufficient sensitivity or specificity.[58] Recently, attention has been focused on molecular biology and proteomic methods to screen for acute rejection. The AlloMap* is a proprietary method for evaluating the profile of gene expression in circulating white cells. It generates a score which can be used to estimate the likelihood of acute cellular rejection at any stage. Recently it has been demonstrated that the AlloMap* can be used as a screening test to safely reduce the number of routine endomyocardial biopsies that are required beyond six months after transplantation[59] and possibly as early as two months post transplantation.[60] Measurement of donor-derived cell-free DNA is another potential biomarker of acute cellular rejection with complementary value to the AlloMap*.[61]

Pathology of rejection

The EMB plays an important role in the diagnosis of acute cellular rejection (ACR), but its contribution to diagnosis of antibody-mediated rejection (AMR) is less well defined. Some biopsies may show features of both ACR and AMR concurrently (mixed acute rejection). The EMB may have an additional role in evaluating long-term microvascular and myocardial changes related to chronic rejection.

ACR is characterized by an interstitial and perivascular infiltration of T-lymphocytes, also infiltrating vascular endothelium ('lymphocytic intimitis') (Figure 61.3a). Plasma cells, macrophages, and eosinophils may be seen in higher grades of rejection. The intensity and distribution of the infiltrate determines the grade of ACR,[62] and is graded as mild (1R), moderate (2R), and severe (3R) (Table 61.1) (Figure 61.3b–d). Myocyte damage (myocytolysis) may occur but is inconspicuous relative to the inflammatory infiltrate. It may be present as an occasional focus in mild ACR but is more frequent in moderate and severe ACR.

AMR develops when donor-specific antibodies are deposited on capillary endothelium, leading to complement activation and the release of inflammatory mediators. Early biopsy changes are microvascular inflammation, with distention of capillaries by swollen endothelial cells and narrowing of capillary lumens by 'plugs' of intravascular (IV) mononuclear cells, shown on immunostaining with CD68 to be macrophages. Immunostaining for complement degradation product C4d shows granular deposits on capillary

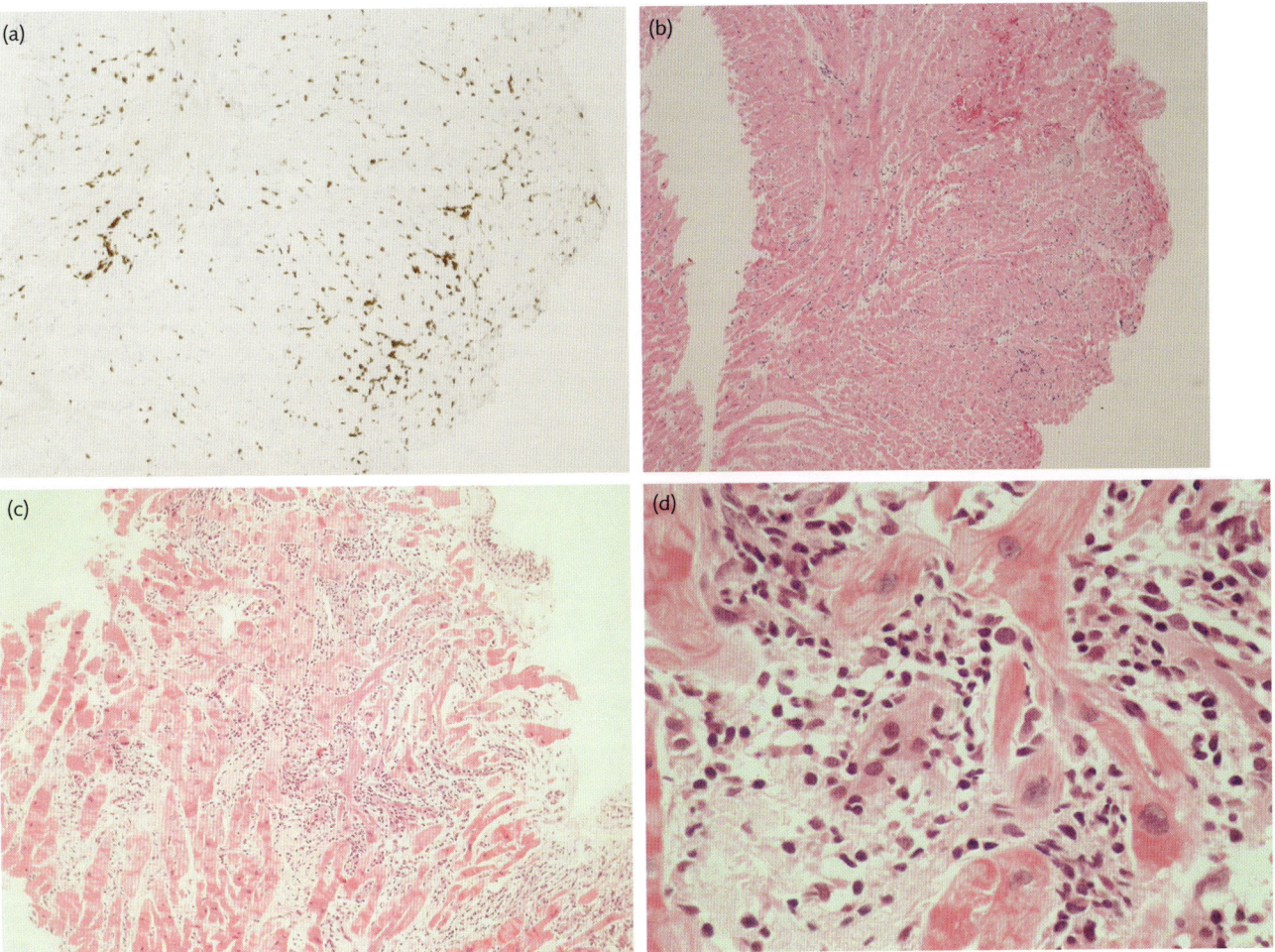

Figure 61.3 Acute cellular rejection (ACR). (a) ACR is mediated by CD3-positive T-lymphocytes. (b) Mild ACR (grade 1R) with a localized perivascular and interstitial lymphocytic infiltrate. (c) Moderate ACR (grade 2R) with a dense infiltrate of lymphocytes causing some disruption of myocardial architecture. (d) Occasional foci of myocytolysis which may dominate the picture in severe ACR (grade 3R) (not shown). (a) CD3 ×100, (b) ×100, (c) ×100, (d) ×400.

Table 61.1 The 2005 revision of the Working Formulation for classification of acute cellular rejection (ACR) of the heart[62]

Grade	Category	Description
Grade 0	No rejection	No myocardial inflammatory infiltrate
Grade 1R	Mild ACR	Multifocal interstitial and/or perivascular mononuclear infiltrates of lymphocytes, some macrophages and occasional eosinophils +/– one focus of myocytolysis
Grade 2R	Moderate ACR	Two or more foci of mononuclear cell infiltrates expanding interstitium and with two or more foci of myocyte damage
Grade 3R	Severe ACR	Diffuse mononuclear cell infiltrates expanding interstitium +/– oedema +/– haemorrhage +/– neutrophils +/– widespread myocyte necrosis +/– vasculitis

R, revised: this avoids confusion with the grades used in the 1990 Working Formulation.
Reproduced from Stewart S, Winters GL, Fishbein MC, *et al*. Revision of the 1990 working formulation for the standardization of nomenclature in the diagnosis of heart rejection. *The Journal of Heart and Lung Transplantation*: the official publication of the International Society for Heart Transplantation 2005;**24**:1710–20.

endothelium forming a 'donut' pattern (**Figure 61.4a–c**). As AMR advances in severity the myocardium develops oedema, vasculitis, haemorrhage, microvascular thrombosis, capillary damage, and myocyte necrosis with neutrophil infiltration and stromal karyorrhectic debris, usually in the clinical setting of profound irretrievable allograft dysfunction (**Figure 61.4d**). Paradoxically, C4d deposition may be only patchy or even negative at this stage because of disruption of capillaries by necrosis.

The diagnosis of cardiac AMR is based on pathology alone, the intensity and extent of histopathological and immunopathological findings determining its grade (**Table 61.2**).[63] Early AMR (pAMR 1) is characterized by either histopathological changes (pAMR1[h+])

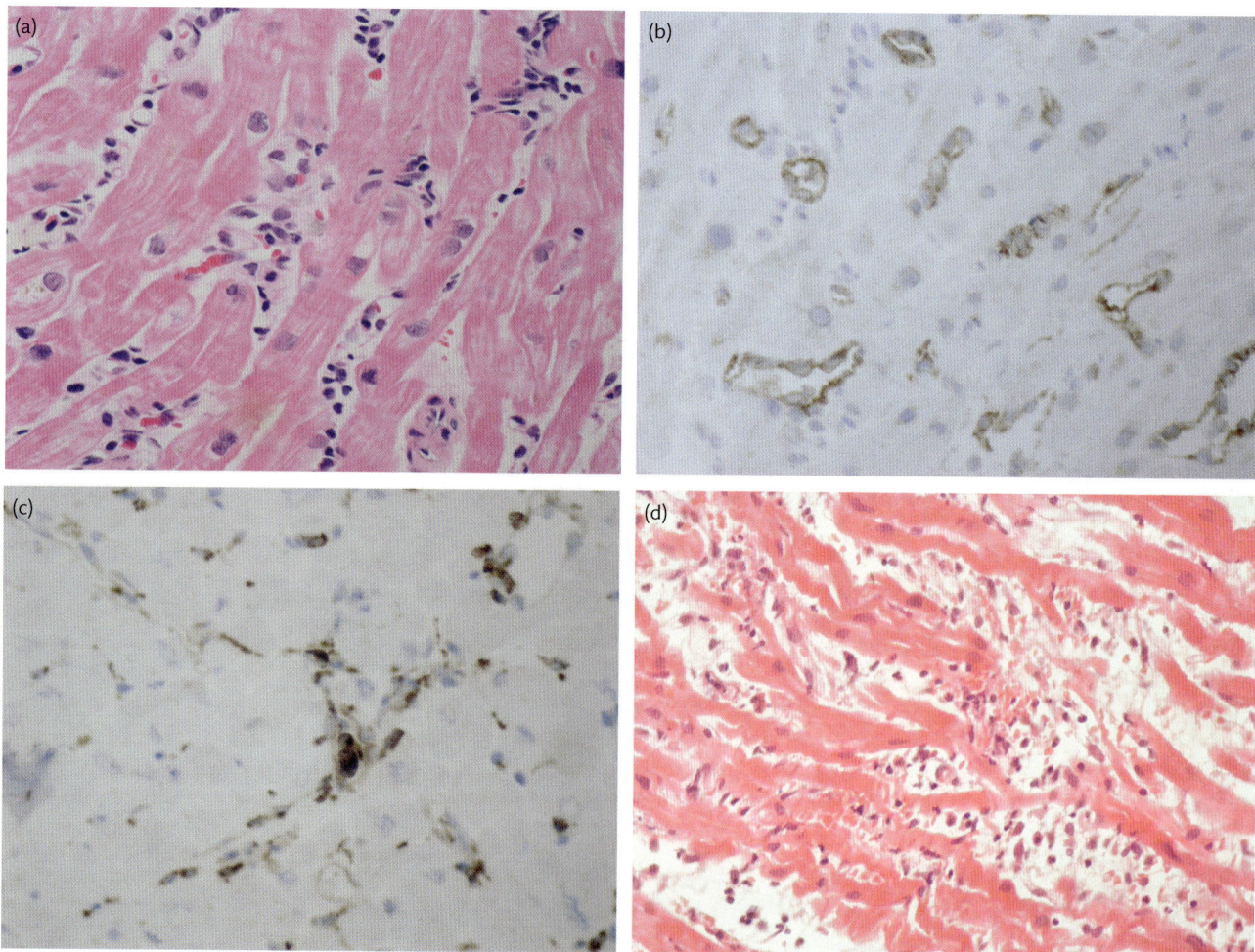

Figure 61.4 Antibody-mediated rejection (AMR). In pAMR2 there is (a) capillary endothelial prominence, intra-luminal mononuclear cells and a sparse interstitial mononuclear cell infiltrate, (b) strong capillary staining for C4d, (c) interstitial and intravascular macrophage accumulation shown on CD68 staining. In pAMR3 (d) there may be interstitial oedema, haemorrhage and a mixed inflammatory cell infiltrate with necrotising vasculitis. (a) ×200, (b) C4d ×200, (c) CD68 ×200, (d) ×200.

Table 61.2 The 2013 Working Formulation for the pathologic diagnosis of cardiac antibody-mediated rejection[63]

Grade	Category	Description
pAMR 0	Negative for pathologic AMR	Both histologic and immunopathologic studies are negative.
pAMR 1 (H+)	Histopathologic AMR alone	Histologic findings positive: Intravascular macrophages in capillaries and venules. Enlarged endothelial cells with large nuclei and expanded cytoplasm appearing to narrow or occlude vascular lumens. Immunopathologic findings negative.
pAMR 1 (I+)	Immunopathologic[a] AMR alone	Immunopathologic findings positive: CD68+: >10% of assessable myocardium shows focal/multifocal/diffuse intravascular macrophages *and/or* C4d+: Multifocal (>50% of assessable myocardium)/diffuse weak or strong[b] capillary positivity. C3d+ (by immunofluorescence staining only): as for C4d+. Histologic findings negative.
pAMR 2	Pathologic AMR	Both histologic *and* immunopathologic findings are present.
pAMR 3	Severe pathologic AMR	Haemorrhage, interstitial oedema, myocyte necrosis, capillary fragmentation, mixed inflammatory infiltrates, endothelial cell pyknosis and/or karyorrhexis *and* immunopathologic findings are present.

[a] May be frozen section immunofluorescence or paraffin section immunoperoxidase staining.
[b] Focal (>10–50%) strong C4d staining is classified as negative but warrants communication with clinician for close follow-up.
Reproduced from Berry GJ, Burke MM, Andersen C, *et al.* The 2013 International Society for Heart and Lung Transplantation Working Formulation for the standardization of nomenclature in the pathologic diagnosis of antibody-mediated rejection in heart transplantation. *The Journal of Heart and Lung Transplantation*: the official publication of the International Society for Heart Transplantation 2013;**32**:1147–62.

or immunopathological findings (pAMR1[i+]). pAMR2 is characterized by both histopathological changes and immunopathological findings. In pAMR3, or severe AMR, there is extensive myocardial damage and often disruption of the microcirculation. Concomitant ACR is frequently found and should be graded separately.

Cardiac allograft vasculopathy (CAV) is a progressive diffuse intimal myofibroblastic proliferation usually inside an intact internal elastic lamina. It affects the entire coronary vascular tree (**Figure 61.5a–d**).[64,65] CAV involving the larger epicardial coronary arteries often exists alongside eccentric, ulcerated atheromatous plaques which may have been inadvertently 'donated' as part of the allograft or developed after transplantation because of pre-existing non-immunological risk factors such as the hyperlipaedaemias at play. Often there may be intimal inflammation in the diffuse component together with microvascular inflammation and capillary C4d deposition in allograft myocardium, and asymptomatic AMR in previous EMBs.[66]

Various imaging methods are used to diagnose and assess the severity of CAV, including an ISHLT-sponsored Working Formulation scheme grading the extent and severity of angiographically detected CAV.[67] Correlation, where possible, with the pathology in the explanted or autopsied heart is often helpful in assessing the relative merits of these techniques as well as the impact of interventions such as stenting—often with little effect as the intimal proliferative process tends to engulf the stent (**Figure 61.5e**).

A current challenge to the histopathologist is biopsy diagnosis of stenotic allograft microvasculopathy (**Figure 61.5f**). A small number of studies have shown that involvement of the microvasculature of the myocardium, including the post-capillary vascular bed, by CAV leads to pruning and diminution in density of the microvascular tree by stenotic medial fibrosis.[68] The result is a reduction in microvascular density and hence coronary flow reserve.[69] The myocardial

remodelling process that results from this, with patchy or diffuse interstitial fibrosis, could represent the substrate for arrhythmic events leading to death. However, universally accepted biopsy diagnostic criteria have yet to be agreed.

Immunosuppression

Many centres use a form of induction therapy with an anti-T-cell antibody to provide additional immunosuppression during the early perioperative period. Agents that have been used for this purpose include monomurab-CD3 (OKT3), anti-thymocyte globulin (ATG), the monoclonal antibodies to the IL-2 receptor (basiliximab and daclizumab) and alemtuzumab (CAMPATH-1H), a humanized antibody against CD52 that can profoundly deplete lymphocytes.

The potential benefits of induction therapy include more reliable immunosuppression in the early postoperative period, lower rates of acute rejection, possible host hyporesponsiveness to alloantigen and, most importantly, renal protection by allowing the delayed introduction of ciclosporin or tacrolimus. Some post-hoc analyses of clinical trials conducted for other purposes suggest that induction therapy may be beneficial. However, there is a concern for the potential adverse effects of non-specific over-immunosuppression, including an increased risk of infection or malignancy.[70]

The use of anti-thymocyte globulin as an induction agent has been found to be related to lower rejection rates, but also with neutral effect on survival and higher risk of infection.[71] Only one large-scale multicentre clinical trial of induction therapy has been conducted in heart transplantation; this compared daclizumab with a placebo control. The daclizumab group had a lower incidence of the composite end-point of moderate or severe cellular rejection, haemodynamically significant allograft dysfunction, redo transplantation, death,

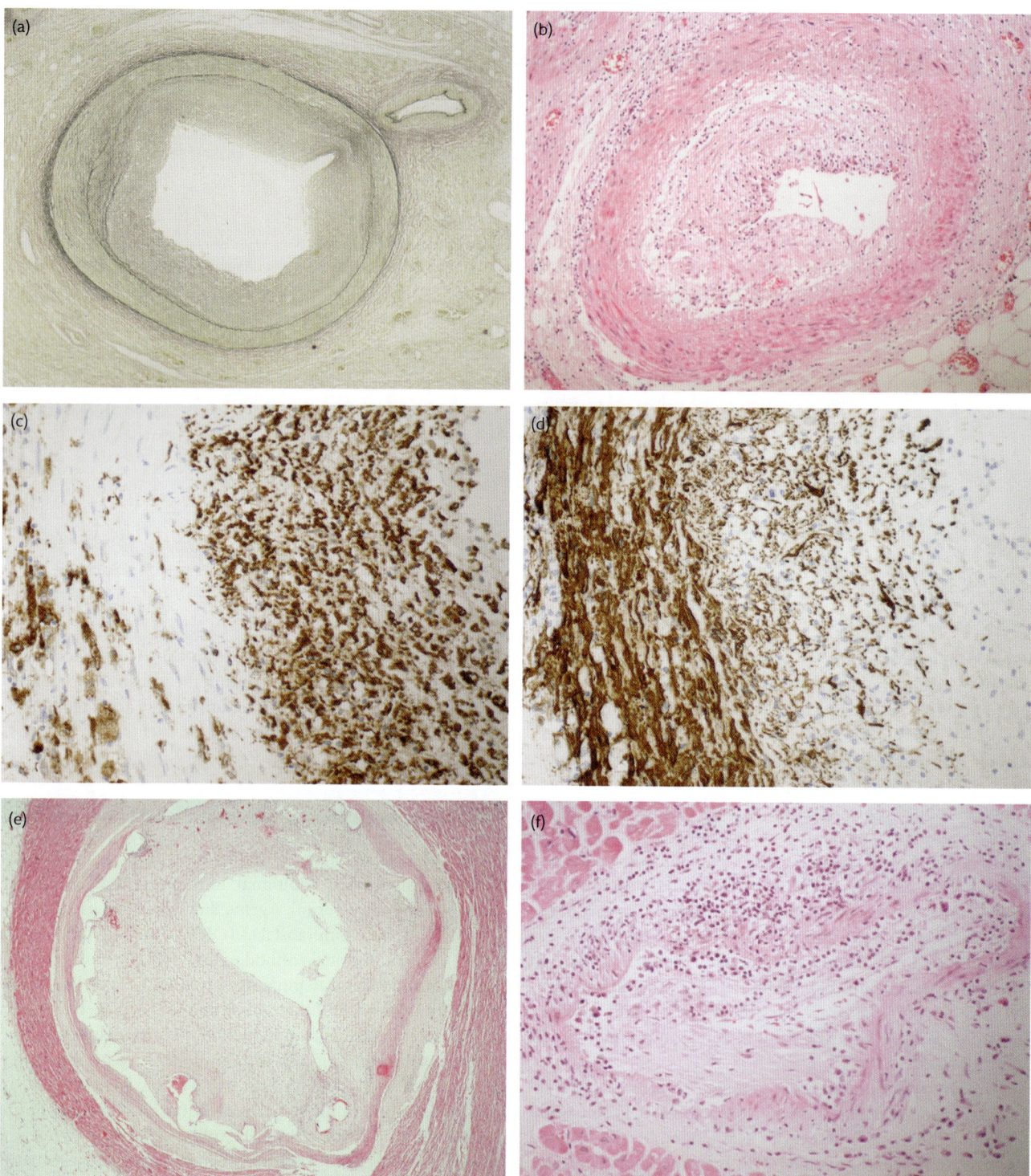

Figure 61.5 Cardiac allograft vasculopathy (CAV). (a) Typical CAV with circumferential thickening of the intima and good preservation of the internal elastic lamina. A small perforating branch of coronary artery (top right of frame) is normal. (b) Active cardiac allograft vasculopathy (CAV) with intimal proliferation due to lymphocytic intimitis. (c) Numerous macrophages inside media and in adventitia and (d) florid myofibroblastic proliferation. (e) Stented coronary artery with diffuse CAV without plaques: there is intimal proliferation causing critical stenosis and sudden death despite insertion some weeks previously of the stent (represented by spaces distributed circumferentially just inside the media). (f) Microvasculopathy: small vessel intimitis in an intramyocardial artery. (a) Verhoeff's Elastic–Van Gieson preparation ×25, (b) ×25, (c) CD68 ×200, (d) smooth muscle actin ×200, (e) ×25, (f) ×100.

or loss to follow-up within six months. However, overall mortality was not different and infection-related deaths were more common in a subgroup of the daclizumab patients who also received cytolytic therapy.[72] Daclizumab is no longer available for clinical use although another IL-2R receptor antagonist, basiliximab, is—although it has a Medicines and Healthcare products Regulatory Agency safety warning regarding its use in heart transplantation. Alemtuzumab has also been used in heart transplant patients combined with

low-dose calcineurin inhibitors and without concomitant steroids; this was associated with reduced risk of rejection, but also with no survival benefit.[73] In current practice, anti-thymocyte globulin is the only available agent to be used in induction therapy. Based on the evidence currently available, the decision about whether to use induction therapy remains a matter of physician preference and, in some centres, is influenced by the risk profile of the recipient.

The calcineurin inhibitors (CNIs) ciclosporin and tacrolimus are the cornerstones of current maintenance immunosuppression regimens. Traditionally these drugs have been used in combination with an anti-proliferative agent and corticosteroids. The introduction of the CNI can be delayed by using induction therapy and this strategy may reduce the incidence of perioperative acute renal injury. After transplantation, CNI target levels gradually decline following the decreasing risk of rejection over time. Tacrolimus is usually the preferred agent, as it has been related to reduced risk of acute rejection compared to ciclosporin, although both CNIs had similar effects on graft and patient survival.[74] Mycophenolate mofetil, an inhibitor of inosine monophosphate dehydrogenase with more selective effect on B and T cells than azathioprine, has been shown to provide more effective prophylaxis against acute rejection.[75] Therefore most centres currently consider the combination of tacrolimus, mycophenolate, and corticosteroids to be the most effective form of maintenance immunosuppression at least for the first 6–12 months after transplantation. After this initial high-risk period, withdrawal of steroids is feasible and reduces the risk of long-term side-effects.[76]

The target of rapamycin (TOR) inhibitors—sirolimus and everolimus—are another important group of immunosuppressive agents. These drugs provide prophylaxis against acute rejection that is similar to mycophenolate.[77] However, the adoption of these drugs as primary immunosuppressive agents after heart transplantation has been limited due to adverse effects, particularly impaired wound healing, increased incidence of postoperative pericardial effusions, and of bacterial and fungal infections. They have several other dermatological and gastrointestinal side-effects. Rarely, sirolimus may trigger a severe form of pneumonitis (Figure 61.6a). The TOR inhibitors potentiate CNI nephrotoxicity; however, a recent study suggested that this effect can be ameliorated by setting lower target levels for ciclosporin therapy when combined with everolimus. The TOR inhibitors have a low inherent nephrotoxicity although their use may increase proteinuria. They have anti-proliferative properties and have been shown to be effective in primary prophylaxis against cardiac allograft vasculopathy as well as in slowing the progression of vasculopathy.[78] These drugs have also been used in non-CNI maintenance immunosuppression regimens to ameliorate chronic nephrotoxicity,[79] although this strategy may be related to increased risk of rejection or immunosuppression-related side-effects, especially when concomitant mycophenolate dose is low.[80]

Ciclosporin, tacrolimus, and sirolimus are all metabolized through the cytochrome P450 3A4 pathway and therefore cause, and are subject to, interaction with other drugs metabolized through that pathway.[81] There are genetic polymorphisms in the P450 system and there is a wide variation between individual dose requirements for these drugs. Consequently, the administration of these three agents is adjusted to control the drug level in the blood (therapeutic drug monitoring).

Adjunctive therapy with statins has been found to improve survival and reduce the risk of serious rejection and CAV after heart transplantation.[82] Routine prophylaxis against cytomegalovirus and *Pneumocystis jirovecii* has reduced the incidence of these opportunistic infections.

Treatment of acute rejection

Acute cellular rejection normally responds to treatment with high-dose intravenous and oral corticosteroids. It is important to ensure that the patient is receiving adequate maintenance immunosuppression and is compliant with therapy. Repeated or late episodes of acute rejection are often an indication to modify the maintenance regimen. Mild cellular rejection (ISHLT grade 1R) with no evidence of allograft dysfunction or heart-related symptoms usually does not warrant treatment. Episodes of steroid-resistant rejection and those associated with haemodynamic compromise are treated more aggressively with combination of corticosteroids and anti-thymocyte globulin.[83] The treatment of acute antibody-mediated rejection involves antibody removal by either plasmapheresis or immunoadsorption coupled with treatment with high-dose polyspecific immunoglobulin, the B-cell antibody rituximab, or cyclophosphamide. Recurrent antibody-mediated rejection episodes may require the use of more aggressive treatment, such as photopheresis and total lymph irradiation, which increases the lifetime risk for lymphoproliferative disorders.[84] Overall, the treatment of antibody-mediated rejection is less standardized than for cellular rejection, the therapeutic response more variable, and the long-term outcome more uncertain.[85]

Survival and long-term outcomes

The ISHLT Heart Transplant Registry demonstrates that despite the increasing complexity of heart transplant recipients, results have improved progressively.[26] In contrast to medical therapy, survival is independent of the severity of the heart failure.[11] Early survival rates tend to be lower in Europe and this is probably related to the risk profile of the cardiac donors that are available.[12] There is heterogeneity of outcomes between diagnostic groups with patients with non-ischaemic dilated cardiomyopathy having the best overall outcome whereas patients with ACHD have a higher perioperative risk.[12,86] However, if the early postoperative risk is factored out, ACHD patients do at least as well in the long term as the other diagnostic groups. The overall outcome of re-transplantation is significantly worse than for de-novo transplants.[87] However, it appears that the outcome for both ACHD and re-transplant cases has improved in the most recent era and this probably reflects both better case selection and perioperative management.[88] Survival after transplantation is similar in patients who have been bridged to transplant with an LVAD (with the exception of ECMO) compared to those undergoing elective transplant and those undergoing heart transplantation following inotropic support.[26] Functional rehabilitation is excellent with 90% of patients deemed capable of normal activity. However, return-to-work data are less encouraging, with >50% of patients not having returned to work or normal activities at one year after transplant.[88] Quality of life, however, is improved after transplantation.[89]

Heart transplant recipients are at risk of several long-term complications. Although the incidence of acute rejection falls rapidly beyond the first few months after transplantation, episodes of late

rejection do occur. These are sometimes unexplained but are often related to periods of under-immunosuppression either because of reductions in maintenance immunosuppression due to drug toxicity, or because of poor adherence to the drug regimen by the patient.[90] Late rejection episodes are often more difficult to treat because clinical surveillance is less frequent and patients often present when the rejection is well established. Perhaps because of late presentation and association with under-immunosuppression, such episodes are often associated with the de-novo formulation of anti-donor HLA antibodies, which complicates treatment.

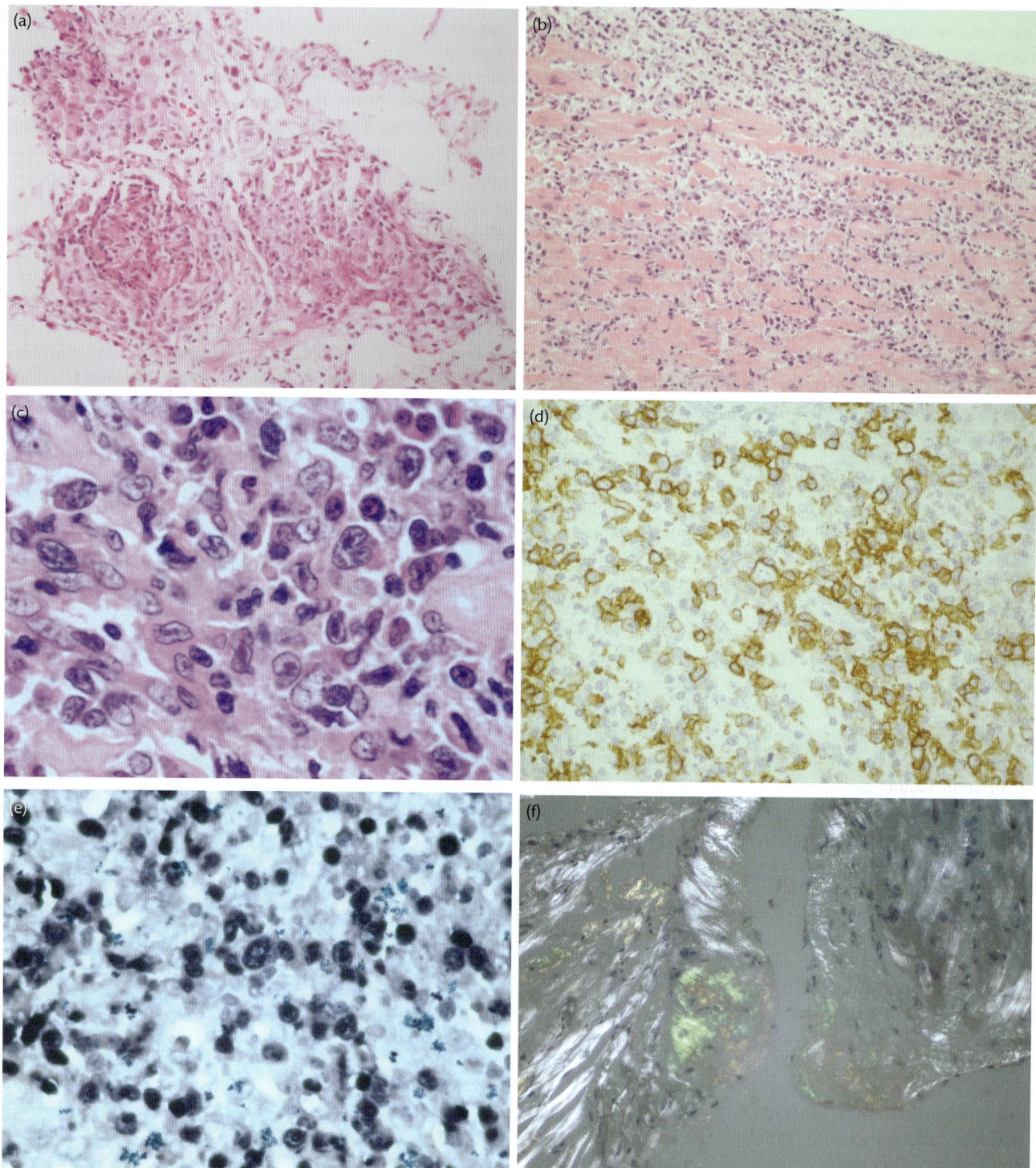

Figure 61.6 Other complications. (a) Sirolimus pulmonary toxicity: there is patchy intra-alveolar macrophage-rich exudation in this transbronchial lung biopsy from a heart transplant recipient receiving sirolimus. (b–c) In Epstein–Barr virus (EBV)-related post-transplant lymphoproliferative disorder in the cardiac allograft, cardiac muscle and endocardium are infiltrated by pleomorphic lymphocytes. (d) The immunophenotype is confirmed as B-cell with immunostaining for CD20. (e) An association with EBV is confirmed by in-situ hybridization for EBV-encoded RNA (EBERs) which marks the nuclei of the tumour cells. (f) Biopsy recurrence of cardiac amyloid 60 months after heart and kidney transplantation for ApoAl Arg60 (variant apolipoprotein Al) amyloidosis. (a) ×200, (b) ×100, (c) ×400, (d) CD20 ×200, (e) EBERs ×200, (f) Congo Red ×200 viewed with polarized light.

CAV used to be the leading cause of late death and is still an important cause of mortality. Occurrence of CAV early after transplantation portends a poor prognosis.[67] Its incidence has been reduced as a result of improved prophylaxis against acute rejection and adjunctive therapy with statins.[82] For patients who do develop disease, percutaneous coronary intervention with standard or drug-eluting stents can be used to treat focal lesions. However, since the disease is often diffuse and has a predilection to affect the secondary and tertiary coronary branches, such intervention is often only palliative. Adjunctive therapy with a TOR inhibitor coupled with intensive management of all modifiable coronary risk factors helps to reduce the progression of the disease. Re-transplantation may be performed in carefully selected cases.

Hypertension is common in orthotopic heart transplant patients and appears to be partly related to the effects of cardiac denervation. CNI inhibitors are also associated with hypertension, which is more of a problem with ciclosporin than with tacrolimus.[91] Treatment can follow conventional lines although caution is required when using an angiotensin converting enzyme inhibitor in those with significant renal impairment, because this and CNIs can both contribute to hyperkalaemia. Some calcium antagonists, notably diltiazem, can also interact with ciclosporin metabolism, requiring therapeutic drug monitoring and dose adjustments.

Dyslipidaemia is common in heart transplant patients. This is partly related to their underlying disease and to the effects of immunosuppressive agents including ciclosporin, tacrolimus, sirolimus, and corticosteroids. Statin therapy is universal after heart transplantation as described above; however, dose escalation and drug switching may be required in patients with refractory dyslipidaemia. In this circumstance, care is needed when treating patients with ciclosporin because serious drug interactions may occur between some of the statins, and there is a risk of rhabdomyolysis and renal failure. In difficult cases, it is safer to switch the patient to tacrolimus to allow conventional doses of statin therapy to be used.

Chronic kidney disease is common after all forms of organ transplantation. It is related to therapy with CNI inhibitors; however, a number of other factors contribute to this problem including preoperative renal dysfunction related to heart failure, acute kidney injury, pre-transplant diabetes, and recipient age.[92] The severity of renal dysfunction varies considerably between patients, but the incidence increases with time and some degree of renal dysfunction is almost universal ten years after transplantation. Management to prevent progression involves tight control of hypertension and the option of switching the patient to a non-CNI immunosuppression regimen.[79] However, the safety of this approach early after heart transplantation has not been established and renal function rarely returns to normal after late conversion.

The incidence of malignancy is increased in heart transplant recipients mainly due to pharmacological immunosuppression.[93] The most common tumours are non-melanoma skin cancer and post-transplant lymphoproliferative disease (PTLD). Skin tumours are related to age and cumulative sun exposure, occurring mainly in fair-skinned patients. PTLD usually presents as non-Hodgkin lymphoma and the risk is related to Epstein–Barr virus exposure, the intensity of immunosuppression, and use of induction therapy (Figure 61.6b–e).[70] The incidence of many other cancers is also increased after transplantation but to a lesser extent.[94]

Recurrence of the original cardiac disease in the allograft may occur. There is an overlap between the risk factors for conventional coronary atherosclerosis and cardiac allograft vasculopathy. Some inflammatory and infiltrative diseases may recur after transplantation, e.g. giant cell myocarditis and amyloidosis (**Figure 61.6f**).

Conclusion

Heart transplantation remains the reference standard treatment for selected patients with advanced heart failure. Unlike medical therapy, outcome is independent of the severity of the heart failure syndrome. However, transplantation is limited by the scarcity of suitable donor hearts. This has led to increasing waiting times and a reliance on mechanical circulatory support to 'bridge' patients to transplantation. The long-term outcome of transplantation is superior to those currently achieved by medical therapy or by long-term mechanical circulatory support. Heart transplant recipients are subject to several long-term complications including an increased risk of malignancy, cardiac allograft vasculopathy, and chronic kidney disease. Nevertheless, most achieve a good level of rehabilitation and an improved quality of life.

REFERENCES

1. Cass MH, Brock R. Heart excision and replacement. *Guys Hosp Rep* 1959;**108**:285–90.
2. Lower RR, Shumway NE. Studies on orthotopic homotransplantation of the canine heart. *Surg Forum* 1960;**11**:18–19.
3. Schnoor M, Schafer T, Luhmann D, Sievers HH. Bicaval versus standard technique in orthotopic heart transplantation: a systematic review and meta-analysis. *J Thor Cardiovasc Surg* 2007;**134**:1322–31.
4. Banner NR, Lyster H. Pharmacological immunosuppression. In: Banner NR, Polak JM, Yacoub MH (eds), *Lung transplantation*, p. 205–42. Cambridge University Press, Cambridge, 2003.
5. Barnard CN. The operation. A human cardiac transplant: an interim report of a successful operation performed at Groote Schuur Hospital, Cape Town. *S Afr Med J* 1967;**41**:1271–4.
6. McRae D. *Every second counts: the race to transplant the first human heart*. Putnam, New York, 2006.
7. Hunt SA. Taking heart—cardiac transplantation past, present, and future. *New Engl J Med* 2006;**355**:231–5.
8. Calne RY, Rolles K, White DJ, *et al.* Cyclosporin A initially as the only immunosuppressant in 34 recipients of cadaveric organs: 32 kidneys, 2 pancreases, and 2 livers. *Lancet* 1979;**2**:1033–6.
9. Banner NR, Yacoub MH. Cyclosporine in thoracic organ transplantation. *Transplant Proc* 2004;**36**:302S–8S.
10. Ponikowski P, Voors AA, Anker SD, *et al.* 2016 ESC Guidelines for the diagnosis and treatment of acute and chronic heart failure: The Task Force for the diagnosis and treatment of acute and chronic heart failure of the European Society of Cardiology (ESC). Developed with the special contribution of the Heart Failure Association (HFA) of the ESC. *Eur J Heart Fail* 2016;**18**:891–975.
11. Banner NR, Rogers CA, Bonser RS. Effect of heart transplantation on survival in ambulatory and decompensated heart failure. *Transplantation* 2008;**86**:1515–22.

12. Thekkudan J, Rogers CA, Thomas HL, *et al.* Trends in adult heart transplantation: a national survey from the United Kingdom Cardiothoracic Transplant Audit 1995–2007. *Eur J Cardiothor Surg* 2010;**37**:80–6.

13. Stehlik J, Stevenson LW, Edwards LB, *et al.* Organ allocation around the world: insights from the ISHLT International Registry for Heart and Lung Transplantation. *J Heart Lung Transplant* 2014;**33**:975–84.

14. Miller LW, Pagani FD, Russell SD, *et al.* Use of a continuous-flow device in patients awaiting heart transplantation. *N Engl J Med* 2007;**357**:885–96.

15. Slaughter MS, Rogers JG, Milano CA, *et al.* Advanced heart failure treated with continuous-flow left ventricular assist device. *N Engl J Med* 2009;**361**:2241–51.

16. Jessup M, Banner N, Brozena S, *et al.* Optimal pharmacologic and non-pharmacologic management of cardiac transplant candidates: approaches to be considered prior to transplant evaluation: International Society for Heart and Lung Transplantation guidelines for the care of cardiac transplant candidates—2006. *J Heart Lung Transplant* 2006;**25**:1003–23.

17. Mehra MR, Canter CE, Hannan MM, *et al.* The 2016 International Society for Heart Lung Transplantation listing criteria for heart transplantation: a 10-year update. *J Heart Lung Transplant* 2016;**35**:1–23.

18. Kolh P, Windecker S, Alfonso F, *et al.* 2014 ESC/EACTS Guidelines on myocardial revascularization: the Task Force on Myocardial Revascularization of the European Society of Cardiology (ESC) and the European Association for Cardio-Thoracic Surgery (EACTS). Developed with the special contribution of the European Association of Percutaneous Cardiovascular Interventions (EAPCI). *Eur J Cardiothorac Surg* 2014;**46**:517–92.

19. Jones RH, Velazquez EJ, Michler RE, *et al.* Coronary bypass surgery with or without surgical ventricular reconstruction. *N Engl J Med* 2009;**360**:1705–17.

20. Mancini DM, Eisen H, Kussmaul W, *et al.* Value of peak exercise oxygen consumption for optimal timing of cardiac transplantation in ambulatory patients with heart failure. *Circulation* 1991;**83**:778–86.

21. Aaronson KD, Schwartz JS, Chen TM, *et al.* Development and prospective validation of a clinical index to predict survival in ambulatory patients referred for cardiac transplant evaluation. *Circulation* 1997;**95**:2660–7.

22. Levy WC, Mozaffarian D, Linker DT, *et al.* The Seattle Heart Failure Model: prediction of survival in heart failure. *Circulation* 2006;**113**:1424–33.

23. Banner NR, Bonser RS, Clark AL, *et al.* UK guidelines for referral and assessment of adults for heart transplantation. *Heart* 2011;**97**:1520–7.

24. Stevenson LW, Miller LW, Desvigne-Nickens P, *et al.* Left ventricular assist device as destination for patients undergoing intravenous inotropic therapy: a subset analysis from REMATCH (Randomized Evaluation of Mechanical Assistance in Treatment of Chronic Heart Failure). *Circulation* 2004;**110**:975–81.

25. Chen JM, Levin HR, Michler RE, *et al.* Reevaluating the significance of pulmonary hypertension before cardiac transplantation: determination of optimal thresholds and quantification of the effect of reversibility on perioperative mortality. *J Thorac Cardiovasc Surg* 1997;**114**:627–34.

26. Lund LH, Edwards LB, Dipchand AI, *et al.* The Registry of the International Society for Heart and Lung Transplantation: Thirty-third Adult Heart Transplantation Report—2016; Focus theme: primary diagnostic indications for transplant. *J Heart Lung Transplant* 2016;**35**:1158–69.

27. Torre-Amione G, Southard RE, Loebe MM, *et al.* Reversal of secondary pulmonary hypertension by axial and pulsatile mechanical circulatory support. *J Heart Lung Transplant* 2010;**29**:195–200.

28. Takayama H, Soni L, Kalesan B, *et al.* Bridge-to-decision therapy with a continuous-flow external ventricular assist device in refractory cardiogenic shock of various causes. *Circ Heart Fail* 2014;**7**:799–806.

29. Lyster H, Banner NR. Intravenous inotropic agents. In: Banner NR, Jessup M (eds), *Advanced heart failure*, pp. 307–24. Elsevier, Philadelphia, 2009.

30. Pagani FD, Lynch W, Swaniker F, *et al.* Extracorporeal life support to left ventricular assist device bridge to heart transplant: a strategy to optimize survival and resource utilization. *Circulation* 1999;**100**:II206–10.

31. Emin A, Rogers CA, Parameshwar J, *et al.* Trends in long-term mechanical circulatory support for advanced heart failure in the UK. *Eur J Heart Fail* 2013;**15**:1185–93.

32. Mehra MR, Naka Y, Uriel N, *et al.* A fully magnetically levitated circulatory pump for advanced heart failure. *N Engl J Med* 2017;**376**:440–50.

33. Dang NC, Topkara VK, Mercando M, *et al.* Right heart failure after left ventricular assist device implantation in patients with chronic congestive heart failure. *J Heart Lung Transplant* 2006;**25**:1–6.

34. Copeland JG, Smith RG, Arabia FA, *et al.* Cardiac replacement with a total artificial heart as a bridge to transplantation. *N Engl J Med* 2004;**351**:859–67.

35. Yacoub M, Mankad P, Ledingham S. Donor procurement and surgical techniques for cardiac transplantation. *Semin Thorac Cardiovasc Surg* 1990;**2**:153–61.

36. Garcia Saez D, Zych B, Sabashnikov A, *et al.* Evaluation of the organ care system in heart transplantation with an adverse donor/recipient profile. *Ann Thorac Surg* 2014;**98**:2099–105; discussion 105–6.

37. Nativi JN, Brown RN, Taylor DO, *et al.* Temporal trends in heart transplantation from high-risk donors: are there lessons to be learned? A multi-institutional analysis. *J Heart Lung Transplant* 2010;**29**:847–52.

38. Dronavalli VB, Rogers CA, Banner NR. Primary cardiac allograft dysfunction-validation of a clinical definition. *Transplantation* 2015;**99**:1919–25.

39. Zaroff JG, Rosengard BR, Armstrong WF, *et al.* Consensus conference report: maximizing use of organs recovered from the cadaver donor: cardiac recommendations, March 28–29, 2001, Crystal City, Va. *Circulation* 2002;**106**:836–41.

40. Zaroff JG, Babcock WD, Shiboski SC, Solinger LL, Rosengard BR. Temporal changes in left ventricular systolic function in heart donors: results of serial echocardiography. *J Heart Lung Transplant* 2003;**22**:383–8.

41. Venkateswaran RV, Steeds RP, Quinn DW, *et al.* The haemodynamic effects of adjunctive hormone therapy in potential heart donors: a prospective randomized double-blind factorially designed controlled trial. *Eur Heart J* 2009;**30**:1771–80.

42. Singh TP, Almond CS, Taylor DO, Graham DA. Decline in heart transplant wait list mortality in the United States following broader regional sharing of donor hearts. *Circ Heart Fail* 2012;**5**:249–58.

43. Stehlik J, Islam N, Hurst D, *et al.* Utility of virtual crossmatch in sensitized patients awaiting heart transplantation. *J Heart Lung Transplant* 2009;**28**:1129–34.

44. Banner NR, Thomas HL, Curnow E, *et al.* The importance of cold and warm cardiac ischemia for survival after heart transplantation. *Transplantation* 2008;**86**:542–7.

45. Ardehali A, Esmailian F, Deng M, *et al.* Ex-vivo perfusion of donor hearts for human heart transplantation (PROCEED II): a prospective, open-label, multicentre, randomised non-inferiority trial. *Lancet* 2015;**385**:2577–84.

46. Dhital KK, Iyer A, Connellan M, *et al.* Adult heart transplantation with distant procurement and ex-vivo preservation of donor hearts after circulatory death: a case series. *Lancet* 2015;**385**:2585–91.

47. Garcia Saez D, Bowles CT, Mohite PN, *et al.* Heart transplantation after donor circulatory death in patients bridged to transplant with implantable left ventricular assist devices. *J Heart Lung Transplant* 2016;**35**:1255–60.

48. Banner NR, Hamour I, Lyster H, *et al.* Postoperative Care of the Heart Transplant Patient. In: O'Donnell JM, Nacul FE (eds), *Surgical intensive care medicine*, 2nd edn, pp. 599–619. Springer, New York, 2010.

49. Chou NK, Chi NH, Ko WJ, *et al.* Extracorporeal membrane oxygenation for perioperative cardiac allograft failure. *Asaio J* 2006;**52**:100–3.

50. Suarez-Barrientos A, Karagiannis G, Banner NR. Postoperative care of the heart transplant patient. In: O'Donnell JM, Nacul FE (eds), *Surgical intensive care medicine*, 3rd edn, pp. 701–30. Springer, New York, 2016.

51. Kobashigawa J, Zuckermann A, Macdonald P, *et al.* Report from a consensus conference on primary graft dysfunction after cardiac transplantation. *J Heart Lung Transplant* 2014;**33**:327–40.

52. Dronavalli VB, Rogers CA, Banner NR. Primary cardiac allograft dysfunction-validation of a clinical definition. *Transplantation* 2015;**99**:1919–25.

53. Fishman JA, Rubin RH. Infection in organ-transplant recipients. *N Engl J Med* 1998;**338**:1741–51.

54. Kohler P, Kuster SP, Bloemberg G, *et al.* Healthcare-associated prosthetic heart valve, aortic vascular graft, and disseminated Mycobacterium chimaera infections subsequent to open heart surgery. *Eur Heart J* 2015;**36**:2745–53.

55. Terasaki PI, Cai J. Human leukocyte antigen antibodies and chronic rejection: from association to causation. *Transplantation* 2008;**86**:377–83.

56. Caves PK, Billingham ME, Schulz WP, Dong E, Jr, Shumway NE. Transvenous biopsy from canine orthotopic heart allografts. *Am Heart J* 1973;**85**:525–30.

57. Hamour IM, Burke MM, Bell AD, *et al.* Limited utility of endomyocardial biopsy in the first year after heart transplantation. *Transplantation* 2008;**85**:969–74.

58. Desruennes M, Corcos T, Cabrol A, *et al.* Doppler echocardiography for the diagnosis of acute cardiac allograft rejection. *J Am Coll Cardiol* 1988;**12**:63–70.

59. Pham MX, Teuteberg JJ, Kfoury AG, *et al.* Gene-expression profiling for rejection surveillance after cardiac transplantation. *N Engl J Med* 2010;**362**:1890–900.

60. Kobashigawa J, Patel J, Azarbal B, *et al.* Randomized pilot trial of gene expression profiling versus heart biopsy in the first year after heart transplant: early invasive monitoring attenuation through gene expression trial. *Circ Heart Fail* 2015;**8**:557–64.

61. De Vlaminck I, Valantine HA, Snyder TM, *et al.* Circulating cell-free DNA enables noninvasive diagnosis of heart transplant rejection. *Sci Transl Med* 2014;**6**:241ra77.

62. Stewart S, Winters GL, Fishbein MC, *et al.* Revision of the 1990 working formulation for the standardization of nomenclature in the diagnosis of heart rejection. *J Heart Lung Transplant* 2005;**24**:1710–20.

63. Berry GJ, Burke MM, Andersen C, *et al.* The 2013 International Society for Heart and Lung Transplantation Working Formulation for the standardization of nomenclature in the pathologic diagnosis of antibody-mediated rejection in heart transplantation. *J Heart Lung Transplant* 2013;**32**:1147–62.

64. Lu WH, Palatnik K, Fishbein GA, *et al.* Diverse morphologic manifestations of cardiac allograft vasculopathy: a pathologic study of 64 allograft hearts. *J Heart Lung Transplant* 2011;**30**:1044–50.

65. Angelini A, Castellani C, Fedrigo M, *et al.* Coronary cardiac allograft vasculopathy versus native atherosclerosis: difficulties in classification. *Virchows Archiv* 2014;**464**:627–35.

66. Loupy A, Toquet C, Rouvier P, *et al.* Late failing heart allografts: pathology of cardiac allograft vasculopathy and association with antibody-mediated rejection. *Am J Transplant* 2016;**16**:111–20.

67. Mehra MR, Crespo-Leiro MG, Dipchand A, *et al.* International Society for Heart and Lung Transplantation working formulation of a standardized nomenclature for cardiac allograft vasculopathy—2010. *J Heart Lung Transplant* 2010;**29**:717–27.

68. Hiemann NE, Wellnhofer E, Knosalla C, *et al.* Prognostic impact of microvasculopathy on survival after heart transplantation: evidence from 9713 endomyocardial biopsies. *Circulation* 2007;**116**:1274–82.

69. Revelo MP, Miller DV, Stehlik J, *et al.* Longitudinal evaluation of microvessel density in survivors vs. nonsurvivors of cardiac pathologic antibody-mediated rejection. *Cardiovasc Pathol* 2012;**21**:445–54.

70. Opelz G, Dohler B. Lymphomas after solid organ transplantation: a collaborative transplant study report. *Am J Transplant* 2004;**4**:222–30.

71. Emin A, Rogers CA, Thekkudan J, Bonser RS, Banner NR. Antithymocyte globulin induction therapy for adult heart transplantation: a UK national study. *J Heart Lung Transplant* 2011;**30**:770–7.

72. Hershberger RE, Starling RC, Eisen HJ, *et al.* Daclizumab to prevent rejection after cardiac transplantation. *N Engl J Med* 2005;**352**:2705–13.

73. Teuteberg JJ, Shullo MA, Zomak R, *et al.* Alemtuzumab induction prior to cardiac transplantation with lower intensity maintenance immunosuppression: one-year outcomes. *Am J Transplant* 2010;**10**:382–8.

74. Grimm M, Rinaldi M, Yonan NA, *et al.* Superior prevention of acute rejection by tacrolimus vs. cyclosporine in heart transplant recipients—a large European trial. *Am J Transplant* 2006;**6**:1387–97.

75. Kobashigawa J, Miller L, Renlund D, *et al.* A randomized active-controlled trial of mycophenolate mofetil in heart transplant recipients. Mycophenolate Mofetil Investigators. *Transplantation* 1998;**66**:507–15.

76. Hamour IM, Lyster HS, Burke MM, Rose ML, Banner NR. Mycophenolate mofetil may allow cyclosporine and steroid sparing in de novo heart transplant patients. *Transplantation* 2007;**83**:570–6.

77. Eisen HJ, Tuzcu EM, Dorent R, *et al.* Everolimus for the prevention of allograft rejection and vasculopathy in cardiac-transplant recipients. *N Engl J Med* 2003;**349**:847–58.

78. Mancini D, Pinney S, Burkhoff D, *et al.* Use of rapamycin slows progression of cardiac transplantation vasculopathy. *Circulation* 2003;**108**:48–53.

79. Lyster H, Leaver N, Hamour I, Palmer A, Banner NR. Transfer from ciclosporin to mycophenolate–sirolimus immunosuppression for chronic renal disease after heart transplantation: safety and efficacy of two regimens. *Nephrol Dial Transplant* 2009;**24**:3872–5.

80. Zuckermann A, Eisen H, See Tai S, *et al.* Sirolimus conversion after heart transplant: risk factors for acute rejection and predictors of renal function response. *Am J Transplant* 2014;**14**:2048–54.

81. Banner NR, Lyster H, Yacoub MH. Clinical immunosuppression using the calcineurin-inhibitors ciclosporin and tacrolimus. In: Pinna LA, Cohen P (eds), *Inhibitors of protein kinases and protein phophatases, Handbook of experimental pharmacology*, pp. 321–59. Springer, Berlin, 2005.

82. Kobashigawa JA, Moriguchi JD, Laks H, *et al.* Ten-year follow-up of a randomized trial of pravastatin in heart transplant patients. *J Heart Lung Transplant* 2005;**24**:1736–40.

83. Hunt SA, Haddad F. The changing face of heart transplantation. *J Am Coll Cardiol* 2008;**52**:587–98.

84. Frist WH, Biggs VJ. Chronic myelogenous leukemia after lymphoid irradiation and heart transplantation. *Ann Thorac Surg* 1994;**57**:214–6.

85. Singh N, Pirsch J, Samaniego M. Antibody-mediated rejection: treatment alternatives and outcomes. *Transplant Rev (Orlando)* 2009;**23**:34–46.

86. Patel ND, Weiss ES, Allen JG, *et al.* Heart transplantation for adults with congenital heart disease: analysis of the United network for organ sharing database. *Annals Thorac Surg* 2009;**88**:814–21; discussion 21–2.

87. Lund LH, Edwards LB, Kucheryavaya AY, *et al.* The registry of the International Society for Heart and Lung Transplantation: thirty-first official adult heart transplant report—2014; focus theme: retransplantation. *J Heart Lung Transplant* 2014;**33**:996–1008.

88. Taylor DO, Stehlik J, Edwards LB, *et al.* Registry of the International Society for Heart and Lung Transplantation: Twenty-sixth Official Adult Heart Transplant Report—2009. *J Heart Lung Transplant* 2009;**28**:1007–22.

89. Grady KL, Jalowiec A, White-Williams C. Improvement in quality of life in patients with heart failure who undergo transplantation. *J Heart Lung Transplant* 1996;**15**:749–57.

90. Butler JA, Peveler RC, Roderick P, *et al.* Modifiable risk factors for non-adherence to immunosuppressants in renal transplant recipients: a cross-sectional study. *Nephrol Dial Transplant* 2004;**19**:3144–9.

91. Taylor DO, Barr ML, Radovancevic B, *et al.* A randomized, multicenter comparison of tacrolimus and cyclosporine immunosuppressive regimens in cardiac transplantation: decreased hyperlipidemia and hypertension with tacrolimus. *J Heart Lung Transplant* 1999;**18**:336–45.

92. Hamour IM, Omar F, Lyster HS, Palmer A, Banner NR. Chronic kidney disease after heart transplantation. *Nephrol Dial Transplant* 2009;**24**:1655–62.

93. Ippoliti G, Rinaldi M, Pellegrini C, Vigano M. Incidence of cancer after immunosuppressive treatment for heart transplantation. *Crit Rev Oncol/Hematol* 2005;**56**:101–13.

94. Crespo-Leiro MG, Alonso-Pulpon L, Vazquez de Prada JA, *et al.* Malignancy after heart transplantation: incidence, prognosis and risk factors. *Am J Transplant* 2008;**8**:1031–9.

62

Revascularization, remodelling, and mitral valve surgery

John Pepper

Introduction

The most common cause of heart failure with reduced ejection fraction (HFrEF) in the industrialized world is coronary heart disease.[1] Patients with an ischaemic aetiology of left ventricular systolic dysfunction have significantly higher mortality rates than those with non-ischaemic aetiologies.[2] This more aggressive course represents the convergence of ischaemic myocardial fibrosis and endothelial dysfunction, which are superimposed on the progressive nature of left ventricular dysfunction, often with co-morbidities such as diabetes or hypertension. The foundation of treatment for HFrEF is guideline-directed medical treatment.[3] This has resulted in a significant improvement in survival and quality of life, but not a return to normal activities. The most commonly considered surgical interventions for patients with HFrEF are coronary artery bypass surgery (CABG), sometimes combined with surgical ventricular reconstruction (SVR) and surgery for mitral regurgitation (MR).

Until recently the treatment of patients with significant coronary artery disease and heart failure was based on randomized trials conducted some 30 years ago. By modern standards of statistical evaluation the results should probably be considered neutral. Each trial managed to find a subgroup, usually not pre-specified, with a positive result. The Coronary Artery Surgery Study (CASS) noted that a subgroup of 78 patients with three-vessel disease and left ventricular ejection fraction (LVEF) of 35–50% had a five-year mortality of 10% when assigned to surgery and 19% when assigned to medical treatment.[4] These values rose to 12% and 35%, respectively, at seven years (*P* = 0.009). Most of these patients had angina, very few had heart failure, and patients with LVEF <35% were excluded. Since then, medical treatment for coronary artery disease has improved considerably. The Clinical Outcomes Utilising Revascularisation and Aggressive Drug Evaluation (COURAGE) trial[5] demonstrated no benefit of revascularization for patients with significant but stable coronary artery disease with objective evidence of myocardial ischaemia and preserved left ventricular function. This trial emphasized the importance of comparing coronary revascularization and modern medical management in stable patients with significant left ventricular dysfunction.

Much of the rationale for current recommendations for coronary artery surgery in patients with ischaemic heart failure is based on the results of the only recent prospective randomized controlled trial, the Surgical Treatment for Ischaemic Heart Failure (STICH) trial.[6]

Surgery in patients with left ventricular systolic dysfunction

The STICH trial[6] enrolled 1212 patients from 96 medical centres in 23 countries with suitable coronary anatomy and LVEF of <35% regardless of myocardial viability. Hypothesis 1, the revascularization hypothesis, sought to compare modern medical management with and without coronary artery surgery. Patients were eligible for medical treatment alone if they did not have stenosis of ≥50% of the diameter of the left main coronary artery and if they did not have Canadian Cardiovascular Society class III or IV angina while receiving medical treatment. The STICH trial demonstrated that coronary bypass surgery reduced cardiovascular death (hazard ratio (HR): 0.81; 95% confidence interval (CI): 0.66–1.00; *P* = 0.05) and the combination of cardiovascular death and cardiovascular hospitalization (0.74; 0.64–0.85; *P* < 0.001) but did not significantly reduce the primary end-point of total mortality (0.86; 0.72–1.04; *P* = 0.12). Subgroup analyses did not identify a statistically positive interaction of coronary artery surgery with any of the pre-specified subgroups of patients.

The results of the STICH trial have been interpreted in different ways. Some have suggested that it is preferable to treat STICH eligible patients medically until they become unstable and only then to proceed to coronary artery surgery. Others have proposed that all patients who would have been eligible for STICH should now be considered for early coronary surgery. This difference of views is reflected in the slightly different guidelines published by the European Society of Cardiology (ESC)[3] and the American College of Cardiology Foundation (ACCF)/American Heart Association (AHA)[7] for the treatment of patients with coronary artery disease and HFrEF.

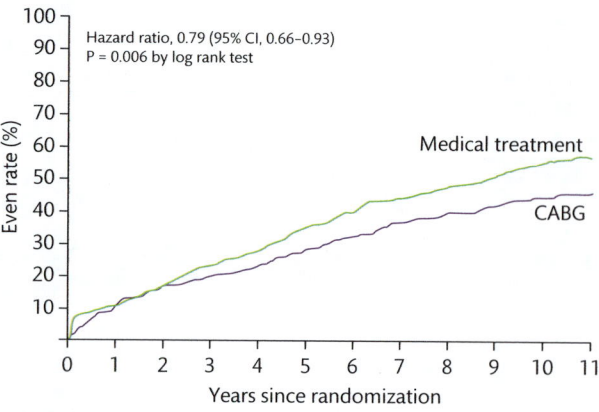

Figure 62.1 Death from cardiovascular causes in the STICH Extension Study. The early risk of coronary artery bypass surgery (CABG) is offset by a durable effect that translates into increasing clinical benefit to at least 10 years.

Velazquez EJ, Lee KL, Jones RH, Al-Khalidi HR, Hill JA, Panza JA, Michler RE, Bonow RO, Doenst T, Petrie MC, Oh JK, She L, Moore VL, Desvigne-Nickens P, Sopko G, Rouleau JL; STICHES Investigators. Coronary-Artery Bypass Surgery in Patients with Ischemic Cardiomyopathy. N Engl J Med 2016;**374**:1511–20.

The ESC guidelines[3] suggest that coronary surgery is recommended (class 1) in patients with two- or three-vessel disease, a life expectancy of more than one year, and good functional capacity to reduce cardiovascular death and admission to hospital for a cardiovascular reason. The ACCF/AHA guidelines[7] recommend (class 2a) coronary surgery to improve survival in patients with mild-to-moderate LV systolic dysfunction and significant multi-vessel coronary artery disease or proximal left anterior descending (LAD) stenosis when viable myocardium is present; and, for patients with severe left ventricular dysfunction (LVEF <35%), heart failure, and significant coronary artery disease, coronary artery surgery or medical treatment is reasonable to improve morbidity and mortality. Both the ESC and ACCF/AHA guidelines recommend coronary surgery for patients with a left main-stem coronary artery obstructed >50%. The ACCF/AHA guidelines also suggest that patients with a left main-stem equivalent coronary lesion should be revascularized.

The result of the recently published STICH Extension Study (STICHES) is helpful and is likely to change our clinical approach to patients with heart failure.[8] Velazquez and colleagues[8] have reported the 10-year outcomes of the revascularization component of STICH. They achieved 98% follow-up from 99 institutions comprising 1212 patients. Coronary surgery was found to confer a substantial survival benefit at 10 years, with a rate of all-cause mortality that was 16% lower than that associated with guideline-directed medical treatment alone (**Figure 62.1**). The initial higher event rate in the surgical group is offset by the benefit at 10 years. This new information substantially supports the class 2a recommendation that coronary surgery is 'probably beneficial' in these patients. Patients with HFrEF should be evaluated for the possibility of coronary revascularization by a multidisciplinary heart team and the shared decision-making should be patient specific.

Subgroup analyses of the STICH trial

Many patients with coronary artery disease and HFrEF were excluded from STICH. These included those in whom coronary surgery was clearly indicated, such as patients with significant left main-stem coronary stenosis or with severe symptoms of angina. It also included those in whom coronary surgery was contraindicated because of the very high operative risk, limited functional capacity, or reduced likelihood of survival. No predetermined subgroup of patients within the STICH trial had a statistically significant interaction with coronary artery surgery. Nevertheless further analyses of subgroups of patients are in progress.

One such subgroup comprises those patients who 'crossed over' from coronary artery surgery to medical treatment in the STICH trial. In most instances the reason for cross-over was the instability of the patient: five patients died before they could have coronary artery surgery. Patients who crossed over to coronary surgery did much better than those who had medical treatment alone. This difference was independent of the baseline risk of individual patients. This suggests that for patients who crossed over in STICH the benefit of coronary surgery on mortality and on cardiovascular end-points was underestimated.

Assessment of myocardial viability and ischaemia

The assessment of myocardial viability was prospectively programmed into the design of the STICH trial.[6] Numerous observation studies and meta-analyses had suggested that viability testing was a powerful tool that could not only predict improvement in ventricular function after coronary surgery but could identify patients with coronary artery disease with HFrEF, with the greatest survival benefit from surgery compared to guideline-directed medical treatment.[9,10] These studies were limited by their retrospective design, heterogeneous methodology to define viability, lack of adjustment for key baseline variables such as age and co-morbidity, and the possibility that selection of patients for surgery might have been influenced in some studies by the results of viability testing. Above all, these studies were carried out before the modern era of medical treatment, with very few patients receiving β-blockers.

In the original trial design, viability testing with single-photon emission computed tomography was required for entry to the study. But due to low recruitment, the protocol was revised to make single-photon emission tomography or viability testing with low-dose dobutamine echocardiography optional but strongly encouraged.[11] Thus only 601 of the 1212 patients enrolled in the revascularization hypothesis arm underwent assessment of myocardial viability. The viability analysis did not identify patients who would preferentially benefit from surgery. Unsurprisingly, over a median 5.1-year follow-up patients with viable tissue represented a cohort with a lower mortality of 37% vs 51% in patients without myocardial viability. But after adjustment for other prognostic variables, myocardial viability was not associated with improved survival, suggesting that patient co-morbidities and the severity of left ventricular remodelling are more important determinants of survival. Furthermore, there was no significant interaction ($P = 0.53$) with respect to mortality between viability status and assignment to surgery or medical treatment. Interestingly, patients in the STICH trial had significantly lower LVEF than most patients in previous retrospective studies and yet had better survival rates with medical treatment than that reported in patients treated medically in the previous studies.[10,12,13] The improved survival with medical treatment in STICH helps to

explain the discordance between this clinical trial result and previous cohort studies.

The implications of the STICH results are that decisions for revascularization in patients with coronary artery disease and HFrEF should not be based on the results of viability testing alone. Coronary surgery should not be withheld from patients whose tests suggest non-viable myocardium if otherwise they have clinical and angiographic features indicating that they are appropriate surgical candidates. Further analysis of imaging data in the STICH trial was performed to assess inducible ischaemia in 399 of 1212 patients in whom stress imaging was performed using single-photon emission computed tomography or dobutamine echocardiography. This analysis failed to show enhanced survival with surgery in any subgroups.[14] This was unexpected and ran counter to the prevailing wisdom from observational studies and previous trials in patients with normal left ventricular systolic function or less severe left ventricular dysfunction. Similarly, circulating levels of brain natriuretic peptide (BNP) and soluble tissue necrosis factor-α receptor-1 (sTNFα-1) were strongly related to survival in both the surgical and medical cohorts, but did not identify those with a survival advantage after surgery.[15]

These results have been interpreted differently in the guidelines. The ESC recommendation (class 3) is that patients without angina and without viable myocardium should not have coronary artery surgery. The ACCF/AHA guidelines recommend that coronary surgery might be considered in patients with ischaemic heart disease, severe left ventricular systolic dysfunction, and operable coronary anatomy whether or not viable myocardium is present (class 2b). The latter guidelines seem to more closely reflect the results of the STICH trial.

More recently, a further substudy of the STICH trial[16] revealed that among patients with ischaemic cardiomyopathy, a lower left ventricular end-systolic volume did not identify patients in whom myocardial viability predicted better outcome with coronary surgery relative to medical treatment. This stands in contrast to retrospective studies which suggested that the severity of left ventricular remodelling determines whether myocardial viability predicts better survival with surgery compared to medical treatment. It had been thought that coronary artery surgery would preferentially benefit patients with a viable myocardium who have a smaller end-systolic volume.

Overall these data suggest that the observed survival benefits of coronary artery surgery in patients with severe left ventricular dysfunction are driven primarily by factors other than biomarkers or objective markers of myocardial viability and ischaemia. Factors associated with higher survival rates after surgery include functional status, as assessed by a 6 min walk, and the interaction of the angiographic severity of coronary artery disease, and severity of adverse left ventricular remodelling as assessed by left ventricular end-systolic volume index. Patients with preserved effort tolerance but with multi-vessel disease, lower ejection fraction, and higher left ventricular end-systolic volume index are more likely to benefit from surgery with respect to long-term survival.

Percutaneous coronary intervention

Percutaneous coronary intervention (PCI) has been less well studied in this setting. There has been no clinical trial comparing revascularization with coronary surgery or PCI of patients with HFrEF. In a retrospective study, Nagendran and colleagues identified 2925 patients with coronary artery disease and left ventricular dysfunction (ejection fraction <35%), of whom 1326 underwent coronary surgery and 1599 received PCI.[17] In a Cox proportional hazard analysis of the propensity-matched subgroups, surgery resulted in significantly lower rates of repeat revascularization and better survival rates compared with PCI at 1, 5, 10, and 15 years. Following the SYNTAX study, the recommendation for patients with multi-vessel disease is invariably surgery, not PCI, especially if the SYNTAX score is >30.[18]

But in clinical practice, the choice of one option over another needs to be personalized and varies according to the patient. The ESC and the ACCF/AHA guidelines recommend (class 2a) that PCI is a reasonable alternative to coronary surgery in patients unsuitable for surgery.

The ventricular reconstruction hypothesis

In patients with HFrEF there are often changes in left ventricular structure and function which include remodelling of the left ventricle from its normal elliptical shape to a more spherical shape, resulting in a less efficient ventricle and a worse prognosis. SVR has been shown, in observational studies, to reverse-remodel the left ventricle and restore some of its original functional capacity.[19,20] The procedure involves removing akinetic or dyskinetic segments of the anterior wall and reshaping the left ventricle to restore it to its original elliptical form. It was uncertain from these observational studies whether SVR combined with coronary artery surgery would result in improved outcomes for patients with ischaemic cardiomyopathy compared with coronary artery surgery alone, especially when combined with medical treatment. This led to the design of Hypothesis 2 of the STICH trial, the only randomized trial to question the role of SVR in patients with HFrEF. Patients were eligible if they had significant coronary artery stenosis amenable to surgical revascularization, severe systolic dysfunction with LVEF <35%, and dominant left ventricular akinesia or dyskinesia amenable to SVR. A total of 1000 patients were randomized to the arm of the trial comparing isolated coronary artery surgery versus coronary surgery and SVR against a background of medical treatment. The primary outcome was a composite of all-cause mortality and hospital readmission for heart failure. Patients who underwent SVR had significantly lower left ventricular end-systolic volumes (LVESV) on short-term follow-up with a reduction of end-systolic volume of 19% versus 6% in those receiving coronary surgery alone. But this reduction in left ventricular volume was small compared to the previous observational studies in which volume reductions of 33% and 72% were achieved.

There was no significant difference between the two treatments for the primary outcome at four-year follow-up. There were also no differences between the two groups in terms of secondary outcomes, including repeat admission to hospital, symptoms, or quality of life.[21] SVR added to coronary artery surgery does not appear to improve quality of life compared with coronary artery surgery alone, but does increase health care costs.[22] There has been much discussion aimed at reconciling the difference between the observational data supporting SVR and the findings of the STICH

trial. A secondary analysis examined the influence of baseline left ventricular volumes and LVEF on outcomes. Contrary to the widely held view by surgeons enthusiastic about SVR that patients with larger, already remodelled, left ventricles would benefit from coronary artery surgery plus SVR compared to isolated coronary artery surgery, patients with smaller baseline left ventricular end-systolic and end-diastolic diameters were more likely to benefit, especially if a postoperative LVESV index (LVESVI) <70 mL/m² can be achieved, suggesting a role for SVR before extensive remodelling has occurred.[23]

Cardiac restraint procedures

Treatments such as the Acorn CoCap and Paracor cardiac support device (CSD) have been evaluated with respect to their usefulness in limiting adverse ventricular remodelling. Dynamic cardiomyoplasty was the precursor of passive prosthetic ventricular support. Unfortunately the results from animal and clinical studies were inconsistent and limited, despite frequently observed clinical benefit. In a canine model of chronic dilated cardiomyopathy, Patel and colleagues[24] suggested that the haemodynamic benefit of cardiomyoplasty was due to the passive effect of the skeletal muscle wrap around the heart. The relief of wall stress produced by girdling of the conditioned muscle wrap was shown to stabilize the remodelling process of heart failure, preventing progressive deterioration of systolic and diastolic function. These studies led to the development of a device that would relieve wall stress, similar to the skeletal muscle wrap.

The device that has been studied most extensively is the CorCap CSD (Acorn Cardiovascular, Inc., St Paul, MN, USA). It is a multifilament polyester mesh implant which is placed around both ventricles to decrease diastolic wall stress without resultant constriction (**Figure 62.2a**). Mann and colleagues[25] assessed the safety and efficacy of the CSD in patients with heart failure. Of the 300 patients enrolled, 193 were randomized to mitral surgery alone or mitral surgery plus CSD. The 107 patients who did not need mitral surgery were randomized to medical treatment or medical treatment plus CSD. The primary end-point was a composite based on changes in clinical status, the need for major cardiac procedures for worsening heart failure, and a change in New York Heart Association (NYHA) class. All patients had LVEF <35%, LVEDD ≥60 mm, and 6 min walk <450 m. The proportional odds ratio for the primary end-point favoured treatment with CSD (1.73; 95% CI: 1.07–2.79; $P = 0.024$). When compared with the baseline, LVEF increased significantly at 12 months ($P = 0.0009$) in the CSD-treated group compared with controls ($P = 0.65$). But the changes in LVEF between groups were not significant ($P = 0.45$). Therefore the CorCap CSD may have a role in preventing adverse remodelling after myocardial infarction.[26] It requires an operation for its insertion but this could be through a small anterior thoracotomy.

The Paracor device is an elastic Nitinol mesh that is designed to mechanically reinforce the heart to retard or hopefully halt the remodelling process (**Figure 62.2a**). It can be deployed in a minimally invasive fashion. Klodell and co-workers have reported their early results.[27] Fifty patients in NYHA class II/III underwent the procedure which was well tolerated. At six months there was a significant improvement in the 6 min walk (+65.7M, $P = 0.002$) and

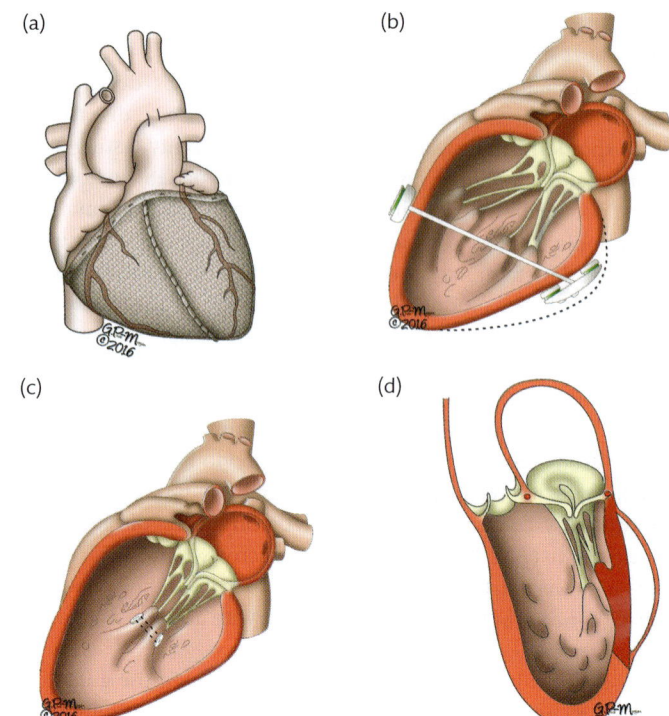

Figure 62.2 Different approaches to achieve mechanical constraint of the left ventricle and thereby reduce or abolish mitral regurgitation. (a) Sleeve around both ventricles by Acorn device or Nitinol sleeve; (b) Coapsys device; (c) approximation sling around papillary muscles; (d) compression patch to the ventricular wall.
Copyright © Gemma Price.

Minnesota Living with Heart Failure scores (−15.7, $P = 0.002$). Long-term functional results are not available because the planned interim analysis of the first 122 patients with a completed six-month follow-up indicated futility to reach the peak VO₂ end-point, and so trial enrolment was stopped.[28]

A third restraint device, the Coapsys device, treats papillary muscle displacement by inward tension on a transventricular strut anchored epicardially (Figure 62.2B). The epicardial anchors are posterior and anterior pads. The posterior pad has two heads that alter the shape of the left ventricle: one is at the level of the mitral annulus; the other is at the level of the posteromedial papillary muscle. The anterior pad is adjustable and can be fixed after confirming placement of the posterior pad under echocardiographic guidance. A PTFE-coated sub-valvular cord connects the pads. Observational studies of the Coapsys device have demonstrated significantly greater left ventricular reshaping than annuloplasty alone.[29] Outcomes of the RESTOR-LV trial were not definitive. The study was terminated when the sponsor failed to secure ongoing funding; 165 patients were randomized. Control and Coapsys both produced a decrease in left ventricular end-diastolic dimension and MR at two years ($P = 0.001$); Coapsys in the RESTOR-MV Trial showed a survival advantage compared with control at two years (87% vs 77%) (HR: 0.421; 95% CI: 0.200–0.886; stratified log-rank test; $P = 0.038$). Survival free from complications (including death, stroke, myocardial infarction, and valve reoperation) was significantly greater with Coapsys at two years (85% vs 71%) (adjusted HR: 0.372; 95% CI: 0.185–0.749).

Although some of these devices have shown promise, it has not been possible to obtain mid-term results in randomized patients.

Ischaemic mitral regurgitation

Definition

Ischaemic mitral regurgitation (IMR) occurs in up to 40% of patients after myocardial infarction. It is usually mild or moderate in severity but is associated with increased incidence of heart failure and death.[30] IMR usually occurs following an inferior myocardial infarction or is associated with an ischemia-induced wall motion abnormality. Subsequent ventricular remodelling displaces the papillary muscles towards the ventricular apex, which, in turn, draws the fixed-length chordae tendineae away from the line of coaptation (Figure 62.3). The retracted chordae tendineae tether the valve leaflets, preventing normal valve closure and resulting in valvular regurgitation. The leaflets are otherwise normal. Clinically, this will be apparent with evidence of prior myocardial infarction by typical ECG findings and/or wall motion abnormalities. Findings on cardiac catheterization or another appropriate imaging technique will confirm the ischaemic aetiology. Echocardiography usually demonstrates the tethering of the leaflets predominantly in the P2 and P3 segments of the posterior leaflet and the resultant regurgitant jet. No evidence of organic mitral valve disease should be present. MR in this setting occurs with less global left ventricular remodelling and dysfunction and especially without any involvement of the antero-septal left ventricular wall. By contrast, in patients with a previous anterior myocardial infarct, MR occurs mainly in the setting of global left ventricular dilatation and severe dysfunction, with tethering of both mitral valve leaflets due to apical displacement of the papillary muscles. Due to the combined effects of ischaemia and MR, these patients may have significant heart failure symptoms and may pose significant clinical management challenges. Because of the complex and dynamic nature of IMR, there is controversy as to the appropriate management of the patients.

Mechanisms underlying IMR

The use of three-dimensional echocardiography in experimental studies has shown that global left ventricular dysfunction alone is insufficient to cause IMR.[31] Displacement and abnormal contraction of the left ventricular wall underlying the papillary muscles, along with decreased shortening of the distance between the papillary muscles, causes mitral leaflet tethering and restricted closure that leads to IMR (Figure 62.3). Isolated annular dilation, such as occurs in patients with lone atrial fibrillation, also impairs coaptation, but relatively mildly unless there is leaflet tethering as well. Tethering geometry may predict the progression of IMR.[32] The posterior location of the papillary muscles explains why IMR is seen predominantly with inferior, as opposed to anterior, myocardial infarction unless the anterior infarction is sufficiently large to cause global dilatation or is associated with anterior dyskinesia causing papillary muscle traction. Investigators using three-dimensional imaging have mapped leaflet tenting relative to papillary muscle displacement by echocardiography and computed tomography, and have shown that asymmetric papillary muscle displacement in the apical direction causes asymmetric leaflet tenting, and is most likely to increase the severity of MR.[33] The substantially increased mortality in patients with IMR is independent of left ventricular size and function, and occurs even in those with mild IMR. IMR also reduces exercise capacity.[34] IMR is a dynamic disease that varies with multiple factors, such as with progressive left ventricular remodelling and dysfunction, with varied haemodynamic loading under exercise conditions, and reduced tethering under anaesthesia. Dynamic increases in IMR can explain reduced survival in patients with apparently mild resting MR,[35] and suggest the need for exercise testing in patients with exertional dyspnoea out of proportion to their resting MR.

The frequent failure of annular ring reduction relates to persistent leaflet tethering by displaced papillary muscles, with continued left ventricular remodelling associated with recurrent MR. The NHLBI-supported trial by the CardioThoracic Surgical Network (CTSN) indicated that 32.6% of the 126 patients who received mitral annuloplasty for severe IMR had recurrent regurgitation within one year, with recurrence predicted by the preoperative degree of tethering.[36] Subannular repair may provide a more comprehensive and lasting reduction in MR,[37] and the best haemodynamics for forward flow as well, guided by computational analysis of this dynamic, interactive system.[38] Importantly, reducing IMR might also slow progression of left ventricular remodelling, ultimately leading to a decrease in volume-overloaded heart failure. Echocardiographic insights into the tethering mechanism and papillary muscle–ventricular unit have led to potential new interventions to resolve postoperative MR by repositioning the papillary muscles (Figure 62.2c). Such interventions

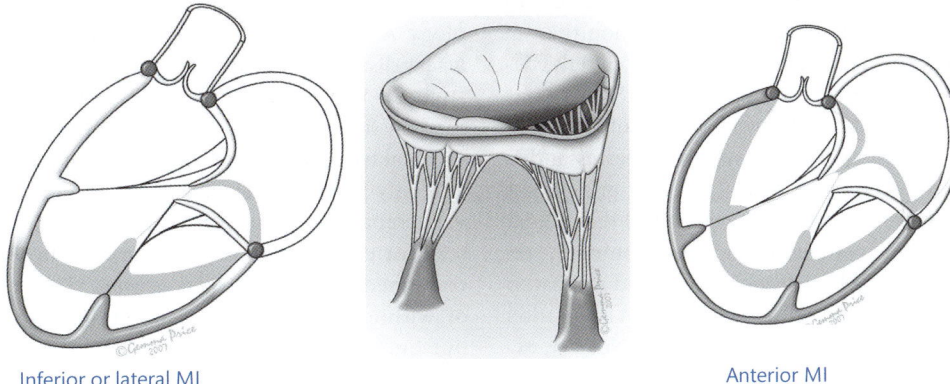

Inferior or lateral MI   Anterior MI

Figure 62.3 Pathophysiology of ischaemic mitral regurgitation. The effect of adverse left ventricular remodelling on the function of the mitral valve. MI, mitral ischaemia.

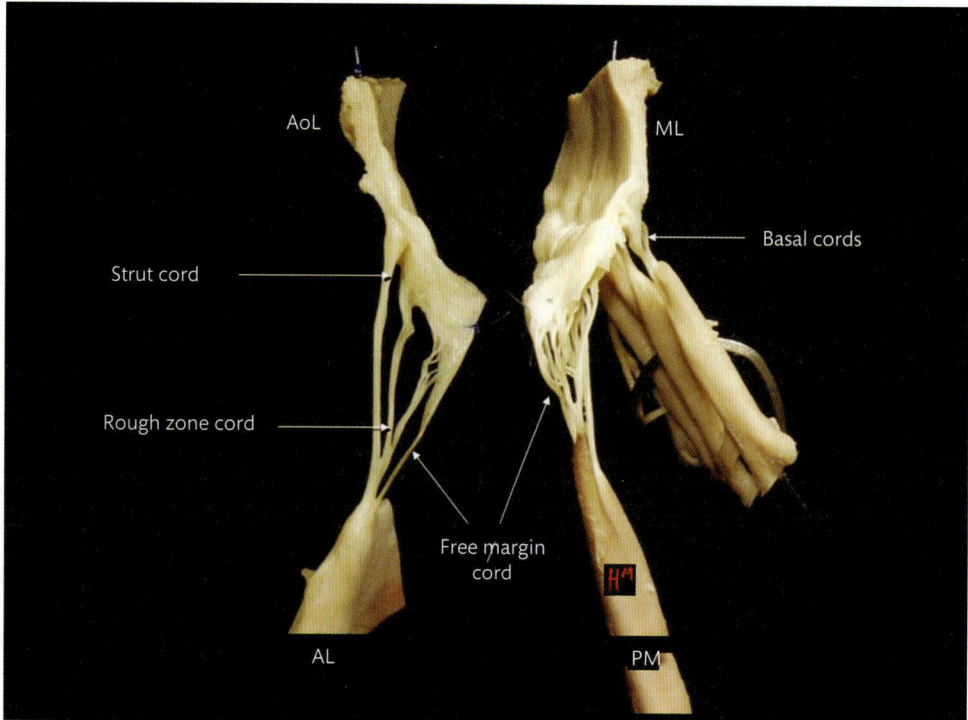

Figure 62.4 The secondary or 'strut' chordae of the mitral valve. AoL, aortic (anterior) leaflet; ML, mitral (posterior) leaflet; AL, anterolateral papillary muscle; PM, posteromedial papillary muscle.
Reproduced from Muresian H. The clinical anatomy of the mitral valve. *Clin Anat* 2009;**22**:85–98.

include direct surgical left ventricular reconstruction or using an adjustable external pericardial patch (**Figure 62.2D**) or polymer injected into the subpapillary muscle of the ventricular wall, or surgical papillary muscle approximation.[39,40] Chordal modification can relieve tethering by cutting the secondary chordae (**Figure 62.4**) that most restrict leaflet motion or by implanting chords to reduce the papillary muscle-to-annulus tethering distance.[41] Saddle-shaped annuloplasty can also reduce leaflet stress and improve coaptation.[42] Papillary muscle resynchronization and leaflet augmentation are additional options for the reduction of MR.[43]

IMR reflects the insufficiency of valve area relative to the remodelling left ventricle. This raises the question of whether the valve can adapt to tethering by increasing its area under the influence of the increased stress, particularly at the chordal attachment zone.[44]

Initial clinical studies have confirmed that the mitral valve area is 35% larger in patients with left ventricular dysfunction than in healthy individuals, and that larger leaflet area in relation to the demands imposed by leaflet tethering corresponds to less MR.[45]

These findings indicate that the mitral valve is a dynamic cellular environment that actively adapts to superimposed stresses and is influenced by ventricular pathology.[46] Adaptive leaflet growth has been reported in other studies,[47] as further evidence of the cellular plasticity of mitral valves. The compensatory adaptation might restore cellular and biomechanical leaflet homeostasis and ultimately valve function, which leads to the question of why leaflet adaptation is often insufficient to alleviate IMR in many patients. Notably, excised leaflets in patients with end-stage heart failure are thicker and stiffer than healthy valves, potentially impairing leaflet coaptation, which requires systolic leaflet stretch and bending. Remodelling of the leaflet, which is beneficial at the early stage after myocardial

infarction, might therefore become counterproductive in the chronic setting after myocardial infarction. Understanding how the valve adapts over time after myocardial infarction could create opportunities for physiological interventions, for example, by modulating transforming growth factor-β, which seems to have a major regulatory role in leaflet homeostasis in IMR.[48]

Mitral valve repair and coronary artery bypass surgery

Many observational and randomized trials comparing coronary artery surgery with PCI have suggested that treatment of the coronary disease is the predominant effect on outcome and that IMR and its associated mortality is mainly driven by ventricular pathology. A retrospective cohort study of 4989 patients with coronary artery disease and moderate or severe IMR from Duke University[49] supports this view. This was a 20-year longitudinal analysis with a median follow-up of 5.4 years. Within this cohort 36% received medical treatment alone, 26% had PCI, 33% had coronary surgery, and only 5% underwent coronary artery surgery with either mitral valve repair or replacement. The adjusted HRs were 0.83 for PCI, 0.56 for coronary bypass surgery, and 0.57 for coronary surgery combined with mitral valve surgery. Thus coronary surgery with or without mitral valve intervention was associated with better outcomes than either PCI or medical treatment. Campwala and colleagues[50] have reported progression of IMR in patients with incomplete coronary revascularization, which may in part explain the better survival of those undergoing coronary surgery compared to PCI.

It has been argued that the correction of MR may be of little benefit due to the underlying ischaemic injury, implying that MR may reflect ischaemia or advanced left ventricular dysfunction and therefore not have an independent impact on survival. Although several retrospective studies using propensity score-matched cohorts of patients showed that coronary surgery combined with mitral repair reduced MR, these studies have not demonstrated a survival advantage.[51-53]

Evidence for repair or replacement in ischaemic mitral regurgitation

The results of surgery for IMR are unproven and unpredictable in improving patient outcomes and have not been tested against medical treatment in a prospective randomized trial. Unfortunately, mitral valve repair is often not durable in IMR due to progression of the underlying left ventricular dysfunction.[54]

There have been several recent prospective randomized trials, all of which have used surrogate end-points. Although this has been criticized, to use mortality as an end-point would require in excess of 4000 patients which exceeds the capacity for timely recruitment. Fattouch and colleagues[55] randomly assigned 102 patients to CABG alone or CABG with mitral valve repair and followed the patients for an average of 32 months. They reported that left ventricular reverse remodelling, the qualitative degree of MR, and NYHA functional class improved with CABG plus mitral valve repair as compared with CABG alone.

In the RIME trial[56] the efficacy of concomitant CABG plus mitral valve repair was compared with CABG alone in patients with moderate ischaemic MR. The primary end-point was peak oxygen consumption—a recognized objective measure of functional capacity and a prognostic indicator in heart failure. Cardiac magnetic resonance (CMR) was employed to measure the main secondary end-point of LVESVI. The severity of MR was quantified both by echocardiography and CMR using established techniques. The addition of mitral valve repair by annuloplasty to coronary artery surgery reduced MR severity, left ventricular volumes, and BNP levels, and these translated into an improvement in functional capacity and symptoms at one year. However, the addition of mitral valve repair to coronary bypass surgery required longer operation times, including time on cardiopulmonary bypass, increased blood transfusion, and intubation times, and resulted in a longer hospital stay. There was also a trend toward higher complication rates in this group, although the differences were not significant.

The results of this study supported the addition of mitral valve repair to coronary artery surgery in patients with moderate ischemic MR undergoing coronary revascularization, but the benefits of the combined procedure must be balanced against a possible increased risk of morbidity in the perioperative period.

More recently the Cardiothoracic Surgical Trials Network (CTSN) has reported on 301 patients randomly assigned to coronary artery surgery or the combined procedure of coronary surgery and mitral valve repair.[57] In those patients who had moderate IMR, the addition of mitral valve repair to coronary artery surgery did not result in a higher degree of left ventricular reverse remodelling using LVESVI as the end-point.

Mitral valve repair was associated with a reduced prevalence of moderate or severe MR but an increased number of untoward events. Thus, at one year, this trial did not show a clinical advantage of adding mitral valve repair to coronary artery surgery. This study has now been updated to an outcome report on two-year outcomes.[58] The conclusion remains the same. Longer-term follow-up may determine whether the lower prevalence of MR translates into a net clinical benefit.

There were also no significant between-group differences in mortality, the composite end-point of cardiac or cerebrovascular events, readmissions, or quality of life. The proportion of patients with residual MR of at least moderate severity was significantly lower with the addition of mitral valve repair; however, patients undergoing repair had more neurological events ($P = 0.03$) than patients undergoing coronary surgery alone. These events included stroke, transient ischaemic attack, and metabolic encephalopathy.

In 2014 a further prospective randomized trial was reported by the CTSN in which 251 patients were randomly assigned with severe IMR to undergo either mitral valve repair or chordal-sparing replacement.[36] This was an efficacy and safety study. The primary end-point was the LVESVI at 12 months. The rate of death was 14.3% in the repair group and 17.6% in the replacement group (HR with repair: 0.79; 95% CI: 0.42–1.47; $P = 0.45$ by the log-rank test). There was no significant between-group difference in LVESVI after adjustment for death (z score: 1.33; $P = 0.18$). As expected the rate of moderate or severe recurrence of MR at 12 months was higher in the repair group than in the replacement group (32.6% vs 2.3%; $P < 0.001$). There were no significant between-group differences in the rate of a composite of major adverse cardiac or cerebrovascular events, in functional status, or in quality of life at 12 months. Replacement provided a more durable correction of MR, but there was no significant between-group difference in clinical outcomes. These findings contradict much of the published literature, which reports advantages to mitral valve repair over replacement, including lower operative mortality, improved left ventricular function, and higher rates of long-term survival. Notably, in a recent meta-analysis,[59] the odds ratios for the studies, comparing replacement to repair, ranged from 0.884 to 17.241 for short-term mortality and the hazard ratios ranged from 0.677 to 3.205 for long-term mortality. This translates into a relative long-term risk of death 35% higher in the replacement group than in the repair group. It should be remembered that patients undergoing mitral valve replacement tend to be older and have more coexisting illnesses than those undergoing repair, so adjustment for baseline differences has been necessary in non-randomized studies.

Conclusion

For patients who are candidates for medical treatment alone or combined with coronary artery surgery, surgery does improve survival and is superior in reducing cardiovascular death and the combination of cardiovascular death and hospital admission for cardiovascular disease. However, coronary surgery carries an up-front risk that disappears by two years after surgery.

For patients who are candidates for revascularization, surgery is superior to PCI in improving survival in patients with three- or

two-vessel disease that includes the proximal LAD. The assessment of myocardial viability or reversible ischaemia does not to appear to be helpful in deciding which patients will improve with coronary bypass surgery.

The addition of SVR to coronary surgery appears to provide no benefit, but in a subgroup of patients with less severe ventricular dilatation, SVR should be considered.

Finally, the addition of mitral valve repair to coronary bypass surgery in patients with moderate-to-severe MR appears to improve survival. But in patients with severe IMR, replacement rather than repair may be a more durable solution.

Acknowledgements

The author would like to thank Gemma Morgan for the artwork and Dr Horia Muresian for permission to use his image of the chordae of the mitral valve.

REFERENCES

1. Gheorghiade M, Sopko G, De Luka L. Navigating the crossroads of coronary artery disease and heart failure. *Circulation* 2006;**114**:1202–13.
2. Felker GM, Shaw LK, O'Connor CM. A standardised definition of ischemic cardiomyopathy for use in clinical research. *J Am Coll Cardiol* 2002;**39**:210–18.
3. McMurray JJ, Adampoulos S, Anker SD, for the ESC Committee for Practice Guidelines. ESC Guidelines for the diagnosis and treatment of acute and chronic heart failure 2012: the Task Force for the Diagnosis and Treatment of Acute and Chronic Heart Failure 2012 of the European Society of Cardiology, developed in collaboration with the Heart Failure Association (HFA) of the ESC. *Eur Heart J* 2012;**33**:1787–847.
4. Passamani E, Davis KB, Gillespie MJ, Killip T. A randomised trial of coronary artery bypass surgery: survival of patients with low ejection fraction. *N Engl J Med* 1985;**312**:1665–71.
5. Boden WE, O'Rourke RA, Teo KK, et al.; COURAGE Trial Research Group. Optimal medical therapy with and without PCI for stable coronary artery disease. *N Engl J Med* 2007;**356**:1503–16.
6. Velazquez EJ, Lee KL, Deja MA, et al.; STICH Investigators. Coronary artery bypass surgery in patients with left ventricular dysfunction. *N Engl J Med* 2011;**364**:1607–16.
7. Yancy CW, Yancy CW, Jessup M, et al. American College of Cardiology Foundation; American Heart Association Task Force on Practice Guidelines. *J Am Coll Cardiol* 2013;**128**:1810–52.
8. Velazquez EJ, Lee KL, Jones RH, et al., for the STICHES Investigators. Coronary-artery bypass surgery in patients with ischemic cardiomyopathy. *N Engl J Med* 2016;**374**:1511–20.
9. Guyton RA, Smith AL. Coronary bypass—survival benefit in heart failure. *N Engl J Med* 2016;**374**:1576–7.
10. Camici PG, Prasad SK, Rimoldi OE. Stunning, hibernation and assessment of myocardial viability. *Circulation* 2008;**117**:103–14.
11. Velazquez EJ, Lee KL, O'Connor CM, et al. Rationale and design of the Surgical Treatment for Ischemic Heart Failure (STICH) Trial. *J Thorac Cardiovasc Surg* 2007;**134**:1540–7.
12. Allman KC, Shaw LJ, Hachamovitch R, Udelson JE. Myocardial viability testing and impact of revascularisation on prognosis in patients with coronary artery disease and left ventricular dysfunction: a meta-analysis. *J Am Coll Cardiol* 2002;**39**:1151–8.
13. Bonow RO, Maurer G, Lee KL, et al.; for the STICH trial investigators. Myocardial viability and survival in ischemic left ventricular dysfunction. *N Engl J Med* 2011;**364**:1617–25.
14. Panza JA, Holly TA, Asch FM, et al. Inducible myocardial ischemia and outcomes in patients with coronary artery disease and left ventricular dysfunction. *J Am Coll Cardiol* 2013;**61**:1860–70.
15. Feldman AM, Mann DL, She L, et al. Prognostic significance of biomarkers in predicting outcome in patients with coronary artery disease and left ventricular dysfunction: results of the biomarker sub-study of the Surgical Treatment of Ischaemic Heart Failure trials. *Circ Heart Fail* 2013;**6**:461–72.
16. Bonow RO, Castelvechio S, Panza JA, et al.; STICH trial investigators. Severity of remodelling, myocardial viability, and survival in ischemic LV dysfunction after surgical revascularisation. *JACC Cardiovasc Imaging* 2015;**8**:1121–9.
17. Nagendran J, Norris CM, Graham MM, et al., for the APPROACH Investigators. Coronary revascularisation for patients with severe left ventricular dysfunction. *Ann Thorac Surg* 2013;**96**:2038–44.
18. Windecker S, Kolh P, Alfonso F, et al. ESC/EACTS guidelines on myocardial revascularisation. *Eur Heart J* 2014;**35**:2541–619.
19. Athanasuleas CL, Stanley AW Jr, Buckberg GD, et al. Surgical anterior ventricular endocardial restoration (SAVER) in the dilated remodelled ventricle after anterior myocardial infarction. RESTORE group. Reconstructive Endoventricular Surgery, returning Torsion Original Radius Elliptical Shape to LV. *J Am Coll Cardiol* 2001;**37**:1210–13.
20. Menicanti L, Castelvecchio S, Rannucci M, et al. Surgical therapy for ischemic heart failure: single center experience with surgical anterior ventricular restoration. *J Thorac Cardiovasc Surg* 2007;**134**:433–41.
21. Jones RH, Velazquez EJ, Michler RE, et al.; STICH Hypothesis 2 Investigators. Coronary bypass surgery with or without surgical ventricular reconstruction. *N Engl J Med* 2009;**360**:1705–17.
22. Mark DB, Knight JD, Velazquez EJ, et al.; Surgical Treatment for Ischemic Heart Failure (STICH) Trial Investigators. Quality of life and economic outcomes with surgical ventricular reconstruction in ischemic heart failure: results from the Surgical Treatment for Ischemic Heart Failure trial. *Am Heart J* 2009;**157**:837–44.
23. Michler RE, Rouleau JL, Al-Khalidi HR, et al.: STICH Investigators. Insights from the STICH trial: change in left ventricular size after coronary artery bypass grafting with and without surgical ventricular reconstruction. *J Thorac Cardiovasc Surg* 2013;**146**:1139–45.
24. Patel HJ, Polidori DJ, Pilla JJ, et al. Stabilisation of chronic remodelling by asynchronous cardiomyoplasty in dilated cardiomyopathy: effects of a conditioned muscle wrap. *Circulation* 1997;**96**:3665–71.
25. Mann DL, Acker MA, Jessup M. Acorn Trial Principal Investigators and Study Coordinators. Clinical evaluation of the CorCap cardiac support device in patients with dilated cardiomyopathy. *Ann Thorac Surg* 2007;**84**:1226–35.
26. Starling RC, Jessup M, Oh K, et al. Sustained benefits of the CorCap cardiac support device on left ventricular remodeling: three year follow-up results from the Acorn Clinical Trial. *Ann Thorac Surg* 2007;**84**:1236–42.
27. Klodell CT, Aranda JM, McGiffin DC, et al. Worldwide surgical experience with the Paracor HeartNet cardiac restraint device. *J Thorac Cardiovasc Surg* 2008;**135**:188–95.

28. Costanzo MR, Ivanhoe RJ, Kao A, *et al.* Prospective evaluation of elastic restraint to lessen the effects of heart failure (PEERLESS-HF) trial. *J Card Fail* 2012;**18**:446–58.

29. Grossi EA, Woo YJ, Schwartz CF, *et al.* Comparison of Coapsys annuloplasty and internal reduction mitral annuloplasty in the randomised treatment of functional ischemic mitral regurgitation: impact on the left ventricle. *J Thorac Cardiovasc Surg* 2006;**131**:1095–8.

30. Aronson D, Goldsher N, Zukermann R, Kapeliovich M. Ischemic mitral regurgitation and risk of heart failure after myocardial infarction. *Arch Intern Med* 2006;**166**:2362–8.

31. Yiu SF, Enriquez-Sarano M, Tribouilloy C, Seward JB, Tajik AJ. Determinants of the degree of functional mitral regurgitation in patients with systolic left ventricular dysfunction: a quantitative clinical study. *Circulation* 2000;**102**:1400–6.

32. Beaudoin J, Levine RA, Yosefy C, *et al.* Severe ischemic mitral regurgitation despite normally contracting subpapillary myocardium. *Circulation* 2012;**126**:138–41.

33. Kim K, Kaji S, An Y, *et al.* Mechanism of asymmetric leaflet tethering in ischemic mitral regurgitation: 3D analysis with multislice CT. *JACC Cardiovasc Imaging* 2012;**5**:230–2.

34. Szymanski C, Levine RA, Tribouilloy C, *et al.* Impact of mitral regurgitation on exercise capacity and clinical outcomes in patients with ischemic left ventricular dysfunction. *Am J Cardiol* 2011;**108**:1714–20.

35. Lancellotti P, Tribouilloy C, Hagendorff A, *et al.* Recommendations for the echocardiographic assessment of native valvular regurgitation: an executive summary from the European Association of Cardiovascular Imaging. *Eur Heart J Cardiovasc Imaging* 2013;**14**:611–44.

36. Acker MA, Parides MK, Perrault LP, *et al.*, for the CTSN. Mitral-valve repair versus replacement for severe ischemic mitral regurgitation. *N Engl J Med* 2014;**370**:23–32.

37. Langer, F, Rodriguez F, Ortiz S, *et al.* Subvalvular repair: the key to repairing ischemic mitral regurgitation? *Circulation* 2005;**112**(Suppl l):I-383–l-389.

38. Kunzelman KS, Reimink MS. Cochran RP. Annular dilatation increases stress in the mitral valve and delays coaptation: a finite element computer model. *Cardiovasc Surg* 1997;**5**:427–34.

39. Solis J, Levine RA, Johnson B, *et al.* Polymer injection therapy to reverse remodel the papillary muscles: efficacy in reducing mitral regurgitation in a chronic ischemic model. *Circ Cardiovasc Interven* 2010;**3**:499–505.

40. Langer F, Schafers HJ. RING plus STRING: papillary muscle repositioning as an adjunctive repair technique for ischemic mitral regurgitation. *J Thorac Cardiovasc Surg* 2007;**133**:247–9.

41. Borger, M A, Murphy PM, Alam A, *et al.* Initial results of the chordal-cutting operation for ischemic mitral regurgitation. *J Thorac Cardiovasc Surg* 2007;**133**:1483–92.

42. Jensen H, Levine RA, Yoganathan AP, *et al.* Saddle-shaped mitral valve annuloplasty rings improve leaflet coaptation geometry. *J Thorac Cardiovasc Surg* 2011;**142**:697–703.

43. Jassar, AS, Minakawa M, Shuto T, *et al.* Posterior leaflet augmentation in ischemic mitral regurgitation increases leaflet coaptation and mobility. *Ann Thorac Surg* 2012;**94**:1438–45.

44. Kunzelman KS, Quick DW, Cochran RP. Altered collagen concentration in mitral valve leaflets: biochemical and finite element analysis. *Ann Thorac Surg* 1998;**66**:S198–S205.

45. Chaput M, Handschumacher MD, Tournoux F, *et al.* Mitral leaflet adaptation to ventricular remodelling: occurrence and adequacy in patients with functional mitral regurgitation. *Circulation* 2008;**118**:845–52.

46. Schoen FJ. Evolving concepts of cardiac valve dynamics: the continuum of development, functional structure, pathobiology, and tissue engineering. *Circulation* 2008;**118**:1864–80.

47. Saito K, Okura H, Watanabe N, *et al.* Influence of chronic tethering of the mitral valve on mitral leaflet size and coaptation in functional mitral regurgitation. *JACC Cardiovasc Imaging* 2012;**5**:337–45.

48. Li C, Gotlieb AI. Transforming growth factor-beta regulates the growth of valve interstitial cells *in vitro. Am J Pathol* 2011;**179**:1746–55.

49. Castleberry AW, Williams JB, Daneshmand MA, *et al.* Surgical revascularization is associated with maximal survival in patients with ischemic mitral regurgitation: a 20-year experience. *Circulation* 2014;**129**:2547–56.

50. Campwala SZ, Wang N, Bansal N, Bansal RC. Mitral regurgitation progression following isolated coronary artery bypass surgery: frequency, risk factors and potential prevention strategies. *Eur J Cardiothorac Surg* 2006;**29**:348.

51. Diodato MD, Moon MR, Pasque MK, *et al.* Repair of ischemic mitral regurgitation does not increase mortality or improve long-term survival in patients undergoing coronary artery revascularisation: a propensity analysis. *Ann Thorac Surg* 2004;**78**:794–9.

52. Magne J, Pibarot P, Dagenais F. Preoperative posterior leaflet angle accurately predicts outcome after restrictive mitral valve annuloplasty for ischaemic mitral regurgitation. *Circulation* 2007;**115**:782–91.

53. Mihaljevic T, Lam BK, Rajeswaran J, *et al.* Impact of mitral valve annuloplasty combined with revascularisation in patients with functional ischemic mitral regurgitation. *J Am Coll Cardiol* 2007;**49**:2191–201.

54. McGee EC, Gillinov AM, Blackstone EH, *et al.* Recurrent mitral regurgitation after annuloplasty for functional ischemic mitral regurgitation. *J Thorac Cardiovasc Surg* 2004;**128**:916–24.

55. Fattouch K, Guccione F, Sampognaro R, *et al.* Efficacy of adding mitral valve annuloplasty to CABG in patients with moderate ischemic mitral regurgitation: a randomized trial. *J Thorac Cardiovasc Surg* 2009;**138**:278–85.

56. Chan KMJ, Punjabi PP, Flather M, *et al.*; for the RIME Investigators. Coronary artery bypass surgery with or without mitral valve annuloplasty in moderate functional ischemic mitral regurgitation. *Circulation* 2012;**126**:2502–10.

57. Smith PK, Puskas JD, Ascheim DD, *et al.*, for the Cardiothoracic Surgical Trials Network Investigators. Surgical treatment of moderate ischemic mitral regurgitation. *N Engl J Med* 2014;**371**:2178–88.

58. Michler RE, Smith PK, Parides MK, *et al.*, for the CTSN. Two-year outcomes of surgical treatment of moderate ischemic mitral regurgitation. *N Engl J Med* 2016;April 3.

59. Vassileva CM, Boley T, Markwell S, Hazelrigg S. Meta-analysis of short-term and long-term survival following repair versus replacement for ischemic mitral regurgitation. *Eur J Cardiothorac Surg* 2011;**39**:295–303.

RECOMMENDED READING

Levine RA, Hagége AA, Judge DP, *et al.*; Leducq Mitral Transatlantic Network. Mitral valve disease—morphology and mechanisms. *Nat Rev Cardiol* 2015;**12**:689–710.

Velazquez EJ, Lee KL, Jones RH, *et al.*; STICHES Investigators. Coronary artery bypass surgery in patients with ischaemic cardiomyopathy. *N Engl J Med* 2016;**374**:1511–20.

63

Mechanical circulatory support

Stephen Pettit

Introduction

Mechanical circulatory support (MCS) describes the use of mechanical pumps to maintain blood flow around the body when the heart is unable to meet this need. MCS may be appropriate in cardiogenic shock, either as a bridge to decision, recovery, heart transplantation, or for long-term support (destination therapy—DT). There are various techniques by which MCS may be delivered and the most appropriate technique will vary depending on the patient, pathology, clinical situation, and experience of the hospital. Adverse events during MCS are frequent despite advances in blood pump technology. Careful patient selection and meticulous care are essential to achieve acceptable long-term survival and quality of life.

Indications for mechanical circulatory support

Cardiogenic shock

Cardiogenic shock is the most common pathophysiological situation in which MCS is appropriate. Cardiogenic shock is initially diagnosed by clinical criteria, but haemodynamic confirmation is required to distinguish cardiogenic shock from other types of shock that may mimic or coexist with cardiogenic shock. Untreated cardiogenic shock is characterized by sustained hypotension (systolic blood pressure <90 mmHg) and poor end-organ perfusion which may be recognized by cool peripheries, oliguria, or an elevated serum lactate concentration.[1] A diagnosis of cardiogenic shock is confirmed if the cardiac output is low (cardiac index <1.8 L/min/m^2) in the absence of low intracardiac filling pressures. Haemodynamic confirmation is most commonly achieved with a pulmonary artery catheter but other methods including echocardiography have been validated.

The majority of patients with cardiogenic shock are hospitalized, but their clinical state can range from near-death to relative stability with pharmacological support. Some patients with advanced heart failure meet the physiological definition of cardiogenic shock, but are able to survive at home with conventional pharmacological therapy for chronic heart failure. The haemodynamic stability, requirement for cardiovascular support, and symptom status of patients with cardiogenic shock may be described using the Interagency Mechanically Assisted Circulatory Support (INTERMACS) profile system (see Table 63.1).[2]

There is significant heterogeneity in risk within INTERMACS profiles. Patients who have frequent hospital admissions with heart failure and those with recurrent ventricular arrhythmias are known to be at greater risk of adverse outcomes. These factors are identified by the profile modifier: 'frequent flyer' (FF) or 'arrhythmias' (A).[3] In addition, patients who have temporary circulatory support are identified by the profile modifier: temporary circulatory support (TCS).

At a population level, the INTERMACS registry has improved understanding of the natural history of cardiogenic shock and has allowed comparison of outcomes with different types of treatment. At an individual patient level, the INTERMACS profile may be used to describe the clinical state of a patient, may help determine whether MCS is likely to improve survival, and determine the timeframe in which MCS is likely to be required.

Basic principles of mechanical circulatory support

The most important function of MCS is maintaining adequate blood flow within the systemic circulation such that oxygen is delivered to vital organs of the body for aerobic cellular respiration. Certain forms of MCS reduce intracardiac filling pressures, thus relieving deleterious wall stress on ventricles that have been injured by the underlying cardiac pathology. MCS confers several additional benefits: it should allow potentially harmful vasoconstrictor and inotropic drugs to be weaned and stopped, it may permit replenishment of tissue ATP stores and clearance of lactic acid, and it may also permit metabolism of cytokines that are released as part of the systemic inflammatory response that accompanies cardiogenic shock.

Through a variety of physiological mechanisms in health, there is balanced cardiac output from left and right ventricles and vasomotor tone in the systemic and pulmonary circulations. Mechanical pumps may be used to maintain blood flow in either the systemic or pulmonary circulations. The clinician must determine whether an individual patient requires left ventricular (LV), right ventricular (RV), or biventricular support. This will depend on the clinical situation, underlying cardiac pathology, and performance of the left and right ventricles. It is normally preferable to maintain blood flow through both systemic and pulmonary circulations, but

Table 63.1 INTERMACS profile system

INTERMACS profile	Brief description	Definition	Modifiers	Time frame in which MCS may be required
1	Critical cardiogenic shock	Life-threatening hypotension and rapidly escalating support with hypoperfusion confirmed by worsening acidosis and lactate levels	A, TCS	Hours
2	Progressive decline	Dependent on inotropic support but ongoing deterioration in nutrition, renal function, fluid retention or major status indicator	A, TCS	Days
3	Stable but inotrope dependent	Clinical stability on inotropic support after repeated failure to wean without symptomatic hypotension, worsening symptoms or end-organ dysfunction	A, TCS, FF	Weeks
4	Resting symptoms	At home on oral therapy but frequently has symptoms at rest or with activities of daily living such as dressing or bathing	A, FF	Months
5	Exertion intolerant	Comfortable at rest but unable to engage in any activity, living predominantly within the house	A, FF	Months
6	Exertion limited	Able to engage in mild activity, but fatigued within few minutes of any physical exertion. Likely to have been hospitalized for heart failure in last year.	A, FF	Months
7	Advanced NHYA class II	Able to engage in moderate activity. No recent hospital admissions for heart failure.	A	Years

INTERMACS, Interagency Registry for Mechanically Assisted Circulatory Support; MCS, mechanical circulatory support; NYHA, New York Heart Association; A, arrhythmia; TCS, temporary circulatory support; FF, frequent flyer.
Source data from Stevenson LW, Pagani FD, Young JB, Jessup M, Miller L, Kormos RL, Naftel DC, Ulisney K, Desvigne-Nickens P, Kirklin JK. INTERMACS profiles of advanced heart failure: the current picture. *J Heart Lung Transplant* 2009;**28**:535–541.

the pulmonary circulation may be bypassed in certain situations with use of veno-arterial extracorporeal membrane oxygenation (VA ECMO).

Types of mechanical circulatory support

Many different blood pumps have been used for MCS. Rather than review MCS historically, this chapter focuses on devices that are used widely in the current era. Selection of an appropriate blood pump will vary according to MCS strategy, but will also be influenced by INTERMACS profile, underlying cardiac pathology, experience of the treating clinicians, and the range of technologies available in the institution.

Intra-aortic balloon counter-pulsation

Intra-aortic balloon pumps (IABPs) are the simplest form of MCS, and can be rapidly placed in a catheter lab or at the bedside. A polyethylene balloon is mounted at the end of a 7.5–8.0F catheter. This is placed in the intra-thoracic descending aorta, typically via the femoral artery. The balloon inflates with the onset of diastole and deflates at the onset of LV systole. Inflation augments mean arterial blood pressure, improving coronary and end-organ perfusion. Deflation reduces LV afterload, therefore improving left ventricular ejection fraction (LVEF) and reducing left ventricular end-diastolic pressure (LVEDP) (**Figure 63.1**).

IABPs tend to be used for short periods of support (days) but may be used for longer (weeks or months) if required to reach definitive treatment such as heart transplantation. Adverse events during support include thromboembolism, vascular access complications, infection, and thrombocytopenia. Significant aortic regurgitation is a contraindication to IABP use. Augmentation of cardiac output is rarely >0.5 L/min, which may not be sufficient for the sickest patients. The IABP is also limited by its dependence on residual cardiac

function and electrical stability. Finally, patients must remain recumbent unless the IABP is placed via the axillary or subclavian artery (non-licensed approaches).

The IABP-SHOCK II trial examined the effectiveness of IABP support following acute myocardial infarction (AMI).[4] Six hundred patients with AMI complicated by cardiogenic shock were randomized to IABP vs conventional therapy. There was no difference in the primary end-point of all-cause mortality at 30 days (39.7% IABP arm and 41.3% in control arm), length of intensive care unit stay, or time to haemodynamic stabilization. As such, the routine use of IABP is no longer recommended (class IIIa indication) in the most recent European guidance in patients with post-myocardial infarction (MI) cardiogenic shock.[5] However, there may be subgroups for whom IABP is helpful. Furthermore,

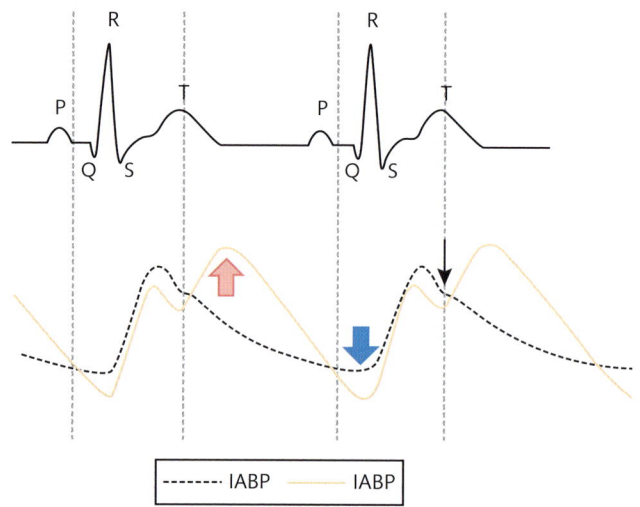

Figure 63.1 Intra-aortic balloon counter-pulsation.
Reproduced with permission from Royal College of Anaesthetists.

no other forms of MCS have been subjected to a randomized controlled trial (RCT) of this quality.

Percutaneous ventricular assist devices

There are several percutaneous devices that can provide greater levels of MCS than IABP without the need for cardiac surgery. These differ with respect to the location of the blood pump which may be situated inside the body (intracorporeal), or situated outside the body (extracorporeal). All these devices require anticoagulation and this is typically achieved with intravenous unfractionated heparin. Depending on the device, MCS may be supplied for days or weeks, but longer periods of MCS are unusual and it is important to identify an exit strategy, particularly if the device cannot be weaned.

Percutaneous ventricular assist devices (intracorporeal)

The Impella family of devices (Abiomed) are miniature intracorporeal blood pumps. These devices are usually placed via the femoral artery, although other methods of arterial access are possible. They are continuous-flow blood pumps which sit across the aortic valve, draining blood from the LV cavity and ejecting blood into the ascending aorta.

The Impella 2.5 and CP (Figure 63.2) may be placed by a cardiologist, but the Impella 5.0 requires surgical cut-down. The Impella 2.5 provides up to 2.5 L/min of blood flow. The Impella CP and 5.0 devices provide up to 4 and 5 L/min of blood flow respectively. These devices have a range of beneficial physiological effects in patients with acute LV failure. In addition to increasing systemic blood flow, they increase mean arterial pressure, reduce LVEDP, and reduce myocardial oxygen demand. They are US Food and Drug Administration (FDA)-approved for short periods of support; up to 4 days for the Impella 2.5 and CP, and up to 6 days for the Impella 5.0, but longer periods of support have been reported.

The major advantage of Impella devices is ease of placement. However, they are prone to displacement, and require regular

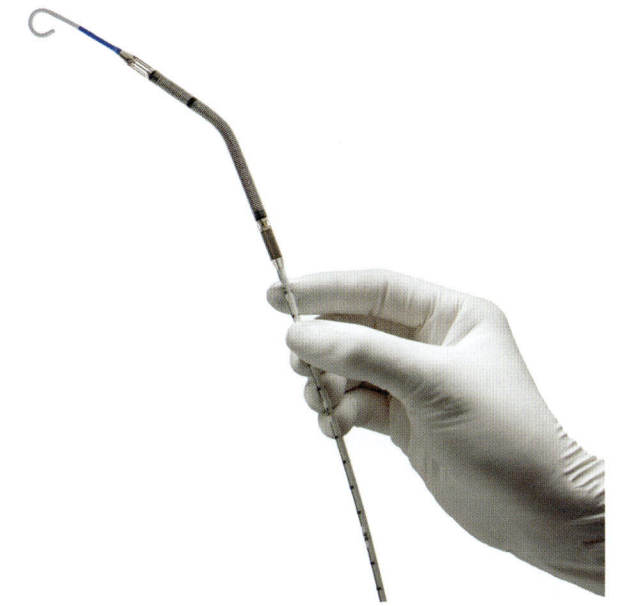

Figure 63.2 Impella® CP Heart Pump.
Courtesy of Abiomed Europe GmbH.

echocardiographic surveillance. Adequate RV function is required as these pumps provide isolated LV support, and significant aortic valve pathology or LV thrombus are contraindications. In the ISAR-SHOCK trial[6] (a small study of 26 patients with cardiogenic shock who were randomized to either Impella 2.5 or IABP support), cardiac index and blood pressure increased more with Impella 2.5 support than with IABP support, but there was no difference in mortality. The Impella-EUROSHOCK Registry reported real-world outcomes with Impella 2.5 in 120 patients with post-MI cardiogenic shock.[7] The 30-day mortality was high at 64.2% despite Impella support, and major adverse events were common, including bleeding that required transfusion (24.2%), haemolysis (7.5%), vascular damage requiring surgery (4.2%), and device malfunction (2.5%). An RCT of the Impella CP vs conventional therapy in acute ST-segment elevation myocardial infarction complicated by cardiogenic shock is currently recruiting patients.[8]

The Impella RP was the first percutaneous intracorporeal RV assist device and is attractive for use in patients with RV dysfunction after durable left ventricular assist device (LVAD) implantation or heart transplantation, as well as shock due to RV dysfunction.[9] This device obtained a CE mark in 2014 and is approved for up to 14 days use in selected patients with right heart failure.

Percutaneous ventricular assist devices (extracorporeal)

TandemHeart (CardiacAssist) is the most widely used extracorporeal percutaneous VAD, and is CE-marked for up to 30 days use, and FDA approved for up to 6 h. Blood is drained from the left atrium via a 21F cannula placed via the femoral vein and through the interatrial septum. Blood is pumped into the descending aorta through a 15–19F cannula placed via the femoral artery. Between 3.5 and 5 L/min of support can be provided, dependent on return cannula size. In addition to increasing systemic blood flow, the TandemHeart increases mean arterial pressure and reduces LVEDP.

The major problem with the TandemHeart is the need for transseptal puncture in a critically ill patient, and cannula displacement may lead to rapid failure of MCS. There is a risk of bleeding and thromboembolism. As with Impella, the TandemHeart provides isolated LV support and adequate RV function is required.

In a single centre trial, 41 patients with post-MI cardiogenic shock were randomized to TandemHeart or IABP.[10] There was no difference in 30-day mortality. TandemHeart led to a greater improvement in cardiac power output, but adverse events were frequent including need for blood transfusion (95%) and limb ischaemia (33%). In a second trial, 33 patients with cardiogenic shock were randomized to TandemHeart or IABP.[11] Again, TandemHeart led to greater improvement in cardiac output, mean arterial pressure and pulmonary capillary wedge pressure, but there was no difference in 30-day mortality.

An extracorporeal right ventricular assist device (RVAD) has been developed for patients who require temporary RV support. Protek Duo (CardiacAssist) is a dual-lumen cannula that may be used with a variety of external continuous flow blood pumps. Protek Duo is placed via the right internal jugular vein and passes through the right heart into the main pulmonary artery. Up to 4 L/min of venous blood is drained from the right atrium through the outer 29 F lumen and is pumped into the pulmonary artery through the tip of the inner 16 F lumen. Clinical experience with this form of MCS is limited, but it may be combined with other forms of MCS to provide short periods of biventricular support.

Peripheral veno-arterial extracorporeal membrane oxygenation

Peripheral VA ECMO is a form of percutaneous MCS. The major difference between VA ECMO and other forms of MCS is that blood bypasses the lungs and therefore needs to be oxygenated before it is returned to the arterial system. A typical circuit is demonstrated in **Figure 63.3**. Deoxygenated blood is drained from the right atrium, passed through an external continuous-flow blood pump, then passed through a membrane oxygenator, then returned to the aorta. The oxygenator also permits carbon dioxide removal. Peripheral VA ECMO is typically delivered with cannulae placed directly in the femoral vessels, including a reperfusion cannula to maintain distal limb perfusion. Other vascular access strategies are possible, including subclavian or axillary arterial return, and cannulae may be placed via an end-to-side vascular graft. Central VA ECMO with open cannulation of the great vessels is also possible but beyond the scope of this chapter.

Peripheral VA ECMO may provide up to 6 L/min of blood flow, depending on cannula size and the amount of flow desired by the treating clinician. The ability to deliver oxygen and remove carbon dioxide is a major advantage in patients with coexistent respiratory failure. Peripheral VA ECMO may be instituted at the bedside or even in the community and has been widely used to facilitate safe transport of very sick patients. Peripheral VA ECMO has also been widely used during cardiac arrest, where it is known as extracorporeal cardiopulmonary resuscitation (ECPR).

Whereas peripheral VA ECMO is excellent for restoring tissue oxygen delivery, it is a highly non-physiological treatment for patients with acute LV failure. Continuous retrograde blood flow in the aorta increases LV afterload. If afterload is too high, then the LV will be unable to eject and this may lead to pulmonary oedema, LV distension, and LV thrombosis. Strategies to maintain LV ejection include avoiding excessive ECMO flow, use of inotropes, an IABP, an Impella, or placement of an LV vent. There are potential problems when LV ejection is maintained, particularly in the context of respiratory failure. LV ejection leads to 'competition' within the aorta between antegrade cardiac output and retrograde ECMO flow. If blood passing through the lungs is not adequately oxygenated, the Harlequin syndrome may arise. In this situation, deoxygenated blood from the LV supplies the upper body and limbs (including the coronary arteries) while oxygenated blood via the ECMO circuit supplies the lower body and limbs. There is also a high risk of bleeding, distal limb ischaemia, and thromboembolism.

Evidence to support use of VA ECMO is currently limited to retrospective, observational studies. In a single-centre study of 71 patients with post-MI cardiogenic shock despite IABP support, 30-day mortality was 39.1% in patients supported with VA ECMO vs 72% in a historical control group supported with IABP alone.[12] In a similar study of 58 patients with post-MI cardiogenic shock despite IABP support, one-year mortality was 36.4% in patients supported with VA ECMO, vs 76% in a historical control group supported with IABP alone.[13] It is uncertain whether the observed mortality differences are due to the use of VA ECMO or other differences, such as baseline characteristics or other aspects of treatment. The same studies have also demonstrated that adverse events during VA ECMO are common; major vascular events requiring surgical intervention are reported to occur in up to 20% of patients and are associated with worse survival.[14] As such, VA ECMO cannot be used for long periods and it is important to identify an exit strategy if VA ECMO cannot be weaned. Several RCTs of VA ECMO are recruiting patients and these trials may clarify the role of VA ECMO in the management of cardiogenic shock.

Extracorporeal ventricular assist devices

Many patients are not suitable for percutaneous MCS. Extracorporeal VADs require sternotomy and direct cannulation of the heart and central vascular system. Both left- and right-sided support can be provided. Blood is drained from atria or ventricles, passes through an external pump, and is returned into the great vessels. The cannulae are tunnelled beneath the sternum and exit through the anterior abdominal wall. The most commonly used pump is a magnetically levitated, centrifugal continuous flow pump called the CentriMag (formerly known as Levitronix), but others include the PVAD (Thoratec) and the Excor (Berlin Heart). A typical biventricular configuration is shown in **Figure 63.4**. If required, a membrane oxygenator may be added to the circuit. All these pumps require anticoagulation and this is typically achieved with intravenous unfractionated heparin in the perioperative period, followed by an oral anticoagulant. In addition, most patients also receive antiplatelet therapy.

Extracorporeal VADs tend to be used as a bridge to heart transplantation in patients who are unsuitable for implantable LVAD support, either because of poor RV function or because they are too unwell (INTERMACS profile 1). The greatest advantages of extracorporeal VADs are the ability to support both the systemic and pulmonary circulation and the ability to provide flow rates of up 9 L/min, irrespective of cardiac rhythm. Patients may receive MCS for several weeks or months while they wait for recovery or definitive treatment, such as upgrade to an implantable LVAD or heart transplantation. Pump heads typically require exchange after 30 days. It is possible for patients to be mobilized during MCS, although it is unusual for these patients to be discharged from the hospital.

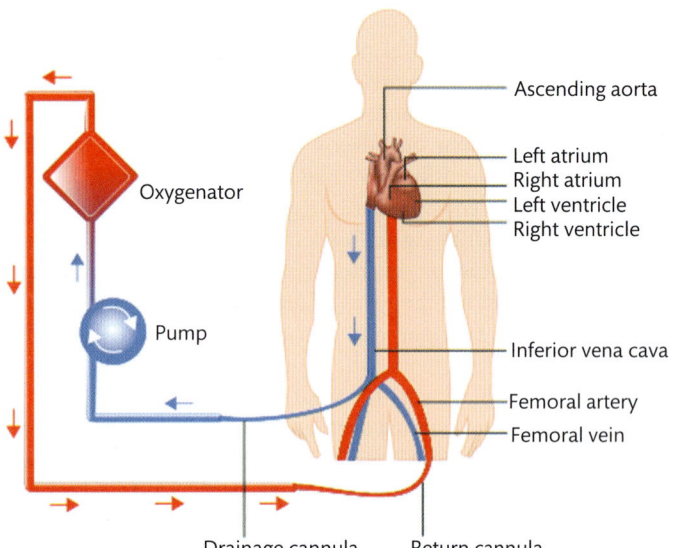

Figure 63.3 Peripheral veno-arterial extracorporeal membrane oxygenation (VA ECMO).

Reproduced with permission from Royal College of Anaesthetists.

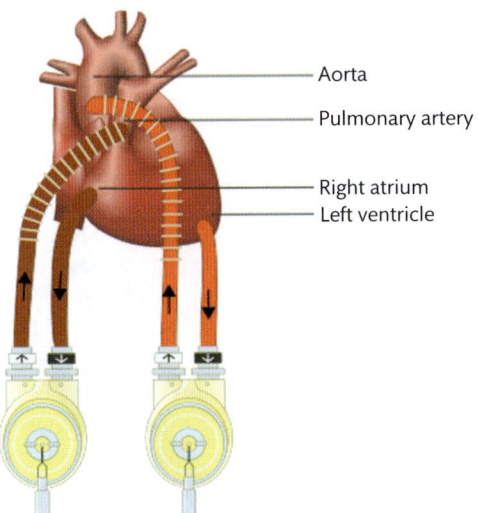

Aorta

Pulmonary artery

Right atrium
Left ventricle

Figure 63.4 Extracorporeal ventricular assist devices.
Reproduced with permission from Royal College of Anaesthetists.

Evidence to support use of the CentriMag VAD is limited to small observational studies with limited follow-up duration. Survival is dependent on the cause of cardiogenic shock and INTERMACS profile at the time of device placement. Excellent outcomes were reported in 27 selected patients with decompensated heart failure who were supported with CentriMag VADs due to failure of medical therapy.[15] Survival to discharge was 74% and one-year survival was 68%. The final treatment for survivors was recovery (*n* = 10), transplantation (*n* = 8), and implantable LVAD (*n* = 6). Other centres have reported outcomes with other causes of cardiogenic shock, including shock after cardiac surgery, heart transplantation, or implantable LVAD placement. Outcomes were less good, with 30-day survival of 30%. Preoperative markers of end-organ dysfunction such as high bilirubin were associated with poor outcomes.[16]

Worldwide experience with the CentriMag VAD was summarized in a systematic review of 53 studies, including a total of 999 patients.[17] There was significant heterogeneity in the type of patients treated and pump configuration (left vs right vs biventricular support). The worst outcomes were observed in post-cardiac surgery cardiogenic shock, with 30-day mortality of 41%. Device failure was rare but adverse events were common despite relatively short periods of support, including bleeding (28%), infection (24%), thrombosis (7%), neurological complications (7%), and haemolysis (3%). Careful patient selection is critical in order to achieve good outcomes with this form of MCS.

Implantable left ventricular assist devices

Implantable LVADs have evolved and become the dominant form of MCS in the twenty-first century. The basic design of implantable LVAD has not changed over the last 30 years. Blood is drained from the left ventricle, passed through a pump and returned to the systemic circulation via an outflow graft that is typically anastomosed to the ascending aorta. Almost all pumps are powered by electricity, supplied by an electrical cable (or driveline) that is tunnelled through the anterior abdominal wall and exits adjacent to the umbilicus. The driveline is connected to a system controller and this is connected to mains electricity or a portable battery pack. The patient must be connected to a power source at all times.

Types of implantable LVAD

First-generation implantable LVADs created pulsatile blood flow, utilizing a complex volume displacement design with a blood chamber, pusher-plate, and valves. Examples included the HeartMate XVE (Thermo Cardiosystems) and Novocor N100 (Baxter). Serious adverse events such as stroke/transient ischaemic attack or device-related infection were very common, occurring in more than half of patients despite support durations of only six months.[18] Additional problems included the need for a large abdominal pump pocket, audible pump operation, and limited mechanical durability. First-generation implantable LVADs are now obsolete, accounting for <0.1% of new implants in the INTERMACS registry since 2010.[19]

Second-generation devices create continuous blood flow, utilizing a small blood chamber with an internal rotor, which spins continuously around a central axle. Although the rotor spins continuously, the device generates more flow in systole than diastole, because flow through the pump is proportional to pressure decrease across the pump, which increases in systole. The HeartMate II (Thoratec) is the mostly widely used second-generation implantable LVAD. Others include the Jarvik 2000 (Jarvik Heart) and the Incor (Berlin Heart). These pumps are smaller than first-generation devices, but HeartMate II required an abdominal pump pocket. In the HeartMate II trial, 200 patients were randomized to a second-generation LVAD (HeartMate II) or a first-generation LVAD (HeartMate XVE).[20] At two years, survival free of disabling stroke or device replacement was significantly higher with the HeartMate II device (46% vs 11%).

Third-generation devices also create continuous blood flow, but have a centrifugal design with a magnetically levitated rotor. The HeartWare HVAD was the first third-generation implantable LVAD and this is shown in **Figure 63.5**. However, this device was withdrawn by the manufacturer in June 2021. The HeartMate III (Abbott) has subsequently entered clinical practice and it features a fully magnetically levitated rotor, wide blood-flow passages and intrinsic pulsatility to reduce shear stress and blood stasis.

Both pumps are small enough to be implanted within the pericardial space and do not require an abdominal pump pocket. Two RCTs have compared second- and third-generation LVADs. In the ENDURANCE trial, 446 patients were randomized to a third-generation LVAD (HeartWare HVAD) or a second-generation LVAD (HeartMate II).[21] At two years, there was no difference in survival free of disabling stroke or need for device replacement (55.4% vs 59.1%). In the final report of the MOMENTUM 3 trial, 1028 patients were randomized to a third-generation LVAD (HeartMate III) or a second-generation LVAD (HeartMate II).[22] At two years, survival free of disabling stroke or need for device replacement was significantly higher with the HeartMate III device (76.9% vs 64.8%). In addition, the number of major bleeding or gastrointestinal bleeding events per patient year were lower with the HeartMate III device.

The HeartWare HVAD was occasionally used for RV support, although it was not designed for this purpose. In a series of 13 transplant-eligible patients with severe biventricular failure, two HeartWare HVADs were used to provide biventricular support.[23] The RVAD inflow cannula was placed in the right atrium in seven patients and right ventricle in six patients. Outcomes were inferior to isolated LVAD support; four patients had RVAD pump thrombosis and six patients died before heart transplantation. The INTERMACS registry also demonstrates worse outcomes with implantable BiVAD support vs isolated LVAD support (approximately 55% vs 85% survival at one-year) and use of implantable BiVAD remains relatively uncommon.[244]

B Fully Magnetically Levitated Centrifugal-Flow Pump

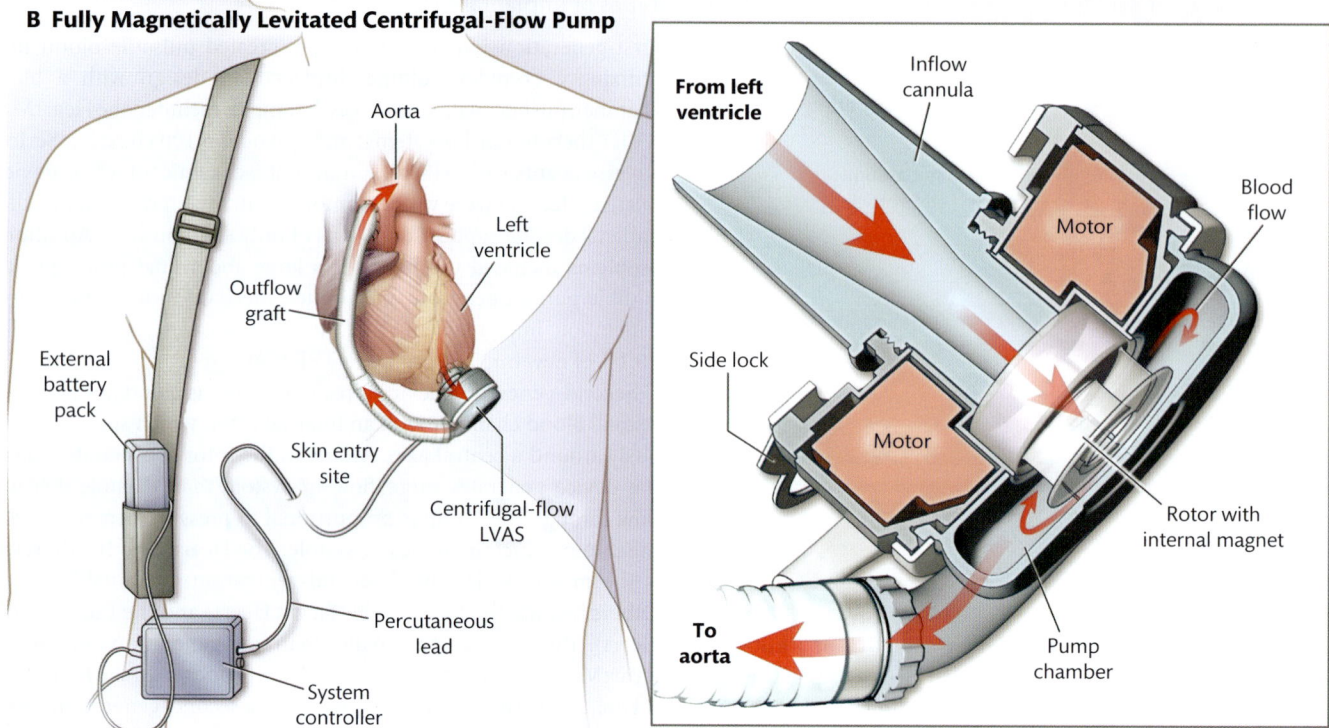

Figure 63.5 The HeartMate III fully magnetically levitated centrifugal-flow pump.
Reproduced from Mehra MR, Naka Y, Uriel N, Goldstein DJ, Cleveland JC Jr, Colombo PC, Walsh MN, Milano CA, Patel CB, Jorde UP, Pagani FD, Aaronson KD, Dean DA, McCants K, Itoh A, Ewald GA, Horstmanshof D, Long JW, Salerno C; MOMENTUM 3 Investigators. A fully magnetically levitated circulatory pump for advanced heart failure. *N Engl J Med* 2017;**376**:440-450

Selection of patients for implantable LVAD support

Implantable LVAD candidates must have advanced heart failure with objective markers of an adverse prognosis, in order to justify the risks of LVAD support. Most patients are in INTERMACS profile 2 or 3, but less 'sick' patients in INTERMACS profiles 4–7 may be supported, particularly if this is required as a bridge to heart transplant candidacy (see Bridge to transplant candidacy). It is generally thought that patients in INTERMACS profile 1 are too sick for implantable LVAD support and better treated with temporary MCS in the first instance.

The ideal heart for LVAD support has a dilated and severely impaired LV which can act as a sump for LVAD inflow. However, the RV must have preserved function and be able to generate sufficient trans-pulmonary blood flow to match performance of the LVAD. Assessment of RV function is difficult because the RV is exquisitely dependent on loading conditions. Systemic venous return will increase significantly after LVAD implantation. Post-LVAD RV failure is a catastrophic problem but is exceptionally difficult to predict. There are associations between post-LVAD RV failure and a huge variety of laboratory tests, echocardiographic variables, and PA catheter derived variables, such as RV stroke work index and pulmonary artery pulsatility index. The predictive ability of individual variables is poor. Several risk scores have been developed for prediction of post-LVAD RV failure, but simple models have modest predictive ability at best and highly complex Bayesian models are not yet usable in regular clinical practice.[25,26]

Other important anatomical requirements for effective LVAD support include a competent aortic valve and absence of an intracardiac shunt, such as a patent foramen ovale, atrial septal defect or ventricular septal defect. If any of these issues are present, then they must be surgically corrected at the time of LVAD implantation. Non-cardiac requirements for successful LVAD support include absence of important co-morbidities or frailty, low bleeding risk, psychological suitability for LVAD support, and a high level of patient motivation. It is important that the LVAD patient has adequate social support, preferably a caregiver who can help them with day-to-day management of the pump and the percutaneous driveline. The process of enabling patients to make an informed decision about receiving highly invasive therapy such as an implantable LVAD is challenging. Multidisciplinary assessment is absolutely vital and patient decision aids may be helpful.[27]

Management of patients with implantable LVAD support

Most patients with implantable LVAD are discharged within three weeks of surgery. Multiple studies have shown a rapid and sustained improvement in heart failure symptoms and quality of life. Within three months of device implantation, more than 75% of LVAD-supported patients have New York Heart Association (NYHA) class I or II heart failure symptoms. There are sustained improvements in 6 min walk distance and quality of life, as measured by the Minnesota Living with Heart Failure Questionnaire and the Kansas City Cardiomyopathy Questionnaire.[28]

Patients require meticulous follow-up to maximize the effectiveness of LVAD support and to minimize the risk of adverse events. Important issues are summarized in Table 63.2. The percutaneous

Table 63.2 Important issues of LVAD support

Anti-platelet therapy	Most patients prescribed aspirin 150–300 mg daily but other antiplatelet agents may be used and the issue of platelet reactivity is controversial.
Anti-coagulation	Most patients are anticoagulated with warfarin, aiming to achieve an INR of 2–3. Close monitoring is required and low molecular weight heparin may be used when INR is sub-therapeutic.
Blood pressure	Most LVAD patients have narrow pulse pressure and BP measurement requires a hand-held Doppler probe. Continuous-flow LVADs are sensitive to afterload. Most patients require vasodilation to maintain a mean arterial pressure of <85 mmHg and optimal LVAD flow.
Drive-line	The driveline exit site must be kept clean and dry to minimize the risk of infection. Many LVAD patients require suppressive antibiotic therapy.
Arrhythmias	Arrhythmias are common. β-Blockade or amiodarone may be helpful. ICDs may be programmed with high rate zones and very long detection to reduce the risk of shocks. Catheter ablation is sometimes indicated for recurrent VT.
Aortic regurgitation	Aortic regurgitation may develop and can lead to ineffective MCS due to recirculation and failure of LV unloading.
Pump thrombosis	Early warning signs of pump thrombosis are rising pump power or a rise in serum lactate dehydrogenase level.

LVAD, left ventricular assist device; INR, international normalized ratio; BP; blood pressure; VT, venous thrombosis; MCS, mechanical circulatory support.

driveline must be kept clean, dry, and fixed to the anterior abdominal wall to prevent traction at the exit site. The system controller must be carefully handled, remain connected to a power supply at all times and any alarms must be attended. Anticoagulation must be taken regularly in order to keep the prothrombin time within the intended range (international normalized ratio of 2–3). Blood pressure must be measured regularly using a handheld Doppler probe and most patients require antihypertensive medication to maintain a mean arterial pressure of <85 mmHg. Good blood pressure control is important to maintain optimum LVAD flow and reduce the risk of adverse events such as intracerebral haemorrhage.[29]

Regular echocardiography is indicated to ensure that pump speed is appropriate and for surveillance of aortic regurgitation. Patients on the transplant waiting list undergo intermittent right heart catheterization to ensure that pulmonary vascular resistance is acceptable. Regular blood tests are arranged to identify anaemia, renal dysfunction, and for surveillance of haemolysis which may be an early sign of pump thrombosis.

Adverse events are inevitable during LVAD support. Low-flow alarms due to 'suction events' are common when patients are relatively dehydrated with low central venous pressure. Ventricular arrhythmias are common, may be remarkably well tolerated, but may result in implantable cardioverter–defibrillator shocks. Infection of the driveline, pump pocket, or pump is relatively common and many patients require long-term antibiotic therapy. Unfortunately, life-threatening adverse events are also relatively common during long periods of support and many are related to the blood–pump interface. Continuous blood flow is associated with acquired Von Willebrand syndrome and this may lead to small bowel angiodysplasia and gastrointestinal bleeding.[30] Pump thrombosis is one of the most feared adverse events and may lead to pump failure, stroke, intracerebral haemorrhage, or systemic thromboembolism. In the most recent INTERMACS registry report, survival free from infection, bleeding, device malfunction, or stroke was approximately 30% at one year, 20% at two years, and only 15% at three years.[24]

Ultimately, a proportion of patients with implantable LVAD will die during support as a consequence of LVAD-related adverse events, and this is a particular issue for destination therapy patients who are not heart transplant candidates. Supportive and palliative care for patients with LVAD is a major challenge, particularly in the home environment. Anticipatory care planning may be helpful while patients are able to contribute to decisions about their healthcare.

Total artificial heart

Total artificial hearts (TAHs) offer complete heart replacement therapy. Many TAHs have been trialled over the last fifty years, but the most widely used device is the SynCardia TAH (SynCardia Systems) with >1700 implants to date. The major advantage of the TAH is the provision of full biventricular support. It may be preferable to biventricular assist devices (BiVADs) in patients with ventricular thrombus, ventricular septal defects, mechanical prosthetic valves, or refractory ventricular arrhythmias. TAH implantation involves excision of the native ventricles, including the atrioventricular and ventriculo-arterial valves. The device is attached to a cuff of atrial tissue and then connected to the great vessels. The artificial blood chambers have a pneumatically driven diaphragm which creates pulsatile flow. The device is powered by a large console, but a portable version is available and patients may be discharged from hospital.

Evidence to support use of the SynCardia TAH is limited to a single large observational study. The device was used in 81 transplant-eligible patients with cardiogenic shock who were unsuitable for implantable LVAD support.[31] Survival to transplantation was achieved in 79% of patients and the mean duration of support was 79.1 days. Post-transplant outcomes were reasonable, with 86% one-year survival and 64% five-year survival. However, complications during TAH support were common with a total of 356 adverse events including bleeding, infection, renal failure, liver failure, and stroke. The relatively high rate of adverse events has limited use of the TAH as a bridge to heart transplantation, particularly in countries such as the UK with longer waiting times for heart transplantation.

Mechanical circulatory support strategy

MCS is limited in duration and exit strategies should be considered before initiating support. MCS may be categorized according to the intention of treatment and with specific reference to whether heart transplantation is a future treatment option. The most common treatment strategies are listed in Table 63.3.

Table 63.3 Mechanical circulatory support: most common treatment strategies

Strategy	Intention of treatment
Salvage	Allow time to make diagnosis and determine treatment options
Bridge to recovery	Allow time for recovery of heart function
Bridge to transplant candidacy	Reverse contraindication and permit listing for heart transplant
Bridge to transplantation	Improve survival and quality of life while waiting for heart transplant
Destination therapy	Improve survival and quality of life

The final strategy may differ from the intended strategy, due to events during MCS that are outside the clinician's control. For example, a patient may be supported as a bridge to transplantation but heart function may recover, or vice versa. Adverse events often affect strategy. For example, a patient may be supported as a bridge to transplantation but sustain a large stroke or develop high levels of anti-HLA antibodies which means that heart transplantation may be inappropriate or impossible to deliver. Clinicians must be aware of changing circumstances and adapt their strategy accordingly.

The evidence base for specific strategies is poor. Destination therapy with an implantable LVAD is the only strategy that has been subjected to RCT. For all other strategies, evidence is limited to observational studies in which outcomes in selected patients are compared to non-randomized control populations. Observational studies are subject to significant bias and likely to overestimate the benefit associated with MCS.

Bridge to decision

Bridge to decision describes support of critically unwell patients who are about to die, in order to allow time to make a diagnosis or determine whether there are options for ongoing treatment. These patients are usually in INTERMACS class I and may be undergoing cardiopulmonary resuscitation at the time when MCS is commenced. Bridge to decision is typically performed using percutaneous or extracorporeal MCS. If the patient is undergoing cardiopulmonary resuscitation or has respiratory failure, then it will be necessary to select a pump which can be used alongside an oxygenator. The most commonly used technique is peripheral VA ECMO.

The evidence base is limited to observational studies. In the most recent summary of the Extracorporeal Life Support Organisation (ELSO) registry, survival to discharge in 3395 adults who had undergone ECPR was only 28%. Futility, which may be defined as progressive multi-organ failure despite MCS, is a major concern. Tools such as the SAVE score (http://www.save-score.com) and the ENCOURAGE risk score may allow clinicians to determine the likelihood of survival with VA ECMO and benchmark their performance against predicted results.[32,33] However, these scoring systems do not allow clinicians to determine whether VA ECMO would improve the absolute chance of survival in individual patients.

Bridge to recovery

'Bridge to recovery' describes support of patients with acute heart failure in whom there is reasonable expectation that heart function will recover and allow MCS to be weaned. The most common pathologies that are supported as a bridge to recovery are primary allograft dysfunction after heart transplantation, acute myocarditis, and reversible forms of cardiomyopathy such as peripartum cardiomyopathy. Bridge to recovery can be performed with almost any MCS technique, with the obvious exception of total artificial hearts. It may be preferable to select a pump that lowers intracardiac filling pressures in order to promote recovery. The clinician must be able to wean the pump in order to determine whether recovery of heart function has occurred. If rapid recovery and weaning is expected, then it may be preferable to avoid a pump that requires direct cannulation of the ventricles.

Once more, the evidence base is limited to observational data. Most centres define recovery by successful withdrawal of MCS. There is great variation in the incidence of recovery. In a recent analysis of the world's largest MCS registry (INTERMACS), the rate of recovery of 13 454 patients supported with a continuous-flow implantable LVAD was 0.9% at one year, 1.9% at two years, and 3.1% at three years. Patients with underlying myocarditis, peripartum cardiomyopathy, or doxorubicin-induced cardiomyopathy had the highest rates of recovery.[34] Higher rates of recovery have been described when recovery is promoted using pharmacological therapy, pump speed alteration, and regular echocardiographic surveillance. In a prospective single-centre study of 20 patients that were selected for recovery potential, 12 (60%) recovered sufficiently to undergo LVAD explant. Survival after LVAD explant was 83.3% at one, two, and three years, but longer-term survival and quality of life is unknown.[35]

Bridge to transplant candidacy

'Bridge to transplant candidacy' describes support of patients with a contraindication to heart transplantation that is likely to be reversed by MCS or to resolve during MCS. Bridge to transplant candidacy is typically performed with an implantable LVAD because long periods of support are required, but other forms of MCS may be used if patients are unsuitable for isolated LVAD support.

The most common bridge to transplant candidacy scenario is severe pulmonary hypertension due to left heart disease with a trans-pulmonary pressure gradient (TPG) or pulmonary vascular resistance (PVR) that are too high to permit safe heart transplantation. A period of durable LVAD support is an effective method of reducing the TPG and PVR. In a case series of 17 consecutive patients who received a continuous flow LVAD as a bridge to transplant candidacy, PVR fell from 5 ± 1.5 Wood units at baseline to 2.0 ± 0.7 Wood units at three months and 1.7 ± 0.4 Wood units at six months. The strategy worked well; all patients reached a PVR that permitted listing for heart transplantation and there was no adverse effect on post-transplant outcomes.[36]

A less common bridge to transplant candidacy scenario is renal dysfunction due to low cardiac output. Data from INTERMACS confirms early improvement in eGFR after LVAD implantation, but this is transient and eGFR is only 6.7% above baseline after one year.[37] The success of using an implantable LVAD to reverse renal dysfunction and achieve transplant candidacy has not been described. Finally, MCS may allow time for contraindications to resolve. Patients who are not candidates for heart transplantation because of recent malignancy may demonstrate sustained remission during MCS. It is also possible that obese patients may lose sufficient weight during MCS to permit listing for heart transplantation. However, analysis of the United Network for Organ Sharing

(UNOS) database showed that only 15.5% of patients with class II obesity (body mass index >30 kg/m²) lost weight during LVAD support and the strategy is not recommended.[38]

Bridge to transplantation

'Bridge to transplantation' describes support of patients without an absolute contraindication to heart transplantation and who are expected to undergo heart transplantation after a period of MCS. The purpose of the strategy is to reduce the likelihood of death, preserve end-organ function, and improve quality of life while waiting for heart transplantation. Bridge to transplantation is preferentially performed with an implantable LVAD because there is a reasonable expectation of survival with an acceptable quality of life for several years. However, not all patients have adequate RV function to permit isolated LVAD support and other forms of MCS may be used.

The outcomes of bridging to heart transplantation with an implantable LVAD in the most recent INTERMACS registry report are shown in **Figure 63.6**.[24] The likelihood of undergoing heart transplantation after a certain period of LVAD support will depend on the availability of donor organs and allocation system in that country, in addition to patient characteristics such as size, blood group, and allosensitization. In the most recent era of a UK-based study, only 10% of patients had undergone heart transplantation after one year and only 14% patients had undergone heart transplantation after two years.[39] Long waiting times for transplantation pose a risk of strategic failure, given the competing risk of adverse events during LVAD support.

The evidence for the strategy of bridging to transplantation is limited. No trial has examined whether long-term survival or quality of life is better than simply waiting for a heart transplant without MCS. The strategy is likely to be reasonable in patients who are inotrope-dependent (INTERMACS class II or III) and expected to deteriorate or die before a donor organ becomes available. The window of opportunity for implantable LVAD support may be limited as a consequence of adverse events or progressive RV failure. However, it remains uncertain whether patients should receive LVAD support when they are 'less sick'. The ROADMAP study suggested

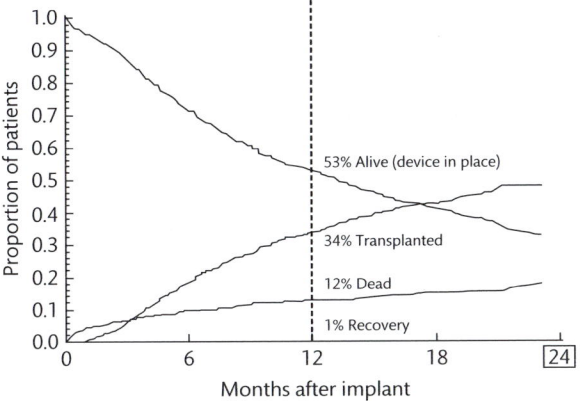

Figure 63.6 INTERMACS registry report.

Reproduced from Anderson M, Goldstein J, Milano C, Morris LD, Kormos RL, Bhama J, Kapur NK, Bansal A, Garcia J, Baker JN, Silvestry S, Holman WL, Douglas PS, O'Neill W. Benefits of a Novel Percutaneous Ventricular Assist Device for Right Heart Failure: The Prospective RECOVER RIGHT Study of the Impella RP Device. *Journal of Heart and Lung Transplantation* 2015,**34**(12):1549–1560 with permission from Elsevier.

that patients in INTERMACS profiles IV–VI did not derive survival benefit from LVAD support compared with those who remained on medical therapy, but that those who received LVAD support were at much greater risk of adverse events compared with those who remained on medical therapy.[40]

There is controversy about whether patients who are 'doing well' with implantable LVAD support should undergo heart transplantation and, if so, when. Most countries believe that waiting list survival with an implantable LVAD is too good to justify the highest priority in organ allocation. However, patients who are 'doing well' remain at risk of adverse events and these are associated with increased waiting list mortality.[41] In a large observational study in the UK, patients with an implantable LVAD who underwent heart transplantation had an increased risk of death in the short term, relating to the transplant operation, but a greatly reduced long-term risk of death. As such, it appears that bridging on to heart transplantation is sensible if a suitable donor heart is available.[39]

Finally, it is recognized that certain LVAD-supported patients are at very high risk of mortality after heart transplantation. Risk scores have been developed to identify these patients and quantify their risk of death after transplantation. The strongest predictors of post-transplant mortality are body mass index >35 kg/m², estimated glomerular filtration rate of <50 mL/min/1.73 m², and need for mechanical ventilation at the time of transplantation.[42] Clinicians might decide that selected patients may have better survival with ongoing MCS, rather than undergoing heart transplantation, or that a donor organ may be better allocated to a recipient with a higher likelihood of deriving more quality-adjusted life-years from that organ.

Destination therapy

Destination therapy (DT) describes support of patients with an absolute permanent contraindication to heart transplantation, such as peripheral vascular disease or microvascular complications of diabetes mellitus. The purpose of the strategy is to improve quality of life and extend survival. DT is almost exclusively performed with implantable LVAD because there is a reasonable expectation of survival with an acceptable quality of life for several years. DT is now the most common indication for implantable LVAD support, constituting 49.8% of all LVAD implants recorded in the INTERMACS registry from 2015 to 2016.[24] However, other forms of MCS have been used for DT in patients who require biventricular support.

DT has a better evidence base than other MCS strategies. An RCT was performed in the late twentieth century with a first-generation pulsatile-flow implantable LVAD (HeartMate XVE, Thoratec).[43] REMATCH included 129 transplant-ineligible patients with NYHA class IV heart failure symptoms, LVEF <25% and either a peak VO₂ of <12 mL/kg/min or dependence on inotropic support. Patients were randomized to LVAD or medical therapy. Survival was significantly better with LVAD than medical therapy (52% vs 25% at one year and 23% vs 8% at two years) (**Figure 63.7**). In addition, patients randomized to LVAD had improved functional state and quality of life.

Implantation of LVAD altered the cause of death in REMATCH. Most LVAD patients died of sepsis or LVAD-related complications, whereas most patients randomized to medical therapy died of progressive pump failure. Only one patient in REMATCH was still alive by 30 months, indicating that these patients were exceptionally sick and that HeartMate XVE was not a good pump for long-term MCS.

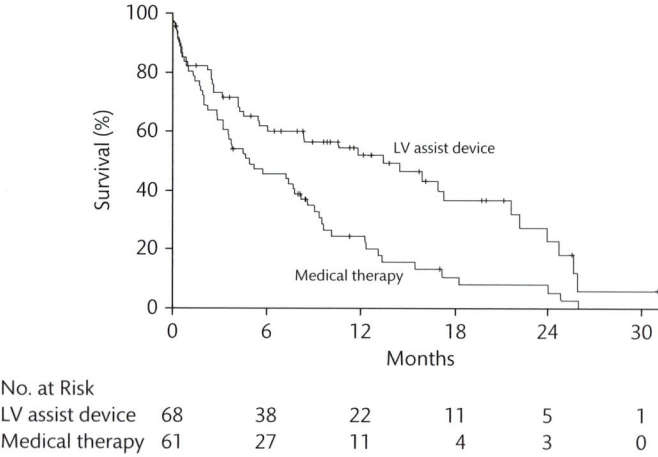

Figure 63.7 Destination therapy.

Reproduced from Rose EA, Gelijns AC, Moskowitz AJ, Heitjan DF, Stevenson LW, Dembitsky W, Long JW, Ascheim DD, Tierney AR, Levitan RG, Watson JT, Meier P, Ronan NS, Shapiro PA, Lazar RM, Miller LW, Gupta L, Frazier OH, Desvigne-Nickens P, Oz MC, Poirier VL, Randomized Evaluation of Mechanical Assistance for the Treatment of Congestive Heart Failure (REMATCH) Study Group. Long-term use of a left ventricular assist device for end-stage heart failure. *N Engl J Med* 2001;**345**:1435–1443.

Two further RCTs have been performed with second- and third-generation implantable LVAD as destination therapy.[20,21] Both trials demonstrated better one-year and two-year survival compared with the outcomes seen in REMATCH, as well as a sustained improvement in NYHA class, 6 min walk distance, and quality of life with LVAD support. However, neither trial included a medical therapy control arm and therefore neither trial assessed the strategy of DT.

There are many unanswered questions in the field of DT. It is uncertain whether implantable LVAD support improves survival and quality of life compared with twenty-first century heart failure therapy. This question may be answered by the ongoing SWEVAD trial (ClinicalTrials.gov NCT02592499). It is uncertain how best to identify ambulant heart failure patients who are sufficiently unwell to justify the risks of implantable LVAD support. It is also uncertain how to identify patients who will not derive net clinical benefit from LVAD support, such as patients who are frail or those who have non-HF related symptoms that will limit their ability to benefit from LVAD support.

Future of mechanical circulatory support

The field of MCS has rapidly developed over the last two decades and major advances are anticipated in the coming decades. Percutaneous LVAD support is finding a role during high-risk cardiovascular procedures, particularly coronary angioplasty and catheter ablation of ventricular tachycardia. A new continuous flow percutaneous LVAD called the HeartMate Percutaneous Heart Pump (PHP, Abbott) was close to clinical practice but has been withdrawn for design modifications. An ambulatory counter-pulsation pump called the iVAS (NuPulse CV) had promising results in a short-term feasibility trial.[44] Implantable LVADs continue to decrease in size. The HeartWare Miniaturized Ventricular Assist Device (MVAD) is being assessed in a CE Mark trial (ClinicalTrials.gov NCT01831544), but this is currently paused for pump design modifications. It is hoped

that size reduction may allow LVADs to be implanted without the need for sternotomy or cardiopulmonary bypass, thus reducing the risk of RV failure. Smaller pumps may also be used for partial LV support or RV support. There are also blood pumps in development that are designed to be placed outside the heart, such as the Aortix device (Procyrion, Houston, USA). Other advances include development of biocompatible internal surfaces to reduce the risk of rheological problems at the blood–pump interface. Adaptations to create pulsatility with continuous flow devices are being developed to reduce the risk of acquired Von Willebrand system. Percutaneous drivelines may be eliminated with trans-cutaneous power delivery systems that use an implanted internal antenna and a wearable external antenna. Wireless power delivery could significantly reduce the risk of driveline and pump pocket infection. Finally, many investigators are exploring whether myocardial recovery during MCS can be improved with adjunctive pharmacological or cell-based therapies. It is hoped that technological developments will increase the number of patients who may benefit from MCS and permit longer periods of support with a lower risk of adverse events. In turn, this should lead to improvement in quality of life for LVAD-supported patients, which is vital as the technology competes with heart transplantation in the twenty-first century.

REFERENCES

1. van Diepen S, Katz JN, Albert NM, *et al.*, American Heart Association Council on Clinical Cardiology; Council on Cardiovascular and Stroke Nursing; Council on Quality of Care and Outcomes Research; and Mission: Lifeline. Contemporary management of cardiogenic shock: a scientific statement from the American Heart Association. *Circulation* 2017;**136**:e232–e268.
2. Stevenson LW, Pagani FD, Young JB, *et al.* INTERMACS profiles of advanced heart failure: the current picture. *J Heart Lung Transplant* 2009;**28**:535–41.
3. Cowger J, Shah P, Stulak J, *et al.* INTERMACS profiles and modifiers: Heterogeneity of patient classification and the impact of modifiers on predicting patient outcome. *J Heart Lung Transplant* 2016;**35**:440–8.
4. Thiele H, Zeymer U, Neumann F-J, *et al.*, IABP-SHOCK II Trial Investigators. Intraaortic balloon support for myocardial infarction with cardiogenic shock. *N Engl J Med* 2012;**367**:1287–96.
5. Roffi M, Patrono C, Collet J-P, *et al.* 2015 ESC Guidelines for the management of acute coronary syndromes in patients presenting without persistent ST-segment elevation: Task Force for the Management of Acute Coronary Syndromes in Patients Presenting without Persistent ST-Segment Elevation of the European Society of Cardiology (ESC). *Eur Heart J* 2016;**37**:267–315.
6. Seyfarth M, Sibbing D, Bauer I, *et al.* A randomized clinical trial to evaluate the safety and efficacy of a percutaneous left ventricular assist device versus intra-aortic balloon pumping for treatment of cardiogenic shock caused by myocardial infarction. *J Am Coll Cardiol* 2008;**52**:1584–8.
7. Lauten A, Engström AE, Jung C, *et al.* Percutaneous left-ventricular support with the Impella-2.5-assist device in acute cardiogenic shock: results of the Impella-EUROSHOCK-registry. *Circ Heart Fail* 2013;**6**:23–30.
8. Udesen NJ, Møller JE, Lindholm MG, *et al.*; DanGer Shock investigators. Rationale and design of DanGer shock: Danish–German cardiogenic shock trial. *Am Heart J* 2019;**214**:60–8.

9. Anderson M, Goldstein J, Milano C, *et al.* Benefits of a novel percutaneous ventricular assist device for right heart failure: the prospective RECOVER RIGHT study of the Impella RP device. *J Heart Lung Transplant* 2015;**34**:1549–60.

10. Thiele H, Sick P, Boudriot E, *et al.* Randomized comparison of intra-aortic balloon support with a percutaneous left ventricular assist device in patients with revascularized acute myocardial infarction complicated by cardiogenic shock. *Eur Heart J* 2005;**26**:1276–83.

11. Burkhoff D, Cohen H, Brunckhorst C, O'Neill WW, TandemHeart Investigators Group. A randomized multicenter clinical study to evaluate the safety and efficacy of the TandemHeart percutaneous ventricular assist device versus conventional therapy with intraaortic balloon pumping for treatment of cardiogenic shock. *Am Heart J* 2006;**152**:469.e1–e8.

12. Sheu J-J, Tsai T-H, Lee F-Y, *et al.* Early extracorporeal membrane oxygenator-assisted primary percutaneous coronary intervention improved 30-day clinical outcomes in patients with ST-segment elevation myocardial infarction complicated with profound cardiogenic shock. *Crit Care Med* 2010;**38**:1810–17.

13. Tsao N-W, Shih C-M, Yeh J-S, *et al.* Extracorporeal membrane oxygenation-assisted primary percutaneous coronary intervention may improve survival of patients with acute myocardial infarction complicated by profound cardiogenic shock. *J Crit Care* 2012;**27**:530.e1–e11.

14. Tanaka D, Hirose H, Cavarocchi N, Entwistle JWC. The impact of vascular complications on survival of patients on venoarterial extracorporeal membrane oxygenation. *Ann Thor Surg* 2016;**101**:1729–34.

15. Worku B, Pak S-W, van Patten D, *et al.* The CentriMag ventricular assist device in acute heart failure refractory to medical management. *J Heart Lung Transplant* 2012;**31**:611–7.

16. Shuhaiber JH, Jenkins D, Berman M, *et al.* The Papworth experience with the Levitronix CentriMag ventricular assist device. *J Heart Lung Transplant* 2008;**27**:158–64.

17. Borisenko O, Wylie G, Payne J, *et al.* Thoratec CentriMag for temporary treatment of refractory cardiogenic shock or severe cardiopulmonary insufficiency: a systematic literature review and meta-analysis of observational studies. *ASAIO J* 2014;**60**:487–97.

18. El-Banayosy A, Arusoglu L, Kizner L, *et al.* Novacor left ventricular assist system versus Heartmate vented electric left ventricular assist system as a long-term mechanical circulatory support device in bridging patients: a prospective study. *J Thor Cardiovasc Surg* 2000;**119**:581–7.

19. Kirklin JK, Naftel DC, Pagani FD, *et al.* Seventh INTERMACS annual report: 15,000 patients and counting. *J Heart Lung Transplant* 2015;**34**:1495–504.

20. Slaughter MS, Rogers JG, Milano CA, *et al.*, HeartMate II Investigators. Advanced heart failure treated with continuous-flow left ventricular assist device. *N Engl J Med* 2009;**361**:2241–51.

21. Rogers JG, Pagani FD, Tatooles AJ, *et al.* Intrapericardial left ventricular assist device for advanced heart failure. *N Engl J Med* 2017;**376**:451–60.

22. Mehra MR, Naka Y, Uriel N, *et al.* A fully magnetically levitated circulatory pump for advanced heart failure. *N Engl J Med* 2019;**380**:1618–27.

23. Shehab S, Macdonald PS, Keogh AM, *et al.* Long-term biventricular HeartWare ventricular assist device support—case series of right atrial and right ventricular implantation outcomes. *J Heart Lung Transplant* 2016;**35**:466–73.

24. Kirklin JK, Pagani FD, Kormos RL, *et al.* Eighth annual INTERMACS report: special focus on framing the impact of adverse events. *J Heart Lung Transplant* 2017;**36**:1080–86.

25. Soliman OI, Akin S, Muslem R, *et al.*, EUROMACS investigators. Derivation and validation of a novel right-sided heart failure model after implantation of continuous flow left ventricular assist devices: The EUROMACS (European Registry for Patients with Mechanical Circulatory Support) Right-Sided Heart Failure Risk Score. *Circulation* 2018;**137**:891–906.

26. Loghmanpour NA, Kormos RL, Kanwar MK, *et al.* A Bayesian model to predict right ventricular failure following left ventricular assist device therapy. *JACC Heart Fail* 2016;**4**:711–21.

27. Thompson JS, Matlock DD, McIlvennan CK, Jenkins AR, Allen LA. Development of a decision aid for patients with advanced heart failure considering a destination therapy left ventricular assist device. *JACC Heart Fail* 2015;**3**:965–76.

28. Rogers JG, Aaronson KD, Boyle AJ, *et al.*, HeartMate II Investigators. Continuous flow left ventricular assist device improves functional capacity and quality of life of advanced heart failure patients. *J Am Coll Cardiol* 2010;**55**:1826–34.

29. Najjar SS, Slaughter MS, Pagani FD, *et al.*, HVAD Bridge to Transplant ADVANCE Trial Investigators. An analysis of pump thrombus events in patients in the HeartWare ADVANCE bridge to transplant and continued access protocol trial. *J Heart Lung Transplant* 2014;**33**:23–34.

30. Proudfoot AG, Davidson SJ, Strueber M. von Willebrand factor disruption and continuous-flow circulatory devices. *J Heart Lung Transplant* 2017;**36**:1155–63.

31. Copeland JG, Smith RG, Arabia FA, *et al.*, CardioWest Total Artificial Heart Investigators. Cardiac replacement with a total artificial heart as a bridge to transplantation. *N Engl J Med* 2004;**351**:859–67.

32. Schmidt M, Burrell A, Roberts L, *et al.* Predicting survival after ECMO for refractory cardiogenic shock: the survival after veno-arterial-ECMO (SAVE)-score. *Eur Heart J* 2015;**36**:2246–56.

33. Muller G, Flecher E, Lebreton G, *et al.* The ENCOURAGE mortality risk score and analysis of long-term outcomes after VA-ECMO for acute myocardial infarction with cardiogenic shock. *Intensive Care Med* 2016;**42**:370–8.

34. Topkara VK, Garan AR, Fine B, *et al.* Myocardial recovery in patients receiving contemporary left ventricular assist devices: results from the Interagency Registry for Mechanically Assisted Circulatory Support (INTERMACS). *Circ Heart Fail* 2016;**9**.

35. Birks EJ, George RS, Hedger M, *et al.* Reversal of severe heart failure with a continuous-flow left ventricular assist device and pharmacological therapy: a prospective study. *Circulation* 2011;**123**:381–90.

36. Kutty RS, Parameshwar J, Lewis C, *et al.* Use of centrifugal left ventricular assist device as a bridge to candidacy in severe heart failure with secondary pulmonary hypertension. *Eur J Cardiothorac Surg* 2013;**43**:1237–42.

37. Brisco MA, Kimmel SE, Coca SG, *et al.* Prevalence and prognostic importance of changes in renal function after mechanical circulatory support. *Circ Heart Fail* 2014;**7**:68–75.

38. Clerkin KJ, Naka Y, Mancini DM, Colombo PC, Topkara VK. The impact of obesity on patients bridged to transplantation with continuous-flow left ventricular assist devices. *JACC Heart Fail* 2016;**4**:761–8.

39. Emin A, Rogers CA, Parameshwar J, *et al.*, Steering Group of the UK Cardiothoracic Transplant Audit, UK VAD Forum. Trends in long-term mechanical circulatory support for advanced heart failure in the UK. *Eur J Heart Fail* 2013;**15**:1185–93.

40. Estep JD, Starling RC, Horstmanshof DA, *et al.*, ROADMAP Study Investigators. Risk assessment and comparative effectiveness of left ventricular assist device and medical management in ambulatory heart failure patients: results from the ROADMAP Study. *J Am Coll Cardiol* 2015;**66**:1747–61.

41. Wever-Pinzon O, Drakos SG, Kfoury AG, *et al.* Morbidity and mortality in heart transplant candidates supported with mechanical circulatory support: is reappraisal of the current United network for organ sharing thoracic organ allocation policy justified? *Circulation* 2013;**127**:452–62.

42. Johnston LE, Grimm JC, Magruder JT, Shah AS. Development of a transplantation risk index in patients with mechanical circulatory support: a decision support tool. *JACC Heart Fail* 2016;**4**:277–86.

43. Rose EA, Gelijns AC, Moskowitz AJ, *et al.*, Randomized Evaluation of Mechanical Assistance for the Treatment of Congestive Heart Failure (REMATCH) Study Group. Long-term use of a left ventricular assist device for end-stage heart failure. *N Engl J Med* 2001;**345**:1435–43.

44. Uriel N, Jeevanandam V, Imamura T, *et al.*; iVAS Investigators. Clinical Outcomes and quality of life with an ambulatory counterpulsation pump in advanced heart failure patients: results of the Multicenter Feasibility Trial. *Circ Heart Fail* 2020;**13**:e006666.

SECTION 15
Disease management

64

Multidisciplinary heart failure management programmes

Ali Vazir and Suzanna Hardman

Introduction

Guidelines and other consensus documents recommend a multidisciplinary approach to the management of people with heart failure.[1–11] The trend and aspiration towards the involvement of a range of health care professionals in the care of a particularly vulnerable patient group does not appear controversial. It seems intuitively obvious that a multidisciplinary team would deliver best care, and it is an approach welcomed by patient groups. But how robust is the evidence for this approach, and which components of multidisciplinary services confer benefit and in what health care contexts? To what extent are they then applicable to other populations and health care environments? The literature is extensive, diverse, complex, lacking in key information and statistically divergent. The variation in turn explains the repeated meta-analyses undertaken, and both published and planned Cochrane reviews. Although there is greater clarity in some areas since the first edition of this textbook was published, the inevitable conclusion is that the literature is largely unchanged and papers continue to conclude with a plea for further research.[12–14]

In this chapter we explore the background to, and evidence for, different models of multidisciplinary working, and conclude by arguing for a more consistent implementation of care programmes for those with heart failure.

Heart failure hospitalization

Heart failure management programmes tend to focus on the care of patients who have been admitted to hospital; this group has a high readmission rate and subsequent mortality, so there is much to be gained by improving hospital care, as perhaps demonstrated by the year-on-year improvements seen in UK National Heart Failure Audit data.[9] Worryingly, however, >50% of heart failure first presentations coincide with the need for an acute admission. The failure to make an early diagnosis and implement best care in the community is then frequently confounded by a failure to optimize management in the hospital setting.[9] This is not intended to underestimate the difficulty, or time involved, in making a robust diagnosis in patients who are often, though not invariably, elderly, and who frequently suffer from a range of other conditions or co-morbidities.

The diagnostic problems are further confounded by the lack of access to natriuretic peptide testing and echocardiography, both in hospitals and in primary care. Although access to both have increased since the National Institute for Health and Care Excellence (NICE) published updated chronic heart failure guidance in 2010 and the first acute heart failure guidance in 2014 (together with related Quality Standards), in the absence of any specialist input, 30% of patients leaving hospital in the audit cycle 2015–16 with a diagnosis of heart failure did so without any record of having undergone echocardiography.[9] Too many patients leave hospital without an adequate diagnosis or even the introduction of basic life-enhancing medication.[9,11]

Following stabilization, introducing and optimizing those drugs which prolong life and reduce hospital readmissions for patients with an ejection fraction of ≤40% (angiotensin converting enzyme (ACE) inhibitors, β-blockers, and mineralocorticoid receptor antagonists (MRAs)) can be time-consuming: optimization of medical therapy in the community following discharge is unusual. Hence an inevitable cycle of inadequate treatment and early readmissions, with psychological and physical deterioration and high mortality, is established. Failures during an admission are confounded by other factors including insufficient discharge planning or poor follow-up. In this context, poor patient self-care behaviour, including increased risk of non-adherence with medication and lifestyle change, or lack of symptom recognition,[15,16] should be no surprise. The management of patients with heart failure can be further complicated by behavioural, psychosocial, and financial considerations. Collectively these factors may contribute to 50% of heart failure exacerbations[3] and more than one-third of hospital readmissions.

Heart failure is one of the commonest causes of either admission or readmission to hospital in adults aged >65 years.[7] About 2% of the National Health Service budget is spent on heart-failure-related care in the UK, although in absolute terms, the UK spends less per patient on heart failure care than France, Germany, or the USA (see **Figure 64.1**).[17] Irrespective of the differentials, heart failure care is expensive across Europe, the USA, and Australia, with a high proportion of the costs attributable to hospitalization.

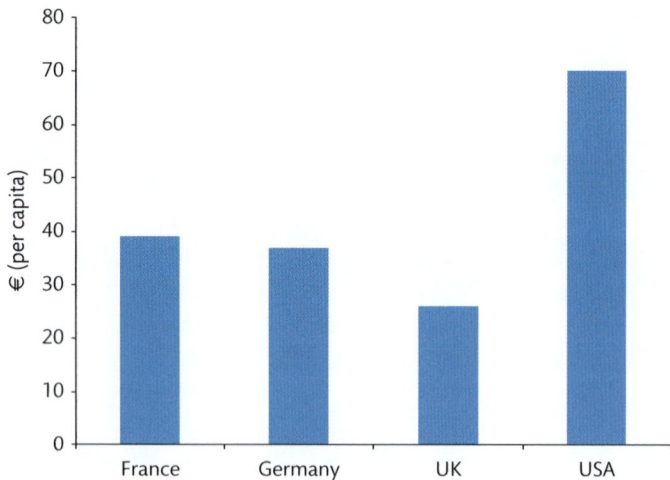

Figure 64.1 Absolute expenditure for heart failure in France, Germany, the UK, and the USA.

Source data from Bundkirchen A, Schwinger RHG. Epidemiology and economic burden of chronic heart failure. *Eur Heart J Suppl* 2004;**6**(D):D57–60.

An additional factor with which people with heart failure (and the teams striving to manage them) have to contend is the unintended consequence of growing awareness of the risks of acute kidney injury (AKI). AKI is a common reason for all disease medication to be stopped, rather than reduced, usually without timely mechanisms to reintroduce being established. This may be one factor among others (such as an increasing tendency to implement new strategies for 'keeping heart failure patients out of hospital', or 'to allow earlier discharge', which have no evidence base) that may account for the substantial year-on-year increase in heart failure-coded admissions across England and Wales. This now averages ≥20% across all acute Trusts over the last two reported heart failure audit cycles.[9,18]

Care after discharge

Inadequately diagnosed and managed, a diagnosis of heart failure continues to carry a high mortality.[18,19] In recent years, there has been a growing interest in the development of effective strategies for the care of patients with heart failure, including the use of heart failure management programmes. These programmes are designed to improve outcomes through a multidisciplinary approach with structured follow-up including: patient education, strategies for patient self-management, outpatient optimization of medical treatment, psychosocial support, and better access to care when needed.[18] The multidisciplinary teams may include any of a wide number of health care professionals, though inclusion of a heart failure nurse is central (and may be the only intervention in some heart failure management programmes). Whereas the latest Cochrane report on the subject emphasizes the increasingly convincing evidence in favour of including a heart failure nurse specialist as a member of the heart failure management programme, there is no evidence that a heart failure nurse alone is sufficient. The content and structure of heart failure management programmes vary from one health care setting to another, but they appear to be most effective where tailored to meet local needs and available infrastructure.[20]

Attempts to understand and to interpret the diverse range of studies relating to heart failure programmes for patients who are being discharged from hospital should recognize the considerable

impact that the quality of inpatient care for heart failure patients will have on immediate and long-term outcomes, and the extent to which any subsequent intervention confers benefit. Where standard inpatient heart failure care is poor, the benefits of the intervention under scrutiny will be exaggerated. In contrast, good standard inpatient clinical care may make it more difficult for any intervention to demonstrate additional benefit (though it should be reflected in mortality outcomes for cohort as a whole).

With a few important exceptions,[21–25] inpatient care before recruitment of patients to clinical trials or registries is not formally optimized (and rarely described) in published reports. The focus of interventions tends to be on outpatient care subsequent to an admission with an emphasis on reducing readmissions. Whereas reducing readmissions is an important consideration, properly constituted care teams in hospital represent an opportunity to reduce early (inpatient) and subsequent mortality; and further to reduce readmissions.

Differences between inpatient care strategies may explain the wide range of mortalities reported from different studies (see **Table 64.1**), where patients with a similarly high risk have had very different rates of adverse outcome. Support for this thesis comes from the National Heart Failure Audit which has shown that one of the best predictors of better long-term outcome for patients who have been admitted to hospital with heart failure is an increasing number of (heart failure) drugs prescribed at the time of discharge (see **Figure 64.2**). There is better outcome for those whose management team includes a cardiologist, for those who are cared for in specialist wards, and for those who remain outside specialist units but receive specialist involvement in their care.[9,26]

In the UK, specialist wards are usually either a cardiology ward or unit, where heart failure patients vie for space with a diversity of other cardiac patients. There are, however, encouraging developments of additional specialist heart failure care, such as the dedicated heart failure unit, recently opened alongside existing cardiac beds at a major London teaching hospital, a strategy which will be carefully evaluated (Dr Lisa Anderson, private communication).

Another difficulty in interpreting the literature is the lack of description of the standard availability of, and access to, heart failure and other services across the wider health community—yet that context may also exert important differential influences on the short- and longer-term patient outcomes, and the ability of any intervention to affect outcome. A further complexity that impacts on an individual's response to a diagnosis of heart failure, including any advice, is the illness beliefs of that person—a complexity we should recognize but which is for the most part beyond the scope of this chapter.[25–28]

Evidence base for multidisciplinary heart failure management programmes: selected studies

Rich *et al.*, USA

One of the first published reports of multidisciplinary heart failure management programmes was a pilot study performed in the early 1990s by Rich *et al.*, exploring the feasibility of a programme in elderly patients.[29] A subsequent randomized controlled trial in 282 patients was powered to show an increase in survival at 90 days

Table 64.1 A range of heart failure studies illustrating wide variation in mortality in usual care

Study	Sample size	Age of patients	Summary findings	Usual care mortality
Home-based intervention				
Rich et al.[29] (USA, 1995)	282	79	Nurse-led education, social service consultation, review of medications and planning for early discharge, as a multidisciplinary intervention, did not significantly alter the combined primary end-point of 'survival for 90 days without re-admissions' when compared with the control group ($P = 0.09$), though the trend was in favour of the intervention.	12.1% at 3 months
Jaarsma et al.[51] (Netherlands, 1999)	179	73	RCT to assess the effect of education and support by nurses on self-care and resource utilization in patients with heart failure. The increase in self-caring behaviour observed in all patients was significantly greater in the intervention group than in the control group, beyond 1 month. No significant effects were found on the use of health care resources.	17% at 9 months
Cline et al.[41] (Sweden, 1998)	190	76	Prospective randomized trial to assess the impact of nurse-led education and nurse follow-up clinics on time to hospitalization, days in hospital and health care costs. Of these outcome measures the intervention only had a significant effect on time to hospitalization ($P < 0.05$), though elsewhere a trend in favour of the intervention was noted.	28% at 12 months
Stewart et al.[31] (Australia, 1998)	97	75	RCT to assess the effect of a home-based intervention involving a pharmacist, nurse, and others as needed, on the combined end-point of 'frequency of re-admissions and out of hospital deaths'. The intervention resulted in a significantly reduced event rate at 6 months ($P = 0.03$).	25% at 6 months
Blue et al.[33] (UK, 2001)	165	75	RCT of nurse-led education beginning in hospital with high-intensity subsequent support and protocol-led uptitration of medicines. Significant reduction in combined primary end-point of 'time to all-cause death or rehospitalization because of worsening HF' in favour of the intervention ($P < 0.05$) at 12 months.	31% at 12 months
Krumholz et al.[36] (USA, 2002)	88	74	RCT of nurse-led education initiative with phone calls to identify deterioration, but not to modify treatment per se. Intervention conferred significant reduction in the primary combined end-point of 're-admission or death at 12 months' and appeared cost-effective.	29.5% at 12 months
Telemonitoring-based intervention				
Goldberg et al.[52] (USA, 2003)	280	59	RCT, in a relatively young cohort, of daily monitoring of weight and symptoms using a technology-based approach. No significant impact on the primary end-point of rehospitalization rate at 180 days, but the intervention conferred mortality benefit in the population studied.	19% at 6 months
Cleland et al.[19] (Europe, 2005)	426	68	RCT of telemonitoring versus telephone support, compared with usual care. The primary end-point was a combined end-point of 'days dead or hospitalized at 12 months', with no significant difference between the groups. However, notably lower mortality with intervention.	48% at 12 months
Dar et al.[44] (UK, 2009)	182	70	RCT of usual care versus telemonitoring. There was no significant difference in the primary end-point of 'days alive and out of hospital at 6 months'.	5.4% at 6 months
Clinic-based intervention				
McDonald et al.[22] (Ireland, 2002)	98	71	RCT of nurse-led heart failure clinics for patient and family, following inpatient optimization of treatment and pre-discharge clinical stability. Significant reduction in the primary combined end-point of 'mortality or HF re-admission' ($P = 0.04$), in context of low overall mortality rate.	6.4% at 3 months
Doughty et al.[38] (New Zealand, 2002)	197	73	Cluster RCT to assess the effect of an integrated heart failure management programme (involving education of patients and their families with follow-up shared between primary and secondary care). No significant impact on on the primary combined end-point of 'death or hospital re-admission'.	24.7% at 12 months
Kasper et al.[40] (USA, 2002)	200	62	RCT of a multidisciplinary input involving a personal treatment plan, devised by a heart failure cardiologist and nurse-implemented, supported by frequent phone calls and GP support for other conditions. There was no significant effect of the intervention on the primary combined end-point of 'all-cause mortality and HF re-admissions'. Some benefit to secondary outcomes.	13.2% at 6 months
Stromberg et al.[34] (Sweden, 2003)	106	78	Patients admitted to hospital with heart failure randomized to either nurse-led heart failure clinics or usual care. Primary end-point of all-cause mortality or all-cause hospital admissions at 12 months significantly reduced ($P < 0.03$).	24% at 3 months, and 37% at 12 months
Jaarsma et al.[39] (Netherlands, 2008)	1023	71	Multicentre RCT of moderate vs high-intensity nurse-led disease management compared with usual care (involving cardiology follow-up). Neither the moderate-intensity nor the high-intensity intervention reduced the primary end-point of 'time to death or rehospitalization because of HF'.	29% at 18 months

HF, heart failure; RCT, randomized controlled trial.

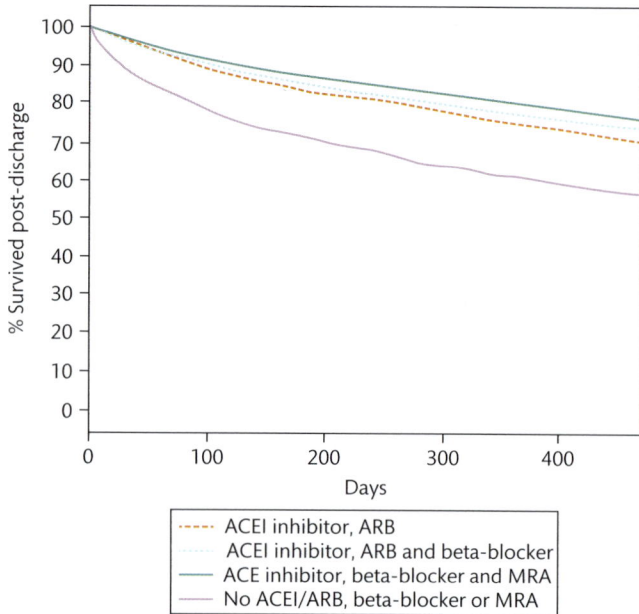

Figure 64.2 Cumulative survival of heart failure patients over the course of a year. Patients on only one core drug have a worse prognosis compared to heart failure patients taking two, whereas those taking three or more core drugs for heart failure have the best survival. This is from the most recently published NICOR HF Audit, published 2017.
Copyright 2017 Healthcare Quality Improvement Partnership.

without readmission. The randomized intervention—nurse-led education with review of medication by a geriatric cardiologist and intensive follow-up at home—did improve the primary end-point, but the results for a range of secondary end-points relating to readmissions were significantly in favour of the intervention, which was cost-effective and improved quality of life when compared with usual care. Other studies of home-based and other multidisciplinary interventions followed, with numerous publications involving many thousands of patients: however, only a small proportion were randomized controlled trials, rarely blinded, and some more statistically robust than others.[13,14]

Stewart *et al.*, Australia

Stewart *et al.*'s work from Adelaide, Australia, examined the impact of a nurse-led intervention, with access to multidisciplinary input, on patients with recurrent hospitalization for heart failure.[30] A home visit was undertaken within 2 weeks of leaving hospital and included a thorough clinical assessment, review of medications, and identification of factors likely to provoke readmission. The visit resulted in a high level of additional input from others (including GPs, cardiologists, and pharmacists) and a range of social support. There were then telephone calls at 3 and 6 months. No detail is reported for inpatient care, but reference to short admissions and the relatively high overall subsequent mortality might suggest that there was no formal programme of inpatient optimization. The intervention significantly reduced the combined primary end-point of the frequency of unplanned readmissions plus all-cause out-of-hospital deaths at 6 months, but there was no impact on out-of-hospital deaths or all-cause mortality at 6 months. The unplanned readmission rates were similar for the two groups, but overall unplanned bed usage was significantly lower in the intervention group.

The background level of care from a range of professionals was high, and services much more accessible than in the UK and some other European countries. Thus, typical follow-up for the patients receiving usual care included both a cardiology outpatient appointment and an appointment with their primary care physician within 14 days, and subsequent regular review by both. The study thus raised a number of interesting questions as to its reproducibility in other, less well-resourced, health care systems.

An interesting finding was a trend towards increased elective bed usage in the intervention group, mostly due to surgical intervention that had earlier been delayed when the patients were unstable. If we assume that this contributed to the well-being of the patients, the finding illustrates the hazards of employing reduced bed usage as a surrogate for good care for patients with heart failure.

Stewart *et al.* had earlier reported a very similar study[32] where the intervention had also reduced the (rather unusual) combined primary end-point of frequency of unplanned readmissions plus all-cause out-of-hospital deaths at 6 months.[41,42] Long-term follow-up of the patients in the two cohorts suggests that the intervention, delivered in the context of a well-resourced and well-supported health care community, continued to deliver considerable late benefits including reduced mortality (**Figure 64.3**), lower readmission rates, and related cumulative bed-day usage, while being highly cost-effective.[43] In discussing these late benefits the authors make an important point, which may be key to an effective multidisciplinary grouping: as the improved outcomes are observed by those involved in the ongoing care of the patients, good practice is reinforced and perpetuated over time.

Blue *et al.*, Scotland

From Scotland came further evidence of the effectiveness of nurse-led interventions, supported by the local heart failure cardiologists, in reducing heart failure readmissions.[44] Patients were not required to receive any predetermined standard of inpatient care, but were

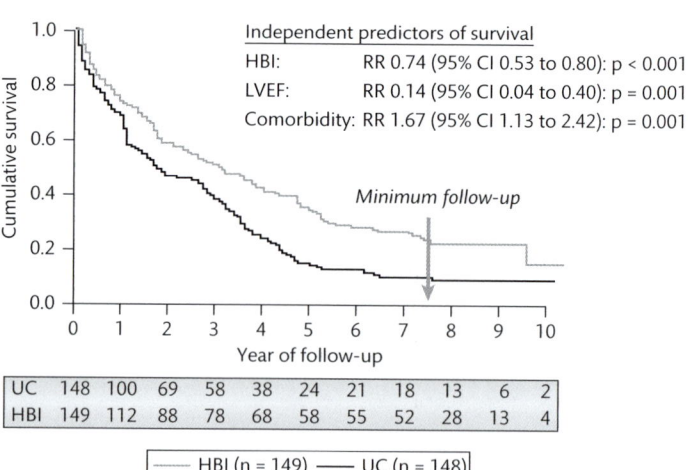

Figure 64.3 All-cause mortality, and the impact of a home-based intervention (HBI), on mortality in a group of patients hospitalized for heart failure and then randomized to either usual care (UC) or HBI with all patients followed up for a minimum of 7.5 years. LVEF, left ventricular ejection fraction; RR, relative risk.
Reproduced from Inglis SC, Pearson S, Treen S, Gallasch T, Horowitz JD, Stewart S. Extending the horizon in chronic heart failure: effects of multidisciplinary, home-based intervention relative to usual care. *Circulation* 2006;**114**(23):2466–73 with permission from Wolters Kluwer.

recruited from a cohort in whom echocardiography confirmed that the heart failure was due to left ventricular systolic dysfunction (LVSD). Patients were randomized either to intervention or to standard care under the admitting physician and subsequently their GP. Those randomized to intervention received input from the heart failure nurse during the index admission and then a home visit within 48 h of discharge; and then subsequent intensive input with visits at 1, 3, and 6 weeks and then at 3, 6, 9, and 12 months. The nurses additionally made 10 phone calls at prespecified time-points and encouraged further contact from the patient and their carers. The nurse input combined education (particularly encouraging the patient's awareness of symptoms) and psychological support. The heart failure nurses also aimed to uptitrate drugs, using written protocols.

The primary end-point was the combination of all-cause mortality or hospital admission for heart failure at 12 months. There was a significant difference in favour of those receiving the intervention; but, very importantly, had the very different inpatient mortalities during the index admission *not* been included, statistical significance would not have been reached.[13] At 12 months heart failure readmissions and related bed usage were both significantly reduced, but there was no impact on all-cause admissions, all-cause hospital bed usage, or all-cause mortality, which was of the order of 30% for the total cohort, and similar to that of Stewart *et al.*[44]

McDonald *et al.*, Ireland

McDonald's group, from Ireland, report a rather different approach, initially as a pilot and subsequently as a randomized controlled trial.[22] Patients with heart failure received inpatient optimization of care, including echocardiography, and medical therapy (then defined for those with impaired systolic function as diuretics, digoxin, and ACE inhibitors at maximally tolerated doses). Patients had to satisfy predefined clinical and stability criteria before discharge. Those randomized to the active intervention received three or more consultations with a nurse specialist and dietician while they were inpatients, and subsequently were telephoned within 3 days of leaving hospital and weekly thereafter. Both the telephone calls and the heart failure clinic appointments at 2, 6, and 12 weeks allowed for clinical reassessment and reinforcement of the educational messages. In clinic appointments, intravenous infusions of diuretics could be administered when necessary. In contrast, following optimization of inpatient care, including predischarge clinical stability, patients in the control group were referred back to their primary physician for any ongoing care.

There was a reduction in the combined primary end-point of death or heart failure readmission at 12 weeks, with the intervention conferring benefit. Although this paper is not without its own statistical quirks,[13] arguably its greatest interest lies in the very low mortality at 3 months (7.1%) for the entire cohort, which perhaps reflects the strategy of inpatient optimization of care.

London

In this context the mortality rates we reported from a randomized controlled trial are of interest. Patients who were hospitalized for heart failure due to LVSD were recruited when stable following a routine strategy of cardiology-led inpatient optimization of care.[23,24,28] The patients were elderly and high risk, with multiple co-morbidities, and were referred from primary care populations with an excess cardiovascular mortality compared with the rest of the UK, London, and similar Primary Care Trusts.

The study was designed to explore the possibility that a low-intensity, nurse-led, self-management intervention using a problem-solving strategy would reduce heart failure readmissions. Following recruitment, those randomized to the intervention were visited by a nurse twice while in hospital and then again at home within 10 days of leaving hospital. Thereafter the nurse phoned the patients once, but was available by phone should the patient initiate further telephone contact.

In all other respects, there was no difference in the heart failure care between the two randomized cohorts, including a hospital-wide, protocol-driven, shared-care strategy involving cardiologists and the admitting physicians, aimed at early diagnosis and subsequent inpatient optimization of ACE inhibitors, diuretics including MRAs, and initiation of β-blockade. Patients were allowed home when they were clinically and biochemically stable without treatment changes for 48 h. Thereafter, all patients had early and continued cardiology review. The broader context was that when the study was designed and undertaken there were no heart failure nurses employed either by the hospital or by the local community, and there were no GPs with a special interest in heart failure.

The results, reported more fully elsewhere,[28] demonstrated no difference in the readmission rates at either 3 or 12 months between the two randomized groups. The all-cause mortality for the total cohort was relatively low at 3 months (and similar to MacDonald *et al.*'s study) and again at 12 months (17.6%). It must be likely that this reflects the early inpatient optimization of care for all.[24,28]

Interestingly, using post-hoc subset analyses, we demonstrated a differential response between those admitted with a pre-existing diagnosis and those admitted with a new diagnosis (incident heart failure). In the latter group, the randomized intervention reduced heart failure readmissions and bed usage at 12 months (see **Figure 64.4**) with, importantly, no mortality penalty, but rather a trend towards lower mortality.[24]

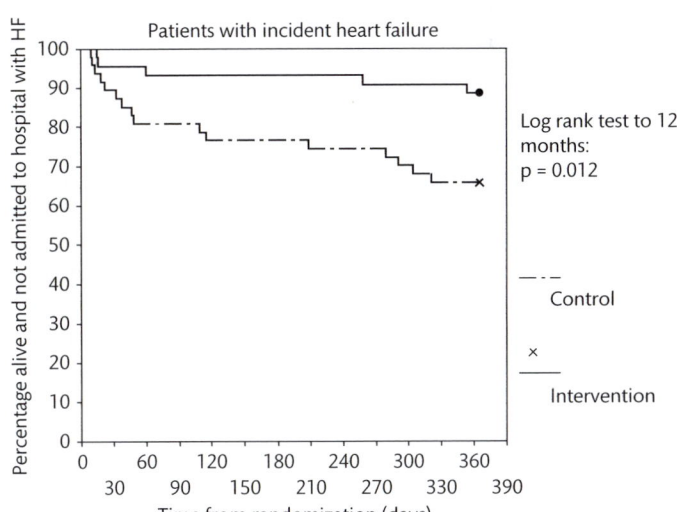

Figure 64.4 Impact of a low-intensity self-management intervention on event-free survival for patients admitted to hospital with incident heart failure (due to left ventricular systolic dysfunction). Results based on post-hoc subset analysis of a randomized controlled blinded trial.

Source data from Zaphiriou A, Mulligan K, Hargrave P, et al. Improved outcomes following hospitalisation in patients with a new diagnosis of heart failure: results from a randomised controlled trial of a novel, nurse-led self-management intervention. *Heart* 2006;**92**:A119–A120.

Other evidence

Thus far we have explored in some detail a few publications from an extensive literature. Elsewhere, papers argue for the benefits of nurse-led heart failure clinics,[45] strategies around patient education,[46,47] the use of nurses and/or pharmacists to effect the uptitration of drugs using agreed protocols and treatment algorithms,[48] either as hospital outpatient-led initiatives[22,45,49–51] or as community-based approaches including programmes in which home visits are key.[30–33,36,41] Many of the studies used phone calls to reinforce care and to provide increased access to additional care. The telephone calls can provide reassurance and allow patients the opportunity to discuss symptoms, treatment and side-effects, particularly when contact with a programme has already been established.[22,24,31,33,39,42]

Phone calls may be less well received where there has been no prior contact, or where the patients are elderly or have some degree of mental impairment. The literature may be especially vulnerable to publication bias in favour of studies with positive outcomes. Patients who are elderly, immobile, or less mentally alert may derive particular benefit from home visits, but this can be a much more costly intervention than clinic-led care. Increasingly in some health care systems, community care is being devolved to other health care professionals who may have little or no specific training in the area of heart failure.

Remote monitoring

Remote monitoring is undoubtedly an emerging model for delivering components of heart failure care, either to a large group of individuals who may not have access to traditional programmes, or as an adjunct to other components of programmes for heart failure care. The subject is dealt with in detail elsewhere, but involves daily monitoring of symptoms and signs measured by patients, family, or caregivers at home, so allowing patients to remain under close supervision[43] in their own home. A range of equipment may be installed in the home, allowing variables such as blood pressure, heart rate, oxygen saturation, weight, symptoms, and medication compliance to be recorded and transmitted. This then allows a designated health care worker to advise remotely on changes in care.

The success of remote monitoring is highly dependent on patient education and the ease with which the equipment can be used, both by those setting it up and by those endeavouring to use it. Central to its effectiveness is patient, and/or carer, education, which is usually time-consuming, and more difficult in those with cognitive impairment. Currently, there is no consensus as to which variables are most helpful to monitor. New equipment, additional monitoring variables, and increasingly sophisticated technologies are under development.[43]

Themes discussed earlier re-emerge from the telemonitoring literature, namely that the extent of any benefit appears greatest where baseline care is less well developed. This may explain in part the differences in outcomes between the Trans-European Network Initiative (TENS-HMS)[19] and those of the Home-HF study.[44]

- 'Usual care' from the TENS-HMS reported the highest 12-month mortality of 48%, but it was also high both in those receiving home telemonitoring, at 29%, and in those receiving nurse telephone support, at 27%.
- In contrast, in the Home-HF study, 6-month mortality rates were 9.8% for the intervention group and 5.4% in the usual care group, though the study was not powered to demonstrate a mortality difference.

Home telemonitoring in TENS-HMS did not reduce readmissions, but the mean duration of stay was shorter by 6 days. In contrast, Home-HF reported no reduction in days alive and out of hospital but there were reduced readmissions via the emergency department and was cost neutral. The message may be simple and appears to be supported by details of the patients studied: namely, that baseline heart failure care for the patients being recruited from three hospitals in north-west London may have been better than that received by their counterparts recruited from hospitals elsewhere in the UK, Germany, and the Netherlands.

A review of increasingly invasive devices, implanted alongside or as part of an existing device, allowing continuous monitoring of an ever-increased range of variables, is dealt with in Chapter 66.

Systematic reviews and meta-analyses

The literature exploring the impact of various interventions ranges from tiny studies to large, well-devised randomized controlled trials with an accompanying range of outcomes, so the extensive literature, not surprisingly, includes systematic reviews and meta-analyses.[13,14,45,46] All recognize the heterogeneity of the studies they include (even in the absence of descriptors of standard care) and so exclude some, and group other, studies in a range of different ways.[13,14,45,46] Holland et al.[45] and McAlister et al.[46] both endeavoured to report on whether multidisciplinary strategies improve outcomes for heart failure patients, with the main emphasis on mortality and readmissions.

- McAlister's group concluded that where follow-up included a specialized multidisciplinary team, both heart failure admissions and mortality were improved, whereas interventions designed to enhance self-care and telephone follow-up or telemonitoring reduced admissions but had no impact on mortality.
- In contrast, Holland's group found that post-discharge interventions combining education with self-management strategies reduced mortality as well as readmissions.

As ever, the answer lies in the detail, much of which goes unpublished in the interest of brevity.[45,46] Nonetheless, some clarity emerges in the most recent Cochrane review in which Takeda et al.[47] reported that case management interventions are associated with a substantial, statistically significant reduction in all-cause mortality at around 12 months of follow-up with an odds ratio of 0.66 (95% CI: 0.47–0.91; $P = 0.91$; $I^2 = 60\%$): however, there is a huge variety of interventions other than the consistent involvement of heart failure specialist nurses.

COACH

So: can the limitations of meta-analyses and structured reviews be overcome by larger studies? The Coordinating study evaluating Outcomes of Advising and Counselling in Heart Failure (COACH)[39] aimed to examine the effect of education and an intense support programme by heart failure nurses on top of frequent visits with a cardiologist following a heart failure hospitalization. The result poses some fundamental questions which challenge earlier accepted conclusions about heart failure care.

As so often, there is no detail in the report surrounding the quality or norm for inpatient care (or whether inpatient optimization is usual). Of note is a reduction from NYHA class III/IV on admission to NHYA class II/III for the vast majority by discharge, though curiously no patients were rendered asymptomatic despite high levels of prescribing of ACE inhibitors/angiotension receptor blockers (83%), diuretics (95%), and β-blockers (66%). These figures of course do not tell us anything about dose levels or timing of uptitration. All patients saw a cardiologist on at least four occasions and additionally as dictated clinically.

On the background of this usual care, there was a three-way randomization to a control group, a basic support group (where there was a nurse-led programme of structured education and outpatient visits, but no home-based intervention), or an intensive nurse-led support programme where contacts with the nurse were monthly over the 18-month study period, and included two home visits and some multidisciplinary input from a physiotherapist, dietician, and social worker. More than 1000 patients from across the Netherlands with a mean age 71 ±11 years, of whom 38% were women, were randomized and then followed for 18 months.

Although there was no significant difference in the primary endpoint of time to death or rehospitalization and the number of days lost to death or hospitalization, the all-cause mortality for the entire cohort (with no significant differences between the groups) was relatively low at around 21–22% at 12 months. The authors concluded that the patients in the control group were already well managed, making it more difficult to improve the outcome with the added intervention. We concur with that conclusion, noting that the mortality rate at 12 months is substantially lower than that in many published studies,[30,31,33] but in keeping with our own.[23] The authors further argue that hospital admissions may be beneficial (where care is thoughtfully and appropriately targeted at the patients' needs), rather than deleterious, noting that in the intervention groups there was an association (albeit non-significant) between lower mortality and more frequent, shorter, hospital admissions.

Conclusions

A critical reading of the literature and recognition of its limitations should not in any way discourage, but rather support, the establishment of effective and responsive multidisciplinary teams for the care of people with known or suspected heart failure. Encouragingly, these aims are consistent with the patients' priorities that emerged from the Health Care Commission within England (see Box 64.1).

Box 64.1 Patient priorities for heart failure service

- Access to quick and accurate diagnosis without delays in the pathway
- Good links between the services, organizations, and professions
- Having a point of contact and someone to coordinate care requirements
- Easy access to specialist advice and medication
- Access to specialist services such as rehabilitation and counselling
- Regular follow-up and ability to seek advice at short notice
- Information
- Honesty about prognosis

Source data from Health Care Commission survey 2007.

To date, the emphasis has been on community-based teams, but a number of studies and emerging audit data argue powerfully, in addition, for an improvement in hospital care. Best outcomes are achieved when patients are actively identified; where ongoing care, including early echocardiography, is led by a (heart failure) cardiologist; and where (ideally) patients can be managed in a specialist ward with access to a range of health care professionals who can ensure rapid stabilization and inpatient optimization of treatment. As the patient recovers, opportunities for education arise and should be embraced—and an admission is the ideal time for first contacts with those who will be involved in patients' care when they leave hospital. The education often involves a heart failure nurse specialist who may subsequently see the patients in clinics or their own homes, but might equally be a number of others.

Discharge planning should include primary care and cardiology review, rehabilitation, uptitration of medication, and ongoing opportunities for individual patients to understand their condition. It is important that the patient knows whom to contact and how to do so in the early days following a hospital admission when they may be most vulnerable (Box 64.2). For some patients, input from others may make the difference between ongoing improvement and an early, unplanned readmission. The nature of this input may be diverse—some needs will be identified before the patient goes home, but others may only become apparent in the days after leaving hospital: this argues for an early home assessment, which, wherever possible, should include any spouse or carer. These themes are now embraced by a range of publications including NICE guidance[3,6] and their related[48,49] standards, European heart failure guidance and standards[49] and guidance from elsewhere.[5] The latest UK Heart Failure Audit suggests that implementation is now beginning to be translated into patient benefit.[9]

Box 64.2 Key information for patients being discharged from hospital, and shared with family, carer, and other health care professionals, as appropriate

The HF summary should include:

1 The HF diagnosis including type, cause if established, and major co-morbidities
2 The echocardiographic evidence to support the HF diagnosis and natriuretic peptide result (including date of both)
3 The cardiologist and other members of the multidisciplinary team that the patient has seen during the admission.
4 Patient's dry weight on discharge and the weight lost during the admission.
5 Blood pressure and heart rate on discharge.
6 ECG: rate and rhythm, QRS duration, whether paced, whether LBBB.
7 Drugs at discharge: where any of BB, ACEi/ARB and MRA not prescribed for LVSD, the reason should be given, and plans for introduction and further uptitration.
8 Haemoglobin, urea and electrolytes, creatinine and eGFR on discharge
9 Follow-up arrangements with the HF team within 2 weeks of discharge (including date, place, time, and with whom), rehabilitation, palliative care, or other, as appropriate. All shared with patient before leaving hospital. If advanced care planning has been discussed this should be included.
10 Care plan including a contact person and contact details for any early queries, and all shared with patient pre-discharge.

Reproduced with permission from the British Society for Heart Failure. *Standards of Heart Failure Care.*

Table 64.2 The multidisciplinary heart failure team[a]

Key members of the hospital HF team	Key members of the community HF team	Other expertise/services periodically required	Comments
Consultant cardiologist with an interest in HF and service lead, and other HF cardiologists (and more junior supervised cardiology trainees)	Consultant cardiologist with an interest in HF and service lead, and other HF cardiologists	Rehabilitation	Rehabilitation ideally should be provided for all, but to date, few benefit
HF specialist nurses	HF specialist nurses	Palliative care	Palliative care teams may upskill the HF team and selectively provide individual input
Adequate administrative/secretarial/audit support	Adequate administrative/secretarial/audit support	Input from health care professionals with other specialist skills, e.g. diabetes, respiratory, haematology, care of the elderly, cardiac surgeons surgeons, tertiary centres and transplant centres	
	General practitioners	Renal	
And ideally: psychology, pharmacists, rehabilitation, elderly care, specialist in echocardiography, and local others	And ideally: psychology, pharmacists, rehabilitation, elderly care and local others	Social services	
		Imaging	
		Pharmacists	
		Electrophysiology and other specialist cardiology	

[a] These components of the team are not intended to be either comprehensive or exclusive but rather a suggested model for those establishing new or improving existing, heart failure (HF) services.

And so we see the emerging need for an established multidisciplinary team, ideally led by the heart failure cardiologist who has been involved with the care of the patient during the index admission, who then continues to support and lead the community team working closely with the primary care physician and heart failure nurse specialists, but with access to many others. The skill in building these teams is to establish mechanisms of support, mutual trust, and learning, so that the patient's changing needs may be met in a timely fashion and delivered in a cost-effective manner across the different health care communities. Table 64.2 summarizes important components of a multidisciplinary heart failure team. The team will include people who may never directly meet many of the patients but their expertise can be drawn upon. It is essential that when discussions occur they include a clinician who knows the patient well.

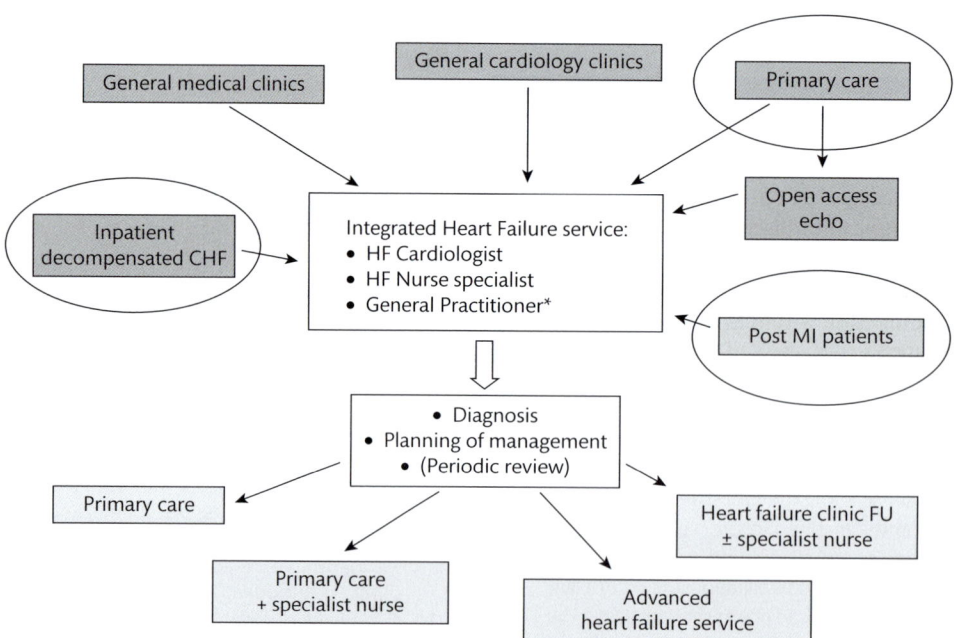

Figure 64.5 Model of an integrated heart failure service, emphasizing the need for multidisciplinary working across the different health care domains. CHF, chronic heart failure; HF, heart failure; MI, myocardial infarction; FU, follow-up.

Source data from McDonagh TA. Lessons from the management of chronic heart failure. *Heart* 2005;**91**(Suppl 2):ii24–7.

Since the first edition of this textbook, heart failure has been recognized across Europe as an area of advanced training, underpinned by a curriculum[50] which aligns well with the UK, where these strategies have been implemented from 2005 onwards. The 2014 acute heart failure guidance from NICE specifies that no hospital should be admitting patients with heart failure unless they have a properly constituted heart failure team, including a specialist heart failure lead. It is perhaps a measure of the difficulty that has been experienced in delivering adequate heart failure care that this needs to be specified. Increasing government awareness of the issues brings the potential of both increased resource to facilitate implementing improved heart failure care, alongside greater penalties where there is a failure to do so. Thus in England strategies such as the Best Practice Tariff and audit data submission for the Care Quality Commission either are, or soon will be, a reality for all involved in the care of people with heart failure.

Rather than having an overriding obsession with length of hospital stay, the heart failure community needs to focus on the quality of care during an index heart failure admission and only then on care in the community, recognizing that for some, timely and planned readmissions may be part of a health care strategy that delivers a much lower mortality rate than we have seen hitherto, and an improved quality of life. Timely access to a range of expertise through a multidisciplinary team is essential for the patient, with the heart failure cardiologist, a heart failure nurse specialist, and the GP ideally at the centre of this care delivery (Figure 64.5). The team will bring in specialist input when necessary, and input from a generalist is also important due to the wide range of co-morbidities seen in patients with heart failure. Over time, continuity of care and (wherever practicable) self-management will reduce the intensity of support needed by some and allow individual patients to re-establish their sense of normality.

REFERENCES

1. McDonagh TA. Lessons from the management of chronic heart failure. *Heart* 2005;**91**(Suppl 2):ii24–7.
2. NHS Information Centre for Health and Social Care. *National Heart Failure Second Audit Report for the audit period between July 2007 and March 2008*. National Clinical Audit Support Programme, 2008. http://www.ic.nhs.uk.
3. National Institute for Health and Care Excellence. *Management of chronic heart failure in adults in primary and secondary care*. 2010, CG 108. http://www.nice.org.uk/guidance/cg108.
4. McDonagh TA, Blue L, Clark AL, *et al.* European Society of Cardiology Heart Failure Association standards for delivering heart failure care. *Eur J Heart Fail* 2011;**13**:235–41.
5. Yancy CW, Jessup M, Bozkurt B, *et al.* Focused Update of the 2013 ACCF/AHA Guideline for the Management of Heart Failure: a report of the American College of Cardiology/ American Heart Association Task Force on Clinical Practice Guidelines and the Herat Failure Society of America. *Circulation* 2017;**136**(6):e137–e161.
6. National Institute for Health and Care Excellence. *Acute heart failure: diagnosis and management*. 2014, CG 187. http://www.nice.org.uk/guidance/cg187.
7. Scottish Intercollegiate Guidelines Network. *Management of chronic heart failure*. SIGN, Edinburgh, 2016 (publication 147). http://www.sign.ac.uk.
8. Ponikowski P, Voors AA, Anker SD, *et al.* ESC Guidelines for the diagnosis and treatment of acute and chronic heart failure The Task Force for the diagnosis and treatment of acute and chronic heart failure of the European Society of Cardiology (ESC) Developed with the special contribution of the Heart Failure Association (HFA) of the ESC Authors/Task Force Members. *Eur Heart J* 2016;**37**:2129–200.
9. NHS Healthcare and Quality Improvement Partnership. *National Heart Failure Ninth Audit Report for the audit period between April 2015 and March 2016*. http://www.ucl.ac.uk/nicor/audits/ heartfailure/additionalfiles.
10. National Institute for Health and Care Excellence. *NICE clinical guidance: Management of chronic heart failure in adults in primary and secondary care*. NICE, 2018.
11. Cleland JG, Swedberg K, Cohen-Solal A, *et al.* The Euro Heart Failure Survey of the EUROHEART survey programme. A survey on the quality of care among patients with heart failure in Europe. The Study Group on Diagnosis of the Working Group on Heart Failure of the European Society of Cardiology. The Medicines Evaluation Group Centre for Health Economics University of York. *Eur J Heart Fail* 2000;**2**(2):123–32.
12. Jonkman NH, Westland H, Groenwold HN *et al.* What are effective program characteristics of self-management interventions in patients with heart failure? An individual patient data meta-analysis. *J Card Fail* 2016;**22**:861–71.
13. Taylor S, Bestall J, Cotter S, *et al.* Clinical service organisation for heart failure. *Cochrane Database Syst Rev* 2005;(2):CD002752.
14. Takeda A, Taylor SJ, Taylor RS, *et al.* Clinical service organisation for heart failure. *Cochrane Database Syst Rev* 2012;(9):CD002752.
15. Evangelista LS, Dracup K. A closer look at compliance research in heart failure patients in the last decade. *Prog Cardiovasc Nurs* 2000;**15**(3):97–103.
16. van der Wal MH, Jaarsma T, van Veldhuisen DJ. Non-compliance in patients with heart failure; how can we manage it? *Eur J Heart Fail* 2005;**7**(1):5–17.
17. Bundkirchen A, Schwinger RHG. Epidemiology and economic burden of chronic heart failure. *Eur Heart J* 2004;**6**(Suppl D): D57–60.
18. National Institute for Cardiovascular Outcomes Research. *National Heart Failure Eighth Audit Report for the audit period between April 2014 and March 2015*. http://www.ucl.ac.uk/nicor/audits/ heartfailure/documents/annualreports/annual_report_2014_15.
19. Cleland JG, Louis AA, Rigby AS, Janssens U, Balk AH. Noninvasive home telemonitoring for patients with heart failure at high risk of recurrent admission and death: the Trans-European Network-Home-Care Management System (TEN-HMS) study. *J Am Coll Cardiol* 2005;**45**(10):1654–64.
20. Yu DS, Thompson DR, Lee DT. Disease management programmes for older people with heart failure: crucial characteristics which improve post-discharge outcomes. *Eur Heart J* 2006;**27**(5):596–612.
21. McDonald K, Ledwidge M, Cahill J, *et al.* Elimination of early rehospitalization in a randomized, controlled trial of multidisciplinary care in a high-risk, elderly heart failure population: the potential contributions of specialist care, clinical stability and optimal angiotensin-converting enzyme inhibitor dose at discharge. *Eur J Heart Fail* 2001;**3**(2):209–15.
22. McDonald K, Ledwidge M, Cahill J, *et al.* Heart failure management: multidisciplinary care has intrinsic benefit above the optimization of medical care. *J Card Fail* 2002;**8**(3):142–8.
23. Zaphiriou A, Mulligan K, Cowie MR, Newman S, Hardman SM. Should we assume that low-intensity interventions benefit

patients admitted to hospital with heart failure in all health care systems? *Circulation* 2005;**112**:2794.

24. Zaphiriou A, Mulligan K, Hagrave P, *et al.* Improved outcomes following hospitalisation in patients with a new diagnosis of heart failure: results from a randomised controlled trial of a novel, nurse-led self-management intervention. *Heart* 2006;**92**:A119–20.

25. Mulligan K, Zaphiriou A, Hargrave P, *et al.* A self-management intervention in heart failure: differential impact on newly diagnosed patients. *Psychol Health* 2006;**21**:109.

26. Griffin EA, Wonderling D, Ludman AJ, *et al.* Cost-effectiveness analysis of natriuretic peptide testing and specialist management in patients with suspected acute heart failure. International Society for Pharmacoeconomics and Outcomes Research, 2017.http://dx.doi.org/10.1016/j.jval.2017.05.007.

27. Mulligan K, Zaphiriou A, Hargrave P, *et al.* Quality of life in heart failure is related to mood and illness beliefs rather than left ventricular dysfunction. *Eur Heart J* 2005;**26**:601.

28. Mulligan K. The design and evaluation of a self-management intervention for patients admitted to hospital with heart failure. PhD thesis, University of London, 2008.

29. Rich MW, Beckham V, Wittenberg C, *et al.* A multidisciplinary intervention to prevent the readmission of elderly patients with congestive heart failure. *N Engl J Med* 1995;**333**(18):1190–5.

30. Stewart S, Marley JE, Horowitz JD. Effects of a multidisciplinary, home-based intervention on unplanned readmissions and survival among patients with chronic congestive heart failure: a randomised controlled study. *Lancet* 1999;**354**(9184):1077–83.

31. Stewart S, Pearson S, Horowitz JD. Effects of a home-based intervention among patients with congestive heart failure discharged from acute hospital care. *Arch Intern Med* 1998;**158**(10):1067–72.

32. Inglis SC, Pearson S, Treen S, *et al.* Extending the horizon in chronic heart failure: effects of multidisciplinary, home-based intervention relative to usual care. *Circulation* 2006;**114**(23):2466–73.

33. Blue L, Lang E, McMurray JJ, *et al.* Randomised controlled trial of specialist nurse intervention in heart failure. *BMJ* 2001;**323**(7315):715–18.

34. Stromberg A, Martensson J, Fridlund B, *et al.* Nurse-led heart failure clinics improve survival and self-care behaviour in patients with heart failure: results from a prospective, randomised trial. *Eur Heart J* 2003;**24**(11):1014–23.

35. Koelling TM, Johnson ML, Cody RJ, Aaronson KD. Discharge education improves clinical outcomes in patients with chronic heart failure. *Circulation* 2005;**111**(2):179–85.

36. Krumholz HM, Amatruda J, Smith GL, *et al.* Randomized trial of an education and support intervention to prevent readmission of patients with heart failure. *J Am Coll Cardiol* 2002;**39**(1):83–9.

37. Blue L, McMurray J. How much responsibility should heart failure nurses take? *Eur J Heart Fail* 2005;**7**(3):351–61.

38. Doughty RN, Wright SP, Pearl A, *et al.* Randomized, controlled trial of integrated heart failure management: The Auckland Heart Failure Management Study. *Eur Heart J* 2002;**23**(2):139–46.

39. Jaarsma T, van der Wal MH, Lesman-Leegte I, *et al.* Effect of moderate or intensive disease management program on outcome in patients with heart failure: Coordinating Study Evaluating Outcomes of Advising and Counseling in Heart Failure (COACH). *Arch Intern Med* 2008;**168**(3):316–24.

40. Kasper EK, Gerstenblith G, Hefter G, *et al.* A randomized trial of the efficacy of multidisciplinary care in heart failure outpatients at high risk of hospital readmission. *J Am Coll Cardiol* 2002;**39**(3):471–80.

41. Cline CM, Israelsson BY, Willenheimer RB, Broms K, Erhardt LR. Cost effective management programme for heart failure reduces hospitalisation. *Heart* 1998;**80**(5):442–6.

42. Riegel B, Carlson B, Kopp Z, *et al.* Effect of a standardized nurse case-management telephone intervention on resource use in patients with chronic heart failure. *Arch Intern Med* 2002;**162**(6):705–12.

43. Clark RA, Inglis SC, McAlister FA, Cleland JG, Stewart S. Telemonitoring or structured telephone support programmes for patients with chronic heart failure: systematic review and meta-analysis. *BMJ* 2007;**334**(7600):942.

44. Dar O, Riley J, Chapman C, *et al.* A randomized trial of home telemonitoring in a typical elderly heart failure population in North West London: results of the Home-HF study. *Eur J Heart Fail* 2009;**11**(3):319–25.

45. Holland R, Battersby J, Harvey I, *et al.* Systematic review of multidisciplinary interventions in heart failure. *Heart* 2005;**91**(7):899–906.

46. McAlister FA, Lawson FM, Teo KK, Armstrong PW. A systematic review of randomized trials of disease management programs in heart failure. *Am J Med* 2001;**110**(5):378–84.

47. Takeda A, Taylor SJ, Taylor RS, *et al.* Clinical service organisation for heart failure. *Cochrane Database Syst Rev* 2012;(9):CD002752.

47. National Institute for Health and Care Excellence. Chronic heart failure quality standards (QS9). http://www.nice.org.uk/guidance/qs9.

48. National Institute for Health and Care Excellence. Acute heart failure quality standard (QS103). http://www.nice.org.uk/guidance/qs103.

50. McDonagh TA, Gardner RS, Lainscak M, *et al.* Heart failure association of the European Society of Cardiology specialist heart failure curriculum. *Eur J Heart Fail* 2014;**16**:151–62.

51. Jaarsma T, Halfens R, Huijer Abu-Saad H, Dracup K, Gorgels T, van Ree J, Stappers J. Effects of education and support on self-care and resource utilization in patients with heart failure. *Eur Heart J* 1999;**20**:673–82.

52. Goldberg LR, Piette JD, Walsh MN, Frank TA, Jaski BE, Smith AL, Rodriguez R, Mancini DM, Hopton LA, Orav EJ, Loh E; WHARF Investigators. Randomized trial of a daily electronic home monitoring system in patients with advanced heart failure: the Weight Monitoring in Heart Failure (WHARF) trial. *Am Heart J* 2003;**146**:705–12.

65

End of life

Miriam J. Johnson

The clinical course of heart failure has been transformed by the development of therapies (medication, devices, and surgery) targeted at the pathophysiological mechanisms underlying its perpetuation and progression. Since the introduction of treatments that target the renin–angiotensin system and cardiac devices, the prognosis has improved and it is likely that the one-year survival figures often quoted[1] are now less bleak. However, given that it is a progressive disease, patients who have not suffered a sudden cardiac death from arrhythmia ultimately enter an end-stage which may be prolonged, and carries a significant daily symptom burden, affecting both themselves and their caregivers. With increasing use of implantable defibrillators, more patients may eventually live to experience such end-stage disease. In addition, co-morbidities, often smoking-related, are common. Co-morbidities add to the symptom load, affect optimum cardiac management, and may be the final cause of death.

End of life care is not always delivered well, particularly in secondary care settings where the emphasis may still be on life-prolonging interventions. The dying phase may not be recognized or acknowledged.[2-4] Despite Hinton's observations 50 years ago[5] that patients with heart failure and renal failure often died in distress, those with non-malignant disease still have unequal access to services skilled in end of life care; most patients seen by hospice services in the UK have cancer. Although this is improving and now 40% of palliative care outpatients have non-cancer conditions, palliative care inpatients are still overwhelmingly those with cancer (85%).[6] In the UK, the Department of Health has declared end of life care to be a national priority.[7] To this end, a national End of Life Strategy emphasized the need to raise the standard of care of the dying to that of the best throughout the National Health Service,[8] and tools such as the Liverpool Care of the Dying Pathway (LCP)[9] and the Gold Standards Framework (GSF)[10] were recommended. However, following controversy surrounding the way in which the LCP was implemented in many healthcare institutions, the consequent and independent Neuberger review recommended that the LCP be replaced by individual care plans. The report also highlighted a number of concerns including the lack of evidence around the recognition of dying and called for further research and clear guidance for clinicians. Continued central drive to improve care for the dying is seen both in the UK and in many other countries[11] but several challenges remain in the care of the patient dying from non-malignant conditions such as heart failure—the main one being the difficulties that clinicians, patients, and their carers may have in recognizing the end stage of the illness.

A growing evidence base demonstrating benefits for patients with heart failure receiving palliative care makes this issue one of increasing importance. A systematic review[12] found 13 interventional and 10 observational studies. Of the five papers reporting on four lower risk-of-bias evaluation phase studies[13-17] of multidisciplinary specialist palliative care showed statistically significant benefit for patient-reported outcomes (symptom burden, depression, functional status, and quality of life), resource use and care costs. However, there were no trials that first identified those most likely to need palliative care, and none were multicentre, limiting generalizability. A recent landmark multicentre randomized controlled trial in Parkinson disease and palliative care in addition to standard care identified the trial population using the equivalent Needs Assessment Tool: Progressive Disease—Parkinson's.[18] They found a larger effect size, probably due to identifying the patient group with the most needs and greatest likelihood of benefit. As most palliative care needs can be met by the usual care team, referral of all patients to specialist palliative care teams is neither necessary nor sustainable.[19] A needs-based integrated approach therefore seems better fit for purpose.

Recognition of end-stage heart failure

'It appears to me a most excellent thing for the physician to cultivate *Prognosis*; for by foreseeing and foretelling … thus a man will be the more esteemed to be a good physician, for he will be the better able to treat those aright who can be saved, having long anticipated everything; and by seeing and announcing beforehand those who will live and those who will die …'.

Source data from Hippocrates (translated by Francis Adams). Book of Prognostics. Dodo Press; 2009 Jan[20]

Hippocrates recognized the importance of prognostication and it remains a vital part of clinical management. Prognostication helps to frame the potential benefits and burdens of medical intervention, both in terms of the individual patient's best interests, but also with regards to the best use of health care resources. Hippocrates stated

strongly that physicians should 'refuse to treat those who are over-mastered by their diseases, realizing that in such cases medicine is powerless'. However, perhaps because of increasing therapeutic possibilities, it is tempting for the clinician to focus on any hope of prolonging a patient's life and to give less attention to the skill of prognostication. The recent greater emphasis on patient choice with regard to place of care and place of death, coupled with recent publications presenting the voices of the patient and caregiver, show that many patients and their caregivers have a poor understanding of what heart failure is, its treatment, and likely clinical course.[21-25] Patients with heart failure therefore have less access to supportive and palliative services, despite a well-documented high psychological morbidity, and less chance to be involved in planning the last stage of their lives, than do patients with cancer.[15]

Trajectories

Performance status is a useful prognostic sign. One of the main difficulties in recognizing the dying phase of patients with heart failure is that the trajectory of their performance status is one of gradual decline interspersed by periods of decompensation followed by recovery to a level almost equal to their pre-decompensation state.[26] Performance will deteriorate more quickly in the last few months of the patient's life, but still follow the pattern of dips and recovery; there may even be an initial indication of recovery from the final episode of deterioration that leads to death. Thus, patients, their caregivers, and clinicians may have been through the cycle of anxiety induced by decompensation followed by relief at restoration several times, and it can be difficult to recognize the one decompensation from which there will be no recovery.

In contrast, the disease trajectory of a patient with lung cancer is said to be more predictable with a rapid decline to death over the last 1–2 months of life.[26] However, in practice, patients with cancer may also follow a declining trajectory interspersed with acute events followed by recovery. Individual patients with heart failure have an even more chaotic trajectory than typically shown[27] and their experience is often characterized by daily fluctuations in how they feel. In addition, many patients have concurrent chronic lung disease and chronic kidney disease, further complicating the clinical situation.

However, despite the difficulties, there are clinical features that make it possible to see the background deterioration in overall stage of heart failure. An in-depth interview study with clinicians (doctors and nurses) caring for people with advanced heart failure showed that patterns of deterioration over time are recognized intuitively as signifying imminent death.[28] It is important to assess this background context when making management decisions about individual patients, in order to allow relevant discussions with the patient and their caregivers about the aims and likely success of various treatment options.

Markers of worsening heart failure

It is important to recognize signs of worsening heart failure that should trigger sensitive conversations with the patient about the stage of their illness and to allow them and their carers to work out together realistic hopes and goals in light of their decline. Awareness of a patient's wishes, such as the wish to be able to die at home and not be readmitted to hospital, is important. Even if the patient dies suddenly at home, the caregiver will be aware of the patient's wishes

and an inappropriate use of an emergency ambulance and futile attempt at cardiopulmonary resuscitation can be avoided. For those who die of progressive heart failure, recognition of this stage allows access to support (social services and financial), symptom control and advanced planning and coordination of care (including out of hours care) in order to allow patients to be cared for in the place of their choosing. Most patients, given the choice, express a wish to die at home, but currently nearly two-thirds will die in hospital.[29] Analysis of English 2009 primary care data showed that only 7% of those who died of heart failure had been recognized as needing a palliative approach to care, compared with nearly half of those dying with cancer.[30] Of the 7%, a third had been placed on the palliative care register within a week before death; a challenging timescale to put sufficient supportive care to allow death at home for those who wish it. A paper examining trends over subsequent years shows that the proportion of heart failure patients placed on the palliative care register had increased to 21.2% by 2014, but continued to lag far behind that for patients with cancer (61.9%).[31]

There are many clinical scoring systems for heart failure that attempt to aid prognostication. They range from the simple New York Heart Association (NYHA) classification to more complex scores including age, aetiology of heart failure, QRS duration and biochemical markers such as brain natriuretic peptide, serum creatinine, and serum sodium.[32-38] More simple systems have been suggested using NYHA status, age, and co-morbidities.[39] However, few seem to help predict the time of death for an individual, although the Gold Standards Framework Prognostic Indicator did identify >80% of heart failure patients with palliative care concerns.[40] In practice, looking at a patient's course in the context of what has been happening over the past 3–6 months is usually adequate. An irreversible decline in health status is indicated in patients with worsening and persistent hypotension, sufficient to render intolerance of cardiac drugs; persistent hyponatraemia and deteriorating renal function; increasing doses of diuretics; repeated hospital admissions with episodes of decompensation (especially those without an apparent precipitating factor); loss of body mass; and worsening fatigue.

A needs-based approach, as distinct from a prognostic-based approach, in identifying the patient who may benefit from palliative care (either general, provided by usual care teams, or specialist, provided by specialist palliative care teams) is discussed below under 'Coordination of care'.

Communication

Patients with heart failure often have inadequate understanding of their disease, the stage of their disease, and the aims of treatment, and thus have little say in their care at the end of life.[21,22,24,41,42] Few patients with heart failure had any discussion regarding prognosis with any health care professional.[43,44] Sensitive communication to explore what patients already understand and what they are able to comprehend is important, both to redress this balance and to ensure informed consent for treatment. There are understandable concerns from clinicians about removing hope, and, indeed, entering such discussions is often difficult for clinician, patient, and carer. However, evidence from the fields of oncology and renal medicine show that although these conversations are hard, on balance, they are welcomed by patients and their carers.[45-47] Interestingly, many

participants in Rogers' study willingly discussed death and dying with the researcher.[24]

Moving a patient's goals from the hopelessly unrealistic to the hopefully achievable may *maintain* hope, and build trust with their clinician—the majority valuing honesty if delivered with concern. However, an individual approach taking cultural aspects into account is important. For example, a study exploring the views of elderly patients with heart failure, who attached less importance to the concept of individual autonomy, showed that many would not want an explicit acknowledgement of the imminence of death.[48] Conversely, patients may wish to discuss issues related to death and dying but their family members feel unable to cope with such a conversation.[49] In addition, some patients may be dealing with their illness using denial, again underlining why a blanket approach is inappropriate, and why it is important to assess the level of information that individual patients can cope with. However, complete denial is unusual, and it is possible to facilitate a discussion, preferably including their caregivers, to establish what their wishes would be 'if the illness got seriously worse' given that they 'aren't as well as they were'.[50]

One particular area of communication that can cause anxiety to clinician, patient, and caregiver is that of cardiopulmonary resuscitation (CPR) decisions. There is a considerable amount of confused thinking about this subject among clinicians and patients.[51] The current British Medical Association advice is clear: clinicians are under no obligation to offer a futile intervention.[52] Although discussion abounds as to what is medically futile or not,[53–56] in the patient dying from end-stage heart failure, an attempt at CPR is highly unlikely to have any clinically meaningful successful outcome.[51] The clinician is therefore not under obligation to offer such an intervention. However, it may be appropriate to discuss *the decision* with the patient, in the context of a general conversation about the current seriousness of the illness. Most are able to understand that only treatments that have a reasonable chance of benefiting them should be employed, rather than those that will not (such as cardiac surgery, further cardiac medication, or insertion of devices and an attempt at CPR). It is therefore part of a more wide-reaching discussion about what can be offered to the patient rather than the stark removal of an option. However, these discussions should be assessed on an individual basis and there is no requirement specifically to talk about CPR if it is considered futile by the medical team and it is likely that a discussion will cause unnecessary distress to the patient.[57]

If the patient is happy for the clinician to discuss their care with the family, it is often useful to mention specifically that 'natural death' will be allowed; some family members are worried that there will be an inappropriate attempt at CPR and are relieved there will not, whereas others have an unrealistic expectation of what an attempted CPR could achieve and would be distressed if an attempt were not made at the time of death. It may be that family members are more concerned that a futile intervention will be attempted inappropriately.[49] The discussion is particularly important for patients who wish to die at home, and clarity with the whole family can often prevent an inappropriate and distressing call to the emergency services. Any conversation should be held with great sensitivity, exploring patient and family expectations of CPR, being aware that wildly overoptimistic views may be held, either as a result of a previously successful CPR much earlier in the illness, or as a result of media portrayals. Any decision and conversation about CPR should be documented in the patient's medical case records and communicated to other staff. Finally, patients and caregiver may change their

opinions about both place of care and CPR, and these decisions should be looked at as an ongoing process.[51,58]

Advance care planning

Discussions about CPR are part of advance care planning (ACP)—a process whereby adults, particularly with advancing disease, but exclusively so, are encouraged to discuss their life goals, personal values, and preferences with regard to medical treatment and care decisions.[59] Despite a growing evidence base, implementation[60] in clinical practice for people with heart failure remains partial or non-existent. An effectiveness systematic review of ACP in heart failure[61] only found eight studies. Only four were randomized controlled trials (RCTs), of which one was a cardiology-led ACP intervention,[62] and three were evaluation phase trials[13,63,64] where ACP was delivered as a component, and in the context, of multidisciplinary specialist palliative care rather than as the primary objective. The authors concluded that there was preliminary benefit with regard to supporting patient-preferred place of care and death, and reduction in hospitalization when ACP was delivered as part of specialist palliative care. A subsequent feasibility non-randomized study from a cardiology-led palliative care service, which included an ACP with medical ceilings of intervention reported findings, like Denvir *et al.*, showed preliminary evidence of benefit with reduction in hospital admission.[62,65]

Care of the dying

The process of recognizing dying follows the principle of assessing a patient's current presentation within the context of their individual illness trajectory.

Almost contemporaneously with the Neuberger Report, the first cluster RCT of the LCP was published.[66] This Italian study failed to show any benefit in their primary outcome measure of overall quality of care toolkit score, although secondary outcomes of respect, dignity and kindness, and control of breathlessness, were improved in the intervention arm, and overall the trial did not achieve adequate statistical power. Medical engagement was poor, reducing the fidelity of the multidisciplinary intervention; and there was a higher rate of family refusals in the control arm which could have allowed selection bias in the control arm, diluting the findings. However, the LCP has been replaced in the UK by individual care plans based around 'Five Priorities' of care: recognition of dying; communication; joint decision-making; support for the family; and compassionate care.[67]

The skills required in caring for the dying heart failure patient are largely the same as those for the cancer patient. The five symptoms commonly encountered in the dying patient remain the same: pain; nausea/vomiting; agitation/distress; breathlessness; excess secretions. The general principles of symptom control should be followed: assessment of the cause of the symptom (so, for example, urinary retention or hypoxia may be a cause of agitation); reverse what can be reversed (catheterize the bladder, give oxygen); and palliate what cannot be reversed (for example, sedation for agitation if no apparent underlying reversible cause or persistent despite attempt at reversal). Care of skin, mouth, bowels, and bladder likewise remain generic skills which should be provided for any patient dying irrespective of disease and will not be discussed here.

However, there are a few issues pertinent to patients with heart failure that need to be borne in mind.

Use of strong opioids

Patients may require strong opioids for ischaemic pain, breathlessness, or severe Cheynes–Stokes respiration (rarely this may be so extreme that the patient may rouse in distress on re-starting breathing after a prolonged apnoeic spell). The evidence base for the use of opioids in breathlessness comes from work primarily in chronic lung disease and cancer, and the few studies in patients with heart failure have produced mixed results.[68–74] Some patients appear to respond better than others, although a pooled data analysis indicated that underlying cause of breathlessness was *not* a predictor of response;[75] a therapeutic trial in the breathless individual with heart failure is therefore appropriate. A phase 3 randomized placebo-controlled trial[74] of modified-release morphine for people with NYHA III/IV symptoms due to heart failure has terminated early due to slow recruitment, but has provided data on longer-term use and toxicities. There were no excess serious adverse events, no evidence of respiratory harm, and transient treatment-emergent (worse or new since baseline) harms during the first week were mild, apart from one, and more common in those with poorer renal function. In this underpowered study there was no benefit for the primary outcome (average breathlessness over previous 24 h); however, all other breathlessness measures improved to a greater extent in the morphine group. A systematic review and meta-analysis of studies of opioids for breathlessness failed to show evidence of respiratory harms.[76]

Strong opioids are poor sedatives because, although they may cause drowsiness, they may also cause agitation if the dose is not carefully titrated against pain or breathlessness, and they should thus not be used simply for sedation.

Clinicians may forget that a parenteral dose of morphine is equivalent to approximately two to three times that dose if given orally. Thus 10 mg parenteral morphine is equivalent to giving 30 mg oral morphine. The implication is that for a patient who is not already taking strong opioids ('opioid naive'), and for whom parenteral morphine is deemed appropriate, an initial small dose of 2.5 mg morphine should be given intravenously or subcutaneously, and the effect monitored.

If repeated doses are needed, then continuous subcutaneous infusion (CSCI) of morphine, starting with a starting dose of 5–10 mg/24 h, may save the patient repeated injections, and the trauma of unsuccessful attempts to find venous access. If the patient is established on oral opioids but can now no longer manage them, the opioids should be converted to CSCI, remembering that the 24 h oral morphine dose is equivalent to approximately one-third of the dose when given parenterally—for example, a patient who has been on 30 mg morphine per day orally would be converted to 10 mg morphine/24 h by CSCI. The response should always be carefully monitored and the dose adjusted according to effect. Overall evidence indicates that doses above an oral daily dose of 30 mg morphine should be adequate and provide the best risk–benefit balance; thus, *if given for breathlessness only*, then 10 mg/24 h of morphine should be considered a top dose.[77–79]

If there is poor renal function, morphine and metabolites may accumulate, leading to agitation, confusion, and hallucinations, and ultimately respiratory depression. The dose should be reduced, the dosing interval increased, and continuous infusion avoided. If there is advanced kidney disease (estimated glomerular filtration rate <25 mL/min), morphine should be avoided altogether and fentanyl or alfentanil for injection used instead.[80] Unless the patient is already established on a fentanyl transdermal patch, e.g. for pain, this formulation is not recommended in the dying patient as the dose–response delay is too cumbersome to manage appropriately if the patches are started in about the last 48 h of life. Renal failure guidelines endorsed by the Department of Health, the Renal Association, and the British Renal Society, advocate an initial immediate stat dose of 25 μg of fentanyl in the opioid naive patient, followed by CSCI of 100–250 μg/24 h if the patient has required three or more doses in a 24 h period.[80]

Oedema

Pulmonary oedema does not seem to occur frequently in the dying patient, presumably because of minimal oral fluid intake at that stage. However, it may still occur and be distressing for all concerned. Furosemide can be given in this situation by CSCI, which is particularly useful when intravenous access is difficult or impossible in a dying patient with little peripheral circulation. The infusion must be sited in an area where there is no peripheral oedema: even in the most oedematous patient, there is usually an area on the upper chest wall that is free of fluid. Diuresis and natriuresis has been demonstrated using this route of administration in a placebo-controlled trial in normal volunteers,[81] in a case series of patients with decompensated heart failure, and in a cohort of patients under the care of an integrated heart failure–palliative care service.[82,83] However, the oral/subcutaneous dose equivalent is not clear, and although the bioavailability has been estimated to be 100% of intravenous injection, an empirical approach is needed with daily review.

If effective, the subcutaneous route of administration may prevent a hospital admission close to the end of life as it is simple to administer CSCI in the patient's home.[83] Commercial development for a US Food and Drug Administration-approved system of administration is underway and a crossover trial of intravenous versus subcutaneous furosemide has been completed (ClinicalTrials.gov NCT02579057). The company has reported 100% bioavailability and equivalent diuresis, but these findings are not yet published after peer review.

There is some evidence that continuous 24 h intravenous infusion generates a more effective diuresis than repeated boluses to the same total dose.[84] It must be remembered, however, that in practice, at this stage, higher doses of loop diuretic may be needed because of diuretic resistance due to renal dysfunction and renal tubule cell hypertrophy. In conjunction with poor peripheral perfusion, frusemide may thus result in limited benefit.

Peripheral oedema is a more common problem than pulmonary oedema and causes discomfort, and increases the risk of complicating pressure sores and cellulitis. Again, parenteral diuretics may help, but the oedema can prove very resistant. Excellent nursing care with attention to pressure-relieving aids and good skin care is mandatory. Itch may also be a problem in patients with end-stage heart failure and the use of aqueous cream with menthol may help both the skin and the itch.

Breathlessness

Even in the absence of pulmonary oedema, breathlessness may be distressing in the patient dying from heart failure and is closely

associated with anxiety. Opioids, and the flow of cool air across the lower part of the face, may be helpful.[85–88]

There is little evidence that oxygen therapy will benefit the patient's *breathlessness*.[89–93] If there is no benefit from oxygen, it should be stopped. However, patients who wish to die at home may feel reassured to have in the home and prevent use of emergency services for that purpose.[89]

When the patient is in the dying phase, breathlessness may require sedation with benzodiazepines. However, there is no robust evidence to support or refute benefit for breathlessness.[94] Therefore, at an earlier stage of the disease, the use of benzodiazepines should be restricted (because of the risk of falls and memory impairment) to intermittent use for panic, or even avoided by using an anxiolytic antidepressant such as mirtazepine. If the patient is semi-conscious but restless due to breathlessness-induced agitation, the effect of a subcutaneous dose of a quick-acting benzodiazepine such as midazolam 2.5–5 mg should be assessed. If it is effective, but the patient requires repeat doses, then CSCI with an initial midazolam dose of 10 mg/24 h should be started and titrated according to effect.

If the patient is still conscious, then the level of sedation and level of relief from distress can be negotiated with them: some patients would rather have some distress but still be awake enough to converse with their family, some wish for 'time out' with the short-term sedation-induced sleep afforded by bolus doses, and still others would rather be asleep continually and unaware of their distress. In the latter case, it is good practice to discuss the situation with the palliative care team. In a patient who is dying over 48–72 h, such deep sedation does not hasten death, but makes the patient comfortable *while* they die.[95] However, if a patient is *not* in the dying phase, then deep sedation is not an appropriate approach for the management of breathlessness. A clear assessment and distinction must be made, and if there is any doubt, a second opinion should be sought. At all stages it is vital to maintain clear communication with the patient's family as sedation is an area of practice which is easily misunderstood.

In patients with troublesome breathlessness but who are not dying, then interventions outlined above are still relevant. Non-pharmacological interventions which use a mixture of activity, exercise, breathing training, and psychological measures should be considered.[96] A series of phase 3 trials has demonstrated benefit in a variety of chronic conditions,[97–101] and, although few patients had heart failure, it is likely that there are common mechanisms at play.

Nausea and excess respiratory secretions ('death rattle')

Patients with heart failure have several reasons to be nauseated, including gut oedema and liver congestion. In the dying patient, drug-related nausea (such as from spironolactone and digoxin) is less of an issue as the patient is often unable to take oral medication. Theoretically, the anti-emetic cyclizine should be avoided in heart failure,[102] but in the dying patient, if it is the only anti-emetic available, it should not be withheld because of potential cardiac adverse effects.

The 'death rattle' can be a problem even if there is no pulmonary oedema. The noise of excess respiratory secretions can be distressing for attendant family and staff, although the patient may not be disturbed by it at this stage.[103–105] Changing patient position may be sufficient to reduce the noise, and occasionally suction can be helpful

if the secretions are severe and the patient is so deeply unconscious that the gag reflex is absent.

The traditionally accepted drug treatment option is anticholinergic medication such as hyoscine butylbromide, hyoscine hydrobromide or glycopyrrhonium. However, the effectiveness of anticholinergics has recently been questioned, although robust clinical trials are difficult in the dying.[106,107] They are an option if the situation appears to be distressing the *patient* and other avenues have failed to help. However, there should be careful review of effectiveness to prevent the continued administration of an unhelpful drug. Anticholinergic drugs could adversely affect cardiac function, but they should not be withheld from a dying patient if a therapeutic trial appeared to show benefit. Of the three options, hyoscine butylbromide and glycopyrrhonium have fewer central effects and reduce the risk of anticholinergic-induced agitation.

Pacemakers and implantable defibrillators

A patient with a pacemaker may request that it be turned off. Although ethically this is accepted as part of withdrawing treatment, it is important to assess fully what is behind the patient's request.[108] It may be because they have the belief that they will not be able to die if it is still functioning or that it will greatly prolong the dying process. Simple reassurance that it is quite possible to die with one functioning may be all that is required. It is also important to counsel the patient and family that the effect of turning the pacemaker to its lowest setting is difficult to predict. If the patient has become totally pacemaker dependent, then death may indeed be hastened or even immediate. However, if the patient is not dependent, little may happen at all, or the symptoms that were present at pacemaker insertion may return just at a time of life when comfort is mandatory.

The issue of reprogramming an implantable cardioverter–defibrillator (ICD) to pacemaker mode only is different, but again comes under the ethical heading of withdrawal of treatment.[109,110] Discharge of an ICD in a patient who is dying is highly unlikely to prolong life, for the same reasons as an attempt at CPR is futile. Even patients who are not imminently dying, but who have end-stage heart failure with an ejection fraction of <30%, are unlikely to have significant survival benefit from an ICD.[111–113] However, there is a risk that the dying patient may receive repeated shocks while fully conscious unless the mode of death is asystole.[114,115] It is therefore important that conversations regarding the likely benefits or otherwise of an active ICD should be started as early as possible in patients with severe heart failure so that there is time while the patient is well enough to attend the pacemaker clinic to have the device reprogrammed. However, frequently this does not happen, either because there is little warning of deterioration, because there is staff reticence to broach the subject or patient reluctance to enter discussion. Local systems should therefore be in place for technicians to reprogramme devices in hospital, hospice, or the patients' homes if that is their preferred place of care and they are too unwell to travel to the clinic. In the hospital and hospice setting, magnets big enough to inactivate ICD discharge should be available to use in an emergency but should not be relied upon as the main solution.

Frank and open discussion with the family, carers, and the patient is an important priority, and the discussions should be meticulously documented. Many people have the misperception that 'turning off' an ICD is synonymous with 'turning off' the patient.[116] As is the case

with decisions about CPR, decisions about ICDs should be seen as potentially changing over the months prior to death.[58]

Although reprogramming an ICD is unlikely to result in immediate death, the same is not true for withdrawing mechanical ventricular support (left ventricular assist devices (LVADs)) where the average time to death is 20 min.[117] It is therefore important to have a clear plan to support patient, family, and staff in this event. Initially used as a bridge to therapy, LVADs are increasingly used as 'destination' therapy and survival is improving.[118] This scenario will therefore become familiar to clinicians. Suggested triggers to initiate discussion about withdrawal of LVAD support include declining quality of life, signs of other organ failure, ongoing sepsis, and impending pump failure.[119]

Coordination of care

One of the main potential problems in caring for the dying is fragmentation of care. Heart failure patients may see clinicians from primary, secondary, tertiary, and voluntary sector care. It is not unusual for a patient to be under the care of a different consultant on each hospital admission and a patient may never be reviewed by a cardiologist. There is a risk that each admission only deals with the immediate problem and does not look at the overall situation. Clinic appointments may also only deal with any immediate problem as there are great time constraints in most clinics. The patient may be seen by a succession of different doctors with varying levels of experience. As a result, the risk is that no overall plan is made with the patient and that there is little helpful communication with the primary care physician. Patients often do not know who they should call if they should run into problems and can 'fall between the stools' of the different areas of the health service.

The NHS Cancer Plan of 2000 recognized this as a problem in oncology and introduced the concept of a 'keyworker'.[120] The keyworker has helped the patients' care to be coordinated throughout their illness and has made information and planning consistent. An additional role is to aid communication, particularly between primary and secondary care. The keyworker may be a nurse specialist, doctor, or district nurse depending on the stage of the illness. The keyworker works closely in conjunction with the multidisciplinary team (MDT) which meets to discuss the management of each patient at diagnosis. Many cardiology units are developing the MDT model, with the MDT including cardiologists, heart failure nurse specialists (HFNSs), and cardiac surgeons. In practice, many HFNSs act as keyworkers and have an important role in providing palliative care.[121] Where they have a remit across primary and secondary care, there are significant benefits in end of life planning.[50]

The MDT approach has also been applied in primary care to coordinate end of life care for patients, initially with cancer, but more recently extended to all patients irrespective of diagnosis. Growing from the realization that most inappropriate admissions to hospital at the end of life were out of hours and triggered by poor symptom control and/or caregiver exhaustion, the GSF[10] has been developed and is now recommended by the Department of Health in the UK. The GSF provides a prompt for the primary care MDT to ensure that there is a designated keyworker, that there is coordination with out-of-hours services, that the preferred place of care is known, that financial assistance has been applied for, and that an overall plan of

> **Box 65.1** Suggested patient clinical features for inclusion in Gold Standards Framework meetings
>
> **Cancer**
> - Any patient whose cancer is metastatic or inoperable
> - Patient thought to be in the last year of life by the care team: the 'surprise' question
>
> **Heart failure (at least two)**
> - Chronic heart failure (CHF) NYHA stage III or IV: CHF symptoms at rest
> - Patient thought to be in the last year of life by the care team: the 'surprise' question
> - Repeated hospital admissions with symptoms of heart failure
> - Difficult physical or psychological symptoms despite optimal tolerated therapy
>
> **General indicators**
> - Weight loss: >10% weight loss over 6 months
> - General physical decline
> - Serum albumin <25 g/L
> - Reduced performance status/Karnofsky score <50%
> - Dependence in most activities of daily living

care has been made. Patients are discussed at the GSF meeting if the clinician 'would not be surprised if the patient died in the next year', in addition to other markers (see **Box 65.1**). In practice, primary care clinicians may feel more nervous of recognizing that their heart failure patients are at end-stage compared to cancer patients about whom they may feel more confident, and this is an area where it is helpful for secondary care clinicians to communicate clearly to their colleagues in primary care when patients are reaching the end-stage of their disease.

Difficulties in identifying a time-point at which patients become 'palliative' have led to a more problem- or needs-based approach to identifying the patient with palliative care needs. This approach can be used at any stage, and alongside active heart failure treatment, and shows promise to foster earlier involvement where necessary and prevent a 'too little, too late' access to palliative care. The GSF identified >80% with palliative care needs, and other tools are available such as the validated Needs Assessment Tool—Progressive Disease: Heart Failure (NAT-PD:HF; a clinical consultation aide-memoire to identify and triage concerns) although care with implementation is important.[122,123] A longitudinal observational study of 272 patients admitted with heart failure found that a Kansas City Cardiomyopathy Questionnaire summary score of <29 identified patients with specialist palliative care needs, defined as severe symptoms on the Edmonton Symptom Assessment Scale (area under receiver operating characteristic curve 0.78).[124] This study also showed a strong association between the NAT-PD:HF assessment and patients identified as having specialist palliative care needs. It is notable that of the 27% identified as having specialist palliative care needs, only 24% actually received such care.

Supporting patients' wishes to die in their preferred place is a challenge for those caring for heart failure patients, but not impossible. Dying at home may be possible if the patient has a family or caregiver who concurs with their wish but is less likely if they do not.[125] Support for patients wishing to die at home may come from social service carers, and be helped by coordination with other services such as hospice-at-home, where available; Marie Curie nurses; and out-of-hours palliative care support telephone lines, which exist in many areas of the UK. Other patients may wish to die in their

local hospice. The hospice service is still patchy in the UK but there is a growing recognition and willingness to accept patients with any diagnosis, not just cancer.[126] Knowledge of local services is important for the primary care and cardiology teams so that the best possible option for the patient can be organized.

Summary conclusions

The most important, and potentially the most difficult, aspect of end of life care for patients with heart failure is the recognition that they are now dying. Recognition of the dying patient remains the first step in providing excellent care for those at the very end of life. Taking the patient's current clinical presentation within the context of their individual disease trajectory is vitally important and requires careful assessment. Coordination of care and communication of management plans between clinical teams, ideally using a keyworker such as the HFNS, may help prevent revolving-door admissions during the last few months of life, and prevent an inappropriate emergency admission around the time of death. Advance planning tools, such as GSF, do exist in primary care, and discussion about the stage of the disease and the possible aims of treatment should be a feature of the growing cardiology MDTs. Although prognostication is important, it seems less useful in identifying the patient who would benefit from palliative care. A needs-based, rather than a prognosis-based, approach to identifying such patients appears to work more effectively.

Sensitive communication tailored to individual patients and their family about their understanding and wishes should allow appropriate planning of services and care for patients who prefer to die at home or in a hospice.

Excellent extended team working and communication skills should result in a patient dying in the place of their choice, with their symptoms well controlled, and their family well supported. That the NHS Darzi Report[7] has raised end of life care to a national UK priority is appropriate. Hinton's observations that 'discomfort was not necessarily greatest in those dying from cancer; patients dying from heart failure, or renal failure, or both, had most physical distress ...'[5] should finally be addressed.

REFERENCES

1. Cowie MR, Wood DA, Coats AJ, et al. Survival of patients with a new diagnosis of heart failure: a population based study. *Heart* 2000;**83**(5):505–10.
2. Mills M, Davies HT, Macrae WA. Care of dying patients in hospital. *BMJ* 1994;**309**(6954):583–6.
3. Rogers A, Karlsen S, Addington-Hall JM. Dying for care: the experiences of terminally ill cancer patients in hospital in an inner city health district. *Palliat Med* 2000;**14**(1):53–4.
4. Kennedy C, Brooks-Young P, Brunton GC, et al. Diagnosing dying: an integrative literature review. *BMJ Support Palliat Care* 2014;**4**(3):263–70.
5. Hinton JM. The physical and mental distress of the dying. *Q J Med* 1963;**32**:1–21.
6. Public Health England. *National survey of patient activity data for specialist palliative care services: MDS full report for the year 2013–2014*. 2013. http://www.endoflifecare-intelligence.org.uk/resources/publications/mdsreport2013.

7. Darzi A. *High quality care for all: NHS Next Stage Review final report*. Department of Health, London, 2008.
8. Department of Health. *End of Life Care Strategy—promoting high quality care for all adults at the end of life*. DH, London, 2008.
9. Ellershaw J, Murphy D, Bloger M, Agar R. *The Liverpool Care Pathway for the Dying Patient (LCP)*. 2007. http://www.endoflifecareforadults.nhs.uk/eolc/files/F2091-LCP_pathway_for_dying_patient_Sep2007.pdf.
10. Thomas K. *The Gold Standards Framework: a programme for community palliative care*. 2009. http://www.goldstandardsframework.nhs.uk/.
11. Centeno C, Clark D, Lynch T, et al. Facts and indicators on palliative care development in 52 countries of the WHO European region: results of an EAPC Task Force. *Palliat Med* 2007;**21**(6):463–71.
12. Datla S, Verberkt CA, Hoye A, Janssen DJA, Johnson MJ. Multidisciplinary palliative care is effective in people with symptomatic heart failure: a systematic review and narrative synthesis. *Palliat Med* 2019;**33**(8):1003–16.
13. Aiken LS, Butner J, Lockhart CA, et al. Outcome evaluation of a randomized trial of the PhoenixCare intervention: program of case management and coordinated care for the seriously chronically ill. *J Palliat Med* 2006;**9**(1):111–26.
14. Brännström M, Boman K. Effects of person-centred and integrated chronic heart failure and palliative home care. PREFER: a randomized controlled study. *Eur J Heart Fail* 2014;**16**(10):1142–51.
15. Rogers JG, Patel CB, Mentz RJ, et al. Palliative care in heart failure: the PAL-HF randomized, controlled clinical trial. *J Am Coll Cardiol* 2017;**70**(3):331–41.
16. Sahlen K-G, Boman K, Brännström M. A cost-effectiveness study of person-centered integrated heart failure and palliative home care: based on a randomized controlled trial. *Palliat Med* 2016;**30**:296–302.
17. Sidebottom AC, Jorgenson A, Richards H, et al. Inpatient palliative care for patients with acute heart failure: outcomes from a randomized trial. *J Palliat Med* 2015;**18**(2):134–42.
18. Kluger BM, Miyasaki J, Katz M, et al. Comparison of integrated outpatient palliative care with standard care in patients with Parkinson disease and related disorders: a randomized clinical trial. *JAMA Neurol* 2020;**77**(5):551–60.
19. Quill TE, Abernethy AP. Generalist plus specialist palliative care—creating a more sustainable model. *N Engl J Med* 2013;**368**(13):1173–5.
20. Hippocrates (transl Francis Adams). *Book of Prognostics*. Dodo Press, 2009.
21. Boyd KJ, Murray SA, Kendall M, et al. Living with advanced heart failure: a prospective, community based study of patients and their carers. *Eur J Heart Fail* 2004;**6**(5):585–91.
22. Buetow SA, Coster GD. Do general practice patients with heart failure understand its nature and seriousness, and want improved information? *Patient Educ Couns* 2001;**45**(3):181–5.
23. Murray SA, Boyd K, Kendall M, et al. Dying of lung cancer or cardiac failure: prospective qualitative interview study of patients and their carers in the community. *BMJ* 2002;**325**(7370):929.
24. Rogers AE, Addington-Hall JM, Abery AJ, et al. Knowledge and communication difficulties for patients with chronic heart failure: qualitative study. *BMJ* 2000;**321**(7261):605–7.
25. Exley C, Field D, Jones L, Stokes T. Palliative care in the community for cancer and end-stage cardiorespiratory disease: the views of patients, lay-carers and health care professionals. *Palliat Med* 2005;**19**(1):76–83.

26. Murray SA, Kendall M, Boyd K, Sheikh A. Illness trajectories and palliative care. *BMJ* 2005;**330**(7498):1007–11.
27. Gott M, Barnes S, Parker C, *et al.* Dying trajectories in heart failure. *Palliat Med* 2007;**21**(2):95–9.
28. Taylor P, Dowding D, Johnson M. Clinical decision making in the recognition of dying: a qualitative interview study. *BMC Palliat Care* 2017;**16**:11.
29. Office for National Statistics. *Mortality statistics: general.* DH1 No 36 2003. 2009. http://www.statistics.gov.uk/downloads/theme_health/Dh1_36_2003/DH1_2003.pdf.
30. Gadoud A, Kane E, Macleod U, *et al.* Palliative care among heart failure patients in primary care: a comparison to cancer patients using English family practice data. *PLoS One* 2014;**9**(11):e113188.
31. Gadoud A, Kane E, Oliver SE, *et al.* Palliative care for non-cancer conditions in primary care: a time trend analysis in the UK (2009–2014). *BMJ Support Palliat Care* 2020 Jan 13. bmjspcare-2019-001833 (online ahead of print).
32. Mancini DM, Eisen H, Kussmaul W, *et al.* Value of peak exercise oxygen consumption for optimal timing of cardiac transplantation in ambulatory patients with heart failure. *Circulation* 1991;**83**(3):778–86.
33. Metra M, Nodari S, Parrinello G, *et al.* The role of plasma biomarkers in acute heart failure. Serial changes and independent prognostic value of NT-proBNP and cardiac troponin-T. *Eur J Heart Fail* 2007;**9**(8):776–86.
34. Metra M, Nodari S, Parrinello G, *et al.* Worsening renal function in patients hospitalised for acute heart failure: clinical implications and prognostic significance. *Eur J Heart Fail* 2008;**10**(2):188–95.
35. Rothenburger M, Wichter T, Schmid C, *et al.* Aminoterminal pro type B natriuretic peptide as a predictive and prognostic marker in patients with chronic heart failure. *J Heart Lung Transplant* 2004;**23**(10):1189–97.
36. Koelling TM, Joseph S, Aaronson KD. Heart failure survival score continues to predict clinical outcomes in patients with heart failure receiving beta-blockers. *J Heart Lung Transplant* 2004;**23**(12):1414–22.
37. Lee DS, Austin PC, Rouleau JL, *et al.* Predicting mortality among patients hospitalized for heart failure: derivation and validation of a clinical model. *JAMA* 2003;**290**(19):2581–7.
38. Levy WC, Mozaffarian D, Linker DT, *et al.* The Seattle Heart Failure Model: prediction of survival in heart failure. *Circulation* 2006;**113**(11):1424–33.
39. Barnes S, Gott M, Payne S, *et al.* Predicting mortality among a general practice-based sample of older people with heart failure. *Chronic Illn* 2008;**4**(1):5–12.
40. Haga K, Murray S, Reid J, *et al.* Identifying community based chronic heart failure patients in the last year of life: a comparison of the Gold Standards Framework Prognostic Indicator Guide and the Seattle Heart Failure Model. *Heart* 2012;**98**(7):579–83.
41. Murray SA, Kendall M, Grant E, *et al.* Patterns of social, psychological, and spiritual decline toward the end of life in lung cancer and heart failure. *J Pain Symptom Manage* 2007;**34**(4):393–402.
42. Rogers A, Addington-Hall JM, McCoy AS, *et al.* A qualitative study of chronic heart failure patients' understanding of their symptoms and drug therapy. *Eur J Heart Fail* 2002;**4**(3):283–7.
43. Barnes S, Gott M, Payne S, *et al.* Communication in heart failure: perspectives from older people and primary care professionals. *Health Soc Care Commun* 2006;**14**(6):482–90.
44. Barclay S, Momen N, Case-Upton S, Kuhn I, Smith E. End-of-life care conversations with heart failure patients: a systematic

literature review and narrative synthesis. *Br J Gen Pract* 2011;**61**(582):e49–e62.
45. Davison SN, Simpson C. Hope and advance care planning in patients with end stage renal disease: qualitative interview study. *BMJ* 2006;**333**(7574):886.
46. Fallowfield LJ, Jenkins VA, Beveridge HA. Truth may hurt but deceit hurts more: communication in palliative care. *Palliat Med* 2002;**16**(4):297–303.
47. Michel DM, Moss AH. Communicating prognosis in the dialysis consent process: a patient-centered, guideline-supported approach. *Adv Chronic Kidney Dis* 2005;**12**(2):196–201.
48. Gott M, Small N, Barnes S, Payne S, Seamark D. Older people's views of a good death in heart failure: implications for palliative care provision. *Soc Sci Med* 2008;**67**(7):1113–21.
49. Small N, Barnes S, Gott M, *et al.* Dying, death and bereavement: a qualitative study of the views of carers of people with heart failure in the UK. *BMC Palliat Care* 2009;**8**:6.
50. Johnson M, Parsons S, Raw J, Williams A, Daley A. Achieving preferred place of death—is it possible for patients with chronic heart failure? *Br J Cardiol* 2009;**16**:194–6.
51. Agard A, Hermeren G, Herlitz J. Should cardiopulmonary resuscitation be performed on patients with heart failure? The role of the patient in the decision-making process. *J Intern Med* 2000;**248**(4):279–86.
52. British Medical Association. *Decisions relating to cardiopulmonary resuscitation: Guidance from the British Medical Association, the Resuscitation Council (UK) and the Royal College of Nursing.* 2016. https://www.bma.org.uk/advice/employment/ethics/ethics-a-to-z/decisions-relating-to-cpr.
53. Schneiderman LJ, Jecker NS, Jonsen AR. Medical futility: its meaning and ethical implications. *Ann Intern Med* 1990;**112**(12):949–54.
54. Schneiderman LJ, Jecker NS, Jonsen AR. Medical futility: response to critiques. *Ann Intern Med* 1996;**125**(8):669–74.
55. Swanson JW, McCrary SV. Medical futility decisions and physicians' legal defensiveness: the impact of anticipated conflict on thresholds for end-of-life treatment. *Soc Sci Med* 1996;**42**(1):125–32.
56. Vayrynen T, Kuisma M, Maatta T, Boyd J. Medical futility in asystolic out-of-hospital cardiac arrest. *Acta Anaesthesiol Scand* 2008;**52**(1):81–7.
57. British Medical Association. *Decisions relating to cardiopulmonary resuscitation: A joint statement from the British Medical Association, the Resuscitation Council (UK) and the Royal College of Nursing*, pp. 1–26. 2007.
58. Withell B. Patient consent and implantable cardioverter defibrillators: some palliative care implications. *Int J Palliat Nurs* 2006;**12**(10):470–5.
59. Sudore RL, Lum HD, You JJ, *et al.* Defining advance care planning for adults: a consensus definition from a multidisciplinary Delphi panel. *J Pain Symptom Manage* 2017;**53**(5):821–832.
60. Jimenez G, Tan WS, Virk AK, *et al.* Overview of systematic reviews of advance care planning: summary of evidence and global lessons. *J Pain Symptom Manage* 2018;**56**(3):436–459.
61. Kernick LA, Hogg KJ, Millerick Y, *et al.* Does advance care planning in addition to usual care reduce hospitalisation for patients with advanced heart failure: a systematic review and narrative synthesis. *Palliat Med* 2018;**32**(10):1539–51.

62. Denvir M, Cudmore S, Highet G, et al. Phase 2 randomised controlled trial and feasibility study of future care planning in patients with advanced heart disease. Sci Rep 2016;6:24619.

63. Wong F, Yuet K. Effects of a transitional palliative care model on patients with end-stage heart failure: a randomised controlled trial. Heart 2016;102(14):1100–8.

64. Rogers JG, Patel CB, Mentz RJ, et al. Palliative care in heart failure: the PAL-HF randomized, controlled clinical trial. J Am Coll Cardiol 2017;70(3):331–41.

65. Johnson MJ, McSkimming P, McConnachie A, et al. The feasibility of a randomised controlled trial to compare the cost-effectiveness of palliative cardiology or usual care in people with advanced heart failure: two exploratory prospective cohorts. Palliat Med 2018;32(6):1133–41.

66. Costantini M, Romoli V, Leo SD, et al. Liverpool Care Pathway for patients with cancer in hospital: a cluster randomised trial. Lancet 2014;383(9913):226–37.

67. Sykes N. One Chance to Get it Right: understanding the new guidance for care of the dying person. Br Med Bull 2015;115(1):143–50.

68. Abernethy AP, Currow DC, Frith P, et al. Randomised, double blind, placebo controlled crossover trial of sustained release morphine for the management of refractory dyspnoea. BMJ 2003;327(7414):523–8.

69. Currow DC, Ward AM, Abernethy AP. Advances in the pharmacological management of breathlessness. Curr Opin Support Palliat Care 2009;3(2):103–6.

70. Jennings L. Systematic review of the use of opioid drugs in the palliative treatment of dyspnoea. Palliat Med 1999;13(4):354.

71. Johnson MJ, McDonagh TA, Harkness A, McKay SE, Dargie HJ. Morphine for the relief of breathlessness in patients with chronic heart failure—a pilot study. Eur J Heart Fail 2002;4(6):753–6.

72. Oxberry SG, Torgerson DJ, Bland JM, et al. Short-term opioids for breathlessness in stable chronic heart failure: a randomized controlled trial. Eur J Heart Fail 2011;13(9):1006–12.

73. Oxberry SG, Bland JM, Clark AL, Cleland JG, Johnson MJ. Repeat dose opioids may be effective for breathlessness in chronic heart failure if given for long enough. J Palliat Med 2013;16(3):250–5.

74. Johnson MJ, Cockayne S, Currow DC, et al. Oral modified release morphine for breathlessness in chronic heart failure: a randomised placebo-controlled trial. ESC HF Open 2019;6:1149–60.

75. Johnson MJ, Bland JM, Oxberry SG, Abernethy AP, Currow DC. Opioids for chronic refractory breathlessness: patient predictors of beneficial response. Eur Respir J 2013;42(3):758–66.

76. Verberkt CA, van den Beuken-van Everdingen MHJ, Schols JMGA, et al. Respiratory adverse effects of opioids for breathlessness: a systematic review and meta-analysis. Eur Respir J 2017;50(5). pii: 1701153.

77. Currow DC, McDonald C, Oaten S, et al. Once daily opioids for chronic dyspnoea: a dose increment and pharmacovigilance study. J Pain Symptom Manage 2011;42(3):388–99.

78. Ekstrom MP, Bornefalk-Hermansson A, Abernethy AP, Currow DC. Safety of benzodiazepines and opioids in very severe respiratory disease: national prospective study. BMJ 2014;348:g445.

79. Bajwah S, Davies JM, Tanash H, et al. Safety of benzodiazepines and opioids in interstitial lung disease: a national prospective study. Eur Respir J 2018;52(6):1801278.

80. Department of Health Renal National Service Framework Team, Marie Curie Palliative Care Institute. Guidelines for LCP Drug Prescribing in Advanced Chronic Kidney Disease (estimated GFR rate <30mls/min). 2008. http://www.renal.org/pages/media/Guidelines/National%20LCP%20Renal%20Symptom%20Control%20Guidelines%20(05.06.08)%20(printable%20pdf).pdf.

81. Verma AK, da Silva JH, Kuhl DR. Diuretic effects of subcutaneous furosemide in human volunteers: a randomized pilot study. Ann Pharmacother 2004;38(4):544–9.

82. Goenaga MA, Millet M, Sanchez E, et al. Subcutaneous furosemide. Ann Pharmacother 2004;38(10):1751.

83. Zacharias H, Raw J, Nunn A, Parsons S, Johnson M. Is there a role for subcutaneous furosemide in the community and hospice management of end-stage heart failure? Palliat Med 2011;25(6):658–63.

84. Dormans TP, van Meyel JJ, Gerlag PG, et al. Diuretic efficacy of high dose furosemide in severe heart failure: bolus injection versus continuous infusion. J Am Coll Cardiol 1996;28(2):376–82.

85. Swan F, Booth S. The role of airflow for the relief of chronic refractory breathlessness. Curr Opin Support Palliat Care 2015;9(3):206–11.

86. Johnson MJ, Abernethy AP, Currow DC. Gaps in the evidence base of opioids for refractory breathlessness. A future work plan? J Pain Symptom Manage 2012;43(3):614–24.

87. Luckett T, Phillips J, Johnson MJ, et al. Contributions of a hand-held fan to self-management of chronic breathlessness. Eur Resp J 2017;50(2):1700262.

88. Barnes-Harris MMM, Swan F, Allgar V, et al. Battery operated fan and chronic breathlessness: does it help? BMJ Support Palliat Care 2019;9(4):478–81.

89. Clark AL, Johnson MJ, Fairhurst C, et al. Long term oxygen therapy for quality of life for people with chronic heart failure: a pragmatic, mixed-methods randomized controlled trial. Health Technol Assess 2015;19:1–148.

90. Currow DC, Agar M, Smith J, Abernethy AP. Does palliative home oxygen improve dyspnoea? A consecutive cohort study. Palliat Med 2009;23(4):309–16.

91. Booth S, Wade R. Oxygen or air for palliation of breathlessness in advanced cancer. J R Soc Med 2003;96(5):215–18.

92. Schwartzstein RM, Lahive K, Pope A, Weinberger SE, Weiss JW. Cold facial stimulation reduces breathlessness induced in normal subjects. Am Rev Respir Dis 1987;136(1):58–61.

93. Uronis HE, Abernethy AP. Oxygen for relief of dyspnea: what is the evidence? Curr Opin Support Palliat Care 2008;2(2):89–94.

94. Simon ST, Higginson IJ, Booth S, Harding R, Bausewein C. Benzodiazepines for the relief of breathlessness in advanced malignant and non-malignant diseases in adults. Cochrane Database Syst Rev 2010;(1):CD007354.

95. de Graeff A, Dean M. Palliative sedation therapy in the last weeks of life: a literature review and recommendations for standards. J Palliat Med 2007;10(1):67–85.

96. Bausewein C, Booth S, Gysels M, Higginson I. Non-pharmacological interventions for breathlessness in advanced stages of malignant and non-malignant diseases. Cochrane Database Syst Rev 2008;(2):CD005623.

97. Farquhar, MC, Prevost AT, McCrone, P. et al. The clinical and cost effectiveness of a Breathlessness Intervention Service for patients with advanced non-malignant disease and their informal carers: mixed findings of a mixed method randomised controlled trial. Trials 2016; 17, 185.

98. Farquhar MC, Prevost A, McCrone P, et al. Is a specialist breathlessness service more effective and cost-effective for patients with advanced cancer and their carers than standard care? Findings of a mixed-method randomised controlled trial. BMC Med 2014;12(1):194.

99. Higginson IJ, Bausewein C, Reilly CC, *et al.* An integrated palliative and respiratory care service for patients with advanced disease and refractory breathlessness: a randomised controlled trial. *Lancet Respir Med* 2014;**2**(12):979–87.

100. Johnson MJ, Kanaan M, Richardson G, *et al.* A randomised controlled trial of three or one breathing technique training sessions for breathlessness in people with malignant lung disease. *BMC Med* 2015;**13**:213.

101. Brighton LJ, Miller S, Farquhar M, *et al.* Holistic services for people with advanced disease and chronic breathlessness: a systematic review and meta-analysis. *Thorax* 2019;**74**:270–81.

102. Tan LB, Bryant S, Murray RG. Detrimental haemodynamic effects of cyclizine in heart failure. *Lancet* 1988;**1**(8585):560–1.

103. Wee B, Coleman P, Hillier R, Holgate S. Death rattle: its impact on staff and volunteers in palliative care. *Palliat Med* 2008;**22**(2):173–6.

104. Wee BL, Coleman PG, Hillier R, Holgate SH. The sound of death rattle. II: How do relatives interpret the sound? *Palliat Med* 2006;**20**(3):177–81.

105. Wee BL, Coleman PG, Hillier R, Holgate SH. The sound of death rattle. I: Are relatives distressed by hearing this sound? *Palliat Med* 2006;**20**(3):171–5.

106. Bennett M, Lucas V, Brennan M, *et al.* Using anti-muscarinic drugs in the management of death rattle: evidence-based guidelines for palliative care. *Palliat Med* 2002;**16**(5):369–74.

107. Wee B, Hillier R. Interventions for noisy breathing in patients near to death. *Cochrane Database Syst Rev* 2008;(1):CD005177.

108. Mueller PS, Hook CC, Hayes DL. Ethical analysis of withdrawal of pacemaker or implantable cardioverter–defibrillator support at the end of life. *Mayo Clin Proc* 2003;**78**(8):959–63.

109. Berger JT. The ethics of deactivating implanted cardioverter defibrillators. *Ann Intern Med* 2005;**142**(8):631–4.

110. Berger JT, Gorski M, Cohen T. Advance health planning and treatment preferences among recipients of implantable cardioverter defibrillators: an exploratory study. *J Clin Ethics* 2006;**17**(1):72–8.

111. Ermis C, Lurie KG, Zhu AX, *et al.* Biventricular implantable cardioverter defibrillators improve survival compared with biventricular pacing alone in patients with severe left ventricular dysfunction. *J Cardiovasc Electrophysiol* 2004;**15**(8):862–6.

112. Setoguchi S, Nohria A, Rassen JA, Stevenson LW, Schneeweiss S. Maximum potential benefit of implantable defibrillators in preventing sudden death after hospital admission because of heart failure. *Can Med Assoc J* 2009;**180**(6):611–16.

113. Marijon E, Trinquart L, Otmani A, *et al.* Competing risk analysis of cause-specific mortality in patients with an implantable cardioverter–defibrillator: the EVADEF cohort study. *Am Heart J* 2009;**157**(2):391–7.

114. Nambisan V, Chao D. Dying and defibrillation: a shocking experience. *Palliat Med* 2004;**18**(5):482–3.

115. Goldstein NE, Lampert R, Bradley E, Lynn J, Krumholz HM. Management of implantable cardioverter defibrillators in end-of-life care. *Ann Intern Med* 2004;**141**(11):835–8.

116. Stromberg A, Fluur C, Miller J, *et al.* ICD recipients' understanding of ethical issues, ICD function, and practical consequences of withdrawing the ICD in the end-of-life. *Pacing Clin Electrophysiol* 2014;**37**(7):834–42.

117. Brush S, Budge D, Alharethi R, *et al.* End-of-life decision making and implementation in recipients of a destination left ventricular assist device. *J Heart Lung Transplant* 2010;**29**(12):1337–41.

118. Long JW, Healy AH, Rasmusson BY, *et al.* Improving outcomes with long-term 'destination' therapy using left ventricular assist devices. *J Thorac Cardiovasc Surg* 2008;**135**(6):1353–60.

119. Lemond L, Allen LA. Palliative care and hospice in advanced heart failure. *Prog Cardiovasc Dis* 2011;**54**(2):168–78.

120. Department of Health. *The NHS cancer plan: a plan for investment, a plan for reform.* DH, London, 2000.

121. Johnson MJ, MacCallum A, Butler J, *et al.* Heart failure specialist nurses' use of palliative care services: a comparison of surveys across England in 2005 and 2010. *Eur J Cardiovasc Nurs* 2012;**11**(2):190–6.

122. Waller A, Girgis A, Davidson PM, *et al.* Facilitating needs-based support and palliative care for people with chronic heart failure: preliminary evidence for the acceptability, inter-rater reliability, and validity of a needs assessment tool. *J Pain Symptom Manage* 2013;**45**:912–25.

123. Janssen DJ, Boyne J, Currow DC, *et al.* Timely recognition of palliative care needs of patients with advanced chronic heart failure: a pilot study of a Dutch translation of the Needs Assessment Tool: Progressive Disease—Heart Failure (NAT:PD-HF). *Eur J Cardiovasc Nurs* 2019;**18**(5):375–88.

124. Campbell RT, Petrie MC, Jackson CE, *et al.* Which patients with heart failure should receive specialist palliative care? *Eur J Heart Fail* 2018;**20**(9):1338–47.

125. Agar M, Currow DC, Shelby-James TM, *et al.* Preference for place of care and place of death in palliative care: are these different questions? *Palliat Med* 2008;**22**(7):787–95.

126. Gibbs LM, Khatri AK, Gibbs JS. Survey of specialist palliative care and heart failure: September 2004. *Palliat Med* 2006;**20**(6):603–9.

66

Monitoring

Martin R. Cowie, Andrew R. Harper, and Arvind Singhal

Introduction

Heart failure is typically a chronic syndrome with the risk of episodic deterioration ('decompensation') that requires adjustment of therapy and/or admission to hospital. Overall, the aims of therapy are to stabilize the syndrome, improve the prognosis and quality of life, and to avoid hospitalization if possible.

International guidelines recommend that patients be enrolled in a disease management programme to help ensure that they receive appropriate multi-professional input to their treatment, education, and monitoring. Management programmes have been designed to help fill the gap that often existed between discharge from hospital and the traditional clinic review—the so-called 'vulnerable' or high-risk period when the risk of clinical deterioration is highest. In the UK, despite such programmes becoming more widespread, only 58% of patients are reviewed by specialist heart failure nurses at any point after leaving hospital,[1] and such review often occurs many weeks after returning home.[2] It is perhaps not surprising that readmission rates remain high: 40% of European patients are readmitted within 12 months of leaving hospital.[3] Not all of these readmissions are necessarily preventable, but wide variation in such readmission rates suggests considerable room for improvement in many local services. As part of a wider National Health Service (NHS) strategy, there has been increased focus on 'telehealth' (healthcare at a distance, i.e. review and monitoring of patients away from traditional healthcare settings) in order to relieve the burden on outpatient departments. In the UK, hospital outpatient appointments have doubled in the past 10 years[4] but the NHS has been set a target of reducing face-to-face outpatient attendances by a third;[5] in order to achieve this the traditional model of outpatient care will have to change, with a greater focus on monitoring at home and in the community, or with review by telemedicine. The COVID-19 pandemic accelerated many of these planned changes while face-to-face clinic appointments were not possible because of social distancing and 'shielding' measures.

This chapter discusses the key elements of monitoring: including what and who should be monitored, the frequency of monitoring, and the different methods of monitoring. Patients are becoming more actively involved in their care, with self-monitoring and management achievable for many, with appropriate professional support.

Advances in digital technologies look promising, but require robust assessment to ensure that integration of such technologies improves the outcome and/or experience of care.

National and international recommendations on monitoring

a. *National Institute for Health and Care Excellence (NICE).* Professional guidelines from NICE in England recommend regular monitoring and clinical assessment for all patients with chronic heart failure, by a member of the specialist heart failure team.[6] Monitoring should include:
   - clinical assessment of functional capacity, fluid status, cardiac rhythm (a minimum of examining the pulse), cognitive status and nutritional status;
   - review of medication, including the need for changes and possible side-effects;
   - assessment of renal function, including measurement of serum electrolytes, creatinine, and estimated glomerular filtration rate (eGFR).

Sensibly, NICE also states that the frequency of monitoring should depend on the clinical status and stability of the patient: the monitoring interval should be short (days to 2 weeks) if the clinical condition or medication has changed, but is needed at least 6-monthly for stable patients. More detailed monitoring is required if patients have significant co-morbidity or if their condition has deteriorated since the previous review. Monitoring of blood pressure and renal function is required after initiation and dose uptitration of angiotensin converting enzyme (ACE) inhibitors, angiotensin receptor blockers, sacubitril–valsartan, and mineralocorticoid receptor antagonists.

The most recent update (2018) also allows for the use of serial N-terminal pro B-type natriuretic peptide (NT-proBNP) monitoring for treatment optimization for patients aged <75 years who have heart failure with reduced ejection fraction (HFrEF) and eGFR >60 mL/min/1.73 m².

Importantly, NICE recognized that patients may wish to be involved in monitoring, and clearly states that such individuals

should be provided with sufficient education and support from their healthcare professionals to do this, with clear guidelines as to what to do in the event of deterioration.

NICE guidelines have not made a recommendation regarding the use of 'telemonitoring' (including structured telephone support) owing to the heterogeneity of type of intervention and trial results making the evidence difficult to interpret. The evidence is discussed below in more detail. NICE has published 'Quality Standards' for heart failure.[7,8] These are concise statements designed to drive measurable improvements in patient safety, patient experience and/or clinical effectiveness. These include three standards related to monitoring (Box 66.1).

b. *Scottish Intercollegiate Guideline Network (SIGN).*

SIGN released their most recent guidance on chronic heart failure in 2016.[9] They are similar to those of NICE, although they specifically excluded appraisal of the evidence on 'tele/video monitoring'. Comprehensive discharge planning was recommended to ensure that links with post-discharge services were in place for all those with symptomatic heart failure. Such comprehensive planning requires communication between primary and secondary care teams, anticipatory care planning, specialist nurse input and (where appropriate) home-based care. Follow-up after discharge by a specialist nurse (with the competence to initiate and adjust medication) was recommended and 'pharmacy input' was highlighted to address the issues of knowledge of drugs and compliance to medication. Feedback to clinicians on possibilities for optimizing drug interventions was also specifically mentioned. No recommendation was made on self-management.

c. *Heart Failure Association of the European Society of Cardiology (ESC).* The ESC also updated its guidance in 2016.[10] It is more supportive of, and specific about, its recommendations on self-monitoring and remote monitoring. It sees multidisciplinary management programmes (with structured follow-up including patient education, optimization of medical treatment, psychosocial support and improved access to care) as fundamental to the delivery of heart failure care (Box 66.2).

Coordinated discharge planning is recommended, starting as soon as a patient is stable in hospital. Providing information and education to support self-care as well as a scheduled outpatient follow-up appointment are stated to reduce the risk of readmission.[10,11]

The ESC guidelines clearly state that monitoring includes self-monitoring, visits to community or hospital clinics, remote monitoring (with or without implanted devices) and 'structured telephone support'. It is recognized that the optimal method of monitoring will depend on local organizations and resources, and will vary depending on the patient. Periods of instability or optimization of medication will require more frequent monitoring, as may older adults, for whom the guideline gives specific recommendations (Box 66.3).[10] The guideline also recommends, based on limited evidence, that referral to primary care for long-term follow-up may be considered for stable patients.

The ESC guideline does not recommend 'broad application' of serial measurement of natriuretic peptides to monitor patients, recognizing the inconsistency of randomized trials of such an approach, which we discuss below.

Similarly, the ESC guideline recognizes the variation in results of randomized trials of remote patient management—with positive results from meta-analysis of small studies, but neutral results from larger randomized trials. The recommendation is made to assess each 'type' of telemedical approach on its own merits. The guideline does, however, give a class IIb (evidence less well established), level B (single randomized trial) recommendation for two technologies: an implantable pulmonary artery pressure monitoring system (CardioMEMS™ device), and call-centre- based remote monitoring of a single manufacturer's implantable defibrillator/resynchronization technology. The relevant trials are discussed further below.

In general, most modern heart failure programmes combine several different approaches to monitoring, and attempt to tailor the monitoring frequency and modality to the needs of the patient

(within what is possible with the resources and skills available locally). Such a tailored approach, matching the model of care to the severity of the condition, is in keeping with current health care policy in the developed world. Meta-analysis suggests that the various types of disease management programmes are similarly effective in terms of reducing mortality and rehospitalizations.[12] A large randomized study from the Netherlands confirms the value of a more tailored approach, reporting that more intensive management for *all* patients is not necessarily better than a less intensive approach tailored to the needs of the individual patients.[13]

Models of monitoring

Traditional periodic monitoring

Historically, patients with heart failure were not taught to self-monitor but were reviewed periodically by a doctor working in either primary or secondary care. Even in the high-risk period after hospital discharge it was traditional to arrange clinic review some weeks after discharge. At that visit the doctor would assess the patient and determine whether changes to treatment were required. In the UK, with very few physicians with a special interest in the condition, many patients would be discharged back to primary care review alone. Such patients might perhaps be reviewed in other clinics, due to co-morbidities such as diabetes, where the heart failure syndrome might or might not be reassessed. It is little surprise that this model of monitoring was associated with poor outcomes, including a high rate of emergency rehospitalizations. Such a model is now considered outdated and sub-standard. NICE has specified an early (2-week) review of patients after discharge from hospital[14] (where the cause for admission was heart failure), although this is currently rarely achieved by cardiology services in England (**Figure 66.1**).[2]

Self-monitoring

There is much that patients and their family can do to monitor how well the heart failure syndrome is controlled. Professional monitoring is likely to be supplemental to this self-monitoring. Self-monitoring should facilitate self-*management*, where a patient adjusts therapy depending on the control of the heart failure

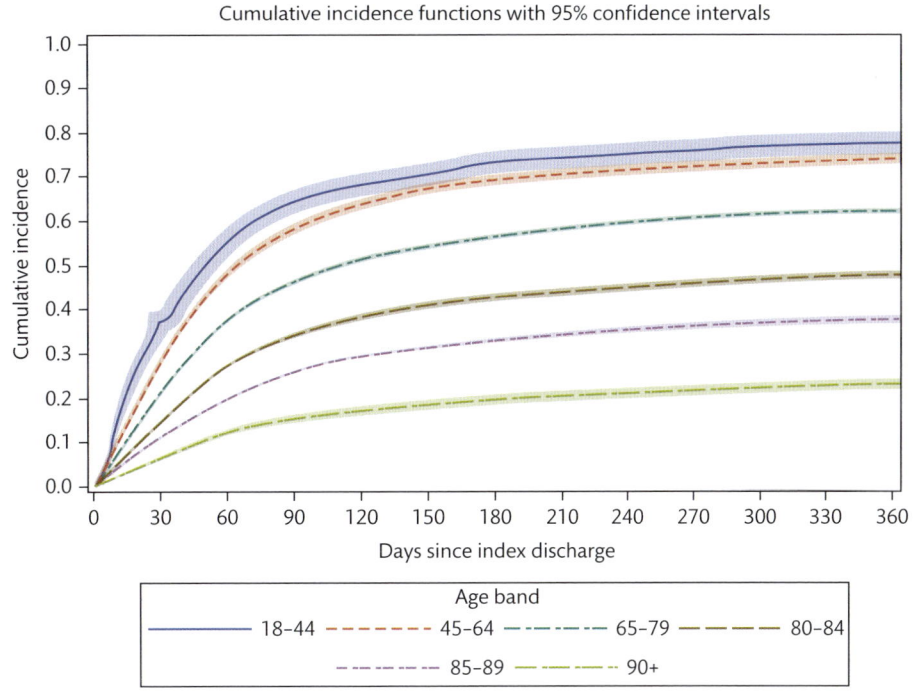

Cumulative incidence functions with 95% confidence intervals

Age band
— 18–44 - - - 45–64 -·-·- 65–79 — — 80–84
-··-··- 85–89 —·—·— 90+

Figure 66.1 Cumulative proportion of patients offered at least one cardiology clinic appointment in the year following a heart failure admission to an English NHS hospital April 2009 to March 2011, by age group.

Reproduced from Bottle A, Goudie R, Bell D, Aylin P, Cowie MR. Use of hospital services by age and comorbidity after an index heart failure admission in England; an observational study. *BMJ Open* 2016;**6**:e010669.

syndrome, particularly by adjusting the dose of diuretic depending on weight changes.

Patients and their families will need advice on how to monitor symptoms easily and on the significance of any changes in symptoms, weight, or other measurements such as blood pressure or pulse. Information (written as well as verbal) on when, and where, to seek professional help can then assist the patient to self-manage.

Patients experience a variety of symptoms, which complicates their ability to recognize the importance of symptoms and to identify their cause as related to heart failure.[15-17] Older age, depression, and cognitive dysfunction may decrease their ability to self-care.

To be effective, self-monitoring requires the local heart failure service to be easily accessible to the patient and their family/carer. Despite the majority of heart failure services providing a telephone advice line (at least during working hours, Monday through Friday), a proportion of patients will be reluctant to use this for fear of interrupting the professional and due to uncertainty regarding the significance of their symptoms. Telemonitoring can be useful in this situation and patients may develop expertise through the timely feedback provided by the monitored data and from the health professional contact triggered by abnormal results.[18]

Remote monitoring

Heart failure typically affects the elderly, and their limited mobility and lack of social support may make hospital clinic attendance problematic. Furthermore, the outbreak of COVID-19 in the UK in Spring 2020 posed significant challenges in attending an outpatient appointment; most face-to-face hospital appointments were cancelled to reduce the risk of transmission. Home visits can bridge the gap, but are costly in terms of travel time for the health professional, limiting the case load that a specialist nurse can take on. Telehealth has the potential to widen access to high-quality care and to provide this care closer to home than when using the traditional hospital-based model. Telemonitoring—the remote monitoring of patients using information technology—has developed rapidly in the past decade. Increasingly, smart phone applications (Apps) are being developed that may be used by patients or their families to assist in self-monitoring and self-care. It may be difficult to establish how well validated these Apps are, and integrating data from these sources is challenging for most healthcare systems. Currently most data from Apps cannot easily be incorporated into electronic health records. Furthermore, clinicians may be reluctant to use this information for fear of generating extra work and uncertainty about the validity of the data. Guidelines are emerging from national and international bodies in an attempt to guide citizens and healthcare professionals in this rapidly expanding, but essentially unregulated, market.

There are several types of remote monitoring, from simple to complex:

1. Structured telephone support from a healthcare professional: patients monitor their symptoms and weight, and report these during a structured telephone call from a healthcare professional;
2. Patient-initiated electronic monitoring with transfer of physiological data and/or symptom record from patients at home (from stand-alone equipment, 'wearable' device, or a smartphone 'App') to the healthcare professional, using a telephone or internet connection;
3. Implanted device monitoring, where a defibrillator or cardiac resynchronization device, or an implanted haemodynamic monitor, can transmit data wirelessly to a near-patient unit connected to a telephone or internet connection and thereby on to the healthcare professional.

What should be monitored?

A summary of what NICE recommends to monitor, as a minimum, has been discussed above. These recommendations are based on expert consensus on good clinical practice, rather than specific randomized controlled trials. The ideal variable to monitor for decompensation would be simple and convenient to measure, reproducible, sensitive and specific to changes in the control of heart failure, and would change rapidly enough to give an early warning that could trigger specific interventions to restabilize the syndrome. No such variable has been identified. In practice, several measurements are relied on to detect decompensation. The patient history, signs and symptoms, supplemented where possible with physiological data, are combined with skilled clinical interpretation.

Symptom monitoring

The signs and symptoms of clinical deterioration of heart failure are typically increasing fluid retention, breathlessness, and effort intolerance, but can include less specific symptoms such as fatigue, cough, and poorer cognition. In many but not all patients and episodes, deterioration is gradual and it should be possible to detect such deterioration if the patient or heart failure team is monitoring the clinical condition. Many patients are aware of symptoms for several weeks but only seek professional help when they become intolerable.[19]

In some patients, and in some episodes, the deterioration may be abrupt and thus could not have been detected earlier by closer monitoring. Such deterioration might occur due to sudden changes in cardiac rhythm (e.g. onset of atrial fibrillation (AF)) or due to incidental chest or urinary tract infection.

Some telemonitoring systems ask patients questions about a range of symptoms which can be useful in identifying deterioration (particularly if combined with daily weight monitoring). From our experience in the Home-HF study,[20] patients often find it difficult to say whether any specific symptom is better or worse than the day before. Changes are often subtle and noticed at different time-points during the day, making it difficult to decide whether they relate to a change in the overall condition, or to differing activities.

The New York Heart Association (NYHA) classification of heart failure provides some structure to symptom monitoring by healthcare professionals by grading the severity of heart failure according to functional limitation, from class I (no symptoms) to class IV (symptoms at rest). It is relatively easy to score but its value is limited by poor sensitivity to small changes and poor reproducibility among clinicians.[21] There is also limited agreement between patients and their clinicians.[22]

Patients tend to measure change in their symptoms by the effect upon their activities of daily living: they may notice a change in their ability to go out shopping, tidy the garden or walk to their friend's house; so behavioural questioning may be more effective at monitoring symptom change. 'Wearables' are sensors externally applied

to the body to measure a physiological signal. Commonly used commercial devices such as FitBit™ or the Apple Watch™ can measure activity, heart rate, and in some cases blood pressure and pulse waveform for arrhythmia detection.[23] Most commercial wearable devices are accurate at measuring activity, but wrist-worn monitors may be less accurate at low speeds and during more sedentary activity. Such systems may be able to send data to the healthcare professional, but integration of such data into the electronic medical record is often not permitted or easily achievable. Wearables have not been extensively studied in heart failure patients, but reduced activity measured by wearables is independently associated with mortality in heart failure.[24,25] They could therefore be used as an objective marker of activity, rather than relying on subjective NYHA classification. They may be used to support and monitor response to exercise training,[26] but the average age at heart failure diagnosis in the UK is 80, and current use of wearables in this age group is low.

The 6 min walk test is a more reliable tool to monitor changes in functional capacity,[27] but is rarely done in routine practice. However, it is of less value where functional capacity is limited by co-morbidity, such as osteoarthritis.

Body weight

An early sign of worsening heart failure in many patients is increasing fluid retention, and in theory daily monitoring of weight using accurate scales should be useful in identifying decompensation early. Such an approach has been standard practice in heart failure management programmes, and has been recommended in many professional guidelines. In the most recent ESC guideline,[10] the professional is advised to provide individualized information, but a recommendation is made that if there is a sudden unexpected weight gain, >2 kg in 3 days, the diuretic dose should be increased and/or the healthcare team contacted. In practice, many patients do use a flexible diuretic regime to control variable fluid retention and/or to ensure the diuresis does not interfere unacceptably with their social commitments.

For more effective monitoring, the weight increase should be the weight above 'dry' weight; that is, the steady weight achieved following any change in diuretic therapy and where there are no signs of fluid overload. To allow for normal weight change, 'dry' weight should be recalculated periodically (every 1–2 months). This is particularly important after discharge from hospital when patients generally feel better and start to eat more, and therefore may put on muscle or fat rather than merely fluid weight. In more advanced heart failure, where cachexia may supervene, a patient's 'dry' weight may decrease and a previously stated target weight may be inappropriate—with the patient remaining very congested at that weight. For weight monitoring to be reliable it requires consistency in its monitoring and patients should be encouraged to wear similar clothing and weigh themselves at the same time each morning.

Despite the widespread use of weight monitoring, its accuracy is limited. Lewin and colleagues recruited patients with established heart failure (70% diagnosed with heart failure with a reduced ejection fraction (HFrEF)) and compared the patients' daily weight diary against clinical examination.[28] They concluded that a weight gain >2 kg over 48–72 h demonstrated good specificity (97%) but poor sensitivity (9%) for predicting clinical deterioration. A weight increase of >2% above dry weight had a similar specificity (94%) with only marginal improvement in sensitivity (17%). Although such weight increase is highly specific for decompensation, these results suggest that *the lack of such a change cannot be taken to exclude decompensation*. Attention must therefore also be directed at assessment of symptoms or other physiological measurements that may reflect overall heart failure status. Patients who are able to self-care should also bear in mind that whereas weight monitoring is useful, they should seek help if they notice an increase in symptoms regardless of any weight change.

Data from a home telemonitoring study in patients with HFrEF also showed that relying only on weight monitoring is unlikely to be of great value in detecting decompensation, even when using more complex calculations of weight change. Weight gain started around 14 days prior to hospital admission with worsening heart failure, but substantial weight gain was seen in only ~20% of patients.[29] Recent evidence suggests that for patients with heart failure and preserved ejection fraction, a rapid weight gain or rise in plasma natriuretic peptide concentration may be more sensitive for impending decompensation than in patients with HFrEF.[30]

It may be that the cause of decompensation influences the number of days over which weight gain occurs. For example, weight gain resulting from worsening left ventricular function or non-adherence to ACE inhibitors or β-blockers may be more insidious, whereas infection, arrhythmias, or non-compliance with diuretic medication may cause a more rapid increase in volume, and may even precipitate heart failure decompensation before any change in weight is noticed.

Despite the above limitations, daily weight measurement is easy to monitor and is still considered the cornerstone of daily monitoring in most heart failure management programmes. It is best combined with monitoring of other variables, including symptoms.

Peripheral oedema/swollen ankles

Monitoring of ankle swelling is a routine component of clinical monitoring for heart failure deterioration. However, perhaps as much as 5 L of excess fluid is present before oedema is noticed by most patients. Patients frequently find it difficult to identify when their ankles are more swollen than usual and may only notice change when it is so severe that they no longer can wear their normal shoes.

In the patient with venous insufficiency, it may be difficult to distinguish dependent oedema resulting from heart failure from the normal state. Often the oedema is asymmetrical, particularly if the patient has had venous harvesting for bypass surgery, and patients often concentrate on the better leg, denying that fluid is building up.

In some patients, particularly those with poor right ventricular function or tricuspid regurgitation, accumulation of fluid may be more marked in the abdomen than in the legs. Patients may notice an increase in girth, with their clothes or belt becoming tighter, or increased pulsation or 'fullness' in their neck as the venous pressure increases. In our experience, it is rare for patients to identify decompensation early through these signs.

Blood pressure

Detection of significant hypotension (including postural hypotension) is important in the clinical review of a patient. It may point towards intravascular fluid depletion due to excessive diuretic usage, or low cardiac output, or sepsis, or inappropriately high dosage of neurohormonal antagonists. For some patients, the control of hypertension is also critical to the control of the heart failure syndrome.

Many patients monitor their own blood pressure at home, and it can be easily monitored remotely.

Arrhythmia

Arrhythmia is common in patients with heart failure. Ventricular arrhythmia may be life-threatening and atrial arrhythmia (e.g. AF) may cause symptom deterioration. Both complicate management decisions. Heart rate monitoring (supplemented by rhythm monitoring if possible and appropriate) may help identify problems that require further investigation.

Single-lead ECG monitoring has been added to external telemonitoring equipment. However, it increases the complexity of monitoring and to date there is no evidence of additional benefit.[31,32] Heart rate monitoring alone is easier and may be sufficient in many cases. Recent developments in technology allow ECG recording from single-lead ECG devices that transmit recordings to smartphones and subsequently the cloud, such as KardiaMobile™. These patient-activated ECG recorders are commonly used for the detection of AF, which in heart failure patients is usually an indication for anticoagulation. NICE 'Medtech Innovation Briefings' provide a framework for 'prescription' of such devices for AF detection, and innovation and technology tariffs offer reimbursement to ensure no net cost to local healthcare services. Some 'smart' watches, such as the Apple™ Watch, have algorithms that analyse pulse waveforms looking for irregular patterns that suggest AF. The Apple heart study[33] showed that such a smart watch algorithm coupled with more extended ECG monitoring resulted in the identification of AF in 34% of patients with an irregular pulse notification who requested and returned the ECG monitor, though the prognostic significance of short, asymptomatic runs of AF is unknown.[34]

Where devices such as cardiac resynchronization therapy (CRT) or a dual-chamber implantable cardioverter defibrillator (ICD) are implanted, device interrogation or remote monitoring can provide potentially continuous information (but more typically reviewed daily or weekly) on both heart rate and rhythm. The evidence that such, more detailed, monitoring can be used to improve the outcome for patients is limited, and is discussed further below.

'Standard' blood tests

Renal function is often abnormal in patients with heart failure, and deterioration is associated with a poor prognosis. Intercurrent illness (such as infection) can have a profound effect on renal function, as can the introduction and uptitration of therapies such as ACE inhibitors, angiotensin receptor blockers, β-blockers, mineralocorticoid receptor antagonists, or sacubitril/valsartan. Regular monitoring of serum biochemistry (especially serum potassium, urea, and creatinine) is important and structured follow-up can ensure that this is not missed. Biochemistry should be checked within two weeks of the introduction or uptitration of new medication and otherwise at a minimum of 6-monthly intervals. Intercurrent illness should trigger a check of heart failure status, including renal function. The introduction of drugs such as non-steroidal anti-inflammatory drugs (either prescribed or over the counter) can markedly impair renal function in patients with heart failure, particularly in combination with renin–angiotensin–aldosterone system inhibition.

Other blood tests may be required as part of routine monitoring: anaemia is increasingly common as heart failure advances, as is diabetes, so a check on the full blood count and plasma glucose

should be made periodically. Thyroid and liver function may be deranged by amiodarone. Urate is often high in patients with heart failure on diuretic therapy, and repeated attacks of acute gout may occur if allopurinol is not used.

Plasma natriuretic peptide serial monitoring

Several randomized trials have assessed whether the serial measurement of plasma natriuretic peptides (NPs) such as BNP or NT-proBNP might aid the management of heart failure. Early studies suggested the clinical outcome was better if a target BNP or NT-proBNP was used to titrate diuretics and ACE inhibitors, but larger randomized trials found little evidence of benefit. The GUIDE-IT study randomized 894 patients with HFrEF to either an NT-proBNP-guided strategy (with a goal of achieving NT-proBNP levels <1000 pg/mL) or usual care, and found no difference in outcomes between the groups.[35] Recent systematic reviews and individual patient data meta-analyses have not demonstrated clear benefit overall;[36,37] however, in patients aged <75 years there is moderate evidence of a reduction in hospitalization with NP monitoring compared with standard clinical monitoring, and an additional reduction in death when compared with no monitoring according to NICE's own literature review and individual patient data meta-analyses.[6] The accompanying recommendation is somewhat guarded as the evidence is described as moderate to low quality: 'Consider measuring NT-proBNP (N-terminal pro-B-type natriuretic peptide) as part of a treatment optimization protocol only in a specialist care setting for people aged under 75 who have heart failure with reduced ejection fraction and an eGFR above 60 mL/min/1.73 m²'.

The current ESC guideline does not recommend routine use of serial monitoring of natriuretic peptides.[10]

The degree to which plasma natriuretic peptides fall during a hospitalization for heart failure is a good indicator of the subsequent risk of readmission, and might be used to target closer follow-up for some patients when the plasma level fails to fall during admission.[38] Home-based testing of natriuretic peptides is now possible, and a pilot study has shown reasonable patient compliance with daily monitoring out to 2 months,[39] but the clinical effectiveness (and value for money) of this approach remains to be determined.

Monitoring adherence to medication

Monitoring adherence to medication is problematic but it is estimated that between 20% and 50% of patients mismanage their medication.[40,41] Patients with heart failure are likely to have multiple co-morbidities, cognitive decline, social isolation, and depression, all of which adversely affect their ability to adhere to medication regimes.

Patients may choose not to comply with medication from concern about side-effects or they may simply forget; they may be unable to refill the drug prescription, or be unsure how to take the medication or of its value. In some countries there may be economic constraints. Non-adherence to medication has been implicated in possibly as many as 30% of hospital admissions with heart failure.[42] Electronic monitoring of medication adherence is possible and may provide insights into particular issues. Some telemonitoring systems also provide reminders to patients regarding their medication, and recent development in smartphone technologies may have value—such as automatic or triggered SMS/text or App-based reminders.

Nutrition

Weight loss indicates a poor prognosis in heart failure. Contributing factors may include inadequate dietary intake, loss of appetite, mal-absorption of nutrients, or gut symptoms.

The simplest method to monitor nutritional status is through the recording of body weight: a decrease of >6% of total body weight within 6 months is suggestive of cachexia. Monitoring of appetite and interest in eating can easily become part of regular monitoring, and may identify potential malnutrition. To date, no specific interventions have shown promise for treating cardiac cachexia over and above standard disease modifying heart failure medication use.

Anxiety, depression, cognitive dysfunction, and frailty

As many as 40% of patients with heart failure may become moderately depressed or anxious.[43,44] Depression is an independent risk factor for mortality,[45] increases symptom reporting,[44] decreases quality of life, and (alongside anxiety) may decrease self-care ability. There is evidence that cognitive behavioural therapy (but not anti-depressants) can improve depression in patients with heart failure, but self-care does not necessarily improve.[46,47] Screening for depression can be performed rapidly using tools such as the Patient Health Questionnaire (two-question initial screen, followed by the more specific nine-question version).[48]

Cognitive decline through age, depression, or chronic illness is also a potential influence on patient outcome and is likely to make self-care more difficult. Traditionally, the Mini-Mental State Examination was recommended for cognitive testing, but this may be time-consuming in routine clinical practice, and more rapid assessments can be provided by using tools such as the six-item Cognitive Impairment Test[49] or the five-item General Practitioner Assessment of Cognition tool.[50]

Frailty is increasingly recognized as a marker of poor outcome, and the need for more health and social care support.[51] NICE suggests that this can be assessed rapidly in the clinic setting by asking a patient to rate their health on a scale from 0 (worst) to 10 (best), with a score of ≤6 indicating frailty, or the 'timed get up and go' test with times of >12 s indicating frailty.[52] Such tests are not reliable if performed when an individual is acutely unwell.

Structured remote monitoring

Telephone monitoring

One of the first large randomized trials of structured telephone support for patients with heart failure—the DIAL trial—enrolled 1518 stable outpatients in Argentina, and used a centralized call-centre together with protocol-driven telephone calls focusing on symptom monitoring, adjustment of medication, and patient education.[53] All telephone calls were nurse-initiated: initially at two-weekly intervals, after which the frequency was based on the clinical condition. The study population was young with a mean age of 65 years and 80% had HFrEF. There was a statistically significant 20% reduction in the number of patients who died or were admitted to hospital with heart failure, driven by a reduction in the number of patients admitted with worsening heart failure. Mortality was unaffected. Importantly, patients were generally on evidence-based medication

at randomization but more patients in the control arm stopped taking their medication or reported non-adherence with other lifestyle advice, demonstrating the potential benefit of regular monitoring on adherence with treatment of proven benefit.

Other studies of telephone monitoring in different healthcare settings provide further evidence of benefit, and, when combined in a recent meta-analysis of 25 studies (9332 participants), demonstrated a 13% reduction in all-cause mortality (95% confidence interval (CI): 2–23) out to 6–12 months, and heart failure-related hospitalizations (15%; 7–23), but not all-cause hospitalization. There was no convincing demonstration of reduction in length of stay for hospitalizations, nor of value for money, but adherence and patient satisfaction appeared good, at least in the randomized trial setting.[54] The limitations of such models are that the telephone calls are primarily initiated by the professional at pre-set times (usually protocol-driven) and they are thus unable to detect more rapid changes in the condition.

Telemonitoring of non-implanted devices

Telemonitoring uses patient-initiated remote electronic monitoring and involves the transmission of information from patients (usually in their home) to health professionals (Figure 66.2).[55] Data transmission can be by landline, broadband, or mobile signal either to a web-based platform or to a specific monitoring interface.

The privacy and security of personal data are of concern to patients, healthcare professionals, and regulators. It is important that the monitoring data are encrypted before being transferred through the home telephone line, mobile phone, or via the internet. Access to any monitoring 'station' should also be secure, with access restricted to those with a legitimate interest in the data and the patient's management. Web-based applications can easily be password-protected, but concerns regarding the storage of data on servers in countries with less stringent data protection rules than in the UK and EU can cause problems.

Telemonitoring enables frequent (usually daily) assessment of clinical variables by a health professional, the possibility of early identification of clinical deterioration, and earlier intervention. Intervention can be as simple as reinforcing the need to adhere to medication and lifestyle measures, or more complex such as increasing diuretic dose, or clinical review by the primary or secondary care physician or heart failure team. In some telemonitoring programmes, patients can activate the system in an emergency, talk to a healthcare professional, and can even summon emergency transfer to the emergency room. Most telemonitoring programmes do not have such a 'panic' button, and are typically operated by a specialist centre Monday through Friday during working hours, or through a call-centre which can triage information on a 24/7 basis.

There is no consensus as to which variables provide the most useful data. There is a balance between accurate patient assessment and overburdening the patient.

A meta-analysis of 18 randomized trials of non-invasive telemonitoring (total of 3860 participants) reported a 20% reduction in all-cause mortality (95% CI: 6–32), and a 29% reduction in heart failure-related hospitalizations (95% CI: 17–40) (but not all-cause hospitalization) typically over 6–12 months after hospital discharge. Not all reported an improvement in quality of life, and there was no evidence that length of stay was reduced. Few studies reported

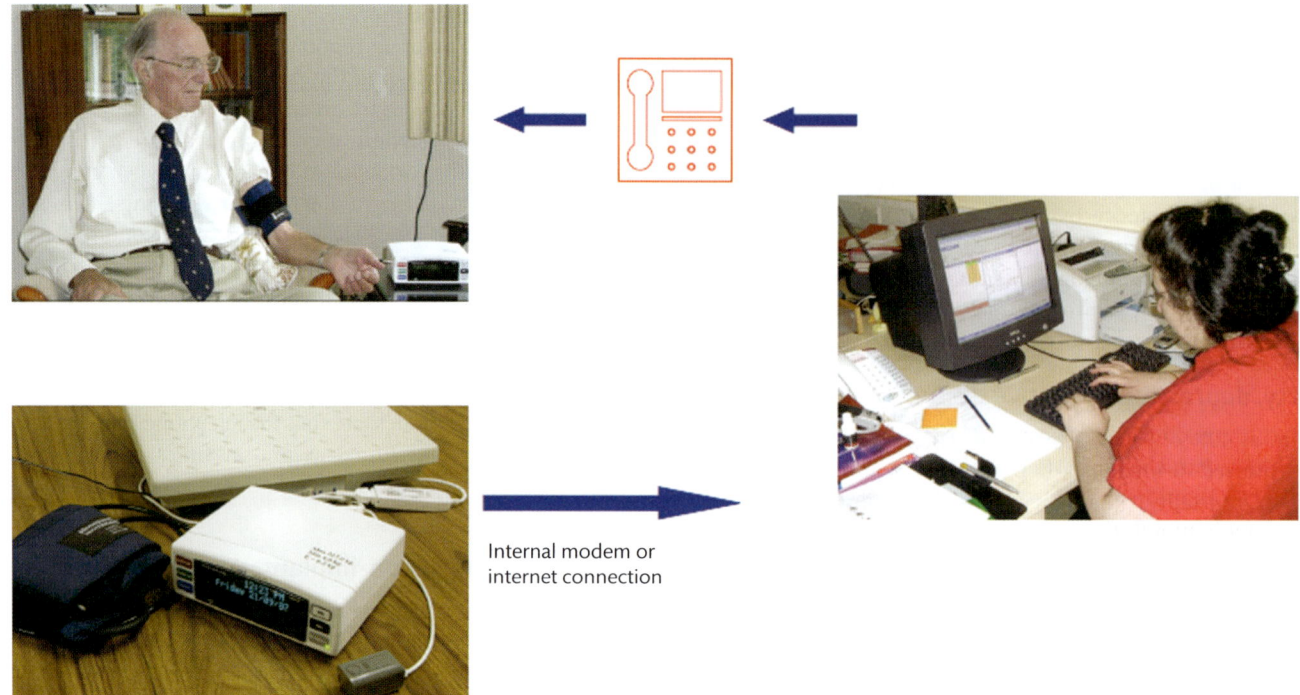

Internal modem or
internet connection

Figure 66.2 The telemonitoring cycle: data collected from the patient is transmitted to the healthcare professional, who views the data and its trends, and may telephone the patient to make a fuller assessment of his condition before giving advice or arranging clinical review.
Reproduced from Riley J, Cowie MR. Telemonitoring in heart failure. *Heart* 2009;**95**:1964–1968 with permission from *BMJ*.

the cost impact of their programmes: but of those who did, more reported an increase in cost, due to the technology and monitoring and the increased medical management.[54]

One of the largest and most recent randomized trials, BEAT-HF, randomized 1437 patients aged ≥50 years who had been hospitalized for heart failure in six academic centres in California, USA. It reported no improvement in mortality or hospitalization over usual care out to 6 months, despite intensive monitoring of blood pressure, heart rate, weight, and symptoms combined with health coaching calls and a nurse telemonitoring centre.[56] There was a small difference in heart-failure-related quality of life, which achieved statistical significance (4 points on the Minnesota Living with Heart Failure questionnaire; $P = 0.02$). This neutral result was similar to the largest European-based randomized trial (Telemedical Interventional Monitoring in Heart Failure study (TIM-HF)) of 710 patients.[57] The larger follow-up study, TIM-HF2, randomized 1571 patients with NYHA II or III heart failure who had been hospitalized for heart failure in the preceding 12 months either to telemonitoring plus usual care or to usual care only. It reported reduced hospitalized days and all-cause mortality in the telemonitoring group, but importantly this study excluded patients with NYHA class I or IV heart failure and those with depression.[58]

In the UK, a more broadly based randomized trial of telemonitoring of 3230 patients with heart failure, chronic lung disease, or diabetes, based in 179 primary care centres in England, demonstrated a reduction in emergency room visits and all-cause hospitalizations,[59] but came at a cost that is currently unaffordable at more than £90,000 per QALY (quality-adjusted life-year).[60]

In a decision-analysis model of cost-effectiveness for patients recently discharged from hospital after a heart failure exacerbation,

another UK analysis based on a network meta-analysis reported an incremental cost-effectiveness of £11,873 per QALY, representing reasonable value for money in the NHS, but, of course, increased expenditure would be needed to reap the benefits.[61]

Important questions remain about the optimal model of remote monitoring, and the patients most likely to benefit. The cost and organizational changes required to run such a service appear large, and may not reflect good value for money at the present time. The less expensive the home monitoring equipment and any associated monitoring charge, and the larger the number of patients who can be monitored by an individual service, the greater the value for money; however, there are likely to be limits to how many patients an individual healthcare professional can follow at any point in time.

In light of the above data, it is perhaps not surprising that current UK and European heart failure guidelines do not support routine remote monitoring for patients with heart failure.[6,9,10] Part of the difficulty with standalone remote monitoring systems is that they still only monitor episodically, rather than continuously, and require patient engagement. Technologies in development may change this over the coming years, as continuous monitoring becomes more easily integrated into 'patches' and 'smart' textiles. The LINK-HF study trialled a multiparameter patch sensor with monitoring of ECG, intrathoracic impedance (an indirect marker of pulmonary fluid content), movement, and temperature. From these physiological data a personalized algorithm was derived that could prospectively predict heart failure decompensation with a sensitivity of 76% and a specificity of 85%, and thereby potentially prevent hospitalization,[62] though further research is required to see if altering therapy in response to these signals is effective at preventing decompensation.

Telemonitoring of devices implanted for therapeutic reasons

Rapid advances in healthcare technology have led to the possibility of remotely monitoring physiological variables using devices implanted for therapeutic reasons, such as cardiac resynchronization therapy (CRT) and/or an implantable cardioverter–defibrillator (ICD). Using a Bluetooth-enabled bedside monitoring device, the patient can be remotely monitored, with the automatic transfer of data to a web-based server via mobile networks. If a patient feels unwell, or has concerns about their heart or device function (e.g. they may be concerned that they have received a shock but are not sure), they can trigger a download from the device to the health professional. Some remote monitoring systems automatically communicate with implanted devices and upload regular reports. Using a web-based system, the professional can monitor device performance and safety, in addition to a large number of physiological variables.

Such remote monitoring reduces rather than eliminates all face-to-face contact, and an annual face-to-face clinic visit to review the implanted device function is still recommended.[63] An audit at our centre demonstrated a 70% reduction in face-to-face pacing clinic visits with the introduction of remote monitoring: in 84% of the remote scheduled pacing checks, no further action was required.[64] A recent survey of cardiologists involved with the European Heart Rhythm Association (EHRA) Electrophysiology Research Network identified a lack of reimbursement (80% of 43 centres) as a major barrier to the introduction of remote monitoring services for patients with implanted devices in Europe.[65] Additional workload was also identified as a significant barrier, although most cardiologists considered remote monitoring as clinically useful, with significant benefits for patients and healthcare organizations.

'Diagnostic' capabilities of such implanted devices include monitoring of intrathoracic impedance, heart rate variability, nocturnal heart rate, patient activity, occurrence of atrial and ventricular arrhythmia, variation in intensity of heart sounds, severity of sleep disordered breathing, and sleeping position (equivalent to detection of orthopnoea).

A further design feature of the modern generation of cardiac implantable electronic devices (CIEDs) has been use of automated 'alerts', sent to either the patient and/or the healthcare professional, when monitored variables exceed pre-determined thresholds considered to indicate heart failure deterioration or a clinical change that may require intervention (e.g. onset of atrial fibrillation, a defibrillator shock, or intrathoracic impedance falling and thus suggesting increased lung congestion). Several studies have explored the use of triggered alerts from monitoring of intrathoracic impedance alone, but this appears to have poor sensitivity and specificity for decompensation and has been shown to drive unnecessary admissions to hospital.[66] The Optimization of Heart Failure Trial Intrathoracic Impedance Monitoring (using such 'alerts') found that this monitoring strategy was not superior to routine care in avoiding death or hospitalization related to cardiovascular causes.[67] In another (non-randomized) trial, such remote notifications reduced time to clinical decision-making, chiefly by the detection of atrial arrhythmia lasting >12 h, but this did not translate into a reduction in the risk of hospitalization.[68]

In contrast to single-variable 'alert-based' monitoring approaches, observational data suggest that use of a combined heart failure

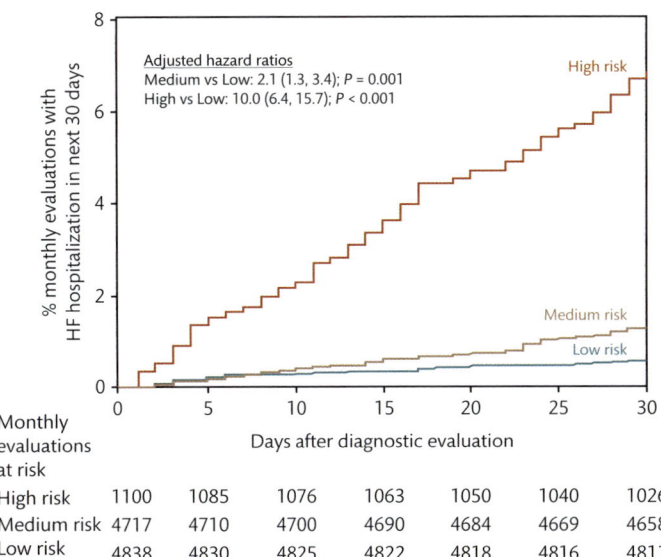

Figure 66.3 Kaplan–Meier curves for time to first heart failure hospitalization after monthly diagnostic evaluation for the different multiparametric risk score groups in a validation set of 1310 patients with an average follow-up duration of 8.1 ± 5.0 months.

Reproduced from Cowie MR, Sarkar S, Koehler J, *et al.* Development and validation of an integrated diagnostic algorithm derived from parameters monitored in implantable devices for identifying patients at risk for heart failure hospitalization in an ambulatory setting. *Eur Heart J* 2013;**34**:2472–80.

diagnostic algorithm might identify patients at higher risk of hospitalization for heart failure within the next 30 days.[69,70] It is possible to identify patients at a much higher risk of decompensation by applying an algorithm to trends in a *number* of variables remotely monitored by CRT or ICD systems (**Figure 66.3**).[70] 'High'-risk individuals at a 10-fold increased risk of decompensation in the next month compared to 'low'-risk individuals can be identified, although the absolute risk remained low—at about 7%. It is important, therefore, that the healthcare professional monitoring the data does not over-react, as this could lead to increased clinical activity (such as clinic review or hospitalization) without necessarily improving outcome.

The Implant-based Multiparameter Telemonitoring of Patients with Heart Failure (IN-TIME) study tested CIED monitoring of tachyarrhythmia, sub-optimal biventricular pacing, increased ventricular extrasystolic activity, and decreased patient activity with daily data downloads sent to a single monitoring centre.[71] Comparing this strategy with usual care for 12 months in 664 patients across 36 centres, there was an improvement in a combined end-point of death from any cause, NYHA class change, and patient global self-assessment. The study demonstrated reduced mortality in the monitored group, although this effect may have been expressed principally in patients with atrial fibrillation. The current ESC guidelines have chosen to select this positive study to make a class IIB, level B recommendation that multiparameter monitoring based on an ICD 'may be considered' in symptomatic patients with HFrEF (LVEF ≤35%) in order to improve clinical outcomes.[10]

Subsequent trials have shown mixed results. The Monitoring Resynchronization devices and cardiac patients (MORE-CARE) was stopped early because of slow enrolment, with 865 of a planned 1720 enrolled.[72] At 24 months follow-up in these patients (who were enrolled within eight weeks of an implant of a CRT-D device),

remote monitoring using an 'alert' for intrathoracic impedance and atrial tachyarrhythmias did not result in any difference in the primary end-point of all-cause mortality or hospitalization for cardiovascular or device-related reasons, although there was a modest cost saving for both patients and the healthcare system. The MultiSENSE study used a multiparameter algorithm combining heart sounds, respiration, thoracic impedance, heart rate, and activity to produce a personalized 'score' (HeartLogic score); a score above the determined threshold had a 70% sensitivity and 86% specificity for predicting heart failure decompensation,[73] but using this score to guide therapy is still under evaluation (NCT03237858).

In the UK, Remote Management of Heart Failure using Implantable Electronic Devices (REM-HF) reported the results of remote monitoring guided management in 1650 patients randomized at nine hospitals, with an average follow-up of more than two years.[74] There was no difference in mortality or hospitalization, or quality of life, between those in the usual care arm, or those who were additionally remotely monitored using their CIED. Subgroup analyses failed to identify a group for which the intervention was effective, including those with a history of atrial fibrillation.

Translating additional physiological information from CIEDs into action that improves outcome is clearly not straightforward, and further work is required to determine which combination of variables might be useful in decision-making, and how such decision-making can be supported to add value at a reasonable cost.

Telemonitoring of implantable haemodynamic monitors

The situation with implanted haemodynamic monitoring may be more promising. The CardioMEMS™ device (a small device implanted in a peripheral pulmonary artery at right heart catheterization) has been the subject of one randomized controlled trial in the USA, showing a 30% reduction in the risk of heart failure hospitalization in NYHA Class III patients when physicians acted on pulmonary pressure collected daily from the patients at home.[75] Extension of the data collection period suggested that the effect was likely to be sustainable.[76] Confirmation in a non-US setting is awaited, with studies in several other countries including the UK underway.[77] Cost-effectiveness may be a challenge in the European setting, where the cost of hospitalizations (avoided) is substantially lower than in the USA.[78]

Another haemodynamic monitoring system, collecting data from the left atrium, has been developed. In 2016, the LAPTOP-HF randomized study (NCT01121107)[79] was stopped early because of concern regarding the risk of implanting the left atrial pressure sensor across the inter-atrial septum. Consequently underpowered, it failed to show a difference in the primary end-point of heart failure and heart-failure-related hospitalizations (relative risk: 0.91; $P = 0.49$). In an analysis using the CHAMPION end-point of heart failure hospitalization alone, data at 12 months suggested that there may be a similar reduction in the heart failure hospitalization risk with pulmonary artery pressure monitoring (hazard ratio: 0.57; $P = 0.003$; 0.40 events per patient year for the treatment group versus 0.70 for controls), but, once again, this requires prospective confirmation. A newer left atrial pressure monitoring device is being studied for safety and efficacy (NCT03775161).

Frequency of monitoring

It is often not possible, or indeed necessary, to follow all patients with the same level of intensity. The period of greatest vulnerability remains the period immediately following hospital discharge. Only a minority of patients is readmitted, but it is best to schedule a review soon after hospital discharge and preferably within 2 weeks. A major difficulty in establishing the frequency of subsequent follow-up is the substantial difference in the intensity of interventions in the randomized trials of heart failure management programmes, with follow-up varying from a single home visit to weekly home visits for older or unstable patients. The positive outcomes of the early studies were largely derived from trials in HFrEF where 'usual' care was very poor. The generalizability to current patients, particularly where 'usual' care has improved, is unclear. More intensive monitoring for all patients, whether with face-to-face meetings (COACH),[13] simple home monitoring (BEAT-HF; TIM-HF),[56,57] or monitoring of CRT/ICD systems (REM-HF)[74] does not appear to add value, and comes with considerable potential organizational disruption.

Who should be monitored more frequently?

A six-monthly clinical review, including a check of symptom control, cardiac rhythm, medication, and blood chemistry may be sufficient when the patient's condition is stable. An annual review by a cardiologist may also be useful. Patients with advanced heart failure, those undergoing therapy changes and those with a history of frequent decompensation are likely to benefit from more frequent monitoring. Patients with multiple co-morbidities or renal failure, the elderly or those on multiple medications may also benefit from more frequent monitoring, but this must be done carefully to prevent too many visits or medication changes.

Patients with CIEDs will require technical checks on the devices.[63] The value of routinely monitoring the physiological variables that such devices can collect remains to be proven. Patients with long-term ventricular assist devices will have follow-up organized by the implanting centre, as will patients after heart transplantation.

Where should monitoring take place?

Current UK government policy promotes healthcare that is easily accessible and adaptive to patient need, with a focus on the delivery of care in the community.[5] A secondary care specialist is usually involved with the initial diagnosis of heart failure and the introduction of medication, but optimization can be safely carried out in primary care if the appropriate interest and expertise is available. This process is best guided by a management plan, shared between primary and secondary care. Once the patient is on optimized medication, the primary care physician and/or community heart failure nurse can continue to monitor the majority of patients with only an annual review by a consultant cardiologist (either in secondary care or a satellite community clinic). If the primary care physician has sufficient expertise, they may be able to take over care of less complicated patients; a Danish randomized study of stable (predominantly NYHA I and II on optimal medical therapy) chronic heart failure patients showed no difference in mortality or hospitalization between patients assigned to extended specialist follow-up or discharge to

primary care.[80] Patients with more complex needs, such as the elderly or those with co-morbidities, and those with more severe heart failure, may benefit from care delivery by a case manager or care co-ordinator (often a community matron) in addition to input from the heart failure multidisciplinary team. Based in primary care, the care co-ordinator is well placed to liaise regularly with the multidisciplinary community health care team and social care services to ensure that the right services are offered at the right time and at the right place.

Who should be involved in monitoring?

Cardiologists and specialist nurses have played a central role in heart failure management in the majority of research studies and are key members of the heart failure team in clinical practice. Not all patients need to be seen at all time-points by a secondary care specialist. Where primary care services are well developed, the general practitioner and community nurse should be involved in the routine monitoring of the stable patient. Monitoring must be incorporated into the activities of the multidisciplinary team,[81] with timely (and accurate) communication between primary, secondary, and tertiary care being vital. Where monitoring also involves technical checks on implanted devices, good communication must be established between those responsible for the technology and the heart failure multidisciplinary team.

Healthcare professional education

Education and training underpin effective monitoring. Sub-specialist heart failure training is now recognized in the UK but there are differences in medical specialist training across Europe. The European Heart Failure Curriculum for Nurses has attempted to provide some standardization, but heart failure education is usually local and country specific. In the UK, nurses and some allied professionals (such as pharmacists) obtain further qualifications to expand their role to include the prescription of medications and so manage their own patient caseload. Training in remote monitoring is essential, as it requires decision making in response to different cues than is usual in traditional face-to-face clinical contacts. There is the risk that more data leads to more frequent, but not necessarily effective, changes in the management plan and increased health care utilization. Remote monitoring cannot replace more traditional care, but where it is used it should be integrated into a multi-professional disease management programme, enabling more patients to access high-quality care.

Conclusions

Monitoring of patients with heart failure happens in a variety of settings. The level of complexity varies from patient to patient, and varies during the course of an individual's illness. Organizations need to develop systems that are adaptive and individualized, adding and removing components as needs change. For patients with advanced heart failure, where transplantation or mechanical circulatory support is not an option, decisions will be needed on when to stop monitoring for the active control of heart failure and move towards monitoring purely for symptom relief and end of life care.

The field of remote monitoring is maturing, but recent results suggest that we need to learn more about integrating the technology into health care decision making. A new generation of technologies, enabling better identification of patients who require specific (and different) intervention, or that provide a new therapeutic target (such as pulmonary artery pressure) show promise, but we are some distance away from the disruptive changes in healthcare delivery that have been promised for so long.

Ultimately, although the health care professionals are important, patients and their families are central to the success of monitoring. Education and support for them is likely to pay dividends.

REFERENCES

1. National Institute for Cardiovascular Outcomes Research (NICOR), Institute of Cardiovascular Science, University College London. *National Heart Failure Audit 2017/18.* https://www.nicor.org.uk/wp-content/uploads/2019/09/Heart-Failure-2019-Report-final.pdf.
2. Bottle A, Goudie R, Bell D, Aylin P, Cowie MR. Use of hospital services by age and comorbidity after an index heart failure admission in England; an observational study. *BMJ Open* 2016;**6**:e010669.
3. Maggioni AP, Dahlstrom U, Filippatos G, *et al.* EURObservational Research Programme: regional differences and 1-year follow-up results of the Heart Failure Pilot Survey (ESC-HF Pilot). *Eur J Heart Fail* 2013;**15**:808–17.
4. NHS Digital. Hospital outpatient activity, 2017–18. National statistics. https://digital.nhs.uk/data-and-information/publications/statistical/hospital-outpatient-activity/2017-18.
5. NHS England. The NHS long term plan. January 2019. Available at: https://www.longtermplan.nhs.uk/publication/nhs-long-term-plan/.
6. National Institute for Health and Care Excellence. *Chronic heart failure in adults: diagnosis and management (NH106).* https://www.nice.org.uk/guidance/ng106.
7. National Institute for Health and Care Excellence. Quality standards for chronic heart failure (QS9). https://www.nice.org.uk/guidance/qs9.
8. National Institute for Health and Care Excellence. *Quality standards for acute heart failure* (QS103). https://www.nice.org.uk/guidance/qs103.
9. Scottish Intercollegiate Guidelines Network (SIGN). *Management of chronic heart failure.* Edinburgh: SIGN; March 2016. SIGN publication no. 147. http://www.sign.ac.uk.
10. Ponikowski P, Voors AA, Anker SD, *et al.* ESC Guidelines for the diagnosis and treatment of acute and chronic heart failure. *Eur Heart J* 2016;**37**:2129–200.
11. Bradley EH, Sipsma H, Horwitz LI, *et al.* Hospital strategy uptake and reductions in unplanned readmission rates for patients with heart failure: a prospective study. *J Gen Intern Med* 2015;**30**:605–11.
12. Roccaforte R, Demers C, Baldassarre F, *et al.* Effectiveness of comprehensive disease management programmes in improving clinical outcomes in heart failure patients. A meta-analysis. *Eur J Heart Fail* 2005;**7**:1133–44.

13. Jaarsma T, van der Wal M, Lesman-Leegte I, *et al.* Effect of moderate or intensive disease management program on outcome in patients with heart failure. *Arch Intern Med* 2008;**168**:316–24.

14. National Institute for Health and Care Excellence. *Acute heart failure: diagnosis and management (CG187).* https://www.nice.org.uk/guidance/cg187.

15. Rogers A, Addington-Hall J, Abery A, *et al.* Knowledge and communication difficulties for patients with chronic heart failure. *BMJ* 2000;**321**:605–7.

16. Horowtiz CR, Rein SB, Leventhal H. A story of maladies, misconceptions and mishaps: Effective management of heart failure. *Social Sci Med* 2004;**58**:631–43.

17. Clark AM, Freydberg CN, McAlister FA, *et al.* Patient and informal caregivers' knowledge of heart failure: necessary but insufficient for effective self-care. *Eur J Heart Fail* 2009;**11**:617–21.

18. Riley JP, Gabe JP, Cowie MR. Does telemonitoring in heart failure empower patients for self-care? A qualitative study. *J Clin Nurs* 2013;**22**:2444–55.

19. Schiff GD, Fung S, Speroff T, McNutt RA. Decompensated heart failure: symptoms, patterns of onset and contributing factors. *Am J Med* 2003;**114**:625–30.

20. Dar O, Riley J, Chapman C, *et al.* A randomized trial of home telemonitoring in a typical elderly heart failure population in North West London: results of the Home-HF study. *Eur J Heart Fail* 2009;**11**:319–25.

21. Raphael C, Briscoe C, Davies J *et al.* Limitations of the New York Heart Association functional classification system and self-reported walking distances in chronic heart failure. *Heart* 2007;**93**:476–82.

22. Goode KM, Nabb S, Cleland JGF, Clark AL. A comparison of patient and physician-rated New York Heart Association Class in a community-based heart failure clinic. *J Card Fail* 2008;**14**:379–87.

23. Singhal A, Cowie MR. The role of wearables in heart failure. *Curr Heart Fail Rep* 2020;**17**:125–32.

24. Loprinzi PD. The effects of free-living physical activity on mortality after congestive heart failure diagnosis. *Int J Cardiol* 2016;**203**:598–9.

25. Izawa KP, Watanabe S, Oka K, *et al.* Usefulness of step counts to predict mortality in Japanese patients with heart failure. *Am J Cardiol* 2013;**111**(12):1767–71.

26. Alharbi M, Straiton N, Gallagher R. Harnessing the potential of wearable activity trackers for heart failure self-care. *Curr Heart Fail Rep* 2017;**14**(1):23–9.

27. Rostagno C, Olivo G, Comeglio M, *et al.* Prognostic values of 6-minute walk corridor test in patients with mild to moderate heart failure: comparison with other methods of functional evaluation. *Eur J Heart Fail* 2003;**5**:247–52.

28. Lewin J, Ledwidge M, O'Loughlin C, McNally C, McDonald K. Clinical deterioration in established heart failure: what is the value of BNP and weight gain in aiding diagnosis. *Eur J Heart Fail* 2005;**7**:953–7.

29. Zhang J, Goode KM, Cuddihy PE, Cleland JFG. Predicting hospitalisation due to worsening heart failure using daily weight measurement: analysis of the Trans-European Network-Home-Care Management System (TEN-HMS) study. *Eur J Heart Fail* 2009;**11**:420–7.

30. Maisel AS, Shah KS, Barnard D, *et al.* How B-type natriuretic peptide (BNP) and body weight changes vary in heart failure with preserved ejection fraction compared with reduced ejection fraction. secondary results of the HABIT (HF Assessment With BNP in the Home) trial. *J Card Fail* 2016;**22**:283–93.

31. Capomolla S, Pinna G, La Rovere M, *et al.* Heart failure case disease management program: a pilot study of home telemonitoring versus usual care. *Eur Heart J* 2004;**6**(Suppl F1):F91–F98.

32. Cleland JGF, Louis AA, Rigby AS, Janssens U, Balk AHMM. Non-invasive home telemonitoring for patients with heart failure at high risk of recurrent admission and death. *J Am Coll Card* 2005;**45**:1654–64.

33. Perez MV, Mahaffey KW, Hedlin H, *et al.* Large-scale assessment of a smartwatch to identify atrial fibrillation. *N Engl J Med* 2019;**381**(20):1909–17.

34. Mulder BA, Van Gelder IC, Rienstra M. Device-detected atrial fibrillation. *Circulation* 2019;**139**(22):2513–15.

35. Felker GM, Anstrom KJ, Adams KF, *et al.* Effect of natriuretic peptide-guided therapy on hospitalization or cardiovascular mortality in high-risk patients with heart failure and reduced ejection fraction: a randomized clinical trial. *JAMA* 2017;**318**(8):713–20.

36. Balion C, McKelvie R, Don-Wauchope AC, *et al.* B-type natriuretic peptide-guided therapy: a systematic review. *Heart Fail Rev* 2014;**19**:553–64.

37. Troughton RW, Frampton CM, Brunner-La Rocca HP, *et al.* Effect of B-type natriuretic peptide-guided treatment of chronic heart failure on total mortality and hospitalization: an individual patient meta-analysis. *Eur Heart J* 2014;**35**:1559–67.

38. Brunner-La Rocca, H-P, Eurlings L, Richards AM, *et al.* Which heart failure patients profit from natriuretic peptide guided therapy? A meta-analysis form individual patient data of randomized trials. *Eur J Heart Fail* 2015;**17**:1252–61.

39. Bettencourt P, Azevedo A, Pimenta J, *et al.* N-terminal-pro-brain natriuretic peptide predicts outcome after hospital discharge in heart failure patients. *Circulation* 2004;**110**;2168–74.

40. Maisel A, Barnard D, Jaski B, *et al.* Primary results of the HABIT Trial (heart failure assessment with BNP in the home). *J Am Coll Cardiol* 2013;**61**:1726–35.

41. Haynes RB, McDonald HP, Garg AX, Monatgue P. Interventions for helping patients to follow prescriptions for medications. *Cochrane Database Syst Rev* 2002;(2):CD000011.

42. Kripalani S, Yao X, Haynes B. Interventions to enhance medication adherence in chronic medical conditions: a systematic review. Arch Intern Med 2007;**167**:540–9.

43. Guck TP, Elsasser GN, Kavan MG *et al.* Depression and congestive heart failure. *Cong Heart Fail* 2003;**9**:163–9.

44. Ramasamy R, Hildebrandt T, O'Hea E, *et al.* Psychological and social factors that correlate with dyspnea in heart failure. *Psychosomatics* 2006;**47**:430–4.

45. Jiang W, Hasselblad V, Krishnan RR, *et al.* Patients with CHF and depression have greater risk of mortality and morbidity than patients without depression. *J Am Coll Cardiol* 2002;**39**:919–21.

46. Freedland KE, Carney RM, Rich MW, Steinmeyer BC, Rubin EH. Cognitive behaviour therapy for depression and self-care in heart failure patients: a randomized clinical trial. *JAMA Intern Med* 2015;**175**:1773–82.

47. Angermann CE, Gelbrich G, Stork S, *et al.* Effect of escitalopram on all-cause mortality and hospitalization in patients with heart failure and depression: the MOOD-HF Randomized Clinical Trial. *JAMA* 2016;**315**:2683–93.

48. Thibault JM, Steiner RW. Efficient identification of adults with depression and dementia. *Am Fam Physician* 2004;**70**:1101–10.

49. Brooke P, Bullock R. validation of a 6 item cognitive impairment test with a view to primary care usage. *Int J Geriat Psych* 1999;**14**:936–40.

50. Brodaty H, Connors MH, Loy C et al. Screening for dementia in primary care: a comparison of the GPCOG and the MMSE. *Dement Gariatr Cogn Disord* 2016;**42**:323–30.

51. Sze S, Zhang J, Pellicori P, Morgan D, Hoye A, Clark AL. Prognostic value of simple frailty and malnutrition screening tools in patients with acute heart failure due to left ventricular systolic dysfunction. *Clin Res Cardiol* 2017;**106**:533–41.

52. National Institute for Health and Care Excellence. *Multimorbidity: clinical assessment and management.* September 2016. https://www.nice.org.uk/guidance/ng56/.

53. Thompson DR, Roebuck A, Stewart S. Effects of a nurse-led, clinic and home-based intervention on recurrent hospital use in chronic heart failure. *Eur J Heart Fail* 2005;**7**:377–84.

54. Inglis SC, Clark RA, Dierckx R, Prieto-Merino D, Cleland JG. Structured telephone support or non-invasive telemonitoring for patients with heart failure. *Cochrane Database Syst Rev* 2015;(10):CD007228.

55. Riley J, Cowie MR. Telemonitoring in Heart failure. *Heart* 2009;**95**:1964–8.

56. Ong MK, Romano PS, Edgington S, et al. Effectiveness of remote patient monitoring after discharge of hospitalized patients with heart failure: the better effectiveness after transition-heart failure (BEAT-HF) Randomized Clinical Trial. *JAMA Intern Med* 2016;**176**:310–18.

57. Koehler F, Winkler S, Schieber M et al. Impact of remote telemedical management on mortality and hospitalizations in ambulatory patients with chronic heart failure: the telemedical interventional monitoring in heart failure study. *Circulation* 2011;**123**:1873–80.

58. Koehler F, Koehler K, Deckward O, et al. Efficacy of telemedical interventional management in patients with heart failure (TIM-HF2): a randomised, controlled, parallel-group, unmasked trial. *Lancet* 2018;**392**(10152):1047–57.

59. Steventon A, Bardsley M, Billings J, et al. Effect of telehealth on use of secondary care and mortality: findings from the Whole System Demonstrator cluster randomised trial. *BMJ* 2012;**344**:e3874.

60. Henderson C, Kanpp M, Fernandez J-L, et al. Cost effectiveness of telehealth for patients with long term conditions (Whole System Demonstrator telehealth questionnaire study): nested economic evaluation in a pragmatic, cluster randomised controlled trial. *BMJ* 2013;**346**:f1035.

61. Thokala P, Baalbaki H, Brennan A, et al. Telemonitoring after discharge from hospital with heart failure: cost-effectiveness modelling of alternative service design. *BMJ Open* 2013;**3**:e003250.

62. Stehlik J, Schmalfuss C, Bozkurt B, et al. Continuous wearable monitoring analytics predict heart failure hospitalization: the LINK-HF Multicenter Study. *Circ Heart Fail* 2020;**13**(3):e006513.

63. Wilkoff BL, Auricchio A, Brugada J, et al. HRS/EHRA Expert consensus on the monitoring of cardiovascular implantable devices (CIEDI): description of techniques, indications, personnel, frequency and ethical considerations. *Europace* 2008;**10**:707–25.

64. Trembath L, Azucena C, Stain N, Cowie MR. Remote monitoring for CRT-D leads to substantial reduction in the need for 'routine' visits to a pacing clinic. *Eur J Heart Fail* 2009;**8** Suppl 2:112.

65. Mairesse GH, Braunschweig F, Klersy K, Cowie MR, Leyva F. Implementation and reimbursement of remote monitoring for cardiac implantable electronic devices in Europe: a survey from the health economics committee of the European Heart Rhythm Association. *Europace* 2015;**17**:814–18.

66. Van Veldhuisen DJ, Braunschweig F, Conraads V, et al. Intrathoracic impedance monitoring, audible patient alerts, and outcome in patients with heart failure. *Circulation* 2011;**124**:1719–26.

67. Bohm M, Drexler H, Oswald H, et al. Fluid status telemedicine alerts for heart failure: a randomized controlled trial. *Eur Heart J* 2016;**37**:3154–63.

68. Crossley GH, Boyle A, Vitense H, Chang Y, Mead RH; CONNECT Investigators: the CONNECT (Clinical Evaluation of Remote Notification to Reduce Time to Clinical Decision) trial: the value of wireless remote monitoring with automatic clinician alerts. *J Am Coll Cardiol* 2011;**57**:1181–9.

69. Whellan DJ, Ousdigian KT, Al-Khatib SM, et al. PARTNERS Study Investigators. Combined heart failure device diagnostics identify patients at higher risk of subsequent heart failure hospitalizations. Results from PARTNERS HF (Program to Access and Review Trending Information and Evaluate Correlation to Symptoms in Patients With Heart Failure) study. *J Am Coll Cardiol* 2010;**55**:1803–10.

70. Cowie MR, Sarkar S, Koehler J, et al. Development and validation of an integrated diagnostic algorithm derived from parameters monitored in implantable devices for identifying patients at risk for heart failure hospitalization in an ambulatory setting. *Eur Heart J* 2013;**34**:2472–80.

71. Hindricks G, Taborsky M, Glikson M, et al. IN-TIME study group. Implant-based multiparameter telemonitoring of patients with heart failure (IN-TIME): a randomised controlled trial. *Lancet* 2014;**384**:583–90.

72. Boriani G, da Costa A, Quesada A, et al. Effects of remote monitoring on clinical outcomes and use of healthcare resources in heart failure patients with biventricular defibrillators: results of the MORE-CARE multicentre randomized controlled trial. *Eur J Heart Fail* 2017;**19**(3):416–25.

73. Boehmer JP, Hariharan R, Devecchi FG, et al. A multisensor algorithm predicts heart failure events in patients with implanted devices: results from the MultiSENSE study. *JACC Hear Fail* 2017;**5**(3):216–25.

74. Morgan JM, Kitt S, Gill J, et al. Remote management of heart failure using implantable electronic devices. *Eur Heart J* 2017;**38**(30):2352–60.

75. Abraham WT, Adamson PB, Bourge RC, et al. Wireless pulmonary artery haemodynamic monitoring in chronic heart failure: a randomised controlled trial. *Lancet* 2011;**377**:658–66.

76. Abraham WT, Stevenson LW, Bourge RC, et al. Sustained efficacy of pulmonary artery pressure to guide adjustment of chronic heart failure therapy: complete follow-up results from the CHAMPION randomised trial. *Lancet* 2016;**387**:453–61.

77. Cowie MR, de Groote P, McKenzie S, et al. Rationale and design of the CardioMEMS Post-Market Multinational Clinical Study: COAST. *ESC Heart Fail* 2020;**7**(3):865–72.

78. Cowie MR, Simon M, Klein L, Thokala P. The cost-effectiveness of real-time pulmonary artery pressure monitoring in heart failure patients: a European perspective. *Eur J Heart Fail* 2017;**19**(5):661–9.

79. Maurer MS, Adamson PB, Costanzo MR, et al. Rationale and design of the Left Atrial Pressure Monitoring to Optimize Heart Failure Therapy Study (LAPTOP-HF). *J Card Fail* 2015;**21**:479–88.

80. Schou M, Gustafsson F, Videbaek L, et al. Extended heart failure clinic follow-up in low-risk patients: a randomized clinical trial (NorthStar). *Eur Heart J* 2013;**34**(6):432–42.

81. McDonagh TA, Blue L, Clark AL, et al. European Society of Cardiology Heart Failure Association standards for delivering heart failure care. *Eur J Heart Fail* 2011;**13**:235–41.

67

Quality improvement in heart failure

Theresa A. McDonagh

Introduction

Over the last thirty years much progress has been made in the diagnosis and treatment of heart failure. Myriad trials have been done. Numerous national and international guidelines have been written to facilitate translation of the evidence into clinical practice. Yet registries repeatedly show that uptake of known disease-modifying therapies (especially for heart failure with reduced ejection fraction (HFrEF)) is far short of the benchmarks set by clinical trials; and real-world outcomes are much poorer than those seen in the clinical trials.

Data from the most recent chronic heart failure treatment trials, incorporating the latest neurohormonal blockade and device therapies, report one-year mortality rates for New York Heart Association class II/III patients with HFrEF of 8–10%,[1] whereas in real world non-selective registries, in which large numbers of consecutive patients are audited, inpatient mortality rates for patients admitted to hospital with heart failure are ~9% (**Figure 67.1**).[2] One-year mortality rates for patients admitted with heart failure are >30%, both in the UK and the USA.[2,3] Real-world patients with heart failure are, of course, very different from those seen in clinical trials. They are older (median age: 79 years in the UK Heart Failure Audit) and have many more co-morbidities. Recent epidemiological data from the UK indicate the average number of co-morbidities at diagnosis is now 5.2.[4] In contrast to the successful clinical trials in heart failure, that were confined to those with HFrEF, up to 30–50% of patients in registries have heart rate with preserved ejection fraction. To date, there are no disease-modifying therapies for this part of the heart failure spectrum. In addition, for patients presenting acutely to hospital with heart failure we have had no new treatments for more than twenty years. It is not just mortality that is a problem: re-admission to hospital after discharge is very frequent, ranging from 25% to 50% in various surveys. Sobering data such as these have led health care professionals to start focusing on 'quality improvement' in heart failure to try and translate evidence-based-medicine for heart failure into improved outcomes for patients.

Quality improvement initiatives to date include:

* setting standards of care for heart failure;
* implementing multi-professional heart failure care;
* specialization and training for heart failure health care professionals;
* auditing and benchmarking.

Standards of care for heart failure

National and international cardiology and heart failure associations have recognized the need to prioritize improved heart failure care. Standards of care documents have been written to try to operationalize how the clinical practice guidelines can best be implemented.[5] The European position paper on standards of care focuses on how to deliver multi-professional heart failure care. It is recognized that the specifics of a heart failure management programme will vary from site to site, depending on geography and location (urban or rural). However, the goal of all services should be the same: 'to provide a seamless system of care across primary and hospital care so that the management of every patient is optimal, no matter where they begin their health care journey'.

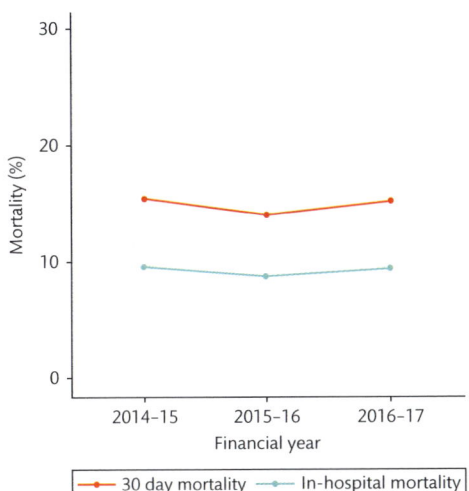

Figure 67.1 Three-year trends of in-hospital mortality and 30-day mortality from admission (2015–2017).
Source data from McDonagh TA. The National Heart Failure Audit Report 2016/17. 2018. www.nicor.ucl.ac.uk.

Delivering multi-professional heart failure care to reduce heart failure rehospitalization and mortality has class 1A evidence in all current heart failure guidelines.[6]

The elements of the heart failure service and how it should operate are crucial. An ideal service should:

- include specialist heart failure cardiologists;
- include specialist heart failure nurses;
- function across sectors of care;
- incorporate heart failure clinics;
- adhere to common guidelines.

Heart failure cardiologists

Evidence for the value of cardiologists has been available for some time. Data from the USA in 1997 showed that specialist cardiology care improved mortality and reduced readmission rates.[7] Consistent data from the UK National Heart Failure Audit (a large real-world registry with >450 000 patient entries over the last nine years) show that patients admitted to hospital under the care of cardiologists have a lower mortality rate than those in general medical wards (**Figure 67.2**).[2,8] In addition, those seen in general medical wards by cardiologists and heart failure nurses have a lower mortality rate. In-hospital mortality rates, adjusted for other known markers of disease severity, are 65% higher for those not admitted under cardiology (P < 0.001). Patients admitted to cardiology wards leave hospital with higher prescription rates for angiotensin converting enzyme inhibitor/β-blockers and mineralocorticoid receptor antagonists for HFrEF than those admitted to general medical wards. These quality care indicators (specifically care delivered by a cardiologist and the use of evidence-based drugs for HFrEF) also translate into improved one-year outcomes compared to general medical care, in both univariate and multivariate analyses (**Figure 67.3**).

That specifically trained heart failure cardiologists have something additional to offer is suggested by research showing that among patients referred by cardiologists for assessment for heart transplantation by the heart failure specialist team, readmission rates to hospital fall markedly with specialist input.[9] Several countries have now introduced heart failure subspecialty training as part of their cardiology training programmes. The USA and the UK have done this for some time. More recently the European Society of Cardiology (ESC) Heart Failure Association (HFA) has introduced a heart failure subspecialist curriculum to serve as a blueprint for European countries to implement.[10]

Heart failure specialist nurses

Many randomized trials of multi-professional care in heart failure have incorporated heart failure specialist nurses. These studies, and meta-analyses thereof, demonstrate that inclusion of specialist heart failure nurses improve both mortality and heart failure hospitalizations.[11]

The role of the heart failure nurse within these programmes is more diverse than that of the cardiologist. Nurses can be involved in nurse-led heart failure clinics, uptitration of therapy, home visits, telephone clinics and/or telemonitoring. A crucial role is that of patient education, particularly in self-management.

The European Society of Cardiology Heart Failure Association has also developed a specialist nursing curriculum to facilitate the adoption of heart failure nurses more widely across Europe.[12]

Function across sectors of care

Ideal heart failure services should involve primary care physicians (general practitioners (GPs)). This is particularly important in health care systems where the GP is the 'gate keeper' to specialist care services. The GP is often the first port of call for patients who have symptoms and signs that may be due to heart failure, and may be the first to be called when a patient deteriorates.

Functioning across sectors of care needs patient pathways to be carefully developed and agreed. It needs to be clear what the GPs should do when diagnosing and treating heart failure. Pathways for suspected heart failure where the GP refers patients to hospital for a firm diagnosis based on natriuretic peptide (NP) concentrations lead to faster and more accurate diagnosis.

Heart failure clinics

Heart failure clinics are an invaluable component of a heart failure service. They should provide access to a heart failure cardiologist. The clinics can be multi-professional and include nurses providing education for patients as well as uptitrating heart failure therapies in a supportive environment with access to a cardiologist. Diagnostic one-stop heart failure clinics to which GPs can refer patients suspected of having heart failure with an abnormal ECG or NP can offer a high-quality, rapid confirmation of the diagnosis.

Follow-up clinics should also be provided. Data on follow-up for stable patients is somewhat lacking. Most guidelines suggest 6-monthly follow-up with biochemistry checks and a yearly ECG to look for a widening QRS duration, for stable patients. Unstable patients or those recently discharged from hospital will require frequent follow-up.

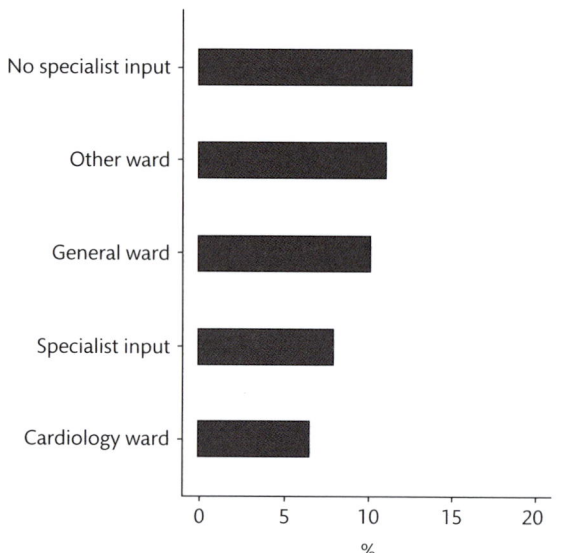

Figure 67.2 In-hospital mortality (2016/17) by ward allocation in the UK National Heart Failure Audit.

Source data from McMurray JJ, Packer M, Desai AS, *et al*. Angiotensin–neprilysin inhibition versus enalapril in heart failure. *N Engl J Med* 2014;**371**(11):993–1004.

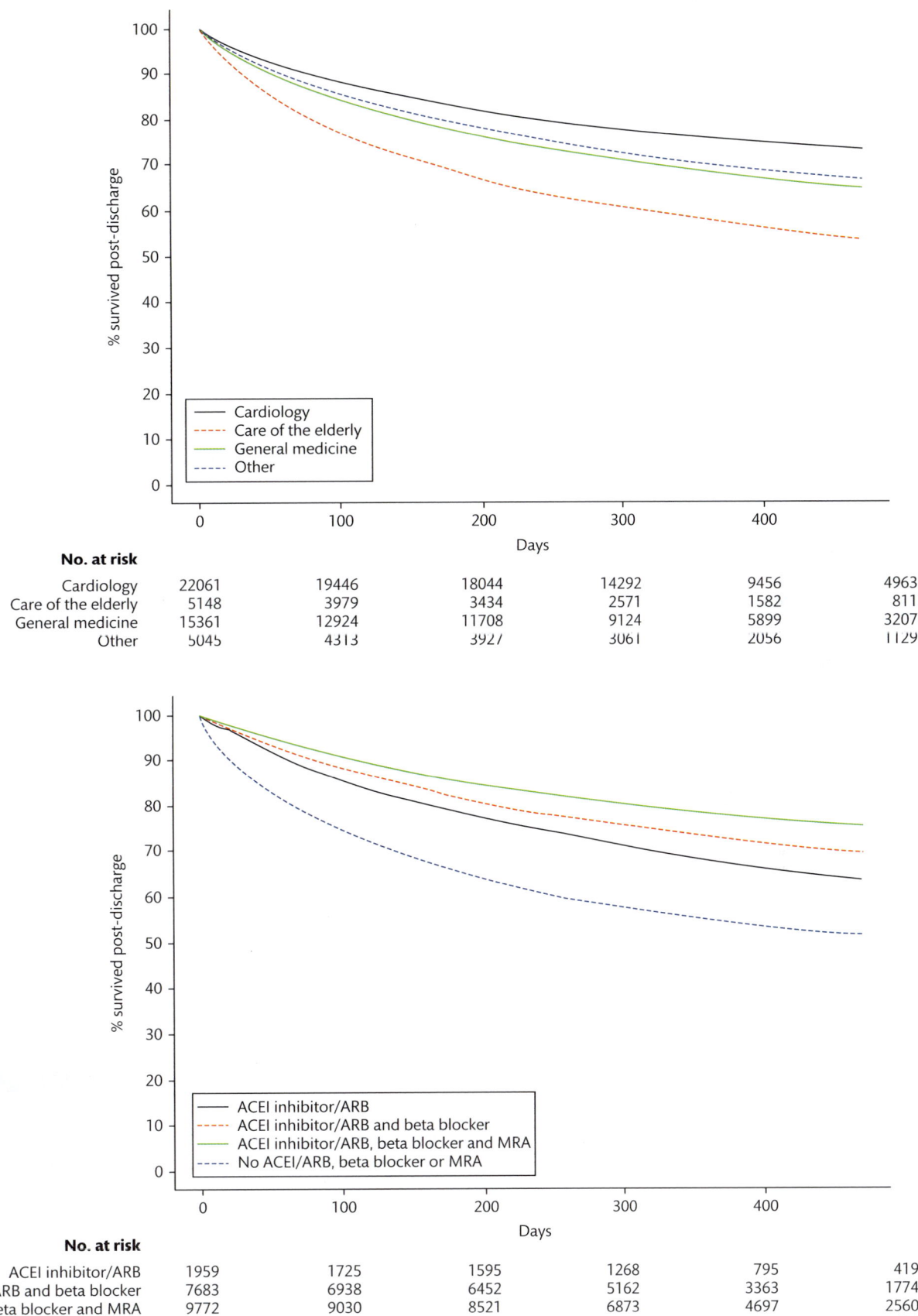

No. at risk						
Cardiology	22061	19446	18044	14292	9456	4963
Care of the elderly	5148	3979	3434	2571	1582	811
General medicine	15361	12924	11708	9124	5899	3207
Other	5045	4313	3927	3061	2056	1129

No. at risk						
ACEI inhibitor/ARB	1959	1725	1595	1268	795	419
ACEI inhibitor/ARB and beta blocker	7683	6938	6452	5162	3363	1774
ACEI inhibitor/ARB, beta blocker and MRA	9772	9030	8521	6873	4697	2560
No ACEI/ARB, beta blocker or MRA	2816	2223	1983	1523	918	456

Figure 67.3 Kaplan–Meier survival curves for all-cause mortality according to admission ward (a) and by number of therapies for HFrEF (b).
Reproduced from McMurray JJ, Packer M, Desai AS, *et al.* Angiotensin-neprilysin inhibition versus enalapril in heart failure. *N Engl J Med* 2014;371(11):993-1004.

Clearly for heart failure services to function they must have access to all the relevant diagnostic and therapeutic options. Of note here, BNP/NT-proBNP testing is invaluable. Access to high-quality echocardiography is a must. Heart failure services are also becoming increasingly dependent on cardiac magnetic resonance testing. Therapeutic pathways should be developed for each service specifically. If all therapies, devices, and advanced heart failure options can be delivered on site, well and good. But for hospitals that do not have cardiac catheterization, device therapy or mechanical support and transplantation on site, good referral pathway should be developed with regional centres to ensure seamless access for patients to all treatment options. It is also important for patients to have access to cardiac rehabilitation and palliative care services.

Guidelines

All members of heart failure services have to adhere to common guidelines. Lengthy international guidelines do not need to be rewritten but the essential diagnostic and treatment pathways need to be abstracted and available in simple form for all health care professionals to follow.

Audit

A key element of quality improvement in heart failure is audit. Many international registries and datasets are available. Audit can be carried out at a local and national level. Many national registries enable the comparison of local data versus the national data to help drive up standards of patient care.

Large unselected registries/audits can facilitate quality improvement. Evidence-based therapies, process indicators, and outcomes can be recorded serially. Bench marks can be set for attainment of the quality indicators and used to drive up standards of care. In many health care systems with national audit programmes, the achievement of key quality indicator targets can be used to determine the level of reimbursement hospitals receive for heart failure admissions. For example, in the UK, data from the National Institute for Cardiovascular Outcomes Research (NICOR) can be used to determine the percentage of patients being discharged from hospital having been seen by a specialist multi-professional heart failure team, which is then used to determine whether the hospital will receive the Best Practice Tariff for heart failure admissions. Similar carrot/stick incentive schemes operate in primary care in the UK (the Quality Outcomes Framework). There are also international examples of these quality improvement initiatives in insurance-base health care systems, for example the 'Get with the Guidelines' initiative in the USA.[13]

Ultimately the goal of heart failure services and quality improvement programmes is to ensure that wherever patients with heart failure begin their health care journey, they see the correct people to make an accurate and timely diagnosis, instigate the most appropriate investigations to ascertain the aetiology and facilitate the introduction of evidence-based therapy, for all patients and not just a selected few (**Figure 67.4**).

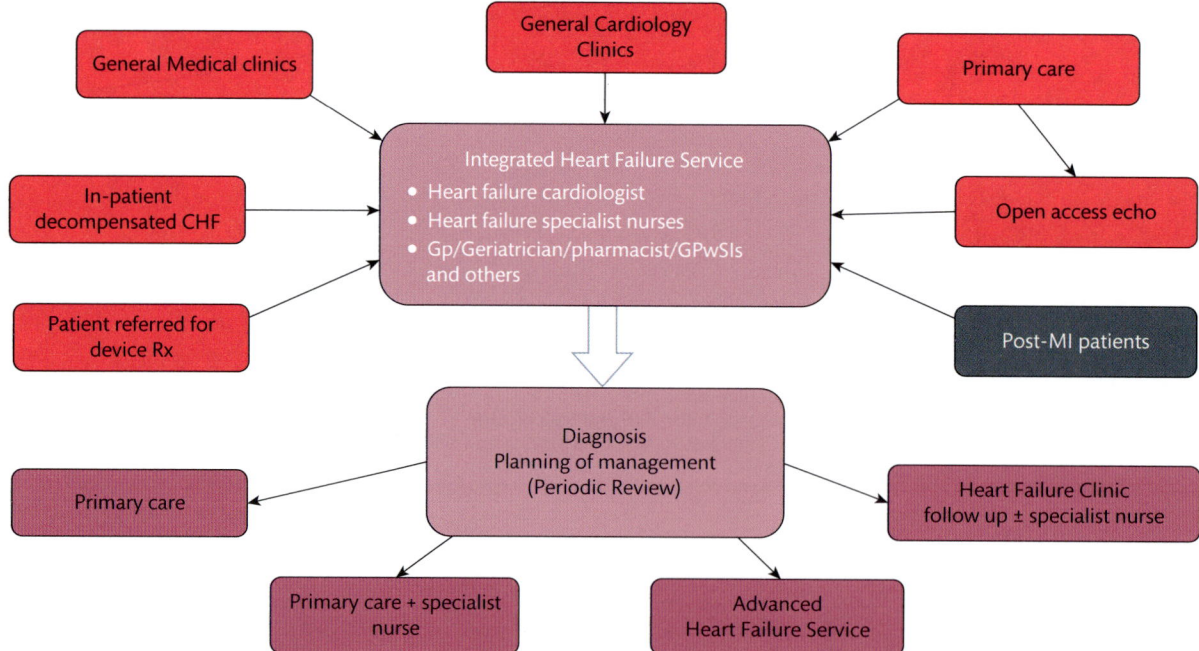

Elements of an Integrated Heart Failure Service

Figure 67.4 The ideal heart failure service.

Reproduced from McDonagh TA, Blue L, Clark AL, *et al*. European Society of Cardiology Heart Failure Association Standards for delivering heart failure care. *Eur J Heart Fail* 2011;**13**(3):235–41 with permission from John Wiley and Sons.

REFERENCES

1. McMurray JJ, Packer M, Desai AS, *et al.* Angiotensin–neprilysin inhibition versus enalapril in heart failure. *N Engl J Med* 2014;**371**(11):993–1004.
2. McDonagh TA. The National Heart Failure Audit Report 2016/17. 2018. www.nicor.ucl.ac.uk.
3. Kociol RD, Greiner MA, Hammill BG, *et al.* Long-term outcomes of medicare beneficiaries with worsening renal function during hospitalization for heart failure. *Am J Cardiol* 2010;**105**(12):1786–93.
4. Conrad N, Judge A, Tran J, *et al.* Temporal trends and patterns in heart failure incidence: a population-based study of 4 million individuals. *Lancet* 2018;**391**(10120):572–80.
5. McDonagh TA, Blue L, Clark AL, *et al.* European Society of Cardiology Heart Failure Association Standards for delivering heart failure care. *Eur J Heart Fail* 2011;**13**(3):235–41.
6. Ponikowski P, Voors AA, Anker SD, *et al.* 2016 ESC Guidelines for the diagnosis and treatment of acute and chronic heart failure: The Task Force for the diagnosis and treatment of acute and chronic heart failure of the European Society of Cardiology (ESC). Developed with the special contribution of the Heart Failure Association (HFA) of the ESC. *Eur J Heart Fail* 2016;**18**(8):891–975.
7. Reis SE, Holubkov R, Edmundowicz D, *et al.* Treatment of patients admitted to the hospital with congestive heart failure: specialty-related disparities in practice patterns and outcomes. *J Am Coll Cardiol* 1997;**30**(3):733–8.
8. Cleland JG, McDonagh T, Rigby AS, *et al.* The national heart failure audit for England and Wales 2008–2009. *Heart* 2011;**97**(11):876–86.
9. Fonarow GC, Stevenson LW, Walden JA, *et al.* Impact of a comprehensive heart failure management program on hospital readmission and functional status of patients with advanced heart failure. *J Am Coll Cardiol* 1997;**30**(3):725–32.
10. McDonagh TA, Gardner RS, Lainscak M, *et al.* Heart failure association of the European Society of Cardiology specialist heart failure curriculum. *Eur J Heart Fail* 2014;**16**(2):151–62.
11. Lambrinou E, Kalogirou F, Lamnisos D, Sourtzi P. Effectiveness of heart failure management programmes with nurse-led discharge planning in reducing re-admissions: a systematic review and meta-analysis. *Int J Nurs Stud* 2012;**49**(5):610–24.
12. Riley JP, Astin F, Crespo-Leiro MG, *et al.* Heart Failure Association of the European Society of Cardiology heart failure nurse curriculum. *Eur J Heart Fail* 2016;**18**(7):736–43.
13. Chen LM, Levine DA, Hayward R, *et al.* Relationship between hospital 30-day mortality rates for heart failure and patterns of early inpatient comfort care. *J Hosp Med* 2018;**13**(3):170–6.

68

Reparative therapies for the failing heart

Richard J. Jabbour and Alexander R. Lyon

Introduction

A significant research effort has been directed at exploring a number of novel biological therapies to repair the failing heart. These range from autologous and allogenic stem cell therapies (unfractionated bone marrow mononuclear stem cells (BMNSCs), mesenchymal stem cells (MSCs), skeletal myoblasts, cardiac progenitor cells (CPCs)), which are delivered exogenously and have been evaluated in phase II and/or phase III clinical trials, to reactivating endogenous myocyte repair mechanisms or direct reprogramming methods, which are still at the preclinical phase. Tissue engineering strategies with engraftment of multicellular preparations incorporated on a structural scaffold to generate a three-dimensional tissue construct are also in preclinical development with one proof-of-principle ongoing phase I study in patients (NCT02057900).[1] These are designed to replace large sections of lost myocardium—for example, following a large anterior myocardial infarction (MI).

Gene therapies have also been assessed using viral vectors to deliver therapeutic genes to the failing myocardium. One type of gene therapy is designed to enhance endogenous stem cell recruitment to the myocardium, thereby effecting a cell therapy approach indirectly. All these biological therapies are being developed to address the unmet need of poor morbidity and mortality in patients with advanced chronic heart failure despite optimal contemporary therapies.

Exogenous stem cell therapy

Exogenous transfer and delivery of cells to a failing heart has the aim of inducing improvement of MI via a number of different mechanisms. Various cell types have been investigated in chronic heart failure including: skeletal myoblasts; BMNSCs; MSCs; cardiac stem cells, and pluripotent stem cell-derived cardiomyocytes (derived from either human adult or embryonic origin).

Despite numerous encouraging preclinical research studies, effective clinical translation with exogenous cell therapy for chronic heart failure has not occurred.[2,3] Some minor changes in structural or symptomatic variables have been seen but it is widely believed that the mechanism of improvement observed in clinical trials is most likely to be paracrine. Exogenously delivered cells do not appear to survive effectively in the host and, to date, regeneration of de-novo myocardium has not been convincingly demonstrated.[3,4] There are various reasons for low cell retention including:

- high washout on first-pass infusion or injection;
- the toxic environment of the failing myocardium;
- increased apoptosis;
- ischaemia;
- matrix detachment.[3,5]

Current evidence from preclinical and clinical studies suggests that the cells are sources of various beneficial growth factors and cytokines that improve function via angiogenesis, beneficial paracrine signalling to failing cardiomyocytes to improve their function, or possibly activation of endogenous CPCs with subsequent differentiation into new myocytes.

The majority of human clinical data has been derived from small, open-label trials, which were underpowered for hard endpoints and prone to bias due to their unblinded design and without effective sham or placebo controls. For example, a meta-analysis of 31 trials, including 1521 patients who were administered a variety of cell types by any delivery route, found an overall mortality benefit, improvement in New York Heart Association (NYHA) class and left ventricular ejection fraction (LVEF). However, if only double-blinded trials (three to seven trials included) were analysed, there was no statistically significant benefit in any endpoint, further underlying the importance of adequately powered, bias-resistant trials.[6] Several phase III trials are ongoing and will provide a more definitive answer as to the efficacy of exogenous cell therapy.

Skeletal myoblasts

One of the first cell types to be investigated was autologous skeletal muscle progenitor cells known as skeletal myoblasts. Despite initial enthusiasm from the scientific community regarding similarities to cardiac muscle, and the ease of providing an autologous source of cells that could be expanded ex-vivo to a very large cell number (one billion) in a matter of 2–3 weeks, data from human trials have been disappointing and concerns exist regarding a higher incidence of ventricular arrhythmias generated after transplant.

The Myoblast Autologous Grafting in Ischemic Cardiomyopathy (MAGIC) Trial was a randomized, placebo-controlled trial that evaluated the efficacy of two different doses of myoblasts (400 million ($n = 33$) or 800 million ($n = 34$)) versus placebo ($n = 30$). All patients had a history of ischaemic heart failure and an indication for coronary artery bypass grafting. Cells were injected in and around the areas of myocardial scar at the time of cardiac surgery and all patients received implantable cardiac defibrillator devices. The trial failed to reach its primary end-point of change in LVEF and a higher number of ventricular arrhythmias occurred in the cell-treated groups. It is now widely believed that arrhythmia generation results from the lack of electrical coupling to host cardiomyocytes since the skeletal myoblasts do not possess gap junction proteins (including connexin-43) that allow efficient electrical coupling with the host myocardium.[7–9]

Bone marrow mononuclear cells

Normal human bone marrow contains small numbers of several stem cell populations, including haematopoietic, endothelial progenitor cells, and mesenchymal stem cells, and once isolated and purified they are collectively known as BMNSCs. BMNSCs are the stem cells that have been most extensively investigated in human clinical trials, with most trials recruiting patients with heart failure secondary to an ischaemic aetiology. A few have specifically recruited non-ischaemic dilated cardiomyopathy (DCM). Several phase I/II clinical trials have been completed and phase III trials are ongoing. A meta-analysis of >20 randomized controlled trials of 1255 patients with heart failure found only a small improvement in LVEF and NYHA class after excluding poorly designed studies.[10] Although no major adverse events have been reported, concerns exist regarding ventricular arrhythmias, particularly following intramyocardial injection, which may partly be due to ineffective electromechanical coupling, or to unwanted cell differentiation.[2,11]

The FOCUS-CCTRN (Effect of transendocardial delivery of autologous bone marrow mononuclear cells on functional capacity, left ventricular function, and perfusion in chronic heart failure) trial was a phase II randomized, double-blind, placebo-controlled study that evaluated the use of BMNSCs in patients with symptomatic chronic ischaemic heart failure (LVEF ≤45%). Sixty-one patients received intramyocardial delivery of autologous BMNSCs and 31 were given a sham procedure. Follow-up after 6 months revealed no significant changes in left ventricular end-systolic volume index, maximal oxygen consumption, or reversibility of ischaemia (determined by single-photon emission computed tomography imaging) at 6 months. An exploratory subgroup analysis revealed an LVEF increase of 1.4% in the BMNSC-treated patients vs a 1.3% decrease in the control group (absolute difference: 2.7%), with the LVEF improvement correlating with the proportion of CD34+ and CD133+ cells contained in BMNSC samples.[12]

One of the largest double-blind, placebo-controlled phase II trials (ixCELL-DCM) randomized 126 patients with post-MI ischaemic cardiomyopathy ineligible for further revascularization to ixmyelocel-T ($n = 60$) or placebo ($n = 66$) with primary composite end-point of all-cause death, cardiovascular admissions to hospital, or unplanned clinic visits to treat acute decompensated heart failure.[13] Ixmyelocel-T consists primarily of a BMNSC population, with a relatively higher population of M2 macrophages and

CD90+ mesenchymal stem cells when compared to unfractionated BMNSCs. Although the trial satisfied the safety primary end-point, the secondary end-points of changes in left ventricular function were minor and not statistically significant. Although the study was well designed with appropriate blinded controls, the fact that only a small number of patients were included and that there was a discordance between the reduction in clinical events and changes in left ventricular remodelling means that larger trials are warranted to ascertain the efficacy of the therapy.

A large number of trials has assessed the benefit and safety of BMNSCs in patients following acute MI where LV function is impaired. This approach may be considered as a strategy for preventing heart failure in high-risk post-MI patients. The numerous trials involving post-MI heart failure have culminated in the largest clinical stem cell trial to date. The Effect of Intracoronary Reinfusion of Bone Marrow-derived Mononuclear Cells on All-Cause Mortality in Acute Myocardial Infarction (BAMI; NCT01569178) randomized phase III trial is ongoing and will recruit in total >3000 patients with heart failure (LVEF <45%) post successful reperfusion therapy for acute ST elevation MI. Autologous BMNSCs will be administered via intracoronary injection 4–7 days post MI and the trial is powered for all-cause mortality as its primary end-point. Notably, however, there is a lack of sham control arm in the study.

The randomized trial of combination cytokine and adult autologous bone marrow progenitor cell administration in patients with non-ischaemic dilated cardiomyopathy (REGENERATE-DCM) clinical trial was the first phase II randomized, placebo controlled trial that assessed the efficacy of granulocyte colony-stimulation factor (G-CSF) with or without intracoronary administration of autologous BMNSCs in patients with idiopathic DCM (no secondary cause). Sixty patients were randomized into four separate groups: saline (placebo) ($n = 15$); peripheral G-CSF ($n = 15$); peripheral G-CSF and IC serum ($n = 15$); and peripheral G-CSF and intracoronary BMNSCs ($n = 15$).

Interestingly, the primary end-point of improvement in LVEF at 3 months post treatment was met only by the combined peripheral G-CSF/BMNSC group with a 5.4% increase in LVEF (32.9% ± 16.5 to 38.3% ± 13.0, $P = 0.01$), which was maintained to one year. This was associated with a decrease in secondary end-points including NYHA class, quality of life, improved exercise capacity (including peak Vo_2) and reduced N-terminal pro B-type natriuretic peptide (NT-proBNP) (by 136.0 pg/mL, $P = 0.0023$). Notably, the trial included a sham intracoronary infusion arm. Although this was a small single-centre trial, the statistically significant improvements in numerous end-points suggest that further validation in larger phase III studies is warranted.[14]

Table 68.1 summarizes some recent trials involving BMNSCs.

Mesenchymal stem cells

In comparison to BMNSCs, there are fewer clinical trials involving MSCs, with encouraging results from some phase II trials leading to several ongoing phase III trials. MSCs can be obtained from bone marrow, as well as umbilical cord blood and adipose tissue.

The Cardiopoietic stem Cell therapy in heart failURE (C-CURE) phase II randomized, open-label trial evaluated the feasibility and safety of autologous bone marrow-derived MSCs in patients with chronic ischaemic heart failure. Cells were subjected to a cardiogenic 'cocktail' pre-treatment to upregulate cardiac-specific transcription

Table 68.1 Summary of selected human clinical trials involving bone marrow stem cells and mesenchymal stem cells

Trial	Phase	Publication date	Details	Registered number	Patients	Aetiology	End-points	Results	Delivery route
BMNSCs									
BAMI	3	Still recruiting	Randomized, open label	NCT01569178	3000	Ischaemic	All-cause death	NA	Intracoronary
ixCELL-DCM	2b	2016	Randomized, double-blind	NCT01670981	126	Ischaemic dilated	All-cause death, cardiovascular hospital admission, unplanned clinic visits	Composite end point met	Intramyocardial
REGENERATE-DCM	2	2015	Randomized, double-blind	NCT01302171	60	Non-ischaemic dilated	LVEF	Improvement in LVEF, NYHA, NT-proBNP	Intracoronary
FOCUS-CCTRN	2	2012	Randomized, double-blind	NCT00824005	92	Ischaemic	LVESV, maximal oxygen consumption, SPECT reversibility	No significant changes	Intramyocardial
REPAIR-AMI	3	2006	Randomized, double-blind	NCT00279175	204	Ischaemic	Change in LV function	Improvement in LV function	Intracoronary
MSCs									
POSEIDON	1/2	2012	Randomized, open label	NCT01087996	31	Ischaemic	Serious adverse events	Low incidence of events	Intramyocardial
C-CURE	2	2013	Randomized, open label	NCT00810238	48	Ischaemic	LVEF	Improvement in LV function	Intramyocardial
PROMETHEUS	1/2	2014	Randomized, double-blind	NCT00587990	9	Ischaemic	Serious adverse events/LV remodelling	Improvement in LV function	Intramyocardial

BMNSCs, bone marrow mononuclear stem cells; MCSs, mesenchymal stem cells; NA, not available; LVEF, left ventricular ejection fraction; NYHA, New York Heart Association; NT-proBNP, N-terminal pro B-type natriuretic peptide; LVESV, left ventricular end-systolic volume; SPECT, single-photon emission computed tomography.

factors.[15] Screening of 320 patients yielded 47 patients who consented and were randomized, 32 patients to the cell therapy arm versus 15 in the control arm (pharmacological therapy), with 21 patients finally receiving an intramyocardial injection of stem cells. No adverse events were observed and in the small number of patients in the cell therapy arm there was a potential signal of efficacy with an improvement in EF (7% absolute increase from 27.5% to 34.5%, $P < 0.0001$), end-systolic volume, and 6 min walk test. It is important to state that the trial was open label with no sham procedure, so a placebo effect cannot be excluded.[16]

The Safety and Efficacy of Autologous Cardiopoietic Cells for Treatment of Ischemic Heart Failure (CHART-1, NCT01768702) trial is a double-blind placebo-controlled phase III trial of the same cell therapy and has recruited a total of 240 patients. It will provide a more robust measure of efficacy using a composite outcome of morbidity and mortality, changes in quality of life, 6 min walk test, and left ventricular structure and function.

The Percutaneous Stem Cell Injection Delivery Effects on Neomyogenesis Pilot (POSEIDON) Study randomized 31 patients with ischaemic cardiomyopathy to intramyocardial delivery of either autologous ($n = 16$) or allogeneic ($n = 15$) MSCs of varying concentrations (20–200 million). This trial addressed the safety and immunological issues regarding the use of allogeneic cells. Both methods were deemed safe, and showed a reduction in infarct size and improvement in ventricular remodelling and functional status. Whereas the study confirmed the initial short term

safety of using allogeneic MSCs in heart failure patients, conclusions on efficacy cannot be drawn at this stage due to the lack of placebo group, small number of patients included, and open-label design.[17]

The Prospective Randomized Study of Mesenchymal Stem Cell Therapy in Patients Undergoing Cardiac Surgery (PROMETHEUS) trial investigated the effects of autologous MSC injection into specific akinetic or hypokinetic myocardial regions deemed unsuitable for surgical revascularization during coronary artery bypass graft surgery. Cardiac magnetic resonance imaging demonstrated after 18 months an overall increase in LVEF by $9.4 \pm 1.7\%$ ($P = 0.0002$) and reduction in scar mass by $47.5 \pm 8.1\%$ ($P < 0.0001$). Notably, at the cell injection sites, there were contractile and perfusion improvements, with a corresponding reduction in scar tissue which contributed to the overall increase in LVEF. It should be noted that although the trial was originally designed as a randomized trial with a total of 45 patients, only the single arm including six patients has so far been published, and thus the results should be interpreted as hypothesis-forming.[18]

An ongoing phase III trial (NCT02032004) is investigating the exogenous administration of allogeneic mesenchymal precursor cells (CEP-41750), a primitive type of MSC, to patients with chronic heart failure (ischaemic/non-ischaemic aetiology), via transendocardial delivery with primary outcome of heart failure major adverse cardiac events.

Table 68.1 summarizes some recent trials involving MSCs.

Resident cardiac progenitor stem cells

Resident cardiac progenitor stem cells, known as CPCs, consist of <1% of the total cardiomyocyte population in adult human hearts, and are divided according to their cell surface markers including c-kit, Isl-1, and Sca-1. Cardiospheres consist of a mixed population of CPCs and together with c-kit cardiac stem cells have reached clinical translation.[9]

c-kit cardiac stem cells

The Administration of Cardiac Stem Cells in Patients With Ischemic Cardiomyopathy: The SCIPIO Trial was a phase I, randomized, open-label trial of autologous c-kit$^+$ cardiac stem cells in patients with ischaemic heart failure (Table 68.2).[19] Cells were obtained from the right atrial appendage at the time of coronary artery bypass grafting. The cells were then harvested and grown *ex vivo* and patients treated via intracoronary injection at least four months after surgery. Out of 33 patients randomized, 20 were treated with cardiac stem cells and a significant improvement in LVEF was found (absolute increase of 12.3% in eight patients at 12 months). It is important to note that this is an open-label trial and subject to potential bias. However, concerns have been raised regarding data integrity and trial randomization by both the editorial board of *The Lancet* and an independent research group, due to inconsistencies in the preclinical science underpinning the trial.[20]

Cardiosphere-derived stem cells

The Cardiosphere-Derived Autologous Stem Cells to Reverse ventricular dysfunction (CADUCEUS) randomized phase I trial assessed the safety of autologous cardiosphere-derived stem cell therapy to patients with ischaemic heart failure (Table 68.2).[21] Out of a total of 31 eligible participants who consented and were randomized, 25 were included in the final analysis (17 in the stem cell group, eight in the control group). CPCs were harvested via percutaneous right ventricular endomyocardial biopsy. On average, 10 endomyocardial biopsies per patient were required to obtain the desired quantity of ventricular myocardium.[22] This may raise potential safety issues in the future both related to the immediate biopsy procedure and to the arrhythmogenic potential. The advantage of this approach is avoiding the need for open chest surgery.

Safety primary end-points included mortality due to ventricular arrhythmias, sudden death, periprocedural MI, and major adverse cardiac events. In addition, magnetic resonance imaging was performed to assess efficacy. After 6 months follow-up, four patients (24%) in the stem cell group had serious adverse events compared with one control (13%; $P = 1.00$). Patients treated with CPC stem cells were reported to have a reduction in scar mass and increase in viability, but these did not translate into an improvement in LVEF or end-systolic volume when compared to controls.

It is important to note that in both SCIPIO and CADUCEUS, a large number of patients was screened (more than 1300 in SCIPIO and 400 in CADUCEUS) with only small numbers of patients actually receiving cell therapy, indicating that there was a highly selected target treatment population and that therefore the results cannot be generalized to all patients with ischaemic heart failure. Further randomized studies with larger numbers of patients and with appropriate sham or placebo controls are needed before any conclusions on efficacy can be made.[9,23]

Future directions in exogenous stem cell therapy

In contrast to the numbers of cells delivered in clinical trials (ranging from 2 million to 200 million), ~1 billion cells are lost in a human MI and therefore larger numbers may be needed to reverse the disease process to a clinically meaningful degree.[24] Replicating this number of cells is expensive and time-consuming with current methods, and may be unachievable using cells acquired from bone marrow or cardiac biopsies. Therefore, other cell sources are being investigated that could yield cardiomyocytes in more clinically

Table 68.2 Summary of selected human clinical trials involving gene therapies and cardiospheres/cardiac stem cells

Trial	Phase	Publication date	Details	Registered number	Patients	Aetiology	End-points	Results	Delivery route
Cardiosphere-derived cells									
CADUCEUS	1	2012	Randomized, open label	NCT00893360	31	Ischaemic	Composite of multiple end-points including MACE, MRI ventricular assessment	Increase in viable mass observed by MRI	Intracoronary
Cardiac stem cells									
SCIPIO	1	2012	Randomized, open label	NCT00474461	33	Ischaemic	Adverse events including death, ventricular tachycardia; MRI ventricular assessment	Improvement in LV function/reduction in LV infarct size	Intracoronary
Gene therapy									
STOP-HF	2	2015	Randomized, double blind	NCT01643590	93	Ischaemic	Composite of 6 min walk distance and QoL questionnaire	Primary end-point not met	Intramyocardial
CUPID	2b	2016	Randomized, double blind	NCT01643330	250	Ischaemic/non-ischaemic	Heart failure hospital admissions/ambulatory treatment for worsening heart failure	Primary end-point not met	Intracoronary

MACE, major adverse cardiac events; MRI, magnetic resonance imaging; LV, left ventricular; QoL, quality of life.

meaningful quantities if cardiomyocyte replacement is the desired therapeutic effect.

Pluripotent stem cells

Human-induced pluripotent stem cells were pioneered by Yamanaka *et al.*, who discovered that delivering four simple transcription factors (Oct4, Sox2, cMyc, and Klf4) to adult cells converted the somatic adult cells to a primitive pluripotent stem cell state.[25] These pluripotent cells could then be differentiated into a variety of cell types including stem cell-derived cardiomyocytes for potential use as a treatment option for cardiovascular disease. Stem cell-derived cardiomyocytes can also be derived from human embryonic stem cells and together with human-induced pluripotent cells show great promise as they have a nearly unlimited proliferation potential. There is the added advantage with human-induced pluripotent cells of decreased risk of immunogenicity since they are an autologous cell source.

However, there are concerns about uncontrolled cell differentiation and teratoma formation. In addition, ethical issues exist surrounding the use of human embryonic stem cells. Stem cell-derived cardiomyocytes have a phenotype that is foetal or immature-like and at present are limited to preclinical testing. A recent preclinical investigation involved the administration of more than one billion embryonic stem cell-derived cardiomyocytes in non-human primates and, for the first time, demonstrated that intramyocardial delivery of human embryonic stem cell-derived cardiomyocytes was able to integrate with the host and form 'new muscle'. The integration process was complicated by the occurrence of non-fatal ventricular arrhythmias, reminiscent of the arrhythmogenesis observed following skeletal myoblast injection.[2] This raises the potential concern that the greater the myocyte differentiation of transplanted cells, the higher the risk of arrhythmogenesis.

Engineered heart tissue

One strategy to improve integration is the creation of exogenous engineered heart tissue.[26] Removing adult cardiomyocytes from their natural three-dimensional, force-generating, environment produces dedifferentiation to an immature phenotype. Engineered heart tissue has been developed to place the stem cells into a three-dimensional fibrin matrix, and use their spontaneous beating activity to provide a continuous mechanical stimulus by being attached to fixed supports.[27] This facilitates the anisotropic rearrangement of the stem cell-derived cardiomyocytes, which then develop more mature calcium-handling characteristics.[28] It is hoped that with the mature phenotype, the tissue will electromechanically couple more effectively to the host, improve survival of the graft, and thereby provide greater clinical effectiveness.

Recently, a first-in-man experiment involving a patient with ischaemic heart failure (LVEF: 26%) confirmed the feasibility of grafting an engineered tissue construct consisting of human embryonic stem cells (CD15+, Isl-1+) and a fibrin scaffold during coronary bypass surgery. The cells were successfully delivered epicardially on to the infarcted area of myocardium during bypass. At 6-month follow-up, the patient was in NYHA class I and a positron emission tomography scan was comparable to baseline.[1] **Box 68.1** summarizes the current barriers to implementing stem cell therapy in humans. **Table 68.3** summarizes the advantages and disadvantages of the potential cell types currently being investigated.

> **Box 68.1** Barriers to implementing stem cell therapy
>
> - Ethical issues
> - Cost
> - Replication
> - Delivery method
> - Immunological rejection
> - Cell survival and integration
> - Safety/teratoma formation

Gene therapy

Improvements in gene transfer technology, viral vector technology, and more efficient methods of myocardial delivery have underpinned the recent interest in cardiac gene therapy for heart failure. These methods allow the direct targeting of the molecular mechanisms that become aberrant in the heart failure syndrome. Gene therapy approaches to the treatment of heart failure are currently under investigation in phase II trials.

SERCA2a

An extensively investigated therapeutic target for heart failure is the cardiac sarcoplasmic reticulum calcium ATPase 2a (SERCA2a). Abnormalities in calcium handling are common in end-stage heart failure and the intracellular accumulation of calcium may lead to arrhythmia formation. SERCA2a is responsible for calcium re-uptake into the sarcoplasmic reticulum in diastole.

Whereas the early Calcium Up-regulation by Percutaneous Administration of Gene Therapy in Cardiac Disease (CUPID) Trial indicated that the approach of using a gene transfer vector based on adeno-associated virus 1 (AAV-1) for delivery of SERCA2a complementary DNA was feasible (and gave a signal of a dose response improvement in functional capacity), the findings were not replicated in the phase II trial (CUPID II, NCT01643330; **Table 68.2**).[29]

The reasons for lack of benefit in CUPID2 are still uncertain, with inadequate gene delivery at an effective dose appearing to be the main issue. Safety at the dose studied (1×10^{13} DNase-resistant viral particles) was confirmed, and further studies at higher doses are warranted. Unfortunately, the neutral result of CUPID2 led to the early termination of recruitment in the two other trials using the same SERCA2a gene therapy product at the same dose (SERCA-LVAD trial, NCT00534703 and the AGENT-HF trial (AAV1.SERCA2a GENe Therapy Trial in Heart Failure), NCT01966887). Hopefully insights from these trials will help guide future trial programmes in cardiac gene therapy for chronic heart failure.

Stromal cell-derived factor-1

Stromal cell-derived factor-1 (SDF-1) is another molecular target that has reached the clinical phase of testing in gene therapy trials. It facilitates tissue repair via a multitude of mechanisms including enhancing cell survival and vasculogenesis as well as facilitating endogenous stem cell recruitment. The Stromal Cell-Derived Factor-1 Plasmid Treatment for Patients with Heart Failure (STOP-HF) was a phase II, double-blind, randomized, placebo-controlled trial which evaluated the safety and efficacy of a single treatment of non-viral DNA plasmid gene therapy that encodes stromal cell-derived factor-1 (JVS-100) administered via endomyocardial injection to patients with ischaemic heart failure (**Table 68.2**). The trial demonstrated the safety of a single endocardial administration of plasmid SDF-1 but

Table 68.3 Summary of advantages and disadvantages of the potential cell types

Cell type	Advantages	Disadvantages
Bone marrow mononuclear stem cells	• Low immunological risk • Relatively easily obtained and safe autologous source • Low cost	• Lack of electrical coupling • Limited differentiation capacity
Mesenchymal stem cells	• Low immunological risk • Relatively easily obtained and safe autologous source • Can be obtained from a variety of tissue sources	• Lack of electrical coupling • Limited differentiation capacity • Relatively difficult to expand and purify
Skeletal myoblasts	• Can be rapidly expanded *ex vivo*	• Pro-arrhythmic • Lack of electrical coupling • Cannot differentiate into cardiomyocytes
Cardiac progenitor cells	• Tissue specific • High proliferative potential	• Myocardial biopsy needed • Relatively difficult to expand and purify
Pluripotent stem cells	• Nearly unlimited proliferation potential • Decreased risk of immunogenicity (human-induced) • High cardiogenic potential	• Theoretical risk of uncontrolled cell differentiation • Theoretical risk of teratoma formation • Ethical issues (embryonic) • Pro-arrhythmic

failed to meet its primary end-point of improved composite score of 6 min walk test and quality-of-life questionnaire at 4 months follow-up. However, subgroup analysis showed an improvement in LVEF in the highest-risk cohort of patients (LVEF <26%).[30]

S100A1

A comprehensive programme of small and large animal heart failure studies has tested the efficacy of using the gene coding for S100 calcium-binding protein A1 (S100A1), again delivered via an AAV vector.[31] The biotech company that developed the approach has partnered with a large pharmaceutical company to develop a clinical trial programme in the near future.

Although the results of some of the gene therapy trials have been disappointing, signals of improvement in the sickest subset of patients allow the opportunity for further work in this area.

Future regenerative strategies

Endogenous cardiac progenitor cell activation

An alternative approach to exogenously replacing lost cardiomyocytes is to activate resident CPCs and their regenerative ability.[9,32] Preclinical reports from murine studies have proposed that de-novo myocytes may develop after MI:[33] higher numbers of peripheral blood c-kit[+] CPCs are found after coronary ligation in an animal MI model.[34] In addition, certain signalling factors, including hepatocyte growth factor and insulin-like growth factor-1, can mobilize and cause resident c-kit[+] CPCs to divide and thus potentially improve outcome after MI.[35]

Epicardial cells are essential during cardiogenesis, by undertaking epithelial–mesenchymal transition to become epicardium-derived cells. The epicardial-derived cells then differentiate into cardiac fibroblasts, coronary smooth muscle cells and, less commonly, endothelial and cardiomyocyte lineages.[36,37] Modulating the pathway might enhance myocardial regeneration, and systemic treatment with the paracrine peptide thymosin β4 resulted in the de-novo generation of murine cardiomyocytes from epicardial progenitor cells following MI.[38]

Collectively, these studies indicate that paracrine factors can mobilize and stimulate endogenous CPCs to form de-novo cardiomyocytes—a 'cell therapy without cells'. The prospect of myocardial regeneration without replacing cells is novel; however, more research is needed to understand this pathway before clinical translation occurs.

Cell cycle re-entry

Foetal cardiomyocytes actively divide and therefore research efforts have started to focus on reverting adult myocytes into a more foetal phenotype with the hope of regenerating myocardium.

In adult rodent cardiomyocytes, various cell cycle mediators and cyclin-dependent protein kinases are downregulated, and certain cell cycle inhibitors actively expressed.[9,32,39] The forced expression of specific cell cycle regulators has been used to try to stimulate cardiomyocyte cell cycle re-entry, with varying degrees of effectiveness. For example, in a murine MI model, transgenic expression of cyclin D2 resulted in the creation of new myocardium and was associated with a progressive reduction in infarct size, over time.[40] By contrast, adenoviral delivery of E2F-1 resulted in apoptosis of adult murine ventricular cells.[41] Critical long-term safety questions must be answered when developing this approach to ensure there is no potential for cardiac tumorigenesis.

Paracrine signalling is important in foetal cardiomyocyte proliferation. The induction of tyrosine kinase receptor signalling pathways via insulin-like growth factor-1 leads to proliferation of adult murine cardiomyocytes followed by improved cardiac structure and function in a dilated cardiomyopathy model.[42] Similarly, p38 mitogen-activated protein kinase inhibition enables cardiomyocyte proliferation.[43]

Neuregulin-1 signalling is important in foetal cardiomyocyte proliferation and adult cell survival. Encouraging preclinical research

led to a single-arm phase I human study administering recombinant human neuregulin-1 to 15 patients. The intervention was safe and resulted in an increase in LVEF which persisted to 12 weeks follow-up.[44,45]

MicroRNAs regulate multiple genes, and may be capable of causing adult cardiomyocytes to proliferate. MicroRNAs can be administered as synthetic small molecules and expressed using the adeno-associated virus.[46] MicroRNAs 590 and 199a specifically augment neonatal cardiomyocyte proliferation and promote regeneration of adult murine cardiomyocytes after MI.[47] The microRNA-17-92 cluster induces cardiomyocyte proliferation[48] whereas the miR-15 family causes the opposite.[49]

Further preclinical work including the identification of the correct type and quantity of paracrine factors to induce cardiac regeneration is needed before proceeding to clinical trials.

Direct reprogramming

Recent research has progressed from the Nobel Prize-winning work of Yamanaka to develop direct reprogramming of somatic cells in numerous cell types.[25] It is now possible to convert fully differentiated adult cells directly into a number of other cell types, circumventing the pluripotent stem cell stage. For example, the conversion of fibroblasts to cardiomyocyte-like cells was enabled by the retroviral delivery of cardiac transcription factor genes (Tbx5, Mef2c, and Gata4) in mice.[50] This was replicated *in vivo* using a murine MI model, and associated with reduced infarct size and improved cardiac function.[51] Other studies have now reported human fibroblast conversion to cardiomyocyte-like cells using various different reprogramming factors.[52,53]

Direct reprogramming has the potential to change the paradigm of replacing lost cells and myocardium by converting fibroblasts, one of the main components of scar tissue, back into normal myocardium. This new paradigm, however, has many challenges that need to be overcome including increasing the maturity and function of the cardiomyocyte-like cells, and improving cell conversion efficiency. In addition, the presence of immature-like cells has the associated concerns of being pro-arrhythmic. The use of viruses to perform the reprogramming process may carry the risk of mutagenesis and malignancy.[9,32] **Figure 68.1** demonstrates the different methods currently being investigated in cardiac regeneration.

Conclusion

The adult human heart has been considered an organ which is fully differentiated with no capacity for regeneration; however, the past few years have seen the science community shift towards considering the heart to be an organ with some limited regenerative capabilities. There are several exciting and novel avenues currently being explored in pursuit of myocardial regeneration either by augmenting the limited self-renewal processes or by replacing lost myocardium with exogenous therapy. Further work is needed in all areas to understand and improve the integration of exogenous cell therapy, and improve the efficiency of endogenous repair mechanisms to enable safe and effective cardiac repair of failing hearts.

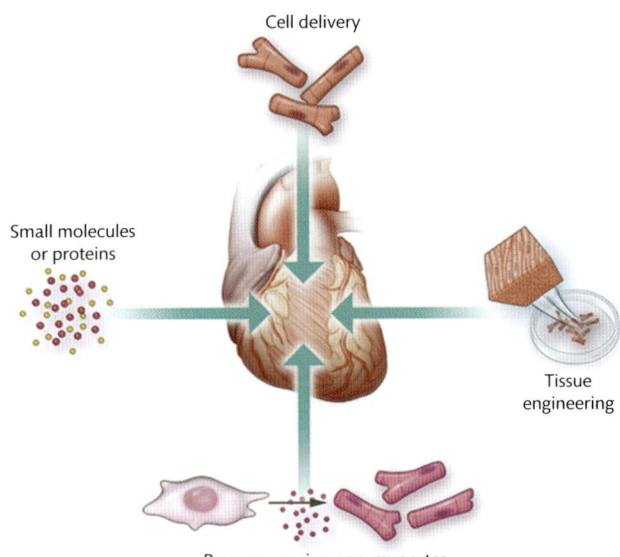

Figure 68.1 Multiple strategies under investigation for cardiac regeneration. Cell therapy delivered by either intracoronary (IC) infusion or intramyocardial (IM) injections has reached human clinical trials; engineered heart tissue combines cells with biomaterials with the aim of creating functional cardiac muscle *ex vivo*; direct reprogramming using viruses aims to convert scar tissue (fibroblasts) into normal myocardium; small molecules including micro-RNAs induce cardiomyocyte proliferation.

Reproduced from Garbern JC and Lee RT. Cardiac stem cell therapy and the promise of heart regeneration. *Cell Stem Cell* 2013 Jun 6;**12**(6):689–98 with permission from Elsevier.

REFERENCES

1. Menasché P, Vanneaux V, Hagège A, *et al.* Human embryonic stem cell-derived cardiac progenitors for severe heart failure treatment: first clinical case report. *Eur Heart J* 2015;**36**:2011–7.
2. Chong JJ, Yang X, Don CW, *et al.* Human embryonic-stem-cell-derived cardiomyocytes regenerate non-human primate hearts. *Nature* 2014;**510**:273–7.
3. Chong JJ, Murry CE. Cardiac regeneration using pluripotent stem cells—progression to large animal models. *Stem Cell Res* 2014;**13**:654–65.
4. Gao J, Dennis JE, Muzic RF, Lundberg M, Caplan AI. The dynamic in vivo distribution of bone marrow-derived mesenchymal stem cells after infusion. *Cells Tissues Organs* 2001;**169**:12–20.
5. Don CW, Murry CE. Improving survival and efficacy of pluripotent stem cell-derived cardiac grafts. *J Cell Mol Med* 2013;**17**:1355–62.
6. Fisher SA, Doree C, Mathur A, Martin-Rendon E. Meta-analysis of cell therapy trials for patients with heart failure. *Circ Res* 2015;**116**:1361–77.
7. Henning RJ. Stem cells in cardiac repair. *Future Cardiol* 2011;**7**:99–117.
8. Menasché P, Alfieri O, Janssens S, *et al.* The Myoblast Autologous Grafting in Ischemic Cardiomyopathy (MAGIC) trial: first randomized placebo-controlled study of myoblast transplantation. *Circulation* 2008;**117**:1189–200.
9. Madonna R, Van Laake LW, Davidson SM, *et al.* Position Paper of the European Society of Cardiology Working Group Cellular Biology of the Heart: cell-based therapies for myocardial repair

and regeneration in ischemic heart disease and heart failure. *Eur Heart J* 2016;**37**:1789–98.

10. Fisher SA, Brunskill SJ, Doree C, *et al*. Stem cell therapy for chronic ischaemic heart disease and congestive heart failure. *Cochrane Database Syst Rev* 2014;(4):CD007888.

11. Nussbaum J, Minami E, Laflamme MA, *et al*. Transplantation of undifferentiated murine embryonic stem cells in the heart: teratoma formation and immune response. *FASEB J* 2007;**21**:1345–57.

12. Perin EC, Willerson JT, Pepine CJ, *et al*., Cardiovascular Cell Therapy Research Network CCTRN. Effect of transendocardial delivery of autologous bone marrow mononuclear cells on functional capacity, left ventricular function, and perfusion in chronic heart failure: the FOCUS-CCTRN trial. *JAMA* 2012;**307**:1717–26.

13. Patel AN, Henry TD, Quyyumi AA, *et al*., ixCELL-DCM Investigators. Ixmyelocel-T for patients with ischaemic heart failure: a prospective randomised double-blind trial. *Lancet* 2016;**387**(10036):2412–21.

14. Hamshere S, Arnous S, Choudhury T, *et al*. Randomized trial of combination cytokine and adult autologous bone marrow progenitor cell administration in patients with non-ischaemic dilated cardiomyopathy: the REGENERATE-DCM clinical trial. *Eur Heart J* 2015;**36**:3061–9.

15. Behfar A, Yamada S, Crespo-Diaz R, *et al*. Guided cardiopoiesis enhances therapeutic benefit of bone marrow human mesenchymal stem cells in chronic myocardial infarction. *J Am Coll Cardiol* 2010;**56**:721–34.

16. Bartunek J, Behfar A, Dolatabadi D, *et al*. Cardiopoietic stem cell therapy in heart failure: the C-CURE (Cardiopoietic stem Cell therapy in heart failURE) multicenter randomized trial with lineage-specified biologics. *J Am Coll Cardiol* 2013;**61**:2329–38.

17. Hare JM, Fishman JE, Gerstenblith G, *et al*. Comparison of allogeneic vs autologous bone marrow-derived mesenchymal stem cells delivered by transendocardial injection in patients with ischemic cardiomyopathy: the POSEIDON randomized trial. *JAMA* 2012;**308**:2369–79.

18. Karantalis V, DiFede DL, Gerstenblith G, *et al*. Autologous mesenchymal stem cells produce concordant improvements in regional function, tissue perfusion, and fibrotic burden when administered to patients undergoing coronary artery bypass grafting. The Prospective Randomized Study of Mesenchymal Stem Cell Therapy in Patients Undergoing Cardiac Surgery (PROMETHEUS) Trial. *Circ Res* 2014;**114**:1302–10.

19. Chugh AR, Beache GM, Loughran JH, *et al*. Administration of cardiac stem cells in patients with ischemic cardiomyopathy: the SCIPIO trial surgical aspects and interim analysis of myocardial function and viability by magnetic resonance. *Circulation* 2012;**126**:S54–S64.

20. The Lancet Editors. Expression of concern: the SCIPIO trial. *Lancet* 2014;**383**:1279.

21. Makkar RR, Smith RR, Cheng K, *et al*. Intracoronary cardiosphere-derived cells for heart regeneration after myocardial infarction (CADUCEUS): a prospective, randomised phase 1 trial. *Lancet* 2012;**379**:895–904.

22. Makkar RR, Smith RR, Czer LS, *et al*. Letter by Makkar et al regarding article, 'Cell therapy for heart failure: a comprehensive overview of experimental and clinical studies, current challenges, and future directions'. *Circ Res* 2014;**115**:e32.

23. Henning RJ. Stem cells for cardiac repair: problems and possibilities. *Future Cardiol* 2013;**9**:875–84.

24. Laflamme MA, Murry CE. Regenerating the heart. *Nat Biotechnol* 2005;**23**:845–56.

25. Takahashi K, Tanabe K, Ohnuki M, *et al*. Induction of pluripotent stem cells from adult human fibroblasts by defined factors. *Cell* 2007;**131**:861–72.

26. Zimmermann WH, Melnychenko I, Wasmeier G, *et al*. Engineered heart tissue grafts improve systolic and diastolic function in infarcted rat hearts. *Nat Med* 2006;**12**:452–8.

27. Kensah G, Roa Lara A, Dahlmann J, *et al*. Murine and human pluripotent stem cell-derived cardiac bodies form contractile myocardial tissue in vitro. *Eur Heart J* 2013;**34**:1134–46.

28. Rao C, Prodromakis T, Kolker L, *et al*. The effect of microgrooved culture substrates on calcium cycling of cardiac myocytes derived from human induced pluripotent stem cells. *Biomaterials* 2013;**34**:2399–411.

29. Greenberg B, Butler J, Felker GM, *et al*. Calcium upregulation by percutaneous administration of gene therapy in patients with cardiac disease (CUPID 2): a randomised, multinational, double-blind, placebo-controlled, phase 2b trial. *Lancet* 2016;**387**:1178–86.

30. Chung ES, Miller L, Patel AN, *et al*. Changes in ventricular remodelling and clinical status during the year following a single administration of stromal cell-derived factor-1 non-viral gene therapy in chronic ischaemic heart failure patients: the STOP-HF randomized Phase II trial. *Eur Heart J* 2015;**36**:2228–38.

31. Pleger ST, Shan C, Ksienzyk J, *et al*. Cardiac AAV9-S100A1 gene therapy rescues post-ischemic heart failure in a preclinical large animal model. *Sci Transl Med* 2011;**3**:92ra64–92ra64.

32. Lin Z, Pu WT. Strategies for cardiac regeneration and repair. *Sci Transl Med* 2014;**6**:239rv1.

33. Hsieh PC, Segers VF, Davis ME, *et al*. Evidence from a genetic fate-mapping study that stem cells refresh adult mammalian cardiomyocytes after injury. *Nat Med* 2007;**13**:970–4.

34. Fazel S, Cimini M, Chen L, *et al*. Cardioprotective c-kit+ cells are from the bone marrow and regulate the myocardial balance of angiogenic cytokines. *J Clin Invest* 2006;**116**:1865–77.

35. Urbanek K, Rota M, Cascapera S, *et al*. Cardiac stem cells possess growth factor-receptor systems that after activation regenerate the infarcted myocardium, improving ventricular function and long-term survival. *Circ Res* 2005;**97**:663–73.

36. Zhou B, Ma Q, Rajagopal S, *et al*. Epicardial progenitors contribute to the cardiomyocyte lineage in the developing heart. *Nature* 2008;**454**:109–13.

37. Zhou B, Honor LB, He H, *et al*. Adult mouse epicardium modulates myocardial injury by secreting paracrine factors. *J Clin Invest* 2011;**121**:1894–904.

38. Smart N, Bollini S, Dubé KN, *et al*. De novo cardiomyocytes from within the activated adult heart after injury. *Nature* 2011;**474**:640–4.

39. Ahuja P, Sdek P, MacLellan WR. Cardiac myocyte cell cycle control in development, disease, and regeneration. *Physiol Rev* 2007;**87**:521–44.

40. Hassink RJ, Pasumarthi KB, Nakajima H, *et al*. Cardiomyocyte cell cycle activation improves cardiac function after myocardial infarction. *Cardiovasc Res* 2008;**78**:18–25.

41. Agah R, Kirshenbaum LA, Abdellatif M, *et al*. Adenoviral delivery of E2F-1 directs cell cycle reentry and p53-independent apoptosis in postmitotic adult myocardium in vivo. *J Clin Invest* 1997;**100**:2722–8.

42. Welch S, Plank D, Witt S, *et al*. Cardiac-specific IGF-1 expression attenuates dilated cardiomyopathy in tropomodulin-overexpressing transgenic mice. *Circ Res* 2002;**90**:641–8.

43. Engel FB, Schebesta M, Duong MT, *et al*. p38 MAP kinase inhibition enables proliferation of adult mammalian cardiomyocytes. *Genes Dev* 2005;**19**:1175–87.

44. Odiete O, Hill MF, Sawyer DB. Neuregulin in cardiovascular development and disease. *Circ Res* 2012;**111**:1376–85.

45. Jabbour A, Hayward CS, Keogh AM, *et al*. Parenteral administration of recombinant human neuregulin-1 to patients with stable chronic heart failure produces favourable acute and chronic haemodynamic responses. *Eur J Heart Fail* 2011;**13**:83–92.

46. Olson EN. MicroRNAs as therapeutic targets and biomarkers of cardiovascular disease. *Sci Transl Med* 2014;**6**:239ps3.

47. Eulalio A, Mano M, Dal Ferro M, *et al*. Functional screening identifies miRNAs inducing cardiac regeneration. *Nature* 2012;**492**:376–81.

48. Chen J, Huang ZP, Seok HY, *et al*. mir-17–92 cluster is required for and sufficient to induce cardiomyocyte proliferation in postnatal and adult hearts. *Circ Res* 2013;**112**:1557–66.

49. Porrello ER, Mahmoud AI, Simpson E, *et al*. Regulation of neonatal and adult mammalian heart regeneration by the miR-15 family. *Proc Natl Acad Sci USA* 2013;**110**:187–92.

50. Ieda M, Fu JD, Delgado-Olguin P, *et al*. Direct reprogramming of fibroblasts into functional cardiomyocytes by defined factors. *Cell* 2010;**142**:375–86.

51. Qian L, Huang Y, Spencer CI, *et al*. In vivo reprogramming of murine cardiac fibroblasts into induced cardiomyocytes. *Nature* 2012;**485**:593–8.

52. Wada R, Muraoka N, Inagawa K, *et al*. Induction of human cardiomyocyte-like cells from fibroblasts by defined factors. *Proc Natl Acad Sci USA* 2013;**110**:12667–72.

53. Nam YJ, Song K, Luo X, *et al*. Reprogramming of human fibroblasts toward a cardiac fate. *Proc Natl Acad Sci USA* 2013;**110**:5588–93.

RECOMMENDED READING

Behfar A, Crespo-Diaz R, Terzic A, Gersh BJ. Cell therapy for heart failure: a comprehensive overview of experimental and clinical studies, current challenges, and future directions. *Nat Rev Cardiol* 2014;**11**:232–46.

Chong JJ, Murry CE. Cardiac regeneration using pluripotent stem cells—progression to large animal models. *Stem Cell Res* 2014;**13**:654–65.

Fisher SA, Brunskill SJ, Doree C, *et al*. Stem cell therapy for chronic ischaemic heart disease and congestive heart failure. *Cochrane Database Syst Rev* 2014;(4):CD007888.

Fisher SA, Doree C, Mathur A, Martin-Rendon E. Meta-analysis of cell therapy trials for patients with heart failure. *Circ Res* 2015;**116**:1361–77.

Gouadon E, Moore-Morris T, Smit NW, *et al*. Concise review: pluripotent stem cell-derived cardiac cells, a promising cell source for therapy of heart failure: where do we stand? *Stem Cells* 2016;**34**:34–43.

Henning RJ. Stem cells in cardiac repair. *Future Cardiol* 2011;**7**:99–117.

Lin Z, Pu WT. Strategies for cardiac regeneration and repair. *Sci Transl Med* 2014;**6**:239rv1.

69

The future

Roy S. Gardner, Theresa A. McDonagh, and Andrew L. Clark

'It's hard to make predictions, especially about the future.' Niels Bohr (attributed)

The outlook for patients with chronic heart failure is incomparably better now than 30 years ago. Nevertheless, the outlook is still poor, particularly after hospitalization, and since heart disease remains the commonest cause of death worldwide, investment in research in heart failure from pharmaceutical and device companies continues apace: the potential financial rewards are great, and so are the potential rewards for patients. Here we consider some of the approaches being tested in heart failure.

Modulation of RAAS

It is often said that the neurohormonal hypothesis, which remains the basis for today's pharmacological therapy, has run its course, and yet, as the results of PARADIGM-HF show, there may be still more to come.

The renin–angiotensin–aldosterone system (RAAS) can now be modulated at all stages of the pathway, and RAAS inhibition is still key to the management of chronic heart failure. The likeliest improvements in manipulating the RAAS probably lie with evermore selective mineralocorticoid receptor antagonists (MRAs), and the use of agents that can prevent (or treat) hyperkalaemia.[1,2] A key question to answer will be whether a patient whose MRA is discontinued for hyperkalaemia gains more from an MRA *plus* a potassium binder than from taking neither drug at all.

TRV027 is a novel agent that acts as a β-arrestin-biased ligand of the AT_1 receptor: it blocks the AT_1 receptor, but stimulates downstream β-arrestin pathways, thereby potentially increasing myocardial contractility.[3] It was developed as a potential therapy for acute heart failure. However, BLAST-AHF,[4] a dose-ranging study in patients presenting with acute heart failure, showed no effect of TRV027 on clinical end-points through to 30 days. The drug is not going to be developed further as a consequence.

Vasodilators in acute heart failure

The failure of expensive vasodilators in patients with acute heart failure to alter clinical or hard end-points extends from nesiritide[5] through serelaxin[6] and now to ularitide.[7] The most recent trial used a strategy of intensive vasodilation based on transdermal nitrates and hydralazine with early renin–angiotensin system inhibition. The effect of vasodilation was again neutral.[8] The rationale behind using vasodilators remains compelling, but the disappointments highlight some of the problems inherent in designing trials for patients with acute heart failure.

The group of patients who might be thought to have most to gain from a vasodilator are those with acute pulmonary oedema, in whom left ventricular filling pressure is high, and, typically, in whom systolic blood pressure is also high. Although the vasodilator studies are designed to capture such patients, the chief requirements require breathlessness at rest or minimal exertion—and that is not the same as acute pulmonary oedema. Patients with acute pulmonary oedema are extremely unwell at presentation, and are not able to give meaningful consent to a trial of a novel therapy: in addition, they frequently present overnight when research teams are not readily available to go through the recruitment procedures. Those procedures themselves often take time, and background therapy will already have had effect before any trial therapy can start. Many studies exclude patients with obvious precipitants for their acute heart failure (such as acute ischaemia or arrhythmia), which unfortunately excludes most—if not all—patients presenting with pulmonary oedema (Table 69.1).

Table 69.1 Recent trials of intravenous vasodilators in patients presenting with 'acute' heart failure

Trial	Drug	Time to enrol	Patient characteristics	Exclusion
ASCEND-HF	Nesiritide	<24 h	Rest/minimal exertion SoB	ACS
TRUE-AHF	Ularitide	Median 6 h	SoB at rest after frusemide	ACS
RELAX-AHF-2	Relaxin	≤16 h	Rest/minimal exertion SoB	ACS, arrhythmia

SoB, shortness of breath; ACS, acute coronary syndrome.

The net result is that trials tend to include patients who are not critically unwell, who are unlikely to be very breathless at rest, and who start trial treatment late after presentation. This is a challenge to clinical triallists. Since there has been no definitive trial of the possible benefits of intravenous nitrates in acute pulmonary oedema, one approach might be to mount a trial using a strategy similar to that of HEAT-PPCI.[9] Patients might have one of two approved therapies—best medical care or best medical care plus intravenous nitrate. There would be no exclusion criteria, and consent taken from patients retrospectively.

Modulating cardiac contractility

Istaroxime

Istaroxime is administered intravenously and has a dual mechanism of action. Like the cardiac glycosides, it inhibits the sodium–potassium ATPase, but in addition it stimulates the sarcoplasmic reticulum calcium adenosine triphosphatase isoform 2a (SERCA2a). It thus acts both as a positive inotrope while having a positive lusitropic effect as the re-uptake of calcium into the sarcoplasmic reticulum is accelerated.

In a study of 120 patients with acute heart failure, istaroxime caused a fall in pulmonary capillary wedge pressure and heart rate, while at the same time increasing blood pressure.[10] A further trial investigating lusitropic effects in more detail is now recruiting patients.[11]

Omecamtiv mecarbil

Omecamtiv is an activator of cardiac myosin. It is not strictly a positive inotrope, but works by prolonging systole. The result in preclinical studies is an increase in cardiac output without an increase in oxygen consumption, unlike with traditional positive inotropes.[12,13]

In ATOMIC-AHF, patients with acute heart failure treated with omecamtiv had a modest improvement in some secondary measures of breathlessness.[14] In GALACTIC-HF, 8256 patients with symptomatic CHF (average ejection fraction 27% and NT-proBNP 2000) were randomised to receive omecamtiv or placebo. The primary end-point of first HF event or cardiovascular death was very slightly lower in the omecamtiv group (hazard ratio 0.92 with a P value of 0.03). There appeared to be significant interactions: those with lower ejection fraction, better renal function and sinus rhythm appeared to gain more. With these equivocal results, it's difficult to picture that omecamtiv will be used widely, but it is possible it may develop a niche role.[15]

Modulating myocyte function

Cyclic guanosine monophosphate (cGMP) is produced by the action of soluble guanylate cyclase (sGC). It causes a fall in intracellular calcium concentrations in smooth muscle, resulting in vasodilation. It also has anti-hypertrophic effects on myocytes.[16] Lower levels of sGC are associated with endothelial dysfunction in both patients with heart failure with reduced ejection fraction (HFrEF) and those with heart failure with normal ejection fraction (HFnEF),[17,18] and so strategies to increase cGMP activity might be helpful. Neprilysin inhibitors prevent the breakdown of natriuretic peptides, which, in turn, activate cGMP.[19]

Cinaciguat is a sGC activator that promotes the formation of cGMP. In exploratory studies, it behaved as a vasodilator in patients with acute heart failure but caused an unacceptably high rate of hypotension.[20] Riociguat is slightly different: it is orally active, and acts as a sGC stimulator—that is, it directly acts on sGC in the same way as its natural stimulator, nitrous oxide. It is licenced for use in pulmonary arterial hypertension.[21]

Vericiguat is another sGC stimulator that has shown promising effects. In SOCRATES-REDUCED, a dose-ranging study, vericiguat reduced the rate of a secondary end-point (cardiovascular death or readmission with acute heart failure) while not affecting the primary end-point (reduction in N-terminal pro B-type natriuretic peptide (NT-proBNP)).[22] Although side-effects were common (particularly hypotension and syncope), the results were sufficiently promising that a large phase III study of vericiguat in patients with heart failure due to reduced left ventricular systolic function (VICTORIA[23]) was launched, powered for the end-point of the composite of cardiovascular death or heart failure hospitalization.

Just over 5000 patients were recruited (average age: 67.5 years; 76% male; left ventricular ejection fraction: 29%) and at just over 10 months follow-up the patients randomized to vericiguat had a significantly lower event rate (35.5% vs 38.5% in the placebo group)[24] with most of the difference being driven by a reduction in hospitalizations. There was no effect on all-cause mortality. Not all the results are published as yet, but there are some strange findings: vericiguat seemed to have no effect on those with the highest NT-proBNP and there seemed to be no effect on left ventricular remodelling.

The future for guanylate cyclase stimulators is not yet clear. Although VICTORIA is formally positive, the effect size is small.

Mitochondrial function

A novel approach is to attempt to modulate mitochondrial function. Mitochondria are abnormal in patients with heart failure (reviewed by Rosca and Hoppel[25]). The end result is decreased energy production and increased production of reactive oxygen species. Improving mitochondrial function is an attractive target, although, due to the intracellular location of the organelles, difficult to achieve.

Cardiolipin is an indispensable component of the inner mitochondrial membrane and is essential for the proper functioning of cytochrome c oxidase (the last complex of the electron transport chain). Elamipretide reduces the breakdown of cardiolipin by inhibiting cardiolipin peroxidase, and might thus improve energy production and reduce free radical production.

In a canine model, subcutaneous elamipretide improved left ventricular function,[26] and in small human studies caused a small reduction in left ventricular volume.[27] Trials of elamipretide in different clinical scenarios are being designed and conducted, including among patients admitted with severe fluid retention and those with normal left ventricular ejection fraction.[28]

Unanswered questions for tested agents

One of the developments in heart failure is the increasing appreciation of the possible value of individualized therapy for different patients. It is possible that some of the agents that have been tested previously and found not to be of great benefit when administered to largely unselected patients with heart failure might have benefits in some subgroups of patients. Examples include:

- Vasopressin antagonists for patients with hyponatraemia. There are no satisfactory treatments for patients with hyponatraemia, and, because the large-scale clinical trial with tolvaptan (EVEREST) was neutral, there is little likelihood of its being widely used.

- Treatments for patients with pulmonary hypertension. 'All-comers' trials may miss potential benefit for some patients. Bosentan was used in the ENABLE study programme in patients with severely symptomatic chronic heart failure, but was ineffective (and, indeed, lead to high rates of early fluid retention).[29] However, there are no treatments specifically for patients with heart failure and significant pulmonary hypertension (which is particularly common in heart failure with normal ejection fraction), and it is possible that endothelin antagonists might be helpful for such patients. Similarly, sildenafil was ineffective in the RELAX trial,[30] but there are ongoing trials with sildenafil in patients with pulmonary hypertension and left ventricular systolic dysfunction.[31,32]

- Ultrafiltration for fluid retention suffers from the problem in reverse: because it has been tried only in populations with severe fluid retention and particularly in those with renal impairment or 'diuretic resistance', we might be missing more beneficial effects in a wider range of patients with fluid retention, particularly in terms of reducing length of stay, a significant problem in Europe if not the USA.

- Although intravenous frusemide has been used for many decades, it might not be the only way to give it parenterally. Subcutaneous frusemide has been reformulated as a preparation with neutral pH, and might be suitable for use among ambulatory patients to try to prevent admission to hospital.[33] A larger study is needed.

- There has been some interest in 'door-to-needle' time for patients presenting with acute heart failure, with some studies suggesting that the quicker furosemide is administered, the better the patients' survival.[34] However, the effect is not seen consistently:[35] we are still learning how to use agents that have been available for decades.

We would hope that investigators are able to carry out trials for therapies that hold promise. Not all agents should be dismissed as a result of a neutral study.

Devices

The success of cardiac resynchronization therapy and implantable defibrillators has generated a huge interest in the potential of devices.

ICDs

The majority of ICDs implanted never discharge. They represent a burden for patients and health care providers alike. Refining patient selection for primary prevention ICDs is a major task: the DANISH study[36] has prompted much speculation that an ICD might not be necessary for patients with a primary diagnosis of non-ischaemic cardiomyopathy, and there has been a general decline in the incidence of sudden death over the last 20 years of clinical trials.[37] Even among patients with an ICD who are reported to die suddenly, interrogation of the device often shows that death was not due to arrhythmia.[38] Although it will be challenging to conduct such trials, new studies are needed to determine what role ICDs now have against the background of hugely improved medical therapy.

Monitoring

A huge amount of effort has centred on ways of detecting incipient decline in a patient's status with the aim of preventing admission to hospital and perhaps improving prognosis. A common thread from the results is that it is possible to pick out signals suggesting that a patient might be about to relapse, but the overwhelming mass of data received makes it almost impossible to pick out the signal from the noise reliably.

A second feature is that patients in the intervention limb of monitoring trials are often treated with higher doses of heart failure medication. What is needed is a way to empower *patients* to take charge of their own condition effectively. A signal that such an approach might be helpful comes from HOMEOSTASIS, in which patients with severe heart failure were implanted with a device measuring left atrial pressure, and made changes to treatment based on the readings using a pre-programmed handheld patient advisor module.[39]

Treating HFrEF?

Mechanical treatments to help support the circulation are now part of clinical practice, even if only for small numbers. Some have developed approaches to try to refashion the failing left ventricle, particularly in those patients with very dilated hearts.

One example is the use of alginate gels to expand and reshape the left ventricle. In animal models, the gel improves left ventricular structure and function,[40] and in AUGMENT-HF, gel injections led to an improvement in exercise capacity and reduction in risk of hospitalization, albeit with a substantial risk of complications.[41]

The ACORN device, designed to prevent resistance to filling during diastole, is a polyester mesh position between apex and atrioventricular groove. Its use is associated with improved haemodynamics, but it appears not to have any effect on long-term survival, limiting its further development.[42] A similar device made from a nitinol mesh has also been tried, but a large trial was halted for futility, despite improvements in some haemodynamic measures.[43]

The Parachute device is implanted in the cavity of the left ventricle with the aim of excluding the akinetic area of the left ventricular in patients with large antero-apical infarcts. The device can be implanted percutaneously, and early results have again suggested that it may lead to haemodynamic and symptomatic improvement. A large study, PARACHUTE IV, is in progress, powered for death or rehospitalization for heart failure.[44] Another device using anchors to exclude scarred antero-apical tissue has to be delivered surgically,[45] and is the subject of ongoing trials.[46]

Many devices have been developed for the treatment of valvular heart disease in heart failure. Transcatheter aortic valve implantation is now well established for selected cases, but the role of devices for managing mitral regurgitation is less than clear cut. Two recent trials have reported conflicting results, with one suggesting that there is no significant role for one device, the MitraClip,[47] whereas a second suggested that the MitraClip was associated with a large reduction in the risk of death in symptomatic patients with moderate-to-severe mitral regurgitation (or worse).[48] There are several percutaneous approaches to the treatment of tricuspid regurgitation in development which may have a role in future. Again, more work is needed to establish the role of devices.

Neural stimulators have attracted a lot of interest, although none has shown convincing evidence of benefit as yet. Vagal nerve stimulators seemed promising, offering the possibility of reversing the sympathetic–parasympathetic nervous system imbalance seen in heart failure, but have fallen by the wayside with the largest trial to date yielding neutral results.[49] Carotid baroreflex stimulators (which are implanted devices with an electrode on the carotid sinus) have shown promise as a method for reversing autonomic system imbalance: a randomized study of just over 400 patients showed that stimulation improved quality of life and exercise capacity while reducing NT-proBNP.[50]

Although treatment of sleep disordered breathing has so far been disappointing in heart failure, with the failure of the SERVE-HF trial,[51] nevertheless interest in periodic respiration remains. A modest-sized study showed that unilateral phrenic nerve stimulation using a transvenous approach (triggered when the onset of periodic respiration was detected) could reduce central sleep apnoea and improve quality of life.[52] More work in a larger population will surely follow.

Another stimulatory approach has been cardiac contractility modulation. An electrode delivers myocardial stimulation without initiating depolarization and appears to affect myocardial biochemistry. Small studies have suggested that there may be an improvement in exercise tolerance and quality of life with cardiac contractility modulation[53] and possibly survival,[54] but a meta-analysis of the available data (in just over 800 patients) suggests that there is no effect on outcomes and a tendency for the system to cause pacemaker and other device malfunction.[55] As so often, more evidence is needed.

At an early stage in development is a method for stimulating cardiopulmonary nerves via the pulmonary artery. The resulting release of noradrenaline improves cardiac performance, although whether this represents any advance on exogenous administration of catecholamines is not clear. Few data are in the public domain as yet, but a small study in patients with acute heart failure showed an increase in left ventricular contractility with stimulation.[56] Further studies are planned.

Devices for treating HFnEF?

One of the features of patients with HFnEF is a rise in left atrial pressure, particularly on exertion.[57,58] Two devices have been developed that create an inter-atrial shunt with the aim of allowing the left atrium to decompress as pressure rises. In an open label study, REDUCE LAP-HF, a device was implanted successfully in most patients, and led to a fall in pulmonary capillary wedge pressure (PCWP) in most patients.[59] There were also improvements in quality of life and modest increases in 6 min walk test distance. The reduction in PCWP was confirmed in a small randomized, sham-controlled study (REDUCE LAP-HF I).[60] Further trials are in progress, but whether such an approach will be useful for many patients with HFnEF is uncertain. Patient selection will be all-important.

Epidemiology revisited

For all the undoubted success of clinical trials in leading to great improvements in treating heart failure, there are some major epidemiological problems that have not been resolved.

Very many research articles on heart failure begin with a series of linked statements to the effect that heart failure is very common; that it is very expensive; and that it is very fatal. However, those of us who treat patients know that long-term survival, even with very severe left ventricular systolic dysfunction, is not a rare occurrence. In CARE-HF, for example, more than 50% of patients were alive at 10 years.[61] Many patients have substantial left ventricular recovery,[62] and we may be doing our patients a disservice by repeating a mantra of doom.[63] Data from the UK suggest that whilst the incidence of new cases of heart failure may be falling, the prevalence has increased by more than 20% between 2002 and 2014.[64] Data from Europe[65] and the USA[66] suggest similarly that the prognosis of patients with heart failure is gradually improving.

We need a more up-to-date appreciation of the basic epidemiology of heart failure: we may be improving prognosis sufficiently that patients with significant left ventricular dysfunction in their 50s and 60s are surviving to develop symptomatic heart failure in their 70s and 80s, by which time, pursuing evermore effective life-prolonging treatments will become self-defeating.

A problem perhaps more obvious in the UK than elsewhere (although presumably as prevalent) is that of missing patients. HFrEF is said to affect 3.5–7.0% of people aged 65–75 years,[67,68] and up to 11% of those aged >80 years.[69,70] Primary care physicians in the UK are financially incentivized to record (and treat) patients with heart failure,[71] and yet the prevalence of heart failure in general practitioner registers is only around 0.7–1%.[72] More work is needed to find the 'missing' patients: they may simply be being treated with loop diuretics for oedema without the diagnosis of heart failure being formally made.[73]

The epidemiology of two major areas of heart failure is curiously underdeveloped.

Acute heart failure is not well defined. To many, the phrase means a patient with acute pulmonary oedema, and it seems that many (or, indeed, most) trials of acute heart failure have been targeted at this population. However, breathlessness at rest is not the commonest symptom at presentation to hospital: most patients have fluid retention and present with peripheral oedema.[74] Thus far, trials of different management strategies in heart failure have been neutral, in large part because of the difficulties in defining the population with sufficient accuracy. We need epidemiological studies to define and refine our understanding of acute heart failure, to define subgroups of patients for whom different therapeutic strategies may be appropriate.

Heart failure with normal ejection (or whichever is your favoured term[75]) remains an enigma. There is something remarkable about a condition said to have a prognosis as bleak as heart failure with reduced ejection when every clinical trial that has ever reported on the subject has found a strong association between increasing ejection fraction and increasing survival. Most trials of patients with HFnEF have struggled to recruit, leading to controversial results, as seen in TOPCAT.[76] More work is needed to define HFnEF robustly and unequivocally. New approaches include using artificial intelligence to help define different phenotypes of patients. None has yet made it into clinical practice.[77,78] It seems beyond doubt that many patients labelled as having HFnEF have other causes for their symptoms.

Conclusions

Heart failure continues to be an exciting field for health care professionals, and is no longer a diagnosis of despair for patients. Even though therapy has advanced enormously, new innovations continue to come forward and continue to offer further hope to patients. Textbooks often struggle to keep pace with developments, and, with the rate of progress, we expect a third edition of this book will become essential within a few years. Even as the present volume was going to press, the first transplant of a genetically engineered pig's heart was implanted into a patient with severe left ventricular dysfunction, opening up a vast potential new area of heart failure treatment.[79]

REFERENCES

1. Pitt B, Anker SD, Bushinsky DA, et al.; PEARL-HF Investigators. Evaluation of the efficacy and safety of RLY5016, a polymeric potassium binder, in a double-blind, placebo-controlled study in patients with chronic heart failure (the PEARL-HF) trial. *Eur Heart J* 2011;**32**:820–8.

2. Kosiborod M, Rasmussen HS, Lavin P, et al. Effect of sodium zirconium cyclosilicate on potassium lowering for 28 days among outpatients with hyperkalemia: the HARMONIZE randomized clinical trial. *JAMA* 2014;**312**:2223–33.

3. Violin JD, DeWire SM, Yamashita D, et al. Selectively engaging β-arrestins at the angiotensin II type 1 receptor reduces blood pressure and increases cardiac performance. *J Pharmacol Exp Ther* 2010;**335**:572–9.

4. Pang PS, Butler J, Collins SP, et al. Biased ligand of the angiotensin II type 1 receptor in patients with acute heart failure: a randomized, double-blind, placebo-controlled, phase IIB, dose ranging trial (BLAST-AHF). *Eur Heart J* 2017;**38**:2364–73.

5. O'Connor CM, Starling RC, Hernandez AF, et al. Effect of nesiritide in patients with acute decompensated heart failure. *N Engl J Med* 2011;**365**:32–43.

6. Metra M, Teerlink JR, Cotter G, et al.; RELAX-AHF-2 Committees Investigators. Effects of serelaxin in patients with acute heart failure. *N Engl J Med* 2019;**381**:716–26.

7. Packer M, O'Connor C, McMurray JJV, et al.; TRUE-AHF Investigators. Effect of ularitide on cardiovascular mortality in acute heart failure. *N Engl J Med* 2017;**376**:1956–64.

8. Kozhuharov N, Goudev A, Flores D, et al. Effect of a strategy of comprehensive vasodilation vs usual care on mortality and heart failure rehospitalization among patients with acute heart failure: the GALACTIC randomized clinical trial. *JAMA* 2019;**322**:2292–302.

9. Shahzad A, Kemp I, Mars C, et al.; HEAT-PPCI trial investigators. Unfractionated heparin versus bivalirudin in primary percutaneous coronary intervention (HEAT-PPCI): an open-label, single centre, randomised controlled trial. *Lancet* 2014;**384**:1849–58.

10. Shah SJ, Blair JE, Filippatos GS, et al.; HORIZON-HF Investigators. Effects of istaroxime on diastolic stiffness in acute heart failure syndromes: results from the hemodynamic, echocardiographic, and neurohormonal effects of istaroxime, a novel intravenous inotropic and lusitropic agent: a randomized controlled trial in patients hospitalized with heart failure (HORIZON-HF) trial. *Am Heart J* 2009;**157**:1035–41.

11. https://clinicaltrials.gov/ct2/show/NCT02617446

12. Malik FI, Hartman JJ, Elias KA, et al. Cardiac myosin activation: a potential therapeutic approach for systolic heart failure. *Science* 2011;**331**:1439–43.

13. Shen YT, Malik FI, Zhao X, et al. Improvement of cardiac function by a cardiac myosin activator in conscious dogs with systolic heart failure. *Circ Heart Fail* 2010;**3**:522–7.

14. Teerlink JR, Felker GM, McMurray JJV, et al.; ATOMIC-AHF Investigators. Acute treatment with omecamtiv mecarbil to increase contractility in acute heart failure: The ATOMIC-AHF Study. *J Am Coll Cardiol* 2016;**67**:1444–55.

15. Teerlink JR, Diaz R, Felker GM, et al. GALACTIC-HF Investigators. Cardiac myosin activation with omecamtiv mecarbil in systolic heart failure. *N Engl J Med* 2021;**384**:105–16.

16. Tsai EJ, Kass DA. Cyclic GMP signaling in cardiovascular pathophysiology and therapeutics. *Pharmacol Ther* 2009;**122**:216–38.

17. Gheorgiade M, Marti CN, Sabbah HN, et al.; Academic Research Team in Heart Failure (ART-HF). Soluble guanylate cyclase: a potential therapeutic target for heart failure. *Heart Fail Rev* 2013;**18**:123–34.

18. Lam CS, Brutsaert DL. Endothelial dysfunction: a pathophysiologic factor in heart failure with preserved ejection fraction. *J Am Coll Cardiol* 2012;**60**:1787–9.

19. Ichiki T, Huntley BK, Sangaralingham SJ, Burnett JC Jr. Pro-atrial natriuretic peptide: a novel guanylyl cyclase-A receptor activator that goes beyond atrial and b-type natriuretic peptides. *JACC Heart Fail* 2015;**3**:715–23.

20. Erdmann E, Semigran MJ, Nieminen MS, et al. Cinaciguat, a soluble guanylate cyclase activator, unloads the heart but also causes hypotension in acute decompensated heart failure. *Eur Heart J* 2013;**34**:57–67.

21. Humbert M, Coghlan JG, Ghofrani HA, et al. Riociguat for the treatment of pulmonary arterial hypertension associated with connective tissue disease: results from PATENT-1 and PATENT-2. *Ann Rheum Dis* 2017;**76**:422–26.

22. Gheorgiade M, Greene SJ, Butler J, et al.; SOCRATES-REDUCED Investigators and Coordinators. Effect of vericiguat, a soluble guanylate cyclase stimulator, on natriuretic peptide levels in patients with worsening chronic heart failure and reduced ejection fraction: the SOCRATES-REDUCED Randomized Trial. *JAMA* 2015;**314**:2251–62.

23. Armstrong PW, Roessig L, Patel MJ, et al. A multicenter, randomized, double-blind, placebo-controlled trial of the efficacy and safety of the oral soluble guanylate cyclase stimulator: the VICTORIA trial. *JACC Heart Fail* 2018;**6**:96–104.

24. Armstrong PW, Pieske B, Anstrom KJ, et al.; VICTORIA Study Group. Vericiguat in patients with heart failure and reduced ejection fraction. *N Engl J Med* 2020;**382**:1883–93.

25. Rosca MG, Hoppel CL. Mitochondrial dysfunction in heart failure. *Heart Fail Rev* 2013;**18**:607–22.

26. Sabbah HN, Gupta RC, Kohli S, et al. Chronic therapy with elamipretide (MTP-131), a novel mitochondria targeting peptide, improves left ventricular and mitochondrial function in dogs with advanced heart failure. *Circ Heart Fail* 2016;**9**:e002206.

27. Daubert MA, Yow E, Dunn G, et al. Effects of a novel tetrapeptide in heart failure with reduced ejection fraction (HFrEF): a phase I randomized, placebo-controlled trial of elamipretide. *J Am Coll Cardiol* 2016;**67**:1283 (abstract).

28. US National Institutes of Health. ClinicalTrials.gov. A study to evaluate the effects of 4 weeks treatment with subcutaneous elamipretide on left ventricular function in subjects with

stable heart failure with preserved ejection fraction. https://clinicaltrials.gov/ct2/show/NCT02814097

29. Packer M, McMurray JJV, Krum H, et al.; ENABLE Investigators and Committees. Long-term effect of endothelin receptor antagonism with bosentan on the morbidity and mortality of patients with severe chronic heart failure: primary results of the enable trials. *JACC Heart Fail* 2017;**5**:317–26.

30. Redfield MM, Chen HH, Borlaug BA, et al. RELAX Trial. Effect of phosphodiesterase-5 inhibition on exercise capacity and clinical status in heart failure with preserved ejection fraction: a randomized clinical trial. *JAMA* 2013;**309**:1268–77.

31. Cooper TJ, Guazzi M, Al-Mohammad A, et al. Sildenafil in Heart failure (SilHF). An investigator-initiated multinational randomized controlled clinical trial: rationale and design. *Eur J Heart Fail* 2013;**15**:119–22.

32. Guglin M, Rajagopalan N, Anaya P, Charnigo R. Sildenafil in heart failure with reactive pulmonary hypertension (Sildenafil HF) clinical trial (rationale and design). *Pulm Circ* 2016; **6**:161–7.

33. Gilotra NA, Princewill O, Marino B, et al. Efficacy of intravenous furosemide versus a novel, pH-neutral furosemide formulation administered subcutaneously in outpatients with worsening heart failure. *JACC Heart Fail* 2018;**6**:65–70.

34. Matsue Y, Damman K, Voors AA, et al. Time-to-furosemide treatment and mortality in patients hospitalized with acute heart failure. *J Am Coll Cardiol* 2017;**69**:3042–51.

35. Park JJ, Kim SH, Oh IY, et al. The effect of door-to-diuretic time on clinical outcomes in patients with acute heart failure. *JACC Heart Fail* 2018;**6**:286–94.

36. Køber L, Thune JJ, Nielsen JC, et al.; DANISH Investigators. Defibrillator implantation in patients with nonischemic systolic heart failure. *N Engl J Med* 2016;**375**:1221–30.

37. Shen L, Jhund PS, Petrie MC, et al. Declining risk of sudden death in heart failure. *N Engl J Med* 2017;**377**:41–51.

38. Nikolaidou T, Ghosh JM, Shah S, et al. Post-mortem ICD interrogation in mode of death classification. *J Cardiovasc Electrophysiol* 2018;**29**:573–83.

39. Ritzema J, Troughton R, Melton I, et al.; Hemodynamically Guided Home Self-Therapy in Severe Heart Failure Patients (HOMEOSTASIS) Study Group. Physician-directed patient self-management of left atrial pressure in advanced chronic heart failure. *Circulation* 2010;**121**:1086–95.

40. Sabbah HN, Wang M, Gupta RC, et al. Augmentation of left ventricular wall thickness with alginate hydrogel implants improves left ventricular function and prevents progressive remodeling in dogs with chronic heart failure. JACC Heart *Fail* 2013;**1**:252–8.

41. Pellicori P, Clark AL. Clinical trials update from the European Society of Cardiology-Heart Failure meeting 2015: AUGMENT-HF, TITRATION, STOP-HF, HARMONIZE, LION HEART, MOOD-HF, and renin-angiotensin inhibitors in patients with heart and renal failure. *Eur J Heart Fail* 2015;**17**:979–83.

42. Mann DL, Kubo SH, Sabbah HN, et al. Beneficial effects of the CorCap cardiac support device: five-year results from the Acorn Trial. *J Thorac Cardiovasc Surg* 2012;**143**:1036–42.

43. Costanzo MR, Ivanhoe RJ, Kao A, et al. Prospective evaluation of elastic restraint to lessen the effects of heart failure (PEERLESS-HF) trial. *J Card Fail* 2012;**18**:446–58.

44. Costa MA, Pencina M, Nikolic S, et al. The PARACHUTE IV trial design and rationale: percutaneous ventricular restoration using the Parachute device in patients with ischemic heart failure and dilated left ventricles. *Am Heart J* 2013;**165**:531–6.

45. Wechsler AS, Sadowski J, Kapelak B, et al. Durability of epicardial ventricular restoration without ventriculotomy. *Eur J Cardiothorac Surg* 2013;**44**:e189–92.

46. Safety and Efficacy Study of the BioVentrix PliCath HF System (CONFIGURE-HF). https://clinicaltrials.gov/ct2/show/NCT01568164

47. Obadia JF, Messika-Zeitoun D, Leurent G, et al.; MITRA-FR Investigators. Percutaneous repair or medical treatment for secondary mitral regurgitation. *N Engl J Med* 2018;**379**(24):2297–306.

48. Stone GW, Lindenfeld J, Abraham WT, et al., for the COAPT Investigators. Transcatheter mitral-valve repair in patients with heart failure. *N Engl J Med* 2018;**379**(24):2307–18.

49. Gold MR, Van Veldhuisen DJ, Hauptman PJ, et al. Vagus nerve stimulation for the treatment of heart failure: the INOVATE-HF Trial. *J Am Coll Cardiol* 2016;**68**:149–58.

50. Zile MR, Lindenfeld J, Weaver FA, et al. Baroreflex activation therapy in patients with heart failure with reduced ejection fraction. *J Am Coll Cardiol* 2020;**76**:1–13.

51. Cowie MR, Woehrle H, Wegscheider K, et al. Adaptive servo-ventilation for central sleep apnea in systolic heart failure. *N Engl J Med* 2015;**373**:1095–105.

52. Costanzo MR, Ponikowski P, Coats A, et al; remedē® System Pivotal Trial Study Group. Phrenic nerve stimulation to treat patients with central sleep apnoea and heart failure. *Eur J Heart Fail* 2018;**20**:1746–54.

53. Abraham WT, Kuck K-H, Goldsmith RL, et al. A randomized controlled trial to evaluate the safety and efficacy of cardiac contractility modulation. *JACC Heart Fail* 2018;**6**:874–83.

54. Anker SD, Borggrefe M, Neuser H, et al. Cardiac contractility modulation improves long-term survival and hospitalizations in heart failure with reduced ejection fraction. *Eur J Heart Fail* 2019;**21**:1103–13.

55. Mando R, Goel A, Habash F, et al. Outcomes of cardiac contractility modulation: a systematic review and meta-analysis of randomized clinical trials. *Cardiovasc Ther* 2019:9769724.

56. Mickelsen S, Molnar G, Marin y Kall C, Ebner A. Early feasibility using a novel neuromodulation device to increase inotropy. *Heart Rhythm* 2018;**15**:S641–S657.

57. Maeder MT, Thompson BR, Brunner-La Rocca HP, Kaye DM. Hemodynamic basis of exercise limitation in patients with heart failure and normal ejection fraction. *J Am Coll Cardiol* 2010;**56**:855–63.

58. Borlaug BA, Nishimura RA, Sorajja P, Lam CS, Redfield MM. Exercise hemodynamics enhance diagnosis of early heart failure with preserved ejection fraction. *Circ Heart Fail* 2010;**3**:588–95.

59. Hasenfuß G, Hayward C, Burkhoff D, et al.; REDUCE LAP-HF study investigators. A transcatheter intracardiac shunt device for heart failure with preserved ejection fraction (REDUCE LAP-HF): a multicentre, open-label, single-arm, phase 1 trial. *Lancet* 2016;**387**:1298–304.

60. Feldman E, Mauri L, Kahwash R, et al. A transcatheter interatrial shunt device for the treatment of heart failure with preserved ejection fraction (REDUCE LAP-HF I): a phase 2, randomized, sham-controlled trial. *Circulation* 2018;**137**:364–75.

61. Cleland JG, Freemantle N, Erdmann E, et al. Long-term mortality with cardiac resynchronization therapy in the Cardiac Resynchronization-Heart Failure (CARE-HF) trial. *Eur J Heart Fail* 2012;**14**:628–34.

62. Kalogeropoulos AP, Fonarow GC, Georgiopoulou V, et al. Characteristics and outcomes of adult outpatients with heart

failure and improved or recovered ejection fraction *JAMA Cardiol* 2016;**1**:510–18.

63. Cleland JGF, Pellicori P, Clark AL, Petrie MC. Time to take the failure out of heart failure: the importance of optimism. *JACC Heart Fail* 2017;**5**:538–40.

64. Conrad N, Judge A, Tran J, *et al*. Temporal trends and patterns in heart failure incidence: a population-based study of 4 million individuals. *Lancet* 2018;**391**(10120):572–80.

65. Merlo M, Pivetta A, Pinamonti B, *et al*. Long-term prognostic impact of therapeutic strategies in patients with idiopathic dilated cardiomyopathy: changing mortality over the last 30 years. *Eur J Heart Fail* 2014;**16**:317–24.

66. Heart Disease and Stroke Statistics—2016 Update: a report from the American Heart Association. *Circulation* 2016;**133**:e38–360.

67. Galasko GI, Senior R, Lahiri A. Ethnic differences in the prevalence and aetiology of left ventricular systolic dysfunction in the community: The Harrow heart failure watch. *Heart* 2005;**91**:595–600.

68. Hedberg P, Lonnberg I, Jonason T, *et al*. Left ventricular systolic dysfunction in 75-year-old men and women; a population-based study. *Eur Heart J* 2001;**22**:676–83.

69. Kannel WB, Belanger AJ. Epidemiology of heart failure. *Am Heart J* 1991;**121**:951–7.

70. Yousaf F, Collerton J, Kingston A, *et al*. Prevalence of left ventricular dysfunction in a UK community sample of very old people: the Newcastle 85+ study. *Heart* 2012;**98**:1418–23.

71. UK Government. *Summary of QoF indicators*. https://www.gov.uk/government/uploads/system/uploads/attachment_data/file/213226/Summary-of-QOF-indicators.pdf.

72. NHS Digital. *Quality and outcomes framework (QOF)—2014–15*. http://content.digital.nhs.uk/catalogue/PUB18887.

73. Cuthbert JJ, Gopal J, Crundall-Goode A, Clark AL. Are there patients missing from community heart failure registers? An audit of clinical practice. *Eur J Prev Cardiol* 2019;**26**:291–8.

74. Shoaib A, Waleed M, Khan S, *et al*. Breathlessness at rest is not the dominant presentation of patients admitted with heart failure. *Eur J Heart Fail* 2014;**16**:1283–91.

75. Sanderson JE. HFNEF, HFpEF, HF-PEF, or DHF: what is in an acronym? *JACC Heart Fail* 2014;**2**:93–4.

76. Pfeffer MA, Claggett B, Assmann SF, *et al*. Regional variation in patients and outcomes in the Treatment of Preserved Cardiac Function Heart Failure With an Aldosterone Antagonist (TOPCAT) trial. *Circulation* 2015;**131**:34–42.

77. Segar MW, Patel KV, Ayers C, *et al*. Phenomapping of patients with heart failure with preserved ejection fraction using machine learning-based unsupervised cluster analysis. *Eur J Heart Fail* 2020;**22**:148–58.

78. Hedman ÅK, Hage C, Sharma A, *et al*. Identification of novel pheno-groups in heart failure with preserved ejection fraction using machine learning. *Heart* 2020;**106**:342–9.

79. Wilson C. How a pig heart was transplanted into a human for the first time. New Scientist 2022 https://www.newscientist.com/article/2304167-how-a-pig-heart-was-transplanted-into-a-human-for-the-first-time/ accessed 14/1/2022.

Index

For the benefit of digital users, indexed terms that span two pages (e.g., 52–53) may, on occasion, appear on only one of those pages.

Tables, figures and boxes are indicated by *t*, *f* and *b* following the page number